# BOWES & CHURCH'S
# FOOD VALUES
# OF PORTIONS COMMONLY USED

# BOWES & CHURCH'S
# FOOD VALUES
# OF PORTIONS COMMONLY USED

### NINETEENTH EDITION

Jean A.T. Pennington, PhD, RD and Judith Spungen, MS, RD

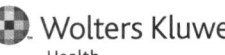
Wolters Kluwer | Lippincott Williams & Wilkins
Health
Philadelphia · Baltimore · New York · London
Buenos Aires · Hong Kong · Sydney · Tokyo

*Acquisitions Editor:* David B. Troy
*Product Manager:* Matt Hauber
*Designer:* Joan Wendt
*Vendor Manager:* Kevin Johnson
*Compositor:* Absolute Service/MDC

19th Edition

351 West Camden Street          530 Walnut Street
Baltimore, MD 21201             Philadelphia, PA 19106

Printed in China

**Library of Congress Cataloging-in-Publication Data**

--------

Library of Congress Cataloging-in-Publication Data

Pennington, Jean A. Thompson.
  Bowes & Church's food values of portions commonly used / Jean A.T. Pennington and Judith Spungen.–19th ed.
    p. ; cm.
  Includes bibliographical references and index.
  ISBN 978-0-7817-8134-3
  1. Nutrition--Tables. 2. Food--Composition--Tables. I. Spungen, Judith. II. Title. III. Title: Bowes and Church's food values of portions commonly used. IV. Title: Food values of portions commonly used.
  [DNLM: 1. Nutritive Value--Tables. 2. Food Analysis--statistics & numerical data--Tables. 3. Nutritional Physiological Phenomena--Tables. QU 145 P414b 2009]
  TX551.P385 2009
  613.2--dc22

                          2009014532

The information provided in this book should be used by the healthcare practitioner under appropriate supervision in accordance with professional standards of care with regard to the unique circumstances that apply in each practice situation. Care has been taken to confirm the accuracy of information presented. The authors, editors, and publisher cannot accept any responsibility for errors or omissions or for any consequences from application of the information in this book and make no warranty, express or implied, with respect to the contents of the book.

The authors have attempted to provide readers with the most accurate food composition data available as of the date of manuscript submission; however, the field of food composition is a dynamic one. The composition of foods varies because of food sampling designs; advances in sample preparation and analytical methodology; genetic, environmental, and processing variables; and changes in product formulations and package sizes. The information in these databases should be used as reasonable approximations of the food component composition of foods. Individual who are on therapeutic diets for medical purposes may need to contact food manufactures for more specific information.

To purchase additional copies of this book, call our customer service department at (800) 638-3030 or fax orders to (301) 223-2320. International customers should call (301) 223-2300.

Visit Lippincott Williams & Wilkins on the Internet: http://www.lww.com. Lippincott Williams & Wilkins customer service representatives are available from 8:30 am to 6:00 pm, EST.

9  8  7  6  5  4  3  2  1

# Dedication

The ninteenth edition of *Bowes & Church's Food Values of Portions Commonly Used* is dedicated to the authors of previous editions:

Anna dePlanter Bowes, MA
Charles F. Church, MD, MS
Helen Nichols Church, BA, RD

Ms. Anna dePlanter Bowes and Dr. Charles F. Church developed the first edition of *Food Values* in 1937 and made it available as a private publication in Philadelphia, Pennsylvania. Ms. Bowes completed editions two through eight, published in 1939, 1940, 1942, 1944, 1946, 1951, and 1956, respectively, as private publications in Philadelphia. Dr. Church and his wife, Ms. Helen Nichols Church, worked together on editions nine through twelve (1963, 1966, 1970, and 1975, respectively). These editions were published by the Lippincott Publishing Company in Philadelphia. To all three previous authors of *Food Values*, we express our gratitude for their devotion to the quality of information in this reference book. We hope that we have carried it forward in their tradition.

The purpose of this book is to supply authoritative data on the nutritional values of foods in a form for quick and easy reference. In teaching nutrition to students of medicine, dentistry, dental hygiene, and public health nursing, food values based on common measures of portions frequently served have been found most useful. This basis of calculation is particularly well suited to the practical study of comparative food values, as well as to the approximate analysis of diets from records of daily food intake. For calculations of diets from weighed portions, the actual weight of each food is given in grams or ounces.

*Anna dePlanter Bowes*
*Charles F. Church*
*November 1937*
*Philadelphia*

# Preface to the Nineteenth Edition

*Bowes & Church's Food Values of Portions Commonly Used* is a reference food composition database intended "to supply authoritative data on the nutritional values of food in a form for quick and easy reference." This was the goal established for the first edition by Ms. Anna dePlanter Bowes and Dr. Charles F. Church in 1937, and has remained the goal for all subsequent editions. The preface to the first edition placed an emphasis on providing nutrient values per typical serving portion (as opposed to 100 grams or one pound as purchased), and indeed, *Bowes & Church Food Values* was the first food composition book in the United States to do this.

The database and accompanying information for this nineteenth edition are intended to assist dietitians and other nutrition professionals in providing dietary information to their patients and clients. The information in this book may also be of use to research nutritionists, students of nutrition and dietetics, and individuals who are on special diets or who want to know more about the composition of foods.

The contents of this publication are identified in the *Features of the Nineteenth Edition*. We have attempted to provide current information for a wide range of commonly consumed foods as well as various foods of interest and curiosity. We gratefully acknowledge the expert reviews of this edition provided by Ms. Sally Schakel, RD, and Ms. Mary Murphy, MS, RD, the industry nutritionists and representatives who responded to our requests for food composition data, and the editorial assistance provided by Mr. David Troy and Mr. Matt Hauber at Lippincott Williams & Wilkins in Baltimore, Maryland.

*Jean A.T. Pennington, PhD, RD*
*Judith Spungen, MS, RD*
*December 2008*
*Chevy Chase, MD, and Reston, VA*

# Contents

## SUPPLEMENTARY DATABASES FOR THE COMPOSITION OF FOODS

# Features of the Nineteenth Edition

## FRONT MATERIAL

The front material provides information on standards for the dietary intake of food components in the United States (US). The standards for macronutrients, vitamins, minerals, electrolyes, water, and energy are those established by the Food and Nutrition Board, Institute of Medicine (IOM), National Academy of Sciences (NAS). The standards for the nutrition labeling of food are those developed by the US Food and Drug Administration (FDA). Also provided are food component definitions, abbreviations and symbols used in the text, reference codes that identify the data sources used for this edition, conversion tables for measures of heat, weight, and volume, and a table of gram-ounce conversion equivalents.

## MAIN DATABASE

The main food composition database provides values for 31 food components for over 6300 foods. The foods are grouped into 32 sections on the basis of food type with considerations for common usage. The foods within each of the 32 sections are arranged in a hierarchical structure and are listed alphabetically. The two-line heading at the top of each page of the main database identifies the food components and units of measurement for the numerical values listed in the two lines of values for each food. For Section 32, Special Dietary Foods, there are four lines of data per food to include the complete profiles that were available for these formulated products. Special Dietary Foods includes infant formulas, formulated products used for medical purposes, and meal replacement or enhancement products typically described as sport, energy, or weight-reduction products.

With regard to food names, upper case is used for brand and trademark names and for proper nouns and adjectives (e.g., French fries, Danish pastry, Brussels sprouts, Chinese cabbage); lower case is otherwise used. Each food is identified by name, description (e.g., color, maturity, preservation method, cooking method), brand name (if applicable), serving portion, and gram weight of the serving portion. The individual food names are bolded, while the descriptive terms are in regular type. Some food names are listed several times with different descriptors. In these cases, the food name is listed once in bold, and its subsequent entries provide only the descriptive terms in regular type. Abbreviations are used as necessary to provide as complete a description as is pos-

sible for each food within the space limitations. The abbreviated words and symbols used with the food names and descriptors are listed in the section *Abbreviations and Symbols*.

Foods are presented primarily in their *as consumed* form, although ingredient items (e.g., flour, baking soda, herbs) are also listed in the database. Where available, brand names are used to help identify commercial products such as ready-to-eat breakfast cereals, desserts, candy bars, soups, and entrees. The serving portions are those provided by food companies or by the US Department of Agriculture (USDA) food composition databases. Foods are assigned to one of the 32 sections, although some foods may be applicable to several food group sections. The index may be used to locate foods for which classification may not be apparent, and the section *Food Name Synonyms and Cross-References* provides a means to locate foods known by several different names. Values for foods such as gelatin desserts, icings, puddings, granola bars, and ice cream may reflect a specific flavor or may be averages for different flavors; the values were averaged if the different flavored items had similar profiles.

## SUPPLEMENTARY DATABASES

The supplementary databases, which follow the main database, provide information on the levels of ethyl alcohol, amines, amino acids, caffeine, carotenoids, coenzyme Q, dietary fiber components, omega-3 and trans fatty acids, flavonoids, glutathione, gluten, three additional minerals, plant acids, plant sterols, purines, resistant starch, individual sugars, total antioxidant capacity, and several additional vitamins or vitamin-like components. The supplementary databases allow efficient use of book space for food components with limited information and/or for food components that occur only in certain types of foods. The foods in the supplementary databases are generally listed by the major food groupings used for the main database. All of the foods in the amino acid database are listed in the main database and are identified by the code numbers used for these foods in the main database. Many of the foods in the other supplementary databases are also listed in the main database and the serving portions, if from the same source, are usually consistent. Where applicable, foods in the supplementary databases are identified by reference codes to link them to foods in the main database. Food components in the supplementary database are listed either per serving portion or per 100 grams of food. Much of the information in the supplementary databases was obtained through computer searches of published literature. The information should be used with discretion as some of it is from older papers and some is from foods produced and analyzed in countries other than the US. Thus, the values may reflect foods that are different than those on the US market and may reflect analytical methods not in use in the US.

## DATA SOURCES

The food component values included in the main and supplementary databases have been obtained from the USDA Database for Standard Reference, Release 21 (2008) (SR21), other USDA databases, scientific literature, food company websites, food companies, and food labels. The data sources for the main database are indicated by the Reference Code in the lower left-hand location of the two lines of data for each food. The data sources for the supplementary databases are indicated in or at the end of each database. The data provided by most food companies were in the form of nutrition labeling data. Labeling values are usually derived from analytical data and are rounded and adjusted to be in compliance with government labeling regulations. Labeling values are therefore not as precise as the original analytical data, but are sufficient for most dietary purposes. Values for vitamins and minerals that were obtained from labeling values were calculated from the percent Daily Values (DVs). (See the section on *Daily Values (DV) for Nutrition Labeling.*) Labeling values less than 2% DV were left blank (rather than as zeros) to avoid underestimating them.

Values for folic acid that were obtained from labeling data were calculated as micrograms of folic acid, rather than micrograms of dietary folate equivalents. It was not possible to determine how much of the folic acid in the foods was naturally occurring versus that added by the manufacturer. Therefore, it is possible that some of the listed folic acid values may underestimate the available folic acid.

International Units (IU) of vitamin E were converted to milligrams of alpha-tocopherol equivalents (ATE) assuming that 1.5 IU of vitamin E is equivalent to 1 milligram of ATE. Although alpha-tocopherol is the primary form of vitamin E, the main database lists ATE because more data were available in this form and it is more similar to the data provided by food companies.

For some food products, the serving size provided by the original source was specified only as a volume measure (fluid ounces, cups) or approximate measure (slice, piece, medium, large, small) rather than as a weight unit (grams or ounces). The gram weights for these foods were estimated. Some of the foods were purchased and weighed; the gram weights for some of the foods were estimated by considering the weight of the proximate nutrients (water, protein, fat, and carbohydrate). In cases where the water weight was not provided, it was esti-

mated from the percent water content of similar foods. For foods where the portion size was provided in fluid ounces without an equivalent weight unit, the gram weight was estimated from the fluid ounce-gram weight equivalent of a similar food. (See *Heat, Weight, & Volume Conversions* and *Gram-Ounce Equivalents.*)

## BACK MATERIAL

The back material includes the scientific names for plants and animals, food name synonyms and cross-references, a bibliography of publications on the composition of foods, a chronology of editions of *Food Values*, and an index. The list of *Food Name Synonyms and Cross-References* is included to assist users in locating foods with various names (including regional names) or various arrangements of the same name (e.g., lima beans versus beans, lima versus butterbeans).

The *Bibliography for Food Composition Data* includes papers concerning food composition that were published between July 2003 (when the eighteenth edition of *Food Values* was submitted to the publisher) and December 2008 (when the nineteenth edition was submitted to the publisher). The references are listed alphabetically by the first author's last name. Key words are listed in bold to identify the foods and food components that are discussed in these papers.

## CHANGES FROM THE EIGHTEENTH EDITION

Updated sources of information were obtained from USDA databases, food companies, food company websites, food labels, and the scientific literature. The format for the main database was altered slightly to include one new component—added sugars. Several new components were added to the supplementary databases: coenzyme Q, proanthocyanidins, resistant starch, serotonin, and total antioxidant capacity. In addition, individual values are provided for flavan-3-ols, flavones, flavonols, and flavanones, rather than summed values as appeared in the eighteenth edition. Like the eighteenth edition, the nineteenth is available as a CD-Rom to allow for electronic searching and retrieving of data. The CD-Rom is accompanied by an instruction manual, which is primarily designed for teaching purposes.

## CAUTIONARY NOTES

The precision and accuracy of the data and the level of detail of food descriptions and serving sizes are limited to that provided by the sources. The collection and aggregation of data from various sources invariably results in some unevenness in food descriptions and some apparent inconsistencies of food component values and serving sizes. The attempt to aggregate generic and brand-specific products causes some unevenness because descriptions for generic foods tend to be less precise, and the foods may not be recognized by data users. Likewise, data for commercial products identified only by brand or trademark names are only useful for database users who are familiar with the products.

Those unfamiliar with the use of food composition databases are requested to note the following:

- The data should be used as approximate guides to the composition of foods. Individuals on special diets for various medical conditions may require more specific composition data from food manufacturers.

- Blank spaces indicate a lack of data and should not be assumed to be zeros.

- The food component values presented here are mean values or are values used for nutrition labeling. Some of the values have large standard deviations and wide ranges. Causes of nutrient variations in foods include soil type, season, geography, genetics, animal diets, processing, method of preparation, changes in product formulations, food sampling designs, and methods of sample preparation and analysis.

- Because of nutrient variation and the fact that the data are collected from various sources (i.e., USDA, scientific literature, websites, food companies, and food labels), apparent inconsistencies may occur. For example, portion sizes, gram weights, and food component values may vary among sources for similar foods.

- The food component values presented for the foods in this edition may not be representative of the entire US food supply. Representativeness depends upon the food sampling designs and the number of samples collected and analyzed. Because the data are collected from various sources, it is not possible to control for sampling design and number of samples or even to evaluate the data based on these variables.

- The mineral content of water varies from one geographic location to anothe1r. The mineral content of beverages made by addition of water to powders or frozen concentrates and of foods cooked in water (e.g., rice, oatmeal, pasta, dry beans, and vegetables) may vary depending on the mineral content of the water used. Likewise, the mineral content of commercial beverages (e.g., beer, carbonated sodas, and juice drinks) depends on the mineral content of the water in the area where the beverages are bottled. Individuals on therapeutic diets may need to obtain information on the mineral content of their home tap water and on the mineral content of the specific beverages they consume.

- Information presented in these databases may not be the same as that provided on food labels because of industry changes in serving sizes or industry product reformulations with different ingredients or different proportions of ingredients.

- As noted above, some of the data in the supplementary databases are from older publications and from countries other than the US. They are provided here for informational purposes, but should be used with caution as they may not reflect foods available from the US market or data obtained from current analytical methods.

## Dietary Reference Intakes (DRIs)—Macronutrients: Recommended Dietary Allowances (RDAs), Adequate Intakes (AIs), and Estimated Average Requirements (EARs)[1]

| Life Stage Group | Carbohydrate (g/day) | Total Fiber (g/day) | Fat (g/day) | n-6 PUFA[2] (g/day) | n-3 PUFA[3] (g/day) | Protein[4] (g/day) | Protein (g/kg/day) |
|---|---|---|---|---|---|---|---|
| **INFANTS** | | | | | | | |
| 0–6 mo | 60 | ND | 31 | 4.4 | 0.5 | 9.1 | |
| 7–12 mo | 95 | ND | 30 | 4.6 | 0.5 | **11** | (1.0) |
| **CHILDREN** | | | | | | | |
| 1–3 yr | **130** (100) | 19 | ND | 7 | 0.7 | **13** | (0.87) |
| 4–8 yr | **130** (100) | 25 | ND | 10 | 0.9 | **19** | (0.76) |
| **MALES** | | | | | | | |
| 9–13 yr | **130** (100) | 31 | ND | 12 | 1.2 | **34** | (0.76) |
| 14–18 yr | **130** (100) | 38 | ND | 16 | 1.6 | **52** | (0.73) |
| 19–30 yr | **130** (100) | 38 | ND | 17 | 1.6 | **56** | (0.66) |
| 31–50 yr | **130** (100) | 38 | ND | 17 | 1.6 | **56** | (0.66) |
| 51–70 yr | **130** (100) | 30 | ND | 14 | 1.6 | **56** | (0.66) |
| >70 yr | **130** (100) | 30 | ND | 14 | 1.6 | **56** | (0.66) |
| **FEMALES** | | | | | | | |
| 9–13 yr | **130** (100) | 26 | ND | 10 | 1.0 | **34** | (0.76) |
| 14–18 yr | **130** (100) | 26 | ND | 11 | 1.1 | **46** | (0.71) |
| 19–30 yr | **130** (100) | 25 | ND | 12 | 1.1 | **46** | (0.66) |
| 31–50 yr | **130** (100) | 25 | ND | 12 | 1.1 | **46** | (0.66) |
| 51–70 yr | **130** (100) | 21 | ND | 11 | 1.1 | **46** | (0.66) |
| >70 yr | **130** (100) | 21 | ND | 11 | 1.1 | **46** | (0.66) |
| **PREGNANCY** | | | | | | | |
| ≤18 yr | **175** (135) | 28 | ND | 13 | 1.4 | **71** | (0.88) |
| 19–30 yr | **175** (135) | 28 | ND | 13 | 1.4 | **71** | (0.88) |
| 31–50 yr | **175** (135) | 28 | ND | 13 | 1.4 | **71** | (0.88) |
| **LACTATION** | | | | | | | |
| ≤18 yr | **210** (160) | 29 | ND | 13 | 1.3 | **71** | (1.05) |
| 19–30 yr | **210** (160) | 29 | ND | 13 | 1.3 | **71** | (1.05) |
| 31–50 yr | **210** (160) | 29 | ND | 13 | 1.3 | **71** | (1.05) |

[1] RDAs are in **bold type**, AIs in unbolded type, and EARs in unbolded type in parentheses. Both RDAs and AIs may be used as goals for individual intake. RDAs are set to meet the needs of almost all (97% to 98%) individuals within a life stage group. For healthy breastfed infants, the AI is the mean intake. The AI for other life stages is believed to cover the needs of all individuals within the group, but lack of data or uncertainty in the data prevent confidence in the percent of individuals covered by this intake. EARs are the average daily intake levels estimated to meet the requirements of half of the healthy individuals in a group.

[2] Primarily linoleic acid; however, approximately 10% of the total n-6 polyunsaturated fatty acids (PUFA) may come from longer-chain n-6 fatty acids.

[3] Primarily alpha-linolenic acid; however, approximately 10% of the total n-3 polyunsaturated fatty acids (PUFA) may come from longer-chain n-3 fatty acids.

[4] Based on g protein/kg body weight for the reference body weight, e.g., for adults 0.8 g protein/kg body weight for the reference body weight.

Source:

National Academy of Sciences. *Dietary Reference Intakes for Energy, Carbohydrate, Fiber, Fat, Fatty Acids, Cholesterol, Protein, and Amino Acids.* National Academy Press: Washington, DC, 2002. Available at www.nap.edu.

## Dietary Reference Intakes (DRIs)—Amino Acids: Recommended Dietary Allowances (RDAs), Adequate Intakes (AIs), and Estimated Average Requirements (EARs)[1]

| Amino Acid | AI[2] 0–6 mo (mg/kg/day) | RDA (EAR) 7–12 mo (mg/kg/day) | RDA (EAR) 1–3 yr (mg/kg/day) | RDA (EAR) 4–8 yr (mg/kg/day) | RDA (EAR) 9–13 yr boys (mg/kg/day) | RDA (EAR) 9–13 yr girls (mg/kg/day) |
|---|---|---|---|---|---|---|
| Histidine | 36 | 32 (22) | 21 (16) | 16 (13) | 17 (13) | 15 (12) |
| Isoleucine | 88 | 43 (30) | 28 (22) | 22 (18) | 22 (18) | 21 (17) |
| Leucine | 156 | 93 (65) | 63 (48) | 49 (40) | 49 (40) | 47 (38) |
| Lysine | 107 | 89 (62) | 58 (45) | 46 (37) | 46 (37) | 43 (35) |
| Methionine and Cysteine | 59 | 43 (30) | 28 (22) | 22 (18) | 22 (18) | 21 (17) |
| Phenylalanine and Tyrosine | 135 | 84 (58) | 54 (41) | 41 (33) | 41 (33) | 38 (31) |
| Threonine | 73 | 49 (34) | 32 (24) | 24 (19) | 24 (19) | 22 (18) |
| Tryptophan | 28 | 13 (9) | 8 (6) | 6 (5) | 6 (5) | 6 (5) |
| Valine | 87 | 58 (39) | 37 (28) | 28 (23) | 28 (23) | 27 (22) |

| Amino Acid | RDA (EAR) 14–18 yr boys (mg/kg/day) | RDA (EAR) 14–18 yr girls (mg/kg/day) | RDA (EAR) ≥19 yr adults (mg/kg/day) | RDA (EAR) pregnancy (mg/kg/day) | RDA (EAR) lactation (mg/kg/day) |
|---|---|---|---|---|---|
| Histidine | 15 (12) | 14 (12) | 14 (11) | 18 (15) | 19 (15) |
| Isoleucine | 21 (17) | 19 (16) | 19 (15) | 25 (20) | 30 (24) |
| Leucine | 47 (38) | 44 (35) | 42 (34) | 56 (45) | 62 (50) |
| Lysine | 43 (35) | 40 (32) | 38 (31) | 51 (41) | 52 (42) |
| Methionine and Cysteine | 21 (17) | 19 (16) | 19 (15) | 25 (20) | 26 (21) |
| Phenylalanine and Tyrosine | 38 (31) | 35 (28) | 33 (27) | 44 (36) | 51 (41) |
| Threonine | 22 (18) | 21 (17) | 20 (16) | 26 (21) | 30 (24) |
| Tryptophan | 6 (5) | 5 (4) | 5 (4) | 7 (5) | 9 (7) |
| Valine | 27 (22) | 24 (20) | 24 (19) | 31 (25) | 35 (28) |

[1] RDAs are in **bold type**, AIs in unbolded type, and EARs in unbolded type in parentheses. Both RDAs and AIs may be used as goals for individual intake. RDAs are set to meet the needs of almost all (97% to 98%) individuals within a life stage group. For healthy breastfed infants, the AI is the mean intake. The AI for other life stages is believed to cover the needs of all individuals within the group, but lack of data or uncertainty in the data prevent confidence in the percent of individuals covered by this intake. EARs are the average daily intake levels estimated to meet the requirements of half of the healthy individuals in a group. [2] In mg/day, the AIs for 0–6 month-old infants are 214 for histidine, 529 for isoleucine, 938 for leucine, 640 for lysine, 353 for methionine and cysteine, 807 for phenylalanine and tyrosine, 436 for threonine, 167 for tryptophan, and 519 for valine.

Source:
National Academy of Sciences. *Dietary Reference Intakes for Energy, Carbohydrate, Fiber, Fat, Fatty Acids, Cholesterol, Protein, and Amino Acids.* National Academy Press: Washington, DC, 2002. Available at www.nap.edu.

# Dietary Reference Intakes (DRIs)—Vitamins: Recommended Dietary Allowances (RDAs) and Adequate Intakes (AIs)[1]

| Life Stage Group | Vit A[2] (mcg/day) | Vit C (mg/day) | Vit D[3] (mcg/day) | Vit E[4] (mg/day) | Vit K (mcg/day) | Thiamin (mg/day) | Riboflavin (mg/day) |
|---|---|---|---|---|---|---|---|
| **INFANTS** | | | | | | | |
| 0–6 mo | 400 | 40 | 5 | 4 | 2.0 | 0.2 | 0.3 |
| 7–12 mo | 500 | 50 | 5 | 5 | 2.5 | 0.3 | 0.4 |
| **CHILDREN** | | | | | | | |
| 1–3 yr | **300** | **15** | 5 | **6** | 30 | **0.5** | **0.5** |
| 4–8 yr | **400** | **25** | 5 | **7** | 55 | **0.6** | **0.6** |
| **MALES** | | | | | | | |
| 9–13 yr | **600** | **45** | 5 | **11** | 60 | **0.9** | **0.9** |
| 14–18 yr | **900** | **75** | 5 | **15** | 75 | **1.2** | **1.3** |
| 19–30 yr | **900** | **90** | 5 | **15** | 120 | **1.2** | **1.3** |
| 31–50 yr | **900** | **90** | 5 | **15** | 120 | **1.2** | **1.3** |
| 51–70 yr | **900** | **90** | 10 | **15** | 120 | **1.2** | **1.3** |
| >70 yr | **900** | **90** | 15 | **15** | 120 | **1.2** | **1.3** |
| **FEMALES** | | | | | | | |
| 9–13 yr | **600** | **45** | 5 | **11** | 60 | **0.9** | **0.9** |
| 14–18 yr | **700** | **65** | 5 | **15** | 75 | **1.0** | **1.0** |
| 19–30 yr | **700** | **75** | 5 | **15** | 90 | **1.1** | **1.1** |
| 31–50 yr | **700** | **75** | 5 | **15** | 90 | **1.1** | **1.1** |
| 51–70 yr | **700** | **75** | 10 | **15** | 90 | **1.1** | **1.1** |
| >70 yr | **700** | **75** | 15 | **15** | 90 | **1.1** | **1.1** |
| **PREGNANCY** | | | | | | | |
| ≤18 yr | **750** | **80** | 5 | **15** | 75 | **1.4** | **1.4** |
| 19–30 yr | **770** | **85** | 5 | **15** | 90 | **1.4** | **1.4** |
| 31–50 yr | **770** | **85** | 5 | **15** | 90 | **1.4** | **1.4** |
| **LACTATION** | | | | | | | |
| ≤18 yr | **1200** | **115** | 5 | **19** | 75 | **1.4** | **1.6** |
| 19–30 yr | **1300** | **120** | 5 | **19** | 90 | **1.4** | **1.6** |
| 31–50 yr | **1300** | **120** | 5 | **19** | 90 | **1.4** | **1.6** |

[1] RDAs are in **bold type**, AIs in unbolded type. Both RDAs and AIs may be used as goals for individual intake. RDAs are set to meet the needs of almost all (97% to 98%) individuals within a life stage group. For healthy breastfed infants, the AI is the mean intake. The AI for other life stages is believed to cover the needs of all individuals within the group, but lack of data or uncertainty in the data prevent confidence in the percent of individuals covered by this intake.

[2] As retinol activity equivalents (RAEs). 1 RAE = 1 mcg retinol, 12 mcg beta-carotene, 24 mcg alpha-carotene, or 24 mcg beta-cryptoxanthin. The RAE for dietary provitamin A carotenoids is two-fold greater than retinol equivalents (RE), whereas the RAE for preformed vitamin A is the same as RE.

[3] Calciferol (vitamin $D_2$ and vitamin $D_3$; 1 mcg calciferol=40 IU vitamin D; RDI assumes the absence of adequate exposure to sunlight).

[4] As alpha-tocopherol. Alpha-tocopherol includes RRR-alpha-tocopherol, the only form of alpha-tocopherol that occurs naturally in foods, and the 2R-stereoisomeric forms of alpha-tocopherol (RRR-, RSR-, RRS-, and RSS-alpha tocopherol) that occur in fortified foods and supplements. It does not include the 2S-stereoisomeric forms of alpha-tocopherol (SRR-, SSR-, and SSS-alpha-tocopherol), also found in fortified foods and supplements.

## *Dietary Reference Intakes (DRIs)—Vitamins: Recommended Dietary Allowances (RDAs) and Adequate Intakes (AIs)[1] (continued)*

| Life Stage Group | Niacin[5] (mg/day) | Vit $B_6$ (mg/day) | Folate[6] (mcg/day) | Vit $B_{12}$[7] (mcg/day) | Pantothenic Acid (mg/day) | Biotin (mcg/day) | Choline[8] (mg/day) |
|---|---|---|---|---|---|---|---|
| **INFANTS** | | | | | | | |
| 0–6 mo | 2 | 0.1 | 65 | 0.4 | 1.7 | 5 | 125 |
| 7–12 mo | 4 | 0.3 | 80 | 0.5 | 1.8 | 6 | 150 |
| **CHILDREN** | | | | | | | |
| 1–3 yr | **6** | **0.5** | **150** | **0.9** | 2 | 8 | 200 |
| 4–8 yr | **8** | **0.6** | **200** | **1.2** | 3 | 12 | 250 |
| **MALES** | | | | | | | |
| 9–13 yr | **12** | **1.0** | **300** | **1.8** | 4 | 20 | 375 |
| 14–18 yr | **16** | **1.3** | **400** | **2.4** | 5 | 25 | 550 |
| 19–30 yr | **16** | **1.3** | **400** | **2.4** | 5 | 30 | 550 |
| 31–50 yr | **16** | **1.3** | **400** | **2.4** | 5 | 30 | 550 |
| 51–70 yr | **16** | **1.7** | **400** | **2.4** | 5 | 30 | 550 |
| >70 yr | **16** | **1.7** | **400** | **2.4** | 5 | 30 | 550 |
| **FEMALES** | | | | | | | |
| 9–13 yr | **12** | **1.0** | **300** | **1.8** | 4 | 20 | 375 |
| 14–18 yr | **14** | **1.2** | **400** | **2.4** | 5 | 25 | 400 |
| 19–30 yr | **14** | **1.3** | **400** | **2.4** | 5 | 30 | 425 |
| 31–50 yr | **14** | **1.3** | **400** | **2.4** | 5 | 30 | 425 |
| 51–70 yr | **14** | **1.5** | **400** | **2.4** | 5 | 30 | 425 |
| >70 yr | **14** | **1.5** | **400** | **2.4** | 5 | 30 | 425 |
| **PREGNANCY** | | | | | | | |
| ≤18 yr | **18** | **1.9** | **600** | **2.6** | 6 | 30 | 450 |
| 19–30 yr | **18** | **1.9** | **600** | **2.6** | 6 | 30 | 450 |
| 31–50 yr | **18** | **1.9** | **600** | **2.6** | 6 | 30 | 450 |
| **LACTATION** | | | | | | | |
| ≤18 yr | **17** | **2.0** | **500** | **2.8** | 7 | 35 | 550 |
| 19–30 yr | **17** | **2.0** | **500** | **2.8** | 7 | 35 | 550 |
| 31–50 yr | **17** | **2.0** | **500** | **2.8** | 7 | 35 | 550 |

[5] As niacin equivalents (NE) except for 0–6 months where the value is for preformed niacin (not NE); 1 mg of niacin = 60 mg of tryptophan.

[6] As dietary folate equivalents (DFE). 1 DFE = 1 mcg food folate = 0.6 mcg of folic acid from fortified food or as a supplement consumed with food = 0.5 mcg of a supplement taken on an empty stomach. In view of evidence linking folate intake with neural tube defects in the fetus, it is recommended that all women capable of becoming pregnant consume 400 mcg per day from supplements or fortified foods in addition to intake of food folate from a varied diet. It is assumed that women will continue consuming 400 mcg per day from supplements or fortified foods until their pregnancy is confirmed and they enter prenatal care, which ordinarily occurs after the end of the periconceptional period—the critical time for formation of the neural tube.

[7] Because 10% to 30% of older people may malabsorb food-bound vitamin $B_{12}$, it is advisable for those older than 50 years to meet their RDA mainly by consuming foods fortified with vitamin $B_{12}$ or a supplement containing vitamin $B_{12}$.

[8] Although AIs have been set for choline, there are few data to assess whether a dietary supply of choline is needed at all stages of the life cycle, and it may be that the choline requirement can be met by endogenous synthesis at some of these stages.

Sources:

National Academy of Sciences. *Dietary Reference Intakes for Calcium, Phosphorus, Magnesium, Vitamin D, and Fluoride,* 1997; *Dietary Reference Intakes for Thiamin, Riboflavin, Niacin, Vitamin B6, Folate, Vitamin B12, Pantothenic Acid, Biotin, and Choline,* 1998; *Dietary Reference Intakes for Vitamin C, Vitamin E, Selenium, and Carotenoids,* 2000; and *Dietary Reference Intakes for Vitamin A, Vitamin K, Arsenic, Boron, Chromium, Copper, Iodine, Iron, Manganese, Molybdenum, Nickel, Silicon, Vanadium, and Zinc,* 2001. National Academy Press: Washington, DC. Available at www.nap.edu.

## Dietary Reference Intakes (DRIs)—Vitamins: Estimated Average Requirements (EARs)[1]

| Life Stage Group | Vit A[2] (µg/day) | Vit C (mg/day) | Vit E[3] (mg/day) | Thiamin (mg/day) | Riboflavin (mg/day) | Niacin[4] (mg/day) | Vit B₆ (mg/day) | Folate[5] (µg/day) | Vit B₁₂ (µg/day) |
|---|---|---|---|---|---|---|---|---|---|
| **INFANTS** | | | | | | | | | |
| 7–12 mo | | | | | | | | | |
| **CHILDREN** | | | | | | | | | |
| 1–3 yr | 210 | 13 | 5 | 0.4 | 0.4 | 5 | 0.4 | 120 | 0.7 |
| 4–8 yr | 275 | 22 | 6 | 0.5 | 0.5 | 6 | 0.5 | 160 | 1.0 |
| **MALES** | | | | | | | | | |
| 9–13 yr | 445 | 39 | 9 | 0.7 | 0.8 | 9 | 0.8 | 250 | 1.5 |
| 14–18 yr | 630 | 63 | 12 | 1.0 | 1.1 | 12 | 1.1 | 330 | 2.0 |
| 19–30 yr | 625 | 75 | 12 | 1.0 | 1.1 | 12 | 1.1 | 320 | 2.0 |
| 31–50 yr | 625 | 75 | 12 | 1.0 | 1.1 | 12 | 1.1 | 320 | 2.0 |
| 51–70 yr | 625 | 75 | 12 | 1.0 | 1.1 | 12 | 1.4 | 320 | 2.0 |
| >70 yr | 625 | 75 | 12 | 1.0 | 1.1 | 12 | 1.4 | 320 | 2.0 |
| **FEMALES** | | | | | | | | | |
| 9–13 yr | 420 | 39 | 9 | 0.7 | 0.8 | 9 | 0.8 | 250 | 1.5 |
| 14–18 yr | 485 | 56 | 12 | 0.9 | 0.9 | 11 | 1.0 | 330 | 2.0 |
| 19–30 yr | 500 | 60 | 12 | 0.9 | 0.9 | 11 | 1.1 | 320 | 2.0 |
| 31–50 yr | 500 | 60 | 12 | 0.9 | 0.9 | 11 | 1.1 | 320 | 2.0 |
| 51–70 yr | 500 | 60 | 12 | 0.9 | 0.9 | 11 | 1.3 | 320 | 2.0 |
| >70 yr | 500 | 60 | 12 | 0.9 | 0.9 | 11 | 1.3 | 320 | 2.0 |
| **PREGNANCY** | | | | | | | | | |
| ≤18 yr | 530 | 66 | 12 | 1.2 | 1.2 | 14 | 1.6 | 520 | 2.2 |
| 19–30 yr | 550 | 70 | 12 | 1.2 | 1.2 | 14 | 1.6 | 520 | 2.2 |
| 31–50 yr | 550 | 70 | 12 | 1.2 | 1.2 | 14 | 1.6 | 520 | 2.2 |
| **LACTATION** | | | | | | | | | |
| ≤18 yr | 885 | 96 | 16 | 1.2 | 1.3 | 13 | 1.7 | 450 | 2.4 |
| 19–30 yr | 900 | 100 | 16 | 1.2 | 1.3 | 13 | 1.7 | 450 | 2.4 |
| 31–50 yr | 900 | 100 | 16 | 1.2 | 1.3 | 13 | 1.7 | 450 | 2.4 |

[1] EARs are the average daily nutrient intake level estimated to meet the requirements of half of the healthy individuals in a group. EARs have not been established for vitamin D, vitamin K, pantothenic acid, biotin, choline, or other vitamins not yet evaluated via the DRI process.

[2] As reinol activity equivalents (RAEs). 1 RAE = 1 µg retinol, 12 µg beta-carotene, 24 µg alpha-carotene, or 24 µg beta-cryptoxanthin. The RAE for dietary provitamin A carotenoids is two-fold greater than retinol equivalents (RE), whereas the RAE for preformed vitamin A is the same as RE.

[3] As alpha-tocopherol. Alpha-tocopherol includes RRR-alpha-tocopherol, the only form of alpha-tocopherol that occurs naturally in foods, and the 2R-stereoisomeric forms of alpha-tocoherol (RRR-, RSR-, RRS-, and RRS-alpha-tocopherol) that occur in fortified foods and supplements. It does not include the 2S-stereoisomeric forms of alpha-tocopherol (SRR-, SSR-, SRS-, and SSS-alpha-tocoherol), also found in fortified foods and supplements.

[4] As niacin equivelants (NE). 1 mg of niacin = 60 mg of tryptophan.

[5] As dietary folate equivalents (DFE). 1 DFE = 1 µg food folate = 0.6 µg of folic acid from fortified food or as a supplement consumed with food = 0.5 µg of a supplement taken on an empty stomach.

Sources:

National Academy of Sciences. *Dietary Reference Intakes for Calcium, Phosphorus, Magnesium, Vitamin D, and Fluoride,* 1997; *Dietary Reference Intakes for Thiamin, Riboflavin, Niacin, Vitamin B₆, Folate, Vitamin B₁₂, Pantothenic Acid, Biotin, and Choline,* 1998; *Dietary Reference Intakes for Vitamin C, Vitamin E, Selenium, and Carotenoids,* 2000; *Dietary Reference Intakes for Vitamin A, Vitamin K, Arsenic, Boron, Chromium, Copper, Iodine, Iron, Manganese, Molybdenum, Nickel, Silicon, Vanadium, and Zinc,* 2001. National Academy Press: Washington, DC. Available at www.nap.edu.

## *Dietary Reference Intakes (DRIs)—Vitamins: Tolerable Upper Intake Levels (ULs)[1]*

| Life Stage Group | Vit A[2] (mcg/day) | Vit C (mg/day) | Vit D (mcg/day) | Vit E[3,4] (mg/day) | Niacin[4] (mg/day) | Vit $B_6$ (mg/day) | Folate[4] (mcg/day) | Choline (g/day) |
|---|---|---|---|---|---|---|---|---|
| **INFANTS** | | | | | | | | |
| 0–6 mo | 600 | ND[5] | 25 | ND | ND | ND | ND | ND |
| 7–12 mo | 600 | ND | 25 | ND | ND | ND | ND | ND |
| **CHILDREN** | | | | | | | | |
| 1–3 yr | 600 | 400 | 50 | 200 | 10 | 30 | 300 | 1.0 |
| 4–8 yr | 900 | 650 | 50 | 300 | 15 | 40 | 400 | 1.0 |
| **ADULTS** | | | | | | | | |
| 9–13 yr | 1700 | 1200 | 50 | 600 | 20 | 60 | 600 | 2.0 |
| 14–18 yr | 2800 | 1800 | 50 | 800 | 30 | 80 | 800 | 3.0 |
| 19–70 yr | 3000 | 2000 | 50 | 1000 | 35 | 100 | 1000 | 3.5 |
| >70 yr | 3000 | 2000 | 50 | 1000 | 35 | 100 | 1000 | 3.5 |
| **PREGNANCY** | | | | | | | | |
| ≤18 yr | 2800 | 1800 | 50 | 800 | 30 | 80 | 800 | 3.0 |
| 19–50 yr | 3000 | 2000 | 50 | 1000 | 35 | 100 | 1000 | 3.5 |
| **LACTATION** | | | | | | | | |
| ≤18 yr | 2800 | 1800 | 50 | 800 | 30 | 80 | 800 | 3.0 |
| 19–50 yr | 3000 | 2000 | 50 | 1000 | 35 | 100 | 1000 | 3.5 |

[1] ULs are the maximum levels of daily intake that are likely to pose no risk of adverse effects. Unless otherwise specified, the UL represents total intake from food, water, and supplements. Due to lack of suitable data, ULs could not be established for vitamin K, thiamin, riboflavin, vitamin $B_{12}$, pantothenic acid, biotin, or the carotenoids. Source of intake should be from food only to prevent high levels of intake. Carotene supplements are advised only to serve as a provitamin A source for individuals at risk of vitamin A deficiency.

[2] As preformed vitamin A only.

[3] As alpha-tocopherol; applies to any form of supplemental alpha-tocopherol.

[4] The Uls for vitamin E, niacin, and folate apply to synthetic forms obtained from supplements, fortified foods, or a combination of the two.

[5] ND = Not determinable due to lack of data of adverse effects and concern with regard to lack of ability to handle excess amounts. In the absence of ULs, extra caution may be warranted in consuming levels above recommended intakes.

Sources:

National Academy of Sciences. *Dietary Reference Intakes for Calcium, Phosphorus, Magnesium, Vitamin D, and Fluoride* (1997); *Dietary Reference Intakes for Thiamin, Riboflavin, Niacin, Vitamin B6, Folate, Vitamin B12, Pantothenic Acid, Biotin, and Choline* (1998); *Dietary Reference Intakes for Vitamin C, Vitamin E, Selenium, and Carotenoids* (2000); and *Dietary Reference Intakes for Vitamin A, Vitamin K, Arsenic, Boron, Chromium, Copper, Iodine, Iron, Manganese, Molybdenum, Nickel, Silicon, Vanadium, and Zinc* (2001). National Academy Press: Washington, DC. Available at www.nap.edu.

## Dietary Reference Intakes (DRIs)—Elements: Recommended Dietary Allowances (RDAs) and Adequate Intakes (AIs)[1]

| Life Stage Group | Ca mg/day | Cr mcg/day | Cu mcg/day | F mg/day | I mcg/day | Fe mg/day | Mg mg/day | Mn mg/day | Mo mcg/day | P mg/day | Se mcg/day | Zn mg/day |
|---|---|---|---|---|---|---|---|---|---|---|---|---|
| **INFANTS** | | | | | | | | | | | | |
| 0–6 mo | 210 | 0.2 | 200 | 0.01 | 110 | 0.27 | 30 | 0.003 | 2 | 100 | 15 | 2 |
| 7–12 mo | 270 | 5.5 | 220 | 0.5 | 130 | **11** | 75 | 0.6 | 3 | 275 | 20 | 3 |
| **CHILDREN** | | | | | | | | | | | | |
| 1–3 yr | 500 | 11 | **340** | 0.7 | **90** | **7** | 80 | 1.2 | **17** | **460** | 20 | 3 |
| 4–8 yr | 800 | 15 | **440** | 1 | **90** | **10** | 130 | 1.5 | **22** | **500** | 30 | 5 |
| **MALES** | | | | | | | | | | | | |
| 9–13 yr | 1300 | 25 | **700** | 2 | **120** | **8** | 240 | 1.9 | **34** | **1250** | 40 | **8** |
| 14–18 yr | 1300 | 35 | **890** | 3 | **150** | **11** | 410 | 2.2 | **43** | **1250** | 55 | **11** |
| 19–30 yr | 1000 | 35 | **900** | 4 | **150** | **8** | 400 | 2.3 | **45** | **700** | 55 | **11** |
| 31–50 yr | 1000 | 35 | **900** | 4 | **150** | **8** | 420 | 2.3 | **45** | **700** | 55 | **11** |
| 51–70 yr | 1200 | 30 | **900** | 4 | **150** | **8** | 420 | 2.3 | **45** | **700** | 55 | **11** |
| >70 yr | 1200 | 30 | **900** | 4 | **150** | **8** | 420 | 2.3 | **45** | **700** | 55 | **11** |
| **FEMALES** | | | | | | | | | | | | |
| 9–13 yr | 1300 | 21 | **700** | 2 | **120** | **8** | 240 | 1.6 | **34** | **1250** | 40 | **8** |
| 14–18 yr | 1300 | 24 | **890** | 3 | **150** | **15** | 360 | 1.6 | **43** | **1250** | 55 | **9** |
| 19–30 yr | 1000 | 25 | **900** | 3 | **150** | **18** | 310 | 1.8 | **45** | **700** | 55 | **8** |
| 31–50 yr | 1000 | 25 | **900** | 3 | **150** | **18** | 320 | 1.8 | **45** | **700** | 55 | **8** |
| 51–70 yr | 1200 | 20 | **900** | 3 | **150** | **8** | 320 | 1.8 | **45** | **700** | 55 | **8** |
| >70 yr | 1200 | 20 | **900** | 3 | **150** | **8** | 320 | 1.8 | **45** | **700** | 55 | **8** |
| **PREGNANCY** | | | | | | | | | | | | |
| ≤18 yr | 1300 | 29 | **1000** | 3 | **220** | **27** | 400 | 2.0 | **50** | **1250** | 60 | **12** |
| 19–30 yr | 1000 | 30 | **1000** | 3 | **220** | **27** | 350 | 2.0 | **50** | **700** | 60 | **11** |
| 31–50 yr | 1000 | 30 | **1000** | 3 | **220** | **27** | 360 | 2.0 | **50** | **700** | 60 | **11** |
| **LACTATION** | | | | | | | | | | | | |
| ≤18 yr | 1300 | 44 | **1300** | 3 | **290** | **10** | 360 | 2.6 | **50** | **1250** | 70 | **13** |
| 19–30 yr | 1000 | 45 | **1300** | 3 | **290** | **9** | 310 | 2.6 | **50** | **700** | 70 | **12** |
| 31–50 yr | 1000 | 45 | **1300** | 3 | **290** | **9** | 320 | 2.6 | **50** | **700** | 70 | **12** |

[1] RDAs are in **bold type**, AIs in unbolded type. Both RDAs and AIs may be used as goals for individual intake. RDAs are set to meet the needs of almost all (97% to 98%) individuals within a life stage group. For healthy breastfed infants, the AI is the mean intake. The AI for other life stages is believed to cover the needs of all individuals within the group, but lack of data or uncertainty in the data prevent confidence in the percent of individuals covered by this intake.

Sources:

National Academy of Sciences. *Dietary Reference Intakes for Calcium, Phosphorus, Magnesium, Vitamin D, and Fluoride* (1997); *Dietary Reference Intakes for Vitamin C, Vitamin E, Selenium, and Carotenoids* (2000); and *Dietary Reference Intakes for Vitamin A, Vitamin K, Arsenic, Boron, Chromium, Copper, Iodine, Iron, Manganese, Molybdenum, Nickel, Silicon, Vanadium, and Zinc* (2001). National Academy Press: Washington, DC. Available at www.nap.edu.

# *Dietary Reference Intakes (DRIs)—Elements: Estimated Average Requirements (EARs)[1]*

| Life Stage Group | Cu (µg/day) | I (µg/day) | Fe (mg/day) | Mg (mg/day) | Mo (µg/day) | P (mg/day) | Se (µg/day) | Zn (mg/day) |
|---|---|---|---|---|---|---|---|---|
| **INFANTS** | | | | | | | | |
| 7–12 mo | | | 6.9 | | | | | 2.5 |
| **CHILDREN** | | | | | | | | |
| 1–3 yr | 260 | 65 | 3.0 | 65 | 13 | 380 | 17 | 2.5 |
| 4–8 yr | 340 | 65 | 4.1 | 110 | 17 | 405 | 23 | 4.0 |
| **MALES** | | | | | | | | |
| 9–13 yr | 540 | 73 | 5.9 | 200 | 26 | 1055 | 35 | 7.0 |
| 14–18 yr | 685 | 95 | 7.7 | 340 | 33 | 1055 | 45 | 8.5 |
| 19–30 yr | 700 | 95 | 6.0 | 330 | 34 | 580 | 45 | 9.4 |
| 31–50 yr | 700 | 95 | 6.0 | 350 | 34 | 580 | 45 | 9.4 |
| 51–70 yr | 700 | 95 | 6.0 | 350 | 34 | 580 | 45 | 9.4 |
| >70 yr | 700 | 95 | 6.0 | 350 | 34 | 580 | 45 | 9.4 |
| **FEMALES** | | | | | | | | |
| 9–13 yr | 540 | 73 | 5.7 | 200 | 26 | 1055 | 35 | 7.0 |
| 14–18 yr | 685 | 95 | 7.9 | 300 | 33 | 1055 | 45 | 7.3 |
| 19–30 yr | 700 | 95 | 8.1 | 255 | 34 | 580 | 45 | 6.8 |
| 31–50 yr | 700 | 95 | 8.1 | 265 | 34 | 580 | 45 | 6.8 |
| 51–70 yr | 700 | 95 | 5.0 | 265 | 34 | 580 | 45 | 6.8 |
| >70 yr | 700 | 95 | 5.0 | 265 | 34 | 580 | 45 | 6.8 |
| **PREGNANCY** | | | | | | | | |
| ≤18 yr | 785 | 160 | 23.0 | 335 | 40 | 1055 | 49 | 10.5 |
| 19–30 yr | 800 | 160 | 22.0 | 290 | 40 | 580 | 49 | 9.5 |
| 31–50 yr | 800 | 160 | 22.0 | 300 | 40 | 580 | 49 | 9.5 |
| **LACTATION** | | | | | | | | |
| ≤18 yr | 985 | 209 | 7.0 | 300 | 35 | 1055 | 59 | 10.9 |
| 19–30 yr | 1000 | 209 | 6.5 | 255 | 36 | 580 | 59 | 10.4 |
| 31–50 yr | 1000 | 209 | 6.5 | 265 | 36 | 580 | 59 | 10.4 |

[1] EARs are the average daily nutrient intake levels estimated to meet the requirements of half of the healthy individuals in a group. EARs have not been established for calcium, chromium, fluoride, manganese, or other elements not yet evaluated via the DRI process.

Sources:
National Academy of Sciences. *Dietary Reference Intakes for Calcium, Phosphorus, Magnesium, Vitamin D, and Fluoride* (1997); *Dietary Reference Intakes for Vitamin C, Vitamin E, Selenium, and Carotenoids* (2000); *Dietary Reference Intakes for Vitamin A, Vitamin K, Arsenic, Boron, Chromium, Copper, Iodine, Iron, Manganese, Molybdenum, Nickel, Silicon, Vanadium, and Zinc* (2001). National Academy Press: Washington, DC. Available at www.nap.edu.

# Dietary Reference Intakes (DRIs)—Elements: Tolerable Upper Intake Levels (ULs)[1]

| Life Stage Group | B (mg/day) | Ca (mg/day) | Cu (mg/day) | F (mg/day) | I (mg/day) | Fe (mg/day) | Mg[2] (mg/day) |
|---|---|---|---|---|---|---|---|
| **INFANTS** | | | | | | | |
| 0–6 mo | ND[3] | ND | ND | 0.7 | ND | 40 | ND |
| 7–12 mo | ND | ND | ND | 0.9 | ND | 40 | ND |
| **CHILDREN** | | | | | | | |
| 1–3 yr | 3 | 2500 | 1 | 1.3 | 200 | 40 | 65 |
| 4–8 yr | 6 | 2500 | 3 | 2.2 | 300 | 40 | 110 |
| **ADULTS** | | | | | | | |
| 9–13 yr | 11 | 2500 | 5 | 10 | 600 | 40 | 350 |
| 14–18 yr | 17 | 2500 | 8 | 10 | 900 | 45 | 350 |
| 19–70 yr | 20 | 2500 | 10 | 10 | 1100 | 45 | 350 |
| >70 yr | 20 | 2500 | 10 | 10 | 1100 | 45 | 350 |
| **PREGNANCY** | | | | | | | |
| ≤18 yr | 17 | 2500 | 8 | 10 | 900 | 45 | 350 |
| 19–50 yr | 20 | 2500 | 10 | 10 | 1100 | 45 | 350 |
| **LACTATION** | | | | | | | |
| ≤18 yr | 17 | 2500 | 8 | 10 | 900 | 45 | 350 |
| 19–50 yr | 20 | 2500 | 10 | 10 | 1100 | 45 | 350 |

[1] ULs are the maximum levels of daily intake that are likely to pose no risk of adverse effects. Unless otherwise specified, the UL represents total intake from food, water, and supplements. Due to lack of suitable data, ULs could not be established for arsenic, chromium, and silicon. In the absence of ULs, extra caution may be warranted in consuming levels above recommended intakes. Although the UL was not determined for arsenic, there is no justification for adding arsenic to food or supplements. Although silicon has not been shown to cause adverse effects in humans, there is no justification for adding silicon to supplements.
[2] The ULs for magnesium represent intake from a pharmacological agent only and do not include intake from food and water.
[3] ND = Not determinable due to lack of data of adverse effects and concern with regard to lack of ability to handle excess amounts. Source of intake should be only from food to prevent high levels of intake.

## *Dietary Reference Intakes (DRIs)—Elements: Tolerable Upper Intake Levels (ULs) (continued)*

| Life Stage Group | Mn (mg/day) | Mo (mcg/day) | Ni (mg/day) | P (g/day) | Se (mcg/day) | V[3] (mg/day) | Zn (mg/day) |
|---|---|---|---|---|---|---|---|
| **INFANTS** | | | | | | | |
| 0–6 mo | ND | ND | ND | ND | 45 | ND | 4 |
| 7–2 mo | ND | ND | ND | ND | 60 | ND | 5 |
| **CHILDREN** | | | | | | | |
| 1–3 yr | 2 | 300 | 0.2 | 3 | 90 | ND | 7 |
| 4–8 yr | 3 | 600 | 0.3 | 3 | 150 | ND | 12 |
| **ADULTS** | | | | | | | |
| 9–13 yr | 6 | 1100 | 0.6 | 4 | 280 | ND | 23 |
| 14–18 yr | 9 | 1700 | 1.0 | 4 | 400 | ND | 34 |
| 19–70 yr | 11 | 2000 | 1.0 | 4 | 400 | 1.8 | 40 |
| >70 yr | 11 | 2000 | 1.0 | 3 | 400 | 1.8 | 40 |
| **PREGNANCY** | | | | | | | |
| ≤18 yr | 9 | 1700 | 1.0 | 3.5 | 400 | ND | 34 |
| 19–50 yr | 11 | 2000 | 1.0 | 3.5 | 400 | ND | 40 |
| **LACTATION** | | | | | | | |
| ≤18 yr | 9 | 1700 | 1.0 | 4 | 400 | ND | 34 |
| 19–50 yr | 11 | 2000 | 1.0 | 4 | 400 | ND | 40 |

[3] Although vanadium in food has not been shown to cause adverse effects in humans, there is no justification for adding vanadium to food, and vanadium supplements should be used with caution. The UL is based on adverse effects in laboratory animals; this data could be used to set a UL for adults, but not for children or adolescents.

Sources:

National Academy of Sciences. *Dietary Reference Intakes for Calcium, Phosphorus, Magnesium, Vitamin C, and Fluoride* (1997); *Dietary Reference Intakes for Vitamin C, Vitamin E, Selenium, and Carotenoids* (2000); and *Dietary Reference Intakes for Vitamin A, Vitamin K, Arsenic, Boron, Chromium Copper, Iodine, Iron, Manganese, Molybdenum, Nickel, Silicon, Vanadium, and Zinc* (2001). National Academy Press: Washington, DC. Available at www.nap.edu.

## *Dietary Reference Intakes (DRIs)—Electrolytes and Water: Adequate Intakes (AIs) and Tolerable Upper Intake Levels (ULs)*

| Life Stage Group | Na AI[1] (g/day) | Na UL[2] (g/day) | Cl AI[1] (g/day) | Cl UL[2] (g/day) | K AI[1] (g/day) | K UL[2] (g/day) | Water AI[1] (L/day) |
|---|---|---|---|---|---|---|---|
| **INFANTS** | | | | | | | |
| 0–6 mo | 0.12 | ND[3] | 0.18 | ND | 0.4 | ND | 0.7 |
| 7–12 mo | 0.37 | ND | 0.57 | ND | 0.7 | ND | 0.8 |
| **CHILDREN** | | | | | | | |
| 1–3 yr | 1.0 | 1.5 | 1.5 | 2.3 | 3.0 | ND | 1.3 |
| 4–8 yr | 1.2 | 1.9 | 1.9 | 2.9 | 3.8 | ND | 1.7 |
| **MALES** | | | | | | | |
| 9–13 yr | 1.5 | 2.2 | 2.3 | 3.4 | 4.5 | ND | 2.4 |
| 14–18 yr | 1.5 | 2.3 | 2.3 | 3.6 | 4.7 | ND | 3.3 |
| 19–30 yr | 1.5 | 2.3 | 2.3 | 3.6 | 4.7 | ND | 3.7 |
| 31–50 yr | 1.5 | 2.3 | 2.3 | 3.6 | 4.7 | ND | 3.7 |
| 51–70 yr | 1.3 | 2.3 | 2.0 | 3.6 | 4.7 | ND | 3.7 |
| >70 yr | 1.2 | 2.3 | 1.8 | 3.6 | 4.7 | ND | 3.7 |
| **FEMALES** | | | | | | | |
| 9–13 yr | 1.5 | 2.2 | 2.3 | 3.4 | 4.5 | ND | 2.1 |
| 14–18 yr | 1.5 | 2.3 | 2.3 | 3.6 | 4.7 | ND | 2.3 |
| 19–30 yr | 1.5 | 2.3 | 2.3 | 3.6 | 4.7 | ND | 2.7 |
| 31–50 yr | 1.5 | 2.3 | 2.3 | 3.6 | 4.7 | ND | 2.7 |
| 51–70 yr | 1.3 | 2.3 | 2.0 | 3.6 | 4.7 | ND | 2.7 |
| >70 yr | 1.2 | 2.3 | 1.8 | 3.6 | 4.7 | ND | 2.7 |
| **PREGNANCY** | | | | | | | |
| ≤18 yr | 1.5 | 2.3 | 2.3 | 3.6 | 4.7 | ND | 3.0 |
| 19–50 yr | 1.5 | 2.3 | 2.3 | 3.6 | 4.7 | ND | 3.0 |
| **LACTATION** | | | | | | | |
| ≤18 yr | 1.5 | 2.3 | 2.3 | 3.6 | 5.1 | ND | 3.8 |
| 19–50 yr | 1.5 | 2.3 | 2.3 | 3.6 | 5.1 | ND | 3.8 |

[1] AIs may be used as a goal for individual intake. For healthy breastfed infants, the AI is the mean intake. The AI for other life stage and gender groups is believed to cover the needs of all individuals in the group, but lack of data prevent being able to specify with confidence the percentage of individuals covered by this intake; therefore, no Recommended Dietary Allowance (RDA) was set.

[2] ULs are the maximum levels of daily intake that are likely to pose no risk for adverse effects. Unless otherwise specified, the UL represents total intake from food, water, and supplements. Due to lack of suitable data, ULs could not be established for potassium, water, and inorganic sulfate. In the absence of ULs, extra caution may be warranted in consuming levels above recommended intakes.

[3] ND = Not determinable due to lack of data of adverse effects in this age group and concern with regard to lack of availability to handle excess amounts. Source of intake should be from food only to prevent high levels of intake.

Source: National Academy of Sciences. *Dietary Reference Intakes for Water, Potassium Sodium, Chloride, and Sulfate* (2004). National Academy Press: Washington, DC. Available at www.nap.edu.

Note: The AIs and ULs for Na and K are presented as g/day in this chart; however, the values in the database are presented as mg/serving. Thus, to compare the food values (or daily intakes from summed food values) with the AIs and ULs, convert the milligrams to grams (move the decimal three places to the left). The AIs for water are presented in this chart as L/day (a volume measure), whereas the values for water in foods in the database are presented as mg/serving (a weight measure). One liter of water weighs 1 kilogram.

## Estimated Energy Requirements (EERs) for Men and Women 30 Years of Age[1]

| Height m (in) | Physical activity level (PAL) | Weight; BMI = 18.5 kg (lb) | Weight; BMI = 24.99 kg (lb) | EER for Men; BMI = 18.5 kcal/day | EER for Men; BMI = 24.99 kcal/day | EER for Women; BMI = 18.5 kcal/day | EER for Women; BMI = 24.99 kcal/day |
|---|---|---|---|---|---|---|---|
| 1.50 (59) | Sedentary | 41.6 (92) | 56.2 (124) | 1848 | 2080 | 1625 | 1762 |
|  | Low Active |  |  | 2010 | 2268 | 1803 | 1956 |
|  | Active |  |  | 2216 | 2506 | 2025 | 2198 |
|  | Very Active |  |  | 2554 | 2898 | 2291 | 2489 |
| 1.65 (65) | Sedentary | 50.4 (111) | 68.0 (150) | 2068 | 2349 | 1816 | 1981 |
|  | Low Active |  |  | 2254 | 2566 | 2016 | 2202 |
|  | Active |  |  | 2490 | 2842 | 2267 | 2477 |
|  | Very Active |  |  | 2880 | 3296 | 2567 | 2807 |
| 1.80 (71) | Sedentary | 59.9 (132) | 81.0 (178) | 2301 | 2636 | 2015 | 2211 |
|  | Low Active |  |  | 2513 | 2884 | 2239 | 2459 |
|  | Active |  |  | 2782 | 3200 | 2519 | 2769 |
|  | Very Active |  |  | 3225 | 3720 | 2855 | 3140 |

[1] For each year below 30, add 7 kcal/day for women and 10 kcal/day for men. For each year above 30, subtract 7 kcal/day for women and 10 kcal/day for men. EERs are derived from the following regression equations based on doubly labeled water data: adult man: EER = $662 - 9.53 \times$ age (yr) + PA $\times$ ($15.91 \times$ Wt [kg] + $539.6 \times$ Ht[m]) adult woman: EER = $354 - 6.91 \times$ age (yr) + PA $\times$ ($9.36 \times$ Wt[kg] + $726 \times$ Ht[m]), where PA refers to the coefficient for Physical Activity Levels (PAL).
PAL = total energy expenditure + basal energy expenditure.
BMI = Body Mass Index
Source:
National Academy of Sciences. *Dietary Reference Intakes for Energy, Carbohydrate, Fiber, Fat, Fatty Acids, Cholesterol, Protein, and Amino Acids.* National Academy Press: Washington, DC, 2002. Available at www.nap.edu.

## Acceptable Macronutrient Distribution Ranges

| Macronutrient | 1–3 yr (% energy) | 4–18 yr (% energy) | ≥18 yr (% energy) |
|---|---|---|---|
| Fat | 30–40 | 25–35 | 20–35 |
| n-6 PUFA[1] | 5–10 | 5–10 | 5–10 |
| n-3 PUFA[2] | 0.6–1.2 | 0.6–1.2 | 0.6–1.2 |
| Carbohydrate | 45–65 | 45–65 | 45–65 |
| Protein | 5–20 | 10–30 | 10–35 |

[1] Primarily linoleic acid; however, approximately 10% of the total n-6 polyunsaturated fatty acids (PUFA) may come from longer-chain n-6 fatty acids.
[2] Primarily alpha-linolenic acid; however, approximately 10% of the total n-3 polyunsaturated fatty acids (PUFA) may come from longer-chain n-3 fatty acids.
[3] The adult category includes pregnant or lactating females regardless of age.
Source:
   National Academy of Sciences. *Dietary Reference Intakes for Energy, Carbohydrate, Fiber, Fat, Fatty Acids, Cholesterol, Protein, and Amino Acids.* National Academy Press: Washington, DC, 2002. Available at www.nap.edu.

## Daily Values (DVs) for Nutrition Labeling[1]

| Mandatory Label Component | Daily Value (DV) |
|---|---|
| Total Fat | 65 g |
| Saturated Fat | 20 g |
| Cholesterol | 300 mg |
| Sodium | 2400 mg |
| Total Carbohydrate | 300 g |
| Dietary Fiber | 25 g |
| Protein | 50 g |
| Vitamin A | 5000 IU[2] |
| Vitamin C | 60 mg |
| Calcium | 1000 mg |
| Iron | 18 mg |

| Voluntary Label Component | Daily Value (DV) |
|---|---|
| Vitamin D | 400 IU[2] |
| Vitamin E | 30 IU[2] |
| Vitamin K | 80 mcg |
| Thiamin | 1.5 mg |
| Riboflavin | 1.7 mg |
| Niacin | 20 mg |
| Vitamin $B_6$ | 2.0 mg |
| Folic Acid | 400 mcg |
| Vitamin $B_{12}$ | 6.0 mcg |
| Biotin | 300 mcg |
| Pantothenic Acid | 10 mg |
| Phosphorus | 1000 mg |
| Iodine | 150 mcg |
| Magnesium | 400 mg |
| Zinc | 15 mg |
| Selenium | 70 mcg |
| Copper | 2.0 mg |
| Manganese | 2.0 mg |
| Chromium | 120 mcg |
| Molybdenum | 75 mcg |
| Chloride | 3400 mg |
| Potassium | 3500 mg |

[1] Daily Values are based on a caloric intake of 2000 kcal per day. This listing is for foods for adults and children four or more years of age.
[2] IU = International Units.
Source:
   The Office of the Federal Register, National Archives and Records Administration. *Code of Federal Regulations, Food and Drugs*, Title 21, Part 101.9, Nutrition labeling of food. Government Printing Office: Washington, DC, 2003. Available at http://www.cfsan.fda.gov/~dms/flg-7a.html.

# Food Component Definitions

## MACRO COMPONENTS IN THE MAIN DATABASE

**WT:** Weight; the mass of the serving of food measured in grams; food weights less than 5 grams were carried to the first decimal point; weights greater than or equal to 5 grams were rounded to the nearest whole number.

**KCAL:** Kilocalories; measure of the energy value of a food when consumed; in nutrition, the term *kilocalories* is used synonymously with *calories* and *Calories*.

**H$_2$O:** Water (hydrogen oxide); molecular weight 18.016; 11.19% hydrogen, 88.81% oxygen; measured in grams.

**CHO:** Total carbohydrate; sum of mono- and disaccharides (sugars) and polysaccharides (starch); usually includes the weight of dietary fiber; composed of carbon, hydrogen, and oxygen; measured in grams.

**TSUGR:** Total sugars; sum of individual sugars (monosaccharides, disaccharides, etc.); measured in grams.

**ASUGR:** Added sugars; sum of individual sugars (monosaccharides, disaccharides, etc.) added to the food as a recipe ingredient during preparation or processing; measured in grams.

**DFIB:** Dietary fiber; includes cellulose, hemicellulose, lignin, pectin, and other nondigestible plant components; measured in grams. The main component of dietary fiber is cellulose $(C_6H_{10}O5)_n$, a nondigestible polysaccharide composed of several hundred to over 10,000 glucose units.

**PRO:** Total protein; sum of the weight of proteins and free amino acids in a food; amino acids are the building blocks of protein molecules and are composed of carbon, hydrogen, oxygen, and nitrogen; each amino acid has an amino (nitrogen) group and an acid group; measured in grams.

**FAT:** Total fat; sum of all fat-soluble components including fatty acids, phospholipids, and sterols; composed of carbon, hydrogen, and oxygen; measured in grams.

**SFA:** Saturated fat/fatty acids; sum of the fatty acids that contain no double carbon bonds; measured in grams.

**MUFA:** Monounsaturated fat/fatty acids; sum of the fatty acids with one double carbon bond; measured in grams.

**PUFA:** Polyunsaturated fat/fatty acids; sum of the fatty acids that contain two or more double carbon bonds; measured in grams.

**CHOL:** Cholesterol; $C_{27}H_{46}O$; molecular weight 386.64; 83.87% carbon, 11.99% hydrogen, 4.14% oxygen; principal sterol of animal fats and oils; measured in milligrams.

## MINERALS/ELECTROLYTES IN THE MAIN DATABASE

**Na:** Sodium (natrium); atomic weight 22.991; atomic number 11, valence 1; part of salt (sodium chloride); measured in milligrams.

**K:** Potassium; atomic weight 39.100; atomic number 19, valence 1; measured in milligrams.

**Ca:** Calcium; atomic weight 40.08; atomic number 20; valence 2; measured in milligrams.

**P:** Phosphorus; atomic weight 30.975; atomic number 15, valences 3, 5; measured in milligrams.

**Mg:** Magnesium; atomic weight 24.32; atomic number 12, valence 2; measured in milligrams.

**Fe:** Iron; atomic weight 55.85; atomic number 26, valences 2, 3; measured in milligrams.

**Zn:** Zinc; atomic weight 65.38; atomic number 30, valence 2; measured in milligrams.

**Cu:** Copper; atomic weight 63.54; atomic number 29, valences 1, 2; measured in milligrams.

**Mn:** Manganese; atomic weight 54.94; atomic number 25, valences 2, 4, 7; measured in milligrams.

**Se:** Selenium; atomic weight 78.96; atomic number 34, valences 2, 4, 6; measured in micrograms.

**Cr:** Chromium; atomic weight 52.01; atomic number 24, valences 2, 3, 6; measured in micrograms; in Section 32 only.

## VITAMINS IN THE MAIN DATABASE

**A (RAE):** Retinol measured in micrograms of Retinol Activity Equivalents (RAE); $C_{20}H_{30}O$; molecular weight 286.44; 83.86% carbon, 10.56% hydrogen, 5.59% oxygen.

**A (IU):** Retinol measured in International Units (IU); $C_{20}H_{30}O$; molecular weight 286.44; 83.86% carbon, 10.56% hydrogen, 5.59% oxygen.

**C:** L-Ascorbic acid; $C_6H_8O_6$; molecular weight 176.12; 40.91% carbon, 4.58% hydrogen, 54.51% oxygen; measured in milligrams.

**E (tocopherol):** Alpha-tocopherol, the most active form of vitamin E is $C_{28}H_{48}O_2$; molecular weight 416.66; 80.71% carbon, 11.61% hydrogen, 7.68% oxygen; measured as milligrams of alpha-tocopherol equivalents (ATE). Beta-tocopherol, which is less biologically active than alpha-tocopherol as vitamin E, is $C_{28}H_{48}O_2$; molecular weight 416.66; 80.71% carbon, 11.61% hydrogen, 7.68% oxygen.

**B$_1$:** Thiamin(e); usually present as thiamin hydrochloride, $C_{12}H_{18}Cl_2N_4OS$; molecular weight 337.28; 42.73% carbon, 5.38% hydrogen, 21.03% chloride, 16.61% nitrogen, 4.74% nitrogen, 9.51% sulfur; measured in milligrams.

**B$_2$:** Riboflavin, $C_{17}H_{20}N_4O_6$; molecular weight 376.36; 54.25% carbon, 5.36% hydrogen, 14.89% nitrogen, 25.51% oxygen; measured in milligrams.

**NIA:** Niacin, nicotinic acid, nicotinamide; $C_6H_6N_2O$; molecular weight 122.12; 59.01% carbon, 4.95% hydrogen, 22.94% nitrogen, 13.10% oxygen; measured in milligrams.

**B$_6$:** Pyridoxal, $C_8H_9NO_3$; molecular weight 167.16; 57.48% C, 5.43% H, 8.38% N, 28.72% O; Pyridoxamine dihydrochloride, $C_8H_{14}Cl_2N_2O_2$; molecular weight 241.12; 39.85 C, 5.85% H, 29.41% Cl, 11.62% N, 13.27% O; and Pyridoxine hydrochloride, $C_8H_{12}ClNO_3$; molecular weight 205.64; 46.72% C, 5.88% H, 17.24% Cl, 6.81% N, 23.34% O; measured in milligrams.

**B$_{12}$:** Cyanocobalamin; cobalt-containing B vitamin; $C_{63}H_{88}CoN_{14}P$; molecular weight 1355.38; 55.83% C, 6.54% H, 4.35% Co, 14.47% N, 16.53% O, 2.28% P; measured in micrograms.

**FOL:** Folacin; Folic acid, $C_{19}H_{19}N_7O_6$; molecular weight 441.40; 51.70% C, 4.34% H, 22.22% N, 21.75% O; Pteroylhexaglutamylglutamic Acid, $C_{49}H_{61}N_{13}O_{24}$; molecular weight 1216.13; 48.39% C, 5.06% H, 14.97% N, 31.58% O; measured as micrograms of dietary folate equivalents (DFE).

**PANT:** Pantothenic acid; $C_9H_{17}NO_5$; molecular weight 219.23; 49.30% carbon, 7.82% hydrogen, 6.39% nitrogen, 36.49% oxygen; measured in milligrams.

## FOOD COMPONENTS IN THE SUPPLEMENTARY DATABASES

**Alcohol, ethyl (ethanol):** $C_2H_5OH$; molecular weight 46.07; 52.14% carbon, 13.13% hydrogen, 34.73% oxygen; alcohol in alcoholic beverages; made from starch, sugar, and other carbohydrates by fermentation with yeast; measured in percent volume and grams.

**Amines**

    **Histamine:** $C_5H_9N_3$; molecular weight 111.15; 54.03% carbon, 8.16% hydrogen, 37.81% nitrogen; measured in milligrams.

    **Serotonin:** $C_{10}H_{12}N_2O$ (5-hyroxy-tryptamine); molecular weight 176.215; measured in milligrams.

    **Tryptamine:** $C_{10}H_{12}N_2$; molecular weight 160.21; 74.96% carbon, 7.55% hydrogen, 17.49% nitrogen; measured in milligrams.

    **Tyramine:** $C_8N_{11}NO$; molecular weight 137.18; 70.04% carbon, 8.08% hydrogen, 10.21% nitrogen, 11.66% oxygen; measured in milligrams.

**Amino Acids**

    **HIS:** L-Histidine; $C_6H_9N_3O_2$; molecular weight 155.16; 46.44% carbon, 5.85% hydrogen, 27.08% nitrogen, 20.62% oxygen; measured in milligrams.

    **ISO:** L-Isoleucine; $C_6H_{13}NO_2$; molecular weight 131.17; 54.94% carbon, 9.99% hydrogen, 10.68% hydrogen, 24.39% oxygen; measured in milligrams.

    **LEU:** L-Leucine; $C_6H_{13}NO_2$; molecular weight 131.17; 54.94% carbon, 9.99% hydrogen, 10.67% nitrogen, 24.40% oxygen; measured in milligrams.

    **LYS:** L-Lysine; $C_6H_{14}N_2O_2$; molecular weight 146.19; 49.29% carbon, 9.65% hydrogen, 19.16% nitrogen, 21.89% oxygen; measured in milligrams.

    **MET:** L-Methionine; $C_5H_{11}NO_2S$; molecular weight 149.21; 40.25% carbon, 7.43% hydrogen, 9.39% nitrogen, 21.45% oxygen, 21.49% sulfur; measured in milligrams.

    **CYS:** L-Cystine; $C_6H_{12}N_2O_4S_2$; molecular weight 240.30; 29.99% carbon, 5.03% hydrogen, 11.66% nitrogen, 26.63% oxygen, 26.69% sulfur; measured in milligrams.

    **PHE:** L-Phenylalanine; $C_9H_{11}NO_2$; molecular weight 165.19; 65.43% carbon, 6.71% hydrogen, 8.48% nitrogen, 19.37% oxygen; measured in milligrams.

    **TYR:** L-Tyrosine; $C_9H_{11}NO_3$; molecular weight 181.19; 59.66% carbon, 6.12% hydrogen, 7.73% nitrogen, 26.49% oxygen; measured in milligrams.

    **THR:** L-Threonine; $C_4H_9NO_3$; molecular weight 119.12; 40.33% carbon, 7.62% hydrogen, 11.76% nitrogen, 40.29% oxygen; measured in milligrams.

    **TRY:** L-Tryptophan; $C_{11}H_{12}N_2O_2$; molecular weight 204.22; 64.69% carbon, 5.92% hydrogen, 13.72% nitrogen, 15.67% oxygen; measured in milligrams.

    **VAL:** L-Valine; $C_5H_{11}NO_2$; molecular weight 117.15; 51.26% carbon, 9.46% hydrogen, 11.96% nitrogen, 27.32% oxygen; measured in milligrams.

    **ARG:** L-Arginine; $C_6H_{14}N_4O_2$; molecular weight 174.20; 41.36% carbon, 8.1% hydrogen, 32.16% nitrogen, 18.37% oxygen; measured in milligrams.

    **TAU:** Taurine; $C_2H_7NO_3S$; molecular weight 125.14; 19.19% carbon, 5.64% hydrogen, 11.19% nitrogen, 38.35% oxygen, 25.62% sulphur; listed only in Section 32 of the main database.

    **CAR:** L-Carnitine; $C_7H_{15}NO_3$; molecular weight 161.20; 52.15% carbon, 9.38% hydrogen, 8.69% nitrogen, 29.78% oxygen; listed only in Section 32 of the main database.

**Caffeine and Theobromine**

    **Caffeine (1,3,7-trimethylxanthine):** $C_6H_{10}N_4O_2$; molecular weight 194.19; 49.48% carbon, 5.19% hydrogen, 28.85% nitrogen, 16.48% oxygen; methylxanthine found in coffee, tea, chocolate, cocoa, and cola beverages; acts as central nervous system stimulant; measured in milligrams.

    **Theobromine (3,7-dimethylxanthine):** $C_7H_8N_4O_2$; molecular weight 180.17; 46.66% carbon, 4.48% hydrogen, 31.10% nitrogen, 17.76% oxygen; principal alkaloid (methylxanthine) of the cacao bean which contains 1.5 to 3% of this compound; also present in coffee and tea; measured in milligrams.

**Carotenoids:** Orange-yellow-red pigments some of which have provitamin A activity; includes alpha-carotene, beta-carotene, beta-cryptoxanthin, lutein and zeaxanthin, and lycopene; measured in micrograms.

    **Alpha-Carotene:** $C_{40}H_{56}$; molecular weight 536.85; 89.49% carbon,10.51% hydrogen; provitamin A; about half as active as beta-carotene as a provitamin A precursor.

    **Beta-Carotene:** $C_{40}H_{56}$; molecular weight 536.85; 89.49% carbon, 10.51% hydrogen; most active/important of the provitamins A.

    **Beta-Cryptoxanthin:** $C_{40}H_{56}O$; molecular weight 552.85; 86.90% carbon, 10.21% hydrogen, 2.89% oxygen; some vitamin A activity.

    **Lutein:** $C_{40}H_{56}O_2$; molecular weight 568.85; 84.45% carbon, 9.92% hydrogen, 5.63% oxygen; carotenoid alcohol (xanthophyll); not a vitamin A precursor.

    **Lycopene:** $C_{40}H_{56}$; molecular weight 536.85; 89.48% carbon, 10.51% hydrogen; not a vitamin A precursor; major source is tomatoes.

**Zeaxanthin:** $C_{40}H_{56}O_2$; molecular weight 568.85; 84.45% carbon, 9.92% hydrogen, 5.63% oxygen; carotenoid alcohol (xanthophylls); not a vitamin A precursor.

**Coenzyme Q (ubiquinone):** $C_{59}H_{40}O_4$; benzoquinone with 10 isoprenyl chemical subunits; the Q refers to the quinine chemical group; also known as Coenzyme Q10, CoQ10, and CoQ; measured in micrograms.

**Dietary Fiber Components**

**Lignin:** Coniferyl, para-coumaryl, and sinapyl alcohols such as matairesinol and secoisolariciresinol found in various plants (e.g., whole grains, beans, peas); most abundant natural aromatic organic polymer in vascular plants; measured in grams.

**Pectin:** Polysaccharide in cell walls of plants; consists primarily of partially methoxylated polygalacturonic acids; molecular weight from 20,000 to 400,000; measured in grams.

**Fatty Acids**

**Omega-3 Fatty Acids:** Polyunsaturated fatty acids with the endmost double bond three carbons back from the end of the carbon chain; sum of available data for alpha-linolenic acid (ALA; 18:3 n-3), eicosapentaenoic acid (EPA; 20:5 n-3), docosapentaenoic acid (DPA; 22:5 n-3), and docosahexaenoic acid (DHA; 22:6 n-3); measured in grams.

**Trans Fatty Acids:** Sum of available data for trans palmitoleic acid (16:1), trans oleic acid (18:1), and trans linoleic acid (18:2); measured in grams.

**Flavonoids**

**Anthocyanins:** Individual values for cyanidin, delphinidin, malvidin, pelargonidin, peonidin, and petunidin; measured in milligrams.

**Flavan-3-ols—Catechins:** Individual values for (−)-epicatechin, (−)-epicatechin 3-gallate, (−)-epigallocatechin, (−)-epigallocatechin 3-gallate, (+)-catechin, (+)-catechin 3-galate, (+)-gallocatechin; measured in milligrams.

**Flavan-3-ols—Theaflavins and Thearubigins:** theaflavin 3,3'digallate, theaflavin 3'-gallate, theaflavin 3-gallate, and thearubigins; measured in milligrams.

**Flavones:** Individual values for apigenin and luteolin; measured in milligrams.

**Flavonols:** Individual values for isorhamnetin, kaempferol, myricetin, and quercetin; measured in milligrams.

**Flavanones:** Individual values for eriodictyol, hesperetin, and narigenin; measured in milligrams.

**Proanthocyanidins:** polymers of flavan-3-ols also know as condensed tannins; presented as monomers, dimmers, trimers, 4–6-mers, 7–10-mers, and polymers; measured in milligrams.

**Isoflavones:** Individual values for the most prominent isoflavones: daidzein, genistein, and glycitein, as well as total isoflavones; measured in milligrams.

**Biochanin A, Coumesterol, and Formononetin:** Compounds that share the estrogenic/antiestrogenic, antioxidant, and antiproliferative activities of the prominent isoflavones (daidzein, genistein, and glycitein).

**Biochanin A:** 4-methyl ether derivative of genistein; reduced to genistein by intestinal bacteria; $C_{16}H_{12}O_5$; measured in milligrams.

**Coumestrol:** The most common coumestan; has a structure similar to and competes with estradiol for cytoplasmic receptors in mammary tumor cells; $C_{15}H_8O_5$; molecular weight 268.21; 67.17% C, 3.01% H, 29.83% O; measured in milligrams.

**Formononetin:** 4-methyl ether derivative of daidzein; reduced to daidzein by intestinal bacteria; $C_{16}H_{12}O_4$; molecular weight 268.26; 71.63% C, 4.51% H, 23.86% C; measured in milligrams.

**Glutathione:** Tripeptide; $C_{10}H_{17}N_3O_6S$; molecular weight 307.33; 39.08% carbon, 5.58% hydrogen, 13.67% nitrogen, 31.24% oxygen, 10.43% sulfur; a bioactive component; measured in milligrams.

**Gluten:** A mixture of plant proteins occurring in cereal grains, especially wheat, and composed chiefly of gliadin and glutenin; allergy to these proteins results in celiac disease and requires a gluten-free or low-gluten diet.

**Minerals**

**Iodine (I):** atomic weight 126.91; atomic number 53, valences 1, 3, 5, 7; measured in micrograms.

**Molybdenum (Mo):** atomic weight 95.95; atomic number 42, valences 2, 3, 4, 6; measured in micrograms.

**Plant Acids**

**Oxalic acid:** $C_2H_2O_4$; molecular weight 126.07; 26.68% carbon, 2.24% hydrogen, 71.08% oxygen; may bind with minerals and prevent complete mineral absorption; measured in milligrams.

**Phytic acid:** $C_{18}H_{24}O_6$; molecular weight 660.08; 10.92% carbon, 2.75% hydrogen, 28.16% phosphorus, 58.18% oxygen; measured in milligrams.

**Salicylic acid:** $C_7H_6O_3$; molecular weight 138.12; 60.87% carbon, 4.38% hydrogen, 34.75% oxygen; measured in micrograms.

**Plant Sterols**

**Phytosterol:** Generic name for sterols from plants; includes stigmasterol, sitosterol, fucosterol, brassicasterol, and campesterol; measured in milligrams.

**Campesterol:** $C_{28}H_{48}O$; molecular weight 400.66; 83.93% carbon, 12.08% hydrogen, 3.99% oxygen; found in rapeseed oil, soybean oil, and wheat germ oil; measured in milligrams.

**Beta-sitosterol:** $C_{29}H_{50}O$; molecular weight 414.69; 83.99% carbon, 12.15% hydrogen, 3.86% oxygen; measured in milligrams.

**Stigmasterol:** $C_{29}H_{48}O$; molecular weight 412.67; 84.40% carbon, 11.72% hydrogen, 3.88% oxygen; measured in milligrams.

**Purines:** Sum of adenine, guanine, and other purines; constituents of nucleic acids; $C_5H_4N_4$; molecular weight 120.11; 50.00% carbon, 3.36% hydrogen, 46.65% nitrogen; measured in milligrams.

**Resistant Starch:** $(C_6H_{12}O_6)_n$; polysaccharide carbohydrate consisting of a large number of glucose monosaccharide units joined together by glycosidic bonds that escapes digestion in the small intestine; measured in milligrams.

**Sugars**

**Galactose:** $C_6H_{12}O_6$; molecular weight 180.16; 40.00% carbon, 6.72% hydrogen, 53.29% oxygen; monosaccharide; measured in grams.

**Glucose (dextrose):** $C_6H_{12}O_6$; molecular weight 180.16; 40.00% carbon, 6.72% hydrogen, 53.29% oxygen; monosaccharide; measured in grams.

**Fructose:** $C_6H_{12}O_6$; molecular weight 180.16; 40.00% carbon, 6.72% hydrogen, 53.29% oxygen; monosaccharide; measured in grams.

**Lactose:** $C_{12}H_{22}O_{11}$; molecular weight 342.30; 42.10% carbon, 6.48% hydrogen, 51.42% oxygen; disaccharide composed of glucose and galactose; major sources are mammal milks; measured in grams.

**Sucrose:** $C_{12}H_{22}O_{11}$; molecular weight 342.30; 42.10% carbon, 6.48% hydrogen, 51.42% oxygen; disaccharide composed of glucose and fructose; major sources are sugar cane and sugar beets; measured in grams.

**Maltose:** $C_{12}H_{22}O_{11}$; molecular weight 342.30; 42.10% carbon, 6.48% hydrogen, 51.42% oxygen; disaccharide composed of 2 glucose molecules; measured in grams.

**Raffinose:** $C_{18}H_{32}O_{16}$; molecular weight 504.46; 42.86% C, 6.39% H, 50.75% O; trisaccharide composed of galactose, glucose, and fructose; measured in grams.

**Stachyose:** $C_{24}H_{42}O_{21}$; molecular weight 666; 43.24% C, 6.31% H, 50.45% H; tetrasaccharide; measured in grams.

**Total Antioxidant Capacity (TAC):** the antioxidant capacity of foods usually measured by the oxygen radical absorbance capacity (ORAC) method; measured in micromoles of Trolox equivalents (TE).

**Vitamins/Vitamin-Like Components**

**Biotin:** $C_{10}H_{16}N_2O_3S$; molecular weight 244.31; 49.16% carbon, 6.6% hydrogen, 11.47% nitrogen, 19.65% oxygen, 13.12% sulfur; richest sources are liver, kidney, pancreas, yeast, milk, and egg yolk; combines with the proteinaceous substance, avidin, in raw egg white and becomes inactive; older names are vitamin H and coenzyme R; measured in micrograms.

**Choline:** $C_5H_{15}NO_2$; molecular weight 121.18; 49.55% carbon, 12.46% hydrogen, 11.56% nitrogen, 26.41% oxygen; measured in milligrams.

**Betaine:** $C_5H_{11}NO_2$; molecular weight 117.15; 51.26% carbon, 9.46% hydrogen, 11.96% nitrogen, 27.32% oxygen; measured in milligrams

**Myo-Inositol:** $C_6H_{12}O_6$; molecular weight 180.16; 40.00% carbon, 6.71% hydrogen, 53.29% oxygen; measured in milligrams.

**Vitamin $D_3$ (Cholecalciferol, 7-dehydrocholesterol):** $C_{27}H_{44}O$; molecular weight 384.62; 84.31% carbon, 11.53% hydrogen, 4.16% oxygen; measured in International Units (IU).

**Vitamin K (Phylloquinone):** $C_{31}H_{46}O_2$; molecular weight 450.68; 82.61% carbon, 10.29% hydrogen, 7.10% oxygen; measured in micrograms.

Sources:
Shils ME, Olson JA, Shike MA, et al. *Modern Nutrition in Health and Disease.* 9th Edition. Lippincott Williams & Wilkins: Baltimore, 1999. *The Merck Index. An Encyclopedia of Chemicals, Drugs, and Biologicals.* 11th Edition. Merck & Co., Inc: Rahway, NJ, 1989.

# Amino Acids and Pathways of Utilization

| Indispensable | Conditionally Indispensable | Dispensable |
|---|---|---|
| Histidine | Arginine | Alanine |
| Isoleucine | Cysteine | Aspartic acid |
| Leucine | Glutamine | Glutamic acid |
| Lysine | Glycine | Serine |
| Methionine | Proline | Taurine |
| Phenylalanine | Tyrosine | |
| Threonine | | |
| Tryptophan | | |
| Valine | | |

Some amino acids are metabolized into other important compounds. Nonprotein pathways of some amino acids are listed below:

| Amino Acid(s) | Metabolic Product(s) |
|---|---|
| Tryptophan | Serotonin, nicotinic acid |
| Tyrosine | Catecholamines, thyroid hormones, melanin |
| Lysine | Carnitine |
| Cysteine | Taurine |
| Arginine | Nitric oxide |
| Glycine | Heme |
| Glycine, arginine, methionine | Creatine |
| Methionine, glycine, serine | Methyl group metabolism |
| Glycine, taurine | Bile acids |
| Glutamic acid, cysteine, glycine | Glutathione |
| Glutamic acid, aspartic acid, glycine | Nucleic acid bases |

Source:
National Academy of Sciences. *Dietary Reference Intakes for Energy, Carbohydrate, Fiber, Fat, Fatty Acids, Cholesterol, Protein, and Amino Acids.* National Academy Press: Washington, DC, 2002. Available at www.nap.edu.

# *Abbreviations and Symbols*[1]

| | | | |
|---|---|---|---|
| AIs | Adequate Intakes | DRIs | Dietary Reference Intakes |
| Al | aluminum | drmstk | drumstick |
| Am | American | drsing | dressing |
| amt | amount | DV | Daily Value |
| apl | apple | Ed | Edition |
| ARG | arginine | EER | estimated energy requirement |
| ASUGR | added sugars | enr | enriched |
| ATE | alpha-tocopherol equivalents | Extr Hlpng | Extra Helping |
| avg | average | F | fluoride/fluorine |
| ban | banana | Fe | iron |
| bbq | barbeque | Fds | Foods |
| Bch-Nut | Beech-Nut | fill | filling |
| Bgnr | Beginner | fl oz | fluid ounce(s) |
| bev | beverage | FOL | folacin/folic acid |
| BIO | biotin | frank | frankfurter |
| bis | biscuit | frzn | frozen (commercially) |
| bkd | baked | g | gram(s) |
| BMI | body mass index | grld | grilled |
| brld | broiled | grn | green |
| broc | broccoli | grn bns | green beans |
| brwn | brown | Grn Gnt Sklt Mls | Green Giant Skillet Meals |
| brwns | browns | grvy | gravy |
| btld | bottled | H | hydrogen |
| C | carbon | $H_2O$ | water |
| Ca | calcium | HIS | histidine |
| cal | calorie(s) | Hlpng | Helping |
| CAR | carnitine | Hlthy | Healthy |
| car | carrots | Hlthy Chc | Healthy Choice |
| cblr | cobbler | Hnz | Heinz |
| cc | cubic centimeter(s) | hydg | hydrogenated |
| ched | cheddar | I | iodine/iodide |
| chkn | chicken | INOS | inositol/myo-inositol |
| CHLN | choline | inst | instant |
| CHO | carbohydrate | ISO | isoleucine |
| choc | chocolate | IU | International Units |
| CHOL | cholesterol | jce | juice |
| chpd | chopped | jr/Jr | junior/Junior |
| chptl | chipotle | K | potassium |
| chry | cherry | KCAL | calorie(s) |
| chs | cheese | Kg | kilogram(s) |
| cinn | cinnamon | L | liter |
| ckd | cooked | lb | pound |
| Cl | chloride | lett | lettuce |
| Cmpbls | Campbell's | LEU | leucine |
| cnd | canned (commercially) | low-cal | low-calorie |
| cntr | center | LYS | lysine |
| Co | Company | mac | macaroni |
| conc | concentrate | marg | margarine |
| cond | condensed | mayo | mayonnaise |
| Cr | chromium | mcg | micrograms |
| Crkr | Crocker | mct | medium-chain triglycerides |
| crm | cream | med | medium |
| crnbrs | cranberries | MET | methionine |
| Cu | copper | mg | milligrams |
| cvrd | covered | Mg | magnesium |
| CYS | cystine | MgCl | magnesium chloride |
| decaf | decaffeinated | min | minute(s) |
| DFE | dietary folate equivalents | Mn | manganese |
| DFIBR | dietary fiber | ml | milliter |
| dia | diameter | Mo | molybdenum |

| | | | |
|---|---|---|---|
| mozz | mozzarella | slds | solids |
| mshd | mashed | smkd | smoked |
| mshrm/mshrms | mushroom/mushrooms | sml | small |
| msqt | mesquite | sndwch | sandwich |
| MUFA | monounsaturated fatty acids | sprd | spread |
| must | mustard | sqzd | squeezed |
| mxd | mixed | Stfrs Hmstl | Stouffer's Homestyle |
| N | nitrogen | Stfrs Ln Csn | Stouffer's Lean Cuisine |
| n-3 | omega three (fatty acids) | Stg | Stage |
| n-6 | omega six (fatty acids) | stk | steak |
| Na | sodium | str/Str | strained/Strained |
| ndls | noodles | sub | submarine sandwich |
| NE | niacin equivalents | Suprm | Supreme |
| nfdm | nonfat dry milk solids | swtnd | sweetened |
| Ni | nickel | swtnr(s) | sweetener(s) |
| NIA | niacin | t | teaspoon |
| O | oxygen | T | tablespoon |
| oz | ounce | TAU | taurine |
| P | phosphorus | TE | trolox equivalents |
| PAL | physical activity level | THR | threonine |
| PANT | panthothenic acid | tom | tomato(es) |
| pckt(s) | pocket(s) | tr | trace |
| pcs | pieces | trpcl | tropical |
| peprs | peppers | TRY | tryptophan |
| PHE | phenylalanine | TSUGR | total sugars |
| pkg | package | TYR | tyrosine |
| pkt | packet | ULs | Tolerable Upper Intake Levels |
| pnt | peanut | US | United States |
| pot | potatoes | V | vanadium |
| prep | prepared | VAL | valine |
| PRO/pro | protein | van | vanilla |
| PUFA | polyunsaturated fatty acids | veg(s) | vegetable(s) |
| pwdr | powder | vit A | vitamin A |
| RAE | retinol activity equivalents | vit $B_1$ | vitamin $B_1$ (thiamine) |
| rasp | raspberry | vit $B_2$ | vitamin $B_2$ (riboflavin) |
| RDAs | Recommended Dietary Allowances | vit $B_6$ | vitamin $B_6$ (pyridoxine) |
| | | vit $B_{12}$ | vitamin $B_{12}$ (cyanocobalamin) |
| RE | retinol equivalents | vit C | vitamin C (ascorbic acid) |
| recon | reconstituted | vit D | vitamin D (calciferol) |
| red | reduced | vit E | vitamin E (tocopherol) |
| red cal | reduced cal | vit K | vitamin K |
| REF | reference code[1] | vol | volume |
| refrig | refrigerated | whpd | whipped |
| reg | regular | wht | wheat |
| rnch | ranch | wrpd | wrapped |
| rsn | raisin | WT | weight |
| rstd | roasted | Wt Wtchrs | Weight Watchers |
| rte | ready-to-eat | w/ | with |
| rtf | ready-to-feed | w/o | without |
| rts | ready-to-serve | Zn | zinc |
| S | sulfur/sulphur | & | and |
| sand | sandwich | ~ | approximately |
| sausg | sausage | " | inch(es) |
| sce | sauce | # | number |
| scrmbld | scrambled | < | less than |
| Se | selenium | ≤ | less than or equal to |
| sec | second | > | greater than |
| serv | serving | ≥ | greater than or equal to |
| SFA | saturated fatty acids | / | per; or |
| Sfwy Grmt Clb | Safeway Select Gourmet Club | % | percent |
| shldr | shoulder | 0 | zero (none) |
| skn | skin | blank space | lack of information |

---

[1] The acronymns and code numbers used for reference codes are explained in the section on *Reference Codes.*

## Reference Codes

The reference code is provided in the lower right-hand position for each food in the main database and indicates the source of the data. The reference codes that are 5-digit numbers represent food names and data from the USDA Database for Standard Reference, Release 21 (2008). The alpha reference codes refer to the food companies and restaurants listed below. Data were obtained from these food companies and restaurants through contact with their nutritionists/representatives, promotional materials, websites, and/or label information.

| Code | Data Source and Location |
|------|--------------------------|
| AANW | A&W |
| ANNA | Annabelle Candy Company |
| AQUA | Aqua Vie |
| ARBY | Arby's |
| ARCH | Archway Cookies, Inc. |
| ARNO | Arnold Foods Company, Inc. |
| ATCO | Ateeco, Inc. |
| AUBN | Au Bon Pain |
| BARB | Barbara's Bakery, Inc. |
| BIGE | Bigelow |
| BNJR | Ben & Jerry's Homemade, Inc. |
| BOBE | Bob Evans |
| BOBO | Boboli (George Weston Bakeries) |
| BOST | Boston Market Corporation |
| BOYE | Boyer Candy Company |
| BRID | Bridgford Foods Corporation |
| BRYS | Breyers Ice Cream Company |
| BSKN | Baskin-Robbins |
| CHEF | Chef Garcia Mexican Foods |
| CELE | Hain Celestial Group, Inc. |
| CHUK | Chukar Cherry Company |
| CLIF | Clif Bar, Inc. |
| CNAG | ConAgra Foods |
| COLA | The Coca-Cola Company |
| CRVL | Carvel Corporation |
| DELM | Del Monte Foods |
| EDYS | Edy's/Dreyer's Grand Ice Cream |
| ENTE | Entenmann's (George Weston Bakeries) |
| EQEX | Equal Exchange |
| FERR | Ferrara Pan Candy Company |
| FLOR | Florida's Natural Growers |
| FRAL | Fralinger's |
| FRIT | Frito-Lay, Inc. |
| FRUI | Fruition Foods, Inc. |
| FUZE | Fuze |
| GARD | Garden of Eatin' (Hain Celestial Group, Inc.) |
| GENI | GeniSoy |
| GENM | General Mills, Inc. |
| GERB | Gerber Products Company |
| GHIR | Ghirardelli Chocolate Company |
| GIRL | Girl Scout Cookies, (Little Brownie Bakers) |
| GODI | Godiva Chocolatier, Inc. |
| GORT | Gorton's, Inc. |
| GOYA | Goya Foods, Inc. |
| GUBA | Gubor Feinste Schoklade GmbH |
| HADA | Harry and David |
| HLCH | Healthy Choice, ConAgra Brands, Inc. |
| HOUS | House Cafe |
| HRSH | Hershey Foods Corporation |
| INOU | In-N-Out Burger |
| JELL | Jelly Belly Candy Company |
| JIMM | Jimmy Dean Foods |
| KAME | KA-ME (Panos Brands) |

| Code | Data Source and Location |
|------|--------------------------|
| KELL | Kellogg's Company |
| KFCN | Kentucky Fried Chicken |
| KRAF | Kraft Foods |
| KRIS | Krispy Kreme |
| LIBO | Liberty Orchards |
| MARI | Mariani Packing Company |
| MARZ | T. Marzetti Company |
| MAUN | Mauna Loa Macadamia Nut Corporation |
| MDJN | Mead Johnson Nutritionals |
| MICA | Michael Angelo's Gourmet Foods, Inc. |
| MIDE | Mi-Del |
| MNTM | The Minute Maid Company |
| MORT | Morton Salt |
| NANC | Nancy's Specialty Foods |
| NBSC | Nabisco |
| NEST | Nestle Clinical Nutrition |
| NTEA | Nestle USA |
| NEWM | Newman's Own, Inc. |
| NTRI | Nutricia North America |
| OCEA | Ocean Spray Cranberries, Inc. |
| ODWA | Odwalla, Inc. |
| ORGA | Organics (Safeway/Safeway Select) |
| PERU | Perugina |
| PNSS | PNS&S Steak Company |
| POPE | Popeyes Louisiana Kitchen |
| PRIE | Priester's Pecan Company |
| PRIV | Promopeddler |
| RSSM | Abbott Labs, Ross Products Division, Medical Foods |
| SAFE | Safeway/Safeway Select |
| SARG | Sargento |
| SCHA | Scharffen Berger Chocolate Maker |
| SEES | See's Candies |
| SHST | Shasta Sales, Inc. |
| SNYD | Snyder's of Hanover, Inc. |
| STAR | Starbucks Corporation |
| STOF | Stouffer's Food Corporation (Nestle USA, Inc.) |
| STOR | Storck USA |
| STRE | Aron Streit, Inc. |
| SUBW | Subway Restaurants |
| SUNN | Sunnyland Farms |
| SUNS | Sunsweet Growers, Inc. |
| TAST | Tasty Baking Company |
| THOM | Thomas' (George Weston Bakeries) |
| THRE | 365 Brand |
| TRAD | Trader Joe's |
| TURK | Turkey Hill Dairy |
| UTZQ | Tuz Quality Foods, Inc. |
| VANS | Van's International Foods |
| WISC | Wisconsin Cheeseman |
| WLCH | Welch's |
| WOLF | Wolferman's |
| WRIG | William Wrigley Jr. Company |

# Heat, Weight, & Volume Conversions

## Heat Measures

| Kilojoules | Kilocalories |
|---|---|
| 1 | 0.239 |
| 4.182 | 1 |

## Weight Measures

| mcg | mg | g | kg | oz | lb |
|---|---|---|---|---|---|
| 1000 | 1 | 0.001 | 0.000001 | 0.000035 | 0.000002 |
| 1,000,000 | 1000 | 1 | 0.001 | 0.035 | 0.002 |
| 1,000,000,000 | 1,000,000 | 1000 | 1 | 35.36 | 2.2 |
| 28,350,000 | 28,350 | 28.35[1] | 0.028 | 1 | 0.0625 |
| 453,590,000 | 453,590 | 453.59[2] | 0.454 | 16 | 1 |

[1] Often rounded to 28 g.
[2] Often rounded to 454 g.

## Volume Measures

| t | T | fl oz | cups | pints | quarts | mL/cc | Liters |
|---|---|---|---|---|---|---|---|
| 0.21 | 0.07 | 0.034 | 0.004 | 0.002 | 0.001 | 1 | 0.001 |
| 1 | 0.33 | 0.17 | 0.021 | 0.011 | 0.005 | 4.9 | 0.005 |
| 3 | 1 | 0.5 | 0.063 | 0.031 | 0.016 | 14.8 | 0.015 |
| 6 | 2 | 1 | 0.125 | 0.063 | 0.03 | 20.6 | 0.021 |
| 12 | 4 | 2 | 0.25 | 0.125 | 0.06 | 59.1 | 0.059 |
| 16 | 5.33 | 2.6 | 0.33 | 0.167 | 0.08 | 78.9 | 0.079 |
| 24 | 8 | 4 | 0.5 | 0.25 | 0.13 | 118.3 | 0.118 |
| 32 | 10.67 | 5.3 | 0.67 | 0.34 | 0.17 | 157.7 | 0.158 |
| 36 | 12 | 6 | 0.75 | 0.38 | 0.19 | 177.4 | 0.177 |
| 42 | 14 | 7 | 0.875 | 0.44 | 0.22 | 207.0 | 0.207 |
| 48 | 16 | 8 | 1 | 0.5 | 0.25 | 236.6 | 0.237 |
| 96 | 32 | 16 | 2 | 1 | 0.5 | 473 | 0.473 |
| 100.8 | 33.6 | 17 | 2.1 | 1.06 | 0.53 | 500 | 0.500 |
| 192 | 64 | 32 | 4 | 2 | 1 | 946 | 0.946 |
| 201.6 | 67.2 | 34 | 4.2 | 2.11 | 1.06 | 1000 | 1.000 |
| 768 | 256 | 128 | 16 | 8 | 4 | 3785 | 3.785 |

## Volume-Weight Relationships

The relationship between volume and weight measures is variable and depends on the density of the food. The weights of 1 level cup of various foods are provided below as examples:

| Food | Weight/cup (g) |
|---|---|
| puffed wheat cereal | 12 |
| shredded wheat cereal | 49 |
| green beans (snap beans), boiled | 125 |
| strawberries, raw whole | 144 |
| green peas, canned | 170 |
| cottage cheese | 210 |
| mayonnaise | 224 |
| water | 237 |
| pickle relish | 240 |
| chicken noodle soup | 241 |
| whole milk | 244 |
| orange juice | 249 |
| macaroni and cheese, cnd | 252 |
| peanut butter | 256 |
| chili con carne, cnd | 256 |

The serving sizes for beverages and some other foods (soups, salad dressings, yogurt, infant formula, medical formulas) are usually provided in fluid ounces, which is a volume measure. The gram weight of one fluid ounce of these beverages and foods varies according to the density of the food. Some examples are provided below in the left-hand box. The volume weight of water is a commonly used reference point for the weight of other fluids. The box on the right below provides the weight of various volumes of water.

| Food | Weight/fl oz (g) | Volume of Water | Weight of Water (g) |
|---|---|---|---|
| yogurt | 28.4 | 1 mL/cc | 1 |
| coffee | 29.5 | 1 T (15 mL/cc) | 15 |
| water | 29.6[1] | 1 fl oz | 29.6[1] |
| tea | 29.7 | 1 cup | 237 |
| whole milk | 30.5 | 1 quart | 948 |
| soy milk | 30.6 | 1 liter | 1000 (1 kg) |
| cola | 30.8 | | |
| fruit punch | 31.0 | | |
| orange juice | 31.1 | | |
| cranberry juice | 31.6 | | |

[1] Often rounded to 30 g.

# Gram-Ounce Equivalents (g-oz)[1]

| g-oz | g-oz | g-oz | g-oz | g-oz | g-oz | g-oz | g-oz | g-oz | g-oz | g-oz |
|------|------|------|------|------|------|------|------|------|------|------|
| 001-0.04 | 044-1.6 | 087-3.1 | 130-4.6 | 173-6.1 | 216-7.6 | 259-9.1 | 302-10.7 | 345-12.2 | 388-13.7 | 431-15.2 |
| 002-0.07 | 045-1.6 | 088-3.1 | 131-4.6 | 174-6.1 | 217-7.7 | 260-9.2 | 303-10.7 | 346-12.2 | 389-13.7 | 432-15.2 |
| 003-0.11 | 046-1.6 | 089-3.1 | 132-4.7 | 175-6.2 | 218-7.7 | 261-9.2 | 304-10.7 | 347-12.2 | 390-13.8 | 433-15.3 |
| 004-0.14 | 047-1.7 | 090-3.2 | 133-4.7 | 176-6.2 | 219-7.7 | 262-9.3 | 305-10.8 | 348-12.3 | 391-13.8 | 434-15.3 |
| 005-0.18 | 048-1.7 | 091-3.2 | 134-4.7 | 177-6.2 | 220-7.8 | 263-9.3 | 306-10.8 | 349-12.3 | 392-13.8 | 435-15.3 |
| 006-0.21 | 049-1.7 | 092-3.3 | 135-4.8 | 178-6.3 | 221-7.8 | 264-9.3 | 307-10.8 | 350-12.4 | 393-13.9 | 436-15.4 |
| 007-0.25 | 050-1.8 | 093-3.3 | 136-4.8 | 179-6.3 | 222-7.8 | 265-9.4 | 308-10.9 | 351-12.4 | 394-13.9 | 437-15.4 |
| 008-0.28 | 051-1.8 | 094-3.3 | 137-4.8 | 180-6.3 | 223-7.9 | 266-9.4 | 309-10.9 | 352-12.4 | 395-13.9 | 438-15.4 |
| 009-0.32 | 052-1.8 | 095-3.4 | 138-4.9 | 181-6.4 | 224-7.9 | 267-9.4 | 310-10.9 | 353-12.5 | 396-14.0 | 439-15.5 |
| 010-0.35 | 053-1.9 | 096-3.4 | 139-4.9 | 182-6.4 | 225-7.9 | 268-9.5 | 311-11.0 | 354-12.5 | 397-14.0 | 440-15.5 |
| 011-0.39 | 054-1.9 | 097-3.4 | 140-4.9 | 183-6.5 | 226-8.0 | 269-9.5 | 312-11.0 | 355-12.5 | 398-14.0 | 441-15.6 |
| 012-0.42 | 055-1.9 | 098-3.5 | 141-5.0 | 184-6.5 | 227-8.0 | 270-9.5 | 313-11.0 | 356-12.6 | 399-14.1 | 442-15.6 |
| 013-0.46 | 056-2.0 | 099-3.5 | 142-5.0 | 185-6.5 | 228-8.0 | 271-9.6 | 314-11.1 | 357-12.6 | 400-14.1 | 443-15.6 |
| 014-0.49 | 057-2.0 | 100-3.5 | 143-5.0 | 186-6.6 | 229-8.1 | 272-9.6 | 315-11.1 | 358-12.6 | 401-14.2 | 444-15.7 |
| 015-0.53 | 058-2.0 | 101-3.6 | 144-5.1 | 187-6.6 | 230-8.1 | 273-9.6 | 316-11.2 | 359-12.7 | 402-14.2 | 445-15.7 |
| 016-0.56 | 059-2.1 | 102-3.6 | 145-5.1 | 188-6.6 | 231-8.2 | 274-9.7 | 317-11.2 | 360-12.7 | 403-14.2 | 446-15.7 |
| 017-0.56 | 060-2.1 | 103-3.6 | 146-5.2 | 189-6.7 | 232-8.2 | 275-9.7 | 318-11.2 | 361-12.7 | 404-14.3 | 447-15.8 |
| 018-0.63 | 061-2.2 | 104-3.7 | 147-5.2 | 190-6.7 | 233-8.2 | 276-9.7 | 319-11.3 | 362-12.8 | 405-14.3 | 448-15.8 |
| 019-0.67 | 062-2.2 | 105-3.7 | 148-5.2 | 191-6.7 | 234-8.3 | 277-9.8 | 320-11.3 | 363-12.8 | 406-14.3 | 449-15.8 |
| 020-0.71 | 063-2.2 | 106-3.7 | 149-5.3 | 192-6.8 | 235-8.3 | 278-9.8 | 321-11.3 | 364-12.8 | 407-14.4 | 450-15.9 |
| 021-0.71 | 064-2.3 | 107-3.8 | 150-5.3 | 193-6.8 | 236-8.3 | 279-9.8 | 322-11.4 | 365-12.9 | 408-14.4 | 451-15.9 |
| 022-0.78 | 065-2.3 | 108-3.8 | 151-5.3 | 194-6.8 | 237-8.4 | 280-9.9 | 323-11.4 | 366-12.9 | 409-14.4 | 452-15.9 |
| 023-0.81 | 066-2.3 | 109-3.8 | 152-5.4 | 195-6.9 | 238-8.4 | 281-9.9 | 324-11.4 | 367-13.0 | 410-14.5 | 453-16.0 |
| 024-0.85 | 067-2.4 | 110-3.9 | 153-5.4 | 196-6.9 | 239-8.4 | 282-10.0 | 325-11.5 | 368-13.0 | 411-14.5 | 454-16.0 |
| 025-0.88 | 068-2.4 | 111-3.9 | 154-5.4 | 197-7.0 | 240-8.5 | 283-10.0 | 326-11.5 | 369-13.0 | 412-14.5 | 455-16.0 |
| 026-0.92 | 069-2.4 | 112-4.0 | 155-5.5 | 198-7.0 | 241-8.5 | 284-10.0 | 327-11.5 | 370-13.1 | 413-14.6 | 456-16.1 |
| 027-0.95 | 070-2.5 | 113-4.0 | 156-5.5 | 199-7.0 | 242-8.5 | 285-10.1 | 328-11.6 | 371-13.1 | 414-14.6 | 457-16.1 |
| 028-0.99 | 071-2.5 | 114-4.0 | 157-5.5 | 200-7.1 | 243-8.6 | 286-10.1 | 329-11.6 | 372-13.1 | 415-14.6 | 458-16.2 |
| 029-1.0 | 072-2.5 | 115-4.1 | 158-5.6 | 201-7.1 | 244-8.6 | 287-10.1 | 330-11.6 | 373-13.2 | 416-14.7 | 459-16.2 |
| 030-1.1 | 073-2.6 | 116-4.1 | 159-5.6 | 202-7.1 | 245-8.6 | 288-10.2 | 331-11.7 | 374-13.2 | 417-14.7 | 460-16.2 |
| 031-1.1 | 074-2.6 | 117-4.1 | 160-5.6 | 203-7.2 | 246-8.7 | 289-10.2 | 332-11.7 | 375-13.2 | 418-14.7 | 461-16.3 |
| 032-1.1 | 075-2.7 | 118-4.2 | 161-5.7 | 204-7.2 | 247-8.7 | 290-10.2 | 333-11.8 | 376-13.3 | 419-14.8 | 462-16.3 |
| 033-1.2 | 076-2.7 | 119-4.2 | 162-5.7 | 205-7.2 | 248-8.7 | 291-10.3 | 334-11.8 | 377-13.3 | 420-14.8 | 463-16.3 |
| 034-1.2 | 077-2.7 | 120-4.2 | 163-5.8 | 206-7.3 | 249-8.8 | 292-10.3 | 335-11.8 | 378-13.3 | 421-14.9 | 464-16.4 |
| 035-1.2 | 078-2.8 | 121-4.3 | 164-5.8 | 207-7.3 | 250-8.8 | 293-10.3 | 336-11.9 | 379-13.4 | 422-14.9 | 465-16.4 |
| 036-1.3 | 079-2.8 | 122-4.3 | 165-5.8 | 208-7.3 | 251-8.9 | 294-10.4 | 337-11.9 | 380-13.4 | 423-14.9 | 466-16.4 |
| 037-1.3 | 080-2.8 | 123-4.3 | 166-5.9 | 209-7.4 | 252-8.9 | 295-10.4 | 338-11.9 | 381-13.4 | 424-15.0 | 467-16.5 |
| 038-1.3 | 081-2.9 | 124-4.4 | 167-5.9 | 210-7.4 | 253-8.9 | 296-10.4 | 339-12.0 | 382-13.5 | 425-15.0 | 468-16.5 |
| 039-1.4 | 082-2.9 | 125-4.4 | 168-5.9 | 211-7.4 | 254-8.9 | 297-10.5 | 340-12.0 | 383-13.5 | 426-15.0 | 469-16.5 |
| 040-1.4 | 083-2.9 | 126-4.4 | 169-6.0 | 212-7.5 | 255-9.0 | 298-10.5 | 341-12.0 | 384-13.5 | 427-15.1 | 470-16.6 |
| 041-1.4 | 084-3.0 | 127-4.5 | 170-6.0 | 213-7.5 | 256-9.0 | 299-10.6 | 342-12.1 | 385-13.6 | 428-15.1 | 471-16.6 |
| 042-1.5 | 085-3.0 | 128-4.5 | 171-6.0 | 214-7.6 | 257-9.1 | 300-10.6 | 343-12.1 | 386-13.6 | 429-15.1 | 472-16.6 |
| 043-1.5 | 086-3.0 | 129-4.6 | 172-6.1 | 215-7.6 | 258-9.1 | 301-10.6 | 344-12.1 | 387-13.7 | 430-15.2 | 473-16.7 |

[1] Calculated on the basis of 1 ounce weighing 28.35 g.

# MAIN DATABASE
# FOR THE COMPOSITION
# OF FOODS

| | WT (g) | KCAL | H₂0 (g) | CHO (g) | TSUG (g) | ASUG (g) | DFIB (g) | Na (mg) | Ca (mg) | Mg (mg) | Zn (mg) | Mn (mg) | A (mcg RAE) | C (mg) | B-1 (mg) | NIA (mg) | B-12 (mcg) | PANT (mg) |
|---|---|---|---|---|---|---|---|---|---|---|---|---|---|---|---|---|---|---|
| | | PRO (g) | FAT (g) | SFA (g) | MUFA (g) | PUFA (g) | CHOL (mg) | K (mg) | P (mg) | Fe (mg) | Cu (mg) | Se (mcg) | A (IU) | E (mg ATE) | B-2 (mg) | B-6 (mg) | FOL (mcg DFE) | REF |

## 1. BEVERAGES
### 1.1 CARBONATED, LOW CALORIE BEVERAGES

| | WT | KCAL/PRO | H₂0/FAT | CHO/SFA | TSUG/MUFA | ASUG/PUFA | DFIB/CHOL | Na/K | Ca/P | Mg/Fe | Zn/Cu | Mn/Se | A(RAE)/A(IU) | C/E | B-1/B-2 | NIA/B-6 | B-12/FOL | PANT/REF |
|---|---|---|---|---|---|---|---|---|---|---|---|---|---|---|---|---|---|---|
| **Cherry Coke Zero** | 355 | 1 | | 0 | | | | 42 | | | | | | | | | | |
| *12 fl oz* | | 0 | 0 | | | | | 50 | 56 | | | | | | | | | COLA68 |
| **club soda** | 355 | 0 | 354.6 | 0 | 0 | | 0 | 75 | 18 | 4 | 0.36 | 0.004 | 0 | 0 | 0 | 0 | 0 | 0 |
| *12 fl oz* | | 0 | 0 | 0 | 0 | 0 | 0 | 7 | 0 | 0.04 | 0.021 | 0 | 0 | 0 | 0 | 0 | 0 | 14121 |
| **club soda**, Seagram's | 355 | 0 | | 0 | 0 | | | | | | | | | | | | | |
| *12 fl oz* | | 0 | | | | | | 27 | | | | | | | | | | COLA70 |
| **Coca-Cola Zero** | 355 | 1 | | 0.2 | | | | 42 | | | | | | | | | | |
| *12 fl oz* | | 0 | 0 | | | | | 46 | 54 | | | | | | | | | COLA74 |
| **Diet Cherry Coke** | 355 | 1 | | 0.2 | | | | 42 | | | | | | | | | | |
| *12 fl oz* | | 0 | 0 | | | | | 28 | 34 | | | | | | | | | COLA4 |
| **Diet Coke** | 355 | 2 | | 0.2 | | | | 42 | | | | | | | | | | |
| *12 fl oz* | | 0 | 0 | | | | | 18 | 27 | | | | | | | | | COLA5 |
| **Diet Coke**, caffeine-free | 355 | 2 | | 0.2 | | | | 42 | | | | | | | | | | |
| *12 fl oz* | | 0 | 0 | | | | | 18 | 27 | | | | | | | | | COLA7 |
| **Diet Coke**, with Splenda | 355 | 2 | | 0.2 | | | | 42 | | | | | | | | | | |
| *12 fl oz* | | 0 | 0 | | | | | 27 | 50 | | | | | | | | | COLA76 |
| **Diet Coke** with lime | 355 | 3 | | 0.2 | | | | 42 | | | | | | | | | | |
| *12 fl oz* | | 0 | 0 | | | | | 28 | 27 | | | | | | | | | COLA75 |
| **diet cola** with aspartame | 355 | 7 | 353.4 | 1.0 | 0 | | 0 | 28 | 11 | 4 | 0.04 | 0.380 | 0 | 0 | 0.02 | 0 | 0 | 0 |
| *12 fl oz* | | 0.4 | 0.1 | 0 | 0 | 0 | 0 | 28 | 32 | 0.39 | 0.007 | 0 | 0 | 0 | 0.08 | 0 | 0 | 14416 |
| **diet cola** with aspartame, caffeine-free - *12 fl oz* | 355 | 4 | 354.1 | 0.5 | 0 | | 0 | 14 | 11 | 0 | 0.04 | 0 | 0 | 0 | 0.02 | 0 | 0 | 0 |
| | | 0.4 | 0 | 0 | 0 | 0 | 0 | 25 | 36 | 0.07 | 0.007 | 0.4 | 0 | 0 | 0.08 | 0 | 0 | 14146 |
| **diet cola** with sodium saccharin | 355 | 0 | 354.3 | 0.4 | 0 | | 0 | 57 | 14 | 4 | 0.11 | 0.032 | 0 | 0 | 0 | 0 | 0 | 0 |
| *12 fl oz* | | 0 | 0 | 0 | 0 | 0 | 0 | 14 | 39 | 0.07 | 0.046 | 0.4 | 0 | 0 | 0 | 0 | 0 | 14166 |
| **diet crème soda**, French vanilla, Barq's - *12 fl oz* | 355 | 2 | | | | | | 66 | | | | | | | | | | |
| | | 0 | 0 | | | | | | 0 | | | | | | | | | COLA1 |
| **diet crème soda**, red, Barq's | 355 | 6 | | 0 | | | | 64 | | | | | | | | | | |
| *12 fl oz* | | 0 | 0 | | | | | 0 | 0 | | | | | | | | | COLA2 |
| **diet ginger ale**, Northern Neck | 355 | 6 | | 0 | | | | 36 | | | | | | | | | | |
| *12 fl oz* | | 0 | 0 | | | | | 20 | 0 | | | | | | | | | COLA77 |
| **diet ginger ale**, raspberry, Seagram's - *12 fl oz* | 355 | 3 | | 0 | 0 | | | 48 | | | | | | | | | | |
| | | 0 | | | | | | 52 | | | | | | | | | | COLA78 |
| **diet ginger ale**, Seagram's | 355 | 3 | | 0 | 0 | | | 45 | | | | | | | | | | |
| *12 fl oz* | | 0 | | | | | | 52 | | | | | | | | | | COLA79 |
| **Diet Inca Kola** | 355 | 2 | | | | | | 51 | | | | | | | | | | |
| *12 fl oz* | | 0 | 0 | | | | | 10 | | | | | | | | | | COLA8 |
| **diet root beer**, Barq's | 355 | 1 | | 0.2 | | | | 72 | | | | | | | | | | |
| *12 fl oz* | | 0 | 0 | | | | | 14 | 0 | | | | | | | | | COLA3 |
| **diet soda** other than cola/pepper w/aspartame - *12 fl oz* | 355 | 0 | 354.3 | 0 | 0 | | 0 | 21 | 14 | 4 | 0 | 0.060 | 0 | 0 | 0 | 0 | 0 | 0 |
| | | 0.4 | 0 | 0 | 0 | 0 | 0 | 7 | 0 | 0.14 | 0.089 | 0 | 0 | 0 | 0 | 0 | 0 | 14143 |
| **diet soda** other than cola/pepper type, w/saccharin - *12 fl oz* | 355 | 0 | 354.3 | 0.4 | | | 0 | 57 | 14 | 4 | 0.18 | 0.060 | 0 | 0 | 0 | 0 | 0 | 0 |
| | | 0 | 0 | 0 | 0 | 0 | 0 | 7 | 0 | 0.14 | 0.089 | 0 | 0 | 0 | 0 | 0 | 0 | 14537 |
| **diet tonic water**, Seagram's | 355 | 4 | | 0 | 0 | | | 48 | | | | | | | | | | |
| *12 fl oz* | | | | | | | | 46 | | | | | | | | | | COLA80 |
| **Fresca** | 355 | 3 | | 0.2 | | | | 36 | | | | | | | | | | |
| *12 fl oz* | | 0 | 0 | | | | | 88 | | | | | | | | | | COLA13 |
| **Fresca**, black cherry | 355 | 4 | | 0 | | | | 36 | | | | | | | | | | |
| *12 fl oz* | | 0 | 0 | | | | | 86 | | | | | | | | | | COLA82 |
| **Fresca**, peach | 355 | 3 | | 0 | | | | 36 | | | | | | | | | | |
| *12 fl oz* | | 0 | 0 | | | | | 86 | | | | | | | | | | COLA83 |
| **orange soda**, Fanta Zero | 355 | 3 | | 0.1 | | | | 36 | | | | | | | | | | |
| *12 fl oz* | | 0 | 0 | | | | | 74 | 0 | | | | | | | | | COLA101 |
| **Pibb Zero** | 355 | 2 | | 0.2 | | | | 46 | | | | | | | | | | |
| *12 fl oz* | | 0 | 0 | | | | | 33 | 44 | | | | | | | | | COLA103 |
| **seltzer water**, black cherry, Seagram's - *12 fl oz* | 355 | 3 | | 0 | 0 | | | | | | | | | | | | | |
| | | 0 | | | | | | 0 | | | | | | | | | | COLA110 |
| **seltzer water**, lemon lime, Seagram's - *12 fl oz* | 355 | 2 | | 0 | 0 | | | | | | | | | | | | | |
| | | 0 | | | | | | 0 | | | | | | | | | | COLA111 |

| | WT (g) | KCAL / PRO (g) | H₂0 (g) / FAT (g) | CHO (g) / SFA (g) | TSUG (g) / MUFA (g) | ASUG (g) / PUFA (g) | DFIB (g) / CHOL (mg) | Na (mg) / K (mg) | Ca (mg) / P (mg) | Mg (mg) / Fe (mg) | Zn (mg) / Cu (mg) | Mn (mg) / Se (mcg) | A (mcg RAE) / A (IU) | C (mg) / E (mg ATE) | B-1 (mg) / B-2 (mg) | NIA (mg) / B-6 (mg) | B-12 (mcg) / FOL (mcg DFE) | PANT (mg) / REF |
|---|---|---|---|---|---|---|---|---|---|---|---|---|---|---|---|---|---|---|
| **seltzer water, orange, Seagram's** | 355 | 2 | | 0 | 0 | | | | | | | | | | | | | |
| *12 fl oz* | | 0 | | | | | | 0 | | | | | | | | | | COLA112 |
| **seltzer water, raspberry, Seagram's** | 355 | 2 | | 0 | 0 | | | | | | | | | | | | | |
| *12 fl oz* | | 0 | | | | | | 0 | | | | | | | | | | COLA113 |
| **seltzer water, Seagram's** | 355 | 0 | | 0 | 0 | | | | | | | | | | | | | |
| *12 fl oz* | | 0 | | | | | | 0 | | | | | | | | | | COLA114 |
| **Sprite Zero** | 355 | 4 | | 0 | | | | 36 | | | | | | | | | | |
| *12 fl oz* | | 0 | 0 | | | | | 110 | 0 | | | | | | | | | COLA115 |
| **Tab** | 355 | 1 | | 0.2 | | | | 42 | | | | | | | | | | |
| *12 fl oz* | | 0 | 0 | | | | | 18 | 45 | | | | | | | | | COLA18 |
| **Vanilla Coke Zero** | 355 | 1 | | 0.2 | | | | 42 | | | | | | | | | | |
| *12 fl oz* | | 0 | 0 | | | | | 46 | 56 | | | | | | | | | COLA120 |

## 1.2 CARBONATED, SUGAR-SWEETENED BEVERAGES

| | WT (g) | KCAL / PRO (g) | H₂0 (g) / FAT (g) | CHO (g) / SFA (g) | TSUG (g) / MUFA (g) | ASUG (g) / PUFA (g) | DFIB (g) / CHOL (mg) | Na (mg) / K (mg) | Ca (mg) / P (mg) | Mg (mg) / Fe (mg) | Zn (mg) / Cu (mg) | Mn (mg) / Se (mcg) | A (mcg RAE) / A (IU) | C (mg) / E (mg ATE) | B-1 (mg) / B-2 (mg) | NIA (mg) / B-6 (mg) | B-12 (mcg) / FOL (mcg DFE) | PANT (mg) / REF |
|---|---|---|---|---|---|---|---|---|---|---|---|---|---|---|---|---|---|---|
| **apple soda, Fanta** | 370 | 182 | | 49.5 | | | | 58 | | | | | | | | | | |
| *12 fl oz* | | 0 | 0 | | | | | 0 | 0 | | | | | | | | | COLA65 |
| **berry soda, Fanta** | 370 | 176 | | 48.0 | | | | 33 | | | | | | | | | | |
| *12 fl oz* | | 0 | 0 | | | | | 51 | 0 | | | | | | | | | COLA66 |
| **black cherry soda, Fanta** | 370 | 165 | | 43.5 | | | | 52 | | | | | | | | | | |
| *12 fl oz* | | 0 | 0 | | | | | 0 | 0 | | | | | | | | | COLA67 |
| **Cherry Coke** | 370 | 156 | | 42.0 | | | | 42 | | | | | | | | | | |
| *12 fl oz* | | 0 | 0 | | | | | 0 | 56 | | | | | | | | | COLA33 |
| **chocolate-flavored soda** | 369 | 155 | 329.1 | 39.5 | 39.5 | 39.5 | 0 | 325 | 15 | 4 | 0.59 | 0.133 | 0 | 0 | 0 | 0 | 0 | 0 |
| *12 fl oz* | | 0 | 0 | 0 | 0 | 0 | 0 | 184 | 4 | 0.37 | 0.048 | 0.4 | 0 | 0 | 0 | 0 | 0 | 14552 |
| **citrus soda, Fanta** | 370 | 136 | | 37.5 | | | | 24 | | | | | | | | | | |
| *12 fl oz* | | 0 | 0 | | | | | 2 | 0 | | | | | | | | | COLA69 |
| **Coca-Cola Blak** | 370 | 69 | | 18.0 | | | | 48 | | | | | | | | | | |
| *12 fl oz* | | 0 | 0 | | | | | 48 | 62 | | | | | | | | | COLA71 |
| **Coca-Cola C2** | 370 | 70 | | 18.0 | 18.0 | | | 45 | | | | | | | | | | |
| *12 fl oz* | | 0 | 0 | | | | | | | | | | | | | | | COLA72 |
| **Coca-Cola Classic** | 370 | 146 | | 40.5 | | | | 50 | | | | | | | | | | |
| *12 fl oz* | | 0 | 0 | | | | | 0 | 62 | | | | | | | | | COLA35 |
| **Coca-Cola Classic, caffeine-free** | 370 | 146 | | 40.5 | | | | 50 | | | | | | | | | | |
| *12 fl oz* | | 0 | 0 | | | | | 0 | 62 | | | | | | | | | COLA36 |
| **Coca-Cola with lime** | 370 | 147 | | 40.5 | | | | 38 | | | | | | | | | | |
| *12 fl oz* | | 0 | 0 | | | | | 51 | 56 | | | | | | | | | COLA73 |
| **cola** | 370 | 137 | 334.1 | 35.4 | 33.2 | 33.2 | 0 | 15 | 7 | 0 | 0.07 | 0.007 | 0 | 0 | 0 | 0 | 0 | 0 |
| *12 fl oz* | | 0.3 | 0.1 | 0 | 0 | 0 | 0 | 7 | 37 | 0.41 | 0.004 | 0.4 | 0 | 0 | 0 | 0 | 0 | 14400 |
| **cola, caffeine-free** | 370 | 152 | 331.6 | 39.1 | 39.1 | 39.1 | 0 | 15 | 7 | 0 | 0.04 | 0 | 0 | 0 | 0 | 0 | 0 | 0 |
| *12 fl oz* | | 0 | 0 | 0 | 0 | 0 | 0 | 11 | 41 | 0.07 | 0 | 0.4 | 0 | 0 | 0 | 0 | 0 | 14147 |
| **cola** with higher caffeine (e.g., Jolt Cola) - *12 fl oz* | 370 | 152 | 331.6 | 39.1 | 39.1 | 39.1 | 0 | 15 | 7 | 0 | 0.04 | 0 | 0 | 0 | 0 | 0 | 0 | 0 |
| | | 0 | 0 | 0 | 0 | 0 | 0 | 11 | 41 | 0.07 | 0 | 0.4 | 0 | 0 | 0 | 0 | 0 | 14148 |
| **cream soda** | 371 | 189 | 321.7 | 49.3 | 49.3 | 49.3 | 0 | 45 | 19 | 4 | 0.26 | 0.048 | 0 | 0 | 0 | 0 | 0 | 0 |
| *12 fl oz* | | 0 | 0 | 0 | 0 | 0 | 0 | 4 | 0 | 0.19 | 0.030 | 0 | 0 | 0 | 0 | 0 | 0 | 14130 |
| **crème soda, French vanilla, Barq's** | 370 | 168 | | 45.0 | | | | 66 | | | | | | | | | | |
| *12 fl oz* | | 0 | 0 | | | | | 0 | 0 | | | | | | | | | COLA30 |
| **crème soda, red, Barq's** | 370 | 172 | | 46.5 | | | | 64 | | | | | | | | | | |
| *12 fl oz* | | 0 | 0 | | | | | 0 | 0 | | | | | | | | | COLA31 |
| **Floatz, Barq's** | 370 | 190 | | 51.0 | | | | 66 | | | | | | | | | | |
| *12 fl oz* | | 0 | 0 | | | | | 3 | 0 | | | | | | | | | COLA81 |
| **ginger ale** | 366 | 124 | 333.9 | 32.1 | 31.8 | 31.8 | 0 | 26 | 11 | 4 | 0.18 | 0.048 | 0 | 0 | 0 | 0 | 0 | 0 |
| *12 fl oz* | | 0 | 0 | 0 | 0 | 0 | 0 | 4 | 0 | 0.66 | 0.066 | 0.4 | 0 | 0 | 0 | 0 | 0 | 14136 |
| **ginger ale, Carver's** | 366 | 141 | | 36.0 | | | | 33 | | | | | | | | | | |
| *12 fl oz* | | 0 | 0 | | | | | 22 | 0 | | | | | | | | | COLA84 |
| **ginger ale, Northern Neck** | 366 | 141 | | 36.0 | | | | 33 | | | | | | | | | | |
| *12 fl oz* | | 0 | 0 | | | | | 22 | 0 | | | | | | | | | COLA85 |
| **ginger ale, raspberry, Seagram's** | 366 | 135 | | 36.0 | 36.0 | | | 45 | | | | | | | | | | |
| *12 fl oz* | | 0 | | | | | | 0 | | | | | | | | | | COLA86 |
| **ginger ale, Seagram's** | 366 | 135 | | 36.0 | 36.0 | | | 45 | | | | | | | | | | |
| *12 fl oz* | | 0 | | | | | | 0 | | | | | | | | | | COLA87 |
| **grape soda** | 372 | 160 | 330.3 | 41.7 | | | 0 | 56 | 11 | 4 | 0.26 | 0.048 | 0 | 0 | 0 | 0 | 0 | 0 |
| *12 fl oz* | | 0 | 0 | 0 | 0 | 0 | 0 | 4 | 0 | 0.30 | 0.082 | 0 | 0 | 0 | 0 | 0 | 0 | 14142 |

| | WT (g) | Macronutrients | | | | | | Minerals | | | | | Vitamins | | | | | |
|---|---|---|---|---|---|---|---|---|---|---|---|---|---|---|---|---|---|---|
| | | KCAL | H₂0 (g) | CHO (g) | TSUG (g) | ASUG (g) | DFIB (g) | Na (mg) | Ca (mg) | Mg (mg) | Zn (mg) | Mn (mg) | A (mcg RAE) | C (mg) | B-1 (mg) | NIA (mg) | B-12 (mcg) | PANT (mg) |
| | | PRO (g) | FAT (g) | SFA (g) | MUFA (g) | PUFA (g) | CHOL (mg) | K (mg) | P (mg) | Fe (mg) | Cu (mg) | Se (mcg) | A (IU) | E (mg ATE) | B-2 (mg) | B-6 (mg) | FOL (mcg DFE) | REF |
| grape soda, Fanta | 370 | 183 | | 49.5 | | | | 45 | | | | | | | | | | |
| *12 fl oz* | | 0 | 0 | | | | | 0 | 0 | | | | | | | | | COLA88 |
| Inca Kola | 370 | 144 | | 39.0 | | | | 46 | | | | | | | | | | |
| *12 fl oz* | | 0 | 0 | | | | | 0 | 0 | | | | | | | | | COLA38 |
| lemon-lime soda | 368 | 147 | 330.4 | 37.3 | 33.0 | | | 33 | 7 | 4 | 0.15 | 0.007 | 0 | 0 | 0 | 0.1 | 0 | 0 |
| *12 fl oz* | | 0.2 | 0.1 | 0 | 0 | 0 | 0 | 4 | 0 | 0.40 | 0.004 | 0 | 0 | 0 | 0 | 0 | 0 | 14145 |
| lemon-lime soda with caffeine | 368 | 151 | 329.3 | 38.3 | 37.5 | 37.5 | | 37 | 7 | 4 | 0.04 | 0 | 0 | 0 | 0 | 0.1 | 0 | 0 |
| *12 fl oz* | | 0.3 | 0 | 0 | 0 | 0 | 0 | 4 | 0 | 0.07 | 0 | 0 | 0 | 0 | 0 | 0 | 0 | 14144 |
| lemon soda, Fanta | 370 | 168 | | 45.0 | | | | 45 | | | | | | | | | | |
| *12 fl oz* | | 0 | 0 | | | | | | 0 | | | | | | | | | COLA97 |
| Manzana Mia | 370 | 148 | | 40.5 | | | | 70 | | | | | | | | | | |
| *12 fl oz* | | 0 | 0 | | | | | 4 | | | | | | | | | | COLA39 |
| Mello Yello | 370 | 177 | | 48.0 | | | | 50 | | | | | | | | | | |
| *12 fl oz* | | 0 | 0 | | | | | 30 | | | | | | | | | | COLA40 |
| Mello Yello cherry | 370 | 177 | | 48.0 | | | | 45 | | | | | | | | | | |
| *12 fl oz* | | 0 | 0 | | | | | 30 | | | | | | | | | | COLA98 |
| Mello Yello melon | 370 | 178 | | 48.0 | | | | 45 | | | | | | | | | | |
| *12 fl oz* | | 0 | 0 | | | | | 30 | | | | | | | | | | COLA99 |
| orange soda | 372 | 179 | 325.9 | 45.8 | | | 0 | 45 | 19 | 4 | 0.37 | 0.048 | 0 | 0 | 0 | 0 | 0 | 0 |
| *12 fl oz* | | 0 | 0 | 0 | 0 | 0 | 0 | 7 | 4 | 0.22 | 0.056 | 0 | 0 | | 0 | 0 | 0 | 14150 |
| orange soda, Fanta | 370 | 166 | | 52.5 | | | | 52 | | | | | | | | | | |
| *12 fl oz* | | 0 | 0 | | | | | | 10 | | | | | | | | | COLA100 |
| peach soda, Fanta | 370 | 165 | | 43.5 | | | | 45 | | | | | | | | | | |
| *12 fl oz* | | 0 | 0 | | | | | | 0 | | | | | | | | | COLA102 |
| pepper-type soda | 368 | 151 | 329.0 | 38.3 | | | 0 | 37 | 11 | 0 | 0.15 | 0.129 | 0 | 0 | 0 | 0 | 0 | 0 |
| *12 fl oz* | | 0 | 0.4 | 0.3 | 0 | 0 | 0 | 4 | 40 | 0.15 | 0.022 | 0.4 | 0 | | 0 | 0 | 0 | 14153 |
| Pibb Xtra | 370 | 146 | | 39.0 | | | | 42 | | | | | | | | | | |
| *12 fl oz* | | 0 | 0 | | | | | 21 | 44 | | | | | | | | | COLA44 |
| pineapple soda, Fanta | 370 | 180 | | 49.5 | | | | 52 | | | | | | | | | | |
| *12 fl oz* | | 0 | 0 | | | | | 0 | 0 | | | | | | | | | COLA104 |
| pink grapefruit soda, Fanta | 370 | 170 | | 45.0 | | | | 45 | | | | | | | | | | |
| *12 fl oz* | | 0 | 0 | | | | | | 0 | | | | | | | | | COLA105 |
| Red Flash | 370 | 158 | | 42.0 | | | | 32 | | | | | | | | | | |
| *12 fl oz* | | 0 | 0 | | | | | 18 | 0 | | | | | | | | | COLA45 |
| red tangerine soda, Fanta | 370 | 184 | | 49.5 | | | | 60 | | | | | | | | | | |
| *12 fl oz* | | 0 | 0 | | | | | 0 | 10 | | | | | | | | | COLA109 |
| root beer | 370 | 152 | 330.4 | 39.2 | 39.2 | 39.2 | 0 | 48 | 18 | 4 | 0.26 | 0.048 | 0 | 0 | 0 | 0 | 0 | 0 |
| *12 fl oz* | | 0 | 0 | 0 | 0 | 0 | 0 | 4 | 0 | 0.19 | 0.026 | 0.4 | 0 | 0 | 0 | 0 | 0 | 14157 |
| root beer, Barq's | 370 | 166 | | 45.0 | | | | 72 | | | | | | | | | | |
| *12 fl oz* | | 0 | 0 | | | | | | 0 | | | | | | | | | COLA32 |
| Sprite | 370 | 144 | | 39.0 | | | | 70 | | | | | | | | | | |
| *12 fl oz* | | 0 | 0 | | | | | 0 | 0 | | | | | | | | | COLA46 |
| strawberry soda, Fanta | 370 | 180 | | 49.5 | | | | 45 | | | | | | | | | | |
| *12 fl oz* | | 0 | 0 | | | | | 0 | 0 | | | | | | | | | COLA116 |
| tonic water | 366 | 124 | 333.4 | 32.2 | 32.2 | 32.2 | 0 | 44 | 4 | 0 | 0.37 | 0.004 | 0 | 0 | 0 | 0 | 0 | 0 |
| *12 fl oz* | | 0 | 0 | 0 | 0 | 0 | 0 | 0 | 0 | 0.04 | 0.022 | 0 | 0 | 0 | 0 | 0 | 0 | 14155 |
| tonic water with lime, Seagram's | 366 | 140 | | 36.0 | 36.0 | | | 45 | | | | | | | | | | |
| *12 fl oz* | | 0 | | | | | | 0 | | | | | | | | | | COLA117 |
| tonic water, Seagram's | 366 | 124 | | 33.0 | 33.0 | | | 45 | | | | | | | | | | |
| *12 fl oz* | | 0 | | | | | | 0 | | | | | | | | | | COLA118 |
| Vanilla Coke | 370 | 150 | | 42.0 | | | | 38 | | | | | | | | | | |
| *12 fl oz* | | 0 | 0 | | | | | 0 | 56 | | | | | | | | | COLA119 |

## 1.3 COCKTAILS (MIXED DRINKS)

| | WT (g) | KCAL | H₂0 (g) | CHO (g) | TSUG (g) | ASUG (g) | DFIB (g) | Na (mg) | Ca (mg) | Mg (mg) | Zn (mg) | Mn (mg) | A (mcg RAE) | C (mg) | B-1 (mg) | NIA (mg) | B-12 (mcg) | PANT (mg) |
|---|---|---|---|---|---|---|---|---|---|---|---|---|---|---|---|---|---|---|
| | | PRO (g) | FAT (g) | SFA (g) | MUFA (g) | PUFA (g) | CHOL (mg) | K (mg) | P (mg) | Fe (mg) | Cu (mg) | Se (mcg) | A (IU) | E (mg ATE) | B-2 (mg) | B-6 (mg) | FOL (mcg DFE) | REF |
| daiquiri (rum, lime juice, sugar) | 60 | 112 | 41.8 | 4.2 | 3.3 | | | 0.1 | 3 | 2 | 1 | 0.02 | 0.009 | 0 | 1 | 0.01 | 0 | 0 | 0.01 |
| *2 fl oz cocktail* | | 0 | 0 | 0 | 0 | 0 | 0 | 13 | 3 | 0.05 | 0.013 | 0.1 | 2 | 0 | 0 | 0 | 1.0 | 14010 |
| daiquiri (rum, lime juice, sugar), canned - *6.8 fl oz can* | 207 | 259 | 154.4 | 32.5 | | | | 0 | 83 | 0 | 2 | 0.06 | 0.010 | 0 | 3 | 0 | 0 | 0 | 0.01 |
| | | 0 | 0 | 0 | | | 0 | 23 | 4 | 0.02 | 0.033 | 0.2 | 4 | | 0 | 0.01 | 2.1 | 14009 |
| pina colada (pineapple jce, rum, sugar, coconut crm) - *4.5 fl oz* | 141 | 245 | 91.6 | 32.0 | 31.5 | | | 0.4 | 8 | 11 | 11 | 0.18 | 0.744 | 0 | 7 | 0.04 | 0.2 | 0 | 0.09 |
| | | 0.6 | 2.7 | 2.3 | 0.1 | 0 | 0 | 100 | 10 | 0.30 | 0.111 | 1.0 | 3 | 0 | 0.02 | 0.06 | 16.9 | 14017 |
| pina colada (pineapple jce, rum, sgr, coconut crm), cnd - *6.8 fl oz* | 222 | 526 | 121.9 | 61.3 | | | | 0.2 | 158 | 2 | 13 | 0.44 | 0.708 | 2 | 3 | 0.04 | 0.2 | 0 | 0.12 |
| | | 1.3 | 16.9 | 14.6 | 1.0 | 0.3 | 0 | 184 | 80 | 0.07 | 0.193 | 1.6 | 53 | | 0.01 | 0.04 | 13.3 | 14015 |

| | WT (g) | KCAL | H₂O (g) | CHO (g) | TSUG (g) | ASUG (g) | DFIB (g) | Na (mg) | Ca (mg) | Mg (mg) | Zn (mg) | Mn (mg) | A (mcg RAE) | C (mg) | B-1 (mg) | NIA (mg) | B-12 (mcg) | PANT (mg) |
|---|---|---|---|---|---|---|---|---|---|---|---|---|---|---|---|---|---|---|
| | | PRO (g) | FAT (g) | SFA (g) | MUFA (g) | PUFA (g) | CHOL (mg) | K (mg) | P (mg) | Fe (mg) | Cu (mg) | Se (mcg) | A (IU) | E (mg ATE) | B-2 (mg) | B-6 (mg) | FOL (mcg DFE) | REF |
| **tequila sunrise** (orange jce, tequila, lime jce, grenadin), cnd | 211 | 232 | 166.3 | 23.8 | | | 0 | 120 | 0 | 15 | 1.27 | 0.030 | 11 | 41 | 0.08 | 0.4 | 0 | 0.19 |
| *6.8 fl oz* | | 0.6 | 0.2 | 0 | | | 0 | 21 | 21 | 0.04 | 0.089 | 0 | 205 | | 0.03 | 0.11 | 23.2 | 14019 |
| **whiskey sour** (lemon juice, whiskey, sgr), cnd - *6.8 fl oz* | 209 | 249 | 160.7 | 28.0 | | | 0.2 | 92 | 0 | 2 | 0.13 | 0.013 | 2 | 3 | 0.02 | 0 | 0 | 0.02 |
| | | 0 | 0 | 0 | | | 0 | 23 | 13 | 0.02 | 0.019 | 0.2 | 27 | | 0.01 | 0 | 0 | 14027 |
| **whiskey sour** (lemon jce, whiskey, sgr), dry mix - *17 g pkt prep* | 103 | 169 | 71.2 | 16.3 | 16.3 | | 0 | 48 | 47 | 3 | 0.04 | 0.007 | 0 | 0 | 0 | 0 | 0 | 0.01 |
| | | 0.1 | 0 | 0 | 0 | 0 | 0 | 4 | 4 | 0.08 | 0.035 | 0.1 | 5 | 0 | 0 | 0 | 0 | 14025 |
| **whiskey sour** (lemon jce, whiskey, sgr), liquid mix - *3.5 fl oz* | 106 | 162 | 76.8 | 13.6 | 13.5 | | 0 | 65 | 1 | 1 | 0.06 | 0.007 | 0 | 2 | 0.01 | 0 | 0 | 0.01 |
| | | 0.1 | 0.1 | 0 | 0 | 0 | 0 | 19 | 5 | 0.08 | 0.008 | 0.2 | 0 | | 0.01 | 0 | 0 | 14029 |
| **whiskey sour mix, dry** | 17 | 65 | 0.1 | 16.5 | 16.5 | | 0 | 47 | 46 | 3 | 0.02 | 0 | 0 | 0 | 0 | 0 | 0 | 0.01 |
| *.56 oz packet* | | 0.1 | 0 | 0 | 0 | 0 | 0 | 3 | 2 | 0.07 | 0.022 | 0.1 | 5 | 0 | 0 | 0 | 0 | 14024 |
| **whiskey sour mix, liquid** | 65 | 57 | 50.8 | 13.9 | 13.9 | 13.9 | 0 | 66 | 1 | 1 | 0.05 | 0 | 0 | 2 | 0.01 | 0 | 0 | 0.01 |
| *2 fl oz* | | 0.1 | 0.1 | 0 | 0 | 0 | 0 | 18 | 4 | 0.07 | 0 | 0.3 | 0 | | 0.01 | 0 | 0 | 14028 |

## 1.4 COFFEE AND COFFEE BEVERAGES

| | WT (g) | KCAL | H₂O (g) | CHO (g) | TSUG (g) | ASUG (g) | DFIB (g) | Na (mg) | Ca (mg) | Mg (mg) | Zn (mg) | Mn (mg) | A (mcg RAE) | C (mg) | B-1 (mg) | NIA (mg) | B-12 (mcg) | PANT (mg) |
|---|---|---|---|---|---|---|---|---|---|---|---|---|---|---|---|---|---|---|
| | | PRO (g) | FAT (g) | SFA (g) | MUFA (g) | PUFA (g) | CHOL (mg) | K (mg) | P (mg) | Fe (mg) | Cu (mg) | Se (mcg) | A (IU) | E (mg ATE) | B-2 (mg) | B-6 (mg) | FOL (mcg DFE) | REF |
| **cappuccino mix**, mocha, decaf, House Café - *.81 oz pkt (makes 8 fl oz)* | 23 | 100 | | 17.0 | 16.0 | | 0 | 70 | 60 | | | | | 0 | | | | |
| | | 2.0 | 2.5 | 1.0 | | | 0 | | 0 | | | | 0 | | | | | HOUS1 |
| **cereal coffee**, from powder w/milk - *1 t powder in 6 fl oz mlk* | 185 | 120 | 161.0 | 10.4 | | | 0.2 | 91 | 220 | 30 | 0.70 | 0.030 | 52 | 2 | 0.07 | 0.5 | 0.65 | 0.57 |
| | | 6.1 | 6.1 | 3.8 | 1.8 | 0.3 | 24 | 318 | 183 | 0.20 | 0.022 | 10.2 | 229 | | 0.30 | 0.08 | 9.2 | 14421 |
| **cereal coffee**, from powder w/wtr - *1 t pwdr in 6 fl oz wtr* | 180 | 11 | 177.1 | 2.3 | 0.1 | 0.1 | 0.7 | 9 | 7 | 9 | 0.02 | 0.034 | 0 | 0 | 0.01 | 0.5 | 0 | 0.04 |
| | | 0.2 | 0.1 | 0 | 0 | 0 | 0 | 74 | 18 | 0.14 | 0.023 | 2.0 | 0 | 0 | 0 | 0.02 | 1.8 | 14237 |
| **coffee and chicory**, from inst pwdr - *1 round t in 6 fl oz water* | 179 | 5 | 177.1 | 1.3 | 0 | | 0 | 13 | 7 | 5 | 0.02 | 0.021 | 0 | 0 | 0 | 0.4 | 0 | 0 |
| | | 0.2 | 0 | 0 | 0 | 0 | 0 | 63 | 5 | 0.09 | 0.018 | 0.2 | 0 | 0 | 0.01 | 0 | 0 | 14223 |
| **coffee and chicory instant powder** | 1.8 | 6 | 0.1 | 1.3 | | | 0 | 5 | 2 | 4 | 0.01 | 0.022 | 0 | 0 | 0 | 0.4 | 0 | 0 |
| *1 round t* | | 0.2 | 0 | 0 | | | 0 | 61 | 5 | 0.09 | 0.001 | 0.2 | 0 | 0.01 | 0 | 0 | 14222 |
| **coffee and cocoa inst pwdr**, decaf w/ whtnr and low-cal swtnr - *1 t* | 6 | 15 | 0.2 | 4.3 | 2.1 | 0 | 0.3 | 30 | 4 | 7 | 0.06 | 0.048 | 0 | 0 | 0 | 0.3 | 0 | 0 |
| | | 0.5 | 0.8 | 0.7 | 0.1 | 0 | 0 | 111 | 27 | 0.18 | 0.034 | 0.2 | 0 | 0 | 0.01 | 0 | 0.3 | 14204 |
| **coffee and cocoa inst pwdr** w/ whtnr and low-cal swtnr - *1 t* | 6 | 15 | 0.2 | 4.3 | 2.1 | 0 | 0.3 | 30 | 4 | 7 | 0.06 | 0.048 | 0 | 0 | 0 | 0.3 | 0 | 0 |
| | | 0.5 | 0.8 | 0.7 | 0.1 | 0 | 0 | 111 | 27 | 0.18 | 0.034 | 0.2 | 0 | 0 | 0.01 | 0 | 0.3 | 43343 |
| **coffee, brewed** | 237 | 2 | 235.6 | 0 | 0 | | 0 | 5 | 5 | 7 | 0.05 | 0.055 | 0 | 0 | 0.03 | 0.5 | 0 | 0.60 |
| *8 fl oz* | | 0.3 | 0 | 0 | 0 | 0 | 0 | 116 | 7 | 0.02 | 0.005 | 0 | 0 | 0.18 | 0 | 4.7 | 14209 |
| **coffee, decaffeinated, brewed** | 237 | 0 | 235.3 | 0 | 0 | | 0 | 5 | 5 | 12 | 0.05 | 0.064 | 0 | 0 | 0 | 0.5 | 0 | 0 |
| *8 fl oz* | | 0.2 | 0 | 0 | 0 | 0 | 0 | 128 | 2 | 0.12 | 0.017 | 0.2 | 0 | 0 | 0 | 0 | 14201 |
| **coffee, decaffeinated**, from instant powder - *8 fl oz* | 237 | 5 | 234.5 | 1.0 | 0 | | 0 | 9 | 9 | 9 | 0.02 | 0.028 | 0 | 0 | 0 | 0.7 | 0 | 0 |
| | | 0.3 | 0 | 0 | 0 | 0 | 0 | 85 | 7 | 0.09 | 0.024 | 0.5 | 0 | 0 | 0.03 | 0 | 14219 |
| **coffee**, from instant powder | 237 | 5 | 234.8 | 0.8 | 0 | | 0 | 9 | 9 | 9 | 0.02 | 0.036 | 0 | 0 | 0 | 0.6 | 0 | 0 |
| *8 fl oz* | | 0.2 | 0 | 0 | 0 | 0 | 0 | 71 | 7 | 0.09 | 0.026 | 0.2 | 0 | 0 | 0 | 0 | 14215 |
| **coffee instant powder** | 1.5 | 4 | 0 | 0.6 | 0 | 0 | 0 | 1 | 2 | 5 | 0.01 | 0.026 | 0 | 0 | 0 | 0.4 | 0 | 0 |
| *1 round t* | | 0.2 | 0 | 0 | 0 | 0 | 0 | 53 | 5 | 0.07 | 0.002 | 0.2 | 0 | 0 | 0 | 0 | 14214 |
| **coffee instant powder**, cappuccino flavor with sugar - *2 round t* | 14 | 57 | 0.2 | 12.0 | 9.7 | 9.0 | 0.2 | 25 | 19 | 6 | 0.04 | 0.028 | 0 | 0 | 0.02 | 0.3 | 0.05 | 0.01 |
| | | 0.4 | 0.8 | 0.5 | 0.2 | 0 | 0 | 116 | 26 | 0.07 | 0.015 | 0.6 | 0 | 0.1 | 0.01 | 0.01 | 0.7 | 14228 |
| **coffee instant powder**, decaf | 1.8 | 4 | 0.1 | 0.8 | 0 | 0 | 0 | 0 | 3 | 6 | 0 | 0.022 | 0 | 0 | 0 | 0.5 | 0 | 0 |
| *1 round t* | | 0.2 | 0 | 0 | 0 | 0 | 0 | 63 | 5 | 0.07 | 0.001 | 0.3 | 0 | 0 | 0.02 | 0 | 14218 |
| **coffee instant powder**, French flvr w/sgr - *2 round t* | 12 | 58 | 0.3 | 7.9 | 5.0 | 5.0 | 0 | 67 | 4 | 3 | 0 | 0.021 | 0 | 0 | 0 | 0.7 | 0 | 0 |
| | | 0.5 | 2.7 | 0.6 | 1.7 | 0.3 | 0 | 142 | 42 | 0.04 | 0.003 | 0.2 | 0 | 0.2 | 0 | 0 | 14229 |
| **coffee instant powder**, mocha flvr w/sgr - *2 round t* | 12 | 55 | 0.2 | 8.9 | 7.0 | 5.0 | 0.2 | 38 | 33 | 8 | 0.12 | 0.053 | 0 | 0 | 0 | 0.3 | 0.05 | 0.01 |
| | | 0.6 | 1.9 | 0.6 | 1.1 | 0.1 | 0 | 124 | 30 | 0 | 0.052 | 0.7 | 1 | 0 | 0.01 | 1.1 | 14224 |
| **espresso**, decaffeinated | 178 | 0 | 174.1 | 0 | 0 | | 0 | 25 | 4 | 142 | 0.09 | 0.089 | 0 | 0 | 0 | 9.3 | 0 | 0.05 |
| *6 fl oz* | | 0.2 | 0.3 | 0.2 | 0 | 0.2 | 0 | 205 | 12 | 0.23 | 0.089 | 0 | 0 | 0.32 | 0 | 1.8 | 14202 |
| **espresso**, from restaurant | 178 | 4 | 174.1 | 0 | 0 | | 0 | 25 | 4 | 142 | 0.09 | 0.089 | 0 | 0 | 0 | 9.3 | 0 | 0.05 |
| *6 fl oz* | | 0.2 | 0.3 | 0.2 | 0 | 0.2 | 0 | 205 | 12 | 0.23 | 0.089 | 0 | 0 | 0.32 | 0 | 1.8 | 14210 |

## 1.5 DISTILLED SPIRITS (HARD LIQUOR)

| | WT (g) | KCAL | H₂O (g) | CHO (g) | TSUG (g) | ASUG (g) | DFIB (g) | Na (mg) | Ca (mg) | Mg (mg) | Zn (mg) | Mn (mg) | A (mcg RAE) | C (mg) | B-1 (mg) | NIA (mg) | B-12 (mcg) | PANT (mg) |
|---|---|---|---|---|---|---|---|---|---|---|---|---|---|---|---|---|---|---|
| | | PRO (g) | FAT (g) | SFA (g) | MUFA (g) | PUFA (g) | CHOL (mg) | K (mg) | P (mg) | Fe (mg) | Cu (mg) | Se (mcg) | A (IU) | E (mg ATE) | B-2 (mg) | B-6 (mg) | FOL (mcg DFE) | REF |
| **distilled spirits**, all types, 100 proof - *1.5 fl oz jigger* | 42 | 124 | 24.2 | 0 | | | 0 | 0 | 0 | 0 | 0.02 | 0.008 | 0 | 0 | 0 | 0 | 0 | 0 |
| | | 0 | 0 | 0 | 0 | 0 | 0 | 1 | 2 | 0.02 | 0.009 | 0 | 0 | 0 | 0 | 0 | 14533 |
| **distilled spirits**, all types, 80 proof - *1.5 fl oz jigger* | 42 | 97 | 28.0 | 0 | 0 | | 0 | 0 | 0 | 0 | 0.02 | 0.008 | 0 | 0 | 0 | 0 | 0 | 0 |
| | | 0 | 0 | 0 | 0 | 0 | 0 | 1 | 2 | 0.02 | 0.009 | 0 | 0 | 0 | 0 | 0 | 14037 |
| **distilled spirits**, all types, 86 proof - *1.5 fl oz jigger* | 42 | 105 | 26.8 | 0 | 0 | | 0 | 0 | 0 | 0 | 0.02 | 0.008 | 0 | 0 | 0 | 0 | 0 | 0 |
| | | 0 | 0 | 0 | 0 | 0 | 0 | 1 | 2 | 0.02 | 0.009 | 0 | 0 | 0 | 0 | 0 | 14550 |

| | WT (g) | KCAL / PRO (g) | H₂0 (g) / FAT (g) | CHO (g) / SFA (g) | TSUG (g) / MUFA (g) | ASUG (g) / PUFA (g) | DFIB (g) / CHOL (mg) | Na (mg) / K (mg) | Ca (mg) / P (mg) | Mg (mg) / Fe (mg) | Zn (mg) / Cu (mg) | Mn (mg) / Se (mcg) | A (mcg RAE) / A (IU) | C (mg) / E (mg ATE) | B-1 (mg) / B-2 (mg) | NIA (mg) / B-6 (mg) | B-12 (mcg) / FOL (mcg DFE) | PANT (mg) / REF |
|---|---|---|---|---|---|---|---|---|---|---|---|---|---|---|---|---|---|---|
| **distilled spirits**, all types, | 42 | 110 | 26.1 | 0 | 0 | | 0 | 0 | 0 | 0 | 0.02 | 0.008 | 0 | 0 | 0 | 0 | 0 | 0 |
| 90 proof - *1.5 fl oz jigger* | | 0 | 0 | 0 | 0 | 0 | 0 | 1 | 2 | 0.02 | 0.009 | 0 | 0 | 0 | 0 | 0 | 0 | 14551 |
| **distilled spirits**, all types, | 42 | 116 | 25.3 | 0 | | | 0 | 0 | 0 | 0 | 0.02 | 0.008 | 0 | 0 | 0 | 0 | 0 | 0 |
| 94 proof - *1.5 fl oz jigger* | | 0 | 0 | 0 | 0 | 0 | 0 | 1 | 2 | 0.02 | 0.009 | 0 | 0 | 0 | 0 | 0 | 0 | 14532 |
| **gin**, 90 proof | 42 | 110 | 26.1 | 0 | 0 | | 0 | 1 | 0 | 0 | 0 | 0 | 0 | 0 | 0 | 0 | 0 | 0 |
| *1.5 fl oz jigger* | | 0 | 0 | 0 | 0 | 0 | 0 | 0 | 0 | 0 | 0.002 | 0 | 0 | 0 | 0 | 0 | 0 | 14049 |
| **rum**, 80 proof | 42 | 97 | 28.0 | 0 | 0 | | 0 | 0 | 0 | 0 | 0.03 | 0.008 | 0 | 0 | 0 | 0 | 0 | 0 |
| *1.5 fl oz jigger* | | 0 | 0 | 0 | 0 | 0 | 0 | 1 | 2 | 0.05 | 0.021 | 0 | 0 | 0 | 0 | 0 | 0 | 14050 |
| **vodka**, 80 proof | 42 | 97 | 28.0 | 0 | 0 | | 0 | 0 | 0 | 0 | 0 | 0 | 0 | 0 | 0 | 0 | 0 | 0 |
| *1.5 fl oz jigger* | | 0 | 0 | 0 | 0 | 0 | 0 | 0 | 2 | 0 | 0.004 | 0 | 0 | 0 | 0 | 0 | 0 | 14051 |
| **whiskey**, 86 proof | 42 | 105 | 26.8 | 0 | 0 | | 0 | 0 | 0 | 0 | 0.01 | 0.003 | 0 | 0 | 0 | 0 | 0 | 0 |
| *1.5 fl oz jigger* | | 0 | 0 | 0 | 0 | 0 | 0 | 0 | 1 | 0.01 | 0.006 | 0 | 0 | 0 | 0 | 0 | 0 | 14052 |

## 1.6 FRUIT DRINKS AND FRUIT-FLAVORED BEVERAGES

| | WT (g) | KCAL / PRO (g) | H₂0 (g) / FAT (g) | CHO (g) / SFA (g) | TSUG (g) / MUFA (g) | ASUG (g) / PUFA (g) | DFIB (g) / CHOL (mg) | Na (mg) / K (mg) | Ca (mg) / P (mg) | Mg (mg) / Fe (mg) | Zn (mg) / Cu (mg) | Mn (mg) / Se (mcg) | A (mcg RAE) / A (IU) | C (mg) / E (mg ATE) | B-1 (mg) / B-2 (mg) | NIA (mg) / B-6 (mg) | B-12 (mcg) / FOL (mcg DFE) | PANT (mg) / REF |
|---|---|---|---|---|---|---|---|---|---|---|---|---|---|---|---|---|---|---|
| **fruit punch drink**, canned/ | 248 | 117 | 218.2 | 29.7 | 28.0 | 14.7 | 0.5 | 94 | 20 | 7 | 0.02 | 0.208 | 5 | 73 | 0.01 | 0.1 | 0 | 0.03 |
| bottled *8 fl oz* | | 0 | 0 | 0 | 0 | 0 | 0 | 77 | 7 | 0.22 | 0.025 | 0.5 | 69 | 0 | 0.06 | 0.03 | 2.5 | 14267 |
| **fruit punch drink**, from frozen | 247 | 114 | 217.7 | 28.8 | 0 | | 0.2 | 12 | 10 | 5 | 0.05 | 0.252 | 2 | 108 | 0.02 | 0.1 | 0 | 0.02 |
| concentrate - *8 fl oz* | | 0.1 | 0 | 0 | 0 | 0 | 0 | 32 | 2 | 0.22 | 0.079 | 0 | 27 | 0 | 0.03 | 0.01 | 2.5 | 14269 |
| **Fuze**, refresh banana colada | 240 | 90 | | 24.0 | 22.0 | | | 15 | 250 | | | | | 30 | | 10.0 | 3.00 | 5.00 |
| *8 fl oz* | | 0 | | | | | | | | | | | 1250 | | | 1.00 | | FUZE1 |
| **Fuze**, slenderize cranberry | 240 | 10 | | 2.0 | 1.0 | | | 5 | | | | | | 60 | | | | |
| apple *8 fl oz* | | 0 | 0 | | | | | | | | | | | | | | | FUZE2 |
| **Fuze**, slenderize cranberry | 240 | 10 | | 2.0 | 1.0 | | | 5 | | | | | | 60 | | | | |
| raspberry - *8 fl oz* | | 0 | 0 | | | | | | | | | | | | | | | FUZE3 |
| **Fuze**, slenderize tropical punch | 240 | 10 | | 1.0 | 0 | | | 5 | | | | | | 60 | | | | |
| *8 fl oz* | | 0 | 0 | | | | | | | | | | | | | | | FUZE4 |
| **grape drink**, canned/bottled | 250 | 152 | 210.5 | 39.4 | 32.6 | 30.1 | 0 | 40 | 130 | 2 | 0.30 | 0.068 | 0 | 78 | 0 | 0 | 0 | 0.01 |
| *8 fl oz* | | 0 | 0 | 0 | 0 | 0 | 0 | 30 | 0 | 0.18 | 0.032 | 0.2 | 0 | 0 | 0.01 | 0 | 0 | 14277 |
| **lemonade-flavored drink**, | 266 | 69 | 247.1 | 17.8 | 17.8 | | 0 | 35 | 24 | 3 | 0.03 | 0 | 0 | 6 | 0 | 0 | 0 | 0 |
| from dry mix - *8 fl oz* | | 0 | 0 | 0 | 0 | 0 | 0 | 3 | 3 | 0.03 | 0.032 | 0 | 0 | 0 | 0 | 0 | 0 | 14297 |
| **lemonade**, from dry mix | 264 | 98 | 236.7 | 25.7 | 25.7 | | 0 | 8 | 74 | 3 | 0.05 | 0 | 0 | 9 | 0.01 | 0 | 0 | 0.02 |
| *8 fl oz* | | 0 | 0 | 0 | 0 | 0 | 0 | 34 | 34 | 0.13 | 0.032 | 0.3 | 3 | 0 | 0.01 | 0.01 | 2.6 | 14288 |
| **lemonade**, from dry mix with | 238 | 7 | 235.9 | 1.6 | 0 | | 0 | 10 | 67 | 2 | 0.02 | 0.002 | 0 | 8 | 0 | 0 | 0 | 0 |
| aspartame - *8 fl oz* | | 0.1 | 0 | 0 | 0 | 0 | 0 | 2 | 31 | 0.12 | 0.026 | 0 | 0 | 0 | 0 | 0 | 0 | 14290 |
| **lemonade**, from frozen | 248 | 99 | 221.6 | 25.8 | 24.8 | | 0 | 10 | 10 | 5 | 0.05 | 0.012 | 0 | 10 | 0.01 | 0 | 0 | 0.03 |
| concentrate - *8 fl oz* | | 0.2 | 0.1 | 0 | 0 | 0 | 0 | 37 | 5 | 0.40 | 0.052 | 0.2 | 2 | 0 | 0.05 | 0.01 | 2.5 | 14293 |
| **lemonade frozen concentrate** | 36.5 | 66 | 19.1 | 17.2 | 16.4 | 11.5 | 0.1 | 1 | 3 | 2 | 0.03 | 0.007 | 0 | 6 | 0.01 | 0 | 0 | 0.02 |
| *1 fl oz* | | 0.1 | 0.1 | 0 | 0 | 0 | 0 | 24 | 3 | 0.26 | 0.022 | 0.1 | 3 | 0 | 0.04 | 0.01 | 1.8 | 14292 |
| **lemonade**, pink, from frozen | 247 | 99 | 220.7 | 25.7 | | | 0.2 | 10 | 10 | 5 | 0.05 | 0.012 | 0 | 10 | 0.01 | 0 | 0 | 0.03 |
| concentrate - *8 fl oz* | | 0.2 | 0.1 | 0 | 0 | 0 | 0 | 37 | 5 | 0.40 | 0.052 | 0 | 5 | 0 | 0.05 | 0.01 | 4.9 | 14543 |
| **limeade**, from frozen concentrate | 247 | 128 | 212.6 | 34.1 | 32.8 | | 0 | 7 | 5 | 5 | 0.02 | 0.002 | 0 | 8 | 0 | 0 | 0 | 0.03 |
| concentrate *8 fl oz* | | 0 | 0 | 0 | 0 | 0 | 0 | 25 | 2 | 0 | 0.040 | 0.2 | 0 | 0 | 0.01 | 0.01 | 2.5 | 14303 |
| **orange breakfast drink**, from | 271 | 133 | 236.2 | 34.3 | 32.0 | | 0.3 | 14 | 141 | 3 | 0.03 | 0.019 | 209 | 80 | 0 | 2.8 | 0 | 0 |
| dry mix - *8 fl oz* | | 0 | 0 | 0 | 0 | 0 | 0 | 68 | 51 | 0 | 0.027 | 0.3 | 694 | 0 | 0.24 | 0.28 | 0 | 14408 |
| **orange breakfast drink**, from | 250 | 112 | 220.2 | 28.3 | 27.6 | | 0 | 25 | 295 | 28 | 0.10 | 0.035 | 0 | 138 | 0.26 | 0.6 | 0 | 0.47 |
| frzn conc - *8 fl oz* | | 0.3 | 0 | 0 | 0 | 0 | 0 | 418 | 82 | 0.20 | 0.250 | 0 | 15 | 0 | 2.60 | 0.18 | 0 | 14427 |
| **orange drink**, canned/bottled | 248 | 122 | 216.9 | 30.6 | 27.4 | 23.1 | 0 | 7 | 12 | 5 | 0.05 | 0.027 | 2 | 142 | 0 | 0 | 0 | 0.04 |
| *8 fl oz* | | 0 | 0.2 | 0 | 0 | 0 | 0 | 45 | 2 | 0.10 | 0 | 0 | 20 | 0 | 0 | 0 | 5.0 | 14323 |
| **orange flavor drink mix**, brkfst type, | 2.5 | 5 | 0 | 2.1 | 0.1 | | 0.1 | 2 | 34 | 7 | 0 | | 150 | 60 | 0 | 2.0 | 0 | 0 |
| low-cal - *amt to make 8 fl oz* | | 0.1 | 0 | 0 | 0 | 0 | 0 | 78 | 16 | 0 | 0 | 0 | 500 | 0 | 0.17 | 0.20 | 0 | 14409 |

## 1.7 LIQUEURS

| | WT (g) | KCAL / PRO (g) | H₂0 (g) / FAT (g) | CHO (g) / SFA (g) | TSUG (g) / MUFA (g) | ASUG (g) / PUFA (g) | DFIB (g) / CHOL (mg) | Na (mg) / K (mg) | Ca (mg) / P (mg) | Mg (mg) / Fe (mg) | Zn (mg) / Cu (mg) | Mn (mg) / Se (mcg) | A (mcg RAE) / A (IU) | C (mg) / E (mg ATE) | B-1 (mg) / B-2 (mg) | NIA (mg) / B-6 (mg) | B-12 (mcg) / FOL (mcg DFE) | PANT (mg) / REF |
|---|---|---|---|---|---|---|---|---|---|---|---|---|---|---|---|---|---|---|
| **liqueur**, coffee, 53 proof | 52 | 170 | 16.1 | 24.3 | 24.1 | 24.1 | 0 | 4 | 1 | 2 | 0.02 | 0.007 | 0 | 0 | 0 | 0.1 | 0 | 0 |
| *1.5 fl oz* | | 0.1 | 0.2 | 0.1 | 0 | 0.1 | 0 | 16 | 3 | 0.03 | 0.021 | 0.2 | 0 | 0 | 0.01 | 0 | 0 | 14414 |
| **liqueur**, coffee, 63 proof | 52 | 160 | 21.5 | 16.7 | 16.7 | 16.7 | 0 | 4 | 1 | 2 | 0.02 | 0.009 | 0 | 0 | 0 | 0.1 | 0 | 0 |
| *1.5 fl oz* | | 0.1 | 0.2 | 0.1 | 0 | 0.1 | 0 | 16 | 3 | 0.03 | 0.021 | 0.2 | 0 | 0 | 0.01 | 0 | 0 | 14534 |
| **liqueur**, coffee with cream, | 47 | 154 | 21.9 | 9.8 | 9.3 | 9.3 | 0 | 43 | 8 | 1 | 0.08 | 0.003 | 81 | 0 | 0.01 | 0 | 0.04 | 0.04 |
| 34 proof - *1.5 fl oz* | | 1.3 | 7.4 | 4.5 | 2.1 | 0.3 | 27 | 15 | 24 | 0.06 | 0.019 | 0.2 | 291 | 0.2 | 0.03 | 0.01 | 0.9 | 14415 |
| **liqueur**, crème de menthe, | 50 | 186 | 14.2 | 20.8 | 20.8 | 20.8 | 0 | 2 | 0 | 0 | 0.02 | 0.020 | 0 | 0 | 0 | 0 | 0 | 0 |
| 72 proof *1.5 fl oz* | | 0 | 0.2 | 0 | 0 | 0.1 | 0 | 0 | 0 | 0.04 | 0.040 | 0.2 | 0 | 0 | 0 | 0 | 0 | 14034 |

| | WT (g) | KCAL / PRO (g) | $H_2O$ (g) / FAT (g) | CHO (g) / SFA (g) | TSUG (g) / MUFA (g) | ASUG (g) / PUFA (g) | DFIB (g) / CHOL (mg) | Na (mg) / K (mg) | Ca (mg) / P (mg) | Mg (mg) / Fe (mg) | Zn (mg) / Cu (mg) | Mn (mg) / Se (mcg) | A (mcg RAE) / A (IU) | C (mg) / E (mg ATE) | B-1 (mg) / B-2 (mg) | NIA (mg) / B-6 (mg) | B-12 (mcg) / FOL (mcg DFE) | PANT (mg) / REF |
|---|---|---|---|---|---|---|---|---|---|---|---|---|---|---|---|---|---|---|

### 1.8 MALT BEVERAGES (BEERS, ALES, STOUTS)

| | WT (g) | KCAL / PRO | $H_2O$ / FAT | CHO / SFA | TSUG / MUFA | ASUG / PUFA | DFIB / CHOL | Na / K | Ca / P | Mg / Fe | Zn / Cu | Mn / Se | A RAE / A IU | C / E | B-1 / B-2 | NIA / B-6 | B-12 / FOL | PANT / REF |
|---|---|---|---|---|---|---|---|---|---|---|---|---|---|---|---|---|---|---|
| beer | 356 | 153 | 327.4 | 12.6 | 0 | 0 | 0 | 14 | 14 | 21 | 0.04 | 0.028 | 0 | 0 | 0.02 | 1.8 | 0.07 | 0.15 |
| *12 fl oz* | | 1.6 | 0 | 0 | 0 | 0 | 0 | 96 | 50 | 0.07 | 0.018 | 2.1 | 0 | 0 | 0.09 | 0.16 | 21.4 | 14003 |
| beer, Bud Light, Anheuser-Busch | 354 | 110 | 336.3 | 6.6 | | | 0 | 11 | 11 | 25 | 0 | 0.021 | | | | | | |
| *12 fl oz* | | 0.9 | 0 | | | | 0 | 92 | 39 | 0 | 0.007 | | | | | | | 14007 |
| beer, Budweiser, Anheuser-Busch | 356 | 146 | 330.3 | 10.6 | | | 0 | 11 | 14 | 25 | 0 | 0.032 | | | | | | |
| *12 fl oz* | | 1.3 | 0 | | | | 0 | 117 | 46 | 0 | 0.011 | | | | | | | 14004 |
| beer, Budweiser Select, light, Anheuser-Busch - *12 fl oz* | 354 | 99 | 337.4 | 3.1 | | | 0 | 11 | 14 | 21 | 0.04 | 0.025 | | | | | | |
| | | 0.7 | 0 | | | | 0 | 92 | | 0 | 0.004 | | | | | | | 14005 |
| beer, light | 354 | 103 | 335.9 | 5.8 | 0.3 | | 0 | 14 | 14 | 18 | 0.04 | 0.021 | 0 | 0 | 0.02 | 1.4 | 0.07 | 0.11 |
| *12 fl oz* | | 0.8 | 0 | 0 | 0 | 0 | 0 | 74 | 42 | 0.11 | 0.021 | 1.4 | 0 | 0 | 0.05 | 0.12 | 21.2 | 14006 |
| beer, Michelob Ultra, light, Anheuser-Busch - *12 fl oz* | 354 | 96 | 337.7 | 2.6 | | | 0 | 11 | 14 | 14 | 0.04 | 0.018 | | | | | | |
| | | 0.6 | 0 | | | | 0 | 60 | 28 | 0 | 0.007 | | | | | | | 14013 |
| malt beverage, no alcohol | 356 | 132 | 324.5 | 28.7 | 28.7 | 0 | 0 | 46 | 25 | 25 | 0.07 | 0.046 | 0 | 2 | 0.06 | 4.0 | 0.07 | 0.13 |
| *12 fl oz* | | 0.7 | 0.4 | 0.1 | 0.1 | 0.2 | 0 | 28 | 57 | 0.21 | 0.028 | 4.3 | 7 | 0 | 0.17 | 0.10 | 49.8 | 14305 |

### 1.9 SPORT AND ENERGY BEVERAGES

| | WT (g) | KCAL / PRO | $H_2O$ / FAT | CHO / SFA | TSUG / MUFA | ASUG / PUFA | DFIB / CHOL | Na / K | Ca / P | Mg / Fe | Zn / Cu | Mn / Se | A RAE / A IU | C / E | B-1 / B-2 | NIA / B-6 | B-12 / FOL | PANT / REF |
|---|---|---|---|---|---|---|---|---|---|---|---|---|---|---|---|---|---|---|
| Gatorade, fruit flavor, Quaker Oats - *8 fl oz* | 240 | 62 | 224.1 | 15.4 | 12.6 | | 0 | 94 | 2 | 0 | 0.02 | 0.031 | 0 | 1 | 0.03 | 0.5 | 0 | 0.13 |
| | | 0 | 0 | 0 | 0 | 0 | 0 | 36 | 24 | 0.12 | 0.014 | 0 | 0 | 0 | 0 | 0.05 | 0 | 14460 |
| Gatorade mix, lemon lime | 16 | 58 | 0.4 | 15.2 | 14.4 | | | 96 | | | | | | | | | | |
| *¾ scoop (amt for 1 serving)* | | 0 | 0 | | | | | 32 | | | | | | | | | | 14131 |
| Powerade Advance, berry | 240 | 99 | | 25.5 | 3.0 | | | 80 | | | | | | | | 3.0 | 0.90 | |
| *8 fl oz* | | 0 | 0 | | | | | 48 | 3 | | | | | | | 0.30 | | COLA106 |
| Powerade, grape | 240 | 98 | | 25.5 | 22.5 | | | 80 | | | | | | | | 3.0 | 0.90 | |
| *8 fl oz* | | 0 | 0 | | | | | 48 | | | | | | | | 0.30 | | COLA108 |
| Powerade, lemon-lime flavor | 240 | 77 | 220.6 | 18.8 | 14.7 | | 0 | 53 | 2 | 0 | 0.02 | 0 | 0 | 0 | 0.03 | 3.8 | 3.29 | 0 |
| *8 fl oz* | | 0 | 0.1 | 0 | 0 | 0.1 | 0 | 43 | 2 | 0.22 | 0 | 0 | 0 | 0 | 0 | 0.37 | 0 | 14461 |
| Powerade Option, black cherry | 240 | 15 | | 3.0 | 3.0 | | | 78 | | | | | | | | 3.0 | 0.90 | |
| *8 fl oz* | | 0 | 0 | | | | | 50 | | | | | | | | 0.30 | | COLA107 |
| Propel Fitness Water, fruit-flavored - *8 fl oz* | 240 | 12 | 237.1 | 2.9 | 2.9 | | 0 | 31 | 2 | 0 | 0 | 0 | 0 | 21 | 0 | 9.8 | 0.02 | 3.77 |
| | | 0 | 0 | 0 | 0 | 0 | 0 | 38 | 0 | 0.07 | 0 | 0 | 0 | 4.0 | 0 | 1.33 | 0 | 14462 |
| Red Bull, sugar-free w/added caffeine and vits, cnd - *8 fl oz* | 240 | 12 | 236.0 | 1.7 | | | | 202 | 31 | 7 | 0 | 0.007 | | | 0.06 | 20.4 | 4.20 | 3.36 |
| | | 0.6 | 0.2 | | | | | 7 | 0 | 0.05 | 0.012 | | | | 1.38 | 2.00 | | 14156 |
| Red Bull w/caffeine and vitamins, canned - *8 fl oz* | 240 | 108 | 212.3 | 26.3 | 24.1 | | 0 | 202 | 31 | 7 | 0 | 0.007 | 0 | 0 | 0.06 | 20.4 | 4.20 | 3.36 |
| | | 0.6 | 0.2 | 0 | 0 | 0 | 0 | 7 | 0 | 0.05 | 0.012 | 0.5 | 0 | 0 | 1.38 | 2.00 | 0 | 14154 |
| thirst quencher beverage, fruit flvrd, low calorie - *8 fl oz* | 240 | 26 | 232.3 | 7.2 | 0 | 0 | 0 | 84 | 0 | 2 | 0.05 | 0 | 0 | 15 | 0 | 0 | 0 | 0 |
| | | 0 | 0 | 0 | 0 | 0 | 0 | 24 | 22 | 0.12 | 0.048 | 0.2 | 0 | 0 | 0 | 0 | 0 | 14383 |
| Vault energy soda | 240 | 178 | | 48.0 | 48.0 | | | 45 | | | | | | | | | | |
| *8 fl oz* | | 0 | 0 | | | | | 30 | | | | | | | | | | COLA121 |
| Vault Zero energy soda | 240 | 6 | | 0.3 | 0.3 | | | 45 | | | | | | | | | | |
| *8 fl oz* | | 0 | 0 | | | | | 42 | | | | | | | | | | COLA122 |

### 1.10 TEA

| | WT (g) | KCAL / PRO | $H_2O$ / FAT | CHO / SFA | TSUG / MUFA | ASUG / PUFA | DFIB / CHOL | Na / K | Ca / P | Mg / Fe | Zn / Cu | Mn / Se | A RAE / A IU | C / E | B-1 / B-2 | NIA / B-6 | B-12 / FOL | PANT / REF |
|---|---|---|---|---|---|---|---|---|---|---|---|---|---|---|---|---|---|---|
| iced tea, canned/bottled, Nestea | 240 | 3 | | 0.3 | | | | 38 | | | | | | | | | | |
| *8 fl oz* | | 0 | | | | | | 32 | | | | | | | | | | COLA90 |
| iced tea, decaffeinated, w/sgr, cnd/btld, Nestea - *8 fl oz* | 255 | 93 | | 25.5 | | | | 36 | | | | | | | | | | |
| | | 0 | | | | | | 32 | | | | | | | | | | COLA91 |
| iced tea, from instant | 237 | 2 | 236.1 | 0.4 | 0 | 0 | 0 | 9 | 7 | 5 | 0.02 | 0.929 | 0 | 0 | 0 | 0.1 | 0 | 0.03 |
| *8 fl oz* | | 0.1 | 0 | 0 | 0 | 0 | 0 | 43 | 2 | 0.02 | 0.026 | 0 | 0 | 0 | 0.01 | 0 | 0 | 14367 |
| iced tea, green, honey lemon w/sgr, cnd/btld, Nestea - *8 fl oz* | 255 | 122 | | 33.0 | | | | 34 | | | | | | | | | | |
| | | 0 | | | | | | 0 | | | | | | | | | | COLA92 |
| iced tea, green, peach w/low-cal swtnrs, Nestea - *8 fl oz* | 240 | 6 | | 0.4 | | | | 48 | | | | | | | | | | |
| | | 0 | | | | | | 30 | | | | | | | | | | COLA93 |
| iced tea, green, peach with sugar, cnd/btld, Nestea - *8 fl oz* | 255 | 130 | | 34.5 | | | | 45 | | | | | | | | | | |
| | | 0 | | | | | | 38 | | | | | | | | | | COLA94 |
| iced tea instant powder, decaffeinated - *1 t* | 11 | 35 | 0.6 | 6.5 | 0.6 | 0 | 0.9 | 8 | 13 | 30 | 0.19 | 14.630 | 0 | 0 | 0 | 1.2 | 0 | 0.50 |
| | | 2.2 | 0 | 0 | 0 | 0 | 0 | 664 | 26 | 0.25 | 0.061 | 0.6 | 0 | 0 | 0.11 | 0.04 | 11.3 | 14353 |
| iced tea instant powder, lemon flavor - *2 round T* | 11 | 38 | 0.5 | 8.6 | 0.5 | 0 | 0.6 | 6 | 3 | 15 | 0.11 | 3.374 | 0 | 0 | 0 | 0.7 | 0 | 0.29 |
| | | 0.8 | 0 | 0 | 0 | 0 | 0 | 380 | 12 | 0.08 | 0.036 | 0.3 | 0 | 0 | 0.06 | 0.02 | 6.7 | 14368 |

| | WT (g) | KCAL / PRO (g) | $H_2O$ (g) / FAT (g) | CHO (g) / SFA (g) | TSUG (g) / MUFA (g) | ASUG (g) / PUFA (g) | DFIB (g) / CHOL (mg) | Na (mg) / K (mg) | Ca (mg) / P (mg) | Mg (mg) / Fe (mg) | Zn (mg) / Cu (mg) | Mn (mg) / Se (mcg) | A (mcg RAE) / A (IU) | C (mg) / E (mg ATE) | B-1 (mg) / B-2 (mg) | NIA (mg) / B-6 (mg) | B-12 (mcg) / FOL (mcg DFE) | PANT (mg) / REF |
|---|---|---|---|---|---|---|---|---|---|---|---|---|---|---|---|---|---|---|
| **iced tea instant powder**, lemon flvr w/saccharin - 4 T (¼ cup) | 14 | 47 | 0.5 | 12.0 | 0.3 | 0 | 0 | 58 | 3 | 18 | 0.12 | 4.252 | 0 | 0 | 0 | 0.5 | 0 | 0.22 |
| | | 0.5 | 0.1 | 0 | 0 | 0 | 0 | 360 | 20 | 1.24 | 0.017 | 0.3 | 0 | 0 | 0.05 | 0.02 | 4.9 | 14375 |
| **iced tea instant powder**, lemon flvr w/sgr - 3 heaping t | 23 | 92 | 0 | 22.7 | 21.9 | 21.9 | 0.2 | 1 | 0 | 1 | 0.01 | 0.324 | 0 | 0 | 0 | 0 | 0 | 0 |
| | | 0 | 0.2 | 0 | 0 | 0.1 | 0 | 39 | 0 | 0.05 | 0.002 | 0.1 | 0 | 0 | 0 | 0 | 0.2 | 14370 |
| **iced tea**, lemon, canned/bottled, Nestea - 8 fl oz | 240 | 86 | 218.8 | 21.8 | 21.8 | | 0 | 50 | 7 | 2 | 0.14 | 0.314 | | | | | | |
| | | 0 | 0 | | | | | 46 | 86 | 0 | 0.019 | | | | | | | 14137 |
| **iced tea**, lemon flavor w/saccharin, from inst - 8 fl oz | 237 | 5 | 235.6 | 1.0 | 0 | | 0 | 14 | 7 | 5 | 0.02 | 0.367 | 0 | 0 | 0 | 0 | 0 | 0.02 |
| | | 0 | 0 | 0 | 0 | 0 | 0 | 33 | 2 | 0.12 | 0.024 | 0 | 0 | 0 | 0 | 0 | 0 | 14376 |
| **iced tea**, lemon flavor w/sgr, cnd/btld, Lipton Brisk - 8 fl oz | 245 | 86 | 223.1 | 21.6 | 21.3 | | 0 | 51 | 2 | 0 | 0.02 | 0.358 | | | | | | |
| | | 0 | 0 | 0 | 0 | | | 47 | 64 | 0 | 0.012 | | | | | | | 14476 |
| **iced tea**, lemon flavor w/sgr, cnd/btld, Arizona - 8 fl oz | 227 | 89 | 204.6 | 22.2 | 21.9 | | 0 | 9 | 7 | 2 | 0.02 | 0.363 | 0 | | | | | |
| | | 0 | 0 | 0 | 0 | | 0 | 23 | 2 | 0 | 0.011 | | 0 | | | | | 14475 |
| **iced tea**, lemon flavor with sugar, from instant - 8 fl oz | 259 | 91 | 236.2 | 22.3 | 21.6 | 21.6 | 0.3 | 5 | 5 | 3 | 0.03 | 0.321 | 0 | 0 | 0 | 0 | 0 | 0 |
| | | 0 | 0.2 | 0 | 0 | 0 | 0 | 39 | 0 | 0.05 | 0.018 | 0.3 | 0 | 0 | 0 | 0 | 0 | 14371 |
| **iced tea**, lemon w/low-cal swtnrs, cnd/btld, Nestea - 8 fl oz | 240 | 3 | | 0 | | | | 48 | | | | | | | | | | |
| | | 0 | | | | | | | 0 | | | | | | | | | COLA20 |
| **iced tea**, lemon with sugar, canned/ bottled, Nestea - 8 fl oz | 255 | 116 | | 31.5 | | | | 34 | | | | | | | | | | |
| | | 0 | | | | | | | 0 | | | | | | | | | COLA95 |
| **iced tea**, raspberry with sugar, cnd/ bottled, Nestea - 8 fl oz | 255 | 117 | | 31.5 | | | | 38 | | | | | | | | | | |
| | | 0 | | | | | | | 0 | | | | | | | | | COLA96 |
| **iced tea** with sugar, canned/ bottled, Nestea - 8 fl oz | 255 | 94 | | 25.5 | | | | 38 | | | | | | | | | | |
| | | 0 | | | | | | | 32 | | | | | | | | | COLA89 |
| **tea bag**, green, rasp, Celestial Seasonings - 1 tea bag | 2 | 0 | 0 | 0 | 0 | | | 0 | | | | | | | | | | |
| | | 0 | 0 | | | | | | | | | | | | | | | CELE1 |
| **tea, black**, brewed 3 minutes - 8 fl oz | 237 | 2 | 236.3 | 0.7 | 0 | | 0 | 7 | 0 | 7 | 0.05 | 0.519 | 0 | 0 | 0 | 0 | 0 | 0.03 |
| | | 0 | 0 | 0 | 0 | 0 | 0 | 88 | 2 | 0.05 | 0.024 | 0 | 0 | 0 | 0.03 | 0 | 11.9 | 14355 |
| **tea, black**, brewed, Constant Comment, Bigelow - 8 fl oz | 240 | 0 | 0 | | | | | 0 | | | | | | | | | | |
| | | 0 | 0 | | | | | | | | | | | | | | | BIGE1 |
| **tea, black**, brewed, vanilla caramel, Bigelow - 8 fl oz | 240 | 0 | | 0 | | | | 0 | | | | | | | | | | |
| | | 0 | 0 | | | | | | | | | | | | | | | BIGE2 |
| **tea, black**, decaffeinated, brewed 3 minutes - 8 fl oz | 237 | 2 | 236.3 | 0.7 | 0 | | 0 | 7 | 0 | 7 | 0.05 | 0.519 | 0 | 0 | 0 | 0 | 0 | 0.03 |
| | | 0 | 0 | 0 | 0 | 0 | 0 | 88 | 2 | 0.05 | 0.024 | 0 | 0 | 0 | 0.03 | 0 | 11.9 | 14352 |
| **tea, chamomile**, brewed - 8 fl oz | 237 | 2 | 236.3 | 0.5 | 0 | | 0 | 2 | 5 | 2 | 0.09 | 0.104 | 2 | 0 | 0.02 | 0 | 0 | 0.03 |
| | | 0 | 0 | 0 | 0 | 0 | 0 | 21 | 0 | 0.19 | 0.036 | 0 | 47 | 0 | 0.01 | 0 | 2.4 | 14545 |
| **tea, herbal** other than chamomile, brewed - 8 fl oz | 237 | 2 | 236.3 | 0.5 | 0 | | 0 | 2 | 5 | 2 | 0.09 | 0.104 | 0 | 0 | 0.02 | 0 | 0 | 0.03 |
| | | 0 | 0 | 0 | 0 | 0 | 0 | 21 | 0 | 0.19 | 0.036 | 0 | 0 | 0 | 0.01 | 0 | 2.4 | 14381 |

## 1.11 WATER

| | WT (g) | KCAL / PRO (g) | $H_2O$ (g) / FAT (g) | CHO (g) / SFA (g) | TSUG (g) / MUFA (g) | ASUG (g) / PUFA (g) | DFIB (g) / CHOL (mg) | Na (mg) / K (mg) | Ca (mg) / P (mg) | Mg (mg) / Fe (mg) | Zn (mg) / Cu (mg) | Mn (mg) / Se (mcg) | A (mcg RAE) / A (IU) | C (mg) / E (mg ATE) | B-1 (mg) / B-2 (mg) | NIA (mg) / B-6 (mg) | B-12 (mcg) / FOL (mcg DFE) | PANT (mg) / REF |
|---|---|---|---|---|---|---|---|---|---|---|---|---|---|---|---|---|---|---|
| **water**, bottled - 8 fl oz | 237 | 0 | 237.0 | 0 | 0 | | 0 | 5 | 24 | 5 | 0 | | 0 | 0 | 0 | 0 | 0 | 0 |
| | | 0 | 0 | 0 | 0 | 0 | 0 | 0 | 0 | 0 | 0.017 | 0 | 0 | 0 | 0 | 0 | 0 | 14555 |
| **water**, bottled, Aqua Vie - 8 fl oz | 237 | 40 | | 11.0 | 11.0 | | | 0 | | | | | | | | | | |
| | | 0 | 0 | | | | | | | | | | | | | | | AQUA1 |
| **water**, bottled, Aquafina - 8 fl oz | 237 | 0 | 236.9 | 0 | | | | 0 | 0 | 0 | 0 | 0 | | | | | | |
| | | 0 | 0 | | | | | 0 | 0 | 0 | 0 | | | | | | | 14433 |
| **water**, bottled, Calistoga - 8 fl oz | 237 | 0 | 237.0 | 0 | | | | 0 | 0 | 0 | | | | | | | | |
| | | 0 | 0 | | | | | 0 | | | | | | | | | | 14437 |
| **water**, bottled, Crystal Geyser - 8 fl oz | 237 | 0 | 237.0 | 0 | | | | 2 | 7 | 0 | | | | | | | | |
| | | 0 | 0 | | | | | 0 | | | | | | | | | | 14438 |
| **water**, bottled, Dannon - 8 fl oz | 237 | 0 | 237.0 | 0 | | | | 0 | 7 | 2 | 0 | 0 | | | | | | |
| | | 0 | 0 | | | | | 0 | 0 | 0 | 0 | | | | | | | 14432 |
| **water**, bottled, Dannon Fluoride To Go - 8 fl oz | 237 | 0 | 236.9 | 0.1 | | | | 2 | 7 | 2 | 0 | 0 | | | | | | |
| | | 0 | 0 | | | | | 0 | 0 | 0.02 | 0 | | | | | | | 14440 |
| **water**, bottled, Dasani - 8 fl oz | 237 | 0 | 236.9 | 0 | | | | 0 | 0 | 0 | 0 | 0 | | | | | | |
| | | 0 | 0 | | | | | 0 | 0 | 0 | 0 | | | | | | | 14434 |
| **water**, bottled, Evian - 8 fl oz | 237 | 0 | 236.9 | 0 | | | | 0 | 19 | 5 | 0 | 0 | | | | | | |
| | | 0 | 0 | | | | | 0 | 0 | 0 | 0 | | | | | | | 14559 |
| **water**, bottled, Naya - 8 fl oz | 237 | 0 | 237.0 | 0 | | | | 2 | 9 | 5 | | | | | | | | |
| | | 0 | 0 | | | | | 0 | | | | | | | | | | 14439 |
| **water**, bottled, Perrier - 8 fl oz | 237 | 0 | 236.8 | 0 | | | 0 | 2 | 33 | 0 | 0 | 0 | 0 | 0 | 0 | 0 | 0 | 0 |
| | | 0 | 0 | 0 | 0 | 0 | 0 | 0 | 0 | 0 | 0 | 0 | 0 | 0 | 0 | 0 | 0 | 14384 |
| **water**, bottled, Poland Spring - 8 fl oz | 237 | 0 | 237.0 | 0 | | | 0 | 2 | 2 | 2 | 0 | 0 | 0 | 0 | 0 | 0 | 0 | 0 |
| | | 0 | 0 | 0 | 0 | 0 | 0 | 0 | 0 | 0.02 | 0 | 0 | 0 | 0 | 0 | 0 | 0 | 14385 |

| | WT (g) | KCAL | H₂0 (g) | CHO (g) | TSUG (g) | ASUG (g) | DFIB (g) | Na (mg) | Ca (mg) | Mg (mg) | Zn (mg) | Mn (mg) | A (mcg RAE) | C (mg) | B-1 (mg) | NIA (mg) | B-12 (mcg) | PANT (mg) |
|---|---|---|---|---|---|---|---|---|---|---|---|---|---|---|---|---|---|---|
| | | PRO (g) | FAT (g) | SFA (g) | MUFA (g) | PUFA (g) | CHOL (mg) | K (mg) | P (mg) | Fe (mg) | Cu (mg) | Se (mcg) | A (IU) | E (mg ATE) | B-2 (mg) | B-6 (mg) | FOL (mcg DFE) | REF |
| **water**, grape/lemon/raspberry/ | 237 | 2 | | 0 | 0 | | | 4 | 0 | | | | | 0 | | | | |
| strawbry, btld, Dasani - *8 fl oz* | | 0 | 0 | | | | | 35 | 0 | | | | | | | | | COLA123 |
| **water**, municipal tap | 237 | 0 | 236.8 | 0 | 0 | | 0 | 7 | 7 | 2 | 0 | 0 | 0 | 0 | 0 | 0 | 0 | 0 |
| *8 fl oz* | | 0 | 0 | 0 | 0 | 0 | 0 | 2 | 0 | 0 | 0.021 | 0 | 0 | 0 | 0 | 0 | 0 | 14429 |
| **water**, well | 237 | 0 | 236.8 | 0 | | | 0 | 12 | 7 | 2 | 0.02 | 0 | | | | | | |
| *8 fl oz* | | 0 | 0 | | | | | 0 | 0 | 0 | 0.038 | | | | | | | 14412 |

## 1.12 WINE

| | WT (g) | KCAL | H₂0 (g) | CHO (g) | TSUG (g) | ASUG (g) | DFIB (g) | Na (mg) | Ca (mg) | Mg (mg) | Zn (mg) | Mn (mg) | A (mcg RAE) | C (mg) | B-1 (mg) | NIA (mg) | B-12 (mcg) | PANT (mg) |
|---|---|---|---|---|---|---|---|---|---|---|---|---|---|---|---|---|---|---|
| | | PRO (g) | FAT (g) | SFA (g) | MUFA (g) | PUFA (g) | CHOL (mg) | K (mg) | P (mg) | Fe (mg) | Cu (mg) | Se (mcg) | A (IU) | E (mg ATE) | B-2 (mg) | B-6 (mg) | FOL (mcg DFE) | REF |
| **sake** | 103 | 138 | 80.8 | 5.2 | 0 | 0 | 0 | 2 | 5 | 6 | 0.02 | | 0 | 0 | 0 | 0 | 0 | |
| *3.5 fl oz* | | 0.5 | 0 | 0 | 0 | 0 | 0 | 26 | 6 | 0.10 | 0.009 | 1.4 | 0 | 0 | 0 | 0 | 0 | 43479 |
| **wine, cooking** | 103 | 52 | 91.6 | 6.5 | 1.6 | 0 | 0 | 645 | 9 | 10 | 0.08 | | 0 | 0 | 0 | 0.1 | 0 | |
| *3.5 fl oz* | | 0.5 | 0 | 0 | 0 | 0 | 0 | 91 | 15 | 0.41 | 0.011 | 0.2 | 0 | 0 | 0.01 | 0.02 | 1.0 | 43154 |
| **wine, dessert, dry** | 103 | 157 | 74.7 | 12.0 | 1.1 | 0 | 0 | 9 | 8 | 9 | 0.07 | 0.123 | 0 | 0 | 0.02 | 0.2 | | 0.03 |
| *3.5 fl oz* | | 0.2 | 0 | 0 | 0 | 0 | 0 | 95 | 9 | 0.25 | 0.046 | 0.5 | 0 | 0 | 0.02 | 0 | | 14536 |
| **wine, dessert, sweet** | 103 | 165 | 72.6 | 14.1 | 8.0 | 0 | 0 | 9 | 8 | 9 | 0.07 | 0.123 | 0 | 0 | 0.02 | 0.2 | | 0.03 |
| *3.5 fl oz* | | 0.2 | 0 | 0 | 0 | 0 | 0 | 95 | 9 | 0.25 | 0.046 | 0.5 | 0 | 0 | 0.02 | 0 | | 14057 |
| **wine, no alcohol** | 102 | 6 | 100.2 | 1.1 | 1.1 | 0 | 0 | 7 | 9 | 10 | 0.08 | | 0 | 0 | 0 | 0.1 | 0 | |
| *3.5 fl oz* | | 0.5 | 0 | 0 | 0 | 0 | 0 | 90 | 15 | 0.41 | 0.011 | 0.2 | 0 | 0 | 0.01 | 0.02 | 1.0 | 14553 |
| **wine, red** | 103 | 88 | 89.1 | 2.7 | 0.6 | 0 | 0 | 4 | 8 | 12 | 0.14 | 0.136 | 0 | 0 | 0.01 | 0.2 | 0 | 0.03 |
| *3.5 fl oz* | | 0.1 | 0 | 0 | 0 | 0 | 0 | 131 | 24 | 0.47 | 0.011 | 0.2 | 2 | 0 | 0.03 | 0.06 | 1.0 | 14096 |
| **wine, red, Burgundy** | 103 | 89 | 88.2 | 3.8 | | | | | | | | | | | | | | |
| *3.5 fl oz* | | 0.1 | 0 | | | | | | | | | | | | | | | 14152 |
| **wine, red, Cabernet Sauvignon** | 103 | 85 | 89.2 | 2.7 | | | | | | | | | | | | | | |
| *3.5 fl oz* | | 0.1 | 0 | | | | | | | | | | | | | | | 14097 |
| **wine, red, claret** | 103 | 85 | 89.0 | 3.1 | | | | | | | | | | | | | | |
| *3.5 fl oz* | | 0.1 | 0 | | | | | | | | | | | | | | | 14105 |
| **wine, red, Merlot** | 103 | 85 | 89.2 | 2.6 | 0.6 | | 0 | 4 | 8 | 12 | 0.14 | 0.136 | | 0 | 0.01 | 0.2 | 0 | 0.03 |
| *3.5 fl oz* | | 0.1 | 0 | | | | | 131 | 24 | 0.47 | 0.011 | 0.2 | | | 0.03 | 0.06 | | 14602 |
| **wine, red, Zinfandel** | 103 | 91 | 88.3 | 2.9 | | | | | | | | | | | | | | |
| *3.5 fl oz* | | 0.1 | 0 | | | | | | | | | | | | | | | 14102 |
| **wine, table, all types** | 103 | 85 | 89.2 | 2.8 | 0.8 | 0 | 0 | 5 | 8 | 11 | 0.13 | 0.128 | 0 | 0 | 0.01 | 0.2 | 0 | 0.04 |
| *3.5 fl oz* | | 0.1 | 0 | 0 | 0 | 0 | 0 | 102 | 21 | 0.38 | 0.007 | 0.2 | 0 | 0 | 0.02 | 0.06 | 1.0 | 14084 |
| **wine, white** | 103 | 84 | 89.5 | 2.7 | 1.0 | 0 | 0 | 5 | 9 | 10 | 0.12 | 0.121 | 0 | 0 | 0.01 | 0.1 | 0 | 0.05 |
| *3.5 fl oz* | | 0.1 | 0 | 0 | 0 | 0 | 0 | 73 | 19 | 0.28 | 0.004 | 0.1 | 0 | 0 | 0.02 | 0.05 | 1.0 | 14106 |
| **wine, white, Pinot Blanc** | 103 | 83 | 89.8 | 2.0 | | | | | | | | | | | | | | |
| *3.5 fl oz* | | 0.1 | 0 | | | | | | | | | | | | | | | 14138 |
| **wine, white, Pinot Gris/Grigio** | 103 | 85 | 89.6 | 2.1 | | | | | | | | | | | | | | |
| *3.5 fl oz* | | 0.1 | 0 | | | | | | | | | | | | | | | 14113 |
| **wine, white, Riesling** | 103 | 82 | 89.2 | 3.9 | | | | | | | | | | | | | | |
| *3.5 fl oz* | | 0.1 | 0 | | | | | | | | | | | | | | | 14132 |
| **wine, white, Sauvignon Blanc** | 103 | 83 | 89.8 | 2.1 | | | | | | | | | | | | | | |
| *3.5 fl oz* | | 0.1 | 0 | | | | | | | | | | | | | | | 14134 |

## 2. CANDY

| | WT (g) | KCAL | H₂0 (g) | CHO (g) | TSUG (g) | ASUG (g) | DFIB (g) | Na (mg) | Ca (mg) | Mg (mg) | Zn (mg) | Mn (mg) | A (mcg RAE) | C (mg) | B-1 (mg) | NIA (mg) | B-12 (mcg) | PANT (mg) |
|---|---|---|---|---|---|---|---|---|---|---|---|---|---|---|---|---|---|---|
| | | PRO (g) | FAT (g) | SFA (g) | MUFA (g) | PUFA (g) | CHOL (mg) | K (mg) | P (mg) | Fe (mg) | Cu (mg) | Se (mcg) | A (IU) | E (mg ATE) | B-2 (mg) | B-6 (mg) | FOL (mcg DFE) | REF |
| **Abba-Zaba**, Annabelle Candy Co | 12 | 50 | | 11.0 | 5.0 | | 1.0 | 20 | | | | | | | | | | |
| *.43 oz bar* | | 1.0 | 1.0 | 1.0 | | | 0 | | | | | | | | | | | ANNA1 |
| **After Eight Mints**, Nestle | 41 | 166 | 2.6 | 31.2 | 27.3 | | 1.0 | 0 | 5 | | | | 0 | 0 | | | | |
| *5 mints* | | 0.7 | 4.9 | 3.4 | | | 0 | | | 0.23 | | | 0 | | | | | 19153 |
| **Almond Joy Bites**, Hershey | 40 | 218 | 0.5 | 23.0 | 20.7 | | 1.7 | 16 | 44 | 15 | 0.32 | 0 | | 0 | 0.02 | 0.1 | | 0.10 |
| *18 pieces* | | 2.2 | 13.8 | 8.2 | 3.5 | 0.6 | 4 | 122 | 52 | 0.53 | 0.072 | 0 | 47 | | 0.06 | 0.02 | | 19248 |
| **Almond Joy**, Hershey | 19 | 91 | 1.6 | 11.3 | 9.2 | | 1.0 | 27 | 12 | | | | | 0 | | | | |
| *.7 oz snack bar* | | 0.8 | 5.1 | 3.3 | 1.0 | 0.2 | 1 | 48 | 21 | 0.24 | | | 8 | | | | | 19065 |
| **Aplets and Cotlets**, Liberty | 56 | 200 | | 41.0 | 32.0 | | | 65 | 0 | | | | | 0 | | | | |
| Orchards - *4 pieces* | | 1.0 | 5.0 | | | | 0 | | 0 | 0 | | | 0 | | | | | LIBO13 |
| **Baby Ruth**, Nestle | 21 | 96 | 1.5 | 13.6 | 11.3 | | 0.4 | 48 | 10 | 9 | 0.15 | 0.074 | 0 | 0 | 0.01 | 0.3 | 0.01 | 0.07 |
| *.7 oz bar* | | 1.1 | 4.5 | 2.5 | 1.2 | 0.6 | 0 | 52 | 20 | 0.13 | 0.047 | 0.5 | 0 | 0.2 | 0.03 | 0.01 | 2.5 | 19111 |
| **Big Hunk**, Annabelle Candy Co | 12 | 50 | | 11.0 | 5.0 | | 0 | 35 | | | | | | | | | | |
| *.43 oz bar* | | 1.0 | 0.5 | 0 | | | 0 | | | | | | | | | | | ANNA2 |

| | WT (g) | KCAL | H₂O (g) | CHO (g) | TSUG (g) | ASUG (g) | DFIB (g) | Na (mg) | Ca (mg) | Mg (mg) | Zn (mg) | Mn (mg) | A (mcg RAE) | C (mg) | B-1 (mg) | NIA (mg) | B-12 (mcg) | PANT (mg) |
|---|---|---|---|---|---|---|---|---|---|---|---|---|---|---|---|---|---|---|
| | | PRO (g) | FAT (g) | SFA (g) | MUFA (g) | PUFA (g) | CHOL (mg) | K (mg) | P (mg) | Fe (mg) | Cu (mg) | Se (mcg) | A (IU) | E (mg ATE) | B-2 (mg) | B-6 (mg) | FOL (mcg DFE) | REF |
| **Bit-O'-Honey**, Nestle | 40 | 150 | 3.3 | 32.0 | 19.2 | | 0.1 | 118 | 14 | 3 | 0.20 | 0.015 | 0 | 0 | 0.02 | 0 | 0.02 | 0.03 |
| *6 pieces (1.4 oz)* | | 0.8 | 3.0 | 2.2 | 0.4 | 0.1 | 0 | 18 | 11 | 0.08 | 0.010 | 0.5 | 0 | 0.1 | 0.02 | 0 | 0.8 | 19068 |
| **bittersweet chocolate**, 70% cacao, | 40 | 230 | | 21.0 | 13.0 | | | 0 | 20 | | | | | 0 | | | | |
| Scharffen Berger - *1.4 oz* | | 4.0 | 14.0 | 9.0 | | | 0 | | | 1.44 | | | 0 | | | | | SCHA1 |
| **bittersweet chocolate** with almonds, | 38 | 200 | | 21.0 | 16.0 | | 3.0 | 0 | 40 | | | | | 0 | | | | |
| Trader Joe's - *3 squares* | | 4.0 | 14.0 | 6.0 | | | 0 | | | 1.44 | | | 0 | | | | | TRAD9 |
| **Butterfinger**, Nestle | 21 | 96 | 0.3 | 15.3 | 9.6 | | 0.4 | 48 | 8 | 10 | 0.21 | 0.103 | 0 | 0 | 0.03 | 0.6 | 0.01 | 0.08 |
| *.7 oz bar* | | 1.1 | 4.0 | 2.0 | 1.1 | 0.7 | 0 | 46 | 20 | 0.17 | 0.041 | 0.6 | 0 | 0.4 | 0.01 | 0.01 | 5.9 | 19069 |
| **butterscotch** | 28 | 109 | 1.5 | 25.3 | 22.5 | 22.5 | 0 | 109 | 1 | 0 | 0.03 | 0 | 8 | 0 | 0 | 0 | 0 | 0 |
| *1 oz (5 pieces)* | | 0 | 0.9 | 0.6 | 0.2 | 0 | 3 | 1 | 0 | 0 | 0 | 0.2 | 28 | 0 | 0 | 0 | 0 | 19070 |
| **butterscotch chips** | 42 | 226 | 0.3 | 28.2 | 28.2 | 26.7 | 0 | 37 | 14 | 2 | 0.05 | 0.001 | 0 | 0 | 0.01 | 0 | 0.04 | 0.06 |
| *¼ cup* | | 0.9 | 12.2 | 10.1 | 1.0 | 0.4 | 0 | 27 | 13 | 0.03 | 0.001 | 0.5 | 0 | 0.3 | 0.03 | 0.01 | 0.4 | 19085 |
| **caramel and chocolate-flavored roll** | 64 | 253 | 4.3 | 55.0 | 36.0 | 31.2 | 0.1 | 28 | 23 | 14 | 0.26 | 0.030 | 0 | 0 | 0.04 | 0.1 | 0 | 0.19 |
| *2.25 oz bar* | | 1.0 | 3.2 | 0.6 | 2.5 | 0.2 | 1 | 74 | 36 | 0.51 | 0.083 | 1.4 | 0 | 0.4 | 0.04 | 0.01 | 7.0 | 19076 |
| **caramel macadamia clusters**, | 40 | 110 | | 15.0 | 13.0 | | 0 | 10 | | | | | | | | | | |
| Mauna Loa - *2 pieces* | | 1.0 | 6.0 | 3.0 | | | 5 | | | | | | | | | | | MAUN6 |
| **Caramello**, Hershey | 45 | 208 | 3.1 | 28.7 | 25.6 | | 0.5 | 55 | 96 | | | | | 1 | | | | |
| *1.6 oz bar* | | 2.8 | 9.5 | 5.7 | 2.4 | 0.3 | 12 | 153 | 68 | 0.49 | | | 136 | | | | | 19075 |
| **caramels** | 71 | 271 | 6.0 | 54.7 | 46.5 | 36.0 | 0 | 174 | 98 | 12 | 0.31 | 0.008 | 9 | 0 | 0.07 | 0.1 | 0.21 | 0.44 |
| *2.5 oz (about 10 pieces)* | | 3.3 | 5.8 | 1.8 | 1.1 | 2.5 | 5 | 152 | 81 | 0.10 | 0.013 | 1.3 | 30 | 0.3 | 0.18 | 0.04 | 2.8 | 19074 |
| **caramels with nuts**, choc-covered | 28 | 132 | 1.7 | 17.0 | 11.6 | 10.6 | 1.2 | 7 | 22 | 23 | 0.52 | | 12 | 0 | 0.01 | 1.3 | 0 | |
| *1 oz* | | 2.7 | 5.9 | 1.3 | 2.6 | 1.6 | 0 | 125 | 46 | 0.48 | 0.162 | 0.8 | 42 | 0.3 | 0.04 | 0.04 | 25.8 | 43031 |
| **carob candy** | 87 | 470 | 1.3 | 49.0 | 29.7 | 0 | 3.3 | 93 | 264 | 31 | 3.07 | 0.122 | 1 | 0 | 0.09 | 0.9 | 0.24 | 0.65 |
| *3 oz bar* | | 7.1 | 27.3 | 25.2 | 0.4 | 0.3 | 1 | 551 | 110 | 1.12 | 0.159 | 4.5 | 9 | 1.4 | 0.15 | 0.11 | 18.3 | 19071 |
| **chewing gum** | 16 | 40 | 0.4 | 10.6 | 10.6 | 10.6 | 0.4 | 0 | 0 | 0 | 0 | 0 | 0 | 0 | 0 | 0 | 0 | 0 |
| *10 Chiclets* | | 0 | 0 | 0 | 0 | 0 | 0 | 0 | 0 | 0 | 0 | 0.1 | 0 | 0 | 0 | 0 | 0 | 19163 |
| **chewing gum**, sugarless | 3 | 8 | 0.1 | 2.8 | 0 | 0 | 0.1 | 0 | 1 | 0 | 0 | | 0 | 0 | 0 | 0 | 0 | |
| *1 piece* | | 0 | 0 | 0 | 0 | 0 | 0 | 0 | 0 | 0 | 0 | 0 | 0 | 0 | 0 | 0 | 0 | 43060 |
| **chocolate bar**, CocoaVia | 22 | 104 | 0.2 | 12.1 | 8.6 | | 1.9 | 2 | 256 | | | | | 9 | | | 0.90 | |
| *.78 oz bar* | | 1.3 | 6.4 | 3.5 | | | 0 | | | 0.76 | | | 7 | 2.7 | | 0.30 | | 19326 |
| **chocolate bar**, crispy, CocoaVia | 20 | 91 | 0.4 | 11.0 | 7.0 | | 1.6 | 8 | 214 | | | | | 8 | | | 0.60 | |
| *.7 oz bar* | | 1.6 | 5.2 | 2.8 | | | 0 | | | 0.69 | | | 5 | 2.0 | | 0.30 | | 19328 |
| **chocolate bar** w/blueberries and | 22 | 104 | 0.6 | 12.2 | 8.6 | | 2.0 | 2 | 217 | | | | | 8 | | | 0.60 | |
| almonds, CocoaVia - *.78 oz bar* | | 1.4 | 6.3 | 2.9 | | | 0 | | | 0.70 | | | 6 | 2.0 | | 0.30 | | 19327 |
| **chocolate candies**, assorted, See's | 34 | 160 | | 20.0 | 16.0 | | | 35 | 20 | | | | | 0 | | | | |
| Candies - *2 pieces* | | 2.0 | 9.0 | 4.5 | | | 10 | | | 0.36 | | | 100 | | | | | SEES4 |
| **chocolate candies**, chocolate, See's | 33 | 160 | | 18.0 | 15.0 | | | 45 | 40 | | | | | 0 | | | | |
| Candies - *2 pieces* | | 2.0 | 10.0 | 4.5 | | | 10 | | | 0.36 | | | 100 | | | | | SEES5 |
| **chocolate-covered almonds**, | 28 | 143 | 0.4 | 12.3 | 7.5 | | 2.9 | 3 | 235 | | | | | 8 | | | 0.60 | |
| CocoaVia - *1 oz pack* | | 2.7 | 10.4 | 3.3 | | | 0 | | | 1.00 | | | 6 | 1.3 | | 0.20 | | 19897 |
| **choc-covered almonds**, Hershey | 41 | 234 | | 19.2 | 15.2 | | 1.8 | 21 | 83 | | | | | 0 | | | | |
| *13 pieces (1.4 oz)* | | 4.9 | 15.2 | 6.2 | | | 5 | | | 1.02 | | | 0 | | | | | 19084 |
| **chocolate-covered caramel**, Riesen | 36 | 170 | | 28.0 | 15.0 | | 0 | 15 | 20 | | | | | 0 | | | | |
| *4 pieces* | | 1.0 | 6.0 | 3.5 | | | 0 | | | 1.26 | | | 0 | | | | | STOR1 |
| **chocolate-covered cherries**, bing, | 42 | 190 | | 28.0 | 24.0 | | 3.0 | 30 | 60 | | | | | 0 | | | | |
| Harry and David - *about 5 pcs* | | 2.0 | 9.0 | 7.0 | | | 5 | | | 0.72 | | | 300 | | | | | HADA2 |
| **chocolate-covered cherries**, Chukar | 42 | 177 | | 26.0 | 19.0 | | 2.0 | 17 | 30 | | | | | 0 | | | | |
| Cherry Co - *3 pieces (1.5 oz)* | | 2.0 | 9.0 | 6.0 | | | 3 | | | 2.34 | | | 100 | | | | | CHUK1 |
| **chocolate-covered macadamia nuts**, | 37 | 220 | | 18.0 | 17.0 | | 1.0 | 25 | 60 | | | | | 0 | | | | |
| Mauna Loa - *9 pieces* | | 3.0 | 15.0 | 6.0 | | | | | | 0.36 | | | 0 | | | | | MAUN1 |
| **Chocolate Decadence**, Harry and | 39 | 180 | | 15.0 | 11.0 | | 2.0 | 20 | | | | | | | | | | |
| David - *1.4 oz piece* | | 2.0 | 14.0 | 8.0 | | | 45 | | | 1.08 | | | 300 | | | | | HADA7 |
| **chocolate**, Mexican | 28 | 119 | 0.4 | 21.7 | 19.4 | 19.2 | 1.1 | 1 | 10 | 27 | 0.35 | 0.126 | 0 | 0 | 0.02 | 0.5 | 0 | 0.05 |
| *1 oz* | | 1.0 | 4.4 | 2.4 | 1.4 | 0.3 | 0 | 111 | 40 | 0.61 | 0.188 | 0.5 | 0 | 0.1 | 0.03 | 0.01 | 1.4 | 19124 |
| **Chocolate Orange**, Terry's | 44 | 240 | | 28.0 | 24.0 | | 3.0 | 5 | | | | | | 0 | | | | |
| *5 pieces* | | 1.0 | 13.0 | 8.0 | | | | | | 1.08 | | | 0 | | | | | KRAT1 |
| **Chunky**, Nestle | 40 | 190 | 1.2 | 24.0 | 21.0 | | 1.0 | 15 | 40 | | | | | 0 | | | | |
| *1.4 oz piece* | | 3.0 | 11.0 | 5.0 | | | 4 | | | 0.36 | | | 0 | | | | | 19119 |
| **Craisins**, milk choc-covered | 40 | 180 | | 28.0 | 25.0 | | 2.0 | 20 | 40 | | | | | 0 | | | | |
| *¼ cup (1.41 oz)* | | 2.0 | 8.0 | 4.0 | | | 5 | | 0 | | | | 0 | | | | | OCEA1 |
| **Crunch**, Nestle | 40 | 200 | 0.3 | 26.8 | 22.0 | | 0.8 | 60 | 40 | | | | | 0 | | | | |
| *4 fun size bars (1.4 oz)* | | 2.0 | 10.4 | 6.4 | | | 5 | 122 | | 0.28 | | | 43 | | | | | 19145 |

Each food has two data lines. The first value in each cell is the upper-line nutrient (WT, KCAL, H2O, CHO, TSUG, ASUG, DFIB, Na, Ca, Mg, Zn, Mn, A mcg RAE, C, B-1, NIA, B-12, PANT); the second value is the lower-line nutrient (PRO, FAT, SFA, MUFA, PUFA, CHOL, K, P, Fe, Cu, Se, A IU, E, B-2, B-6, FOL, REF).

| Food | WT (g) | KCAL / PRO (g) | H2O (g) / FAT (g) | CHO (g) / SFA (g) | TSUG (g) / MUFA (g) | ASUG (g) / PUFA (g) | DFIB (g) / CHOL (mg) | Na (mg) / K (mg) | Ca (mg) / P (mg) | Mg (mg) / Fe (mg) | Zn (mg) / Cu (mg) | Mn (mg) / Se (mcg) | A (mcg RAE) / A (IU) | C (mg) / E (mg ATE) | B-1 (mg) / B-2 (mg) | NIA (mg) / B-6 (mg) | B-12 (mcg) / FOL (mcg DFE) | PANT (mg) / REF |
|---|---|---|---|---|---|---|---|---|---|---|---|---|---|---|---|---|---|---|
| dark chocolate, 45–59% cacao | 28 | 152 | 0.3 | 17.3 | 13.4 |  | 2.0 | 7 | 16 | 41 | 0.56 | 0.397 | 1 |  | 0.01 | 0.2 | 0.06 | 0.08 |
| 1 oz |  | 1.4 | 8.6 | 5.2 | 2.7 | 0.3 | 2 | 157 | 58 | 2.25 | 0.288 | 0.8 | 14 |  | 0.01 | 0.01 |  | 19902 |
| dark chocolate, 60–69% cacao | 28 | 162 | 0.4 | 14.7 | 10.3 |  | 2.2 | 3 | 17 | 49 | 0.74 | 0.371 | 1 |  | 0.01 | 0.2 | 0.05 | 0.08 |
| 1 oz |  | 1.7 | 10.7 | 6.2 | 3.2 | 0.3 | 2 | 159 | 73 | 1.77 | 0.349 | 2.4 | 14 |  | 0.01 | 0.01 |  | 19903 |
| dark chocolate, 70–85% cacao | 28 | 168 | 0.4 | 12.8 | 6.7 |  | 3.1 | 6 | 20 | 64 | 0.93 | 0.545 | 1 |  | 0.01 | 0.3 | 0.08 | 0.12 |
| 1 oz |  | 2.2 | 12.0 | 6.9 | 3.6 | 0.4 | 1 | 200 | 86 | 3.33 | 0.494 | 1.9 | 11 |  | 0.02 | 0.01 |  | 19904 |
| dark chocolate, bittersweet, Trader Joe's - 3 squares (1.34 oz) | 38 | 200 |  | 24.0 | 20.0 |  | 2.0 | 0 | 20 |  |  |  |  | 0 |  |  |  |  |
|  |  | 2.0 | 12.0 | 7.0 |  |  | 0 |  |  | 1.44 |  |  | 0 |  |  |  |  | TRAD8 |
| dark chocolate candies, See's Candies - 2 pieces | 34 | 160 |  | 19.0 | 16.0 |  | 2.0 | 40 | 20 |  |  |  |  | 0 |  |  |  |  |
|  |  | 2.0 | 10.0 | 4.5 |  |  | 10 |  |  | 0.72 |  |  | 100 |  |  |  |  | SEES2 |
| dark chocolate chips, semi-sweet | 42 | 201 | 0.3 | 26.5 | 22.9 | 22.7 | 2.5 | 5 | 13 | 48 | 0.68 | 0.336 | 0 |  | 0.02 | 0.2 | 0 | 0.04 |
| ¼ cup |  | 1.8 | 12.6 | 7.5 | 4.2 | 0.4 | 0 | 153 | 55 | 1.31 | 0.294 | 1.8 | 0 | 0.1 | 0.04 | 0.01 | 5.5 | 19080 |
| dark chocolate-covered coffee beans - 28 pieces | 40 | 216 | 0.6 | 24.0 | 17.0 |  | 3.0 | 10 | 40 | 43 | 0.53 | 0.223 | 0 | 0 | 0.01 | 0.2 | 0 | 0.04 |
|  |  | 3.0 | 12.0 | 6.0 | 0 | 0 | 5 | 137 | 54 | 1.08 | 0.225 | 1.1 | 0 | 0.1 | 0.11 | 0.02 | 1.2 | 19268 |
| dark chocolate-covered espresso beans, Starbucks - 28 pieces | 41 | 190 |  | 23.0 | 18.0 |  | 3.0 | 10 | 40 |  |  |  |  | 0 |  |  |  |  |
|  |  | 3.0 | 12.0 | 7.0 |  |  | 5 |  |  | 0.72 |  |  | 0 |  |  |  |  | STAR25 |
| dark choc-covered, macadamias, Mauna Loa - 9 pieces (1.3 oz) | 37 | 200 |  | 18.0 | 14.0 |  | 3.0 | 0 |  |  |  |  |  |  |  |  |  |  |
|  |  | 2.0 | 16.0 | 7.0 |  |  | 0 |  |  |  |  |  |  |  |  |  |  | MAUN4 |
| dark chocolate, Dove | 37 | 192 | 0.6 | 22.0 | 17.1 |  | 2.8 | 1 | 14 |  |  |  |  | 0 |  |  |  |  |
| 1.3 oz bar |  | 1.9 | 12.0 | 7.1 |  |  | 3 |  |  | 1.18 |  |  | 50 |  |  |  |  | 19255 |
| chocolate-covered peanuts, | 40 | 208 | 0.8 | 19.9 | 15.0 | 12.4 | 1.9 | 16 | 42 | 38 | 1.04 | 0.378 | 16 | 0 | 0.05 | 1.7 | 0.21 | 0.30 |
| 10 pieces |  | 5.2 | 13.4 | 5.8 | 5.2 | 1.7 | 4 | 201 | 85 | 0.52 | 0.218 | 2.2 | 52 | 1.0 | 0.07 | 0.04 | 20.4 | 19126 |
| chocolate-covered, peanuts, Goobers - 1.38 oz package | 39 | 200 | 0.7 | 20.7 | 16.8 |  | 3.8 | 14 | 35 |  |  |  |  | 0 |  |  |  |  |
|  |  | 3.8 | 13.3 | 4.7 |  |  | 5 | 196 |  | 0.43 |  |  | 27 |  |  |  |  | 19105 |
| chocolate-covered raisins, | 45 | 176 | 5.0 | 30.8 | 28.0 | 17.8 | 1.4 | 16 | 39 | 20 | 0.56 | 0.161 | 13 | 0 | 0.04 | 0.2 | 0.17 | 0.12 |
| ¼ cup |  | 1.8 | 6.7 | 4.6 | 1.4 | 0.3 | 1 | 231 | 64 | 0.77 | 0.168 | 1.2 | 41 | 0.1 | 0.07 | 0.03 | 3.2 | 19127 |
| chocolate-covered, raisins, Raisinets - 1.58 oz package | 45 | 190 | 2.9 | 32.0 | 26.6 |  | 1.0 | 15 | 38 |  |  |  |  | 1 |  |  |  |  |
|  |  | 2.0 | 7.6 | 5.0 |  |  | 5 |  |  | 0.54 |  |  | 35 |  |  |  |  | 19149 |
| dark chocolate, Hershey Special Dark - 2.6 oz bar | 73 | 406 | 0.7 | 44.2 | 34.7 |  | 4.7 | 4 | 22 | 23 | 0.01 | 0 | 0 | 0 | 0 |  |  | 0 |
|  |  | 4.0 | 23.7 |  | 3.8 | 0.3 | 4 | 366 | 37 | 1.55 | 0.015 | 0.2 |  |  | 0.01 | 0 |  | 19164 |
| dark chocolate, organic Equal Exchange - 1.4 oz | 40 | 220 |  | 18.0 | 11.0 |  | 5.0 | 5 | 20 |  |  |  |  | 0 |  |  |  |  |
|  |  | 3.0 | 17.0 | 10.0 |  |  | 0 |  |  | 6.30 |  |  | 0 |  |  |  |  | EQEX1 |
| dark chocolate pecan clusters, Priester's Pecan Co - 2 oz | 57 | 330 |  | 24.0 | 18.0 |  | 4.0 | 20 | 40 |  |  |  |  |  |  |  |  |  |
|  |  | 4.0 | 27.0 | 9.0 |  |  | 5 |  |  | 1.80 |  |  |  |  |  |  |  | PRIE1 |
| dark chocolate pecan clusters, Sunnyland Farms - .88 oz piece | 25 | 130 |  | 13.0 | 100.0 |  |  | 15 | 20 |  |  |  |  | 0 |  |  |  |  |
|  |  | 2.0 | 9.0 | 3.0 |  |  | 0 |  |  | 0.72 |  |  | 0 |  |  |  |  | SUNN1 |
| dark chocolate, sweet | 41 | 207 | 0.2 | 24.4 | 21.1 | 20.9 | 2.3 | 7 | 10 | 46 | 0.62 | 0.203 | 0 | 0 | 0.01 | 0.3 | 0 | 0.03 |
| 1.45 oz bar |  | 1.6 | 14.0 | 8.2 | 4.6 | 0.4 | 0 | 119 | 60 | 1.13 | 0.235 | 1.1 | 0 | 0.1 | 0.10 | 0.02 | 1.2 | 19081 |
| dark chocolate, Swiss, Trader Joe's - 4 sections (1.48 oz) | 42 | 210 |  | 27.0 | 21.0 |  | 5.0 | 0 | 0 |  |  |  |  | 0 |  |  |  |  |
|  |  | 2.0 | 12.0 | 7.0 |  |  | 0 |  |  | 2.70 |  |  | 200 |  |  |  |  | TRAD7 |
| dark chocolate w/white mint filling, Ghirardelli - 3 squares (1.6 oz) | 45 | 210 |  | 29.0 | 2.5 |  | 2.0 | 0 | 20 |  |  |  |  | 0 |  |  |  |  |
|  |  | 1.0 | 12.0 | 6.0 |  |  | 0 |  |  | 1.80 |  |  | 0 |  |  |  |  | GHIR1 |
| dark chocolate with almonds, Perugina - ⅛ bar (1.16 oz) | 33 | 180 |  | 17.0 | 14.0 |  | 2.0 | 5 | 20 |  |  |  |  | 0 |  |  |  |  |
|  |  | 2.0 | 13.0 | 7.0 |  |  | 0 |  |  | 0.72 |  |  | 0 |  |  |  |  | PERU1 |
| dark chocolate with raspberries, Godiva - 1.48 oz bar | 42 | 220 |  | 28.0 | 22.0 |  | 0 | 10 | 20 |  |  |  |  | 2 |  |  |  |  |
|  |  | 2.0 | 11.0 | 4.0 |  |  | 3 |  |  | 1.80 |  |  | 0 |  |  |  |  | GODI1 |
| dark chocolate with truffle center, Private Selection - 6 pieces | 40 | 240 |  | 20.0 | 16.0 |  | 2.0 | 5 | 20 |  |  |  |  | 0 |  |  |  |  |
|  |  | 2.0 | 17.0 | 10.0 |  |  | 5 |  |  | 2.70 |  |  | 0 |  |  |  |  | PRIV1 |
| deluxe Easter mix, Wisconsin Cheeseman - ¼ cup | 43 | 160 |  | 37.0 | 29.0 |  | 0 | 40 | 0 |  |  |  |  | 0 |  |  |  |  |
|  |  |  | 2.0 | 1.5 |  |  | 0 |  | 0 |  |  |  | 0 |  |  |  |  | WISC1 |
| divinity, homemade | 11 | 40 | 1.0 | 9.8 | 8.7 |  | 0 | 4 | 1 | 0 | 0.01 | 0 | 0 | 0 | 0 | 0 | 0 | 0 |
| .4 oz piece |  | 0.1 | 0 | 0 | 0 | 0 | 0 | 3 | 0 | 0 | 0.001 | 0.3 | 0 | 0 | 0.01 | 0 | 0 | 19384 |
| Fifth Avenue, Hershey | 56 | 270 | 1.3 | 35.1 | 26.4 |  | 1.7 | 126 | 41 | 35 | 0.63 | 0.028 | 8 | 0 | 0.08 | 2.2 | 0.10 | 0.30 |
| 2 oz bar |  | 4.9 | 13.4 | 3.7 | 5.9 | 1.9 | 3 | 194 | 79 | 0.67 | 0.118 | 0.3 | 29 | 1.5 | 0.05 | 0.06 | 20.2 | 19098 |
| fondant, chocolate-covered | 43 | 157 | 3.3 | 34.6 | 33.0 | 33.0 | 0.9 | 11 | 7 | 27 | 0.19 | 0.172 | 0 | 0 | 0.01 | 0.2 | 0 | 0.01 |
| 1 large patty (1.5 oz) |  | 0.9 | 4.0 | 2.3 | 1.3 | 0.1 | 0 | 72 | 41 | 0.67 | 0.185 | 0.7 | 0 | 0.1 | 0.02 | 0 | 1.3 | 19083 |
| fondant, homemade | 16 | 60 | 1.1 | 14.9 | 14.2 | 14.2 | 0 | 2 | 0 | 0 | 0.01 | 0 | 0 | 0 | 0 | 0 | 0 | 0 |
| .56 oz piece |  | 0 | 0 | 0 | 0 | 0 | 0 | 1 | 0 | 0 | 0 | 0.1 | 0 | 0 | 0 | 0 | 0 | 19099 |
| fruit and nut squares, soft | 56 | 218 | 7.8 | 41.3 | 25.7 | 24.0 | 1.3 | 73 | 10 | 14 | 0.30 | 0.302 | 0 | 0 | 0.03 | 0.1 | 0 | 0.06 |
| 4 pieces |  | 1.3 | 5.3 | 0.5 | 0.7 | 3.8 | 0 | 46 | 30 | 0.52 | 0.170 | 0.8 | 2 | 0.1 | 0.02 | 0.05 | 6.2 | 19866 |
| Fruit Delights, Liberty Orchards | 56 | 200 |  | 41.0 | 32.0 |  | 0 | 65 | 0 |  |  |  |  | 0 |  |  |  |  |
| 4 pieces |  | 1.0 | 5.0 |  |  |  | 0 |  | 0 |  |  |  | 0 |  |  |  |  | LIBO14 |

| | WT (g) | KCAL / PRO (g) | H₂O (g) / FAT (g) | CHO (g) / SFA (g) | TSUG (g) / MUFA (g) | ASUG (g) / PUFA (g) | DFIB (g) / CHOL (mg) | Na (mg) / K (mg) | Ca (mg) / P (mg) | Mg (mg) / Fe (mg) | Zn (mg) / Cu (mg) | Mn (mg) / Se (mcg) | A (mcg RAE) / A (IU) | C (mg) / E (mg ATE) | B-1 (mg) / B-2 (mg) | NIA (mg) / B-6 (mg) | B-12 (mcg) / FOL (mcg DFE) | PANT (mg) / REF |
|---|---|---|---|---|---|---|---|---|---|---|---|---|---|---|---|---|---|---|
| **fruit snacks**, mixed berry, Nabisco | 30 | 90 | | 22.0 | 17.0 | | | 15 | | | | | | 60 | | | | |
| *12 pieces (1.06 oz)* | | 1.0 | 0 | | | | | | | | | | | | | | | NBSC22 |
| **fudge**, chocolate, homemade | 17 | 70 | 1.7 | 13.0 | 12.4 | 12.1 | 0.3 | 8 | 8 | 6 | 0.19 | 0.072 | 7 | 0 | 0 | 0 | 0.02 | 0.02 |
| *.6 oz piece* | | 0.4 | 1.8 | 1.1 | 0.5 | 0.1 | 2 | 23 | 12 | 0.30 | 0.056 | 0.4 | 27 | 0 | 0.01 | 0 | 0.7 | 19100 |
| **fudge**, chocolate marshmallow, homemade - .7 oz piece | 20 | 91 | 1.6 | 14.3 | 12.8 | | 0.3 | 17 | 9 | 7 | 0.12 | 0.046 | 15 | 0 | 0 | 0 | 0.01 | 0.02 |
| | | 0.5 | 3.5 | 2.1 | 1.0 | 0.1 | 5 | 29 | 13 | 0.19 | 0.043 | 0.4 | 55 | 0.1 | 0.02 | 0 | 1.0 | 19379 |
| **fudge**, chocolate marshmallow with nuts, homemade - .78 oz piece | 22 | 104 | 1.6 | 14.8 | | | 0.5 | 17 | 11 | 10 | 0.17 | 0.103 | 15 | 0 | 0.01 | 0.1 | 0.01 | 0.03 |
| | | 0.7 | 4.6 | 2.3 | 1.2 | 0.9 | 5 | 37 | 19 | 0.24 | 0.070 | 0.5 | 50 | | 0.02 | 0.01 | 2.4 | 19301 |
| **fudge**, chocolate with nuts, homemade - .67 oz piece | 19 | 88 | 1.5 | 12.9 | 12.0 | 11.7 | 0.5 | 7 | 11 | 10 | 0.27 | 0.168 | 7 | 0 | 0.01 | 0.1 | 0.01 | 0.04 |
| | | 0.8 | 3.6 | 1.2 | 0.7 | 1.4 | 2 | 35 | 22 | 0.37 | 0.100 | 0.6 | 27 | 0 | 0.02 | 0.02 | 3.0 | 19101 |
| **fudge**, peanut butter, homemade | 16 | 62 | 1.7 | 12.4 | 11.7 | | 0.1 | 19 | 7 | 3 | 0.08 | 0.026 | 1 | 0 | 0 | 0.2 | 0.02 | 0.04 |
| *.6 oz piece* | | 0.6 | 1.1 | 0.3 | 0.5 | 0.3 | 0 | 19 | 11 | 0.04 | 0.009 | 0.4 | 5 | 0.2 | 0.01 | 0.01 | 1.4 | 19102 |
| **fudge**, vanilla, homemade | 16 | 61 | 1.7 | 13.1 | 12.8 | 12.5 | 0 | 8 | 6 | 0 | 0.02 | 0 | 7 | 0 | 0 | 0 | 0.01 | 0.02 |
| *.56 oz piece* | | 0.2 | 0.9 | 0.5 | 0.2 | 0 | 2 | 8 | 5 | 0 | 0.001 | 0.3 | 27 | 0 | 0.01 | 0 | 0.2 | 19103 |
| **fudge**, vanilla with nuts, homemade | 15 | 65 | 1.2 | 11.2 | 10.6 | 10.4 | 0.1 | 6 | 7 | 4 | 0.08 | 0.070 | 6 | 0 | 0 | 0 | 0.01 | 0.03 |
| *.53 oz piece* | | 0.4 | 2.1 | 0.6 | 0.4 | 1.0 | 2 | 15 | 11 | 0.06 | 0.033 | 0.3 | 23 | 0 | 0.01 | 0.01 | 1.8 | 19104 |
| **gumdrops** | 36 | 143 | 0.4 | 35.6 | 21.2 | 21.2 | 0 | 16 | 1 | 0 | 0 | 0.004 | 0 | 0 | 0 | 0 | 0 | 0 |
| *10 gumdrops* | | 0 | 0 | 0 | 0 | 0 | 0 | 2 | 0 | 0.14 | 0.004 | 0.3 | 0 | 0 | 0 | 0 | 0 | 19106 |
| **gumdrops**, low-calorie with sorbitol | 36 | 58 | 4.2 | 31.7 | 25.2 | 0 | 6.5 | 3 | 0 | 0 | 0 | 0 | 0 | 0 | 0 | 0 | 0 | 0 |
| *10 gumdrops* | | 0 | 0.1 | 0 | 0 | 0 | 0 | 0 | 0 | 0 | 0 | 0.2 | 0 | 0 | 0 | 0 | 0 | 43057 |
| **gummy bears** | 36 | 143 | 0.4 | 35.6 | 21.2 | 21.2 | 0 | 16 | 1 | 0 | 0 | 0.004 | 0 | 0 | 0 | 0 | 0 | 0 |
| *10 gummy bears* | | 0 | 0 | 0 | 0 | 0 | 0 | 2 | 0 | 0.14 | 0.004 | 0.3 | 0 | 0 | 0 | 0 | 0 | 19106 |
| **gummy bears**, Black Forest | 40 | 140 | | 31.0 | 20.0 | | 0 | 30 | | | | | | 0 | | | | |
| *20 gummy bears* | | 3.0 | 0 | 0 | | | 0 | | 0 | | | | 0 | | | | | FERR1 |
| **halvah** | 49 | 230 | 1.8 | 29.6 | | | 2.2 | 96 | 16 | 107 | 2.12 | 0.428 | 0 | 0 | 0.21 | 1.4 | 0.02 | 0.09 |
| *1.75 oz bar* | | 6.1 | 10.5 | 2.0 | 4.0 | 4.2 | 0 | 92 | 297 | 2.22 | 0.589 | 5.6 | 1 | | 0.04 | 0.17 | 31.8 | 19117 |
| **hard candy** | 28 | 110 | 0.4 | 27.4 | 17.6 | 17.6 | 0 | 11 | 1 | 1 | 0 | 0.003 | 0 | 0 | 0 | 0 | 0 | 0 |
| *1 oz (5 pieces)* | | 0 | 0.1 | 0 | 0 | 0 | 0 | 1 | 1 | 0.08 | 0.008 | 0.2 | 0 | 0 | 0 | 0 | 0 | 19107 |
| **hard candy**, low-calorie w/sorbitol | 28 | 105 | 0.4 | 26.2 | 26.0 | 0 | 0 | 0 | 0 | 0 | 0 | 0 | 0 | 0 | 0 | 0 | 0 | |
| *1 oz (5 pieces)* | | 0 | 0 | 0 | 0 | 0 | 0 | 0 | 0 | 0 | 0 | 0.2 | 0 | 0 | 0 | 0 | 0 | 43058 |
| **Heath Bites** | 39 | 207 | 0.3 | 24.7 | 23.4 | | 0.8 | 96 | 34 | 2 | 0.04 | 0 | | 0 | 0.01 | 0 | | 0 |
| *15 pieces* | | 1.5 | 11.8 | 6.1 | 3.4 | 1.0 | 7 | 82 | 28 | 0.30 | 0.012 | 0 | 90 | | 0.04 | 0 | | 19243 |
| **Hundred Grand**, Nestle | 43 | 201 | 2.6 | 30.5 | 22.3 | | 0.4 | 87 | 33 | 11 | 0.43 | 0.074 | 16 | 0 | 0.02 | 0.1 | 0.12 | 0.08 |
| *1.5 oz bar* | | 1.1 | 8.3 | 5.1 | 2.6 | 0.6 | 5 | 70 | 37 | 0.15 | 0.080 | 1.1 | 55 | 0.2 | 0.05 | 0.01 | 2.2 | 19144 |
| **jelly beans** | 28 | 105 | 1.8 | 26.2 | 19.6 | 19.6 | 0.1 | 14 | 1 | 1 | 0.01 | 0.010 | 0 | 0 | 0 | 0 | 0 | 0 |
| *1 oz (10 large or 25 small)* | | 0 | 0 | 0 | 0 | 0 | 0 | 10 | 1 | 0.04 | 0.008 | 0.3 | 0 | 0 | 0 | 0 | 0 | 19108 |
| **jelly beans**, Lifesaver | 40 | 150 | | 37.0 | 32.0 | | | 10 | | | | | | | | | | |
| *32 pieces (1.41 oz)* | | 0 | 0 | | | | | | | | | | | | | | | WRIG1 |
| **jelly beans**, various flavors, Jelly Belly - 35 pieces (1.41 oz) | 40 | 140 | | 37.0 | 28.0 | | 0 | 15 | | | | | | 0 | | | | |
| | | 0 | 0 | 0 | | | 0 | | | 0 | | | 0 | | | | | JELL1 |
| **jelly beans**, Wisconsin Cheeseman | 40 | 150 | | 37.0 | 23.0 | | 0 | 15 | | | | | | 0 | | | | |
| *17 pieces (1.41 oz)* | | 0 | 0 | 0 | | | 0 | | | 0 | | | 0 | | | | | WISC2 |
| **Kit Kat** Big Kat, Hershey | 79 | 411 | 0.9 | 50.3 | 42.6 | | 1.5 | 51 | 109 | 2 | 0.06 | 0 | | 1 | 0.04 | 0.1 | | 0.03 |
| *2.8 oz bar* | | 4.9 | 22.0 | 14.2 | 3.9 | 0.4 | 7 | 232 | 88 | 0.66 | 0.008 | 0 | 73 | | 0.13 | 0 | | 19250 |
| **Kit Kat** Bites, Hershey | 39 | 199 | 0.4 | 25.2 | 19.3 | | 0.9 | 26 | 51 | 0 | 0 | 0 | | 0 | 0.01 | 0 | | 0 |
| *15 pieces* | | 2.5 | 10.3 | 6.7 | 1.8 | 0.2 | 3 | 116 | 37 | 0.34 | 0 | 0 | 33 | | 0.06 | 0 | | 19237 |
| **Kit Kat**, Hershey | 78 | 404 | 1.3 | 50.4 | 38.0 | | 0.8 | 42 | 98 | 29 | 0.07 | 0.078 | 19 | 0 | 0.09 | 0.4 | 0.44 | 0.50 |
| *2.8 oz bar* | | 5.1 | 20.3 | 14.0 | 4.6 | 0.7 | 9 | 180 | 105 | 0.78 | 0.172 | 3.9 | 63 | 0.3 | 0.16 | 0.02 | 14.0 | 19109 |
| **kona coffee crunch chocolate bar**, Mauna Loa - 1.8 oz bar | 50 | 250 | | 29.0 | 23.0 | | 2.0 | 15 | | | | | | | | | | |
| | | 2.0 | 17.0 | 9.0 | | | | | | | | | | | | | | MAUN15 |
| **Krackel**, Hershey | 56 | 287 | 0.7 | 35.8 | 29.4 | | 1.2 | 110 | 88 | 7 | 0.27 | 0 | | 0 | 0.03 | 0.1 | | 0.24 |
| *2 oz bar* | | 3.7 | 14.9 | 8.9 | 3.5 | 0.3 | 6 | 182 | 69 | 0.59 | 0.011 | 2.0 | 57 | | 0.11 | 0.02 | | 19110 |
| **Look**, Annabelle Candy Co | 12 | 50 | | 9.0 | 5.0 | | 0 | 25 | | | | | | | | | | |
| *.43 oz bar* | | 1.0 | 1.0 | 1.0 | | | 0 | | | | | | | | | | | ANNA3 |
| **M&M's**, almond | 37 | 188 | 0.9 | 22.2 | 18.2 | | 2.1 | 17 | 57 | 43 | 0.69 | 0.381 | 9 | 0 | 0.04 | 0.4 | 0.08 | 0.11 |
| *1.31 oz bag* | | 2.8 | 10.3 | 3.5 | 4.2 | 1.4 | 3 | 141 | 75 | 0.64 | 0.204 | 1.0 | 33 | 3.5 | 0.12 | 0.02 | 4.4 | 42227 |
| **M&M's**, crispy | 47 | 223 | 0.8 | 34.0 | 27.7 | | 0.9 | 64 | 42 | | | | | 0 | | | | |
| *1.6 oz bag* | | 2.0 | 9.1 | 5.5 | | | 6 | | | | 0.40 | | 78 | | | | | 19292 |
| **M&M's**, peanut butter | 46 | 243 | 0.9 | 26.2 | 21.7 | | 1.8 | 98 | 40 | 37 | 0.69 | 0.443 | 13 | 0 | 0.07 | 2.0 | 0.09 | 0.28 |
| *1.63 oz bag* | | 4.7 | 13.5 | 8.5 | 2.0 | 0.2 | 3 | 152 | 88 | 0.49 | 0.208 | 1.3 | 46 | 0.6 | 0.03 | 0.04 | 20.7 | 42148 |
| **M&M's**, peanut | 49 | 252 | 1.2 | 29.6 | 24.9 | | 1.8 | 24 | 50 | 34 | 0.86 | 0.325 | 11 | 0 | 0.03 | 1.6 | 0.16 | 0.31 |
| *1.74 oz package (25 pieces)* | | 4.7 | 12.8 | 5.0 | 4.0 | 1.7 | 4 | 170 | 93 | 0.57 | 0.247 | 2.0 | 39 | 1.4 | 0.05 | 0.04 | 27.0 | 19140 |

| Food | WT (g) | KCAL / PRO (g) | $H_2O$ / FAT (g) | CHO / SFA (g) | TSUG / MUFA (g) | ASUG / PUFA (g) | DFIB (g) / CHOL (mg) | Na / K (mg) | Ca / P (mg) | Mg / Fe (mg) | Zn / Cu (mg) | Mn / Se (mg / mcg) | A (mcg RAE) / A (IU) | C (mg) / E (mg ATE) | B-1 / B-2 (mg) | NIA / B-6 (mg) | B-12 (mcg) / FOL (mcg DFE) | PANT (mg) / REF |
|---|---|---|---|---|---|---|---|---|---|---|---|---|---|---|---|---|---|---|
| **M&M's, plain** | 48 | 236 | 0.8 | 34.2 | 30.6 | | 1.3 | 29 | 50 | 21 | 0.77 | 0.158 | 27 | 0 | 0.04 | 0.1 | 0.25 | 0.16 |
| *1.69 oz package (69 pieces)* | | 2.1 | 10.1 | 6.3 | 2.5 | 0.4 | 7 | 125 | 70 | 0.53 | 0.165 | 1.6 | 97 | 0.2 | 0.10 | 0.01 | 3.8 | 19141 |
| **M&M's, plain mini** | 42 | 211 | 0.5 | 28.7 | 26.3 | | 1.1 | 29 | 49 | | | | | 0 | | | | |
| *1.5 oz* | | 2.0 | 9.8 | 6.1 | | | 6 | | | 0.52 | | | 94 | | | | | 19157 |
| **M&M's, plain mini baking bits** | 14 | 70 | 0.2 | 9.6 | 8.8 | | 0.4 | 10 | 16 | | | | | 0 | | | | |
| *.5 oz* | | 0.7 | 3.3 | 2.0 | | | 2 | | | 0.17 | | | 31 | | | | | 19146 |
| **M&M's, plain semi-sweet chocolate mini baking bits - 1 T** | 14 | 72 | 0.2 | 9.2 | 7.4 | | 0.9 | 0 | 5 | | | | | 0 | | | | |
| | | 0.6 | 3.7 | 2.2 | | | 0 | | | 0.41 | | | 10 | | | | | 19139 |
| **macadamia brittle, Mauna Loa** | 28 | 130 | | 18.0 | 15.0 | | 1.0 | 200 | | | | | | | | | | |
| *1 oz* | | 1.0 | 7.0 | 2.0 | | | 5 | | | | | | | | | | | MAUN7 |
| **Mallo Cup, Boyer Candy Co** | 45 | 200 | | 28.0 | 25.0 | | | 40 | 40 | | | | | 0 | | | | |
| *2 pieces (1.6 oz)* | | 2.0 | 10.0 | 7.0 | | | 10 | | | 0.36 | | | 0 | | | | | BOYE1 |
| **Mars Almond** | 50 | 234 | 2.2 | 31.4 | 26.0 | | 1.0 | 85 | 84 | 36 | 0.56 | 0.184 | 8 | 0 | 0.02 | 0.5 | 0.18 | 0.20 |
| *1.76 oz bar* | | 4.0 | 11.5 | 3.6 | 5.3 | 2.0 | 8 | 162 | 117 | 0.55 | 0.125 | 0.8 | 28 | 3.9 | 0.16 | 0.03 | 4.5 | 19115 |
| **marshmallow, miniature** | 7 | 22 | 1.1 | 5.7 | 4.0 | 4.0 | 0 | 6 | 0 | 0 | 0 | 0.001 | 0 | 0 | 0 | 0 | 0 | 0 |
| *10 pieces* | | 0.1 | 0 | 0 | 0 | 0 | 0 | 0 | 1 | 0.02 | 0.007 | 0.1 | 0 | 0 | 0 | 0 | 0.1 | 19116 |
| **marshmallow, miniature, Safeway** | 30 | 100 | | 24.0 | 18.0 | | 0 | 30 | | | | | | 0 | | | | |
| *⅔ cup* | | 0 | 0 | | | | 0 | | | 0 | | | 0 | | | | | SAFE51 |
| **marshmallow, regular** | 7 | 22 | 1.1 | 5.7 | 4.0 | 4.0 | 0 | 6 | 0 | 0 | 0 | 0.001 | 0 | 0 | 0 | 0 | 0 | 0 |
| *1 piece* | | 0.1 | 0 | 0 | 0 | 0 | 0 | 0 | 1 | 0.02 | 0.007 | 0.1 | 0 | 0 | 0 | 0 | 0.1 | 19116 |
| **milk chocolate** | 42 | 225 | 0.6 | 24.9 | 21.6 | 18.5 | 1.4 | 33 | 79 | 26 | 0.97 | 0.198 | 25 | 0 | 0.05 | 0.2 | 0.32 | 0.20 |
| *¼ cup* | | 3.2 | 12.5 | 7.8 | 3.0 | 0.6 | 10 | 156 | 87 | 0.99 | 0.206 | 1.9 | 82 | 0.2 | 0.13 | 0.02 | 4.6 | 19120 |
| **milk chocolate block w/decoration, Mauna Loa - ⅛ pkg (1.34 oz)** | 38 | 210 | | 22.0 | 20.0 | | | 35 | 80 | | | | | 0 | | | | |
| | | 3.0 | 12.0 | 7.0 | | | 10 | | | 0.36 | | | 0 | | | | | MAUN2 |
| **milk chocolate candies, See's** | 34 | 160 | | 20.0 | 17.0 | | | 40 | 40 | | | | | 0 | | | | |
| *2 pieces* | | 2.0 | 9.0 | 4.5 | | | 10 | | | 0.36 | | | 100 | | | | | SEES1 |
| **milk chocolate chips** | 42 | 225 | 0.6 | 24.9 | 21.6 | 18.5 | 1.4 | 33 | 79 | 26 | 0.97 | 0.198 | 25 | 0 | 0.05 | 0.2 | 0.32 | 0.20 |
| *¼ cup* | | 3.2 | 12.5 | 7.8 | 3.0 | 0.6 | 10 | 156 | 87 | 0.99 | 0.206 | 1.9 | 82 | 0.2 | 0.13 | 0.02 | 4.6 | 19120 |
| **milk chocolate-covered coffee beans** | 40 | 220 | 1.0 | 22.1 | 20.3 | 17.7 | 2.3 | 28 | 68 | 26 | 0.81 | 0.214 | 20 | 0 | 0.04 | 0.1 | 0.26 | 0.18 |
| *28 pieces* | | 3.0 | 13.3 | 7.3 | 5.5 | 0.5 | 8 | 165 | 75 | 0.92 | 0.197 | 1.7 | 64 | 0.2 | 0.13 | 0.01 | 4.0 | 19279 |
| **milk choc-covered, macadamias, Mauna Loa - ¼ cup (1 oz)** | 28 | 150 | | 15.0 | 13.0 | | 1.0 | 10 | | | | | | | | | | |
| | | 2.0 | 10.0 | 4.5 | | | 5 | | | | | | | | | | | MAUN3 |
| **milk chocolate, Dove** | 37 | 202 | 0.6 | 22.1 | 20.5 | | 0.9 | 23 | 59 | | | | | 0 | | | | |
| *1.3 oz bar* | | 2.2 | 11.7 | 7.1 | | | 7 | | | 0.41 | | | 108 | | | | | 19254 |
| **milk chocolate Kisses, caramel-filled, Hershey - 8 pieces** | 38 | 180 | | 24.0 | 21.0 | | 0 | 60 | 60 | | | | | 0 | | | | |
| | | 2.0 | 8.0 | 5.0 | | | 10 | | | 0 | | | 0 | | | | | HRSH97 |
| **milk chocolate with almond bites, Hershey - 17 pieces** | 39 | 214 | 0.5 | 19.9 | 17.4 | | 1.4 | 29 | 86 | 23 | 0.52 | 0.004 | | 1 | 0.03 | 0.2 | | 0.18 |
| | | 3.8 | 13.9 | 6.8 | 5.6 | 0.9 | 7 | 184 | 89 | 0.58 | 0.078 | 1.3 | 69 | | 0.15 | 0.03 | | 19236 |
| **milk chocolate with almonds** | 44 | 231 | 0.7 | 23.5 | 19.3 | 16.3 | 2.7 | 33 | 99 | 40 | 0.59 | 0.275 | 23 | 0 | 0.03 | 0.3 | 0.29 | 0.20 |
| *1.55 oz bar* | | 4.0 | 15.1 | 7.8 | 5.3 | 1.3 | 8 | 195 | 116 | 0.72 | 0.186 | 1.8 | 77 | 1.4 | 0.19 | 0.02 | 5.7 | 19132 |
| **milk chocolate with almonds, Hershey - 2.8 oz package** | 78 | 450 | | 36.0 | 30.0 | | 3.0 | 50 | 150 | | | | | 0 | | | | |
| | | 10.0 | 30.0 | 13.0 | | | 10 | | | 1.44 | | | | | | | | 19130 |
| **milk chocolate with crisped rice** | 44 | 225 | 0.7 | 26.3 | 22.5 | 20.7 | 1.5 | 38 | 82 | 27 | 1.01 | 0.210 | 29 | 0 | 0.06 | 0.3 | 0.35 | 0.21 |
| *1.55 oz bar* | | 3.4 | 12.9 | 7.0 | 3.8 | 0.3 | 10 | 163 | 91 | 1.17 | 0.215 | 2.0 | 95 | 0.2 | 0.14 | 0.02 | 9.2 | 19134 |
| **milk chocolate with macadamia nuts, Mauna Loa - 1.8 oz bar** | 50 | 280 | | 25.0 | 25.0 | | 1.0 | 40 | | | | | | | | | | |
| | | 4.0 | 19.0 | 10.0 | | | 10 | | | | | | | | | | | MAUN14 |
| **milk/dark chocolate candies, nuts/chews, See's Candies - 3 pieces** | 47 | 240 | | 25.0 | 18.0 | | 2.0 | 50 | 60 | | | | | 0 | | | | |
| | | 4.0 | 16.0 | 6.0 | | | 10 | | | 0.72 | | | 100 | | | | | SEES3 |
| **milk/dark chocolate candies, soft centers, See's Candies - 2 pcs** | 39 | 170 | | 25.0 | 22.0 | | | 40 | 20 | | | | | 1 | | | | |
| | | 1.0 | 9.0 | 5.0 | | | 10 | | | 0.36 | | | 100 | | | | | SEES6 |
| **Milky Way** | 18 | 83 | 1.3 | 12.3 | 10.6 | | 0.1 | 49 | 25 | | | | | 0 | | | | |
| *.6 oz bar* | | 0.8 | 3.5 | 2.4 | | | 4 | | | 0.06 | | | 47 | | | | | 19256 |
| **Milky Way, dark chocolate** | 50 | 222 | 3.6 | 35.6 | 28.9 | | 1.4 | 84 | 26 | 29 | 0.44 | 0.196 | 21 | 0 | 0.02 | 0.1 | 0.02 | 0.04 |
| *1.76 oz bar* | | 1.6 | 8.8 | 5.7 | 2.3 | 0.3 | 5 | 98 | 38 | 0.60 | 0.172 | 1.2 | 78 | 0.2 | 0.03 | 0.01 | 3.5 | 42196 |
| **Milky Way, dark chocolate** | 44 | 202 | 3.1 | 29.7 | 23.8 | | 1.2 | 108 | 37 | | | | | 0 | | | | |
| *5 pieces* | | 1.7 | 9.0 | 6.1 | | | 7 | | | 0.53 | | | 108 | | | | | 19258 |
| **Milky Way Pop'ables** | 39 | 177 | 2.3 | 27.8 | 23.8 | | 0.4 | 57 | 35 | | | | | 0 | | | | |
| *13 pieces* | | 1.3 | 7.0 | 3.5 | | | 4 | | | 0.20 | | | 53 | | | | | 19307 |
| **Mini-Mints, Harry and David** | 42 | 250 | | 21.0 | 19.0 | | 1.0 | 25 | 40 | | | | | 0 | | | | |
| *4 pieces (1.48 oz)* | | 2.0 | 18.0 | 12.0 | | | 5 | | | 0.72 | | | 100 | | | | | HADA6 |
| **Moose Munch bar, Harry and David - 2 oz bar** | 56 | 300 | | 28.0 | 23.0 | | 2.0 | 45 | 80 | | | | | | | | | |
| | | 4.0 | 22.0 | 12.0 | | | 5 | | | 0.72 | | | | | | | | HADA9 |
| **Mounds, Hershey** | 53 | 258 | 4.8 | 31.1 | 24.5 | | 2.0 | 77 | 11 | 29 | 0.58 | 0.502 | 0 | 0 | 0.03 | 0.1 | 0 | 0.13 |
| *1.9 oz bar* | | 2.4 | 14.1 | 10.9 | 0.2 | 0.1 | 1 | 170 | 48 | 1.11 | 0.212 | 3.5 | 0 | 0.1 | 0.03 | 0.05 | 3.2 | 19142 |

| | WT (g) | KCAL / PRO (g) | H₂0 (g) / FAT (g) | CHO (g) / SFA (g) | TSUG (g) / MUFA (g) | ASUG (g) / PUFA (g) | DFIB (g) / CHOL (mg) | Na (mg) / K (mg) | Ca (mg) / P (mg) | Mg (mg) / Fe (mg) | Zn (mg) / Cu (mg) | Mn (mg) / Se (mcg) | A (mcg RAE) / A (IU) | C (mg) / E (mg ATE) | B-1 (mg) / B-2 (mg) | NIA (mg) / B-6 (mg) | B-12 (mcg) / FOL (mcg DFE) | PANT (mg) / REF |
|---|---|---|---|---|---|---|---|---|---|---|---|---|---|---|---|---|---|---|
| **Mr. Goodbar**, Hershey | 49 | 264 | 0.2 | 26.6 | 23.1 | | 1.9 | 20 | 54 | 23 | 0.46 | 0 | 17 | 0 | 0.07 | 1.7 | 0.16 | 0.21 |
| *1.75 oz bar* | | 5.0 | 16.3 | 6.9 | 4.0 | 2.1 | 5 | 193 | 80 | 0.68 | 0.083 | 0 | 61 | 1.6 | 0.07 | 0.03 | 18.6 | 19143 |
| nougat with almonds | 14 | 56 | 0.3 | 12.9 | 11.7 | 11.4 | 0.5 | 5 | 4 | 4 | 0.06 | 0.043 | 0 | 0 | 0 | 0.1 | 0 | 0.01 |
| *.5 oz piece* | | 0.5 | 0.2 | 0.2 | 0 | 0 | 0 | 15 | 8 | 0.08 | 0.019 | 0.4 | 0 | 0.4 | 0.02 | 0 | 0.7 | 43046 |
| **Oh Henry!**, Nestle | 57 | 263 | 1.3 | 37.3 | 26.3 | | 1.1 | 110 | 39 | 29 | 0.68 | 0.305 | 0 | 0 | 0.08 | 1.5 | 0.11 | 0.31 |
| *2 oz bar* | | 4.4 | 13.1 | 5.5 | 3.2 | 1.5 | 4 | 148 | 80 | 0.28 | 0.201 | 1.8 | 0 | 1.3 | 0.07 | 0.05 | 25.1 | 19118 |
| **Party Mix** (choc-covered nuts, raisins), | 30 | 150 | | 17.0 | 12.0 | | 1.0 | 15 | 30 | | | | 0 | | | | | |
| Sunnyland Farms - *16 pcs* | | 2.0 | 9.0 | 4.0 | | | 3 | | | 0.36 | | | 0 | | | | | SUNN2 |
| peanut bar | 45 | 235 | 0.7 | 21.3 | 19.0 | 17.9 | 1.8 | 70 | 35 | 50 | 1.77 | 0.559 | 0 | 0 | 0.05 | 3.6 | | 0.37 |
| *1.6 oz bar* | | 7.0 | 15.2 | 2.1 | 7.5 | 4.8 | 0 | 183 | 139 | 0.44 | 0.348 | 2.1 | 0 | 1.8 | 0.06 | 0.07 | 33.8 | 19147 |
| peanut brittle | 28 | 136 | 0.2 | 19.9 | 14.4 | 14.1 | 0.7 | 125 | 8 | 12 | 0.24 | 0.166 | 11 | 0 | 0.04 | 0.7 | | 0.15 |
| *1 oz* | | 2.1 | 5.3 | 1.2 | 2.3 | 1.3 | 3 | 47 | 30 | 0.34 | 0.071 | 0.7 | 40 | 0.7 | 0.01 | 0.02 | 12.9 | 19148 |
| peanut butter chips | 168 | 889 | 4.5 | 78.8 | 64.3 | 57.8 | 8.4 | 420 | 185 | 185 | 3.36 | 2.352 | 0 | 1 | 0.39 | 13.8 | 0.34 | 1.77 |
| *1 cup* | | 30.7 | 50.1 | 22.0 | 21.6 | 3.4 | 2 | 848 | 521 | 2.86 | 0.672 | 6.6 | 2 | 2.3 | 0.34 | 0.29 | 129.4 | 19086 |
| **Pecan Fiddlesticks**, Priester's | 57 | 280 | | 31.0 | 23.0 | | 1.0 | 40 | 60 | | | | | | | | | |
| Pecan Company - *2 oz* | | 3.0 | 16.0 | 4.0 | | | 5 | | | | | | | | | | | PRIE2 |
| pralines, homemade | 39 | 189 | 4.0 | 23.2 | 21.8 | | 1.4 | 19 | 17 | 19 | 0.65 | 0.656 | 0 | 0 | 0.08 | 0.2 | 0 | 0.13 |
| *1.4 oz piece* | | 1.3 | 10.1 | 0.9 | 5.7 | 3.0 | 0 | 85 | 41 | 0.50 | 0.193 | 0.7 | 7 | 0.2 | 0.02 | 0.03 | 2.3 | 19216 |
| **Reese's Bites**, Hershey | 39 | 203 | 0.6 | 21.5 | 18.7 | | 1.2 | 70 | 44 | 25 | 0.41 | 0.254 | | 0 | 0.06 | 1.7 | | 0.22 |
| *16 pieces* | | 4.4 | 11.6 | 7.0 | 2.8 | 0.7 | 3 | 149 | 76 | 0.33 | 0.117 | 0.6 | 23 | 0.08 | 0.08 | 0.04 | | 19238 |
| **Reese's Fast Break**, Hershey | 56 | 277 | 0.9 | 35.8 | 30.0 | | 2.0 | 180 | 20 | 34 | 0.81 | 0.407 | 8 | 0 | 0.07 | 1.6 | 0.10 | 0.30 |
| *2 oz bar* | | 5.0 | 13.0 | 4.5 | 4.5 | 2.4 | 5 | 144 | 87 | 0.36 | 0.180 | 2.1 | 27 | 1.4 | 0.06 | 0.03 | 15.7 | 19896 |
| **Reese's** Nutrageous, Hershey | 34 | 176 | 0.5 | 18.0 | 13.7 | | 1.3 | 48 | 23 | 23 | 0.44 | 0 | | 0 | 0.06 | 1.8 | | 0.18 |
| *2 bars (1.2 oz)* | | 3.8 | 10.9 | 3.0 | 4.3 | 2.8 | 1 | 124 | 60 | 0.42 | 0.092 | 0.1 | 12 | | 0.03 | 0.03 | | 19239 |
| **Reese's** Peanut Butter Cups, | 45 | 232 | 0.6 | 24.9 | 21.2 | | 1.6 | 141 | 35 | 28 | 0.58 | 0 | 8 | 0 | 0.07 | 2.0 | 0.12 | 0.28 |
| Hershey - *2 pieces (1.6 oz)* | | 4.6 | 13.7 | 4.8 | 5.9 | 2.5 | 3 | 154 | 72 | 0.54 | 0.108 | 0.6 | 25 | 0.1 | 0.05 | 0.05 | 22.5 | 19150 |
| **Reese's** Pieces, Hershey | 46 | 229 | 0.5 | 27.5 | 24.5 | | 1.4 | 89 | 32 | 40 | 0.53 | 0.506 | 0 | 0 | 0.08 | 2.8 | 0.05 | 0.28 |
| *1.6 oz package (58 pieces)* | | 5.7 | 11.4 | 7.6 | 2.1 | 0.9 | 0 | 165 | 95 | 0.23 | 0.189 | 0.4 | 0 | 0.5 | 0.10 | 0.05 | 25.3 | 19151 |
| **Reesesticks**, Hershey | 42 | 219 | 0.7 | 23.3 | 16.9 | | 1.4 | 111 | 29 | 21 | 0.42 | 0 | 6 | 0 | 0.05 | 1.5 | 0.06 | 0.18 |
| *1.5 oz piece* | | 4.0 | 13.2 | 5.5 | 4.5 | 2.0 | 3 | 124 | 60 | 0.55 | 0.084 | 0.3 | 24 | 1.2 | 0.04 | 0.03 | 16.8 | 19249 |
| **Rolo** caramels w/milk chocolate, | 54 | 256 | 2.5 | 36.7 | 34.5 | | 0.5 | 102 | 78 | 0 | 0 | 0 | 18 | 0 | 0.01 | 0 | 0.18 | 0 |
| Hershey - *1.9 oz pkg (9 pieces)* | | 2.7 | 11.3 | 7.9 | 1.1 | 0.1 | 6 | 102 | 38 | 0.23 | 0 | 0 | 65 | 0.6 | 0.06 | 0 | 0 | 19152 |
| **semi-sweet chocolate chips**, Nestle | 14 | 70 | | 9.0 | 8.0 | | | 0 | 0 | | | | 0 | | | | | |
| *1 T* | | | 4.0 | 2.5 | | | 0 | | 0 | | | | 0 | | | | | NTEA30 |
| sesame crunch | 35 | 181 | 0.8 | 17.6 | 10.9 | 10.8 | 2.7 | 58 | 224 | 88 | 1.32 | 0.563 | 0 | 0 | 0.16 | 1.3 | 0 | 0.01 |
| *20 pieces* | | 4.1 | 11.7 | 1.6 | 4.4 | 5.1 | 0 | 107 | 144 | 1.49 | 0.332 | 1.4 | 2 | 0.1 | 0.06 | 0.17 | 17.8 | 19154 |
| **Skittles** Candies | 57 | 231 | 2.2 | 51.7 | 43.2 | | 0 | 9 | 0 | 1 | 0.01 | 0.036 | 0 | 38 | 0 | 0 | 0 | 0.01 |
| *2 oz package (54 pieces)* | | 0.1 | 2.5 | 2.3 | 0 | 0 | 0 | 7 | 1 | 0 | 0.021 | 0.6 | 0 | 0.1 | 0.01 | 0 | 0 | 19370 |
| **Skittles** Sours | 51 | 202 | 2.0 | 44.3 | 37.3 | | 0 | 7 | 0 | | | | | 31 | | | | |
| *1.8 oz bag* | | 0.1 | 2.0 | 1.9 | | | 0 | | | 0.01 | | | 0 | | | | | 19369 |
| **Skittles** Tropical | 62 | 251 | 2.4 | 56.3 | 47.0 | | 0 | 9 | 0 | | | | | 42 | | | | |
| *2.1 oz bag* | | 0.1 | 2.7 | | | | 0 | | | 0 | | | 0 | | | | | 19368 |
| **Skittles**, wild berry | 62 | 251 | 2.4 | 56.4 | 47.1 | | 0 | 9 | 0 | | | | | 42 | | | | |
| *2.1 oz bag* | | 0.1 | 2.6 | 2.6 | | | 0 | | | 0 | | | 0 | | | | | 19363 |
| **Skor Toffee Bar**, Hershey | 39 | 209 | 0.6 | 24.1 | 23.4 | | 0.5 | 124 | 4 | | 0.07 | 0 | | 0 | 0.01 | 0.1 | | 0.02 |
| *1.4 oz bar* | | 1.2 | 12.6 | 7.3 | 3.6 | 0.5 | 21 | 60 | 24 | 0.22 | 0.016 | 0 | 280 | | 0.04 | | | 19136 |
| **Snickers** | 57 | 271 | 3.2 | 34.5 | 28.8 | | 1.3 | 140 | 53 | 41 | 1.42 | 0.199 | 26 | 0 | 0.03 | 2.1 | 0.09 | 0.34 |
| *2 oz bar* | | 4.3 | 13.6 | 5.2 | 4.5 | 1.7 | 7 | 184 | 108 | 0.41 | 0.154 | 4.4 | 96 | 0.9 | 0.07 | 0.05 | 17.7 | 19155 |
| **Snickers** Almond | 50 | 236 | 2.7 | 32.3 | 27.0 | | 1.3 | 78 | 66 | | | | 0 | | | | | |
| *1.76 oz bar* | | 2.7 | 11.2 | 4.3 | | | 6 | | | 0.42 | | | 83 | | | | | 19302 |
| **Snickers** Cruncher | 47 | 229 | 2.1 | 29.5 | 21.9 | | 0.9 | 89 | 42 | | | | 0 | | | | | |
| *1.66 oz bar* | | 3.2 | 11.5 | 6.0 | | | 4 | | | 0.32 | | | 56 | | | | | 19359 |
| **Snickers** Munch Bar | 40 | 214 | 1.2 | 17.5 | 12.3 | | 1.9 | 143 | 22 | | | | 0 | | | | | |
| *1.42 oz bar* | | 6.1 | 14.5 | 3.5 | | | 10 | | | 0.41 | | | 126 | | | | | 19295 |
| **Snickers** Pop'ables | 39 | 187 | 2.3 | 23.8 | 20.2 | | 0.9 | 87 | 37 | | | | 0 | | | | | |
| *13 pieces* | | 2.8 | 9.5 | 3.9 | | | 5 | | | 0.28 | | | 68 | | | | | 19306 |
| **Starburst** Fruit Chews | 59 | 241 | 5.0 | 48.7 | 34.3 | | 0 | 1 | 0 | 1 | 0 | 0.009 | 0 | 35 | 0 | 0 | 0 | 0.02 |
| *2.07 oz package (6 pieces)* | | 0.2 | 4.8 | 4.6 | 0 | 0 | 0 | 1 | 3 | 0.01 | 0.007 | 0.5 | 1 | 0.2 | 0 | 0 | 0.6 | 19156 |
| **Starburst** Fruit Chews, fruit and | 40 | 163 | 3.5 | 33.0 | 23.2 | | 0 | 1 | 0 | | | | | 23 | | | | |
| crème - *8 pieces* | | 0.2 | 3.3 | 3.2 | | | 0 | | | 0 | | | 0 | | | | | 19309 |
| **Starburst** Fruit Chews, tropical | 40 | 164 | 3.4 | 33.1 | 23.3 | | 0 | 1 | 0 | | | | | 24 | | | | |
| fruits - *8 pieces* | | 0.2 | 3.3 | 3.2 | | | 0 | | | 0 | | | 0 | | | | | 19313 |

| Item | WT (g) | KCAL | H₂0 (g) | CHO (g) | TSUG (g) | ASUG (g) | DFIB (g) | Na (mg) | Ca (mg) | Mg (mg) | Zn (mg) | Mn (mg) | A (mcg RAE) | C (mg) | B-1 (mg) | NIA (mg) | B-12 (mcg) | PANT (mg) |
|---|---|---|---|---|---|---|---|---|---|---|---|---|---|---|---|---|---|---|
| | | PRO (g) | FAT (g) | SFA (g) | MUFA (g) | PUFA (g) | CHOL (mg) | K (mg) | P (mg) | Fe (mg) | Cu (mg) | Se (mcg) | A (IU) | E (mg ATE) | B-2 (mg) | B-6 (mg) | FOL (mcg DFE) | REF |
| **Starburst** Sour Fruit Chews | 59 | 236 | 6.4 | 47.0 | 33.1 | | 0 | 53 | 0 | | | | | 33 | | | | |
| *2.07 oz pack* | | 0.2 | 4.6 | 4.4 | | | 0 | | | 0.01 | | | 0 | | | | | 19315 |
| **Surprise Apple** (orange-flavored dark choc), Gubor - *6 pieces* | 42 | 220 | | 20.0 | 19.0 | | 3.0 | 5 | 10 | | | | | 0 | | | | |
| | | 2.5 | 15.0 | 9.0 | | | 4 | | | 1.62 | | | 0 | | | | | GUBO1 |
| **Symphony,** Hershey | 42 | 223 | 0.4 | 24.4 | 22.7 | | 0.7 | 42 | 105 | | | | | 1 | | | | |
| *1.5 oz bar* | | 3.6 | 12.8 | 7.7 | 3.3 | 0.3 | 10 | 184 | 87 | 0.38 | | | 96 | | | | | 19093 |
| **taffy,** creamy mint sticks, Fralinger's - *5 pieces* | 42 | 170 | | 38.0 | 38.0 | | | 0 | | | | | | | | | | |
| | | 0 | 2.0 | | | | | | | | | | | | | | | FRAL2 |
| **taffy,** holiday, Harry and David *about 5 pieces* | 40 | 160 | | 33.0 | 28.0 | | 0 | 260 | | | | | | | | | | |
| | | 0 | 3.0 | 0.5 | | | 0 | | | | | | | | | | | HADA4 |
| **taffy,** homemade *.53 oz piece* | 15 | 60 | 0.7 | 13.7 | 10.3 | | 0 | 8 | 1 | 0 | 0.03 | 0 | 4 | 0 | 0 | 0 | 0 | 0 |
| | | 0 | 0.5 | 0.3 | 0.1 | 0 | 1 | 0 | 0 | 0 | 0 | 0.1 | 15 | 0 | 0 | 0 | 0 | 19382 |
| **taffy,** peanut butter, Fralinger's *5 pieces* | 42 | 170 | | 28.0 | 17.0 | | | 100 | | | | | | | | | | |
| | | 2.0 | 6.0 | | | | | | | | | | | | | | | FRAL5 |
| **taffy,** rum and butter toffee flavor Fralinger's - *5 pieces* | 42 | 150 | | 30.0 | 19.0 | | | 40 | | | | | | | | | | |
| | | | 2.5 | | | | | | | | | | | | | | | FRAL4 |
| **taffy,** salt water, Fralinger's *5 pieces* | 42 | 150 | | 32.0 | 20.0 | | | 30 | | | | | | | | | | |
| | | 0 | 2.5 | | | | | | | | | | | | | | | FRAL1 |
| **taffy** with filled centers, Fralinger's - *5 pieces* | 42 | 150 | | 31.0 | 19.0 | | | 35 | | | | | | | | | | |
| | | 0 | 3.0 | | | | | | | | | | | | | | | FRAL3 |
| **Three Musketeers** *2.13 oz bar* | 60 | 257 | 3.5 | 46.3 | 40.1 | | 0.9 | 116 | 32 | 17 | 0.33 | 0.096 | 12 | 0 | 0.02 | 0.1 | 0.10 | 0.14 |
| | | 1.6 | 7.6 | 5.2 | 1.4 | 0.2 | 3 | 80 | 41 | 0.40 | 0.093 | 1.1 | 43 | 0.6 | 0.03 | 0.01 | 2.4 | 19159 |
| **Three Musketeers** Pop'ables *15 pieces* | 41 | 182 | 2.2 | 31.1 | 27.5 | | 0.5 | 71 | 25 | | | | | 0 | | | | |
| | | 1.1 | 6.2 | 4.1 | | | 3 | | | 0.24 | | | 41 | | | | | 19308 |
| **toffee,** homemade *.42 oz piece* | 12 | 67 | 0.1 | 7.8 | 7.6 | | 0 | 16 | 4 | 0 | 0.01 | 0 | 38 | 0 | 0 | 0 | 0.01 | 0.02 |
| | | 0.1 | 3.9 | 2.5 | 1.1 | 0.1 | 12 | 6 | 4 | 0 | 0 | 0.1 | 138 | 0.1 | 0.01 | 0 | 0.2 | 19383 |
| **toffee** w/macadamias, mlk choc-cvrd, Mauna Loa - *7 pcs (1.4 oz)* | 40 | 210 | | 23.0 | 21.0 | | 1.0 | 70 | | | | | | | | | | |
| | | 2.0 | 13.0 | 5.0 | | | 5 | | | | | | | | | | | MAUN5 |
| **Tootsie Roll** *6 pieces* | 40 | 155 | 2.7 | 35.1 | 22.5 | | 0 | 18 | 14 | 9 | 0.16 | 0.019 | 0 | 0 | 0.02 | 0.1 | 0 | 0.12 |
| | | 0.6 | 1.3 | 0.4 | 0.8 | 0.1 | 1 | 46 | 23 | 0.32 | 0.052 | 0.9 | 0 | 0.3 | 0.03 | 0 | 4.4 | 19064 |
| **truffles,** homemade *.42 oz piece* | 12 | 61 | 1.6 | 5.4 | 4.6 | | 0.3 | 8 | 19 | 6 | 0.19 | 0.042 | 17 | 0 | 0.01 | 0 | 0.06 | 0.05 |
| | | 0.7 | 4.1 | 2.2 | 1.5 | 0.1 | 6 | 36 | 21 | 0.21 | 0.044 | 0.4 | 62 | 0.2 | 0.03 | 0 | 1.1 | 19138 |
| **truffles,** milk chocolate, Harry and David - *2 pieces* | 37 | 200 | | 18.0 | 16.0 | | 1.0 | 15 | 20 | | | | | | | | | |
| | | 2.0 | 16.0 | 11.0 | | | 0 | | | 0.72 | | | | | | | | HADA5 |
| **truffles,** mocha double choc Wisconsin Cheeseman - *2 pcs (1.2 oz)* | 34 | 170 | | 20.0 | 18.0 | | | 45 | 40 | | | | | 0 | | | | |
| | | 2.0 | 6.0 | 0 | | | 10 | | | 0.36 | | | 100 | | | | | WISC3 |
| **Twix Cookie Bar,** caramel *2 bars* | 58 | 291 | 2.5 | 37.7 | 28.0 | | 0.6 | 115 | 61 | 16 | 0.61 | 0.158 | 12 | 0 | 0.09 | 0.6 | 0.19 | 0.15 |
| | | 2.8 | 14.4 | 11.0 | 1.7 | 0.4 | 4 | 108 | 61 | 0.47 | 0.114 | 2.5 | 45 | 0.4 | 0.12 | 0.01 | 22.0 | 19160 |
| **Twix Cookie Bar,** peanut butter *2 bars* | 58 | 311 | 1.1 | 31.4 | 21.0 | | 1.8 | 131 | 44 | 35 | 0.93 | 0.546 | 12 | 0 | 0.06 | 1.4 | 0.15 | 0.27 |
| | | 5.3 | 18.9 | 9.1 | 7.1 | 2.0 | 3 | 153 | 100 | 0.77 | 0.168 | 7.5 | 43 | 2.0 | 0.08 | 0.07 | 8.7 | 19161 |
| **Twizzlers,** Cherry Bits, Hershey *1.4 oz bag (8 pieces)* | 40 | 135 | 6.0 | 31.8 | | | 0 | 104 | 5 | | | | | 0 | | | | |
| | | 1.2 | 0.7 | 0.1 | 0.2 | 0 | 0 | 6 | 19 | 0.22 | | | 0 | | | | | 19067 |
| **Twizzlers Nibs,** Cherry Bits *27 pieces* | 40 | 139 | 6.0 | 31.7 | 20.5 | | 0.2 | 78 | 3 | | | | | 0 | | | | |
| | | 0.9 | 1.1 | 0.2 | 0.8 | 0.1 | 0 | 15 | 10 | 0.11 | | | 0 | | | | | 19092 |
| **Twizzlers,** Strawberry Twists, Hershey - *2.5 oz package* | 71 | 248 | | 56.6 | 28.1 | | 0 | 204 | 0 | | | | | 0 | | | | |
| | | 1.8 | 1.6 | 0 | | | 0 | | | 0.36 | | | 0 | | | | | 19112 |
| **U-No,** chocolate center, Annabelle Candy Co - *.43 oz bar* | 12 | 70 | | 6.0 | 6.0 | | 0 | 15 | | | | | | | | | | |
| | | 1.0 | 5.0 | 3.0 | | | 0 | | | | | | | | | | | ANNA4 |
| **Whatchamacallit,** Hershey *1.7 oz bar* | 48 | 237 | 1.5 | 30.4 | 23.5 | | 0.9 | 144 | 57 | 13 | 0.21 | 0.158 | 18 | 0 | 0.05 | 1.2 | 0.18 | 0.12 |
| | | 3.9 | 11.4 | 8.2 | 1.8 | 0.4 | 6 | 145 | 66 | 0.54 | 0.058 | 0.3 | 64 | 0.6 | 0.10 | 0.02 | 8.6 | 19162 |
| **white chocolate chips** *¼ cup* | 42 | 226 | 0.5 | 24.9 | 24.8 | 21.4 | 0.1 | 38 | 84 | 5 | 0.31 | 0.003 | 4 | 0 | 0.03 | 0.3 | 0.24 | 0.26 |
| | | 2.5 | 13.5 | 8.2 | 3.8 | 0.4 | 9 | 120 | 74 | 0.10 | 0.025 | 1.9 | 13 | 0.4 | 0.12 | 0.02 | 2.9 | 19087 |
| **yogurt candy chips** *¼ cup* | 42 | 219 | 0.8 | 26.9 | 26.2 | 22.6 | 0 | 37 | 86 | 8 | 0.29 | 0.001 | 0 | 0 | 0.03 | 0.1 | 0.27 | 0.25 |
| | | 2.5 | 11.3 | 10.1 | 0.2 | 0.2 | 0 | 122 | 66 | 0.06 | 0.003 | 2.0 | 2 | 0.5 | 0.11 | 0.02 | 3.4 | 19079 |
| **York Bites** *15 pieces* | 39 | 154 | 3.5 | 31.8 | 29.2 | | 0.8 | 18 | 4 | 0 | 0 | 0 | 0 | 0 | 0 | 0 | | 0 |
| | | 0.7 | 2.9 | 1.7 | 0.2 | 0 | 0 | 42 | 1 | 0.37 | 0 | 0 | 3 | 0 | 0 | 0 | | 19181 |
| **York Peppermint Pattie,** Hershey *1.5 oz patty* | 43 | 165 | 3.9 | 34.8 | 27.4 | | 0.9 | 12 | 5 | | | | | 0 | | | | |
| | | 0.9 | 3.1 | 1.9 | 0.2 | 0 | 0 | 48 | 0 | 0.40 | | | 3 | | | | | 19091 |

| | WT (g) | KCAL / PRO (g) | H₂0 (g) / FAT (g) | CHO (g) / SFA (g) | TSUG (g) / MUFA (g) | ASUG (g) / PUFA (g) | DFIB (g) / CHOL (mg) | Na (mg) / K (mg) | Ca (mg) / P (mg) | Mg (mg) / Fe (mg) | Zn (mg) / Cu (mg) | Mn (mg) / Se (mcg) | A (mcg RAE) / A (IU) | C (mg) / E (mg ATE) | B-1 (mg) / B-2 (mg) | NIA (mg) / B-6 (mg) | B-12 (mcg) / FOL (mcg DFE) | PANT (mg) / REF |
|---|---|---|---|---|---|---|---|---|---|---|---|---|---|---|---|---|---|---|

## 3. CEREALS AND GRAINS, COOKED

| Food | WT | KCAL/PRO | H₂O/FAT | CHO/SFA | TSUG/MUFA | ASUG/PUFA | DFIB/CHOL | Na/K | Ca/P | Mg/Fe | Zn/Cu | Mn/Se | A(RAE)/A(IU) | C/E | B-1/B-2 | NIA/B-6 | B-12/FOL | PANT/REF |
|---|---|---|---|---|---|---|---|---|---|---|---|---|---|---|---|---|---|---|
| **amaranth grain**, boiled | 246 | 251 | 184.9 | 46.0 | | | 5.2 | 15 | 116 | 160 | 2.12 | 2.101 | | | 0.04 | 0.6 | | |
| 1 cup | | 9.3 | 3.9 | | | | | 332 | 364 | 5.17 | 0.367 | 13.5 | | 0.5 | 0.05 | 0.28 | | 20002 |
| **amaranth**, whole grain, dry | 195 | 723 | 22.0 | 127.2 | 3.3 | | 13.1 | 8 | 310 | 484 | 5.60 | 6.499 | 0 | 8 | 0.23 | 1.8 | 0 | 2.84 |
| 1 cup | | 26.4 | 13.7 | 2.8 | 3.3 | 5.4 | 0 | 991 | 1086 | 14.84 | 1.024 | 36.5 | 4 | 2.3 | 0.39 | 1.15 | 159.9 | 20001 |
| **barley cereal**, scotch, regular/quick, dry, Quaker - 1 oz | 28 | 97 | 2.7 | 21.4 | 0.2 | | 2.9 | 2 | 8 | 17 | 0.41 | 0.353 | 0 | 0 | 0.07 | 1.3 | 0 | 0.08 |
| | | 3.0 | 0.6 | 0.1 | 0.1 | 0.3 | 0 | 73 | 59 | 0.56 | 0.106 | | 6 | | 0.03 | 0.07 | 6.4 | 8232 |
| **barley**, pearled, cooked | 157 | 193 | 108.0 | 44.3 | 0.4 | 0 | 6.0 | 5 | 17 | 35 | 1.29 | 0.407 | 0 | 0 | 0.13 | 3.2 | 0 | 0.21 |
| 1 cup | | 3.5 | 0.7 | 0.1 | 0.1 | 0.3 | 0 | 146 | 85 | 2.09 | 0.165 | 13.5 | 11 | 0 | 0.10 | 0.18 | 25.1 | 20006 |
| **barley**, whole grain, dry | 184 | 651 | 17.4 | 135.2 | 1.5 | 0 | 31.8 | 22 | 61 | 245 | 5.10 | 3.575 | 2 | 0 | 1.19 | 8.5 | 0 | 0.52 |
| 1 cup | | 23.0 | 4.2 | 0.9 | 0.5 | 2.0 | 0 | 832 | 486 | 6.62 | 0.916 | 69.4 | 40 | 1.0 | 0.52 | 0.59 | 35.0 | 20004 |
| **buckwheat groats**, dry | 170 | 583 | 16.6 | 121.6 | 1.5 | | 17.0 | 2 | 31 | 393 | 4.08 | 2.210 | 0 | 0 | 0.17 | 11.9 | 0 | 2.10 |
| 1 cup | | 22.5 | 5.8 | 1.3 | 1.8 | 1.8 | 0 | 782 | 590 | 3.74 | 1.870 | 14.1 | 0 | | 0.72 | 0.36 | 51.0 | 20008 |
| **buckwheat groats**, roasted, cooked | 168 | 155 | 127.1 | 33.5 | 1.5 | | 4.5 | 7 | 12 | 86 | 1.02 | 0.677 | 0 | 0 | 0.07 | 1.6 | 0 | 0.60 |
| 1 cup | | 5.7 | 1.0 | 0.2 | 0.3 | 0.3 | 0 | 148 | 118 | 1.34 | 0.245 | 3.7 | 0 | 0.2 | 0.07 | 0.13 | 23.5 | 20010 |
| **buckwheat groats**, roasted, dry | 164 | 567 | 13.8 | 122.9 | | | 16.9 | 18 | 28 | 362 | 3.97 | 2.654 | 0 | 0 | 0.37 | 8.4 | 0 | 2.02 |
| 1 cup | | 19.2 | 4.4 | 1.0 | 1.4 | 1.4 | 0 | 525 | 523 | 4.05 | 1.023 | 13.8 | 0 | | 0.44 | 0.58 | 68.9 | 20009 |
| **bulgur**, cooked | 182 | 151 | 141.5 | 33.8 | 0.2 | 0 | 8.2 | 9 | 18 | 58 | 1.04 | 1.108 | 0 | 0 | 0.10 | 1.8 | 0 | 0.63 |
| 1 cup | | 5.6 | 0.4 | 0.1 | 0.1 | 0.2 | 0 | 124 | 73 | 1.75 | 0.136 | 1.1 | 4 | 0 | 0.05 | 0.15 | 32.8 | 20013 |
| **corn grits**, butter flavor, inst, enr, prep, Quaker - 1 pkt prep | 141 | 100 | 116.3 | 19.8 | 0.2 | | 1.3 | 348 | 111 | 8 | 0.11 | 0.024 | 11 | 0 | 0.16 | 2.1 | 0 | 0.11 |
| | | 2.1 | 1.5 | 0.6 | 0.3 | 0.1 | 0 | 39 | 23 | 7.63 | 0.027 | 0 | 214 | | 0.17 | 0.03 | | 8238 |
| **corn grits**, butter flavor, inst, enr, dry, Quaker - 1 oz packet | 28 | 102 | 1.9 | 21.0 | 0.2 | | 1.3 | 367 | 115 | 8 | 0.11 | 0.025 | 11 | 0 | 0.17 | 2.2 | 0 | 0.12 |
| | | 2.3 | 1.5 | 0.7 | 0.3 | 0.1 | 0 | 41 | 24 | 8.10 | 0.020 | 0 | 228 | | 0.18 | 0.04 | | 8221 |
| **corn grits**, cheddar cheese flvr, inst, enr, dry, Quaker - 1 oz pkt | 28 | 102 | 2.1 | 20.5 | 0.6 | | 1.2 | 522 | 13 | 10 | 0.21 | 0.076 | 1 | 0 | 0.16 | 2.2 | 0 | 0.11 |
| | | 2.3 | 1.7 | 0.5 | 0.4 | 0.2 | 1 | 48 | 39 | 8.10 | 0.031 | 4.4 | 4 | 0.1 | 0.18 | 0.04 | 71.4 | 8094 |
| **corn grits**, cheddar cheese flvr, inst, enr, prep, Quaker - 1 pkt prep | 142 | 102 | 116.8 | 19.9 | 0.6 | | 1.1 | 508 | 16 | 11 | 0.21 | 0.074 | 1 | 0 | 0.16 | 2.1 | 0 | 0.11 |
| | | 2.3 | 1.6 | 0.4 | 0.4 | 0.2 | 0 | 47 | 38 | 7.85 | 0.037 | 4.4 | 4 | 0.1 | 0.18 | 0.04 | 69.6 | 8095 |
| **corn grits**, instant, enriched, dry, Quaker - 1 oz packet | 28 | 96 | 2.4 | 22.1 | 0.1 | | 1.3 | 305 | 6 | 10 | 0.19 | 0.087 | 0 | 0 | 0.18 | 2.5 | 0 | 0.12 |
| | | 2.4 | 0.3 | 0 | 0 | 0.1 | 0 | 41 | 31 | 8.51 | 0.028 | 4.8 | 1 | 0 | 0.21 | 0.06 | 83.2 | 8092 |
| **corn grits**, instant, enriched, prepared, Quaker - 1 cup | 245 | 167 | 201.9 | 36.9 | 0.1 | | 2.2 | 514 | 15 | 17 | 0.32 | 0.147 | 0 | 0 | 0.28 | 4.0 | 0 | 0.20 |
| | | 3.9 | 0.5 | 0 | 0.1 | 0.1 | 0 | 69 | 51 | 14.23 | 0.061 | 7.8 | 2 | 0 | 0.33 | 0.10 | 139.6 | 8093 |
| **corn grits** w/imitation bacon bits, inst, enr, dry, Quaker - 1 oz pkt | 28 | 98 | 2.0 | 21.7 | 0.1 | | 1.5 | 341 | 11 | 10 | 0.26 | 0.028 | 0 | 0 | 0.18 | 2.3 | 0 | 0.11 |
| | | 2.8 | 0.5 | 0.1 | 0.1 | 0.2 | 0 | 71 | 39 | 8.10 | 0.020 | 4.5 | 0 | 0 | 0.20 | 0.06 | 78.4 | 8096 |
| **corn grits** w/imitation bacon bits, inst, enr, prep, Quaker - 1 pkt prep | 141 | 97 | 115.9 | 20.6 | 0.1 | | 1.4 | 413 | 6 | 7 | 0.16 | 0.027 | 0 | 0 | 0.17 | 2.3 | 0 | 0.12 |
| | | 2.7 | 0.5 | 0.1 | 0.1 | 0.2 | 0 | 56 | 25 | 7.80 | 0.039 | 0 | 0 | 0 | 0.19 | 0.04 | 45.1 | 8097 |
| **corn grits**, white, quick, dry, Quaker - 1 oz | 28 | 97 | 2.9 | 22.2 | 0.3 | | 1.3 | 1 | 1 | 14 | 0.26 | 0.062 | | 0 | 0.16 | 1.3 | 0 | 0.09 |
| | | 2.4 | 0.4 | 0.1 | 0.1 | 0.2 | 0 | 41 | 46 | 0.99 | 0.031 | | 0 | 0 | 0.09 | 0.08 | 72.5 | 8314 |
| **corn grits**, white, quick, enriched, cooked - 1 cup | 242 | 143 | 206.5 | 31.1 | 0.2 | | 0.7 | 540 | 7 | 12 | 0.17 | 0.044 | 0 | 0 | 0.20 | 1.7 | 0 | 0.19 |
| | | 3.4 | 0.5 | 0.1 | 0.1 | 0.2 | 0 | 51 | 27 | 1.45 | 0.044 | 7.5 | 0 | 0 | 0.13 | 0.05 | 135.5 | 8161 |
| **corn grits**, white, regular, dry, Quaker - 1 oz | 28 | 97 | 2.9 | 22.2 | 0.3 | | 1.3 | 1 | 1 | 14 | 0.26 | 0.062 | 0 | 0 | 0.16 | 1.3 | 0 | 0.09 |
| | | 2.4 | 0.4 | 0.1 | 0.1 | 0.2 | 0 | 41 | 46 | 0.99 | 0.031 | | 0 | | 0.09 | 0.08 | | 8316 |
| **corn grits**, white, regular/quick, enriched, cooked - 1 cup | 242 | 143 | 206.5 | 31.1 | 0.2 | 0 | 0.7 | 5 | 7 | 12 | 0.17 | 0.044 | 0 | 0 | 0.20 | 1.7 | 0 | 0.19 |
| | | 3.4 | 0.5 | 0.1 | 0.1 | 0.2 | 0 | 51 | 27 | 1.45 | 0.044 | 7.5 | 0 | 0 | 0.13 | 0.05 | 133.1 | 8091 |
| **corn grits**, white, regular/quick, unenriched, cooked - 1 cup | 242 | 143 | 206.5 | 31.1 | 0.2 | | 0.7 | 5 | 7 | 12 | 0.17 | 0.044 | 0 | 0 | 0.04 | 0.4 | 0 | 0.19 |
| | | 3.4 | 0.5 | 0.1 | 0.1 | 0.2 | 0 | 51 | 27 | 0.39 | 0.044 | 7.5 | 2 | 0.01 | 0.05 | 2.4 | | 8162 |
| **corn grits**, yellow, quick, dry, Quaker - 1 oz | 28 | 94 | 3.3 | 21.8 | 0.3 | | 1.6 | 1 | 1 | 11 | 0.20 | 0.028 | | 0 | 0.14 | 1.2 | 0 | 0.09 |
| | | 2.3 | 0.5 | 0.1 | 0.2 | 0.2 | 0 | 47 | 35 | 1.15 | 0.020 | | 159 | | 0.10 | 0.07 | | 8315 |
| **corn grits**, yellow, quick, enriched, cooked - 1 cup | 242 | 143 | 206.5 | 31.1 | 0.2 | | 0.7 | 540 | 7 | 12 | 0.17 | 0.044 | 5 | 0 | 0.20 | 1.7 | 0 | 0.19 |
| | | 3.4 | 0.5 | 0.1 | 0.1 | 0.2 | 0 | 51 | 27 | 1.45 | 0.044 | 6.5 | 75 | 0 | 0.13 | 0.05 | 135.5 | 8165 |
| **corn grits**, yellow, regular/quick, enriched, cooked - 1 cup | 242 | 143 | 206.5 | 31.1 | 0.2 | 0 | 0.7 | 5 | 7 | 12 | 0.17 | 0.044 | 5 | 0 | 0.20 | 1.7 | 0 | 0.19 |
| | | 3.4 | 0.5 | 0.1 | 0.1 | 0.2 | 0 | 51 | 27 | 1.45 | 0.044 | 6.5 | 75 | 0 | 0.13 | 0.05 | 135.5 | 8164 |
| **corn grits**, yellow, regular/quick, unenriched, cooked - 1 cup | 242 | 143 | 206.5 | 31.1 | 0.2 | | 0.7 | 5 | 7 | 12 | 0.17 | 0.044 | 5 | 0 | 0.04 | 0.4 | 0 | 0.19 |
| | | 3.4 | 0.5 | 0.1 | 0.1 | 0.2 | 0 | 51 | 27 | 0.39 | 0.044 | 6.5 | 75 | 0 | 0.01 | 0.05 | 2.4 | 8166 |
| **corn**, whole grain, dry - 3.5 oz | 100 | 365 | 10.4 | 74.3 | 0.6 | 0 | 7.3 | 35 | 7 | 127 | 2.21 | 0.485 | 11 | 0 | 0.38 | 3.6 | 0 | 0.42 |
| | | 9.4 | 4.7 | 0.7 | 1.3 | 2.2 | 0 | 287 | 210 | 2.71 | 0.314 | 15.5 | 214 | 0.5 | 0.20 | 0.62 | 19.0 | 20014 |
| **couscous**, cooked | 157 | 176 | 113.9 | 36.5 | 0.2 | 0 | 2.2 | 8 | 13 | 13 | 0.41 | 0.132 | 0 | 0 | 0.10 | 1.5 | 0 | 0.58 |
| 1 cup | | 6.0 | 0.3 | 0 | 0 | 0.1 | 0 | 91 | 35 | 0.60 | 0.064 | 43.2 | 0 | 0.2 | 0.04 | 0.08 | 23.6 | 20029 |
| **Cream of Rice cereal**, cooked | 244 | 127 | 213.5 | 27.8 | 0 | | 0.2 | 2 | 7 | 7 | 0.39 | 0.351 | 0 | 0 | 0 | 1.0 | 0 | 0.19 |
| 1 cup | | 2.2 | 0.2 | 0.1 | 0.1 | 0.1 | 0 | 49 | 41 | 0.49 | 0.083 | 7.3 | 0 | 0 | 0 | 0.07 | 7.3 | 8101 |
| **Maltex cereal**, cooked | 249 | 189 | 201.7 | 39.4 | 0.3 | | 2.2 | 12 | 22 | 57 | 1.87 | 0 | 0 | 0 | 0.21 | 2.1 | 0 | 0.35 |
| 1 cup | | 5.7 | 1.1 | 0.2 | 0.1 | 0.4 | 0 | 266 | 177 | 1.79 | 0.349 | 36.1 | 0 | 1.1 | 0.09 | 0.07 | 19.9 | 8115 |

| Food | WT (g) | KCAL / PRO (g) | H₂O (g) / FAT (g) | CHO (g) / SFA (g) | TSUG (g) / MUFA (g) | ASUG (g) / PUFA (g) | DFIB (g) / CHOL (mg) | Na (mg) / K (mg) | Ca (mg) / P (mg) | Mg (mg) / Fe (mg) | Zn (mg) / Cu (mg) | Mn (mg) / Se (mcg) | A (mcg RAE) / A (IU) | C (mg) / E (mg ATE) | B-1 (mg) / B-2 (mg) | NIA (mg) / B-6 (mg) | B-12 (mcg) / FOL (mcg DFE) | PANT (mg) / REF |
|---|---|---|---|---|---|---|---|---|---|---|---|---|---|---|---|---|---|---|
| **Maypo cereal**, cooked | 240 | 170 | 198.5 | 31.9 | 15.0 | | 5.8 | 10 | 125 | 50 | 1.49 | | 701 | 29 | 0.72 | 9.4 | 2.88 | 0.34 |
| *1 cup* | | 5.8 | 2.4 | 0.4 | 0.7 | 0.9 | 0 | 211 | 247 | 8.40 | 0.158 | 18.5 | 2338 | 0.2 | 0.72 | 0.96 | 9.6 | 8119 |
| millet, cooked | 174 | 207 | 124.3 | 41.2 | 0.2 | 0 | 2.3 | 3 | 5 | 77 | 1.58 | 0.473 | 0 | 0 | 0.18 | 2.3 | 0 | 0.30 |
| *1 cup* | | 6.1 | 1.7 | 0.3 | 0.3 | 0.9 | 0 | 108 | 174 | 1.10 | 0.280 | 1.6 | 5 | 0 | 0.14 | 0.19 | 33.1 | 20032 |
| **millet**, dry | 200 | 756 | 17.3 | 145.7 | | | 17.0 | 10 | 16 | 228 | 3.36 | 3.264 | 0 | 0 | 0.84 | 9.4 | 0 | 1.70 |
| *1 cup* | | 22.0 | 8.4 | 1.4 | 1.5 | 4.3 | 0 | 390 | 570 | 6.02 | 1.500 | 5.4 | | 0.1 | 0.58 | 0.77 | 170.0 | 20031 |
| **MultiGrain oatmeal**, dry, Quaker | 40 | 133 | 4.4 | 29.4 | 0.2 | | 4.8 | 1 | 14 | 46 | 1.28 | 1.048 | 0 | 0 | 0.12 | 1.4 | 0 | 0.20 |
| *½ cup (amount for 1 serving)* | | 4.5 | 1.0 | 0.2 | 0.2 | 0.5 | 0 | 164 | 138 | 1.19 | 0.176 | 17.8 | 4 | 0.3 | 0.05 | 0.10 | 10.4 | 8200 |
| **MultiGrain oatmeal**, prep with water, Quaker - *1 cup* | 234 | 143 | 195.6 | 31.6 | | | 5.1 | 7 | 19 | 51 | 1.43 | 1.128 | 0 | | 0.12 | 1.5 | 0 | 0.22 |
| | | 4.9 | 1.1 | 0.2 | 0.2 | 0.5 | 0 | 176 | 150 | 1.31 | 0.201 | | 2 | | 0.06 | 0.10 | 18.7 | 8249 |
| **Nestum cereal** (wheat with honey), prepared, Nestle - *1 cup* | 240 | 175 | 195.6 | 38.9 | 7.0 | | 1.0 | 79 | 259 | 19 | 0.26 | 0.250 | 374 | 15 | 0.38 | 5.1 | 0.41 | 0.68 |
| | | 3.4 | 0.6 | 0 | 0.2 | 0.3 | 0 | 60 | 134 | 12.19 | 0.360 | 10.3 | 1270 | 3.4 | 0.58 | 0.13 | 24.0 | 43306 |
| **oat bran cereal**, dry, Quaker/Mother's | 40 | 146 | 3.6 | 25.2 | 0.6 | | 5.7 | 2 | 32 | 96 | 1.68 | 2.280 | | 0 | 0.39 | 0.3 | 0 | 0.34 |
| *½ cup (amt for 1 srvng)* | | 6.8 | 3.2 | 0.6 | 1.0 | 1.2 | 0 | 232 | 278 | 3.23 | 0.120 | 0 | 40 | | 0.12 | 0.04 | 15.2 | 8231 |
| **oat bran cereal**, prepared w/wtr, Quaker/Mother's - *1 cup* | 234 | 101 | 208.4 | 17.5 | | | 4.0 | 7 | 26 | 70 | 1.24 | 1.589 | 2 | 0 | 0.27 | 0.2 | 0 | 0.24 |
| | | 4.8 | 2.2 | 0.4 | 0.7 | 0.8 | 0 | 161 | 194 | 2.27 | 0.096 | | 28 | | 0.08 | 0.03 | 11.7 | 8236 |
| **oat bran**, cooked | 219 | 88 | 184.0 | 25.1 | | | 5.7 | 2 | 22 | 88 | 1.16 | 2.111 | 0 | 0 | 0.35 | 0.3 | 0 | 0.48 |
| *1 cup* | | 7.0 | 1.9 | 0.4 | 0.6 | 0.7 | 0 | 201 | 261 | 1.93 | 0.145 | 16.9 | 0 | | 0.07 | 0.05 | 13.1 | 20034 |
| **oatmeal**, apl spice, inst, prep, Nutrition for Women - *1 pkt prep* | 166 | 178 | 121.6 | 34.9 | 16.0 | | 3.2 | 319 | 402 | 37 | 0.86 | 1.099 | 339 | 0 | 0.30 | 4.3 | 1.34 | 0.19 |
| | | 5.0 | 2.0 | 0.3 | 0.7 | 0.6 | 0 | 138 | 134 | 7.10 | 0.131 | 9.5 | 1125 | 5.3 | 0.36 | 0.79 | 260.6 | 8433 |
| **oatmeal**, apples and cinnamon, inst prepared, Quaker - *1 pkt prep* | 149 | 130 | 117.1 | 26.5 | 12.1 | | 2.7 | 165 | 110 | 28 | 0.64 | 0.854 | 322 | 0 | 0.29 | 4.1 | 0 | 0.16 |
| | | 2.7 | 1.5 | 0.2 | 0.5 | 0.4 | 0 | 109 | 94 | 3.84 | 0.082 | 7.6 | 1070 | 0.1 | 0.35 | 0.43 | 140.1 | 8125 |
| **oatmeal**, baked apple, instant, prep, Quaker - *1 packet prepared* | 159 | 153 | 121.3 | 30.9 | 14.0 | | 2.9 | 229 | 224 | 33 | 0.75 | 1.011 | 331 | 0 | 0.30 | 4.2 | 0 | 0.18 |
| | | 3.2 | 1.8 | 0.3 | 0.6 | 0.5 | 0 | 121 | 111 | 3.98 | 0.097 | 7.0 | 1103 | 0.2 | 0.35 | 0.44 | 143.1 | 8426 |
| **oatmeal**, cinnamon roll, instant, prep, Quaker Express - *1 pkt prep* | 173 | 209 | 122.4 | 41.3 | 16.8 | | 3.6 | 249 | 112 | 50 | 1.12 | 1.543 | 332 | 0 | 0.30 | 4.2 | 0 | 0.25 |
| | | 4.8 | 2.7 | 0.5 | 0.9 | 0.8 | 0 | 142 | 171 | 3.98 | 0.121 | 12.3 | 1104 | 0.2 | 0.35 | 0.44 | 141.9 | 8430 |
| **oatmeal**, cinnamon spice, instant, prepared - *1 packet prepared* | 161 | 172 | 118.8 | 34.6 | 15.2 | | 2.9 | 243 | 111 | 40 | 0.90 | 1.248 | 324 | 0 | 0.29 | 4.1 | 0 | 0.20 |
| | | 3.9 | 2.1 | 0.4 | 0.8 | 0.6 | 0 | 113 | 135 | 3.88 | 0.103 | 0 | 1077 | 0.2 | 0.35 | 0.43 | 138.5 | 8129 |
| **oatmeal**, cinnamon spice, instant, prepared, Quaker - *1 pkt prep* | 165 | 177 | 121.8 | 35.5 | 15.5 | | 3.0 | 249 | 114 | 41 | 0.92 | 1.279 | 332 | 0 | 0.30 | 4.2 | 0 | 0.21 |
| | | 4.0 | 2.2 | 0.4 | 0.8 | 0.6 | 0 | 116 | 139 | 3.98 | 0.106 | 0 | 1104 | 0.2 | 0.35 | 0.44 | 141.9 | 8423 |
| **oatmeal**, French vanilla, instant, prep, Quaker - *1 packet prep* | 162 | 165 | 121.7 | 32.7 | 12.8 | | 2.9 | 249 | 113 | 40 | 0.91 | 1.260 | 332 | 0 | 0.29 | 4.2 | 0 | 0.21 |
| | | 3.9 | 2.1 | 0.4 | 0.8 | 0.6 | 0 | 113 | 136 | 3.97 | 0.104 | 9.1 | 1103 | 0.2 | 0.36 | 0.44 | 142.6 | 8425 |
| **oatmeal**, fruit and cream, instant, dry, Quaker - *1.2 oz packet* | 35 | 135 | 2.2 | 26.2 | 10.9 | | 2.0 | 178 | 110 | 28 | 0.61 | 0.834 | 330 | 0 | 0.33 | 4.4 | 0.02 | 0.14 |
| | | 2.8 | 2.6 | 0.6 | 0.8 | 0.4 | 0 | 99 | 104 | 3.96 | 0.065 | 5.6 | 1100 | 0.2 | 0.37 | 0.44 | 143.8 | 8225 |
| **oatmeal**, fruit and cream, instant, prep, Quaker - *1 pkt prep* | 155 | 112 | 128.5 | 21.0 | 8.8 | | 1.7 | 146 | 91 | 23 | 0.50 | 0.671 | 265 | 0 | 0.24 | 3.4 | 0.02 | 0.11 |
| | | 2.2 | 2.1 | 0.4 | 0.7 | 0.4 | 0 | 79 | 84 | 3.19 | 0.060 | 4.5 | 884 | 0.1 | 0.28 | 0.35 | 116.2 | 8227 |
| **oatmeal**, golden brown sgr, inst, prep, Nutrition for Women - *1 pkt prep* | 165 | 173 | 121.8 | 33.1 | 12.9 | | 2.8 | 328 | 394 | 46 | 0.96 | 1.256 | 332 | 0 | 0.30 | 4.2 | 1.32 | 0.20 |
| | | 5.3 | 2.2 | 0.4 | 0.8 | 0.6 | 0 | 145 | 150 | 6.96 | 0.124 | 10.6 | 1104 | 5.2 | 0.35 | 0.77 | 255.8 | 8432 |
| **oatmeal**, golden brown sgr, inst, prep, Quaker Express - *1 pkt prep* | 173 | 209 | 122.3 | 41.7 | 17.6 | | 3.5 | 294 | 112 | 48 | 1.07 | 1.484 | 332 | 0 | 0.30 | 4.2 | 0 | 0.24 |
| | | 4.6 | 2.6 | 0.4 | 0.9 | 0.8 | 0 | 135 | 164 | 3.98 | 0.121 | 11.4 | 1104 | 0.2 | 0.35 | 0.44 | 141.9 | 8434 |
| **oatmeal**, honey nut, instant, prepared, Quaker - *1 pkt prep* | 162 | 173 | 121.5 | 31.3 | 12.9 | | 2.8 | 238 | 109 | 42 | 0.91 | 1.230 | 316 | 0 | 0.28 | 4.0 | 0 | 0.21 |
| | | 4.0 | 3.6 | 0.5 | 0.9 | 1.8 | 0 | 115 | 134 | 3.81 | 0.128 | 8.7 | 1055 | 0.3 | 0.34 | 0.42 | 136.1 | 8428 |
| **oatmeal**, instant, dry | 28 | 105 | 2.9 | 18.9 | 0.4 | 0 | 2.8 | 72 | 99 | 39 | 0.99 | 0.818 | 300 | 0 | 0.57 | 4.6 | 0 | 0.31 |
| *1 oz packet* | | 3.6 | 1.8 | 0.4 | 0.6 | 0.7 | 0 | 101 | 119 | 8.20 | 0.105 | 7.5 | 1000 | 0.1 | 0.34 | 0.45 | 129.9 | 8122 |
| **oatmeal**, instant, prepared | 234 | 159 | 196.6 | 27.3 | 1.1 | 0 | 4.0 | 115 | 187 | 61 | 1.45 | 1.306 | 435 | 0 | 0.61 | 7.1 | 0 | 0.74 |
| *1 cup* | | 5.5 | 3.2 | 0.6 | 0.9 | 1.0 | 0 | 143 | 180 | 13.95 | 0.154 | 11.7 | 1453 | 0.2 | 0.50 | 0.68 | 166.1 | 8123 |
| **oatmeal**, maple and brown sugar, inst, prep, Quaker - *1 pkt prep* | 155 | 157 | 116.5 | 31.1 | 12.6 | | 2.8 | 253 | 108 | 39 | 0.87 | 1.189 | 318 | 0 | 0.28 | 4.0 | 0 | 0.19 |
| | | 3.7 | 2.0 | 0.3 | 0.7 | 0.6 | 0 | 107 | 129 | 3.81 | 0.099 | 9.0 | 1056 | 0.2 | 0.34 | 0.42 | 138.0 | 8131 |
| **oatmeal**, quick, dry, Quaker | 40 | 148 | 3.7 | 27.3 | 0.6 | | 3.8 | 1 | 19 | 108 | 1.28 | 1.720 | 0 | 0 | 0.22 | 0.3 | 0 | 0.28 |
| *½ cup* | | 5.5 | 2.7 | 0.4 | 0.8 | 0.9 | 0 | 143 | 183 | 1.86 | 0.148 | 13.6 | 0 | 0.3 | 0.05 | 0.04 | 12.8 | 8402 |
| **oatmeal**, quick/regular, cooked | 234 | 166 | 195.6 | 28.1 | 0.6 | 0 | 4.0 | 9 | 21 | 63 | 2.34 | 1.357 | 0 | 0 | 0.18 | 0.5 | 0 | 0.73 |
| *1 cup* | | 5.9 | 3.6 | 0.7 | 1.0 | 1.3 | 0 | 164 | 180 | 2.11 | 0.173 | 12.6 | 0 | 0.2 | 0.04 | 0.01 | 14.0 | 8121 |
| **oatmeal**, quick/regular, dry | 27 | 102 | 2.9 | 18.3 | 0.3 | 0 | 2.7 | 2 | 14 | 37 | 0.98 | 0.980 | 0 | 0 | 0.12 | 0.3 | 0 | 0.30 |
| *⅓ cup (.95 oz)* | | 3.6 | 1.8 | 0.3 | 0.5 | 0.6 | 0 | 98 | 111 | 1.15 | 0.106 | 7.8 | 0 | 0.1 | 0.04 | 0.03 | 8.6 | 8120 |
| **oatmeal**, raisin and spice, instant, prepared, Quaker - *1 pkt prep* | 162 | 162 | 122.3 | 32.9 | 15.7 | | 2.6 | 245 | 113 | 36 | 0.75 | 1.014 | 330 | 0 | 0.29 | 4.2 | 0 | 0.16 |
| | | 3.4 | 1.8 | 0.3 | 0.6 | 0.6 | 0 | 156 | 115 | 3.97 | 0.112 | 9.4 | 1103 | 0.2 | 0.35 | 0.44 | 140.9 | 8437 |
| **oatmeal**, raisins and spice, instant, prepared - *1 packet prepared* | 158 | 158 | 119.3 | 32.1 | 15.3 | | 2.5 | 239 | 111 | 35 | 0.73 | 0.989 | 322 | 0 | 0.29 | 4.1 | 0 | 0.16 |
| | | 3.3 | 1.8 | 0.3 | 0.6 | 0.6 | 0 | 152 | 112 | 3.87 | 0.109 | | 1076 | 0.2 | 0.34 | 0.43 | 137.5 | 8133 |
| **oatmeal**, raisins, dates, walnuts, inst, prep, Quaker - *1 pkt prep* | 161 | 187 | 113.7 | 37.8 | | | 3.4 | 333 | 150 | 47 | 1.03 | 1.367 | 438 | 0 | 0.43 | 5.8 | 0 | 0.23 |
| | | 4.6 | 2.8 | 0.5 | 0.9 | 1.1 | 0 | 180 | 151 | 5.57 | 0.140 | | 1457 | | 0.49 | 0.59 | 188.4 | 8235 |

| Food | WT (g) | KCAL | H₂O (g) | CHO (g) | TSUG (g) | ASUG (g) | DFIB (g) | Na (mg) | Ca (mg) | Mg (mg) | Zn (mg) | Mn (mg) | A (mcg RAE) | C (mg) | B-1 (mg) | NIA (mg) | B-12 (mcg) | PANT (mg) |
|---|---|---|---|---|---|---|---|---|---|---|---|---|---|---|---|---|---|---|
|  |  | PRO (g) | FAT (g) | SFA (g) | MUFA (g) | PUFA (g) | CHOL (mg) | K (mg) | P (mg) | Fe (mg) | Cu (mg) | Se (mcg) | A (IU) | E (mg ATE) | B-2 (mg) | B-6 (mg) | FOL (mcg DFE) | REF |
| oatmeal, treasure hunt, instant, prepared, Quaker - 1 pkt prep | 166 | 179 | 122.1 | 36.3 | 17.0 |  | 2.7 | 257 | 108 | 43 | 0.85 | 1.160 | 334 | 0 | 0.28 | 4.2 | 0 | 0.19 |
|  |  | 3.6 | 2.2 | 0.5 | 0.7 | 0.6 | 0 | 105 | 126 | 3.80 | 0.093 | 9.0 | 1111 | 0.2 | 0.36 | 0.44 | 142.8 | 8427 |
| oatmeal, vanilla cinn, prep, Nutrition for Women - 1 pkt prep | 162 | 168 | 120.2 | 32.1 | 13.1 |  | 2.8 | 287 | 389 | 40 | 0.94 | 1.204 | 327 | 0 | 0.29 | 4.1 | 1.31 | 0.20 |
|  |  | 5.2 | 2.1 | 0.4 | 0.7 | 0.6 | 0 | 118 | 143 | 6.89 | 0.123 | 10.0 | 1090 | 5.2 | 0.35 | 0.76 | 252.7 | 8431 |
| oats, whole grain, dry - 1 cup | 156 | 607 | 12.8 | 103.4 |  |  | 16.5 | 3 | 84 | 276 | 6.19 | 7.669 | 0 | 0 | 1.19 | 1.5 | 0 | 2.10 |
|  |  | 26.3 | 10.8 | 1.9 | 3.4 | 4.0 | 0 | 669 | 816 | 7.36 | 0.977 |  | 0 |  | 0.22 | 0.19 | 87.4 | 20038 |
| quinoa, dry - 1 cup | 170 | 626 | 22.6 | 109.1 |  |  | 11.9 | 8 | 80 | 335 | 5.27 | 3.456 | 2 | 0 | 0.61 | 2.6 | 0 | 1.31 |
|  |  | 24.0 | 10.3 | 1.2 | 2.7 | 5.6 | 0 | 957 | 777 | 7.77 | 1.003 | 14.4 | 24 | 4.1 | 0.54 | 0.83 | 312.8 | 20035 |
| Ralston cereal, cooked - 1 cup | 253 | 134 | 217.8 | 28.3 |  |  | 6.1 | 5 | 13 | 58 | 1.42 |  | 0 | 0 | 0.20 | 2.0 | 0.10 | 0.33 |
|  |  | 5.6 | 0.8 | 0.1 | 0.1 | 0.4 | 0 | 154 | 147 | 1.64 | 0.200 |  | 0 |  | 0.18 | 0.11 | 17.7 | 8135 |
| rice, brown, long grain, boiled - 1 cup | 195 | 216 | 142.5 | 44.8 | 0.7 | 0 | 3.5 | 10 | 20 | 84 | 1.23 | 1.765 | 0 | 0 | 0.19 | 3.0 | 0 | 0.56 |
|  |  | 5.0 | 1.8 | 0.4 | 0.6 | 0.6 | 0 | 84 | 162 | 0.82 | 0.195 | 19.1 | 0 | 0.1 | 0.05 | 0.28 | 7.8 | 20037 |
| rice, brown, medium grain, boiled - 1 cup | 195 | 218 | 142.3 | 45.8 |  |  | 3.5 | 2 | 20 | 86 | 1.21 | 2.139 | 0 | 0 | 0.20 | 2.6 | 0 | 0.76 |
|  |  | 4.5 | 1.6 | 0.3 | 0.6 | 0.6 | 0 | 154 | 150 | 1.03 | 0.158 |  | 0 |  | 0.02 | 0.29 | 7.8 | 20041 |
| rice medley, frozen, Green Giant - 10 oz package | 283 | 250 |  | 48.0 | 3.0 |  | 3.0 | 930 | 40 |  |  |  |  | 5 |  |  |  |  |
|  |  | 7.0 | 3.5 | 0.5 |  |  | 0 |  |  |  | 1.08 |  | 200 |  |  |  |  | GENM3 |
| rice pilaf, frozen, Green Giant - 10 oz package | 283 | 200 |  | 40.0 | 3.0 |  | 3.0 | 1080 | 60 |  |  |  |  | 4 |  |  |  |  |
|  |  | 5.0 | 3.0 | 1.5 |  |  | 5 |  |  |  | 3.60 |  | 1750 |  |  |  |  | GENM5 |
| rice, white and wild, frozen, Green Giant - 10 oz package | 283 | 260 |  | 48.0 | 3.0 |  | 3.0 | 1260 | 60 |  |  |  |  | 4 |  |  |  |  |
|  |  | 6.0 | 5.0 | 1.0 |  |  | 0 |  |  |  | 1.08 |  | 100 |  |  |  |  | GENM6 |
| rice, white, enriched, dry - ½ cup | 98 | 358 | 11.4 | 78.4 | 0.1 | 0 | 1.3 | 5 | 27 | 24 | 1.07 | 1.066 | 0 | 0 | 0.56 | 4.1 | 0 | 0.99 |
|  |  | 7.0 | 0.6 | 0.2 | 0.2 | 0.2 | 0 | 113 | 113 | 4.22 | 0.216 | 14.8 | 0 | 0.1 | 0.05 | 0.16 | 379.3 | 20044 |
| rice, white, glutinous, enriched, boiled - 1 cup | 174 | 169 | 133.3 | 36.7 | 0.1 | 0 | 1.7 | 9 | 3 | 9 | 0.71 | 0.456 | 0 | 0 | 0.03 | 0.5 | 0 | 0.37 |
|  |  | 3.5 | 0.3 | 0.1 | 0.1 | 0.1 | 0 | 17 | 14 | 0.24 | 0.085 | 9.7 | 0 | 0.1 | 0.02 | 0.05 | 1.7 | 20055 |
| rice, white, long grain, enriched, boiled - 1 cup | 186 | 242 | 127.3 | 52.4 | 0.1 | 0 | 0.7 | 2 | 19 | 22 | 0.91 | 0.878 | 0 | 0 | 0.30 | 2.7 | 0 | 0.73 |
|  |  | 5.0 | 0.5 | 0.1 | 0.2 | 0.1 | 0 | 65 | 80 | 2.23 | 0.128 | 14.0 | 0 | 0.1 | 0.02 | 0.17 | 180.4 | 20045 |
| rice, white, long grain, enriched, instant, boiled - 1 cup | 165 | 193 | 118.8 | 41.4 | 0 | 0 | 1.0 | 7 | 13 | 8 | 0.81 | 0.566 | 0 | 0 | 0.12 | 2.9 | 0 | 0.09 |
|  |  | 3.6 | 0.8 | 0 | 0.1 | 0 | 0 | 15 | 61 | 2.92 | 0.061 | 7.9 | 0 |  | 0.01 | 0.08 | 194.7 | 20049 |
| rice, white, long grain, enriched, parboiled, boiled - 1 cup | 175 | 215 | 123.1 | 45.6 | 0.2 | 0 | 1.6 | 4 | 33 | 16 | 0.65 | 0.619 | 0 | 0 | 0.37 | 4.0 | 0 | 0.57 |
|  |  | 5.1 | 0.6 | 0.1 | 0.1 | 0.2 | 0 | 98 | 96 | 3.17 | 0.123 | 16.3 | 0 |  | 0.03 | 0.27 | 238.0 | 20047 |
| rice, white, medium grain, enriched, boiled - 1 cup | 186 | 242 | 127.6 | 53.2 |  |  | 0.6 | 0 | 6 | 24 | 0.78 | 0.701 | 0 | 0 | 0.31 | 3.4 | 0 | 0.76 |
|  |  | 4.4 | 0.4 | 0.1 | 0.1 | 0.1 | 0 | 54 | 69 | 2.77 | 0.071 | 14.0 | 0 |  | 0.03 | 0.09 | 180.4 | 20051 |
| rice, white, short grain, enriched, boiled - 1 cup | 186 | 242 | 127.5 | 53.4 |  |  |  | 0 | 2 | 15 | 0.74 | 0.664 | 0 | 0 | 0.31 | 2.8 | 0 | 0.74 |
|  |  | 4.4 | 0.4 | 0.1 | 0.1 | 0.1 | 0 | 48 | 61 | 2.72 | 0.134 | 14.0 | 0 |  | 0.03 | 0.11 | 184.1 | 20053 |
| Roman Meal cereal, cooked - 1 cup | 241 | 147 | 199.3 | 33.0 |  |  | 8.2 | 2 | 29 | 108 | 1.78 |  | 0 | 0 | 0.24 | 3.1 | 0 | 0.37 |
|  |  | 6.5 | 1.0 | 0.1 |  |  | 0 | 301 | 214 | 2.12 | 0.321 |  | 0 |  | 0.12 | 0.11 | 24.1 | 8137 |
| Roman Meal cereal with oats, cooked - 1 cup | 240 | 170 | 195.6 | 34.1 |  |  | 7.0 | 10 | 26 | 74 | 1.94 |  | 0 | 0 | 0.31 | 3.3 | 0 | 0.25 |
|  |  | 7.2 | 1.9 | 0.2 |  |  | 0 | 257 | 235 | 1.39 | 0.149 |  | 22 |  | 0.22 | 0.38 | 24.0 | 8155 |
| rye, whole grain, dry - 1 cup | 169 | 566 | 18.5 | 117.9 | 1.8 | 0 | 24.7 | 10 | 56 | 204 | 6.30 | 4.529 | 2 | 0 | 0.53 | 7.2 | 0 | 2.46 |
|  |  | 24.9 | 4.2 | 0.5 | 0.5 | 1.9 | 0 | 446 | 632 | 4.51 | 0.760 | 59.7 | 19 | 2.2 | 0.42 | 0.50 | 101.4 | 20062 |
| sorghum grain, dry - 1 cup | 192 | 651 | 17.7 | 143.3 |  |  | 12.1 | 12 | 54 |  |  |  | 0 | 0 | 0.46 | 5.6 | 0 |  |
|  |  | 21.7 | 6.3 | 0.9 | 1.9 | 2.6 | 0 | 672 | 551 | 8.45 |  |  | 0 |  | 0.27 |  |  | 20067 |
| wheat cereal, apl, ban, maple, inst, enr, prep, Crm of Wht - 1 pkt prep | 150 | 132 | 117.4 | 29.0 |  |  | 0.4 | 242 | 40 | 9 | 0.22 |  | 375 | 0 | 0.45 | 4.9 | 0 | 0.12 |
|  |  | 2.4 | 0.4 | 0.1 |  |  | 0 | 56 | 20 | 8.10 | 0.057 |  | 1251 |  | 0.30 | 0.45 | 165.0 | 8111 |
| wheat cereal, cinnamon, enr, dry Creamy Wheat, Quaker - ¼ cup | 44 | 152 | 5.3 | 32.8 | 0.1 |  | 1.6 | 1 | 15 | 6 | 0.24 | 0.119 | 0 | 0 | 0.19 | 1.5 | 0 | 0.16 |
|  |  | 5.3 | 0.3 | 0.1 |  |  | 0 | 46 | 39 | 13.20 | 0.031 | 0 | 2 |  | 0.11 | 0.02 |  | 8317 |
| wheat cereal, dry, Malt-O-Meal - 3 T (1.2 oz) | 35 | 127 | 3.4 | 26.0 | 0.2 |  | 1.4 | 4 | 132 |  |  |  | 0 |  | 0.58 | 4.6 |  |  |
|  |  | 4.7 | 0.4 | 0.1 | 0.1 | 0.3 | 0 | 49 |  | 13.86 |  |  | 35 |  | 0.34 | 0.65 | 582.0 | 8488 |
| wheat cereal, enriched, cooked - 1 cup | 233 | 112 | 204.8 | 24.4 | 0.1 | 0 | 0.7 | 5 | 9 | 5 | 0.19 | 0.217 | 0 | 0 | 0.14 | 1.1 | 0 | 0.13 |
|  |  | 3.3 | 0.2 | 0 | 0 | 0.1 | 0 | 30 | 28 | 1.16 | 0.037 | 21.2 | 0 |  | 0.10 | 0.02 | 132.8 | 8113 |
| wheat cereal, enriched, dry, Creamy Wheat, Quaker - ¼ cup | 44 | 154 | 5.1 | 33.5 | 0.1 |  | 1.3 | 1 | 5 | 7 | 0.27 | 0.123 | 0 | 0 | 0.19 | 1.5 | 0 | 0.19 |
|  |  | 4.8 | 0.4 | 0.1 | 0 | 0.2 | 0 | 43 | 37 | 13.20 | 0.053 |  | 0 |  | 0.11 | 0.02 | 108.2 | 8230 |
| wheat cereal, enr, prep, Creamy Wheat, Quaker - 1 cup | 233 | 119 | 202.7 | 26.2 |  |  | 0.9 | 7 | 9 | 7 | 0.23 | 0.096 | 0 | 0 | 0.16 | 1.8 | 0 | 0.12 |
|  |  | 3.6 | 0.2 | 0 | 0.1 | 0.1 | 0 | 33 | 30 | 11.02 | 0.035 |  | 0 |  | 0.11 | 0.02 | 86.2 | 8237 |
| wheat cereal, inst, enr, prep, Crm of Wht Mix & Eat - 1 pkt prep | 142 | 102 | 116.6 | 21.4 |  |  | 0.4 | 241 | 20 | 7 | 0.24 |  | 376 | 0 | 0.43 | 5.0 | 0 | 0.13 |
|  |  | 2.7 | 0.3 | 0 | 0 | 0.2 | 0 | 38 | 20 | 8.09 | 0.041 |  | 1252 |  | 0.28 | 0.57 | 164.7 | 8109 |
| wheat cereal, instant, enr, prep Cream of Wheat - 1 cup | 240 | 149 | 202.6 | 31.4 | 0.2 |  | 1.4 | 10 | 154 | 14 | 0.41 | 0 | 557 | 0 | 0.56 | 7.4 | 0 | 0.17 |
|  |  | 4.4 | 0.6 | 0.1 | 0.1 | 0.3 | 0 | 48 | 43 | 11.90 | 0.103 | 8.4 | 1855 |  | 0.50 | 0.74 | 242.4 | 8107 |
| wheat cereal, quick, enr, ckd, Cream of Wheat - 1 cup | 239 | 129 | 207.0 | 26.8 |  |  | 1.2 | 139 | 50 | 12 | 0.33 |  | 0 | 0 | 0.24 | 1.4 | 0 | 0.17 |
|  |  | 3.6 | 0.5 | 0.1 | 0.1 | 0.3 | 0 | 45 | 100 | 10.28 | 0.067 | 30.6 | 0 | 0 | 0.03 | 176.9 |  | 8105 |

| | WT | Macronutrients | | | | | | Minerals | | | | | Vitamins | | | | | |
|---|---|---|---|---|---|---|---|---|---|---|---|---|---|---|---|---|---|---|
| | (g) | KCAL | $H_2O$ (g) | CHO (g) | TSUG (g) | ASUG (g) | DFIB (g) | Na (mg) | Ca (mg) | Mg (mg) | Zn (mg) | Mn (mg) | A (mcg RAE) | C (mg) | B-1 (mg) | NIA (mg) | B-12 (mcg) | PANT (mg) |
| | | PRO (g) | FAT (g) | SFA (g) | MUFA (g) | PUFA (g) | CHOL (mg) | K (mg) | P (mg) | Fe (mg) | Cu (mg) | Se (mcg) | A (IU) | E (mg ATE) | B-2 (mg) | B-6 (mg) | FOL (mcg DFE) | REF |
| **wheat cereal**, regular, enr, cooked, | 242 | 126 | 210.8 | 26.6 | 0.1 | | 1.2 | 7 | 111 | 10 | 0.31 | 0 | 0 | 0 | 0.17 | 1.5 | 0 | 0.18 |
| Cream of Wheat - *1 cup* | | 3.7 | 0.5 | 0.1 | 0.1 | 0.3 | 0 | 41 | 41 | 9.97 | 0.085 | 7.0 | 0 | 0 | 0.07 | 0.04 | 62.9 | 8103 |
| **Wheatena cereal**, cooked | 243 | 136 | 207.5 | 28.7 | | | 6.6 | 5 | 10 | 49 | 1.68 | 1.997 | 0 | 0 | 0.02 | 1.3 | 0 | 0.10 |
| *1 cup* | | 4.9 | 1.2 | 0.2 | 0.2 | 0.6 | 0 | 187 | 146 | 1.36 | 0.126 | | 0 | | 0.05 | 0.05 | 17.0 | 8143 |
| **Whole Wheat Hot Natural Cereal**, | 242 | 150 | 202.3 | 33.2 | 0.2 | | 3.9 | 0 | 17 | 53 | 1.16 | | 0 | 0 | 0.17 | 2.2 | 0 | |
| cooked - *1 cup* | | 4.8 | 1.0 | 0.1 | 0.1 | 0.5 | 0 | 172 | 167 | 1.50 | 0.201 | 31.0 | 0 | 0.6 | 0.12 | 0.18 | 33.9 | 8145 |
| **wild rice**, boiled | 164 | 166 | 121.2 | 35.0 | 1.2 | 0 | 3.0 | 5 | 5 | 52 | 2.20 | 0.462 | 0 | 0 | 0.09 | 2.1 | 0 | 0.25 |
| *1 cup* | | 6.5 | 0.6 | 0.1 | 0.1 | 0.3 | 0 | 166 | 134 | 0.98 | 0.198 | 1.3 | 5 | 0.4 | 0.14 | 0.22 | 42.6 | 20089 |

## 4. CEREALS, READY-TO-EAT

| | | | | | | | | | | | | | | | | | | |
|---|---|---|---|---|---|---|---|---|---|---|---|---|---|---|---|---|---|---|
| **All-Bran** Buds, Kellogg's | 30 | 75 | 0.9 | 24.0 | 8.1 | | 12.9 | 203 | 19 | 62 | 1.50 | 2.461 | 153 | 6 | 0.36 | 5.1 | 6.00 | 0.45 |
| *⅓ cup (1.1 oz)* | | 2.1 | 0.6 | 0.1 | 0.2 | 0.4 | 0 | 300 | 150 | 4.50 | 0.144 | 8.7 | 510 | 0.5 | 0.42 | 2.01 | 677.4 | 8005 |
| **All-Bran**, Kellogg's | 31 | 81 | 0.7 | 23.0 | 4.9 | | 9.1 | 75 | 121 | 112 | 3.84 | 2.297 | 163 | 6 | 0.70 | 4.6 | 5.83 | 0.33 |
| *½ cup (1.1 oz)* | | 4.1 | 1.5 | 0.2 | 0.2 | 0.7 | 0 | 316 | 356 | 5.46 | 0.322 | 2.9 | 542 | 0.4 | 0.84 | 3.72 | 681.4 | 8001 |
| **All-Bran** with extra fiber, Kellogg's | 26 | 50 | 0.8 | 20.0 | 0.1 | | 13.0 | 124 | 108 | 88 | 1.56 | 1.887 | 160 | 6 | 0.39 | 5.2 | 6.24 | 0.41 |
| *½ cup (.92 oz)* | | 2.9 | 0.9 | 0.2 | 0.2 | 0.6 | 0 | 273 | 234 | 4.68 | 0.156 | 2.4 | 532 | 0.6 | 0.44 | 2.08 | 178.1 | 8253 |
| **All-Bran** Yogurt Bites, Kellogg's | 56 | 192 | 1.3 | 44.1 | 7.3 | | 10.1 | 235 | 36 | 85 | 3.92 | | | 6 | 0.39 | 5.0 | 6.16 | 0 |
| *1¼ cup (2 oz)* | | 6.2 | 2.9 | 1.7 | 0.3 | 0.8 | 0 | 292 | 248 | 4.48 | 0.224 | | 509 | 0 | 0.45 | 2.02 | | 8518 |
| **Alpen**, Barbara's Bakery | 55 | 200 | | 41.0 | 11.0 | | 4.0 | 30 | 60 | 60 | 3.75 | | | 15 | 0.38 | 5.0 | | |
| *⅔ cup* | | 6.0 | 3.0 | 0 | | | 0 | 240 | 200 | 8.10 | | | 1250 | | 0.42 | 0.50 | | BARB5 |
| **Alpen**, Weetabix Co | 113 | 398 | 8.4 | 85.5 | 22.6 | | 10.3 | 241 | 166 | 106 | 3.39 | | 0 | 10 | 0.45 | 2.4 | 0.14 | |
| *1 cup (4 oz)* | | 12.7 | 3.7 | 0.6 | 1.5 | 1.0 | 0 | 642 | 419 | 3.39 | 0.339 | 19.5 | 0 | 0.6 | 0.45 | 0.32 | 33.9 | 43218 |
| **Alpha-Bits**, frosted, Post | 32 | 130 | 0.4 | 26.7 | 12.5 | | 1.3 | 212 | 10 | 25 | 1.50 | | | 0 | 0.37 | 5.0 | 1.50 | |
| *1 cup (1.1 oz)* | | 2.7 | 1.3 | 0.3 | | | 0 | 62 | 67 | 2.70 | 0.099 | | 750 | | 0.43 | 0.50 | 165.4 | 8325 |
| **Alpha-Bits**, marshmallow, Post | 29 | 115 | 0.4 | 25.1 | 12.6 | | 0.5 | 206 | 4 | 12 | 1.50 | | | 0 | 0.37 | 5.0 | 1.50 | |
| *1 cup (1 oz)* | | 1.7 | 1.0 | 0.2 | | | 0 | 29 | 38 | 2.70 | 0.029 | | 750 | | 0.43 | 0.50 | 166.2 | 8326 |
| **Apple Cinnamon O's**, organic, | 30 | 110 | | 24.0 | 11.0 | | 2.0 | 85 | 100 | | | | | 15 | 0.38 | 5.0 | 1.50 | |
| Barbara's Bakery - *¾ cup* | | 3.0 | 1.5 | 0 | | | 0 | 85 | 0 | 8.10 | | | 1250 | | 0.42 | 0.50 | | BARB6 |
| **Apple Cinnamon Squares**, | 55 | 182 | 5.2 | 44.1 | 11.7 | | 4.7 | 20 | 21 | 48 | 1.49 | 1.701 | 0 | 0 | 0.38 | 5.0 | 1.49 | 0.35 |
| Kellogg's - *¾ cup (1.9 oz)* | | 4.0 | 1.0 | 0.2 | 0.3 | 0.5 | 0 | 166 | 154 | 16.23 | 0.110 | 2.3 | 0 | 0.3 | 0.44 | 0.50 | 179.9 | 8254 |
| **Apple Jacks**, Kellogg's | 30 | 117 | 0.9 | 27.0 | 12.5 | | 0.5 | 133 | 3 | 6 | 2.26 | 0.163 | 241 | 18 | 0.52 | 8.1 | 1.80 | 0.10 |
| *1 cup (1.1 oz)* | | 1.3 | 0.4 | 0.1 | 0.1 | 0.1 | 0 | 32 | 23 | 5.60 | 0.028 | 1.7 | 819 | 0 | 0.66 | 0.76 | 197.7 | 8003 |
| **Apple Zaps**, Quaker | 30 | 118 | 0.8 | 26.6 | 14.1 | | 0.7 | 135 | 3 | 15 | 4.12 | 0.105 | 165 | 7 | 0.41 | 5.5 | 0 | 0.10 |
| *¾ cup (1.1 oz)* | | 1.1 | 1.0 | 0.3 | 0.2 | 0.2 | 0 | 52 | 45 | 4.95 | 0.042 | 0 | 550 | | 0.46 | 0.55 | 710.1 | 8293 |
| **Apple Zings**, Malt-O-Meal | 33 | 130 | 0.7 | 28.8 | 14.2 | | 0.9 | 170 | 142 | 12 | 4.75 | 0.270 | 277 | 20 | 0.44 | 6.6 | 2.13 | |
| *1 cup (1.2 oz)* | | 1.8 | 0.9 | 0.1 | 0.4 | 0.3 | 0 | 46 | 41 | 5.64 | 0.043 | 4.7 | 921 | 0.1 | 0.65 | 0.86 | 192.1 | 8493 |
| **Banana Nut Crunch**, Post | 59 | 249 | 2.7 | 43.7 | 12.0 | | 4.0 | 253 | 21 | 48 | 1.50 | | | 0 | 0.38 | 5.0 | 1.50 | |
| *1 cup (2.1 oz)* | | 5.0 | 6.1 | 0.8 | | | 0 | 171 | 183 | 16.20 | 0.226 | | 750 | | 0.42 | 0.50 | 161.7 | 8320 |
| **Basic 4**, General Mills | 55 | 210 | 2.2 | 44.0 | 14.0 | | 3.2 | 320 | 250 | 32 | 3.75 | 0.547 | 150 | 0 | 0.37 | 5.0 | 1.50 | 0.27 |
| *1 cup (1.9 oz)* | | 4.0 | 3.0 | 0.5 | 1.0 | 0.5 | 0 | 150 | 100 | 4.50 | 0.080 | 9.4 | 500 | 0.6 | 0.42 | 0.50 | 162.8 | 8262 |
| **Blueberry Morning**, Post | 55 | 211 | 4.0 | 43.4 | 11.4 | | 2.1 | 266 | 15 | 24 | 0.90 | | | 0 | 0.37 | 5.0 | 1.50 | |
| *1¼ cups (1.9 oz)* | | 3.6 | 2.5 | 0.3 | | | 0 | 91 | 70 | 1.80 | 0.074 | | 750 | | 0.42 | 0.50 | 162.8 | 8321 |
| **Blueberry Muffin Tops Cereal**, | 30 | 133 | 0.3 | 24.0 | 10.6 | | 1.4 | 124 | 107 | 12 | 4.11 | 0.128 | 189 | 11 | 0.47 | 6.2 | 2.31 | 0.08 |
| Malt-O-Meal - *¾ cup (1.1 oz)* | | 1.5 | 3.4 | 0.6 | 1.3 | 1.4 | 0 | 47 | 87 | 5.01 | 0.051 | 5.0 | 630 | 0.3 | 0.47 | 0.73 | 252.0 | 8487 |
| **Boo Berry**, General Mills | 30 | 120 | 0.6 | 26.6 | 14.0 | | 0.3 | 190 | 20 | 0 | 3.75 | 0.012 | 1 | 6 | 0.38 | 5.0 | 1.50 | 0.03 |
| *1 cup (1.1 oz)* | | 1.0 | 1.0 | 0.2 | 0.5 | 0 | 0 | 35 | 20 | 4.50 | 0.017 | 2.0 | 18 | 0.2 | 0.43 | 0.50 | 165.9 | 8273 |
| **Bran, 100%**, Post | 29 | 83 | 0.8 | 22.7 | 7.1 | | 8.3 | 121 | 22 | 81 | 3.75 | | | 0 | 0.37 | 5.0 | 0 | |
| *⅓ cup (1 oz)* | | 3.7 | 0.6 | 0.1 | | | 0 | 275 | 236 | 8.10 | 0.266 | | 750 | | 0.43 | 0.50 | 166.2 | 8343 |
| **Bran Flakes**, high fiber, | 29 | 113 | 0.7 | 23.4 | 5.7 | | 4.3 | 195 | 13 | 49 | 3.89 | 1.890 | | 17 | 0.45 | 8.8 | 8.21 | 0.39 |
| Malt-O-Meal *¾ cup (1 oz)* | | 3.1 | 0.7 | 0.2 | 0.1 | 0.4 | 0 | 173 | 140 | 10.21 | 0.151 | 18.3 | 1714 | 7.7 | 0.59 | 2.81 | | 8490 |
| **Bran Flakes**, Post | 30 | 96 | 1.1 | 24.1 | 5.7 | | 5.3 | 220 | 17 | 64 | 1.50 | | | 0 | 0.38 | 5.0 | 1.50 | |
| *¾ cup (1.1 oz)* | | 2.8 | 0.7 | 0.1 | | | 0 | 185 | 152 | 8.10 | 0.193 | | 750 | | 0.43 | 0.50 | 165.9 | 8322 |
| **Bran flakes**, Ralston | 29 | 90 | 0.7 | 23.1 | 5.0 | | 4.9 | 236 | 13 | 55 | 18.66 | 1.005 | 154 | 70 | 1.37 | 26.3 | | 8.64 |
| *¾ cup (1 oz)* | | 3.0 | 1.0 | 0.1 | 0.1 | 0.4 | | 183 | 155 | 19.62 | 0.156 | 2.7 | 514 | 23.3 | 2.11 | 1.97 | | 8504 |
| **Breakfast O's**, organic, Barbara's | 30 | 120 | | 22.0 | 1.0 | | 3.0 | 125 | 0 | 40 | | | | 0 | | | | |
| Bakery - *1 cup (1.1 oz)* | | 4.0 | 2.0 | 0 | | | 0 | 80 | | 0.72 | | | 0 | | | | | BARB7 |
| **Brown Rice Crisps**, organic, Barbara's | 30 | 120 | | 25.0 | 2.0 | | 1.0 | 125 | 0 | | | | | 0 | | | | |
| Bakery - *1 cup (1.1 oz)* | | 2.0 | 1.0 | 0 | | | 0 | 110 | | 0.36 | | | 0 | | | | | BARB8 |
| **Brown Sugar Bliss Oatmeal**, | 49 | 188 | 1.2 | 39.0 | | | 3.6 | 249 | 146 | 51 | 5.88 | 1.387 | 235 | 2 | 0.59 | 7.8 | 0 | 0.30 |
| Quaker - *1 cup (1.7 oz)* | | 4.3 | 2.7 | 0.6 | 0.8 | 0.7 | 0 | 160 | 155 | 4.95 | 0.167 | 1.1 | 784 | | 0.67 | 0.78 | 734.0 | 8360 |

| Food | WT (g) | KCAL / PRO (g) | $H_2O$ / FAT (g) | CHO / SFA (g) | TSUG / MUFA (g) | ASUG / PUFA (g) | DFIB / CHOL (g / mg) | Na / K (mg) | Ca / P (mg) | Mg / Fe (mg) | Zn / Cu (mg) | Mn / Se (mg / mcg) | A (mcg RAE) / A (IU) | C (mg) / E (mg ATE) | B-1 / B-2 (mg) | NIA / B-6 (mg) | B-12 (mcg) / FOL (mcg DFE) | PANT (mg) / REF |
|---|---|---|---|---|---|---|---|---|---|---|---|---|---|---|---|---|---|---|
| Cap'n Crunch Crunchberries, Quaker - ¾ cup (.92 oz) | 26 | 105 | 0.6 | 22.1 | 11.6 |  | 0.6 | 182 | 4 | 14 | 4.18 | 0.166 | 2 | 0 | 0.42 | 5.5 | 0 | 0.10 |
|  |  | 1.1 | 1.5 | 1.0 | 0.2 | 0.2 | 0 | 49 | 43 | 5.02 | 0.039 | 0 | 37 | 0.2 | 0.47 | 0.55 | 676.5 | 8011 |
| Cap'n Crunch Peanut Butter Crunch, Quaker) - ¾ cup (.95 oz) | 27 | 112 | 0.7 | 21.3 | 8.9 |  | 0.7 | 200 | 2 | 19 | 4.13 | 0.194 | 2 | 0 | 0.41 | 5.5 | 0 | 0.13 |
|  |  | 1.9 | 2.5 | 1.1 | 0.7 | 0.6 | 0 | 64 | 53 | 4.96 | 0.054 | 0 | 41 | 0.2 | 0.47 | 0.55 | 709.8 | 8012 |
| Cap'n Crunch, Quaker ¾ cup (.95 oz) | 27 | 109 | 0.7 | 22.9 | 11.8 |  | 0.7 | 202 | 3 | 15 | 4.32 | 0.176 | 2 | 0 | 0.43 | 5.7 | 0 | 0.10 |
|  |  | 1.2 | 1.6 | 1.1 | 0.2 | 0.2 | 0 | 50 | 45 | 5.19 | 0.040 | 1.8 | 40 | 0.2 | 0.49 | 0.57 | 710.1 | 8010 |
| Cheerios, apple cinnamon, General Mills - ¾ cup (1.1 oz) | 30 | 120 | 0.7 | 25.0 | 13.0 |  | 1.2 | 120 | 100 | 16 | 3.75 | 0.454 | 150 | 6 | 0.38 | 5.0 | 1.50 | 0.16 |
|  |  | 2.0 | 1.5 | 0 | 1.0 | 0.5 | 0 | 60 | 60 | 4.50 | 0.050 | 11.2 | 500 | 0.2 | 0.43 | 0.50 | 336.3 | 8263 |
| Cheerios, berry burst, General Mills - 1 cup (1.1 oz) | 30 | 110 | 0.6 | 24.0 | 9.3 |  | 2.2 | 180 | 111 | 32 | 4.17 | 0.771 | 167 | 21 | 0.42 | 5.6 | 1.67 | 0.26 |
|  |  | 3.0 | 1.2 | 0 | 0.8 | 0.4 | 0 | 78 | 60 | 5.00 | 0.073 | 11.2 | 556 | 0.2 | 0.47 | 0.56 | 373.8 | 8239 |
| Cheerios, frosted, General Mills 1 cup (1.1 oz) | 30 | 118 | 0.7 | 25.0 | 12.9 |  | 1.3 | 214 | 107 | 17 | 4.02 | 0.423 | 161 | 6 | 0.40 | 5.4 | 1.61 | 0.16 |
|  |  | 2.1 | 1.1 | 0.2 | 0.4 | 0.4 | 0 | 59 | 64 | 4.82 | 0.049 | 4.7 | 536 | 0.1 | 0.46 | 0.54 | 360.3 | 8267 |
| Cheerios, General Mills 1 cup (1.1 oz) | 30 | 110 | 1.1 | 22.4 | 1.2 |  | 3.0 | 200 | 122 | 36 | 4.76 | 1.017 | 260 | 7 | 0.58 | 5.7 | 1.86 | 0.32 |
|  |  | 3.4 | 1.8 | 0.3 | 0.6 | 0.6 | 0 | 183 | 130 | 9.53 | 0.074 | 8.5 | 866 | 0.2 | 0.48 | 0.53 | 493.2 | 8013 |
| Cheerios, honey nut, General Mills 1 cup (1.1 oz) | 30 | 118 | 0.7 | 23.2 | 9.6 |  | 2.1 | 204 | 107 | 34 | 4.02 | 0.823 | 161 | 6 | 0.40 | 5.4 | 1.61 | 0.25 |
|  |  | 3.2 | 1.6 | 0 | 0.5 | 0.5 | 0 | 123 | 107 | 4.82 | 0.076 | 7.0 | 536 | 0.3 | 0.46 | 0.54 | 360.3 | 8045 |
| Cheerios, multi-grain, General Mills 1 cup (1.1 oz) | 30 | 114 | 0.8 | 25.0 | 6.2 |  | 2.8 | 207 | 104 | 25 | 15.52 | 0.504 | 155 | 16 | 1.55 | 20.7 | 6.21 | 10.34 |
|  |  | 2.1 | 1.0 | 0.2 | 0.3 | 0.4 | 0 | 88 | 83 | 18.62 | 0.041 | 5.0 | 517 | 14.0 | 1.76 | 2.07 | 699.6 | 8087 |
| Cinn-Raisin Crunch, Kashi ¾ cup (1.8 oz) | 50 | 165 | 2.5 | 41.0 | 12.5 |  | 7.6 | 104 | 16 | 31 | 1.50 | 1.197 |  |  |  |  |  | 0.20 |
|  |  | 4.0 | 1.4 | 0.2 | 0.5 | 0.7 | 0 | 221 | 68 | 1.30 | 0.157 |  | 36 | 0.4 |  |  |  | 8461 |
| Cinnamon Crunch, Quaker ¾ cup (1 oz) | 27 | 107 | 0.7 | 22.6 |  |  | 1.1 | 210 | 9 | 17 | 3.71 | 0.265 | 149 | 6 | 0.37 | 4.9 | 0 | 0.10 |
|  |  | 1.4 | 1.6 | 0.4 | 0.3 | 0.2 | 0 | 55 | 52 | 4.46 | 0.043 |  | 495 |  | 0.42 | 0.49 | 639.1 | 8364 |
| Cinnamon Grahams, General Mills ¾ cup (1.1 oz) | 30 | 113 | 0.8 | 25.8 | 11.4 |  | 1.0 | 237 | 100 | 8 | 3.75 | 0 | 150 | 6 | 0.38 | 5.0 | 1.50 | 0 |
|  |  | 1.5 | 0.8 | 0.2 | 0.3 | 0.3 | 0 | 44 | 20 | 4.50 | 0.026 | 1.3 | 500 | 0.1 | 0.43 | 0.50 | 165.9 | 8139 |
| Cinnamon Mini Swirlz, Kellogg's 1 cup (1.1 oz) | 30 | 122 | 0.5 | 24.9 | 3.3 |  | 1.0 | 116 | 7 | 11 | 1.50 |  |  | 15 | 0.39 | 5.0 | 1.50 |  |
|  |  | 1.7 | 2.1 | 0.3 | 0.8 | 0.6 | 0 | 45 | 40 | 1.80 | 0 |  | 500 | 0 | 0.42 | 0.51 | 165.9 | 8520 |
| Cinnamon Oat Crunch, Mother's ¾ cup (1 oz) | 27 | 103 | 0.7 | 21.4 | 6.8 |  | 2.2 | 113 | 20 | 29 | 0.69 | 0.813 | 0 | 0 | 0.08 | 0.6 | 0 | 0.16 |
|  |  | 2.8 | 1.3 | 0.2 | 0.4 | 0.4 | 0 | 145 | 97 | 0.97 | 0.076 | 1.7 | 2 |  | 0.07 | 0.03 | 9.7 | 8353 |
| Cinnamon Oatmeal Squares, Quaker - 1 cup (2.1 oz) | 60 | 227 | 1.5 | 47.5 | 12.7 |  | 4.9 | 264 | 117 | 67 | 4.14 | 1.896 | 166 | 7 | 0.41 | 5.5 | 0 | 0.38 |
|  |  | 6.3 | 2.7 | 0.5 | 0.9 | 0.9 | 0 | 215 | 209 | 16.96 | 0.186 | 3.8 | 552 | 1.5 | 0.47 | 0.55 | 733.2 | 8215 |
| Cinnamon Toast Crunch, General Mills - ¾ cup (1.1 oz) | 30 | 130 | 0.8 | 23.9 | 9.9 |  | 1.1 | 210 | 135 | 13 | 5.11 | 0.442 | 297 | 7 | 0.60 | 7.1 | 1.58 | 0.16 |
|  |  | 1.6 | 2.8 | 0.4 | 1.0 | 0.9 | 0 | 46 | 48 | 5.48 | 0.051 | 2.1 | 990 | 0.6 | 0.61 | 0.54 | 188.1 | 8272 |
| Cinnamon Toasters, Malt-O-Meal ¾ cup (1.1 oz) | 30 | 129 | 0.7 | 23.7 | 10.4 |  | 1.4 | 138 | 116 | 14 | 4.56 | 0.482 | 140 | 6 | 0.43 | 7.0 | 1.48 | 0.14 |
|  |  | 1.7 | 3.0 | 0.5 | 1.2 | 1.2 | 0 | 45 | 101 | 4.92 | 0.056 | 8.8 | 468 | 0.3 | 0.57 | 0.91 | 195.9 | 8494 |
| Coco-Roos, Malt-O-Meal ¾ cup (1.1 oz) | 30 | 119 | 0.6 | 26.8 | 14.0 |  | 0.5 | 170 | 122 | 7 | 5.16 | 0.032 | 178 | 6 | 0.36 | 5.8 | 1.86 | 0.03 |
|  |  | 1.1 | 0.8 | 0.1 | 0.5 | 0.1 | 0 | 58 | 42 | 5.85 | 0.036 | 2.0 | 618 | 0.1 | 0.59 | 0.76 | 200.1 | 8206 |
| Cocoa Blasts, Quaker 1 cup (1.2 oz) | 33 | 130 | 0.8 | 29.3 | 15.9 |  | 0.8 | 135 | 2 | 17 | 4.12 | 0.125 | 157 | 7 | 0.41 | 5.5 | 0 | 0.10 |
|  |  | 1.2 | 1.2 | 0.3 | 0.2 | 0.2 | 0 | 62 | 50 | 4.95 | 0.059 | 2.1 | 550 | 0.3 | 0.47 | 0.55 | 709.8 | 8294 |
| Cocoa Bumpers, Mother's ¾ cup (1 oz) | 29 | 109 | 0.7 | 25.4 | 12.1 |  | 0.9 | 158 | 40 | 17 | 0.31 | 0.107 | 2 | 0 | 0.04 | 0.4 | 0 | 0.10 |
|  |  | 1.5 | 0.5 | 0.1 | 0.1 | 0.2 | 0 | 228 | 48 | 1.53 | 0.055 |  | 48 |  | 0.18 | 0.01 | 3.8 | 8355 |
| Cocoa Krispies, Kellogg's ¾ cup (1.1 oz) | 31 | 118 | 0.9 | 26.7 | 10.5 |  | 0.6 | 197 | 5 | 12 | 1.49 | 0.341 | 153 | 15 | 0.46 | 5.0 | 2.15 | 0.08 |
|  |  | 1.6 | 0.9 | 0.6 | 0.1 | 0.1 | 0 | 61 | 32 | 6.88 | 0.103 | 5.0 | 508 | 0.1 | 0.70 | 1.02 | 334.8 | 8014 |
| Cocoa Pebbles, Post ¾ cup (1 oz) | 29 | 115 | 0.8 | 25.5 | 12.8 |  | 0.5 | 157 | 3 | 11 | 1.50 |  |  | 0 | 0.37 | 5.0 | 1.50 |  |
|  |  | 1.0 | 1.2 | 1.1 |  |  | 0 | 42 | 23 | 1.80 | 0.062 |  | 750 |  | 0.43 | 0.50 | 166.2 | 8323 |
| Cocoa Puffs, General Mills 1 cup (1.1 oz) | 30 | 120 | 0.5 | 26.0 | 14.0 |  | 1.5 | 160 | 100 | 8 | 3.75 | 0.147 | 0 | 6 | 0.38 | 5.0 | 1.50 | 0.05 |
|  |  | 1.0 | 1.5 | 0 | 1.0 | 0 | 0 | 60 | 20 | 4.50 | 0.040 | 2.0 | 8 | 0.2 | 0.43 | 0.50 | 165.9 | 8271 |
| Colossal Crunch, berry, Malt-O-Meal - ¾ cup (1.1 oz) | 30 | 124 | 0.5 | 25.8 | 12.4 |  | 1.0 | 247 | 4 | 20 | 3.81 | 0.164 | 0 | 1 | 0.76 | 8.0 | 0 | 0.13 |
|  |  | 1.5 | 1.6 | 0 | 0.4 | 0.2 | 0 | 34 | 59 | 4.68 | 0.051 | 3.6 | 0 | 0.2 | 0.52 | 0.91 | 483.0 | 8347 |
| Colossal Crunch, Malt-O-Meal ¾ cup (1.1 oz) | 30 | 124 | 0.4 | 26.0 | 12.2 |  | 0.2 | 197 | 2 | 18 | 3.23 | 0.105 | 0 | 0 | 0.40 | 7.0 | 0 | 0.12 |
|  |  | 1.3 | 1.6 | 0.3 | 0.4 | 0.1 | 0 | 27 | 52 | 4.10 | 0.044 | 3.0 | 0 | 0.4 | 0.52 | 0.98 | 204.3 | 8346 |
| Cookie Crisp, choc chip/vanilla, General Mills - 1 cup (1.1 oz) | 30 | 120 | 0.7 | 26.0 | 13.0 |  | 1.2 | 170 | 100 | 8 | 3.75 | 0.288 | 146 | 6 | 0.38 | 5.0 | 1.50 | 0.13 |
|  |  | 1.0 | 1.5 | 0 | 0.5 | 0 | 0 | 40 | 40 | 4.50 | 0.034 | 2.2 | 500 | 0.3 | 0.43 | 0.50 | 165.9 | 8017 |
| Cookie Crisp, peanut butter, General Mills ¾ cup (1.1 oz) | 30 | 130 | 0.8 | 22.8 | 13.0 |  | 1.0 | 135 | 100 | 8 | 3.75 |  |  | 6 | 0.38 | 5.0 | 1.50 |  |
|  |  | 2.0 | 3.5 | 0.5 | 1.0 | 0.5 | 0 | 60 | 20 | 4.50 |  |  | 500 |  | 0.43 | 0.50 | 165.9 | 8516 |
| Corn Biscuits, Ralston 1 cup (1.1 oz) | 31 | 114 | 1.1 | 26.6 | 2.9 |  | 0.8 | 332 | 117 | 5 | 5.31 | 0.069 | 95 | 6 | 0.47 | 6.8 |  | 0.04 |
|  |  | 1.8 | 0.3 | 0.1 | 0 | 0.1 | 0 | 28 | 12 | 11.89 | 0.023 | 0.7 | 363 | 0 | 0.53 | 0.69 |  | 8505 |
| Corn Bursts, Malt-O-Meal 1 cup (1.1 oz) | 31 | 122 | 0.3 | 29.0 | 13.5 |  | 0.6 | 124 | 2 | 1 | 1.77 | 0.043 | 270 | 19 | 0.88 | 11.9 | 1.78 | 0.05 |
|  |  | 1.2 | 0.1 | 0.1 | 0 | 0 | 0 | 18 | 6 | 2.03 | 0.028 | 2.0 | 936 | 0 | 0.95 | 1.46 | 226.0 | 8083 |
| Corn Chex, General Mills 1 cup (1.1 oz) | 30 | 110 | 0.8 | 25.5 | 3.0 |  | 1.2 | 280 | 100 | 15 | 3.75 | 0.056 | 136 | 6 | 0.38 | 5.0 | 1.50 | 0.11 |
|  |  | 2.0 | 0.5 | 0.1 | 0.1 | 0.2 | 0 | 45 | 22 | 9.00 | 0.037 | 2.9 | 500 | 0.1 | 0.43 | 0.50 | 336.0 | 8019 |

| | WT (g) | KCAL | H₂O (g) | CHO (g) | TSUG (g) | ASUG (g) | DFIB (g) | Na (mg) | Ca (mg) | Mg (mg) | Zn (mg) | Mn (mg) | A (mcg RAE) | C (mg) | B-1 (mg) | NIA (mg) | B-12 (mcg) | PANT (mg) |
|---|---|---|---|---|---|---|---|---|---|---|---|---|---|---|---|---|---|---|
| | | PRO (g) | FAT (g) | SFA (g) | MUFA (g) | PUFA (g) | CHOL (mg) | K (mg) | P (mg) | Fe (mg) | Cu (mg) | Se (mcg) | A (IU) | E (mg ATE) | B-2 (mg) | B-6 (mg) | FOL (mcg DFE) | REF |
| **Corn Flakes**, Country, General Mills | 30 | 110 | 0.7 | 25.2 | 2.0 | | 1.2 | 270 | 250 | 7 | 3.75 | 0.031 | 136 | 6 | 0.38 | 5.0 | 1.50 | |
| *1 cup (1.1 oz)* | | 2.0 | 0.5 | 0.2 | 0.1 | 0.2 | 0 | 50 | 20 | 8.40 | 0.030 | 1.5 | 500 | | 0.43 | 0.50 | 336.0 | 8269 |
| **Corn Flakes**, honey crisp, Quaker | 30 | 112 | 0.8 | 26.6 | | | 0.9 | 261 | 0 | 5 | 0.08 | 0.018 | | 15 | 0.38 | 5.0 | 0 | 0.08 |
| *1 cup (1.1 oz)* | | 1.7 | 0.2 | 0 | 0.1 | 0.1 | 0 | 27 | 14 | 4.50 | 0.015 | 0 | 750 | | 0.42 | 0.50 | | 8396 |
| **Corn Flakes**, Kellogg's | 30 | 108 | 1.1 | 26.1 | 3.2 | | 0.8 | 217 | 1 | 3 | 0.05 | 0.049 | 137 | 7 | 0.64 | 7.3 | 2.84 | 0.02 |
| *1 cup (1.1 oz)* | | 2.0 | 0.2 | 0.1 | 0 | | 0 | 24 | 11 | 8.70 | 0.032 | 2.5 | 537 | 0 | 0.79 | 1.03 | 237.6 | 8020 |
| **Corn Flakes**, Malt-O-Meal | 30 | 114 | 0.9 | 26.3 | 2.3 | | 0.9 | 306 | 1 | 5 | 0.11 | 0.017 | 363 | 20 | 0.50 | 5.9 | | 0.02 |
| *1 cup (1.1 oz)* | | 2.0 | 0.1 | 0 | 0 | 0.1 | 0 | 27 | 18 | 8.58 | 0.042 | 2.4 | 1257 | 0 | 0.52 | 0.63 | 186.3 | 8497 |
| **Corn Flakes**, organic, Barbara's | 30 | 110 | | 25.0 | 3.0 | | 1.0 | 140 | 0 | 40 | | | | 0 | | | | |
| Bakery - *1 cup (1.1 oz)* | | 2.0 | 1.0 | 0 | | | 0 | 100 | 80 | 0.36 | | | 0 | | | | | BARB20 |
| **Corn Flakes**, Post Toasties | 28 | 101 | 1.0 | 24.3 | 1.8 | | 1.3 | 266 | 1 | 4 | 0.13 | | | 0 | 0.38 | 5.0 | 1.50 | |
| *1 cup (1 oz)* | | 1.9 | 0 | 0 | | | 0 | 33 | 15 | 5.40 | 0.009 | | 750 | | 0.43 | 0.50 | 166.3 | 8338 |
| **Corn Flakes**, Ralston | 31 | 111 | 1.0 | 27.3 | 2.4 | | 0.8 | 220 | 1 | 2 | 0.06 | 0.029 | 180 | 20 | 1.39 | 6.5 | | 0.03 |
| *1 cup (1.1 oz)* | | 1.8 | 0.3 | 0.1 | 0 | 0.1 | | 27 | 10 | 6.01 | 0.023 | 0.7 | 656 | 0 | 0.54 | 0.59 | | 8506 |
| **Corn Flakes** with bananas, Kelloggs | 26 | 108 | 0.8 | 21.8 | 6.5 | | 0.7 | 118 | 8 | 6 | 0.08 | 0.059 | 121 | 7 | 0.34 | 5.5 | 1.30 | 0 |
| *¾ cup (.9 oz)* | | 0.8 | 2.2 | 2.0 | 0.2 | 0.1 | 0 | 48 | 8 | 1.56 | 0.049 | | 434 | 0 | 0.36 | 0.52 | 146.4 | 8472 |
| **Corn Pops**, Kellogg's | 31 | 117 | 0.9 | 27.9 | 14.8 | | 0.2 | 120 | 5 | 2 | 1.52 | 0.076 | 143 | 7 | 0.37 | 5.0 | 1.52 | 0.09 |
| *1 cup (1.1 oz)* | | 1.1 | 0.2 | 0.1 | 0.1 | 0.1 | 0 | 26 | 10 | 1.92 | 0.012 | 2.0 | 500 | 0 | 0.43 | 0.50 | 169.3 | 8068 |
| **Count Chocula**, General Mills | 30 | 120 | 0.6 | 26.5 | 13.0 | | 1.2 | 190 | 100 | 9 | 3.75 | 0.293 | 1 | 6 | 0.38 | 5.0 | 1.50 | 0.14 |
| *1 cup (1.1 oz)* | | 1.0 | 1.0 | 0.2 | 0.5 | 0.2 | 0 | 55 | 20 | 4.50 | 0.040 | 2.0 | 15 | 0.2 | 0.43 | 0.50 | 165.9 | 8270 |
| **Cracklin' Oat Bran**, Kellogg's | 55 | 221 | 1.6 | 39.5 | 17.6 | | 7.0 | 170 | 33 | 85 | 1.71 | 0.110 | 253 | 17 | 0.44 | 5.6 | 1.71 | |
| *¾ cup (1.9 oz)* | | 4.4 | 7.6 | 3.4 | 2.6 | 1.6 | 0 | 248 | 218 | 2.04 | 0.220 | 5.9 | 842 | 0.3 | 0.50 | 0.55 | 183.7 | 8023 |
| **Cran-Vanilla Crunch**, Kellogg's | 55 | 205 | 1.9 | 47.3 | 18.2 | | 2.6 | 235 | 15 | 26 | 1.49 | | | 0 | 0.38 | 5.0 | 1.49 | |
| *1¼ cups (1.9 oz)* | | 3.3 | 1.2 | 0.7 | 0.1 | 0.4 | 0 | 96 | 86 | 4.40 | 0 | | 500 | | 0.44 | 0.50 | 162.8 | 8521 |
| **Cranberry Macadamia Nut**, Quaker | 60 | 245 | 2.6 | 46.2 | 17.2 | | 3.6 | 251 | 76 | 39 | 2.99 | 1.002 | 232 | 11 | 0.46 | 6.5 | 0 | 0.25 |
| *1 cup (2.1 oz)* | | 4.0 | 5.9 | 1.0 | 3.9 | 0.5 | 0 | 134 | 107 | 10.29 | 0.168 | 0.8 | 773 | | 0.56 | 0.67 | 533.4 | 8400 |
| **Crispix Cinnamon Crunch**, | 30 | 120 | 0.9 | 26.1 | 9.1 | | 0.2 | 179 | 9 | 5 | 1.56 | 0.093 | 150 | 6 | 0.39 | 5.1 | 1.53 | 0.09 |
| Kellogg's - *3.4 cup (1.1 oz)* | | 1.4 | 1.1 | 0.2 | 0.6 | 0.3 | 0 | 37 | 21 | 5.88 | 0.027 | | 500 | 0.1 | 0.45 | 0.51 | 341.4 | 8374 |
| **Crispix**, Kellogg's | 29 | 109 | 1.0 | 25.2 | 3.3 | | 0.3 | 222 | 4 | 7 | 2.28 | 0.289 | 262 | 9 | 1.27 | 8.5 | 2.09 | 0.06 |
| *1 cup (1.1 oz)* | | 1.8 | 0.4 | 0.1 | 0.1 | 0.1 | 0 | 33 | 28 | 9.61 | 0.042 | 3.6 | 897 | 0 | 1.25 | 0.98 | 336.4 | 8259 |
| **Crispy Brown Rice**, gluten-free, | 32 | 124 | 1.0 | 27.5 | 2.9 | | 2.3 | 4 | 9 | 28 | 0.48 | | 0 | 0 | 0.03 | 0.7 | 0 | |
| Erewhon - *1 cup (1.1 oz)* | | 2.3 | 1.1 | 0.2 | 0.3 | 0.5 | 0 | 76 | 91 | 0.37 | 0.077 | 4.9 | 0 | 0 | 0.01 | 0.03 | 6.1 | 43510 |
| **Crispy Corn**, Quaker | 30 | 113 | 0.8 | 25.0 | 6.1 | | 1.3 | 240 | 113 | 27 | 4.12 | 0.378 | 165 | 7 | 0.41 | 5.5 | 0 | 0.17 |
| *1 cup (1.1 oz)* | | 2.2 | 0.9 | 0.2 | 0.2 | 0.4 | 0 | 84 | 99 | 8.62 | 0.063 | | 550 | | 0.46 | 0.55 | 710.1 | 8358 |
| **Crispy Hexagons**, Ralston | 28 | 106 | 1.1 | 24.3 | 2.7 | | 0.4 | 228 | 2 | 4 | 2.08 | 0.183 | 220 | 12 | 2.11 | 8.4 | | 0.06 |
| *1 cup (1 oz)* | | 1.7 | 0.3 | 0.1 | 0.1 | 0.1 | 0 | 28 | 18 | 9.71 | 0.037 | 0.6 | 753 | 0 | 1.00 | 2.16 | | 8507 |
| **Crispy Rice**, Malt-O-Meal | 33 | 126 | 1.1 | 28.5 | 3.0 | | 0.3 | 297 | 2 | 8 | 0.36 | 0.376 | 289 | 20 | 0.56 | 6.5 | 2.03 | 0.27 |
| *1 cup (1.2 oz)* | | 2.1 | 0.4 | 0.2 | 0.1 | 0.1 | 0 | 41 | 40 | 11.58 | 0.067 | 4.8 | 964 | 0 | 0.66 | 0.95 | 680.1 | 8348 |
| **Crispy Rice**, Ralston | 28 | 102 | 1.0 | 24.1 | 2.1 | | 0.2 | 214 | 1 | 6 | 0.36 | 0.308 | 197 | 18 | 0.57 | 8.1 | 1.53 | 0.09 |
| *1 cup (1 oz)* | | 1.9 | 0.4 | 0.1 | 0.1 | 0.1 | 0 | 31 | 27 | 9.16 | 0.042 | 5.0 | 657 | 0 | 0.79 | 0.54 | 287.6 | 8025 |
| **Crispy Wheats**, organic, Barbara's | 30 | 110 | | 25.0 | 5.0 | | 3.0 | 180 | 20 | 24 | 3.75 | | | 15 | 0.38 | 5.0 | 1.50 | |
| Bakery - *¾ cup* | | 3.0 | 0.5 | 0 | | | 0 | 130 | 100 | 8.10 | | | 1250 | | 0.42 | 0.50 | | BARB21 |
| **Cruncheroos**, Kellogg's | 30 | 110 | 0.9 | 22.0 | 1.3 | | 3.0 | 240 | 122 | 32 | 4.59 | | | 7 | 0.46 | 6.1 | 1.83 | |
| *1 cup (1.1 oz)* | | 4.0 | 1.5 | 0 | 0.8 | 0.8 | 0 | 90 | 150 | 9.99 | 0.090 | | 610 | | 0.52 | 0.61 | 118.5 | 8375 |
| **Crunchy Bran**, Quaker | 27 | 90 | 0.5 | 22.7 | 5.6 | | 4.7 | 235 | 19 | 16 | 4.13 | 0.216 | 2 | 0 | 0.14 | 5.5 | 0 | 0.11 |
| *¾ cup (.95 oz)* | | 1.7 | 1.1 | 0.5 | 0.2 | 0.3 | 0 | 65 | 50 | 8.36 | 0.043 | 3.2 | 42 | 0.2 | 0.47 | 0.55 | 709.8 | 8018 |
| **Dyno-Bites**, cocoa, Malt-O-Meal | 29 | 117 | 0.4 | 25.9 | 13.1 | | 0.3 | 177 | 2 | 7 | 1.58 | 0.194 | 300 | 0 | 0.46 | 11.6 | 2.38 | 0.17 |
| *¾ cup (1 oz)* | | 1.2 | 0.9 | 0.7 | 0.1 | 0.1 | 0 | 52 | 20 | 1.97 | 0.056 | 2.6 | 1000 | 0 | 0.67 | 0.96 | 243.3 | 8495 |
| **Dyno-Bites**, fruity, Malt-O-Meal | 27 | 109 | 0.3 | 24.3 | 11.5 | | 0.3 | 173 | 1 | 4 | 1.62 | 0.171 | 294 | 0 | 0.39 | 7.2 | 1.86 | 0.16 |
| *¾ cup (1 oz)* | | 1.1 | 0.9 | 0.2 | 0.6 | 0.1 | 0 | 21 | 18 | 2.06 | 0.035 | | 980 | 0.3 | 0.68 | 0.74 | 226.8 | 8501 |
| **Eggo Crunch**, maple, Kellogg's | 33 | 124 | 0.8 | 27.4 | 13.2 | | 1.9 | 158 | 55 | 13 | 1.48 | 0 | | 15 | 0.36 | 5.0 | 1.48 | |
| *1 cup (1.2 oz)* | | 2.2 | 1.5 | 0.5 | 0.5 | 0.4 | 0 | 70 | 78 | 4.49 | 0.033 | 0.1 | 500 | 0 | 0.43 | 0.50 | 165.7 | 8524 |
| **Fiber 7 Flakes**, Health Valley | 30 | 106 | 0.9 | 23.4 | 0.6 | | 4.2 | 16 | 21 | 43 | 0.87 | 0.969 | 32 | 1 | 0.16 | 2.1 | 0.64 | 0.22 |
| *½ cup (1.1 oz)* | | 4.3 | 0.4 | 0.1 | 0.1 | 0.2 | 0 | 138 | 98 | 0.76 | 0.143 | 5.7 | 106 | 0.3 | 0.18 | 0.21 | 67.8 | 8290 |
| **Fiber One**, General Mills | 30 | 60 | 1.0 | 25.0 | 0 | | 14.2 | 105 | 100 | 40 | 3.75 | 0.587 | 1 | 6 | 0.38 | 5.0 | 1.50 | 0.24 |
| *½ cup (1.1 oz)* | | 2.0 | 1.0 | 0.1 | 0.1 | 0.4 | 0 | 180 | 150 | 4.50 | 0.094 | 2.7 | 12 | 0.3 | 0.43 | 0.50 | 165.9 | 8244 |
| **Frankenberry**, General Mills | 30 | 120 | 0.6 | 26.7 | 14.0 | | 0.3 | 190 | 20 | 3 | 3.75 | 0.022 | 1 | 6 | 0.38 | 5.0 | 1.50 | 0.03 |
| *1 cup (1.1 oz)* | | 1.0 | 1.0 | 0.2 | 0.5 | 0.3 | 0 | 35 | 20 | 4.50 | 0.021 | 5.9 | 18 | 0.2 | 0.43 | 0.50 | 165.9 | 8268 |
| **French Toast Crunch**, General Mills | 30 | 131 | 0.6 | 23.3 | 10.3 | | 0.9 | 216 | 94 | 8 | 3.52 | 0.025 | 134 | 6 | 0.35 | 4.7 | 1.41 | 0.05 |
| *¾ cup (1.1 oz)* | | 1.9 | 3.3 | 0.2 | 2.3 | 0.5 | 0 | 42 | 38 | 4.22 | 0.014 | 1.2 | 469 | 0.6 | 0.40 | 0.47 | 155.4 | 8086 |
| **Froot Loops**, Kellogg's | 30 | 118 | 0.9 | 26.2 | 13.5 | | 0.9 | 141 | 23 | 7 | 1.41 | 0.168 | 145 | 14 | 0.36 | 4.7 | 1.41 | 0.10 |
| *1 cup (1.1 oz)* | | 1.0 | 1.2 | 0.6 | 0.3 | 0.4 | 0 | 33 | 19 | 4.23 | 0.027 | 1.8 | 483 | 0 | 0.39 | 0.48 | 155.7 | 8030 |

| | WT | Macronutrients | | | | | | Minerals | | | | | Vitamins | | | | | |
|---|---|---|---|---|---|---|---|---|---|---|---|---|---|---|---|---|---|---|
| | (g) | KCAL | $H_2$0 (g) | CHO (g) | TSUG (g) | ASUG (g) | DFIB (g) | Na (mg) | Ca (mg) | Mg (mg) | Zn (mg) | Mn (mg) | A (mcg RAE) | C (mg) | B-1 (mg) | NIA (mg) | B-12 (mcg) | PANT (mg) |
| | | PRO (g) | FAT (g) | SFA (g) | MUFA (g) | PUFA (g) | CHOL (mg) | K (mg) | P (mg) | Fe (mg) | Cu (mg) | Se (mcg) | A (IU) | E (mg ATE) | B-2 (mg) | B-6 (mg) | FOL (mcg DFE) | REF |
| **Froot Loops**, marshmallow blasted, | 30 | 118 | 0.8 | 27.0 | 15.9 | | 0.4 | 108 | 3 | 8 | 1.86 | 0.187 | 146 | 15 | 0.39 | 5.0 | 1.50 | 0.02 |
| Kellogg's - *1 cup (1.1 oz)* | | 1.2 | 0.7 | 0.4 | 0.1 | 0.2 | 0 | 26 | 17 | 4.50 | 0.034 | 2.7 | 500 | 0.1 | 0.42 | 0.51 | 165.9 | 8376 |
| **Froot Loops**, marshmallow, rainbow | 30 | 117 | 0.8 | 26.7 | 15.9 | | 0.4 | 107 | 3 | 7 | 1.50 | | | 15 | 0.39 | 5.0 | 1.50 | |
| breeze, Kellogg's - *1 cup (1.1 oz)* | | 1.2 | 0.7 | 0.4 | 0.1 | 0.2 | 0 | 25 | 17 | 4.50 | | | 500 | | 0.42 | 0.48 | | 8526 |
| **Froot Loops**, ⅓ less sugar, | 32 | 126 | 0.8 | 27.5 | 10.1 | | 1.0 | 180 | 5 | 12 | 1.92 | 0.264 | 155 | 15 | 0.51 | 6.7 | 1.60 | 0.05 |
| Kellogg's - 1¼ cups (1.1 oz) | | 2.0 | 1.1 | 0.4 | 0.2 | 0.2 | 0 | 44 | 29 | 6.08 | 0.047 | 2.8 | 516 | 0.1 | 0.58 | 0.64 | 224.6 | 8468 |
| **Frosted Chex**, General Mills | 30 | 110 | 0.7 | 26.8 | 10.0 | | 0 | 180 | 100 | 11 | 3.75 | 0.266 | 150 | 6 | 0.38 | 5.0 | 1.50 | 0.13 |
| *¾ cup (1.1 oz)* | | 1.1 | 0.5 | 0.1 | 0.2 | 0.2 | 0 | 30 | 28 | 9.00 | 0.027 | 2.8 | 500 | 0.1 | 0.43 | 0.50 | 338.7 | 8514 |
| **Frosted Flakes**, *⅓ less sugar,* | 31 | 117 | 0.9 | 28.0 | 8.4 | | 0.3 | 178 | 2 | 3 | 0.29 | 0.059 | 173 | 7 | 0.43 | 5.9 | 1.77 | 0.07 |
| Kellogg's - *1 cup (1.1 oz)* | | 1.6 | 0.1 | 0 | 0 | 0 | 0 | 26 | 12 | 7.13 | 0.078 | 2.6 | 608 | 0.1 | 0.56 | 0.59 | 198.4 | 8469 |
| **Frosted Flakes**, Kellogg's | 31 | 114 | 1.0 | 28.2 | 12.0 | | 0.6 | 143 | 1 | 2 | 0.04 | 0.013 | 183 | 8 | 0.64 | 8.3 | 2.48 | 0.07 |
| *¾ cup (1.1 oz)* | | 1.3 | 0.1 | 0 | 0 | 0 | 0 | 23 | 13 | 7.26 | 0.011 | 1.4 | 608 | 0 | 0.59 | 0.91 | 196.8 | 8069 |
| **Frosted Flakes**, Malt-O-Meal | 40 | 155 | 0.8 | 36.4 | 15.0 | | 0.8 | 229 | 0 | 3 | 0.07 | 0.026 | 474 | 25 | 0.87 | 15.9 | 2.22 | 0.08 |
| *1 cup (1.4 oz)* | | 2.0 | 0.2 | 0.1 | 0 | 0.1 | 0 | 27 | 14 | 5.73 | 0.016 | 1.8 | 1580 | 0 | 1.28 | 1.60 | 322.8 | 8409 |
| **Frosted Krispies**, Kellogg's | 30 | 115 | 0.9 | 26.7 | 11.7 | | 0.1 | 193 | 3 | 8 | 0 | 0.225 | 223 | 6 | 0.39 | 5.1 | 1.50 | 0.21 |
| *¾ cup (1.1 oz)* | | 1.5 | 0.3 | 0.1 | 0.1 | 0.1 | 0 | 27 | 28 | 5.40 | 0 | 4.6 | 742 | 0 | 0.42 | 0.51 | 168.9 | 8032 |
| **Frosted Mini-Wheats**, bite size, | 55 | 189 | 3.3 | 44.6 | 11.1 | | 5.5 | 4 | 18 | 65 | 1.76 | | 0 | 0 | 0.41 | 5.4 | 1.62 | |
| Kellogg's - *1 cup (1.9 oz)* | | 5.6 | 0.9 | 0.2 | 0.1 | 0.6 | 0 | 190 | 162 | 15.40 | 0.176 | 2.3 | 0 | 0 | 0.46 | 0.54 | 176.0 | 8319 |
| **Frosted Mini-Wheats**, Kellogg's | 51 | 175 | 3.1 | 41.8 | 10.7 | | 5.1 | 5 | 17 | 47 | 1.53 | 1.422 | 0 | 0 | 0.51 | 5.1 | 1.53 | 0.38 |
| *1 cup (1.8 oz)* | | 4.6 | 0.8 | 0.2 | 0.1 | 0.5 | 0 | 180 | 153 | 16.32 | 0 | 2.1 | 0 | 0.3 | 0.51 | 0.51 | 167.3 | 8031 |
| **Frosted Oats**, Quaker | 55 | 218 | 1.4 | 45.1 | 20.6 | | 2.4 | 475 | 14 | 34 | 8.71 | 1.062 | 349 | 14 | 0.56 | 11.6 | 0 | 0.17 |
| *1 cup (1.9 oz)* | | 3.3 | 3.3 | 0.7 | 1.0 | 0.5 | 0 | 101 | 134 | 10.46 | 0.082 | | 1162 | | 0.98 | 1.16 | 1489.0 | 8359 |
| **Frosted Whole Wheat**, | 55 | 213 | 2.4 | 45.6 | 9.8 | | 5.8 | 10 | 15 | 58 | 3.35 | | | 1 | 0.42 | 8.9 | 1.46 | |
| Malt-O-Meal - *1 cup (1.9 oz)* | | 5.2 | 1.1 | 0.2 | 0.2 | 0.7 | 1 | 187 | 171 | 21.29 | 0.192 | | 55 | | 0.57 | 0.81 | | 8500 |
| **Fruit & Fibre** (dates, raisins, | 55 | 212 | 4.7 | 41.9 | 16.4 | | 5.3 | 280 | 24 | 66 | 1.50 | | | 0 | 0.37 | 5.0 | 1.50 | |
| walnuts), Post - *1 cup (1.9 oz)* | | 3.9 | 3.1 | 0.4 | | | 0 | 244 | 162 | 5.40 | 0.260 | | 750 | | 0.42 | 0.50 | 162.8 | 8327 |
| **Fruit Harvest**, apple cinnamon, | 52 | 206 | 1.6 | 43.2 | 19.2 | | 3.1 | 255 | 22 | 37 | 1.25 | 0.798 | 125 | | 0.31 | 4.2 | 1.25 | 0.32 |
| Kellogg's - *1 cup (1.8 oz)* | | 3.6 | 2.6 | 0.3 | 1.7 | 0.6 | 0 | 165 | 89 | 3.64 | 0.154 | | 416 | | 0.36 | 0.42 | 134.7 | 8456 |
| **Fruit Harvest**, banana berry, | 30 | 119 | 0.9 | 25.5 | 8.7 | | 1.6 | 136 | 10 | 16 | 1.50 | 0.406 | 150 | 1 | 0.39 | 5.1 | 1.50 | 0.14 |
| Kellogg's - *¾ cup (1.1 oz)* | | 1.6 | 1.8 | 1.4 | 0.2 | 0.2 | 0 | 86 | 43 | 4.50 | 0.074 | | 500 | 0.1 | 0.42 | 0.51 | 165.9 | 8470 |
| **Fruit Harvest**, peach/strawberry, | 30 | 110 | 0.9 | 26.1 | 9.0 | | 1.5 | 165 | 7 | 15 | 0.90 | 0.558 | 120 | 1 | 0.30 | 3.6 | 1.14 | 0.21 |
| Kellogg's - *¾ cup (1.1 oz)* | | 2.1 | 0.4 | 0.1 | 0.1 | 0.2 | 0 | 84 | 51 | 3.30 | 0.070 | 2.1 | 399 | 0.1 | 0.30 | 0.36 | 131.1 | 8457 |
| **Fruit Harvest**, strawberry/blueberry, | 29 | 107 | 0.9 | 25.2 | 9.9 | | 1.3 | 137 | 8 | 15 | 1.74 | 0.442 | 171 | 1 | 0.43 | 5.2 | 1.62 | 0.21 |
| Kellogg's - *¾ cup (1 oz)* | | 1.7 | 0.3 | 0.1 | 0.1 | 0.2 | 0 | 82 | 52 | 4.93 | 0.055 | 2.0 | 569 | 0.1 | 0.46 | 0.55 | 181.0 | 8458 |
| **Fruitangy Oh's**, Quaker | 31 | 122 | 0.8 | 27.0 | 13.4 | | 0.8 | 152 | 3 | 18 | 3.88 | 0.205 | 311 | 12 | 0.39 | 5.2 | 0 | 0.11 |
| *1 cup (1.1 oz)* | | 1.5 | 1.1 | 0.3 | 0.5 | 0.3 | 0 | 59 | 55 | 4.65 | 0.046 | 2.0 | 1034 | 0.3 | 0.44 | 0.51 | 172.0 | 8297 |
| **Fruity Brontosaurus Blasts**, Quaker | 31 | 117 | 0.8 | 27.7 | 13.6 | | 0.4 | 183 | 2 | 6 | 0.20 | 0.192 | 250 | 9 | 0.22 | 6.1 | 0 | 0.21 |
| *1 cup (1.1 oz)* | | 1.2 | 0.8 | 0.1 | 0.6 | 0.1 | 0 | 15 | 20 | 2.97 | 0.022 | | 831 | | 0.52 | 0.62 | 140.4 | 8357 |
| **Fruity Ocean Adventure**, Quaker | 31 | 122 | 0.8 | 27.0 | 13.4 | | 0.9 | 79 | 4 | 19 | 4.74 | 0.267 | 190 | 8 | 0.47 | 6.3 | 0 | 0 |
| *1 cup (1.1 oz)* | | 1.5 | 1.2 | 0.3 | 0.3 | 0.3 | 0 | 60 | 58 | 5.69 | 0.050 | 0 | 632 | | 0.54 | 0.63 | 815.6 | 8401 |
| **Fruity Pebbles**, Post | 27 | 108 | 0.8 | 23.7 | 11.9 | | 0.2 | 158 | 1 | 5 | 1.50 | | | 0 | 0.38 | 5.0 | 1.50 | |
| *¾ cup (.95 oz)* | | 1.0 | 1.1 | 0.2 | | | 0 | 30 | 16 | 1.80 | 0.032 | | 750 | | 0.42 | 0.50 | 166.3 | 8324 |
| **Golden Crisp**, Post | 27 | 107 | 0.8 | 24.5 | 14.6 | | 0 | 40 | 4 | 16 | 1.50 | | | 0 | 0.38 | 5.0 | 1.50 | |
| *¾ cup (.95 oz)* | | 1.5 | 0.4 | 0.1 | | | 0 | 34 | 37 | 1.80 | 0.059 | | 750 | | 0.42 | 0.50 | 166.3 | 8328 |
| **Golden Grahams**, General Mills | 30 | 120 | 0.7 | 26.0 | 10.0 | | 1.0 | 270 | 100 | 8 | 3.75 | 0.413 | 150 | 6 | 0.38 | 5.0 | 1.50 | 0.11 |
| *¾ cup (1.1 oz)* | | 1.0 | 1.0 | 0.1 | 0.5 | 0.3 | 0 | 60 | 40 | 4.50 | 0.042 | 1.7 | 500 | 0.2 | 0.43 | 0.50 | 165.9 | 8035 |
| **Golden Puffs**, Malt-O-Meal | 37 | 147 | 1.0 | 33.2 | 19.0 | | 1.0 | 65 | 4 | 17 | 2.70 | 0.315 | 446 | 10 | 0.64 | 9.3 | 2.47 | 0.12 |
| *1 cup (1.3 oz)* | | 2.1 | 0.3 | 0.1 | 0.1 | 0.1 | 0 | 57 | 52 | 2.93 | 0.062 | 10.1 | 1489 | 0.2 | 0.80 | 0.76 | 276.4 | 8478 |
| **GoLean Crunch Honey almond** | 53 | 202 | 1.9 | 35.5 | 12.2 | | 8.6 | 138 | 54 | 38 | 0.42 | | | 0 | | | | |
| **flax,** Kashi - *1 cup* | | 8.8 | 4.4 | 0.4 | 2.2 | 1.9 | 0 | 258 | 110 | 1.59 | | | 9 | | | | | 8560 |
| **GoLean Crunch**, Kashi | 53 | 200 | 2.1 | 36.0 | 13.0 | | 8.1 | 204 | 46 | 44 | 0.48 | 0.064 | 0 | 0 | 0.03 | 0.2 | 0 | 0.35 |
| *1 cup (1.9 oz)* | | 9.3 | 3.1 | 0.2 | 1.7 | 1.1 | 0 | 300 | 113 | 1.86 | 0.159 | 11.1 | 5 | 0.3 | 0.02 | 0.02 | 24.4 | 8386 |
| **GoLean**, Kashi | 52 | 148 | 1.1 | 30.2 | 6.2 | | 10.2 | 86 | 73 | 86 | 0.36 | 1.195 | 3 | 0 | 0.22 | 1.2 | 0 | 0.69 |
| *1 cup (1.8 oz)* | | 13.6 | 1.0 | 0.2 | 0.2 | 0.6 | 0 | 482 | 247 | 2.60 | 1.087 | 6.0 | 50 | 0.2 | 0.09 | 0.22 | 22.4 | 8393 |
| **Good Friends**, Kashi | 53 | 167 | 1.1 | 43.4 | 9.0 | | 11.8 | 129 | 18 | 60 | 1.40 | 1.801 | 3 | 0 | 0.11 | 2.1 | 0 | 0.54 |
| *1 cup (1.9 oz)* | | 5.0 | 1.9 | 0.2 | 0.5 | 0.9 | 0 | 262 | 125 | 1.59 | 0.205 | 16.4 | 63 | 0.4 | 0.06 | 0.14 | 22.8 | 8390 |
| **Grain Shop**, organic, Barbara's | 30 | 80 | | 24.0 | 6.0 | | 8.0 | 120 | 0 | | | | | 0 | | | | |
| Bakery - *½ cup* | | 3.0 | 1.0 | 0 | | | 0 | 180 | | 1.44 | | | 0 | | | | | BARB33 |
| **granola**, cocoa beach, Kashi | 55 | 226 | 2.2 | 33.6 | 10.9 | | 7.0 | 118 | 28 | | | | | 0 | | | | |
| *½ cup* | | 6.1 | 9.2 | 1.8 | 4.5 | 3.0 | 0 | 150 | | 1.49 | | | 6 | | | | | 8563 |
| **granola**, homemade | 61 | 298 | 3.3 | 32.5 | 12.2 | 6.5 | 5.5 | 15 | 48 | 107 | 2.46 | 2.472 | 1 | 1 | 0.45 | 1.3 | 0 | 0.95 |
| *½ cup (2.2 oz)* | | 9.1 | 14.7 | 2.5 | 5.8 | 5.6 | 0 | 329 | 278 | 2.58 | 0.387 | 17.0 | 12 | 6.8 | 0.18 | 0.18 | 50.0 | 8037 |

| | WT (g) | KCAL | H₂O (g) | CHO (g) | TSUG (g) | ASUG (g) | DFIB (g) | Na (mg) | Ca (mg) | Mg (mg) | Zn (mg) | Mn (mg) | A (mcg RAE) | C (mg) | B-1 (mg) | NIA (mg) | B-12 (mcg) | PANT (mg) |
|---|---|---|---|---|---|---|---|---|---|---|---|---|---|---|---|---|---|---|
| | | PRO (g) | FAT (g) | SFA (g) | MUFA (g) | PUFA (g) | CHOL (mg) | K (mg) | P (mg) | Fe (mg) | Cu (mg) | Se (mcg) | A (IU) | E (mg ATE) | B-2 (mg) | B-6 (mg) | FOL (mcg DFE) | REF |
| **granola**, lowfat, Kellogg's | 49 | 190 | 1.7 | 39.9 | 13.7 | | 3.0 | 107 | 19 | 37 | 3.77 | | 225 | 1 | 0.39 | 5.0 | 5.98 | |
| ½ cup (1.7 oz) | | 3.9 | 2.5 | 0.6 | 1.1 | 0.8 | 0 | 122 | 118 | 1.81 | 0.294 | 8.5 | 750 | 1.2 | 0.44 | 2.01 | 673.3 | 8189 |
| **granola**, mountain medley, Kashi | 55 | 218 | 1.6 | 36.6 | 12.1 | | 6.3 | 110 | 18 | | | | | 0 | | | | |
| ½ cup | | 6.1 | 7.2 | 1.2 | 4.0 | 2.0 | 0 | 140 | | 1.26 | | | 0 | | | | | 8566 |
| **granola**, orchard spice, Kashi | 55 | 222 | 1.6 | 36.8 | 11.0 | | 6.3 | 129 | 22 | | | | | 0 | | | | |
| ½ cup | | 6.1 | 7.4 | 0.9 | 3.8 | 2.6 | 0 | 153 | | 1.32 | | | 0 | | | | | 8564 |
| **granola**, summer berry, Kashi | 55 | 215 | 2.2 | 36.6 | 9.4 | | 6.8 | 132 | 21 | | | | | 0 | | | | |
| ½ cup | | 6.6 | 6.4 | 0.9 | 3.0 | 2.5 | 0 | 129 | | 1.43 | | | 4 | | | | | 8565 |
| **granola** with almonds, Quaker Sun Country - ½ cup (2 oz) | 57 | 266 | 0.8 | 38.3 | 11.6 | | 3.0 | 19 | 49 | 52 | 1.14 | 1.528 | 0 | 0 | 0.18 | 0.5 | 0.04 | 0.32 |
| | | 6.7 | 10.3 | 1.3 | 3.3 | 1.8 | 0 | 221 | 168 | 2.48 | 0.165 | 9.9 | 0 | 2.2 | 0.10 | 0.07 | 19.4 | 8212 |
| **granola** with fruit, lowfat, Nature Valley - ⅔ cup (1.9 oz) | 55 | 212 | 3.7 | 44.0 | 18.4 | | 2.8 | 207 | 20 | 24 | 0.61 | 1.104 | 0 | 0 | 0.09 | 0.9 | 0 | |
| | | 4.4 | 2.5 | 0.5 | 1.2 | 0.6 | 0 | 153 | 150 | 1.10 | 0.120 | 9.5 | 0 | 0.8 | 0.03 | 0.06 | 7.2 | 8277 |
| **granola** w/raisins, lowfat, 100% natural, Quaker - ⅔ cup (1.9 oz) | 55 | 215 | 1.9 | 44.6 | 18.5 | | 3.1 | 139 | 35 | 47 | 1.07 | 1.150 | 1 | 0 | 0.19 | 1.2 | 0.05 | 0.37 |
| | | 4.3 | 3.0 | 1.4 | 0.8 | 0.6 | 0 | 227 | 147 | 1.46 | 0.170 | 1.4 | 10 | 0.4 | 0.11 | 0.10 | 14.3 | 8220 |
| **granola** with raisins, lowfat, Kellogg's - ⅔ cup (2.1 oz) | 60 | 230 | 2.1 | 49.0 | 17.4 | | 3.8 | 148 | 23 | 44 | 3.78 | | 225 | 1 | 0.36 | 5.0 | 6.00 | 0.37 |
| | | 4.7 | 3.0 | 0.8 | 1.2 | 1.0 | 0 | 184 | 140 | 1.80 | 0.360 | 10.4 | 750 | 1.3 | 0.42 | 1.98 | 672.6 | 8284 |
| **Grape Nuts Flakes**, Post | 29 | 106 | 0.9 | 23.6 | 5.1 | | 2.6 | 140 | 11 | 30 | 1.20 | | | 0 | 0.37 | 5.0 | 1.50 | |
| ¾ cup (1 oz) | | 2.9 | 0.8 | 0.2 | | | 0 | 99 | 88 | 8.10 | 0.145 | | 750 | | 0.43 | 0.50 | 166.2 | 8330 |
| **Great Grains**, crunchy pecan, Post | 53 | 216 | 3.1 | 37.8 | 8.1 | | 3.7 | 214 | 15 | 46 | 1.20 | | | 0 | 0.38 | 5.0 | 1.50 | |
| ⅔ cup (1.9 oz) | | 4.9 | 6.3 | 0.7 | | | 0 | 170 | 118 | 2.70 | 0.179 | | 750 | | 0.45 | 0.50 | 163.2 | 8331 |
| **Great Grains**, raisin, date, pecan, Post - ⅔ cup (1.9 oz) | 54 | 204 | 4.7 | 39.5 | 13.3 | | 4.0 | 156 | 17 | 45 | 1.20 | | | 0 | 0.38 | 5.0 | 1.50 | |
| | | 4.3 | 4.5 | 0.6 | | | 0 | 176 | 106 | 3.60 | 0.166 | | 750 | | 0.43 | 0.50 | 162.5 | 8332 |
| **Groovy Grahams**, Mother's | 30 | 112 | 0.8 | 25.9 | 13.4 | | 0.9 | 261 | 41 | 17 | 0.31 | 0.114 | 2 | 0 | 0.04 | 0.5 | 0 | 0.12 |
| ¾ cup (1.1 oz) | | 1.6 | 0.5 | 0.1 | 0.1 | 0.2 | 0 | 226 | 49 | 1.49 | 0.036 | | 44 | | 0.21 | 0.02 | 4.2 | 8354 |
| **Harmony**, General Mills | 55 | 201 | 1.6 | 43.4 | 13.2 | | 2.2 | 355 | 600 | 24 | 7.48 | 0.747 | 150 | 30 | 1.50 | 10.0 | 4.18 | |
| 1¼ cups (1.9 oz) | | 6.1 | 1.2 | 0.3 | 0.4 | 0.3 | 0 | 91 | 100 | 9.02 | 0.080 | 12.0 | 500 | 13.5 | 0.85 | 1.00 | 672.7 | 8398 |
| **Healthy Choice**, almond crnch w/ raisins, Kellogg's - 1 cup (1.9 oz) | 55 | 198 | 3.2 | 43.2 | 15.5 | | 4.6 | 215 | 27 | 49 | 1.43 | 1.205 | 142 | 0 | 0.50 | 6.7 | 1.98 | 3.30 |
| | | 4.8 | 2.6 | 0.4 | 1.2 | 0.8 | 0 | 198 | 130 | 6.00 | 0.165 | 4.6 | 474 | 1.9 | 0.55 | 0.66 | 179.3 | 8195 |
| **Heart-to-Heart**, Kashi | 33 | 118 | 0.9 | 25.1 | 4.6 | | 4.7 | 79 | 8 | 9 | 1.48 | | 62 | 30 | 0.16 | 0.6 | 6.01 | 0.21 |
| ¾ cup (1.2 oz) | | 4.3 | 1.7 | 0.3 | | 1.0 | 0 | 102 | 33 | 1.82 | 0.100 | 9.4 | 1250 | 13.5 | 0.06 | 2.01 | 669.9 | 8387 |
| **Heart-to-Heart**, wild blueberry, Kashi - 1¼ cups (1.9 oz) | 55 | 204 | 1.6 | 41.8 | 12.1 | | 3.9 | 133 | 25 | 47 | 1.49 | | 63 | 30 | | | 6.00 | |
| | | 6.0 | 2.6 | 0.5 | 0.7 | 1.4 | 0 | 116 | 145 | 1.82 | | | 1258 | 20.1 | — | 1.98 | | 8538 |
| **Honey Bunches of Oats**, almond, Post - ¾ cup (1.1 oz) | 31 | 126 | 0.9 | 24.2 | 6.5 | | 1.4 | 187 | 11 | 21 | 0.30 | | | 0 | 0.38 | 5.0 | 1.50 | |
| | | 2.4 | 2.6 | 0.3 | | | 0 | 70 | 60 | 8.10 | 0.069 | | 750 | | 0.42 | 0.50 | 166.2 | 8334 |
| **Honey Buzzers**, Malt-O-Meal | 29 | 115 | 0.5 | 25.4 | 10.8 | | 0.8 | 206 | 4 | 9 | 2.15 | 0.175 | 313 | 1 | 0.54 | 6.3 | 2.12 | 0.02 |
| 1⅓ cups (1 oz) | | 1.8 | 0.6 | 0.2 | 0.2 | 0.2 | 0 | 35 | 29 | 2.28 | 0.048 | 3.1 | 1044 | 0.1 | 0.59 | 0.62 | 518.2 | 8476 |
| **Honey Crunch 'n Oats**, organic, Barbara's Bakery - ½ cup | 30 | 110 | | 25.0 | 6.0 | | 3.0 | 105 | 0 | | 3.75 | | | 6 | 0.38 | 5.0 | | |
| | | 2.0 | 1.5 | 0 | | | 0 | 110 | | 4.50 | | | 500 | | 0.42 | 0.50 | | BARB40 |
| **Honey Crunch Corn Flakes**, Kellogg's - ¾ cup (1.1 oz) | 30 | 116 | 0.9 | 26.1 | 9.9 | | 1.0 | 210 | 7 | 7 | 0.09 | 0.045 | 151 | 6 | 0.38 | 5.0 | 1.50 | 0.07 |
| | | 2.0 | 0.6 | 0.1 | 0.3 | 0.2 | 0 | 31 | 18 | 1.86 | 0.030 | 1.5 | 501 | 0.2 | 0.45 | 0.51 | 165.9 | 8309 |
| **Honey Graham Cereal**, Malt-O-Meal - ¾ cup (1.1 oz) | 30 | 114 | 1.1 | 24.8 | 9.3 | | 1.6 | 273 | 357 | 11 | 4.01 | 0.198 | 122 | 6 | 0.33 | 6.6 | 0.85 | 0.08 |
| | | 1.5 | 0.9 | 0.2 | 0.4 | 0.4 | 0 | 47 | 191 | 4.95 | 0.028 | 4.4 | 405 | 0.1 | 0.43 | 0.80 | 186.3 | 8481 |
| **Honey Graham Oh!s**, Quaker | 27 | 111 | 0.7 | 22.6 | 11.6 | | 0.5 | 166 | 3 | 12 | 4.96 | 0.140 | 199 | 2 | 0.50 | 6.6 | 0 | 0.09 |
| ¾ cup (.95 oz) | | 1.1 | 2.0 | 1.6 | 0.2 | 0.2 | 0 | 44 | 39 | 5.95 | 0.035 | 1.3 | 662 | 0.2 | 0.56 | 0.66 | 676.6 | 8211 |
| **Honey Graham**, Quaker | 30 | 118 | 0.8 | 25.1 | 11.5 | | 0.8 | 248 | 10 | 18 | 4.42 | 0.162 | 177 | 7 | 0.44 | 5.9 | 0.02 | 0.15 |
| ¾ cup (1.1 oz) | | 1.7 | 1.6 | 0.4 | 0.2 | 0.2 | 0 | 70 | 57 | 5.30 | 0.054 | 0.9 | 590 | | 0.50 | 0.59 | 761.1 | 8361 |
| **Honey Nut Chex**, General Mills | 30 | 120 | 0.7 | 25.8 | 9.0 | | 0.3 | 220 | 100 | 5 | 3.75 | 0.434 | 1 | 6 | 0.38 | 5.0 | 1.50 | 0.20 |
| ¾ cup (1.1 oz) | | 2.0 | 0.5 | 0.1 | 0.2 | 0.2 | 0 | 35 | 20 | 9.00 | 0.042 | 0.5 | 20 | 0.2 | 0.43 | 0.50 | 336.0 | 8057 |
| **Honey Nut Clusters**, General Mills | 55 | 210 | 1.2 | 46.0 | 17.0 | | 3.0 | 280 | 20 | 24 | 4.50 | 1.026 | 0 | 6 | 0.37 | 5.0 | 1.50 | 0.35 |
| 1 cup (1.9 oz) | | 4.0 | 2.5 | 0 | 1.5 | 0.5 | 0 | 135 | 80 | 4.50 | 0.080 | 5.9 | 3 | 1.3 | 0.42 | 0.50 | 162.8 | 8243 |
| **Honey Nut O's**, organic, Barbara's Bakery - ¾ cup | 30 | 120 | | 24.0 | 11.0 | | 2.0 | 80 | 80 | 24 | 3.75 | | | 15 | 0.38 | 5.0 | 1.50 | |
| | | 3.0 | 2.0 | 0 | | | 0 | 80 | 0 | 8.10 | | | 1250 | | 0.42 | 0.50 | | BARB41 |
| **Honey Nut Oats**, Quaker | 55 | 212 | 1.4 | 46.5 | 21.3 | | 2.4 | 443 | 15 | 35 | 8.10 | 1.056 | | 13 | 0.52 | 10.8 | 0 | 0.17 |
| 1 cup (1.9 oz) | | 3.3 | 2.0 | 0.3 | 0.8 | 0.5 | 0 | 105 | 139 | 9.72 | 0.082 | | 1081 | | 0.92 | 1.08 | | 8395 |
| **Honey Puffs**, Kashi | 30 | 114 | 0.9 | 24.8 | 6.9 | | 2.0 | 6 | 9 | 34 | 0.75 | 0.945 | 0 | 0 | 0.03 | 0.8 | 0 | 0.29 |
| 1 cup (1.1 oz) | | 3.0 | 1.0 | 0.1 | 0.2 | 0.3 | 0 | 79 | 79 | 0.70 | 0.112 | 8.5 | 1 | 0.3 | 0.04 | 0.07 | 7.8 | 8389 |
| **Honey Roundup**, Mother's | 30 | 115 | 0.8 | 26.3 | 10.7 | | 0.9 | 176 | 7 | 19 | 0.38 | 0.276 | | 0 | 0.05 | 0.3 | 0 | 0.12 |
| ¾ cup (1.1 oz) | | 1.6 | 0.6 | 0.1 | 0.2 | 0.2 | 0 | 71 | 59 | 0.53 | 0.045 | | 41 | | 0.02 | 0.02 | | 8394 |
| **Honeycomb**, Post | 29 | 115 | 0.4 | 25.8 | 11.1 | | 0.7 | 215 | 5 | 11 | 1.50 | | | 0 | 0.37 | 5.0 | 1.50 | |
| 1⅓ cups (1 oz) | | 1.5 | 0.6 | 0.2 | | | 0 | 35 | 27 | 2.70 | 0.020 | | 750 | | 0.43 | 0.50 | 166.2 | 8335 |
| **Just Right**, fruit and nut, Kellogg's - 1 cup (2.1 oz) | 60 | 220 | 3.5 | 49.0 | 15.0 | | 3.1 | 275 | 21 | 31 | 0.78 | 0.857 | 149 | 0 | 0.36 | 5.0 | 6.00 | 0 |
| | | 4.2 | 2.0 | 0.3 | 0.9 | 0.8 | 0 | 161 | 107 | 16.20 | 0.120 | 3.1 | 497 | 1.3 | 0.42 | 1.98 | 673.2 | 8283 |

| | WT (g) | KCAL / PRO (g) | H₂0 (g) / FAT (g) | CHO (g) / SFA (g) | TSUG (g) / MUFA (g) | ASUG (g) / PUFA (g) | DFIB (g) / CHOL (mg) | Na (mg) / K (mg) | Ca (mg) / P (mg) | Mg (mg) / Fe (mg) | Zn (mg) / Cu (mg) | Mn (mg) / Se (mcg) | A (mcg RAE) / A (IU) | C (mg) / E (mg ATE) | B-1 (mg) / B-2 (mg) | NIA (mg) / B-6 (mg) | B-12 (mcg) / FOL (mcg DFE) | PANT (mg) / REF |
|---|---|---|---|---|---|---|---|---|---|---|---|---|---|---|---|---|---|---|
| **Just Right** with crunchy nuggets, Kellogg's - *1 cup (1.9 oz )* | 55 | 204 | 1.8 | 46.0 | 11.7 | | 2.8 | 338 | 14 | 34 | 0.88 | 1.149 | 376 | 0 | 0.38 | 5.0 | 1.49 | 0 |
| | | 4.2 | 1.5 | 0.1 | 0.3 | 1.0 | 0 | 121 | 106 | 16.23 | 0.055 | 2.8 | 1250 | 1.5 | 0.44 | 0.50 | 166.6 | 8242 |
| **Kaboom**, General Mills *1¼ cups (1.1 oz)* | 30 | 120 | 0.7 | 26.2 | 6.0 | | 1.0 | 190 | 100 | 16 | 3.75 | 0.096 | 150 | 6 | 0.38 | 5.0 | 1.50 | 0.11 |
| | | 1.0 | 1.0 | 0.1 | 0.3 | 0.4 | 0 | 40 | 40 | 8.40 | 0.048 | 6.0 | 500 | 0.2 | 0.43 | 0.50 | 336.0 | 8278 |
| **King Vitaman**, Quaker *1½ cups (1.1 oz)* | 31 | 120 | 0.6 | 26.4 | 6.3 | | 1.1 | 259 | 3 | 26 | 3.94 | 0.282 | 297 | 12 | 0.39 | 5.2 | 1.55 | 0.17 |
| | | 2.0 | 1.1 | 0.5 | 0.2 | 0.4 | 0 | 85 | 79 | 8.99 | 0.065 | 2.0 | 1039 | 1.4 | 0.44 | 0.52 | 699.0 | 8047 |
| **Kix**, berry berry, General Mills *¾ cup (1.1 oz)* | 30 | 120 | 0.7 | 26.0 | 9.0 | | 1.0 | 160 | 40 | 0 | 3.75 | 0.084 | 150 | 6 | 0.38 | 5.0 | 1.50 | 0.08 |
| | | 1.0 | 1.5 | 0.4 | 0.9 | 0 | 0 | 40 | 40 | 4.50 | 0.028 | 6.0 | 500 | 0.2 | 0.43 | 0.50 | 165.9 | 8274 |
| **Kix**, General Mills *1⅓ cups (1.1 oz)* | 30 | 110 | 0.8 | 24.8 | 2.9 | | 2.7 | 199 | 171 | 15 | 5.23 | 0.339 | 263 | 8 | 0.59 | 7.3 | 1.71 | 0.16 |
| | | 2.3 | 1.0 | 0.2 | 0.3 | 0.4 | 0 | 56 | 57 | 9.60 | 0.043 | 2.6 | 904 | 0.1 | 0.60 | 0.69 | 397.2 | 8048 |
| **Life**, oat cinnamon, Quaker *¾ cup (1.1 oz)* | 32 | 119 | 1.4 | 25.4 | 8.4 | | 2.0 | 153 | 112 | 28 | 4.41 | 0.810 | 1 | 0 | 0.44 | 5.9 | 0 | 0.16 |
| | | 2.9 | 1.3 | 0.2 | 0.4 | 0.4 | 0 | 83 | 120 | 7.42 | 0.074 | 0.8 | 11 | 0.2 | 0.50 | 0.59 | | 8210 |
| **Life**, oat, Quaker *¾ cup (1.1 oz)* | 32 | 119 | 1.4 | 24.9 | 6.2 | | 2.1 | 164 | 112 | 30 | 4.06 | 0.874 | 1 | 0 | 0.41 | 5.6 | 0 | 0.18 |
| | | 3.2 | 1.4 | 0.3 | 0.5 | 0.5 | 0 | 91 | 132 | 8.99 | 0.086 | 1.0 | 13 | 0.2 | 0.48 | 0.56 | 452.2 | 8049 |
| **Lucky Charms**, chocolate, General Mills - *1 cup (1.1 oz)* | 30 | 120 | 0.7 | 26.4 | 15.0 | | 1.0 | 160 | 100 | 16 | 3.75 | | | 6 | 0.38 | 5.0 | 1.50 | |
| | | 1.0 | 1.0 | | | | 0 | 50 | 40 | 4.50 | | | 500 | | 0.43 | 0.50 | 336.0 | 8513 |
| **Lucky Charms**, General Mills *1 cup (1.1 oz)* | 30 | 122 | 1.0 | 24.9 | 12.0 | | 1.4 | 204 | 120 | 18 | 4.87 | 0.562 | 168 | 7 | 0.52 | 6.7 | 1.78 | 0.20 |
| | | 2.1 | 1.1 | 0.2 | 0.4 | 0.4 | 0 | 55 | 71 | 5.52 | 0.050 | 4.9 | 558 | 0.1 | 0.57 | 0.58 | 375.9 | 8050 |
| **Marshmallow Mateys**, Malt-O-Meal - *1 cup (1.1 oz)* | 30 | 118 | 0.5 | 25.0 | 12.8 | | 1.4 | 220 | 137 | 18 | 4.35 | 0.508 | 268 | 9 | 0.50 | 6.0 | 2.19 | 0.03 |
| | | 2.2 | 1.1 | 0.2 | 0.4 | 0.4 | 0 | 59 | 75 | 5.79 | 0.075 | 4.5 | 891 | 0.1 | 0.56 | 0.79 | 375.9 | 8138 |
| **Marshmallow Safari**, Quaker *¾ cup (1.1 oz)* | 30 | 119 | 0.6 | 25.3 | 14.2 | | 1.3 | 192 | 26 | 17 | 3.75 | 0.579 | 300 | 12 | 0.38 | 5.0 | 0 | 0.11 |
| | | 1.7 | 1.5 | 0.4 | 0.8 | 0.4 | 0 | 42 | 58 | 4.50 | 0.063 | 5.9 | 1000 | 0.1 | 0.42 | 0.50 | 165.9 | 8298 |
| **Mighty Bites**, cinnamon, Kashi *1 cup (1.2 oz)* | 33 | 117 | 0.9 | 23.1 | 5.3 | | 3.0 | 162 | 150 | 40 | 3.76 | | | 15 | 0.36 | 5.0 | 1.65 | |
| | | 5.6 | 1.3 | 0.3 | 0.5 | 0.5 | 0 | 111 | 111 | 8.25 | | | 500 | 2.0 | 0.43 | 0.50 | 165.7 | 8540 |
| **Mighty Bites**, honey crunch, Kashi *1 cup (1.2 oz)* | 33 | 116 | 0.9 | 22.8 | 5.6 | | 3.0 | 159 | 150 | 40 | 3.76 | 0 | | 15 | 0.36 | 5.0 | 1.48 | 0 |
| | | 5.6 | 1.3 | 0.3 | 0.5 | 0.5 | 0 | 109 | 112 | 9.90 | 0 | 0 | 500 | 2.0 | 0.43 | 0.50 | | 8541 |
| **millet, puffed** *1 cup (.7 oz)* | 21 | 74 | 0.5 | 16.8 | 0.1 | | 0.6 | 1 | 2 | 22 | 0.33 | | 0 | 0 | 0.08 | 0.9 | 0 | |
| | | 2.7 | 0.7 | 0.1 | 0.2 | 0.4 | 0 | 8 | 56 | 0.59 | 0.147 | 0.6 | 0 | 0.1 | 0.06 | 0.08 | 16.6 | 43483 |
| **Mini Swirlz**, peanut butter, Kellogg's - *1 cup* | 30 | 131 | 0.8 | 22.5 | 11.4 | | 1.2 | 200 | 5 | | 3.00 | | | 15 | 0.39 | 5.0 | 1.50 | |
| | | 2.4 | 3.9 | 0.8 | 1.7 | 1.0 | 0 | 30 | 7 | 4.50 | | | 500 | 0 | 0.42 | 0.51 | 103.8 | 8558 |
| **Mini-Wheats**, frstd, maple and brown sgr, Kellogg's - *24 bscts* | 52 | 185 | 3.1 | 42.6 | 12.5 | | 5.0 | 1 | 17 | 46 | 1.51 | 1.525 | 0 | 0 | 0.36 | 5.0 | 1.51 | 0.38 |
| | | 4.2 | 0.8 | 0.2 | 0.1 | 0.5 | 0 | 176 | 148 | 16.22 | 0.177 | | 0 | | 0.42 | 0.52 | 159.6 | 8459 |
| **Mini-Wheats**, frosted strawberry delight, Kellogg's *24 biscuits* | 52 | 180 | 3.1 | 43.2 | 12.2 | | 5.0 | 0 | 16 | 45 | 1.51 | | | 0 | 0.36 | 5.0 | 1.51 | |
| | | 4.3 | 0.9 | 0.2 | 0.2 | 0.6 | 0 | 172 | 147 | 16.12 | 0.156 | | 0 | 0.2 | 0.42 | 0.52 | | 8557 |
| **Mini-Wheats**, strawberry delight, Kellogg's - *24 biscuits (1.8 oz)* | 52 | 180 | 3.1 | 43.2 | 12.2 | | 5.0 | 0 | 16 | | 1.51 | | | | 0.36 | 5.0 | 1.51 | |
| | | 4.3 | 0.9 | 0.2 | 0.2 | 0.6 | 0 | | | 16.12 | 0.156 | | | | 0.42 | 0.52 | 162.8 | 8542 |
| **Mini-Wheats**, vanilla crème, Kellogg's - *24 biscuits (1.8 oz)* | 52 | 180 | 3.1 | 43.2 | 12.5 | | 5.0 | 1 | 17 | 61 | 1.66 | | | 0 | 0.42 | 5.2 | 1.51 | |
| | | 4.2 | 0.9 | 0.2 | 0.2 | 0.5 | 0 | 172 | 153 | 16.12 | 0.156 | | 0 | 0 | 0.47 | 0.52 | 165.4 | 8525 |
| **MiniSwirlz**, fudge ripple, Kellogg's - *1 cup (1.1 oz)* | 30 | 117 | 0.8 | 25.2 | 12.3 | | 0.9 | 135 | 6 | 12 | 3.00 | | | 15 | 0.39 | 5.0 | 1.50 | |
| | | 1.8 | 1.4 | 0.3 | 0.5 | 0.3 | 0 | 49 | 40 | 4.50 | 0.030 | | 500 | | 0.42 | 0.51 | 165.9 | 8536 |
| **Muesli**, dried fruit and nuts *1 cup (3 oz)* | 85 | 289 | 4.9 | 66.1 | 26.4 | | 6.2 | 196 | 0 | 66 | 3.10 | 1.850 | 139 | 0 | 0.77 | 10.3 | 3.10 | 3.91 |
| | | 8.2 | 4.2 | 0.7 | 2.0 | 1.1 | 0 | 413 | 207 | 7.44 | 0.332 | 14.7 | 464 | 6.1 | 0.88 | 1.04 | 340.0 | 42184 |
| **Mueslix**, raisin almond crunch w/ dates, Kellogg's - *⅔ cup (1.9 oz)* | 55 | 196 | 4.8 | 40.2 | 17.0 | | 4.0 | 170 | 32 | 49 | 3.74 | 1.197 | 90 | 0 | 0.44 | 5.5 | 6.05 | 2.53 |
| | | 5.0 | 3.0 | 0.4 | 1.6 | 1.0 | 0 | 240 | 100 | 4.51 | 0.110 | 9.5 | 300 | 4.0 | 0.44 | 2.04 | 682.6 | 8286 |
| **Multi-Bran Chex**, General Mills *1 cup (1.7 oz)* | 49 | 161 | 1.2 | 41.2 | 10.1 | | 5.9 | 304 | 104 | 63 | 3.91 | 1.558 | 144 | 6 | 0.39 | 5.2 | 1.56 | |
| | | 3.4 | 1.3 | 0.2 | 0.3 | 0.4 | 0 | 186 | 127 | 16.89 | 0.189 | 3.9 | 521 | 0.2 | 0.44 | 0.52 | 694.8 | 8345 |
| **Natural Cereal**, 100%, oats and honey, Quaker - *½ cup (1.8 oz)* | 51 | 219 | 1.1 | 37.0 | 13.2 | | 3.5 | 26 | 60 | 57 | 1.38 | 1.346 | 0 | 0 | 0.19 | 1.1 | 0.12 | 0.46 |
| | | 5.3 | 6.6 | 4.0 | 1.3 | 0.9 | 1 | 236 | 187 | 1.37 | 0.184 | 1.0 | 4 | 0.8 | 0.14 | 0.11 | 17.8 | 8054 |
| **Natural Cereal**, 100%, oats, honey, raisins, Quaker - *½ cup (1.8 oz)* | 51 | 213 | 1.8 | 37.7 | 15.2 | | 3.3 | 28 | 55 | 52 | 1.22 | 1.193 | 0 | 0 | 0.18 | 1.0 | 0.11 | 0.41 |
| | | 4.8 | 5.8 | 3.6 | 1.2 | 0.8 | 1 | 247 | 168 | 1.32 | 0.178 | 7.0 | 4 | 0.7 | 0.13 | 0.11 | 15.8 | 8218 |
| **Oat Bran Flakes**, Common Sense, Kellogg's - *¾ cup (1.1 oz)* | 30 | 105 | 0.9 | 23.1 | 6.0 | | 3.9 | 210 | 16 | 45 | 15.60 | 1.195 | 235 | 63 | 1.65 | 21.0 | 6.03 | 10.50 |
| | | 3.3 | 1.0 | 0.2 | 0.5 | 0.3 | 0 | 120 | 105 | 18.90 | 0.090 | 5.1 | 781 | 12.6 | 1.80 | 2.10 | 681.9 | 8258 |
| **Oat Bran Flakes**, Health Valley *1 cup (1.7 oz)* | 47 | 166 | 1.6 | 36.9 | 9.2 | | 6.1 | 17 | 18 | 79 | 1.19 | | 0 | 0 | 0.25 | 3.2 | 0 | |
| | | 5.0 | 0.7 | 0.1 | 0.2 | 0.2 | 0 | 151 | 238 | 2.35 | 0.084 | 17.6 | 4 | 0.18 | 0.05 | 21.6 | 43495 |
| **Oat Bran**, Quaker *1¼ cups (2 oz)* | 57 | 212 | 2.3 | 42.7 | 9.3 | | 5.6 | 207 | 109 | 96 | 3.96 | 2.194 | 165 | 7 | 0.41 | 5.5 | 0 | 0.48 |
| | | 7.1 | 2.9 | 0.5 | 0.9 | 1.2 | 0 | 250 | 295 | 17.07 | 0.182 | 4.0 | 550 | 1.4 | 0.47 | 0.55 | 706.8 | 8216 |
| **Oatmeal Crisp**, almond, General Mills - *1 cup (1.9 oz)* | 55 | 220 | 1.6 | 42.5 | 16.0 | | 4.1 | 250 | 20 | 60 | 3.75 | 1.448 | 0 | 6 | 0.37 | 5.0 | 1.50 | 0.39 |
| | | 5.0 | 4.5 | 0.5 | 2.0 | 1.5 | 0 | 180 | 150 | 4.50 | 0.120 | 9.5 | 3 | 1.9 | 0.42 | 0.50 | 162.8 | 8202 |
| **Oatmeal Crisp**, apple, General Mills - *1 cup (1.9 oz)* | 55 | 210 | 1.4 | 46.2 | 19.0 | | 4.0 | 270 | 20 | 40 | 3.75 | 1.324 | 0 | 6 | 0.37 | 5.0 | 1.50 | 0.39 |
| | | 4.0 | 2.0 | 0.5 | 1.0 | 0.5 | 0 | 170 | 100 | 4.50 | 0.080 | 9.5 | 3 | 0.5 | 0.42 | 0.50 | 162.8 | 8190 |
| **Oatmeal Crisp**, raisin, General Mills - *1 cup (1.9 oz)* | 55 | 210 | 2.6 | 44.0 | 18.0 | | 3.4 | 220 | 20 | 40 | 3.75 | 1.223 | 0 | 0 | 0.37 | 5.0 | 1.50 | 0.40 |
| | | 5.0 | 2.0 | 0.5 | 1.0 | 0.5 | 0 | 180 | 100 | 4.50 | 0.080 | 9.5 | 0 | 1.4 | 0.42 | 0.50 | 162.8 | 8245 |

| | WT | Macronutrients | | | | | | Minerals | | | | | Vitamins | | | | | |
|---|---|---|---|---|---|---|---|---|---|---|---|---|---|---|---|---|---|---|
| | (g) | KCAL | H₂0 (g) | CHO (g) | TSUG (g) | ASUG (g) | DFIB (g) | Na (mg) | Ca (mg) | Mg (mg) | Zn (mg) | Mn (mg) | A (mcg RAE) | C (mg) | B-1 (mg) | NIA (mg) | B-12 (mcg) | PANT (mg) |
| | | PRO (g) | FAT (g) | SFA (g) | MUFA (g) | PUFA (g) | CHOL (mg) | K (mg) | P (mg) | Fe (mg) | Cu (mg) | Se (mcg) | A (IU) | E (mg ATE) | B-2 (mg) | B-6 (mg) | FOL (mcg DFE) | REF |
| **Oatmeal Crisp**, triple berry, | 55 | 210 | 1.4 | 44.6 | 16.0 | | 4.7 | 260 | 20 | 40 | 3.75 | | | 6 | 0.37 | 5.0 | 1.50 | |
| General Mills - *1 cup (1.9 oz)* | | 5.0 | 2.5 | 0.5 | 1.0 | 0.5 | 0 | 190 | 150 | 4.50 | | | 0 | | 0.42 | 0.50 | 162.8 | 8515 |
| **Oatmeal Squares**, Quaker | 56 | 212 | 1.5 | 43.9 | 9.0 | | 4.0 | 269 | 113 | 66 | 4.24 | 1.814 | 167 | 6 | 0.39 | 5.6 | 0 | 0.34 |
| *1 cup (2 oz)* | | 6.2 | 2.4 | 0.5 | 0.8 | 1.0 | 0 | 205 | 206 | 17.07 | 0.179 | 3.9 | 555 | 1.4 | 0.48 | 0.55 | 739.8 | 8214 |
| **Optimum**, Nature's Path | 55 | 190 | 2.0 | 40.4 | 16.0 | | 10.0 | 200 | 250 | 137 | 1.70 | 2.348 | 0 | 1 | 0.18 | 3.2 | 6.00 | 0.63 |
| *1 cup (1.9 oz)* | | 8.0 | 2.5 | 0 | 0.5 | 1.7 | 0 | 413 | 261 | 2.70 | 0.623 | 20.7 | 0 | 0.3 | 0.15 | 0.32 | 672.7 | 8502 |
| **Optimum Slim**, Nature's Path | 30 | 98 | 1.2 | 20.7 | 5.5 | | 6.0 | 136 | 136 | 74 | 0.91 | 1.138 | 0 | 0 | 0.10 | 1.5 | 0 | 0.36 |
| *½ cup (1.1 oz)* | | 4.9 | 1.4 | 0 | 0.3 | 0.9 | 0 | 287 | 126 | 1.47 | 0.341 | 10.4 | 0 | 0.3 | 0.11 | 0.15 | 24.6 | 8503 |
| **Oreo O's**, Post | 27 | 112 | 0.7 | 21.5 | 11.4 | | 1.5 | 128 | 5 | 15 | 1.50 | | | 0 | 0.38 | 5.0 | 1.50 | |
| *¾ cup (.95 oz)* | | 1.3 | 2.4 | 0.4 | | | 0 | 49 | 32 | 1.80 | 0.081 | | 750 | | 0.42 | 0.50 | 166.3 | 8336 |
| **Organic Promise**, autumn wheat, | 54 | 191 | 2.1 | 44.8 | 7.2 | | 6.0 | 5 | 0 | | | | 0 | 0 | | | | |
| Kashi - *1 cup (1.9 oz)* | | 5.2 | 1.1 | 0.2 | 0.2 | 0.7 | 0 | 180 | | 1.57 | | | 0 | | | | | 8462 |
| **Organic Promise**, cinnamon harvest, | 54 | 184 | 3.2 | 43.7 | 8.9 | | 5.6 | 5 | 0 | | | | | 0 | | | | |
| Kashi - *1 cup (1.9 oz)* | | 4.5 | 1.1 | 0.2 | 0.2 | 0.6 | 0 | 169 | | 1.51 | | | 0 | | | | | 8539 |
| **Organic Promise**, cranberry | 29 | 116 | 0.9 | 25.5 | 7.2 | | 2.9 | 21 | | | | | | | | | | |
| sunshine, Kashi - *1 cup (1 oz)* | | 1.6 | 0.9 | 0.1 | 0.2 | 0.5 | 0 | 83 | | 0.41 | | | | | | | | 8467 |
| **Organic Promise**, strawberry fields, | 54 | 199 | 1.3 | 47.0 | 15.8 | | 1.9 | 338 | 9 | | | | | 12 | | | | |
| Kashi - *1 cup (1.9 oz)* | | 4.2 | 0.2 | 0 | 0 | 0 | 0 | 66 | | 0.79 | | | 10 | | | | | 8463 |
| **Organic Wild Puffs**, Barbara's | 27 | 100 | | 23.0 | 12.0 | | 0.5 | 40 | 0 | | 3.75 | | | 15 | 0.38 | 5.0 | 1.50 | |
| Bakery - *1 cup* | | 2.0 | 0.5 | 0 | | | 0 | 50 | | 8.10 | | | 1250 | | 0.42 | 0.50 | | BARB43 |
| **Organic Wild Puffs**, caramel, | 30 | 110 | | 25.0 | 9.0 | | 0.5 | 160 | 40 | 32 | 3.75 | | | 15 | 0.38 | 5.0 | 1.50 | |
| Barbara's Bakery - *¾ cup* | | 2.0 | 1.0 | 0 | | | 0 | 85 | 40 | 8.10 | | | 1250 | | 0.42 | 0.50 | | BARB44 |
| **Organic Wild Puffs**, cocoa, | 30 | 110 | | 25.0 | 9.0 | | 1.0 | 190 | 40 | 40 | 3.75 | | | 15 | 0.38 | 5.0 | 1.50 | |
| Barbara's Bakery - *1 cup* | | 2.0 | 1.0 | 0 | | | 0 | 100 | 40 | 8.10 | | | 1250 | | 0.42 | 0.50 | | BARB45 |
| **Organic Wild Puffs**, fruit punch, | 30 | 110 | | 26.0 | 9.0 | | 1.0 | 55 | 40 | 36 | | | | 15 | 0.38 | 5.0 | 1.50 | |
| Barbara's Bakery - *1 cup* | | 2.0 | 1.0 | 0 | | | 0 | 95 | 40 | 8.10 | | | 1250 | | 0.42 | 0.50 | | BARB46 |
| **Peanut Butter Bumpers**, Mother's | 30 | 121 | 0.8 | 23.5 | 8.9 | | 0.9 | 242 | 30 | 22 | 0.43 | 0.201 | 2 | 0 | 0.04 | 0.9 | 0 | 0.15 |
| *¾ cup (1.1 oz)* | | 2.5 | 2.2 | 0.4 | 0.9 | 0.7 | 0 | 194 | 64 | 1.21 | 0.045 | 0.2 | 44 | | 0.15 | 0.03 | 7.2 | 8351 |
| **Peanut Butter Toast Crunch**, | 30 | 130 | 0.6 | 22.8 | 13.0 | | 1.0 | 135 | 100 | 8 | 3.75 | 0.317 | 150 | 6 | 0.38 | 5.0 | 1.50 | 0.14 |
| General Mills - *¾ cup (1.1 oz)* | | 2.0 | 3.5 | 0.5 | 2.0 | 1.0 | 0 | 60 | 20 | 4.50 | 0.048 | 4.6 | 500 | 0.6 | 0.43 | 0.50 | 165.9 | 8517 |
| **Product 19**, Kellogg's | 30 | 100 | 0.9 | 24.9 | 4.0 | | 1.0 | 207 | 5 | 16 | 15.30 | 0.338 | 214 | 61 | 1.50 | 20.0 | 6.00 | 10.08 |
| *1 cup (1.1 oz)* | | 2.3 | 0.4 | 0.1 | 0.1 | 0.2 | 0 | 50 | 40 | 18.09 | 0.036 | 3.6 | 750 | 13.5 | 1.71 | 2.07 | 675.9 | 8058 |
| **puffed rice** | 14 | 56 | 0.4 | 12.6 | | | 0.2 | 0 | 1 | 4 | 0.14 | 0.210 | 0 | 0 | 0.36 | 4.9 | 0 | 0.04 |
| *1 cup (.49 oz)* | | 0.9 | 0.1 | 0 | | | 0 | 16 | 14 | 4.44 | 0.024 | 1.5 | 0 | | 0.25 | 0.01 | 2.7 | 8156 |
| **Puffed Rice**, Malt-O-Meal | 15 | 60 | 0.1 | 13.5 | 0.1 | | 0.2 | 1 | 1 | 4 | 0.17 | 0.187 | | 0 | 0.56 | 7.8 | | 0.16 |
| *1 cup (.53 oz)* | | 1.2 | 0.1 | 0 | 0 | 0.1 | 0 | 15 | 17 | 6.68 | 0.034 | 2.6 | 15 | 0 | 0.39 | 0.03 | | 8492 |
| **Puffed Rice**, Quaker | 14 | 54 | 0.5 | 12.3 | 0 | | 0.2 | 1 | 1 | 4 | 0.15 | 0.132 | 0 | 0 | 0.06 | 0.5 | 0 | 0.05 |
| *1 cup (.49 oz)* | | 1.0 | 0.1 | 0 | 0 | 0 | 0 | 16 | 17 | 0.40 | 0.132 | 1.5 | 0 | 0 | 0.04 | 0 | 36.3 | 8066 |
| **puffed wheat** | 12 | 44 | 0.4 | 9.6 | | | 0.5 | 0 | 3 | 17 | 0.28 | 0.211 | 0 | 0 | 0.31 | 4.2 | 0 | 0.06 |
| *1 cup (.42 oz)* | | 1.8 | 0.1 | 0 | | | 0 | 42 | 43 | 3.80 | 0.049 | 14.8 | 0 | | 0.22 | 0.02 | 3.8 | 8157 |
| **Puffed Wheat**, Kellogg's | 12 | 39 | 0.5 | 9.2 | 0 | | 1.8 | 0 | 5 | | | | | 0 | | | 0 | |
| *1 cup (.5 oz)* | | 1.8 | 0.2 | 0 | 0.1 | 0.1 | 0 | 57 | 51 | 0 | | | 0 | | | | | 8379 |
| **Puffed Wheat**, Malt-O-Meal | 15 | 59 | 0.3 | 11.8 | 0.2 | | 1.1 | 2 | 4 | 22 | 0.46 | 0.644 | | 0 | 0.58 | 9.6 | | 0.16 |
| *1 cup (.5 oz)* | | 2.3 | 0.3 | 0.1 | 0.1 | 0.2 | 0 | 62 | 60 | 7.95 | 0.068 | 11.7 | 15 | 0.2 | 0.50 | 0.05 | | 8483 |
| **Puffed Wheat**, Quaker | 15 | 55 | 0.6 | 11.5 | 0.2 | | 1.4 | 1 | 4 | 20 | 0.46 | 0.300 | 0 | 0 | 0.09 | 0.8 | 0 | 0.07 |
| *1¼ cups (.53 oz)* | | 2.4 | 0.3 | 0.1 | 0 | 0.2 | 0 | 55 | 50 | 0.66 | 0.092 | 18.5 | 0 | 0 | 0.06 | 0.02 | 38.8 | 8146 |
| **puffed wheat**, sugar-coated | 28 | 111 | 0.8 | 25.5 | 15.1 | | 0 | 42 | 4 | 17 | 1.56 | 0.288 | 234 | 0 | 0.39 | 5.2 | 1.56 | 0.07 |
| *⅞ cup* | | 1.5 | 0.4 | 0.1 | 0.1 | 0.2 | 0 | 35 | 38 | 1.87 | 0.062 | 13.6 | 778 | 0.1 | 0.44 | 0.52 | 172.5 | 8073 |
| **Puffins**, Barbara's Bakery | 27 | 90 | | 23.0 | 5.0 | | 5.0 | 190 | 0 | | | | | 6 | | | | |
| *¾ cup* | | 2.0 | 1.0 | 0 | | | 0 | 85 | | 0.36 | | | 0 | | | | | BARB2 |
| **Puffins**, cinnamon, Barbara's | 30 | 100 | | 26.0 | 6.0 | | 6.0 | 150 | 0 | | | | | 9 | | | | |
| Bakery - *⅔ cup* | | 2.0 | 1.0 | 0 | | | 0 | 45 | | 0.18 | | | 0 | | | | | BARB47 |
| **Puffins**, honey rice, Barbara's | 30 | 120 | | 25.0 | 6.0 | | 2.0 | 125 | 20 | | 0.60 | | | 0 | | | | |
| Bakery - *¾ cup* | | 2.0 | 1.5 | 0 | | | 0 | 90 | | 1.08 | | | 0 | | | | | BARB48 |
| **Puffins**, peanut butter, Barbara's | 30 | 110 | | 23.0 | 6.0 | | 2.0 | 230 | 20 | | | | | 0 | | | | |
| Bakery - *¾ cup* | | 3.0 | 2.0 | 0.5 | | | 0 | 105 | | 1.08 | | | 100 | | | | | BARB49 |
| **Puffs**, Kashi | 19 | 75 | 0.6 | 15.2 | 0.6 | | 1.3 | 2 | 8 | 29 | 0.58 | 0.646 | 0 | 0 | 0.02 | 0.6 | 0 | 0.22 |
| *1 cup (.7 oz)* | | 2.3 | 0.6 | 0.1 | 0.2 | 0.2 | 0 | 63 | 46 | 0.53 | 0.086 | 6.8 | 1 | 0.2 | 0.03 | 0.06 | 6.1 | 8388 |
| **Raisin Bran Crunch**, Kellogg's | 53 | 188 | 2.8 | 45.0 | 20.0 | | 4.0 | 209 | 19 | 47 | 1.59 | 0.939 | 163 | 1 | 0.37 | 5.3 | 1.54 | 0.30 |
| *1 cup (1.9 oz)* | | 3.2 | 1.0 | 0.2 | 0.4 | 0.4 | 0 | 213 | 137 | 4.50 | 0.159 | 1.9 | 541 | 0.2 | 0.42 | 0.48 | 164.3 | 8380 |
| **Raisin Bran**, Kellogg's | 59 | 190 | 5.2 | 45.6 | 17.6 | | 6.5 | 342 | 28 | 74 | 2.05 | 1.677 | 261 | 0 | 0.66 | 8.6 | 3.02 | 0.54 |
| *1 cup (2.1 oz)* | | 5.1 | 1.3 | 0.2 | 0.2 | 0.4 | 0 | 335 | 215 | 7.53 | 0.247 | 2.1 | 868 | 0.4 | 0.94 | 1.05 | 248.4 | 8060 |

| Food | WT (g) | KCAL / PRO (g) | H₂O (g) / FAT (g) | CHO (g) / SFA (g) | TSUG (g) / MUFA (g) | ASUG (g) / PUFA (g) | DFIB (g) / CHOL (mg) | Na (mg) / K (mg) | Ca (mg) / P (mg) | Mg (mg) / Fe (mg) | Zn (mg) / Cu (mg) | Mn (mg) / Se (mcg) | A (mcg RAE) / A (IU) | C (mg) / E (mg ATE) | B-1 (mg) / B-2 (mg) | NIA (mg) / B-6 (mg) | B-12 (mcg) / FOL (mcg DFE) | PANT (mg) / REF |
|---|---|---|---|---|---|---|---|---|---|---|---|---|---|---|---|---|---|---|
| **Raisin Bran**, Malt-O-Meal | 59 | 213 | 5.0 | 45.4 | 17.9 | | 8.0 | 392 | 27 | 84 | 6.55 | 3.021 | 223 | 8 | 0.55 | 13.9 | 1.93 | 0.58 |
| *1 cup (2.1 oz)* | | 5.3 | 1.2 | 0.3 | 0.2 | 0.6 | 1 | 341 | 239 | 5.79 | 0.289 | 20.4 | 743 | 0.4 | 0.80 | 0.87 | 262.6 | 8484 |
| **Raisin Bran**, Para Su Familia, | 55 | 170 | 4.5 | 42.0 | 11.0 | | 6.8 | 300 | 700 | 40 | 7.50 | | 150 | 0 | 0.37 | 10.0 | 1.50 | |
| General Mills - *1⅓ cups (1.9 oz)* | | 4.0 | 1.0 | | | | 0 | 270 | 100 | 18.00 | 0.120 | | 500 | | 0.85 | 1.00 | 672.7 | 8371 |
| **Raisin Bran**, Post | 59 | 187 | 4.8 | 45.3 | 16.6 | | 7.1 | 289 | 32 | 93 | 4.61 | 1.894 | 225 | 5 | 0.97 | 7.7 | 3.21 | 0.12 |
| *1 cup (2.1 oz)* | | 5.5 | 1.5 | 0.2 | 0.3 | 0.6 | 0 | 362 | 232 | 14.16 | 0.311 | 3.5 | 750 | 0.5 | 1.00 | 1.07 | 333.9 | 8061 |
| **Raisin Nut Bran**, General Mills | 55 | 200 | 4.1 | 42.0 | 15.0 | | 5.4 | 250 | 20 | 40 | 3.75 | 1.241 | 0 | 0 | 0.37 | 5.0 | 1.50 | 0.32 |
| *1 cup (1.9 oz)* | | 4.0 | 3.5 | 0.5 | 1.5 | 0.5 | 0 | 200 | 150 | 4.50 | 0.160 | 3.9 | 4 | 0.9 | 0.42 | 0.50 | 162.8 | 8261 |
| **Raisin Squares Mini-Wheats**, | 55 | 188 | 4.3 | 43.9 | 12.1 | | 4.8 | 3 | 21 | 43 | 1.54 | 1.273 | 0 | 0 | 0.39 | 5.2 | 1.60 | 0 |
| Kellogg's - *¾ cup (1.9 oz)* | | 5.2 | 0.8 | 0.2 | 0.1 | 0.4 | 0 | 265 | 156 | 15.40 | 0.138 | 2.3 | 0 | 0.4 | 0.44 | 0.52 | 169.4 | 8287 |
| **Reese's Peanut Butter Puffs**, | 30 | 130 | 0.8 | 22.8 | 12.0 | | 1.2 | 200 | 100 | 8 | 3.75 | 0.090 | 145 | 6 | 0.38 | 5.0 | 1.50 | 0.10 |
| General Mills - *¾ cup* | | 2.0 | 3.5 | 0.5 | 1.5 | 1.0 | 0 | 65 | 60 | 4.50 | 0.035 | 2.0 | 500 | 0.8 | 0.43 | 0.50 | 165.9 | 8194 |
| **Rice Chex**, General Mills | 31 | 118 | 0.8 | 26.5 | 2.3 | | 0.3 | 276 | 115 | 28 | 4.31 | 0.764 | 172 | 7 | 0.43 | 5.7 | 1.72 | 0.36 |
| *1¼ cups (1.1 oz)* | | 2.0 | 0.5 | 0.1 | 0.2 | 0.2 | 0 | 52 | 35 | 10.33 | 0.063 | 1.2 | 574 | 0.2 | 0.49 | 0.57 | 389.4 | 8064 |
| **Rice Krispies**, berry, Kellogg's | 30 | 115 | 0.9 | 26.4 | 9.3 | | 0.1 | 218 | 2 | 9 | 0.33 | | | 6 | 0.39 | 5.0 | 1.50 | |
| *1 cup (1.1 oz)* | | 1.6 | 0.3 | 0.1 | 0.1 | 0.1 | 0 | 30 | 32 | 5.40 | 0.060 | | 500 | | 0.42 | 0.51 | 168.9 | 8519 |
| **Rice Krispies**, Kellogg's | 33 | 128 | 1.4 | 28.1 | 3.1 | | 0.3 | 299 | 2 | 9 | 0.42 | 0.454 | 187 | 9 | 0.60 | 7.0 | 3.13 | 0.20 |
| *1¼ cups (1.2 oz)* | | 2.3 | 0.3 | 0.1 | 0.1 | 0.1 | 0 | 37 | 42 | 11.35 | 0.057 | 6.0 | 623 | 0 | 0.73 | 0.99 | 301.3 | 8065 |
| **Rice Krispies** Treats, Kellogg's | 30 | 120 | 1.0 | 25.4 | 9.3 | | 0.1 | 166 | 3 | 7 | 0.24 | | 152 | 6 | 0.39 | 5.1 | 1.50 | |
| *¾ cup (1.1 oz)* | | 1.4 | 1.4 | 0.3 | 0.5 | 0.2 | 0 | 23 | 24 | 1.86 | 0.030 | 3.6 | 504 | 0.1 | 0.42 | 0.51 | 169.5 | 8288 |
| **Robots**, Kellogg's | 29 | 113 | 0.9 | 24.9 | 11.0 | | 0.8 | 157 | 5 | 15 | 1.51 | | | 15 | 0.38 | 5.0 | 1.51 | |
| *1 cup (1 oz)* | | 1.7 | 0.9 | 0.1 | 0.4 | 0.2 | 0 | | 37 | 4.50 | | | 500 | | 0.43 | 0.49 | 166.2 | 8527 |
| **Scooby-Doo**, berry bones, Kellogg's | 32 | 124 | 0.9 | 27.5 | 11.8 | | 0.8 | 226 | 6 | 15 | 1.66 | 0.143 | 166 | 17 | 0.42 | 5.4 | 1.66 | 0.06 |
| *1 cup (1.1 oz)* | | 1.9 | 0.9 | 0.1 | 0.2 | 0.5 | 0 | 47 | 33 | 1.98 | 0.032 | 2.7 | 552 | 0.1 | 0.48 | 0.54 | 183.4 | 8466 |
| **Seven in the Morning**, Kashi | 50 | 178 | 1.5 | 40.5 | 2.5 | | 5.8 | 224 | 20 | 70 | 1.52 | 1.918 | 0 | 0 | 0.12 | 2.3 | 0 | 0.55 |
| *½ cup (1.8 oz)* | | 6.0 | 1.4 | 0.3 | 0.3 | 0.8 | 0 | 188 | 149 | 11.50 | 0.212 | 27.0 | 4 | 0.4 | 0.08 | 0.15 | 16.0 | 8464 |
| **Seven Whole Grain Flakes**, Kashi | 50 | 175 | 1.7 | 40.9 | 4.3 | | 5.6 | 152 | 15 | 50 | 1.25 | | | 0 | | | | |
| *1 cup (1.8 oz)* | | 5.5 | 1.0 | 0.2 | 0.2 | 0.6 | 0 | 160 | 142 | 1.50 | | | 0 | | | | | 8537 |
| **Shredded Oats**, bite size, Barbara's | 58 | 220 | | 46.0 | 12.0 | | 5.0 | 260 | 20 | 60 | 1.50 | | | 21 | 0.15 | 1.2 | | |
| Bakery - *1¼ cups* | | 6.0 | 2.5 | 0.5 | | | 0 | 230 | 150 | 1.80 | 0.200 | | 0 | | 0.07 | | | BARB53 |
| **Shredded Oats**, vanilla almond, bite | 55 | 220 | | 42.0 | 15.0 | | 4.0 | 210 | 20 | 60 | | | | 21 | 0.15 | 0.8 | | |
| size, Barbara's Bakery - *1 cup* | | 7.0 | 3.0 | 0.5 | | | 0 | 150 | 150 | 1.80 | | | 0 | | 0.07 | | | BARB54 |
| **Shredded Spoonfuls**, Barbara's | 32 | 120 | | 24.0 | 5.0 | | 4.0 | 200 | | | | | | 5 | | | | |
| Bakery - *¾ cup* | | 4.0 | 1.5 | 0 | | | 0 | 125 | | 0.72 | | | 0 | | | | | BARB1 |
| **Shredded Wheat**, Barbara's Bakery | 40 | 140 | | 31.0 | 0 | | 5.0 | 0 | 20 | 60 | 1.20 | | | 0 | 0.09 | 2.0 | | |
| *2 biscuits* | | 4.0 | 1.0 | 0 | | | 0 | 160 | 150 | 1.08 | 0.200 | | 0 | | 0.03 | 0.08 | | BARB55 |
| **shredded wheat**, frosted | 24 | 92 | 0.9 | 19.5 | 5.5 | | 1.8 | 5 | 6 | 21 | 0.52 | 0.684 | 0 | 0 | 0.17 | 2.3 | 0.69 | 0.15 |
| *1 rectangular biscuit (.85 oz)* | | 2.4 | 0.9 | 0.1 | 0.4 | 0.3 | 0 | 61 | 57 | 0.83 | 0.075 | 9.8 | 0 | 0.4 | 0.20 | 0.23 | 71.3 | 8081 |
| **Shredded Wheat**, frosted, bite size, | 52 | 183 | 3.1 | 43.6 | 11.6 | | 5.0 | 10 | 7 | 48 | 1.50 | | | 0 | 0.37 | 5.0 | 1.50 | |
| Post - *1 cup (1.8 oz)* | | 4.1 | 1.0 | 0.2 | | | 0 | 170 | 144 | 1.80 | 0.090 | | 0 | | 0.43 | 0.50 | 162.8 | 8339 |
| **Shredded Wheat Miniatures**, | 53 | 180 | 2.7 | 42.4 | 1.1 | | 6.9 | 0 | 22 | | 1.86 | | | | 0.26 | 3.6 | | |
| Kellogg's - *1 cup (1.9 oz)* | | 5.8 | 1.1 | 0.2 | 0.2 | 0.7 | 0 | 240 | 205 | 15.90 | 0.212 | | | | 0.32 | 0.37 | 109.7 | 8384 |
| **Shredded Wheat n' Bran**, Post | 59 | 197 | 2.7 | 47.1 | 0.6 | | 7.9 | 3 | 27 | 81 | 1.93 | | | 0 | 0.15 | 3.7 | 0 | |
| *1¼ cups (2.1 oz)* | | 7.4 | 0.8 | 0.1 | | | 0 | 248 | 235 | 2.47 | 0.236 | | 0 | | 0.07 | 0.19 | 27.1 | 8341 |
| **Shredded Wheat**, Post | 24 | 81 | 1.5 | 18.9 | 0.2 | | 2.9 | 1 | 12 | 32 | 0.72 | 0.605 | 0 | 2 | 0.06 | 1.3 | 0 | 0.07 |
| *1 rectangular biscuit (.85 oz)* | | 2.7 | 0.5 | 0.1 | 0.1 | 0.3 | 0 | 90 | 89 | 0.71 | 0.087 | 0.7 | 0 | 0 | 0.03 | 0.28 | 10.3 | 8147 |
| **Shredded Wheat**, spoon size, Post | 49 | 167 | 2.0 | 40.7 | 0.4 | | 5.6 | 3 | 21 | 57 | 1.31 | | | 0 | 0.13 | 2.7 | 0 | |
| *1 cup (1.7 oz)* | | 5.0 | 0.5 | 0.1 | | | 0 | 203 | 175 | 1.56 | 0.162 | | 0 | | 0.06 | 0.20 | 20.6 | 8342 |
| **Smacks**, Kellogg's | 27 | 104 | 0.7 | 24.0 | 15.1 | | 1.0 | 50 | 6 | 16 | 0.35 | 0.378 | 153 | 6 | 0.38 | 5.0 | 1.51 | 0.10 |
| *¾ cup (.95 oz)* | | 1.7 | 0.5 | 0.1 | 0.2 | 0.2 | 0 | 41 | 46 | 0.35 | 0.054 | 13.1 | 509 | 0.1 | 0.43 | 0.51 | 168.5 | 8071 |
| **Smart Start Healthy Heart**, | 50 | 183 | 1.8 | 39.5 | 14.0 | | 4.4 | 117 | 18 | 68 | 3.15 | | | 12 | 0.30 | 4.2 | 1.25 | 2.10 |
| Kellogg's - *1 cup (1.8 oz)* | | 5.0 | 1.9 | 0.4 | 0.6 | 1.0 | 0 | 316 | 208 | 3.75 | | | 1042 | 11.2 | 0.35 | 0.40 | 138.0 | 8528 |
| **Smart Start Healthy Heart**, maple | 60 | 220 | 2.1 | 47.4 | 16.8 | | 5.1 | 140 | 22 | 79 | 3.78 | | | 15 | 0.36 | 5.0 | 1.50 | 2.52 |
| brown sgr, Kellogg's - *1¼ cups* | | 6.0 | 2.2 | 0.4 | 0.7 | 1.1 | 0 | 380 | 254 | 4.50 | 0.162 | 0.1 | 1250 | 13.5 | 0.42 | 0.48 | | 8529 |
| **Smart Start**, Kellogg's | 50 | 182 | 1.5 | 43.0 | 14.0 | | 2.7 | 275 | 12 | 24 | 15.00 | | 376 | 15 | 1.50 | 20.0 | 6.00 | 10.00 |
| *1 cup (1.8 oz)* | | 3.5 | 0.7 | 0.1 | 0.1 | 0.5 | 0 | 90 | 80 | 18.00 | 0.100 | 10.7 | 1250 | 13.5 | 1.70 | 2.00 | 673.5 | 8318 |
| **Smorz**, Kellogg's | 30 | 122 | 0.8 | 24.9 | 12.9 | | 0.8 | 137 | 7 | 9 | 1.50 | 0.138 | 155 | 15 | 0.39 | 5.0 | 1.50 | 0.08 |
| *1 cup (1.1 oz)* | | 1.5 | 2.1 | 0.9 | 0.3 | 1.2 | 0 | 29 | 20 | 4.50 | 0.053 | 2.1 | 500 | 0.1 | 0.42 | 0.51 | 166.8 | 8530 |
| **Special K**, fruit and yogurt, | 32 | 122 | 1.0 | 27.5 | 10.6 | | 1.5 | 137 | 10 | 15 | 0.45 | 0.433 | 72 | 7 | 0.16 | 2.2 | 0.67 | 0.23 |
| Kellogg's - *¾ cup (1.1 oz)* | | 2.2 | 0.9 | 0.5 | 0.1 | 0.4 | 0 | 53 | 49 | 2.59 | 0.072 | 7.5 | 240 | 0.2 | 0.19 | 0.22 | 73.9 | 8531 |
| **Special K**, Kellogg's | 31 | 117 | 0.9 | 22.0 | 4.0 | | 0.7 | 224 | 9 | 19 | 0.90 | 0.859 | 230 | 21 | 0.53 | 7.1 | 6.04 | |
| *1 cup (1.1 oz)* | | 7.0 | 0.5 | 0.1 | 0.1 | 0.2 | 0 | 61 | 68 | 8.37 | 0.062 | 17.0 | 767 | 4.7 | 0.59 | 1.98 | 675.8 | 8067 |

| | WT (g) | KCAL / PRO (g) | H₂0 (g) / FAT (g) | CHO (g) / SFA (g) | TSUG (g) / MUFA (g) | ASUG (g) / PUFA (g) | DFIB (g) / CHOL (mg) | Na (mg) / K (mg) | Ca (mg) / P (mg) | Mg (mg) / Fe (mg) | Zn (mg) / Cu (mg) | Mn (mg) / Se (mcg) | A (mcg RAE) / A (IU) | C (mg) / E (mg ATE) | B-1 (mg) / B-2 (mg) | NIA (mg) / B-6 (mg) | B-12 (mcg) / FOL (mcg DFE) | PANT (mg) / REF |
|---|---|---|---|---|---|---|---|---|---|---|---|---|---|---|---|---|---|---|
| **Special K, Low Carb Lifestyle,** | 29 | 101 | 0.9 | 13.9 | 1.9 | | 4.9 | 110 | 39 | 68 | 1.39 | 0.290 | 225 | 21 | 0.52 | 7.0 | 2.09 | 0.36 |
| Kellogg's - ¾ cup (1 oz) | | 9.8 | 2.8 | 0.6 | 0.7 | 1.6 | 0 | 322 | 195 | 8.12 | 0.145 | 7.5 | 750 | 4.7 | 0.61 | 0.67 | 234.3 | 8471 |
| **Special K Red Berries, Kellogg's** | 31 | 114 | 0.9 | 25.0 | 10.0 | | 1.0 | 220 | 19 | 12 | 0.50 | 0.439 | 225 | 21 | 0.52 | 7.0 | 2.11 | 0.15 |
| *1 cup (1.1 oz)* | | 3.8 | 0.3 | 0.1 | 0.1 | 0.2 | 0 | 75 | 50 | 8.12 | 0.053 | 4.0 | 750 | 4.7 | 0.62 | 0.70 | 234.0 | 8383 |
| **SpongeBob SquarePants, Kellogg's** | 30 | 118 | 0.8 | 26.1 | 12.6 | | 0.6 | 121 | 5 | 11 | 1.62 | | | 14 | 0.26 | 6.4 | 1.29 | |
| *1 cup (1.1 oz)* | | 1.5 | 1.1 | 0.2 | 0.5 | 0.1 | 0 | 41 | 35 | 4.80 | | | 339 | | 0.63 | 0.51 | 200.1 | 8532 |
| **Star Wars, Kellogg's** | 29 | 109 | 0.8 | 24.4 | 12.5 | | 1.5 | 182 | 7 | 21 | 1.51 | | | 6 | 0.38 | 5.0 | 1.45 | |
| *1 cup (1 oz)* | | 1.7 | 1.0 | 0.1 | 0.5 | 0.3 | 0 | 52 | 56 | 1.80 | 0.029 | | 750 | | 0.43 | 0.49 | 166.2 | 8533 |
| **Strawberry Squares Mini-Wheats,** | 50 | 168 | 3.8 | 40.0 | 9.3 | | 4.8 | 15 | 22 | 60 | 1.55 | 1.158 | 0 | 0 | 0.38 | 5.0 | 1.50 | 0 |
| Kellogg's - *1 cup (1.8 oz)* | | 4.6 | 1.0 | 0.2 | 0.2 | 0.6 | 0 | 172 | 150 | 16.20 | 0.135 | 2.0 | 0 | 0.3 | 0.42 | 0.50 | 148.0 | 8289 |
| **Sweet Crunch/Quisp, Quaker** | 27 | 109 | 0.5 | 23.0 | 11.7 | | 0.6 | 200 | 2 | 15 | 4.13 | 0.178 | 12 | 0 | 0.41 | 5.5 | 0 | 0.10 |
| *1 cup (.95 oz)* | | 1.2 | 1.6 | 1.2 | 0.2 | 0.2 | 0 | 50 | 45 | 4.95 | 0.057 | 1.8 | 40 | 0 | 0.47 | 0.55 | 710.1 | 8059 |
| **Sweet Puffs, Quaker** | 34 | 133 | 0.8 | 29.9 | 16.1 | | 1.2 | 80 | 3 | 19 | 0.42 | 0.303 | 0 | 0 | 0.05 | 1.5 | 0.05 | 0.11 |
| *1 cup (1.2 oz)* | | 2.3 | 0.7 | 0.1 | 0.1 | 0.3 | 0 | 50 | 48 | 0.65 | 0.078 | 2.2 | 1 | 0.4 | 0.04 | 0.02 | 6.5 | 8299 |
| **Tasteeos, Ralston** | 28 | 111 | 1.0 | 20.8 | 1.3 | | 3.0 | 239 | 100 | 34 | 4.01 | 0.756 | 144 | 4 | 0.47 | 6.7 | 1.48 | 0.11 |
| *1 cup (1 oz)* | | 3.3 | 1.7 | 0.3 | 0.5 | 0.5 | 0 | 86 | 146 | 8.40 | 0.092 | 13.2 | 479 | 0.1 | 0.53 | 0.64 | 313.6 | 8074 |
| **Team Cheerios, General Mills** | 27 | 100 | 0.6 | 22.4 | 10.0 | | 1.8 | 180 | 100 | 16 | 7.50 | 0.400 | 150 | 6 | 0.90 | 10.0 | 3.00 | 5.00 |
| *¾ cup (1 oz)* | | 2.0 | 1.0 | 0.2 | 0.2 | 0.5 | 0 | 65 | 60 | 10.80 | 0.040 | 4.2 | 500 | 6.1 | 1.02 | 1.20 | 403.9 | 8088 |
| **Tiger Power, Kellogg's** | 30 | 105 | 0.8 | 21.3 | 7.6 | | 2.5 | 253 | 91 | 25 | 1.35 | | | 14 | 0.33 | 4.6 | 1.35 | |
| *1 cup (1.1 oz)* | | 5.7 | 0.6 | 0.1 | 0.1 | 0.4 | 0 | 112 | 98 | 4.08 | | | 454 | | 0.39 | 0.45 | 150.6 | 8534 |
| **Toasted Honey Crunch, Kellogg's** | 58 | 225 | 1.7 | 49.9 | 18.6 | | 2.3 | 316 | 10 | 19 | 1.51 | | | 4 | 0.35 | 5.0 | 1.51 | 0 |
| *1¼ cups (2 oz)* | | 3.5 | 1.3 | 0.5 | 0.1 | 0.8 | 0 | 78 | 64 | 4.52 | 0.116 | | 500 | | 0.41 | 0.52 | 161.8 | 8535 |
| **Toasted Oat Bran, brown sugar,** | 28 | 104 | 1.1 | 21.0 | 4.3 | | 2.5 | 177 | 18 | 40 | 0.83 | 0.955 | | 0 | 0.11 | 0.5 | 0 | 0.21 |
| Mother's - *1 oz* | | 3.3 | 1.4 | 0.2 | 0.5 | 0.5 | 0 | 137 | 128 | 1.15 | 0.078 | 1.2 | 20 | | 0.05 | 0.04 | | 8352 |
| **Toasted Oatmeal, honey nut,** | 49 | 188 | 1.2 | 39.8 | 12.3 | | 2.7 | 228 | 165 | 36 | 6.74 | 1.039 | 159 | 2 | 0.69 | 9.0 | 0 | 0.25 |
| Quaker - *1 cup (1.7 oz)* | | 4.4 | 2.0 | 0.6 | 0.6 | 0.5 | 0 | 111 | 118 | 8.64 | 0.103 | 0.5 | 530 | 3.2 | 0.76 | 0.88 | 696.8 | 8219 |
| **Toasted Oats/Oatmmm's, Quaker** | 28 | 106 | 1.0 | 21.8 | 2.2 | | 1.8 | 267 | 11 | 27 | 3.85 | 0.823 | 154 | 6 | 0.19 | 5.1 | 0 | 0.13 |
| *1 oz* | | 2.6 | 1.4 | 0.3 | 0.5 | 0.4 | 0 | 81 | 108 | 8.27 | 0.059 | 0 | 514 | | 0.45 | 0.51 | 662.8 | 8362 |
| **Toasty O's, apple cinnamon,** | 40 | 164 | 0.8 | 33.0 | 16.5 | | 2.0 | 216 | 167 | 26 | 5.56 | | 345 | 10 | 0.60 | 8.0 | 2.48 | 0.04 |
| Malt-O-Meal - *1 cup (1.4 oz)* | | 2.8 | 2.3 | 0.4 | 1.2 | 0.6 | 0 | 80 | 83 | 6.72 | 0.080 | 15.0 | 1148 | 0.2 | 0.79 | 1.10 | 470.8 | 8408 |
| **Toasty O's, honey nut, Malt-O-Meal** | 30 | 117 | 0.6 | 24.5 | 11.6 | | 1.7 | 251 | 119 | 31 | 4.88 | 1.232 | 282 | 9 | 0.45 | 7.0 | 0.70 | 0.16 |
| *1 cup (1.1 oz)* | | 2.9 | 0.6 | 0.1 | 0.2 | 0.3 | 0 | 93 | 107 | 5.12 | 0.081 | 7.6 | 940 | 0.5 | 0.71 | 0.80 | 445.2 | 8491 |
| **Toasty O's, Malt-O-Meal** | 30 | 121 | 0.6 | 22.4 | 1.2 | | 3.2 | 269 | 122 | 36 | 4.41 | 0.090 | 65 | 6 | 0.47 | 5.7 | 1.84 | 0.02 |
| *1 cup (1.1 oz)* | | 3.9 | 1.8 | 0.4 | 0.6 | 0.7 | 0 | 95 | 112 | 9.81 | 0.096 | 11.2 | 218 | 0.2 | 0.60 | 0.72 | 261.3 | 8350 |
| **Tony's Cinnamon Krunchers,** | 29 | 130 | 0.9 | 22.9 | 10.4 | | 0.3 | 154 | 6 | 7 | 0.29 | 0.247 | 150 | 6 | 0.38 | 4.9 | 1.51 | 0.17 |
| Kellogg's - ¾ cup (1 oz) | | 1.2 | 3.5 | 0.6 | 1.2 | 0 | 0 | 23 | 22 | 4.64 | 0.027 | | 500 | 0.3 | 0.43 | 0.49 | 167.6 | 8460 |
| **Tootie Fruities, Malt-O-Meal** | 32 | 128 | 0.5 | 28.1 | 14.6 | | 0.8 | 148 | 130 | 11 | 4.00 | 0.268 | 398 | 22 | 0.51 | 5.7 | 1.85 | 0.09 |
| *1 cup (1.1 oz)* | | 1.6 | 1.1 | 0.2 | 0.5 | 0.3 | 0 | 42 | 36 | 4.96 | 0.032 | 4.0 | 1322 | 0.1 | 0.72 | 0.82 | 223.7 | 8349 |
| **Total, corn, General Mills** | 30 | 112 | 0.8 | 25.7 | 3.3 | | 0.8 | 209 | 1000 | 8 | 15.00 | 0.029 | 117 | 60 | 1.50 | 20.0 | 6.00 | 9.90 |
| *1⅓ cups (1.1 oz)* | | 1.8 | 0.5 | 0.1 | 0.1 | 0.1 | 0 | 28 | 110 | 18.00 | 0 | 1.5 | 428 | 13.5 | 1.70 | 2.00 | 675.9 | 8246 |
| **Total, General Mills** | 30 | 100 | 0.8 | 23.2 | 5.0 | | 2.7 | 190 | 1000 | 24 | 15.00 | | 150 | 60 | 1.50 | 20.0 | 6.00 | 10.00 |
| *¾ cup (1.1 oz)* | | 2.0 | 0.5 | 0.1 | 0.1 | 0.2 | 0 | 90 | 80 | 18.00 | 0.080 | 1.2 | 500 | 13.5 | 1.70 | 2.00 | 675.9 | 8077 |
| **Total, raisin bran, General Mills** | 55 | 170 | 4.8 | 42.0 | 19.0 | | 5.0 | 240 | 1000 | 32 | 15.00 | 0.816 | 150 | 0 | 1.50 | 20.0 | 6.00 | 10.00 |
| *1 cup (1.9 oz)* | | 3.0 | 1.0 | 0.2 | 0.1 | 0.5 | 0 | 310 | 100 | 18.00 | 0.120 | 3.9 | 500 | 13.5 | 1.70 | 2.00 | 672.7 | 8247 |
| **Trix, General Mills** | 30 | 120 | 0.6 | 26.0 | 13.0 | | 1.0 | 169 | 94 | 8 | 3.52 | 0.024 | 141 | 6 | 0.35 | 4.7 | 1.41 | 0.04 |
| *1 cup* | | 1.0 | 1.5 | 0.2 | 0.7 | 0.5 | 0 | 33 | 38 | 4.22 | 0.014 | 2.0 | 469 | 0.4 | 0.40 | 0.47 | 155.4 | 8078 |
| **Uncle Sam Cereal** | 55 | 237 | 2.4 | 36.2 | 0.9 | | 11.2 | 113 | 52 | 113 | 2.13 | 1.986 | 0 | 34 | 1.25 | 9.0 | 0 | 0.34 |
| *1 cup (1.9 oz)* | | 8.8 | 6.4 | 0.7 | 1.1 | 4.6 | 0 | 245 | 206 | 2.22 | 0.414 | 48.6 | 0 | 0.4 | 1.45 | 0.53 | 29.2 | 8435 |
| **Waffelos** | 30 | 122 | 0.8 | 25.9 | | | | 125 | 8 | 6 | 0.24 | | 397 | 16 | 0.39 | 5.3 | 1.59 | 0.05 |
| *1 cup (1.1 oz)* | | 1.7 | 1.3 | | | | 0 | 26 | 244 | 4.77 | 0.034 | | 1323 | | 0.45 | 0.54 | 3.3 | 8079 |
| **Weetabix** | 18 | 67 | 0.9 | 13.9 | 0.4 | | 2.1 | 70 | 18 | 17 | 0.31 | | 0 | 0 | 0.19 | 1.0 | 0 | |
| *.6 oz biscuit* | | 2.1 | 0.5 | 0.1 | 0.1 | 0.2 | 0 | 98 | 31 | 0.93 | 0.041 | 1.1 | 0 | 0.3 | 0.18 | 0.08 | 8.3 | 42237 |
| **Weetabix, crispy flakes & fiber,** | 55 | 170 | | 44.0 | 10.0 | | 11.0 | 320 | 20 | | 3.75 | | | 15 | 0.38 | 5.0 | | |
| Barbara's Bakery - 1¼ cups | | 6.0 | 1.5 | 0 | | | 0 | 310 | | 4.50 | | | 0 | | 0.42 | 0.50 | | BARB60 |
| **Weetabix, organic, Barbara's** | 35 | 120 | | 28.0 | 2.0 | | 4.0 | 130 | 0 | | 3.75 | | | 15 | 0.38 | 5.0 | | |
| Bakery - *2 biscuits* | | 4.0 | 1.0 | 0 | | | 0 | 120 | | 4.50 | | | 0 | | 0.42 | 0.50 | | BARB62 |
| **Weetabix, organic crispy flakes,** | 30 | 110 | | 24.0 | 4.0 | | 4.0 | 180 | | | 3.75 | | | 15 | 0.38 | 5.0 | | |
| Barbara's Bakery - ¾ cup | | 3.0 | 0.5 | 0 | | | 0 | 150 | | 4.50 | | | 0 | | 0.42 | 0.50 | | BARB61 |
| **wheat and malted barley flakes** | 28 | 102 | 0.9 | 22.8 | 4.9 | | 2.5 | 135 | 11 | 29 | 1.16 | 0.573 | 217 | 0 | 0.36 | 4.8 | 1.45 | 0.18 |
| ⅞ cup | | 2.8 | 0.8 | 0.2 | 0.2 | 0.3 | 0 | 95 | 85 | 7.82 | 0.140 | 2.7 | 724 | 0.3 | 0.41 | 0.48 | 160.4 | 8039 |
| **wheat and malted barley nuggets** | 28 | 101 | 0.8 | 22.4 | 3.5 | | 2.5 | 153 | 11 | 29 | 1.55 | 0.906 | 148 | 0 | 0.28 | 4.1 | 1.77 | 0.24 |
| ¼ cup | | 3.5 | 0.5 | 0.1 | 0.1 | 0.2 | 0 | 95 | 85 | 10.66 | 0.105 | 2.5 | 495 | 0.2 | 0.20 | 0.67 | 224.0 | 8038 |

| | WT (g) | KCAL / PRO (g) | H₂0 (g) / FAT (g) | CHO (g) / SFA (g) | TSUG (g) / MUFA (g) | ASUG (g) / PUFA (g) | DFIB (g) / CHOL (mg) | Na (mg) / K (mg) | Ca (mg) / P (mg) | Mg (mg) / Fe (mg) | Zn (mg) / Cu (mg) | Mn (mg) / Se (mcg) | A (mcg RAE) / A (IU) | C (mg) / E (mg ATE) | B-1 (mg) / B-2 (mg) | NIA (mg) / B-6 (mg) | B-12 (mcg) / FOL (mcg DFE) | PANT (mg) / REF |
|---|---|---|---|---|---|---|---|---|---|---|---|---|---|---|---|---|---|---|
| **Wheat Bran Flakes**, Kellogg's | 28 | 89 | 0.8 | 22.1 | 4.8 | | 4.9 | 200 | 15 | 53 | 14.56 | | 218 | 58 | 1.46 | 19.3 | 5.80 | 9.66 |
| Complete - ⅔ cup | | 2.8 | 0.6 | 0.1 | 0.1 | 0.3 | 0 | 165 | 134 | 17.36 | 0.140 | 2.9 | 724 | 13.0 | 1.65 | 1.96 | 652.7 | 8028 |
| **Wheat Chex**, General Mills | 30 | 108 | 0.8 | 24.3 | 3.0 | | 3.2 | 252 | 60 | 24 | 2.25 | 1.072 | 90 | 4 | 0.22 | 3.0 | 0.90 | 0.28 |
| *1 cup (1.1 oz)* | | 3.0 | 0.6 | 0.1 | 0.1 | 0.2 | 0 | 114 | 90 | 8.64 | 0.096 | 1.5 | 300 | 0.2 | 0.26 | 0.30 | 404.1 | 8082 |
| **Wheaties**, General Mills | 30 | 110 | 0.8 | 24.2 | 4.0 | | 3.0 | 210 | 20 | 32 | 7.50 | 1.001 | 150 | 6 | 0.75 | 10.0 | 3.00 | 0.26 |
| *1 cup (1.1 oz)* | | 3.0 | 1.0 | 0.1 | 0.3 | 0.4 | 0 | 105 | 100 | 8.40 | 0.080 | 1.4 | 500 | 0.4 | 0.85 | 1.00 | 336.3 | 8089 |
| **Wheaties** Raisin Bran, General | 55 | 183 | 3.9 | 44.6 | 18.2 | | 5.0 | 251 | 0 | 42 | 7.48 | 1.443 | 150 | 0 | 0.75 | 10.0 | 3.03 | 0.36 |
| Mills - *1 cup (1.9 oz)* | | 3.9 | 0.9 | 0.2 | 0.1 | 0.4 | 0 | 227 | 140 | 7.48 | 0.176 | 3.9 | 500 | 0.3 | 0.85 | 1.00 | 324.5 | 8026 |
| **Whole Grain Nuggets**, Kashi | 58 | 206 | 1.7 | 47.0 | 2.9 | | 6.8 | 260 | 24 | 49 | | | 0 | | | | | |
| *½ cup* | | 6.8 | 1.6 | 0.3 | 0.3 | 0.9 | 0 | | 157 | 13.92 | | | 0 | | | | | 8567 |

# 5. CHEESE, CHEESE PRODUCTS, AND CHEESE SUBSTITUTES
## 5.1 CHEESE

| | WT (g) | KCAL / PRO (g) | H₂0 (g) / FAT (g) | CHO (g) / SFA (g) | TSUG (g) / MUFA (g) | ASUG (g) / PUFA (g) | DFIB (g) / CHOL (mg) | Na (mg) / K (mg) | Ca (mg) / P (mg) | Mg (mg) / Fe (mg) | Zn (mg) / Cu (mg) | Mn (mg) / Se (mcg) | A (mcg RAE) / A (IU) | C (mg) / E (mg ATE) | B-1 (mg) / B-2 (mg) | NIA (mg) / B-6 (mg) | B-12 (mcg) / FOL (mcg DFE) | PANT (mg) / REF |
|---|---|---|---|---|---|---|---|---|---|---|---|---|---|---|---|---|---|---|
| **American processed cheese** | 28 | 105 | 11.0 | 0.4 | 0.1 | 0 | 0 | 417 | 155 | 8 | 0.80 | 0.002 | 71 | 0 | 0.01 | 0 | 0.20 | 0.13 |
| *1 oz* | | 6.2 | 8.8 | 5.5 | 2.5 | 0.3 | 26 | 47 | 144 | 0.05 | 0.004 | 4.0 | 269 | 0.1 | 0.10 | 0.02 | 2.2 | 1042 |
| **American processed cheese**, nonfat, | 21 | 31 | 12.2 | 2.5 | 1.4 | | 0 | 273 | 150 | | 0.52 | | | 0 | | | | |
| Kraft Free Singles - *1 slice* | | 4.8 | 0.2 | 0.1 | | | 3 | 50 | 194 | 0.01 | | | 455 | | 0.06 | | | 1190 |
| **American processed cheese**, | 28 | 67 | 14.5 | 3.0 | 2.2 | 0 | 0 | 444 | 148 | 9 | 0.66 | | 71 | 0 | 0.02 | 0.1 | 0.31 | |
| reduced fat - *1 oz* | | 4.9 | 3.9 | 2.5 | 1.2 | 0.1 | 15 | 92 | 232 | 0.06 | 0.008 | 3.5 | 269 | 0.1 | 0.13 | 0.02 | 5.0 | 42258 |
| **blue cheese** | 28 | 99 | 11.9 | 0.7 | 0.1 | 0 | 0 | 391 | 148 | 6 | 0.74 | 0.003 | 55 | 0 | 0.01 | 0.3 | 0.34 | 0.48 |
| *1 oz* | | 6.0 | 8.0 | 5.2 | 2.2 | 0.2 | 21 | 72 | 108 | 0.09 | 0.011 | 4.1 | 214 | 0.1 | 0.11 | 0.05 | 10.1 | 1004 |
| **brick cheese** | 28 | 104 | 11.5 | 0.8 | 0.1 | 0 | 0 | 157 | 189 | 7 | 0.73 | 0.003 | 82 | 0 | 0 | 0 | 0.35 | 0.08 |
| *1 oz* | | 6.5 | 8.3 | 5.3 | 2.4 | 0.2 | 26 | 38 | 126 | 0.12 | 0.007 | 4.1 | 302 | 0.1 | 0.10 | 0.02 | 5.6 | 1005 |
| **brie cheese** | 28 | 94 | 13.6 | 0.1 | 0.1 | 0 | 0 | 176 | 52 | 6 | 0.67 | 0.010 | 49 | 0 | 0.02 | 0.1 | 0.46 | 0.19 |
| *1 oz* | | 5.8 | 7.8 | 4.9 | 2.2 | 0.2 | 28 | 43 | 53 | 0.14 | 0.005 | 4.1 | 166 | 0.1 | 0.15 | 0.07 | 18.2 | 1006 |
| **camembert cheese** | 28 | 84 | 14.5 | 0.1 | 0.1 | 0 | 0 | 236 | 109 | 6 | 0.67 | 0.011 | 67 | 0 | 0.01 | 0.2 | 0.36 | 0.38 |
| *1 oz* | | 5.5 | 6.8 | 4.3 | 2.0 | 0.2 | 20 | 52 | 97 | 0.09 | 0.006 | 4.1 | 230 | 0.1 | 0.14 | 0.06 | 17.4 | 1007 |
| **caraway cheese** | 28 | 105 | 11.0 | 0.9 | | | 0 | 193 | 188 | 6 | 0.82 | 0.006 | 76 | 0 | 0.01 | 0.1 | 0.08 | 0.25 |
| *1 oz* | | 7.1 | 8.2 | 5.2 | 2.3 | 0.2 | 26 | 26 | 137 | 0.18 | 0.007 | 4.1 | 295 | | 0.13 | 0.02 | 5.0 | 1008 |
| **cheddar cheese** | 28 | 113 | 10.3 | 0.4 | 0.1 | 0 | 0 | 174 | 202 | 8 | 0.87 | 0.003 | 74 | 0 | 0.01 | 0 | 0.23 | 0.12 |
| *1 oz* | | 7.0 | 9.3 | 5.9 | 2.6 | 0.3 | 29 | 27 | 143 | 0.19 | 0.009 | 3.9 | 281 | 0.1 | 0.11 | 0.02 | 5.0 | 1009 |
| **cheddar cheese/colby cheese**, | 28 | 111 | 10.9 | 0.5 | 0.1 | 0 | 0 | 6 | 197 | 8 | 0.87 | 0.003 | 74 | 0 | 0.01 | 0 | 0.23 | 0.09 |
| low sodium - *1 oz* | | 6.8 | 9.1 | 5.8 | 2.6 | 0.3 | 28 | 31 | 136 | 0.20 | 0.010 | 4.1 | 279 | 0.1 | 0.11 | 0.02 | 5.0 | 1169 |
| **cheddar cheese/colby cheese**, | 28 | 48 | 17.7 | 0.5 | 0.1 | 0 | 0 | 171 | 116 | 4 | 0.51 | 0.002 | 17 | 0 | 0 | 0 | 0.14 | 0.05 |
| lowfat - *1 oz* | | 6.8 | 2.0 | 1.2 | 0.6 | 0.1 | 6 | 18 | 136 | 0.12 | 0.006 | 4.1 | 58 | 0 | 0.06 | 0.01 | 3.1 | 1168 |
| **cheshire cheese** | 28 | 108 | 10.5 | 1.3 | | | 0 | 196 | 180 | 6 | 0.78 | 0.003 | 65 | 0 | 0.01 | 0 | 0.23 | 0.12 |
| *1 oz* | | 6.5 | 8.6 | 5.5 | 2.4 | 0.2 | 29 | 27 | 130 | 0.06 | 0.012 | 4.1 | 276 | | 0.08 | 0.02 | 5.0 | 1010 |
| **colby cheese** | 28 | 110 | 10.7 | 0.7 | 0.1 | 0 | 0 | 169 | 192 | 7 | 0.86 | 0.003 | 74 | 0 | 0 | 0 | 0.23 | 0.06 |
| *1 oz* | | 6.7 | 9.0 | 5.7 | 2.6 | 0.3 | 27 | 36 | 128 | 0.21 | 0.012 | 4.1 | 278 | 0.1 | 0.11 | 0.02 | 5.0 | 1011 |
| **cottage cheese**, <5% fat | 226 | 163 | 183.1 | 15.1 | 4.2 | 0 | 0 | 746 | 194 | 25 | 1.06 | 0.050 | 5 | 0 | 0.05 | 0.3 | 1.04 | 1.01 |
| *1 cup* | | 23.4 | 0.7 | 0.4 | 0.2 | 0 | 16 | 310 | 429 | 0.34 | 0.068 | 21.2 | 18 | 0 | 0.51 | 0.04 | 20.3 | 1014 |
| **cottage cheese**, 1% fat | 226 | 163 | 186.4 | 6.1 | 6.1 | 0 | 0 | 918 | 138 | 11 | 0.86 | 0.007 | 25 | 0 | 0.05 | 0.3 | 1.42 | 0.49 |
| *1 cup* | | 28.0 | 2.3 | 1.5 | 0.7 | 0.1 | 9 | 194 | 303 | 0.32 | 0.063 | 20.3 | 93 | 0 | 0.37 | 0.15 | 27.1 | 1016 |
| **cottage cheese**, 2% fat | 226 | 194 | 182.4 | 8.3 | 8.3 | 0 | 0 | 746 | 206 | 16 | 0.93 | 0.016 | 45 | 0 | 0.09 | 0.2 | 1.02 | 0.57 |
| *1 cup* | | 26.7 | 5.5 | 2.2 | 1.0 | 0.2 | 23 | 190 | 368 | 0.34 | 0.068 | 22.4 | 167 | 0.1 | 0.45 | 0.05 | 22.6 | 1015 |
| **cottage cheese**, 4% fat, creamed | 226 | 219 | 180.0 | 10.4 | 5.4 | 4.9 | 0.5 | 777 | 120 | 16 | 0.75 | 0.007 | 86 | 3 | 0.07 | 0.3 | 1.20 | 0.41 |
| with fruit - *1 cup* | | 24.2 | 8.7 | 5.2 | 2.3 | 0.3 | 29 | 203 | 255 | 0.36 | 0.090 | 17.4 | 330 | 0.1 | 0.32 | 0.15 | 24.9 | 1013 |
| **cottage cheese**, creamed, large curd | 225 | 220 | 179.5 | 7.6 | 6.0 | 0 | 0 | 819 | 187 | 18 | 0.90 | 0.005 | 83 | 0 | 0.06 | 0.2 | 0.97 | 1.25 |
| *1 cup* | | 25.0 | 9.7 | 3.9 | 1.8 | 0.3 | 38 | 234 | 358 | 0.16 | 0.065 | 21.8 | 315 | 0.2 | 0.37 | 0.10 | 27.0 | 1012 |
| **cottage cheese**, creamed, small curd | 225 | 220 | 179.5 | 7.6 | 6.0 | 0 | 0 | 819 | 187 | 18 | 0.90 | 0.005 | 83 | 0 | 0.06 | 0.2 | 0.97 | 1.25 |
| *1 cup* | | 25.0 | 9.7 | 3.9 | 1.8 | 0.3 | 38 | 234 | 358 | 0.16 | 0.065 | 21.8 | 315 | 0.2 | 0.37 | 0.10 | 27.0 | 1012 |
| **cream cheese** | 15 | 51 | 8.2 | 0.6 | 0.5 | 0 | 0 | 48 | 15 | 1 | 0.08 | 0.002 | 54 | 0 | 0 | 0 | 0.04 | 0.09 |
| *1 T* | | 0.9 | 5.1 | 2.9 | 1.3 | 0.2 | 16 | 21 | 16 | 0.06 | 0.003 | 0.4 | 190 | 0.1 | 0.02 | 0.01 | 1.6 | 1017 |
| **cream cheese**, fat-free | 28 | 29 | 20.1 | 2.1 | 1.5 | 0 | 0 | 197 | 98 | 6 | 0.42 | 0.005 | 3 | 0 | 0.01 | 0.1 | 0.27 | 0.24 |
| *1 oz* | | 4.4 | 0.3 | 0.2 | 0.1 | 0 | 3 | 78 | 146 | 0.05 | 0.010 | 1.4 | 15 | 0 | 0.07 | 0.01 | 9.8 | 1186 |
| **cream cheese**, lowfat | 28 | 56 | 18.7 | 2.3 | 1.6 | 0 | 0 | 132 | 41 | 2 | 0.16 | 0.003 | 45 | 0 | 0.01 | 0 | 0.26 | 0.24 |
| *1 oz* | | 2.2 | 4.3 | 2.5 | 1.1 | 0.2 | 15 | 69 | 43 | 0.05 | 0.009 | 1.1 | 155 | 0.1 | 0.05 | 0.01 | 5.3 | 43274 |
| **edam cheese** | 28 | 100 | 11.6 | 0.4 | 0.4 | 0 | 0 | 270 | 205 | 8 | 1.05 | 0.003 | 68 | 0 | 0.01 | 0 | 0.43 | 0.08 |
| *1 oz* | | 7.0 | 7.8 | 4.9 | 2.3 | 0.2 | 25 | 53 | 150 | 0.12 | 0.010 | 4.1 | 231 | 0.1 | 0.11 | 0.02 | 4.5 | 1018 |
| **feta cheese** | 28 | 74 | 15.5 | 1.1 | 1.1 | 0 | 0 | 312 | 138 | 5 | 0.81 | 0.008 | 35 | 0 | 0.04 | 0.3 | 0.47 | 0.27 |
| *1 oz* | | 4.0 | 6.0 | 4.2 | 1.3 | 0.2 | 25 | 17 | 94 | 0.18 | 0.009 | 4.2 | 118 | 0.1 | 0.24 | 0.12 | 9.0 | 1019 |

| | WT (g) | KCAL | H2O (g) | CHO (g) | TSUG (g) | ASUG (g) | DFIB (g) | Na (mg) | Ca (mg) | Mg (mg) | Zn (mg) | Mn (mg) | A (mcg RAE) | C (mg) | B-1 (mg) | NIA (mg) | B-12 (mcg) | PANT (mg) |
|---|---|---|---|---|---|---|---|---|---|---|---|---|---|---|---|---|---|---|
| | | PRO (g) | FAT (g) | SFA (g) | MUFA (g) | PUFA (g) | CHOL (mg) | K (mg) | P (mg) | Fe (mg) | Cu (mg) | Se (mcg) | A (IU) | E (mg ATE) | B-2 (mg) | B-6 (mg) | FOL (mcg DFE) | REF |
| **fontina cheese** | 28 | 109 | 10.6 | 0.4 | 0.4 | 0 | 0 | 224 | 154 | 4 | 0.98 | 0.004 | 73 | 0 | 0.01 | 0 | 0.47 | 0.12 |
| *1 oz* | | 7.2 | 8.7 | 5.4 | 2.4 | 0.5 | 32 | 18 | 97 | 0.06 | 0.007 | 4.1 | 256 | 0.1 | 0.06 | 0.02 | 1.7 | 1020 |
| **gjetost cheese** | 28 | 130 | 3.8 | 11.9 | | | 0 | 168 | 112 | 20 | 0.32 | 0.011 | 94 | 0 | 0.09 | 0.2 | 0.68 | 0.94 |
| *1 oz* | | 2.7 | 8.3 | 5.4 | 2.2 | 0.3 | 26 | 395 | 124 | 0.15 | 0.022 | 4.1 | 312 | | 0.39 | 0.08 | 1.4 | 1021 |
| **goat milk cheese, hard** | 28 | 127 | 8.1 | 0.6 | 0.6 | 0 | 0 | 97 | 251 | 15 | 0.45 | 0.071 | 136 | 0 | 0.04 | 0.7 | 0.03 | 0.11 |
| *1 oz* | | 8.5 | 10.0 | 6.9 | 2.3 | 0.2 | 29 | 13 | 204 | 0.53 | 0.176 | 1.5 | 489 | 0.1 | 0.33 | 0.02 | 1.1 | 1156 |
| **goat milk cheese, semi-soft** | 28 | 102 | 12.7 | 0.7 | 0.7 | 0 | 0 | 144 | 83 | 8 | 0.18 | 0.026 | 114 | 0 | 0.02 | 0.3 | 0.06 | 0.05 |
| *1 oz* | | 6.0 | 8.4 | 5.8 | 1.9 | 0.2 | 22 | 44 | 105 | 0.45 | 0.158 | 1.1 | 410 | 0.1 | 0.19 | 0.02 | 0.6 | 1157 |
| **goat milk cheese, soft** | 28 | 75 | 17.0 | 0.2 | 0.2 | 0 | 0 | 103 | 39 | 4 | 0.26 | 0.028 | 81 | 0 | 0.02 | 0.1 | 0.05 | 0.19 |
| *1 oz* | | 5.2 | 5.9 | 4.1 | 1.3 | 0.1 | 13 | 7 | 72 | 0.53 | 0.205 | 0.8 | 289 | 0.1 | 0.11 | 0.07 | 3.4 | 1159 |
| **gouda cheese** | 28 | 100 | 11.6 | 0.6 | 0.6 | 0 | 0 | 229 | 196 | 8 | 1.09 | 0.003 | 46 | 0 | 0.01 | 0 | 0.43 | 0.10 |
| *1 oz* | | 7.0 | 7.7 | 4.9 | 2.2 | 0.2 | 32 | 34 | 153 | 0.07 | 0.010 | 4.1 | 158 | 0.1 | 0.09 | 0.02 | 5.9 | 1022 |
| **gruyere cheese** | 28 | 116 | 9.3 | 0.1 | 0.1 | 0 | 0 | 94 | 283 | 10 | 1.09 | 0.005 | 76 | 0 | 0.02 | 0 | 0.45 | 0.16 |
| *1 oz* | | 8.3 | 9.1 | 5.3 | 2.8 | 0.5 | 31 | 23 | 169 | 0.05 | 0.009 | 4.1 | 265 | 0.1 | 0.08 | 0.02 | 2.8 | 1023 |
| **limburger cheese** | 28 | 92 | 13.6 | 0.1 | 0.1 | 0 | 0 | 224 | 139 | 6 | 0.59 | 0.011 | 95 | 0 | 0.02 | 0 | 0.29 | 0.33 |
| *1 oz* | | 5.6 | 7.6 | 4.7 | 2.4 | 0.1 | 25 | 36 | 110 | 0.04 | 0.006 | 4.1 | 323 | 0.1 | 0.14 | 0.02 | 16.2 | 1024 |
| **Mexican cheese, quesa asadero** | 28 | 100 | 11.8 | 0.8 | 0.8 | 0 | 0 | 183 | 185 | 7 | 0.85 | 0.010 | 15 | 0 | 0.01 | 0.1 | 0.28 | 0.06 |
| *1 oz* | | 6.3 | 7.9 | 5.0 | 2.3 | 0.2 | 29 | 24 | 124 | 0.14 | 0.007 | 4.1 | 53 | 0.1 | 0.06 | 0.01 | 2.2 | 1166 |
| **Mexican cheese, queso anejo** | 28 | 104 | 10.7 | 1.3 | 1.3 | 0 | 0 | 317 | 190 | 8 | 0.82 | 0.010 | 15 | 0 | 0.01 | 0 | 0.39 | 0.07 |
| *1 oz* | | 6.0 | 8.4 | 5.3 | 2.4 | 0.3 | 29 | 24 | 124 | 0.13 | 0.002 | 4.1 | 52 | 0.1 | 0.06 | 0.01 | 0.3 | 1165 |
| **Mexican cheese, queso chihuahua** | 28 | 105 | 11.0 | 1.6 | 1.6 | 0 | 0 | 173 | 182 | 8 | 0.98 | 0.020 | 16 | 0 | 0.01 | 0 | 0.29 | 0.08 |
| *1 oz* | | 6.0 | 8.3 | 5.3 | 2.4 | 0.2 | 29 | 15 | 124 | 0.13 | 0.007 | 4.1 | 54 | 0.1 | 0.06 | 0.02 | 0.6 | 1167 |
| **monterey cheese, lowfat** | 28 | 88 | 12.9 | 0.2 | 0.2 | 0 | 0 | 158 | 197 | 8 | 0.84 | | 40 | 0 | 0.01 | 0 | 0.23 | |
| *1 oz* | | 7.9 | 6.0 | 3.9 | 1.6 | 0.2 | 18 | 23 | 124 | 0.20 | 0.009 | 4.1 | 154 | 0.1 | 0.10 | 0.02 | 5.0 | 42155 |
| **monterey jack cheese** | 28 | 104 | 11.5 | 0.2 | 0.1 | 0 | 0 | 150 | 209 | 8 | 0.84 | 0.003 | 55 | 0 | 0 | 0 | 0.23 | 0.06 |
| *1 oz slice* | | 6.9 | 8.5 | 5.3 | 2.5 | 0.3 | 25 | 23 | 124 | 0.20 | 0.009 | 4.1 | 215 | 0.1 | 0.11 | 0.02 | 5.0 | 1025 |
| **mozzarella cheese, nonfat** | 28 | 42 | 16.9 | 1.0 | 0.4 | 0 | 0.5 | 208 | 269 | 9 | 1.10 | | 36 | 0 | 0.01 | 0 | 0.26 | |
| *1 oz* | | 8.9 | 0 | 0 | 0 | 0 | 5 | 30 | 184 | 0.09 | 0.010 | 5.3 | 135 | 0 | 0.08 | 0.02 | 2.8 | 42304 |
| **mozzarella cheese, part skim** | 28 | 71 | 15.1 | 0.8 | 0.3 | 0 | 0 | 173 | 219 | 6 | 0.77 | 0.003 | 36 | 0 | 0.01 | 0 | 0.23 | 0.02 |
| *1 oz* | | 6.8 | 4.5 | 2.8 | 1.3 | 0.1 | 18 | 24 | 130 | 0.06 | 0.007 | 4.0 | 135 | 0 | 0.08 | 0.02 | 2.5 | 1028 |
| **mozzarella cheese, part skim, low** moisture - *1 oz* | 28 | 85 | 13.0 | 1.1 | 0.2 | 0 | 0 | 148 | 205 | 7 | 0.88 | 0.003 | 38 | 0 | 0.03 | 0 | 0.65 | 0.03 |
| | | 7.3 | 5.6 | 3.5 | 1.6 | 0.2 | 15 | 27 | 147 | 0.07 | 0.008 | 4.6 | 145 | 0.1 | 0.09 | 0.02 | 2.8 | 1029 |
| **mozzarella cheese, reduced fat,** shredded, Sargento - *¼ cup* | 28 | 80 | | 0 | 0 | | 0 | 200 | 200 | | | | | 0 | | | | |
| | | 8.0 | 4.5 | | | | 10 | | | 0 | | | 300 | | | | | SARG1 |
| **mozzarella cheese, whole milk** | 28 | 84 | 14.0 | 0.6 | 0.3 | 0 | 0 | 176 | 141 | 6 | 0.82 | 0.008 | 50 | 0 | 0.01 | 0 | 0.64 | 0.04 |
| *1 oz* | | 6.2 | 6.3 | 3.7 | 1.8 | 0.2 | 22 | 21 | 99 | 0.12 | 0.003 | 4.8 | 189 | 0.1 | 0.08 | 0.01 | 2.0 | 1026 |
| **mozzarella cheese, whole milk,** low moisture - *1 oz* | 28 | 89 | 13.5 | 0.7 | 0.3 | 0 | 0 | 116 | 161 | 6 | 0.69 | 0.003 | 55 | 0 | 0 | 0 | 0.20 | 0.02 |
| | | 6.0 | 6.9 | 4.4 | 2.0 | 0.2 | 25 | 21 | 115 | 0.06 | 0.006 | 4.5 | 209 | 0.1 | 0.08 | 0.02 | 2.2 | 1027 |
| **muenster cheese** | 28 | 103 | 11.7 | 0.3 | 0.3 | 0 | 0 | 176 | 201 | 8 | 0.79 | 0.002 | 83 | 0 | 0 | 0 | 0.41 | 0.05 |
| *1 oz* | | 6.6 | 8.4 | 5.4 | 2.4 | 0.2 | 27 | 38 | 131 | 0.11 | 0.009 | 4.1 | 283 | 0.1 | 0.09 | 0.02 | 3.4 | 1030 |
| **muenster cheese, lowfat** | 28 | 77 | 14.1 | 1.0 | 1.0 | 0 | 0 | 168 | 148 | 8 | 0.79 | | 49 | 0 | 0 | 0 | 0.41 | |
| *1 oz* | | 6.9 | 4.9 | 3.1 | 1.4 | 0.2 | 18 | 38 | 131 | 0.11 | 0.009 | 4.1 | 166 | 0.1 | 0.10 | 0.02 | 3.4 | 42303 |
| **Neufchatel cheese** | 28 | 71 | 17.7 | 1.0 | 0.9 | | 0 | 94 | 33 | 3 | 0.23 | 0.003 | 67 | 0 | 0.01 | 0.1 | 0.08 | 0.16 |
| *1 oz* | | 2.6 | 6.4 | 3.6 | 1.6 | 0.3 | 21 | 43 | 39 | 0.04 | 0.008 | 0.8 | 235 | 0.1 | 0.04 | 0.01 | 3.9 | 1031 |
| **parmesan cheese, grated** | 5 | 22 | 1.0 | 0.2 | 0 | 0 | 0 | 76 | 55 | 2 | 0.19 | 0.004 | 6 | 0 | 0 | 0 | 0.11 | 0.02 |
| *1 T* | | 1.9 | 1.4 | 0.9 | 0.4 | 0.1 | 4 | 6 | 36 | 0.05 | 0.012 | 0.9 | 22 | 0 | 0.02 | 0 | 0.5 | 1032 |
| **parmesan cheese, hard** | 28 | 110 | 8.2 | 0.9 | 0.2 | 0 | 0 | 449 | 332 | 12 | 0.77 | 0.006 | 30 | 0 | 0.01 | 0.1 | 0.34 | 0.13 |
| *1 oz* | | 10.0 | 7.2 | 4.6 | 2.1 | 0.2 | 19 | 26 | 194 | 0.23 | 0.009 | 6.3 | 112 | 0.1 | 0.09 | 0.03 | 2.0 | 1033 |
| **pimiento cheese, processed** | 28 | 105 | 10.9 | 0.5 | 0.2 | 0 | 0 | 400 | 172 | 6 | 0.83 | 0.004 | 69 | 1 | 0.01 | 0 | 0.20 | 0.14 |
| *1 oz* | | 6.2 | 8.7 | 5.5 | 2.5 | 0.3 | 26 | 45 | 208 | 0.12 | 0.009 | 4.1 | 293 | 0.1 | 0.10 | 0.02 | 2.2 | 1043 |
| **port de salut cheese** | 28 | 99 | 12.7 | 0.2 | 0.2 | 0 | 0 | 150 | 182 | 7 | 0.73 | 0.003 | 88 | 0 | 0 | 0 | 0.42 | 0.06 |
| *1 oz* | | 6.7 | 7.9 | 4.7 | 2.6 | 0.2 | 34 | 38 | 101 | 0.12 | 0.006 | 4.1 | 306 | 0.1 | 0.07 | 0.01 | 5.0 | 1034 |
| **provolone cheese** | 43 | 151 | 17.6 | 0.9 | 0.2 | 0 | 0 | 377 | 325 | 12 | 1.39 | 0.004 | 101 | 0 | 0.01 | 0.1 | 0.63 | 0.20 |
| *1.5 oz* | | 11.0 | 11.4 | 7.3 | 3.2 | 0.3 | 30 | 59 | 213 | 0.22 | 0.011 | 6.2 | 378 | 0.1 | 0.14 | 0.03 | 4.3 | 1035 |
| **ricotta cheese, part nonfat** | 124 | 171 | 92.3 | 6.4 | 0.4 | 0 | 0 | 155 | 337 | 19 | 1.66 | 0.012 | 133 | 0 | 0.03 | 0.1 | 0.36 | 0.30 |
| *½ cup* | | 14.1 | 9.8 | 6.1 | 2.9 | 0.3 | 38 | 155 | 227 | 0.55 | 0.042 | 20.7 | 476 | 0.1 | 0.23 | 0.02 | 16.1 | 1037 |
| **ricotta cheese, whole milk** | 124 | 216 | 88.9 | 3.8 | 0.3 | 0 | 0 | 104 | 257 | 14 | 1.44 | 0.007 | 149 | 0 | 0.02 | 0.1 | 0.42 | 0.26 |
| *½ cup* | | 14.0 | 16.1 | 10.3 | 4.5 | 0.5 | 63 | 130 | 196 | 0.47 | 0.026 | 18.0 | 552 | 0.1 | 0.24 | 0.05 | 14.9 | 1036 |
| **romano cheese** | 28 | 108 | 8.7 | 1.0 | 0.2 | 0 | 0 | 336 | 298 | 11 | 0.72 | 0.006 | 27 | 0 | 0.01 | 0 | 0.31 | 0.12 |
| *1 oz* | | 8.9 | 7.5 | 4.8 | 2.2 | 0.2 | 29 | 24 | 213 | 0.22 | 0.008 | 4.1 | 116 | 0.1 | 0.10 | 0.02 | 2.0 | 1038 |
| **roquefort cheese (from sheep milk)** | 28 | 103 | 11.0 | 0.6 | | | 0 | 507 | 185 | 8 | 0.58 | 0.008 | 82 | 0 | 0.01 | 0.2 | 0.18 | 0.48 |
| *1 oz* | | 6.0 | 8.6 | 5.4 | 2.4 | 0.4 | 25 | 25 | 110 | 0.16 | 0.010 | 4.1 | 293 | | 0.16 | 0.03 | 13.7 | 1039 |

| | WT (g) | KCAL / PRO (g) | H₂O (g) / FAT (g) | CHO (g) / SFA (g) | TSUG (g) / MUFA (g) | ASUG (g) / PUFA (g) | DFIB (g) / CHOL (mg) | Na (mg) / K (mg) | Ca (mg) / P (mg) | Mg (mg) / Fe (mg) | Zn (mg) / Cu (mg) | Mn (mg) / Se (mcg) | A (mcg RAE) / A (IU) | C (mg) / E (mg ATE) | B-1 (mg) / B-2 (mg) | NIA (mg) / B-6 (mg) | B-12 (mcg) / FOL (mcg DFE) | PANT (mg) / REF |
|---|---|---|---|---|---|---|---|---|---|---|---|---|---|---|---|---|---|---|
| **Swiss cheese** | 28 | 106 | 10.4 | 1.5 | 0.4 | 0 | 0 | 54 | 221 | 11 | 1.22 | 0.001 | 62 | 0 | 0.02 | 0 | 0.94 | 0.12 |
| *1 oz* | | 7.5 | 7.8 | 5.0 | 2.0 | 0.3 | 26 | 22 | 159 | 0.06 | 0.012 | 5.1 | 232 | 0.1 | 0.08 | 0.02 | 1.7 | 1040 |
| **Swiss cheese**, lowfat | 28 | 50 | 16.7 | 1.0 | 0.4 | | 0 | 73 | 269 | 10 | 1.09 | | 11 | 0 | 0.01 | 0 | 0.47 | |
| *1 oz* | | 8.0 | 1.4 | 0.9 | 0.4 | 0.1 | 10 | 31 | 169 | 0.05 | 0.008 | 3.6 | 43 | 0 | 0.10 | 0.02 | 1.7 | 43589 |
| **Swiss cheese**, processed | 28 | 94 | 11.8 | 0.6 | 0.3 | 0 | 0 | 384 | 216 | 8 | 1.01 | 0.004 | 55 | 0 | 0 | 0 | 0.34 | 0.07 |
| *1 oz* | | 6.9 | 7.0 | 4.5 | 2.0 | 0.2 | 24 | 60 | 213 | 0.17 | 0.008 | 4.5 | 209 | 0.1 | 0.08 | 0.01 | 1.7 | 1044 |
| **Swiss cheese**, processed, lowfat | 28 | 48 | 16.5 | 1.2 | 0.4 | 0 | 0 | 400 | 192 | 7 | 0.93 | | 11 | 0 | 0.01 | 0 | 0.22 | |
| *1 oz* | | 7.1 | 1.4 | 0.9 | 0.4 | 0.1 | 10 | 50 | 232 | 0.12 | 0.009 | 4.9 | 43 | 0 | 0.11 | 0.02 | 2.5 | 43379 |
| **tilsit cheese**, whole milk | 28 | 95 | 12.0 | 0.5 | | | 0 | 211 | 196 | 4 | 0.98 | 0.004 | 70 | 0 | 0.02 | 0.1 | 0.59 | 0.10 |
| *1 oz* | | 6.8 | 7.3 | 4.7 | 2.0 | 0.2 | 29 | 18 | 140 | 0.06 | 0.007 | 4.1 | 293 | | 0.10 | 0.02 | 5.6 | 1041 |

## 5.2 CHEESE PRODUCTS AND CHEESE SUBSTITUTES

| | WT (g) | KCAL / PRO (g) | H₂O (g) / FAT (g) | CHO (g) / SFA (g) | TSUG (g) / MUFA (g) | ASUG (g) / PUFA (g) | DFIB (g) / CHOL (mg) | Na (mg) / K (mg) | Ca (mg) / P (mg) | Mg (mg) / Fe (mg) | Zn (mg) / Cu (mg) | Mn (mg) / Se (mcg) | A (mcg RAE) / A (IU) | C (mg) / E (mg ATE) | B-1 (mg) / B-2 (mg) | NIA (mg) / B-6 (mg) | B-12 (mcg) / FOL (mcg DFE) | PANT (mg) / REF |
|---|---|---|---|---|---|---|---|---|---|---|---|---|---|---|---|---|---|---|
| **American cheese food**, cold pack | 28 | 93 | 12.1 | 2.3 | | | 0 | 270 | 139 | 8 | 0.84 | 0.003 | 45 | 0 | 0.01 | 0 | 0.36 | 0.27 |
| *1 oz* | | 5.5 | 6.8 | 4.3 | 2.0 | 0.2 | 18 | 102 | 112 | 0.24 | 0.008 | 4.5 | 197 | | 0.12 | 0.04 | 1.4 | 1045 |
| **American processed cheese food** | 28 | 92 | 12.1 | 2.2 | 2.1 | 0 | 0 | 354 | 160 | 9 | 0.89 | 0.020 | 56 | 0 | 0.02 | 0 | 0.35 | 0.27 |
| *1 oz* | | 5.2 | 7.1 | 4.2 | 2.0 | 0.3 | 22 | 81 | 123 | 0.16 | 0.024 | 4.5 | 213 | 0.1 | 0.14 | 0.02 | 2.0 | 1046 |
| **cheese 'n salsa dip**, lowfat, medium Old El Paso - *2 T (1 oz)* | 29 | 30 | | 3.0 | 0 | | 0 | 260 | 20 | | | | | 0 | | | | |
| | | 0.5 | 1.5 | 1.0 | | | 2 | | | 0 | | | 0 | | | | | GENM22 |
| **cheese 'n salsa dip**, mild/medium Old El Paso - *2 T (1 oz)* | 29 | 40 | | 3.0 | 0 | | 0 | 300 | 20 | | | | | 0 | | | | |
| | | 0.5 | 3.0 | 1.0 | | | 2 | | | 0 | | | 0 | | | | | GENM23 |
| **cheese fondue** (table wine, Swiss cheese, flour) - *½ cup* | 108 | 247 | 66.5 | 4.1 | | | 0 | 143 | 514 | 25 | 2.12 | 0.107 | 118 | 0 | 0.03 | 0.2 | 0.90 | 0.25 |
| | | 15.4 | 14.5 | 9.4 | 3.8 | 0.5 | 49 | 113 | 330 | 0.42 | 0.028 | 9.7 | 447 | | 0.21 | 0.06 | 11.9 | 1163 |
| **cheese sauce**, homemade | 30 | 59 | 20.1 | 1.6 | | | 0 | 148 | 93 | 6 | 0.38 | 0.012 | 50 | 0 | 0.01 | 0.1 | 0.10 | 0.07 |
| *2 T* | | 3.1 | 4.5 | 2.4 | 1.4 | 0.4 | 11 | 43 | 69 | 0.10 | 0.006 | 2.0 | 182 | | 0.07 | 0.01 | 3.3 | 1164 |
| **cheese sauce**, ready-to-serve | 63 | 110 | 44.4 | 4.3 | 0.3 | | 0.3 | 522 | 116 | 6 | 0.62 | 0.006 | 50 | 0 | 0 | 0 | 0.09 | 0.08 |
| *¼ cup* | | 4.2 | 8.4 | 3.8 | 2.4 | 1.6 | 18 | 19 | 99 | 0.13 | 0.011 | 2.0 | 199 | | 0.07 | 0.01 | 2.5 | 6930 |
| **cheese spread**, American | 28 | 81 | 13.3 | 2.4 | 2.0 | 0 | 0 | 377 | 157 | 8 | 0.73 | 0.006 | 48 | 0 | 0.01 | 0 | 0.11 | 0.19 |
| *1 oz* | | 4.6 | 5.9 | 3.7 | 1.7 | 0.2 | 15 | 68 | 199 | 0.09 | 0.009 | 3.2 | 183 | 0.1 | 0.12 | 0.03 | 2.0 | 1048 |
| **cheese spread**, Cheez Whiz, Kraft | 33 | 91 | 17.0 | 3.0 | 2.2 | | 0.1 | 541 | 118 | | 0.54 | | | 0 | | | | |
| *2 T* | | 4.0 | 6.9 | 4.3 | | | 25 | 79 | 266 | 0.06 | | | 214 | | 0.08 | | | 1188 |
| **cheese spread**, Cheez Whiz Light, Kraft - *2 T* | 35 | 75 | 18.0 | 5.7 | 2.9 | | 0.1 | 597 | 146 | | 0.83 | | | 0 | | | | |
| | | 5.7 | 3.3 | 2.2 | | | 12 | 104 | 330 | 0.06 | | | 220 | | 0.12 | | | 1189 |
| **cheese spread**, Velveeta, Kraft | 28 | 85 | 12.8 | 2.7 | 2.3 | | 0 | 420 | 130 | | 0.52 | | | 0 | | | | |
| *1 oz* | | 4.6 | 6.2 | 4.0 | | | 22 | 94 | 242 | 0.05 | | | 310 | | 0.10 | | | 1191 |
| **cheese spread**, Velveeta Light, reduced fat, Kraft - *1 oz* | 28 | 62 | 14.4 | 3.3 | 2.4 | | 0 | 444 | 161 | | 0.70 | | | 0 | | | | |
| | | 5.5 | 3.0 | 2.0 | | | 12 | 97 | 287 | 0.04 | | | 275 | | 0.18 | | | 1192 |
| **mozzarella cheese substitute** | 28 | 69 | 13.3 | 6.6 | 6.6 | 0 | 0 | 192 | 171 | 11 | 0.54 | 0.008 | 122 | 0 | 0.01 | 0.1 | 0.23 | 0.02 |
| *1 oz* | | 3.2 | 3.4 | 1.0 | 1.7 | 0.5 | 0 | 127 | 163 | 0.11 | 0.031 | 5.4 | 408 | 0 | 0.12 | 0.01 | 3.1 | 1161 |
| **soy cheese** | 28 | 42 | 19.9 | 1.9 | 0.4 | 0 | 0 | 6 | 53 | 64 | 0.48 | 0.249 | 1 | 0 | 0 | 0.1 | 0 | 0.03 |
| *1 oz* | | 3.5 | 2.3 | 0.3 | 0.5 | 1.3 | 0 | 56 | 62 | 1.57 | 0.106 | 4.7 | 12 | 0.2 | 0.04 | 0.02 | 6.2 | 43299 |
| **Swiss cheese food** | 28 | 90 | 12.2 | 1.3 | | | 0 | 435 | 202 | 8 | 0.99 | 0.003 | 66 | 0 | 0 | 0 | 0.64 | 0.14 |
| *1 oz* | | 6.1 | 6.8 | 4.3 | 1.9 | 0.2 | 23 | 80 | 147 | 0.17 | 0.008 | 4.5 | 240 | | 0.11 | 0.01 | 1.7 | 1047 |

## 6. CREAMS AND CREAMERS (CREAM SUBSTITUTES)

| | WT (g) | KCAL / PRO (g) | H₂O (g) / FAT (g) | CHO (g) / SFA (g) | TSUG (g) / MUFA (g) | ASUG (g) / PUFA (g) | DFIB (g) / CHOL (mg) | Na (mg) / K (mg) | Ca (mg) / P (mg) | Mg (mg) / Fe (mg) | Zn (mg) / Cu (mg) | Mn (mg) / Se (mcg) | A (mcg RAE) / A (IU) | C (mg) / E (mg ATE) | B-1 (mg) / B-2 (mg) | NIA (mg) / B-6 (mg) | B-12 (mcg) / FOL (mcg DFE) | PANT (mg) / REF |
|---|---|---|---|---|---|---|---|---|---|---|---|---|---|---|---|---|---|---|
| **cream**, half & half | 15 | 20 | 12.1 | 0.6 | 0 | 0 | 0 | 6 | 16 | 2 | 0.08 | 0 | 15 | 0 | 0.01 | 0 | 0.05 | 0.04 |
| *1 T (½ fl oz container)* | | 0.4 | 1.7 | 1.1 | 0.5 | 0.1 | 6 | 20 | 14 | 0.01 | 0.002 | 0.3 | 53 | 0 | 0.02 | 0.01 | 0.4 | 1049 |
| **cream**, light (coffee/table) | 15 | 29 | 11.1 | 0.5 | 0 | 0 | 0 | 6 | 14 | 1 | 0.04 | 0 | 27 | 0 | 0 | 0 | 0.03 | 0.04 |
| *1 T* | | 0.4 | 2.9 | 1.8 | 0.8 | 0.1 | 10 | 18 | 12 | 0.01 | 0.001 | 0.1 | 98 | 0.1 | 0.02 | 0 | 0.3 | 1050 |
| **creamer**, liquid, light | 30 | 21 | 25.9 | 2.7 | 2.7 | 2.7 | 0 | 18 | 0 | 0 | 0.02 | | 0 | 0 | 0 | 0 | 0 | |
| *1 fl oz* | | 0.2 | 1.0 | 0.3 | 0.6 | 0.1 | 0 | 53 | 22 | 0.17 | 0 | 0.3 | 2 | 0.1 | 0 | 0 | 0 | 42141 |
| **creamer**, liquid/frozen, hydrogenated veg oils - *1 T (½ fl oz)* | 15 | 20 | 11.6 | 1.7 | 1.7 | 1.7 | 0 | 12 | 1 | 0 | 0 | 0 | 0 | 0 | 0 | 0 | 0 | 0 |
| | | 0.2 | 1.5 | 0.3 | 1.1 | 0 | 0 | 29 | 10 | 0 | 0 | 0.2 | 2 | 0.1 | 0 | 0 | 0 | 1067 |
| **creamer**, liquid/frozen, lauric acid oils - *1 T (½ fl oz)* | 15 | 20 | 11.6 | 1.7 | | | 0 | 12 | 1 | 0 | 0 | 0.006 | 1 | 0 | 0 | 0 | 0 | 0 |
| | | 0.2 | 1.5 | 1.4 | 0 | 0 | 0 | 29 | 10 | 0 | 0.004 | 0.2 | 13 | 0 | 0 | 0 | 0 | 1068 |
| **creamer**, powdered | 6 | 33 | 0.1 | 3.3 | 3.3 | 3.3 | 0 | 11 | 1 | 0 | 0.03 | 0.013 | 0 | 0 | 0 | 0 | 0 | 0 |
| *1 T* | | 0.3 | 2.1 | 2.0 | 0.1 | 0 | 0 | 49 | 25 | 0.07 | 0.007 | 0 | 2 | 0 | 0.01 | 0 | 0 | 1069 |
| **creamer**, powdered, light | 6 | 26 | 0.4 | 4.4 | 4.4 | 4.4 | 0 | 14 | 0 | 0 | 0 | 0 | 0 | 0 | 0 | 0 | 0 | |
| *1 T* | | 0.1 | 0.9 | 0.2 | 0.7 | 0 | 0 | 54 | 8 | 0 | 0.001 | 0 | 1 | 0 | 0 | 0 | 0.1 | 42136 |
| **sour cream**, cultured | 24 | 46 | 17.9 | 0.7 | 0.8 | 0 | 0 | 19 | 26 | 2 | 0.09 | 0.003 | 39 | 0 | 0.01 | 0 | 0.07 | 0.08 |
| *2 T* | | 0.5 | 4.7 | 2.8 | 1.2 | 0.2 | 12 | 34 | 28 | 0.04 | 0.005 | 0.6 | 138 | 0.1 | 0.04 | 0.01 | 1.7 | 1056 |

| | WT (g) | KCAL | $H_2O$ (g) | CHO (g) | TSUG (g) | ASUG (g) | DFIB (g) | Na (mg) | Ca (mg) | Mg (mg) | Zn (mg) | Mn (mg) | A (mcg RAE) | C (mg) | B-1 (mg) | NIA (mg) | B-12 (mcg) | PANT (mg) |
|---|---|---|---|---|---|---|---|---|---|---|---|---|---|---|---|---|---|---|
| | | PRO (g) | FAT (g) | SFA (g) | MUFA (g) | PUFA (g) | CHOL (mg) | K (mg) | P (mg) | Fe (mg) | Cu (mg) | Se (mcg) | A (IU) | E (mg ATE) | B-2 (mg) | B-6 (mg) | FOL (mcg DFE) | REF |
| **sour cream**, cultured, fat-free, Breakstone's Free - 2 T | 32 | 29 | 24.9 | 4.8 | 2.3 | | 0 | 23 | 45 | | | | | 0 | | | | |
| | | 1.5 | 0.4 | 0.3 | | | 3 | 70 | 37 | 0.02 | | | 217 | | | | | 1194 |
| **sour cream**, cultured, imitation, 1 oz | 28 | 58 | 19.9 | 1.9 | 1.9 | 0 | 0 | 29 | 1 | 2 | 0.33 | 0.031 | 0 | 0 | 0 | 0 | 0 | 0 |
| | | 0.7 | 5.5 | 5.0 | 0.2 | 0 | 0 | 45 | 13 | 0.11 | 0.016 | 0.7 | 0 | 0.2 | 0 | 0 | 0 | 1074 |
| **sour cream**, cultured, reduced-fat, 1 T | 15 | 20 | 12.0 | 0.6 | 0 | 0 | 0 | 6 | 16 | 2 | 0.08 | 0 | 15 | 0 | 0.01 | 0 | 0.04 | 0.05 |
| | | 0.4 | 1.8 | 1.1 | 0.5 | 0.1 | 6 | 19 | 14 | 0.01 | 0.002 | 0.3 | 56 | 0.1 | 0.02 | 0 | 1.6 | 1055 |
| **sour cream**, cultured, reduced-fat, Breakstone's - 2 T | 31 | 47 | 23.6 | 2.2 | 2.0 | | 0 | 18 | 50 | | | | | 0 | | | | |
| | | 1.4 | 3.7 | 2.4 | | | 16 | 65 | 34 | 0.02 | | | 326 | | | | | 1193 |
| **sour cream**, fat-free, 2 T | 30 | 22 | 24.2 | 4.7 | 0.1 | 0 | 0 | 42 | 38 | 3 | 0.15 | | 22 | 0 | 0.01 | 0 | 0.09 | |
| | | 0.9 | 0 | 0 | 0 | 0 | 3 | 39 | 28 | 0 | 0.005 | 1.6 | 76 | 0 | 0.04 | 0.01 | 3.3 | 1180 |
| **sour cream**, light, 2 T | 30 | 41 | 23.4 | 2.1 | 0.1 | 0 | 0 | 21 | 42 | 3 | 0.15 | | 27 | 0 | 0.01 | 0 | 0.13 | |
| | | 1.0 | 3.2 | 2.0 | 0.9 | 0.1 | 10 | 64 | 21 | 0.02 | 0.005 | 0.9 | 98 | 0.1 | 0.04 | 0.01 | 3.3 | 1179 |
| **sour cream**, reduced fat, 2 T | 30 | 54 | 21.3 | 2.1 | 0.1 | 0 | 0 | 21 | 42 | 3 | 0.08 | | 36 | 0 | 0.01 | 0 | 0.09 | |
| | | 2.1 | 4.2 | 2.6 | 1.2 | 0.2 | 10 | 63 | 26 | 0.02 | 0.003 | 1.2 | 131 | 0.1 | 0.07 | 0.01 | 3.3 | 1178 |
| **soy creamer**, French vanilla, Silk, 1 T | 15 | 20 | 10.9 | 3.0 | 3.0 | | 0 | 10 | 0 | | | | | 0 | | | | |
| | | 0 | 1.0 | 0 | | | 0 | | | | 0 | | 0 | | | | | 16261 |
| **soy creamer**, hazelnut, Silk, 1 T | 15 | 20 | 10.9 | 3.0 | 3.0 | | 0 | 10 | 0 | | | | | | 30 | | | |
| | | 0 | 1.0 | 0 | | | 0 | | | | 0 | | 0 | | | | | 16262 |
| **soy creamer**, Silk, 1 T | 15 | 15 | 12.9 | 1.0 | 0 | | 0 | 10 | 0 | | | | | 0 | | | | |
| | | 0 | 1.0 | 0 | | | 0 | | | | 0 | | 0 | | | | | 16260 |
| **whipped topping**, from mix, prepared with whole milk - 1 T | 4 | 8 | 2.7 | 0.7 | 0.7 | 0.5 | 0 | 3 | 4 | 0 | 0.01 | 0 | 1 | 0 | 0 | 0 | 0.01 | 0.01 |
| | | 0.1 | 0.5 | 0.4 | 0 | 0 | 0 | 6 | 3 | 0 | 0 | 0.2 | 5 | 0 | 0 | 0 | 0.2 | 1071 |
| **whipped topping**, frozen, 1 T | 4 | 13 | 2.0 | 0.9 | 0.9 | 0.9 | 0 | 1 | 0 | 0 | 0 | 0.002 | 0 | 0 | 0 | 0 | 0 | 0 |
| | | 0 | 1.0 | 0.9 | 0.1 | 0 | 0 | 1 | 0 | 0 | 0.001 | 0.1 | 6 | 0 | 0 | 0 | 0 | 1073 |
| **whipped topping**, pressurized, 1 T | 4 | 11 | 2.4 | 0.6 | 0.6 | 0.6 | 0 | 2 | 0 | 0 | 0 | 0.002 | 0 | 0 | 0 | 0 | 0 | 0 |
| | | 0 | 0.9 | 0.8 | 0.1 | 0 | 0 | 1 | 1 | 0 | 0.001 | 0.1 | 3 | 0 | 0 | 0 | 0 | 1072 |
| **whipping cream**, heavy fluid, 1 T | 15 | 52 | 8.7 | 0.4 | 0 | 0 | 0 | 6 | 10 | 1 | 0.03 | 0 | 62 | 0 | 0 | 0 | 0.03 | 0.04 |
| | | 0.3 | 5.6 | 3.5 | 1.6 | 0.2 | 21 | 11 | 9 | 0 | 0.001 | 0.1 | 220 | 0.2 | 0.02 | 0 | 0.6 | 1053 |
| **whipping cream**, light fluid, 1 T | 15 | 44 | 9.5 | 0.4 | 0 | 0 | 0 | 5 | 10 | 1 | 0.04 | 0 | 42 | 0 | 0 | 0 | 0.03 | 0.04 |
| | | 0.3 | 4.6 | 2.9 | 1.4 | 0.1 | 17 | 15 | 9 | 0 | 0.001 | 0.1 | 152 | 0.1 | 0.02 | 0 | 0.6 | 1052 |
| **whipping cream**, pressurized, 1 T | 3 | 8 | 1.8 | 0.4 | 0.2 | 0.2 | 0 | 4 | 3 | 0 | 0.01 | 0 | 6 | 0 | 0 | 0 | 0.01 | 0.01 |
| | | 0.1 | 0.7 | 0.4 | 0.2 | 0 | 2 | 4 | 3 | 0 | 0 | 0 | 21 | 0 | 0 | 0 | 0.1 | 1054 |

# 7. DESSERTS
## 7.1 BROWNIES AND BARS

| | WT (g) | KCAL | $H_2O$ (g) | CHO (g) | TSUG (g) | ASUG (g) | DFIB (g) | Na (mg) | Ca (mg) | Mg (mg) | Zn (mg) | Mn (mg) | A (mcg RAE) | C (mg) | B-1 (mg) | NIA (mg) | B-12 (mcg) | PANT (mg) |
|---|---|---|---|---|---|---|---|---|---|---|---|---|---|---|---|---|---|---|
| | | PRO (g) | FAT (g) | SFA (g) | MUFA (g) | PUFA (g) | CHOL (mg) | K (mg) | P (mg) | Fe (mg) | Cu (mg) | Se (mcg) | A (IU) | E (mg ATE) | B-2 (mg) | B-6 (mg) | FOL (mcg DFE) | REF |
| **brownie**, 1 brownie (2¾" × ⅞") | 56 | 227 | 7.6 | 35.8 | 20.5 | 19.8 | 1.2 | 175 | 16 | 17 | 0.40 | 0.072 | 11 | 0 | 0.14 | 1.0 | 0.04 | 0.31 |
| | | 2.7 | 9.1 | 2.4 | 5.0 | 1.3 | 10 | 83 | 57 | 1.26 | 0.125 | 3.5 | 39 | 0.1 | 0.12 | 0.02 | 40.3 | 18151 |
| **brownie**, choc chunk, from mix, Betty Crckr Suprm - 1 brwnie | 40 | 180 | | 25.0 | 17.0 | | 1.0 | 95 | | | | | | | 0.03 | 0.4 | | |
| | | 1.0 | 9.0 | 2.0 | | | 20 | 95 | | 1.08 | | | | | 0.03 | | | GENM24 |
| **brownie**, dark choc fudge, from mix, Betty Crckr Suprm - 1 brwnie | 38 | 170 | | 24.0 | 16.0 | | 1.0 | 105 | | | | | | | 0.03 | 0.4 | | |
| | | 2.0 | 7.0 | 1.5 | | | 20 | | | 0.72 | | | | | 0.03 | | | GENM25 |
| **brownie**, dark choc w/Hrshy syrp, fr mix, Bty Crkr Suprm -1 brwnie | 42 | 170 | | 25.0 | 17.0 | | 0.5 | 105 | | | | | | | 0.03 | 0.4 | | |
| | | 2.0 | 7.0 | 1.5 | | | 20 | 95 | | 1.08 | | | | | 0.03 | | | GENM26 |
| **brownie**, frosted, from mix, Betty Crocker Suprm - 1 brwnie | 48 | 170 | | 23.0 | 15.0 | | 0.5 | 105 | | | | | | | 0.03 | 0.4 | | |
| | | 2.0 | 8.0 | 1.5 | | | 20 | 85 | | 0.72 | | | | | 0.03 | | | GENM27 |
| **brownie**, homemade, 1 brownie (2¾" × ⅞") | 56 | 261 | 7.1 | 28.1 | | | | 192 | 32 | 30 | 0.54 | 0.329 | 99 | 0 | 0.08 | 0.5 | 0.09 | 0.18 |
| | | 3.5 | 16.3 | 4.1 | 6.1 | 5.3 | 41 | 99 | 74 | 1.03 | 0.217 | 6.4 | 463 | | 0.11 | 0.05 | 21.8 | 18154 |
| **brownie**, Little Debbie, 1 twin wrapped pkg (2 pcs) | 61 | 247 | 8.3 | 39.0 | 22.3 | | 1.3 | 190 | 18 | 19 | 0.44 | 0.078 | 12 | 0 | 0.16 | 1.0 | 0.04 | 0.33 |
| | | 2.9 | 9.9 | 2.6 | 5.5 | 1.4 | 10 | 91 | 62 | 1.37 | 0.137 | 3.8 | 42 | 0.1 | 0.13 | 0.02 | 43.9 | 18151 |
| **brownie**, turtle, from mix, Betty Crocker Suprm - 1 brwnie | 40 | 170 | | 23.0 | 15.0 | | 0.5 | 105 | | | | | | | 0.03 | 0.4 | | |
| | | 2.0 | 8.0 | 1.5 | | | 20 | 85 | | 0.72 | | | | | 0.03 | | | GENM37 |
| **brownie**, walnut, from mix, Betty Crocker Suprm - ½ pkg (1.6 oz) | 39 | 170 | | 22.0 | 15.0 | | 0.5 | 95 | | | | | | | 0.03 | 0.4 | | |
| | | 2.0 | 9.0 | 1.5 | | | 20 | | | 1.08 | | | | | 0.03 | | | GENM38 |
| **Sunkist Lemon bar**, from mix, Betty Crocker - 1 bar | 40 | 140 | | 24.0 | 17.0 | | | 90 | | | | | | | 0.03 | 0.4 | | |
| | | 2.0 | 4.0 | 1.0 | | | 40 | 20 | | 0.36 | | | | | 0.07 | | | GENM43 |

## 7.2 CAKES AND SNACK CAKES

| | WT (g) | KCAL | $H_2O$ (g) | CHO (g) | TSUG (g) | ASUG (g) | DFIB (g) | Na (mg) | Ca (mg) | Mg (mg) | Zn (mg) | Mn (mg) | A (mcg RAE) | C (mg) | B-1 (mg) | NIA (mg) | B-12 (mcg) | PANT (mg) |
|---|---|---|---|---|---|---|---|---|---|---|---|---|---|---|---|---|---|---|
| | | PRO (g) | FAT (g) | SFA (g) | MUFA (g) | PUFA (g) | CHOL (mg) | K (mg) | P (mg) | Fe (mg) | Cu (mg) | Se (mcg) | A (IU) | E (mg ATE) | B-2 (mg) | B-6 (mg) | FOL (mcg DFE) | REF |
| **angel food cake** | 28 | 72 | 9.3 | 16.2 | | | 0.4 | 210 | 39 | 3 | 0.02 | 0.024 | 0 | 0 | 0.03 | 0.2 | 0.02 | 0.06 |
| *1/12 cake (1 oz)* | | 1.7 | 0.2 | 0 | 0 | 0.1 | 0 | 26 | 91 | 0.15 | 0.022 | 2.0 | 0 | | 0.14 | 0.01 | 16.0 | 18086 |
| **angel food cake**, from mix | 50 | 128 | 16.4 | 29.4 | 15.3 | 15.1 | 0.1 | 254 | 42 | 4 | 0.06 | 0.032 | 0 | 0 | 0.05 | 0.1 | 0.02 | 0.06 |
| *1/12 cake of 10″ diameter cake* | | 3.0 | 0.2 | 0 | 0 | 0.1 | 0 | 68 | 116 | 0.12 | 0.034 | 7.6 | 0 | 0 | 0.10 | 0 | 14.5 | 18088 |
| **angel food cake mix**, white, | 38 | 140 | | 32.0 | 23.0 | | | 320 | 60 | | | | | | | | | |
| SuperMoist - *1/12 pkg (1.3 oz)* | | 3.0 | 0 | 0 | 0 | 0 | 0 | 40 | | | | | | | 0.10 | | | GENM44 |
| **Boston cream pie/cake**, frozen | 92 | 232 | 41.8 | 39.5 | 33.2 | 28.9 | 1.3 | 132 | 21 | 6 | 0.15 | 0.046 | 22 | 0 | 0.38 | 0.2 | 0.15 | 0.28 |
| *1/6 of 19.5 oz cake* | | 2.2 | 7.8 | 2.2 | 4.2 | 0.9 | 34 | 36 | 45 | 0.35 | 0.039 | 3.8 | 75 | 0.1 | 0.25 | 0.02 | 16.6 | 18090 |
| **butter pecan cake**, from mix, | 77 | 240 | | 34.0 | 18.0 | | | 290 | 80 | | | | | | 0.12 | 0.8 | | |
| SuperMoist - *1/12 cake* | | 3.0 | 11.0 | 2.0 | 3.0 | 4.0 | 55 | 35 | | 0.72 | | | | | 0.10 | | | GENM45 |
| **carrot cake**, from mix, SuperMoist | 83 | 320 | | 41.0 | 22.0 | | 0 | 340 | 100 | | | | | | 0.12 | 0.8 | | |
| *1/10 cake* | | 4.0 | 16.0 | 2.5 | 4.0 | 7.0 | 65 | 45 | | 1.08 | | | | | 0.14 | | | GENM46 |
| **carrot mini cake**, frozen, Entenman | 39 | 160 | | 22.0 | 15.0 | | | 140 | 0 | | | | | 0 | | | | |
| *1 minicake (1.4 oz)* | | 1.0 | 7.0 | 1.5 | | | 20 | | | 0.36 | | | 0 | | | | | ENTE1 |
| **cheesecake** | 80 | 257 | 36.5 | 20.4 | | | 0.3 | 166 | 41 | 9 | 0.41 | 0.112 | 114 | 0 | 0.02 | 0.2 | 0.14 | 0.46 |
| *1/6 of 17 oz cake* | | 4.4 | 18.0 | 7.9 | 6.9 | 1.3 | 44 | 72 | 74 | 0.50 | 0.016 | 4.2 | 438 | | 0.15 | 0.04 | 16.0 | 18147 |
| **cheesecake**, choc mousse, frzn Harry | 113 | 420 | | 40.0 | 28.0 | | 3.0 | 300 | 40 | | | | | | | | | |
| and David - *1/4 cake (4 oz)* | | 7.0 | 26.0 | 13.0 | | | 75 | | | 2.70 | | | 500 | | | | | HADA3 |
| **cheesecake**, from mix, no-bake type | 99 | 271 | 43.8 | 35.1 | | | 1.9 | 376 | 170 | 19 | 0.46 | 0.119 | 95 | 0 | 0.12 | 0.5 | 0.31 | 0.61 |
| *1/8 of 9″ cake* | | 5.4 | 12.6 | 6.6 | 4.5 | 0.8 | 29 | 209 | 232 | 0.47 | 0.029 | 4.7 | 362 | | 0.26 | 0.05 | 37.6 | 18148 |
| **cherry chip cake**, from mix, | 83 | 290 | | 40.0 | 21.0 | | 1.0 | 360 | 60 | | | | | | 0.15 | 0.8 | | |
| SuperMoist - *1/10 cake* | | 4.0 | 13.0 | 3.0 | 4.5 | 3.0 | 65 | 50 | | 1.08 | | | | | 0.14 | | | GENM51 |
| **cherry fudge cake** with chocolate | 71 | 187 | 32.7 | 27.0 | 23.4 | 18.6 | 0.9 | 160 | 34 | 13 | 0.20 | 0.048 | 55 | 10 | 0.02 | 0.5 | 0.15 | 0.33 |
| icing - *1/8 of 20 oz cake* | | 1.7 | 8.9 | 3.6 | 3.1 | 1.7 | 30 | 118 | 75 | 0.78 | 0.040 | 2.4 | 312 | 0.5 | 0.13 | 0.04 | 9.2 | 18095 |
| **chocolate cake**, butter recipe, from | 76 | 260 | | 34.0 | 18.0 | | 1.0 | 460 | 40 | | | | | | 0.09 | 0.8 | | |
| mix, SuperMoist - *1/12 cake* | | 4.0 | 12.0 | 6.0 | 4.0 | 0.5 | 75 | 130 | | 1.80 | | | 300 | | 0.14 | | | GENM52 |
| **chocolate cake**, homemade | 95 | 352 | 23.2 | 50.7 | | | 1.5 | 299 | 57 | 30 | 0.66 | 0.266 | | 0 | 0.13 | 1.1 | 0.15 | 0.29 |
| *1/12 of 9″ cake* | | 5.0 | 14.3 | 5.2 | 5.7 | 2.6 | 55 | 133 | 101 | 1.53 | 0.197 | 11.3 | 133 | | 0.20 | 0.04 | 37.0 | 18101 |
| **chocolate cake** with chocolate icing | 64 | 235 | 14.7 | 34.9 | | | 1.8 | 214 | 28 | 22 | 0.44 | 0.205 | 17 | 0 | 0.02 | 0.4 | 0.09 | 0.13 |
| *1/8 of 18 oz cake* | | 2.6 | 10.5 | 3.1 | 5.6 | 1.2 | 27 | 128 | 78 | 1.41 | 0.155 | 2.1 | 54 | | 0.09 | 0.03 | 14.7 | 18096 |
| **chocolate creme-filled snack cake** | 50 | 200 | 9.3 | 30.2 | 18.9 | 16.6 | 1.6 | 194 | 58 | 18 | 0.52 | 0.242 | 0 | 1 | 0.02 | 0.5 | 0.03 | 0.04 |
| with icing - *1.8 oz snack cake* | | 1.8 | 8.0 | 2.4 | 4.3 | 0.9 | 0 | 88 | 44 | 1.80 | 0.152 | 1.7 | 1 | 0.5 | 0.04 | 0.07 | 17.5 | 18127 |
| **chocolate cupcake** with chocolate | 60 | 210 | | 36.0 | 26.0 | | 2.0 | 260 | 20 | | | | | 0 | | | | |
| icing, Tastykake - *2 cupcakes* | | 2.0 | 7.0 | 2.0 | | | 5 | | | 1.08 | | | 0 | | | | | TAST1 |
| **chocolate cupcake** with icing, | 43 | 131 | 9.8 | 28.9 | | | 1.8 | 178 | 15 | 11 | 0.24 | 0.096 | 0 | 0 | 0.02 | 0.3 | 0 | 0.10 |
| lowfat - *1.5 oz cupcake* | | 1.8 | 1.6 | 0.5 | 0.8 | 0.2 | 0 | 96 | 79 | 0.66 | 0.076 | 2.4 | 0 | | 0.06 | 0 | 9.5 | 18452 |
| **chocolate cupcakes** w/crm filling & | 67 | 250 | | 40.0 | 27.0 | | 1.0 | 240 | 20 | | | | | 0 | | | | |
| choc icing, Tstykake - *2 cupcakes* | | 2.0 | 10.0 | 2.5 | | | 10 | | | 1.08 | | | 0 | | | | | TAST2 |
| **chocolate devil's food cake**, from | 80 | 270 | | 34.0 | 18.0 | | 1.0 | 380 | 40 | | | | | | 0.09 | 0.8 | | |
| mix, SuperMoist - *1/12 cake* | | 4.0 | 14.0 | 2.5 | 4.0 | 6.0 | 55 | 130 | | 1.80 | | | | | 0.14 | | | GENM57 |
| **chocolate fudge cake**, from mix, | 80 | 270 | | 34.0 | 18.0 | | 1.0 | 370 | 40 | | | | | | 0.09 | 0.8 | | |
| SuperMoist - *1/12 cake* | | 4.0 | 14.0 | 2.5 | 4.0 | 6.0 | 55 | 105 | | 1.44 | | | | | 0.10 | | | GENM54 |
| **coffeecake**, cinnamon with crumb | 63 | 263 | 13.8 | 29.4 | | | 1.3 | 221 | 34 | 14 | 0.51 | 0.284 | 21 | 0 | 0.13 | 1.1 | 0.11 | 0.41 |
| topping - *1/9 of 20 oz cake* | | 4.3 | 14.7 | 3.7 | 8.2 | 2.0 | 20 | 77 | 68 | 1.20 | 0.079 | 10.8 | 70 | | 0.14 | 0.02 | 51.0 | 18104 |
| **coffeecake**, cinn w/crumb topping, | 56 | 178 | 17.1 | 29.6 | 16.5 | 15.7 | 0.7 | 236 | 76 | 10 | 0.25 | 0.174 | 20 | 0 | 0.09 | 0.9 | 0.08 | 0.15 |
| from mix - *1/8 of 8″ × 5¾″ cake* | | 3.1 | 5.4 | 1.0 | 2.2 | 1.8 | 27 | 63 | 120 | 0.80 | 0.083 | 9.4 | 68 | 0.1 | 0.10 | 0.03 | 40.9 | 18108 |
| **coffeecake**, cream/neufchatel | 76 | 258 | 24.5 | 33.7 | | | 0.8 | 258 | 45 | 11 | 0.45 | 0.131 | 65 | 0 | 0.08 | 0.5 | 0.26 | 0.30 |
| cheese - *1/6 of 16 oz cake* | | 5.3 | 11.6 | 4.1 | 5.4 | 1.3 | 65 | 220 | 77 | 0.49 | 0.040 | 10.1 | 218 | | 0.10 | 0.04 | 40.3 | 18103 |
| **coffeecake**, crème-filled with choc | 90 | 298 | 26.2 | 48.4 | | | 1.8 | 291 | 34 | 14 | 0.40 | 0.171 | 33 | 0 | 0.07 | 0.8 | 0.18 | 0.35 |
| icing - *1/6 of 19 oz cake* | | 4.5 | 9.7 | 2.5 | 5.1 | 1.3 | 62 | 70 | 68 | 0.46 | 0.063 | 13.0 | 111 | | 0.07 | 0.04 | 52.2 | 18105 |
| **coffeecake** with fruit | 50 | 156 | 15.8 | 25.8 | | | 1.2 | 192 | 22 | 8 | 0.32 | 0.120 | 4 | 0 | 0.02 | 1.3 | 0.01 | 0.33 |
| *1/8 of 14 oz cake* | | 2.6 | 5.1 | 1.2 | 2.8 | 0.7 | 4 | 45 | 59 | 1.22 | 0.015 | 8.2 | 70 | | 0.10 | 0.02 | 33.5 | 18106 |
| **French vanilla cake**, from mix, | 77 | 240 | | 34.0 | 18.0 | | | 290 | 80 | | | | | | 0.12 | 0.8 | | |
| SuperMoist - *1/12 cake* | | 3.0 | 11.0 | 2.0 | 3.0 | 4.0 | 55 | 35 | | 0.72 | | | | | 0.14 | | | GENM61 |
| **fruitcake** | 43 | 139 | 10.9 | 26.5 | 12.8 | 11.2 | 1.6 | 116 | 14 | 7 | 0.12 | 0.095 | 3 | 0 | 0.02 | 0.3 | 0 | 0.10 |
| *1.5 oz piece* | | 1.2 | 3.9 | 0.5 | 1.8 | 1.4 | 2 | 66 | 22 | 0.89 | 0.022 | 0.9 | 12 | 0.4 | 0.04 | 0.02 | 13.8 | 18110 |
| **German chocolate cake**, from mix, | 80 | 270 | | 34.0 | 18.0 | | 0.5 | 360 | 40 | | | | | | 0.12 | 0.8 | | |
| SuperMoist - *1/12 cake* | | 3.0 | 14.0 | 2.5 | 4.0 | 6.0 | 55 | 80 | | 1.08 | | | | | 0.14 | | | GENM63 |

| | WT (g) | KCAL / PRO (g) | H₂0 (g) / FAT (g) | CHO (g) / SFA (g) | TSUG (g) / MUFA (g) | ASUG (g) / PUFA (g) | DFIB (g) / CHOL (mg) | Na (mg) / K (mg) | Ca (mg) / P (mg) | Mg (mg) / Fe (mg) | Zn (mg) / Cu (mg) | Mn (mg) / Se (mcg) | A (mcg RAE) / A (IU) | C (mg) / E (mg ATE) | B-1 (mg) / B-2 (mg) | NIA (mg) / B-6 (mg) | B-12 (mcg) / FOL (mcg DFE) | PANT (mg) / REF |
|---|---|---|---|---|---|---|---|---|---|---|---|---|---|---|---|---|---|---|
| **gingerbread**, from mix, Betty Crocker Classic - ⅛ cake | 82 | 220 | | 39.0 | 19.0 | | | 360 | 40 | | | | | | 0.12 | 0.8 | | |
| | | 3.0 | 6.0 | 1.5 | | | 25 | 140 | | 1.80 | | | | | 0.10 | | | GENM64 |
| **gingerbread**, homemade - ⅑ of 8″ square cake | 74 | 263 | 20.7 | 36.4 | | | | 242 | 53 | 52 | 0.29 | 0.505 | 10 | 0 | 0.14 | 1.3 | 0.04 | 0.28 |
| | | 2.9 | 12.1 | 3.1 | 5.3 | 3.1 | 24 | 325 | 40 | 2.13 | 0.144 | 12.1 | 36 | | 0.12 | 0.14 | 37.7 | 18116 |
| **golden vanilla cake**, from mix, SuperMoist - 1/12 cake | 77 | 240 | | 34.0 | 18.0 | | | 290 | 80 | | | | | | 0.12 | 0.8 | | |
| | | 3.0 | 11.0 | 2.0 | 3.0 | 4.0 | 55 | 35 | | 0.72 | | | | | 0.14 | | | GENM65 |
| **Kreamies snack cake**, banana, Tastykake - 1 cake | 43 | 170 | | 25.0 | 18.0 | | 0 | 100 | 20 | | | | | 0 | | | | |
| | | 1.0 | 8.0 | 2.0 | | | 5 | | | 0.36 | | | 0 | | | | | TAST3 |
| **Kreamies snack cake**, chocolate, Tastykake - 1 cake | 43 | 190 | | 26.0 | 18.0 | | 0 | 130 | 40 | | | | | 0 | | | | |
| | | 2.0 | 9.0 | 2.5 | | | 15 | | | 0.72 | | | 0 | | | | | TAST4 |
| **Krimpets snack cake**, butterscotch, Tastykake - 2 cakes | 57 | 210 | | 37.0 | 26.0 | | 0 | 170 | 20 | | | | | 0 | | | | |
| | | 2.0 | 6.0 | 2.0 | | | 50 | | | 0.36 | | | 100 | | | | | TAST5 |
| **Krimpets snack cake**, choc with kreme fill, Tastykake - 2 cakes | 57 | 190 | | 36.0 | 25.0 | | 0 | 150 | 20 | | | | | 0 | | | | |
| | | 2.0 | 4.0 | 1.5 | | | 50 | | | 0.36 | | | 100 | | | | | TAST6 |
| **Krimpets snack cake** with jelly filling, Tastykake - 2 cakes | 57 | 180 | | 34.0 | 21.0 | | 0 | 220 | 20 | | | | | 1 | | | | |
| | | 2.0 | 4.0 | 1.0 | | | 60 | | | 1.08 | | | 100 | | | | | TAST7 |
| **lemon cake**, from mix, SuperMoist - 1/12 cake | 75 | 240 | | 34.0 | 18.0 | | | 290 | 80 | | | | | | 0.12 | 0.8 | | |
| | | 3.0 | 11.0 | 2.0 | 3.0 | 4.0 | 55 | 35 | | 0.72 | | | | | 0.14 | | | GENM66 |
| **milk chocolate cake**, from mix, SuperMoist - 1/12 cake | 77 | 240 | | 34.0 | 18.0 | | 1.0 | 290 | 80 | | | | | | 0.09 | 0.8 | | |
| | | 4.0 | 11.0 | 2.0 | 3.0 | 4.0 | 55 | 110 | | 1.44 | | | | | 0.14 | | | GENM67 |
| **pineapple cake**, from mix, Betty Crocker Classic - ⅙ cake | 127 | 390 | | 65.0 | 43.0 | | | 330 | 40 | | | | | | 0.09 | 0.8 | | |
| | | 3.0 | 13.0 | 3.5 | 4.0 | 1.5 | 35 | 80 | | 0.72 | | | 200 | | 0.10 | | | GENM70 |
| **pineapple upside-down cake**, homemade - ⅑ of 8″ sq cake | 115 | 367 | 37.1 | 58.1 | | | 0.9 | 367 | 138 | 15 | 0.36 | 0.402 | 71 | 1 | 0.18 | 1.4 | 0.09 | 0.23 |
| | | 4.0 | 13.9 | 3.4 | 6.0 | 3.8 | 25 | 129 | 94 | 1.70 | 0.100 | 10.8 | 291 | | 0.18 | 0.04 | 44.8 | 18119 |
| **pound cake**, fat-free - 1 oz slice | 28 | 79 | 8.7 | 17.1 | 9.6 | 9.1 | 0.3 | 95 | 12 | 3 | 0.09 | 0.038 | 8 | 0 | 0.04 | 0.2 | 0 | 0.10 |
| | | 1.5 | 0.3 | 0.1 | 0 | 0.1 | 0 | 31 | 41 | 0.58 | 0.016 | 1.5 | 27 | | 0.08 | 0 | 19.6 | 18451 |
| **pound cake**, from mix, Betty Crocker Classic - ⅛ cake | 82 | 260 | | 45.0 | 26.0 | | 1.0 | 210 | 40 | | | | | | 0.12 | 0.8 | | |
| | | 3.0 | 8.0 | 2.0 | 2.5 | 0.5 | 55 | 40 | | 1.08 | | | | | 0.14 | | | GENM71 |
| **pound cake**, made with butter - 1/10 of 10.6 oz cake | 30 | 116 | 7.4 | 14.6 | | | 0.2 | 119 | 10 | 3 | 0.14 | 0.027 | 45 | 0 | 0.04 | 0.4 | 0.08 | 0.13 |
| | | 1.6 | 6.0 | 3.5 | 1.8 | 0.3 | 66 | 36 | 41 | 0.41 | 0.010 | 2.6 | 182 | | 0.07 | 0.01 | 18.6 | 18120 |
| **pound cake**, made with veg shortening - 1/10 of 10.6 oz cake | 30 | 117 | 6.9 | 15.8 | | | 0.3 | 120 | 19 | 4 | 0.12 | 0.026 | 10 | 0 | 0.04 | 0.4 | 0.04 | 0.09 |
| | | 1.6 | 5.4 | 1.4 | 3.0 | 0.7 | 17 | 32 | 40 | 0.49 | 0.016 | 2.0 | 35 | | 0.08 | 0.01 | 16.5 | 18121 |
| **pound snack cake** - 1.1 oz snack cake | 30 | 117 | 6.9 | 15.8 | | | 0.3 | 120 | 19 | 4 | 0.12 | 0.026 | 10 | 0 | 0.04 | 0.4 | 0.04 | 0.09 |
| | | 1.6 | 5.4 | 1.4 | 3.0 | 0.7 | 17 | 32 | 40 | 0.49 | 0.016 | 2.0 | 35 | | 0.08 | 0.01 | 16.5 | 18121 |
| **rainbow chip cake**, from mix, SuperMoist - 1/10 cake | 83 | 300 | | 40.0 | 20.0 | | 0.5 | 370 | 60 | | | | | | 0.15 | 1.2 | | |
| | | 4.0 | 14.0 | 3.0 | 4.0 | 5.0 | 65 | 50 | | 1.08 | | | | | 0.17 | | | GENM72 |
| **shortcake**, biscuit-type, homemade - 1 oz shortcake | 28 | 97 | 8.0 | 13.6 | | | | 142 | 57 | 4 | 0.13 | 0.092 | 5 | 0 | 0.09 | 0.7 | 0.02 | 0.07 |
| | | 1.7 | 4.0 | 1.1 | 1.7 | 1.0 | 1 | 30 | 40 | 0.71 | 0.021 | 4.8 | 20 | | 0.08 | 0.01 | 23.2 | 18126 |
| **Snowball**, Tastykake - 1 snowball | 60 | 210 | | 36.0 | 29.0 | | | 200 | 0 | | | | | 0 | | | | |
| | | 2.0 | 7.0 | 2.5 | | | 15 | | | 0.72 | | | 0 | | | | | TAST8 |
| **spice cake**, from mix, SuperMoist - 1/12 cake | 77 | 240 | | 34.0 | 18.0 | | | 290 | 80 | | | | | | 0.12 | 0.8 | | |
| | | 3.0 | 11.0 | 2.0 | 3.0 | 4.0 | 55 | 40 | | 1.08 | | | | | 0.14 | | | GENM74 |
| **sponge cake** - 1/12 of 16 oz cake | 38 | 110 | 11.3 | 23.2 | 13.9 | 13.5 | 0.2 | 93 | 27 | 4 | 0.19 | 0.080 | 17 | 0 | 0.09 | 0.7 | 0.09 | 0.18 |
| | | 2.1 | 1.0 | 0.3 | 0.4 | 0.2 | 39 | 38 | 52 | 1.03 | 0.024 | 3.5 | 59 | 0.1 | 0.10 | 0.02 | 27.0 | 18133 |
| **sponge cake**, homemade - 1/12 of 16 oz cake | 38 | 113 | 11.2 | 21.9 | | | | 87 | 16 | 3 | 0.22 | 0.063 | 29 | 0 | 0.06 | 0.5 | 0.14 | 0.21 |
| | | 2.8 | 1.6 | 0.5 | 0.6 | 0.2 | 65 | 54 | 38 | 0.60 | 0.021 | 7.0 | 98 | | 0.11 | 0.02 | 20.1 | 18134 |
| **sponge snack cake**, crème-filled - 1.5 oz snack cake | 43 | 161 | 8.4 | 27.5 | 16.0 | 16.2 | 0.4 | 172 | 10 | 3 | 0.26 | 0.131 | 2 | 0 | 0.08 | 0.7 | 0.08 | 0.10 |
| | | 1.5 | 5.0 | 1.8 | 2.1 | 0.8 | 18 | 31 | 80 | 0.58 | 0.064 | 1.5 | 7 | 0.3 | 0.07 | 0 | 23.2 | 18128 |
| **strawberry cake**, from mix, SuperMoist - 1/12 cake | 77 | 240 | | 34.0 | 18.0 | | | 290 | 80 | | | | | | 0.12 | 0.8 | | |
| | | 3.0 | 11.0 | 2.0 | 3.0 | 4.0 | 55 | 35 | | 0.72 | | | | | 0.14 | | | GENM75 |
| **white cake**, from mix, SuperMoist - 1/12 cake | 72 | 230 | | 33.0 | 17.0 | | | 300 | 40 | | | | | | 0.12 | 0.8 | | |
| | | 3.0 | 10.0 | 2.0 | 2.5 | 4.0 | 35 | 35 | | 0.72 | | | | | 0.10 | | | GENM76 |
| **white cake**, homemade - 1/12 of 9″ cake | 74 | 264 | 17.2 | 42.3 | 26.3 | 25.0 | 0.6 | 242 | 96 | 9 | 0.24 | 0.146 | 11 | 0 | 0.14 | 1.1 | 0.06 | 0.14 |
| | | 4.0 | 9.2 | 2.4 | 3.9 | 2.3 | 1 | 70 | 69 | 1.12 | 0.044 | 9.6 | 38 | 0.1 | 0.18 | 0.02 | 44.4 | 18139 |
| **white cake** with coconut icing, homemade - 1/12 of 9″ cake | 112 | 399 | 23.2 | 70.8 | 64.3 | 61.4 | 1.1 | 318 | 101 | 13 | 0.37 | 0.310 | 13 | 0 | 0.14 | 1.2 | 0.07 | 0.19 |
| | | 4.9 | 11.5 | 4.4 | 4.1 | 2.4 | 1 | 111 | 78 | 1.30 | 0.075 | 12.0 | 47 | 0.1 | 0.21 | 0.03 | 57.1 | 18102 |
| **yellow cake**, butter recipe, from mix, SuperMoist - 1/12 cake | 77 | 240 | | 34.0 | 18.0 | | | 290 | 80 | | | | | | 0.12 | 0.8 | | |
| | | 3.0 | 11.0 | 2.0 | 3.0 | 4.0 | 55 | 35 | | 0.72 | | | | | 0.14 | | | GENM78 |
| **yellow cake**, from mix, SuperMoist - 1/12 cake | 77 | 240 | | 34.0 | 18.0 | | | 290 | 80 | | | | | | 0.12 | 0.8 | | |
| | | 3.0 | 11.0 | 2.0 | 3.0 | 4.0 | 55 | 35 | | 0.72 | | | | | 0.14 | | | GENM79 |
| **yellow cake**, homemade - 1/12 of 8″ cake | 68 | 245 | 17.1 | 36.0 | | | 0.5 | 233 | 99 | 8 | 0.31 | 0.129 | 27 | 0 | 0.12 | 1.0 | 0.11 | 0.21 |
| | | 3.6 | 9.9 | 2.7 | 4.2 | 2.4 | 37 | 62 | 80 | 1.12 | 0.038 | 9.3 | 95 | | 0.16 | 0.02 | 34.7 | 18146 |

| | WT (g) | KCAL / PRO (g) | H₂O (g) / FAT (g) | CHO (g) / SFA (g) | TSUG (g) / MUFA (g) | ASUG (g) / PUFA (g) | DFIB (g) / CHOL (mg) | Na (mg) / K (mg) | Ca (mg) / P (mg) | Mg (mg) / Fe (mg) | Zn (mg) / Cu (mg) | Mn (mg) / Se (mcg) | A (mcg RAE) / A (IU) | C (mg) / E (mg ATE) | B-1 (mg) / B-2 (mg) | NIA (mg) / B-6 (mg) | B-12 (mcg) / FOL (mcg DFE) | PANT (mg) / REF |
|---|---|---|---|---|---|---|---|---|---|---|---|---|---|---|---|---|---|---|
| yellow cake mix | 56 | 242 | 2.1 | 43.7 | 24.3 | 23.4 | 0.6 | 368 | 76 | 6 | 0.15 | 0.107 | 0 | 0 | 0.11 | 1.0 | 0.06 | 0.20 |
| 2 oz | | 2.5 | 6.5 | 1.0 | 2.7 | 2.5 | 1 | 46 | 174 | 0.84 | 0.040 | 1.7 | 1 | 0.5 | 0.11 | 0.04 | 95.8 | 18144 |
| yellow cake with chocolate icing | 64 | 243 | 14.0 | 35.5 | | | 1.2 | 216 | 24 | 19 | 0.40 | 0.166 | 21 | 0 | 0.08 | 0.8 | 0.11 | 0.18 |
| ⅛ of 18 oz cake | | 2.4 | 11.1 | 3.0 | 6.1 | 1.4 | 35 | 114 | 103 | 1.33 | 0.120 | 2.2 | 70 | | 0.10 | 0.02 | 20.5 | 18140 |
| yellow cake with vanilla icing | 64 | 239 | 14.1 | 37.6 | | | 0.2 | 220 | 40 | 4 | 0.16 | 0.061 | 12 | 0 | 0.06 | 0.3 | 0.10 | 0.22 |
| ⅛ of 18 oz cake | | 2.2 | 9.3 | 1.5 | 3.9 | 3.3 | 35 | 34 | 92 | 0.68 | 0.022 | 3.5 | 40 | | 0.04 | 0.02 | 25.6 | 18141 |

## 7.3 COOKIES

| | WT (g) | KCAL / PRO (g) | H₂O (g) / FAT (g) | CHO (g) / SFA (g) | TSUG (g) / MUFA (g) | ASUG (g) / PUFA (g) | DFIB (g) / CHOL (mg) | Na (mg) / K (mg) | Ca (mg) / P (mg) | Mg (mg) / Fe (mg) | Zn (mg) / Cu (mg) | Mn (mg) / Se (mcg) | A (mcg RAE) / A (IU) | C (mg) / E (mg ATE) | B-1 (mg) / B-2 (mg) | NIA (mg) / B-6 (mg) | B-12 (mcg) / FOL (mcg DFE) | PANT (mg) / REF |
|---|---|---|---|---|---|---|---|---|---|---|---|---|---|---|---|---|---|---|
| Almond Joy cookie, Hershey | 28 | 150 | | 17.0 | 13.0 | | | 55 | 20 | | | | | | | | 0 | |
| 2 cookies | | 1.0 | 9.0 | 4.5 | | | 0 | | 0 | | | | 0 | | | | | HRSH98 |
| animal crackers | 57 | 254 | 2.2 | 42.2 | 7.9 | 7.5 | 0.6 | 224 | 25 | 10 | 0.36 | 0.241 | 0 | 0 | 0.20 | 2.0 | 0.03 | 0.21 |
| 2 oz box (23 pieces) | | 3.9 | 7.9 | 2.0 | 4.4 | 1.1 | 0 | 57 | 65 | 1.57 | 0.089 | 4.0 | 0 | 0.1 | 0.19 | 0.01 | 94.0 | 18150 |
| anisette sponge | 11 | 40 | 2.1 | 6.6 | | | 0.1 | 16 | 5 | 1 | 0.13 | 0.026 | 18 | 0 | 0.03 | 0.2 | 0.08 | 0.12 |
| 1 piece | | 1.2 | 1.0 | 0.4 | 0.5 | 0.2 | 24 | 12 | 19 | 0.39 | 0.010 | | 61 | | 0.05 | 0.01 | 11.6 | 18423 |
| apple 'n raisin cookie, Archway | 26 | 113 | 2.5 | 17.2 | 8.8 | | 0.6 | 137 | 9 | | | | | 0 | 0.07 | 0.4 | | |
| Gourmet - 1 cookie | | 1.3 | 4.3 | 0.9 | 1.7 | 0.6 | 2 | 60 | | 0.65 | | | 3 | | 0.04 | | | 18549 |
| apricot filled cookie, Archway | 25 | 100 | 3.7 | 16.5 | 7.5 | | 0.6 | 80 | 5 | | | | | | 0.07 | 0.6 | | |
| Home Style - 1 cookie | | 1.1 | 3.3 | 1.3 | 1.0 | 0.3 | 2 | 34 | | 0.59 | | | 15 | | 0.04 | | | 18517 |
| arrowroot cookie | 57 | 254 | 2.2 | 42.2 | 7.9 | 7.5 | 0.6 | 224 | 25 | 10 | 0.36 | 0.241 | 0 | 0 | 0.20 | 2.0 | 0.03 | 0.21 |
| 2 oz box (23 pieces) | | 3.9 | 7.9 | 2.0 | 4.4 | 1.1 | 0 | 57 | 65 | 1.57 | 0.089 | 4.0 | 0 | 0.1 | 0.19 | 0.01 | 94.0 | 18150 |
| arrowroot cookie, Nabisco | 7 | 30 | | 5.0 | 2.0 | | 0 | 45 | 0 | | | | | | | | 0 | |
| .25 oz cookie | | 0 | 1.0 | | | | 0 | | 0 | | | | 0 | | | | | NBSC155 |
| arrowroot cookie, wheat-free, Mi-Del - 14 cookies | 29 | 130 | | 22.0 | 8.0 | | 5.0 | 90 | 40 | | | | | 0 | | | | |
| | | 2.0 | 3.0 | 1.0 | | | 10 | | | 1.08 | | | 100 | | | | | MIDE1 |
| Breakfast Treat | 11 | 40 | 2.1 | 6.6 | | | 0.1 | 16 | 5 | 1 | 0.13 | 0.026 | 18 | 0 | 0.03 | 0.2 | 0.08 | 0.12 |
| 1 piece | | 1.2 | 1.0 | 0.4 | 0.5 | 0.2 | 24 | 12 | 19 | 0.39 | 0.010 | | 61 | | 0.05 | 0.01 | 11.6 | 18423 |
| butter cookie | 28 | 131 | 1.3 | 19.3 | 5.7 | 5.4 | 0.2 | 98 | 8 | 3 | 0.11 | 0.048 | 46 | 0 | 0.10 | 0.9 | 0.10 | 0.14 |
| 5 cookies (1 oz) | | 1.7 | 5.3 | 3.1 | 1.5 | 0.3 | 33 | 31 | 29 | 0.62 | 0.056 | 2.4 | 168 | 0.2 | 0.09 | 0.01 | 35.0 | 18155 |
| Cameo sandwich cookie, Nabisco | 28 | 130 | | 21.0 | 10.0 | | 0 | 105 | | | | | | | | | | |
| 1 oz cookie | | 1.0 | 5.0 | 1.0 | | | 0 | | | | | | | | | | | NBSC156 |
| cherry-filled cookie, Archway | 25 | 101 | 3.8 | 16.2 | 7.8 | | 0.5 | 87 | 6 | | | | | 0 | 0.07 | 0.5 | | |
| Home Style - 1 cookie | | 1.2 | 3.5 | 1.4 | 1.1 | 0.3 | 5 | 34 | | 0.57 | | | 13 | | 0.06 | | | 18520 |
| chocolate chip candy blasts cookie, Chips Ahoy - .56 oz cookie | 17 | 90 | | 11.0 | 5.0 | | 0 | 55 | 0 | | | | | | | | 0 | |
| | | 1.0 | 4.5 | 2.0 | | | 0 | | | 0.36 | | | 0 | | | | | NBSC108 |
| chocolate chip cookie, Chips Ahoy | 32 | 160 | | 21.0 | 10.0 | | 1.0 | 105 | | | | | | | | | 0 | |
| 1.1 oz cookie | | 2.0 | 8.0 | 2.5 | | | 0 | | | 0.72 | | | 0 | | | | | NBSC103 |
| chocolate chip cookie, Chips Ahoy | 33 | 160 | | 22.0 | 11.0 | | 1.0 | 110 | 0 | | | | | | | | 0 | |
| 1.2 oz cookie | | 2.0 | 8.0 | 2.5 | | | 0 | | | 0.72 | | | 0 | | | | | NBSC104 |
| chocolate chip cookie, Chips Ahoy | 27 | 120 | | 18.0 | 10.0 | | 1.0 | 80 | | | | | | | | | 0 | |
| Chewy - .95 oz cookie | | 1.0 | 6.0 | 3.0 | | | 0 | | | 0.36 | | | 0 | | | | | NBSC100 |
| chocolate chip cookie, Chips Ahoy | 28 | 130 | | 19.0 | 10.0 | | 1.0 | 100 | 0 | | | | | | | | 0 | |
| Soft Baked - 1 oz cookie | | 1.0 | 5.0 | 3.0 | | | 0 | | | 0.72 | | | 0 | | | | | NBSC101 |
| chocolate chip cookie dough, refrig | 28 | 135 | 2.5 | 17.0 | 10.0 | | 0.6 | 85 | | | | | | | | | | |
| Pillsbury - 1 oz cookie | | 1.0 | 7.0 | 2.0 | 2.5 | 0.5 | 5 | | | 0.72 | | | | | | | | 18630 |
| chocolate chip cookie, from mix, Betty Crocker - 2 cookies | 32 | 170 | | 22.0 | 13.0 | | 1.0 | 140 | | | | | | | 0.06 | 0.4 | | |
| | | 2.0 | 8.0 | 5.0 | | | 25 | 50 | | 0.36 | | | 200 | | 0.03 | | | GENM84 |
| chocolate chip cookie, from refrig | 12 | 59 | 0.4 | 8.2 | | | 0.2 | 28 | 3 | 3 | 0.07 | 0.057 | 2 | 0 | 0.02 | 0.2 | 0.01 | 0.02 |
| dough - 1 cookie | | 0.6 | 2.7 | 0.9 | 1.4 | 0.3 | 3 | 24 | 9 | 0.30 | 0.024 | 0.7 | 7 | | 0.02 | 0 | 8.4 | 18164 |
| chocolate chip cookie, higher fat | 12 | 57 | 0.8 | 7.7 | 4.2 | 4.1 | 0.3 | 36 | 3 | 5 | 0.08 | 0.044 | 0 | 0 | 0.02 | 0.2 | 0 | 0.03 |
| 1 cookie (2¼″ diameter) | | 0.6 | 2.8 | 1.2 | 0.9 | 0.3 | 0 | 18 | 10 | 0.38 | 0.032 | 0.5 | 0 | 0.3 | 0.02 | 0 | 8.3 | 18159 |
| chocolate chip cookie, homemade | 16 | 78 | 0.9 | 9.3 | | | | 55 | 6 | 9 | 0.15 | 0.106 | 22 | 0 | 0.03 | 0.2 | 0.01 | 0.04 |
| w/butter - 1 cookie (2¼″ dia) | | 0.9 | 4.5 | 2.3 | 1.3 | 0.7 | 11 | 35 | 16 | 0.40 | 0.062 | 1.8 | 95 | | 0.03 | 0.01 | 7.5 | 18378 |
| chocolate chip cookie, homemade | 16 | 78 | 0.9 | 9.3 | | | 0.4 | 58 | 6 | 9 | 0.15 | 0.106 | 23 | 0 | 0.03 | 0.2 | 0.01 | 0.04 |
| w/margarine - 1 cookie (2¼″ dia) | | 0.9 | 4.5 | 1.3 | 1.7 | 1.3 | 5 | 36 | 16 | 0.39 | 0.061 | 1.8 | 109 | | 0.03 | 0.01 | 7.5 | 18165 |
| chocolate chip cookie, ice box, | 24 | 119 | 1.2 | 15.6 | 8.2 | | 0.5 | 65 | 3 | | | | | 0 | 0.06 | 0.5 | | |
| Archway Home Style - 1 cookie | | 1.0 | 5.9 | 1.9 | 2.1 | 0.3 | 3 | 30 | | 0.63 | | | 4 | | 0.04 | | | 18522 |
| chocolate chip cookie, lower fat | 10 | 45 | 0.4 | 7.3 | | | 0.4 | 38 | 2 | 3 | 0.07 | 0.045 | 0 | 0 | 0.03 | 0.3 | 0 | 0.03 |
| 1 cookie (2¼″ diameter) | | 0.6 | 1.5 | 0.4 | 0.6 | 0.5 | 0 | 12 | 8 | 0.31 | 0.025 | 0.6 | 0 | | 0.03 | 0.03 | 11.5 | 18158 |
| chocolate chip cookie, mini, Chips | 35 | 170 | | 24.0 | 10.0 | | 1.0 | 115 | 0 | | | | | | | | 0 | |
| Ahoy Go-Pak - 1.2 oz pak | | 2.0 | 8.0 | 2.5 | | | 0 | | | 1.08 | | | 0 | | | | | NBSC110 |

| | WT (g) | KCAL / PRO (g) | H₂0 (g) / FAT (g) | CHO (g) / SFA (g) | TSUG (g) / MUFA (g) | ASUG (g) / PUFA (g) | DFIB (g) / CHOL (mg) | Na (mg) / K (mg) | Ca (mg) / P (mg) | Mg (mg) / Fe (mg) | Zn (mg) / Cu (mg) | Mn (mg) / Se (mcg) | A (mcg RAE) / A (IU) | C (mg) / E (mg ATE) | B-1 (mg) / B-2 (mg) | NIA (mg) / B-6 (mg) | B-12 (mcg) / FOL (mcg DFE) | PANT (mg) / REF |
|---|---|---|---|---|---|---|---|---|---|---|---|---|---|---|---|---|---|---|
| chocolate chip cookie, mini, Chips Ahoy Snak Sak - 1.1 oz Snak Sak | 31 | 150 | | 21.0 | 9.0 | | 1.0 | 100 | 0 | | | | | 0 | | | | |
| | | 2.0 | 8.0 | 2.5 | | | 0 | | | 0.72 | | | 0 | | | | NBSC111 |
| chocolate chip cookie, reduced fat, Chips Ahoy - 1.1 oz cookie | 32 | 140 | | 23.0 | 11.0 | | 1.0 | 150 | 0 | | | | | 0 | | | | |
| | | 2.0 | 5.0 | 2.0 | | | 0 | | | 0.72 | | | 0 | | | | NBSC1 |
| chocolate chip cookie, soft type | 15 | 68 | 1.3 | 9.8 | 5.7 | | 0.4 | 41 | 3 | 5 | 0.09 | 0.063 | 0 | | 0.02 | 0.3 | 0.01 | 0.05 |
| 1 cookie | | 0.7 | 3.1 | 1.5 | 1.1 | 0.4 | | 21 | 11 | 0.45 | 0.037 | 0.4 | 0 | 0.3 | 0.01 | 0 | 9.6 | 18160 |
| chocolate chip cookie, sugar-free, Archway Hm Styl - 1 cookie | 24 | 117 | 1.2 | 15.9 | 0.2 | | 0.3 | 64 | 63 | | | | | 0 | 0.06 | 0.5 | | |
| | | 1.1 | 5.5 | 1.5 | 2.2 | 0.3 | 0 | 18 | | 0.51 | | | 2 | | 0.04 | | | 18565 |
| chocolate chip cookie, whole grain, Chips Ahoy - 1.2 oz cookie | 33 | 150 | | 22.0 | 10.0 | | 2.0 | 110 | 0 | | | | | 0 | | | | |
| | | 2.0 | 8.0 | 2.5 | | | 0 | | | 0.72 | | | 0 | | | | NBSC109 |
| chocolate chip drop cookie, Archway Hm Styl - .9 oz cookie | 25 | 102 | 4.0 | 15.8 | 7.2 | | 0.4 | 98 | 4 | | | | | 0 | 0.06 | 0.5 | | |
| | | 1.0 | 3.8 | 1.3 | 1.4 | 0.2 | 3 | 24 | | 0.55 | | | 3 | | 0.04 | | | 18521 |
| chocolate chunk cookie, Chips Ahoy - .56 oz cookie | 17 | 80 | | 11.0 | 6.0 | | 1.0 | 55 | 0 | | | | | 0 | | | | |
| | | 1.0 | 4.5 | 1.5 | | | 0 | | | 0.36 | | | 0 | | | | NBSC107 |
| chocolate cookie, mini, 100-cal pk, Barbara's Bakery - 1 pkg | 25 | 100 | | 18.0 | 8.0 | | | 150 | 0 | | | | | 0 | | | | |
| | | 1.0 | 2.0 | 1.0 | | | 5 | | | 0.72 | | | 0 | | | | BARB19 |
| chocolate devil's food cookie, fat-free, Archway Hm Styl - 1 cookie | 20 | 68 | 2.6 | 15.9 | 8.2 | | 0.6 | 79 | 2 | | | | | 0 | 0.06 | 0.4 | | |
| | | 1.0 | 0.2 | 0.1 | 0.1 | 0.1 | 0 | 54 | | 0.53 | | | 0 | | 0.04 | | | 18553 |
| chocolate devil's food cookie, fat-free, Snackwell's - 1 cookie | 16 | 49 | 2.8 | 11.9 | 6.9 | | 0.3 | 28 | 5 | 4 | 0.07 | | 0 | | 0.01 | 0.2 | 0.01 | 0.01 |
| | | 0.8 | 0.2 | 0.1 | 0 | 0 | 0 | 18 | 11 | 0.44 | 0.027 | 0.3 | 0 | | 0.03 | 0 | | 18651 |
| chocolate sandwich cookie with crème filling - 1 cookie | 17 | 82 | 0.3 | 11.2 | 10.8 | 10.6 | 0.9 | 55 | 6 | 7 | 0.10 | 0.063 | 0 | 0 | 0.02 | 0.2 | 0.01 | 0.03 |
| | | 0.6 | 4.5 | 1.3 | 2.5 | 0.5 | 0 | 41 | 15 | 0.53 | 0.054 | 0.5 | 1 | 0 | 0.03 | 0.01 | 4.4 | 18167 |
| chocolate sandwich cookie w/crème fill, choc-covered - 1 cookie | 10 | 47 | 0.2 | 7.1 | 4.1 | 3.5 | 0.3 | 50 | 2 | 5 | 0.09 | 0.068 | 0 | 0 | 0.01 | 0.2 | 0 | 0.03 |
| | | 0.6 | 2.0 | 0.6 | 0.9 | 0.4 | 0 | 22 | 10 | 0.87 | 0.036 | 0.4 | 0 | 0.3 | 0.01 | 0 | 11.1 | 18166 |
| chocolate sandwich cookie with extra crème filling - 1 cookie | 13 | 65 | 0.2 | 8.9 | 6.0 | 5.6 | 0.4 | 46 | 2 | 5 | 0.10 | 0.065 | 0 | 0 | 0.01 | 0.3 | 0 | 0.02 |
| | | 0.6 | 3.2 | 0.7 | 2.1 | 0.3 | 0 | 18 | 9 | 1.01 | 0.044 | 1.1 | 0 | 0.2 | 0.02 | 0 | 9.4 | 18168 |
| chocolate wafer | 28 | 121 | 1.3 | 20.3 | 8.3 | 7.8 | 1.0 | 162 | 9 | 15 | 0.31 | 0.195 | 1 | 0 | 0.06 | 0.8 | 0.03 | 0.11 |
| 5 wafers (1 oz) | | 1.8 | 4.0 | 1.2 | 1.4 | 1.2 | 1 | 59 | 37 | 1.12 | 0.130 | 1.6 | 3 | 0.2 | 0.07 | 0.01 | 26.9 | 18157 |
| crème sandwich cookie, Snack Well's - .92 oz | 26 | 110 | | 20.0 | 10.0 | | 0 | 130 | 0 | | | | | 0 | | | | |
| | | 1.0 | 3.0 | 0.5 | | | 0 | | | 0.36 | | | 0 | | | | NBSC159 |
| devil's food cookie, fat-free, Snack Well's - .56 oz | 16 | 50 | | 12.0 | 7.0 | | 0 | 30 | 0 | | | | | 0 | | | | |
| | | 1.0 | 0 | 0 | | | 0 | | | 0.36 | | | 0 | | | | NBSC160 |
| double chocolate chunk cookie, from mix, Bty Crckr - 2 cookies | 30 | 140 | | 21.0 | 13.0 | | 0.5 | 120 | | | | | | | 0.03 | 0.4 | | |
| | | 2.0 | 6.0 | 2.0 | | | 10 | 70 | | 0.72 | | | | | 0.03 | | | GENM89 |
| Double Dutch Girl Scout Cookie | 24 | 110 | | 16.0 | 8.0 | | | 85 | 40 | | | | | 1 | | | | |
| 2 cookies | | 0 | 6.0 | 1.5 | | | 0 | | | | | | 0 | | | | GIRL1 |
| Dutch cocoa cookie, Archway Home Style - 1 cookie | 24 | 103 | 2.2 | 16.7 | 8.5 | | 0.6 | 92 | 3 | | | | | 0.06 | 0.5 | | | |
| | | 1.1 | 3.6 | 0.9 | 1.4 | 0.3 | 2 | 57 | | 0.81 | | | 3 | | 0.04 | | | 18528 |
| fig bar | 31 | 108 | 5.1 | 22.0 | 14.4 | 9.2 | 1.4 | 108 | 20 | 8 | 0.12 | 0.106 | 3 | 0 | 0.05 | 0.6 | 0.03 | 0.11 |
| 2 square bars | | 1.1 | 2.3 | 0.3 | 0.9 | 0.9 | 0 | 64 | 19 | 0.90 | 0.046 | 1.0 | 10 | 0.2 | 0.07 | 0.02 | 16.4 | 18170 |
| fig bar, apple cinnamon, Barbara's Bakery - 1 bar | 19 | 60 | | 14.0 | 9.0 | | 1.0 | 25 | 0 | | | | | 1 | | | | |
| | | 1.0 | 0 | 0 | | | 0 | | | 0.36 | | | 0 | | | | BARB22 |
| fig bar, Barbara's Bakery | 19 | 60 | | 14.0 | 8.0 | | | 20 | 0 | | | | | 5 | | | | |
| 1 bar | | 0 | 0.5 | 0 | | | 0 | | | 1.44 | | | 0 | | | | BARB23 |
| fig bar, blueberry, Barbara's Bakery - 1 bar | 19 | 70 | | 15.0 | 9.0 | | | 20 | 0 | | | | | 1 | | | | |
| | | 0 | 0.5 | 0 | | | 0 | | | 0.36 | | | 0 | | | | BARB24 |
| fig bar, raspberry, Barbara's Bakery - 1 bar | 19 | 60 | | 14.0 | 9.0 | | 1.0 | 25 | 0 | | | | | 1 | | | | |
| | | 0 | 0 | 0 | | | 0 | | | 0.36 | | | 0 | | | | BARB25 |
| fig bar, Safeway Select | 35 | 120 | | 23.0 | 11.0 | | 2.0 | 110 | 20 | | | | | | | 0.4 | | |
| 2 bars | | 1.0 | 3.0 | 1.0 | | | 0 | | | 0.72 | | | 0 | | 0.07 | | 8.0 | SAFE45 |
| fig bar, wheat-free, Barbara's Bakery - 1 bar | 19 | 60 | | 13.0 | 8.0 | | 1.0 | 25 | 0 | | | | | 5 | | | | |
| | | 0 | 0 | 0 | | | 0 | | | 0.36 | | | 0 | | | | BARB26 |
| fig bar, whole wheat, Barbara's Bakery - 1 bar | 19 | 60 | | 13.0 | 8.0 | | 1.0 | 25 | 0 | | | | | 5 | | | | |
| | | 1.0 | 0 | 0 | | | 0 | | | 0.72 | | | 0 | | | | BARB27 |
| Fig Newton, fat-free, Nabisco | 29 | 90 | | 22.0 | 12.0 | | 1.0 | 125 | 40 | | | | | 0 | | | | |
| 2 square bars (1 oz) | | 1.0 | 0 | 0 | | | 0 | | | 0.72 | | | 0 | | | | NBSC115 |
| Fig Newton Mini, whole grain, Nabisco - 1.34 oz | 38 | 130 | | 26.0 | 14.0 | | 2.0 | 140 | 150 | | | | | 0 | | | | |
| | | 2.0 | 3.0 | 0.5 | | | | | | 2.70 | | | 750 | | | | NBSC119 |
| Fig Newton, Nabisco | 31 | 110 | | 22.0 | 13.0 | | 1.0 | 120 | 20 | | | | | 0 | | | | |
| 2 bars | | 1.0 | 2.2 | 0 | | | 0 | | | 0.72 | | | 0 | | | | NBSC21 |
| Fig Newton, whole grain, Nabisco | 31 | 110 | | 22.0 | 13.0 | | 2.0 | 115 | 20 | | | | | 0 | | | | |
| 2 square bars (1.1 oz) | | 1.0 | 2.0 | 0.5 | | | 0 | | | 0.36 | | | 0 | | | | NBSC116 |

| Food | WT (g) | KCAL / PRO (g) | H₂O (g) / FAT (g) | CHO (g) / SFA (g) | TSUG (g) / MUFA (g) | ASUG (g) / PUFA (g) | DFIB (g) / CHOL (mg) | Na (mg) / K (mg) | Ca (mg) / P (mg) | Mg (mg) / Fe (mg) | Zn (mg) / Cu (mg) | Mn (mg) / Se (mcg) | A (mcg RAE) / A (IU) | C (mg) / E (mg ATE) | B-1 (mg) / B-2 (mg) | NIA (mg) / B-6 (mg) | B-12 (mcg) / FOL (mcg DFE) | PANT (mg) / REF |
|---|---|---|---|---|---|---|---|---|---|---|---|---|---|---|---|---|---|---|
| **fortune cookie** | 8 | 30 | 0.6 | 6.7 | 3.6 | 3.6 | 0.1 | 22 | 1 | 1 | 0.01 | 0.015 | 0 | 0 | 0.01 | 0.1 | 0 | 0.02 |
| *1 cookie* | | 0.3 | 0.2 | 0.1 | 0.1 | 0 | 0 | 3 | 3 | 0.12 | 0.005 | 0.2 | 0 | 0 | 0.01 | 0 | 8.4 | 18171 |
| **frosty lemon cookie**, Archway | 26 | 112 | 3.1 | 16.8 | 8.7 | | 0.2 | 95 | 11 | | | | | 0 | 0.06 | 0.5 | | |
| Home Style - *1 cookie* | | 1.1 | 4.4 | 1.5 | 1.5 | 0.2 | 0 | 24 | | 0.42 | | | 0 | | 0.05 | | | 18529 |
| **fruit and honey bar**, Archway | 26 | 106 | 3.1 | 18.0 | 9.8 | | 0.5 | 107 | 6 | | | | | 0 | 0.07 | 0.6 | | |
| Home Style - *1 cookie* | | 1.2 | 3.3 | 0.7 | 1.3 | 0.2 | 4 | 49 | | 0.57 | | | 3 | | 0.05 | | | 18531 |
| **fudge cookie**, cake type | 21 | 73 | 2.5 | 16.4 | | | 0.6 | 40 | 7 | 7 | 0.12 | 0.068 | 0 | 0 | 0.05 | 0.3 | 0.02 | 0.05 |
| *1 cookie* | | 1.0 | 0.8 | 0.2 | 0.4 | 0.1 | 0 | 29 | 17 | 0.52 | 0.061 | 0.8 | 0 | | 0.04 | 0.01 | 14.1 | 18156 |
| **ginger cookie**, mini, 100-cal pak, | 25 | 100 | | 19.0 | 9.0 | | | 150 | 0 | | | | | 0 | | | | |
| Barbara's Bakery - *1 pkg* | | 1.0 | 2.0 | 1.0 | | | 5 | | | 0.72 | | | 0 | | | | | BARB32 |
| **gingersnap** | 7 | 29 | 0.4 | 5.4 | 1.4 | 1.3 | 0.2 | 46 | 5 | 3 | 0.04 | 0.109 | 0 | 0 | 0.01 | 0.2 | 0 | 0.03 |
| *1 small cookie* | | 0.4 | 0.7 | 0.2 | 0.4 | 0.1 | 0 | 24 | 6 | 0.45 | 0.021 | 0.4 | 0 | 0.1 | 0.02 | 0.01 | 10.2 | 18172 |
| **gingersnap**, Nabisco | 28 | 120 | | 23.0 | 11.0 | | 0 | 190 | 20 | | | | | 0 | | | | |
| *1 oz* | | 1.0 | 2.5 | 0 | | | 0 | | | 1.08 | | | 0 | | | | | NBSC144 |
| **gingersnap**, reduced fat, Archway | 32 | 136 | 1.7 | 24.4 | 11.6 | | 0.4 | 130 | 20 | | | | | | 0.10 | 0.9 | | |
| Home Style - *5 cookies* | | 1.5 | 3.6 | 0.8 | 1.1 | 0.5 | 0 | 99 | | 4.02 | | | 1 | | 0.07 | | | 18562 |
| **graham cracker** | 14 | 59 | 0.6 | 10.8 | 4.4 | 4.3 | 0.4 | 85 | 3 | 4 | 0.11 | 0.113 | 0 | 0 | 0.03 | 0.6 | 0 | 0.08 |
| *2 crackers (2½" sq)* | | 1.0 | 1.4 | 0.2 | 0.6 | 0.5 | 0 | 19 | 15 | 0.52 | 0.028 | 1.4 | 0 | 0 | 0.04 | 0.01 | 9.2 | 18173 |
| **graham cracker**, choc, Honey Maid, | 31 | 130 | | 24.0 | 9.0 | | 1.0 | 190 | 150 | | | | | 0 | | | | |
| Nabisco - *8 small sections* | | 2.0 | 3.0 | 0.5 | | | 0 | | | 1.44 | | | 0 | | | | | NBSC152 |
| **graham cracker**, chocolate-covered | 14 | 68 | 0.4 | 9.3 | 5.8 | 5.7 | 0.4 | 41 | 8 | 8 | 0.14 | 0.102 | 1 | 0 | 0.02 | 0.3 | 0 | 0.03 |
| *2½" square* | | 0.8 | 3.2 | 1.9 | 1.1 | 0.1 | 0 | 29 | 19 | 0.50 | 0.060 | 2.0 | 2 | 0 | 0.03 | 0.01 | 3.8 | 18174 |
| **graham cracker**, chocolate-covered, | 27 | 126 | 0.8 | 19.4 | 7.2 | | | 96 | | | | | | | | | | |
| Keebler - *3 squares* | | 1.9 | 4.5 | 0.8 | | | | | | | | | | | | | | 18608 |
| **graham cracker**, cinn, Honey Maid, | 31 | 130 | | 25.0 | 11.0 | | 1.0 | 150 | 150 | | | | | 0 | | | | |
| Nabisco - *8 small sections (1.1 oz)* | | 2.0 | 2.5 | 0 | | | 0 | | | 1.08 | | | 0 | | | | | NBSC153 |
| **graham cracker**, cinn, lowfat, Honey | 31 | 120 | | 26.0 | 12.0 | | 1.0 | 170 | 150 | | | | | 0 | | | | |
| Maid, Nabisco - *8 small sections* | | 2.0 | 1.5 | 0 | | | 0 | | | 1.08 | | | 0 | | | | | NBSC151 |
| **graham cracker**, Honey Maid, | 31 | 130 | | 25.0 | 8.0 | | 0 | 190 | 150 | | | | | 0 | | | | |
| Nabisco - *8 small sections* | | 2.0 | 3.0 | 0.5 | | | 0 | | | 1.08 | | | 0 | | | | | NBSC149 |
| **graham cracker**, Nabisco | 31 | 159 | 1.0 | 19.6 | 10.0 | | 0.3 | 69 | 13 | 2 | 0.09 | | | | 0.05 | 0.8 | 0.03 | |
| *8 small sections* | | 1.1 | 8.4 | 1.6 | 5.8 | 0.4 | 3 | 21 | 26 | 0.55 | 0.016 | | 3 | | 0.06 | 0.01 | | 18618 |
| **graham cracker stick**, choc, Honey | 31 | 130 | | 25.0 | 10.0 | | 1.0 | 170 | 20 | | | | | 0 | | | | |
| Maid, Nabisco - *1.1 oz* | | 2.0 | 3.0 | 1.0 | | | 0 | | | 1.44 | | | 0 | | | | | NBSC150 |
| **graham cracker stick**, cinn, Honey | 31 | 130 | | 25.0 | 9.0 | | 1.0 | 170 | 20 | | | | | 0 | | | | |
| Maid, Nabisco - *1.1 oz* | | 2.0 | 3.0 | 0.5 | | | 0 | | | 1.08 | | | 0 | | | | | NBSC146 |
| **graham cracker stick**, Honey Maid, | 31 | 130 | | 25.0 | 9.0 | | 1.0 | 180 | 0 | | | | | 0 | | | | |
| Nabisco - *1.1 oz* | | 2.0 | 3.0 | 0.5 | | | 0 | | | 1.08 | | | 0 | | | | | NBSC145 |
| **graham cracker stick**, lowfat, Honey | 31 | 120 | | 25.0 | 8.0 | | 1.0 | 190 | 150 | | | | | 0 | | | | |
| Maid, Nabisco - *1.1 oz* | | 2.0 | 2.0 | 0 | | | 0 | | | 1.08 | | | 0 | | | | | NBSC147 |
| **hermit**, Archway Home Style | 25 | 98 | 3.0 | 17.6 | 8.6 | | 0.4 | 164 | 14 | | | | | 0 | 0.08 | 0.6 | | |
| *1 cookie* | | 1.3 | 2.4 | 0.6 | 1.0 | 0.2 | 2 | 43 | | 0.70 | | | 4 | | 0.06 | | | 18525 |
| **holiday shape cookie**, from refrig | 26 | 120 | | 15.0 | 8.0 | | 0 | 85 | 0 | | | | | 0 | | | | |
| dough, Pillsbury - *.9 oz cookie* | | 1.0 | 6.0 | 1.5 | | | 2 | | | 0.36 | | | 0 | | | | | GENM94 |
| **ice cream cone**, cake/wafer | 4 | 17 | 0.2 | 3.2 | 0.2 | 0.2 | 0.1 | 6 | 1 | 1 | 0.03 | 0.023 | 0 | 0 | 0.01 | 0.2 | 0 | 0.02 |
| *(cone only) - 1 cone* | | 0.3 | 0.3 | 0 | 0.1 | 0.1 | 0 | 4 | 4 | 0.14 | 0.008 | 0.2 | 0 | 0 | 0.01 | 0 | 11.6 | 18271 |
| **ice cream cone**, sugar, rolled | 10 | 40 | 0.3 | 8.4 | 2.6 | 2.5 | 0.2 | 32 | 4 | 3 | 0.08 | 0.073 | 0 | 0 | 0.05 | 0.5 | 0 | 0.04 |
| *(cone only) - 1 cone* | | 0.8 | 0.4 | 0.1 | 0.1 | 0 | 0 | 14 | 10 | 0.44 | 0.027 | 0.5 | 0 | 0 | 0.04 | 0.01 | 23.6 | 18272 |
| **ice cream cone**, waffle (cone only) | 4 | 17 | 0.2 | 3.2 | 0.2 | 0.2 | 0.1 | 6 | 1 | 1 | 0.03 | 0.023 | 0 | 0 | 0.01 | 0.2 | 0 | 0.02 |
| *1 cone* | | 0.3 | 0.3 | 0 | 0.1 | 0.1 | 0 | 4 | 4 | 0.14 | 0.008 | 0.2 | 0 | 0 | 0.01 | 0 | 11.6 | 18271 |
| **ladyfinger** | 11 | 40 | 2.1 | 6.6 | | | 0.1 | 16 | 5 | 1 | 0.13 | 0.026 | 18 | 0 | 0.03 | 0.2 | 0.08 | 0.12 |
| *1 ladyfinger* | | 1.2 | 1.0 | 0.4 | 0.5 | 0.2 | 24 | 12 | 19 | 0.39 | 0.010 | | 61 | | 0.05 | 0.01 | 11.6 | 18423 |
| **ladyfinger** with lemon juice and | 11 | 40 | 2.1 | 6.6 | 2.8 | 2.7 | 0.1 | 16 | 5 | 1 | 0.13 | 0.026 | 0 | 0 | 0.03 | 0.2 | 0.08 | 0.12 |
| rind - *1 ladyfinger* | | 1.2 | 1.0 | 0.4 | 0.5 | 0.2 | 24 | 12 | 19 | 0.39 | 0.010 | 2.3 | 6 | 0.1 | 0.05 | 0.01 | 8.4 | 18175 |
| **lemon crème sandwich cookie**, | 32 | 130 | | 23.0 | 0 | | 2.0 | 135 | 0 | | | | | 0 | | | | |
| sgr-free, SnackWell's - *1.1 oz* | | 1.0 | 6.0 | 2.0 | | | 0 | | | 0.72 | | | 0 | | | | | NBSC158 |
| **macadamia nut chocolate chip** | 28 | 140 | | 16.0 | 6.0 | | 1.0 | 85 | | | | | | | | | | |
| **cookie**, Mauna Loa - *4 cookies* | | 1.0 | 8.0 | 1.5 | | | 0 | | | | | | | | | | | MAUN12 |
| **macadamia nut Hawaiian crunch** | 28 | 140 | | 16.0 | 5.0 | | 1.0 | 105 | | | | | | | | | | |
| **cookie**, Mauna Loa - *4 cookies* | | 1.0 | 8.0 | 1.0 | | | 5 | | | | | | | | | | | MAUN13 |

| | WT (g) | KCAL / PRO (g) | H2O (g) / FAT (g) | CHO (g) / SFA (g) | TSUG (g) / MUFA (g) | ASUG (g) / PUFA (g) | DFIB (g) / CHOL (mg) | Na (mg) / K (mg) | Ca (mg) / P (mg) | Mg (mg) / Fe (mg) | Zn (mg) / Cu (mg) | Mn (mg) / Se (mcg) | A (mcg RAE) / A (IU) | C (mg) / E (mg ATE) | B-1 (mg) / B-2 (mg) | NIA (mg) / B-6 (mg) | B-12 (mcg) / FOL (mcg DFE) | PANT (mg) / REF |
|---|---|---|---|---|---|---|---|---|---|---|---|---|---|---|---|---|---|---|
| macaroon, Archway Home Style | 22 | 101 | 2.5 | 13.5 | 9.9 | | 1.1 | 53 | 1 | | | | | 0 | 0 | 0 | | |
| 1 cookie | | 0.7 | 5.0 | 4.4 | 0.4 | 0.2 | 0 | 27 | | 0.18 | | | 0 | | 0.01 | | | 18524 |
| macaroon, homemade | 24 | 97 | 2.5 | 17.3 | 17.0 | 16.2 | 0.4 | 59 | 2 | 5 | 0.17 | 0.227 | 0 | 0 | 0 | 0 | 0.01 | 0.06 |
| 1 cookie (2″ diameter) | | 0.9 | 3.0 | 2.7 | 0.1 | 0 | 0 | 37 | 10 | 0.18 | 0.034 | 2.5 | 0 | 0 | 0.03 | 0.02 | 1.0 | 18169 |
| Mallomar, Nabisco | 27 | 120 | | 18.0 | 2.0 | | 1.0 | 40 | 0 | | | | 0 | | | | | |
| .95 oz cookie | | 1.0 | 5.0 | 3.0 | | | 0 | | | 0.72 | | | 0 | | | | | NBSC113 |
| marshmallow pie | 13 | 55 | 1.3 | 8.8 | 5.8 | 5.1 | 0.3 | 22 | 6 | 5 | 0.08 | 0.037 | | 0 | 0.01 | 0.1 | 0.02 | 0.06 |
| 1 small cookie (1¾″ × ¾″) | | 0.5 | 2.2 | 0.6 | 1.2 | 0.3 | 0 | 24 | 13 | 0.33 | 0.034 | 0.6 | 1 | 0 | 0.03 | 0.01 | 4.9 | 18176 |
| molasses cookie | 20 | 86 | 1.2 | 14.8 | 3.5 | 3.5 | 0.2 | 92 | 15 | 10 | 0.09 | 0.251 | | 0 | 0.07 | 0.6 | 0 | 0.08 |
| 1 cookie | | 1.1 | 2.6 | 0.6 | 1.4 | 0.3 | 0 | 69 | 19 | 1.29 | 0.075 | 1.1 | 0 | 0 | 0.05 | 0.02 | 29.2 | 18177 |
| molasses cookie, Archway | 27 | 100 | | 18.0 | 10.0 | | 0 | 140 | 0 | | | | 0 | | | | | |
| 1 oz cookie | | 1.0 | 3.0 | 0.5 | | | 10 | | | 1.08 | | | 0 | | | | | ARCH1 |
| molasses cookie, Archway Home Style - 1 cookie | 26 | 105 | 3.0 | 18.0 | 9.5 | | 0.3 | 150 | 8 | | | | 0 | 0 | 0.08 | 0.7 | | |
| | | 1.1 | 3.1 | 0.7 | 1.3 | 0.3 | 6 | 30 | | 1.22 | | | 4 | | 0.06 | | | 18535 |
| molasses cookie, dark, Archway Home Style - 1 cookie | 28 | 114 | 2.8 | 19.4 | 9.8 | | 0.3 | 155 | 12 | | | | 0 | 0 | 0.09 | 0.8 | | |
| | | 1.2 | 3.5 | 0.8 | 1.4 | 0.3 | 0 | 97 | | 1.27 | | | 2 | | 0.06 | | | 18526 |
| molasses cookie, iced, Archway Home Style - 1 cookie | 28 | 118 | 2.9 | 19.4 | 10.8 | | 0.3 | 148 | 7 | | | | | | 0.07 | 0.7 | | |
| | | 1.0 | 4.0 | 1.2 | 1.3 | 0.7 | 3 | 35 | | 1.15 | | | 3 | | 0.05 | | | 18532 |
| molasses cookie, Little Debbie | 20 | 86 | 1.2 | 14.8 | 3.5 | 3.5 | 0.2 | 92 | 15 | 10 | 0.09 | 0.251 | 0 | 0 | 0.07 | 0.6 | 0 | 0.08 |
| 1 cookie | | 1.1 | 2.6 | 0.6 | 1.4 | 0.3 | 0 | 69 | 19 | 1.29 | 0.075 | 1.1 | 0 | 0 | 0.05 | 0.02 | 29.2 | 18177 |
| molasses cookie, old fashioned, Archway Hm Styl - 1 cookie | 26 | 106 | 2.7 | 18.3 | 9.4 | | 0.3 | 146 | 8 | | | | 0 | 0 | 0.08 | 0.7 | | |
| | | 1.1 | 3.1 | 0.7 | 1.2 | 0.3 | 6 | | | 1.30 | | | 3 | | 0.06 | | | 18539 |
| Nilla Wafer, mini, Nabisco | 30 | 140 | | 21.0 | 11.0 | | 0 | 115 | 20 | | | | | | | | | |
| 1.1 oz | | 1.0 | 6.0 | 1.5 | | | 5 | | | 0.72 | | | | | | | | NBSC123 |
| Nilla Wafer, Nabisco | 30 | 140 | | 21.0 | 11.0 | | 0 | 115 | 20 | | | | 0 | | | | | |
| 1.1 oz | | 1.0 | 6.0 | 1.5 | | | 5 | | | 0.72 | | | 0 | | | | | NBSC121 |
| Nilla Wafer, reduced fat, Nabisco | 29 | 120 | | 24.0 | 12.0 | | 0 | 110 | 0 | | | | 0 | | | | | |
| 1 oz | | 1.0 | 2.0 | 0 | | | 0 | | | 0.72 | | | 0 | | | | | NBSC122 |
| Nutter Butter Sandwich Cookie Bite, choc-cvrd, Nabisco - 1.3 oz | 36 | 180 | | 24.0 | 15.0 | | 1.0 | 85 | 20 | | | | 0 | | | | | |
| | | 2.0 | 9.0 | 4.5 | | | 0 | | | 0.72 | | | 0 | | | | | NBSC124 |
| Nutter Butter Sandwich Cookie Bite, Nabisco - 1.2 oz | 35 | 170 | | 24.0 | 10.0 | | 1.0 | 135 | 0 | | | | 0 | | | | | |
| | | 3.0 | 7.0 | 1.5 | | | 0 | | | 0.72 | | | 0 | | | | | NBSC127 |
| Nutter Butter Sand Cookie, choc-cvrd, Nabisco - .63 oz cookie | 18 | 90 | | 12.0 | 7.0 | | 0 | 45 | 0 | | | | 0 | | | | | |
| | | 1.0 | 4.5 | 2.0 | | | 0 | | | 0.36 | | | 0 | | | | | NBSC126 |
| Nutter Butter Sandwich Cookie, Nabisco - 1 oz cookie | 28 | 130 | | 19.0 | 8.0 | | 1.0 | 110 | 20 | | | | 0 | | | | | |
| | | 2.0 | 6.0 | 1.0 | | | 0 | | | 0.72 | | | 0 | | | | | NBSC125 |
| Nutty Bar, Little Debbie | 57 | 312 | 1.7 | 31.5 | 19.4 | | | 127 | | | | | | 1 | | | | |
| 1 bar | | 4.6 | 18.7 | 3.6 | | | | | | | | | | | | | | 18612 |
| oatmeal choc chip cookie, from mix, Bty Crckr - 2 cookies | 35 | 160 | | 22.0 | 12.0 | | 1.0 | 120 | | | | | | | 0.03 | 0.4 | | |
| | | 2.0 | 8.0 | 4.5 | | | 25 | 55 | | 0.36 | | | 200 | | 0.03 | | | GENM96 |
| oatmeal choc chip cookie, from refrig dough, Pillsbury - 1 oz cookie | 29 | 130 | | 17.0 | 10.0 | | 1.0 | 100 | 0 | | | | 0 | | | | | |
| | | 1.0 | 6.0 | 2.0 | | | 5 | | | 0.36 | | | 0 | | | | | GENM97 |
| oatmeal cookie | 18 | 81 | | 12.4 | 4.4 | 3.4 | 0.5 | 69 | 7 | 6 | 0.14 | 0.151 | 1 | 0 | 0.05 | 0.4 | 0 | 0.07 |
| 1 cookie | | 1.1 | 3.3 | 1.8 | 0.5 | | | 26 | 25 | 0.46 | 0.024 | 1.8 | 3 | 0 | 0.04 | 0.01 | 17.1 | 18178 |
| oatmeal cookie, apl filled, Archway Home Style - 1 cookie | 25 | 98 | 3.7 | 16.8 | 8.1 | | 0.4 | 83 | 8 | | | | | | 0.07 | 0.5 | | |
| | | 1.1 | 2.9 | 0.7 | 1.2 | 0.3 | 2 | 45 | | 0.60 | | | 2 | | 0.04 | | | 18516 |
| oatmeal cookie, Archway Home Style 1 cookie | 25 | 105 | 2.6 | 17.0 | 8.6 | | 0.7 | 98 | 9 | | | | 0 | | 0.08 | 0.5 | | |
| | | 1.4 | 3.5 | 0.8 | 1.4 | 0.3 | 2 | 55 | | 0.61 | | | 4 | | 0.04 | | | 18537 |
| oatmeal cookie, date-filled, Archway Hm Styl - 1 cookie | 25 | 100 | 3.4 | 17.0 | 8.6 | | 0.5 | 83 | 7 | | | | | | 0.07 | 0.5 | | |
| | | 1.2 | 3.0 | 0.7 | 1.2 | 0.3 | 2 | 40 | | 0.56 | | | 3 | | 0.04 | | | 18527 |
| oatmeal cookie, fat-free | 28 | 91 | 3.5 | 22.0 | 11.7 | 7.5 | 2.0 | 83 | 11 | 10 | 0.18 | 0.222 | 0 | 0 | 0.04 | 0.3 | 0 | 0.10 |
| 2 cookies (1 oz) | | 1.7 | 0.4 | 0.1 | 0.1 | 0.2 | 0 | 59 | 29 | 0.61 | 0.060 | 2.2 | 0 | 0 | 0.07 | 0.02 | 19.9 | 18456 |
| oatmeal cookie, from mix, Betty Crocker - 2 cookies | 32 | 150 | | 22.0 | 11.0 | | 1.0 | 140 | | | | | | | 0.06 | 0.4 | | |
| | | 2.0 | 6.0 | 3.5 | | | 25 | 40 | | 0.72 | | | 200 | | 0.03 | | | GENM98 |
| oatmeal cookie, from refrigerated dough - 1 cookie | 12 | 57 | 0.7 | 7.9 | | | 0.3 | 39 | 4 | 4 | 0.09 | 0.114 | 0 | 0 | 0.02 | 0.2 | 0 | 0.03 |
| | | 0.7 | 2.5 | 0.6 | 1.4 | 0.4 | 3 | 20 | 14 | 0.29 | 0.015 | 1.2 | 8 | 0 | 0.02 | 0.01 | 4.9 | 18183 |
| oatmeal cookie, homemade | 15 | 67 | 0.9 | 10.0 | | | | 90 | 16 | 6 | 0.14 | 0.159 | 24 | 0 | 0.04 | 0.2 | 0.01 | 0.05 |
| 1 cookie (2⅝″ diameter) | | 1.0 | 2.7 | 0.5 | 1.2 | 0.8 | 5 | 27 | 25 | 0.40 | 0.025 | 2.6 | 114 | 0 | 0.03 | 0.01 | 7.2 | 18377 |
| oatmeal cookie, iced, Archway Home Style - 1 cookie | 28 | 122 | 2.8 | 18.7 | 10.4 | | 0.6 | 106 | 9 | | | | 0 | | 0.08 | 0.5 | | |
| | | 1.4 | 4.6 | 1.3 | 1.6 | 0.8 | 2 | 52 | | 0.61 | | | 4 | | 0.04 | | | 18533 |
| oatmeal cookie, mini, 100-cal pks, Barbara's Bakery - 1 package | 25 | 100 | | 19.0 | 9.0 | | | 140 | 0 | | | | 0 | | | | | |
| | | 1.0 | 2.0 | 1.0 | | | 5 | | | 0.72 | | | 0 | | | | | BARB42 |

| | WT (g) | | Macronutrients | | | | | Minerals | | | | | Vitamins | | | | |
|---|---|---|---|---|---|---|---|---|---|---|---|---|---|---|---|---|---|
| | | KCAL | H₂0 (g) | CHO (g) | TSUG (g) | ASUG (g) | DFIB (g) | Na (mg) | Ca (mg) | Mg (mg) | Zn (mg) | Mn (mg) | A (mcg RAE) | C (mg) | B-1 (mg) | NIA (mg) | B-12 (mcg) | PANT (mg) |
| | | PRO (g) | FAT (g) | SFA (g) | MUFA (g) | PUFA (g) | CHOL (mg) | K (mg) | P (mg) | Fe (mg) | Cu (mg) | Se (mcg) | A (IU) | E (mg ATE) | B-2 (mg) | B-6 (mg) | FOL (mcg DFE) | REF |
| **oatmeal cookie**, Ruth's, Archway | 26 | 111 | 2.6 | 17.2 | 8.9 | | 0.7 | 114 | 8 | | | | | 0 | 0.07 | 0.4 | | |
| Home Style - *1 cookie* | | 1.5 | 4.1 | 0.9 | 1.5 | 0.6 | 4 | 48 | | 0.72 | | | 9 | | 0.04 | | | 18545 |
| **oatmeal cookie**, soft type | 15 | 61 | 1.6 | 9.9 | | | 0.4 | 52 | 14 | 4 | 0.07 | 0.063 | 1 | 0 | 0.03 | 0.3 | 0 | 0.07 |
| *1 cookie* | | 0.9 | 2.2 | 0.5 | 1.2 | 0.3 | 1 | 20 | 31 | 0.42 | 0.082 | 1.6 | 5 | | 0.03 | 0.01 | 7.8 | 18179 |
| **oatmeal cookie**, sgr-free, | 24 | 106 | 1.2 | 16.1 | 0.3 | | 0.5 | 74 | 5 | | | | | 0 | 0.06 | 0.4 | | |
| Archway Hm Styl - *1 cookie* | | 1.3 | 5.0 | 1.2 | 1.9 | 0.3 | 0 | 21 | | 0.47 | | | 0 | | 0.04 | | | 18513 |
| **oatmeal pecan cookie**, Archway | 28 | 132 | 2.6 | 16.9 | 7.8 | | 0.9 | 97 | 7 | | | | | | 0.08 | 0.5 | | |
| Gourmet - *1 cookie* | | 1.5 | 6.5 | 2.1 | 2.4 | 0.6 | 2 | 41 | | 0.60 | | | 3 | | 0.04 | | | 18560 |
| **oatmeal raisin cookie**, Archway | 26 | 106 | 3.0 | 18.0 | 10.3 | | 0.7 | 88 | 10 | | | | | 0 | 0.07 | 0.4 | | |
| Home Style - *1 cookie* | | 1.3 | 3.1 | 0.7 | 1.3 | 0.3 | 2 | 74 | | 0.62 | | | 4 | | 0.04 | | | 18538 |
| **oatmeal raisin cookie**, fat-free, | 31 | 108 | 3.8 | 24.7 | 14.6 | | 0.7 | 179 | 10 | | | | | | 0.08 | 0.6 | | |
| Archway Hm Styl - *1 cookie* | | 1.3 | 0.5 | 0.1 | 0.2 | 0.2 | 14 | 86 | | 0.77 | | | 2 | | 0.05 | | | 18555 |
| **oatmeal raisin cookie**, homemade | 15 | 65 | 1.0 | 10.3 | | | | 81 | 15 | 6 | 0.13 | 0.148 | 21 | 0 | 0.04 | 0.2 | 0.01 | 0.05 |
| *1 cookie (2⅜" diameter)* | | 1.0 | 2.4 | 0.5 | 1.0 | 0.8 | 5 | 36 | 24 | 0.40 | 0.027 | 2.3 | 102 | | 0.02 | 0.01 | 6.4 | 18184 |
| **Oreo sandwich cookie**, Carb Well, | 24 | 100 | | 16.0 | 0 | | 3.0 | 105 | 20 | | | | | 0 | | | | |
| Nabisco - *.85 oz* | | 2.0 | 5.0 | 1.5 | | | 0 | | | 0.36 | | | 0 | | | | | NBSC140 |
| **Oreo sandwich cookie**, choc | 30 | 150 | | 21.0 | 14.0 | | 1.0 | 130 | 0 | | | | | 0 | | | | |
| crème, Nabisco - *1.1 oz* | | 1.0 | 7.0 | 2.5 | | | 0 | | | 1.44 | | | 0 | | | | | NBSC139 |
| **Oreo sandwich cookie**, choc fudge- | 19 | 100 | | 13.0 | 9.0 | | 1.0 | 70 | 0 | | | | | 0 | | | | |
| covered, Nabisco - *.67 oz* | | 1.0 | 5.0 | 1.0 | | | 0 | | | 0.72 | | | 0 | | | | | NBSC143 |
| **Oreo sandwich cookie**, double choc | 29 | 140 | | 20.0 | 13.0 | | 1.0 | 120 | 0 | | | | | 0 | | | | |
| mint 'n crème, Nabisco - *1 oz* | | 1.0 | 7.0 | 1.5 | | | 0 | | | 1.08 | | | 0 | | | | | NBSC141 |
| **Oreo sandwich cookie**, Double Stuf | 30 | 150 | | 20.0 | 14.0 | | 1.0 | 130 | 0 | | | | | 0 | | | | |
| choc crème, Nabisco - *1.1 oz* | | 1.0 | 7.0 | 2.5 | | | 0 | | | 1.44 | | | 0 | | | | | NBSC133 |
| **Oreo sandwich cookie**, Double Stuf | 43 | 210 | | 29.0 | 20.0 | | 1.0 | 200 | 0 | | | | | 0 | | | | |
| choc, Nabisco - *1.5 oz* | | 2.0 | 10.0 | 2.5 | | | 0 | | | 1.80 | | | 0 | | | | | NBSC135 |
| **Oreo sandwich cookie**, fudge mint- | 18 | 90 | | 12.0 | 8.0 | | 1.0 | 70 | 0 | | | | | 0 | | | | |
| covered, Nabisco - *.63 oz* | | 1.0 | 4.5 | 1.0 | | | 0 | | | 0.72 | | | 0 | | | | | NBSC142 |
| **Oreo sandwich cookie**, golden, | 35 | 170 | | 25.0 | 12.0 | | 0 | 120 | 0 | | | | | 0 | | | | |
| Nabisco - *1.2 oz* | | 1.0 | 7.0 | 2.0 | | | 0 | | | 0.72 | | | 0 | | | | | NBSC130 |
| **Oreo sandwich cookie**, golden w/ | 34 | 170 | | 24.0 | 12.0 | | 1.0 | 135 | 0 | | | | | 0 | | | | |
| choc crème, Nabisco - *1.2 oz* | | 1.0 | 7.0 | 2.0 | | | 0 | | | 0.72 | | | 0 | | | | | NBSC138 |
| **Oreo sandwich cookie**, mini bite | 29 | 140 | | 21.0 | 11.0 | | 1.0 | 160 | 0 | | | | | 0 | | | | |
| size, Nabisco - *1 oz* | | 1.0 | 6.0 | 1.0 | | | 0 | | | 1.44 | | | 0 | | | | | NBSC136 |
| **Oreo sandwich cookie**, mint milk | 18 | 90 | | 12.0 | 9.0 | | 0 | 60 | 0 | | | | | 0 | | | | |
| choc-covered, Nabisco - *.63 oz* | | 1.0 | 4.5 | 2.5 | | | 0 | | | 0.72 | | | 0 | | | | | NBSC134 |
| **Oreo sandwich cookie**, Nabisco | 34 | 160 | | 25.0 | 14.0 | | 1.0 | 190 | 0 | | | | | 0 | | | | |
| *1.2 oz* | | 2.0 | 7.0 | 2.0 | | | 0 | | | 1.80 | | | 0 | | | | | NBSC128 |
| **Oreo sandwich cookie**, reduced fat, | 34 | 150 | | 26.0 | 14.0 | | 1.0 | 190 | 0 | | | | | 0 | | | | |
| Nabisco - *1.2 oz* | | 2.0 | 4.5 | 1.0 | | | 0 | | | 1.80 | | | 0 | | | | | NBSC137 |
| **Oreo sandwich cookie**, white fudge- | 20 | 100 | | 13.0 | 10.0 | | 0 | 65 | 20 | | | | | 0 | | | | |
| covered, Nabisco - *.71 oz* | | 1.0 | 5.0 | 3.0 | | | 0 | | | 0.36 | | | 0 | | | | | NBSC131 |
| **Oreo sandwich cookie**, Double | 29 | 140 | | 21.0 | 13.0 | | 1.0 | 120 | 0 | | | | | 0 | | | | |
| Stuf, Nabisco - *1 oz* | | 1.0 | 7.0 | 2.5 | | | 0 | | | 1.08 | | | 0 | | | | | NBSC129 |
| **peanut butter chunky cookie**, | 17 | 90 | | 10.0 | 6.0 | | 0 | 85 | 0 | | | | | 0 | | | | |
| Chips Ahoy - *.56 oz cookie* | | 1.0 | 5.0 | 2.5 | | | 0 | | | 0.36 | | | 0 | | | | | NBSC105 |
| **peanut butter cookie** | 15 | 72 | 0.9 | 8.8 | 4.8 | 4.2 | 0.3 | 62 | 5 | 7 | 0.08 | 0.042 | 0 | 0 | 0.03 | 0.6 | 0.01 | 0.09 |
| *1 cookie* | | 1.4 | 3.5 | 0.7 | 1.9 | 0.8 | 0 | 25 | 13 | 0.38 | 0.030 | 0.9 | 2 | 0.3 | 0.03 | 0.01 | 15.0 | 18185 |
| **peanut butter cookie**, Archway | 21 | 101 | 1.3 | 12.3 | 6.8 | | 0.6 | 85 | 7 | | | | | 0 | 0.05 | 0.9 | | |
| Home Style - *1 cookie* | | 1.9 | 5.1 | 1.1 | 2.1 | 0.9 | 8 | 44 | | 0.57 | | | 13 | | 0.04 | | | 18541 |
| **peanut butter cookie**, from mix, | 32 | 140 | | 19.0 | 11.0 | | 1.0 | 150 | | | | | | | 0.03 | 0.4 | | |
| Betty Crocker - *2 cookies* | | 3.0 | 6.0 | 1.0 | | | 10 | 25 | | 0.36 | | | | | 0.03 | | | GENM99 |
| **peanut butter cookie**, from refrig | 12 | 60 | 0.5 | 6.9 | | | 0.1 | 52 | 13 | 5 | 0.09 | 0.055 | 2 | 0 | 0.02 | 0.5 | 0.01 | 0.04 |
| dough - *1 cookie* | | 1.1 | 3.3 | 0.7 | 1.7 | 0.6 | 4 | 41 | 32 | 0.22 | 0.020 | 0.6 | 6 | | 0.02 | 0.01 | 8.3 | 18188 |
| **peanut butter cookie**, from refrig | 29 | 130 | | 16.0 | 9.0 | | 0 | 135 | 0 | | | | | 0 | | | | |
| dough, Pillsbury - *1 oz* | | 2.0 | 6.0 | 1.5 | | | 5 | | | 0.36 | | | 0 | | | | | GENM100 |
| **peanut butter cookie**, homemade | 20 | 95 | 1.2 | 11.8 | | | | 104 | 8 | 8 | 0.16 | 0.114 | 27 | 0 | 0.04 | 0.7 | 0.02 | 0.07 |
| *1 cookie (3" diameter)* | | 1.8 | 4.8 | 0.9 | 2.2 | 1.4 | 6 | 46 | 23 | 0.45 | 0.037 | 3.0 | 129 | | 0.04 | 0.02 | 16.2 | 18189 |
| **peanut butter cookie**, Ruth's Golden, | 28 | 121 | 3.1 | 18.2 | 9.4 | | 0.8 | 109 | 10 | | | | | | 0.08 | 0.5 | | |
| Archway Gourmet - *1 cookie* | | 1.6 | 4.6 | 0.9 | 1.6 | 1.2 | 2 | 65 | | 0.64 | | | 6 | | 0.05 | | | 18564 |
| **peanut butter cookie**, soft type | 15 | 69 | 1.7 | 8.7 | | | 0.3 | 50 | 2 | 5 | 0.08 | 0.064 | 0 | 0 | 0.04 | 0.3 | 0 | 0.05 |
| *1 cookie* | | 0.8 | 3.7 | 0.9 | 2.1 | 0.5 | 0 | 16 | 13 | 0.13 | 0.012 | 0.7 | 0 | | 0.02 | | 16.5 | 18186 |

| | WT (g) | Macronutrients | Minerals | Vitamins |
|---|---|---|---|---|

| Food | WT (g) | KCAL / PRO | H₂0 / FAT | CHO / SFA | TSUG / MUFA | ASUG / PUFA | DFIB / CHOL | Na / K | Ca / P | Mg / Fe | Zn / Cu | Mn / Se | A(mcg RAE) / A(IU) | C / E(mg ATE) | B-1 / B-2 | NIA / B-6 | B-12 / FOL(mcg DFE) | PANT / REF |
|---|---|---|---|---|---|---|---|---|---|---|---|---|---|---|---|---|---|---|
| **peanut butter sandwich cookie** | 14 | 67 | 0.4 | 9.2 | 5.0 | 4.7 | 0.3 | 52 | 7 | 7 | 0.15 | 0.128 | 0 | 0 | 0.05 | 0.5 | 0.03 | 0.13 |
| *1 cookie* | | 1.2 | 3.0 | 0.7 | 1.6 | 0.5 | 0 | 27 | 26 | 0.36 | 0.033 | 1.1 | 1 | 0.3 | 0.04 | 0.02 | 13.0 | 18190 |
| **pecan ice box cookie, Archway** | 24 | 120 | 1.6 | 14.6 | 6.8 | | 0.3 | 76 | 3 | | | | | 0 | 0.07 | 0.6 | | |
| Home Style - *1 cookie* | | 1.1 | 6.4 | 1.4 | 2.8 | 0.6 | 7 | 18 | | 0.52 | | | 4 | | 0.05 | | | 18543 |
| **pecan shortbread cookie** | 14 | 76 | 0.5 | 8.2 | | | 0.3 | 39 | 4 | 3 | 0.08 | 0.086 | 0 | 0 | 0.04 | 0.3 | 0 | 0.05 |
| *1 cookie (2" diameter)* | | 0.7 | 4.6 | 1.1 | 2.6 | 0.6 | 5 | 10 | 12 | 0.34 | 0.021 | 0.4 | 0 | | 0.03 | 0 | 14.3 | 18193 |
| **raisin cookie, soft type** | 15 | 60 | 2.0 | 10.2 | 7.1 | 4.9 | 0.2 | 51 | 7 | 3 | 0.05 | 0.046 | 1 | 0 | 0.03 | 0.3 | 0 | 0.04 |
| *1 cookie* | | 0.6 | 2.0 | 0.5 | 1.1 | 0.3 | 0 | 21 | 12 | 0.34 | 0.062 | 0.4 | 4 | 0.3 | 0.03 | 0.01 | 7.2 | 18191 |
| **raspberry-filled cookie, Archway** | 25 | 100 | 3.7 | 16.5 | 7.9 | | 0.6 | 84 | 5 | | | | | | 0.08 | 0.5 | | |
| Home Style - *1 cookie* | | 1.1 | 3.3 | 1.3 | 1.0 | 0.3 | 2 | 30 | | 0.58 | | | 4 | | 0.04 | | | 18544 |
| **Raspberry Newton, Nabisco** | 29 | 100 | | 21.0 | 13.0 | | 0 | 110 | 0 | | | | | 0 | | | | |
| *2 square bars (1 oz)* | | 1.0 | 1.5 | 0 | | | 0 | | | 0.36 | | | 0 | | | | | NBSC117 |
| **rocky road cookie, Archway** | 28 | 129 | 2.2 | 18.5 | 9.8 | | 0.7 | 79 | 5 | | | | | 0 | 0.06 | 0.5 | | |
| Gourmet - *1 cookie* | | 1.4 | 5.5 | 1.4 | 1.9 | 1.0 | 3 | 67 | | 0.82 | | | 3 | | 0.05 | | | 18563 |
| **rocky road cookie, sgr-free, Archway** | 24 | 112 | 1.8 | 15.5 | 0.2 | | 0.7 | 68 | 42 | | | | | | 0.06 | 0.4 | | |
| Home Style - *1 cookie* | | 1.4 | 4.9 | 1.2 | 1.7 | 1.0 | 0 | 62 | | 0.76 | | | 5 | | 0.05 | | | 18514 |
| **Samoa, Girl Scout Cookies** | 31 | 150 | | 20.0 | 12.0 | | | 55 | 20 | | | | | 0 | | | | |
| *2 cookies* | | 1.0 | 8.0 | 4.5 | | | 0 | | | 0.36 | | | 0 | | | | | GIRL2 |
| **shortbread cookie** | 8 | 40 | 0.3 | 5.2 | 1.2 | 1.1 | 0.1 | 36 | 3 | 1 | 0.04 | 0.034 | 1 | 0 | 0.03 | 0.3 | 0.01 | 0.02 |
| *1 cookie (1⅝" square)* | | 0.5 | 1.9 | 0.5 | 1.1 | 0.3 | 2 | 8 | 9 | 0.22 | 0.012 | 0.6 | 7 | 0 | 0.03 | 0.01 | 9.0 | 18192 |
| **shortbread cookie, Lorna Doone** | 29 | 140 | | 20.0 | 6.0 | | 0 | 150 | 0 | | | | | 0 | | | | |
| *1 oz* | | 1.0 | 7.0 | 2.0 | | | 0 | | | 0.72 | | | 0 | | | | | NBSC154 |
| **shortbread cookie, strawbry-fill,** | 25 | 100 | 3.7 | 16.5 | 7.9 | | 0.6 | 84 | 5 | | | | | | 0.08 | 0.5 | | |
| Archway Hm Styl - *1 cookie* | | 1.1 | 3.3 | 1.3 | 1.0 | 0.3 | 2 | 30 | | 0.58 | | | 4 | | 0.04 | | | 18547 |
| **shortbread cookie, sugar-free,** | 30 | 130 | | 21.0 | 0 | | 2.0 | 140 | 0 | | | | | 0 | | | | |
| SnackWell's - *1.1 oz* | | 2.0 | 6.0 | 1.5 | | | 5 | | | 1.08 | | | 0 | | | | | NBSC157 |
| **Snackimal, choc chip, Barbara's** | 30 | 120 | | 19.0 | 8.0 | | | 80 | 0 | | | | | 0 | | | | |
| Bakery - *10 cookies* | | 1.0 | 4.0 | 0 | | | 0 | | | 0.72 | | | 0 | | | | | BARB56 |
| **Snackimal, oatmeal, wheat-free,** | 30 | 120 | | 17.0 | 6.0 | | 1.0 | 130 | 40 | | | | | 0 | | | | |
| Barbara's Bakery - *10 cookies* | | 1.0 | 5.0 | 0 | | | 0 | | | 1.44 | | | 0 | | | | | BARB57 |
| **Snackimal, snickerdoodle,** | 30 | 120 | | 19.0 | 5.0 | | | 65 | 0 | | | | | 0 | | | | |
| Barbara's Bakery - *10 cookies* | | 2.0 | 4.0 | 0 | | | 0 | | | 0.72 | | | 0 | | | | | BARB58 |
| **Snackimal, vanilla, Barbara's** | 30 | 110 | | 17.0 | 5.0 | | | 65 | 40 | | | | | 0 | | | | |
| Bakery - *10 cookies* | | 2.0 | 4.0 | 0 | | | 0 | | | 1.44 | | | 0 | | | | | BARB59 |
| **Social Tea Biscuit, Nabisco** | 31 | 140 | | 24.0 | 7.0 | | 1.0 | 150 | 0 | | | | | 0 | | | | |
| *1.1 oz* | | 2.0 | 4.0 | 1.0 | | | 0 | | | 1.08 | | | 0 | | | | | NBSC161 |
| **Strawberry Newton Mini, whole** | 38 | 130 | | 27.0 | 15.0 | | 2.0 | 140 | 150 | | | | | 0 | | | | |
| grain, Nabisco - *1.34 oz* | | 2.0 | 3.0 | 0.5 | | | 0 | | | 2.70 | | | 750 | | | | | NBSC120 |
| **Strawberry Newton, Nabisco** | 29 | 100 | | 21.0 | 13.0 | | 0 | 110 | 0 | | | | | 0 | | | | |
| *2 square bars (1 oz)* | | 1.0 | 1.5 | 0 | | | 0 | | | 0.36 | | | 0 | | | | | NBSC118 |
| **sugar cookie** | 15 | 72 | 0.7 | 10.2 | 5.7 | 5.2 | 0.1 | 54 | 3 | 2 | 0.06 | 0.002 | 4 | 0 | 0.03 | 0.4 | 0.03 | 0.04 |
| *1 cookie* | | 0.8 | 3.2 | 0.8 | 1.8 | 0.4 | 8 | 9 | 12 | 0.32 | 0.011 | 0.3 | 14 | 0 | 0.03 | 0.01 | 12.3 | 18204 |
| **sugar cookie, Archway Home Style** | 24 | 99 | 2.5 | 16.6 | | | 0.4 | 154 | 6 | | | | | 0 | 0.08 | 0.6 | | |
| *1 cookie* | | 1.2 | 3.1 | 0.7 | 1.2 | 0.3 | 4 | 21 | | 0.59 | | | 5 | | 0.06 | | | 18548 |
| **sugar cookie, from mix, Betty** | 33 | 160 | | 21.0 | 12.0 | | 0 | 120 | | | | | | | 0.06 | 0.4 | | |
| Crocker - *2 cookies* | | 2.0 | 8.0 | 4.0 | | | 25 | 20 | | 0.36 | | | 200 | | 0.03 | | | GENM101 |
| **sugar cookie, from refrig dough** | 15 | 73 | 0.8 | 9.8 | 3.6 | 3.6 | 0.1 | 70 | 14 | 1 | 0.04 | 0.043 | 2 | 0 | 0.03 | 0.4 | 0.01 | 0.02 |
| *1 cookie* | | 0.7 | 3.5 | 0.9 | 2.0 | 0.4 | 5 | 24 | 28 | 0.28 | 0.006 | 0.5 | 6 | 0 | 0.02 | 0 | 17.2 | 18206 |
| **sugar cookie, from refrig dough,** | 29 | 130 | | 18.0 | 10.0 | | 0 | 95 | 0 | | | | | 0 | | | | |
| Pillsbury - *2 cookies* | | 1.0 | 6.0 | 1.5 | | | 10 | | | 0.36 | | | 0 | | | | | GENM102 |
| **sugar cookie, homemade w/** | 14 | 66 | 1.2 | 8.4 | 3.5 | 3.4 | 0.2 | 69 | 10 | 2 | 0.06 | 0.044 | 33 | 0 | 0.04 | 0.3 | 0.01 | 0.03 |
| margarine - *1 cookie - (3" dia)* | | 0.8 | 3.3 | 0.7 | 1.4 | 1.0 | 4 | 11 | 13 | 0.33 | 0.011 | 2.5 | 144 | 0.4 | 0.04 | 0 | 13.7 | 18208 |
| **sugar drop cookie, soft, Archway** | 28 | 111 | 4.6 | 17.7 | 8.6 | | 0.2 | 111 | 11 | | | | | | 0.08 | 0.6 | | |
| Home Style - *1 oz* | | 1.3 | 3.9 | 0.9 | 1.6 | 0.3 | 11 | 27 | | 0.55 | | | 6 | | 0.06 | | | 18546 |
| **sugar wafer with crème filling** | 28 | 143 | 0.3 | 19.6 | 9.9 | 9.8 | 0.2 | 41 | 5 | 3 | 0.10 | 0.077 | 0 | 0 | 0.03 | 0.7 | 0 | 0.05 |
| *8 small wafers (1 oz)* | | 1.1 | 6.8 | 1.0 | 2.9 | 2.6 | 0 | 17 | 16 | 0.55 | 0.025 | 0.7 | 0 | 0.5 | 0.05 | 0 | 23.5 | 18209 |
| **sugar wafer with crème filling,** | 28 | 140 | | 21.0 | 13.0 | | | 40 | 0 | | | | | 0 | | | | |
| Biscos - *8 small wafers (1 oz)* | | 1.0 | 6.0 | 1.5 | | | 0 | | | 0.36 | | | 0 | | | | | NBSC112 |
| **Tagalong, Girl Scout Cookies** | 27 | 140 | | 13.0 | 8.0 | | 1.0 | 95 | 0 | | | | | 0 | | | | |
| *2 cookies* | | 2.0 | 10.0 | 4.0 | | | 0 | | | 0.72 | | | 0 | | | | | GIRL3 |
| **Teddy Graham**, choc, Nabisco | 30 | 130 | | 22.0 | 8.0 | | 2.0 | 160 | 100 | | | | | 0 | | | | |
| *1.1 oz* | | 2.0 | 4.5 | 1.0 | | | 0 | | | 1.08 | | | 0 | | | | | NBSC164 |

| | WT (g) | KCAL | H₂0 (g) | CHO (g) | TSUG (g) | ASUG (g) | DFIB (g) | Na (mg) | Ca (mg) | Mg (mg) | Zn (mg) | Mn (mg) | A (mcg RAE) | C (mg) | B-1 (mg) | NIA (mg) | B-12 (mcg) | PANT (mg) |
|---|---|---|---|---|---|---|---|---|---|---|---|---|---|---|---|---|---|---|
| | | PRO (g) | FAT (g) | SFA (g) | MUFA (g) | PUFA (g) | CHOL (mg) | K (mg) | P (mg) | Fe (mg) | Cu (mg) | Se (mcg) | A (IU) | E (mg ATE) | B-2 (mg) | B-6 (mg) | FOL (mcg DFE) | REF |
| **Teddy Graham**, chocolatey chip, Nabisco - *1.1 oz* | 30 | 130 | | 23.0 | 8.0 | | 1.0 | 170 | 100 | | | | | 0 | | | | |
| | | 1.0 | 4.5 | 1.0 | | | 0 | | | 0.72 | | | 0 | | | | | NBSC166 |
| **Teddy Graham**, cinn, Nabisco *1.1 oz* | 30 | 130 | | 23.0 | 8.0 | | 1.0 | 150 | 100 | | | | | 0 | | | | |
| | | 2.0 | 4.0 | 1.0 | | | 0 | | | 0.72 | | | 0 | | | | | NBSC163 |
| **Teddy Graham**, honey, Nabisco *1.1 oz* | 30 | 130 | | 23.0 | 7.0 | | 1.0 | 150 | 100 | | | | | 0 | | | | |
| | | 2.0 | 4.0 | 1.0 | | | 0 | | | 0.72 | | | 0 | | | | | NBSC165 |
| **Teddy Graham**, mini-cinn cubs, Nabisco - *.78 oz* | 22 | 100 | | 16.0 | 4.0 | | 1.0 | 115 | 100 | | | | | 0 | | | | |
| | | 1.0 | 3.0 | | | | 0 | | | 0.72 | | | 0 | | | | | NBSC162 |
| **Trefoil**, Girl Scout Cookies *4 cookies* | 28 | 130 | | 17.0 | 5.0 | | 0 | 85 | 0 | | | | | 0 | | | | |
| | | 2.0 | 6.0 | 1.5 | | | 0 | | | 0.72 | | | 0 | | | | | GIRL4 |
| **Twirl**, Nabisco *1.1 oz cookie* | 30 | 130 | | 20.0 | 14.0 | | 0 | 75 | 0 | | | | | 0 | | | | |
| | | 1.0 | 6.0 | 1.0 | | | 0 | | | 0.72 | | | 0 | | | | | NBSC114 |
| **vanilla sandwich with crème filling** *1 round cookie (1¾" diameter)* | 10 | 48 | 0.2 | 7.2 | 3.9 | 3.9 | 0.2 | 35 | 3 | 1 | 0.04 | 0.029 | 0 | 0 | 0.03 | 0.3 | 0 | 0.04 |
| | | 0.4 | 2.0 | 0.3 | 0.8 | 0.8 | 0 | 9 | 8 | 0.22 | 0.011 | 0.3 | 0 | 0.2 | 0.02 | 0 | 8.2 | 18210 |
| **vanilla wafer**, 12–17% fat *7 wafers (1 oz)* | 28 | 123 | 1.4 | 20.6 | 10.5 | 8.2 | 0.5 | 87 | 13 | 4 | 0.10 | 0.073 | 2 | 0 | 0.08 | 0.9 | 0.04 | 0.11 |
| | | 1.4 | 4.3 | 1.1 | 1.8 | 1.1 | 14 | 27 | 29 | 0.67 | 0.028 | 3.2 | 8 | 0.1 | 0.09 | 0.02 | 26.9 | 18212 |
| **vanilla wafer**, 18–21% fat *5 wafers (1 oz)* | 28 | 132 | 1.2 | 19.9 | | | 0.6 | 86 | 7 | 3 | 0.09 | 0.108 | 0 | 0 | 0.10 | 0.8 | 0.01 | 0.08 |
| | | 1.2 | 5.4 | 1.4 | 3.1 | 0.7 | 0 | 30 | 18 | 0.62 | 0.035 | 3.2 | 0 | 0.06 | 0.01 | 19.0 | 18213 |
| **vanilla wafer**, Keebler *8 wafers* | 31 | 147 | 1.3 | 21.6 | 8.5 | | | 120 | | | | | | | | | | |
| | | 1.6 | 6.0 | 1.1 | | | | | | | | | | | | | | 18609 |
| **vanilla wafer**, Streit's *3 cookies* | 30 | 170 | | 18.0 | 13.0 | | 0 | 15 | 0 | | | | | 0 | | | | |
| | | 1.0 | 11.0 | 2.0 | 2.0 | 7.0 | 0 | | | 0.36 | | | 0 | | | | | STRE1 |
| **white choc chip macadamia nut cookie**, Mauna Loa - *4 cookies* | 28 | 140 | | 15.0 | 9.0 | | 0 | 90 | | | | | | | | | | |
| | | 2.0 | 8.0 | 1.5 | | | 0 | | | | | | | | | | | MAUN11 |
| **white fudge & choc chunk cookie**, Chips Ahoy - *1 oz cookie* | 28 | 120 | | 19.0 | 11.0 | | 1.0 | 150 | 20 | | | | | 0 | | | | |
| | | 1.0 | 5.0 | 3.0 | | | 0 | | | 0.72 | | | 0 | | | | | NBSC102 |
| **white fudge chunky cookie**, Chips Ahoy - *.56 oz cookie* | 17 | 80 | | 11.0 | 6.0 | | 0 | 60 | 0 | | | | | 0 | | | | |
| | | 1.0 | 4.5 | 1.5 | | | 0 | | | 0.36 | | | 0 | | | | | NBSC106 |
| **windmill cookie**, old fashioned, Archway Hm Styl - *1 cookie* | 20 | 94 | 0.6 | 14.4 | 6.5 | | 0.4 | 94 | 7 | | | | | 0 | 0.07 | 0.6 | | |
| | | 1.0 | 3.5 | 0.8 | 1.6 | 0.3 | 0 | 23 | | 0.61 | | | 0 | | 0.05 | | | 18540 |

## 7.4 DOUGHNUTS

| | WT (g) | KCAL | H₂0 (g) | CHO (g) | TSUG (g) | ASUG (g) | DFIB (g) | Na (mg) | Ca (mg) | Mg (mg) | Zn (mg) | Mn (mg) | A (mcg RAE) | C (mg) | B-1 (mg) | NIA (mg) | B-12 (mcg) | PANT (mg) |
|---|---|---|---|---|---|---|---|---|---|---|---|---|---|---|---|---|---|---|
| | | PRO (g) | FAT (g) | SFA (g) | MUFA (g) | PUFA (g) | CHOL (mg) | K (mg) | P (mg) | Fe (mg) | Cu (mg) | Se (mcg) | A (IU) | E (mg ATE) | B-2 (mg) | B-6 (mg) | FOL (mcg DFE) | REF |
| **apple fritter**, Krispy Kreme *3.6 oz fritter* | 101 | 380 | | 46.0 | 23.0 | | 2.0 | 290 | 100 | | | | | 1 | | | | |
| | | 4.0 | 21.0 | 5.0 | | | 5 | | | 1.44 | | | 0 | | | | | KRIS29 |
| **cruller**, chocolate-glazed, Krispy Kreme - *2.4 oz cruller* | 69 | 290 | | 37.0 | 25.0 | | | 240 | 20 | | | | | 0 | | | | |
| | | 2.0 | 15.0 | 3.5 | | | 15 | | | 1.08 | | | 0 | | | | | KRIS27 |
| **cruller**, glazed *3" diameter cruller* | 41 | 169 | 7.3 | 24.4 | 14.4 | 14.1 | 0.5 | 141 | 11 | 5 | 0.11 | 0.088 | 1 | 0 | 0.07 | 0.9 | 0.02 | 0.09 |
| | | 1.3 | 7.5 | 1.9 | 4.3 | 0.9 | 5 | 32 | 50 | 0.99 | 0.029 | 0.9 | 3 | 0.1 | 0.09 | 0.01 | 27.1 | 18253 |
| **cruller**, glazed, Krispy Kreme *1.9 oz cruller* | 54 | 240 | | 26.0 | 14.0 | | | 240 | 20 | | | | | 0 | | | | |
| | | 2.0 | 14.0 | 3.5 | | | 15 | | | 1.08 | | | 0 | | | | | KRIS8 |
| **doughnut** *3¼" diameter doughnut* | 47 | 196 | 10.8 | 21.4 | 10.6 | 10.0 | 0.8 | 262 | 12 | 8 | 0.32 | 0.136 | 1 | 1 | 0.11 | 0.9 | 0.03 | 0.10 |
| | | 2.8 | 11.1 | 3.3 | 6.0 | 1.2 | 4 | 53 | 123 | 1.41 | 0.034 | 4.8 | 5 | 0.9 | 0.07 | 0.01 | 54.0 | 18248 |
| **doughnut**, caramel kreme crunch, Krispy Kreme - *3.3 oz doughnut* | 92 | 350 | | 43.0 | 25.0 | | | 170 | 100 | | | | | 1 | | | | |
| | | 4.0 | 19.0 | 5.0 | | | 5 | | | 1.44 | | | 0 | | | | | KRIS11 |
| **doughnut**, chocolate coating/icing - *3" diameter doughnut* | 43 | 194 | 7.2 | 22.1 | 11.5 | 9.1 | 0.8 | 178 | 10 | 13 | 0.42 | 0.275 | 2 | 1 | 0.07 | 0.7 | 0.04 | 0.05 |
| | | 2.1 | 10.9 | 5.8 | 3.7 | 0.8 | 8 | 86 | 90 | 1.72 | 0.112 | 2.9 | 7 | 0.9 | 0.05 | 0.01 | 38.7 | 18249 |
| **doughnut**, choc, glazed/sugared *3" doughnut* | 42 | 175 | 6.8 | 24.1 | 13.4 | 13.0 | 0.9 | 143 | 89 | 14 | 0.24 | 0.155 | 5 | 0 | 0.02 | 0.2 | 0.04 | 0.14 |
| | | 1.9 | 8.4 | 2.2 | 4.7 | 1.0 | 24 | 45 | 68 | 0.95 | 0.080 | 1.7 | 16 | 0.1 | 0.03 | 0.01 | 27.3 | 18251 |
| **doughnut**, choc icing, custard-fill, Krispy Kreme - *3 oz doughnut* | 86 | 300 | | 35.0 | 19.0 | | | 140 | 80 | | | | | 1 | | | | |
| | | 3.0 | 17.0 | 4.0 | | | 5 | | | 1.08 | | | 0 | | | | | KRIS5 |
| **doughnut**, choc icing, glazed, Krispy Kreme - *2.3 oz doughnut* | 66 | 250 | | 33.0 | 21.0 | | | 100 | 60 | | | | | 1 | | | | |
| | | 3.0 | 12.0 | 3.0 | | | 5 | | | 0.72 | | | 0 | | | | | KRIS2 |
| **doughnut**, choc icing, kreme-filled, Krispy Kreme - *3 oz doughnut* | 86 | 350 | | 38.0 | 23.0 | | | 140 | 80 | | | | | 1 | | | | |
| | | 3.0 | 20.0 | 5.0 | | | 5 | | | 1.08 | | | 0 | | | | | KRIS4 |
| **doughnut**, choc icing, Krispy Kreme - *2.5 oz doughnut* | 71 | 270 | | 36.0 | 20.0 | | | 320 | 20 | | | | | 0 | | | | |
| | | 3.0 | 14.0 | 3.0 | | | 20 | | | 1.44 | | | 0 | | | | | KRIS26 |
| **doughnut**, choc icing w/sprinkles, Krispy Kreme - *2.5 oz doughnut* | 71 | 260 | | 38.0 | 24.0 | | | 100 | 60 | | | | | 1 | | | | |
| | | 3.0 | 12.0 | 3.0 | | | 5 | | | 0.72 | | | 0 | | | | | KRIS3 |
| **doughnut**, cinnamon apple-filled, Krispy Kreme - *2.9 oz doughnut* | 81 | 290 | | 32.0 | 14.0 | | | 150 | 100 | | | | | 1 | | | | |
| | | 3.0 | 16.0 | 4.0 | | | 5 | | | 1.08 | | | 0 | | | | | KRIS9 |
| **doughnut**, cinnamon twist, Krispy Kreme - *2.1 oz doughnut* | 59 | 230 | | 33.0 | 19.0 | | 1.0 | 85 | 80 | | | | | 1 | | | | |
| | | 3.0 | 9.0 | 2.5 | | | 5 | | | 1.08 | | | 0 | | | | | KRIS19 |

| Food | WT (g) | KCAL / PRO (g) | H₂O (g) / FAT (g) | CHO (g) / SFA (g) | TSUG (g) / MUFA (g) | ASUG (g) / PUFA (g) | DFIB (g) / CHOL (mg) | Na (mg) / K (mg) | Ca (mg) / P (mg) | Mg (mg) / Fe (mg) | Zn (mg) / Cu (mg) | Mn (mg) / Se (mcg) | A (mcg RAE) / A (IU) | C (mg) / E (mg ATE) | B-1 (mg) / B-2 (mg) | NIA (mg) / B-6 (mg) | B-12 (mcg) / FOL (mcg DFE) | PANT (mg) / REF |
|---|---|---|---|---|---|---|---|---|---|---|---|---|---|---|---|---|---|---|
| doughnut, crumb, Entenmann's 2.1 oz doughnut | 60 | 260 | | 34.0 | 19.0 | | | 240 | 60 | | | | | 0 | | | | |
|  | | 3.0 | 13.0 | 3.0 | | | 15 | | | 0.72 | | | 0 | | | | | ENTE2 |
| doughnut, dulce de leche, Krispy Kreme - 2.7 oz doughnut | 75 | 290 | | 30.0 | 12.0 | | | 160 | 100 | | | | | 1 | | | | |
|  | | 3.0 | 18.0 | 4.5 | | | 5 | | | 1.44 | | | 0 | | | | | KRIS28 |
| doughnut, glazed, blueberry, Krispy Kreme - 2.8 oz doughnut | 80 | 330 | | 43.0 | 28.0 | | | 290 | 20 | | | | | 0 | | | | |
|  | | 3.0 | 17.0 | 4.0 | | | 20 | | | 1.44 | | | 0 | | | | | KRIS16 |
| doughnut, glazed, choc, Krispy Kreme - 2.9 oz doughnut | 81 | 300 | | 41.0 | 26.0 | | 2.0 | 310 | 0 | | | | | 0 | | | | |
|  | | 3.0 | 15.0 | 3.5 | | | 5 | | | 1.80 | | | 0 | | | | | KRIS13 |
| doughnut, glazed, cinnamon, Krispy Kreme - 1.9 oz doughnut | 54 | 210 | | 24.0 | 12.0 | | | 100 | 60 | | | | | 1 | | | | |
|  | | 2.0 | 12.0 | 3.0 | | | 5 | | | 0.72 | | | 0 | | | | | KRIS17 |
| doughnut, glazed, Entenmann's 2.1 oz doughnut | 60 | 260 | | 32.0 | 19.0 | | | 250 | 60 | | | | | 0 | | | | |
|  | | 3.0 | 14.0 | 3.5 | | | 15 | | | 0.72 | | | 0 | | | | | ENTE3 |
| doughnut, glazed, kreme-filled, Krispy Kreme - 3 oz doughnut | 86 | 340 | | 38.0 | 23.0 | | | 140 | 80 | | | | | 1 | | | | |
|  | | 3.0 | 20.0 | 5.0 | | | 5 | | | 1.08 | | | 0 | | | | | KRIS15 |
| doughnut, glazed, Krispy Kreme 1.8 oz doughnut | 52 | 200 | | 22.0 | 10.0 | | | 95 | 60 | | | | | 1 | | | | |
|  | | 2.0 | 12.0 | 3.0 | | | 5 | | | 0.72 | | | 0 | | | | | KRIS1 |
| doughnut, glazed, lemon-filled, Krispy Kreme - 3 oz doughnut | 85 | 290 | | 35.0 | 18.0 | | | 135 | 80 | | | | | 1 | | | | |
|  | | 3.0 | 16.0 | 4.0 | | | 5 | | | 1.08 | | | 0 | | | | | KRIS6 |
| doughnut, glazed, raspberry-filled, Krispy Kreme - 3 oz doughnut | 85 | 300 | | 38.0 | 22.0 | | | 130 | 80 | | | | | 1 | | | | |
|  | | 3.0 | 16.0 | 4.0 | | | 5 | | | 1.44 | | | 0 | | | | | KRIS7 |
| doughnut, glazed, sour crème, Krispy Kreme -2.8 oz doughnut | 80 | 340 | | 42.0 | 27.0 | | | 310 | 20 | | | | | 0 | | | | |
|  | | 3.0 | 18.0 | 4.5 | | | 20 | | | 1.44 | | | 0 | | | | | KRIS21 |
| doughnut hole, glazed blueberry, Krispy Kreme - 4 pieces | 51 | 210 | | 24.0 | 11.0 | | 0 | 250 | 20 | | | | | 0 | | | | |
|  | | 2.0 | 11.0 | 2.5 | | | 15 | | | 1.08 | | | 0 | | | | | KRIS31 |
| doughnut hole, glazed chocolate, Krispy Kreme - 4 pieces | 56 | 210 | | 28.0 | 17.0 | | | 230 | 20 | | | | | 0 | | | | |
|  | | 2.0 | 11.0 | 2.5 | | | 15 | | | 1.08 | | | 0 | | | | | KRIS33 |
| doughnut hole, glazed, Krispy Kreme - 4 pieces | 56 | 210 | | 28.0 | 17.0 | | | 230 | 20 | | | | | 0 | | | | |
|  | | 2.0 | 11.0 | 2.5 | | | 15 | | | 1.08 | | | 0 | | | | | KRIS32 |
| doughnut, key lime pie, Krispy Kreme - 3.3 oz doughnut | 92 | 320 | | 40.0 | 24.0 | | | 150 | 80 | | | | | 1 | | | | |
|  | | 3.0 | 17.0 | 4.5 | | | 5 | | | 1.08 | | | 0 | | | | | KRIS12 |
| doughnut, Krispy Kreme 2 oz doughnut | 57 | 230 | | 25.0 | 9.0 | | | 320 | 20 | | | | | 0 | | | | |
|  | | 3.0 | 13.0 | 3.0 | | | 20 | | | 1.44 | | | 0 | | | | | KRIS14 |
| doughnut, maple icing, glazed, Krispy Kreme -2.3 oz doughnut | 66 | 240 | | 32.0 | 20.0 | | | 100 | 60 | | | | | 1 | | | | |
|  | | 2.0 | 12.0 | 3.0 | | | 5 | | | 0.72 | | | 0 | | | | | KRIS20 |
| doughnut, New York cheesecake, Krispy Kreme -3.2 oz doughnut | 90 | 320 | | 35.0 | 17.0 | | | 190 | 80 | | | | | 1 | | | | |
|  | | 4.0 | 19.0 | 5.0 | | | 10 | | | 1.08 | | | 100 | | | | | KRIS10 |
| doughnut, old fashion, Entenmann's 1.8 oz doughnut | 50 | 230 | | 24.0 | 10.0 | | | 260 | 0 | | | | | 0 | | | | |
|  | | 3.0 | 14.0 | 3.5 | | | 15 | | | 0.72 | | | 0 | | | | | ENTE5 |
| doughnut, powdered, blueberry-fill, Krispy Kreme -2.9 oz doughnut | 81 | 290 | | 33.0 | 14.0 | | | 140 | 80 | | | | | 1 | | | | |
|  | | 3.0 | 16.0 | 4.0 | | | 5 | | | 1.08 | | | 0 | | | | | KRIS23 |
| doughnut, powdered, Krispy Kreme - 2.5 oz doughnut | 71 | 280 | | 37.0 | 19.0 | | | 320 | 40 | | | | | 0 | | | | |
|  | | 3.0 | 14.0 | 3.0 | | | 20 | | | 1.44 | | | 0 | | | | | KRIS25 |
| doughnut, powdered, strawbry-fill, Krispy Kreme -2.9 oz doughnut | 81 | 290 | | 33.0 | 13.0 | | | 135 | 80 | | | | | 1 | | | | |
|  | | 3.0 | 16.0 | 4.0 | | | 5 | | | 1.08 | | | 0 | | | | | KRIS24 |
| doughnut, powdered sugar, Tastykake - 4 mini donuts | 53 | 210 | | 27.0 | 14.0 | | | 210 | 20 | | | | | 0 | | | | |
|  | | 3.0 | 10.0 | 2.0 | | | 20 | | | 1.08 | | | 0 | | | | | TAST9 |
| doughnut, rich frosted, Entenmann's - 2 oz doughnut | 57 | 280 | | 27.0 | 16.0 | | 1.0 | 210 | 0 | | | | | 0 | | | | |
|  | | 2.0 | 19.0 | 5.0 | | | 10 | | | 1.44 | | | 0 | | | | | ENTE4 |
| doughnut, sugar, Krispy Kreme 1.7 oz doughnut | 49 | 200 | | 21.0 | 10.0 | | 0 | 95 | 60 | | | | | 1 | | | | |
|  | | 2.0 | 12.0 | 3.0 | | | 5 | | | 0.72 | | | 0 | | | | | KRIS22 |
| doughnut, yeast-raised, glazed 3¾" doughnut | 60 | 239 | 13.6 | 30.4 | 14.2 | 13.2 | 1.3 | 232 | 28 | 11 | 0.75 | 0.231 | 3 | 1 | 0.19 | 1.6 | 0.07 | 0.13 |
|  | | 3.7 | 11.5 | 3.3 | 6.0 | 1.7 | 18 | 60 | 83 | 2.25 | 0.057 | 9.4 | 14 | 0.9 | 0.11 | 0.02 | 93.0 | 18255 |
| doughnut, yst-raised w/crème filling 1 oval doughnut (3½" × 2½") | 85 | 307 | 32.5 | 25.5 | 12.4 | 9.6 | 0.7 | 263 | 21 | 17 | 0.68 | 0.191 | 9 | 0 | 0.29 | 1.9 | 0.12 | 0.56 |
|  | | 5.4 | 20.8 | 4.6 | 10.3 | 2.6 | 20 | 68 | 65 | 1.56 | 0.096 | 9.2 | 34 | 0.2 | 0.13 | 0.06 | 92.6 | 18254 |
| doughnut, yeast-raised w/jelly filling 1 oval doughnut (3½" × 2½") | 85 | 289 | 30.3 | 33.2 | 17.9 | 15.9 | 0.8 | 249 | 21 | 17 | 0.64 | 0.174 | 14 | 0 | 0.27 | 1.8 | 0.19 | 0.74 |
|  | | 5.0 | 15.9 | 4.1 | 8.7 | 2.0 | 22 | 67 | 72 | 1.50 | 0.116 | 10.6 | 60 | 0.4 | 0.12 | 0.08 | 88.4 | 18256 |
| doughnut, yeast-raised, wheat, glazed/sgrd - 3" doughnut | 45 | 162 | 13.4 | 19.2 | 9.7 | 9.1 | 1.0 | 160 | 22 | 10 | 0.31 | 0.389 | 1 | 0 | 0.10 | 0.8 | 0.08 | 0.20 |
|  | | 2.8 | 8.7 | 1.4 | 3.6 | 3.2 | 9 | 67 | 47 | 0.50 | 0.050 | 8.7 | 5 | 0.8 | 0.11 | 0.04 | 10.8 | 18252 |
| doughnut, yeast-raised, glazed/ sugared - 3" doughnut | 45 | 192 | 8.8 | 22.9 | | | 0.7 | 181 | 27 | 8 | 0.20 | 0.150 | 1 | 0 | 0.10 | 0.7 | 0.11 | 0.20 |
|  | | 2.3 | 10.3 | 2.7 | 5.7 | 1.3 | .14 | 46 | 53 | 0.48 | 0.045 | 4.3 | 4 | | 0.09 | 0.01 | 31.5 | 18250 |

## 7.5 FROZEN DESSERTS

| | WT (g) | KCAL / PRO (g) | H₂0 (g) / FAT (g) | CHO (g) / SFA (g) | TSUG (g) / MUFA (g) | ASUG (g) / PUFA (g) | DFIB (g) / CHOL (mg) | Na (mg) / K (mg) | Ca (mg) / P (mg) | Mg (mg) / Fe (mg) | Zn (mg) / Cu (mg) | Mn (mg) / Se (mcg) | A (mcg RAE) / A (IU) | C (mg) / E (mg ATE) | B-1 (mg) / B-2 (mg) | NIA (mg) / B-6 (mg) | B-12 (mcg) / FOL (mcg DFE) | PANT (mg) / REF |
|---|---|---|---|---|---|---|---|---|---|---|---|---|---|---|---|---|---|---|
| **Creamsicle Pop**, Good Humor | 44 | 25 | 36.2 | 6.4 | 1.2 | | 0.1 | 18 | 60 | | | | | 0 | | | | |
| *1 pop* | | 0.8 | 0.4 | 0.2 | | | 1 | | | 0.12 | | | 10 | | | | | 19891 |
| **Creamsicle Pop**, sugar-free, Good | 80 | 39 | 67.1 | 9.6 | 0.3 | | 6.0 | 5 | 18 | | | | | 0 | | | | |
| Humor - *2 pops* | | 1.1 | 1.9 | 1.6 | | | 0 | | | 0.02 | | | 0 | | | | | 19892 |
| **Frappuccino ice cream bar**, lowfat, | 81 | 120 | | 22.0 | 16.0 | | 3.0 | 50 | 100 | | | | | 0 | | | | |
| Starbucks - *1 bar* | | 4.0 | 1.5 | 1.0 | | | 5 | | | 0 | | | 200 | | | | | STAR26 |
| **frozen yogurt**, flavors other than | 174 | 221 | 123.9 | 37.6 | 37.3 | 27.6 | 0 | 110 | 174 | 17 | 0.49 | | 85 | 1 | 0.07 | 0.1 | 0.12 | |
| chocolate - *1 cup* | | 5.2 | 6.3 | 4.0 | 1.7 | 0.2 | 23 | 271 | 155 | 0.80 | 0.016 | 3.3 | 306 | 0.2 | 0.31 | 0.07 | 7.0 | 42187 |
| **frozen yogurt**, lowfat, cherry | 87 | 170 | | 32.0 | 22.0 | | | 65 | 200 | | | | | 0 | | | | |
| garcia, Ben & Jerry's - *½ cup* | | 4.0 | 3.0 | 2.0 | | | 20 | | | 0.36 | | | 100 | | | | | BNJR5 |
| **frozen yogurt**, lowfat, choc fudge | 87 | 190 | | 35.0 | 23.0 | | 1.0 | 100 | 150 | | | | | 0 | | | | |
| brownie Ben & Jerry's - *½ cup* | | 5.0 | 2.5 | 1.5 | | | 15 | | | 1.80 | | | 0 | | | | | BNJR6 |
| **frozen yogurt**, nonfat w/low-cal | 72 | 77 | 52.9 | 14.2 | 9.1 | 0 | 0.7 | 58 | 114 | 29 | 0.35 | | 1 | 1 | 0.03 | 0.1 | 0.35 | |
| sweetener, choc - *½ cup* | | 3.2 | 0.6 | 0.4 | 0.2 | 0 | 3 | 244 | 93 | 0.03 | 0.146 | 2.0 | 12 | 0.1 | 0.13 | 0.03 | 8.6 | 42185 |
| **frozen yogurt**, soft serve, choc | 72 | 115 | 45.9 | 17.9 | | | 1.6 | 71 | 106 | 19 | 0.35 | 0.087 | 32 | 0 | 0.03 | 0.2 | 0.21 | 0.49 |
| *½ cup* | | 2.9 | 4.3 | 2.6 | 1.3 | 0.2 | 4 | 188 | 100 | 0.90 | 0.094 | 1.7 | 115 | | 0.15 | 0.05 | 7.9 | 19393 |
| **frozen yogurt**, soft serve, vanilla | 72 | 117 | 47.0 | 17.4 | 17.3 | 12.8 | 0 | 63 | 103 | 10 | 0.30 | 0.009 | 42 | 1 | 0.03 | 0.2 | 0.21 | 0.46 |
| *½ cup* | | 2.9 | 4.0 | 2.5 | 1.1 | 0.2 | 1 | 152 | 93 | 0.22 | 0.029 | 2.4 | 153 | 0.1 | 0.16 | 0.06 | 4.3 | 19293 |
| **frozen yogurt**, whole fat, chocolate | 72 | 91 | 51.3 | 15.6 | 15.4 | 11.4 | 0.9 | 45 | 72 | 18 | 0.20 | | 28 | 0 | 0.03 | 0.1 | 0.05 | |
| *½ cup* | | 2.2 | 2.6 | 1.6 | 0.7 | 0.1 | 9 | 168 | 64 | 0.33 | 0.039 | 1.4 | 98 | 0.1 | 0.13 | 0.03 | 8.6 | 42186 |
| **fruit and cream bar**, Breyers | 54 | 60 | | 12.0 | 12.0 | | 0 | 30 | 20 | | | | | 1 | | | | |
| Pure Fruit - *1.75 fl oz bar* | | 1.0 | 0.5 | 0 | | | 0 | | | 0 | | | 100 | | | | | BRYS31 |
| **fruit juice bar** | 92 | 80 | 72.0 | 18.6 | 16.1 | 0 | 0.9 | 4 | 5 | 4 | 0.05 | 0.152 | 1 | 9 | 0.01 | 0.1 | 0 | 0.04 |
| *3 fl oz bar* | | 1.1 | 0.1 | 0 | 0 | 0 | 0 | 49 | 6 | 0.17 | 0 | 0.2 | 17 | 0 | 0.02 | 0.02 | 6.4 | 19263 |
| **fruit juice bar**, coconut, | 123 | 150 | | 31.0 | 27.0 | | 1.0 | 45 | | | | | | | | | | |
| Breyers Pure Fruit - *4 fl oz* | | 0 | 2.5 | 2.0 | | | | | | | | | | | | | | BRYS9 |
| **fruit juice bar**, lime, Breyers | 123 | 110 | | 27.0 | 25.0 | | | 10 | | | | | | 5 | | | | |
| Pure Fruit - *4 fl oz bar* | | 0 | 0 | | | | | | | | | | | | | | | BRYS10 |
| **fruit juice bar**, pineapple, Breyers | 123 | 100 | | 26.0 | 25.0 | | | 5 | | | | | | 1 | | | | |
| Pure Fruit - *4 fl oz* | | 0 | 0 | | | | | | | | | | | | | | | BRYS8 |
| **fruit juice bar**, strawberry, Breyers | 123 | 100 | | 25.0 | 24.0 | | | 10 | | | | | | 9 | | | | |
| Pure Fruit - *4 fl oz* | | 0 | 0 | | | | 0 | | | | | | | | | | | BRYS7 |
| **fruit jce bar**, strawbry, trpcl, rspbry, | 54 | 25 | | 5.0 | 2.0 | | | 0 | | | | | | 1 | | | | |
| Breyers Pure Frt - *1.75 fl oz bar* | | 0 | 0 | | | | | | | | | | | | | | | BRYS30 |
| **fruit juice bar** with aspartame | 51 | 12 | 47.5 | 3.2 | | | 0 | 3 | 1 | 1 | 0.02 | 0.011 | 0 | 0 | 0 | 0.1 | 0 | 0 |
| *1 bar* | | 0.3 | 0.1 | 0 | | | 0 | 13 | 0 | 0.07 | 0.009 | 0.1 | 1 | 0 | 0 | 0 | 0 | 19217 |
| **fudge bar**, Breyers Carb Smart | 63 | 100 | | 9.0 | 3.0 | | 1.0 | 50 | 60 | | | | | 0 | | | | |
| *3 fl oz bar* | | 2.0 | 7.0 | 4.5 | | | 20 | | | 0.36 | | | 200 | | | | | BRYS37 |
| **fudge bar**, Klondike Slim-A-Bear | 74 | 92 | 47.0 | 22.3 | 5.3 | | 4.4 | 89 | 102 | | | | | 1 | | | | |
| *3.5 fl oz bar* | | 3.2 | 1.4 | 0.7 | | | 5 | | | 0.53 | | | 36 | | | | | 19874 |
| **Fudgesicle**, fat-free, Good Humor | 51 | 65 | 33.6 | 13.7 | 10.3 | | 0.9 | 48 | 81 | | | | | 1 | | | | |
| *1.75 fl oz bar* | | 2.8 | 0.3 | 0.2 | | | 2 | | | 0.46 | | | 2 | | | | | 19872 |
| **Fudgesicle**, no added sugar, | 84 | 88 | 60.4 | 18.7 | 3.3 | | 1.3 | 86 | 85 | 13 | 0.34 | 0.008 | 6 | 1 | 0.04 | 0.1 | 0.32 | |
| Good Humor - *1 pop* | | 3.0 | 0.8 | 0.5 | 0.1 | 0.1 | 2 | 165 | 89 | 0.79 | 0.015 | 2.4 | 21 | 0.3 | 0.15 | 0.04 | 4.2 | 19871 |
| **ice cream bar**, mangos 'n cream, | 79 | 120 | | 22.0 | 16.0 | | 1.0 | 45 | 80 | | | | | 2 | | | | |
| Goya - *3.75 fl oz bar* | | 3.0 | 3.0 | 2.0 | | | 10 | | | 0 | | | 500 | | | | | BRYS15 |
| **ice cream bar**, strawberries 'n | 79 | 100 | | 17.0 | 13.0 | | 0 | 40 | 80 | | | | | 9 | | | | |
| cream, Goya - *3.75 fl oz bar* | | 2.0 | 3.0 | 2.0 | | | 10 | | | 0 | | | 200 | | | | | BRYS14 |
| **ice cream bar**, van w/choc coating, | 54 | 170 | | 9.0 | 5.0 | | 2.0 | 45 | 350 | | | | | 0 | | | | |
| Breyers Carb Smart - *3 fl oz bar* | | 2.0 | 15.0 | 11.0 | | | 15 | | | 0 | | | 200 | | | | | BRYS36 |
| **ice cream bar**, van w/choc almond | 54 | 290 | | 24.0 | 20.0 | | 2.0 | 65 | 150 | | | | | 0 | | | | |
| coating, Breyers - *3 fl oz bar* | | 5.0 | 20.0 | 11.0 | | | 25 | | | 0.36 | | | 200 | | | | | BRYS12 |
| **ice cream bar**, van w/dark choc | 54 | 260 | | 25.0 | 21.0 | | 1.0 | 45 | 100 | | | | | 0 | | | | |
| coating, Breyers - *3 fl oz bar* | | 4.0 | 17.0 | 11.0 | | | 30 | | | 0 | | | 200 | | | | | BRYS13 |
| **ice cream**, black cherry, Turkey | 66 | 140 | | 18.0 | 16.0 | | 0 | 30 | 80 | | | | | 0 | | | | |
| Hill - *½ cup* | | 2.0 | 7.0 | 4.5 | | | 25 | | | 0 | | | 300 | | | | | TURK1 |
| **ice cream**, black raspberry choc, | 68 | 160 | | 20.0 | 19.0 | | 0 | 35 | 80 | | | | | 0 | | | | |
| Breyers - *½ cup* | | 2.0 | 7.0 | 4.5 | | | 20 | | | 0 | | | 200 | | | | | BRYS41 |

| | WT (g) | Macronutrients KCAL | $H_2O$ (g) | CHO (g) | TSUG (g) | ASUG (g) | DFIB (g) | Minerals Na (mg) | Ca (mg) | Mg (mg) | Zn (mg) | Mn (mg) | Vitamins A (mcg RAE) | C (mg) | B-1 (mg) | NIA (mg) | B-12 (mcg) | PANT (mg) |
|---|---|---|---|---|---|---|---|---|---|---|---|---|---|---|---|---|---|---|
| | | PRO (g) | FAT (g) | SFA (g) | MUFA (g) | PUFA (g) | CHOL (mg) | K (mg) | P (mg) | Fe (mg) | Cu (mg) | Se (mcg) | A (IU) | E (mg ATE) | B-2 (mg) | B-6 (mg) | FOL (mcg DFE) | REF |
| **ice cream**, brownie mud pie, | 68 | 140 | | 23.0 | 18.0 | | 1.0 | 95 | 80 | | | | | 0 | | | | |
| Breyers - *½ cup* | | 3.0 | 4.5 | 3.0 | | | 10 | | | 0.72 | | | 200 | | | | | BRYS26 |
| **ice cream**, butter pecan, Breyers All | 68 | 160 | | 14.0 | 14.0 | | 0 | 110 | 100 | | | | | 0 | | | | |
| Natural - *½ cup* | | 3.0 | 10.0 | 4.5 | | | 20 | | | 0 | | | 200 | | | | | BRYS22 |
| **ice cream cake**, choc chip w/choc cake, | 117 | 290 | | 41.0 | 28.0 | | 2.0 | 340 | 100 | | | | | 2 | | | | |
| Baskin Robbins - *4.1 oz slice* | | 4.0 | 15.0 | 6.0 | | | 40 | | | 1.08 | | | 300 | | | | | BSKN1 |
| **ice cream cake**, mint choc chip w/choc | 117 | 290 | | 36.0 | 28.0 | | 2.0 | 240 | 100 | | | | | 2 | | | | |
| cake, Baskin Robbins - *4.1 oz* | | 5.0 | 14.0 | 6.0 | | | 45 | | | 1.80 | | | 300 | | | | | BSKN2 |
| **ice cream cake**, van w/choc cake, | 117 | 270 | | 39.0 | 27.0 | | 2.0 | 340 | 100 | | | | | 1 | | | | |
| Baskin Robbins - *4.1 oz slice* | | 4.0 | 14.0 | 4.0 | | | 45 | | | 1.44 | | | 400 | | | | | BSKN3 |
| **ice cream**, cherry garcia, Ben & | 68 | 250 | | 26.0 | 22.0 | | | 50 | 150 | | | | | 0 | | | | |
| Jerry's - *½ cup* | | 4.0 | 14.0 | 10.0 | | | 60 | | | 0.72 | | | 500 | | | | | BNJR1 |
| **ice cream**, cherry vanilla, Breyers | 68 | 140 | | 17.0 | 16.0 | | 0 | 40 | 100 | | | | | 0 | | | | |
| *½ cup* | | 3.0 | 7.0 | 4.0 | | | 20 | | | 0 | | | 200 | | | | | BRYS39 |
| **ice cream**, chocolate | 66 | 143 | 36.8 | 18.6 | 16.7 | 14.4 | 0.8 | 50 | 72 | 19 | 0.38 | 0.092 | 78 | 0 | 0.03 | 0.1 | 0.19 | 0.37 |
| *½ cup* | | 2.5 | 7.3 | 4.5 | 2.1 | 0.3 | 22 | 164 | 71 | 0.61 | 0.089 | 1.6 | 275 | 0.2 | 0.13 | 0.04 | 10.6 | 19270 |
| **ice cream**, chocolate, 98% fat-free, | 68 | 92 | 43.0 | 20.5 | 13.8 | | 3.9 | 51 | 86 | | | | | 0 | | | | |
| Breyers - *½ cup* | | 2.6 | 1.5 | 0.9 | | | 5 | | | 0.57 | | | 173 | | | | | 19894 |
| **ice cream**, chocolate, Breyers Carb | 68 | 120 | | 10.0 | 4.0 | | 3.0 | 55 | 80 | | | | | 0 | | | | |
| Smart - *½ cup* | | 2.0 | 8.0 | 5.0 | | | 20 | | | 0.36 | | | 200 | | | | | BRYS29 |
| **ice cream**, chocolate chip, Breyers | 68 | 160 | | 17.0 | 17.0 | | 0 | 40 | 100 | | | | | 0 | | | | |
| *½ cup* | | 3.0 | 9.0 | 5.0 | | | 20 | | | 0 | | | 200 | | | | | BRYS40 |
| **ice cream**, chocolate chip cookie | 68 | 270 | | 32.0 | 24.0 | | 0 | 85 | 150 | | | | | 0 | | | | |
| dough, Ben & Jerry's - *½ cup* | | 4.0 | 15.0 | 10.0 | | | 65 | | | 0.72 | | | 500 | | | | | BNJR2 |
| **ice cream**, chocolate chip, Edy's | 65 | 170 | | 18.0 | 15.0 | | 0 | 45 | 60 | | | | | 0 | | | | |
| Grand - *½ cup* | | 3.0 | 9.0 | 6.0 | | | 25 | | | 0 | | | 400 | | | | | EDYS21 |
| **ice cream**, chocolate, extra creamy, | 68 | 120 | | 18.0 | 13.0 | | 1.0 | 55 | 100 | | | | | 0 | | | | |
| Breyers All Natural - *½ cup* | | 4.0 | 4.0 | 2.5 | | | 30 | | | 0.72 | | | 300 | | | | | BRYS21 |
| **ice cream**, chocolate, Goya | 68 | 130 | | 21.0 | 16.0 | | 1.0 | 50 | 100 | | | | | 0 | | | | |
| *½ cup* | | 3.0 | 4.0 | 2.5 | | | 10 | | | 0.72 | | | 300 | | | | | BRYS17 |
| **ice cream**, chocolate, light | 67 | 135 | 41.2 | 17.2 | 16.6 | 15.5 | 0.5 | 48 | 107 | 13 | 0.29 | 0.068 | 48 | 1 | 0.02 | 0.1 | 0.09 | 0.16 |
| *½ cup* | | 3.4 | 4.8 | 2.9 | 1.4 | 0.2 | 19 | 114 | 56 | 0.46 | 0.069 | 1.5 | 284 | 0.1 | 0.09 | 0.02 | 2.7 | 19114 |
| **ice cream**, chocolate, rich | 148 | 377 | 83.7 | 30.7 | 25.7 | 20.6 | 1.3 | 84 | 210 | 47 | 0.95 | 0.256 | 297 | 1 | 0.04 | 0.3 | 0.27 | 0.50 |
| *1 cup* | | 7.0 | 25.1 | 15.4 | 7.1 | 1.0 | 89 | 352 | 170 | 1.51 | 0.259 | 3.1 | 1055 | 0.7 | 0.25 | 0.05 | 7.4 | 43541 |
| **ice cream**, chunky monkey, Ben & | 68 | 300 | | 30.0 | 28.0 | | 1.0 | 45 | 150 | | | | | 1 | | | | |
| Jerry's - *½ cup* | | 5.0 | 18.0 | 10.0 | | | 55 | | | 0.72 | | | 500 | | | | | BNJR3 |
| **ice cream**, coffee, Breyers | 68 | 140 | | 15.0 | 15.0 | | 0 | 40 | 100 | | | | | 0 | | | | |
| *½ cup* | | 3.0 | 8.0 | 4.5 | | | 20 | | | 0 | | | 200 | | | | | BRYS38 |
| **ice cream**, coffee, Breyers All | 68 | 140 | | 15.0 | 15.0 | | 0 | 40 | 0 | | | | | 6 | | | | |
| Natural Organic - *½ cup* | | 4.0 | 7.0 | 4.5 | | | 25 | | | 0 | | | 0 | | | | | BRYS24 |
| **ice cream**, dulce de leche, | 68 | 130 | | 22.0 | 17.0 | | 0 | 105 | 100 | | | | | 0 | | | | |
| Goya - *½ cup* | | 3.0 | 3.0 | 2.0 | | | 10 | | | 0 | | | 200 | | | | | BRYS18 |
| **ice cream**, eggnog, Edys' Grand | 65 | 140 | | 18.0 | 15.0 | | 0 | 35 | 60 | | | | | 0 | | | | |
| *½ cup* | | 2.0 | 7.0 | 4.0 | | | 25 | | | 0 | | | 400 | | | | | EDYS22 |
| **ice cream**, French chocolate, fat- | 68 | 90 | | 22.0 | 13.0 | | 4.0 | 55 | 100 | | | | | 0 | | | | |
| free, Breyers - *½ cup* | | 3.0 | 0 | 0 | | | 0 | | | 0.72 | | | 200 | | | | | BRYS25 |
| **ice cream**, French chocolate, light, | 68 | 137 | 38.5 | 20.2 | 16.3 | | 0.7 | 51 | 107 | | | | | 1 | | | | |
| Breyers - *½ cup* | | 3.6 | 5.0 | 2.9 | | | 28 | | | 0.58 | | | 303 | | | | | 19893 |
| **ice cream**, French vanilla, light, | 68 | 118 | 42.6 | 17.7 | 14.4 | | 0.1 | 50 | 105 | | | | | 1 | | | | |
| Breyers - *½ cup* | | 3.3 | 3.8 | 2.2 | | | 36 | | | 0.14 | | | 333 | | | | | 19876 |
| **ice cream**, French vanilla, soft | 86 | 191 | 51.4 | 19.1 | 18.2 | 16.1 | 0.6 | 52 | 113 | 10 | 0.45 | 0.004 | 139 | 1 | 0.04 | 0.1 | 0.43 | 0.44 |
| serve - *½ cup* | | 3.5 | 11.2 | 6.4 | 3.0 | 0.4 | 78 | 152 | 100 | 0.18 | 0.026 | 2.6 | 507 | 0.5 | 0.16 | 0.04 | 7.7 | 19090 |
| **ice cream**, low/reduced calorie | 65 | 101 | 42.6 | 13.9 | 4.2 | 0 | 0.5 | 62 | 88 | 6 | 0.20 | 0.004 | 56 | 1 | 0.02 | 0 | 0.34 | 0.17 |
| with aspartame - *½ cup* | | 2.6 | 4.8 | 2.6 | 1.2 | 0.5 | 18 | 127 | 49 | 0.12 | 0.020 | 1.2 | 196 | 0.2 | 0.08 | 0.02 | 2.6 | 19260 |
| **ice cream**, mint chocolate chip, | 68 | 133 | 40.2 | 19.3 | 17.3 | | 0.4 | 46 | 109 | | | | | 1 | | | | |
| light, Breyers - *½ cup* | | 3.2 | 4.8 | 3.0 | | | 10 | | | 0.35 | | | 275 | | | | | 19879 |
| **ice cream**, Phish Food, Ben & | 68 | 280 | | 37.0 | 22.0 | | 1.0 | 85 | 100 | | | | | 0 | | | | |
| Jerry's - *½ cup* | | 4.0 | 13.0 | 9.0 | | | 30 | | | 1.80 | | | 400 | | | | | BNJR4 |
| **Ice Cream Poppers**, Heath, Breyers | 111 | 410 | | 32.0 | 31.0 | | 1.0 | 120 | 100 | | | | | 0 | | | | |
| *27 pieces* | | 3.0 | 30.0 | 21.0 | | | 20 | | | 0.72 | | | 200 | | | | | BRYS32 |
| **Ice Cream Poppers**, Hershey's, | 111 | 430 | | 31.0 | 27.0 | | 1.0 | 65 | 150 | | | | | 0 | | | | |
| Breyers - *27 pieces* | | 5.0 | 31.0 | 22.0 | | | 25 | | | 0.36 | | | 200 | | | | | BRYS33 |

| | WT (g) | KCAL | H₂O (g) | CHO (g) | TSUG (g) | ASUG (g) | DFIB (g) | Na (mg) | Ca (mg) | Mg (mg) | Zn (mg) | Mn (mg) | A (mcg RAE) | C (mg) | B-1 (mg) | NIA (mg) | B-12 (mcg) | PANT (mg) |
|---|---|---|---|---|---|---|---|---|---|---|---|---|---|---|---|---|---|---|
| | PRO (g) | FAT (g) | SFA (g) | MUFA (g) | PUFA (g) | CHOL (mg) | | K (mg) | P (mg) | Fe (mg) | Cu (mg) | Se (mcg) | A (IU) | E (mg ATE) | B-2 (mg) | B-6 (mg) | FOL (mcg DFE) | REF |
| **Ice Cream Poppers**, Oreo, Breyers | 111 | 410 | | 38.0 | 28.0 | | 1.0 | 190 | 80 | | | | | 0 | | | | |
| *27 pieces* | 4.0 | 27.0 | 18.0 | | | 15 | | | | 1.80 | | | 200 | | | | | BRYS34 |
| **Ice Cream Poppers**, Reese's Pnt | 111 | 470 | | 35.0 | 31.0 | | 1.0 | 110 | 100 | | | | | 0 | | | | |
| Butter Cup, Breyers - *27 pieces* | 5.0 | 34.0 | 23.0 | | | 20 | | | | 0 | | | 200 | | | | | BRYS35 |
| **ice cream**, rocky road, Breyers All | 68 | 160 | | 19.0 | 17.0 | | 1.0 | 65 | 80 | | | | | 0 | | | | |
| Natural - *½ cup* | 3.0 | 9.0 | 5.0 | | | 20 | | | | 0.72 | | | 200 | | | | | BRYS23 |
| **ice cream sandwich**, choc, Klondike | 64 | 136 | 29.8 | 28.2 | 13.8 | | 3.1 | 120 | 92 | | | | | 0 | | | | |
| Slim-A-Bear - *2.3 oz* | 4.0 | 1.6 | 0.5 | | | 3 | | | | 0.63 | | | 242 | | | | | 19888 |
| **ice cream sandwich**, mint, Klondike | 64 | 134 | 29.9 | 28.3 | 14.0 | | 2.8 | 122 | 91 | | | | | 0 | | | | |
| Slim-A-Bear - *2.3 oz* | 3.8 | 1.5 | 0.5 | | | 3 | | | | 0.24 | | | 184 | | | | | 19889 |
| **ice cream sandwich**, van, Klondike | 64 | 135 | 29.9 | 28.3 | 14.0 | | 2.8 | 122 | 91 | | | | | 0 | | | | |
| Slim-A-Bear - *2.3 oz* | 3.8 | 1.5 | 0.5 | | | 3 | | | | 0.24 | | | 184 | | | | | 19887 |
| **ice cream sandwich**, van w/choc | 198 | 460 | | 68.0 | 41.0 | | 1.0 | 300 | 80 | | | | | 0 | | | | |
| chip cookies, Mrs. Fields - *7 oz* | 5.0 | 19.0 | 11.0 | | | 20 | | | | 1.80 | | | 200 | | | | | BRYS11 |
| **ice cream**, spumoni, Edy's Grand | 65 | 150 | | 16.0 | 13.0 | | 0 | 40 | 60 | | | | | 0 | | | | |
| *½ cup* | 3.0 | 8.0 | 4.5 | | | 25 | | | | 0 | | | 400 | | | | | EDYS23 |
| **ice cream**, spumoni, Safeway | 67 | 150 | | 16.0 | 12.0 | | | 40 | 80 | | | | | 0 | | | | |
| Select - *½ cup* | 2.0 | 9.0 | 5.0 | | | 30 | | | | 0 | | | 300 | | | | | SAFE49 |
| **ice cream**, strawberry | 66 | 127 | 39.6 | 18.2 | | | 0.6 | 40 | 79 | 9 | 0.22 | 0.051 | 63 | 5 | 0.03 | 0.1 | 0.20 | 0.48 |
| *½ cup* | 2.1 | 5.5 | 3.4 | | | 19 | | 124 | 66 | 0.14 | 0.024 | 1.3 | 211 | | 0.17 | 0.03 | 7.9 | 19271 |
| **ice cream sundae**, caramel, Carvel | 377 | 900 | | 109.0 | 81.0 | | 0 | 490 | 400 | | | | | 4 | | | | |
| *large* | 10.0 | 45.0 | 31.0 | | | 200 | | | | 0 | | | 1750 | | | | | CRVL3 |
| **ice cream sundae**, hot fudge, | 402 | 900 | | 99.0 | 84.0 | | 2.0 | 380 | 350 | | | | | 4 | | | | |
| Carvel - *large* | 11.0 | 50.0 | 32.0 | | | 195 | | | | 0 | | | 1750 | | | | | CRVL1 |
| **ice cream sundae**, strawberry, | 358 | 770 | | 86.0 | 73.0 | | 1.0 | 300 | 350 | | | | | 27 | | | | |
| Carvel - *large* | 10.0 | 43.0 | 29.0 | | | 195 | | | | 0.36 | | | 1750 | | | | | CRVL2 |
| **ice cream sundae, tin roof**, Breyers | 68 | 150 | | 21.0 | 15.0 | | 1.0 | 90 | 80 | | | | | 0 | | | | |
| *½ cup* | 3.0 | 6.0 | 3.5 | | | 10 | | | | 0 | | | 200 | | | | | BRYS27 |
| **ice cream**, triple chocolate, Breyers | 68 | 150 | | 17.0 | 15.0 | | 1.0 | 60 | 80 | | | | | 0 | | | | |
| All Natural - *½ cup* | 3.0 | 8.0 | 4.5 | | | 20 | | | | 1.08 | | | 200 | | | | | BRYS19 |
| **ice cream**, vanilla, 98% fat-free, | 68 | 93 | 43.1 | 20.7 | 14.2 | | 3.7 | 50 | 83 | | | | | 1 | | | | |
| Breyers - *½ cup* | 2.2 | 1.5 | 1.0 | | | 5 | | | | 0.06 | | | 182 | | | | | 19877 |
| **ice cream**, vanilla, Breyers Carb | 68 | 110 | | 10.0 | 4.0 | | 3.0 | 30 | 90 | | | | | 0 | | | | |
| Smart - *½ cup* | 2.0 | 8.0 | 5.0 | | | 20 | | | | 0 | | | 200 | | | | | BRYS28 |
| **ice cream**, vanilla, chocolate, and strawberry, light, Breyers | 68 | 109 | 43.1 | 17.7 | 15.3 | | 0.3 | 47 | 107 | | | | | 1 | | | | |
| *½ cup* | 3.2 | 3.0 | 1.8 | | | 10 | | | | 0.21 | | | 284 | | | | | 19878 |
| **ice cream**, vanilla, extra creamy, | 68 | 120 | | 17.0 | 14.0 | | 0 | 50 | 100 | | | | | 0 | | | | |
| Breyers All Natural - *½ cup* | 3.0 | 4.0 | 2.0 | | | 30 | | | | 0 | | | 300 | | | | | BRYS20 |
| **ice cream**, vanilla, fat-free | 68 | 94 | 43.8 | 20.4 | 4.3 | 2.6 | 0.7 | 66 | 101 | 14 | 0.72 | | 136 | 0 | 0.03 | 0.1 | 0.31 | |
| *½ cup* | 3.0 | 0 | 0 | 0 | 0 | 0 | 205 | 102 | 0 | 0.019 | 2.0 | 475 | 0 | 0.17 | 0.03 | 4.8 | 19867 |
| **ice cream**, vanilla, fat-free, | 68 | 90 | | 21.0 | 21.0 | | | 50 | 100 | | | | | 0 | | | | |
| Breyers - *½ cup* | 3.0 | 0 | 0 | | | 0 | | | | 0 | | | 300 | | | | | BRYS2 |
| **ice cream**, vanilla, Goya | 68 | 120 | | 18.0 | 13.0 | | 0 | 50 | 100 | | | | | 0 | | | | |
| *½ cup* | 3.0 | 3.5 | 2.5 | | | 10 | | | | 0 | | | 300 | | | | | BRYS16 |
| **ice cream**, vanilla, light, Breyers | 68 | 110 | 44.1 | 17.2 | 15.5 | | 0.1 | 48 | 115 | | | | | 1 | | | | |
| *½ cup* | 3.3 | 3.1 | 1.9 | | | 10 | | | | 0.04 | | | 297 | | | | | 19875 |
| **ice cream**, vanilla, low/reduced cal (½ the fat) - *½ cup* | 66 | 109 | 41.9 | 17.0 | 14.6 | | 0.2 | 49 | 106 | 9 | 0.48 | 0.003 | 84 | 1 | 0.03 | 0.1 | 0.31 | 0.32 |
| | 3.2 | 3.2 | 1.9 | 0.8 | 0.1 | 18 | 137 | 68 | 0.13 | 0.011 | 1.3 | 296 | 0.1 | 0.17 | 0.03 | 4.0 | 19088 |
| **ice cream**, vanilla, low/reduced cal (½ the fat), soft serve - *½ cup* | 88 | 111 | 61.2 | 19.2 | 9.5 | 5.7 | 0 | 62 | 138 | 12 | 0.47 | 0.007 | 26 | 1 | 0.05 | 0.1 | 0.44 | 0.39 |
| | 4.3 | 2.3 | 1.4 | 0.7 | 0.1 | 11 | 194 | 106 | 0.05 | 0.024 | 3.2 | 91 | 0.1 | 0.17 | 0.04 | 4.4 | 19096 |
| **ice cream**, vanilla, regular (10% fat) - *½ cup* | 66 | 137 | 40.3 | 15.6 | 14.0 | 12.0 | 0.5 | 53 | 84 | 9 | 0.46 | 0.005 | 78 | 0 | 0.03 | 0.1 | 0.26 | 0.38 |
| | 2.3 | 7.3 | 4.5 | 2.0 | 0.3 | 29 | 131 | 69 | 0.06 | 0.015 | 1.2 | 278 | 0.2 | 0.16 | 0.03 | 3.3 | 19095 |
| **ice cream**, vanilla, rich (16% fat) | 107 | 266 | 61.2 | 23.9 | 22.1 | 18.4 | 0 | 65 | 125 | 12 | 0.50 | 0.004 | 195 | 0 | 0.04 | 0.1 | 0.42 | 0.49 |
| *½ cup* | 3.7 | 17.3 | 11.1 | 4.8 | 0.7 | 98 | 168 | 112 | 0.36 | 0.009 | 3.7 | 699 | 0.5 | 0.18 | 0.05 | 8.6 | 19089 |
| **ice pop** | 59 | 47 | 47.5 | 11.3 | 8.1 | 7.9 | 0 | 4 | 0 | 1 | 0.09 | 0 | 0 | 0 | 0 | 0 | 0 | 0 |
| *2 fl oz bar* | 0 | 0.1 | 0 | 0 | 0 | 0 | 9 | 0 | 0.32 | 0 | 0.1 | 0 | 0 | 0 | 0 | 0 | 19283 |
| **ice pop** with low-calorie | 55 | 13 | 51.7 | 3.3 | 0.8 | 0.2 | 0 | 6 | 0 | 1 | 0.26 | 0 | 0 | 6 | 0 | 0 | 0 | 0 |
| sweetener - *1.75 fl oz pop* | 0 | 0 | 0 | 0 | 0 | 0 | 6 | 0 | 0.37 | 0 | 0 | 0 | 0 | 0 | 0 | 0 | 43514 |
| **Italian ice**, from restaurant | 116 | 61 | 100.2 | 15.7 | | | 0 | 5 | 1 | 1 | 0.03 | 0.023 | | 1 | 0.01 | 0.8 | 0 | 0.01 |
| *½ cup* | 0 | 0 | 0 | 0 | 0 | 0 | 7 | 0 | 0.10 | 0.012 | 0.1 | 194 | | 0.01 | | 5.8 | 19281 |
| **lime ice** | 99 | 127 | 66.2 | 32.3 | 32.3 | 32.3 | 0 | 22 | 2 | 1 | 0.02 | 0.020 | 0 | 1 | 0 | 0 | 0 | 0 |
| *½ cup* | 0.4 | 0 | 0 | 0 | 0 | 0 | 3 | 1 | 0.16 | 0.013 | 0.1 | 0 | 0 | 0 | 0 | 0 | 19280 |

| | WT (g) | KCAL / PRO (g) | H2O (g) / FAT (g) | CHO (g) / SFA (g) | TSUG (g) / MUFA (g) | ASUG (g) / PUFA (g) | DFIB (g) / CHOL (mg) | Na (mg) / K (mg) | Ca (mg) / P (mg) | Mg (mg) / Fe (mg) | Zn (mg) / Cu (mg) | Mn (mg) / Se (mcg) | A (mcg RAE) / A (IU) | C (mg) / E (mg ATE) | B-1 (mg) / B-2 (mg) | NIA (mg) / B-6 (mg) | B-12 (mcg) / FOL (mcg DFE) | PANT (mg) / REF |
|---|---|---|---|---|---|---|---|---|---|---|---|---|---|---|---|---|---|---|
| orange juice bar | 74 | 70 | 56.3 | 17.1 | 14.8 | 0 | 0.1 | 6 | 7 | 6 | 0.01 | 0.006 | 1 | 19 | 0.01 | 0.1 | 0 | 0.05 |
| *1 bar* | | 0.4 | 0 | 0 | 0 | 0 | 0 | 74 | 10 | 0.35 | 0.016 | 0.1 | 16 | 0 | 0.02 | 0.01 | 13.3 | 43346 |
| **pineapple coconut ice** | 99 | 112 | 72.6 | 23.7 | | | 0.7 | 35 | 0 | 5 | 0.11 | 0.159 | 0 | 13 | 0.01 | 0 | 0 | 0.04 |
| *½ cup* | | 0 | 2.6 | 2.3 | 0.1 | 0 | 0 | 17 | 9 | 3.49 | 0.044 | 0.9 | 0 | 0 | 0.02 | 1.0 | | 19387 |
| **popsicle**, cherry/grape, sgr free, | 55 | 12 | 51.7 | 2.8 | 0.8 | | 0 | 6 | 0 | 1 | 0.26 | 0 | | 6 | | | | |
| Good Humor - *1.75 fl oz bar* | | 0 | 0 | 0 | 0 | | 0 | 6 | 0 | 0.37 | | | 0 | | | | | 19873 |
| **praline caramel frozen dessert**, | 71 | 121 | 42.7 | 22.9 | 18.7 | | 0.7 | 63 | 94 | | | | | 0 | | | | |
| low fat, Hlthy Chc - *½ cup* | | 2.6 | 2.1 | 1.0 | 0.8 | 0.3 | 5 | | | | 0.05 | | 377 | | | | | 19259 |
| **sherbet**, berry patch, Safeway | 89 | 140 | | 29.0 | 22.0 | | 0 | 30 | 40 | | | | | 1 | | | | |
| Select - *½ cup* | | 1.0 | 1.5 | 1.0 | | | 5 | | | 0 | | | 0 | | | | | SAFE54 |
| **sherbet**, orange | 74 | 107 | 48.9 | 22.5 | 18.0 | 15.4 | 1.0 | 34 | 40 | 6 | 0.36 | 0.008 | 9 | 2 | 0.02 | 0 | 0.10 | 0.17 |
| *½ cup* | | 0.8 | 1.5 | 0.9 | 0.4 | 0.1 | 1 | 71 | 30 | 0.10 | 0.021 | 1.1 | 34 | 0 | 0.07 | 0.02 | 3.0 | 19097 |
| **sorbet**, Jamaican Me Crazy, | 97 | 130 | | 33.0 | 28.0 | | 4.0 | 10 | 0 | | | | | 4 | | | | |
| Ben & Jerry's - *½ cup* | | 0 | 0 | 0 | | | 0 | | | 0 | | | 100 | | | | | BNJR7 |
| **sorbet**, strawberry kiwi swirl, | 97 | 110 | | 28.0 | 24.0 | | 1.0 | 10 | 0 | | | | | 5 | | | | |
| Ben & Jerry's - *½ cup* | | 0 | 0 | 0 | | | 0 | | | 0 | | | 0 | | | | | BNJR8 |

## 7.6 GELATIN DESSERTS

| | WT (g) | KCAL / PRO (g) | H2O (g) / FAT (g) | CHO (g) / SFA (g) | TSUG (g) / MUFA (g) | ASUG (g) / PUFA (g) | DFIB (g) / CHOL (mg) | Na (mg) / K (mg) | Ca (mg) / P (mg) | Mg (mg) / Fe (mg) | Zn (mg) / Cu (mg) | Mn (mg) / Se (mcg) | A (mcg RAE) / A (IU) | C (mg) / E (mg ATE) | B-1 (mg) / B-2 (mg) | NIA (mg) / B-6 (mg) | B-12 (mcg) / FOL (mcg DFE) | PANT (mg) / REF |
|---|---|---|---|---|---|---|---|---|---|---|---|---|---|---|---|---|---|---|
| **gelatin dessert**, from mix | 117 | 23 | 110.8 | 4.9 | 0 | 0 | 0 | 56 | 4 | 1 | 0 | 0 | 0 | 0 | 0 | 0 | 0 | 0 |
| w/aspartame, all flvrs - *½ cup* | | 1.0 | 0 | 0 | 0 | 0 | 0 | 1 | 80 | 0.01 | 0.008 | 0 | 0 | 0 | 0 | 0 | 0 | 19176 |
| **gelatin dessert**, from mix with | 135 | 84 | 113.9 | 19.2 | 18.2 | 18.2 | 0 | 101 | 4 | 1 | 0.01 | 0.003 | 0 | 0 | 0 | 0 | 0 | 0 |
| sugar, all flavors - *½ cup* | | 1.6 | 0 | 0 | 0 | 0 | 0 | 1 | 30 | 0.03 | 0.032 | 1.5 | 0 | 0 | 0.01 | 0 | 1.4 | 19173 |
| **gelatin dessert mix**, cherry, sgr-free, | 2.5 | 10 | 0 | 0 | 0 | | 0 | 65 | 0 | | | | | 0 | | | | |
| Safeway - *¼ pkg (makes ½ cup)* | | 1.0 | 0 | 0 | | | 0 | | | 0 | | | 0 | | | | | SAFE46 |
| **gelatin dessert mix**, rasp, sgr-free, | 2.5 | 5 | 0 | 0 | 0 | | 0 | 30 | 0 | | | | | 0 | | | | |
| Safeway - *¼ pkg (makes ½ cup)* | | 1.0 | 0 | 0 | | | 0 | | | 0 | | | 0 | | | | | SAFE47 |
| **gelatin dessert mix** with aspartame, | 10 | 34 | 0.7 | 3.3 | | | 0 | 16 | 0 | 0 | 0.01 | 0.005 | 0 | 0 | 0 | 0 | 0 | 0.01 |
| all flvrs - *.35 oz packet* | | 5.5 | 0 | 0 | | | 0 | 1 | 129 | 0 | 0.102 | 2.6 | 0 | | 0.01 | 0 | 1.4 | 19704 |
| **gelatin dessert mix** with sugar, | 85 | 324 | 0.8 | 76.9 | 73.1 | 73.1 | 0 | 396 | 3 | 2 | 0.01 | 0.009 | 0 | 0 | 0 | 0 | 0 | 0.01 |
| all flavors - *3 oz packet* | | 6.6 | 0 | 0 | 0 | 0 | 0 | 6 | 120 | 0.11 | 0.100 | 5.7 | 0 | 0 | 0.03 | 0 | 2.6 | 19172 |

## 7.7 PASTRIES, SWEET ROLLS, COBBLERS, STRUDELS, AND TURNOVERS

| | WT (g) | KCAL / PRO (g) | H2O (g) / FAT (g) | CHO (g) / SFA (g) | TSUG (g) / MUFA (g) | ASUG (g) / PUFA (g) | DFIB (g) / CHOL (mg) | Na (mg) / K (mg) | Ca (mg) / P (mg) | Mg (mg) / Fe (mg) | Zn (mg) / Cu (mg) | Mn (mg) / Se (mcg) | A (mcg RAE) / A (IU) | C (mg) / E (mg ATE) | B-1 (mg) / B-2 (mg) | NIA (mg) / B-6 (mg) | B-12 (mcg) / FOL (mcg DFE) | PANT (mg) / REF |
|---|---|---|---|---|---|---|---|---|---|---|---|---|---|---|---|---|---|---|
| **apple crisp**, homemade | 141 | 227 | 88.7 | 43.5 | 27.7 | | 2.0 | 495 | 49 | 11 | 0.25 | 0.183 | 41 | 3 | 0.12 | 1.2 | 0 | 0.13 |
| *½ cup* | | 2.5 | 4.8 | 1.0 | 1.9 | 1.6 | 0 | 110 | 39 | 1.16 | 0.100 | 4.9 | 200 | 0.5 | 0.11 | 0.06 | 33.8 | 19186 |
| **apple strudel** | 71 | 195 | 30.9 | 29.2 | 18.3 | 14.3 | 1.6 | 191 | 11 | 6 | 0.13 | 0.135 | 4 | 1 | 0.03 | 0.2 | 0.16 | 0.19 |
| *2.5 oz piece* | | 2.3 | 8.0 | 1.5 | 2.3 | 3.8 | 4 | 106 | 23 | 0.30 | 0.021 | 4.3 | 21 | 1.0 | 0.02 | 0.03 | 30.5 | 18354 |
| **apple turnover**, from refrig dough, | 57 | 180 | | 24.0 | 12.0 | | 0 | 260 | 0 | | | | | 0 | | | | |
| Pillsbury - *2 oz turnover* | | 2.0 | 8.0 | 2.0 | | | 0 | | | | 0.72 | | 0 | | | | | GENM105 |
| **apple turnover**, frozen, Pepperidge | 89 | 284 | 37.3 | 31.2 | 10.8 | | 1.6 | 176 | | | | | | | | | | |
| Farm - *3.1 oz turnover* | | 3.7 | 16.0 | 4.0 | | | | | | | 1.22 | | | | | | | 18628 |
| **cherry turnover**, from refrig dough, | 57 | 180 | | 24.0 | 12.0 | | 0 | 250 | 0 | | | | | 0 | | | | |
| Pillsbury - *2 oz turnover* | | 2.0 | 8.0 | 2.0 | | | 0 | | | | 0.72 | | 0 | | | | | GENM106 |
| **cinnamon bun**, Krispy Kreme | 67 | 260 | | 28.0 | 13.0 | | | 125 | 80 | | | | | 1 | | | | |
| *2.4 oz bun* | | 3.0 | 16.0 | 4.0 | | | 5 | | | | 1.08 | | 0 | | | | | KRIS18 |
| **cinnamon roll minis**, Eggo Toaster | 47 | 120 | | 20.0 | 6.0 | | | 200 | 40 | | | | | 0 | 0.15 | 2.0 | 0.60 | |
| Swirlz, Kelloggs - *1.7 oz roll* | | 2.0 | 3.0 | 0.5 | | | 5 | 25 | 100 | 1.80 | | | 500 | | 0.17 | 0.20 | | KELL8 |
| **cream puff shell**, homemade | 66 | 239 | 26.7 | 15.0 | 0.3 | 0 | 0.5 | 368 | 24 | 8 | 0.48 | 0.139 | 183 | 0 | 0.14 | 1.0 | 0.26 | 0.41 |
| *1 shell* | | 5.9 | 17.1 | 7.3 | 4.9 | 0.5 | 129 | 64 | 79 | 1.33 | 0.034 | 15.8 | 765 | 1.9 | 0.24 | 0.05 | 49.5 | 18237 |
| **cream puff with custard filling**, | 130 | 335 | 69.6 | 29.8 | 12.3 | 9.6 | 0.5 | 443 | 86 | 16 | 0.78 | 0.146 | 185 | 0 | 0.16 | 1.1 | 0.47 | 0.67 |
| homemade - *1 cream puff* | | 8.7 | 20.2 | 4.8 | 8.5 | 5.4 | 174 | 150 | 142 | 1.52 | 0.046 | 20.0 | 768 | 1.9 | 0.36 | 0.08 | 67.6 | 18238 |
| **croissant** | 57 | 231 | 13.2 | 26.1 | 6.4 | 5.6 | 1.5 | 424 | 21 | 9 | 0.43 | 0.188 | 117 | 0 | 0.22 | 1.2 | 0.09 | 0.49 |
| *1 medium croissant* | | 4.7 | 12.0 | 6.6 | 3.1 | 0.6 | 38 | 67 | 60 | 1.16 | 0.046 | 12.9 | 424 | 0.5 | 0.14 | 0.03 | 74.1 | 18239 |
| **croissant**, apple | 57 | 145 | 26.0 | 21.1 | | | 1.4 | 156 | 17 | 7 | 0.59 | 0.120 | 54 | 0 | 0.13 | 0.9 | 0.11 | 0.34 |
| *1 medium croissant* | | 4.2 | 5.0 | 2.8 | 1.4 | 0.4 | 18 | 51 | 33 | 0.63 | 0.023 | 10.8 | 217 | | 0.09 | 0.02 | 50.2 | 18240 |
| **croissant**, cheese | 57 | 236 | 12.0 | 26.8 | 6.5 | 6.0 | 1.5 | 316 | 30 | 14 | 0.54 | 0.194 | 116 | 0 | 0.30 | 1.2 | 0.18 | 0.48 |
| *1 medium croissant* | | 5.2 | 11.9 | 6.1 | 3.7 | 1.4 | 32 | 75 | 74 | 1.23 | 0.057 | 15.3 | 459 | 0.8 | 0.19 | 0.04 | 58.7 | 18241 |
| **Danish pastry**, cinnamon | 65 | 262 | 15.8 | 29.0 | 12.9 | 11.7 | 0.8 | 241 | 46 | 12 | 0.47 | 0.235 | 4 | 0 | 0.20 | 1.9 | 0.06 | 0.26 |
| *1 pastry (4¼″ diameter)* | | 4.6 | 14.6 | 3.7 | 8.1 | 1.9 | 14 | 81 | 70 | 1.27 | 0.065 | 11.0 | 16 | 0.3 | 0.17 | 0.02 | 59.8 | 18244 |
| **Danish pastry**, cream/neufchatel | 71 | 266 | 22.3 | 26.4 | 4.9 | 3.4 | 0.7 | 320 | 25 | 11 | 0.50 | 0.249 | 25 | 0 | 0.13 | 1.4 | 0.12 | 0.22 |
| cheese - *1 pastry (4¼″ diameter)* | | 5.7 | 15.5 | 4.8 | 8.0 | 1.8 | 11 | 70 | 77 | 1.14 | 0.063 | 13.4 | 91 | 0.2 | 0.18 | 0.03 | 60.4 | 18245 |
| **Danish pastry**, fruit | 71 | 263 | 19.2 | 33.9 | 19.5 | 13.6 | 1.3 | 251 | 33 | 11 | 0.38 | 0.180 | 11 | 3 | 0.19 | 1.4 | 0.06 | 0.45 |
| *1 pastry (4¼″ diameter)* | | 3.8 | 13.1 | 3.5 | 7.1 | 1.7 | 81 | 59 | 63 | 1.26 | 0.046 | 10.5 | 36 | 0.2 | 0.16 | 0.03 | 49.0 | 18246 |

| Food | WT (g) | KCAL | H₂0 (g) | CHO (g) | TSUG (g) | ASUG (g) | DFIB (g) | Na (mg) | Ca (mg) | Mg (mg) | Zn (mg) | Mn (mg) | A (mcg RAE) | C (mg) | B-1 (mg) | NIA (mg) | B-12 (mcg) | PANT (mg) |
|---|---|---|---|---|---|---|---|---|---|---|---|---|---|---|---|---|---|---|
| | | PRO (g) | FAT (g) | SFA (g) | MUFA (g) | PUFA (g) | CHOL (mg) | K (mg) | P (mg) | Fe (mg) | Cu (mg) | Se (mcg) | A (IU) | E (mg ATE) | B-2 (mg) | B-6 (mg) | FOL (mcg DFE) | REF |
| **Danish pastry**, lemon | 71 | 263 | 19.2 | 33.9 | | | 1.3 | 251 | 33 | 11 | 0.38 | 0.180 | 38 | 3 | 0.05 | 0.5 | 0.06 | 0.45 |
| *1 pastry (4¼″ diameter)* | | 3.8 | 13.1 | 2.0 | 4.2 | 1.1 | 28 | 59 | 63 | 0.53 | 0.046 | | 124 | | 0.07 | 0.03 | 11.4 | 18433 |
| **Danish pastry**, nut | 65 | 280 | 13.3 | 29.7 | 16.8 | 15.2 | 1.3 | 236 | 61 | 21 | 0.57 | 0.549 | 6 | 1 | 0.14 | 1.5 | 0.14 | 0.46 |
| *1 pastry (4¼″ diameter)* | | 4.6 | 16.4 | 3.8 | 8.9 | 2.8 | 30 | 62 | 72 | 1.17 | 0.127 | 9.2 | 23 | 0.5 | 0.16 | 0.07 | 79.3 | 18247 |
| **Danish pastry**, raspberry | 71 | 263 | 19.2 | 33.9 | | | 1.3 | 251 | 33 | 11 | 0.38 | 0.180 | 43 | 3 | 0.05 | 0.5 | 0.06 | 0.45 |
| *1 pastry (4¼″ diameter)* | | 3.8 | 13.1 | 2.0 | 4.2 | 1.1 | 28 | 59 | 63 | 0.53 | 0.046 | | 142 | | 0.07 | 0.03 | 11.4 | 18435 |
| **éclair** w/custard filling, choc glaze, frzn, Wt Wtchrs -*1 éclair* | 59 | 142 | 27.9 | 23.8 | 9.9 | | 1.2 | 177 | 28 | | | | | 0 | | | | |
| | | 2.6 | 4.1 | 0.8 | 1.2 | 1.7 | 28 | | | 0.41 | | | 44 | | | | | 18640 |
| **éclair** w/custard filling, choc glaze, homemade - *1 éclair (5″ long)* | 100 | 262 | 52.4 | 24.2 | 6.6 | 5.4 | 0.6 | 337 | 63 | 15 | 0.61 | 0.128 | 199 | 0 | 0.12 | 0.8 | 0.34 | 0.49 |
| | | 6.4 | 15.7 | 4.1 | 6.5 | 3.9 | 127 | 117 | 107 | 1.18 | 0.058 | 15.6 | 828 | 2.0 | 0.27 | 0.06 | 63.0 | 18257 |
| **honey bun**, glazed, Tastykake | 78 | 330 | | 39.0 | 19.0 | | | 220 | 80 | | | | | | | | | |
| *1 bun* | | 3.0 | 18.0 | 4.0 | | | 0 | | | 1.44 | | | 0 | 2 | | | | TAST10 |
| **honey bun**, iced, Tastykake | 92 | 400 | | 46.0 | 21.0 | | 1.0 | 260 | 60 | | | | | | | | | |
| *1 bun* | | 4.0 | 22.0 | 5.0 | | | 0 | | | 1.44 | | | 0 | 4 | | | | TAST11 |
| **puff pastry**, frozen | 40 | 223 | 3.0 | 18.3 | 0.3 | 0 | 0.6 | 101 | 4 | 6 | 0.22 | 0.198 | 0 | 0 | 0.13 | 1.5 | 0 | 0 |
| *1 pastry* | | 3.0 | 15.4 | 2.2 | 3.5 | 8.9 | 0 | 25 | 24 | 1.04 | 0.046 | 9.8 | 0 | 0.2 | 0.10 | 0.01 | 34.8 | 18211 |
| **sweet roll**, caramel, from refrig dough, Pillsbury - *1.7 oz roll* | 49 | 170 | | 24.0 | 10.0 | | 0.5 | 320 | 0 | | | | 0 | | | | | |
| | | 2.0 | 7.0 | 1.5 | | | 0 | | | 1.08 | | | 0 | | | | | GENM107 |
| **sweet roll**, cheese (cream/neufchatel) - *1 roll* | 66 | 238 | 19.4 | 28.8 | | | 0.8 | 236 | 78 | 13 | 0.42 | 0.139 | | 0 | 0.10 | 0.5 | 0.20 | 0.27 |
| | | 4.7 | 12.1 | 4.0 | 6.0 | 1.3 | 50 | 90 | 65 | 0.50 | 0.063 | 7.9 | 168 | | 0.09 | 0.05 | 33.7 | 18355 |
| **sweet roll**, cinn w/crm chs icing, from rfrg dgh, Pillsbury - *1.6 oz roll* | 44 | 150 | | 23.0 | 10.0 | | 0.5 | 340 | 0 | | | | 0 | | | | | |
| | | 2.0 | 5.0 | 1.5 | | | 0 | | | 0.72 | | | 0 | | | | | GENM111 |
| **sweet roll**, cinn w/icing, from refrig dough, Pillsbury - *1 roll* | 44 | 145 | 12.3 | 23.0 | 10.0 | | 0.5 | 340 | | | | | | | | | | |
| | | 2.0 | 5.0 | 1.5 | | | 0 | | | 0.72 | | | 0 | | | | | 18635 |
| **sweet roll**, cinn w/icing, red fat, from rfrg dgh, Pillsbury - *1.6 oz roll* | 44 | 140 | | 24.0 | 10.0 | | 0.5 | 340 | 0 | | | | 0 | | | | | |
| | | 2.0 | 3.5 | 2.5 | 0.5 | 0 | 0 | | | 0.72 | | | 0 | | | | | GENM115 |
| **sweet roll**, cinnamon raisin | 60 | 223 | 14.9 | 30.5 | 19.0 | 16.2 | 1.4 | 230 | 43 | 10 | 0.35 | 0.180 | 37 | 1 | 0.19 | 1.4 | 0.08 | 0.24 |
| *1 roll* | | 3.7 | 9.8 | 1.8 | 2.9 | 4.5 | 40 | 67 | 46 | 0.96 | 0.053 | 10.2 | 128 | 1.2 | 0.16 | 0.06 | 63.6 | 18356 |
| **sweet roll**, cinnamon with icing, from refrig dough - *1 roll* | 30 | 109 | 6.8 | 16.8 | | | | 250 | 10 | 4 | 0.10 | 0.125 | 0 | 0 | 0.12 | 1.1 | 0.02 | 0.08 |
| | | 1.6 | 4.0 | 1.0 | 2.2 | 0.5 | 0 | 19 | 104 | 0.80 | 0.021 | 5.3 | 1 | | 0.07 | 0.01 | 26.7 | 18358 |
| **toaster pastry**, apl cinn Danish, Pop-Tarts Pastry Swirls - *1 pastry* | 62 | 256 | 10.4 | 37.0 | 11.0 | | 0.9 | 190 | 20 | | | | 0 | | | | | |
| | | 3.0 | 11.0 | 3.0 | 3.6 | 4.4 | 0 | | | 1.08 | | | 0 | | | | | 18508 |
| **toaster pastry**, apple cinnamon, Pop-Tarts - *1 pastry* | 52 | 205 | 6.5 | 37.5 | 17.5 | | 0.6 | 174 | 12 | 6 | 0.34 | | | 0 | 0.15 | 2.0 | | 0 |
| | | 2.3 | 5.3 | 0.9 | 3.1 | 1.4 | 0 | 47 | 28 | 1.82 | 0.021 | | 500 | | 0.17 | 0.20 | | 18475 |
| **toaster pastry**, apple strudel, Pop-Tarts - *1 pastry* | 50 | 200 | | 35.0 | 16.0 | | | 170 | 0 | | | | | 0 | 0.15 | 2.0 | | |
| | | 2.0 | 6.0 | 2.0 | | | 0 | | | 1.80 | | | 500 | | 0.17 | 0.20 | | KELL9 |
| **toaster pastry**, apple/blueberry/cherry/strawberry - *1 pastry* | 52 | 203 | 7.5 | 36.0 | 14.9 | 7.5 | 0.6 | 174 | 6 | 6 | 0.18 | 0.162 | 159 | 0 | 0.19 | 2.7 | 0 | 0.14 |
| | | 2.4 | 5.5 | 1.4 | 3.3 | 0.6 | 0 | 39 | 37 | 2.00 | 0.031 | 2.7 | 535 | 0.4 | 0.28 | 0.23 | 42.1 | 18362 |
| **toaster pastry**, blueberry, frosted, Pop-Tarts - *1 pastry* | 50 | 196 | 6.2 | 35.9 | 15.6 | | 0.6 | 199 | 12 | 8 | 0.62 | | | 0 | 0.14 | 1.9 | 0 | 0 |
| | | 2.3 | 5.0 | 1.0 | 3.4 | 0.6 | 0 | 48 | 42 | 1.75 | 0.075 | | 481 | | 0.16 | 0.19 | | 18477 |
| **toaster pastry**, blueberry, Pop-Tarts *1 pastry* | 52 | 212 | 6.5 | 35.6 | 16.1 | | 0.6 | 207 | 12 | 8 | 0.66 | | | 0 | 0.15 | 2.0 | 0 | 0 |
| | | 2.4 | 6.9 | 1.1 | 3.4 | 2.5 | 0 | 49 | 46 | 1.82 | 0.078 | | 500 | | 0.17 | 0.20 | | 18476 |
| **toaster pastry**, brown sugar cinn | 50 | 206 | 5.4 | 34.0 | | | 0.5 | 212 | 17 | 12 | 0.32 | 0.161 | 148 | 0 | 0.19 | 2.3 | 0.11 | 0.13 |
| *1 pastry* | | 2.6 | 7.1 | 1.8 | 4.0 | 0.9 | 0 | 57 | 66 | 2.02 | 0.066 | 6.3 | 493 | | 0.29 | 0.21 | 21.0 | 18361 |
| **toaster pastry**, brwn sgr cinn, frosted, lowfat, Pop-Tarts - *1 pastry* | 50 | 188 | 5.2 | 39.2 | 18.1 | | 0.6 | 210 | 7 | 5 | 0.15 | | | 0 | 0.15 | 2.0 | | 0 |
| | | 2.4 | 2.8 | 0.6 | 1.4 | 0.6 | 0 | 30 | 22 | 1.80 | 0.050 | | 500 | | 0.15 | 0.20 | | 18494 |
| **toaster pastry**, brown sugar cinn, frosted, Pop-Tarts - *1 pastry* | 50 | 211 | 5.2 | 34.2 | 15.4 | | 0.6 | 184 | 14 | 8 | 1.21 | | | 0 | 0.15 | 2.0 | 0 | 0 |
| | | 2.5 | 7.4 | 1.1 | 3.9 | 2.4 | 0 | 56 | 46 | 1.80 | 0.040 | | 500 | | 0.17 | 0.20 | | 18479 |
| **toaster pastry**, brown sugar cinn, Pop-Tarts - *1 pastry* | 50 | 219 | 5.2 | 32.2 | 12.7 | | 0.8 | 214 | 16 | 8 | 0.61 | | | 0 | 0.15 | 2.0 | 0 | 0 |
| | | 2.7 | 9.2 | 1.0 | 3.6 | 4.6 | 0 | 68 | 32 | 1.80 | 0.040 | | 500 | | 0.17 | 0.20 | | 18478 |
| **toaster pastry**, cheese Danish, Pop-Tarts Pastry Swirls - *1 pastry* | 62 | 252 | 10.4 | 36.6 | 12.0 | | 0.3 | 180 | 40 | | | | 0 | | | | | |
| | | 3.0 | 11.0 | 3.0 | 3.6 | 4.4 | 1 | | | 1.08 | | | 0 | | | | | 18510 |
| **toaster pastry**, cherry, frosted, Pop-Tarts - *1 pastry* | 52 | 204 | 6.5 | 37.4 | 18.7 | | 0.5 | 220 | 13 | 7 | 0.76 | | | 0 | 0.15 | 2.0 | 0 | 0 |
| | | 2.2 | 5.3 | 1.0 | 3.5 | 0.8 | 0 | 49 | 42 | 1.82 | 0.099 | | 500 | | 0.17 | 0.20 | | 18481 |
| **toaster pastry**, cherry, Pop-Tarts *1 pastry* | 52 | 204 | 6.5 | 37.0 | 16.5 | | 0.6 | 220 | 15 | 8 | 0.64 | | | 0 | 0.15 | 2.0 | 0 | 0 |
| | | 2.4 | 5.4 | 0.9 | 3.0 | 1.6 | 0 | 59 | 44 | 1.82 | 0.078 | | 500 | | 0.17 | 0.20 | | 18480 |
| **toaster pastry**, choc van crème, frosted, Pop-Tarts - *1 pastry* | 52 | 203 | 6.5 | 36.8 | 19.4 | | 0.5 | 229 | 16 | 11 | 0.62 | | | 0 | 0.15 | 2.0 | 0 | 0 |
| | | 2.6 | 5.3 | 1.0 | 3.2 | 1.0 | 0 | 62 | 36 | 1.82 | 0.052 | | 500 | | 0.17 | 0.21 | | 18483 |
| **toaster pastry**, choc fudge, frosted, lowfat, Pop-Tarts - *1 pastry* | 52 | 190 | 6.5 | 39.5 | 18.8 | | 0.6 | 249 | 14 | 15 | 0.26 | | | 0 | 0.16 | 2.0 | 0 | |
| | | 2.7 | 3.0 | 0.5 | 1.2 | 0.9 | 0 | 62 | 40 | 1.82 | 0.104 | | 500 | | 0.16 | 0.21 | | 18495 |

| | WT (g) | KCAL | H₂O (g) | CHO (g) | TSUG (g) | ASUG (g) | DFIB (g) | Na (mg) | Ca (mg) | Mg (mg) | Zn (mg) | Mn (mg) | A (mcg RAE) | C (mg) | B-1 (mg) | NIA (mg) | B-12 (mcg) | PANT (mg) |
|---|---|---|---|---|---|---|---|---|---|---|---|---|---|---|---|---|---|---|
| | | PRO (g) | FAT (g) | SFA (g) | MUFA (g) | PUFA (g) | CHOL (mg) | K (mg) | P (mg) | Fe (mg) | Cu (mg) | Se (mcg) | A (IU) | E (mg ATE) | B-2 (mg) | B-6 (mg) | FOL (mcg DFE) | REF |
| **toaster pastry**, chocolate fudge, frosted, Pop-Tarts - *1 pastry* | 52 | 201 | 6.5 | 37.3 | 19.8 | | 0.6 | 203 | 20 | 15 | 0.26 | | | 0 | 0.16 | 2.0 | 0 | 0 |
| | | 2.7 | 4.8 | 1.0 | 2.7 | 1.1 | 0 | 82 | 44 | 1.82 | 0.104 | | 500 | | 0.16 | 0.21 | | 18482 |
| **toaster pastry**, grape, frosted, Pop-Tarts - *1 pastry* | 52 | 203 | 6.5 | 37.6 | 18.4 | | 0.5 | 198 | 12 | 11 | 0.68 | | | 0 | 0.15 | 2.0 | 0 | 0 |
| | | 2.3 | 5.1 | 0.9 | 3.1 | 1.1 | 0 | 60 | 46 | 1.82 | 0.052 | | 500 | | 0.17 | 0.21 | | 18484 |
| **toaster pastry**, raspberry, frosted, Pop-Tarts - *1 pastry* | 52 | 205 | 6.5 | 37.2 | 18.4 | | 0.5 | 211 | 11 | 8 | 0.63 | | | 0 | 0.15 | 2.0 | 0 | 0 |
| | | 2.2 | 5.5 | 1.0 | 3.2 | 1.3 | 0 | 44 | 46 | 1.82 | 0.042 | | 500 | | 0.17 | 0.21 | | 18486 |
| **toaster pastry**, s'mores, Pop-Tarts *1 pastry* | 52 | 204 | 6.5 | 36.2 | 19.0 | | 0.7 | 199 | 15 | 11 | 0.21 | | | 0 | 0.16 | 2.0 | 0 | 0 |
| | | 3.2 | 5.5 | 1.5 | 3.1 | 0.9 | 0 | 65 | 39 | 1.82 | 0.052 | | 500 | | 0.16 | 0.21 | | 18487 |
| **toaster pastry**, strawbry Danish, Pop-Tarts Pastry Swirls - *1 pastry* | 62 | 254 | 10.1 | 37.2 | 16.0 | | 1.1 | 170 | 20 | | | | | 0 | | | | |
| | | 3.0 | 11.0 | 3.0 | 3.6 | 4.4 | 0 | | | | 1.08 | | 0 | | | | | 18509 |
| **toaster pastry**, strawberry, frosted, lowfat, Pop-Tarts - *1 pastry* | 52 | 191 | 6.5 | 40.3 | 20.7 | | 0.6 | 201 | 5 | 4 | 0.16 | | | 0 | 0.16 | 2.0 | 0 | 0 |
| | | 2.1 | 3.0 | 0.6 | 1.4 | 1.0 | 0 | 25 | 20 | 1.82 | 0 | | 500 | | 0.16 | 0.21 | | 18497 |
| **toaster pastry**, strawberry, frosted, Pop-Tarts - *1 pastry* | 52 | 203 | 6.5 | 37.6 | 19.5 | | 0.5 | 169 | 11 | 5 | 0.16 | | | 0 | 0.16 | 2.0 | 0 | 0 |
| | | 2.3 | 5.0 | 1.4 | 2.9 | 0.7 | 0 | 44 | 27 | 1.82 | 0 | | 500 | | 0.16 | 0.21 | | 18489 |
| **toaster pastry**, strawberry, lowfat, Pop-Tarts - *1 pastry* | 52 | 192 | 6.5 | 39.8 | 18.6 | | 0.6 | 220 | 6 | 5 | 0.16 | | 25 | 0 | 0.16 | 2.0 | 0 | 0 |
| | | 2.3 | 2.9 | 0.6 | 1.5 | 0.7 | 0 | 28 | 22 | 1.82 | 0 | | 500 | | 0.16 | 0.21 | | 18496 |
| **toaster pastry**, strawberry, Pop-Tarts - *1 pastry* | 52 | 205 | 6.5 | 36.9 | 17.2 | | 0.6 | 185 | 12 | 6 | 0.16 | | | 0 | 0.16 | 2.0 | 0 | 0 |
| | | 2.4 | 5.5 | 1.5 | 3.2 | 0.8 | 0 | 48 | 29 | 1.82 | 0 | | 500 | | 0.16 | 0.21 | | 18488 |
| **toaster pastry**, wild berry, frosted, Pop-Tarts - *1 pastry* | 54 | 210 | 6.8 | 39.4 | 21.0 | | 0.5 | 168 | 11 | 5 | 0.16 | | | 0 | 0.16 | 2.0 | 0 | 0 |
| | | 2.3 | 5.0 | 1.4 | 2.9 | 0.7 | 0 | 44 | 26 | 1.78 | 0 | | 500 | | 0.16 | 0.22 | | 18490 |
| **toaster strudel pastry** (avg for 11 flavors), frzn, Pillsbury *1.9 oz strudel* | 54 | 190 | | 25.2 | 8.5 | | 0.5 | 200 | 0 | | | | | 0 | | | | |
| | | 2.5 | 9.5 | 4.0 | | | 8 | | | 0.90 | | | 0 | | | | | GENM117 |

## 7.8 PIES, PIE CRUSTS, AND PIE FILLINGS

| | WT (g) | KCAL | H₂O (g) | CHO (g) | TSUG (g) | ASUG (g) | DFIB (g) | Na (mg) | Ca (mg) | Mg (mg) | Zn (mg) | Mn (mg) | A (mcg RAE) | C (mg) | B-1 (mg) | NIA (mg) | B-12 (mcg) | PANT (mg) |
|---|---|---|---|---|---|---|---|---|---|---|---|---|---|---|---|---|---|---|
| | | PRO (g) | FAT (g) | SFA (g) | MUFA (g) | PUFA (g) | CHOL (mg) | K (mg) | P (mg) | Fe (mg) | Cu (mg) | Se (mcg) | A (IU) | E (mg ATE) | B-2 (mg) | B-6 (mg) | FOL (mcg DFE) | REF |
| **apple pie** *⅛ of 9″ pie* | 125 | 296 | 65.2 | 42.5 | 19.6 | 13.4 | 2.0 | 332 | 14 | 9 | 0.20 | 0.227 | 40 | 4 | 0.04 | 0.3 | 0.01 | 0.15 |
| | | 2.4 | 13.8 | 4.7 | 5.5 | 2.7 | 0 | 81 | 30 | 0.56 | 0.057 | 1.2 | 155 | 1.9 | 0.03 | 0.05 | 53.8 | 18301 |
| **apple pie**, Dutch *4.8 oz slice* | 137 | 397 | 56.3 | 61.0 | 30.2 | | 2.2 | 274 | 19 | 11 | 0.26 | 0.319 | 25 | 8 | 0.26 | 1.5 | 0 | 0.13 |
| | | 3.0 | 15.8 | 3.2 | 7.9 | 2.9 | 0 | 104 | 40 | 1.25 | 0.203 | 3.0 | 112 | 1.3 | 0.09 | 0.05 | 43.8 | 18944 |
| **apple pie**, Dutch, frzn, Marie Callender's - *1/10 of 13 oz pie* | 128 | 320 | | 45.0 | 29.0 | | 4.0 | 180 | 20 | | | | | 0 | | | | |
| | | 2.0 | 16.0 | 2.5 | | | 0 | | | 1.08 | | | 0 | | | | | CNAG312 |
| **apple pie filling**, canned *⅛ can* | 74 | 74 | 54.3 | 19.3 | 10.2 | 4.0 | 0.7 | 35 | 3 | 1 | 0.03 | 0.020 | 1 | 1 | 0.01 | 0 | 0 | 0.03 |
| | | 0.1 | 0.1 | 0 | 0 | 0 | 0 | 33 | 5 | 0.21 | 0.041 | 0.2 | 18 | 0 | 0.01 | 0.01 | 0 | 19312 |
| **apple pie**, homemade *⅛ of 9″ pie* | 155 | 411 | 73.3 | 57.5 | | | | 327 | 11 | 11 | 0.29 | 0.287 | 17 | 3 | 0.23 | 1.9 | 0 | 0.14 |
| | | 3.7 | 19.4 | 4.7 | 8.4 | 5.2 | 0 | 122 | 43 | 1.74 | 0.082 | 12.1 | 90 | | 0.17 | 0.05 | 58.9 | 18302 |
| **apple pie**, Tastykake *1 snack pie* | 113 | 270 | | 40.0 | 19.0 | | 2.0 | 310 | 20 | | | | | 1 | | | | |
| | | 2.0 | 11.0 | 2.5 | | | 0 | | | 1.08 | | | 0 | | | | | TAST12 |
| **banana cream pie**, from mix *⅛ of 9″ pie* | 92 | 231 | 46.8 | 29.1 | | | 0.6 | 267 | 67 | 11 | 0.30 | 0.098 | 87 | 0 | 0.09 | 0.7 | 0.19 | 0.24 |
| | | 3.1 | 11.9 | 6.4 | 4.2 | 0.7 | 27 | 104 | 154 | 0.42 | 0.040 | 4.5 | 375 | | 0.13 | 0.03 | 28.5 | 18303 |
| **banana cream pie**, homemade *⅛ of 9″ pie* | 144 | 387 | 69.0 | 47.4 | 17.4 | 12.7 | 1.0 | 346 | 108 | 23 | 0.69 | 0.219 | 88 | 2 | 0.20 | 1.5 | 0.36 | 0.56 |
| | | 6.3 | 19.6 | 5.4 | 8.2 | 4.7 | 73 | 238 | 132 | 1.50 | 0.075 | 13.1 | 341 | 0.6 | 0.30 | 0.19 | 54.7 | 18304 |
| **banana cream pie**, Tastykake *1 snack pie* | 120 | 360 | | 52.0 | 28.0 | | 1.0 | 380 | 80 | | | | | 0 | | | | |
| | | 4.0 | 15.0 | 4.0 | | | 20 | | | 1.08 | | | 0 | | | | | TAST13 |
| **blueberry pie** *⅛ of 9″ pie* | 125 | 290 | 65.6 | 43.6 | 12.4 | 9.6 | 1.2 | 406 | 10 | 6 | 0.20 | 0.220 | 55 | 3 | 0.01 | 0.4 | 0.01 | 0.17 |
| | | 2.2 | 12.5 | 2.1 | 5.3 | 4.4 | 0 | 62 | 29 | 0.38 | 0.057 | 1.8 | 251 | 1.3 | 0.04 | 0.05 | 53.8 | 18305 |
| **blueberry pie filling**, canned *½ cup* | 131 | 237 | 71.6 | 58.1 | 49.5 | 32.7 | 3.4 | 16 | 35 | 13 | 0.13 | 0.282 | 1 | 1 | 0.03 | 0.1 | 0 | 0.12 |
| | | 0.5 | 0.3 | 0 | 0 | 0 | 0 | 151 | 16 | 1.05 | 0.147 | 0.5 | 29 | 0.3 | 0.04 | 0.04 | 1.3 | 44158 |
| **blueberry pie**, homemade *⅛ of 9″ pie* | 147 | 360 | 75.3 | 49.2 | | | | 272 | 10 | 12 | 0.29 | 0.441 | 3 | 1 | 0.22 | 1.8 | 0 | 0.18 |
| | | 4.0 | 17.5 | 4.3 | 7.5 | 4.5 | 0 | 74 | 44 | 1.81 | 0.098 | 10.9 | 62 | | 0.19 | 0.05 | 52.9 | 18306 |
| **blueberry pie**, Tastykake *1 snack pie* | 113 | 300 | | 48.0 | 25.0 | | 2.0 | 310 | 20 | | | | | 2 | | | | |
| | | 3.0 | 11.0 | 2.5 | | | 0 | | | 1.08 | | | 0 | | | | | TAST14 |
| **cherry pie** *⅛ of 9″ pie* | 125 | 325 | 57.8 | 49.2 | 17.9 | 12.7 | 1.0 | 308 | 15 | 10 | 0.22 | 0.175 | 65 | 1 | 0.03 | 0.2 | 0.01 | 0.40 |
| | | 2.5 | 13.8 | 3.2 | 7.3 | 2.6 | 0 | 101 | 36 | 0.60 | 0.050 | 1.5 | 334 | 1.0 | 0.04 | 0.05 | 50.0 | 18308 |
| **cherry pie filling**, canned *⅛ can* | 74 | 85 | 52.7 | 20.7 | | | 0.4 | 13 | 8 | 5 | 0.04 | 0.022 | 7 | 3 | 0.02 | 0.1 | 0 | 0.05 |
| | | 0.3 | 0.1 | 0 | 0 | 0 | 0 | 78 | 11 | 0.18 | 0.059 | 0.3 | 152 | | 0.01 | 0.03 | 3.0 | 19314 |
| **cherry pie filling**, low-calorie, canned - *½ cup* | 132 | 70 | 114.5 | 15.8 | 12.1 | 0 | 1.6 | 16 | 15 | 11 | 0.09 | 0.075 | 13 | 4 | 0.03 | 0.5 | 0 | 0 |
| | | 1.1 | 0.2 | 0 | 0 | 0 | 0 | 156 | 20 | 0.44 | 0.111 | 0.1 | 275 | 0 | 0.05 | 0.04 | 5.3 | 43098 |
| **cherry pie**, homemade *⅛ of 9″ pie* | 180 | 486 | 82.4 | 69.3 | | | | 344 | 18 | 16 | 0.36 | 0.360 | 52 | 2 | 0.27 | 2.3 | 0 | 0.22 |
| | | 5.0 | 22.0 | 5.4 | 9.6 | 5.8 | 0 | 139 | 54 | 3.33 | 0.139 | 14.0 | 736 | | 0.22 | 0.06 | 73.8 | 18309 |
| **cherry pie**, Tastykake *1 snack pie* | 113 | 290 | | 45.0 | 23.0 | | 2.0 | 310 | 20 | | | | | 2 | | | | |
| | | 3.0 | 11.0 | 2.5 | | | 0 | | | 1.08 | | | 0 | | | | | TAST15 |
| **cherry snack pie**, fried *1 snack pie (5″ × 3¾″)* | 128 | 404 | 48.1 | 54.5 | | | 3.3 | 479 | 28 | 13 | 0.29 | 0.287 | 12 | 2 | 0.18 | 1.8 | 0.10 | 0.14 |
| | | 3.8 | 20.6 | 3.1 | 9.5 | 6.9 | 0 | 83 | 55 | 1.56 | 0.060 | 3.1 | 220 | | 0.14 | 0.04 | 37.1 | 18444 |

| | WT | Macronutrients | | | | | | Minerals | | | | | Vitamins | | | | | |
|---|---|---|---|---|---|---|---|---|---|---|---|---|---|---|---|---|---|---|
| | (g) | KCAL | $H_2O$ (g) | CHO (g) | TSUG (g) | ASUG (g) | DFIB (g) | Na (mg) | Ca (mg) | Mg (mg) | Zn (mg) | Mn (mg) | A (mcg RAE) | C (mg) | B-1 (mg) | NIA (mg) | B-12 (mcg) | PANT (mg) |
| | | PRO (g) | FAT (g) | SFA (g) | MUFA (g) | PUFA (g) | CHOL (mg) | K (mg) | P (mg) | Fe (mg) | Cu (mg) | Se (mcg) | A (IU) | E (mg ATE) | B-2 (mg) | B-6 (mg) | FOL (mcg DFE) | REF |
| **chocolate creme pie** | 113 | 344 | 49.2 | 38.0 | | | 2.3 | 154 | 41 | 24 | 0.26 | 0.226 | 0 | 0 | 0.04 | 0.8 | 0.01 | 0.44 |
| *1/6 of 8″ pie* | | 2.9 | 21.9 | 5.6 | 12.6 | 2.7 | 6 | 144 | 77 | 1.21 | 0.056 | 8.5 | 0 | | 0.12 | 0.02 | 19.2 | 18310 |
| **chocolate mousse pie**, from mix | 95 | 247 | 47.2 | 28.1 | | | | 437 | 73 | 30 | 0.57 | 0.119 | 118 | 0 | 0.05 | 0.6 | 0.20 | 0.19 |
| *1/8 of 9″ pie* | | 3.3 | 14.6 | 7.8 | 4.8 | 0.8 | 33 | 271 | 219 | 1.03 | 0.193 | 5.8 | 392 | | 0.14 | 0.03 | 39.9 | 18312 |
| **coconut cream pie** | 64 | 191 | 27.6 | 23.8 | 23.2 | 21.0 | 0.8 | 163 | 19 | 13 | 0.30 | 0.280 | 17 | 0 | 0.03 | 0.1 | 0.08 | 0.15 |
| *1/6 of 7″ pie* | | 1.3 | 10.6 | 4.5 | 4.6 | 1.0 | 0 | 42 | 54 | 0.51 | 0.044 | 3.4 | 58 | 0.1 | 0.05 | 0.04 | 5.1 | 18313 |
| **coconut cream pie**, from mix | 94 | 259 | 46.7 | 26.8 | | | 0.5 | 309 | 68 | 16 | 0.36 | 0.179 | 89 | 1 | 0.03 | 0.1 | 0.20 | 0.24 |
| *1/8 of 9″ pie* | | 2.6 | 16.5 | 8.4 | 6.2 | 1.1 | 22 | 133 | 159 | 0.38 | 0.075 | 4.7 | 381 | | 0.10 | 0.04 | 21.6 | 18314 |
| **coconut cream pie**, Tastykake | 113 | 370 | | 42.0 | 19.0 | | 2.0 | 420 | 60 | | | | | 0 | | | | |
| *1 snack pie* | | 4.0 | 20.0 | 6.0 | | | 55 | | | 0.72 | | | 100 | | | | | TAST16 |
| **coconut custard pie** | 104 | 270 | 51.2 | 31.4 | | | 1.9 | 348 | 84 | 19 | 0.71 | 0.218 | 27 | 1 | 0.09 | 0.4 | 0.09 | 0.25 |
| *1/6 of 8″ pie* | | 6.1 | 13.7 | 6.1 | 5.7 | 1.2 | 36 | 182 | 127 | 0.83 | 0.066 | 6.7 | 114 | | 0.15 | 0.01 | 19.8 | 18316 |
| **egg custard pie** | 105 | 220 | 63.9 | 21.8 | 12.2 | 8.9 | 1.7 | 252 | 84 | 12 | 0.55 | 0.063 | 60 | 1 | 0.04 | 0.3 | 0.45 | 0.70 |
| *1/6 of 8″ pie* | | 5.8 | 12.2 | 2.5 | 5.0 | 3.9 | 35 | 111 | 118 | 0.61 | 0.025 | 7.5 | 214 | 1.0 | 0.22 | 0.05 | 21.0 | 18317 |
| **fruit snack pie**, fried | 128 | 404 | 48.1 | 54.5 | 27.4 | 19.1 | 3.3 | 479 | 28 | 13 | 0.29 | 0.287 | 6 | 2 | 0.18 | 1.8 | 0.10 | 0.14 |
| *1 snack pie (5″ × 3¾″)* | | 3.8 | 20.6 | 3.1 | 9.5 | 6.9 | 0 | 83 | 55 | 1.56 | 0.060 | 3.1 | 35 | 2.2 | 0.14 | 0.04 | 37.1 | 18319 |
| **lemon meringue pie** | 133 | 356 | 55.5 | 62.8 | 31.7 | 31.0 | 1.6 | 194 | 74 | 20 | 0.65 | 0.080 | 68 | 4 | 0.08 | 0.9 | 0.23 | 1.05 |
| *1/6 of 8″ pie* | | 2.0 | 11.6 | 2.3 | 3.6 | 4.9 | 60 | 118 | 140 | 0.81 | 0.001 | 4.0 | 230 | 1.4 | 0.28 | 0.04 | 46.6 | 18320 |
| **lemon meringue pie**, homemade | 127 | 362 | 55.0 | 49.7 | | | | 307 | 15 | 8 | 0.36 | 0.163 | 55 | 4 | 0.15 | 1.2 | 0.15 | 0.27 |
| *1/8 of 9″ pie* | | 4.8 | 16.4 | 4.0 | 7.1 | 4.2 | 67 | 83 | 53 | 1.27 | 0.053 | 14.7 | 203 | | 0.20 | 0.03 | 45.7 | 18321 |
| **lemon pie**, Tastykake | 113 | 300 | | 44.0 | 22.0 | | 1.0 | 320 | 20 | | | | | 0 | | | | |
| *1 snack pie* | | 3.0 | 14.0 | 3.5 | | | 40 | | | 1.08 | | | 100 | | | | | TAST17 |
| **lemon snack pie**, fried | 128 | 404 | 48.1 | 54.5 | | | 3.3 | 479 | 28 | 13 | 0.29 | 0.287 | 3 | 0 | 0.18 | 1.8 | 0.10 | 0.14 |
| *1 snack pie (5″ × 3¾″)* | | 3.8 | 20.6 | 3.1 | 9.5 | 6.9 | 0 | 83 | 55 | 1.56 | 0.060 | 3.1 | 41 | | 0.14 | 0.04 | 37.1 | 18445 |
| **mince pie**, homemade | 165 | 477 | 61.7 | 79.2 | 46.7 | 25.6 | 4.3 | 419 | 36 | 23 | 0.36 | 0.434 | 2 | 10 | 0.25 | 2.0 | 0 | 0.16 |
| *1/8 of 9″ pie* | | 4.3 | 17.8 | 4.4 | 7.7 | 4.7 | 0 | 335 | 69 | 2.46 | 0.186 | 10.9 | 36 | 0.2 | 0.17 | 0.11 | 59.4 | 18322 |
| **peach pie** | 117 | 261 | 63.6 | 38.5 | 7.2 | 5.6 | 0.9 | 316 | 9 | 7 | 0.11 | 0.178 | 12 | 1 | 0.07 | 0.2 | 0 | 0.13 |
| *1/6 of 8″ pie* | | 2.2 | 11.7 | 1.8 | 5.0 | 4.4 | 0 | 146 | 26 | 0.58 | 0.062 | 1.5 | 164 | 1.1 | 0.04 | 0.03 | 55.0 | 18323 |
| **pecan pie** | 113 | 460 | 20.6 | 67.4 | 31.4 | 31.3 | 2.4 | 271 | 25 | 25 | 0.98 | 0.802 | 58 | 0 | 0.23 | 1.5 | 0.14 | 0.44 |
| *1/6 of 8″ pie* | | 5.1 | 18.9 | 3.0 | 9.4 | 4.0 | 47 | 112 | 94 | 1.05 | 0.208 | 7.9 | 198 | 0.9 | 0.09 | 0.04 | 48.6 | 18324 |
| **pecan pie**, homemade | 122 | 503 | 23.8 | 63.7 | | | | 320 | 39 | 32 | 1.24 | 0.869 | 100 | 0 | 0.23 | 1.0 | 0.21 | 0.58 |
| *1/8 of 9″ pie* | | 6.0 | 27.1 | 4.9 | 13.6 | 7.0 | 106 | 162 | 115 | 1.81 | 0.257 | 14.6 | 436 | | 0.22 | 0.07 | 41.5 | 18325 |
| **pie crust**, chocolate cookie, Ready | 182 | 881 | 9.1 | 117.4 | 47.9 | | 4.9 | 915 | 58 | 73 | 3.82 | 3.336 | 0 | 0 | 0.61 | 5.6 | 0 | 0.31 |
| Crust - *6.4 oz crust* | | 11.1 | 40.8 | 8.6 | 26.4 | 3.7 | 0 | 340 | 218 | 7.83 | 1.401 | 4.6 | 0 | 3.3 | 0.48 | 0.08 | 196.6 | 18943 |
| **pie crust**, chocolate wafer, | 28 | 142 | 2.0 | 15.2 | 6.2 | 5.8 | 0.4 | 188 | 8 | 11 | 0.23 | 0.145 | 59 | 0 | 0.04 | 0.6 | 0.01 | 0.08 |
| homemade - *1/8 of 9″ crust* | | 1.4 | 8.7 | 1.9 | 4.1 | 2.2 | 0 | 47 | 29 | 0.84 | 0.097 | 1.2 | 258 | 0.8 | 0.06 | 0 | 25.2 | 18398 |
| **pie crust**, from mix | 20 | 100 | 2.1 | 10.1 | | | 0.4 | 146 | 12 | 3 | 0.08 | 0.061 | 0 | 0 | 0.06 | 0.5 | 0 | 0.03 |
| *1/8 of 9″ crust* | | 1.3 | 6.1 | 1.5 | 3.5 | 0.8 | 0 | 12 | 17 | 0.43 | 0.015 | 4.4 | 0 | | 0.04 | 0.01 | 22.2 | 18333 |
| **pie crust**, frozen | 16 | 81 | 1.1 | 9.0 | 0.7 | 0.5 | 0.5 | 75 | 3 | 3 | 0.08 | | 0 | 0 | 0.05 | 0.6 | 0 | 0.07 |
| *1/8 of 9″ crust* | | 1.0 | 4.6 | 1.5 | 2.2 | 0.6 | 0 | 18 | 13 | 0.45 | 0.016 | 1.1 | 0 | 0.1 | 0.02 | 0.01 | 16.3 | 18335 |
| **pie crust**, graham cracker, Ready | 183 | 917 | 8.0 | 117.7 | 33.2 | | 3.5 | 763 | 53 | 42 | 2.29 | 2.355 | 0 | 0 | 0.34 | 5.9 | 0 | 0.33 |
| Crust - *6.5 oz crust* | | 9.3 | 45.4 | 9.1 | 31.0 | 3.1 | 0 | 207 | 214 | 4.76 | 0.408 | 4.8 | 0 | 3.4 | 0.39 | 0.14 | 177.5 | 18942 |
| **pie crust**, graham, homemade | 30 | 148 | 1.3 | 19.6 | 11.5 | 11.4 | 0.4 | 171 | 6 | 5 | 0.14 | 0.139 | 58 | 0 | 0.03 | 0.6 | 0.01 | 0.07 |
| *1/8 of 9″ crust* | | 1.3 | 7.5 | 1.6 | 3.4 | 2.1 | 0 | 26 | 20 | 0.65 | 0.038 | 1.8 | 248 | 0.7 | 0.05 | 0.01 | 10.8 | 18330 |
| **pie crust**, graham, ready-to-use, | 28 | 150 | | 18.0 | 8.0 | | 0 | 115 | | | | | | | | | | |
| Nabisco - *1/6 crust (1 oz)* | | 1.0 | 8.0 | 1.5 | | | 0 | | | 0.72 | | | | | | | | NBSC148 |
| **pie crust**, homemade | 23 | 121 | 2.3 | 10.9 | 0 | 0 | 0.4 | 125 | 2 | 3 | 0.10 | 0.099 | 0 | 0 | 0.09 | 0.8 | 0 | 0.04 |
| *1/8 of 9″ crust* | | 1.5 | 8.0 | 2.0 | 3.5 | 2.1 | 0 | 15 | 15 | 0.66 | 0.021 | 4.9 | 0 | 0.1 | 0.06 | 0.01 | 24.4 | 18336 |
| **pie crust**, Nilla, ready-to-use, | 31 | 159 | 1.0 | 19.6 | 10.0 | | 0.3 | 69 | 13 | 2 | 0.09 | | | | 0.05 | 0.8 | 0.03 | |
| Nabisco - *8 small sections* | | 1.1 | 8.4 | 1.6 | 5.8 | 0.4 | 3 | 21 | 26 | 0.55 | 0.016 | | 3 | | 0.06 | 0.01 | | 18618 |
| **pie crust**, Oreo, ready-to-use, | 28 | 130 | | 19.0 | 9.0 | | 1.0 | 170 | | | | | | | | | | |
| Nabisco - *1/6 pie crust (1 oz)* | | 1.0 | 7.0 | 1.5 | | | 0 | | | 1.44 | | | | | | | | NBSC132 |
| **pie crust**, refrigerated, baked | 198 | 1002 | 15.8 | 115.9 | | | 2.8 | 935 | 24 | 18 | 0.44 | 0.414 | | | 0.28 | 2.5 | 0 | 0.58 |
| *7 oz crust* | | 6.8 | 56.8 | 22.0 | 23.4 | 7.4 | | 164 | 103 | 2.28 | 0.101 | 8.9 | | 0.1 | 0.07 | 0.04 | 93.1 | 18946 |
| **pie crust**, vanilla wafer, homemade | 22 | 117 | 1.9 | 11.0 | 1.6 | 1.5 | 0 | 113 | 9 | 2 | 0.05 | 0.039 | 59 | 0 | 0.04 | 0.5 | 0.02 | 0.07 |
| *1/8 of 9″ crust* | | 0.8 | 8.0 | 1.6 | 3.4 | 2.4 | 9 | 17 | 17 | 0.36 | 0.015 | 1.7 | 258 | 0.7 | 0.05 | 0.01 | 17.4 | 18401 |
| **pumpkin pie** | 109 | 265 | 54.9 | 38.0 | 20.6 | 11.5 | 2.0 | 254 | 70 | 15 | 0.43 | 0.247 | 488 | 0 | 0.19 | 1.2 | 0.38 | 0.49 |
| *1/6 of 8″ pie* | | 4.3 | 10.6 | 2.2 | 5.0 | 1.9 | 28 | 182 | 88 | 0.98 | 0.161 | 5.9 | 3743 | 0.8 | 0.14 | 0.07 | 40.3 | 18326 |
| **pumpkin pie**, homemade | 155 | 316 | 90.7 | 40.9 | | | | 349 | 146 | 29 | 0.71 | 0.307 | 660 | 3 | 0.14 | 1.2 | 0.14 | 0.69 |
| *1/8 of 9″ pie* | | 7.0 | 14.4 | 4.9 | 5.7 | 2.8 | 65 | 288 | 152 | 1.97 | 0.102 | 11.0 | 12431 | | 0.31 | 0.07 | 43.4 | 18327 |
| **pumpkin pie mix**, canned | 270 | 281 | 193.0 | 71.3 | | | 22.4 | 562 | 100 | 43 | 0.73 | 1.083 | 1120 | 9 | 0.04 | 1.0 | 0 | 3.07 |
| *1 cup* | | 2.9 | 0.4 | 0.2 | 0 | 0 | 0 | 373 | 122 | 2.86 | 0.184 | 3.0 | 22405 | | 0.32 | 0.43 | 94.5 | 11426 |
| **vanilla cream pie**, homemade | 126 | 350 | 59.2 | 41.1 | 16.0 | 11.6 | 0.8 | 328 | 113 | 16 | 0.67 | 0.161 | 105 | 1 | 0.18 | 1.2 | 0.38 | 0.52 |
| *1/8 of 9″ pie* | | 6.0 | 18.1 | 5.1 | 7.6 | 4.3 | 78 | 159 | 131 | 1.29 | 0.049 | 12.0 | 386 | 0.6 | 0.27 | 0.06 | 46.6 | 18328 |

| | WT (g) | KCAL | H₂0 (g) | CHO (g) | TSUG (g) | ASUG (g) | DFIB (g) | Na (mg) | Ca (mg) | Mg (mg) | Zn (mg) | Mn (mg) | A (mcg RAE) | C (mg) | B-1 (mg) | NIA (mg) | B-12 (mcg) | PANT (mg) |
|---|---|---|---|---|---|---|---|---|---|---|---|---|---|---|---|---|---|---|
| | | PRO (g) | FAT (g) | SFA (g) | MUFA (g) | PUFA (g) | CHOL (mg) | K (mg) | P (mg) | Fe (mg) | Cu (mg) | Se (mcg) | A (IU) | E (mg ATE) | B-2 (mg) | B-6 (mg) | FOL (mcg DFE) | REF |

## 7.9 PUDDINGS AND CUSTARDS

| Food | WT (g) | KCAL / PRO | H₂0 / FAT | CHO / SFA | TSUG / MUFA | ASUG / PUFA | DFIB / CHOL | Na / K | Ca / P | Mg / Fe | Zn / Cu | Mn / Se | A(RAE) / A(IU) | C / E | B-1 / B-2 | NIA / B-6 | B-12 / FOL | PANT / REF |
|---|---|---|---|---|---|---|---|---|---|---|---|---|---|---|---|---|---|---|
| **banana pudding**, from instant mix | 140 | 147 | 104.3 | 27.6 | | | 0 | 414 | 143 | 17 | 0.46 | 0.004 | 64 | 1 | 0.05 | 0.1 | 0.42 | 0.37 |
| with 2% milk - ½ cup | | 3.9 | 2.4 | 1.4 | 0.6 | 0.2 | 8 | 183 | 302 | 0.08 | 0.014 | 2.8 | 238 | | 0.19 | 0.05 | 5.6 | 19121 |
| **banana pudding**, from inst | 147 | 169 | 108.1 | 28.9 | 25.5 | 19.1 | 0 | 435 | 147 | 16 | 0.47 | 0.007 | 35 | 1 | 0.05 | 0.1 | 0.44 | 0.39 |
| mix w/whl milk - ½ cup | | 4.0 | 4.2 | 2.5 | 1.2 | 0.2 | 16 | 188 | 315 | 0.09 | 0.018 | 2.6 | 154 | | 0.20 | 0.05 | 5.9 | 19319 |
| **banana pudding**, from regular | 140 | 141 | 106.3 | 25.8 | | | 0 | 230 | 153 | 18 | 0.49 | 0.006 | 70 | 1 | 0.04 | 0.1 | 0.35 | 0.39 |
| mix with 2% milk - ½ cup | | 4.1 | 2.4 | 1.4 | 0.6 | 0.1 | 10 | 192 | 116 | 0.07 | 0.014 | 2.9 | 249 | | 0.20 | 0.05 | 5.6 | 19122 |
| **banana pudding**, from reg | 140 | 155 | 104.8 | 25.6 | 22.4 | 16.0 | 0 | 230 | 150 | 18 | 0.48 | 0.007 | 36 | 1 | 0.04 | 0.1 | 0.35 | 0.38 |
| mix w/whl milk - ½ cup | | 4.0 | 4.2 | 2.5 | 1.1 | 0.2 | 17 | 188 | 115 | 0.07 | 0.017 | 2.7 | 154 | | 0.20 | 0.05 | 5.6 | 19321 |
| **chocolate mousse**, homemade | 202 | 454 | 127.1 | 32.5 | 29.9 | | 1.2 | 77 | 194 | 40 | 1.29 | 0.119 | 283 | 0 | 0.09 | 0.3 | 0.95 | 1.08 |
| ½ cup | | 8.4 | 32.3 | 18.5 | 10.2 | 1.8 | 283 | 289 | 236 | 1.11 | 0.152 | 14.9 | 1028 | 1.0 | 0.41 | 0.12 | 30.3 | 19182 |
| **chocolate pudding**, from inst | 147 | 154 | 109.6 | 27.8 | | | 0.6 | 417 | 153 | 28 | 0.63 | 0.091 | 68 | 1 | 0.05 | 0.2 | 0.46 | 0.40 |
| mix w/lowfat milk - ½ cup | | 4.6 | 2.8 | 1.6 | 0.8 | 0.2 | 9 | 247 | 350 | 0.59 | 0.100 | 3.4 | 250 | | 0.22 | 0.06 | 7.4 | 19123 |
| **chocolate pudding**, from inst | 147 | 163 | 108.2 | 27.6 | | | 1.5 | 417 | 150 | 26 | 0.62 | 0.062 | 38 | 1 | 0.05 | 0.1 | 0.44 | 0.40 |
| mix w/whl milk - ½ cup | | 4.6 | 4.6 | 2.7 | 1.4 | 0.3 | 16 | 244 | 351 | 0.43 | 0.094 | 2.5 | 176 | | 0.21 | 0.06 | 5.9 | 19185 |
| **chocolate pudding**, from regular | 142 | 155 | 105.3 | 27.8 | | | 0.4 | 148 | 159 | 30 | 0.65 | 0.061 | 67 | 1 | 0.05 | 0.1 | 0.36 | 0.40 |
| mix with 2% milk - ½ cup | | 4.7 | 2.8 | 1.7 | 0.8 | 0.1 | 10 | 237 | 136 | 0.51 | 0.104 | 3.1 | 250 | | 0.25 | 0.05 | 5.7 | 19190 |
| **chocolate pudding**, from reg | 142 | 169 | 104.1 | 27.5 | 17.0 | 10.5 | 1.1 | 136 | 151 | 28 | 0.71 | 0.136 | 34 | 0 | 0.05 | 0.2 | 0.43 | 0.45 |
| mix w/whl milk - ½ cup | | 4.6 | 4.5 | 2.6 | 1.2 | 0.3 | 13 | 226 | 132 | 0.50 | 0.141 | 5.3 | 124 | 0.1 | 0.24 | 0.04 | 5.7 | 19189 |
| **chocolate pudding**, ready-to-eat | 142 | 202 | 98.6 | 32.7 | 24.4 | 20.3 | 0 | 216 | 72 | 26 | 0.48 | 0.168 | 20 | 0 | 0.03 | 0.2 | 0.13 | 0.35 |
| 5 oz serving | | 3.0 | 6.5 | 1.8 | 3.9 | 0.1 | 1 | 261 | 80 | 1.80 | 0.131 | 0 | 65 | 0.4 | 0.10 | 0.03 | 4.3 | 19183 |
| **chocolate rennin dessert**, from | 136 | 116 | 109.3 | 18.3 | | | 0.7 | 71 | 171 | 27 | 0.69 | 0.090 | 68 | 1 | 0.05 | 0.1 | 0.45 | 0.40 |
| mix with 2% milk - ½ cup | | 4.4 | 2.8 | 1.7 | 0.8 | 0.1 | 10 | 248 | 133 | 0.41 | 0.110 | 3.1 | 231 | | 0.21 | 0.06 | 6.8 | 19213 |
| **chocolate rennin dessert**, from | 136 | 131 | 107.8 | 18.1 | | | 0.7 | 69 | 169 | 27 | 0.68 | 0.092 | 37 | 1 | 0.05 | 0.1 | 0.44 | 0.39 |
| mix w/whl milk - ½ cup | | 4.4 | 4.5 | 2.7 | 1.3 | 0.2 | 16 | 243 | 132 | 0.41 | 0.113 | 2.9 | 150 | | 0.21 | 0.06 | 6.8 | 19221 |
| **coconut cream pudding**, from | 147 | 157 | 109.4 | 28.2 | | | 0.1 | 362 | 150 | 21 | 0.49 | 0.028 | 66 | 1 | 0.05 | 0.1 | 0.44 | 0.40 |
| inst mix w/2% milk - ½ cup | | 4.3 | 3.4 | 2.0 | 0.9 | 0.3 | 9 | 194 | 295 | 0.22 | 0.037 | 2.9 | 220 | | 0.20 | 0.06 | 5.9 | 19191 |
| **coconut cream pudding**, from | 147 | 172 | 107.9 | 28.1 | | | 0.1 | 362 | 147 | 21 | 0.49 | 0.028 | 35 | 1 | 0.05 | 0.1 | 0.44 | 0.39 |
| inst mix w/whl milk - ½ cup | | 4.3 | 5.1 | 3.1 | 1.4 | 0.4 | 16 | 190 | 294 | 0.22 | 0.038 | 2.9 | 154 | | 0.20 | 0.05 | 5.9 | 19323 |
| **coconut cream pudding**, from | 140 | 146 | 105.8 | 24.9 | | | 0.3 | 228 | 158 | 22 | 0.52 | 0.052 | 69 | 1 | 0.04 | 0.1 | 0.36 | 0.41 |
| reg mix w/2% milk - ½ cup | | 4.3 | 3.5 | 2.5 | 0.7 | 0.1 | 10 | 223 | 125 | 0.28 | 0.035 | 3.2 | 238 | | 0.20 | 0.20 | 5.6 | 19219 |
| **coconut cream pudding**, from | 140 | 160 | 104.4 | 24.8 | | | 0.3 | 227 | 155 | 22 | 0.50 | 0.052 | 36 | 1 | 0.04 | 0.1 | 0.35 | 0.40 |
| reg mix w/whl milk - ½ cup | | 4.2 | 5.3 | 3.6 | 1.2 | 0.2 | 17 | 220 | 123 | 0.28 | 0.038 | 3.2 | 154 | | 0.20 | 0.20 | 5.6 | 19325 |
| **egg custard**, from mix with | 133 | 148 | 99.4 | 23.2 | | | 0 | 118 | 193 | 25 | 0.69 | 0.007 | 81 | 1 | 0.07 | 0.2 | 0.60 | 0.85 |
| 2% milk - ½ cup | | 5.4 | 3.6 | 1.8 | 1.1 | 0.3 | 64 | 298 | 184 | 0.47 | 0.020 | 6.1 | 290 | | 0.28 | 0.09 | 12.0 | 19205 |
| **egg custard**, from mix with | 133 | 161 | 98.0 | 23.0 | | | 0 | 117 | 190 | 25 | 0.68 | 0.009 | 49 | 1 | 0.07 | 0.2 | 0.59 | 0.85 |
| whole milk - ½ cup | | 5.4 | 5.2 | 2.8 | 1.6 | 0.3 | 70 | 294 | 181 | 0.47 | 0.021 | 5.9 | 196 | | 0.28 | 0.09 | 12.0 | 19170 |
| **egg custard**, homemade | 141 | 148 | 111.2 | 15.1 | 16.0 | | 0 | 86 | 151 | 16 | 0.76 | 0.014 | 69 | 0 | 0.05 | 0.1 | 0.55 | 0.80 |
| ½ cup | | 7.1 | 6.5 | 3.1 | 1.9 | 0.6 | 118 | 209 | 159 | 0.49 | 0.039 | 12.4 | 247 | 0.3 | 0.34 | 0.07 | 14.1 | 19168 |
| **flan**, from mix, Goya | 133 | 60 | | 13.0 | 11.0 | | | 110 | 0 | | | | | 0 | | | | |
| ½ cup | | 0 | 0.5 | 0 | | | 0 | | | 0 | | | 0 | | | | | GOYA2 |
| **flan**, from mix, with 2% milk | 133 | 137 | 100.7 | 25.0 | | | 0 | 150 | 150 | 16 | 0.48 | 0.004 | 69 | 1 | 0.04 | 0.1 | 0.35 | 0.38 |
| ½ cup | | 4.0 | 2.3 | 1.4 | 0.6 | 0.1 | 9 | 217 | 114 | 0.08 | 0.013 | 7.0 | 239 | | 0.20 | 0.05 | 5.3 | 19231 |
| **flan**, from mix, with whole milk | 133 | 150 | 99.3 | 24.8 | | | 0 | 149 | 148 | 16 | 0.47 | 0.007 | 39 | 1 | 0.04 | 0.1 | 0.35 | 0.38 |
| ½ cup | | 3.9 | 4.0 | 2.4 | 1.1 | 0.1 | 16 | 213 | 112 | 0.08 | 0.015 | 6.9 | 150 | | 0.19 | 0.05 | 5.3 | 19232 |
| **flan**, homemade | 153 | 223 | 104.1 | 34.7 | 35.4 | | 0 | 81 | 127 | 14 | 0.72 | 0.015 | 70 | 0 | 0.05 | 0.1 | 0.55 | 0.79 |
| ½ cup | | 6.9 | 6.2 | 2.8 | 1.9 | 0.6 | 138 | 181 | 147 | 0.58 | 0.043 | 13.3 | 246 | 0.4 | 0.32 | 0.07 | 13.8 | 19094 |
| **lemon pudding**, from instant mix | 147 | 157 | 109.0 | 29.7 | | | 0 | 394 | 148 | 16 | 0.49 | 0.004 | 68 | 1 | 0.05 | 0.1 | 0.44 | 0.39 |
| with 2% milk - ½ cup | | 4.1 | 2.5 | 1.4 | 0.7 | 0.1 | 9 | 191 | 304 | 0.09 | 0.013 | 2.9 | 250 | | 0.20 | 0.05 | 5.9 | 19204 |
| **lemon pudding**, from inst mix | 147 | 169 | 107.6 | 29.5 | | | 0 | 392 | 146 | 16 | 0.47 | 0.004 | 35 | 1 | 0.05 | 0.1 | 0.44 | 0.39 |
| w/whl milk - ½ cup | | 4.0 | 4.3 | 2.6 | 1.2 | 0.2 | 16 | 187 | 301 | 0.09 | 0.016 | 2.6 | 154 | | 0.20 | 0.05 | 5.9 | 19331 |
| **lemon pudding**, from reg mix | 146 | 159 | 107.5 | 35.3 | 19.7 | | 0 | 92 | 12 | 1 | 0.15 | 0.007 | 22 | 0 | 0.01 | 0 | 0.09 | 0.18 |
| egg yolk, w/sgr, wtr - ½ cup | | 0.9 | 1.6 | 0.6 | 0.7 | 0.2 | 72 | 9 | 23 | 0.19 | 0.019 | 3.5 | 85 | 0.1 | 0.03 | 0.02 | 5.8 | 19333 |
| **Pudding Snacks**, choc van, sgr-free, | 106 | 60 | | 13.0 | 0 | | | 180 | 100 | | | | | 0 | | | | |
| red-cal, Jell-O - 1 snack cup | | 2.0 | 1.5 | 1.0 | | | 0 | | | 0.36 | | | 0 | | | | | KRAF1 |
| **rice pudding**, from regular mix | 144 | 160 | 105.7 | 30.0 | | | 0.1 | 157 | 151 | 19 | 0.55 | 0.082 | 66 | 1 | 0.11 | 0.6 | 0.35 | 0.41 |
| with 2% milk - ½ cup | | 4.7 | 2.3 | 1.4 | 0.6 | 0.1 | 9 | 187 | 125 | 0.53 | 0.026 | 2.7 | 248 | | 0.20 | 0.05 | 5.8 | 19208 |
| **rice pudding**, from regular mix | 144 | 174 | 104.3 | 29.8 | | | 0.1 | 156 | 148 | 19 | 0.55 | 0.085 | 42 | 1 | 0.11 | 0.6 | 0.35 | 0.41 |
| with whole milk - ½ cup | | 4.7 | 4.1 | 2.4 | 1.1 | 0.1 | 16 | 184 | 122 | 0.53 | 0.029 | 2.6 | 166 | | 0.20 | 0.05 | 5.8 | 19195 |
| **rice pudding**, ready-to-eat | 142 | 168 | 104.1 | 27.5 | 20.0 | | 1.3 | 175 | 74 | 11 | 0.70 | 0.179 | 31 | 0 | 0.03 | 0.2 | 0.26 | 0.50 |
| 5 oz serving | | 5.0 | 3.8 | 2.5 | 0.6 | 0.2 | 26 | 85 | 97 | 0.16 | 0.036 | 6.8 | 112 | 0.1 | 0.10 | 0.06 | 5.7 | 19193 |

| | WT (g) | KCAL / PRO (g) | $H_2O$ (g) / FAT (g) | CHO (g) / SFA (g) | TSUG (g) / MUFA (g) | ASUG (g) / PUFA (g) | DFIB (g) / CHOL (mg) | Na (mg) / K (mg) | Ca (mg) / P (mg) | Mg (mg) / Fe (mg) | Zn (mg) / Cu (mg) | Mn (mg) / Se (mcg) | A (mcg RAE) / A (IU) | C (mg) / E (mg ATE) | B-1 (mg) / B-2 (mg) | NIA (mg) / B-6 (mg) | B-12 (mcg) / FOL (mcg DFE) | PANT (mg) / REF |
|---|---|---|---|---|---|---|---|---|---|---|---|---|---|---|---|---|---|---|
| **tapioca pudding**, from regular | 141 | 148 | 105.8 | 27.6 | | | 0 | 171 | 148 | 17 | 0.49 | 0.010 | 66 | 1 | 0.04 | 0.1 | 0.35 | 0.39 |
| mix with 2% milk - ½ cup | | 4.1 | 2.4 | 1.4 | 0.6 | 0.1 | 8 | 188 | 116 | 0.08 | 0.017 | 2.8 | 226 | | 0.20 | 0.05 | 5.6 | 19209 |
| **tapioca pudding**, from reg mix | 141 | 162 | 104.3 | 27.4 | | | 0 | 169 | 145 | 17 | 0.48 | 0.013 | 35 | 1 | 0.04 | 0.1 | 0.35 | 0.38 |
| with whole milk - ½ cup | | 4.0 | 4.1 | 2.4 | 1.1 | 0.2 | 17 | 185 | 114 | 0.08 | 0.018 | 2.7 | 152 | | 0.20 | 0.05 | 5.6 | 19199 |
| **tapioca pudding**, ready-to-eat | 142 | 185 | 102.0 | 30.8 | 21.2 | 20.7 | 0 | 206 | 101 | 9 | 0.31 | 0.016 | 0 | 0 | 0.03 | 0.1 | 0.30 | 0.33 |
| 5 oz serving | | 2.8 | 5.5 | 1.4 | 3.6 | 0.1 | 1 | 131 | 85 | 0.16 | 0.026 | 0 | 0 | 0.2 | 0.14 | 0.03 | 4.3 | 19218 |
| **vanilla pudding**, from instant mix | 142 | 162 | 104.4 | 28.0 | 25.6 | 18.7 | 0 | 406 | 143 | 17 | 0.47 | 0.010 | 36 | 1 | 0.05 | 0.1 | 0.43 | 0.37 |
| with whole milk - ½ cup | | 3.8 | 4.1 | 2.5 | 1.2 | 0.2 | 16 | 182 | 280 | 0.10 | 0.034 | 2.3 | 149 | | 0.19 | 0.05 | 5.7 | 19203 |
| **vanilla pudding**, from regular mix | 140 | 141 | 106.2 | 25.9 | | | 0 | 223 | 151 | 17 | 0.48 | 0.006 | 67 | 1 | 0.04 | 0.1 | 0.35 | 0.39 |
| with 2% milk - ½ cup | | 4.1 | 2.4 | 1.4 | 0.6 | 0.1 | 10 | 192 | 116 | 0.08 | 0.018 | 2.9 | 224 | | 0.20 | 0.05 | 5.6 | 19212 |
| **vanilla pudding**, from regular mix | 140 | 157 | 104.5 | 26.2 | 23.9 | 17.5 | 0.1 | 216 | 139 | 13 | 0.49 | 0.006 | 35 | | 0.05 | 0.1 | 0.43 | 0.44 |
| with whole milk - ½ cup | | 4.0 | 4.1 | 2.3 | 1.0 | 0.3 | 13 | 179 | 112 | 0.06 | 0.018 | 4.6 | 125 | 0.1 | 0.23 | 0.04 | 5.6 | 19207 |
| **vanilla pudding**, ready-to-eat | 113 | 147 | 81.0 | 25.5 | 22.8 | 19.6 | 0 | 160 | 55 | 5 | 0.18 | 0.012 | 2 | 0 | 0.02 | 0.1 | 0.17 | 0.17 |
| 4 oz serving | | 1.6 | 4.3 | 1.1 | 2.6 | 0.1 | 1 | 73 | 46 | 0.10 | 0.020 | 0 | 7 | 0.3 | 0.08 | 0.02 | 2.3 | 19201 |
| **vanilla rennin dessert**, from mix | 133 | 102 | 109.2 | 16.4 | | | 0 | 61 | 161 | 17 | 0.48 | 0.004 | 68 | 1 | 0.05 | 0.1 | 0.44 | 0.39 |
| with 2% milk - ½ cup | | 4.1 | 2.4 | 1.4 | 0.6 | 0.1 | 9 | 189 | 126 | 0.07 | 0.016 | 2.8 | 226 | | 0.20 | 0.05 | 6.6 | 19214 |
| **vanilla rennin dessert**, from mix | 133 | 118 | 107.7 | 16.2 | | | 0 | 61 | 158 | 16 | 0.47 | 0.005 | 36 | 1 | 0.05 | 0.1 | 0.44 | 0.38 |
| with whole milk - ½ cup | | 4.0 | 4.1 | 2.5 | 1.1 | 0.2 | 17 | 186 | 124 | 0.07 | 0.019 | 2.5 | 153 | | 0.20 | 0.05 | 6.6 | 19223 |

## 7.10 SAUCES, SYRUPS, AND TOPPINGS FOR DESSERTS

| | WT (g) | KCAL / PRO (g) | $H_2O$ (g) / FAT (g) | CHO (g) / SFA (g) | TSUG (g) / MUFA (g) | ASUG (g) / PUFA (g) | DFIB (g) / CHOL (mg) | Na (mg) / K (mg) | Ca (mg) / P (mg) | Mg (mg) / Fe (mg) | Zn (mg) / Cu (mg) | Mn (mg) / Se (mcg) | A (mcg RAE) / A (IU) | C (mg) / E (mg ATE) | B-1 (mg) / B-2 (mg) | NIA (mg) / B-6 (mg) | B-12 (mcg) / FOL (mcg DFE) | PANT (mg) / REF |
|---|---|---|---|---|---|---|---|---|---|---|---|---|---|---|---|---|---|---|
| **butterscotch/caramel dessert** | 41 | 103 | 13.1 | 27.0 | | | 0.4 | 143 | 22 | 3 | 0.08 | 0.020 | 11 | 0 | 0 | 0 | 0.04 | 0.06 |
| topping - 2 T | | 0.6 | 0 | 0 | 0 | 0 | 0 | 34 | 19 | 0.08 | 0.010 | 0 | 37 | | 0.04 | 0.01 | 0.8 | 19364 |
| **chocolate fudge dessert topping** | 38 | 133 | 8.3 | 23.9 | 13.2 | 12.2 | 1.1 | 131 | 19 | 18 | 0.32 | 0.141 | 0 | 0 | 0.01 | 0.1 | 0.02 | 0.05 |
| 2 T | | 1.7 | 3.4 | 1.5 | 1.5 | 0.1 | 0 | 108 | 37 | 0.49 | 0.132 | 0.9 | 1 | 1.0 | 0.03 | 0.01 | 1.5 | 19348 |
| **chocolate syrup** | 39 | 109 | 12.1 | 25.4 | 19.4 | 19.2 | 1.0 | 28 | 5 | 25 | 0.28 | 0.149 | 0 | 0 | 0 | 0.1 | 0 | 0.01 |
| 2 T | | 0.8 | 0.4 | 0.2 | 0.1 | 0 | 0 | 87 | 50 | 0.82 | 0.200 | 0.5 | 0 | 0 | 0.02 | 0 | 0.8 | 14181 |
| **chocolate syrup, lite**, Hershey | 35 | 50 | 21.8 | 12.1 | 10.0 | | 0 | 35 | 4 | 13 | 0.17 | 0.097 | 0 | 0 | 0 | 0.1 | 0 | 0.01 |
| 2 T | | 0.5 | 0.3 | 0 | 0 | 0 | 0 | 65 | 19 | 0 | 0.097 | 0.4 | 0 | 0 | 0.01 | 0 | 0.7 | 19345 |
| **dessert glaze**, homemade | 27 | 92 | 4.1 | 22.6 | 21.7 | | 0 | 2 | 5 | 1 | 0.02 | 0.004 | 1 | 0 | 0 | 0 | 0.01 | 0.01 |
| 1/12 recipe yield (~1 oz) | | 0.1 | 0.1 | 0.1 | 0 | 0 | 0 | 8 | 4 | 0.01 | 0.002 | 0.3 | 4 | | 0.01 | 0 | 0.3 | 19375 |
| **icing/frosting**, choc, | 41 | 163 | 7.0 | 25.9 | 23.7 | | 0.4 | 75 | 3 | 9 | 0.12 | 0.098 | 0 | 0 | 0.01 | 0 | 0 | 0.01 |
| ready-to-spread, 2 T | | 0.5 | 7.2 | 2.3 | 3.7 | 0.9 | 0 | 80 | 32 | 0.58 | 0.082 | 0.3 | 0 | 0.6 | 0.01 | 0 | 0.4 | 19226 |
| **icing/frosting**, chocolate, from mix | 42 | 170 | 6.0 | 29.8 | | | 0.8 | 63 | 5 | 13 | 0.26 | 0.108 | 33 | 0 | 0 | 0 | 0 | 0.01 |
| made w/butter - 1/12 pkg prep | | 0.5 | 5.4 | 2.3 | 1.0 | 0.1 | 10 | 59 | 21 | 0.39 | 0.096 | 0.5 | 134 | | 0.01 | 0.03 | 1.3 | 19241 |
| **icing/frosting**, chocolate, from mix | 42 | 170 | 5.9 | 29.8 | | | 0.8 | 68 | 5 | 13 | 0.26 | | 34 | 0 | 0 | 0 | 0 | 0.01 |
| made w/margarine - 1/12 pkg prep | | 0.5 | 5.4 | 0.7 | 1.7 | 1.2 | 0 | 60 | 21 | 0.39 | 0.095 | 0.5 | 165 | | 0.01 | 0.03 | 0 | 19372 |
| **icing/frosting**, choc, ready-to-spread, | 33 | 130 | | 21.0 | 17.0 | | 0.5 | 95 | | | | | | | | | | |
| Betty Crocker - 2 T (1.2 oz) | | 0 | 5.0 | 1.5 | | | 0 | 75 | | 0.36 | | | | | | | | GENM123 |
| **icing/frosting**, coconut, ready-to- | 41 | 178 | 8.6 | 21.6 | 16.4 | 15.6 | 1.0 | 80 | 5 | 8 | 0.17 | 0.276 | 0 | 0 | 0.01 | 0.1 | 0 | 0.06 |
| spread - 2 T | | 0.6 | 9.8 | 3.5 | 4.4 | 1.3 | 0 | 76 | 26 | 0.22 | 0.051 | 1.0 | 2 | 0.4 | 0.01 | 0.02 | 0.8 | 19227 |
| **icing/frosting**, cream cheese, | 33 | 137 | 5.0 | 22.2 | 21.0 | | 0 | 63 | 1 | 1 | 0.01 | 0.004 | 0 | 0 | 0 | 0 | 0 | 0 |
| ready-to-spread - 1/12 tub | | 0 | 5.7 | 1.5 | 1.2 | 2.0 | | 12 | 1 | 0.05 | 0.007 | 0.2 | 0 | | 0 | 0 | 0 | 19228 |
| **icing/frosting**, van, from mix | 43 | 178 | 5.2 | 31.9 | | | 0 | 49 | 3 | 1 | 0 | | 34 | 0 | 0 | 0 | 0 | 0.01 |
| made w/marg - 1/12 pkg prep | | 0.1 | 5.5 | 0.7 | 1.7 | 1.2 | 0 | 4 | 3 | 0 | 0.012 | 0.3 | 169 | | 0 | 0 | 0 | 19371 |
| **icing/frosting**, vanilla, ready-to- | 38 | 159 | 5.7 | 25.8 | 24.0 | 23.8 | 0 | 70 | 1 | 0 | 0.03 | 0 | 0 | 0 | 0 | 0.1 | 0 | 0.02 |
| spread - 2 T | | 0 | 6.2 | 1.1 | 1.8 | 3.0 | 0 | 13 | 7 | 0.06 | 0 | 0 | 0 | 0.6 | 0.11 | 0 | 3.0 | 19230 |
| **icing/frosting**, van, whpd, ready- | 24 | 110 | | 15.0 | 13.0 | | | 25 | | | | | | | | | | |
| to-spread, Bty Crckr - 2 T | | 0 | 5.0 | 1.5 | | | | | | | | | | | | | | GENM125 |
| **icing/frosting mix**, white fluffy, | 26 | 100 | | 24.0 | 23.0 | | | 55 | | | | | | | | | | |
| Betty Crocker - 3 T (6 T prep) | | 0.5 | 0 | 0 | | | 0 | 30 | | | | | | | | | | GENM122 |
| **icing/frosting**, white fluffy, from | 26 | 63 | 9.2 | 16.3 | | | 0 | 41 | 1 | 1 | 0.01 | 0.001 | 0 | 0 | 0 | 0.2 | 0 | 0.01 |
| mix made w/wtr - 1/12 pkg prep | | 0.4 | 0 | 0 | | | 0 | 20 | 1 | 0.02 | 0.007 | 0.7 | 0 | | 0.01 | 0 | 0.5 | 19247 |
| **marshmallow cream dessert** | 28 | 90 | 5.5 | 22.1 | 13.1 | 13.1 | 0 | 22 | 1 | 1 | 0.01 | 0.002 | 0 | 0 | 0 | 0 | 0 | 0 |
| topping - 1 oz | | 0.2 | 0.1 | 0 | 0 | 0 | 0 | 1 | 2 | 0.06 | 0.027 | 0.5 | 0 | 0 | 0 | 0 | 0.3 | 19365 |
| **nuts in syrup dessert topping** | 41 | 184 | 6.0 | 23.8 | 15.1 | 14.4 | 0.9 | 17 | 14 | 22 | 0.43 | 0.495 | 0 | 0 | 0.07 | 0.2 | 0 | 0.08 |
| 2 T | | 1.8 | 9.0 | 0.8 | 2.0 | 5.6 | 0 | 62 | 48 | 0.43 | 0.221 | 0.9 | 3 | 0.1 | 0.05 | 0.07 | 10.7 | 19367 |
| **Oreo Crunchies topping**, Nabisco | 11 | 52 | 0.2 | 7.7 | 4.0 | | 0.4 | 58 | 3 | 5 | 0.14 | | | | 0.01 | 0.2 | 0 | 0 |
| .4 oz | | 0.5 | 2.4 | 0.5 | 0.3 | 0.1 | | 21 | 11 | 0.54 | 0.030 | | 0 | | 0.02 | 0 | | 18619 |
| **pineapple dessert topping** | 42 | 106 | 13.9 | 27.9 | 8.8 | 7.2 | 0.2 | 18 | 3 | 3 | 0.02 | 0.029 | 0 | 1 | 0.02 | 0 | 0 | 0.01 |
| 2 T | | 0 | 0 | 0 | 0 | 0 | 0 | 18 | 1 | 0.05 | 0.022 | 0.3 | 7 | 0 | 0.01 | 0.01 | 0.8 | 19366 |
| **strawberry dessert topping** | 42 | 107 | 13.9 | 27.8 | 11.5 | 11.2 | 0.3 | 9 | 3 | 2 | 0.03 | 0.070 | 0 | 6 | 0 | 0.1 | 0 | 0.02 |
| 2 T | | 0.1 | 0 | 0 | 0 | 0 | 0 | 21 | 2 | 0.12 | 0.013 | 0.3 | 8 | 0 | 0.01 | 0.01 | 2.5 | 19137 |

| | WT (g) | Macronutrients | | | | | | Minerals | | | | | Vitamins | | | | | |
|---|---|---|---|---|---|---|---|---|---|---|---|---|---|---|---|---|---|---|
| | | KCAL | H₂0 (g) | CHO (g) | TSUG (g) | ASUG (g) | DFIB (g) | Na (mg) | Ca (mg) | Mg (mg) | Zn (mg) | Mn (mg) | A (mcg RAE) | C (mg) | B-1 (mg) | NIA (mg) | B-12 (mcg) | PANT (mg) |
| | | PRO (g) | FAT (g) | SFA (g) | MUFA (g) | PUFA (g) | CHOL (mg) | K (mg) | P (mg) | Fe (mg) | Cu (mg) | Se (mcg) | A (IU) | E (mg ATE) | B-2 (mg) | B-6 (mg) | FOL (mcg DFE) | REF |

## 8. EGGS, EGG DISHES, AND EGG SUBSTITUTES

| | WT | KCAL | H₂0 | CHO | TSUG | ASUG | DFIB | Na | Ca | Mg | Zn | Mn | A | C | B-1 | NIA | B-12 | PANT |
|---|---|---|---|---|---|---|---|---|---|---|---|---|---|---|---|---|---|---|
| chicken egg, boiled, hard | 50 | 78 | 37.3 | 0.6 | 0.6 | 0 | 0 | 62 | 25 | 5 | 0.52 | 0.013 | 84 | 0 | 0.03 | 0 | 0.56 | 0.70 |
| 1 large egg | | 6.3 | 5.3 | 1.6 | 2.0 | 0.7 | 212 | 63 | 86 | 0.60 | 0.006 | 15.4 | 293 | 0.5 | 0.26 | 0.06 | 22.0 | 1129 |
| chicken egg, dried | 5 | 31 | 0.1 | 0.1 | | | 0 | 27 | 11 | 2 | 0.29 | 0.008 | 31 | 0 | 0.02 | 0 | 0.53 | 0.34 |
| 1 T | | 2.4 | 2.2 | 0.7 | 0.9 | 0.3 | 101 | 26 | 36 | 0.41 | 0.014 | 6.1 | 102 | | 0.06 | 0.02 | 9.6 | 1134 |
| chicken egg, fried | 46 | 90 | 31.8 | 0.4 | 0.4 | 0 | 0 | 94 | 27 | 6 | 0.55 | 0.019 | 91 | 0 | 0.03 | 0 | 0.64 | 0.72 |
| 1 large egg | | 6.3 | 7.0 | 2.0 | 2.9 | 1.2 | 210 | 68 | 96 | 0.91 | 0.051 | 15.7 | 335 | 0.6 | 0.24 | 0.07 | 23.5 | 1128 |
| chicken egg omelet, plain | 61 | 96 | 46.3 | 0.4 | 0.4 | 0 | 0 | 98 | 29 | 6 | 0.57 | 0.020 | 95 | 0 | 0.04 | 0 | 0.66 | 0.74 |
| 1 large egg | | 6.5 | 7.3 | 2.0 | 3.0 | 1.4 | 217 | 70 | 99 | 0.95 | 0.054 | 16.3 | 349 | 0.7 | 0.25 | 0.07 | 23.8 | 1130 |
| chicken egg, poached | 50 | 71 | 37.8 | 0.4 | 0.4 | 0 | 0 | 147 | 26 | 6 | 0.55 | 0.020 | 70 | 0 | 0.03 | 0 | 0.64 | 0.72 |
| 1 large egg | | 6.3 | 5.0 | 1.5 | 1.9 | 0.7 | 211 | 66 | 95 | 0.92 | 0.051 | 15.8 | 242 | 0.5 | 0.20 | 0.06 | 17.5 | 1131 |
| chicken egg, raw | 50 | 72 | 37.9 | 0.4 | 0.4 | 0 | 0 | 70 | 26 | 6 | 0.56 | 0.019 | 70 | 0 | 0.03 | 0 | 0.64 | 0.72 |
| 1 large egg | | 6.3 | 5.0 | 1.5 | 1.9 | 0.7 | 212 | 67 | 96 | 0.92 | 0.051 | 15.8 | 244 | 0.5 | 0.24 | 0.07 | 23.5 | 1123 |
| chicken egg, scrambled with milk | 61 | 102 | 44.6 | 1.3 | 1.1 | 0 | 0 | 171 | 43 | 7 | 0.61 | 0.013 | 87 | 0 | 0.03 | 0 | 0.47 | 0.61 |
| 1 large egg | | 6.8 | 7.4 | 2.2 | 2.9 | 1.3 | 215 | 84 | 104 | 0.73 | 0.009 | 13.7 | 321 | 0.7 | 0.27 | 0.07 | 18.3 | 1132 |
| chicken egg white, raw | 33 | 16 | 28.9 | 0.2 | 0.2 | 0 | 0 | 55 | 2 | 4 | 0.01 | 0.004 | 0 | 0 | 0 | 0 | 0.03 | 0.06 |
| white of 1 large egg | | 3.6 | 0.1 | 0 | 0 | 0 | 0 | 54 | 5 | 0.03 | 0.008 | 6.6 | 0 | 0 | 0.14 | 0 | 1.3 | 1124 |
| chicken egg yolk, raw | 17 | 54 | 8.9 | 0.6 | 0.1 | 0 | 0 | 8 | 22 | 1 | 0.39 | 0.009 | 65 | 0 | 0.03 | 0 | 0.33 | 0.51 |
| yolk of 1 large egg | | 2.7 | 4.5 | 1.6 | 2.0 | 0.7 | 210 | 19 | 66 | 0.46 | 0.013 | 9.5 | 245 | 0.4 | 0.09 | 0.06 | 24.8 | 1125 |
| duck egg, raw | 70 | 130 | 49.6 | 1.0 | 0.7 | 0 | 0 | 102 | 45 | 12 | 0.99 | 0.027 | 136 | 0 | 0.11 | 0.1 | 3.78 | 1.30 |
| 1 egg | | 9.0 | 9.6 | 2.6 | 4.6 | 0.9 | 619 | 155 | 154 | 2.70 | 0.043 | 25.5 | 472 | 0.9 | 0.28 | 0.18 | 56.0 | 1138 |
| egg substitute, frozen | 60 | 96 | 43.9 | 1.9 | 1.9 | 0 | 0 | 119 | 44 | 9 | 0.59 | 0.004 | 7 | 0 | 0.07 | 0.1 | 0.20 | 1.00 |
| ¼ cup | | 6.8 | 6.7 | 1.2 | 1.5 | 3.7 | 1 | 128 | 43 | 1.19 | 0.013 | 24.8 | 135 | 1.0 | 0.23 | 0.08 | 9.6 | 1142 |
| egg substitute, liquid | 47 | 39 | 38.9 | 0.3 | 0.3 | 0 | 0 | 83 | 25 | 4 | 0.61 | 0.003 | 8 | 0 | 0.05 | 0.1 | 0.14 | 1.27 |
| 1.5 fl oz | | 5.6 | 1.6 | 0.3 | 0.4 | 0.8 | 0 | 155 | 57 | 0.99 | 0.011 | 11.7 | 169 | 0.1 | 0.14 | 0 | 7.0 | 1143 |
| egg substitute, powdered | 10 | 44 | 0.4 | 2.2 | 2.2 | 0 | 0 | 80 | 33 | 6 | 0.18 | 0.008 | 37 | 0 | 0.02 | 0.1 | 0.35 | 0.34 |
| .35 oz | | 5.6 | 1.3 | 0.4 | 0.5 | 0.2 | 57 | 74 | 48 | 0.32 | 0.021 | 12.8 | 123 | 0.1 | 0.18 | 0.01 | 12.5 | 1144 |
| goose egg, raw | 144 | 266 | 101.4 | 1.9 | 1.4 | 0 | 0 | 199 | 86 | 23 | 1.92 | 0.055 | 269 | 0 | 0.21 | 0.3 | 7.34 | 2.53 |
| 1 egg | | 20.0 | 19.1 | 5.2 | 8.3 | 2.4 | 1227 | 302 | 300 | 5.24 | 0.089 | 53.1 | 936 | 1.9 | 0.55 | 0.34 | 109.4 | 1139 |
| quail egg, raw | 9 | 14 | 6.7 | 0 | 0 | 0 | 0 | 13 | 6 | 1 | 0.13 | 0.003 | 14 | 0 | 0.01 | 0 | 0.14 | 0.16 |
| 1 egg | | 1.2 | 1.0 | 0.3 | 0.4 | 0.1 | 76 | 12 | 20 | 0.33 | 0.006 | 2.9 | 49 | 0.1 | 0.07 | 0.01 | 5.9 | 1140 |
| turkey egg, raw | 79 | 135 | 57.3 | 0.9 | | | 0 | 119 | 78 | 10 | 1.25 | 0.030 | 131 | 0 | 0.09 | 0 | 1.34 | 1.49 |
| 1 egg | | 10.8 | 9.4 | 2.9 | 3.6 | 1.3 | 737 | 112 | 134 | 3.24 | 0.049 | 27.1 | 438 | | 0.37 | 0.10 | 56.1 | 1141 |

## 9. ENTREES AND MEALS
### 9.1 CANNED ENTREES

| | WT | KCAL | H₂0 | CHO | TSUG | ASUG | DFIB | Na | Ca | Mg | Zn | Mn | A | C | B-1 | NIA | B-12 | PANT |
|---|---|---|---|---|---|---|---|---|---|---|---|---|---|---|---|---|---|---|
| baked beans with beef | 266 | 322 | 189.7 | 45.0 | | | | 1267 | 120 | 66 | 3.19 | 1.596 | 29 | 5 | 0.14 | 2.5 | 0 | 0.49 |
| 1 cup (9.1 oz) | | 17.0 | 9.2 | 4.5 | 3.7 | 0.5 | 59 | 851 | 215 | 4.26 | 0.798 | 25.5 | 567 | | 0.12 | 0.23 | 114.0 | 16007 |
| baked beans with frankurters | 259 | 368 | 179.6 | 39.9 | 16.9 | 13.3 | 17.9 | 1114 | 124 | 73 | 4.84 | 1.088 | 10 | 6 | 0.15 | 2.3 | 0.88 | 0.36 |
| 1 cup (9.1 oz) | | 17.5 | 17.0 | 6.1 | 7.3 | 2.2 | 16 | 609 | 269 | 4.48 | 0.552 | 16.8 | 225 | 0.4 | 0.15 | 0.12 | 77.7 | 16008 |
| beef ravioli in tomato and meat sauce, Chef Boyardee - 8.6 oz | 244 | 224 | 193.1 | 33.1 | 4.7 | | 1.2 | 910 | 27 | | | | 0 | | | | | |
| | | 8.1 | 6.5 | 2.8 | 2.7 | 0.3 | 7 | | | 1.63 | | | 273 | | | | | 22515 |
| beef ravioli, mini in tom and meat sce, Chef Boyardee - 8.9 oz | 252 | 232 | 200.9 | 31.1 | 4.9 | | 2.5 | 935 | 30 | | | | 0 | | | | | |
| | | 8.2 | 8.2 | 3.5 | 3.4 | 0.4 | 8 | | | 2.57 | | | 416 | | | | | 22517 |
| beef stew | 232 | 220 | 189.1 | 15.7 | 2.2 | 0 | 3.5 | 947 | 28 | 32 | 1.90 | 0.332 | 204 | 10 | 0.17 | 2.9 | 0.86 | 0.50 |
| 8.2 oz | | 11.5 | 12.5 | 5.2 | 5.5 | 0.5 | 37 | 404 | 128 | 1.65 | 0.183 | 1.6 | 3860 | 0.3 | 0.14 | 0.30 | 25.5 | 22905 |
| beef stew, Dinty Moore | 236 | 222 | 192.5 | 16.1 | 2.3 | | 2.6 | 984 | 19 | 24 | 2.60 | | | 3 | | | | |
| 1 cup (8.3 oz) | | 11.3 | 13.1 | 5.6 | 6.3 | 0.7 | 38 | 396 | | 1.65 | 0 | | 3988 | | | | | 22694 |
| Beefaroni, Chef Boyardee | 212 | 195 | 167.8 | 28.8 | 4.1 | | 1.1 | 791 | 23 | | | | 0 | | | | | |
| 7.5 oz | | 7.0 | 5.7 | 2.5 | 2.4 | 0.3 | 6 | | | 1.42 | | | 237 | | | | | 22516 |
| chili con carne, Hormel | 236 | 194 | 191.6 | 17.9 | 3.4 | | 3.1 | 970 | 50 | 38 | 2.60 | | | 0 | | | | |
| 1 cup (8.3 oz) | | 17.0 | 6.6 | 2.2 | 2.2 | 0.8 | 35 | 349 | | 2.60 | 0.236 | | 2384 | | | | | 22705 |
| chili con carne (no beans) | 222 | 262 | 172.4 | 13.5 | | | | 864 | 67 | 44 | 2.49 | 0.613 | | 4 | 0.07 | 2.8 | 2.26 | 0.35 |
| 7.8 oz | | 16.7 | 15.8 | 5.0 | 5.5 | 1.0 | 47 | 411 | 171 | 4.46 | 0.417 | 14.4 | | | 0.25 | 0.29 | | 22911 |
| chili con carne (no beans), Chef-Mate - 1 cup (8.8 oz) | 250 | 368 | 176.4 | 20.0 | 3.8 | | 3.8 | 1400 | 80 | 45 | 4.50 | 0.408 | | 0 | 0.14 | 4.8 | 1.82 | 0.78 |
| | | 22.5 | 22.5 | 7.6 | 9.8 | 1.2 | 55 | 530 | 162 | 5.00 | 0.360 | | 2375 | | 0.27 | 0.34 | | 22216 |
| chili con carne with beans | 222 | 269 | 165.0 | 25.4 | | | 8.7 | 941 | 84 | 64 | 2.31 | 0.526 | | 3 | 0.12 | 2.2 | 1.44 | 0.36 |
| 7.8 oz | | 15.7 | 11.7 | 3.9 | 4.8 | 0.9 | 29 | 608 | 215 | 5.79 | 0.602 | 22.6 | 884 | | 0.22 | 0.28 | 57.7 | 22904 |

Column key — each food occupies two lines. The header shows *upper-line label / lower-line label*.

| Food | WT (g) | KCAL / PRO | H₂O / FAT | CHO / SFA | TSUG / MUFA | ASUG / PUFA | DFIB / CHOL | Na / K | Ca / P | Mg / Fe | Zn / Cu | Mn / Se | A mcg RAE / A IU | C / E mg ATE | B-1 / B-2 | NIA / B-6 | B-12 / FOL DFE | PANT / REF |
|---|---|---|---|---|---|---|---|---|---|---|---|---|---|---|---|---|---|---|
| chili con carne with beans, Chef-Mate - 1 cup (8.9 oz) | 253 | 420 | 175.8 | 34.2 | 3.8 | | 7.6 | 1280 | 71 | 46 | 3.87 | 0.407 | | 0 | 0.11 | 3.5 | 1.44 | 0.66 |
| | | 17.7 | 24.0 | 10.1 | 10.7 | 1.4 | 40 | 511 | 167 | 3.80 | 0.329 | | 1012 | | 0.20 | 0.23 | | 22215 |
| chili con carne with beans, Hormel - 1 cup (8.7 oz) | 247 | 240 | 187.8 | 33.7 | 4.6 | | 8.4 | 1163 | 69 | 59 | 2.72 | | | 0 | | | | |
| | | 16.6 | 4.4 | 1.8 | 1.7 | 0.9 | 25 | 662 | | 3.21 | 0.247 | | 968 | | | | | 22719 |
| chili con carne with beans, Nalley - 9.1 oz | 258 | 281 | 192.5 | 11.9 | | | 12.9 | 1231 | | | | | | | | | | |
| | | 40.2 | 8.0 | 2.8 | 3.0 | 0.8 | 26 | | | 4.59 | | | 0 | | | | | 22513 |
| chili con carne with beans, Old El Paso - 8 oz | 228 | 249 | 175.3 | 21.7 | | | 9.8 | 588 | | | | | | 0 | | | | |
| | | 17.6 | 10.3 | 2.1 | 4.3 | 2.2 | 36 | | | 2.69 | | | 0 | | | | | 22514 |
| chili con carne with beans, Stagg Classic - 1 cup (8.7 oz) | 247 | 324 | 180.9 | 29.2 | 7.1 | | 7.4 | 825 | 91 | 64 | 2.72 | | | 2 | | | | |
| | | 17.2 | 16.3 | 6.7 | 6.9 | 1.1 | 42 | 785 | | 3.95 | 0.247 | | 1161 | | | | | 22716 |
| chili con carne with beans, Stagg Country - 1 cup (8.7 oz) | 247 | 319 | 182.2 | 29.0 | 5.9 | | 5.9 | 1131 | 57 | 52 | 2.47 | | | 2 | | | | |
| | | 15.5 | 15.8 | 6.8 | 7.5 | 0.7 | 40 | 558 | | 3.46 | 0.247 | | 514 | | | | | 22717 |
| chili con carne with beans, Stagg Dynamite - 1 cup (8.7 oz) | 247 | 333 | 178.1 | 30.7 | 6.6 | | 8.2 | 862 | 104 | 69 | 2.72 | | | 3 | | | | |
| | | 18.3 | 15.4 | 5.7 | 6.8 | 0.9 | 44 | 778 | | 4.45 | 0.247 | | 1252 | | | | | 22714 |
| chili con carne with beans, Stagg Ranchhouse - 1 cup (8.7 oz) | 247 | 284 | 183.0 | 31.6 | 5.7 | | 8.6 | 813 | 114 | 82 | 1.98 | | | 5 | | | | |
| | | 19.2 | 8.9 | 2.6 | 4.1 | 2.0 | 47 | 867 | | 4.20 | 0.494 | | 1082 | | | | | 22715 |
| chili con carne with beans, Stagg Silverado - 1 cup (8.7 oz) | 247 | 227 | 189.1 | 33.1 | 7.2 | | 8.2 | 865 | 89 | 72 | 2.72 | | | 5 | | | | |
| | | 18.0 | 2.8 | 1.0 | 0.9 | 0.9 | 40 | 815 | | 3.70 | 0.494 | | 1247 | | | | | 22718 |
| chili with beans (no meat) 1 cup (9 oz) | 256 | 287 | 193.3 | 30.5 | 3.0 | 0 | 11.3 | 1336 | 120 | 115 | 5.12 | 0.343 | 44 | 4 | 0.12 | 0.9 | 0 | 3.64 |
| | | 14.6 | 14.1 | 6.0 | 6.0 | 0.9 | 44 | 934 | 394 | 8.78 | 0.300 | 3.3 | 863 | 1.3 | 0.27 | 0.34 | 58.9 | 16059 |
| chili with beans, vegetarian, Hormel - 1 cup (8.7 oz) | 247 | 205 | 192.5 | 38.0 | 6.2 | | 9.9 | 778 | 96 | 82 | 1.73 | | | 1 | | | | |
| | | 11.9 | 0.7 | 0.1 | 0.1 | 0.4 | 0 | 803 | | 3.46 | 0.494 | | 1941 | | | | | 22720 |
| corned beef hash 1 cup (8.3 oz) | 236 | 387 | 166.0 | 21.9 | 0.8 | 0 | 2.6 | 1003 | 45 | 31 | 3.30 | 0.198 | 0 | 2 | 0.16 | 3.7 | 0.97 | 0.95 |
| | | 20.6 | 24.2 | 10.2 | 12.4 | 0.7 | 76 | 406 | 132 | 2.36 | 0 | 17.7 | 0 | 0.1 | 0.12 | 0.55 | 16.5 | 22908 |
| corned beef hash, Chef-Mate 1 cup (8.9 oz) | 253 | 455 | 163.9 | 27.8 | 2.0 | | 2.8 | 1619 | 20 | 38 | 7.51 | 0.111 | 0 | | 0.22 | 6.3 | 2.45 | 1.23 |
| | | 21.0 | 30.4 | 13.9 | 14.7 | 1.1 | 71 | 536 | 240 | 1.44 | 0.339 | | 0 | | 0.30 | 0.58 | | 22217 |
| corned beef hash, Hormel 1 cup (8.3 oz) | 236 | 387 | 166.0 | 21.9 | 0.8 | | 2.6 | 1003 | 45 | 31 | 3.30 | | | 2 | | | | |
| | | 20.6 | 24.2 | 10.2 | 12.4 | 0.7 | 76 | 406 | | 2.36 | 0 | | 0 | | | | | 22698 |
| macaroni and cheese 8.9 oz serving | 252 | 207 | 205.1 | 29.0 | 1.3 | 0 | 1.3 | 1061 | 88 | 23 | 1.13 | 0.564 | 43 | 0 | 0.25 | 3.0 | 0.38 | 0.19 |
| | | 8.5 | 6.2 | 2.2 | 1.5 | 0.8 | 15 | 212 | 118 | 2.27 | 0.746 | 23.9 | 164 | 0.1 | 0.29 | 0.09 | 55.4 | 22247 |
| pasta with franks in tomato sauce 1 cup (8.9 oz) | 252 | 262 | 197.1 | 30.0 | 8.1 | 3.3 | 2.3 | 1215 | 45 | 35 | 1.31 | 0.325 | 25 | 10 | 0.20 | 2.9 | 0.48 | 0.60 |
| | | 9.3 | 11.6 | 3.7 | 4.8 | 1.5 | 23 | 481 | 108 | 2.29 | 0.343 | 20.2 | 333 | 1.9 | 0.17 | 0.18 | 52.9 | 22522 |
| pasta with meatballs in tomato sce 1 cup (8.9 oz) | 252 | 260 | 196.2 | 31.0 | 10.0 | 5.4 | 6.8 | 1053 | 28 | 35 | 1.84 | 0.393 | 35 | 8 | 0.19 | 3.3 | 0.58 | 0.52 |
| | | 10.9 | 10.3 | 4.0 | 4.2 | 0.6 | 20 | 416 | 116 | 2.34 | 0.214 | 19.2 | 499 | 1.9 | 0.16 | 0.17 | 93.2 | 22907 |
| roast beef hash, Hormel 1 cup (8.3 oz) | 236 | 385 | 165.5 | 22.9 | 0.6 | | 3.5 | 793 | 42 | 33 | 3.30 | | | 2 | | | | |
| | | 21.3 | 23.6 | 9.9 | 11.3 | 0.6 | 73 | 432 | | 2.36 | 0.236 | | 0 | | | | | 22721 |
| spaghetti and meatballs in tom sce, Chef Boyardee - 8.5 oz | 240 | 240 | 188.5 | 28.6 | 7.1 | | 3.4 | 864 | 26 | | | | | 1 | | | | |
| | | 10.5 | 9.3 | 3.8 | 3.9 | 0.8 | 17 | | | 1.97 | | | 0 | | | | | 22518 |
| turkey chili with beans, Hormel 1 cup (8.7 oz) | 247 | 203 | 194.8 | 25.6 | 5.7 | | 6.4 | 1198 | 116 | 69 | 2.72 | | | 1 | | | | |
| | | 18.7 | 2.8 | 0.7 | 0.4 | 1.2 | 35 | 682 | | 3.46 | 0.247 | | 1650 | | | | | 22706 |

## 9.2 FROZEN BREAKFASTS

| Food | WT (g) | KCAL / PRO | H₂O / FAT | CHO / SFA | TSUG / MUFA | ASUG / PUFA | DFIB / CHOL | Na / K | Ca / P | Mg / Fe | Zn / Cu | Mn / Se | A-RAE / A-IU | C / E | B-1 / B-2 | NIA / B-6 | B-12 / FOL | PANT / REF |
|---|---|---|---|---|---|---|---|---|---|---|---|---|---|---|---|---|---|---|
| biscuit with sausage, Jimmy Dean 2 biscuits (3.4 oz) | 96 | 385 | 32.2 | 23.1 | | | 1.4 | 881 | 76 | | | | | | | | | |
| | | 9.5 | 28.2 | 8.6 | | | 32 | | | 1.58 | | | | | | | | 22364 |
| burrito, breakfast w/ham and cheese - 3.5 oz entrée | 99 | 212 | 53.3 | 27.8 | | | 1.4 | 405 | | | | | | | | | | |
| | | 9.6 | 6.9 | 2.0 | 2.1 | 1.8 | 192 | | | 3.17 | | | 0 | | | | | 22679 |
| eggs, scrmbld, sausage, hash browns - 6.2 oz meal | 177 | 361 | 117.4 | 17.2 | | | 1.4 | 772 | | | | | | | | | | |
| | | 12.6 | 26.9 | 7.3 | 12.7 | 3.6 | 283 | | | 1.66 | | | 0 | | | | | 22595 |
| French toast, cinn swirl w/sausage 5.5 oz entrée | 156 | 415 | 79.2 | 38.2 | | | 2.3 | 502 | | | | | | | | | | |
| | | 13.1 | 23.2 | 7.3 | 9.4 | 3.4 | 98 | | | 2.54 | | | 0 | | | | | 22592 |
| Toaster Scrambles Pastry, chs, egg, bacon, Pillsbury - 1.66 oz entrée | 47 | 180 | | 15.0 | 1.0 | | 0 | 330 | 0 | | | | | 0 | | | | |
| | | 4.0 | 12.0 | 3.5 | | | 25 | | | 0.72 | | | 0 | | | | | GENM128 |
| Toaster Scrambles Pastry, chs, egg, ham, Pillsbury - 1.66 oz entrée | 47 | 180 | | 15.0 | 1.0 | | 0 | 340 | 0 | | | | | 0 | | | | |
| | | 4.0 | 11.0 | 3.0 | | | 25 | | | 0.72 | | | 0 | | | | | GENM129 |
| Toaster Scrambles Pastry, chs, egg, sausg, Pillsbury - 1.66 oz entrée | 47 | 180 | | 15.0 | 1.0 | | 0 | 320 | 0 | | | | | 0 | | | | |
| | | 4.0 | 12.0 | 3.0 | | | 25 | | | 0.72 | | | 0 | | | | | GENM130 |

## 9.3 FROZEN ENTREES AND SANDWICHES

| Food | WT (g) | KCAL / PRO | H₂O / FAT | CHO / SFA | TSUG / MUFA | ASUG / PUFA | DFIB / CHOL | Na / K | Ca / P | Mg / Fe | Zn / Cu | Mn / Se | A-RAE / A-IU | C / E | B-1 / B-2 | NIA / B-6 | B-12 / FOL | PANT / REF |
|---|---|---|---|---|---|---|---|---|---|---|---|---|---|---|---|---|---|---|
| beef and cheddar pocket sandwich, Hot Pockets - 5 oz pocket | 142 | 403 | 62.5 | 39.2 | | | | 906 | 337 | | | | | 0 | | | | |
| | | 16.3 | 20.2 | 8.8 | 6.7 | 1.2 | 53 | | | 2.93 | | | 0 | | | | | 22534 |
| beef, creamed chipped, Stouffer's 4.4 oz entrée | 125 | 138 | 97.3 | 8.8 | 4.2 | | 0.5 | 589 | 101 | | | | | 0 | 0.06 | 1.2 | | |
| | | 9.4 | 7.1 | 4.1 | 1.9 | 0.4 | 31 | 230 | | 0.86 | | | 0 | | 0.20 | | | 22579 |

| | WT (g) | KCAL / PRO (g) | H₂O (g) / FAT (g) | CHO (g) / SFA (g) | TSUG (g) / MUFA (g) | ASUG (g) / PUFA (g) | DFIB (g) / CHOL (mg) | Na (mg) / K (mg) | Ca (mg) / P (mg) | Mg (mg) / Fe (mg) | Zn (mg) / Cu (mg) | Mn (mg) / Se (mcg) | A (mcg RAE) / A (IU) | C (mg) / E (mg ATE) | B-1 (mg) / B-2 (mg) | NIA (mg) / B-6 (mg) | B-12 (mcg) / FOL (mcg DFE) | PANT (mg) / REF |
|---|---|---|---|---|---|---|---|---|---|---|---|---|---|---|---|---|---|---|
| **beef macaroni,** Healthy Choice | 240 | 211 | 187.7 | 33.5 | 9.1 | | 4.6 | 444 | 46 | 36 | 1.22 | 0.547 | 55 | 58 | 0.28 | 3.1 | 0.12 | 0.41 |
| *8.5 oz entrée* | | 14.1 | 2.2 | 0.7 | 1.2 | 0.3 | 14 | 365 | 134 | 2.71 | 0.307 | 24.2 | 514 | 1.7 | 0.16 | 0.19 | 158.4 | 22402 |
| **beef pot pie** | 198 | 436 | 114.9 | 43.7 | | | 1.6 | 723 | 28 | 26 | 2.18 | 0.410 | | 1 | 0.39 | 3.2 | 0.63 | 0.29 |
| *7 oz individual pot pie* | | 14.4 | 22.6 | 8.2 | 10.5 | 2.9 | 42 | 228 | 133 | 2.48 | 0.059 | 10.5 | | 0.5 | 0.17 | 0.26 | 55.4 | 22529 |
| **beef pot roast w/whpd pot,** Stouffer's Lean Cuisine - *9 oz entrée* | 255 | 184 | 211.5 | 21.1 | 3.6 | | 3.1 | 768 | 71 | | | | | 3 | 0.18 | 3.0 | | |
| | | 12.7 | 5.5 | 1.4 | 2.6 | 1.0 | 20 | 895 | | 1.58 | | | 946 | | 0.15 | | | 22578 |
| **beef shepherd's pie,** Sfwy Slct Grmt Club - *1 cup (¼ pkg)* | 227 | 360 | | 17.0 | 0 | | 4.0 | 890 | 100 | | | | | 0 | | | | |
| | | 28.0 | 20.0 | 9.0 | | | 75 | | | 2.16 | | | 100 | | | | | SAFE41 |
| **burrito,** bean and cheese | 143 | 302 | 75.9 | 46.3 | 2.0 | | 14.6 | 589 | 60 | 37 | 0.97 | 0.519 | 70 | 0 | 0.48 | 3.1 | | |
| *5 oz burrito* | | 9.9 | 8.5 | 2.2 | 3.2 | 2.1 | | 310 | 94 | 3.98 | 0.209 | 16.2 | 270 | | 0.20 | 0.12 | 145.9 | 22918 |
| **burrito,** beef and bean | 139 | 332 | 70.2 | 42.9 | 4.9 | | 5.8 | 816 | 47 | 44 | 1.38 | 0.669 | 15 | 1 | 0.55 | 4.0 | | 0.01 |
| *4.9 oz burrito* | | 10.1 | 13.4 | 4.1 | 5.3 | 1.9 | 11 | 307 | 100 | 4.11 | 0.293 | 14.9 | 295 | | 0.33 | 0.13 | 171.0 | 22917 |
| **burrito,** beef and bean w/grn chili, mild, Patio - *4.9 oz entrée* | 140 | 2 90 | 76.7 | 42.2 | 7.4 | | 4.9 | 713 | 29 | | | | 0 | | | | | |
| | | 9.1 | 9.4 | 3.4 | 3.5 | 2.2 | 7 | | | 3.28 | | | 0 | | | | | 22584 |
| **cabbage, stuffed,** whpd pot, Stfrs Ln Csn - *9.5 oz entrée* | 269 | 196 | 224.0 | 24.4 | 5.8 | | 4.0 | 710 | 89 | | | | | 1 | 0.22 | 2.6 | | |
| | | 10.8 | 6.1 | 1.7 | 3.0 | 0.9 | 13 | 732 | | 1.51 | | | 113 | | 0.11 | | | 22585 |
| **calzone,** sauge peprni, Madalena's Masterpie - *8 oz calzone* | 227 | 500 | | 42.0 | 5.0 | | 0 | 1340 | 350 | | | | | 5 | | | | |
| | | 26.0 | 27.0 | 11.0 | | | 65 | | | 3.60 | | | 500 | | | | | FRUI1 |
| **cheesy rice and broccoli,** Green Giant - *10 oz entrée* | 283 | 270 | | 52.0 | 4.0 | | 2.0 | 970 | 100 | | | | | 21 | | | | |
| | | 7.0 | 4.5 | 1.5 | | | 5 | | | 0.36 | | | 3500 | | | | | GENM132 |
| **chicken al'orange,** rice, veg, Stfrs Ln Csn - *9 oz entrée* | 255 | 230 | | 33.0 | 9.0 | | 2.0 | 300 | 20 | | | | | 9 | | | | |
| | | 20.0 | 1.5 | 0.5 | 0 | 0.5 | 40 | 430 | | 0.36 | | | 2250 | | | | | STOF21 |
| **chicken,** broc, ched pckt sndwch, Croissant Pockets - *4.5 oz pocket* | 128 | 301 | 64.0 | 38.9 | | | 1.4 | 652 | | | | | | 6 | | | | |
| | | 11.4 | 11.0 | 3.4 | 4.4 | 1.7 | 37 | | | 3.80 | | | 339 | | | | | 22535 |
| **chicken fajita kit,** Tyson *3.8 (½ pkg yield)* | 107 | 128 | 76.6 | 17.4 | 2.2 | | 1.8 | 368 | 21 | | | | | 20 | | | | |
| | | 6.8 | 3.6 | 0.9 | 1.1 | 1.6 | 12 | | | 1.13 | | | 717 | | | | | 22687 |
| **chicken,** grvy, rstd pot, veg, cherry crisp, Hlthy Chc - *11.35 oz meal* | 321 | 280 | | 37.0 | 19.0 | | 5.0 | 600 | 40 | | | | | 12 | | | | |
| | | 18.0 | 6.0 | 2.5 | 2.0 | 1.5 | 40 | | | 1.44 | | | 500 | | | | | HLCH13 |
| **chicken,** grn bns, mushrooms, rice, Stfrs Ln Csn - *8.5 oz entrée* | 240 | 230 | | 25.0 | 6.0 | | 1.0 | 520 | 20 | | | | | 2 | | | | |
| | | 21.0 | 5.0 | 1.0 | 1.0 | 1.5 | 50 | 540 | | 0.36 | | | 100 | | | | | STOF23 |
| **chicken marsala,** mshrms, grn bns, Sfwy Grmt Clb - *5 oz (¼ pkg)* | 140 | 160 | | 4.0 | 3.0 | | 0 | 330 | 0 | | | | | 0 | | | | |
| | | 22.0 | 4.5 | 2.0 | | | 65 | | | 0.72 | | | 0 | | | | | SAFE43 |
| **chicken pot pie** | 217 | 464 | 127.3 | 50.0 | | | 2.6 | 825 | 63 | 30 | 1.22 | 0.484 | 577 | 1 | 0.50 | 4.8 | 0.69 | 1.02 |
| *7.7 oz individual pot pie* | | 13.2 | 23.5 | 7.8 | 8.0 | 3.0 | 52 | 269 | 178 | 2.39 | 0.065 | 15.4 | 2285 | 0.3 | 0.24 | 0.26 | 108.5 | 22906 |
| **chicken pot pie,** Banquet *7 oz individual pot pie* | 198 | 380 | 126.5 | 35.7 | 5.6 | | 3.4 | 842 | 30 | | | | | | | | | |
| | | 11.1 | 21.5 | 8.3 | 9.2 | 3.7 | 30 | | | 1.01 | | | 1370 | | | | | 22525 |
| **chicken pot pie,** Marie Callender's *1 cup (8.3 oz)* | 234 | 550 | 136.2 | 44.9 | 1.8 | | 2.3 | 826 | 37 | | | | | 0 | | | | |
| | | 16.0 | 34.1 | 9.6 | 13.4 | 4.1 | 21 | | | 3.39 | | | 1753 | | | | | 22526 |
| **chicken pot pie,** Stouffer's *10 oz individual pot pie* | 283 | 733 | 150.6 | 63.9 | 10.6 | | 4.0 | 1177 | 144 | | | | | 1 | 0.65 | 6.8 | | |
| | | 20.3 | 43.9 | 17.8 | 16.0 | 6.2 | 62 | 464 | | 2.89 | | | 1013 | | 0.57 | | | 22527 |
| **chicken, veg, vermicelli,** Stfs Ln Csn - *10.5 oz entrée* | 297 | 232 | 242.1 | 26.5 | 4.5 | | 3.9 | 633 | 163 | | | | | 3 | 0.27 | 6.6 | | |
| | | 19.8 | 5.0 | 1.9 | 1.8 | 1.1 | 30 | 692 | | 1.43 | | | 1568 | | 0.24 | | | 22577 |
| **chicken w/almonds,** rice, grn bns, car, broc, Stfrs Ln Csn - *8.5 oz entrée* | 240 | 280 | | 44.0 | 13.0 | | 2.0 | 650 | 40 | | | | | 6 | | | | |
| | | 16.0 | 4.5 | 0.5 | 1.0 | 1.0 | 30 | 330 | | 1.80 | | | 1250 | | | | | STOF22 |
| **chicken wings,** glazed, bbq, microwaved - *3.4 oz* | 96 | 238 | 51.7 | 3.7 | 2.0 | | 0.9 | 804 | 36 | 26 | 1.49 | 0 | 19 | 0 | 0.08 | 6.8 | 0.46 | 0.68 |
| | | 24.3 | 13.3 | 3.5 | 6.0 | 2.5 | 150 | 244 | 261 | 2.63 | 0.047 | 40.0 | 65 | 0.4 | 0.28 | 0.20 | 11.5 | 5313 |
| **chicken wings,** glazed, bbq, oven-heated - *2.6 oz* | 74 | 179 | 42.4 | 2.5 | 1.4 | | 0.4 | 414 | 21 | 16 | 0.96 | 0 | 16 | 0 | 0.09 | 4.5 | 0.41 | 0.45 |
| | | 16.5 | 11.0 | 2.9 | 5.0 | 2.1 | 101 | 161 | 172 | 1.46 | 0 | 25.3 | 51 | 0.3 | 0.19 | 0.14 | 7.4 | 5320 |
| **eggplant chicken Bolognese,** Michael Angelo's - *12 oz entrée* | 340 | 390 | | 29.0 | 4.0 | | 5.0 | 1070 | 600 | | | | | 18 | | | | |
| | | 28.0 | 18.0 | 6.0 | | | 70 | | | 1.80 | | | 2500 | | | | | MICA1 |
| **eggplant parmesan,** tom sce, mozz chs, Michael Angelo's - *6 oz (½ pkg)* | 170 | 280 | | 23.0 | 5.0 | | 4.0 | 330 | 40 | | | | | 0 | | | | |
| | | 5.0 | 19.0 | 3.0 | | | 40 | | | 1.62 | | | 0 | | | | | MICA2 |
| **enchilada,** chicken, rice, chs sce, Stouffer's - *10 oz entrée* | 283 | 424 | 188.3 | 61.0 | 5.7 | | 3.7 | 855 | 300 | | | | | 4 | | | | |
| | | 15.3 | 13.3 | 7.4 | 2.7 | 0.9 | 51 | 243 | | 2.18 | | | 484 | | | | | 22615 |
| **enchilada,** chkn suiza, sour crm sce, chs, Wt Wtchrs - *9 oz entrée* | 255 | 311 | 184.6 | 45.1 | 33.2 | | 3.3 | 727 | 189 | | | | | 4 | | | | |
| | | 13.5 | 8.4 | 3.6 | 2.3 | 1.3 | 33 | | | 0.76 | | | 469 | | | | | 22671 |
| **enchilada,** chkn suiza, sour crm sce, rice, Stfrs Ln Csn - *9 oz entrée* | 255 | 268 | 190.9 | 46.9 | 6.5 | | 3.3 | 507 | 158 | | | | | 3 | 0.20 | 1.7 | | |
| | | 10.6 | 4.1 | 1.6 | 1.2 | 1.0 | 20 | 349 | | 1.02 | | | 258 | | 0.15 | | | 22611 |
| **fish fillet,** macaroni and cheese, Stouffer's - *9 oz entrée* | 255 | 410 | | 45.0 | 7.0 | | 1.0 | 980 | 150 | | | | | 0 | | | | |
| | | 20.0 | 17.0 | 6.0 | | | 60 | | | 0.72 | | | 0 | | | | | STOF24 |

| Food | WT (g) | KCAL / PRO (g) | H₂O (g) / FAT (g) | CHO (g) / SFA (g) | TSUG (g) / MUFA (g) | ASUG (g) / PUFA (g) | DFIB (g) / CHOL (mg) | Na (mg) / K (mg) | Ca (mg) / P (mg) | Mg (mg) / Fe (mg) | Zn (mg) / Cu (mg) | Mn (mg) / Se (mcg) | A (mcg RAE) / A (IU) | C (mg) / E (mg ATE) | B-1 (mg) / B-2 (mg) | NIA (mg) / B-6 (mg) | B-12 (mcg) / FOL (mcg DFE) | PANT (mg) / REF |
|---|---|---|---|---|---|---|---|---|---|---|---|---|---|---|---|---|---|---|
| **ham and cheese pocket sandwich,** | 133 | 356 | 61.4 | 36.2 | | | | 1052 | 190 | | | | | | | | | |
| Red Baron - 4.7 oz pocket | | 14.9 | 16.9 | 6.2 | 6.1 | 1.8 | 41 | | | | | | 0 | | | | | 22540 |
| **ham 'n cheese pocket sandwich,** | 128 | 340 | 57.5 | 38.4 | | | | 666 | 251 | | | | | | | | | |
| Hot Pockets - 4.5 oz pocket | | 14.8 | 14.2 | 5.8 | 4.4 | 1.5 | 50 | | | 2.61 | | | 0 | | | | | 22537 |
| **lasagna,** cheese, heated | 297 | 386 | 216.2 | 41.1 | 12.6 | | 5.0 | 843 | 330 | 62 | 2.70 | 0.585 | 116 | 51 | 0.34 | 4.0 | 1.69 | 0.61 |
| 10.5 oz entrée | | 19.4 | 15.8 | 6.3 | 4.7 | 3.0 | 39 | 541 | 318 | 3.77 | 0.324 | 77.8 | 386 | 2.6 | 0.46 | 0.20 | | 22910 |
| **lasagna** with meat and sauce, | 215 | 249 | 159.7 | 27.0 | 4.7 | | 2.4 | 671 | 148 | | | | 1 | | 0.13 | 1.4 | | |
| Stouffer's - 7.6 oz (⅓ pkg) | | 17.3 | 8.1 | 4.1 | 2.8 | 0.5 | 28 | 340 | | 1.31 | | | 331 | | 0.11 | | | 22570 |
| **lasagna** with meat and tom sauce, | 309 | 312 | 236.0 | 41.7 | | | 4.0 | 559 | 334 | 59 | 2.66 | 0.658 | | 55 | 0.12 | 3.8 | 1.39 | 0.33 |
| lowfat - 10.9 oz entree | | 21.0 | 6.9 | 3.0 | 2.2 | 0.9 | 22 | 464 | 105 | 3.00 | 0.516 | 40.2 | | | 0.39 | 0.38 | | 22915 |
| **lasagna** with meat sauce | 255 | 324 | 185.4 | 32.8 | 5.4 | | 3.1 | 714 | 260 | 48 | 2.55 | 0.408 | | 55 | 0.15 | 3.3 | 1.89 | 0.27 |
| 9 oz entrée | | 21.1 | 12.1 | 5.7 | 4.5 | 0.9 | 38 | 403 | 191 | 2.17 | 1.076 | 41.6 | | | 0.37 | 0.18 | | 22916 |
| **macaroni and beef in tom sauce,** | 283 | 258 | 220.5 | 37.4 | 11.0 | | 4.8 | 569 | 85 | | | | | 2 | 0.20 | 3.3 | | |
| Stfrs Ln Csn - 10 oz entrée | | 17.2 | 4.4 | 1.7 | 1.7 | 0.6 | 17 | 773 | | 1.78 | | | 272 | | 0.08 | | | 22576 |
| **macaroni and cheese,** Sfwy Grmt | 240 | 360 | | 34.0 | 1.0 | | 1.0 | 790 | 250 | | | | | 0 | | | | |
| Club - 1 cup | | 13.0 | 18.0 | 12.0 | | | 60 | | | 1.80 | | | 500 | | | | | SAFE50 |
| **nachos,** stuffed, cheese, Totino's | 84 | 200 | | 28.0 | 2.0 | | 1.0 | 450 | 60 | | | | | 0 | | | | |
| 6 nachos | | 7.0 | 7.0 | 2.5 | | | 10 | | | 1.44 | | | 100 | | | | | GENM133 |
| **peppers stuffed** w/beef in tom sce, | 220 | 161 | 184.5 | 19.2 | 6.0 | | 2.6 | 625 | 37 | | | | | 26 | 0.13 | 1.4 | | |
| Stouffer's - 7.8 ozsce, (½ pkg) | | 8.2 | 5.7 | 2.2 | 2.2 | 0.4 | 18 | 348 | | 1.50 | | | 198 | | 0.11 | | | 22569 |
| **pierogies,** broc, cheddar, Mrs. Ts | 120 | 200 | | 33.0 | 2.0 | | 2.0 | 560 | 40 | | | | | 12 | | | | |
| 3 pierogies | | 6.0 | 4.5 | 1.0 | | | 5 | | | 1.80 | | | 300 | | | | | ATCO2 |
| **pierogies,** cheddar, bacon, Mrs. Ts | 85 | 140 | | 25.0 | 1.0 | | 1.0 | 450 | 20 | | | | | 5 | | | | |
| 4 mini pierogies | | 5.0 | 3.0 | 1.0 | | | 5 | | | 1.08 | | | 100 | | | | | ATCO11 |
| **pierogies,** cheddar, jalapeno, | 120 | 180 | | 34.0 | 2.0 | | 1.0 | 540 | 40 | | | | | 9 | | | | |
| Mrs. Ts - 3 pierogies | | 6.0 | 2.5 | 1.0 | | | 10 | | | 1.80 | | | 100 | | | | | ATCO4 |
| **pierogies,** potato, 4 cheese blend, | 120 | 230 | | 36.0 | 2.0 | | 1.0 | 570 | 40 | | | | | 9 | | | | |
| Mrs. Ts - 3 pierogies | | 6.0 | 7.0 | 1.0 | | | 10 | | | 1.44 | | | 0 | | | | | ATCO6 |
| **pierogies,** potato, 4 cheese blend, | 85 | 160 | | 27.0 | 1.0 | | 1.0 | 390 | 40 | | | | | 5 | | | | |
| Mrs. Ts - 4 mini pierogies | | 4.0 | 4.5 | 1.0 | | | 5 | | | 1.08 | | | 0 | | | | | ATCO5 |
| **pierogies,** potato, Am cheese, | 120 | 210 | | 32.0 | 1.0 | | 1.0 | 570 | 80 | | | | | 5 | | | | |
| Mrs. Ts - 3 pierogies | | 8.0 | 6.0 | 3.0 | | | 15 | | | 1.44 | | | 100 | | | | | ATCO1 |
| **pierogies,** potato, cheddar, Mrs. | 120 | 180 | | 34.0 | 1.0 | | 1.0 | 530 | 40 | | | | | 6 | | | | |
| Ts - 3 pierogies | | 6.0 | 2.5 | 1.0 | | | 5 | | | 1.44 | | | 100 | | | | | ATCO10 |
| **pierogies,** potato, cheddar, Mrs. | 85 | 130 | | 25.0 | 1.0 | | 1.0 | 360 | 20 | | | | | 5 | | | | |
| Ts - 4 mini pierogies | | 4.0 | 1.5 | 0.5 | | | 5 | | | 1.08 | | | 100 | | | | | ATCO9 |
| **pierogies,** potato, onion, Mrs. Ts | 120 | 170 | | 34.0 | 1.0 | | 1.0 | 420 | 20 | | | | | 9 | | | | |
| 3 pierogies | | 5.0 | 2.0 | 0 | | | 5 | | | 1.44 | | | 100 | | | | | ATCO7 |
| **pierogies,** sauerkraut, Mrs. Ts | 120 | 150 | | 30.0 | 1.0 | | 3.0 | 770 | 20 | | | | | 9 | | | | |
| 3 pierogies | | 4.0 | 1.5 | 0 | | | 5 | | | 1.44 | | | 100 | | | | | ATCO12 |
| **pierogies,** sour cream, chive, | 120 | 210 | | 34.0 | 2.0 | | 1.0 | 510 | 40 | | | | | 9 | | | | |
| Mrs. Ts - 3 pierogies | | 6.0 | 5.0 | 2.0 | | | 15 | | | 1.80 | | | 400 | | | | | ATCO13 |
| **pizza rolls,** pepperoni, Totino's | 85 | 220 | | 24.0 | 2.0 | | 1.0 | 460 | 40 | | | | | 0 | | | | |
| 6 rolls | | 7.0 | 11.0 | 2.5 | | | 10 | | | 1.80 | | | 300 | | | | | GENM164 |
| **pizza rolls,** sausage, Totino's | 85 | 210 | | 24.0 | 3.0 | | 1.0 | 410 | 40 | | | | | 0 | | | | |
| 6 rolls | | 8.0 | 10.0 | 2.5 | | | 10 | | | 1.44 | | | 200 | | | | | GENM165 |
| **pork, roasted,** grvy, garlic, mshd pot, | 425 | 490 | | 38.0 | 3.0 | | 3.0 | 1730 | 100 | | | | | 2 | | | | |
| Boston Market - 15 oz entrée | | 30.0 | 24.0 | 8.0 | | | 80 | 35 | 0 | 2.70 | | | 300 | | | | | BOST34 |
| **Quiche Florentine,** Nancy's | 170 | 410 | | 35.0 | 6.0 | | 1.0 | 560 | 400 | | | | | 0 | | | | |
| Specialty Foods - 6 oz quiche | | 19.0 | 23.0 | 13.0 | | | 195 | | | 2.70 | | | 1250 | | | | | NANC1 |
| **rice bowl** with chicken | 340 | 428 | 234.9 | 76.4 | 13.8 | | 2.4 | 1132 | 44 | 48 | 1.29 | 0.704 | 109 | 10 | 0.25 | 7.7 | 1.09 | 1.21 |
| 12 oz entrée | | 19.2 | 5.3 | 1.1 | 1.7 | 1.4 | 54 | 418 | 320 | 1.19 | 0.102 | 24.1 | 2071 | 0.8 | 0.19 | 0.54 | 74.8 | 22958 |
| **salisbury steak,** grvy, mac and chs, | 272 | 277 | 217.8 | 20.3 | 5.3 | | 4.1 | 443 | 46 | | | | | 5 | 0.11 | 3.7 | | |
| Stfrs Hmstl - 9.6 oz entrée | | 17.3 | 14.1 | 4.9 | 5.2 | 2.6 | 38 | 517 | | 2.01 | | | 193 | | 0.14 | | | 22583 |
| **spaghetti Bolognese,** Hlthy Chc | 283 | 255 | 220.2 | 43.1 | 7.4 | 3.3 | 5.1 | 473 | 51 | 42 | 1.44 | 0.603 | 25 | 15 | 0.35 | 0.5 | 0.17 | 0.20 |
| 10 oz entrée | | 14.3 | 2.9 | 1.0 | 0.9 | 0.9 | 17 | 408 | 139 | 3.54 | 0.354 | 33.7 | 492 | 1.4 | 3.77 | 0.20 | 203.8 | 22401 |
| **spaghetti** w/meat sce, Stfrs Ln Csn | 326 | 284 | 256.9 | 48.6 | 8.4 | | 4.6 | 548 | 101 | | | | | 3 | 0.33 | 3.9 | | |
| 11.5 oz entrée | | 14.1 | 3.5 | 1.1 | 1.3 | 0.9 | 13 | 574 | | 2.38 | | | 447 | | 0.20 | | | 22580 |
| **spaghetti** w/meatballs and sce, | 269 | 250 | 210.0 | 33.0 | 6.5 | | 4.0 | 568 | 100 | | | | | 3 | 0.24 | 4.3 | | |
| Stfrs Ln Csn - 9.5 oz entrée | | 18.0 | 5.1 | 2.0 | 1.9 | 0.8 | 24 | 511 | | 2.18 | | | 256 | | 0.16 | | | 22572 |
| **Swedish meatballs** w/pasta, | 326 | 510 | | 43.0 | 4.0 | | 3.0 | 1150 | 60 | | | | | 0 | | | | |
| Stouffer's - 11.5 oz entrée | | 25.0 | 26.0 | 10.0 | | | 100 | | | 2.70 | | | 0 | | | | | STOF27 |

| | WT (g) | Macronutrients | | | | | | Minerals | | | | | Vitamins | | | | | |
|---|---|---|---|---|---|---|---|---|---|---|---|---|---|---|---|---|---|---|
| | | KCAL | H₂0 (g) | CHO (g) | TSUG (g) | ASUG (g) | DFIB (g) | Na (mg) | Ca (mg) | Mg (mg) | Zn (mg) | Mn (mg) | A (mcg RAE) | C (mg) | B-1 (mg) | NIA (mg) | B-12 (mcg) | PANT (mg) |
| | | PRO (g) | FAT (g) | SFA (g) | MUFA (g) | PUFA (g) | CHOL (mg) | K (mg) | P (mg) | Fe (mg) | Cu (mg) | Se (mcg) | A (IU) | E (mg ATE) | B-2 (mg) | B-6 (mg) | FOL (mcg DFE) | REF |
| Swedish meatballs w/pasta, Stfrs Ln Csn - *9.1 oz entrée* | 258 | 273 | 194.7 | 31.3 | 4.5 | | 2.6 | 614 | 114 | | | | | 0 | 0.23 | 4.2 | | |
| | | 22.1 | 6.8 | 2.8 | 2.6 | 0.9 | 49 | 560 | | 2.58 | | | 0 | | 0.28 | | | 22573 |
| **turkey and gravy** - *5 oz package* | 142 | 95 | 120.8 | 6.5 | | | 0 | 787 | 20 | 11 | 0.99 | 0.007 | 18 | 0 | 0.03 | 2.6 | 0.34 | 0.30 |
| | | 8.3 | 3.7 | 1.2 | 1.4 | 0.7 | 26 | 87 | 115 | 1.32 | 0.031 | 27.3 | 60 | 0 | 0.18 | 0.14 | 5.7 | 5286 |
| **turkey breast**, gravy, stuffing, mshd pot, Stouffer's - *9.63 oz entrée* | 272 | 300 | | 34.0 | 5.0 | | 2.0 | 1190 | 40 | | | | | 0 | | | | |
| | | 16.0 | 11.0 | 3.0 | | | 35 | | | 0.72 | | | 0 | | | | | STOF28 |
| **turkey pot pie** - *13.7 oz pot pie* | 387 | 681 | 254.3 | 68.5 | | | 4.3 | 1354 | | | | | | | | | | |
| | | 25.2 | 34.1 | 11.1 | 13.4 | 5.3 | 62 | | | 3.87 | | | 6838 | | | | | 22528 |

## 9.4 FROZEN MEALS

| | WT (g) | KCAL / PRO | H₂0 / FAT | CHO / SFA | TSUG / MUFA | ASUG / PUFA | DFIB / CHOL | Na / K | Ca / P | Mg / Fe | Zn / Cu | Mn / Se | A (mcg RAE) / A (IU) | C / E | B-1 / B-2 | NIA / B-6 | B-12 / FOL | PANT / REF |
|---|---|---|---|---|---|---|---|---|---|---|---|---|---|---|---|---|---|---|
| **beef**, msqt, bbq sce, rstd pot, corn-car-peas, Hlthy Chc - *11 oz meal* | 312 | 343 | 233.3 | 45.1 | 15.7 | | 5.9 | 402 | 37 | | | | | 16 | | | | |
| | | 22.3 | 8.2 | 2.7 | 2.9 | 1.7 | 53 | | | 2.34 | | | 936 | | | | | 22923 |
| **beef Oriental** w/veg and rice, Stouffer's - *9 oz meal* | 255 | 189 | 208.3 | 28.2 | 7.9 | | 4.1 | 536 | 31 | | | | | 5 | 0.18 | 3.8 | | |
| | | 12.6 | 2.8 | 1.1 | 1.1 | 0.3 | 23 | 724 | | 1.17 | | | 1104 | | 0.10 | | | 22582 |
| **beef pot roast**, grvy, rstd pot, car, apl rsn crsp, Hlthy Chc - *11 oz meal* | 311 | 320 | | 39.0 | 24.0 | | 6.0 | 550 | 20 | | | | | 18 | | | | |
| | | 19.0 | 9.0 | 3.0 | 3.0 | 1.0 | 45 | | | 1.80 | | | 1250 | | | | | HLCH10 |
| **beef ribs**, bbq sce, pot, veg, Healthy Choice - *11 oz meal* | 311 | 360 | | 47.0 | 18.0 | | 8.0 | 580 | 20 | | | | | 0 | | | | |
| | | 22.0 | 9.0 | 3.0 | 4.0 | 1.5 | 55 | | | 1.80 | | | 1000 | | | | | HLCH11 |
| **beef**, sliced, gravy, mshd pot, car, Freeze Queen - *9 oz meal* | 255 | 207 | 207.1 | 25.5 | | | 3.6 | 648 | | | | | 530 | | | | | |
| | | 15.3 | 4.8 | 1.3 | 1.2 | 1.7 | 31 | | | | | | 10582 | | | | | 22710 |
| **beef**, sliced, gravy, mshd pot, peas, Banquet - *9 oz meal* | 255 | 224 | 205.2 | 16.5 | 3.6 | | 4.1 | 806 | 43 | | | | | 7 | | | | |
| | | 22.4 | 7.5 | 3.1 | 3.1 | 0.7 | 48 | | | 2.52 | | | 191 | | | | | 22691 |
| **beef stroganoff** w/ndls, car, peas, Marie Callender's - *13 oz meal* | 368 | 420 | 280.9 | 39.6 | 6.2 | | 7.4 | 1343 | 77 | | | | | 0 | | | | |
| | | 24.6 | 18.0 | 7.2 | 5.5 | 4.1 | 63 | | | 2.06 | | | 2050 | | | | | 22677 |
| **beef tips**, msqt, jalapeno ched pot, corn mdly, Stfrs - *14 oz meal* | 396 | 440 | | 50.0 | 9.0 | | 8.0 | 1740 | 100 | | | | | 120 | | | | |
| | | 19.0 | 18.0 | 6.0 | | | 40 | | | 2.70 | | | 1000 | | | | | STOF25 |
| **Burgundy beef stew**, Sfwy Grmt Clb - *10 oz (½ pkg)* | 288 | 250 | | 38.0 | 10.0 | | 3.0 | 860 | 40 | | | | | 18 | | | | |
| | | 13.0 | 9.0 | 1.5 | | | 25 | | | 2.70 | | | 7500 | | | | | SAFE42 |
| **chicken alfredo pasta**, Grn Gnt Sklt Mls - *1½ ups prep* | 207 | 270 | | 39.0 | 7.0 | | 3.0 | 760 | 150 | | | | | 15 | | | | |
| | | 17.0 | 6.0 | 2.5 | | | 30 | | | 1.80 | | | 750 | | | | | GENM138 |
| **chicken cheesy pasta**, Grn Gnt Sklt Mls - *1¼ cups prep* | 224 | 270 | | 41.0 | 9.0 | | 4.0 | 760 | 100 | | | | | 5 | | | | |
| | | 17.0 | 6.0 | 3.0 | | | 35 | | | 1.80 | | | 1500 | | | | | GENM139 |
| **chicken**, fried, mshd pot, corn, Banquet - *8 oz meal* | 228 | 388 | 152.5 | 30.4 | 0.8 | | 4.1 | 604 | 135 | | | | | 3 | | | | |
| | | 21.9 | 19.8 | 4.4 | 8.1 | 5.3 | 68 | | | 1.62 | | | 130 | | | | | 22571 |
| **chicken garlic pasta**, Grn Gnt Sklt Mls - *1 cup (8 oz) prep* | 227 | 230 | | 33.0 | 5.0 | | 4.0 | 840 | 60 | | | | | 15 | | | | |
| | | 13.0 | 6.0 | 2.5 | | | 30 | | | 1.44 | | | 1250 | | | | | GENM143 |
| **chicken**, ginger, spinach, rice, Sfwy Grmt Clb - *10.5 oz (½ pkg)* | 297 | 350 | | 49.0 | 15.0 | | 2.0 | 310 | 80 | | | | | 12 | | | | |
| | | 24.0 | 6.0 | 1.5 | | | 55 | | | 2.70 | | | 4500 | | | | | SAFE48 |
| **chicken lo mein stir fry**, Grn Gnt Sklt Mls - *1 cup (8 oz) prep* | 227 | 190 | | 31.0 | 7.0 | | 3.0 | 740 | 40 | | | | | 24 | | | | |
| | | 12.0 | 2.0 | 0 | | | 20 | | | 1.80 | | | 1000 | | | | | GENM140 |
| **chkn**, msqt bbq, rice, mxd veg, apl rsn cblr, Hlthy Chc - *10.5 oz meal* | 298 | 277 | 231.4 | 42.2 | 14.4 | | 6.6 | 447 | 30 | | | | | 9 | | | | |
| | | 16.9 | 4.4 | 1.2 | 1.8 | 1.1 | 33 | | | 1.49 | | | 2086 | | | | | 22713 |
| **chicken nuggets**, mac and chs, corn, Kid Cuisine - *9.1 oz meal* | 257 | 457 | 164.3 | 50.8 | 28.1 | | 7.5 | 843 | 85 | | | | | 0 | | | | |
| | | 18.5 | 20.0 | 5.6 | 7.9 | 4.9 | 57 | | | 2.78 | | | 463 | | | | | 22690 |
| **chicken**, orange chkn, broc, fried rice, Sfwy Grmt Clb - *11 oz (½ pkg)* | 311 | 350 | | 56.0 | 13.0 | | 3.0 | 790 | 40 | | | | | 30 | | | | |
| | | 19.0 | 5.0 | 1.0 | | | 35 | | | 2.70 | | | 4000 | | | | | SAFE53 |
| **chicken teriyaki**, rice, mxd veg, apl chry compote, Hlthy Chc *11 oz meal* | 312 | 250 | 253.4 | 35.7 | 13.8 | | 9.4 | 596 | 31 | | | | | 44 | | | | |
| | | 15.7 | 4.8 | 1.6 | 1.7 | 1.4 | 22 | | | 0.59 | | | 250 | | | | | 22587 |
| **enchilada**, chkn, grn chili sce, rice, corn, Hlthy Chc - *11.3 oz meal* | 320 | 352 | 239.1 | 58.2 | 2.3 | | 4.8 | 573 | 58 | | | | | | | | | |
| | | 12.1 | 7.8 | 3.3 | 2.3 | 2.1 | 35 | | | 0.99 | | | 406 | | | | | 22588 |
| **lo mein stir fry**, Grn Gnt Create A Meal - *1¼ cup prep* | 283 | 270 | | 28.0 | 7.0 | | 2.0 | 780 | 40 | | | | | 18 | | | | |
| | | 24.0 | 7.0 | 1.5 | | | 50 | | | 1.80 | | | 1000 | | | | | GENM147 |
| **meatloaf**, brwn sce, mshd pot, grn bns, apl crisp, Hlthy Chc *12 oz meal* | 340 | 296 | 273.7 | 36.7 | 13.6 | | 6.5 | 496 | 102 | | | | | 26 | | | | |
| | | 17.6 | 8.8 | 2.1 | 2.3 | 1.3 | 37 | | | 2.82 | | | 248 | | | | | 22920 |
| **meatloaf**, grvy, mshd pot, vegs, Mar Clndrs - *14 oz meal* | 397 | 480 | | 39.0 | 6.0 | | | 1080 | 80 | | | | | 2 | | | | |
| | | 31.0 | 22.0 | 9.0 | | | 60 | | | 6.30 | | | 1500 | | | | | CNAG257 |
| **meatloaf**, grvy, pot, grn bns, Sfwy Grmt Clb - *10.5 oz (½ pkg)* | 297 | 230 | | 31.0 | 4.0 | | 6.0 | 600 | 150 | | | | | 30 | | | | |
| | | 15.0 | 6.0 | 2.0 | | | 20 | | | 4.50 | | | 750 | | | | | SAFE52 |
| **salisbury stk**, grvy, msh pot, corn, Banquet Extr Hlpng *16.5 oz meal* | 468 | 646 | 348.8 | 46.4 | 6.0 | | 9.8 | 2363 | 84 | | | | | 0 | | | | |
| | | 24.0 | 40.5 | 15.0 | 16.8 | 6.5 | 66 | | | 3.37 | | | 0 | | | | | 22689 |

| Food | WT (g) | KCAL / PRO (g) | $H_20$ (g) / FAT (g) | CHO (g) / SFA (g) | TSUG (g) / MUFA (g) | ASUG (g) / PUFA (g) | DFIB (g) / CHOL (mg) | Na (mg) / K (mg) | Ca (mg) / P (mg) | Mg (mg) / Fe (mg) | Zn (mg) / Cu (mg) | Mn (mg) / Se (mcg) | A (mcg RAE) / A (IU) | C (mg) / E (mg ATE) | B-1 (mg) / B-2 (mg) | NIA (mg) / B-6 (mg) | B-12 (mcg) / FOL (mcg DFE) | PANT (mg) / REF |
|---|---|---|---|---|---|---|---|---|---|---|---|---|---|---|---|---|---|---|
| **salisbury stk**, grvy, mshd pot, | 269 | 339 | 204.1 | 26.6 | 2.5 | | 4.0 | 1036 | 56 | | | | | 0 | | | | |
| corn, Banquet - *9.5 oz meal* | | 15.2 | 19.1 | 9.4 | 7.0 | 1.9 | 30 | | | 1.32 | | | 0 | | | | | 22711 |
| **salisbury stk**, mshrm grvy, pot, | 354 | 360 | | 45.0 | 19.0 | | 5.0 | 580 | 80 | | | | | 21 | | | | |
| vegs, apl dessert - *12.5 oz meal* | | 23.0 | 9.0 | 3.5 | 4.0 | 1.0 | 45 | | | 2.70 | | | 500 | | | | | HLCH15 |
| **salisbury stk**, grvy, rstd pot, w/veg | 354 | 333 | 276.5 | 44.9 | 20.5 | | 7.1 | 573 | 88 | | | | | 42 | | | | |
| Hlthy Chc - *12.5 oz meal* | | 21.3 | 7.6 | 3.1 | 3.1 | 1.4 | 32 | | | 2.76 | | | 1239 | | | | | 22921 |
| **steak tips Dijon**, pot, grn bns, Stfrs | 340 | 310 | | 44.0 | 11.0 | | 5.0 | 820 | 150 | | | | | 15 | | | | |
| Ln Csn - *12 oz meal* | | 18.0 | 7.0 | 3.0 | 2.5 | 1.0 | 35 | 1080 | | 3.60 | | | 750 | | | | | STOF26 |
| **sweet and sour stir fry**, Grn Gnt Crt | 283 | 280 | | 36.0 | 29.0 | | 3.0 | 540 | 40 | | | | | 24 | | | | |
| A Ml - *1¼ cups prep (10 oz)* | | 22.0 | 7.0 | 1.0 | | | 55 | | | 1.44 | | | 2250 | | | | | GENM150 |
| **Szechuan stir fry**, Grn Gnt Create | 283 | 190 | | 10.0 | 4.0 | | 3.0 | 900 | 40 | | | | | 30 | | | | |
| A Meal - *1¼ cups prep (10 oz)* | | 18.0 | 9.0 | 2.5 | | | 40 | | | 1.80 | | | 1750 | | | | | GENM151 |
| **teriyaki stir fry**, Grn Gnt Create A | 283 | 180 | | 10.0 | 3.0 | | 3.0 | 850 | 40 | | | | | 42 | | | | |
| Meal - *1¼ cups (10 oz)* | | 3.0 | 6.0 | 1.0 | | | 50 | | | 1.44 | | | 400 | | | | | GENM152 |
| **turkey**, grvy, drsing, mshd pot, | 262 | 259 | 204.9 | 28.5 | 5.0 | | 8.1 | 1051 | 58 | | | | | 7 | | | | |
| corn, Banquet - *9.2 oz meal* | | 15.5 | 9.1 | 2.2 | 3.9 | 2.6 | 37 | | | 1.76 | | | 341 | | | | | 22607 |
| **turkey**, grvy, drsing, mshd pot, grn bns, | 397 | 393 | 304.1 | 45.1 | 8.9 | | 4.0 | 1235 | 95 | | | | | 4 | | | | |
| crnbrs, Mar Clndrs - *14 oz meal* | 32.4 | 9.4 | 2.5 | 2.9 | 3.0 | 67 | | | 0.79 | | | 488 | | | | | 22924 | |
| **turkey** mdlons, mshrms, sce, rice, | 240 | 202 | 188.9 | 35.8 | 0.7 | | 2.4 | 516 | 19 | | | | | 1 | | | | |
| vegs, Wt Wtchrs - *8.5 oz meal* | | 12.0 | 1.2 | 0.5 | 0.5 | 0.5 | 53 | | | 0.72 | | | 326 | | | | | 22672 |
| **turkey**, stuffing, mshd pot, grvy, mxd | 422 | 540 | 300.3 | 68.9 | 20.3 | | 5.5 | 1772 | 114 | 76 | 2.03 | 0.663 | | 3 | 0.58 | 12.9 | 1.39 | 0.98 |
| veg, micro ckd - *14.9 oz meal* | | 29.4 | 16.4 | 3.8 | 5.2 | 4.6 | 59 | 971 | 447 | 3.33 | 0.236 | 33.3 | 359 | 1.0 | 1.06 | 0.75 | 122.4 | 22957 |

## 9.5 FROZEN PIZZA

| Food | WT (g) | KCAL / PRO (g) | $H_20$ (g) / FAT (g) | CHO (g) / SFA (g) | TSUG (g) / MUFA (g) | ASUG (g) / PUFA (g) | DFIB (g) / CHOL (mg) | Na (mg) / K (mg) | Ca (mg) / P (mg) | Mg (mg) / Fe (mg) | Zn (mg) / Cu (mg) | Mn (mg) / Se (mcg) | A (mcg RAE) / A (IU) | C (mg) / E (mg ATE) | B-1 (mg) / B-2 (mg) | NIA (mg) / B-6 (mg) | B-12 (mcg) / FOL (mcg DFE) | PANT (mg) / REF |
|---|---|---|---|---|---|---|---|---|---|---|---|---|---|---|---|---|---|---|
| **cheese**, Jeno's Crisp 'N Tasty | 195 | 440 | | 50.0 | 6.0 | | 1.0 | 1040 | 250 | | | | | 0 | | | | |
| *6.9 oz pizza* | | 16.0 | 20.0 | 4.5 | | | 10 | | | 2.70 | | | 500 | | | | | GENM155 |
| **cheese**, regular crust, heated | 103 | 276 | 47.7 | 29.9 | 3.7 | | 2.3 | 460 | 184 | 24 | 1.36 | 0.300 | 68 | 1 | 0.22 | 2.3 | 0.80 | 0.23 |
| *3.6 oz slice* | | 10.7 | 12.6 | 4.4 | 4.4 | 2.0 | 14 | 157 | 184 | 2.34 | 0.234 | 22.1 | 352 | 1.0 | 0.27 | 0.09 | 67.0 | 21224 |
| **cheese**, rising crust, heated | 139 | 361 | 60.4 | 45.7 | 7.1 | | 3.5 | 773 | 246 | 36 | 1.83 | 0.595 | 96 | 3 | 0.33 | 2.8 | 0.97 | 0.36 |
| *4.9 oz slice* | | 17.2 | 12.2 | 5.3 | 3.1 | 1.9 | 22 | 243 | 331 | 2.46 | 0.354 | 48.4 | 499 | 1.0 | 0.34 | 0.13 | 87.6 | 21225 |
| **combination**, Jeno's Crisp 'N Tasty | 198 | 490 | | 49.0 | 5.0 | | 1.0 | 1160 | 100 | | | | | 0 | | | | |
| *7 oz pizza* | | 16.0 | 25.0 | 6.0 | | | 20 | | | 2.70 | | | 400 | | | | | GENM158 |
| **meat and veg**, reg crust, heated | 136 | 375 | 63.5 | 34.2 | | | 3.0 | 755 | 207 | 34 | 2.33 | 0.439 | | 5 | 0.29 | 3.2 | 0.84 | 0.45 |
| *4.8 oz slice* | | 15.3 | 19.6 | 6.5 | 7.9 | 3.4 | 22 | 284 | 246 | 1.85 | 0.231 | 12.2 | | | 0.32 | 0.20 | | 21226 |
| **meat and veg**, rising crust, heated | 149 | 404 | 65.9 | 42.9 | | | 3.4 | 954 | 231 | 40 | 2.79 | 0.481 | | 6 | 0.37 | 3.2 | 1.19 | 0.65 |
| *5.3 oz slice* | | 18.8 | 17.5 | 6.3 | 6.4 | 2.7 | 28 | 282 | 314 | 2.03 | 0.313 | 17.3 | | | 0.31 | 0.21 | | 21227 |
| **pepperoni** | 146 | 432 | 62.0 | 41.6 | | | 3.2 | 902 | 220 | 35 | 2.16 | 0.466 | 0 | 3 | 0.33 | 3.6 | 0.83 | 0.40 |
| *5.1 oz serving* | | 16.4 | 22.2 | 7.0 | 10.0 | 3.4 | 22 | 289 | 302 | 3.52 | 0.153 | 28.6 | 0 | | 0.34 | 0.14 | | 22903 |
| **sausage**, Jeno's Crisp 'N Tasty | 198 | 460 | | 49.0 | 5.0 | | 1.0 | 1130 | 150 | | | | | 0 | | | | |
| *7 oz pizza* | | 17.0 | 22.0 | 5.0 | | | 20 | | | 2.70 | | | 400 | | | | | GENM168 |
| **supreme**, Jeno's Crisp 'N Tasty | 204 | 480 | | 49.0 | 5.0 | | 1.0 | 1150 | 100 | | | | | 0 | | | | |
| *7.2 oz pizza* | | 16.0 | 25.0 | 6.0 | | | 20 | | | 2.70 | | | 400 | | | | | GENM169 |

## 9.6 HOMEMADE AND UNSPECIFIED ENTREES

| Food | WT (g) | KCAL / PRO (g) | $H_20$ (g) / FAT (g) | CHO (g) / SFA (g) | TSUG (g) / MUFA (g) | ASUG (g) / PUFA (g) | DFIB (g) / CHOL (mg) | Na (mg) / K (mg) | Ca (mg) / P (mg) | Mg (mg) / Fe (mg) | Zn (mg) / Cu (mg) | Mn (mg) / Se (mcg) | A (mcg RAE) / A (IU) | C (mg) / E (mg ATE) | B-1 (mg) / B-2 (mg) | NIA (mg) / B-6 (mg) | B-12 (mcg) / FOL (mcg DFE) | PANT (mg) / REF |
|---|---|---|---|---|---|---|---|---|---|---|---|---|---|---|---|---|---|---|
| **acorn stew**, Apache | 100 | 95 | 79.8 | 9.2 | 0.3 | | 0.7 | 130 | 14 | 12 | 1.60 | 0.140 | 0 | 0 | 0.18 | 2.1 | 0.68 | 0.21 |
| *3.5 oz* | | 6.8 | 3.5 | 1.3 | 1.7 | 0.3 | 20 | 110 | 62 | 1.00 | 0.030 | 8.3 | 0 | 0.3 | 0.12 | 0.06 | 44.0 | 35182 |
| **agutuk** with caribou, Alaskan | 100 | 258 | 55.2 | 0.9 | | | | 95 | 16 | 20 | 3.83 | 0.060 | | 2 | 0.18 | 4.3 | 4.83 | 1.95 |
| *3.5 oz* | | 21.7 | 18.6 | 5.1 | 8.7 | 3.6 | 89 | 228 | 170 | 4.55 | 0.190 | | 559 | | 0.66 | 0.23 | | 35003 |
| **agutuk** with fish and shortening, | 100 | 470 | 34.0 | 10.5 | | | | 24 | | 16 | 0.47 | | | | 0.06 | 1.4 | | |
| Alaskan - *3.5 oz* | | 9.0 | 43.5 | 8.6 | 15.6 | 17.3 | 26 | 206 | 134 | 0.20 | 0.030 | | 257 | 4.0 | 0.06 | | | 35002 |
| **agutuk** with fish, berries, and seal | 100 | 353 | 47.3 | 13.4 | | | 0.5 | 21 | 8 | 7 | 0.18 | 0.130 | | 3 | 0.04 | 0.6 | | 0.02 |
| oil, Alaskan - *3.5 oz* | | 3.4 | 31.8 | 7.7 | 14.4 | 8.4 | 10 | 70 | 46 | 0.30 | 0.030 | | 696 | 2.4 | 0.05 | 0.01 | | 35001 |
| **corned beef** and potatoes in | 100 | 224 | 52.5 | 29.4 | 1.8 | | 1.5 | 511 | 27 | 22 | 0.88 | 0.310 | | | 0.28 | 2.5 | 0.23 | |
| tortilla, homemade - *3.5 oz* | | 7.9 | 8.3 | 3.4 | 3.3 | 0.9 | 11 | 275 | 82 | 1.80 | 0.066 | 11.3 | | 0.2 | 0.14 | 0.21 | | 35186 |
| **dumpling and mutton stew**, | 100 | 101 | 79.2 | 8.0 | 0.2 | | | 46 | 14 | 8 | 1.85 | 0.064 | 0 | 0 | 0.06 | 2.0 | 0.82 | 0.16 |
| Navajo - *3.5 oz* | | 8.7 | 3.8 | 1.7 | 1.5 | 0.3 | 28 | 82 | 63 | 1.79 | 0.053 | 10.2 | 0 | 0.4 | 0.09 | 0.04 | | 35144 |
| **hominy and mutton stew**, Navajo | 100 | 83 | 81.6 | 9.4 | 0.1 | | 2.0 | 45 | 8 | 20 | 1.19 | 0.089 | 0 | 0 | 0.03 | 1.5 | 0.64 | |
| *3½ oz* | | 6.7 | 2.1 | 0.7 | 0.9 | 0.3 | 13 | 118 | 82 | 0.81 | 0.047 | 4.1 | 0 | 0.4 | 0.07 | 0.09 | | 35145 |
| **mutton, corn, and squash stew**, | 100 | 103 | 76.1 | 7.3 | 0.6 | | 1.7 | 49 | 38 | 21 | 1.87 | 0.087 | 0 | 0 | 0.03 | 2.0 | 1.16 | 0.27 |
| Navajo - *3.5 oz* | | 8.6 | 4.3 | 1.7 | 1.7 | 0.4 | 43 | 199 | 111 | 1.21 | 0.063 | 8.4 | 0 | 0.4 | 0.11 | 0.11 | | 35146 |

| | WT (g) | KCAL | H₂O (g) | CHO (g) | TSUG (g) | ASUG (g) | DFIB (g) | Na (mg) | Ca (mg) | Mg (mg) | Zn (mg) | Mn (mg) | A (mcg RAE) | C (mg) | B-1 (mg) | NIA (mg) | B-12 (mcg) | PANT (mg) |
|---|---|---|---|---|---|---|---|---|---|---|---|---|---|---|---|---|---|---|
| | | PRO (g) | FAT (g) | SFA (g) | MUFA (g) | PUFA (g) | CHOL (mg) | K (mg) | P (mg) | Fe (mg) | Cu (mg) | Se (mcg) | A (IU) | E (mg ATE) | B-2 (mg) | B-6 (mg) | FOL (mcg DFE) | REF |
| **scrapple** (cornmeal, pork), | 56 | 119 | 35.0 | 7.9 | 0.1 | 0 | 0.2 | 369 | 4 | 7 | 0.59 | | 351 | 1 | 0.06 | 1.3 | 0.17 | |
| homemade - *2 oz* | | 4.5 | 7.8 | 2.6 | 3.4 | 0.9 | 27 | 88 | 43 | 1.06 | 0.119 | 9.7 | 1168 | 0.1 | 0.16 | 0.07 | 2.8 | 7951 |
| **tamale**, Navajo, homemade | 100 | 153 | 68.1 | 18.1 | 1.0 | | 3.1 | 427 | 29 | 22 | 1.48 | 0.174 | 0 | 2 | 0.05 | 1.6 | 0.54 | 0.20 |
| *3.5 oz* | | 6.3 | 6.1 | 2.4 | 2.7 | 0.7 | 17 | 131 | 99 | 1.22 | 0.063 | 6.0 | 0 | 0 | 0.08 | 0.14 | | 35147 |
| **tortellini** with cheese filling | 81 | 249 | 24.7 | 38.1 | 0.8 | 0 | 1.5 | 279 | 123 | 17 | 0.83 | | 31 | 0 | 0.25 | 2.2 | 0.13 | |
| *¾ cup* | | 10.9 | 5.9 | 2.9 | 1.7 | 0.4 | 34 | 72 | 172 | 1.22 | 0.065 | 19.4 | 116 | 0.1 | 0.25 | 0.03 | 94.8 | 22901 |

## 9.7 PACKAGED ENTREES (SHELF-STABLE OR REFRIGERATED)

| | WT (g) | KCAL | H₂O (g) | CHO (g) | TSUG (g) | ASUG (g) | DFIB (g) | Na (mg) | Ca (mg) | Mg (mg) | Zn (mg) | Mn (mg) | A (mcg RAE) | C (mg) | B-1 (mg) | NIA (mg) | B-12 (mcg) | PANT (mg) |
|---|---|---|---|---|---|---|---|---|---|---|---|---|---|---|---|---|---|---|
| | | PRO (g) | FAT (g) | SFA (g) | MUFA (g) | PUFA (g) | CHOL (mg) | K (mg) | P (mg) | Fe (mg) | Cu (mg) | Se (mcg) | A (IU) | E (mg ATE) | B-2 (mg) | B-6 (mg) | FOL (mcg DFE) | REF |
| **Chicken Helper**, ched and | 231 | 300 | | 27.0 | 5.0 | | 1.0 | 790 | 100 | | | | 0 | | 0.22 | 10.0 | | |
| broc, prep - *1 cup* | | 27.0 | 10.0 | 3.0 | | | 65 | 410 | | 1.80 | | | 200 | | 0.26 | | | GENM177 |
| **Chicken Helper**, chicken and | 213 | 290 | | 25.0 | 3.0 | | 1.0 | 820 | 20 | | | | 0 | | 0.15 | 8.0 | | |
| stuffing, prep - *1 cup* | | 27.0 | 9.0 | 2.0 | | | 60 | 250 | | 1.80 | | | 200 | | 0.17 | | | GENM180 |
| **Chicken Helper**, fettuccini alfredo, | 243 | 340 | | 32.0 | 7.0 | | 1.0 | 840 | 100 | | | | | | 0.30 | 10.0 | | |
| prep - *1 cup* | | 28.0 | 12.0 | 3.5 | | | 65 | 400 | | 1.44 | | | 500 | | 0.34 | | | GENM181 |
| **fajitas**, prep, Old El Paso Dinner | 208 | 320 | | 34.0 | 3.0 | | 2.0 | 1090 | 80 | | | | | 12 | | | | |
| Kit - *2 fajitas* | | 25.0 | 10.0 | 2.0 | | | 55 | | | 1.80 | | | 200 | | | | | GENM188 |
| **gordita** w/ranch sce, prep, Old El | 142 | 340 | | 33.0 | 1.0 | | 1.0 | 920 | 60 | | | | | | | | | |
| Paso Dinner Kit - *1 gordita* | | 22.0 | 13.0 | 3.0 | | | 50 | | | 1.80 | | | 300 | | | | | GENM189 |
| **Hamburger Helper**, cheeseburger | 229 | 300 | | 27.0 | 6.0 | | 1.0 | 870 | 100 | | | | | | 0.22 | 4.0 | | |
| mac, prep - *1 cup* | | 20.0 | 13.0 | 5.0 | | | 50 | | | 1.80 | | | 200 | | 0.26 | | | GENM191 |
| **Hamburger Helper**, chili mac, | 239 | 280 | | 27.0 | 3.0 | | 1.0 | 710 | 20 | | | | | | 0.15 | 5.0 | | |
| prep - *1 cup* | | 19.0 | 11.0 | 4.0 | | | 50 | 380 | | 2.70 | | | 500 | | 0.17 | | | GENM192 |
| **Hamburger Helper**, four cheese | 220 | 320 | | 31.0 | 6.0 | | 1.0 | 830 | 100 | | | | | | 0.22 | 5.0 | | |
| lasagna, prep - *1 cup* | | 22.0 | 12.0 | 5.0 | | | 60 | 450 | | 1.80 | | | 300 | | 0.34 | | | GENM193 |
| **Hamburger Helper**, rice oriental, | 235 | 300 | | 31.0 | 1.0 | | 2.0 | 980 | 60 | | | | | | 0.15 | 4.0 | | |
| prep - *1 cup* | | 19.0 | 11.0 | 4.0 | | | 55 | 310 | | 2.70 | | | | | 0.14 | | | GENM194 |
| **Hamburger Helper**, stroganoff, | 210 | 310 | | 26.0 | 7.0 | | 1.0 | 870 | 150 | | | | | | 0.22 | 5.0 | | |
| prep - *1 cup* | | 23.0 | 13.0 | 5.0 | | | 60 | 480 | | 1.80 | | | 200 | | 0.34 | | | GENM195 |
| **herb chicken veg rice**, dry, Bowl | 68 | 260 | | 49.0 | 2.0 | | 2.0 | 780 | 20 | | | | | | 0.15 | 2.0 | | |
| Appetit - *2.4 oz bowl* | | 7.0 | 5.0 | 1.5 | | | 15 | 160 | | 1.80 | | | 500 | | 0.17 | | | GENM174 |
| **tacos**, soft with ground beef, prep, Old | 176 | 380 | | 33.0 | 3.0 | | 1.0 | 1280 | 100 | | | | | 1 | | | | |
| El Paso Dinner Kit - *2 tacos* | | 22.0 | 18.0 | 7.0 | | | 60 | | | 2.70 | | | 400 | | | | | GENM199 |
| **Tuna Helper**, creamy pasta, prep | 246 | 310 | | 37.0 | 6.0 | | 1.0 | 850 | 150 | | | | | | 0.30 | 4.0 | | |
| *1 cup* | | 13.0 | 12.0 | 3.5 | | | 15 | 300 | | 1.08 | | | 750 | | 0.26 | | | GENM201 |
| **Tuna Helper**, tetrazzini, prep | 239 | 310 | | 33.0 | 5.0 | | 1.0 | 790 | 80 | | | | | | 0.30 | 6.0 | | |
| *1 cup* | | 15.0 | 13.0 | 3.0 | | | 15 | 270 | | 1.44 | | | 500 | | 0.17 | | | GENM203 |
| **Tuna Helper**, tuna melt, prep | 238 | 300 | | 38.0 | 8.0 | | 1.0 | 1030 | 150 | | | | | | 0.30 | 5.0 | | |
| *1 cup* | | 14.0 | 10.0 | 3.0 | | | 15 | 360 | | 1.08 | | | 500 | | 0.34 | | | GENM204 |

## 10. FAST FOODS AND RESTAURANT FOODS
### 10.1 GENERIC FAST FOODS

| | WT (g) | KCAL | H₂O (g) | CHO (g) | TSUG (g) | ASUG (g) | DFIB (g) | Na (mg) | Ca (mg) | Mg (mg) | Zn (mg) | Mn (mg) | A (mcg RAE) | C (mg) | B-1 (mg) | NIA (mg) | B-12 (mcg) | PANT (mg) |
|---|---|---|---|---|---|---|---|---|---|---|---|---|---|---|---|---|---|---|
| | | PRO (g) | FAT (g) | SFA (g) | MUFA (g) | PUFA (g) | CHOL (mg) | K (mg) | P (mg) | Fe (mg) | Cu (mg) | Se (mcg) | A (IU) | E (mg ATE) | B-2 (mg) | B-6 (mg) | FOL (mcg DFE) | REF |
| **animal crackers** | 67 | 299 | 2.5 | 50.5 | | | | 273 | 11 | 11 | 0.30 | 0.326 | 7 | 1 | 0.25 | 2.5 | 0.05 | 0.21 |
| *1 box* | | 4.1 | 9.0 | 3.5 | 3.8 | 1.0 | 11 | 56 | 64 | 1.47 | 0.051 | 4.7 | 27 | 0.3 | 0.24 | 0.02 | 122.6 | 21029 |
| **bagel** w/egg, sausage patty, cheese | 219 | 646 | 98.9 | 49.6 | 6.3 | | 0.4 | 1204 | 206 | 44 | 2.30 | 0.392 | 140 | 1 | 0.67 | 6.3 | 2.10 | 1.96 |
| *7.7 oz sandwich* | | 28.4 | 37.2 | 14.0 | 13.2 | 5.7 | 291 | 269 | 405 | 3.88 | 0.716 | 52.1 | 464 | 1.4 | 0.48 | 0.20 | 175.2 | 21410 |
| **bagel** w/ham, egg, cheese | 191 | 483 | 88.7 | 52.4 | 7.0 | | 0.4 | 1259 | 185 | 40 | 2.39 | 0.376 | 185 | 0 | 0.71 | 6.0 | 1.39 | 1.45 |
| *6.7 oz sandwich* | | 26.7 | 18.5 | 7.9 | 5.7 | 3.3 | 243 | 262 | 397 | 4.14 | 0.437 | 50.4 | 672 | 1.2 | 0.60 | 0.15 | 192.9 | 21409 |
| **bagel** w/steak, egg, cheese | 217 | 612 | 97.4 | 49.9 | 6.4 | | 0.4 | 1150 | 202 | 48 | 4.80 | 0.408 | 180 | 0 | 0.51 | 7.3 | 2.76 | 1.66 |
| *7.7 oz sandwich* | | 34.6 | 30.5 | 11.8 | 10.8 | 4.0 | 282 | 315 | 443 | 4.47 | 0.731 | 54.5 | 664 | 1.2 | 0.55 | 0.29 | 158.4 | 21411 |
| **biscuit** w/egg | 136 | 373 | 68.1 | 31.9 | | | 0.8 | 891 | 82 | 19 | 0.99 | 0.261 | 180 | 0 | 0.30 | 2.2 | 0.63 | 0.89 |
| *4.8 oz serving* | | 11.6 | 22.1 | 4.7 | 9.1 | 6.4 | 245 | 238 | 388 | 2.90 | 0.061 | 27.3 | 620 | | 0.49 | 0.11 | 80.2 | 21002 |
| **biscuit** w/egg, bacon | 150 | 458 | 70.0 | 28.6 | 3.3 | 1.5 | 0.8 | 999 | 189 | 24 | 1.64 | 0.279 | 93 | 3 | 0.14 | 2.4 | 1.03 | 1.22 |
| *5.3 oz serving* | | 17.0 | 31.1 | 8.0 | 13.4 | 7.5 | 352 | 250 | 238 | 3.74 | 0.112 | 30.9 | 340 | 2.0 | 0.22 | 0.14 | 81.0 | 21003 |
| **biscuit** w/egg, cheese | 146 | 340 | 82.2 | 25.9 | | | | 804 | 225 | 22 | 1.65 | 0.219 | 201 | 1 | 0.26 | 2.1 | 1.14 | 0.88 |
| *5.2 oz serving* | | 15.6 | 19.4 | 6.6 | 8.3 | 2.6 | 291 | 188 | 302 | 2.98 | 0.110 | 33.7 | 669 | | 0.57 | 0.13 | 140.2 | 21104 |
| **biscuit** w/egg, cheese, bacon | 144 | 433 | 61.9 | 35.2 | 2.5 | | 0.3 | 1175 | 148 | 22 | 1.57 | 0.196 | 108 | 0 | 0.39 | 3.4 | 1.24 | 1.11 |
| *5.1 oz serving* | | 17.3 | 25.2 | 8.1 | 11.6 | 2.8 | 239 | 189 | 523 | 2.26 | 0.393 | 33.6 | 360 | 1.5 | 0.36 | 0.16 | 108.0 | 21007 |
| **biscuit** w/egg, ham | 192 | 442 | 108.7 | 31.4 | 4.2 | 1.6 | 0.8 | 1382 | 221 | 31 | 2.23 | 0.305 | 117 | 0 | 0.67 | 2.0 | 1.19 | 1.67 |
| *6.8 oz serving* | | 20.4 | 27.0 | 5.9 | 11.0 | 7.7 | 300 | 319 | 317 | 4.55 | 0.138 | 36.9 | 430 | 2.1 | 0.60 | 0.27 | 88.3 | 21004 |

| Food | WT (g) | KCAL / PRO (g) | H₂0 (g) / FAT (g) | CHO (g) / SFA (g) | TSUG (g) / MUFA (g) | ASUG (g) / PUFA (g) | DFIB (g) / CHOL (mg) | Na (mg) / K (mg) | Ca (mg) / P (mg) | Mg (mg) / Fe (mg) | Zn (mg) / Cu (mg) | Mn (mg) / Se (mcg) | A (mcg RAE) / A (IU) | C (mg) / E (mg ATE) | B-1 (mg) / B-2 (mg) | NIA (mg) / B-6 (mg) | B-12 (mcg) / FOL (mcg DFE) | PANT (mg) / REF |
|---|---|---|---|---|---|---|---|---|---|---|---|---|---|---|---|---|---|---|
| **biscuit w/egg, sausage** | 180 | 562 | 80.1 | 37.9 | 1.7 | 2.1 | 0.4 | 1210 | 92 | 23 | 1.62 | 0.248 | 77 | 0 | 0.51 | 4.4 | 1.35 | 1.69 |
| *6.3 oz serving* | | 20.0 | 37.4 | 11.6 | 18.0 | 5.3 | 290 | 268 | 562 | 3.42 | 0.439 | 40.7 | 356 | 1.7 | 0.47 | 0.12 | 118.8 | 21005 |
| **biscuit w/egg, steak** | 148 | 410 | 77.7 | 21.3 | | | | 888 | 138 | 25 | 2.80 | 0.244 | 206 | 0 | 0.36 | 3.1 | 1.41 | 1.08 |
| *5.2 oz serving* | | 17.9 | 28.4 | 8.6 | 11.7 | 5.8 | 272 | 306 | 225 | 5.30 | 0.107 | 31.4 | 704 | | 0.52 | 0.18 | 75.5 | 21006 |
| **biscuit w/ham** | 113 | 386 | 32.1 | 43.8 | 2.6 | 2.4 | 0.8 | 1433 | 160 | 23 | 1.65 | 0.362 | 31 | 0 | 0.51 | 3.5 | 0.03 | 0.41 |
| *4 oz serving* | | 13.4 | 18.4 | 4.8 | 4.8 | 1.0 | 25 | 197 | 554 | 2.72 | 0.036 | 19.3 | 133 | 1.4 | 0.32 | 0.14 | 59.9 | 21008 |
| **biscuit w/sausage** | 124 | 460 | 40.7 | 37.2 | 2.0 | 2.2 | 0.5 | 1009 | 58 | 16 | 0.88 | 0.222 | 1 | 0 | 0.48 | 4.3 | 0.74 | 0.58 |
| *4.4 oz serving* | | 12.0 | 30.3 | 9.2 | 15.1 | 3.9 | 35 | 190 | 423 | 2.31 | 0.316 | 18.6 | 16 | 1.0 | 0.27 | 0.08 | 93.0 | 21009 |
| **brownie** | 60 | 243 | 7.6 | 39.0 | | | | 153 | 25 | 16 | 0.55 | 0.109 | 3 | 3 | 0.07 | 0.6 | 0.16 | 0.33 |
| *1 brownie (20 square)* | | 2.7 | 10.1 | 3.1 | 3.8 | 2.6 | 10 | 83 | 88 | 1.29 | 0 | 3.8 | 11 | | 0.13 | 0.02 | 26.4 | 21027 |
| **burrito, apple/cherry** | 74 | 231 | 26.4 | 35.0 | | | | 212 | 16 | 7 | 0.40 | 0.130 | 21 | 1 | 0.17 | 1.9 | 0.51 | 0.95 |
| *1 small* | | 2.5 | 9.5 | 4.6 | 3.4 | 1.1 | 4 | 104 | 15 | 1.07 | 0.081 | 6.9 | 406 | | 0.18 | 0.07 | 39.2 | 21069 |
| **burrito, bean** | 217 | 447 | 114.0 | 71.4 | | | | 985 | 113 | 87 | 1.52 | 0.868 | | 2 | 0.63 | 4.1 | 1.08 | 2.00 |
| *2 burritos* | | 14.1 | 13.5 | 6.9 | 4.7 | 1.2 | 4 | 653 | 98 | 4.51 | 0.378 | 21.9 | 332 | | 0.61 | 0.30 | | 21060 |
| **burrito, bean and cheese** | 186 | 378 | 100.3 | 55.0 | | | | 1166 | 214 | 80 | 1.64 | 0.432 | 99 | 2 | 0.22 | 3.6 | 0.89 | 1.60 |
| *2 burritos* | | 15.1 | 11.7 | 6.8 | 2.5 | 1.8 | 28 | 497 | 180 | 2.27 | 0.352 | 16.9 | 1250 | | 0.71 | 0.24 | 104.2 | 21061 |
| **burrito, bean and chili pepper** | 204 | 412 | 110.9 | 58.1 | | | | 1044 | 100 | 71 | 3.41 | 0.783 | 10 | 1 | 0.45 | 4.4 | 1.16 | 1.88 |
| *2 burritos* | | 16.4 | 14.7 | 7.6 | 5.4 | 1.0 | 33 | 579 | 114 | 4.55 | 0.333 | 18.4 | 204 | | 0.71 | 0.29 | 136.7 | 21062 |
| **burrito, bean and meat** | 231 | 508 | 119.9 | 66.0 | | | | 1335 | 106 | 83 | 3.83 | 0.832 | 32 | 2 | 0.53 | 5.4 | 1.73 | 2.24 |
| *2 burritos* | | 22.5 | 17.8 | 8.3 | 7.0 | 1.2 | 49 | 656 | 141 | 4.90 | 0.377 | 30.5 | 635 | | 0.83 | 0.37 | 145.5 | 21063 |
| **burrito, bean, cheese, and beef** | 203 | 331 | 131.8 | 39.7 | | | | 991 | 130 | 51 | 2.35 | 0.396 | | 5 | 0.30 | 3.9 | 1.10 | 1.66 |
| *2 burritos* | | 14.6 | 13.3 | 7.1 | 4.5 | 1.0 | 124 | 410 | 140 | 3.74 | 0.329 | 17.7 | 800 | | 0.71 | 0.22 | 85.3 | 21064 |
| **burrito, bean, cheese, and** | 336 | 662 | 187.4 | 85.2 | | | | 2060 | 289 | 97 | 6.08 | 0.813 | 185 | 7 | 0.54 | 7.7 | 1.98 | 2.89 |
| chili pepper - *2 burritos* | | 33.3 | 23.0 | 11.2 | 8.5 | 1.3 | 158 | 810 | 286 | 7.69 | 0.588 | 44.4 | 1596 | | 1.21 | 0.40 | 178.1 | 21065 |
| **burrito, beef** | 220 | 524 | 109.1 | 58.5 | | | | 1492 | 84 | 81 | 4.73 | 0.785 | 13 | 1 | 0.24 | 6.4 | 1.96 | 2.99 |
| *2 burritos* | | 26.6 | 20.8 | 10.5 | 7.4 | 0.9 | 64 | 739 | 174 | 6.09 | 0.409 | 36.7 | 277 | | 0.92 | 0.31 | 193.6 | 21066 |
| **burrito, beef and chili pepper** | 201 | 426 | 109.4 | 49.4 | | | | 1116 | 86 | 60 | 4.32 | 0.746 | 24 | 2 | 0.40 | 5.1 | 1.29 | 1.87 |
| *2 burritos* | | 21.5 | 16.5 | 8.0 | 6.1 | 1.0 | 54 | 498 | 141 | 4.44 | 0.316 | 23.9 | 462 | | 0.80 | 0.30 | 138.7 | 21067 |
| **burrito, beef, cheese, and** | 304 | 632 | 167.8 | 63.7 | | | | 2092 | 222 | 70 | 7.90 | 0.608 | 198 | 4 | 0.61 | 8.3 | 2.07 | 3.01 |
| chili pepper - *2 burritos* | | 40.9 | 24.8 | 10.4 | 9.9 | 2.2 | 170 | 973 | 316 | 7.81 | 0.362 | 33.4 | 973 | | 1.25 | 0.36 | 197.6 | 21068 |
| **cheese and deli meats sub** | 228 | 456 | 131.8 | 51.0 | | | | 1651 | 189 | 68 | 2.58 | 0.531 | 71 | 12 | 1.00 | 5.5 | 1.09 | 0.89 |
| *8 oz sub* | | 21.8 | 18.6 | 6.8 | 8.2 | 2.3 | 36 | 394 | 287 | 2.51 | 0.303 | 30.8 | 424 | | 0.80 | 0.14 | 109.4 | 21124 |
| **cheeseburger, large, double meat,** | 258 | 704 | 131.8 | 39.7 | | | | 1148 | 240 | 52 | 6.68 | 0.317 | | 1 | 0.36 | 7.2 | 3.41 | 0.85 |
| lettuce, tom - *1 sandwich* | | 38.0 | 43.7 | 17.7 | 17.4 | 4.7 | 142 | 596 | 395 | 5.91 | 0.206 | 28.9 | 348 | | 0.49 | 0.41 | 92.9 | 21100 |
| **cheeseburger, large, ham,** | 254 | 726 | 127.1 | 33.0 | | | | 1712 | 302 | 51 | 6.63 | 0.373 | | 7 | 0.53 | 9.2 | 2.87 | 1.04 |
| lettuce, tom - *1 sandwich* | | 39.5 | 48.2 | 21.1 | 18.9 | 3.9 | 122 | 538 | 531 | 5.03 | 0.246 | 32.5 | 505 | | 0.56 | 0.38 | 99.1 | 21099 |
| **cheeseburger, large, lettuce, tom** | 219 | 451 | 130.4 | 36.8 | 8.8 | | 3.1 | 843 | 208 | 42 | 4.75 | 0.399 | | 4 | 0.32 | 7.3 | 2.21 | |
| *1 sandwich* | | 25.4 | 22.7 | 8.5 | 7.7 | 0.7 | 74 | 460 | 261 | 4.07 | 0.197 | | 565 | | 0.62 | | | 21098 |
| **cheeseburger, large, triple meat** | 304 | 942 | 133.5 | 49.1 | 10.0 | | 1.5 | 1936 | 529 | 64 | 9.18 | 0.441 | | 0 | 0.45 | 13.0 | 4.74 | 1.18 |
| *1 sandwich* | | 55.3 | 58.3 | 24.4 | 19.9 | 1.9 | 192 | 699 | 596 | 6.78 | 0.237 | | | | 0.83 | 0.64 | | 21101 |
| **cheeseburger, reg** | 113 | 305 | 51.7 | 28.8 | 5.9 | | 2.1 | 710 | 139 | 26 | 2.50 | 0.287 | 68 | 0 | 0.36 | 4.0 | 1.48 | 0.47 |
| *1 sandwich* | | 15.2 | 14.6 | 6.6 | 5.7 | 1.7 | 44 | 208 | 160 | 2.54 | 0.111 | 25.7 | 330 | 0.1 | 0.21 | 0.42 | 44.1 | 21090 |
| **cheeseburger, reg, double meat** | 155 | 477 | 65.4 | 32.2 | 6.2 | | 1.1 | 963 | 279 | 33 | 4.26 | 0.281 | | 0 | 0.29 | 6.8 | 2.14 | 0.53 |
| *1 sandwich* | | 26.6 | 27.0 | 11.0 | 9.0 | 0.9 | 85 | 335 | 284 | 3.67 | 0.126 | | | | 0.44 | 0.29 | | 21092 |
| **cheeseburger, reg, double meat,** | 160 | 488 | 61.9 | 47.8 | 8.8 | | 1.6 | 942 | 306 | 34 | 3.52 | 0.402 | | 0 | 0.41 | 7.4 | 1.63 | 0.40 |
| 3-piece bun - *1 sandwich* | | 24.2 | 22.3 | 8.4 | 6.9 | 0.7 | 66 | 304 | 254 | 4.26 | 0.139 | | | | 0.48 | 0.22 | | 21094 |
| **cheeseburger, reg, double meat, 3-pc** | 228 | 650 | 106.2 | 53.1 | | | | 921 | 169 | 36 | 4.13 | 0.274 | | 3 | 0.57 | 8.3 | 2.07 | 0.64 |
| bun, lettuce, tom - *1 sandwich* | | 29.7 | 35.3 | 12.8 | 12.6 | 6.4 | 93 | 390 | 349 | 4.72 | 0.162 | 39.4 | 372 | 2.0 | 0.43 | 0.27 | 132.2 | 21095 |
| **cheeseburger, reg, double meat,** | 166 | 417 | 85.0 | 35.2 | | | | 1051 | 171 | 30 | 3.49 | 0.299 | | 2 | 0.35 | 8.1 | 1.93 | 0.43 |
| lettuce, tom - *1 sandwich* | | 21.2 | 21.1 | 8.7 | 7.8 | 2.7 | 60 | 335 | 242 | 3.42 | 0.149 | 23.6 | 398 | | 0.28 | 0.18 | 88.0 | 21093 |
| **cheeseburger, reg, lettuce, tom** | 154 | 359 | 85.0 | 28.1 | | | | 976 | 182 | 26 | 2.62 | 0.293 | | 2 | 0.32 | 6.4 | 1.23 | 0.34 |
| *1 sandwich* | | 17.8 | 19.8 | 9.2 | 7.2 | 1.5 | 52 | 229 | 216 | 2.65 | 0.123 | 20.5 | 431 | | 0.23 | 0.15 | 95.5 | 21091 |
| **chicken, breaded, fried, dark meat** | 148 | 431 | 72.5 | 15.7 | | | | 755 | 36 | 37 | 3.24 | 0.127 | 67 | 0 | 0.13 | 7.2 | 0.83 | 2.46 |
| *drumstick and thigh* | | 30.1 | 26.7 | 7.0 | 10.9 | 6.3 | 166 | 445 | 240 | 1.60 | 0.118 | 35.1 | 222 | | 0.43 | 0.33 | 37.0 | 21035 |
| **chicken, breaded, fried, light meat** | 163 | 494 | 74.5 | 19.6 | | | | 975 | 60 | 37 | 1.55 | 0.155 | 57 | 0 | 0.15 | 12.0 | 0.67 | 2.59 |
| *side breast and wing* | | 35.7 | 29.5 | 7.8 | 12.2 | 6.8 | 148 | 566 | 306 | 1.48 | 0.101 | 35.4 | 192 | | 0.29 | 0.57 | 44.0 | 21036 |
| **chicken fillet sandwich** | 182 | 515 | 86.1 | 38.7 | | | | 957 | 60 | 35 | 1.87 | 0.473 | | 9 | 0.33 | 6.8 | 0.38 | 0.60 |
| *1 sandwich* | | 24.1 | 29.4 | 8.5 | 10.4 | 8.4 | 60 | 353 | 233 | 4.68 | 0.231 | 40.4 | 100 | | 0.24 | 0.20 | 149.2 | 21102 |
| **chicken fillet sandwich w/cheese** | 228 | 632 | 104.9 | 41.6 | | | | 1238 | 258 | 43 | 2.90 | 0.381 | 164 | 3 | 0.41 | 9.1 | 0.46 | 1.35 |
| *1 sandwich* | | 29.4 | 38.8 | 12.4 | 13.7 | 9.9 | 78 | 333 | 406 | 3.63 | 0.171 | 48.1 | 620 | | 0.46 | 0.41 | 155.0 | 21103 |
| **chili con carne** | 253 | 256 | 194.1 | 21.9 | | | | 1007 | 68 | 46 | 3.57 | 0.397 | 83 | 2 | 0.13 | 2.5 | 1.14 | 3.59 |
| *8.9 oz (1 cup)* | | 24.6 | 8.3 | 3.4 | 3.4 | 0.5 | 134 | 691 | 197 | 5.19 | 0.595 | 44.0 | 1662 | | 1.14 | 0.33 | 55.7 | 21042 |

| | WT (g) | KCAL | H₂0 (g) | CHO (g) | TSUG (g) | ASUG (g) | DFIB (g) | Na (mg) | Ca (mg) | Mg (mg) | Zn (mg) | Mn (mg) | A (mcg RAE) | C (mg) | B-1 (mg) | NIA (mg) | B-12 (mcg) | PANT (mg) |
|---|---|---|---|---|---|---|---|---|---|---|---|---|---|---|---|---|---|---|
| | | PRO (g) | FAT (g) | SFA (g) | MUFA (g) | PUFA (g) | CHOL (mg) | K (mg) | P (mg) | Fe (mg) | Cu (mg) | Se (mcg) | A (IU) | E (mg ATE) | B-2 (mg) | B-6 (mg) | FOL (mcg DFE) | REF |
| **chimichanga**, beef | 174 | 425 | 88.2 | 42.8 | | | | 910 | 63 | 63 | 4.96 | 0.557 | 7 | 5 | 0.49 | 5.8 | 1.51 | 2.05 |
| *1 chimichanga* | | 19.6 | 19.7 | 8.5 | 8.1 | 1.1 | 9 | 586 | 124 | 4.54 | 0.423 | 23.7 | 146 | | 0.64 | 0.28 | 120.1 | 21070 |
| **chimichanga**, beef, cheese | 183 | 443 | 96.4 | 39.3 | | | | 957 | 238 | 60 | 3.37 | 0.489 | 132 | 3 | 0.38 | 4.7 | 1.30 | 1.79 |
| *1 chimichanga* | | 20.1 | 23.4 | 11.2 | 9.4 | 0.7 | 51 | 203 | 187 | 3.84 | 0.351 | 23.1 | 540 | | 0.86 | 0.22 | 131.8 | 21071 |
| **chimichanga**, beef, cheese, red chilies | 180 | 364 | 106.5 | 38.3 | | | | 895 | 218 | 41 | 4.63 | 0.391 | 50 | 2 | 0.23 | 3.5 | 1.28 | 1.48 |
| *1 chimichanga* | | 14.7 | 17.6 | 8.4 | 7.1 | 0.5 | 50 | 329 | 146 | 3.15 | 0.563 | 24.7 | 702 | | 0.95 | 0.16 | 129.6 | 21073 |
| **chimichanga**, beef, red chilies | 190 | 424 | 103.1 | 45.8 | | | | 1168 | 70 | 65 | 3.02 | 0.616 | 13 | 0 | 0.28 | 5.3 | 1.08 | 2.18 |
| *1 chimichanga* | | 18.1 | 19.1 | 8.3 | 7.8 | 1.1 | 10 | 614 | 112 | 4.18 | 0.275 | 24.3 | 262 | | 0.66 | 0.23 | 131.1 | 21072 |
| **chocolate chip cookies** | 55 | 233 | 2.9 | 36.2 | | | | 188 | 20 | 16 | 0.34 | 0.237 | 11 | 1 | 0.09 | 1.4 | 0.10 | 0.14 |
| *1 box* | | 2.9 | 12.1 | 5.3 | 5.1 | 1.0 | 12 | 82 | 52 | 1.47 | 0.184 | 3.3 | 52 | 0.4 | 0.19 | 0.03 | 45.1 | 21030 |
| **cinnamon roll**, mini | 50 | 202 | 9.8 | 26.7 | 9.0 | | 1.1 | 277 | 27 | 6 | 0.27 | 0.280 | | 0 | 0.13 | 1.6 | 0.06 | 0.25 |
| *2 rolls* | | 3.5 | 9.0 | 2.4 | 4.6 | 1.2 | 10 | 66 | 90 | 1.27 | 0.035 | 5.8 | | 0.6 | 0.15 | 0.02 | | 21388 |
| **clams**, breaded, fried | 115 | 451 | 33.6 | 38.8 | | | | 834 | 21 | 31 | 1.63 | 0.308 | 37 | 0 | 0.21 | 2.9 | 1.10 | 0.30 |
| *¾ cup* | | 12.8 | 26.4 | 6.6 | 11.4 | 6.8 | 87 | 266 | 238 | 3.05 | 0.095 | 9.5 | 122 | | 0.26 | 0.03 | 65.6 | 21043 |
| **coleslaw** | 99 | 147 | 73.3 | 12.8 | | | | 267 | 34 | 9 | 0.20 | 0.124 | 36 | 8 | 0.04 | 0.1 | 0.18 | 0.15 |
| *¾ cup* | | 1.5 | 11.0 | 1.6 | 2.4 | 6.4 | 5 | 177 | 36 | 0.72 | 0.042 | 1.0 | 338 | | 0.03 | 0.11 | 38.6 | 21127 |
| **corn**, yellow, on cob, boiled, buttered | 146 | 155 | 105.2 | 31.9 | | | | 29 | 4 | 41 | 0.91 | 0 | 34 | 7 | 0.25 | 2.2 | 0 | 0.36 |
| *1 ear* | | 4.5 | 3.4 | 1.6 | 1.0 | 0.6 | 6 | 359 | 108 | 0.88 | 0 | 1.0 | 391 | | 0.10 | 0.32 | 43.8 | 21128 |
| **corndog** | 175 | 460 | 81.7 | 55.8 | | | | 973 | 102 | 18 | 1.31 | 0.192 | 60 | 0 | 0.28 | 4.2 | 0.44 | 1.35 |
| *1 corndog* | | 16.8 | 18.9 | 5.2 | 9.1 | 3.5 | 79 | 262 | 166 | 6.18 | 0.245 | 22.2 | 206 | | 0.70 | 0.28 | 134.8 | 21120 |
| **crabcake** | 60 | 160 | 32.0 | 5.1 | | | 0.2 | 491 | 202 | 25 | 2.12 | 0.282 | 93 | 0 | 0.06 | 1.2 | 4.40 | 0.27 |
| *2.1 oz cake* | | 11.2 | 10.4 | 2.2 | 4.3 | 3.1 | 82 | 162 | 227 | 1.12 | 0.366 | 25.3 | 313 | | 0.08 | 0.15 | 35.4 | 21046 |
| **croissant** w/egg, cheese | 127 | 368 | 57.7 | 24.3 | | | | 551 | 244 | 22 | 1.75 | 0.226 | | 0 | 0.19 | 1.5 | 0.77 | 1.05 |
| *1 sandwich* | | 12.8 | 24.7 | 14.1 | 7.5 | 1.4 | 216 | 174 | 348 | 2.20 | 0.091 | 24.5 | 1001 | | 0.38 | 0.10 | 54.6 | 21011 |
| **croissant** w/egg, cheese, bacon | 129 | 413 | 56.7 | 23.6 | | | | 889 | 151 | 23 | 1.90 | 0.222 | 142 | 2 | 0.35 | 2.2 | 0.86 | 1.07 |
| *1 sandwich* | | 16.2 | 28.4 | 15.4 | 9.2 | 1.8 | 215 | 201 | 276 | 2.19 | 0.099 | 24.5 | 472 | | 0.34 | 0.12 | 52.9 | 21012 |
| **croissant** w/egg, cheese, ham | 154 | 480 | 78.8 | 24.5 | | | | 1095 | 146 | 26 | 2.20 | 0.223 | 132 | 12 | 0.52 | 3.2 | 1.02 | 1.26 |
| *1 sandwich* | | 19.2 | 34.0 | 17.7 | 11.5 | 2.4 | 216 | 276 | 340 | 2.16 | 0.128 | 27.6 | 457 | | 0.31 | 0.23 | 52.4 | 21013 |
| **croissant** w/egg, cheese, sausage | 160 | 523 | 73.4 | 24.7 | | | | 1115 | 144 | 24 | 2.14 | 0.253 | | 0 | 0.99 | 4.0 | 0.90 | 1.31 |
| *1 sandwich* | | 20.3 | 38.2 | 18.2 | 14.3 | 3.0 | 216 | 283 | 290 | 3.04 | 0.109 | 20.6 | 422 | | 0.32 | 0.11 | 46.4 | 21014 |
| **Danish pastry**, cheese | 91 | 353 | 30.8 | 28.7 | | | | 319 | 70 | 15 | 0.63 | 0.350 | 45 | 3 | 0.26 | 2.5 | 0.23 | 0.57 |
| *3.2 oz pastry* | | 5.8 | 24.6 | 5.1 | 15.6 | 2.4 | 20 | 116 | 80 | 1.85 | 0.086 | 17.2 | 155 | | 0.21 | 0.05 | 82.8 | 21015 |
| **Danish pastry**, cinnamon | 88 | 349 | 18.4 | 46.9 | | | | 326 | 37 | 14 | 0.48 | 0.370 | 5 | 3 | 0.26 | 2.2 | 0.22 | 0.55 |
| *3.1 oz pastry* | | 4.8 | 16.7 | 3.5 | 10.6 | 1.6 | 27 | 96 | 74 | 1.80 | 0.075 | 15.0 | 18 | | 0.19 | 0.05 | 82.7 | 21016 |
| **Danish pastry**, fruit | 94 | 335 | 27.3 | 45.1 | | | | 333 | 22 | 14 | 0.48 | 0.193 | 25 | 2 | 0.29 | 1.8 | 0.24 | 0.59 |
| *3.3 oz pastry* | | 4.8 | 15.9 | 3.3 | 10.1 | 1.6 | 19 | 110 | 69 | 1.40 | 0.055 | 13.9 | 86 | | 0.21 | 0.06 | 42.3 | 21017 |
| **egg drop soup**, Chinese Restaurant | 241 | 65 | 223.8 | 10.3 | | | | 892 | 17 | 5 | 0.22 | 0.027 | | | 0.05 | 0.4 | 0.07 | 0.29 |
| *8 fl oz* | | 2.8 | 1.5 | 0.4 | 0.5 | 0.6 | 55 | 53 | 36 | 0.63 | 0.046 | 1.0 | | | 0.05 | 0.05 | | 27000 |
| **eggs**, scrambled | 94 | 199 | 62.7 | 2.0 | 1.5 | 0 | 0 | 211 | 54 | 13 | 1.56 | 0.040 | 165 | 3 | 0.08 | 0.2 | 0.95 | 0.88 |
| *2 eggs* | | 13.0 | 15.2 | 5.8 | 5.5 | 1.9 | 400 | 138 | 227 | 2.43 | 0.063 | 21.2 | 637 | 0.9 | 0.49 | 0.18 | 27.3 | 21018 |
| **enchilada**, cheese, beef | 192 | 323 | 128.4 | 30.5 | | | | 1319 | 228 | 83 | 2.69 | 0.584 | 98 | 1 | 0.10 | 2.5 | 1.02 | 1.44 |
| *1 enchilada* | | 11.9 | 17.6 | 9.0 | 6.1 | 1.4 | 40 | 574 | 167 | 3.07 | 0.518 | 9.8 | 1135 | | 0.40 | 0.27 | 67.2 | 21075 |
| **enchilada**, cheese, sour cream | 163 | 319 | 103.1 | 28.5 | | | | 784 | 324 | 51 | 2.51 | 0.240 | 99 | 1 | 0.08 | 1.9 | 0.75 | 1.52 |
| *1 enchilada* | | 9.6 | 18.8 | 10.6 | 6.3 | 0.8 | 44 | 240 | 134 | 1.32 | 0.259 | 10.1 | 1161 | | 0.42 | 0.39 | 86.4 | 21074 |
| **enchirito**, cheese, beef, beans | 193 | 344 | 121.0 | 33.8 | | | | 1251 | 218 | 71 | 2.76 | 0.384 | 89 | 5 | 0.17 | 3.0 | 1.62 | 1.83 |
| *1 enchirito* | | 17.9 | 16.1 | 7.9 | 6.5 | 0.3 | 50 | 560 | 224 | 2.39 | 0.270 | 8.1 | 1015 | | 0.69 | 0.21 | 119.7 | 21076 |
| **English muffin**, toasted, buttered | 63 | 189 | 20.6 | 30.4 | | | | 386 | 103 | 13 | 0.42 | 0.209 | 32 | 1 | 0.25 | 2.6 | 0.02 | 0.14 |
| *1 muffin* | | 4.9 | 5.8 | 2.4 | 1.5 | 1.3 | 13 | 69 | 85 | 1.59 | 0.064 | 11.7 | 136 | 0.1 | 0.32 | 0.04 | 84.4 | 21019 |
| **English muffin**, toasted w/cheese, sausage - 1 muffin sandwich | 115 | 389 | 43.6 | 29.1 | 2.3 | 1.2 | 0.6 | 768 | 241 | 24 | 1.37 | 0.327 | 66 | 0 | 0.55 | 4.8 | 0.91 | 0.80 |
| | | 15.3 | 23.8 | 9.4 | 9.1 | 3.6 | 49 | 206 | 193 | 3.61 | 0.290 | 29.1 | 259 | 0.7 | 0.23 | 0.10 | 86.2 | 21020 |
| **English muffin**, toasted w/egg, cheese, Canadian bacon - 1 muffin sandwich | 137 | 303 | 73.3 | 29.4 | 2.5 | | 0.5 | 762 | 264 | 23 | 1.42 | 0.258 | 133 | 2 | 0.52 | 4.4 | 1.11 | 1.10 |
| | | 18.5 | 12.4 | 5.1 | 3.9 | 1.8 | 230 | 208 | 269 | 2.90 | 0.164 | 41.5 | 444 | 1.2 | 0.40 | 0.10 | 146.6 | 21021 |
| **English muffin**, toasted w/egg, chs, sauge - 1 muffin sandwich | 165 | 472 | 80.6 | 28.8 | 2.5 | | 0.3 | 776 | 277 | 28 | 1.65 | 0.317 | 112 | 0 | 0.64 | 5.3 | 1.57 | 1.78 |
| | | 22.1 | 29.9 | 11.0 | 11.2 | 4.6 | 269 | 243 | 297 | 4.34 | 0.348 | 48.2 | 371 | 1.6 | 0.45 | 0.12 | 141.9 | 21022 |
| **fish fillet**, battered/breaded, fried | 91 | 211 | 48.7 | 15.4 | | | 0.5 | 484 | 16 | 22 | 0.40 | 0.168 | 10 | 0 | 0.10 | 1.9 | 1.01 | 0.18 |
| *3.2 oz fillet* | | 13.3 | 11.2 | 2.6 | 2.3 | 5.7 | 31 | 291 | 156 | 1.92 | 0.041 | 8.3 | 35 | | 0.10 | 0.09 | 18.2 | 21047 |
| **fish sandwich**, tartar sauce | 158 | 431 | 74.8 | 41.0 | | | | 615 | 84 | 33 | 1.00 | 0.365 | | 3 | 0.33 | 3.4 | 1.07 | 0.58 |
| *5.6 oz sandwich* | | 16.9 | 22.8 | 5.2 | 7.7 | 8.2 | 55 | 340 | 212 | 2.61 | 0.191 | 79.9 | 109 | 0.9 | 0.22 | 0.11 | 113.8 | 21105 |
| **fish sandwich**, tartar sauce, cheese | 183 | 523 | 82.7 | 47.6 | | | | 939 | 185 | 37 | 1.17 | 0.362 | | 3 | 0.46 | 4.2 | 1.08 | 0.44 |
| *6.5 oz sandwich* | | 20.6 | 28.6 | 8.1 | 8.9 | 9.4 | 68 | 353 | 311 | 3.50 | 0.119 | 88.6 | 432 | 1.8 | 0.42 | 0.11 | 133.6 | 21106 |

| | WT (g) | Macronutrients | | | | | | Minerals | | | | | Vitamins | | | | | |
|---|---|---|---|---|---|---|---|---|---|---|---|---|---|---|---|---|---|---|
| | | KCAL / PRO (g) | $H_2O$ (g) / FAT (g) | CHO (g) / SFA (g) | TSUG (g) / MUFA (g) | ASUG (g) / PUFA (g) | DFIB (g) / CHOL (mg) | Na (mg) / K (mg) | Ca (mg) / P (mg) | Mg (mg) / Fe (mg) | Zn (mg) / Cu (mg) | Mn (mg) / Se (mcg) | A (mcg RAE) / A (IU) | C (mg) / E (mg ATE) | B-1 (mg) / B-2 (mg) | NIA (mg) / B-6 (mg) | B-12 (mcg) / FOL (mcg DFE) | PANT (mg) / REF |
| **frankfurter in bun** | 114 | 282 | 61.5 | 21.0 | | | | 780 | 27 | 15 | 2.30 | 0.106 | 0 | 0 | 0.27 | 4.2 | 0.59 | 0.59 |
| *4 oz sandwich* | | 12.1 | 16.9 | 5.9 | 8.0 | 2.0 | 51 | 166 | 113 | 2.69 | 0.089 | 30.2 | 0 | | 0.32 | 0.06 | 70.7 | 21118 |
| **frankfurter in bun with chili** | 114 | 296 | 54.5 | 31.3 | | | | 480 | 19 | 10 | 0.78 | 0.114 | 3 | 3 | 0.22 | 3.7 | 0.30 | 0.55 |
| *4 oz sandwich* | | 13.5 | 13.4 | 4.9 | 6.6 | 1.2 | 51 | 166 | 192 | 3.28 | 0.103 | 13.0 | 58 | | 0.40 | 0.05 | 88.9 | 21119 |
| **French fries** | 134 | 427 | 53.3 | 50.3 | 0.9 | 0 | 4.7 | 260 | 17 | 46 | 0.98 | 0.320 | 0 | 4 | 0.23 | 3.3 | 0 | 0.83 |
| *20–25 fries (regular size)* | | 5.0 | 22.8 | 5.3 | 13.3 | 4.0 | 0 | 737 | 185 | 1.84 | 0.196 | 1.2 | 0 | 1.0 | 0.09 | 0.51 | 40.2 | 21138 |
| **French toast sticks** | 141 | 479 | 47.3 | 58.1 | 26.4 | 25.9 | 2.0 | 603 | 75 | 27 | 0.72 | 0.550 | 0 | 0 | 0.40 | 3.6 | 0 | 0.47 |
| *5 oz (5 sticks)* | | 8.5 | 25.0 | 5.6 | 13.4 | 3.6 | 0 | 157 | 123 | 2.71 | 0.120 | 17.2 | 7 | 1.2 | 0.25 | 0.07 | 298.9 | 21024 |
| **French toast with butter** | 135 | 356 | 68.5 | 36.0 | | | | 513 | 73 | 16 | 0.59 | 0.209 | 136 | 0 | 0.58 | 3.9 | 0.36 | 0.54 |
| *2 slices* | | 10.3 | 18.8 | 7.7 | 7.1 | 2.4 | 116 | 177 | 146 | 1.89 | 0.065 | 20.9 | 473 | | 0.50 | 0.05 | 102.6 | 21023 |
| **frijoles with cheese** | 167 | 225 | 115.4 | 28.7 | | | | 882 | 189 | 85 | 1.74 | 0.503 | 35 | 2 | 0.13 | 1.5 | 0.68 | 1.10 |
| *1 cup* | | 11.4 | 7.8 | 4.1 | 2.6 | 0.7 | 37 | 605 | 175 | 2.24 | 0.341 | 2.8 | 456 | | 0.33 | 0.20 | 111.9 | 21077 |
| **griddle cake sandwich, sausage** | 135 | 429 | 54.1 | 42.2 | 15.2 | 14.4 | 1.4 | 995 | 85 | 19 | 1.03 | 0.267 | 0 | 0 | 0.28 | 4.2 | 0.36 | 0.52 |
| *4.7 oz sandwich* | | 11.4 | 24.0 | 7.3 | 10.2 | 3.5 | 32 | 196 | 427 | 1.92 | 0.107 | 20.5 | 0 | 0 | 0.21 | 0.15 | 135.0 | 21306 |
| **griddle cake sandwich, egg, cheese,** | 168 | 457 | 77.0 | 44.0 | 16.1 | 15.2 | 1.3 | 1263 | 183 | 35 | 2.28 | | 106 | 3 | 0.21 | 2.2 | 0.66 | 0.88 |
| *bacon - 5 oz sandwich* | | 20.2 | 22.2 | 7.1 | 7.9 | 3.0 | 247 | 262 | 304 | 2.77 | 0.158 | 41.5 | 390 | 0.9 | 0.50 | 0.14 | 137.8 | 21307 |
| **griddle cake sandwich, egg, cheese,** | 199 | 579 | 93.6 | 43.9 | 15.7 | 14.8 | 1.2 | 1297 | 191 | 28 | 2.05 | 0.285 | 115 | 0 | 0.34 | 4.2 | 1.05 | 1.17 |
| *sausage - 7 oz sandwich* | | 21.4 | 35.3 | 11.2 | 13.4 | 4.5 | 263 | 291 | 611 | 3.00 | 0.157 | 34.0 | 428 | 1.1 | 0.58 | 0.25 | 139.3 | 21305 |
| **ham and cheese sandwich** | 146 | 352 | 74.2 | 33.3 | | | | 771 | 130 | 16 | 1.37 | 0.139 | 96 | 3 | 0.31 | 2.7 | 0.54 | 1.04 |
| *1 sandwich* | | 20.7 | 15.5 | 6.4 | 6.7 | 1.4 | 58 | 291 | 152 | 3.24 | 0.182 | 23.1 | 320 | 0.3 | 0.48 | 0.20 | 78.8 | 21116 |
| **ham, egg, and cheese sandwich** | 143 | 347 | 73.1 | 30.9 | | | | 1005 | 212 | 26 | 1.99 | 0.243 | 166 | 3 | 0.43 | 4.2 | 1.23 | 0.94 |
| *1 sandwich* | | 19.2 | 16.3 | 7.4 | 5.7 | 1.7 | 246 | 210 | 346 | 3.10 | 0.122 | 32.5 | 562 | | 0.56 | 0.16 | 98.7 | 21117 |
| **hamburger, ¼ lb** | 176 | 414 | 98.0 | 32.3 | | | | 665 | 77 | 35 | 3.94 | 0.282 | | 2 | 0.33 | 5.9 | 1.92 | 0.58 |
| *6.1 oz sandwich* | | 20.9 | 22.1 | 8.4 | 9.2 | 1.8 | 70 | 387 | 188 | 3.98 | 0.160 | 27.1 | 252 | | 0.30 | 0.26 | 93.3 | 21113 |
| **hamburger, large** | 172 | 440 | 84.0 | 38.1 | 6.3 | | 1.9 | 643 | 150 | 41 | 5.23 | 0.332 | 3 | 1 | 0.28 | 8.0 | 2.86 | 0.68 |
| *6.1 oz sandwich* | | 27.0 | 20.0 | 8.2 | 9.3 | 2.0 | 69 | 387 | 208 | 2.98 | 0.174 | 42.7 | 57 | 0.1 | 0.35 | 0.25 | 53.3 | 21202 |
| **hamburger, large, double meat,** | 226 | 540 | 121.5 | 40.3 | | | | 791 | 102 | 50 | 5.67 | 0.249 | | 1 | 0.36 | 7.6 | 4.07 | 0.54 |
| *lettuce, tomato - 8 oz sandwich* | | 34.3 | 26.6 | 10.5 | 10.3 | 2.8 | 122 | 570 | 314 | 5.85 | 0.219 | 25.5 | 102 | | 0.38 | 0.54 | 110.7 | 21114 |
| **hamburger, large, triple meat** | 259 | 692 | 135.6 | 28.6 | | | | 712 | 65 | 54 | 10.75 | 0.233 | 8 | 1 | 0.31 | 11.0 | 4.92 | 0.67 |
| *9.1 oz sandwich* | | 50.0 | 41.5 | 15.9 | 18.2 | 2.7 | 142 | 785 | 394 | 8.31 | 0.197 | 55.7 | 158 | | 0.54 | 0.62 | 106.2 | 21115 |
| **hamburger, reg** | 90 | 232 | 41.5 | 25.9 | 4.7 | | 1.6 | 442 | 67 | 21 | 1.85 | 0.244 | 3 | 0 | 0.31 | 3.7 | 1.08 | 0.33 |
| *3.2 oz sandwich* | | 11.8 | 9.1 | 3.6 | 4.2 | 1.0 | 26 | 165 | 100 | 2.28 | 0.095 | 22.2 | 46 | 0.1 | 0.17 | 0.10 | 50.4 | 21108 |
| **hamburger, reg, double meat** | 176 | 519 | 75.1 | 42.4 | 7.3 | | 1.6 | 729 | 180 | 35 | 5.05 | 0.382 | 0 | 0 | 0.38 | 9.4 | 2.53 | 0.55 |
| *6.2 oz sandwich* | | 30.1 | 25.3 | 9.7 | 9.7 | 0.7 | 83 | 398 | 239 | 5.07 | 0.160 | | 0 | | 0.44 | 0.36 | | 21110 |
| **hamburger, reg, lettuce, tomato** | 110 | 279 | 54.4 | 27.3 | | | | 504 | 63 | 22 | 2.06 | 0.253 | | 2 | 0.23 | 3.7 | 0.88 | 0.30 |
| *3.9 oz sandwich* | | 12.9 | 13.5 | 4.1 | 5.3 | 2.6 | 26 | 227 | 124 | 2.63 | 0.102 | 20.6 | 82 | | 0.20 | 0.12 | 74.8 | 21109 |
| **hamburger, reg w/condiment** | 90 | 232 | 41.5 | 25.9 | 4.7 | | 1.6 | 442 | 67 | 21 | 1.85 | 0.244 | 3 | 0 | 0.31 | 3.7 | 1.08 | 0.33 |
| *3.2 oz sandwich* | | 11.8 | 9.1 | 3.6 | 4.2 | 1.0 | 26 | 165 | 100 | 2.28 | 0.095 | 22.2 | 46 | 0.1 | 0.17 | 0.10 | 50.4 | 21108 |
| **hot and sour soup,** Chinese | 233 | 91 | 211.2 | 10.1 | 1.0 | | | 876 | 44 | 21 | 0.51 | 0.198 | | 0 | 0.06 | 1.2 | 0.23 | 0.53 |
| *restaurant - 8 fl oz* | | 6.0 | 2.8 | 0.5 | 0.7 | 0.7 | 49 | 128 | 75 | 1.49 | 0.061 | 0.9 | | | 0.07 | 0.15 | | 27001 |
| **hush puppies** | 78 | 257 | 25.2 | 34.9 | | | | 965 | 69 | 16 | 0.43 | 0.267 | 9 | 0 | 0 | 2.0 | 0.17 | 0.22 |
| *5 pieces* | | 4.9 | 11.6 | 2.7 | 7.8 | 0.4 | 135 | 188 | 190 | 1.43 | 0.204 | 8.0 | 94 | | 0.02 | 0.10 | 83.5 | 21129 |
| **ice milk,** soft serve in cone | 103 | 164 | 67.4 | 24.1 | 16.9 | 11.8 | 0.1 | 92 | 153 | 15 | 0.57 | 0.021 | 60 | 1 | 0.05 | 0.3 | 0.21 | 0.27 |
| *1 cone* | | 3.9 | 6.1 | 3.5 | 1.8 | 0.4 | 28 | 169 | 139 | 0.15 | 0.019 | 3.8 | 211 | 0.4 | 0.26 | 0.06 | 17.5 | 21028 |
| **nachos w/cheese** | 113 | 346 | 45.7 | 36.3 | | | | 816 | 272 | 55 | 1.79 | 0.224 | | 1 | 0.19 | 1.5 | 0.82 | 1.31 |
| *6–8 nachos* | | 9.1 | 19.0 | 7.8 | 8.0 | 2.2 | 18 | 172 | 276 | 1.28 | 0.140 | 15.7 | 559 | | 0.37 | 0.20 | | 21078 |
| **nachos w/cheese and jalapenos** | 204 | 608 | 87.1 | 60.1 | | | | 1736 | 620 | 108 | 2.90 | 0.439 | 573 | 1 | 0.12 | 2.8 | 1.02 | 2.45 |
| *6–8 nachos* | | 16.8 | 34.1 | 14.0 | 14.4 | 4.0 | 84 | 294 | 394 | 2.45 | 0.173 | 14.1 | 4062 | | 0.49 | 0.24 | 18.4 | 21079 |
| **nachos w/cheese, beans, ground** | 255 | 569 | 142.7 | 55.8 | | | | 1800 | 385 | 97 | 3.65 | 0.423 | 3402 | 5 | 0.23 | 3.3 | 1.02 | 2.52 |
| *beef, peppers - 6–8 nachos* | | 19.8 | 30.7 | 12.5 | 11.0 | 5.7 | 20 | 451 | 388 | 2.78 | 0.745 | 13.8 | 3402 | 5 | 0.69 | 0.41 | 38.2 | 21080 |
| **nachos w/cinnamon and sugar** | 109 | 592 | 1.1 | 63.4 | | | | 439 | 85 | 20 | 0.59 | 0.493 | 5 | 8 | 0.19 | 3.9 | 1.72 | 1.90 |
| *6–8 nachos* | | 7.2 | 36.0 | 18.2 | 11.8 | 4.1 | 39 | 78 | 33 | 2.89 | 0.156 | 6.6 | 108 | | 0.45 | 0.17 | 7.6 | 21081 |
| **noodles,** crunchy, Chinese restaurant | 45 | 234 | 2.2 | 23.4 | | | | 170 | 9 | 9 | 0.28 | 0.163 | | | 0.09 | 1.1 | | |
| *1 cup* | | 4.6 | 14.3 | 2.2 | 3.4 | 7.6 | | 40 | 39 | 0.79 | 0.055 | | | | 0.05 | | | 20118 |
| **onion rings,** breaded, fried | 83 | 276 | 30.8 | 31.3 | | | | 430 | 73 | 16 | 0.35 | 0.296 | 1 | 1 | 0.08 | 0.9 | 0.12 | 0.20 |
| *8–9 rings* | | 3.7 | 15.5 | 7.0 | 6.7 | 0.7 | 14 | 129 | 86 | 0.85 | 0.069 | 2.9 | 8 | 0.3 | 0.10 | 0.06 | 84.7 | 21130 |
| **oysters,** battered/breaded, fried | 139 | 368 | 66.7 | 39.9 | | | | 677 | 28 | 24 | 15.64 | 0.424 | 108 | 4 | 0.31 | 4.4 | 1.01 | 1.06 |
| *6 oysters* | | 12.5 | 17.9 | 4.6 | 6.9 | 4.6 | 108 | 182 | 196 | 4.46 | 0.796 | 92.2 | 363 | | 0.35 | 0.03 | 43.1 | 21048 |
| **pancakes w/butter and syrup** | 232 | 520 | 115.4 | 90.9 | | | | 1104 | 128 | 49 | 1.02 | 0.322 | 81 | 3 | 0.39 | 3.4 | 0.23 | 0.67 |
| *2 pancakes* | | 8.3 | 14.0 | 5.9 | 5.3 | 2.0 | 58 | 251 | 476 | 2.62 | 0.151 | 19.3 | 281 | 1.4 | 0.56 | 0.12 | 62.6 | 21025 |
| **pizza,** cheese, reg crust | 103 | 272 | 45.1 | 33.6 | 4.1 | 1.1 | 1.8 | 551 | 182 | 25 | 1.41 | 0.327 | 71 | 0 | 0.35 | 3.4 | 0.57 | 0.36 |
| *3.6 oz slice* | | 12.3 | 9.8 | 4.3 | 2.4 | 1.8 | 22 | 159 | 218 | 2.20 | 0.123 | 25.2 | 369 | 0.9 | 0.52 | 0.12 | 132.9 | 21299 |

| | WT (g) | KCAL / PRO (g) | H₂O (g) / FAT (g) | CHO (g) / SFA (g) | TSUG (g) / MUFA (g) | ASUG (g) / PUFA (g) | DFIB (g) / CHOL (mg) | Na (mg) / K (mg) | Ca (mg) / P (mg) | Mg (mg) / Fe (mg) | Zn (mg) / Cu (mg) | Mn (mg) / Se (mcg) | A (mcg RAE) / A (IU) | C (mg) / E (mg ATE) | B-1 (mg) / B-2 (mg) | NIA (mg) / B-6 (mg) | B-12 (mcg) / FOL (mcg DFE) | PANT (mg) / REF |
|---|---|---|---|---|---|---|---|---|---|---|---|---|---|---|---|---|---|---|
| **pizza, cheese, thick crust** | 106 | 288 | 46.0 | 33.2 | 3.4 | 0.4 | 1.6 | 565 | 197 | 25 | 1.46 | 0.334 | 73 | 0 | 0.38 | 3.7 | 0.59 | 0.47 |
| *3.7 oz slice* | | 12.7 | 11.6 | 5.0 | 3.1 | 2.5 | 25 | 166 | 229 | 2.44 | 0.117 | 29.5 | 382 | 0.9 | 0.28 | 0.06 | 161.1 | 21300 |
| **pizza, cheese, thin crust** | 63 | 192 | 25.7 | 16.7 | 1.9 | 0.1 | 1.3 | 366 | 189 | 16 | 1.03 | 0.149 | 45 | 0 | 0.16 | 1.3 | 0.50 | 0.19 |
| *2.2 oz slice* | | 8.9 | 9.9 | 4.4 | 2.9 | 1.8 | 22 | 110 | 180 | 0.52 | 0.078 | 17.9 | 237 | 0.8 | 0.13 | 0.05 | 85.0 | 21301 |
| **pizza, meat and veg, reg crust** | 136 | 332 | 68.5 | 34.5 | 5.1 | 1.3 | 3.0 | 801 | 163 | 31 | 1.69 | 0.371 | 83 | 0 | 0.35 | 4.2 | 0.92 | 0.62 |
| *4.8 oz slice* | | 15.0 | 14.8 | 6.0 | 5.2 | 2.6 | 37 | 250 | 249 | 2.53 | 0.188 | 31.4 | 428 | 1.2 | 0.36 | 0.13 | 118.3 | 21304 |
| **pizza, pepperoni, reg crust** | 108 | 298 | 45.9 | 34.0 | 4.1 | 1.1 | 1.6 | 683 | 168 | 26 | 1.54 | 0.367 | 76 | 0 | 0.37 | 4.0 | 0.69 | 0.47 |
| *3.8 oz slice* | | 13.3 | 12.1 | 5.3 | 3.7 | 2.2 | 29 | 186 | 216 | 2.38 | 0.127 | 28.6 | 394 | 0.9 | 0.36 | 0.17 | 141.5 | 21302 |
| **pizza, pepperoni, thick crust** | 106 | 301 | 44.8 | 32.2 | 3.2 | 0.3 | 1.9 | 654 | 170 | 26 | 1.53 | 0.354 | 68 | 0 | 0.33 | 3.9 | 0.66 | 0.50 |
| *3.7 oz slice* | | 13.2 | 13.2 | 5.3 | 4.0 | 2.8 | 30 | 181 | 216 | 2.31 | 0.126 | 30.8 | 367 | 0.9 | 0.29 | 0.10 | 151.6 | 21303 |
| **potato, baked w/cheese sce** | 296 | 474 | 194.6 | 46.5 | | | | 382 | 311 | 65 | 1.89 | 0.515 | 252 | 26 | 0.24 | 3.3 | 0.18 | 1.30 |
| *1 potato* | | 14.6 | 28.7 | 10.6 | 10.7 | 6.0 | 18 | 1166 | 320 | 3.02 | 0.630 | 7.7 | 835 | | 0.21 | 0.71 | 26.6 | 21131 |
| **potato, baked w/cheese sce, bacon** | 299 | 451 | 194.4 | 44.4 | | | | 972 | 308 | 69 | 2.15 | 0.505 | 188 | 29 | 0.27 | 4.0 | 0.33 | 1.29 |
| *1 potato* | | 18.4 | 25.9 | 10.1 | 9.7 | 4.8 | 30 | 1178 | 347 | 3.14 | 0.646 | 9.6 | 628 | | 0.24 | 0.75 | 29.9 | 21132 |
| **potato, baked w/cheese sce, broc** | 339 | 403 | 237.4 | 46.6 | | | | 485 | 336 | 78 | 2.03 | 0.803 | 268 | 48 | 0.27 | 3.6 | 0.34 | 1.42 |
| *1 potato* | | 13.7 | 21.4 | 8.5 | 7.7 | 4.2 | 20 | 1441 | 346 | 3.32 | 0.647 | 5.8 | 1695 | | 0.27 | 0.78 | 61.0 | 21133 |
| **potato, baked w/cheese sce, chili** | 395 | 482 | 276.8 | 55.9 | | | | 699 | 411 | 111 | 3.79 | 0.675 | 186 | 32 | 0.28 | 4.2 | 0.24 | 2.57 |
| *1 potato* | | 23.2 | 21.8 | 13.0 | 6.8 | 0.9 | 32 | 1572 | 498 | 6.12 | 0.826 | 5.5 | 766 | | 0.36 | 0.95 | 47.4 | 21134 |
| **potato, baked w/sour cream, chives** | 302 | 393 | 209.7 | 50.0 | | | | 181 | 106 | 69 | 0.91 | 0.580 | 266 | 34 | 0.27 | 3.7 | 0.21 | 1.48 |
| *1 potato* | | 6.7 | 22.3 | 10.0 | 7.9 | 3.3 | 24 | 1383 | 184 | 3.11 | 0.686 | 3.3 | 1347 | | 0.18 | 0.79 | 33.2 | 21135 |
| **potato, hashed brown** | 72 | 235 | 29.9 | 23.2 | 0.2 | | 1.9 | 373 | 12 | 14 | 0.24 | 0.105 | 0 | 2 | 0.10 | 1.2 | 0 | 0.20 |
| *½ cup serving* | | 1.9 | 15.6 | 3.6 | 8.3 | 2.7 | 0 | 256 | 79 | 0.48 | 0.119 | 0.4 | 0 | 0.7 | 0.06 | 0.16 | 14.4 | 21026 |
| **potato, mashed** | 240 | 199 | 190.1 | 38.7 | | | | 545 | 50 | 43 | 0.77 | 0.281 | 26 | 1 | 0.22 | 2.9 | 0.12 | 1.15 |
| *1 cup* | | 5.5 | 2.9 | 1.1 | 0.8 | 0.7 | 5 | 706 | 132 | 1.13 | 0.233 | 1.2 | 98 | | 0.12 | 0.55 | 19.2 | 21139 |
| **potato salad** | 95 | 108 | 74.8 | 12.9 | | | | 312 | 13 | 8 | 0.19 | 0.070 | 28 | 1 | 0.07 | 0.3 | 0.11 | 0.35 |
| *⅓ cup* | | 1.5 | 5.7 | 1.0 | 1.6 | 2.9 | 57 | 256 | 53 | 0.69 | 0.075 | 0.9 | 95 | | 0.10 | 0.14 | 23.8 | 21140 |
| **roast beef sandwich** | 139 | 346 | 67.6 | 33.4 | | | | 792 | 54 | 31 | 3.39 | 0.125 | 11 | 2 | 0.38 | 5.9 | 1.22 | 0.83 |
| *1 sandwich* | | 21.5 | 13.8 | 3.6 | 6.8 | 1.7 | 51 | 316 | 239 | 4.23 | 0.097 | 29.2 | 210 | | 0.31 | 0.26 | 68.1 | 21121 |
| **roast beef sandwich with cheese** | 176 | 473 | 76.6 | 45.4 | | | | 1633 | 183 | 40 | 5.37 | 0.312 | 58 | 0 | 0.39 | 5.9 | 2.06 | 0.69 |
| *1 sandwich* | | 32.2 | 18.0 | 9.0 | 3.7 | 3.5 | 77 | 345 | 401 | 5.05 | 0.199 | 34.3 | 194 | | 0.46 | 0.33 | 79.2 | 21122 |
| **roast beef sub** | 216 | 410 | 127.4 | 44.3 | | | | 845 | 41 | 67 | 4.38 | 0.432 | 30 | 6 | 0.41 | 6.0 | 1.81 | 0.78 |
| *8 oz sub* | | 28.6 | 13.0 | 7.1 | 1.8 | 2.6 | 73 | 330 | 192 | 2.81 | 0.361 | 25.7 | 413 | | 0.41 | 0.32 | 88.6 | 21125 |
| **salad, veg, no dressing** | 207 | 33 | 197.7 | 6.7 | | | | 54 | 27 | 23 | 0.43 | 0.304 | 118 | 48 | 0.06 | 1.1 | 0 | 0.25 |
| *1½ cups* | | 2.6 | 0.1 | 0 | 0 | 0.1 | 0 | 356 | 81 | 1.30 | 0.104 | 0.8 | 2352 | | 0.10 | 0.17 | 76.6 | 21052 |
| **salad, veg w/cheese, egg,** | 217 | 102 | 196.3 | 4.8 | | | | 119 | 100 | 24 | 1.00 | 0.273 | 104 | 10 | 0.09 | 1.0 | 0.30 | 0.52 |
| no dressing - *1½ cups* | | 8.8 | 5.8 | 3.0 | 1.8 | 0.5 | 98 | 371 | 132 | 0.67 | 0.089 | 7.4 | 822 | | 0.17 | 0.11 | 84.6 | 21053 |
| **salad, veg w/chicken, no dressing** | 218 | 105 | 189.8 | 3.7 | | | | 209 | 37 | 33 | 0.89 | 0.249 | 52 | 17 | 0.11 | 5.9 | 0.20 | 0.59 |
| *1½ cups* | | 17.4 | 2.2 | 0.6 | 0.7 | 0.6 | 72 | 447 | 170 | 1.09 | 0.094 | 15.5 | 935 | | 0.13 | 0.44 | 67.6 | 21054 |
| **salad, veg w/pasta, seafood, no** | 417 | 379 | 335.1 | 32.0 | | | | 1572 | 71 | 50 | 1.67 | 0.667 | 317 | 38 | 0.29 | 3.5 | 1.71 | 0.38 |
| dressing - *1½ cups* | | 16.4 | 20.8 | 2.6 | 4.8 | 9.1 | 50 | 600 | 204 | 3.17 | 0.363 | 44.6 | 6247 | | 0.21 | 0.33 | 250.2 | 21055 |
| **salad, veg w/shrimp, no dressing** | 236 | 106 | 210.3 | 6.6 | | | | 489 | 59 | 38 | 1.27 | 0.142 | 40 | 9 | 0.12 | 1.2 | 3.78 | 0.50 |
| *1½ cups* | | 14.5 | 2.5 | 0.5 | 0.7 | 0.5 | 179 | 404 | 160 | 0.90 | 0.160 | 38.2 | 791 | | 0.17 | 0.14 | 87.3 | 21056 |
| **salad, veg w/turkey, ham, cheese,** | 326 | 267 | 268.8 | 4.7 | | | | 743 | 235 | 49 | 3.13 | 0.359 | 147 | 16 | 0.39 | 6.0 | 0.85 | 0.91 |
| no dressing - *1½ cups* | | 26.0 | 16.1 | 8.2 | 5.2 | 1.4 | 140 | 401 | 401 | 1.96 | 0.166 | 36.8 | 1053 | | 0.39 | 0.42 | 101.1 | 21057 |
| **scallops, breaded, fried** | 144 | 386 | 69.1 | 38.5 | | | | 919 | 19 | 32 | 1.08 | 0.298 | 42 | 0 | 0.20 | 0 | 0.43 | 0.50 |
| *6 scallops* | | 15.8 | 19.4 | 4.9 | 12.6 | 0.6 | 108 | 294 | 292 | 2.04 | 0.216 | 38.9 | 138 | | 0.85 | 0.07 | 61.9 | 21058 |
| **shake, chocolate** | 250 | 318 | 178.8 | 51.2 | 46.5 | 34.2 | 4.8 | 242 | 282 | 42 | 1.02 | 0.098 | 65 | 1 | 0.15 | 0.4 | 0.85 | 0.98 |
| *12 fl oz* | | 8.5 | 9.2 | 5.8 | 2.7 | 0.4 | 32 | 500 | 255 | 0.78 | 0.162 | 4.2 | 232 | 0.3 | 0.61 | 0.12 | 12.5 | 14346 |
| **shake, strawberry** | 282 | 319 | 209.0 | 53.3 | | | 1.1 | 234 | 319 | 37 | 1.02 | 0.042 | 73 | 2 | 0.13 | 0.5 | 0.87 | 1.39 |
| *12 fl oz* | | 9.6 | 7.9 | 4.9 | | | 31 | 513 | 282 | 0.31 | 0.062 | 5.9 | 338 | | 0.55 | 0.12 | 8.5 | 14428 |
| **shake, vanilla** | 250 | 370 | 174.1 | 49.0 | 34.1 | 20.4 | 2.2 | 202 | 288 | 32 | 1.42 | 0.088 | 228 | 0 | 0.06 | 0.5 | 0.55 | 1.41 |
| *12 fl oz* | | 8.4 | 16.3 | 9.9 | 4.5 | 0.8 | 58 | 415 | 245 | 1.15 | 0.258 | 8.0 | 760 | 0.6 | 1.65 | 0.15 | 0 | 14347 |
| **shrimp, breaded, fried** | 164 | 454 | 78.4 | 40.0 | | | | 1446 | 84 | 39 | 1.21 | 0.333 | 36 | 0 | 0.21 | 0 | 0.15 | 0.48 |
| *6–8 shrimp* | | 18.9 | 24.9 | 5.4 | 17.4 | 0.6 | 200 | 184 | 344 | 2.95 | 0.144 | 68.4 | 120 | | 0.90 | 0.07 | 136.1 | 21059 |
| **steak sandwich,** lettuce, tomato, | 204 | 459 | 104.2 | 52.0 | | | | 798 | 92 | 49 | 4.53 | 0.367 | | 6 | 0.41 | 7.3 | 1.57 | 0.92 |
| mayo - *1 sandwich* | | 30.3 | 14.1 | 3.8 | 5.3 | 3.3 | 73 | 524 | 298 | 5.16 | 0.220 | 42.0 | 367 | | 0.37 | 0.37 | | 21123 |
| **sundae, caramel** | 155 | 304 | 87.6 | 49.3 | | | 0 | 195 | 189 | 28 | 0.82 | 0.093 | 70 | 3 | 0.06 | 0.9 | 0.60 | 0.37 |
| *1 sundae* | | 7.3 | 9.3 | 4.5 | 3.0 | 1.0 | 25 | 318 | 217 | 0.22 | 0.082 | 5.0 | 264 | | 0.29 | 0.05 | 12.4 | 21032 |
| **sundae, hot fudge** | 158 | 284 | 94.3 | 47.7 | | | 0 | 182 | 207 | 33 | 0.95 | 0.126 | 58 | 2 | 0.06 | 1.1 | 0.65 | 0.33 |
| *1 sundae* | | 5.6 | 8.6 | 5.0 | 2.3 | 0.8 | 21 | 395 | 228 | 0.58 | 0.130 | 5.2 | 221 | 0.7 | 0.30 | 0.13 | 9.5 | 21033 |
| **sundae, strawberry** | 153 | 268 | 93.2 | 44.6 | | | 0 | 92 | 161 | 24 | 0.66 | 0.168 | 57 | 2 | 0.06 | 0.9 | 0.64 | 0.44 |
| *1 sundae* | | 6.3 | 7.8 | 3.7 | 2.7 | 1.0 | 21 | 271 | 155 | 0.32 | 0.077 | 4.4 | 222 | 0.8 | 0.28 | 0.08 | 18.4 | 21034 |

| | WT (g) | KCAL | H₂O (g) | CHO (g) | TSUG (g) | ASUG (g) | DFIB (g) | Na (mg) | Ca (mg) | Mg (mg) | Zn (mg) | Mn (mg) | A (mcg RAE) | C (mg) | B-1 (mg) | NIA (mg) | B-12 (mcg) | PANT (mg) |
|---|---|---|---|---|---|---|---|---|---|---|---|---|---|---|---|---|---|---|
| | | PRO (g) | FAT (g) | SFA (g) | MUFA (g) | PUFA (g) | CHOL (mg) | K (mg) | P (mg) | Fe (mg) | Cu (mg) | Se (mcg) | A (IU) | E (mg ATE) | B-2 (mg) | B-6 (mg) | FOL (mcg DFE) | REF |
| **taco** | 263 | 571 | 153.6 | 41.1 | | | | 1233 | 339 | 108 | 6.05 | 0.676 | | 3 | 0.24 | 4.9 | 1.60 | 2.60 |
| *6 oz taco (small)* | | 31.8 | 31.6 | 17.5 | 10.1 | 1.5 | 87 | 729 | 313 | 3.71 | 0.316 | 36.0 | 1315 | | 0.68 | 0.37 | 152.5 | 21082 |
| **taco** | 263 | 571 | 153.6 | 41.1 | | | | 1233 | 339 | 108 | 6.05 | 0.676 | | 3 | 0.24 | 4.9 | 1.60 | 2.60 |
| *9.3 oz taco (large)* | | 31.8 | 31.6 | 17.5 | 10.1 | 1.5 | 87 | 729 | 313 | 3.71 | 0.316 | 36.0 | 1315 | | 0.68 | 0.37 | 152.5 | 21082 |
| **taco salad** | 198 | 279 | 143.3 | 23.6 | | | | 762 | 192 | 51 | 2.69 | 0.331 | | 4 | 0.10 | 2.5 | 0.63 | 1.35 |
| *1½ cups* | | 13.2 | 14.8 | 6.8 | 5.2 | 1.7 | 44 | 416 | 143 | 2.28 | 0.224 | 4.4 | 588 | | 0.36 | 0.22 | 112.9 | 21083 |
| **taco salad** w/chili con carne | 261 | 290 | 200.4 | 26.6 | | | | 885 | 245 | 52 | 3.29 | 0.337 | | 3 | 0.16 | 2.5 | 0.73 | 1.44 |
| *1½ cups* | | 17.4 | 13.1 | 6.0 | 4.5 | 1.5 | 5 | 392 | 154 | 2.66 | 0.300 | 7.6 | 1574 | | 0.50 | 0.52 | 112.2 | 21084 |
| **tostada, beans, beef, cheese** | 225 | 333 | 158.5 | 29.7 | | | | 871 | 189 | 68 | 3.17 | 0.360 | | 4 | 0.09 | 2.9 | 1.12 | 1.87 |
| *1 tostada* | | 16.1 | 16.9 | 11.5 | 3.5 | 0.6 | 74 | 490 | 173 | 2.45 | 0.315 | 20.9 | 1276 | | 0.50 | 0.25 | 85.5 | 21086 |
| **tostada, beans, cheese** | 144 | 223 | 95.4 | 26.5 | | | | 543 | 210 | 59 | 1.90 | 0.367 | | 1 | 0.10 | 1.3 | 0.69 | 1.14 |
| *1 tostada* | | 9.6 | 9.9 | 5.4 | 3.1 | 0.7 | 30 | 403 | 117 | 1.89 | 0.206 | 3.5 | 622 | | 0.33 | 0.16 | 43.2 | 21085 |
| **tostada, beef, cheese** | 163 | 315 | 101.1 | 22.8 | | | | 896 | 217 | 64 | 3.68 | 0.504 | | 3 | 0.10 | 3.1 | 1.17 | 1.89 |
| *1 tostada* | | 19.0 | 16.3 | 10.4 | 3.3 | 1.0 | 41 | 572 | 179 | 2.87 | 0.264 | 19.1 | 712 | | 0.55 | 0.23 | 117.4 | 21087 |
| **tostada** with guacamole | 261 | 360 | 189.3 | 32.0 | | | | 799 | 423 | 73 | 4.07 | 0.352 | | 4 | 0.13 | 2.0 | 0.99 | 2.01 |
| *2 tostadas* | | 12.5 | 23.3 | 9.9 | 8.5 | 3.1 | 39 | 650 | 232 | 1.62 | 0.253 | 7.0 | 1751 | | 0.57 | 0.26 | 117.4 | 21088 |
| **tuna salad sub** | 256 | 584 | 139.0 | 55.4 | | | | 1293 | 74 | 79 | 1.87 | 0.512 | | 4 | 0.46 | 11.3 | 1.61 | 1.87 |
| *9 oz sub* | | 29.7 | 28.0 | 5.3 | 13.4 | 7.3 | 49 | 335 | 220 | 2.64 | 0.428 | 60.2 | 187 | | 0.33 | 0.23 | 135.7 | 21126 |
| **wonton soup,** Chinese Restaurant | 223 | 71 | 203.3 | 11.7 | 0.8 | | | 905 | 11 | 7 | 0.27 | 0.076 | 0 | | 0.05 | 1.3 | 0.20 | 0.31 |
| *8 fl oz* | | 4.6 | 0.6 | 0.1 | 0.2 | 0.2 | 9 | 71 | 40 | 0.47 | 0.054 | 2.5 | 22 | | 0.04 | 0.17 | | 27002 |

## 10.2 A&W

| | WT (g) | KCAL | H₂O (g) | CHO (g) | TSUG (g) | ASUG (g) | DFIB (g) | Na (mg) | Ca (mg) | Mg (mg) | Zn (mg) | Mn (mg) | A (mcg RAE) | C (mg) | B-1 (mg) | NIA (mg) | B-12 (mcg) | PANT (mg) |
|---|---|---|---|---|---|---|---|---|---|---|---|---|---|---|---|---|---|---|
| | | PRO (g) | FAT (g) | SFA (g) | MUFA (g) | PUFA (g) | CHOL (mg) | K (mg) | P (mg) | Fe (mg) | Cu (mg) | Se (mcg) | A (IU) | E (mg ATE) | B-2 (mg) | B-6 (mg) | FOL (mcg DFE) | REF |
| **Cheese Curds** | 142 | 570 | | 27.0 | 3.0 | | 2.0 | 1220 | 800 | | | | | 0 | | | | |
| *5 oz* | | 27.0 | 40.0 | 21.0 | | | 105 | | | 1.80 | | | 1750 | | | | | AANW24 |
| **Cheese Fries** | 170 | 380 | | 50.0 | 0 | | 4.0 | 870 | 40 | | | | | 18 | | | | |
| *6 oz* | | 4.0 | 19.0 | 5.0 | | | 5 | | | 0 | | | 0 | | | | | AANW21 |
| **cheeseburger,** bacon | 223 | 570 | | 41.0 | 9.0 | | 2.0 | 1200 | 200 | | | | | 6 | | | | |
| *7.9 oz sandwich* | | 27.0 | 33.0 | 10.0 | | | 90 | | | 2.70 | | | 750 | | | | | AANW4 |
| **cheeseburger,** bacon double | 303 | 800 | | 47.0 | 10.0 | | 2.0 | 1610 | 300 | | | | | 6 | | | | |
| *10.7 oz sandwich* | | 45.0 | 48.0 | 17.0 | | | 165 | | | 4.50 | | | 1000 | | | | | AANW2 |
| **cheeseburger,** double | 288 | 720 | | 46.0 | 10.0 | | 2.0 | 1370 | 300 | | | | | 6 | | | | |
| *10.2 oz sandwich* | | 41.0 | 42.0 | 15.0 | | | 150 | | | 4.50 | | | 1000 | | | | | AANW3 |
| **cheeseburger,** kids | 175 | 460 | | 39.0 | 9.0 | | 2.0 | 1080 | 200 | | | | | 1 | | | | |
| *6.2 oz sandwich* | | 23.0 | 24.0 | 8.0 | | | 70 | | | 2.70 | | | 300 | | | | | AANW6 |
| **chicken, crispy, sandwich** | 219 | 590 | | 54.0 | 8.0 | | 3.0 | 1170 | 100 | | | | | 6 | | | | |
| *7.7 oz sandwich* | | 31.0 | 29.0 | 4.5 | | | 65 | | | 2.70 | | | 500 | | | | | AANW8 |
| **chicken, grilled, sandwich** | 213 | 440 | | 34.0 | 9.0 | | 2.0 | 860 | 80 | | | | | 6 | | | | |
| *7.5 oz sandwich* | | 36.0 | 19.0 | 3.5 | | | 90 | | | 1.80 | | | 500 | | | | | AANW7 |
| **Chicken Strips** | 159 | 500 | | 32.0 | 0 | | 2.0 | 1050 | 60 | | | | | 0 | | | | |
| *3 pieces (5.6 oz)* | | 28.0 | 29.0 | 5.0 | | | 55 | | | 2.70 | | | 0 | | | | | AANW9 |
| **Chili Bowl** | 225 | 190 | | 22.0 | 9.0 | | 5.0 | 640 | 80 | | | | | 1 | | | | |
| *7.9 oz* | | 12.0 | 6.0 | 2.0 | | | 20 | | | 2.70 | | | 1500 | | | | | AANW25 |
| **Chili Cheese Fries** | 198 | 400 | | 51.0 | 2.0 | | 5.0 | 990 | 40 | | | | | 18 | | | | |
| *7 oz* | | 8.0 | 19.0 | 5.0 | | | 10 | | | 0.72 | | | 400 | | | | | AANW22 |
| **Chili Fries** | 170 | 370 | | 49.0 | 2.0 | | 5.0 | 780 | 20 | | | | | 18 | | | | |
| *6 oz* | | 8.0 | 16.0 | 4.5 | | | 10 | | | 0.72 | | | 400 | | | | | AANW20 |
| **diet root beer** | 592 | 0 | | 0 | 0 | | 0 | 50 | 0 | | | | | 0 | | | | |
| *20 fl oz (medium)* | | 0 | 0 | 0 | | | 0 | | | 0 | | | 0 | | | | | AANW43 |
| **diet root beer float** | 794 | 350 | | 60.0 | 34.0 | | 0 | 200 | 150 | | | | | 0 | | | | |
| *large* | | 4.0 | 10.0 | 6.0 | | | 75 | | | 0 | | | 750 | | | | | AANW50 |
| **diet root beer float** | 468 | 170 | | 30.0 | 17.0 | | 0 | 105 | 80 | | | | | 0 | | | | |
| *medium* | | 2.0 | 5.0 | 3.0 | | | 40 | | | 0 | | | 400 | | | | | AANW49 |
| **diet root beer float** | 411 | 170 | | 30.0 | 17.0 | | 0 | 100 | 80 | | | | | 0 | | | | |
| *small* | | 2.0 | 5.0 | 3.0 | | | 40 | | | 0 | | | 400 | | | | | AANW48 |
| **dipping sauce,** bbq | 28 | 40 | | 10.0 | 6.0 | | 0 | 230 | 0 | | | | | 0 | | | | |
| *1 oz* | | 0 | 0 | 0 | | | 0 | | | 0.36 | | | 0 | | | | | AANW11 |
| **dipping sauce,** honey mustard | 28 | 100 | | 12.0 | 6.0 | | 0 | 170 | 0 | | | | | 0 | | | | |
| *1 oz* | | 0 | 6.0 | 1.5 | | | 0 | | | 0 | | | 0 | | | | | AANW12 |
| **dipping sauce,** ranch | 28 | 160 | | 2.0 | 1.0 | | 0 | 240 | 0 | | | | | 0 | | | | |
| *1 oz* | | 0 | 17.0 | 2.5 | | | 15 | | | 0 | | | 0 | | | | | AANW10 |
| **dipping sauce,** sweet and sour | 28 | 45 | | 12.0 | 7.0 | | 0 | 120 | 0 | | | | | 1 | | | | |
| *1 oz* | | 0 | 0 | 0 | | | 0 | | | 0 | | | 0 | | | | | AANW13 |

| WT (g) | KCAL | H₂O (g) | CHO (g) | TSUG (g) | ASUG (g) | DFIB (g) | Na (mg) | Ca (mg) | Mg (mg) | Zn (mg) | Mn (mg) | A (mcg RAE) | C (mg) | B-1 (mg) | NIA (mg) | B-12 (mcg) | PANT (mg) |
|---|---|---|---|---|---|---|---|---|---|---|---|---|---|---|---|---|---|
| | PRO (g) | FAT (g) | SFA (g) | MUFA (g) | PUFA (g) | CHOL (mg) | K (mg) | P (mg) | Fe (mg) | Cu (mg) | Se (mcg) | A (IU) | E (mg ATE) | B-2 (mg) | B-6 (mg) | FOL (mcg DFE) | REF |
| **frankfurter in bun** 90 | 280 | | 22.0 | 4.0 | | 1.0 | 710 | 40 | | | | 0 | | | | | |
| *3.2 oz sandwich* | 11.0 | 17.0 | 6.0 | | | 35 | | | 1.44 | | | 100 | | | | | AANW14 |
| **frankfurter in bun w/cheese** 126 | 320 | | 25.0 | 4.0 | | 1.0 | 910 | 60 | | | | | 1 | | | | |
| *(Chs Dog) - 4.4 oz sandwich* | 11.0 | 20.0 | 7.0 | | | 40 | | | 1.44 | | | 100 | | | | | AANW17 |
| **frankfurter in bun w/chili, chs** 154 | 350 | | 27.0 | 5.0 | | 2.0 | 1070 | 80 | | | | | 1 | | | | |
| *(Coney Chs Dog) - 5.4 oz sand* | 13.0 | 21.0 | 8.0 | | | 45 | | | 1.80 | | | 200 | | | | | AANW16 |
| **frankfurter in bun w/chili** 126 | 310 | | 24.0 | 5.0 | | 2.0 | 870 | 60 | | | | | 1 | | | | |
| *(Cone Dog) - 4.4 oz sandwich* | 13.0 | 18.0 | 7.0 | | | 40 | | | 1.80 | | | 200 | | | | | AANW15 |
| **French fries** 113 | 310 | | 45.0 | 0 | | 4.0 | 460 | 0 | | | | | 18 | | | | |
| *4 oz (kids size)* | 3.0 | 13.0 | 3.5 | | | 0 | | | 0 | | | 0 | | | | | AANW19 |
| **French fries** 156 | 430 | | 61.0 | 1.0 | | 6.0 | 640 | 0 | | | | | 27 | | | | |
| *5.5 oz (large)* | 5.0 | 18.0 | 4.5 | | | 0 | | | 0 | | | 0 | | | | | AANW18 |
| **hamburger, kids** 161 | 420 | | 35.0 | 8.0 | | 2.0 | 900 | 150 | | | | | 1 | | | | |
| *5.7 oz sandwich* | 21.0 | 22.0 | 7.0 | | | 55 | | | 2.70 | | | 100 | | | | | AANW5 |
| **hamburger, Papa Burger** 288 | 720 | | 46.0 | 10.0 | | 2.0 | 1390 | 300 | | | | | 6 | | | | |
| *10.2 oz sandwich* | 41.0 | 42.0 | 15.0 | | | 145 | | | 4.50 | | | 100 | | | | | AANW1 |
| **ice cream, vanilla, in cone** 157 | 260 | | 41.0 | 29.0 | | 0 | 145 | 200 | | | | | 0 | | | | |
| *5.5 oz (medium)* | 7.0 | 7.0 | 4.0 | | | 25 | | | 0.36 | | | 750 | | | | | AANW32 |
| **onion rings** 113 | 350 | | 45.0 | 3.0 | | 2.0 | 710 | 20 | | | | | 0 | | | | |
| *4 oz* | 5.0 | 16.0 | 3.5 | | | 0 | | | 0.36 | | | 0 | | | | | AANW23 |
| **Polar Swirl, M&M** 340 | 710 | | 107.0 | 93.0 | | 2.0 | 290 | 450 | | | | | 0 | | | | |
| *12 oz (medium)* | 15.0 | 25.0 | 16.0 | | | 55 | | | 1.08 | | | 1500 | | | | | AANW26 |
| **Polar Swirl, Oreo** 340 | 690 | | 107.0 | 79.0 | | 3.0 | 570 | 400 | | | | | 0 | | | | |
| *12 oz (medium)* | 14.0 | 24.0 | 11.0 | | | 50 | | | 3.60 | | | 1500 | | | | | AANW27 |
| **Polar Swirl, Reese's** 340 | 740 | | 97.0 | 85.0 | | 3.0 | 380 | 400 | | | | | 0 | | | | |
| *12 oz (medium)* | 18.0 | 31.0 | 14.0 | | | 55 | | | 1.08 | | | 1500 | | | | | AANW28 |
| **root beer** 617 | 290 | | 76.0 | 76.0 | | 0 | 50 | 0 | | | | | 0 | | | | |
| *20 oz (medium)* | 0 | 0 | 0 | | | 0 | | | 0 | | | 0 | | | | | AANW40 |
| **root beer float** 794 | 640 | | 136.0 | 110.0 | | 0 | 200 | 150 | | | | | 0 | | | | |
| *large* | 4.0 | 10.0 | 6.0 | | | 75 | | | 0 | | | 750 | | | | | AANW47 |
| **root beer float** 468 | 350 | | 77.0 | 64.0 | | 0 | 105 | 80 | | | | | 0 | | | | |
| *medium* | 2.0 | 5.0 | 3.0 | | | 40 | | | 0 | | | 400 | | | | | AANW46 |
| **root beer float** 411 | 330 | | 70.0 | 57.0 | | 0 | 100 | 80 | | | | | 0 | | | | |
| *small* | 2.0 | 5.0 | 3.0 | | | 40 | | | 0 | | | 400 | | | | | AANW45 |
| **Root Beer Freeze** 510 | 480 | | 89.0 | 42.0 | | 0 | 230 | 300 | | | | | 0 | | | | |
| *18 oz (medium)* | 10.0 | 10.0 | 6.0 | | | 40 | | | 0.72 | | | 1250 | | | | | AANW33 |
| **shake, chocolate** 475 | 700 | | 100.0 | 60.0 | | 2.0 | 200 | 300 | | | | | 0 | | | | |
| *16.8 oz (medium)* | 11.0 | 29.0 | 18.0 | | | 125 | | | 1.44 | | | 1500 | | | | | AANW31 |
| **shake, strawberry** 475 | 670 | | 90.0 | 52.0 | | 0 | 180 | 400 | | | | | 0 | | | | |
| *16.8 oz (medium)* | 11.0 | 29.0 | 18.0 | | | 115 | | | 1.08 | | | 1250 | | | | | AANW29 |
| **shake, vanilla** 475 | 720 | | 97.0 | 57.0 | | 0 | 210 | 450 | | | | | 0 | | | | |
| *16.8 oz (medium)* | 12.0 | 31.0 | 19.0 | | | 135 | | | 1.44 | | | 1250 | | | | | AANW30 |
| **sundae, carmel** 189 | 340 | | 57.0 | 13.0 | | 0 | 250 | 200 | | | | | 0 | | | | |
| *6.7 oz (medium)* | 8.0 | 9.0 | 4.0 | | | 35 | | | 0.36 | | | 1000 | | | | | AANW38 |
| **sundae, chocolate** 189 | 320 | | 53.0 | 15.0 | | 0 | 180 | 200 | | | | | 0 | | | | |
| *6.7 oz (medium)* | 8.0 | 8.0 | 4.0 | | | 30 | | | 0.36 | | | 750 | | | | | AANW36 |
| **sundae, hot fudge** 189 | 350 | | 54.0 | 15.0 | | 1.0 | 140 | 200 | | | | | 0 | | | | |
| *6.7 oz (medium)* | 8.0 | 11.0 | 6.0 | | | 30 | | | 0.36 | | | 750 | | | | | AANW37 |
| **sundae, strawberry** 189 | 300 | | 47.0 | 12.0 | | 0 | 140 | 200 | | | | | 0 | | | | |
| *6.7 oz (medium)* | 7.0 | 8.0 | 4.0 | | | 30 | | | 0.36 | | | 750 | | | | | AANW34 |
| **sundae, vanilla** 189 | 310 | | 52.0 | 18.0 | | 0 | 140 | 200 | | | | | 0 | | | | |
| *6.7 oz (medium)* | 7.0 | 8.0 | 4.0 | | | 30 | | | 0.36 | | | 750 | | | | | AANW35 |

## 10.3 ARBY'S

| WT (g) | KCAL | H₂O (g) | CHO (g) | TSUG (g) | ASUG (g) | DFIB (g) | Na (mg) | Ca (mg) | Mg (mg) | Zn (mg) | Mn (mg) | A (mcg RAE) | C (mg) | B-1 (mg) | NIA (mg) | B-12 (mcg) | PANT (mg) |
|---|---|---|---|---|---|---|---|---|---|---|---|---|---|---|---|---|---|
| | PRO (g) | FAT (g) | SFA (g) | MUFA (g) | PUFA (g) | CHOL (mg) | K (mg) | P (mg) | Fe (mg) | Cu (mg) | Se (mcg) | A (IU) | E (mg ATE) | B-2 (mg) | B-6 (mg) | FOL (mcg DFE) | REF |
| **apple turnover** 128 | 377 | | 65.0 | 41.0 | | 2.0 | 201 | 10 | | | | | 2 | | | | |
| *4.5 oz turnover* | 4.0 | 16.0 | 5.0 | | | 0 | | | 1.26 | | | 50 | | | | | ARBY180 |
| **Arby's Melt on bun** 146 | 355 | | 40.0 | 4.0 | | 2.0 | 1047 | 90 | | | | | 0 | | | | |
| *5.2 oz sandwich* | 18.0 | 14.0 | 5.0 | | | 30 | | | 2.70 | | | 100 | | | | | ARBY100 |
| **Arby's sauce** 14 | 15 | | 4.0 | 1.0 | | 0 | 177 | 0 | | | | | 1 | | | | |
| *.49 oz* | 0 | 0 | 0 | | | 0 | | | 0 | | | 0 | | | | | ARBY82 |

| | WT (g) | KCAL / PRO (g) | H₂O (g) / FAT (g) | CHO (g) / SFA (g) | TSUG (g) / MUFA (g) | ASUG (g) / PUFA (g) | DFIB (g) / CHOL (mg) | Na (mg) / K (mg) | Ca (mg) / P (mg) | Mg (mg) / Fe (mg) | Zn (mg) / Cu (mg) | Mn (mg) / Se (mcg) | A (mcg RAE) / A (IU) | C (mg) / E (mg ATE) | B-1 (mg) / B-2 (mg) | NIA (mg) / B-6 (mg) | B-12 (mcg) / FOL (mcg DFE) | PANT (mg) / REF |
|---|---|---|---|---|---|---|---|---|---|---|---|---|---|---|---|---|---|---|
| **Bacon Beef'n Cheddar on bun** | 212 | 521 | | 45.0 | 9.0 | | 2.0 | 1573 | 80 | | | | | 2 | | | | |
| *7.5 oz sandwich* | | 27.0 | 27.0 | 9.0 | | | 64 | | | 4.14 | | | 150 | | | | | ARBY101 |
| **bacon, egg, Swiss chs on sourdough** | 116 | 437 | | 40.0 | 5.0 | | 2.0 | 1220 | 300 | | | | | 0 | | | | |
| *bread - 4.1 oz sandwich* | | 20.0 | 16.0 | 5.0 | | | 174 | | | 2.52 | | | 350 | | | | | ARBY102 |
| **BBQ Bacon'n Jack** | 169 | 302 | | 36.0 | 5.0 | | 2.0 | 921 | 60 | | | | | 0 | | | | |
| *6 oz sandwich* | | 16.0 | 12.0 | 4.0 | | | 30 | | | 3.06 | | | 100 | | | | | ARBY103 |
| **Beef'n Cheddar on bun** | 195 | 445 | | 44.0 | 8.0 | | 2.0 | 1274 | 80 | | | | | 2 | | | | |
| *6.9 oz sandwich* | | 22.0 | 21.0 | 6.0 | | | 51 | | | 3.96 | | | 150 | | | | | ARBY104 |
| **biscuit** | 82 | 273 | | 28.0 | 3.0 | | 1.0 | 786 | 30 | | | | | 0 | | | | |
| *2.9 oz biscuit* | | 5.0 | 15.0 | 4.0 | | | 1 | | | | | | 150 | | | | | ARBY110 |
| **biscuit w/bacon** | 95 | 340 | | 29.0 | 3.0 | | 1.0 | 1028 | 30 | | | | | 0 | | | | |
| *3.4 oz sandwich* | | 9.0 | 21.0 | 6.0 | | | 13 | | | 0.18 | | | 150 | | | | | ARBY1 |
| **biscuit w/bacon, egg, Swiss cheese** | 158 | 461 | | 30.0 | 4.0 | | 1.0 | 1446 | 150 | | | | | 0 | | | | |
| *5.6 oz sandwich* | | 17.0 | 28.0 | 8.0 | | | 169 | | | 0.90 | | | 400 | | | | | ARBY105 |
| **biscuit w/chicken fingers** | 132 | 417 | | 39.0 | 3.0 | | 1.0 | 1240 | 120 | | | | | 0 | | | | |
| *4.7 oz sandwich* | | 15.0 | 23.0 | 5.0 | | | 17 | | | 0.72 | | | 150 | | | | | ARBY106 |
| **biscuit w/ham** | 125 | 316 | | 29.0 | 4.0 | | 1.0 | 1240 | 40 | | | | | 1 | | | | |
| *4.4 oz sandwich* | | 13.0 | 17.0 | 4.0 | | | 13 | | | 0.36 | | | 150 | | | | | ARBY3 |
| **biscuit w/ham, egg, Swiss chs** | 188 | 437 | | 31.0 | 4.0 | | 1.0 | 1658 | 150 | | | | | 1 | | | | |
| *6.6 oz sandwich* | | 20.0 | 23.0 | 6.0 | | | 169 | | | 1.26 | | | 400 | | | | | ARBY107 |
| **biscuit w/sausage** | 122 | 436 | | 28.0 | 3.0 | | 1.0 | 1160 | 30 | | | | | 0 | | | | |
| *4.3 oz sandwich* | | 10.0 | 31.0 | 9.0 | | | 32 | | | | | | 150 | | | | | ARBY4 |
| **biscuit w/sausage, egg, Swiss** | 185 | 557 | | 30.0 | 3.0 | | 1.0 | 1579 | 150 | | | | | 0 | | | | |
| *cheese - 6.5 oz sandwich* | | 18.0 | 38.0 | 11.0 | | | 187 | | | 0.72 | | | 400 | | | | | ARBY109 |
| **biscuit w/sausage, gravy** | 238 | 961 | | 107.0 | 19.0 | | 1.0 | 3755 | 30 | | | | | 0 | | | | |
| *8.4 oz sandwich* | | 7.0 | 68.0 | 14.0 | | | 12 | | | | | | 150 | | | | | ARBY108 |
| **BLT sandwich** | 294 | 779 | | 75.0 | 18.0 | | 6.0 | 1571 | 170 | | | | | 17 | | | | |
| *10.4 oz sandwich* | | 23.0 | 45.0 | 11.0 | | | 51 | | | 4.68 | | | 800 | | | | | ARBY5 |
| **blueberry muffin** | 85 | 320 | | 49.0 | 26.0 | | 1.0 | 490 | 20 | | | | | | | | | |
| *3 oz muffin* | | 4.0 | 12.0 | 2.0 | | | 20 | | | 0.36 | | | | | | | | ARBY111 |
| **Cheddar Fries** | 170 | 465 | | 51.0 | 0 | | 5.0 | 1311 | 70 | | | | | 6 | | | | |
| *6 oz (medium)* | | 6.0 | 28.0 | 6.0 | | | 2 | | | 1.98 | | | 600 | | | | | ARBY19 |
| **cherry turnover** | 128 | 377 | | 65.0 | 41.0 | | 2.0 | 201 | 10 | | | | | 2 | | | | |
| *4.5 oz turnover* | | 4.0 | 15.0 | 5.0 | | | 0 | | | 1.26 | | | 50 | | | | | ARBY99 |
| **chicken, bacon, Swiss, crispy** | 214 | 624 | | 52.0 | 13.0 | | 2.0 | 1320 | 190 | | | | | 1 | | | | |
| *on bun - 7.6 oz sandwich* | | 36.0 | 29.0 | 7.0 | | | 68 | | | 2.34 | | | 150 | | | | | ARBY122 |
| **chicken, bacon, Swiss, grilled** | 209 | 462 | | 38.0 | 9.0 | | 2.0 | 1333 | 180 | | | | | 2 | | | | |
| *on bun - 7.4 oz sandwich* | | 38.0 | 17.0 | 4.0 | | | 25 | | | 2.88 | | | 300 | | | | | ARBY121 |
| **chicken cordon bleu sand, crispy** | 243 | 650 | | 49.0 | 11.0 | | 2.0 | 1548 | 190 | | | | | 1 | | | | |
| *8.6 oz sandwich* | | 40.0 | 31.0 | 6.0 | | | 74 | | | 2.52 | | | 150 | | | | | ARBY112 |
| **chicken cordon bleu sand, grilled** | 238 | 488 | | 35.0 | 7.0 | | 2.0 | 1561 | 180 | | | | | 2 | | | | |
| *8.4 oz sandwich* | | 42.0 | 19.0 | 4.0 | | | 32 | | | 3.06 | | | 300 | | | | | ARBY113 |
| **chicken fillet sandwich, crispy** | 238 | 576 | | 50.0 | 11.0 | | 3.0 | 901 | 90 | | | | | 10 | | | | |
| *8.4 oz sandwich* | | 30.0 | 30.0 | 5.0 | | | 52 | | | 2.34 | | | 500 | | | | | ARBY114 |
| **chicken fillet sandwich, grilled** | 233 | 414 | | 36.0 | 7.0 | | 3.0 | 913 | 90 | | | | | 11 | | | | |
| *8.2 oz sandwich* | | 32.0 | 17.0 | 3.0 | | | 9 | | | 3.06 | | | 650 | | | | | ARBY115 |
| **chicken salad w/pecans sandwich** | 322 | 769 | | 79.0 | 17.0 | | 9.0 | 1240 | 180 | | | | | 30 | | | | |
| *11.4 oz sandwich* | | 30.0 | 39.0 | 10.0 | | | 74 | | | 4.32 | | | 200 | | | | | ARBY116 |
| **chicken sand, SW Chipotle, crispy** | 269 | 680 | | 51.0 | 11.0 | | 3.0 | 1228 | 240 | | | | | 10 | | | | |
| *9.5 oz sandwich* | | 38.0 | 37.0 | 10.0 | | | 77 | | | 2.52 | | | 750 | | | | | ARBY117 |
| **chicken sand, SW Chipotle, grilled** | 264 | 517 | | 37.0 | 7.0 | | 3.0 | 1241 | 240 | | | | | 11 | | | | |
| *9.3 oz sandwich* | | 39.0 | 25.0 | 8.0 | | | 34 | | | 3.06 | | | 900 | | | | | ARBY118 |
| **Chicken Tenders** | 100 | 289 | | 21.0 | 0 | | 1.0 | 907 | 170 | | | | | 1 | | | | |
| *3.5 oz (2 kids meal pieces)* | | 19.0 | 14.0 | 2.0 | | | 32 | | | 1.44 | | | 50 | | | | | ARBY120 |
| **Chicken Tenders** | 218 | 630 | | 47.0 | 0 | | 3.0 | 1977 | 370 | | | | | 1 | | | | |
| *7.7 oz (5 pieces)* | | 42.0 | 31.0 | 5.0 | | | 70 | | | 2.88 | | | 150 | | | | | ARBY119 |
| **chocolate chip cookie** | 45 | 202 | | 26.0 | 16.0 | | 1.0 | 213 | 10 | | | | | | | | | |
| *1.6 oz cookie* | | 2.0 | 10.0 | 4.0 | | | 15 | | | 1.26 | | | 150 | | | | | ARBY123 |
| **Chocolate Twist, TJ Cinnamons** | 71 | 250 | | 34.0 | 12.0 | | 2.0 | 110 | 40 | | | | | | | | | |
| *2.5 oz Twist* | | 4.0 | 12.0 | 4.0 | | | 5 | | | 1.62 | | | 500 | | | | | ARBY124 |
| **cinnamon roll, TJ Cinnamons** | 149 | 507 | | 73.0 | 31.0 | | 4.0 | 373 | 180 | | | | | 4 | | | | |
| *5.3 oz roll* | | 10.0 | 10.0 | 4.0 | | | 7 | | | 4.50 | | | 500 | | | | | ARBY125 |

| Food / serving | WT (g) | KCAL / PRO (g) | H₂O / FAT (g) | CHO / SFA (g) | TSUG / MUFA (g) | ASUG / PUFA (g) | DFIB / CHOL (g/mg) | Na / K (mg) | Ca / P (mg) | Mg / Fe (mg) | Zn / Cu (mg) | Mn / Se (mg/mcg) | A (mcg RAE) / A (IU) | C / E (mg / mg ATE) | B-1 / B-2 (mg) | NIA / B-6 (mg) | B-12 / FOL (mcg / mcg DFE) | PANT (mg) / REF |
|---|---|---|---|---|---|---|---|---|---|---|---|---|---|---|---|---|---|---|
| **Cinnamon Twist,** TJ Cinnamons | 71 | 260 | | 33.0 | 11.0 | | 1.0 | 190 | 40 | | | | | | | | | |
| *2.5 oz Twist* | | 3.0 | 14.0 | 5.0 | | | 5 | | | 1.62 | | | 300 | | | | | ARBY126 |
| **Corned Beef Reuben** | 309 | 606 | | 55.0 | 6.0 | | 3.0 | 1849 | 360 | | | | | 3 | | | | |
| *10.9 oz sandwich* | | 34.0 | 33.0 | 9.0 | | | 83 | | | 5.22 | | | 200 | | | | | ARBY127 |
| **croissant** | 57 | 190 | | 21.0 | 2.0 | | 1.0 | 190 | 20 | | | | | 1 | | | | |
| *2 oz croissant* | | 3.0 | 10.0 | 6.0 | | | 30 | | | 0.90 | | | | | | | | ARBY134 |
| **croissant w/bacon, egg** | 120 | 337 | | 23.0 | 3.0 | | 1.0 | 651 | 40 | | | | | 1 | | | | |
| *4.2 oz sandwich* | | 11.0 | 22.0 | 10.0 | | | 187 | | | 1.80 | | | 150 | | | | | ARBY128 |
| **croissant w/bacon, egg, Swiss chs** | 133 | 378 | | 23.0 | 3.0 | | 1.0 | 850 | 140 | | | | | 1 | | | | |
| *4.7 oz sandwich* | | 14.0 | 22.0 | 10.0 | | | 198 | | | 1.80 | | | 250 | | | | | ARBY129 |
| **croissant w/egg, ham, Swiss chs** | 163 | 434 | | 25.0 | 4.0 | | 1.0 | 1282 | 150 | | | | | 1 | | | | |
| *5.8 oz sandwich* | | 22.0 | 24.0 | 10.0 | | | 343 | | | 2.88 | | | 400 | | | | | ARBY130 |
| **croissant w/ham, Swiss cheese** | 113 | 274 | | 22.0 | 3.0 | | 1.0 | 842 | 120 | | | | | 1 | | | | |
| *4 oz sandwich* | | 13.0 | 12.0 | 7.0 | | | 53 | | | 1.44 | | | 100 | | | | | ARBY131 |
| **croissant w/sausage, egg** | 147 | 433 | | 23.0 | 3.0 | | 1.0 | 784 | 40 | | | | | 1 | | | | |
| *5.2 oz sandwich* | | 12.0 | 32.0 | 13.0 | | | 206 | | | 1.62 | | | 150 | | | | | ARBY132 |
| **croissant w/sausage, egg,** | 160 | 475 | | 23.0 | 3.0 | | 1.0 | 982 | 140 | | | | | 1 | | | | |
| Swiss chs - *5.6 oz sandwich* | | 15.0 | 32.0 | 13.0 | | | 216 | | | 1.62 | | | 250 | | | | | ARBY133 |
| **Curly Fries** | 106 | 338 | | 39.0 | 0 | | 4.0 | 791 | 40 | | | | | 5 | | | | |
| *3.7 oz (small)* | | 4.0 | 20.0 | 4.0 | | | | | | 1.80 | | | 350 | | | | | ARBY21 |
| **Curly Fries** | 128 | 406 | | 47.0 | 0 | | 5.0 | 949 | 50 | | | | | 6 | | | | |
| *4.5 oz (medium)* | | 5.0 | 24.0 | 4.0 | | | 0 | | | 1.98 | | | 450 | | | | | ARBY22 |
| **Curly Fries** | 198 | 631 | | 73.0 | 0 | | 7.0 | 1476 | 80 | | | | | 10 | | | | |
| *7 oz (large)* | | 8.0 | 37.0 | 7.0 | | | 0 | | | 3.24 | | | 650 | | | | | ARBY20 |
| **dipping sauce, bbq** | 28 | 44 | | 11.0 | 8.0 | | 0 | 343 | 10 | | | | | 1 | | | | |
| *1 oz* | | 0 | 0 | 0 | | | 0 | | | 0.18 | | | 100 | | | | | ARBY84 |
| **dipping sauce, Bronco Berry** | 57 | 122 | | 30.0 | 28.0 | | 0 | 36 | 0 | | | | | 3 | | | | |
| *2 oz* | | 0 | 0 | 0 | | | 0 | | | 0.18 | | | 100 | | | | | ARBY85 |
| **dipping sauce, Buffalo** | 57 | 20 | | 3.0 | 1.0 | | 0 | 1600 | | | | | | | | | | |
| *2 oz* | | 0 | 1.0 | 0 | | | 0 | | | | | | | | | | | ARBY135 |
| **dipping sauce, Cool Ranch** | 43 | 158 | | 2.0 | 1.0 | | 0 | 277 | 20 | | | | | | | | | |
| Sour Crm - *1.5 oz* | | 1.0 | 16.0 | 4.0 | | | 0 | | | | | | | | | | | ARBY136 |
| **dipping sauce, Honey Mustard** | 28 | 129 | | 6.0 | 5.0 | | 0 | 151 | 0 | | | | | 0 | | | | |
| *1 oz* | | 0 | 12.0 | 2.0 | | | 9 | | | 0.18 | | | 0 | | | | | ARBY86 |
| **egg and Swiss chs on sourdough** | 107 | 392 | | 40.0 | 5.0 | | 2.0 | 1058 | 300 | | | | | 0 | | | | |
| bread - *3.8 oz sandwich* | | 17.0 | 12.0 | 3.0 | | | 166 | | | 2.34 | | | 350 | | | | | ARBY137 |
| **fish sandwich on bun** | 229 | 569 | | 63.0 | 9.0 | | 3.0 | 995 | 60 | | | | | 10 | | | | |
| *8.1 oz sandwich* | | 22.0 | 26.0 | 7.0 | | | 60 | | | 3.06 | | | 450 | | | | | ARBY138 |
| **French dip and Swiss on French roll** | 224 | 473 | | 38.0 | 2.0 | | 3.0 | 1679 | 250 | | | | | 6 | | | | |
| *7.9 oz sandwich* | | 32.0 | 18.0 | 7.0 | | | 79 | | | 2.70 | | | 200 | | | | | ARBY139 |
| **French dip on French roll** | 198 | 391 | | 37.0 | 2.0 | | 3.0 | 1282 | 40 | | | | | 6 | | | | |
| *7 oz sandwich* | | 26.0 | 16.0 | 6.0 | | | 58 | | | 2.70 | | | | | | | | ARBY140 |
| **French dip sub w/au jus** | 281 | 448 | | 48.0 | 3.0 | | 2.0 | 2803 | 70 | | | | | 1 | | | | |
| *9.9 oz sub* | | 29.0 | 17.0 | 7.0 | | | 59 | | | 4.32 | | | 0 | | | | | ARBY16 |
| **French Toastix** | 124 | 312 | | 44.0 | 11.0 | | 1.0 | 492 | 50 | | | | | | | | | |
| *4.4 oz piece* | | 6.0 | 13.0 | 2.0 | | | 0 | | | 1.26 | | | | | | | | ARBY18 |
| **French Toastix syrup** | 28 | 78 | | 20.0 | 11.0 | | 0 | 25 | 0 | | | | | | | | | |
| *1 oz* | | 0 | 0 | 0 | | | 0 | | | 0 | | | | | | | | ARBY17 |
| **fries, homestyle** | 113 | 302 | | 44.0 | 1.0 | | 3.0 | 549 | 30 | | | | | 7 | | | | |
| *4 oz (small)* | | 3.0 | 20.0 | 4.0 | | | 0 | | | 0.90 | | | | | | | | ARBY26 |
| **fries, homestyle** | 142 | 377 | | 55.0 | 1.0 | | 4.0 | 686 | 30 | | | | | 8 | | | | |
| *5 oz (medium)* | | 4.0 | 25.0 | 4.0 | | | 0 | | | 1.08 | | | | | | | | ARBY25 |
| **fries, homestyle** | 213 | 566 | | 82.0 | 1.0 | | 6.0 | 1029 | 50 | | | | | 13 | | | | |
| *7.5 oz (large)* | | 6.0 | 37.0 | 7.0 | | | 0 | | | 1.62 | | | | | | | | ARBY24 |
| **fruit cup** | 57 | 35 | | 9.0 | 8.0 | | 1.0 | 0 | 0 | | | | | 4 | | | | |
| *2 oz* | | 0 | 0 | 0 | | | 0 | | | 0 | | | 0 | | | | | ARBY141 |
| **ham and cheese sandwich** | 112 | 228 | | 28.0 | 6.0 | | 2.0 | 916 | 160 | | | | | 1 | | | | |
| *4 oz sandwich* | | 14.0 | 5.0 | 1.0 | | | 23 | | | 1.98 | | | 100 | | | | | ARBY142 |
| **ham and Swiss cheese sandwich** | 359 | 705 | | 75.0 | 19.0 | | 5.0 | 2103 | 370 | | | | | 11 | | | | |
| *12.7 oz sandwich* | | 36.0 | 31.0 | 8.0 | | | 63 | | | 5.40 | | | 650 | | | | | ARBY60 |
| **ham and Swiss cheese sub** | 276 | 498 | | 45.0 | 6.0 | | 3.0 | 1826 | 280 | | | | | 10 | | | | |
| *9.7 oz sub* | | 29.0 | 18.0 | 4.0 | | | 55 | | | 3.42 | | | 550 | | | | | ARBY143 |

| | WT (g) | KCAL / PRO (g) | H₂O (g) / FAT (g) | CHO (g) / SFA (g) | TSUG (g) / MUFA (g) | ASUG (g) / PUFA (g) | DFIB (g) / CHOL (mg) | Na (mg) / K (mg) | Ca (mg) / P (mg) | Mg (mg) / Fe (mg) | Zn (mg) / Cu (mg) | Mn (mg) / Se (mcg) | A (mcg RAE) / A (IU) | C (mg) / E (mg ATE) | B-1 (mg) / B-2 (mg) | NIA (mg) / B-6 (mg) | B-12 (mcg) / FOL (mcg DFE) | PANT (mg) / REF |
|---|---|---|---|---|---|---|---|---|---|---|---|---|---|---|---|---|---|---|
| **Ham and Swiss Melt** on bun | 138 | 275 | | 35.0 | 6.0 | | 1.0 | 1118 | 160 | | | | | 1 | | | | |
| *4.9 oz sandwich* | | 18.0 | 6.0 | 2.0 | | | 27 | | | 2.52 | | | 100 | | | | | ARBY144 |
| **ham, egg, Swiss cheese** on sourdough | 189 | 679 | | 42.0 | 6.0 | | 2.0 | 2104 | 320 | | | | | 1 | | | | |
| *bread - 6.7 oz sandwich* | | 34.0 | 35.0 | 11.0 | | | 354 | | | 3.60 | | | 500 | | | | | ARBY147 |
| **Ham n'Cheese** on bun | 167 | 304 | | 35.0 | 7.0 | | 1.0 | 1420 | 160 | | | | | 1 | | | | |
| *5.9 oz sandwich* | | 23.0 | 7.0 | 2.0 | | | 35 | | | 2.70 | | | 100 | | | | | ARBY146 |
| **Horsey sauce** | 14 | 62 | | 3.0 | 1.0 | | 0 | 173 | 0 | | | | | 0 | | | | |
| *.49 oz* | | 0 | 5.0 | 1.0 | | | 5 | | | 0 | | | 0 | | | | | ARBY87 |
| **iced tea**, sweetened | 454 | 120 | | 32.0 | 31.0 | | 0 | 15 | | | | | | | | | | |
| *~15 fl oz* | | 0 | 0 | 0 | | | 0 | | | | | | | | | | | ARBY148 |
| **Italian sub** | 277 | 622 | | 48.0 | 6.0 | | 3.0 | 1986 | 280 | | | | | 12 | | | | |
| *9.8 oz sub* | | 24.0 | 33.0 | 7.0 | | | 51 | | | 3.24 | | | 600 | | | | | ARBY32 |
| **Jalapeno Bites** | 44 | 611 | | 58.0 | 5.0 | | 4.0 | 1052 | 70 | | | | | 1 | | | | |
| *10 bites (large)* | | 11.0 | 43.0 | 18.0 | | | 56 | | | 1.80 | | | 1450 | | | | | ARBY33 |
| **Mocha Chill**, TJ Cinnamons | 354 | 306 | | 48.0 | 46.0 | | 1.0 | 214 | 390 | | | | | 3 | | | | |
| *~15 fl oz* | | 11.0 | 7.0 | 4.0 | | | 29 | | | 0.18 | | | 0 | | | | | ARBY149 |
| **Mozzarella Sticks** | 274 | 852 | | 76.0 | 9.0 | | 4.0 | 2740 | 760 | | | | | 1 | | | | |
| *8 sticks (large)* | | 36.0 | 56.0 | 26.0 | | | 90 | | | 1.98 | | | 1600 | | | | | ARBY40 |
| **Onion Petals** | 283 | 828 | | 88.0 | 18.0 | | 5.0 | 831 | 60 | | | | | 1 | | | | |
| *10 oz (large)* | | 10.0 | 57.0 | 9.0 | | | 2 | | | 1.98 | | | 1400 | | | | | ARBY42 |
| **Pecan Sticky Bun**, TJ Cinnamons | 184 | 688 | | 91.0 | 45.0 | | 5.0 | 420 | 190 | | | | | 5 | | | | |
| *6.5 oz bun* | | 12.0 | 22.0 | 5.0 | | | 7 | | | 5.04 | | | 500 | | | | | ARBY150 |
| **Philly Beef and Swiss cheese sub** | 307 | 670 | | 46.0 | 5.0 | | 4.0 | 1942 | 310 | | | | | 9 | | | | |
| *10.8 oz sub* | | 36.0 | 35.0 | 11.0 | | | 90 | | | 4.68 | | | 250 | | | | | ARBY43 |
| **potato**, baked, w/broccoli, cheddar | 398 | 535 | | 73.0 | 1.0 | | 8.0 | 784 | 180 | | | | | 85 | | | | |
| *cheese - 14 oz* | | 12.0 | 22.0 | 11.0 | | | 48 | | | 3.96 | | | 1750 | | | | | ARBY46 |
| **potato**, baked, w/butter, sour crm | 320 | 495 | | 65.0 | 0 | | 6.0 | 167 | 90 | | | | | 32 | | | | |
| *11.3 oz* | | 8.0 | 24.0 | 15.0 | | | 56 | | | 3.42 | | | 900 | | | | | ARBY47 |
| **potato**, baked, w/sour cream | 306 | 393 | | 65.0 | 0 | | 6.0 | 50 | 90 | | | | | 32 | | | | |
| *10.8 oz* | | 8.0 | 12.0 | 7.0 | | | 25 | | | 3.42 | | | 450 | | | | | ARBY152 |
| **Potato Bites**, loaded | 144 | 707 | | 54.0 | 0 | | 5.0 | 1601 | 370 | | | | | 25 | | | | |
| *10 bites (large)* | | 23.0 | 44.0 | 14.0 | | | 27 | | | 2.16 | | | 450 | | | | | ARBY151 |
| **Potato Cakes** | 150 | 369 | | 39.0 | 0 | | 3.0 | 587 | 30 | | | | | 3 | | | | |
| *5.3 oz (3 cakes)* | | 3.0 | 28.0 | 5.0 | | | 0 | | | 0.72 | | | | | | | | ARBY44 |
| **potato**, deluxe, baked, w/sour crm, | 361 | 645 | | 67.0 | 0 | | 6.0 | 346 | 290 | | | | | 33 | | | | |
| *butter, chs, bacon bits - 12.7 oz* | | 20.0 | 32.0 | 19.0 | | | 91 | | | 3.60 | | | 1250 | | | | | ARBY153 |
| **roast beef and Swiss chs sandwich** | 264 | 777 | | 73.0 | 16.0 | | 5.0 | 1743 | 360 | | | | | 6 | | | | |
| *9.3 oz sandwich* | | 37.0 | 41.0 | 13.0 | | | 89 | | | 6.30 | | | 550 | | | | | ARBY48 |
| **roast beef sandwich** on bun | 125 | 272 | | 34.0 | 5.0 | | 2.0 | 740 | 60 | | | | | 0 | | | | |
| *4.4 oz sandwich (junior)* | | 16.0 | 10.0 | 4.0 | | | 29 | | | 3.06 | | | 0 | | | | | ARBY53 |
| **roast beef sandwich** on bun | 154 | 320 | | 34.0 | 5.0 | | 2.0 | 953 | 60 | | | | | 0 | | | | |
| *5.4 oz sandwich (regular)* | | 21.0 | 14.0 | 5.0 | | | 44 | | | 3.60 | | | | | | | | ARBY54 |
| **roast beef sandwich** on bun | 198 | 398 | | 40.0 | 10.0 | | 2.0 | 1060 | 70 | | | | | 6 | | | | |
| *7 oz sandwich (super)* | | 21.0 | 19.0 | 6.0 | | | 44 | | | 3.78 | | | 350 | | | | | ARBY55 |
| **roast beef sandwich** on bun | 210 | 415 | | 34.0 | 5.0 | | 2.0 | 1379 | 60 | | | | | 1 | | | | |
| *7.4 oz sandwich (medium)* | | 31.0 | 21.0 | 9.0 | | | 73 | | | 4.68 | | | 0 | | | | | ARBY154 |
| **roast beef sandwich** on bun | 281 | 547 | | 41.0 | 6.0 | | 3.0 | 1869 | 70 | | | | | 1 | | | | |
| *9.9 oz sandwich (large)* | | 42.0 | 28.0 | 12.0 | | | 102 | | | 6.30 | | | 0 | | | | | ARBY155 |
| **roast beef sub** | 300 | 723 | | 46.0 | 4.0 | | 3.0 | 2210 | 280 | | | | | 7 | | | | |
| *10.6 oz sub* | | 35.0 | 42.0 | 11.0 | | | 89 | | | 5.04 | | | 450 | | | | | ARBY56 |
| **salad, Chicken Club** | 409 | 504 | | 32.0 | 4.0 | | 5.0 | 1235 | 390 | | | | | 35 | | | | |
| *14.4 oz salad* | | 33.0 | 26.0 | 8.0 | | | 209 | | | 3.78 | | | 4050 | | | | | ARBY160 |
| **salad dressing**, buttermilk ranch | 64 | 296 | | 4.0 | 1.0 | | 0 | 692 | 20 | | | | | 3 | | | | |
| *2.3 oz* | | 1.0 | 31.0 | 5.0 | | | 21 | | | 0.36 | | | 100 | | | | | ARBY157 |
| **salad dressing**, light buttermilk | 64 | 112 | | 13.0 | 5.0 | | 1.0 | 472 | 40 | | | | | 1 | | | | |
| *ranch - 2.3 oz* | | 1.0 | 6.0 | 1.0 | | | 1 | | | 0.36 | | | 0 | | | | | ARBY158 |
| **salad dressing**, Santa Fe Ranch | 64 | 71 | | 9.0 | 0 | | 1.0 | 25 | 20 | | | | | | | | | |
| *2.3 oz* | | 1.0 | 3.0 | 0 | | | 0 | | | 0.36 | | | | | | | | ARBY159 |
| **salad, Martha's Vineyard** w/grilled | 330 | 277 | | 24.0 | 17.0 | | 5.0 | 454 | 200 | | | | | 34 | | | | |
| *chicken - 11.6 oz salad* | | 26.0 | 8.0 | 4.0 | | | 72 | | | 1.62 | | | 3200 | | | | | ARBY161 |
| **salad, Santa Fe** w/chicken fingers | 372 | 499 | | 42.0 | 6.0 | | 7.0 | 1231 | 420 | | | | | 37 | | | | |
| *13.1 oz salad* | | 30.0 | 23.0 | 8.0 | | | 59 | | | 3.60 | | | 6600 | | | | | ARBY162 |

| Food | WT (g) | KCAL / PRO (g) | H2O (g) / FAT (g) | CHO (g) / SFA (g) | TSUG (g) / MUFA (g) | ASUG (g) / PUFA (g) | DFIB (g) / CHOL (mg) | Na (mg) / K (mg) | Ca (mg) / P (mg) | Mg (mg) / Fe (mg) | Zn (mg) / Cu (mg) | Mn (mg) / Se (mcg) | A (mcg RAE) / A (IU) | C (mg) / E (mg ATE) | B-1 (mg) / B-2 (mg) | NIA (mg) / B-6 (mg) | B-12 (mcg) / FOL (mcg DFE) | PANT (mg) / REF |
|---|---|---|---|---|---|---|---|---|---|---|---|---|---|---|---|---|---|---|
| **salad, Santa Fe** w/grilled chicken | 357 | 305 | | 21.0 | 8.0 | | 6.0 | 621 | 260 | | | | | 39 | | | | |
| *12.6 oz salad* | | 30.0 | 11.0 | 6.0 | | | 78 | | | 2.52 | | | 6600 | | | | | ARBY163 |
| **sausage, egg, Swiss cheese on sourdough bread** | 147 | 514 | | 40.0 | 5.0 | | 2.0 | 1232 | 200 | | | | | 0 | | | | |
| *5.2 oz sandwich* | | 19.0 | 27.0 | 8.0 | | | 186 | | | 2.34 | | | 250 | | | | | ARBY164 |
| **shake, chocolate** | 397 | 507 | | 83.0 | 81.0 | | 0 | 357 | 510 | | | | | 5 | | | | |
| *14 oz (regular)* | | 13.0 | 13.0 | 8.0 | | | 34 | | | 0.54 | | | 400 | | | | | ARBY90 |
| **shake, chocolate** | 510 | 660 | | 110.0 | 106.0 | | 1.0 | 455 | 650 | | | | | 7 | | | | |
| *18 oz (large)* | | 17.0 | 17.0 | 10.0 | | | 43 | | | 0.72 | | | 500 | | | | | ARBY165 |
| **shake, jamocha** | 397 | 498 | | 81.0 | 78.0 | | 0 | 393 | 510 | | | | | 5 | | | | |
| *14 oz (regular)* | | 13.0 | 13.0 | 8.0 | | | 34 | | | 0.54 | | | 400 | | | | | ARBY91 |
| **shake, jamocha** | 510 | 647 | | 107.0 | 102.0 | | 1.0 | 509 | 650 | | | | | 7 | | | | |
| *18 oz (large)* | | 17.0 | 17.0 | 10.0 | | | 43 | | | 0.72 | | | 500 | | | | | ARBY166 |
| **shake, strawberry** | 397 | 498 | | 81.0 | 77.0 | | 0 | 363 | 510 | | | | | 7 | | | | |
| *14 oz (regular)* | | 13.0 | 13.0 | 8.0 | | | 34 | | | 0.72 | | | 400 | | | | | ARBY92 |
| **shake, strawberry** | 510 | 646 | | 107.0 | 101.0 | | 1.0 | 464 | 650 | | | | | 9 | | | | |
| *18 oz (large)* | | 16.0 | 17.0 | 10.0 | | | 43 | | | 1.08 | | | 500 | | | | | ARBY167 |
| **shake, vanilla** | 369 | 437 | | 66.0 | 65.0 | | 0 | 350 | 510 | | | | | 5 | | | | |
| *13 oz (regular)* | | 13.0 | 13.0 | 8.0 | | | 34 | | | 0.36 | | | 400 | | | | | ARBY93 |
| **shake, vanilla** | 468 | 555 | | 83.0 | 82.0 | | 0 | 445 | 640 | | | | | 7 | | | | |
| *16.5 oz (large)* | | 16.0 | 17.0 | 10.0 | | | 43 | | | 0.36 | | | 500 | | | | | ARBY94 |
| **Sourdough Ham Melt** | 165 | 22 | | 3.0 | 3.0 | | 0 | 140 | 0 | | | | | 1 | | | | |
| *5.8 oz sandwich* | | 0 | 1.0 | 0 | | | 0 | | | 0.18 | | | 200 | | | | | ARBY95 |
| **Sourdough Roast Beef Melt** | 166 | 380 | | 39.0 | 5.0 | | 2.0 | 1280 | 190 | | | | | 1 | | | | |
| *5.9 oz sandwich* | | 19.0 | 13.0 | 3.0 | | | 31 | | | 2.16 | | | 100 | | | | | ARBY96 |
| **Spicy Three Pepper sauce** | 14 | 105 | | 0 | 0 | | 0 | 74 | 0 | | | | | 0 | | | | |
| *.49 oz* | | 0 | 11.0 | 2.0 | | | 9 | | | 0 | | | 0 | | | | | ARBY179 |
| **Swiss Melt with roast beef** on bun | 146 | 303 | | 37.0 | 6.0 | | 2.0 | 919 | 60 | | | | | 0 | | | | |
| *5.2 oz sandwich* | | 16.0 | 12.0 | 4.0 | | | 29 | | | 3.06 | | | 0 | | | | | ARBY98 |
| **Tangy Southwest sauce** | 57 | 333 | | 5.0 | 4.0 | | 0 | 371 | 0 | | | | | 2 | | | | |
| *2 oz* | | 1.0 | 35.0 | 5.0 | | | 29 | | | 0.18 | | | 150 | | | | | ARBY89 |
| **turkey and cheese sandwich** | 112 | 235 | | 28.0 | 6.0 | | 2.0 | 798 | 160 | | | | | 0 | | | | |
| *4 oz sandwich (mini)* | | 17.0 | 4.0 | 1.0 | | | 33 | | | 1.80 | | | 100 | | | | | ARBY168 |
| **turkey and Swiss cheese sandwich** | 359 | 725 | | 75.0 | 17.0 | | 5.0 | 1788 | 360 | | | | | 10 | | | | |
| *12.7 oz sandwich* | | 45.0 | 30.0 | 8.0 | | | 91 | | | 5.22 | | | 650 | | | | | ARBY61 |
| **Turkey Ranch and Bacon sandwich** | 382 | 834 | | 75.0 | 17.0 | | 5.0 | 2258 | 330 | | | | | 11 | | | | |
| *13.5 oz sandwich* | | 49.0 | 38.0 | 11.0 | | | 109 | | | 5.40 | | | 800 | | | | | ARBY62 |
| **Turkey Reuben** on rye bread | 309 | 611 | | 56.0 | 6.0 | | 3.0 | 1429 | 370 | | | | | 4 | | | | |
| *10.9 oz sandwich* | | 44.0 | 30.0 | 8.0 | | | 94 | | | 4.32 | | | 200 | | | | | ARBY169 |
| **turkey sub** | 285 | 633 | | 47.0 | 5.0 | | 3.0 | 2029 | 280 | | | | | 7 | | | | |
| *10.1 oz sub* | | 35.0 | 30.0 | 6.0 | | | 75 | | | 3.42 | | | 450 | | | | | ARBY97 |
| **wrap, bacon, egg, potato, Am cheese** | 188 | 515 | | 50.0 | 2.0 | | 2.0 | 1367 | 230 | | | | | 1 | | | | |
| *6.6 oz wrap* | | 16.0 | 29.0 | 8.0 | | | 165 | | | 3.24 | | | 350 | | | | | ARBY170 |
| **wrap, bacon, lett, tom, mayo** | 249 | 648 | | 45.0 | 4.0 | | 5.0 | 1530 | 40 | | | | | 17 | | | | |
| *8.8 oz wrap* | | 23.0 | 44.0 | 11.0 | | | 51 | | | 5.22 | | | 800 | | | | | ARBY171 |
| **wrap, chicken, jack and ched chs, lett, onion, rnch sce** - *8.9 oz wrap* | 251 | 567 | | 42.0 | 3.0 | | 4.0 | 1451 | 240 | | | | | 8 | | | | |
| | | 36.0 | 29.0 | 9.0 | | | 88 | | | 4.50 | | | 600 | | | | | ARBY173 |
| **wrap, chicken salad, pecans** | 277 | 638 | | 48.0 | 3.0 | | 8.0 | 1199 | 50 | | | | | 30 | | | | |
| *9.8 oz wrap* | | 30.0 | 38.0 | 10.0 | | | 74 | | | 4.86 | | | 200 | | | | | ARBY172 |
| **wrap, corned beef Reuben** | 280 | 577 | | 42.0 | 6.0 | | 1.0 | 1721 | 200 | | | | | 3 | | | | |
| *9.9 oz wrap* | | 38.0 | 29.0 | 8.0 | | | 83 | | | 2.34 | | | 200 | | | | | ARBY177 |
| **wrap, ham, egg, pot, Am chs** | 228 | 568 | | 51.0 | 3.0 | | 2.0 | 1929 | 310 | | | | | 2 | | | | |
| *8 oz wrap* | | 24.0 | 31.0 | 10.0 | | | 183 | | | 3.60 | | | 600 | | | | | ARBY174 |
| **wrap, roast turkey Reuben** | 280 | 581 | | 43.0 | 6.0 | | 1.0 | 1301 | 210 | | | | | 4 | | | | |
| *9.9 oz wrap* | | 48.0 | 27.0 | 6.0 | | | 94 | | | 1.62 | | | 200 | | | | | ARBY178 |
| **wrap, sausage, egg, pot, Am chs** | 225 | 689 | | 50.0 | 2.0 | | 2.0 | 1849 | 310 | | | | | 1 | | | | |
| *7.9 oz wrap* | | 21.0 | 45.0 | 15.0 | | | 202 | | | 3.24 | | | 600 | | | | | ARBY175 |
| **wrap, trky, ched, bacon, onion, tom, lett** - *11.2 oz wrap* | 317 | 700 | | 44.0 | 3.0 | | 4.0 | 2215 | 190 | | | | | 8 | | | | |
| | | 49.0 | 37.0 | 11.0 | | | 109 | | | 5.76 | | | 700 | | | | | ARBY176 |

| WT (g) | KCAL | H₂O (g) | CHO (g) | TSUG (g) | ASUG (g) | DFIB (g) | Na (mg) | Ca (mg) | Mg (mg) | Zn (mg) | Mn (mg) | A (mcg RAE) | C (mg) | B-1 (mg) | NIA (mg) | B-12 (mcg) | PANT (mg) |
|---|---|---|---|---|---|---|---|---|---|---|---|---|---|---|---|---|---|
| | PRO (g) | FAT (g) | SFA (g) | MUFA (g) | PUFA (g) | CHOL (mg) | K (mg) | P (mg) | Fe (mg) | Cu (mg) | Se (mcg) | A (IU) | E (mg ATE) | B-2 (mg) | B-6 (mg) | FOL (mcg DFE) | REF |

## 10.4 AU BON PAIN

| WT (g) | KCAL/PRO | H₂O/FAT | CHO/SFA | TSUG/MUFA | ASUG/PUFA | DFIB/CHOL | Na/K | Ca/P | Mg/Fe | Zn/Cu | Mn/Se | A RAE / A IU | C / E | B-1/B-2 | NIA/B-6 | B-12/FOL | PANT/REF |
|---|---|---|---|---|---|---|---|---|---|---|---|---|---|---|---|---|---|
| **apple spice muffin** | 420 | | 65.0 | 32.0 | | 3.0 | 450 | 80 | | | | | 2 | | | | |
| *5.6 oz muffin* | 7.0 | 15.0 | 1.5 | | | 20 | | | 1.80 | | | 100 | | | | | AUBN163 |
| **bagel**, asiago cheese | 360 | | 55.0 | 4.0 | | 3.0 | 590 | 100 | | | | | 0 | | | | |
| *4.6 oz bagel* (129) | 15.0 | 4.0 | 2.5 | | | 10 | | | 3.60 | | | 100 | | | | | AUBN164 |
| **bagel**, cinnamon crisp | 370 | | 84.0 | 18.0 | | 3.0 | 380 | 40 | | | | | 0 | | | | |
| *4.6 oz bagel* (129) | 10.0 | 5.0 | 1.0 | | | 0 | | | 3.60 | | | 0 | | | | | AUBN7 |
| **bagel**, cinnamon raisin | 320 | | 67.0 | 4.0 | | 3.0 | 440 | 20 | | | | | 1 | | | | |
| *4.2 oz bagel* (119) | 11.0 | 1.0 | 0 | | | 0 | | | 3.60 | | | 0 | | | | | AUBN8 |
| **bagel**, Dutch apple | 430 | | 87.0 | 25.0 | | 3.0 | 460 | 40 | | | | | 0 | | | | |
| *5.2 oz bagel* (146) | 11.0 | 4.0 | 1.0 | | | 0 | | | 3.60 | | | 0 | | | | | AUBN9 |
| **bagel**, everything | 350 | | 64.0 | 4.0 | | 3.0 | 990 | 80 | | | | | 0 | | | | |
| *4.3 oz bagel* (123) | 13.0 | 5.0 | 0 | | | 0 | | | 3.60 | | | 0 | | | | | AUBN10 |
| **bagel**, focaccia | 300 | | 57.0 | 4.0 | | 3.0 | 460 | 20 | | | | | 0 | | | | |
| *3.9 oz bagel* (110) | 11.0 | 3.0 | 0.5 | | | 0 | | | 3.60 | | | 0 | | | | | AUBN165 |
| **bagel**, French toast | 400 | | 79.0 | 17.0 | | 2.0 | 650 | 20 | | | | | 0 | | | | |
| *4.5 oz bagel* (127) | 9.0 | 8.0 | 2.5 | | | 5 | | | 2.70 | | | 0 | | | | | AUBN12 |
| **bagel**, honey 9 grain | 330 | | 68.0 | 4.0 | | 6.0 | 540 | 20 | | | | | 0 | | | | |
| *4.8 oz bagel* (135) | 13.0 | 1.5 | 0 | | | 0 | | | 3.60 | | | 0 | | | | | AUBN13 |
| **bagel**, jalapeno cheddar | 350 | | 55.0 | 4.0 | | 2.0 | 650 | 150 | | | | | 0 | | | | |
| *4.8 oz bagel* (135) | 17.0 | 10.0 | 6.0 | | | 30 | | | 2.70 | | | 400 | | | | | AUBN14 |
| **bagel**, onion dill | 350 | | 72.0 | 5.0 | | 4.0 | 530 | 40 | | | | | 1 | | | | |
| *4.5 oz bagel* (128) | 13.0 | 1.0 | 0 | | | 0 | | | 4.50 | | | 0 | | | | | AUBN166 |
| **bagel**, sesame seed | 330 | | 61.0 | 4.0 | | 3.0 | 440 | 80 | | | | | 0 | | | | |
| *4.1 oz bagel* (116) | 12.0 | 4.5 | 1.0 | | | 0 | | | 4.50 | | | 0 | | | | | AUBN16 |
| **bagel** with egg | 400 | | 63.0 | 5.0 | | 3.0 | 730 | 40 | | | | | 0 | | | | |
| *7.1 oz sandwich* (201) | 25.0 | 4.0 | 1.0 | | | 120 | | | 1.08 | | | 300 | | | | | AUBN3 |
| **bagel** with egg and bacon | 480 | | 63.0 | 5.0 | | 3.0 | 960 | 40 | | | | | 0 | | | | |
| *7.6 oz sandwich* (215) | 30.0 | 12.0 | 3.5 | | | 130 | | | 1.44 | | | 300 | | | | | AUBN4 |
| **bagel** with egg and cheese | 480 | | 63.0 | 5.0 | | 3.0 | 870 | 200 | | | | | 0 | | | | |
| *7.9 oz sandwich* (223) | 31.0 | 11.0 | 5.0 | | | 140 | | | 1.08 | | | 500 | | | | | AUBN5 |
| **bagel** with egg, cheese, and bacon | 560 | | 63.0 | 5.0 | | 3.0 | 1100 | 200 | | | | | 0 | | | | |
| *8.4 oz sandwich* (237) | 35.0 | 18.0 | 7.0 | | | 155 | | | 1.44 | | | 500 | | | | | AUBN6 |
| **baguette**, Artisan | 245 | | 53.0 | 0 | | 1.0 | 477 | 0 | | | | | 2 | | | | |
| *3.5 oz slice* (100) | 8.0 | 0 | 0 | | | 0 | | | 1.26 | | | 0 | | | | | AUBN17 |
| **baguette**, Artisan honey multigrain | 250 | | 48.0 | 1.0 | | 4.0 | 390 | 0 | | | | | 2 | | | | |
| *3.5 slice* (100) | 9.0 | 2.5 | 0 | | | 0 | | | 1.26 | | | | | | | | AUBN167 |
| **banana walnut muffin** | 440 | | 60.0 | 24.0 | | 3.0 | 450 | 80 | | | | | 1 | | | | |
| *5 oz muffin* (142) | 9.0 | 19.0 | 2.0 | | | 20 | | | 1.44 | | | 100 | | | | | AUBN72 |
| **biscotti** | 371 | | 60.0 | 32.0 | | 1.0 | 353 | 80 | | | | | 0 | | | | |
| *3.5 oz piece* (100) | 8.0 | 10.6 | 2.2 | | | 129 | | | 0.36 | | | 0 | | | | | AUBN168 |
| **black forest cake** | 270 | | 41.0 | 29.0 | | 1.0 | 250 | 150 | | | | | 0 | | | | |
| *3.5 oz slice* (100) | 6.0 | 9.0 | 7.0 | | | 40 | | | 0.72 | | | 200 | | | | | AUBN169 |
| **blueberry muffin** | 510 | | 76.0 | 33.0 | | 5.0 | 550 | 100 | | | | | 2 | | | | |
| *5.8 oz muffin* (164) | 9.0 | 19.0 | 2.0 | | | 20 | | | 1.80 | | | 0 | | | | | AUBN73 |
| **boule**, raisin pecan | 170 | | 26.0 | 7.0 | | 3.0 | 190 | 20 | | | | | 0 | | | | |
| *2 oz* (57) | 4.0 | 5.0 | 0.5 | | | 0 | | | 1.44 | | | 0 | | | | | AUBN170 |
| **bread bowl** | 640 | | 127.0 | 3.0 | | 6.0 | 1830 | 150 | | | | | 36 | | | | |
| *9.2 oz bowl* (260) | 28.0 | 3.0 | 0 | | | 0 | | | 1.44 | | | 0 | | | | | AUBN18 |
| **breadstick**, rosemary garlic | 200 | | 33.0 | 2.0 | | 2.0 | 1430 | 60 | | | | | 2 | | | | |
| *2.3 oz breadstick* (65) | 6.0 | 5.0 | 0.5 | | | 0 | | | 1.44 | | | 100 | | | | | AUBN171 |
| **brownie**, blondie with nuts | 570 | | 57.0 | 31.0 | | 2.0 | 460 | 60 | | | | | 0 | | | | |
| *4 oz brownie* (113) | 6.0 | 36.0 | 14.0 | | | 65 | | | 3.60 | | | 1250 | | | | | AUBN26 |
| **brownie**, cheesecake | 410 | | 62.0 | 44.0 | | 1.0 | 400 | 60 | | | | | 0 | | | | |
| *4 oz brownie* (113) | 5.0 | 16.0 | 3.5 | | | 75 | | | 2.70 | | | 200 | | | | | AUBN27 |
| **brownie**, chocolate chip | 420 | | 63.0 | 34.0 | | 1.0 | 400 | 60 | | | | | 0 | | | | |
| *4 oz brownie* (113) | 5.0 | 18.0 | 3.5 | | | 75 | | | 4.50 | | | 300 | | | | | AUBN28 |
| **brownie**, hazelnut mocha | 450 | | 58.0 | 32.0 | | 3.0 | 360 | 80 | | | | | 0 | | | | |
| *4 oz brownie* (113) | 6.0 | 23.0 | 4.0 | | | 70 | | | 4.50 | | | 300 | | | | | AUBN172 |
| **brownie**, rocky road | 440 | | 61.0 | 33.0 | | 2.0 | 440 | 80 | | | | | 0 | | | | |
| *4 oz brownie* (113) | 6.0 | 20.0 | 4.0 | | | 75 | | | 4.50 | | | 500 | | | | | AUBN173 |

| | WT (g) | KCAL | H₂O (g) | CHO (g) | TSUG (g) | ASUG (g) | DFIB (g) | Na (mg) | Ca (mg) | Mg (mg) | Zn (mg) | Mn (mg) | A (mcg RAE) | C (mg) | B-1 (mg) | NIA (mg) | B-12 (mcg) | PANT (mg) |
|---|---|---|---|---|---|---|---|---|---|---|---|---|---|---|---|---|---|---|
| | | PRO (g) | FAT (g) | SFA (g) | MUFA (g) | PUFA (g) | CHOL (mg) | K (mg) | P (mg) | Fe (mg) | Cu (mg) | Se (mcg) | A (IU) | E (mg ATE) | B-2 (mg) | B-6 (mg) | FOL (mcg DFE) | REF |
| **butter crumb cake** | 170 | 690 | | 85.0 | 41.0 | | 2.0 | 610 | 100 | | | | | 0 | | | | |
| *6 oz slice* | | 9.0 | 35.0 | 17.0 | | | 135 | | | 3.60 | | | 1250 | | | | | AUBN32 |
| **calzone**, breakfast | 191 | 470 | | 35.0 | 7.0 | | 1.0 | 1040 | 150 | | | | | 6 | | | | |
| *6.8 oz calzone* | | 25.0 | 25.0 | 11.0 | | | 185 | | | 2.70 | | | 750 | | | | | AUBN174 |
| **cannoli**, Au Bon Pain | 100 | 250 | | 44.0 | 30.0 | | 1.0 | 65 | 150 | | | | | 4 | | | | |
| *3.5 oz canoli* | | 8.0 | 5.0 | 3.0 | | | 20 | | | 1.08 | | | 200 | | | | | AUBN175 |
| **carrot nut muffin** | 163 | 520 | | 66.0 | 38.0 | | 4.0 | 800 | 60 | | | | | 5 | | | | |
| *5.8 oz muffin* | | 8.0 | 25.0 | 5.0 | | | 55 | | | 1.44 | | | 8500 | | | | | AUBN74 |
| **cheese bread** | 57 | 150 | | 23.0 | 0 | | 1.0 | 270 | 20 | | | | | 0 | | | | |
| *2 oz slice* | | 6.0 | 4.0 | 2.0 | | | 10 | | | 1.08 | | | 100 | | | | | AUBN176 |
| **cheese sandwich**, grilled | 213 | 700 | | 84.0 | 12.0 | | 3.0 | 1080 | 400 | | | | | 2 | | | | |
| *7.5 oz sandwich* | | 25.0 | 32.0 | 17.0 | | | 85 | | | 4.50 | | | 1250 | | | | | AUBN177 |
| **cheese toasts**, basil pesto | 55 | 140 | | 28.0 | 0 | | 1.0 | 270 | 20 | | | | | 1 | | | | |
| *3 pieces* | | 5.0 | 1.0 | 0 | | | 0 | | | 3.60 | | | 0 | | | | | AUBN178 |
| **cheesecake**, New York | 133 | 430 | | 29.0 | 24.0 | | 0 | 250 | 80 | | | | | 0 | | | | |
| *4.7 oz slice* | | 9.0 | 31.0 | 18.0 | | | 200 | | | 1.80 | | | 1500 | | | | | AUBN179 |
| **chicken, Arizona, sandwich** on | 400 | 750 | | 75.0 | 8.0 | | 5.0 | 1150 | 350 | | | | | 36 | | | | |
| *ciabatta - 14.1 oz sandwich* | | 50.0 | 28.0 | 9.0 | | | 120 | | | 12.60 | | | 1500 | | | | | AUBN180 |
| **chicken, Arizona, sandwich** on | 340 | 680 | | 61.0 | 5.0 | | 5.0 | 1550 | 350 | | | | | 15 | | | | |
| *tom bread - 12 oz sandwich* | | 42.0 | 30.0 | 10.0 | | | 125 | | | 9.00 | | | 1500 | | | | | AUBN181 |
| **chicken curry salad sandwich** | 262 | 470 | | 38.0 | 10.0 | | 2.0 | 770 | 40 | | | | | 6 | | | | |
| *9.3 oz sandwich* | | 21.0 | 27.0 | 10.0 | | | 100 | | | 2.70 | | | 1000 | | | | | AUBN182 |
| **chicken, grilled, sandwich** | 199 | 540 | | 56.0 | 8.0 | | 2.0 | 850 | 40 | | | | | 4 | | | | |
| *7 oz sandwich* | | 23.0 | 27.0 | 4.0 | | | 55 | | | 3.60 | | | 0 | | | | | AUBN183 |
| **chicken, grld, blue cheese, onion** | 327 | 672 | | 64.0 | 6.0 | | 3.0 | 1901 | 250 | | | | | 9 | | | | |
| *sandwich - 11.5 oz sandwich* | | 37.0 | 29.0 | 9.3 | | | 104 | | | 5.40 | | | 750 | | | | | AUBN184 |
| **chicken, grld, gouda, onion, chptl** | 312 | 660 | | 68.0 | 4.0 | | 3.0 | 980 | 250 | | | | | 6 | | | | |
| *mayo sand - 11 oz sandwich* | | 40.0 | 25.0 | 8.0 | | | 110 | | | 1.80 | | | 200 | | | | | AUBN185 |
| **chicken tarragon w/romaine sand** | 300 | 630 | | 57.0 | 4.0 | | 2.0 | 1280 | 40 | | | | | 9 | | | | |
| *10.6 oz sandwich* | | 32.0 | 29.0 | 4.5 | | | 90 | | | 8.10 | | | 400 | | | | | AUBN187 |
| **chicken, Thai salad sandwich** | 388 | 590 | | 70.0 | 12.0 | | 4.0 | 850 | 700 | | | | | 18 | | | | |
| *13.7 oz sandwich* | | 32.0 | 18.0 | 2.5 | | | 60 | | | 1.44 | | | 1000 | | | | | AUBN186 |
| **chocolate cake muffin**, lowfat | 117 | 320 | | 74.0 | 48.0 | | 4.0 | 590 | 20 | | | | | 0 | | | | |
| *4.2 oz muffin* | | 4.0 | 2.0 | 0.5 | | | 20 | | | 16.20 | | | 0 | | | | | AUBN75 |
| **chocolate chip cookie** | 57 | 260 | | 37.0 | 22.0 | | 0 | 250 | 20 | | | | | 0 | | | | |
| *2 oz cookie* | | 3.0 | 11.0 | 5.0 | | | 25 | | | 1.80 | | | 300 | | | | | AUBN43 |
| **chocolate chunk macadamia nut** | 61 | 280 | | 34.0 | 19.0 | | 2.0 | 190 | 20 | | | | | 0 | | | | |
| *cookie - 2.2 oz cookie* | | 3.0 | 16.0 | 7.0 | | | 30 | | | 1.08 | | | 300 | | | | | AUBN44 |
| **chocolate chunk muffin** | 152 | 590 | | 83.0 | 46.0 | | 5.0 | 480 | 150 | | | | | 0 | | | | |
| *5.3 oz muffin* | | 10.0 | 20.0 | 6.0 | | | 25 | | | 3.60 | | | 0 | | | | | AUBN188 |
| **chocolate pound cake** | 130 | 490 | | 57.0 | 35.0 | | 2.0 | 550 | 20 | | | | | 0 | | | | |
| *4.6 oz slice* | | 6.0 | 27.0 | 6.0 | | | 95 | | | 2.70 | | | 100 | | | | | AUBN189 |
| **confetti cookie with M&M's** | 69 | 310 | | 42.0 | 25.0 | | 1.0 | 290 | 20 | | | | | 0 | | | | |
| *2.4 oz cookie* | | 3.0 | 14.0 | 5.0 | | | 25 | | | 1.08 | | | 200 | | | | | AUBN190 |
| **corn muffin** | 163 | 460 | | 69.0 | 29.0 | | 2.0 | 550 | 80 | | | | | 2 | | | | |
| *5.8 oz muffin* | | 9.0 | 16.0 | 3.0 | | | 60 | | | 0.72 | | | 100 | | | | | AUBN76 |
| **corn muffin**, southwest | 163 | 530 | | 61.0 | 29.0 | | 1.0 | 850 | 60 | | | | | 0 | | | | |
| *5.8 oz muffin* | | 8.0 | 29.0 | 4.5 | | | 90 | | | 1.80 | | | 100 | | | | | AUBN191 |
| **cranberry walnut muffin** | 163 | 500 | | 61.0 | 26.0 | | 5.0 | 460 | 80 | | | | | 5 | | | | |
| *5.8 oz muffin* | | 10.0 | 24.0 | 2.0 | | | 20 | | | 1.44 | | | 0 | | | | | AUBN77 |
| **cream cheese**, honey walnut | 57 | 140 | | 12.0 | 12.0 | | 0 | 150 | 40 | | | | | 0 | | | | |
| *2 oz* | | 3.0 | 9.0 | 6.0 | | | 30 | | | 0 | | | 300 | | | | | AUBN192 |
| **cream cheese**, vegetable | 57 | 140 | | 3.0 | 1.0 | | 0 | 380 | 40 | | | | | 0 | | | | |
| *2 oz* | | 6.0 | 12.0 | 7.0 | | | 40 | | | 0.72 | | | 1250 | | | | | AUBN193 |
| **crème puff**, chocolate caramel | 129 | 510 | | 74.0 | 33.0 | | 4.0 | 230 | 40 | | | | | 1 | | | | |
| *4.6 oz crème puff* | | 8.0 | 22.0 | 7.0 | | | 35 | | | 1.80 | | | 300 | | | | | AUBN194 |
| **croissant** | 76 | 260 | | 28.0 | 3.0 | | 1.0 | 190 | 20 | | | | | 2 | | | | |
| *2.7 oz croissant* | | 5.0 | 15.0 | 8.0 | | | 40 | | | 1.44 | | | 500 | | | | | AUBN58 |
| **croissant**, almond | 133 | 570 | | 50.0 | 17.0 | | 4.0 | 270 | 80 | | | | | 2 | | | | |
| *4.7 oz croissant* | | 12.0 | 38.0 | 15.0 | | | 125 | | | 2.70 | | | 1000 | | | | | AUBN59 |
| **croissant**, apple | 101 | 230 | | 31.0 | 11.0 | | 2.0 | 230 | 20 | | | | | 45 | | | | |
| *3.4 oz croissant* | | 4.0 | 10.0 | 6.0 | | | 25 | | | 1.44 | | | 300 | | | | | AUBN60 |

| | WT (g) | KCAL | H₂O (g) | CHO (g) | TSUG (g) | ASUG (g) | DFIB (g) | Na (mg) | Ca (mg) | Mg (mg) | Zn (mg) | Mn (mg) | A (mcg RAE) | C (mg) | B-1 (mg) | NIA (mg) | B-12 (mcg) | PANT (mg) |
|---|---|---|---|---|---|---|---|---|---|---|---|---|---|---|---|---|---|---|
| | | PRO (g) | FAT (g) | SFA (g) | MUFA (g) | PUFA (g) | CHOL (mg) | K (mg) | P (mg) | Fe (mg) | Cu (mg) | Se (mcg) | A (IU) | E (mg ATE) | B-2 (mg) | B-6 (mg) | FOL (mcg DFE) | REF |
| **croissant,** chocolate | 91 | 330 | | 42.0 | 16.0 | | 3.0 | 180 | 40 | | | | | 2 | | | | |
| *3.2 oz croissant* | | 6.0 | 17.0 | 10.0 | | | 30 | | | 2.70 | | | 400 | | | | | AUBN61 |
| **croissant,** cinnamon raisin | 110 | 330 | | 52.0 | 20.0 | | 2.0 | 220 | 40 | | | | | 4 | | | | |
| *3.9 oz croissant* | | 7.0 | 12.0 | 6.0 | | | 40 | | | 1.80 | | | 400 | | | | | AUBN62 |
| **croissant,** raspberry cheese | 103 | 330 | | 41.0 | 17.0 | | 1.0 | 250 | 40 | | | | | 4 | | | | |
| *3.6 oz croissant* | | 6.0 | 16.0 | 10.0 | | | 55 | | | 1.80 | | | 500 | | | | | AUBN195 |
| **croissant,** sweet cheese | 103 | 340 | | 37.0 | 13.0 | | 1.0 | 270 | 40 | | | | | 2 | | | | |
| *3.6 oz croissant* | | 7.0 | 19.0 | 11.0 | | | 65 | | | 1.44 | | | 500 | | | | | AUBN66 |
| **croissant** with ham and cheese | 120 | 350 | | 34.0 | 4.0 | | 1.0 | 550 | 100 | | | | | 4 | | | | |
| *4.2 oz croissant* | | 14.0 | 18.0 | 10.0 | | | 60 | | | 1.80 | | | 400 | | | | | AUBN63 |
| **croissant** with spinach and cheese | 102 | 250 | | 25.0 | 3.0 | | 2.0 | 280 | 100 | | | | | 4 | | | | |
| *3.6 oz croissant* | | 8.0 | 14.0 | 8.0 | | | 35 | | | 1.80 | | | 3250 | | | | | AUBN65 |
| **Danish pastry,** cherry | 107 | 370 | | 44.0 | 16.0 | | 1.0 | 300 | 60 | | | | | 6 | | | | |
| *3.8 oz pastry* | | 7.0 | 19.0 | 8.0 | | | 85 | | | 1.80 | | | 500 | | | | | AUBN196 |
| **Danish pastry,** lemon | 108 | 370 | | 44.0 | 15.0 | | 1.0 | 300 | 60 | | | | | 6 | | | | |
| *3.8 oz pastry* | | 7.0 | 19.0 | 8.0 | | | 85 | | | 1.80 | | | 500 | | | | | AUBN86 |
| **Danish pastry,** sweet cheese | 107 | 380 | | 44.0 | 15.0 | | 1.0 | 310 | 60 | | | | | 6 | | | | |
| *3.8 oz pastry* | | 7.0 | 20.0 | 9.0 | | | 90 | | | 1.80 | | | 500 | | | | | AUBN88 |
| **egg BLT breakfast sandwich** | 349 | 790 | | 61.0 | 2.0 | | 3.0 | 1050 | 60 | | | | | 18 | | | | |
| *12.3 oz sandwich* | | 41.0 | 41.0 | 18.0 | | | 260 | | | 2.70 | | | 3500 | | | | | AUBN197 |
| **eggplant and mozzarella sandwich** | 382 | 750 | | 75.0 | 7.0 | | 7.0 | 1370 | 400 | | | | | 24 | | | | |
| *13.5 oz sandwich* | | 27.0 | 37.0 | 13.0 | | | 60 | | | 10.80 | | | 500 | | | | | AUBN198 |
| **English toffee cookie** | 46 | 210 | | 26.0 | 15.0 | | 1.0 | 240 | 20 | | | | | 0 | | | | |
| *1.6 oz cookie* | | 2.0 | 11.0 | 4.0 | | | 20 | | | 0.36 | | | 400 | | | | | AUBN47 |
| **focaccia** | 127 | 310 | | 58.0 | 2.0 | | 2.0 | 640 | 80 | | | | | 0 | | | | |
| *4.5 oz piece* | | 10.0 | 3.5 | 1.0 | | | 0 | | | 3.60 | | | 0 | | | | | AUBN22 |
| **frittata,** arugula and tomato | 210 | 290 | | 27.0 | 3.0 | | 2.0 | 210 | 250 | | | | | 12 | | | | |
| *7.4 oz piece* | | 17.0 | 13.0 | 7.0 | | | 260 | | | 1.80 | | | 1750 | | | | | AUBN199 |
| **frittata,** ciabatta | 255 | 700 | | 86.0 | 6.0 | | 3.0 | 1400 | 250 | | | | | 12 | | | | |
| *9 oz piece* | | 26.0 | 29.0 | 14.0 | | | 170 | | | 12.60 | | | 750 | | | | | AUBN200 |
| **frittata,** ham and cheese | 168 | 320 | | 26.0 | 2.0 | | 1.0 | 860 | 200 | | | | | 1 | | | | |
| *5.9 oz piece* | | 23.0 | 14.0 | 7.0 | | | 290 | | | 3.60 | | | 500 | | | | | AUBN201 |
| **gingerbread man** | 77 | 280 | | 50.0 | 21.0 | | 1.0 | 230 | 40 | | | | | 0 | | | | |
| *2.7 oz cookie* | | 4.0 | 7.0 | 2.0 | | | 10 | | | 1.80 | | | 300 | | | | | AUBN48 |
| **ham and cheese sandwich** | 331 | 630 | | 74.0 | 22.0 | | 3.0 | 2370 | 350 | | | | | 12 | | | | |
| *11.7 oz sandwich* | | 42.0 | 16.0 | 9.0 | | | 85 | | | 9.00 | | | 1000 | | | | | AUBN202 |
| **hummus,** roasted red pepper | 57 | 100 | | 8.0 | 0 | | 2.0 | 210 | 0 | | | | | 0 | | | | |
| *2 oz* | | 4.0 | 6.0 | 0 | | | 0 | | | 0.72 | | | 0 | | | | | AUBN203 |
| **key lime crumb cake** | 107 | 400 | | 50.0 | 28.0 | | 1.0 | 270 | 20 | | | | | 1 | | | | |
| *3.8 oz square* | | 4.0 | 20.0 | 4.0 | | | 55 | | | 1.44 | | | 200 | | | | | AUBN204 |
| **key lime sugar cookie** | 61 | 250 | | 39.0 | 19.0 | | 1.0 | 190 | 0 | | | | | 0 | | | | |
| *2.2 oz cookie* | | 3.0 | 9.0 | 4.0 | | | 35 | | | 1.08 | | | 300 | | | | | AUBN205 |
| **lavash** (bread) | 113 | 320 | | 62.0 | 1.0 | | 2.0 | 190 | 250 | | | | | 0 | | | | |
| *4 oz piece* | | 15.0 | 1.0 | 0 | | | 0 | | | 1.44 | | | 0 | | | | | AUBN206 |
| **lemon pound cake** | 139 | 520 | | 64.0 | 40.0 | | 0 | 460 | 20 | | | | | 2 | | | | |
| *4.9 oz slice* | | 5.0 | 27.0 | 6.0 | | | 85 | | | 1.44 | | | 100 | | | | | AUBN207 |
| **macaroon,** cranberry almond, | 79 | 320 | | 42.0 | 33.0 | | 3.0 | 190 | 40 | | | | | 0 | | | | |
| *choc-dipped - 2.8 oz macaroon* | | 4.0 | 16.0 | 8.0 | | | 0 | | | 1.08 | | | 0 | | | | | AUBN208 |
| **Mandarin orange choc cookie** | 61 | 240 | | 38.0 | 20.0 | | 1.0 | 210 | 20 | | | | | 0 | | | | |
| *2.2 oz cookie* | | 3.0 | 9.0 | 4.0 | | | 30 | | | 1.80 | | | 300 | | | | | AUBN209 |
| **marble pound cake** | 130 | 480 | | 58.0 | 34.0 | | 1.0 | 490 | 20 | | | | | 0 | | | | |
| *4.6 oz slice* | | 5.0 | 26.0 | 5.0 | | | 90 | | | 1.80 | | | 100 | | | | | AUBN210 |
| **molasses cookie** | 61 | 240 | | 40.0 | 21.0 | | 1.0 | 220 | 0 | | | | | 0 | | | | |
| *2.2 oz cookie* | | 3.0 | 8.0 | 4.0 | | | 25 | | | 1.44 | | | 300 | | | | | AUBN211 |
| **mozzarella chicken sandwich** | 381 | 680 | | 58.0 | 4.0 | | 3.0 | 1370 | 250 | | | | | 15 | | | | |
| *13.4 oz sandwich* | | 41.0 | 30.0 | 10.0 | | | 120 | | | 8.10 | | | 1500 | | | | | AUBN212 |
| **mozzarella, tom, basil pesto, onion** | 300 | 638 | | 66.0 | 4.0 | | 3.0 | 1045 | 500 | | | | | 9 | | | | |
| *sandwich - 10.5 oz sandwich* | | 23.0 | 30.0 | 11.3 | | | 52 | | | 5.40 | | | 1750 | | | | | AUBN213 |
| **multigrain bread,** Artisan | 69 | 165 | | 31.0 | 0 | | 2.0 | 342 | 20 | | | | | 2 | | | | |
| *2.3 oz slice* | | 5.0 | 1.8 | 0 | | | 0 | | | 1.62 | | | 0 | | | | | AUBN23 |
| **oatmeal raisin cookie** | 57 | 230 | | 37.0 | 23.0 | | 2.0 | 190 | 20 | | | | | 0 | | | | |
| *2 oz cookie* | | 3.0 | 8.0 | 4.0 | | | 35 | | | 1.08 | | | 200 | | | | | AUBN50 |

| | WT (g) | KCAL | H₂O (g) | CHO (g) | TSUG (g) | ASUG (g) | DFIB (g) | Na (mg) | Ca (mg) | Mg (mg) | Zn (mg) | Mn (mg) | A (mcg RAE) | C (mg) | B-1 (mg) | NIA (mg) | B-12 (mcg) | PANT (mg) |
|---|---|---|---|---|---|---|---|---|---|---|---|---|---|---|---|---|---|---|
| | | PRO (g) | FAT (g) | SFA (g) | MUFA (g) | PUFA (g) | CHOL (mg) | K (mg) | P (mg) | Fe (mg) | Cu (mg) | Se (mcg) | A (IU) | E (mg ATE) | B-2 (mg) | B-6 (mg) | FOL (mcg DFE) | REF |
| **olive bread** | 57 | 130 | | 24.0 | 0 | | 1.0 | 320 | 0 | | | | | 0 | | | | |
| *2 oz slice* | | 4.0 | 1.5 | 0 | | | 0 | | | 1.44 | | | 0 | | | | | AUBN214 |
| **panini** with barbequed chicken | 424 | 930 | | 95.0 | 13.0 | | 5.0 | 1650 | 300 | | | | | 9 | | | | |
| *15 oz sandwich* | | 47.0 | 41.0 | 11.0 | | | 105 | | | 12.60 | | | 750 | | | | | AUBN215 |
| **panini** with Mediterranean vegs | 345 | 610 | | 80.0 | 8.0 | | 6.0 | 1450 | 150 | | | | | 48 | | | | |
| *12.2 oz sandwich* | | 22.0 | 24.0 | 8.0 | | | 25 | | | 12.60 | | | 4000 | | | | | AUBN216 |
| **panini** with steak | 416 | 960 | | 79.0 | 9.0 | | 6.0 | 2240 | 500 | | | | | 15 | | | | |
| *14.7 oz sandwich* | | 49.0 | 51.0 | 16.0 | | | 110 | | | 12.60 | | | 750 | | | | | AUBN217 |
| **pastry**, almond Artisan | 117 | 464 | | 41.0 | 12.0 | | 2.0 | 140 | 100 | | | | | 9 | | | | |
| *4.1 oz pastry* | | 10.0 | 30.0 | 14.0 | | | 125 | | | 0.72 | | | 1000 | | | | | AUBN218 |
| **pastry**, blueberry cheese Artisan | 130 | 410 | | 44.0 | 14.0 | | 1.0 | 150 | 60 | | | | | 9 | | | | |
| *4.6 oz pastry* | | 8.0 | 23.0 | 13.0 | | | 105 | | | 0.72 | | | 750 | | | | | AUBN219 |
| **pastry**, crème de fleur | 157 | 550 | | 71.0 | 32.0 | | 1.0 | 540 | 60 | | | | | 4 | | | | |
| *5.6 oz pastry* | | 12.0 | 26.0 | 15.0 | | | 110 | | | 0.72 | | | 750 | | | | | AUBN85 |
| **pastry**, Danish apple nun | 95 | 260 | | 35.0 | 21.0 | | 0 | 135 | 40 | | | | | 2 | | | | |
| *3.4 oz pastry* | | 3.0 | 13.0 | 3.5 | | | 30 | | | 1.08 | | | 0 | | | | | AUBN220 |
| **pastry**, Danish pretzel | 159 | 630 | | 95.0 | 65.0 | | 1.0 | 310 | 100 | | | | | 6 | | | | |
| *6 oz pastry* | | 10.0 | 26.0 | 11.0 | | | 55 | | | 2.70 | | | 500 | | | | | AUBN221 |
| **pastry**, hurricane | 184 | 790 | | 111.0 | 62.0 | | 2.0 | 230 | 60 | | | | | 0 | | | | |
| *6.5 oz pastry* | | 4.0 | 38.0 | 8.0 | | | 10 | | | 2.70 | | | 200 | | | | | AUBN222 |
| **pastry**, strawberry puff | 89 | 260 | | 31.0 | 20.0 | | 1.0 | 130 | 40 | | | | | 12 | | | | |
| *3.1 oz pastry* | | 3.0 | 15.0 | 7.0 | | | 45 | | | 0.72 | | | 400 | | | | | AUBN223 |
| **pizza**, apple, bacon, goat cheese | 401 | 830 | | 85.0 | 18.0 | | 3.0 | 1630 | 700 | | | | | 9 | | | | |
| *14 oz pizza* | | 41.0 | 50.0 | 21.0 | | | | | | 2.70 | | | 1000 | | | | | AUBN224 |
| **pizza**, chicken supreme | 391 | 690 | | 43.0 | 4.0 | | 2.0 | 1360 | 600 | | | | | 5 | | | | |
| *13.8 oz pizza* | | 40.0 | 41.0 | 22.0 | | | 165 | | | 3.60 | | | 750 | | | | | AUBN225 |
| **pizza**, mozzarella | 227 | 500 | | 39.0 | 4.0 | | 2.0 | 670 | 500 | | | | | 5 | | | | |
| *8 oz pizza* | | 21.0 | 30.0 | 13.0 | | | 65 | | | 2.70 | | | 1000 | | | | | AUBN226 |
| **pizzetta**, cordon bleu | 284 | 470 | | 53.0 | 2.0 | | 5.0 | 870 | 40 | | | | | 9 | | | | |
| *10 oz pizzetta* | | 38.0 | 11.0 | 2.5 | | | 90 | | | 1.80 | | | 500 | | | | | AUBN227 |
| **pizzetta**, Shanghai chicken | 212 | 420 | | 66.0 | 7.0 | | 6.0 | 1210 | 40 | | | | | 4 | | | | |
| *7.5 oz pizzetta* | | 16.0 | 6.0 | 1.5 | | | 25 | | | 5.40 | | | 500 | | | | | AUBN228 |
| **pizzetta**, spicy barbeque shrimp | 227 | 440 | | 68.0 | 10.0 | | 8.0 | 1300 | 150 | | | | | 2 | | | | |
| *8 oz pizzetta* | | 13.0 | 11.0 | 5.0 | | | 60 | | | 1.08 | | | 3000 | | | | | AUBN229 |
| **pizzetta**, spinach and portobello | 241 | 470 | | 61.0 | 3.0 | | 7.0 | 670 | 100 | | | | | 9 | | | | |
| *8.5 oz pizzetta* | | 13.0 | 20.0 | 7.0 | | | 15 | | | 2.70 | | | 1500 | | | | | AUBN230 |
| **pizzetta**, steak and chipotle pesto | 198 | 430 | | 58.0 | 1.0 | | 5.0 | 980 | 150 | | | | | 12 | | | | |
| *7 oz pizzetta* | | 16.0 | 14.0 | 7.0 | | | 40 | | | 6.30 | | | 1000 | | | | | AUBN231 |
| **pork** (barbecued pulled) sandwich | 295 | 610 | | 83.0 | 15.0 | | 6.0 | 1610 | 60 | | | | | 5 | | | | |
| *10.4 oz sandwich* | | 29.0 | 18.0 | 6.0 | | | 75 | | | 3.60 | | | 3000 | | | | | AUBN232 |
| **portabello and goat cheese sand** | 295 | 560 | | 63.0 | 4.0 | | 6.0 | 1000 | 100 | | | | | 15 | | | | |
| *10.4 oz sandwich* | | 20.0 | 27.0 | 8.0 | | | 35 | | | 2.70 | | | 1750 | | | | | AUBN233 |
| **prosciutto breakfast sandwich** | 273 | 660 | | 67.0 | 4.0 | | 3.0 | 1580 | 200 | | | | | 0 | | | | |
| *9.7 oz sandwich* | | 40.0 | 25.0 | 8.0 | | | 185 | | | 4.50 | | | 500 | | | | | AUBN234 |
| **prosciutto mozzarella sandwich** | 359 | 880 | | 71.0 | 5.0 | | 4.0 | 2270 | 400 | | | | | 9 | | | | |
| *12.7 oz sandwich* | | 40.0 | 49.0 | 17.0 | | | 110 | | | 12.60 | | | 750 | | | | | AUBN235 |
| **pumpkin muffin** | 163 | 470 | | 66.0 | 34.0 | | 3.0 | 500 | 60 | | | | | 2 | | | | |
| *5.8 oz muffin* | | 8.0 | 14.0 | 2.0 | | | 65 | | | 2.70 | | | 7500 | | | | | AUBN79 |
| **raisin bran muffin** | 163 | 410 | | 74.0 | 40.0 | | 9.0 | 590 | 100 | | | | | 0 | | | | |
| *5.8 oz muffin* | | 10.0 | 9.0 | 2.0 | | | 30 | | | 2.70 | | | 0 | | | | | AUBN80 |
| **raspberry cookie** | 63 | 280 | | 32.0 | 14.0 | | 1.0 | 125 | 0 | | | | | 0 | | | | |
| *2.2 oz cookie* | | 3.0 | 16.0 | 9.0 | | | 50 | | | 0 | | | 0 | | | | | AUBN236 |
| **roast beef and herb cheese on roll** | 354 | 600 | | 74.0 | 7.0 | | 4.0 | 1730 | 100 | | | | | 9 | | | | |
| *12.5 oz sandwich* | | 37.0 | 18.0 | 7.0 | | | 90 | | | 12.60 | | | 750 | | | | | AUBN237 |
| **salmon (smoked) wasabi sandwich** | 201 | 490 | | 77.0 | 6.0 | | 3.0 | 1250 | 40 | | | | | 1 | | | | |
| *7.1 oz sandwich* | | 18.0 | 11.0 | 4.0 | | | 45 | | | 3.60 | | | 400 | | | | | AUBN238 |
| **scone**, cinnamon | 113 | 430 | | 48.0 | 16.0 | | 1.0 | 360 | 40 | | | | | 0 | | | | |
| *4 oz scone* | | 9.0 | 24.0 | 14.0 | | | 130 | | | 1.80 | | | 500 | | | | | AUBN130 |
| **scone**, orange | 120 | 410 | | 51.0 | 16.0 | | 2.0 | 370 | 40 | | | | | 2 | | | | |
| *4.3 oz scone* | | 9.0 | 20.0 | 11.0 | | | 130 | | | 1.80 | | | 500 | | | | | AUBN239 |
| **shortbread cookie** | 64 | 310 | | 34.0 | 10.0 | | 1.0 | 270 | 0 | | | | | 0 | | | | |
| *2.3 oz cookie* | | 3.0 | 18.0 | 9.0 | | | 25 | | | 0.72 | | | 500 | | | | | AUBN53 |

| Food | WT (g) | KCAL / PRO (g) | H₂0 (g) / FAT (g) | CHO (g) / SFA (g) | TSUG (g) / MUFA (g) | ASUG (g) / PUFA (g) | DFIB (g) / CHOL (mg) | Na (mg) / K (mg) | Ca (mg) / P (mg) | Mg (mg) / Fe (mg) | Zn (mg) / Cu (mg) | Mn (mg) / Se (mcg) | A (mcg RAE) / A (IU) | C (mg) / E (mg ATE) | B-1 (mg) / B-2 (mg) | NIA (mg) / B-6 (mg) | B-12 (mcg) / FOL (mcg DFE) | PANT (mg) / REF |
|---|---|---|---|---|---|---|---|---|---|---|---|---|---|---|---|---|---|---|
| shortbread cookie, choc-dipped | 71 | 350 | | 38.0 | 14.0 | | 1.0 | 280 | 0 | | | | | 0 | | | | |
| *2.5 oz cookie* | | 3.0 | 20.0 | 9.0 | | | 25 | | | 0.72 | | | 500 | 0 | | | | AUBN54 |
| steak and gorgonzola on onion roll | 401 | 780 | | 76.0 | 6.0 | | 6.0 | 1790 | 300 | | | | | 12 | | | | |
| *14 oz sandwich* | | 40.0 | 39.0 | 10.0 | | | 90 | | | 4.50 | | | 1500 | | | | | AUBN240 |
| steak chimichurri sandwich | 383 | 920 | | 78.0 | 7.0 | | 5.0 | 2540 | 350 | | | | | 24 | | | | |
| *13.5 oz sandwich* | | 47.0 | 47.0 | 19.0 | | | 130 | | | 12.60 | | | 1500 | | | | | AUBN241 |
| steak, Swiss chs, onion, mshrms, | 298 | 690 | | 68.0 | 5.0 | | 4.0 | 1180 | 450 | | | | | 5 | | | | |
| *jalapeno sand - 10.5 oz sand* | | 43.0 | 28.0 | 12.0 | | | 75 | | | 2.70 | | | 300 | | | | | AUBN242 |
| strawberry, chocolate-coated | 23 | 30 | | 4.0 | 3.0 | | 0 | 5 | 0 | | | | | 12 | | | | |
| *1 strawberry* | | 0 | 1.5 | 0 | | | 0 | | | 0 | | | 0 | | | | | AUBN243 |
| strudel, apple | 134 | 410 | | 49.0 | 22.0 | | 1.0 | 340 | 0 | | | | | 2 | | | | |
| *4.8 oz piece* | | 5.0 | 23.0 | 7.0 | | | 0 | | | 1.44 | | | 750 | | | | | AUBN153 |
| strudel, cherry | 113 | 340 | | 34.0 | 10.0 | | 1.0 | 300 | 0 | | | | | 1 | | | | |
| *4 oz piece* | | 4.0 | 20.0 | 6.0 | | | 0 | | | 1.08 | | | 1250 | | | | | AUBN154 |
| sun-dried tomato bread | 57 | 130 | | 27.0 | 1.0 | | 2.0 | 370 | 20 | | | | | 2 | | | | |
| *2 oz slice* | | 5.0 | 0 | 0 | | | 0 | | | 0.72 | | | 0 | | | | | AUBN244 |
| sweet roll, cinnamon | 114 | 350 | | 53.0 | 21.0 | | 2.0 | 240 | 40 | | | | | 4 | | | | |
| *4 oz roll* | | 7.0 | 12.0 | 7.0 | | | 40 | | | 1.80 | | | 400 | | | | | AUBN83 |
| sweet roll, pecan | 133 | 520 | | 61.0 | 29.0 | | 2.0 | 270 | 80 | | | | | 4 | | | | |
| *4.7 oz roll* | | 7.0 | 28.0 | 9.0 | | | 30 | | | 2.70 | | | 500 | | | | | AUBN87 |
| tart, pear | 100 | 270 | | 38.0 | 20.0 | | 2.0 | 170 | 40 | | | | | 6 | | | | |
| *3.5 oz tart* | | 3.0 | 13.0 | 7.0 | | | 45 | | | 0.36 | | | 500 | | | | | AUBN245 |
| tiramisu | 100 | 310 | | 39.0 | 30.0 | | 2.0 | 130 | 150 | | | | | 0 | | | | |
| *3.5 oz piece* | | 7.0 | 15.0 | 8.0 | | | 70 | | | 0.36 | | | 100 | | | | | AUBN246 |
| triple berry muffin, lowfat | 123 | 290 | | 61.0 | 31.0 | | 2.0 | 310 | 60 | | | | | 4 | | | | |
| *4.4 oz muffin* | | 5.0 | 2.0 | 0.5 | | | 25 | | | 0.72 | | | 0 | | | | | AUBN81 |
| tuna, cheddar, roasted pepper | 291 | 553 | | 62.0 | 4.0 | | 3.0 | 1411 | 250 | | | | | 18 | | | | |
| *sandwich - 10.2 oz sandwich* | | 37.0 | 18.0 | 6.2 | | | 22 | | | 4.50 | | | 6500 | | | | | AUBN250 |
| tuna melt sandwich | 373 | 800 | | 60.0 | 4.0 | | 4.0 | 1420 | 60 | | | | | 18 | | | | |
| *13.2 oz sandwich* | | 44.0 | 45.0 | 13.0 | | | 105 | | | 7.20 | | | 3000 | | | | | AUBN248 |
| tuna salad sandwich | 298 | 550 | | 57.0 | 3.0 | | 5.0 | 910 | 60 | | | | | 9 | | | | |
| *10.5 oz sandwich* | | 29.0 | 27.0 | 3.0 | | | 55 | | | 1.80 | | | 3000 | | | | | AUBN249 |
| tuna, spicy, on multigrain bread | 332 | 690 | | 72.0 | 4.0 | | 8.0 | 1170 | 60 | | | | | 42 | | | | |
| *12 oz sandwich* | | 30.0 | 33.0 | 4.0 | | | 20 | | | 9.00 | | | 2500 | | | | | AUBN247 |
| turkey and chutney ciabatta | 319 | 710 | | 78.0 | 13.0 | | 3.0 | 1520 | 40 | | | | | 15 | | | | |
| *sandwich - 11.3 oz sandwich* | | 36.0 | 27.0 | 4.5 | | | 70 | | | 12.60 | | | 200 | | | | | AUBN252 |
| turkey and Swiss sandwich | 391 | 850 | | 72.0 | 3.0 | | 4.0 | 1640 | 400 | | | | | 12 | | | | |
| *13.8 oz sandwich* | | 50.0 | 41.0 | 14.0 | | | 105 | | | 12.60 | | | 1000 | | | | | AUBN253 |
| turkey, Baja, sandwich | 403 | 910 | | 69.0 | 3.0 | | 4.0 | 1810 | 250 | | | | | 9 | | | | |
| *14.2 oz sandwich* | | 48.0 | 47.0 | 13.0 | | | 120 | | | 12.60 | | | 1000 | | | | | AUBN251 |
| turkey club sand on French bread | 330 | 830 | | 57.0 | 2.0 | | 2.0 | 1810 | 300 | | | | | 6 | | | | |
| *11.6 oz sandwich* | | 47.0 | 46.0 | 15.0 | | | 125 | | | 9.00 | | | 1000 | | | | | AUBN255 |
| turkey club sandwich on focaccia | 393 | 830 | | 58.0 | 4.0 | | 3.0 | 2070 | 350 | | | | | 9 | | | | |
| *13.9 oz sandwich* | | 55.0 | 42.0 | 14.0 | | | 130 | | | 10.80 | | | 1250 | | | | | AUBN254 |
| turkey, guacamole, Swiss on | 397 | 760 | | 77.0 | 3.0 | | 6.0 | 1260 | 400 | | | | | 30 | | | | |
| *baguette - 14 oz sandwich* | | 51.0 | 28.0 | 12.0 | | | 85 | | | 4.50 | | | 500 | | | | | AUBN257 |
| turkey melt sandwich | 394 | 1030 | | 78.0 | 10.0 | | 3.0 | 2300 | 350 | | | | | 4 | | | | |
| *13.9 oz sandwich* | | 56.0 | 57.0 | 17.0 | | | 145 | | | 12.60 | | | 500 | | | | | AUBN256 |
| white bread, Artisan French | 57 | 130 | | 27.0 | 0 | | 1.0 | 340 | 0 | | | | | 1 | | | | |
| *2 oz slice* | | 4.0 | 0 | 0 | | | 0 | | | 0.72 | | | 0 | | | | | AUBN25 |
| wrap, chicken Caesar | 269 | 590 | | 67.0 | 4.0 | | 3.0 | 850 | 400 | | | | | 12 | | | | |
| *9.5 oz wrap* | | 31.0 | 22.0 | 5.0 | | | 60 | | | 2.70 | | | 1750 | | | | | AUBN258 |
| wrap, chicken salsa | 327 | 440 | | 68.0 | 3.0 | | 8.0 | 1440 | 40 | | | | | 12 | | | | |
| *11.5 oz wrap* | | 29.0 | 8.0 | 1.5 | | | 50 | | | 2.70 | | | 1250 | | | | | AUBN259 |
| wrap, chopped Cobb salad | 312 | 561 | | 65.0 | 2.0 | | 6.0 | 1280 | 100 | | | | | 18 | | | | |
| *11 oz wrap* | | 32.0 | 20.0 | 7.0 | | | 120 | | | 1.44 | | | 2000 | | | | | AUBN260 |
| wrap, fields and feta | 354 | 560 | | 79.0 | 6.0 | | 5.0 | 770 | 450 | | | | | 42 | | | | |
| *12.5 oz wrap* | | 23.0 | 17.0 | 4.0 | | | 10 | | | 5.40 | | | 4000 | | | | | AUBN261 |
| wrap, Mediterranean | 340 | 571 | | 80.0 | 4.0 | | 9.0 | 990 | 100 | | | | | 21 | | | | |
| *12 oz wrap* | | 19.0 | 22.0 | 2.5 | | | 5 | | | 3.60 | | | 1250 | | | | | AUBN263 |
| wrap, Mediterranean chicken | 373 | 570 | | 75.0 | 7.0 | | 4.0 | 980 | 350 | | | | | 21 | | | | |
| *13.2 oz wrap* | | 32.0 | 16.0 | 2.5 | | | 40 | | | 2.70 | | | 3500 | | | | | AUBN262 |

| | WT (g) | KCAL / PRO (g) | H₂0 (g) / FAT (g) | CHO (g) / SFA (g) | TSUG (g) / MUFA (g) | ASUG (g) / PUFA (g) | DFIB (g) / CHOL (mg) | Na (mg) / K (mg) | Ca (mg) / P (mg) | Mg (mg) / Fe (mg) | Zn (mg) / Cu (mg) | Mn (mg) / Se (mcg) | A (mcg RAE) / A (IU) | C (mg) / E (mg ATE) | B-1 (mg) / B-2 (mg) | NIA (mg) / B-6 (mg) | B-12 (mcg) / FOL (mcg DFE) | PANT (mg) / REF |
|---|---|---|---|---|---|---|---|---|---|---|---|---|---|---|---|---|---|---|
| **wrap**, Riviera chopped | 283 | 550 | | 83.0 | 17.0 | | 4.0 | 530 | 400 | | | | | 21 | | | | |
| *10 oz wrap* | | 20.0 | 16.0 | 4.5 | | | 15 | | | 2.70 | | | 3500 | | | | | AUBN264 |
| **wrap**, Riviera tuna | 319 | 630 | | 73.0 | 9.0 | | 4.0 | 650 | 350 | | | | | 21 | | | | |
| *11.3 oz wrap* | | 26.0 | 27.0 | 5.0 | | | 40 | | | 2.70 | | | 5000 | | | | | AUBN265 |
| **wrap**, Sonoma | 347 | 630 | | 80.0 | 12.0 | | 5.0 | 1070 | 350 | | | | | 30 | | | | |
| *12.2 oz wrap* | | 35.0 | 19.0 | 6.0 | | | 45 | | | 3.60 | | | 2000 | | | | | AUBN266 |
| **wrap**, southwest tuna | 418 | 794 | | 68.0 | 5.0 | | 7.0 | 1060 | 350 | | | | | 27 | | | | |
| *14.8 oz wrap* | | 44.0 | 25.0 | 7.0 | | | 30 | | | 1.80 | | | 7000 | | | | | AUBN267 |
| **wrap**, Thai chicken | 411 | 610 | | 86.0 | 10.0 | | 5.0 | 990 | 300 | | | | | 24 | | | | |
| *14.5 oz wrap* | | 33.0 | 6.0 | 1.5 | | | 45 | | | 3.60 | | | 5500 | | | | | AUBN268 |

## 10.5 BOB EVANS

| | WT (g) | KCAL / PRO (g) | H₂0 (g) / FAT (g) | CHO (g) / SFA (g) | TSUG (g) / MUFA (g) | ASUG (g) / PUFA (g) | DFIB (g) / CHOL (mg) | Na (mg) / K (mg) | Ca (mg) / P (mg) | Mg (mg) / Fe (mg) | Zn (mg) / Cu (mg) | Mn (mg) / Se (mcg) | A (mcg RAE) / A (IU) | C (mg) / E (mg ATE) | B-1 (mg) / B-2 (mg) | NIA (mg) / B-6 (mg) | B-12 (mcg) / FOL (mcg DFE) | PANT (mg) / REF |
|---|---|---|---|---|---|---|---|---|---|---|---|---|---|---|---|---|---|---|
| **apple dumpling pie a la mode** | 383 | 792 | | 108.0 | 50.0 | | 4.0 | 405 | | | | | | | | | | |
| *9 oz slice* | | 8.0 | 38.0 | 12.0 | | | 40 | | | | | | | | | | | BOBE38 |
| **bean soup** | 283 | 205 | | 27.0 | 1.0 | | 7.0 | 1111 | | | | | | | | | | |
| *10 fl oz bowl* | | 14.0 | 5.0 | 2.0 | | | 12 | | | | | | | | | | | BOBE42 |
| **blackberry cobbler** | 227 | 567 | | 80.0 | 42.0 | | 5.0 | 400 | | | | | | | | | | |
| *8 oz piece* | | 5.0 | 27.0 | 8.0 | | | 8 | | | | | | | | | | | BOBE39 |
| **BLT sandwich** | 252 | 641 | | 27.0 | 6.0 | | 2.0 | 1070 | | | | | | | | | | |
| *8.9 oz sandwich* | | 19.0 | 39.0 | 15.0 | | | 279 | | | | | | | | | | | BOBE24 |
| **burrito**, border scramble | 460 | 846 | | 78.0 | 8.0 | | 11.0 | 1949 | | | | | | | | | | |
| *16.2 oz* | | 40.0 | 43.0 | 17.0 | | | 87 | | | | | | | | | | | BOBE10 |
| **cheddar cheese potato soup** | 404 | 371 | | 24.0 | 4.0 | | 2.0 | 1474 | | | | | | | | | | |
| *14.3 fl oz bowl* | | 13.0 | 25.0 | 10.0 | | | 42 | | | | | | | | | | | BOBE43 |
| **cheese sandwich**, grilled | 135 | 392 | | 25.0 | 4.0 | | 2.0 | 782 | | | | | | | | | | |
| *4.8 oz sandwich* | | 9.0 | 17.0 | 7.0 | | | 30 | | | | | | | | | | | BOBE29 |
| **cheeseburger** | 220 | 641 | | 32.0 | 4.0 | | 3.0 | 1232 | | | | | | | | | | |
| *7.8 oz sandwich* | | 36.0 | 42.0 | 18.0 | | | 126 | | | | | | | | | | | BOBE21 |
| **cheeseburger** with bacon | 235 | 712 | | 32.0 | 4.0 | | 3.0 | 1340 | | | | | | | | | | |
| *8.3 oz sandwich* | | 38.0 | 49.0 | 21.0 | | | 136 | | | | | | | | | | | BOBE20 |
| **chicken, fried, club sandwich** | 264 | 699 | | 45.0 | 4.0 | | 3.0 | 1609 | | | | | | | | | | |
| *9.3 oz sandwich* | | 42.0 | 38.0 | 13.0 | | | 111 | | | | | | | | | | | BOBE28 |
| **chicken, grilled, club sandwich** | 243 | 606 | | 31.0 | 4.0 | | 2.0 | 1485 | | | | | | | | | | |
| *8.6 oz sandwich* | | 41.0 | 35.0 | 12.0 | | | 118 | | | | | | | | | | | BOBE30 |
| **chicken salad sandwich** | 206 | 649 | | 53.0 | 8.0 | | 6.0 | 1282 | | | | | | | | | | |
| *7.2 oz sandwich* | | 22.0 | 38.0 | 6.0 | | | 62 | | | | | | | | | | | BOBE25 |
| **chili with sausage** | 298 | 376 | | 26.0 | 2.0 | | 10.0 | 962 | | | | | | | | | | |
| *10.5 fl oz bowl* | | 22.0 | 24.0 | 9.0 | | | 59 | | | | | | | | | | | BOBE44 |
| **coconut cream pie** | 203 | 555 | | 67.0 | 41.0 | | 2.0 | 457 | | | | | | | | | | |
| *7.2 oz slice* | | 9.0 | 29.0 | 18.0 | | | 17 | | | | | | | | | | | BOBE40 |
| **fish sandwich** | 330 | 836 | | 75.0 | 1.0 | | 2.0 | 1702 | | | | | | | | | | |
| *11.6 oz sandwich* | | 39.0 | 37.0 | 11.0 | | | 90 | | | | | | | | | | | BOBE26 |
| **hamburger** | 192 | 539 | | 31.0 | 4.0 | | 3.0 | 756 | | | | | | | | | | |
| *6.8 oz sandwich* | | 31.0 | 32.0 | 11.0 | | | 96 | | | | | | | | | | | BOBE22 |
| **meatloaf sandwich** | 470 | 844 | | 58.0 | 5.0 | | 3.0 | 2491 | | | | | | | | | | |
| *16.6 oz sandwich* | | 36.0 | 48.0 | 19.0 | | | 140 | | | | | | | | | | | BOBE31 |
| **omelet**, bacon and cheese | 293 | 953 | | 6.0 | 2.0 | | 1.0 | 1603 | | | | | | | | | | |
| *10.3 oz* | | 49.0 | 80.0 | 28.0 | | | 826 | | | | | | | | | | | BOBE1 |
| **omelet**, Border Scramble | 438 | 893 | | 14.0 | 7.0 | | 2.0 | 1129 | | | | | | | | | | |
| *15.5 oz* | | 43.0 | 73.0 | 23.0 | | | 798 | | | | | | | | | | | BOBE2 |
| **omelet**, Farmer's Market | 435 | 911 | | 15.0 | 5.0 | | 2.0 | 1826 | | | | | | | | | | |
| *15.3 oz* | | 42.0 | 74.0 | 26.0 | | | 810 | | | | | | | | | | | BOBE3 |
| **omelet**, Garden Harvest | 450 | 795 | | 17.0 | 6.0 | | 3.0 | 1324 | | | | | | | | | | |
| *15.9 oz* | | 33.0 | 64.0 | 22.0 | | | 782 | | | | | | | | | | | BOBE4 |
| **omelet**, ham and cheese | 326 | 761 | | 3.0 | 0 | | 1.0 | 1419 | | | | | | | | | | |
| *11.5 oz* | | 44.0 | 62.0 | 19.0 | | | 798 | | | | | | | | | | | BOBE5 |
| **omelet**, sausage and cheese | 323 | 935 | | 3.0 | 0 | | 1.0 | 1171 | | | | | | | | | | |
| *11.4 oz* | | 46.0 | 80.0 | 26.0 | | | 807 | | | | | | | | | | | BOBE6 |
| **omelet**, three cheese | 268 | 770 | | 4.0 | 0 | | 1.0 | 1028 | | | | | | | | | | |
| *9.4 oz* | | 35.0 | 67.0 | 24.0 | | | 796 | | | | | | | | | | | BOBE7 |
| **omelet**, turkey Florentine | 407 | 834 | | 6.0 | 3.0 | | 1.0 | 1686 | | | | | | | | | | |
| *14.4 oz* | | 47.0 | 66.0 | 22.0 | | | 827 | | | | | | | | | | | BOBE8 |

| | WT (g) | KCAL | H₂0 (g) | CHO (g) | TSUG (g) | ASUG (g) | DFIB (g) | Na (mg) | Ca (mg) | Mg (mg) | Zn (mg) | Mn (mg) | A (mcg RAE) | C (mg) | B-1 (mg) | NIA (mg) | B-12 (mcg) | PANT (mg) |
|---|---|---|---|---|---|---|---|---|---|---|---|---|---|---|---|---|---|---|
| | | PRO (g) | FAT (g) | SFA (g) | MUFA (g) | PUFA (g) | CHOL (mg) | K (mg) | P (mg) | Fe (mg) | Cu (mg) | Se (mcg) | A (IU) | E (mg ATE) | B-2 (mg) | B-6 (mg) | FOL (mcg DFE) | REF |
| **omelet**, western | 394 | 782 | | 8.0 | 3.0 | | 2.0 | 1420 | | | | | | | | | | |
| *13.9 oz* | | 44.0 | 63.0 | 19.0 | | | 798 | | | | | | | | | | | BOBE9 |
| **pasta** w/chicken parmesan | 701 | 845 | | 87.0 | 11.0 | | 6.0 | 2973 | | | | | | | | | | |
| *24.7 oz* | | 48.0 | 34.0 | 10.0 | | | 103 | | | | | | | | | | | BOBE17 |
| **pasta** w/green peppers, onion | 627 | 548 | | 82.0 | 15.0 | | 7.0 | 2350 | | | | | | | | | | |
| *22.1 oz* | | 15.0 | 19.0 | 4.0 | | | 2 | | | | | | | | | | | BOBE19 |
| **pasta** w/Italian sausage and | 627 | 812 | | 75.0 | 12.0 | | 6.0 | 2854 | | | | | | | | | | |
| *peppers - 22.1 oz* | | 33.0 | 41.0 | 12.0 | | | 40 | | | | | | | | | | | BOBE18 |
| **pork loin sandwich** | 457 | 719 | | 41.0 | 9.0 | | 3.0 | 3403 | | | | | | | | | | |
| *16.1 oz sandwich* | | 28.0 | 38.0 | 17.0 | | | 144 | | | | | | | | | | | BOBE32 |
| **pot roast sandwich** | 245 | 605 | | 58.0 | 7.0 | | 3.0 | 1361 | | | | | | | | | | |
| *8.6 oz sandwich* | | 31.0 | 28.0 | 11.0 | | | 81 | | | | | | | | | | | BOBE34 |
| **pumpkin pie** | 217 | 575 | | 71.0 | 51.0 | | 1.0 | 313 | | | | | | | | | | |
| *7.7 oz slice* | | 7.0 | 30.0 | 14.0 | | | 53 | | | | | | | | | | | BOBE41 |
| **salad**, chili and cheese taco | 822 | 1019 | | 140.0 | 23.0 | | 17.0 | 2379 | | | | | | | | | | |
| *29 oz salad* | | 32.0 | 51.0 | 14.0 | | | 71 | | | | | | | | | | | BOBE11 |
| **salad**, Cobb w/grilled chicken | 560 | 469 | | 10.0 | 4.0 | | 3.0 | 1180 | | | | | | | | | | |
| *19.7 oz salad* | | 41.0 | 30.0 | 12.0 | | | 293 | | | | | | | | | | | BOBE12 |
| **salad**, country spinach | 335 | 509 | | 12.0 | 4.0 | | 4.0 | 1183 | | | | | | | | | | |
| *11.8 oz salad* | | 41.0 | 35.0 | 9.0 | | | 274 | | | | | | | | | | | BOBE13 |
| **salad**, cranberry pecan chicken | 588 | 783 | | 49.0 | 33.0 | | 5.0 | 1816 | | | | | | | | | | |
| *20.7 oz salad* | | 28.0 | 46.0 | 15.0 | | | 79 | | | | | | | | | | | BOBE14 |
| **salad**, wildfire fried chicken | 548 | 617 | | 65.0 | 19.0 | | 8.0 | 1131 | | | | | | | | | | |
| *19.3 oz salad* | | 27.0 | 29.0 | 8.0 | | | 62 | | | | | | | | | | | BOBE15 |
| **salad**, wildfire grilled chicken | 563 | 541 | | 49.0 | 19.0 | | 7.0 | 1041 | | | | | | | | | | |
| *19.9 oz salad* | | 31.0 | 26.0 | 8.0 | | | 82 | | | | | | | | | | | BOBE16 |
| **sausage breakfast burger** | 209 | 600 | | 32.0 | 4.0 | | 1.0 | 1120 | | | | | | | | | | |
| *7.4 oz sandwich* | | 28.0 | 39.0 | 15.0 | | | 307 | | | | | | | | | | | BOBE35 |
| **sausage sandwich** | 172 | 493 | | 31.0 | 3.0 | | 1.0 | 1248 | | | | | | | | | | |
| *6.1 oz sandwich* | | 21.0 | 30.0 | 11.0 | | | 53 | | | | | | | | | | | BOBE36 |
| **sausage sandwich** | 248 | 715 | | 31.0 | 3.0 | | 1.0 | 1746 | | | | | | | | | | |
| *8.8 oz sandwich* | | 34.0 | 46.0 | 18.0 | | | 92 | | | | | | | | | | | BOBE27 |
| **steak burger** | 358 | 1139 | | 35.0 | 8.0 | | 3.0 | 2308 | | | | | | | | | | |
| *12.6 oz sandwich* | | 47.0 | 89.0 | 35.0 | | | 193 | | | | | | | | | | | BOBE23 |
| **turkey bacon melt sandwich** | 254 | 613 | | 53.0 | 3.0 | | 3.0 | 1824 | | | | | | | | | | |
| *9 oz sandwich* | | 33.0 | 29.0 | 12.0 | | | 88 | | | | | | | | | | | BOBE37 |
| **turkey sandwich** | 411 | 696 | | 46.0 | 7.0 | | 2.0 | 2439 | | | | | | | | | | |
| *14.5 oz sandwich* | | 24.0 | 36.0 | 12.0 | | | 80 | | | | | | | | | | | BOBE33 |
| **vegetable beef soup** | 283 | 180 | | 18.0 | 7.0 | | 3.0 | 627 | | | | | | | | | | |
| *10 fl oz bowl* | | 10.0 | 8.0 | 3.0 | | | 24 | | | | | | | | | | | BOBE45 |

## 10.6 BOSTON MARKET

| | WT (g) | KCAL | H₂0 (g) | CHO (g) | TSUG (g) | ASUG (g) | DFIB (g) | Na (mg) | Ca (mg) | Mg (mg) | Zn (mg) | Mn (mg) | A (mcg RAE) | C (mg) | B-1 (mg) | NIA (mg) | B-12 (mcg) | PANT (mg) |
|---|---|---|---|---|---|---|---|---|---|---|---|---|---|---|---|---|---|---|
| | | PRO (g) | FAT (g) | SFA (g) | MUFA (g) | PUFA (g) | CHOL (mg) | K (mg) | P (mg) | Fe (mg) | Cu (mg) | Se (mcg) | A (IU) | E (mg ATE) | B-2 (mg) | B-6 (mg) | FOL (mcg DFE) | REF |
| **apple pie** | 170 | 420 | | 56.0 | 24.0 | | 2.0 | 650 | | | | | | | | | | |
| *6 oz slice* | | 3.0 | 20.0 | 4.0 | | | 0 | | | | | | | | | | | BOST32 |
| **apples with cinnamon** | 145 | 210 | | 47.0 | 42.0 | | 3.0 | 15 | | | | | | | | | | |
| *5.1 oz* | | 0 | 3.0 | 0 | | | 0 | | | | | | | | | | | BOST10 |
| **beef sirloin**, roasted | 142 | 300 | | 2.0 | 0 | | 1.0 | 440 | | | | | | | | | | |
| *5 oz* | | 38.0 | 15.0 | 6.0 | | | 125 | | | | | | | | | | | BOST5 |
| **beef sirloin sandwich** | 374 | 920 | | 70.0 | 4.0 | | 3.0 | 1260 | | | | | | | | | | |
| *13 oz sandwich* | | 64.0 | 43.0 | 12.0 | | | 200 | | | | | | | | | | | BOST23 |
| **chicken**, dark meat | 134 | 280 | | 3.0 | 2.0 | | 0 | 660 | | | | | | | | | | |
| *4.7 oz* | | 31.0 | 15.0 | 4.5 | | | 155 | | | | | | | | | | | BOST2 |
| **chicken noodle soup** | 283 | 180 | | 16.0 | 2.0 | | 1.0 | 220 | | | | | | | | | | |
| *6 fl oz* | | 13.0 | 7.0 | 2.0 | | | 55 | | | | | | | | | | | BOST18 |
| **chicken sandwich** | 321 | 700 | | 68.0 | 4.0 | | 3.0 | 1560 | | | | | | | | | | |
| *11.3 oz sandwich* | | 44.0 | 29.0 | 7.0 | | | 90 | | | | | | | | | | | BOST20 |
| **chicken tortilla soup** w/toppings | 227 | 340 | | 24.0 | 2.0 | | 1.0 | 1310 | | | | | | | | | | |
| *6 fl oz* | | 12.0 | 22.0 | 7.0 | | | 45 | | | | | | | | | | | BOST17 |
| **chicken**, white meat | 110 | 330 | | 3.0 | 2.0 | | 0 | 960 | | | | | | | | | | |
| *3.9 oz* | | 50.0 | 12.0 | 4.0 | | | 165 | | | | | | | | | | | BOST1 |
| **chocolate cake** | 145 | 600 | | 75.0 | 55.0 | | 2.0 | 210 | | | | | | | | | | |
| *5.1 oz piece* | | 5.0 | 32.0 | 7.0 | | | 65 | | | | | | | | | | | BOST33 |

Each food item is listed on two lines. The first line gives the top-row nutrients (KCAL, $H_2O$, CHO, TSUG, ASUG, DFIB, Na, Ca, Mg, Zn, Mn, A[mcg RAE], C, B-1, NIA, B-12, PANT); the second line (serving description) gives the bottom-row nutrients (PRO, FAT, SFA, MUFA, PUFA, CHOL, K, P, Fe, Cu, Se, A[IU], E, B-2, B-6, FOL, REF).

| Food | WT (g) | KCAL / PRO (g) | $H_2O$ / FAT (g) | CHO / SFA (g) | TSUG / MUFA (g) | ASUG / PUFA (g) | DFIB / CHOL | Na / K (mg) | Ca / P (mg) | Mg / Fe (mg) | Zn / Cu (mg) | Mn / Se | A(RAE) / A(IU) | C / E | B-1 / B-2 | NIA / B-6 | B-12 / FOL | PANT / REF |
|---|---|---|---|---|---|---|---|---|---|---|---|---|---|---|---|---|---|---|
| chocolate chip cookie | 78 | 370 | | 49.0 | 28.0 | | 2.0 | 340 | | | | | | | | | | |
| 2.8 oz cookie | | 4.0 | 19.0 | 9.0 | | | 20 | | | | | | | | | | | BOST30 |
| chocolate chip fudge brownie | 147 | 580 | | 81.0 | 61.0 | | 3.0 | 390 | | | | | | | | | | |
| 5.2 oz brownie | | 9.0 | 23.0 | 5.0 | | | 90 | | | | | | | | | | | BOST31 |
| coleslaw | 108 | 190 | | 9.0 | 5.0 | | 2.0 | 135 | | | | | | | | | | |
| 3.8 oz | | 2.0 | 16.0 | 2.5 | | | 15 | | | | | | | | | | | BOST15 |
| corn with butter blend | 176 | 170 | | 37.0 | 10.0 | | 2.0 | 95 | | | | | | | | | | |
| 6.2 oz | | 6.0 | 4.0 | 1.0 | | | 0 | | | | | | | | | | | BOST7 |
| cornbread | 45 | 130 | | 21.0 | 8.0 | | 0 | 220 | | | | | | | | | | |
| 1.6 oz piece | | 1.0 | 3.5 | 1.0 | | | 5 | | | | | | | | | | | BOST27 |
| cranberry walnut relish | 85 | 140 | | 30.0 | 27.0 | | 2.0 | 0 | | | | | | | | | | |
| 3 oz | | 1.0 | 2.0 | 0 | | | 0 | | | | | | | | | | | BOST14 |
| green beans with butter blend | 91 | 60 | | 7.0 | 1.0 | | 3.0 | 180 | | | | | | | | | | |
| 3.2 oz | | 2.0 | 3.5 | 1.5 | | | 0 | | | | | | | | | | | BOST9 |
| macaroni and cheese | 221 | 330 | | 39.0 | 9.0 | | 1.0 | 1290 | | | | | | | | | | |
| 7.8 oz | | 14.0 | 12.0 | 7.0 | | | 30 | | | | | | | | | | | BOST11 |
| meatloaf, beef, baked | 218 | 480 | | 23.0 | 6.0 | | 2.0 | 970 | | | | | | | | | | |
| 7.7 oz | | 29.0 | 33.0 | 13.0 | | | 125 | | | | | | | | | | | BOST4 |
| meatloaf sandwich | 434 | 940 | | 96.0 | 11.0 | | 6.0 | 2080 | | | | | | | | | | |
| 15.3 oz sandwich | | 49.0 | 45.0 | 18.0 | | | 155 | | | | | | | | | | | BOST22 |
| pecan pie | 106 | 470 | | 59.0 | 33.0 | | 2.0 | 190 | | | | | | | | | | |
| 3.7 oz slice | | 5.0 | 24.0 | 6.0 | | | 70 | | | | | | | | | | | BOST28 |
| potatoes au gratin | 140 | 180 | | 16.0 | 3.0 | | 1.0 | 310 | | | | | | | | | | |
| 4.9 oz | | 6.0 | 11.0 | 5.0 | | | 25 | | | | | | | | | | | BOST6 |
| potatoes, mashed | 221 | 210 | | 29.0 | 2.0 | | 3.0 | 660 | | | | | | | | | | |
| 7.8 oz | | 4.0 | 9.0 | 6.0 | | | 25 | | | | | | | | | | | BOST12 |
| pumpkin pie | 104 | 240 | | 36.0 | 22.0 | | 1.0 | 200 | | | | | | | | | | |
| 3.7 oz slice | | 4.0 | 15.0 | 4.0 | | | 30 | | | | | | | | | | | BOST29 |
| salad, Caesar | 206 | 500 | | 12.0 | 8.0 | | 3.0 | 1190 | | | | | | | | | | |
| 7.3 oz salad | | 13.0 | 45.0 | 11.0 | | | 45 | | | | | | | | | | | BOST24 |
| salad, Caesar side | 71 | 40 | | 3.0 | 2.0 | | 1.0 | 75 | | | | | | | | | | |
| 2.5 oz salad | | 3.0 | 2.0 | 1.5 | | | 0 | | | | | | | | | | | BOST16 |
| salad, chopped with dressing | 563 | 580 | | 31.0 | 16.0 | | 9.0 | 2010 | | | | | | | | | | |
| 19.9 oz salad | | 11.0 | 48.0 | 9.0 | | | 10 | | | | | | | | | | | BOST26 |
| salad dressing, Caesar | 71 | 360 | | 4.0 | 2.0 | | 1.0 | 910 | | | | | | | | | | |
| 2.5 oz | | 2.0 | 38.0 | 6.0 | | | 30 | | | | | | | | | | | BOST25 |
| spinach, creamed | 191 | 280 | | 12.0 | 1.0 | | 4.0 | 580 | | | | | | | | | | |
| 6.7 oz | | 9.0 | 23.0 | 15.0 | | | 70 | | | | | | | | | | | BOST8 |
| spinach with garlic butter sauce | 170 | 130 | | 9.0 | 1.0 | | 5.0 | 200 | | | | | | | | | | |
| 6 oz | | 5.0 | 9.0 | 6.0 | | | 20 | | | | | | | | | | | BOST19 |
| sweet potato casserole | 198 | 460 | | 77.0 | 39.0 | | 3.0 | 210 | | | | | | | | | | |
| 7 oz | | 4.0 | 17.0 | 6.0 | | | 20 | | | | | | | | | | | BOST13 |
| turkey, roasted | 142 | 180 | | 0 | 0 | | 0 | 620 | | | | | | | | | | |
| 5 oz | | 38.0 | 3.0 | 1.0 | | | 70 | | | | | | | | | | | BOST3 |
| turkey sandwich | 397 | 530 | | 55.0 | 3.0 | | 2.0 | 1050 | | | | | | | | | | |
| 14 oz sandwich | | 41.0 | 17.0 | 6.0 | | | 80 | | | | | | | | | | | BOST21 |

## 10.7 BURGER KING

| Food | WT (g) | KCAL / PRO (g) | $H_2O$ / FAT (g) | CHO / SFA (g) | TSUG / MUFA (g) | ASUG / PUFA (g) | DFIB / CHOL | Na / K (mg) | Ca / P (mg) | Mg / Fe (mg) | Zn / Cu (mg) | Mn / Se | A(RAE) / A(IU) | C / E | B-1 / B-2 | NIA / B-6 | B-12 / FOL | PANT / REF |
|---|---|---|---|---|---|---|---|---|---|---|---|---|---|---|---|---|---|---|
| cheeseburger | 133 | 380 | 59.3 | 31.5 | 6.0 | | 3.7 | 801 | 124 | 32 | 3.19 | 0.386 | 0 | | 0.40 | 4.5 | | 0.31 |
| 4.7 oz sandwich | | 19.4 | 19.7 | 9.1 | 7.6 | 2.0 | 60 | 237 | 190 | 3.32 | 0.146 | 32.5 | | 0.1 | 0.32 | 0.12 | | 21251 |
| cheeseburger, Double Whopper | 426 | 1133 | 227.0 | 57.6 | 15.4 | | 6.8 | 1649 | 332 | 81 | 14.91 | 0.596 | 1 | | 1.14 | 12.8 | | 0.85 |
| 15 oz sandwich | | 61.6 | 72.7 | 29.8 | 26.8 | 12.7 | 200 | 805 | 545 | 22.58 | 0.332 | 72.4 | | 0.3 | 0.89 | 0.48 | 178.9 | 21255 |
| cheeseburger, Whopper | 395 | 988 | 216.9 | 66.0 | 16.2 | | 4.0 | 1789 | 324 | 71 | 6.32 | 0.711 | 1 | | 0.84 | 10.1 | | 0.71 |
| 13.9 oz sandwich | | 44.2 | 60.6 | 22.8 | 20.0 | 14.9 | 142 | 668 | 446 | 7.90 | 0.209 | 72.7 | | 0.3 | 0.79 | 0.29 | 284.4 | 21253 |
| chicken sandwich | 204 | 583 | 92.9 | 49.7 | 5.5 | | 4.9 | 1204 | 82 | 49 | 2.86 | 0.796 | 0 | | 0.57 | 9.6 | | 0.88 |
| 7.2 oz sandwich | | 25.6 | 31.4 | 6.9 | 11.1 | 11.4 | 63 | 377 | 271 | 4.28 | 0.029 | 47.7 | | | 0.33 | 0.31 | 97.9 | 21259 |
| chicken tenders | 77 | 223 | 35.5 | 13.4 | 0.1 | | 1.8 | 555 | 12 | 19 | 0.45 | 0.156 | 1 | | 0.10 | 5.8 | | 0.46 |
| 2.7 oz (5 pieces) | | 13.3 | 12.8 | 3.3 | 7.3 | 1.6 | 40 | 203 | 175 | 0.47 | 0.039 | 23.8 | | 0.6 | 0.08 | 0.27 | 6.9 | 21256 |
| chicken tenders | 123 | 355 | 56.7 | 21.4 | 0.1 | | 2.8 | 887 | 18 | 31 | 0.71 | 0.248 | 1 | | 0.16 | 9.2 | | 0.74 |
| 4.3 oz (8 pieces) | | 21.2 | 20.5 | 5.2 | 11.7 | 2.6 | 64 | 323 | 279 | 0.75 | 0.062 | 38.0 | | 1.0 | 0.13 | 0.43 | 11.1 | 21256 |
| Chicken Whopper sandwich | 272 | 588 | 155.9 | 50.8 | 9.2 | | 4.1 | 1178 | 90 | 57 | 3.26 | 0.517 | 1 | | 0.84 | 12.2 | | 1.03 |
| 9.6 oz sandwich | | 32.0 | 28.6 | 6.0 | 8.4 | 12.9 | 84 | 498 | 405 | 14.96 | 0.038 | 75.1 | | | 0.41 | 0.43 | 165.9 | 21257 |

| | WT (g) | Macronutrients | | | | | | Minerals | | | | | Vitamins | | | | | |
|---|---|---|---|---|---|---|---|---|---|---|---|---|---|---|---|---|---|---|
| | | KCAL | H₂0 (g) | CHO (g) | TSUG (g) | ASUG (g) | DFIB (g) | Na (mg) | Ca (mg) | Mg (mg) | Zn (mg) | Mn (mg) | A (mcg RAE) | C (mg) | B-1 (mg) | NIA (mg) | B-12 (mcg) | PANT (mg) |
| | | PRO (g) | FAT (g) | SFA (g) | MUFA (g) | PUFA (g) | CHOL (mg) | K (mg) | P (mg) | Fe (mg) | Cu (mg) | Se (mcg) | A (IU) | E (mg ATE) | B-2 (mg) | B-6 (mg) | FOL (mcg DFE) | REF |
| **croissant** with egg and cheese | 112 | 317 | 52.0 | 27.8 | 4.5 | | 0.8 | 728 | 259 | 19 | 1.16 | 0.254 | 0 | | 0.27 | 2.3 | 0.59 | 0.93 |
| *4 oz Croissan'wich* | | 11.6 | 17.7 | 5.3 | 7.5 | 3.3 | 156 | 188 | 279 | 2.13 | 0.083 | 24.9 | | 1.2 | 0.48 | 0.13 | | 21385 |
| **croissant** with sausage and cheese | 107 | 402 | 37.5 | 24.6 | 3.6 | | 0.7 | 837 | 114 | 20 | 1.53 | 0.275 | 0 | | 0.35 | 4.4 | 0.59 | 0.70 |
| *3.8 oz Croissan'wich* | | 14.7 | 27.2 | 9.2 | 12.9 | 3.3 | 46 | 219 | 169 | 2.00 | 0.077 | 22.4 | | 1.0 | 0.34 | 0.19 | | 21384 |
| **croissant** with sausage, egg, cheese | 157 | 506 | 70.5 | 27.7 | 4.5 | | 1.1 | 1079 | 264 | 28 | 2.06 | 0.308 | 0 | | 0.38 | 4.7 | 1.10 | 1.27 |
| *5.5 oz Croissan'wich* | | 19.3 | 35.3 | 11.7 | 15.6 | 6.1 | 188 | 309 | 344 | 2.67 | 0.113 | 37.5 | | 1.6 | 0.51 | 0.29 | | 21383 |
| **French fries** | 74 | 245 | 27.1 | 29.7 | 0.5 | | 2.1 | 337 | 7 | 22 | 0.81 | 0.179 | 1 | | 0.13 | 1.7 | | 0.29 |
| *2.6 oz serving (small)* | | 2.6 | 12.9 | 3.2 | 8.2 | 0.8 | | 350 | 106 | 0.95 | 0.107 | 0.9 | | 0.6 | 0.02 | 0.13 | | 21249 |
| **French fries** | 117 | 387 | 42.9 | 46.9 | 0.8 | | 3.4 | 532 | 11 | 35 | 1.29 | 0.283 | 1 | | 0.20 | 2.7 | | 0.46 |
| *4.1 oz serving (medium)* | | 4.1 | 20.4 | 5.1 | 12.9 | 1.3 | | 553 | 167 | 1.51 | 0.170 | 1.4 | | 0.9 | 0.04 | 0.20 | | 21249 |
| **French fries** | 160 | 530 | 58.7 | 64.1 | 1.1 | | 4.6 | 728 | 14 | 48 | 1.76 | 0.387 | 1 | | 0.28 | 3.7 | | 0.62 |
| *5.6 oz serving (large)* | | 5.6 | 27.8 | 7.0 | 17.7 | 1.8 | | 757 | 229 | 2.06 | 0.232 | 1.9 | | 1.2 | 0.05 | 0.28 | | 21249 |
| **French fries** | 194 | 642 | 71.1 | 77.8 | 1.3 | | 5.6 | 883 | 17 | 58 | 2.13 | 0.469 | 1 | | 0.34 | 4.5 | | 0.76 |
| *6.8 oz serving (king)* | | 6.8 | 33.8 | 8.5 | 21.5 | 2.2 | | 918 | 277 | 2.50 | 0.281 | 2.3 | | 1.5 | 0.06 | 0.34 | | 21249 |
| **French toast sticks** | 113 | 394 | 37.9 | 46.6 | 11.2 | | 1.6 | 484 | 60 | 21 | 0.58 | 0.441 | 0 | | 0.32 | 2.9 | 0 | 0.38 |
| *4 oz (5 sticks)* | | 6.8 | 20.0 | 4.5 | 10.7 | 2.9 | 0 | 125 | 98 | 2.17 | 0.096 | 13.8 | | 1.0 | 0.20 | 0.06 | | 21386 |
| **hamburger** | 121 | 333 | 54.1 | 32.8 | 5.9 | | 2.4 | 551 | 62 | 29 | 2.60 | 0.336 | 0 | | 0.40 | 4.8 | | 0.27 |
| *4.3 oz sandwich* | | 17.2 | 14.7 | 6.1 | 6.4 | 1.5 | 42 | 220 | 144 | 3.05 | 0.113 | 30.1 | 0 | | 0.27 | 0.12 | 107.7 | 21250 |
| **hamburger**, Double Whopper | 401 | 1011 | 221.7 | 55.1 | 14.1 | | 5.6 | 1159 | 140 | 72 | 12.03 | 0.802 | 1 | | 0.77 | 13.0 | | 0.76 |
| *14 oz sandwich* | | 55.9 | 62.8 | 23.1 | 24.5 | 12.1 | 184 | 770 | 445 | 11.23 | 0.481 | 80.6 | | | 0.76 | 0.46 | 240.6 | 21254 |
| **hamburger**, Whopper | 304 | 708 | 171.5 | 56.4 | 12.8 | | 5.5 | 952 | 119 | 55 | 8.60 | 0.547 | 1 | | 0.65 | 8.7 | | 0.53 |
| *10.7 oz sandwich* | | 32.6 | 39.0 | 12.9 | 14.2 | 10.3 | 91 | 514 | 274 | 13.28 | 0.040 | 55.3 | | 0.5 | 0.53 | 0.28 | 212.8 | 21252 |
| **Hash Brown Rounds** | 75 | 277 | 27.1 | 25.9 | 0.2 | | 2.2 | 383 | 12 | 14 | 0.24 | 0.110 | 0 | 1 | 0.12 | 1.4 | 0 | 0.22 |
| *2.6 oz* | | 2.2 | 18.3 | 4.4 | 10.3 | 2.4 | 0 | 274 | 82 | 0.52 | 0.074 | 0.3 | 0 | 0.8 | 0.07 | 0.17 | | 21387 |
| **Hash Brown Rounds** | 128 | 472 | 46.2 | 44.2 | 0.3 | | 3.7 | 654 | 20 | 24 | 0.41 | 0.188 | 0 | 2 | 0.20 | 2.3 | 0 | 0.38 |
| *4.5 oz* | | 3.7 | 31.2 | 7.6 | 17.6 | 4.1 | 0 | 467 | 141 | 0.88 | 0.125 | 0.5 | 0 | 1.4 | 0.11 | 0.29 | | 21387 |
| **shake**, vanilla | 397 | 667 | 270.5 | 75.5 | 46.3 | | 0 | 397 | 413 | 48 | 2.66 | 0.242 | 0 | | | 0.4 | 1.43 | 2.46 |
| *14 fl oz (medium)* | | 12.7 | 34.7 | 21.2 | 9.8 | 1.7 | 123 | 607 | 385 | 1.67 | 0.754 | 12.7 | | 1.3 | 0.71 | 0.12 | | 21141 |

## 10.8 CHICKEN OUT ROTISSERIE

| | WT (g) | KCAL / PRO | H₂0 / FAT | CHO / SFA | TSUG / MUFA | ASUG / PUFA | DFIB / CHOL | Na / K | Ca / P | Mg / Fe | Zn / Cu | Mn / Se | | | | | | REF |
|---|---|---|---|---|---|---|---|---|---|---|---|---|---|---|---|---|---|---|
| **applesauce**, chunky cinnamon | 227 | 241 | | 52.0 | 13.0 | | 5.0 | 36 | | | | | | | | | | |
| *8 oz* | | 1.0 | 4.0 | 2.0 | | | 9 | | | | | | | | | | | CKOT76 |
| **apricot chicken salad** | 221 | 610 | | 23.0 | 17.0 | | 3.0 | 930 | | | | | | | | | | |
| *7.8 oz salad* | | 49.0 | 36.0 | 6.0 | | | 135 | | | | | | | | | | | CKOT62 |
| **baked potato corn chowder** | 369 | 545 | | 64.0 | 9.0 | | 5.0 | 1330 | | | | | | | | | | |
| *13 oz* | | 12.0 | 29.0 | 18.0 | | | 80 | | | | | | | | | | | CKOT67 |
| **broccoli and carrots**, boiled | 227 | 48 | | 10.0 | 4.0 | | 4.0 | 62 | | | | | | | | | | |
| *8 oz* | | 3.0 | 0 | 0 | | | 0 | | | | | | | | | | | CKOT72 |
| **brown rice with grilled vegetables** | 227 | 170 | | 25.0 | 7.0 | | 2.0 | 25 | | | | | | | | | | |
| *8 oz* | | 3.0 | 7.0 | 1.0 | | | 340 | | | | | | | | | | | CKOT73 |
| **chicken**, BBQ pulled | 227 | 539 | | 39.0 | 31.0 | | 0 | 2710 | | | | | | | | | | |
| *8 oz* | | 72.0 | 8.0 | 2.0 | | | 197 | | | | | | | | | | | CKOT65 |
| **chicken bean chili** | 369 | 548 | | 79.0 | 26.0 | | 19.0 | 2263 | | | | | | | | | | |
| *13 oz* | | 43.0 | 8.0 | 1.0 | | | 54 | | | | | | | | | | | CKOT68 |
| **chicken breast**, pulled rotisserie | 255 | 452 | | 5.0 | 4.0 | | 0 | 958 | | | | | | | | | | |
| *9 oz* | | 82.0 | 9.0 | 3.0 | | | 224 | | | | | | | | | | | CKOT66 |
| **chicken gravy** | 57 | 45 | | 3.0 | 0 | | 0 | 105 | | | | | | | | | | |
| *2 oz* | | 1.0 | 3.0 | 2.0 | | | 10 | | | | | | | | | | | CKOT75 |
| **chicken noodle soup** | 369 | 211 | | 9.0 | 3.0 | | 1.0 | 396 | | | | | | | | | | |
| *13 oz* | | 30.0 | 6.0 | 2.0 | | | 80 | | | | | | | | | | | CKOT69 |
| **chicken salad**, lowfat | 227 | 320 | | 14.0 | 5.0 | | 1.0 | 1110 | | | | | | | | | | |
| *8 oz salad* | | 48.0 | 6.0 | 1.5 | | | 130 | | | | | | | | | | | CKOT63 |
| **chicken salad**, signature | 227 | 680 | | 14.0 | 9.0 | | 1.0 | 1275 | | | | | | | | | | |
| *8 oz salad* | | 39.0 | 51.0 | 8.0 | | | 125 | | | | | | | | | | | CKOT64 |
| **coleslaw** | 227 | 226 | | 18.0 | 13.0 | | 3.0 | 417 | | | | | | | | | | |
| *8 oz* | | 2.0 | 17.0 | 3.0 | | | 9 | | | | | | | | | | | CKOT79 |
| **cranberry relish** | 227 | 285 | | 69.0 | 66.0 | | 3.0 | 64 | | | | | | | | | | |
| *8 oz* | | 1.0 | 2.0 | 0 | | | 45 | | | | | | | | | | | CKOT77 |
| **creamed spinach** | 227 | 320 | | 16.0 | 7.0 | | 3.0 | 1190 | | | | | | | | | | |
| *8 oz* | | 9.0 | 25.0 | 14.0 | | | 75 | | | | | | | | | | | CKOT78 |
| **fruit salad** | 227 | 110 | | 29.0 | 25.0 | | 3.0 | 10 | | | | | | | | | | |
| *8 oz* | | 1.0 | 0 | 0 | | | 0 | | | | | | | | | | | CKOT81 |

| | WT (g) | KCAL / PRO (g) | H₂0 (g) / FAT (g) | CHO (g) / SFA (g) | TSUG (g) / MUFA (g) | ASUG (g) / PUFA (g) | DFIB (g) / CHOL (mg) | Na (mg) / K (mg) | Ca (mg) / P (mg) | Mg (mg) / Fe (mg) | Zn (mg) / Cu (mg) | Mn (mg) / Se (mcg) | A (mcg RAE) / A (IU) | C (mg) / E (mg ATE) | B-1 (mg) / B-2 (mg) | NIA (mg) / B-6 (mg) | B-12 (mcg) / FOL (mcg DFE) | PANT (mg) / REF |
|---|---|---|---|---|---|---|---|---|---|---|---|---|---|---|---|---|---|---|
| **green beans, red peppers and** | 227 | 130 | | 12.0 | 4.0 | | 4.0 | 310 | | | | | | | | | | |
| caramelized onions - *8 oz* | | 2.0 | 9.0 | 1.0 | | | 0 | | | | | | | | | | | CKOT80 |
| **macaroni and cheese** | 227 | 355 | | 56.0 | 5.0 | | 3.0 | 635 | | | | | | | | | | |
| *8 oz* | | 13.0 | 8.0 | 2.5 | | | 10 | | | | | | | | | | | CKOT82 |
| **mashed potatoes,** red-skin | 227 | 334 | | 44.0 | 3.0 | | 4.0 | 1317 | | | | | | | | | | |
| *8 oz* | | 5.0 | 16.0 | 10.0 | | | 42 | | | | | | | | | | | CKOT87 |
| **mashed sweet potatoes** | 227 | 423 | | 102.0 | 54.0 | | 4.0 | 120 | | | | | | | | | | |
| *8 oz* | | 4.0 | 1.0 | 0 | | | 0 | | | | | | | | | | | CKOT83 |
| **pasta salad,** Caesar | 227 | 457 | | 49.0 | 8.0 | | 5.0 | 551 | | | | | | | | | | |
| *8 oz* | | 14.0 | 23.0 | 5.0 | | | 21 | | | | | | | | | | | CKOT74 |
| **pasta salad,** tri-colored orzo | 227 | 370 | | 50.0 | 13.0 | | 4.0 | 170 | | | | | | | | | | |
| *8 oz* | | 9.0 | 15.0 | 2.5 | | | 5 | | | | | | | | | | | CKOT84 |
| **peas, corn, carrots,** boiled | 227 | 176 | | 34.0 | 7.0 | | 8.0 | 528 | | | | | | | | | | |
| *8 oz* | | 8.0 | 3.0 | 1.0 | | | 6 | | | | | | | | | | | CKOT85 |
| **potato chips,** 40% reduced fat, | 43 | 200 | | 27.0 | 1.0 | | 2.0 | 160 | | | | | | | | | | |
| Cape Cod - *1.5 oz package* | | 3.0 | 9.0 | 0.5 | | | 0 | | | | | | | | | | | CKOT91 |
| **potato salad** with eggs | 227 | 395 | | 29.0 | 3.0 | | 3.0 | 640 | | | | | | | | | | |
| *8 oz* | | 8.0 | 27.0 | 6.0 | | | 175 | | | | | | | | | | | CKOT86 |
| **sesame ginger green beans** | 227 | 97 | | 7.0 | 1.0 | | 3.0 | 753 | | | | | | | | | | |
| *8 oz* | | 3.0 | 7.0 | 1.0 | | | 0 | | | | | | | | | | | CKOT88 |
| **stuffing,** apple cornbread | 227 | 453 | | 58.0 | 7.0 | | 2.0 | 1612 | | | | | | | | | | |
| *8 oz* | | 9.0 | 21.0 | 10.0 | | | 38 | | | | | | | | | | | CKOT71 |
| **vegetable medley,** steamed | 227 | 30 | | 6.0 | 2.0 | | 2.0 | 25 | | | | | | | | | | |
| *8 oz* | | 2.0 | 0 | 0 | | | 0 | | | | | | | | | | | CKOT89 |
| **vegetable primavera soup** | 369 | 330 | | 45.0 | 20.0 | | 10.0 | 1580 | | | | | | | | | | |
| *13 oz* | | 26.0 | 7.0 | 1.0 | | | 45 | | | | | | | | | | | CKOT70 |
| **zucchini and yellow squash,** boiled | 227 | 45 | | 5.0 | 3.0 | | 2.0 | 125 | | | | | | | | | | |
| *8 oz* | | 2.0 | 3.0 | 2.0 | | | 10 | | | | | | | | | | | CKOT90 |

## 10.9 CHICK-FIL-A

| | WT (g) | KCAL / PRO (g) | H₂0 (g) / FAT (g) | CHO (g) / SFA (g) | TSUG (g) / MUFA (g) | ASUG (g) / PUFA (g) | DFIB (g) / CHOL (mg) | Na (mg) / K (mg) | Ca (mg) / P (mg) | Mg (mg) / Fe (mg) | Zn (mg) / Cu (mg) | Mn (mg) / Se (mcg) | A (mcg RAE) / A (IU) | C (mg) / E (mg ATE) | B-1 (mg) / B-2 (mg) | NIA (mg) / B-6 (mg) | B-12 (mcg) / FOL (mcg DFE) | PANT (mg) / REF |
|---|---|---|---|---|---|---|---|---|---|---|---|---|---|---|---|---|---|---|
| **bagel with chicken, egg, cheese** | 215 | 500 | | 49.0 | 9.0 | | 3.0 | 1280 | 150 | | | | | 0 | | | | |
| *7.6 oz bagel* | | 30.0 | 20.0 | 6.0 | | | 290 | | | 3.60 | | | 400 | | | | | CKFL66 |
| **biscuit** | 86 | 310 | | 41.0 | 4.0 | | 2.0 | 700 | 60 | | | | | 0 | | | | |
| *3 oz biscuit* | | 5.0 | 13.0 | 6.0 | | | 0 | | | 1.08 | | | 100 | | | | | CKFL67 |
| **biscuit and gravy** | 199 | 420 | | 51.0 | 5.0 | | 2.0 | 1370 | 80 | | | | | 0 | | | | |
| *7 oz biscuit* | | 8.0 | 20.0 | 8.0 | | | 10 | | | 1.44 | | | 100 | | | | | CKFL68 |
| **biscuit with bacon, egg, cheese** | 174 | 520 | | 44.0 | 6.0 | | 2.0 | 1360 | 150 | | | | | 0 | | | | |
| *6.1 oz biscuit* | | 21.0 | 29.0 | 13.0 | | | 270 | | | 2.70 | | | 500 | | | | | CKFL69 |
| **Chick-n-Minis** | 94 | 260 | | 29.0 | 6.0 | | 1.0 | 590 | 20 | | | | | 1 | | | | |
| *3.3 oz (3 pieces)* | | 13.0 | 10.0 | 2.5 | | | 40 | | | 1.80 | | | 100 | | | | | CKFL83 |
| **Chick-n-Strips** | 215 | 470 | | 22.0 | 4.0 | | 3.0 | 1390 | 60 | | | | | 0 | | | | |
| *7.6 oz (4 strips)* | | 44.0 | 23.0 | 4.5 | | | 125 | | | 3.60 | | | 100 | | | | | CKFL84 |
| **Chick-n-Strips** salad | 388 | 450 | | 26.0 | 7.0 | | 6.0 | 1160 | 200 | | | | | 42 | | | | |
| *13.7 oz salad* | | 39.0 | 22.0 | 6.0 | | | 105 | | | 3.60 | | | 8000 | | | | | CKFL85 |
| **chicken** and fruit salad | 347 | 210 | | 20.0 | 14.0 | | 4.0 | 860 | 150 | | | | | 90 | | | | |
| *12.3 oz salad* | | 22.0 | 6.0 | 3.5 | | | 50 | | | 1.80 | | | 7000 | | | | | CKFL70 |
| **chicken** biscuit | 150 | 450 | | 48.0 | 5.0 | | 3.0 | 1310 | 80 | | | | | 0 | | | | |
| *5.3 oz biscuit* | | 19.0 | 20.0 | 8.0 | | | 30 | | | 1.80 | | | 100 | | | | | CKFL71 |
| **chicken** breakfast burrito | 184 | 410 | | 41.0 | 3.0 | | 4.0 | 890 | 250 | | | | | 9 | | | | |
| *6.5 oz burrito* | | 22.0 | 18.0 | 7.0 | | | 245 | | | 4.50 | | | 750 | | | | | CKFL72 |
| **Chicken Caesar Cool Wrap** | 232 | 480 | | 45.0 | 5.0 | | 8.0 | 1810 | 500 | | | | | 9 | | | | |
| *8.2 oz wrap* | | 40.0 | 16.0 | 7.0 | | | 70 | | | 3.60 | | | 2500 | | | | | CKFL73 |
| **chicken** club sandwich, chargrilled | 250 | 380 | | 34.0 | 10.0 | | 7.0 | 1650 | 200 | | | | | 9 | | | | |
| *8.8 oz sandwich* | | 36.0 | 12.0 | 5.0 | | | 75 | | | 2.70 | | | 2250 | | | | | CKFL74 |
| **Chicken** Cool Wrap, chargrilled | 291 | 410 | | 49.0 | 7.0 | | 9.0 | 1510 | 200 | | | | | 24 | | | | |
| *10.3 oz wrap* | | 33.0 | 12.0 | 4.0 | | | 50 | | | 4.50 | | | 6500 | | | | | CKFL75 |
| **Chicken** Cool Wrap, spicy | 277 | 400 | | 47.0 | 6.0 | | 9.0 | 1320 | 200 | | | | | 21 | | | | |
| *9.8 oz wrap* | | 35.0 | 12.0 | 4.0 | | | 60 | | | 4.50 | | | 4000 | | | | | CKFL76 |
| **chicken** garden salad | 298 | 170 | | 10.0 | 5.0 | | 4.0 | 860 | 150 | | | | | 42 | | | | |
| *10.5 oz salad* | | 22.0 | 6.0 | 3.5 | | | 50 | | | 1.44 | | | 8000 | | | | | CKFL77 |

| | WT (g) | KCAL | H₂0 (g) | CHO (g) | TSUG (g) | ASUG (g) | DFIB (g) | Na (mg) | Ca (mg) | Mg (mg) | Zn (mg) | Mn (mg) | A (mcg RAE) | C (mg) | B-1 (mg) | NIA (mg) | B-12 (mcg) | PANT (mg) |
|---|---|---|---|---|---|---|---|---|---|---|---|---|---|---|---|---|---|---|
| | | PRO (g) | FAT (g) | SFA (g) | MUFA (g) | PUFA (g) | CHOL (mg) | K (mg) | P (mg) | Fe (mg) | Cu (mg) | Se (mcg) | A (IU) | E (mg ATE) | B-2 (mg) | B-6 (mg) | FOL (mcg DFE) | REF |
| **chicken** nuggets | 170 | 400 | | 15.0 | 4.0 | | 3.0 | 1250 | 40 | | | | | 0 | | | | |
| *6 oz (12 pieces)* | | 40.0 | 19.0 | 4.0 | | | 105 | | | 1.80 | | | 100 | | | | | CKFL78 |
| **chicken** salad sandwich | 233 | 500 | | 53.0 | 13.0 | | 4.0 | 1220 | 150 | | | | | 5 | | | | |
| *8.2 oz sandwich* | | 29.0 | 20.0 | 3.5 | | | 95 | | | 3.60 | | | 1750 | | | | | CKFL79 |
| **chicken** sandwich | 179 | 430 | | 39.0 | 7.0 | | 3.0 | 1370 | 150 | | | | | 0 | | | | |
| *6.3 oz sandwich* | | 31.0 | 17.0 | 3.5 | | | 65 | | | 2.70 | | | 0 | | | | | CKFL80 |
| **chicken** sandwich, chargrilled | 220 | 260 | | 33.0 | 9.0 | | 7.0 | 1300 | 60 | | | | | 9 | | | | |
| *7.8 oz sandwich* | | 27.0 | 3.0 | 0.5 | | | 50 | | | 2.70 | | | 2000 | | | | | CKFL81 |
| **chicken** southwest salad | 326 | 240 | | 17.0 | 6.0 | | 5.0 | 750 | 150 | | | | | 42 | | | | |
| *11.5 oz salad* | | 25.0 | 9.0 | 4.0 | | | 60 | | | 1.80 | | | 7500 | | | | | CKFL82 |
| **Cinnamon Cluster** | 105 | 400 | | 61.0 | 28.0 | | 3.0 | 280 | 60 | | | | | 0 | | | | |
| *3.7 oz* | | 8.0 | 15.0 | 6.0 | | | 35 | | | 1.80 | | | 100 | | | | | CKFL86 |
| **hash browns** | 77 | 280 | | 25.0 | 0 | | 2.0 | 410 | 20 | | | | | 6 | | | | |
| *2.7 oz* | | 3.0 | 19.0 | 4.0 | | | 0 | | | 0.72 | | | 0 | | | | | CKFL87 |
| **sausage biscuit** | 149 | 590 | | 42.0 | 4.0 | | 2.0 | 1250 | 80 | | | | | 0 | | | | |
| *5.2 oz biscuit* | | 16.0 | 41.0 | 16.0 | | | 50 | | | 1.80 | | | 200 | | | | | CKFL88 |
| **sausage breakfast burrito** | 184 | 480 | | 38.0 | 3.0 | | 4.0 | 870 | 250 | | | | | 9 | | | | |
| *6.5 oz burrito* | | 21.0 | 27.0 | 11.0 | | | 250 | | | 4.50 | | | 750 | | | | | CKFL89 |

## 10.10 DOMINO'S

| | WT (g) | KCAL | H₂0 (g) | CHO (g) | TSUG (g) | ASUG (g) | DFIB (g) | Na (mg) | Ca (mg) | Mg (mg) | Zn (mg) | Mn (mg) | A (mcg RAE) | C (mg) | B-1 (mg) | NIA (mg) | B-12 (mcg) | PANT (mg) |
|---|---|---|---|---|---|---|---|---|---|---|---|---|---|---|---|---|---|---|
| | | PRO (g) | FAT (g) | SFA (g) | MUFA (g) | PUFA (g) | CHOL (mg) | K (mg) | P (mg) | Fe (mg) | Cu (mg) | Se (mcg) | A (IU) | E (mg ATE) | B-2 (mg) | B-6 (mg) | FOL (mcg DFE) | REF |
| **pizza**, cheese, Deep Dish Crust | 106 | 290 | 44.6 | 36.0 | 3.5 | | 2.4 | 595 | 157 | 26 | 1.45 | 0.381 | 83 | 0 | 0.24 | 4.5 | 0.50 | 0.56 |
| *3.7 oz slice* | | 12.0 | 11.0 | 4.3 | 3.1 | 2.0 | 15 | 174 | 214 | 3.14 | 0.110 | 37.7 | 360 | 0.9 | 0.26 | | | 21278 |
| **pizza**, cheese, Hand-Tossed Crust | 106 | 272 | 47.0 | 36.5 | 3.8 | | 1.5 | 507 | 142 | 25 | 1.22 | 0.316 | 65 | 0 | 0.18 | 3.4 | 0.45 | 0.48 |
| *3.7 oz slice* | | 11.6 | 8.9 | 3.8 | 2.1 | 1.7 | 14 | 161 | 198 | 2.44 | 0.140 | 27.5 | 319 | 1.0 | 0.23 | 0.12 | | 21277 |
| **pizza**, cheese, Thin Crust | 39 | 123 | 15.5 | 10.9 | 1.2 | | 0.8 | 194 | 87 | 10 | 0.65 | 0.101 | 37 | 0 | 0.03 | 0.4 | 0.31 | 0.16 |
| *1.4 oz slice* | | 5.1 | 6.6 | 2.6 | 1.6 | 1.4 | 8 | 72 | 117 | 0.28 | 0.039 | 13.8 | 160 | 0.6 | 0.04 | | | 21279 |
| **pizza**, Extravaganzza, Hand-Tossed | 151 | 368 | 76.7 | 38.8 | 5.0 | | 3.0 | 689 | 171 | 33 | 1.92 | 0.393 | 77 | 0 | 0.20 | 4.9 | 0.83 | 0.76 |
| Crust - *5.3 oz slice* | | 15.6 | 16.8 | 6.6 | 5.5 | 2.2 | 30 | 263 | 278 | 3.50 | 0.168 | 36.2 | 343 | 1.2 | 0.33 | | | 21282 |
| **pizza**, pepperoni, Hand-Tossed | 120 | 324 | 52.1 | 38.7 | 4.1 | | 1.8 | 608 | 146 | 30 | 1.48 | 0.380 | 56 | 0 | 0.21 | 4.3 | 0.66 | 0.66 |
| Crust - *4.2 oz slice* | | 13.9 | 12.6 | 5.1 | 3.8 | 2.1 | 26 | 211 | 222 | 2.83 | 0.146 | 34.2 | 282 | 1.2 | 0.27 | 0.18 | | 21280 |
| **pizza**, pepperoni, Deep Dish Crust | 127 | 366 | 51.9 | 41.0 | 4.1 | | 2.7 | 668 | 142 | 32 | 1.92 | 0.467 | 89 | 0 | 0.20 | 5.0 | 0.71 | 0.76 |
| *4.5 oz slice* | | 15.4 | 15.6 | 6.2 | 5.1 | 2.6 | 22 | 224 | 257 | 3.30 | 0.147 | 46.7 | 382 | 1.1 | 0.31 | | | 21281 |

## 10.11 IN-N-OUT BURGER

| | WT (g) | KCAL | H₂0 (g) | CHO (g) | TSUG (g) | ASUG (g) | DFIB (g) | Na (mg) | Ca (mg) | Mg (mg) | Zn (mg) | Mn (mg) | A (mcg RAE) | C (mg) | B-1 (mg) | NIA (mg) | B-12 (mcg) | PANT (mg) |
|---|---|---|---|---|---|---|---|---|---|---|---|---|---|---|---|---|---|---|
| | | PRO (g) | FAT (g) | SFA (g) | MUFA (g) | PUFA (g) | CHOL (mg) | K (mg) | P (mg) | Fe (mg) | Cu (mg) | Se (mcg) | A (IU) | E (mg ATE) | B-2 (mg) | B-6 (mg) | FOL (mcg DFE) | REF |
| **cheeseburger**, double-double, onion, | 330 | 590 | | 41.0 | 10.0 | | 3.0 | 1520 | 350 | | | | | 12 | | | | |
| must, ketchup - *11.6 oz sand* | | 37.0 | 32.0 | 17.0 | | | 115 | | | 5.40 | | | 1250 | | | | | INOU5 |
| **cheeseburger**, double-double, onion, | 330 | 670 | | 39.0 | 10.0 | | 3.0 | 1440 | 350 | | | | | 9 | | | | |
| spread - *11.6 oz sandwich* | | 37.0 | 41.0 | 18.0 | | | 120 | | | 5.40 | | | 1000 | | | | | INOU4 |
| **cheeseburger**, double-double, wrpd | 362 | 520 | | 11.0 | 7.0 | | 3.0 | 1160 | 350 | | | | | 12 | | | | |
| in lett (no bun) - *12.8 oz sand* | | 33.0 | 39.0 | 17.0 | | | 120 | | | 4.50 | | | 1250 | | | | | INOU6 |
| **cheeseburger**, onion, must, | 268 | 400 | | 41.0 | 10.0 | | 3.0 | 1080 | 200 | | | | | 12 | | | | |
| ketchup - *9.5 oz sandwich* | | 22.0 | 18.0 | 9.0 | | | 60 | | | 3.60 | | | 1000 | | | | | INOU2 |
| **cheeseburger**, onion, spread | 268 | 480 | | 39.0 | 10.0 | | 3.0 | 1000 | 200 | | | | | 9 | | | | |
| *9.5 oz sandwich* | | 22.0 | 27.0 | 10.0 | | | 60 | | | 3.60 | | | 750 | | | | | INOU1 |
| **cheeseburger**, onion, wrpd in lettuce | 300 | 330 | | 11.0 | 7.0 | | 3.0 | 720 | 200 | | | | | 12 | | | | |
| (no bun) - *10.6 oz sandwich* | | 18.0 | 25.0 | 9.0 | | | 60 | | | 2.70 | | | 1000 | | | | | INOU3 |
| **French fries** | 125 | 400 | | 54.0 | 0 | | 2.0 | 245 | 20 | | | | | 0 | | | | |
| *4.4 oz* | | 7.0 | 18.0 | 5.0 | | | 0 | | | 1.80 | | | 0 | | | | | INOU7 |
| **hamburger**, onion, mustard, | 243 | 310 | | 41.0 | 10.0 | | 3.0 | 730 | 40 | | | | | 12 | | | | |
| ketchup - *8.6 oz sandwich* | | 16.0 | 10.0 | 4.0 | | | 35 | | | 3.60 | | | 750 | | | | | INOU9 |
| **hamburger**, onion, spread | 243 | 390 | | 39.0 | 10.0 | | 3.0 | 650 | 40 | | | | | 9 | | | | |
| *8.6 oz sandwich* | | 16.0 | 19.0 | 5.0 | | | 40 | | | 3.60 | | | 500 | | | | | INOU8 |
| **hamburger**, onion, wrappd in lettuce | 275 | 240 | | 11.0 | 7.0 | | 3.0 | 370 | 40 | | | | | 12 | | | | |
| (no bun) - *9.7 oz sandwich* | | 13.0 | 17.0 | 4.0 | | | 40 | | | 2.70 | | | 750 | | | | | INOU10 |
| **iced tea** | 475 | 0 | 0 | 0 | 0 | | 0 | 0 | 0 | | | | | 0 | | | | |
| *16 fl oz* | | 0 | 0 | 0 | | | 0 | | | 0 | | | 0 | | | | | INOU15 |
| **lemonade** | 475 | 198 | | 40.0 | 38.0 | | 0 | 20 | 0 | | | | | 0 | | | | |
| *16 fl oz* | | 0 | 0 | 0 | | | 0 | | | 0 | | | 400 | | | | | INOU14 |
| **shake**, chocolate | 312 | 690 | | 83.0 | 62.0 | | 0 | 350 | 300 | | | | | 0 | | | | |
| *15 fl oz* | | 9.0 | 36.0 | 24.0 | | | 95 | | | 0.72 | | | 750 | | | | | INOU11 |

| | WT (g) | KCAL / PRO (g) | H₂0 (g) / FAT (g) | CHO (g) / SFA (g) | TSUG (g) / MUFA (g) | ASUG (g) / PUFA (g) | DFIB (g) / CHOL (mg) | Na (mg) / K (mg) | Ca (mg) / P (mg) | Mg (mg) / Fe (mg) | Zn (mg) / Cu (mg) | Mn (mg) / Se (mcg) | A (mcg RAE) / A (IU) | C (mg) / E (mg ATE) | B-1 (mg) / B-2 (mg) | NIA (mg) / B-6 (mg) | B-12 (mcg) / FOL (mcg DFE) | PANT (mg) / REF |
|---|---|---|---|---|---|---|---|---|---|---|---|---|---|---|---|---|---|---|
| shake, strawberry | 312 | 690 | | 91.0 | 75.0 | | 0 | 280 | 300 | | | | | 0 | | | | |
| 15 fl oz | | 9.0 | 33.0 | 22.0 | | | 85 | | | 0 | | | 750 | | | | | INOU13 |
| shake, vanilla | 312 | 680 | | 78.0 | 57.0 | | 0 | 390 | 300 | | | | | 0 | | | | |
| 15 fl oz | | 9.0 | 37.0 | 25.0 | | | 90 | | | 0 | | | 750 | | | | | INOU12 |

## 10.12 KENTUCKY FRIED CHICKEN

| | WT (g) | KCAL / PRO (g) | H₂0 (g) / FAT (g) | CHO (g) / SFA (g) | TSUG (g) / MUFA (g) | ASUG (g) / PUFA (g) | DFIB (g) / CHOL (mg) | Na (mg) / K (mg) | Ca (mg) / P (mg) | Mg (mg) / Fe (mg) | Zn (mg) / Cu (mg) | Mn (mg) / Se (mcg) | A (mcg RAE) / A (IU) | C (mg) / E (mg ATE) | B-1 (mg) / B-2 (mg) | NIA (mg) / B-6 (mg) | B-12 (mcg) / FOL (mcg DFE) | PANT (mg) / REF |
|---|---|---|---|---|---|---|---|---|---|---|---|---|---|---|---|---|---|---|
| **BBQ baked beans** | 130 | 200 | | 39.0 | 18.0 | | 9.0 | 680 | | | | | | | | | | |
| 4.6 oz | | 8.0 | 1.5 | 0 | | | 0 | | | | | | | | | | | KFCN71 |
| biscuit | 54 | 180 | | 23.0 | 2.0 | | 1.0 | 530 | | | | | | | | | | |
| 1.9 oz biscuit | | 4.0 | 8.0 | 6.0 | | | 0 | | | | | | | | | | | KFCN74 |
| chicken and biscuit bowl | 470 | 780 | | 84.0 | 5.0 | | 6.0 | 2440 | | | | | | | | | | |
| 16.6 oz | | 28.0 | 37.0 | 14.0 | | | 55 | | | | | | | | | | | KFCN67 |
| chicken pot pie | 369 | 690 | | 57.0 | 14.0 | | 3.0 | 1760 | | | | | | | | | | |
| 13 oz | | 27.0 | 40.0 | 31.0 | | | 95 | | | | | | | | | | | KFCN66 |
| coleslaw | 130 | 180 | | 22.0 | 18.0 | | 3.0 | 270 | | | | | | | | | | |
| 4.6 oz | | 1.0 | 10.0 | 1.5 | | | 5 | | | | | | | | | | | KFCN73 |
| cornbread muffin | 52 | 210 | | 27.0 | 11.0 | | 1.0 | 160 | | | | | | | | | | |
| 1.8 oz muffin | | 3.0 | 10.0 | 2.0 | | | 40 | | | | | | | | | | | KFCN79 |
| **Crispy chicken strips** | 152 | 380 | | 12.0 | 0 | | 1.0 | 720 | | | | | | | | | | |
| 3 pieces | | 33.0 | 22.0 | 6.0 | | | 80 | | | | | | | | | | | KFCN62 |
| **Extra Crispy chicken breast** | 181 | 490 | | 17.0 | 0 | | 0 | 1080 | | | | | | | | | | |
| 6.4 oz breast | | 38.0 | 31.0 | 7.0 | | | 120 | | | | | | | | | | | KFCN58 |
| **Extra Crispy chicken drumstick** | 58 | 150 | | 6.0 | 0 | | 0 | 360 | | | | | | | | | | |
| 2 oz drumstick | | 11.0 | 9.0 | 2.0 | | | 50 | | | | | | | | | | | KFCN59 |
| **Extra Crispy chicken thigh** | 113 | 370 | | 12.0 | 0 | | 0 | 840 | | | | | | | | | | |
| 4 oz thigh | | 18.0 | 27.0 | 6.0 | | | 85 | | | | | | | | | | | KFCN60 |
| **Extra Crispy chicken wing** | 48 | 150 | | 6.0 | 0 | | 1.0 | 320 | | | | | | | | | | |
| 1.7 oz wing | | 11.0 | 10.0 | 2.0 | | | 50 | | | | | | | | | | | KFCN57 |
| macaroni and cheese | 137 | 180 | | 20.0 | 4.0 | | 2.0 | 880 | | | | | | | | | | |
| 4.8 oz | | 6.0 | 9.0 | 3.0 | | | 5 | | | | | | | | | | | KFCN69 |
| macaroni salad | 107 | 180 | | 20.0 | 6.0 | | 1.0 | 400 | | | | | | | | | | |
| 3.8 oz | | 3.0 | 9.0 | 2.0 | | | 5 | | | | | | | | | | | KFCN76 |
| mashed potatoes and gravy | 153 | 130 | | 20.0 | 0 | | 1.0 | 550 | | | | | | | | | | |
| 5.4 oz | | 2.0 | 4.5 | 1.0 | | | 0 | | | | | | | | | | | KFCN68 |
| **Mean Greens** | 128 | 30 | | 4.0 | 1.0 | | 2.0 | 400 | | | | | | | | | | |
| 4.5 oz | | 3.0 | 0 | 0 | | | 0 | | | | | | | | | | | KFCN75 |
| **Original Recipe chicken breast** | 166 | 370 | | 7.0 | 0 | | 0 | 1050 | | | | | | | | | | |
| 5.9 oz breast | | 38.0 | 21.0 | 5.0 | | | 120 | | | | | | | | | | | KFCN54 |
| **Original Recipe chicken drumstick** | 50 | 110 | | 2.0 | 0 | | 0 | 290 | | | | | | | | | | |
| 1.8 oz drumstick | | 10.0 | 7.0 | 1.5 | | | 55 | | | | | | | | | | | KFCN55 |
| **Original Recipe chicken strips** | 146 | 310 | | 11.0 | 1.0 | | 2.0 | 990 | | | | | | | | | | |
| 3 pieces | | 32.0 | 15.0 | 5.0 | | | 80 | | | | | | | | | | | KFCN61 |
| **Original Recipe chicken thigh** | 98 | 260 | | 6.0 | 0 | | 0 | 670 | | | | | | | | | | |
| 3.5 oz thigh | | 16.0 | 19.0 | 5.0 | | | 85 | | | | | | | | | | | KFCN56 |
| **Original Recipe chicken wing** | 42 | 110 | | 3.0 | 0 | | 0 | 310 | | | | | | | | | | |
| 1.5 oz wing | | 9.0 | 7.0 | 1.5 | | | 45 | | | | | | | | | | | KFCN53 |
| pie, pecan | 95 | 410 | | 52.0 | 22.0 | | 1.0 | 220 | | | | | | | | | | |
| 3.4 oz slice | | 4.0 | 21.0 | 6.0 | | | 70 | | | | | | | | | | | KFCN81 |
| pie, strawberry cream cheese | 78 | 270 | | 31.0 | 22.0 | | 0 | 220 | | | | | | | | | | |
| 2.8 oz slice | | 3.0 | 15.0 | 10.0 | | | 5 | | | | | | | | | | | KFCN80 |
| **Popcorn Chicken** | 85 | 290 | | 16.0 | 0 | | 2.0 | 850 | | | | | | | | | | |
| kid size | | 16.0 | 19.0 | 3.5 | | | 40 | | | | | | | | | | | KFCN63 |
| **Popcorn Chicken** | 160 | 550 | | 30.0 | 0 | | 3.0 | 1600 | | | | | | | | | | |
| large | | 29.0 | 35.0 | 6.0 | | | 80 | | | | | | | | | | | KFCN65 |
| **Popcorn Chicken** | 116 | 400 | | 22.0 | 0 | | 3.0 | 1160 | | | | | | | | | | |
| regular | | 21.0 | 26.0 | 4.5 | | | 60 | | | | | | | | | | | KFCN64 |
| potato salad | 128 | 200 | | 24.0 | 5.0 | | 3.0 | 540 | | | | | | | | | | |
| 4.5 oz | | 2.0 | 10.0 | 2.0 | | | 5 | | | | | | | | | | | KFCN72 |
| potato wedges | 102 | 260 | | 33.0 | 0 | | 3.0 | 740 | | | | | | | | | | |
| 3.6 oz | | 4.0 | 13.0 | 2.5 | | | 0 | | | | | | | | | | | KFCN70 |
| red beans with sausage and rice | 144 | 160 | | 26.0 | 0 | | 4.0 | 340 | | | | | | | | | | |
| 5.1 oz | | 24.0 | 2.5 | 0.5 | | | 5 | | | | | | | | | | | KFCN78 |
| three bean salad | 87 | 70 | | 14.0 | 7.0 | | 3.0 | 170 | | | | | | | | | | |
| 3.1 oz | | 3.0 | 0 | 0 | | | 0 | | | | | | | | | | | KFCN77 |

| | WT (g) | KCAL / PRO (g) | H₂O (g) / FAT (g) | CHO (g) / SFA (g) | TSUG (g) / MUFA (g) | ASUG (g) / PUFA (g) | DFIB (g) / CHOL (mg) | Na (mg) / K (mg) | Ca (mg) / P (mg) | Mg (mg) / Fe (mg) | Zn (mg) / Cu (mg) | Mn (mg) / Se (mcg) | A (mcg RAE) / A (IU) | C (mg) / E (mg ATE) | B-1 (mg) / B-2 (mg) | NIA (mg) / B-6 (mg) | B-12 (mcg) / FOL (mcg DFE) | PANT (mg) / REF |
|---|---|---|---|---|---|---|---|---|---|---|---|---|---|---|---|---|---|---|

### 10.13 LITTLE CAESAR'S PIZZA

| | WT (g) | | | | | | | | | | | | | | | | | |
|---|---|---|---|---|---|---|---|---|---|---|---|---|---|---|---|---|---|---|
| **pizza, cheese, deep dish crust** | 102 | 268 | 45.8 | 30.7 | 3.7 | | 1.3 | 441 | 228 | 28 | 1.55 | 0.317 | 78 | 0 | 0.45 | 3.0 | 0.44 | 0.58 |
| *3.6 oz slice* | | 12.9 | 10.4 | 4.3 | 2.8 | 1.8 | 23 | 163 | 225 | 2.36 | 0.118 | 30.6 | 341 | 0.8 | 0.28 | | | 21290 |
| **pizza, cheese, regular crust** | 89 | 236 | 38.6 | 28.0 | 3.6 | | 1.5 | 404 | 207 | 25 | 1.43 | 0.286 | 69 | 0 | 0.34 | 2.9 | 0.36 | 0.40 |
| *3.1 oz slice* | | 11.9 | 8.5 | 3.7 | 2.1 | 1.3 | 21 | 151 | 206 | 2.08 | 0.112 | 27.9 | 320 | 0.5 | 0.26 | | | 21287 |
| **pizza, cheese, thin crust** | 48 | 148 | 19.8 | 11.0 | 1.3 | | 0.8 | 218 | 203 | 13 | 1.02 | 0.101 | 59 | 0 | 0.07 | 0.4 | 0.34 | 0.20 |
| *1.7 oz slice* | | 7.8 | 8.2 | 3.5 | 2.1 | 1.5 | 19 | 85 | 143 | 0.31 | 0.039 | 13.5 | 260 | 0.6 | 0.09 | | | 21292 |
| **pizza, meat and veg, reg crust** | 115 | 279 | 58.8 | 26.6 | 4.3 | | 2.4 | 665 | 192 | 28 | 1.78 | 0.305 | 55 | 0 | 0.33 | 4.1 | 0.70 | 0.66 |
| *4.1 oz slice* | | 13.9 | 13.1 | 5.2 | 4.7 | 2.0 | 36 | 224 | 238 | 2.43 | 0.163 | 31.2 | 243 | 1.0 | 0.30 | | | 21289 |
| **pizza, pepperoni, deep dish crust** | 104 | 276 | 46.8 | 30.2 | 3.5 | | 1.6 | 512 | 209 | 28 | 1.63 | 0.329 | 68 | 0 | 0.39 | 3.9 | 0.48 | 0.50 |
| *3.7 oz slice* | | 13.4 | 11.2 | 4.5 | 3.3 | 1.8 | 27 | 180 | 224 | 2.39 | 0.126 | 32.1 | 328 | 0.8 | 0.29 | | | 21291 |
| **pizza, pepperoni, regular crust** | 90 | 246 | 38.3 | 27.9 | 3.4 | | 1.5 | 466 | 189 | 25 | 1.49 | 0.304 | 64 | 0 | 0.30 | 3.4 | 0.47 | 0.48 |
| *3.2 oz slice* | | 12.2 | 9.5 | 4.1 | 2.8 | 1.4 | 25 | 160 | 202 | 2.11 | 0.112 | 28.8 | 298 | 0.7 | 0.28 | | | 21288 |

### 10.14 MCDONALD'S

| | WT (g) | | | | | | | | | | | | | | | | | |
|---|---|---|---|---|---|---|---|---|---|---|---|---|---|---|---|---|---|---|
| **apple dippers** | 68 | 33 | 59.5 | 8.2 | 6.3 | | | 0 | 42 | | | | 1 | 188 | | 0 | | |
| *2.4 oz* | | 0 | 0 | | | | | | | 0.07 | | | 5 | 0.1 | | | | 21342 |
| **apple dippers w/lowfat caramel sce - 3.1 oz** | 89 | 99 | 64.2 | 23.2 | 15.3 | | | 36 | 57 | | 0.06 | | 11 | 188 | 0.02 | 0 | 0 | 0.08 |
| | | 0.4 | 0.7 | 0.4 | 0.2 | 0 | 3 | | | 0.10 | | | 36 | 0.1 | 0.03 | 0.01 | | 21366 |
| **apple pie** | 77 | 249 | 28.5 | 33.6 | 13.3 | | 1.5 | 153 | 15 | 5 | 0.18 | 0.136 | | 25 | 0.23 | 2.0 | | 0.18 |
| *2.7 oz pie* | | 2.4 | 12.1 | 3.1 | 7.1 | 0.8 | | 49 | 28 | 1.53 | 0.043 | | | 1.5 | 0.16 | 0.04 | | 21324 |
| **Big Breakfast** (eggs, sausg, hash | 266 | 758 | 134.8 | 46.6 | 2.5 | | 2.9 | 1460 | 136 | 40 | 2.58 | 0.317 | 186 | 1 | 0.61 | 6.0 | 1.52 | 1.98 |
| brown, bis) - *9.3 oz breakfast* | | 27.0 | 51.5 | 17.0 | 19.6 | 8.5 | 460 | 551 | 681 | 4.63 | 0.218 | | 622 | | 0.94 | 0.46 | | 21341 |
| **Big Mac** | 215 | 553 | 110.3 | 43.2 | 8.5 | | 3.4 | 989 | 249 | 43 | 4.11 | 0.443 | | 1 | 0.38 | 7.3 | 1.89 | |
| *7.6 oz sandwich* | | 25.4 | 32.2 | 8.2 | 7.5 | 0.7 | 77 | 389 | 262 | 4.30 | 0.211 | | 404 | | 0.45 | | | 21237 |
| **Big N'Tasty** | 232 | 524 | 133.9 | 38.5 | 8.8 | | 3.2 | 735 | 151 | 42 | 4.78 | 0.422 | | 4 | 0.33 | 7.7 | 2.27 | |
| *8.2 oz sandwich* | | 24.7 | 31.7 | 8.6 | 9.7 | 6.9 | 77 | 464 | 227 | 4.36 | 0.209 | | 371 | | 0.60 | | | 21351 |
| **Big N'Tasty w/cheese** | 247 | 573 | 140.1 | 39.7 | 9.5 | | 3.2 | 956 | 225 | 44 | 5.11 | 0.427 | | 4 | 0.34 | 7.8 | 2.42 | |
| *8.7 oz sandwich* | | 27.2 | 36.0 | 10.8 | 10.7 | 7.1 | 91 | 492 | 282 | 4.40 | 0.215 | | 608 | | 0.66 | | | 21353 |
| **biscuit, McDonald's** | 69 | 237 | 21.2 | 30.2 | 2.0 | | 1.4 | 672 | 52 | 8 | 0.29 | 0.182 | 4 | 0 | 0.33 | 2.8 | 0.08 | 0.29 |
| *2.4 oz biscuit* | | 4.3 | 11.0 | 6.4 | 2.6 | 1.5 | 0 | 83 | 305 | 1.88 | 0.057 | | 14 | 0.8 | 0.25 | 0.03 | | 21317 |
| **biscuit, McDonald's** | 90 | 310 | 27.6 | 39.4 | 2.7 | | 1.8 | 877 | 68 | 10 | 0.38 | 0.238 | 5 | 0 | 0.43 | 3.7 | 0.11 | 0.38 |
| *3.2 oz biscuit (large)* | | 5.5 | 14.4 | 8.3 | 3.4 | 2.0 | 0 | 108 | 398 | 2.46 | 0.074 | | 18 | 1.1 | 0.32 | 0.04 | | 21460 |
| **biscuit w/bacon, egg, cheese** | 152 | 462 | 64.3 | 33.8 | 3.3 | | 1.4 | 1312 | 166 | 18 | 1.37 | 0.208 | | 3 | 0.40 | 3.0 | | 0.98 |
| *5.4 oz sandwich* | | 20.4 | 28.5 | 12.6 | 8.4 | 4.0 | 254 | 184 | 509 | 3.24 | 0.111 | | 606 | | 0.63 | 0.14 | | 21360 |
| **biscuit w/sausage** | 112 | 421 | 38.9 | 30.5 | 2.2 | | 1.3 | 980 | 62 | 15 | 0.96 | 0.195 | 9 | 0 | 0.45 | 4.8 | 0.44 | 0.58 |
| *4 oz sandwich* | | 10.8 | 28.4 | 11.9 | 9.9 | 3.8 | 32 | 198 | 362 | 2.25 | 0.083 | | 29 | 0.8 | 0.31 | 0.14 | | 21361 |
| **biscuit w/sausage, egg** | 162 | 504 | 72.3 | 31.2 | 2.3 | | 1.3 | 1076 | 94 | 21 | 1.68 | 0.211 | 104 | 0 | 0.50 | 4.8 | 0.97 | 1.16 |
| *5.7 oz sandwich* | | 18.3 | 36.1 | 14.0 | 12.6 | 5.1 | 246 | 267 | 491 | 3.29 | 0.126 | | 347 | 1.6 | 0.62 | 0.23 | | 21362 |
| **burrito, sausage** | 113 | 296 | 55.8 | 24.2 | 1.4 | | 1.2 | 763 | 203 | 19 | 1.33 | 0.215 | 97 | 1 | 0.18 | 1.9 | 0.61 | 0.88 |
| *4 oz burrito* | | 13.0 | 17.1 | 6.1 | 6.5 | 2.4 | 173 | 155 | 247 | 1.84 | 0.092 | | 382 | 0.2 | 0.33 | 0.41 | | 21340 |
| **caramel sauce, lowfat** | 28 | 88 | 6.3 | 20.0 | 12.1 | | | 48 | 20 | 2 | 0.08 | 0.003 | 13 | | 0.02 | 0 | | 0.11 |
| *1 oz packet* | | 0.5 | 0.9 | 0.5 | 0.2 | | 3 | 33 | 25 | 0.04 | 0.005 | | 41 | 0 | 0.04 | 0.01 | | 21343 |
| **cheeseburger** | 121 | 318 | 54.4 | 33.7 | 7.5 | | 1.3 | 757 | 202 | 24 | 2.31 | 0.278 | | 1 | 0.27 | 4.9 | 1.04 | |
| *4.3 oz sandwich* | | 15.7 | 14.3 | 5.4 | 4.4 | 0.4 | 42 | 242 | 169 | 2.84 | 0.117 | | 294 | | 0.31 | | | 21233 |
| **cheeseburger, double** | 173 | 458 | 82.6 | 34.3 | 8.1 | | 1.4 | 1137 | 277 | 35 | 4.15 | 0.291 | | 1 | 0.28 | 6.7 | 2.04 | |
| *6.1 oz sandwich* | | 25.8 | 25.9 | 10.5 | 8.6 | 0.8 | 83 | 375 | 280 | 3.68 | 0.161 | | 526 | | 0.43 | | | 21344 |
| **Chicken, crispy, Classic Sandwich** | 232 | 529 | 120.6 | 59.1 | 12.5 | | 3.2 | 1188 | 79 | 63 | 1.53 | 0.998 | 42 | 6 | 0.46 | 12.9 | | 2.38 |
| *8.2 oz sandwich* | | 28.0 | 20.1 | 3.3 | 7.4 | 8.6 | 60 | 527 | 374 | 3.29 | 0.202 | | 766 | | 0.40 | | | 21403 |
| **Chicken, crispy, Club Sandwich** | 272 | 680 | 130.6 | 61.5 | 13.6 | | 3.3 | 1646 | 250 | | | | | 10 | 0.48 | 12.9 | | 2.48 |
| *9.6 oz sandwich* | | 41.8 | 32.0 | 9.1 | 11.5 | 9.7 | 103 | | | 3.59 | | | 944 | | 0.46 | | | 21405 |
| **Chicken, crispy, Ranch BLT Sand** | 245 | 598 | 119.1 | 61.1 | 13.5 | | 3.4 | 1561 | 86 | | | | | 11 | 0.47 | 12.9 | | 2.36 |
| *8.6 oz sandwich* | | 36.0 | 23.4 | 4.8 | 9.2 | 7.9 | 74 | | | 3.48 | | | 750 | | 0.40 | | | 21407 |
| **Chicken, grilled, Classic Sandwich** | 229 | 419 | 131.2 | 51.0 | 11.5 | | 3.2 | 1237 | 85 | 64 | 1.58 | 0.818 | | 7 | 0.45 | 14.9 | 0.34 | 2.12 |
| *8 oz sandwich* | | 32.4 | 9.8 | 2.0 | 2.6 | 4.7 | 78 | 522 | 447 | 3.39 | 0.167 | | 776 | 1.2 | 0.44 | 0.70 | | 21402 |
| **Chicken, grilled, Club Sandwich** | 269 | 594 | 141.3 | 53.5 | 12.6 | | 3.2 | 1695 | 256 | | | | | 12 | 0.46 | 15.0 | | 2.22 |
| *9.4 oz sandwich* | | 46.2 | 21.7 | 7.8 | 6.7 | 5.8 | 124 | | | 3.69 | | | 955 | | 0.50 | | | 21404 |
| **Chicken, grilled, Ranch BLT** | 242 | 494 | 129.7 | 53.0 | 12.6 | | 3.4 | 1612 | 92 | | | | | 12 | 0.45 | 14.9 | | 2.10 |
| Sandwich - *8.5 oz sandwich* | | 40.4 | 13.1 | 3.5 | 4.5 | 4.1 | 92 | | | 3.58 | | | 762 | | 0.44 | | | 21406 |
| **Chicken McNugget sauce,** | 28 | 46 | 16.2 | 10.3 | 9.6 | | 0.4 | 255 | 3 | 4 | 0.05 | 0.027 | 3 | 0 | 0.01 | 0.2 | | 0.05 |
| barbeque - *1 oz packet* | | 0.4 | 0.3 | 0 | 0.1 | 0.1 | | 55 | 8 | 0.11 | 0.010 | | 66 | 0.3 | 0.01 | 0.02 | | 21310 |

| | WT (g) | KCAL / PRO (g) | H₂0 / FAT (g) | CHO / SFA (g) | TSUG / MUFA (g) | ASUG / PUFA (g) | DFIB / CHOL (g/mg) | Na / K (mg) | Ca / P (mg) | Mg / Fe (mg) | Zn / Cu (mg) | Mn / Se (mg/mcg) | A (mcg RAE) / A (IU) | C (mg) / E (mg ATE) | B-1 / B-2 (mg) | NIA / B-6 (mg) | B-12 (mcg) / FOL (mcg DFE) | PANT (mg) / REF |
|---|---|---|---|---|---|---|---|---|---|---|---|---|---|---|---|---|---|---|
| **Chicken McNugget sauce,** honey | 14 | 49 | 1.9 | 12.1 | 10.4 | | | 1 | 1 | 0 | 0.02 | 0.011 | | 0 | 0.01 | 0 | | 0.01 |
| *.5 oz packet* | | 0 | 0 | 0 | 0 | 0 | | 4 | 1 | 0.04 | 0.005 | | | 0 | 0.01 | | | 21312 |
| **Chicken McNugget sauce,** honey mustard - *.5 oz packet* | 14 | 23 | 8.8 | 4.0 | 3.1 | | 0.4 | 54 | 3 | 2 | 0.04 | 0.015 | 0 | 0 | 0 | 0 | 0.02 | 0.04 |
| | | 0.2 | 0.8 | 0.1 | 0.2 | 0.4 | | 7 | 5 | 0.06 | 0.005 | | 0 | 0.1 | 0.01 | 0 | | 21316 |
| **Chicken McNugget sauce,** hot mustard - *1 oz packet* | 28 | 53 | 16.4 | 8.1 | 6.1 | | 1.4 | 253 | 9 | 7 | 0.10 | 0.062 | 0 | 0 | 0.01 | 0.1 | 0.06 | 0.05 |
| | | 0.7 | 2.0 | 0.3 | 0.5 | 1.0 | | 23 | 16 | 0.24 | 0.010 | | 0 | 0.2 | 0.02 | 0.02 | | 21313 |
| **Chicken McNugget sauce,** sweet'n sour - *1 oz packet* | 28 | 48 | 16.1 | 11.0 | 10.0 | | 0 | 156 | 2 | 2 | 0.02 | 0.013 | 2 | 0 | 0.05 | 0.1 | | 0.03 |
| | | 0.2 | 0.3 | 0 | 0.1 | 0.1 | | 28 | 4 | 0.18 | 0.010 | | 47 | 0.2 | 0.01 | 0.01 | | 21315 |
| **Chicken McNuggets** | 108 | 314 | 51.2 | 18.6 | 0 | | 0.9 | 683 | 15 | 24 | 0.64 | 0.111 | | 1 | 0.17 | 8.0 | 0.36 | 0.95 |
| *3.8 oz (6 pieces)* | | 16.2 | 19.5 | 3.4 | 8.8 | 6.4 | 48 | 271 | 359 | 0.98 | 0.040 | | 0 | | 0.12 | 0.43 | | 21309 |
| **Chicken Selects** (breast strips) | 221 | 670 | 97.5 | 39.4 | 0 | | 0.4 | 1695 | 44 | 53 | 1.15 | 0.378 | | 0 | 0.13 | 18.6 | 0.42 | 2.85 |
| *7.8 oz (5 pieces)* | | 38.1 | 40.0 | 5.7 | 18.0 | 14.6 | 88 | 643 | 608 | 1.33 | 0.128 | | 44 | 0.21 | 1.15 | | 21308 |
| chocolate chip cookie | 57 | 274 | 2.4 | 37.8 | 19.3 | | 1.1 | 167 | 19 | 23 | 0.44 | 0.316 | 74 | | 0.13 | 1.1 | 0.11 | 0.31 |
| *2 oz box* | | 3.2 | 13.0 | 6.5 | 3.4 | 0.7 | 37 | 111 | 60 | 2.22 | 0.157 | | 245 | 0.4 | 0.13 | 0.06 | | 21325 |
| cinnamon roll | 99 | 394 | 20.1 | 52.5 | 24.4 | | 1.9 | 374 | 56 | 19 | 0.80 | 0.468 | 125 | 0 | 0.31 | 2.4 | | 0.80 |
| *3.4 oz roll* | | 7.1 | 18.0 | 4.4 | 9.0 | 2.8 | 57 | 139 | 103 | 1.70 | 0.079 | | 416 | 1.8 | 0.27 | 0.10 | | 21322 |
| **Deluxe Brkfst** (eggs, bsct, sausg, hash brns, pncks) - *15.2 oz meal* | 437 | 1245 | 200.6 | 128.8 | 43.2 | | 4.4 | 1910 | 218 | 57 | 3.02 | 0.568 | | 1 | 0.90 | 8.2 | 1.53 | 2.69 |
| | | 33.0 | 66.6 | 20.3 | 22.8 | 12.3 | 476 | 743 | 944 | 6.56 | 0.319 | | 1127 | | 1.20 | 0.54 | | 21363 |
| **Double Quarter Pounder** w/cheese | 280 | 734 | 141.0 | 40.4 | 9.8 | | 2.8 | 1333 | 297 | 59 | 9.32 | 0.372 | | 2 | 0.36 | 11.8 | 4.70 | |
| *9.9 oz sandwich* | | 47.5 | 45.4 | 18.1 | 16.4 | 1.3 | 160 | 678 | 462 | 6.10 | 0.255 | | 560 | | 0.85 | | | 21345 |
| **Egg McMuffin** | 138 | 297 | 76.2 | 28.3 | 2.8 | | 1.5 | 854 | 273 | 26 | 1.59 | 0.298 | | 2 | 0.36 | 4.3 | 0.91 | 1.15 |
| *1 McMuffin* | | 17.5 | 12.6 | 4.4 | 3.8 | 2.5 | 228 | 217 | 268 | 2.97 | 0.141 | | 548 | 0.8 | 0.51 | 0.20 | 109.0 | 21357 |
| eggs, scrambled | 101 | 195 | 67.6 | 1.9 | 0.3 | | | 194 | 67 | 12 | 1.44 | 0.032 | 184 | | 0.10 | 0.1 | 1.09 | 1.17 |
| *3.6 oz (2 eggs)* | | 15.2 | 14.8 | 4.1 | 5.3 | 2.2 | 431 | 140 | 264 | 2.10 | 0.090 | | 612 | 1.5 | 0.61 | 0.18 | | 21320 |
| **English muffin** | 57 | 162 | 20.7 | 25.3 | 1.5 | | 1.5 | 276 | 166 | 13 | 0.46 | 0.260 | 0 | | 0.25 | 2.7 | 0 | 0.26 |
| *2 oz muffin* | | 5.3 | 4.5 | 0.9 | 1.1 | 2.3 | 0 | 73 | 68 | 1.82 | 0.070 | | 129 | 0.3 | 0.19 | 0.04 | | 21408 |
| **Filet-O-Fish sandwich** | 156 | 429 | 72.0 | 42.8 | 4.1 | | 1.6 | 757 | 179 | 31 | 0.78 | 0.317 | | 0 | 0.39 | 3.7 | 1.15 | |
| *5.5 oz sandwich* | | 17.1 | 21.0 | 4.1 | 6.0 | 8.8 | 44 | 273 | 184 | 2.31 | 0.097 | | 137 | | 0.28 | | | 21232 |
| **French fries** | 68 | 215 | 27.0 | 26.5 | 0.1 | | 2.9 | 154 | 12 | 22 | 0.30 | 0.152 | | 5 | 0.22 | 1.9 | | 0.44 |
| *2.4 oz serving (small)* | | 2.6 | 11.0 | 1.4 | 5.3 | 3.2 | 0 | 381 | 90 | 0.58 | 0.080 | | 0 | 0.02 | 0.35 | | | 21238 |
| fruit and walnut salad | 264 | 312 | 200.5 | 43.8 | 32.9 | | | 84 | 172 | 34 | 0.74 | | | 384 | 0.10 | 0.3 | 0.16 | 0.42 |
| *9.3 oz salad* | | 4.8 | 13.3 | 1.8 | 2.1 | 8.5 | 5 | | 129 | 0.90 | 0.322 | | 84 | | 0.15 | 0.25 | | 21369 |
| fruit yogurt parfait | 310 | 279 | 242.4 | 54.8 | 36.9 | | 2.8 | 118 | 270 | 37 | 0.93 | 0.378 | | 45 | 0.10 | 0.6 | 0.62 | 1.23 |
| *11 oz* | | 7.7 | 3.5 | 0 | 0 | 0.1 | 16 | 512 | 220 | 1.12 | 0.127 | | 192 | | 0.36 | | | 21381 |
| fruit yogurt parfait w/granola | 338 | 355 | 252.2 | 70.0 | 43.4 | | 3.4 | 196 | 291 | 47 | 1.22 | 0.686 | | 47 | 0.16 | 0.8 | 0.64 | 1.41 |
| *12 oz* | | 9.2 | 4.4 | 0.1 | 0.4 | 0.3 | 17 | 564 | 284 | 1.52 | 0.172 | | 199 | | 0.39 | | | 21380 |
| hamburger | 105 | 265 | 48.0 | 32.2 | 6.9 | | 1.4 | 532 | 127 | 21 | 1.96 | 0.270 | | 1 | 0.26 | 4.8 | 0.87 | |
| *3.8 oz sandwich* | | 13.0 | 9.8 | 3.1 | 3.3 | 0.2 | 28 | 213 | 112 | 2.77 | 0.110 | | 58 | | 0.25 | | | 21228 |
| hashed browns | 53 | 139 | 27.9 | 13.9 | 0 | | 1.5 | 290 | 7 | 11 | 0.18 | 0.088 | 0 | | 0.06 | 1.2 | | 0.23 |
| *1.9 oz* | | 1.2 | 8.7 | 1.2 | 4.5 | 2.6 | 0 | 207 | 57 | 0.30 | 0.046 | | 0 | | 0.01 | 0.13 | | 21319 |
| **ice cream,** van (red fat) in cone | 90 | 146 | 57.3 | 23.7 | 17.5 | | 0.1 | 60 | 116 | 12 | 0.45 | 0.034 | | | 0.04 | 0.4 | 0.52 | 0.66 |
| *3.2 oz cone* | | 3.8 | 4.4 | 2.2 | 1.1 | 0.3 | 14 | 174 | 100 | 0.32 | 0.021 | | 289 | 0 | 0.22 | 0.05 | | 21333 |
| **McChicken Sandwich** w/o mayo | 133 | 319 | 63.1 | 41.2 | 5.5 | | 1.9 | 759 | 128 | 27 | 1.00 | 0.391 | | 1 | 0.31 | 5.8 | 0.23 | |
| *4.7 oz sandwich* | | 14.7 | 11.3 | 2.2 | 4.5 | 3.8 | 29 | 245 | 200 | 2.37 | 0.097 | | 73 | | 0.29 | | | 21356 |
| **McDonaldland cookies** | 57 | 255 | 2.3 | 41.5 | 13.8 | | 0.9 | 275 | 10 | 10 | 0.34 | 0.294 | 0 | | 0.21 | 2.1 | | 0.25 |
| *2 oz box* | | 3.7 | 8.7 | 1.8 | 4.6 | 1.2 | | 56 | 63 | 1.92 | 0.055 | | 0 | 1.1 | 0.17 | 0.07 | | 21326 |
| **McFlurry,** M&M | 348 | 616 | 214.9 | 93.3 | 84.8 | | 0.7 | 188 | 470 | 59 | 1.88 | 0.160 | | | 0.18 | 0.5 | 2.09 | 2.54 |
| *12.3 oz* | | 14.0 | 22.5 | 11.8 | 5.8 | 1.0 | 56 | 724 | 404 | 0.94 | 0.153 | | 1086 | 0.3 | 0.85 | 0.18 | | 21338 |
| **McFlurry,** Oreo | 337 | 556 | 215.3 | 86.1 | 71.4 | | 0.3 | 253 | 435 | 47 | 1.68 | 0.142 | | | 0.16 | 0.9 | 1.95 | 2.43 |
| *11.9 oz* | | 13.4 | 19.1 | 8.7 | 5.8 | 1.2 | 51 | 667 | 374 | 2.06 | 0.101 | | 1089 | 0.3 | 0.77 | 0.20 | | 21339 |
| **McGriddles,** bacon, egg, cheese | 168 | 457 | 77.0 | 44.0 | 16.1 | | 1.3 | 1263 | 183 | | | | | 3 | 0.21 | 2.2 | | |
| *5.9 oz entrée* | | 20.2 | 22.2 | 7.1 | 7.9 | 3.0 | 247 | | | 2.77 | | | 526 | | 0.50 | | | 21327 |
| **McGriddles,** sausage | 135 | 421 | 54.1 | 42.2 | 15.2 | | 1.4 | 995 | 85 | 19 | 1.03 | 0.267 | | 0 | 0.28 | 4.2 | 0.36 | 0.52 |
| *4.7 oz entrée* | | 11.4 | 24.0 | 7.3 | 10.2 | 3.5 | 32 | 196 | 427 | 1.92 | 0.107 | | 0 | | 0.21 | 0.15 | | 21328 |
| **McGriddles,** sausage, egg, cheese | 199 | 563 | 93.6 | 43.9 | 15.7 | | 1.2 | 1297 | 191 | 28 | 2.05 | 0.285 | | 0 | 0.34 | 4.2 | 1.05 | 1.17 |
| *7 oz entrée* | | 21.4 | 35.3 | 11.2 | 13.4 | 4.5 | 263 | 291 | 611 | 3.00 | 0.157 | | 525 | | 0.58 | | | 21329 |
| pancakes and sausage | 264 | 776 | 107.4 | 102.4 | 45.7 | | 2.1 | 935 | 135 | 37 | 1.32 | 0.391 | | 0 | 0.57 | 5.2 | 0.37 | 1.36 |
| *9.3 oz entrée* | | 15.5 | 34.9 | 7.3 | 9.0 | 6.5 | 50 | 391 | 451 | 3.22 | 0.174 | | 533 | | 0.47 | 0.23 | | 21364 |
| pancakes w/margarine and syrup | 228 | 620 | 92.6 | 105.1 | 46.9 | | 2.1 | 645 | 130 | 30 | 0.66 | 0.390 | | 0 | 0.46 | 3.3 | 0.02 | 1.09 |
| *8 oz entree* | | 9.2 | 18.4 | 1.9 | 2.0 | 4.8 | 21 | 285 | 404 | 2.92 | 0.150 | | 549 | | 0.41 | 0.12 | | 21365 |
| **peanuts** for sundaes | 7 | 45 | 0 | 1.1 | 0.3 | | | 0 | 3 | 14 | 0.19 | 0.140 | | | 0.01 | 1.2 | | 0.07 |
| *.3 oz pack* | | 2.0 | 3.7 | 0.6 | 1.8 | 1.0 | | 44 | 25 | 0.10 | 0.029 | | | 0.6 | 0.01 | 0.05 | | 21337 |

| | WT (g) | KCAL | H₂O (g) | CHO (g) | TSUG (g) | ASUG (g) | DFIB (g) | Na (mg) | Ca (mg) | Mg (mg) | Zn (mg) | Mn (mg) | A (mcg RAE) | C (mg) | B-1 (mg) | NIA (mg) | B-12 (mcg) | PANT (mg) |
|---|---|---|---|---|---|---|---|---|---|---|---|---|---|---|---|---|---|---|
| | | PRO (g) | FAT (g) | SFA (g) | MUFA (g) | PUFA (g) | CHOL (mg) | K (mg) | P (mg) | Fe (mg) | Cu (mg) | Se (mcg) | A (IU) | E (mg ATE) | B-2 (mg) | B-6 (mg) | FOL (mcg DFE) | REF |
| **Quarter Pounder** | 171 | 417 | 86.1 | 37.9 | 8.8 | | 2.7 | 730 | 144 | 38 | 4.60 | 0.340 | | 2 | 0.31 | 7.6 | 2.19 | |
| *6.1 oz sandwich* | | 24.1 | 19.8 | 6.9 | 7.2 | 0.5 | 67 | 388 | 212 | 4.12 | 0.183 | | 96 | | 0.59 | | | 21234 |
| **Quarter Pounder w/cheese** | 199 | 513 | 97.3 | 39.7 | 9.8 | | 2.8 | 1152 | 287 | 44 | 5.23 | 0.346 | | 2 | 0.33 | 7.7 | 2.51 | |
| *7.05 oz sandwich* | | 29.0 | 28.3 | 11.2 | 9.2 | 0.9 | 94 | 436 | 320 | 4.18 | 0.193 | | 557 | | 0.70 | | | 21235 |
| **salad, bacon ranch** | 223 | 136 | 194.5 | 9.4 | 4.8 | | 3.3 | 294 | 140 | 22 | | | | 30 | 0.10 | 0.5 | 0.22 | |
| *7.9 oz salad* | | 9.2 | 8.1 | 3.4 | 2.4 | 0.7 | 27 | 448 | 100 | 1.49 | | | 6447 | | 0.13 | | | 21378 |
| **salad, bacon ranch w/crispy chkn** | 323 | 355 | 249.9 | 19.6 | 4.9 | | 3.2 | 953 | 149 | | | | | 31 | 0.19 | 9.8 | 1.81 | |
| *11.4 oz salad* | | 28.5 | 20.3 | 5.2 | 8.0 | 5.2 | 71 | | | 1.97 | | | 8027 | | 0.23 | | | 21377 |
| **salad, bacon ranch w/grilled chkn** | 321 | 260 | 261.4 | 11.7 | 5.6 | | 3.2 | 1005 | 154 | | | | | 33 | 0.18 | 11.9 | 1.56 | |
| *11.3 oz salad* | | 33.0 | 10.1 | 4.0 | 3.3 | 1.4 | 90 | | | 2.09 | | | 6459 | | 0.27 | | | 21376 |
| **salad, Caesar** | 213 | 94 | 191.1 | 9.1 | 4.4 | | 3.4 | 177 | 183 | 19 | | | | 30 | 0.09 | 0.5 | 0 | |
| *7.5 oz salad* | | 6.8 | 4.4 | 2.5 | 1.0 | 0.3 | 11 | 460 | 168 | 1.30 | | 0.4 | 6441 | | 0.08 | | | 21372 |
| **salad, Caesar w/crispy chicken,** | 313 | 326 | 246.6 | 19.4 | 4.6 | | 3.4 | 836 | 191 | | | | | 31 | 0.19 | 9.8 | 1.78 | |
| *11 oz salad* | | 26.0 | 16.6 | 4.4 | 6.6 | 4.8 | 56 | 795 | | 1.78 | | | 8019 | | 0.18 | | | 21371 |
| **salad, chicken, grilled, Caesar** | 163 | 116 | 135.2 | 6.0 | 2.6 | | 1.8 | 465 | 104 | | | | | 17 | 0.09 | 6.2 | 0.80 | |
| *5.7 oz salad* | | 16.0 | 3.3 | 1.6 | 1.0 | 0.5 | 39 | 416 | | 0.99 | | | 3381 | | 0.11 | | | 21370 |
| **salad dressing, balsamic vin lowfat,** Newman's Own - 2 fl oz | 47 | 40 | 31.0 | 11.6 | 3.2 | | 0.2 | 734 | 4 | 1 | 0.01 | 0.019 | | 2 | 0 | 0 | 0 | 0 |
| | | 0.1 | 2.8 | 0.4 | 1.0 | 1.3 | 0 | 9 | 0 | 0.13 | 0.005 | 0 | 52 | 0 | 0 | 0 | | 21348 |
| **salad dressing, cobb, Newman's** Own - 2 fl oz | 62 | 122 | 41.2 | 9.6 | 4.8 | | 0.2 | 440 | 31 | 2 | 0.19 | 0 | | 0 | 0.01 | 0 | 0.03 | 0.01 |
| | | 1.0 | 9.0 | 1.7 | 2.3 | 4.9 | 8 | 12 | 19 | 0.12 | 0 | 0.2 | 58 | 0 | 0.01 | 0 | | 21346 |
| **salad dressing, creamy Caesar,** Newman's Own - 2 fl oz | 59 | 188 | 32.4 | 4.0 | 1.8 | | 0.1 | 502 | 61 | 3 | 0.20 | | | 0 | 0.01 | 0 | 0.05 | 0.06 |
| | | 2.1 | 18.6 | 3.5 | 4.6 | 9.6 | 21 | 16 | 38 | 0.17 | 0.071 | 0.1 | 84 | 15.4 | 0.02 | 0.64 | | 21347 |
| **salad dressing, ranch,** | 22 | 69 | 11.3 | 3.7 | 1.4 | | 0.1 | 210 | 17 | 1 | 0.01 | 0.004 | | 0 | 0 | 0 | 0 | 0.02 |
| *1.5 fl oz packet* | | 0.6 | 5.8 | 1.0 | 3.4 | 1.4 | 7 | 26 | 17 | 0.06 | 0.002 | 0.1 | 15 | | 0.03 | 0.01 | | 21349 |
| **salad, side,** | 206 | 41 | 193.5 | 8.9 | 4.6 | | 3.3 | 25 | 49 | | | | | 32 | 0.09 | 0.4 | 0 | |
| *7.3 oz salad* | | 2.1 | 0.4 | 0 | 0 | 0.2 | 0 | 453 | | 1.34 | | | 5871 | | 0.08 | | | 21379 |
| **sauce, creamy ranch,** | 43 | 201 | 17.8 | 1.5 | 1.5 | | 0 | 304 | 12 | 1 | 0.06 | 0.009 | 0 | 0 | 0.01 | 0 | 0.10 | 0.08 |
| *1.5 oz* | | 0.5 | 22.4 | 3.4 | 4.8 | 12.1 | 9 | 34 | 13 | 0.11 | 0.016 | | 0 | 1.5 | 0.03 | 0.02 | | 21311 |
| **sauce, spicy buffalo,** | 43 | 61 | 32.7 | 0.8 | 0 | | 0.6 | 920 | 4 | 3 | 0.03 | 0.020 | 22 | 0 | 0.01 | 0.2 | 0 | 0.04 |
| *1.5 oz* | | 0.2 | 6.6 | 1.0 | 1.4 | 3.6 | 0 | 43 | 5 | 0.15 | 0.016 | | 442 | 1.2 | 0.02 | 0.10 | | 21314 |
| **Sausage and Egg McMuffin** | 164 | 449 | 81.9 | 28.3 | 2.6 | | 1.5 | 938 | 282 | 30 | 2.00 | 0.310 | | 0 | 0.43 | 4.8 | 1.15 | 1.34 |
| *1 McMuffin* | | 20.6 | 29.2 | 9.9 | 10.8 | 4.5 | 253 | 280 | 280 | 3.23 | 0.154 | | 549 | 0.8 | 0.56 | 0.24 | | 21359 |
| **Sausage McMuffin** | 114 | 380 | 44.4 | 28.0 | 2.2 | | 1.6 | 790 | 255 | 24 | 1.46 | 0.290 | | 0 | 0.40 | 4.8 | 0.51 | 0.63 |
| *1 McMuffin* | | 14.4 | 24.0 | 8.3 | 8.8 | 3.7 | 44 | 214 | 186 | 2.33 | 0.104 | | 296 | 0.3 | 0.33 | 0.17 | | 21358 |
| **sausage patty,** | 43 | 174 | 17.7 | 0.6 | 0.2 | | | 310 | 10 | 7 | 0.68 | 0.014 | | 0 | 0.13 | 2.0 | 0.36 | 0.30 |
| *1.5 oz* | | 6.5 | 17.0 | 5.5 | 7.2 | 2.1 | 32 | 115 | 60 | 0.39 | 0.026 | | 0 | 0 | 0.07 | 0.11 | | 21323 |
| **shake, chocolate** | 250 | 318 | 178.8 | 51.2 | 46.5 | 34.2 | 4.8 | 242 | 282 | 42 | 1.02 | 0.098 | 65 | 1 | 0.15 | 0.4 | 0.85 | 0.98 |
| *12 fl oz* | | 8.5 | 9.2 | 5.8 | 2.7 | 0.4 | 32 | 500 | 255 | 0.78 | 0.162 | 4.2 | 232 | 0.3 | 0.61 | 0.12 | 12.5 | 14346 |
| **shake, chocolate, triple thick** | 333 | 543 | 209.7 | 92.8 | 78.7 | | 0.7 | 236 | 406 | 53 | 1.66 | 0.166 | 303 | | 0.13 | 0.4 | 1.80 | 2.23 |
| *16 fl oz* | | 12.3 | 15.0 | 7.7 | 3.7 | 0.7 | 47 | 753 | 350 | 1.80 | 0.163 | | 1006 | 0 | 0.71 | 0.17 | | 21331 |
| **shake, strawberry** | 333 | 526 | 214.6 | 89.2 | 79.2 | | 0 | 163 | 406 | 40 | 1.43 | 0.087 | 303 | 1 | 0.13 | 0.4 | 1.83 | 2.23 |
| *16 fl oz* | | 11.7 | 14.8 | 7.5 | 3.6 | 0.7 | 47 | 613 | 333 | 0.30 | 0.047 | | 1012 | 0 | 0.70 | 0.17 | | 21332 |
| **shake, vanilla** | 250 | 370 | 174.1 | 49.0 | 34.1 | 20.4 | 2.2 | 202 | 288 | 32 | 1.42 | 0.088 | 228 | 0 | 0.06 | 0.5 | 0.55 | 1.41 |
| *12 fl oz* | | 8.4 | 16.3 | 9.9 | 4.5 | 0.8 | 58 | 415 | 245 | 1.15 | 0.258 | 8.0 | 760 | 0.6 | 1.65 | 0.15 | 0 | 14347 |
| **shake, vanilla, triple thick** | 333 | 519 | 215.4 | 88.6 | 68.0 | | 0 | 176 | 403 | 40 | 1.43 | 0.027 | | | 0.13 | 0.4 | 1.83 | 2.22 |
| *16 fl oz* | | 11.6 | 14.8 | 7.5 | 3.6 | 0.7 | 47 | 586 | 333 | 0.23 | 0.043 | | 1012 | 0 | 0.70 | 0.16 | | 21330 |
| **sundae, hot caramel** | 182 | 342 | 104.2 | 60.7 | 42.8 | | 0 | 146 | 231 | 22 | 0.82 | 0.016 | 167 | | 0.07 | 0.2 | 0.93 | 1.24 |
| *6.4 oz sundae* | | 6.5 | 8.9 | 4.5 | 2.2 | 0.4 | 29 | 339 | 204 | 0.15 | 0.027 | | 559 | 0 | 0.41 | 0.09 | | 21335 |
| **sundae, hot fudge** | 179 | 333 | 105.3 | 53.8 | 48.1 | | 0.7 | 168 | 249 | 34 | 1.00 | 0.118 | 145 | | 0.08 | 0.3 | 0.98 | 1.34 |
| *6.3 oz sundae* | | 7.4 | 10.6 | 6.4 | 1.9 | 0.4 | 23 | 440 | 229 | 1.49 | 0.091 | | 483 | 0.3 | 0.40 | 0.09 | | 21336 |
| **sundae, strawberry** | 178 | 281 | 114.0 | 50.0 | 45.1 | | 0 | 84 | 196 | 20 | 0.69 | 0.126 | 144 | 3 | 0.07 | 0.2 | 0.87 | 1.09 |
| *6.3 oz sundae* | | 5.7 | 7.0 | 3.6 | 1.7 | 0.3 | 23 | 308 | 162 | 0.18 | 0.027 | | 482 | 0 | 0.35 | 0.09 | | 21334 |

## 10.15 PAPA JOHN'S

| | WT (g) | KCAL | H₂O (g) | CHO (g) | TSUG (g) | ASUG (g) | DFIB (g) | Na (mg) | Ca (mg) | Mg (mg) | Zn (mg) | Mn (mg) | A (mcg RAE) | C (mg) | B-1 (mg) | NIA (mg) | B-12 (mcg) | PANT (mg) |
|---|---|---|---|---|---|---|---|---|---|---|---|---|---|---|---|---|---|---|
| | | PRO (g) | FAT (g) | SFA (g) | MUFA (g) | PUFA (g) | CHOL (mg) | K (mg) | P (mg) | Fe (mg) | Cu (mg) | Se (mcg) | A (IU) | E (mg ATE) | B-2 (mg) | B-6 (mg) | FOL (mcg DFE) | REF |
| **pizza, cheese, regular crust** | 117 | 304 | 51.7 | 38.3 | 6.2 | | 2.2 | 676 | 194 | 28 | 1.45 | 0.395 | 70 | 0 | 0.53 | 3.6 | 0.80 | 0.21 |
| *4.1 oz slice* | | 13.5 | 10.8 | 4.5 | 2.9 | 2.3 | 22 | 161 | 238 | 2.30 | 0.146 | 32.3 | 343 | 1.3 | 1.43 | 0.14 | 127.5 | 21283 |
| **pizza, cheese, thin crust** | 87 | 257 | 37.7 | 22.8 | 3.3 | | 2.0 | 459 | 207 | 19 | 1.09 | 0.183 | 73 | 0 | 0.41 | 0.8 | 0.72 | 0.12 |
| *3.1 oz slice* | | 10.7 | 13.6 | 5.4 | 5.2 | 1.4 | 24 | 139 | 213 | 0.44 | 0.130 | 25.2 | 339 | 1.5 | 0.19 | | | 21286 |
| **pizza, pepperoni, regular crust** | 123 | 338 | 53.6 | 36.9 | 6.0 | | 1.5 | 825 | 187 | 28 | 1.65 | 0.428 | 71 | 0 | 0.53 | 4.0 | 0.97 | 0.33 |
| *4.3 oz slice* | | 14.7 | 14.6 | 6.0 | 4.8 | 2.7 | 32 | 184 | 241 | 2.44 | 0.157 | 36.0 | 362 | 1.4 | 0.60 | 0.20 | 125.5 | 21284 |
| **pizza, The Works, regular crust** | 153 | 367 | 77.4 | 40.8 | 7.4 | | 3.8 | 872 | 151 | 32 | 1.50 | 0.431 | 47 | 0 | 0.36 | 4.9 | 1.10 | 0.50 |
| *5.4 oz slice* | | 15.7 | 15.6 | 5.8 | 5.6 | 2.9 | 32 | 245 | 245 | 2.30 | 0.228 | 41.0 | 263 | 1.6 | 0.45 | | 140.8 | 21285 |

| | WT (g) | Macronutrients | | | | | | Minerals | | | | | Vitamins | | | | | |
|---|---|---|---|---|---|---|---|---|---|---|---|---|---|---|---|---|---|---|
| | | KCAL | H₂0 (g) | CHO (g) | TSUG (g) | ASUG (g) | DFIB (g) | Na (mg) | Ca (mg) | Mg (mg) | Zn (mg) | Mn (mg) | A (mcg RAE) | C (mg) | B-1 (mg) | NIA (mg) | B-12 (mcg) | PANT (mg) |
| | | PRO (g) | FAT (g) | SFA (g) | MUFA (g) | PUFA (g) | CHOL (mg) | K (mg) | P (mg) | Fe (mg) | Cu (mg) | Se (mcg) | A (IU) | E (mg ATE) | B-2 (mg) | B-6 (mg) | FOL (mcg DFE) | REF |

## 10.16 PIZZA HUT

| | WT (g) | KCAL / PRO | H₂0 / FAT | CHO / SFA | TSUG / MUFA | ASUG / PUFA | DFIB / CHOL | Na / K | Ca / P | Mg / Fe | Zn / Cu | Mn / Se | A(RAE) / A(IU) | C / E | B-1 / B-2 | NIA / B-6 | B-12 / FOL | PANT / REF |
|---|---|---|---|---|---|---|---|---|---|---|---|---|---|---|---|---|---|---|
| **pizza, cheese, regular crust** | 106 | 287 | 45.9 | 33.1 | 3.6 | | 1.9 | 726 | 222 | 23 | 1.75 | 0.326 | 87 | 0 | 0.28 | 3.5 | 0.74 | 0.30 |
| *3.7 oz slice* | | 12.6 | 11.5 | 5.3 | 3.1 | 1.9 | 25 | 183 | 264 | 2.07 | 0.098 | 21.7 | 461 | 0.7 | 0.27 | 0.12 | | 21271 |
| **pizza, cheese, reg crust, 14"** | 100 | 271 | 43.2 | 31.6 | 3.2 | | 1.1 | 632 | 189 | 21 | 1.46 | 0.310 | 69 | 0 | 0.37 | 3.6 | 0.71 | 0.33 |
| *diameter - 3.5 oz slice* | | 11.8 | 10.9 | 4.4 | 2.6 | 1.8 | 26 | 157 | 227 | 1.96 | 0.091 | 13.3 | 311 | 0.6 | 0.27 | 0.12 | 149.0 | 21293 |
| **pizza, cheese, thick crust,** | 95 | 266 | 41.1 | 28.5 | 2.5 | | 0.9 | 533 | 178 | 20 | 1.21 | 0.262 | 68 | 0 | 0.38 | 3.1 | 0.75 | 0.22 |
| *14" diameter - 3.4 oz slice* | | 11.4 | 11.8 | 4.7 | 3.0 | 2.7 | 28 | 140 | 214 | 1.54 | | 16.9 | 307 | 0.7 | 0.26 | 0.06 | 144.4 | 21294 |
| **pizza, cheese, Thin n' Crispy** | 85 | 258 | 33.0 | 24.3 | 2.3 | | 1.4 | 666 | 236 | 20 | 1.59 | 0.252 | 91 | 0 | 0.19 | 2.5 | 0.76 | 0.27 |
| *2.8 oz slice* | | 13.0 | 12.0 | 5.9 | 3.2 | 1.4 | 29 | 162 | 269 | 1.45 | 0.082 | 19.6 | 318 | 0.7 | 0.23 | 0.09 | | 21273 |
| **pizza, cheese, Thin n' Crispy,** | 76 | 225 | 29.8 | 22.1 | 1.9 | | 0.8 | 595 | 200 | 19 | 1.14 | 0.201 | 74 | 0 | 0.25 | 4.1 | 0.66 | 0.18 |
| *14" diameter - 2.7 oz slice* | | 11.6 | 10.1 | 4.9 | 2.7 | 1.3 | 31 | 135 | 230 | 1.10 | 0.125 | 16.0 | 336 | 0.5 | 0.23 | 0.06 | 102.6 | 21295 |
| **pizza, pepperoni, reg crust,** | 101 | 290 | 40.9 | 32.8 | 3.2 | | 2.6 | 751 | 140 | 22 | 1.47 | 0.364 | 48 | 0 | 0.41 | 4.4 | 0.73 | 0.40 |
| *14" diameter - 3.6 oz slice* | | 12.3 | 12.1 | 4.8 | 3.7 | 2.1 | 29 | 186 | 199 | 2.15 | 0.097 | 16.2 | 255 | 0.7 | 0.33 | 0.15 | 160.6 | 21296 |
| **pizza, pepperoni, regular crust** | 116 | 325 | 48.0 | 36.6 | 4.3 | | 2.0 | 929 | 180 | 27 | 1.95 | 0.423 | 66 | 0 | 0.37 | 4.7 | 0.79 | 0.54 |
| *4.1 oz slice* | | 14.9 | 13.2 | 6.0 | 4.7 | 2.4 | 30 | 240 | 253 | 2.48 | 0.121 | 24.7 | 237 | 0.9 | 0.31 | 0.18 | | 21274 |
| **pizza, pepperoni, thick crust,** | 85 | 253 | 34.8 | 25.4 | 2.1 | | 1.3 | 568 | 119 | 19 | 1.06 | 0.269 | 41 | 0 | 0.33 | 2.8 | 0.71 | 0.27 |
| *14" diameter - 3.5 oz slice* | | 10.4 | 12.2 | 4.2 | 3.5 | 2.8 | 27 | 139 | 167 | 1.40 | | 16.8 | 195 | 0.8 | 0.26 | 0.08 | 121.6 | 21297 |
| **pizza, Super Supreme, regular** | 139 | 338 | 69.8 | 35.6 | 5.2 | | 2.8 | 958 | 179 | 32 | 2.02 | 0.450 | 50 | 0 | 0.37 | 5.0 | 0.86 | 0.61 |
| *crust - 4.9 oz slice* | | 15.2 | 14.9 | 6.3 | 5.5 | 2.4 | 28 | 324 | 278 | 2.78 | 0.177 | 27.1 | 190 | 1.1 | 0.34 | 0.20 | | 21276 |
| **pizza, Super Supreme, reg crust,** | 127 | 315 | 62.4 | 33.0 | 3.9 | | 2.9 | 836 | 132 | 29 | 1.46 | 0.362 | 41 | 1 | 0.47 | 3.0 | 1.07 | 0.54 |
| *14" diameter - 4.5 oz slice* | | 14.4 | 13.9 | 5.4 | 4.8 | 2.4 | 36 | 264 | 232 | 1.94 | 0.189 | 18.4 | 198 | 0.8 | 0.37 | 0.12 | 105.4 | 21298 |

## 10.17 POPEYE'S

| | WT (g) | KCAL / PRO | H₂0 / FAT | CHO / SFA | TSUG / MUFA | ASUG / PUFA | DFIB / CHOL | Na / K | Ca / P | Mg / Fe | Zn / Cu | Mn / Se | A(RAE) / A(IU) | C / E | B-1 / B-2 | NIA / B-6 | B-12 / FOL | PANT / REF |
|---|---|---|---|---|---|---|---|---|---|---|---|---|---|---|---|---|---|---|
| **biscuit** | 60 | 240 | | 26.0 | 2.0 | | 1.0 | 490 | | | | | | | | | | |
| *2.1 oz* | | 4.0 | 13.0 | 7.0 | | | 0 | | | | | | | | | | | POPE29 |
| **Cajun rice** | 117 | 170 | | 22.0 | 1.0 | | 2.0 | 530 | | | | | | | | | | |
| *4.1 oz* | | 8.0 | 6.0 | 2.0 | | | 60 | | | | | | | | | | | POPE35 |
| **Cajun wings** | 244 | 595 | | 19.0 | 0 | | 0 | 1274 | | | | | | | | | | |
| *6 pieces* | | 34.0 | 43.0 | 15.0 | | | 260 | | | | | | | | | | | POPE14 |
| **chicken biscuit** | 102 | 350 | | 30.0 | 0 | | | 930 | | | | | | | | | | |
| *3.6 oz biscuit* | | 13.0 | 20.0 | 9.0 | | | 35 | | | | | | | | | | | POPE18 |
| **chicken bowl** | 368 | 570 | | 44.0 | 2.0 | | 8.0 | 1600 | | | | | | | | | | |
| *13 oz bowl* | | 35.0 | 29.0 | 10.0 | | | 100 | | | | | | | | | | | POPE19 |
| **chicken nuggets** | 71 | 220 | | 13.0 | 0 | | | 500 | | | | | | | | | | |
| *6 pieces* | | 15.0 | 12.0 | 5.0 | | | 40 | | | | | | | | | | | POPE11 |
| **chicken sausage jambalaya** | 151 | 220 | | 20.0 | 3.0 | | 1.0 | 760 | | | | | | | | | | |
| *5.3 oz* | | 10.0 | 11.0 | 3.0 | | | 32 | | | | | | | | | | | POPE25 |
| **coleslaw** | 138 | 260 | | 14.0 | 15.0 | | 9.0 | 260 | | | | | | | | | | |
| *4.9 oz* | | | 23.0 | 3.5 | | | 15 | | | | | | | | | | | POPE36 |
| **corn-on-the-cob** | 284 | 190 | | 37.0 | 7.0 | | 4.0 | 0 | | | | | | | | | | |
| *10 oz ear* | | 6.0 | 2.0 | 0.5 | | | 0 | | | | | | | | | | | POPE31 |
| **crispy chicken sandwich** | 227 | 560 | | 56.0 | 12.0 | | 3.0 | 1690 | | | | | | | | | | |
| *8 oz sandwich* | | 33.0 | 23.0 | 8.0 | | | 75 | | | | | | | | | | | POPE20 |
| **Delta mini** | 101 | 300 | | 30.0 | 4.0 | | 1.0 | 780 | | | | | | | | | | |
| *3.6 oz* | | 15.0 | 13.0 | 4.0 | | | 30 | | | | | | | | | | | POPE17 |
| **deluxe mild/spicy chicken sandwich** | 265 | 630 | | 53.0 | 5.0 | | 3.0 | 1480 | | | | | | | | | | |
| *w/mayo - 9.4 oz sandwich* | | 35.0 | 31.0 | 8.0 | | | 71 | | | | | | | | | | | POPE21 |
| **etouffee, chicken** | 151 | 160 | | 6.0 | 1.0 | | 2.0 | 870 | | | | | | | | | | |
| *5.3 oz* | | 12.0 | 10.0 | 3.0 | | | 20 | | | | | | | | | | | POPE27 |
| **etouffee, crawfish** | 151 | 180 | | 25.0 | 0 | | 2.0 | 640 | | | | | | | | | | |
| *5.3 oz* | | 7.0 | 5.0 | 1.0 | | | 48 | | | | | | | | | | | POPE28 |
| **French fries** | 88 | 310 | | 35.0 | 1.0 | | 3.0 | 660 | | | | | | | | | | |
| *3.1 oz* | | 4.0 | 17.0 | 7.0 | | | 7 | | | | | | | | | | | POPE30 |
| **green beans** | 100 | 70 | | 14.0 | 1.0 | | 2.0 | 400 | | | | | | | | | | |
| *3.5 oz* | | 2.0 | 1.0 | 0 | | | 5 | | | | | | | | | | | POPE37 |
| **loaded chicken wrap** | 170 | 400 | | 44.0 | 0 | | 4.0 | 1100 | | | | | | | | | | |
| *6 oz wrap* | | 19.0 | 17.0 | 6.0 | | | 35 | | | | | | | | | | | POPE16 |
| **mashed potatoes** | 113 | 100 | | 17.0 | 3.0 | | | 380 | | | | | | | | | | |
| *4 oz* | | 1.0 | 3.0 | 1.0 | | | 0 | | | | | | | | | | | POPE32 |
| **mashed potatoes and gravy** | 142 | 120 | | 18.0 | 0 | | 2.0 | 570 | | | | | | | | | | |
| *5 oz* | | 3.0 | 4.0 | 2.0 | | | 5 | | | | | | | | | | | POPE33 |

| | WT (g) | KCAL | H₂0 (g) | CHO (g) | TSUG (g) | ASUG (g) | DFIB (g) | Na (mg) | Ca (mg) | Mg (mg) | Zn (mg) | Mn (mg) | A (mcg RAE) | C (mg) | B-1 (mg) | NIA (mg) | B-12 (mcg) | PANT (mg) |
|---|---|---|---|---|---|---|---|---|---|---|---|---|---|---|---|---|---|---|
| | | PRO (g) | FAT (g) | SFA (g) | MUFA (g) | PUFA (g) | CHOL (mg) | K (mg) | P (mg) | Fe (mg) | Cu (mg) | Se (mcg) | A (IU) | E (mg ATE) | B-2 (mg) | B-6 (mg) | FOL (mcg DFE) | REF |
| mild chicken breast | 179 | 350 | | 8.0 | 0 | | 0 | 1130 | | | | | | | | | | |
| 6.3 oz | | 33.0 | 20.0 | 7.0 | | | 179 | | | | | | | | | | | POPE4 |
| mild chicken leg | 63 | 110 | | 3.0 | 0 | | 0 | 280 | | | | | | | | | | |
| 2.2 oz | | 11.0 | 7.0 | 2.5 | | | 92 | | | | | | | | | | | POPE2 |
| mild chicken strips | 94 | 130 | | 3.0 | 0 | | 0 | 620 | | | | | | | | | | |
| 2 pieces (3.3 oz) | | 25.0 | 2.5 | 1.0 | | | 50 | | | | | | | | | | | POPE5 |
| mild chicken tenders | 174 | 375 | | 24.0 | 0 | | 0 | 1620 | | | | | | | | | | |
| 3 pieces | | 33.0 | 17.0 | 7.0 | | | 84 | | | | | | | | | | | POPE12 |
| mild chicken thigh | 111 | 280 | | 7.0 | 0 | | 0 | 710 | | | | | | | | | | |
| 3.9 oz | | 16.0 | 20.0 | 7.0 | | | 135 | | | | | | | | | | | POPE3 |
| mild chicken wing | 59 | 150 | | 5.0 | 0 | | 0 | 690 | | | | | | | | | | |
| 2.1 oz | | 9.0 | 10.0 | 3.5 | | | 59 | | | | | | | | | | | POPE1 |
| naked chicken strips | 118 | 220 | | 2.0 | 0 | | 0 | 720 | | | | | | | | | | |
| 3 pieces | | 30.0 | 10.0 | 4.0 | | | 80 | | | | | | | | | | | POPE15 |
| Po Boy sandwich | 113 | 330 | | 36.0 | 10.0 | | 0 | 560 | | | | | | | | | | |
| 4 oz sandwich | | 8.0 | 17.0 | 3.0 | | | 10 | | | | | | | | | | | POPE22 |
| red beans and rice | 174 | 320 | | 31.0 | 2.0 | | 17.0 | 710 | | | | | | | | | | |
| 6.1 oz | | 10.0 | 19.0 | 6.0 | | | 20 | | | | | | | | | | | POPE34 |
| shrimp, butterfly | 102 | 310 | | 22.0 | 0 | | 2.0 | 800 | | | | | | | | | | |
| 3.6 oz | | 13.0 | 19.0 | 8.0 | | | 90 | | | | | | | | | | | POPE24 |
| shrimp, popcorn | 85 | 280 | | 22.0 | 0 | | | 1110 | | | | | | | | | | |
| 3 oz | | 12.0 | 16.0 | 6.0 | | | 95 | | | | | | | | | | | POPE23 |
| smothered chicken | 151 | 210 | | 24.0 | 0 | | 1.0 | 743 | | | | | | | | | | |
| 5.3 oz | | 10.0 | 8.0 | 2.0 | | | 23 | | | | | | | | | | | POPE26 |
| spicy chicken breast | 179 | 360 | | 8.0 | 0 | | 1.0 | 760 | | | | | | | | | | |
| 6.3 oz | | 31.0 | 22.0 | 8.0 | | | 170 | | | | | | | | | | | POPE9 |
| spicy chicken leg | 63 | 100 | | 3.0 | 0 | | 0 | 230 | | | | | | | | | | |
| 2.2 oz | | 9.0 | 5.0 | 2.0 | | | 71 | | | | | | | | | | | POPE7 |
| spicy chicken strips | 94 | 150 | | 5.0 | 0 | | 0 | 820 | | | | | | | | | | |
| 3.3 oz (2 pieces) | | 23.0 | 4.0 | 1.5 | | | 55 | | | | | | | | | | | POPE10 |
| spicy chicken tenders | 174 | 405 | | 30.0 | 0 | | 0 | 2160 | | | | | | | | | | |
| 2 pieces | | 33.0 | 17.0 | 7.0 | | | 84 | | | | | | | | | | | POPE13 |
| spicy chicken thigh | 111 | 300 | | 7.0 | 0 | | 0 | 490 | | | | | | | | | | |
| 3.9 oz | | 15.0 | 24.0 | 8.0 | | | 131 | | | | | | | | | | | POPE8 |
| spicy chicken wing | 59 | 140 | | 5.0 | 0 | | 0 | 290 | | | | | | | | | | |
| 2.1 oz | | 8.0 | 9.0 | 3.5 | | | 79 | | | | | | | | | | | POPE6 |
| turnover, cinnamon apple | 86 | 250 | | 34.0 | 11.0 | | 2.0 | 320 | | | | | | | | | | |
| 3 oz turnover | | 3.0 | 12.0 | 4.0 | | | 5 | | | | | | | | | | | POPE38 |

## 10.18 STARBUCKS

| | WT (g) | KCAL | H₂0 (g) | CHO (g) | TSUG (g) | ASUG (g) | DFIB (g) | Na (mg) | Ca (mg) | Mg (mg) | Zn (mg) | Mn (mg) | A (mcg RAE) | C (mg) | B-1 (mg) | NIA (mg) | B-12 (mcg) | PANT (mg) |
|---|---|---|---|---|---|---|---|---|---|---|---|---|---|---|---|---|---|---|
| | | PRO (g) | FAT (g) | SFA (g) | MUFA (g) | PUFA (g) | CHOL (mg) | K (mg) | P (mg) | Fe (mg) | Cu (mg) | Se (mcg) | A (IU) | E (mg ATE) | B-2 (mg) | B-6 (mg) | FOL (mcg DFE) | REF |
| **Caffe Americano** | 475 | 15 | | 3.0 | 0 | | 0 | 10 | 20 | | | | | 0 | | | | |
| grande (16 fl oz) | | 1.0 | 0 | 0 | | | 0 | | | 0 | | | 0 | | | | | STAR1 |
| **Caffe Latte** with whole milk | 480 | 220 | | 18.0 | 16.0 | | 0 | 140 | 400 | | | | | 0 | | | | |
| grande (16 fl oz) | | 12.0 | 11.0 | 7.0 | | | 35 | | | 0 | | | 400 | | | | | STAR2 |
| **Caffe Mocha** w/whole milk and | 480 | 360 | | 42.0 | 32.0 | | 2.0 | 125 | 350 | | | | | 0 | | | | |
| whpd crm - grande (16 fl oz) | | 13.0 | 19.0 | 10.0 | | | 55 | | | 3.60 | | | 500 | | | | | STAR3 |
| **cappuccino** with whole milk | 480 | 140 | | 11.0 | 9.0 | | 0 | 85 | 250 | | | | | 0 | | | | |
| grande (16 fl oz) | | 7.0 | 7.0 | 4.0 | | | 20 | | | 0 | | | 200 | | | | | STAR4 |
| **caramel apple spice** cider w/whipped | 480 | 380 | | 76.0 | 68.0 | | 0 | 30 | 250 | | | | | 0 | | | | |
| cream - grande (16 fl oz) | | 0 | 8.0 | 4.5 | | | 25 | | | 1.44 | | | 300 | | | | | STAR19 |
| **Caramel Macchiato** w/whole milk | 480 | 270 | | 34.0 | 31.0 | | 0 | 130 | 350 | | | | | 0 | | | | |
| grande (16 fl oz) | | 10.0 | 10.0 | 6.0 | | | 30 | | | 0 | | | 300 | | | | | STAR5 |
| **espresso** | 30 | 5 | | 1.0 | 0 | | 0 | 0 | 0 | | | | | 0 | | | | |
| solo (1 fl oz) | | 0 | 0 | 0 | | | 0 | | | 0 | | | 0 | | | | | STAR6 |
| **Frappuccino**, caramel, light | 480 | 160 | | 30.0 | 21.0 | | 3.0 | 230 | 150 | | | | | 0 | | | | |
| grande (16 fl oz) | | 5.0 | 1.5 | 0 | | | 5 | | | 0 | | | 0 | | | | | STAR13 |
| **Frappuccino**, caramel w/whipped | 480 | 380 | | 57.0 | 48.0 | | 0 | 240 | 200 | | | | | 0 | | | | |
| cream - grande (16 fl oz) | | 6.0 | 15.0 | 9.0 | | | 55 | | | 0 | | | 500 | | | | | STAR10 |
| **Frappuccino**, cinn dolce w/whpd | 480 | 370 | | 55.0 | 47.0 | | 0 | 240 | 200 | | | | | 0 | | | | |
| crm - grande (16 fl oz) | | 6.0 | 14.0 | 9.0 | | | 55 | | | 0 | | | 500 | | | | | STAR11 |
| **Frappuccino**, mocha, light | 480 | 140 | | 29.0 | 19.0 | | 3.0 | 230 | 150 | | | | | 0 | | | | |
| grande (16 fl oz) | | 6.0 | 1.0 | 0 | | | 0 | | | 0.72 | | | 0 | | | | | STAR14 |

| | WT (g) | KCAL · PRO (g) | H₂O (g) · FAT (g) | CHO (g) · SFA (g) | TSUG (g) · MUFA (g) | ASUG (g) · PUFA (g) | DFIB (g) · CHOL (mg) | Na (mg) · K (mg) | Ca (mg) · P (mg) | Mg (mg) · Fe (mg) | Zn (mg) · Cu (mg) | Mn (mg) · Se (mcg) | A (mcg RAE) · A (IU) | C (mg) · E (mg ATE) | B-1 (mg) · B-2 (mg) | NIA (mg) · B-6 (mg) | B-12 (mcg) · FOL (mcg DFE) | PANT (mg) · REF |
|---|---|---|---|---|---|---|---|---|---|---|---|---|---|---|---|---|---|---|
| Frappuccino, mocha w/whipped | 480 | 380 | | 57.0 | 47.0 | | 0 | 240 | 200 | | | | | 0 | | | | |
| cream - *grande (16 fl oz)* | | 6.0 | 15.0 | 9.0 | | | 55 | | | 0.72 | | | 500 | | | | | STAR27 |
| Frappuccino, van, light | 480 | 190 | | 42.0 | 32.0 | | 3.0 | 240 | 150 | | | | | | | | | |
| *grande (16 fl oz)* | | 6.0 | 1.0 | 0 | | | 0 | | | | | | 0 | | | | | STAR12 |
| Frappuccino, van w/whipped | 480 | 430 | | 70.0 | 60.0 | | 0 | 240 | 200 | | | | | 0 | | | | |
| cream *grande (16 fl oz)* | | 6.0 | 14.0 | 9.0 | | | 55 | | | 0 | | | 500 | | | | | STAR9 |
| hot chocolate w/whole milk and | 480 | 400 | | 49.0 | 40.0 | | 2.0 | 150 | 400 | | | | | 0 | | | | |
| whpd crm - *grande (16 fl oz)* | | 14.0 | 20.0 | 11.0 | | | 60 | | | 3.60 | | | 500 | | | | | STAR20 |
| Iced Caffe Latte w/whole milk | 480 | 150 | | 12.0 | 10.0 | | 0 | 95 | 250 | | | | | 0 | | | | |
| *grande (16 fl oz)* | | 8.0 | 7.0 | 4.5 | | | 25 | | | 0 | | | 200 | | | | | STAR7 |
| Iced Caffe Mocha w/whole milk and | 480 | 330 | | 38.0 | 28.0 | | 2.0 | 85 | 250 | | | | | 0 | | | | |
| whpd crm - *grande (16 fl oz)* | | 9.0 | 19.0 | 10.0 | | | 60 | | | 3.60 | | | 500 | | | | | STAR8 |
| iced tea, Tazo black/green, | 475 | 80 | | 21.0 | 20.0 | | 0 | 10 | 0 | | | | | 0 | | | | |
| sweetened - *grande (16 fl oz)* | | 0 | 0 | 0 | | | 0 | | | 0 | | | 0 | | | | | STAR16 |
| iced tea, Tazo passion, sweetened, | 475 | 80 | | 21.0 | 20.0 | | 0 | 10 | 0 | | | | | 0 | | | | |
| *grande (16 fl oz)* | | 0 | 0 | 0 | | | 0 | | | 0 | | | 0 | | | | | STAR18 |
| Latte, cinn dolce, w/whole milk and | 480 | 370 | | 41.0 | 39.0 | | 0 | 140 | 350 | | | | | 0 | | | | |
| whpd crm - *grande (16 fl oz)* | | 11.0 | 17.0 | 10.0 | | | 60 | | | 0 | | | 500 | | | | | STAR22 |
| Latte, van, skinny | 480 | 130 | | 19.0 | 17.0 | | 0 | 170 | 400 | | | | | 0 | | | | |
| *grande (16 fl oz)* | | 12.0 | 0 | 0 | | | 5 | | | 0 | | | 750 | | | | | STAR23 |
| Latte, van w/whole milk | 480 | 280 | | 36.0 | 33.0 | | 0 | 135 | 350 | | | | | 0 | | | | |
| *grande (16 fl oz)* | | 11.0 | 11.0 | 6.0 | | | 35 | | | 0 | | | 300 | | | | | STAR24 |
| lemonade w/Tazo Zen green tea | 475 | 190 | | 47.0 | 45.0 | | 1.0 | 5 | 0 | | | | | 9 | | | | |
| *grande (16 fl oz)* | | 0 | 0 | 0 | | | 0 | | | 0 | | | 0 | | | | | STAR15 |
| white chocolate mocha w/whl mlk and | 480 | 500 | | 62.0 | 59.0 | | 0 | 240 | 500 | | | | | 0 | | | | |
| whpd crm - *grande (16 fl oz)* | | 15.0 | 22.0 | 14.0 | | | 55 | | | 0 | | | 500 | | | | | STAR17 |
| white hot chocolate w/whl mlk and | 480 | 520 | | 63.0 | 61.0 | | 0 | 260 | 500 | | | | | 0 | | | | |
| whpd crm - *grande (16 fl oz)* | | 16.0 | 24.0 | 15.0 | | | 60 | | | 0 | | | 750 | | | | | STAR21 |

## 10.19 SUBWAY

| | WT (g) | KCAL · PRO (g) | H₂O (g) · FAT (g) | CHO (g) · SFA (g) | TSUG (g) · MUFA (g) | ASUG (g) · PUFA (g) | DFIB (g) · CHOL (mg) | Na (mg) · K (mg) | Ca (mg) · P (mg) | Mg (mg) · Fe (mg) | Zn (mg) · Cu (mg) | Mn (mg) · Se (mcg) | A (mcg RAE) · A (IU) | C (mg) · E (mg ATE) | B-1 (mg) · B-2 (mg) | NIA (mg) · B-6 (mg) | B-12 (mcg) · FOL (mcg DFE) | PANT (mg) · REF |
|---|---|---|---|---|---|---|---|---|---|---|---|---|---|---|---|---|---|---|
| 6-inch sub, chicken and bacon | 297 | 580 | | 47.0 | 7.0 | | 6.0 | 1390 | 300 | | | | | 24 | | | | |
| ranch - *10.5 oz sub* | | 36.0 | 30.0 | 11.0 | | | 99 | | | 4.50 | | | 750 | | | | | SUBW73 |
| 6-inch sub, cold cut combo | 249 | 410 | | 47.0 | 8.0 | | 5.0 | 1530 | 200 | | | | | 21 | | | | |
| *8.8 oz sub* | | 21.0 | 17.0 | 7.0 | | | 60 | | | 5.40 | | | 500 | | | | | SUBW74 |
| 6-inch sub, double chicken and bcn | 377 | 710 | | 48.0 | 8.0 | | 6.0 | 1890 | 300 | | | | | 27 | | | | |
| ranch w/chs - *13.3 oz sub* | | 55.0 | 35.0 | 13.0 | | | 160 | | | 5.40 | | | 750 | | | | | SUBW102 |
| 6-inch sub, double cold cut combo | 320 | 550 | | 49.0 | 8.0 | | 5.0 | 2360 | 250 | | | | | 24 | | | | |
| w/cheese - *11.3 oz sub* | | 31.0 | 28.0 | 10.0 | | | 110 | | | 6.30 | | | 750 | | | | | SUBW103 |
| 6-inch sub, double ham | 281 | 350 | | 49.0 | 9.0 | | 5.0 | 2020 | 80 | | | | | 21 | | | | |
| *9.9 oz sub* | | 28.0 | 7.0 | 2.5 | | | 50 | | | 5.40 | | | 400 | | | | | SUBW95 |
| 6-inch sub, double Italian BMT | 306 | 630 | | 49.0 | 10.0 | | 5.0 | 2850 | 150 | | | | | 21 | | | | |
| with cheese - *10.8 oz sub* | | 34.0 | 35.0 | 14.0 | | | 100 | | | 5.40 | | | 500 | | | | | SUBW105 |
| 6-inch sub, double meatball | 575 | 860 | | 82.0 | 18.0 | | 11.0 | 2480 | 250 | | | | | 48 | | | | |
| marinara w/chs - *20.3 oz sub* | | 37.0 | 42.0 | 18.0 | | | 85 | | | 9.00 | | | 750 | | | | | SUBW106 |
| 6-inch sub, double oven roasted | 309 | 400 | | 51.0 | 11.0 | | 6.0 | 1160 | 80 | | | | | 36 | | | | |
| chicken - *10.9 oz sub* | | 38.0 | 8.0 | 2.5 | | | 45 | | | 4.50 | | | 400 | | | | | SUBW96 |
| 6-inch sub, double roast beef | 281 | 360 | | 46.0 | 9.0 | | 5.0 | 1300 | 80 | | | | | 21 | | | | |
| *9.9 oz sub* | | 29.0 | 7.0 | 3.5 | | | 40 | | | 8.10 | | | 400 | | | | | SUBW97 |
| 6-inch sub, double steak and | 632 | 540 | | 52.0 | 12.0 | | 7.0 | 1510 | 150 | | | | | 30 | | | | |
| cheese *22.3 oz sub* | | 46.0 | 18.0 | 8.0 | | | 105 | | | 9.00 | | | 1000 | | | | | SUBW104 |
| 6-inch sub, double Subway Club | 347 | 420 | | 50.0 | 10.0 | | 5.0 | 2080 | 80 | | | | | 21 | | | | |
| *12.2 oz sub* | | 39.0 | 8.0 | 3.5 | | | 65 | | | 7.20 | | | 400 | | | | | SUBW98 |
| 6-inch sub, double Subway Melt | 330 | 490 | | 51.0 | 9.0 | | 5.0 | 2500 | 150 | | | | | 21 | | | | |
| with cheese - *11.6 oz sub* | | 40.0 | 17.0 | 8.0 | | | 80 | | | 5.40 | | | 500 | | | | | SUBW107 |
| 6-inch sub, double sweet onion | 373 | 480 | | 65.0 | 23.0 | | 6.0 | 1820 | 100 | | | | | 30 | | | | |
| chicken teriyaki - *13.2 oz sub* | | 43.0 | 7.0 | 2.0 | | | 100 | | | 5.40 | | | 500 | | | | | SUBW99 |
| 6-inch sub, double tuna | 320 | 790 | | 45.0 | 7.0 | | 5.0 | 1330 | 150 | | | | | 21 | | | | |
| *11.3 oz sub* | | 32.0 | 55.0 | 11.0 | | | 80 | | | 6.30 | | | 500 | | | | | SUBW108 |
| 6-inch sub, double turkey breast | 281 | 330 | | 48.0 | 8.0 | | 5.0 | 1500 | 80 | | | | | 21 | | | | |
| *9.9 oz sub* | | 28.0 | 5.0 | 1.5 | | | 40 | | | 5.40 | | | 400 | | | | | SUBW100 |
| 6-inch sub, double turkey breast | 300 | 360 | | 50.0 | 9.0 | | 5.0 | 1930 | 80 | | | | | 21 | | | | |
| and ham - *10.6 oz sub* | | 31.0 | 7.0 | 2.0 | | | 50 | | | 5.40 | | | 400 | | | | | SUBW101 |

| | WT | Macronutrients | | | | | | Minerals | | | | | Vitamins | | | | | |
|---|---|---|---|---|---|---|---|---|---|---|---|---|---|---|---|---|---|---|
| | (g) | KCAL | $H_20$ (g) | CHO (g) | TSUG (g) | ASUG (g) | DFIB (g) | Na (mg) | Ca (mg) | Mg (mg) | Zn (mg) | Mn (mg) | A (mcg RAE) | C (mg) | B-1 (mg) | NIA (mg) | B-12 (mcg) | PANT (mg) |
| | | PRO (g) | FAT (g) | SFA (g) | MUFA (g) | PUFA (g) | CHOL (mg) | K (mg) | P (mg) | Fe (mg) | Cu (mg) | Se (mcg) | A (IU) | E (mg ATE) | B-2 (mg) | B-6 (mg) | FOL (mcg DFE) | REF |
| **6-inch sub, Italian BMT** | 243 | 450 | | 47.0 | 8.0 | | 5.0 | 1770 | 150 | | | | | 21 | | | | |
| *8.6 oz sub* | | 23.0 | 21.0 | 8.0 | | | 55 | | | 4.50 | | | 500 | | | | | SUBW75 |
| **6-inch sub, meatball marinara** | 377 | 560 | | 63.0 | 13.0 | | 8.0 | 1590 | 200 | | | | | 36 | | | | |
| *13.3 oz sub* | | 24.0 | 24.0 | 11.0 | | | 45 | | | 7.20 | | | 750 | | | | | SUBW76 |
| **6-inch sub, prime rib** | 278 | 400 | | 48.0 | 9.0 | | 6.0 | 1110 | 150 | | | | | 24 | | | | |
| *9.8 oz sub* | | 29.0 | 12.0 | 6.0 | | | 60 | | | 7.20 | | | 750 | | | | | SUBW78 |
| **6-inch sub, spicy Italian** | 227 | 480 | | 45.0 | 8.0 | | 5.0 | 1660 | 80 | | | | | 21 | | | | |
| *8 oz sub* | | 21.0 | 25.0 | 9.0 | | | 55 | | | 4.50 | | | 400 | | | | | SUBW77 |
| **6-inch sub, Subway Melt** | 254 | 380 | | 48.0 | 8.0 | | 5.0 | 1600 | 150 | | | | | 21 | | | | |
| *8.9 oz sub* | | 25.0 | 12.0 | 5.0 | | | 45 | | | 4.50 | | | 500 | | | | | SUBW79 |
| **6-inch sub, tuna** | 250 | 530 | | 44.0 | 7.0 | | 5.0 | 1010 | 150 | | | | | 21 | | | | |
| *8.8 oz sub* | | 22.0 | 31.0 | 7.0 | | | 45 | | | 5.40 | | | 500 | | | | | SUBW80 |
| **Flatbread sandwich, chicken** | 303 | 520 | | 47.0 | 3.0 | | 4.0 | 1330 | 400 | | | | | 18 | | | | |
| Florentine - *10.7 oz sub* | | 35.0 | 22.0 | 8.0 | | | 85 | | | 3.60 | | | 1250 | | | | | SUBW81 |
| **Flatbread sandwich, steak and** | 260 | 440 | | 48.0 | 4.0 | | 3.0 | 1370 | 250 | | | | | 12 | | | | |
| **bacon** melt - *9.2 oz sub* | | 27.0 | 16.0 | 6.0 | | | 55 | | | 3.60 | | | 500 | | | | | SUBW82 |
| **Footlong sub, ham** | 448 | 570 | | 93.0 | 16.0 | | 11.0 | 2520 | 150 | | | | | 42 | | | | |
| *15.8 oz sub* | | 37.0 | 10.0 | 3.5 | | | 50 | | | 9.00 | | | 750 | | | | | SUBW87 |
| **Footlong sub, roast beef** | 448 | 580 | | 90.0 | 16.0 | | 11.0 | 1800 | 150 | | | | | 42 | | | | |
| *15.8 oz sub* | | 38.0 | 10.0 | 4.5 | | | 40 | | | 12.60 | | | 750 | | | | | SUBW89 |
| **Footlong sub, roasted chicken** | 477 | 630 | | 95.0 | 17.0 | | 11.0 | 1660 | 150 | | | | | 54 | | | | |
| breast - *16.8 oz sub* | | 47.0 | 11.0 | 3.5 | | | 45 | | | 8.10 | | | 750 | | | | | SUBW88 |
| **Footlong sub, Subway Club** | 514 | 640 | | 94.0 | 16.0 | | 11.0 | 2580 | 150 | | | | | 42 | | | | |
| *18.1 oz sub* | | 48.0 | 12.0 | 4.5 | | | 65 | | | 10.80 | | | 750 | | | | | SUBW90 |
| **Footlong sub, sweet onion chicken** | 562 | 750 | | 118.0 | 37.0 | | 11.0 | 2400 | 150 | | | | | 48 | | | | |
| teriyaki - *19.8 oz sub* | | 52.0 | 10.0 | 3.0 | | | 100 | | | 9.00 | | | 750 | | | | | SUBW91 |
| **Footlong sub, turkey breast** | 448 | 560 | | 92.0 | 14.0 | | 11.0 | 2000 | 150 | | | | | 42 | | | | |
| *15.8 oz sub* | | 37.0 | 9.0 | 2.5 | | | 40 | | | 9.00 | | | 750 | | | | | SUBW92 |
| **Footlong sub, turkey breast and** | 467 | 580 | | 93.0 | 15.0 | | 11.0 | 2420 | 150 | | | | | 42 | | | | |
| **ham** *16.5 oz sub* | | 40.0 | 10.0 | 3.0 | | | 50 | | | 9.00 | | | 750 | | | | | SUBW93 |
| **Footlong sub, Veggie Delite** | 335 | 450 | | 88.0 | 13.0 | | 11.0 | 1000 | 150 | | | | | 42 | | | | |
| *11.8 oz sub* | | 18.0 | 6.0 | 2.0 | | | 0 | | | 8.10 | | | 750 | | | | | SUBW94 |

## 10.20 TACO BELL

| | | | | | | | | | | | | | | | | | | |
|---|---|---|---|---|---|---|---|---|---|---|---|---|---|---|---|---|---|---|
| **burrito**, bean | 198 | 404 | 109.0 | 55.0 | | | 7.7 | 1216 | 232 | 61 | 1.70 | 0.733 | 6 | | 0.40 | 3.4 | 0 | 0.33 |
| *7 oz burrito* | | 15.6 | 13.6 | 4.8 | 5.9 | 1.7 | 18 | 533 | 337 | 4.57 | 0.335 | 20.6 | 133 | 1.0 | 0.30 | 0.24 | 134.6 | 21264 |
| **burrito**, Supreme, beef | 247 | 467 | 149.7 | 52.0 | | | 7.9 | 1418 | 230 | 62 | 2.59 | 0.813 | 10 | | 0.38 | 4.3 | 1.24 | 0.44 |
| *8.7 oz burrito* | | 19.9 | 19.9 | 7.5 | 8.1 | 2.0 | 40 | 605 | 336 | 5.58 | 0.279 | 23.7 | 203 | 1.1 | 0.37 | 0.26 | 168.0 | 21265 |
| **burrito**, Supreme, chicken | 247 | 442 | 150.7 | 50.7 | | | 5.9 | 1393 | 232 | 69 | 1.61 | 0.667 | 10 | | 0.43 | 9.6 | 0.82 | 1.40 |
| *8.7 oz burrito* | | 24.3 | 15.9 | 5.8 | 6.3 | 2.0 | 52 | 652 | 403 | 3.85 | 0.247 | 23.7 | 203 | 1.0 | 0.42 | 0.31 | 158.1 | 21266 |
| **burrito**, Supreme, steak | 247 | 452 | 151.2 | 50.2 | | | 5.9 | 1319 | 249 | 67 | 3.41 | 0.677 | 10 | | 0.62 | 5.6 | 1.48 | 0.54 |
| *8.7 oz burrito* | | 22.6 | 18.0 | 6.6 | 7.0 | 1.9 | 52 | 563 | 324 | 4.94 | 0.284 | 24.9 | 178 | 0.9 | 0.45 | 0.25 | 133.4 | 21267 |
| **nachos** | 90 | 329 | 30.9 | 32.7 | | | 3.4 | 463 | 80 | 47 | 1.03 | 0.229 | 1 | | 0.11 | 0.8 | 0 | 0.28 |
| *3.2 oz serving* | | 4.6 | 20.0 | 4.2 | 11.4 | 2.3 | 4 | 164 | 255 | 1.01 | 0.111 | 3.1 | 17 | 0.9 | 0.12 | 0.16 | 11.7 | 21268 |
| **nachos**, Supreme | 194 | 477 | 104.3 | 44.8 | | | 8.0 | 834 | 142 | 89 | 2.64 | 0.524 | 8 | | 0.20 | 1.9 | 0.76 | 0.49 |
| *6.8 oz serving* | | 14.7 | 26.5 | 7.7 | 13.6 | 2.8 | 37 | 469 | 382 | 4.15 | 0.225 | 13.0 | 136 | 1.4 | 0.28 | 0.34 | 56.3 | 21269 |
| **taco**, beef | 78 | 184 | 43.6 | 14.0 | | | 2.8 | 349 | 62 | 26 | 1.73 | 0.215 | 3 | | 0.07 | 1.5 | 0.75 | 0.14 |
| *2.75 oz taco* | | 8.4 | 10.5 | 3.6 | 4.2 | 1.6 | 24 | 168 | 139 | 1.47 | 0.058 | 7.2 | 60 | 0.5 | 0.15 | 0.11 | 16.4 | 21260 |
| **taco salad** | 475 | 808 | 319.8 | 71.7 | | | 14.2 | 1724 | 451 | 128 | 5.56 | 1.216 | 14 | | 0.71 | 7.1 | 1.90 | 0.97 |
| *16.8 oz salad* | | 31.8 | 43.6 | 14.2 | 18.9 | 3.6 | 90 | 1088 | 489 | 8.41 | 0.717 | 34.2 | 294 | 2.6 | 0.50 | 0.49 | 256.5 | 21270 |
| **taco**, soft, beef | 99 | 217 | 55.2 | 19.5 | | | 2.6 | 626 | 115 | 20 | 1.62 | 0.306 | 4 | | 0.15 | 2.6 | 0.77 | 0.20 |
| *3.5 oz taco* | | 11.7 | 10.2 | 4.2 | 4.3 | 1.0 | 28 | 179 | 161 | 2.41 | 0.074 | 10.9 | 78 | 0.4 | 0.21 | 0.09 | 70.3 | 21261 |
| **taco**, soft, chicken | 99 | 200 | 55.9 | 19.4 | | | 1.8 | 600 | 104 | 22 | 0.78 | 0.211 | 1 | | 0.21 | 6.3 | 0.37 | 0.74 |
| *3.5 oz taco* | | 14.2 | 7.2 | 2.6 | 2.8 | 1.0 | 37 | 235 | 222 | 1.70 | 0.074 | 12.6 | 25 | 0.3 | 0.16 | 0.15 | 68.3 | 21262 |
| **taco**, soft, steak | 127 | 286 | 72.2 | 21.9 | | | 2.0 | 700 | 149 | 27 | 2.73 | 0.279 | 1 | | 0.39 | 3.8 | 1.22 | 0.33 |
| *4.5 oz taco* | | 15.0 | 15.4 | 4.3 | 5.0 | 4.4 | 39 | 232 | 197 | 2.82 | 0.144 | 16.6 | 29 | 0.5 | 0.25 | 0.11 | 66.0 | 21263 |

## 10.21 WENDY'S

| | | | | | | | | | | | | | | | | | | |
|---|---|---|---|---|---|---|---|---|---|---|---|---|---|---|---|---|---|---|
| **cheeseburger**, Classic Double | 310 | 747 | 173.1 | 36.3 | | | 3.4 | 1308 | 180 | 59 | 9.46 | 0.412 | | 2 | 0.75 | 10.9 | 5.95 | 1.11 |
| *10.9 oz sandwich* | | 51.2 | 44.0 | 18.3 | 17.8 | 4.0 | 158 | 663 | 415 | 9.11 | 0.232 | 61.7 | | | 0.78 | 0.59 | | 21243 |
| **cheeseburger**, Classic Single | 236 | 522 | 135.7 | 33.5 | | | 3.3 | 1123 | 177 | 45 | 6.09 | 0.382 | | 1 | 0.61 | 7.5 | 3.63 | 0.69 |
| *8.3 oz sandwich* | | 35.1 | 27.4 | 12.3 | 10.4 | 3.3 | 90 | 441 | 297 | 5.52 | 0.177 | 45.1 | | | 0.60 | 0.25 | | 21240 |

| | WT (g) | KCAL / PRO (g) | H₂0 (g) / FAT (g) | CHO (g) / SFA (g) | TSUG (g) / MUFA (g) | ASUG (g) / PUFA (g) | DFIB (g) / CHOL (mg) | Na (mg) / K (mg) | Ca (mg) / P (mg) | Mg (mg) / Fe (mg) | Zn (mg) / Cu (mg) | Mn (mg) / Se (mcg) | A (mcg RAE) / A (IU) | C (mg) / E (mg ATE) | B-1 (mg) / B-2 (mg) | NIA (mg) / B-6 (mg) | B-12 (mcg) / FOL (mcg DFE) | PANT (mg) / REF |
|---|---|---|---|---|---|---|---|---|---|---|---|---|---|---|---|---|---|---|
| **cheeseburger**, Junior | 129 | 330 | 62.0 | 32.2 | | | 1.8 | 851 | 119 | 28 | 2.81 | 0.312 | 1 | | 0.47 | 4.0 | 1.68 | 0.39 |
| *4.6 oz sandwich* | | 16.8 | 14.8 | 6.7 | 5.7 | 1.5 | 46 | 230 | 173 | 3.59 | 0.141 | 28.3 | | | 0.22 | 1.23 | | 21242 |
| **chicken fillet sandwich** | 230 | 492 | 126.4 | 49.6 | | | 3.0 | 922 | 53 | 55 | 1.40 | 0.529 | 1 | | 0.68 | 7.6 | 0.76 | 1.21 |
| *8.1 oz sandwich* | | 31.7 | 18.6 | 3.7 | 6.7 | 7.1 | 71 | 524 | 370 | 3.45 | 0.310 | 56.1 | | | 0.30 | 0.43 | | 21244 |
| **Chicken Grill Sandwich** | 188 | 337 | 112.2 | 35.5 | | | 2.1 | 803 | 47 | 45 | 1.07 | 0.368 | 2 | | 0.74 | 7.8 | 0.62 | |
| *6.6 oz sandwich* | | 27.7 | 9.4 | 1.9 | 2.7 | 3.4 | 75 | 415 | 316 | 2.91 | 0.141 | 58.8 | | | 0.49 | 0.27 | | 21245 |
| **Chicken Nuggets** | 60 | 200 | 25.9 | 9.2 | | | 0.6 | 407 | 14 | 14 | 0.38 | 0.117 | 1 | | 0.05 | 3.6 | 0.20 | 0.54 |
| *2.1 oz kid's meal (4 pieces)* | | 9.6 | 13.9 | 3.0 | 6.8 | 3.5 | 30 | 142 | 172 | 0.44 | 0.097 | 15.0 | | | 0.07 | 0.15 | | 21246 |
| **Chicken Nuggets** | 75 | 250 | 32.3 | 11.5 | | | 0.8 | 509 | 18 | 18 | 0.47 | 0.146 | 1 | | 0.06 | 4.5 | 0.25 | 0.68 |
| *2.6 oz (5 pieces)* | | 11.9 | 17.4 | 3.7 | 8.5 | 4.3 | 38 | 177 | 215 | 0.55 | 0.122 | 18.8 | | | 0.09 | 0.19 | | 21246 |
| **French fries** | 91 | 290 | 35.3 | 35.9 | | | 3.4 | 157 | 14 | 31 | 0.48 | 0.233 | 5 | | 0.16 | 2.3 | | 0.60 |
| *3.2 oz serving (kid's meal size)* | | 3.5 | 14.8 | 2.9 | 7.8 | 3.4 | | 523 | 125 | 1.76 | 0.140 | 0.7 | | | 0.06 | 0.36 | | 21247 |
| **French fries** | 142 | 453 | 55.1 | 56.0 | | | 5.3 | 244 | 21 | 48 | 0.75 | 0.364 | 7 | | 0.25 | 3.5 | | 0.93 |
| *5 oz serving (medium)* | | 5.5 | 23.0 | 4.5 | 12.1 | 5.3 | | 816 | 195 | 2.74 | 0.219 | 1.1 | | | 0.09 | 0.56 | | 21247 |
| **French fries** | 159 | 507 | 61.7 | 62.7 | | | 5.9 | 273 | 24 | 54 | 0.84 | 0.407 | 8 | | 0.28 | 3.9 | | 1.04 |
| *5.6 oz serving (Biggie)* | | 6.2 | 25.8 | 5.1 | 13.5 | 5.9 | | 914 | 218 | 3.07 | 0.245 | 1.3 | | | 0.10 | 0.62 | | 21247 |
| **French fries** | 190 | 606 | 73.7 | 74.9 | | | 7.0 | 327 | 28 | 65 | 1.01 | 0.486 | 10 | | 0.34 | 4.7 | | 1.25 |
| *6.7 oz serving (Great Biggie)* | | 7.4 | 30.8 | 6.1 | 16.2 | 7.1 | | 1092 | 260 | 3.67 | 0.293 | 1.5 | | | 0.12 | 0.74 | | 21247 |
| **frosty dairy dessert** | 113 | 149 | 78.3 | 26.7 | | | 3.7 | 111 | 145 | 23 | 0.50 | 0.071 | 0 | | 0.07 | 0.4 | 0.67 | 0.68 |
| *6 fl oz (junior)* | | 3.9 | 2.9 | 1.8 | 0.8 | 0.1 | 18 | 209 | 127 | 1.18 | 0.085 | 3.7 | | | 0.81 | 0 | | 21248 |
| **frosty dairy dessert** | 227 | 300 | 157.2 | 53.6 | | | 7.5 | 222 | 291 | 45 | 1.00 | 0.143 | 0 | | 0.14 | 0.8 | 1.34 | 1.36 |
| *12 fl oz (small)* | | 7.9 | 5.9 | 3.7 | 1.6 | 0.3 | 36 | 420 | 254 | 2.36 | 0.170 | 7.5 | | | 1.63 | 0 | | 21248 |
| **frosty dairy dessert** | 298 | 393 | 206.4 | 70.4 | | | 9.8 | 292 | 381 | 60 | 1.31 | 0.188 | 0 | | 0.18 | 1.0 | 1.76 | 1.79 |
| *16 fl oz (medium)* | | 10.4 | 7.7 | 4.9 | 2.1 | 0.3 | 48 | 551 | 334 | 3.10 | 0.224 | 9.8 | | | 2.15 | 0 | | 21248 |
| **hamburger**, Classic Single | 218 | 464 | 127.3 | 36.7 | | | 2.8 | 861 | 74 | 39 | 5.38 | 0.408 | 1 | | 0.60 | 7.0 | 3.16 | 0.73 |
| *7.7 oz sandwich* | | 27.5 | 23.1 | 8.0 | 8.9 | 3.4 | 76 | 425 | 225 | 5.95 | 0.303 | 39.7 | | | 0.45 | 0.25 | | 21239 |
| **hamburger**, Junior | 117 | 284 | 56.5 | 33.3 | | | 2.0 | 631 | 53 | 25 | 2.46 | 0.329 | 1 | | 0.49 | 4.5 | 1.49 | 0.40 |
| *4.2 oz sandwich* | | 14.8 | 10.2 | 4.1 | 4.1 | 1.3 | 32 | 205 | 125 | 3.92 | 0.137 | 27.0 | | | 0.27 | 0.15 | | 21241 |
| **iced tea**, no ice | 356 | 4 | 355.3 | 0 | | | | 11 | 7 | 4 | 0.04 | 0.484 | | | 0.06 | 0 | | 0.03 |
| *12 fl oz* | | 0.8 | 0 | 0 | 0 | 0 | | 50 | 4 | 0 | 0.028 | 0 | | | 0.09 | 0 | | 14601 |

# 11. FATS, OILS, SHORTENINGS, AND SPREADS
## 11.1 ANIMAL FATS

| | WT (g) | KCAL / PRO (g) | H₂0 (g) / FAT (g) | CHO (g) / SFA (g) | TSUG (g) / MUFA (g) | ASUG (g) / PUFA (g) | DFIB (g) / CHOL (mg) | Na (mg) / K (mg) | Ca (mg) / P (mg) | Mg (mg) / Fe (mg) | Zn (mg) / Cu (mg) | Mn (mg) / Se (mcg) | A (mcg RAE) / A (IU) | C (mg) / E (mg ATE) | B-1 (mg) / B-2 (mg) | NIA (mg) / B-6 (mg) | B-12 (mcg) / FOL (mcg DFE) | PANT (mg) / REF |
|---|---|---|---|---|---|---|---|---|---|---|---|---|---|---|---|---|---|---|
| **bacon fat** | 13 | 116 | 0 | 0 | 0 | | | 0 | 20 | 0 | 0 | 0.01 | 0 | 0 | 0 | 0 | 0 | 0 |
| *1 T* | | 0 | 12.9 | 5.1 | 5.8 | 1.4 | 12 | 0 | 0 | 0 | 0 | 0 | 0 | 0.1 | 0 | 0 | 0 | 4609 |
| **beef fat**, cooked | 28 | 190 | 5.2 | 0 | 0 | | | 0 | 6 | 5 | 2 | 0.35 | 0 | 0 | 0 | 0.01 | 0.4 | 0.25 | 0.06 |
| *1 oz* | | 3.0 | 19.7 | 8.0 | 8.5 | 0.7 | 27 | 28 | 18 | 0.30 | 0.011 | 2.3 | 0 | 0 | 0.01 | 0.04 | 0 | 13020 |
| **beef suet**, raw | 28 | 239 | 1.1 | 0 | 0 | | | 0 | 2 | 1 | 0 | 0.06 | 0 | 0 | 0 | 0 | 0.1 | 0.08 | 0.01 |
| *1 oz* | | 0.4 | 26.3 | 14.6 | 8.8 | 0.9 | 19 | 4 | 4 | 0.05 | 0.002 | 0.1 | 0 | 0.4 | 0 | 0.01 | 0.3 | 13335 |
| **beef tallow**, raw | 13 | 117 | 0 | 0 | 0 | | | 0 | 0 | 0 | 0 | 0 | 0 | 0 | 0 | 0 | 0 | 0 | 0 |
| *1 T* | | 0 | 13.0 | 6.5 | 5.4 | 0.5 | 14 | 0 | 0 | 0 | 0 | 0 | 0 | 0.4 | 0 | 0 | 0 | 4001 |
| **chicken fat**, raw | 13 | 117 | 0 | 0 | 0 | | | 0 | 0 | 0 | 0 | 0 | 0 | 0 | 0 | 0 | 0 | 0 | 0 |
| *1 T* | | 0 | 13.0 | 3.9 | 5.8 | 2.7 | 11 | 0 | 0 | 0 | 0 | 0 | 0 | 0.4 | 0 | 0 | 0 | 4542 |
| **duck fat**, raw | 13 | 115 | 0 | 0 | 0 | | | 0 | 0 | 0 | 0 | 0 | 0 | 0 | 0 | 0 | 0 | 0 | 0 |
| *1 T* | | 0 | 13.0 | 4.3 | 6.4 | 1.7 | 13 | 0 | 0 | 0 | 0 | 0 | 0 | 0.4 | 0 | 0 | 0 | 4574 |
| **goose fat**, raw | 13 | 117 | 0 | 0 | 0 | | | 0 | 0 | 0 | 0 | 0 | 0 | 0 | 0 | 0 | 0 | 0 | 0 |
| *1 T* | | 0 | 13.0 | 3.6 | 7.4 | 1.4 | 13 | 0 | 0 | 0 | 0 | 0 | 0 | 0.4 | 0 | 0 | 0 | 4576 |
| **lamb fat**, cooked | 28 | 164 | 7.3 | 0 | 0 | | | 0 | 16 | 6 | 4 | 0.49 | 0.001 | 0 | 0 | 0.02 | 2.2 | 0.66 | 0.16 |
| *1 oz* | | 3.4 | 16.6 | 7.6 | 6.8 | 1.3 | 32 | 54 | 32 | 0.36 | 0.025 | 5.3 | 0 | 0 | 0.05 | 0.01 | 0.8 | 17006 |
| **lard** (pork fat), raw | 13 | 117 | 0 | 0 | 0 | | | 0 | 0 | 0 | 0 | 0.01 | 0 | 0 | 0 | 0 | 0 | 0 | 0 |
| *1 T* | | 0 | 13.0 | 5.1 | 5.9 | 1.5 | 12 | 0 | 0 | 0 | 0 | 0 | 0 | 0.1 | 0 | 0 | 0 | 4002 |
| **mutton tallow**, raw | 13 | 117 | 0 | 0 | 0 | | | 0 | 0 | 0 | 0 | 0 | 0 | 0 | 0 | 0 | 0 | 0 | 0 |
| *1 T* | | 0 | 13.0 | 6.1 | 5.3 | 1.0 | 13 | 0 | 0 | 0 | 0 | 0 | 0 | 0.4 | 0 | 0 | 0 | 4520 |
| **pork backfat**, raw | 28 | 227 | 2.2 | 0 | 0 | | | 0 | 3 | 1 | 1 | 0.10 | 0.001 | 1 | 0 | 0.02 | 0.3 | 0.05 | 0.03 |
| *1 oz* | | 0.8 | 24.8 | 9.0 | 11.7 | 2.9 | 16 | 18 | 11 | 0.05 | 0.005 | 2.2 | 4 | 0 | 0.01 | 0.01 | 0.3 | 10004 |
| **pork fat**, cooked | 28 | 178 | 6.2 | 0 | 0 | | | 0 | 8 | 12 | 3 | 0.27 | 0 | 8 | 0 | 0.06 | 0.9 | 0.35 | 0.13 |
| *1 oz* | | 2.5 | 18.5 | 6.6 | 7.6 | 2.6 | 23 | 47 | 32 | 0.18 | 0.012 | 3.8 | 27 | 0.1 | 0.03 | 0.06 | 0 | 10007 |
| **pork fat**, raw | 28 | 186 | 6.7 | 0 | 0 | | | 0 | 6 | 10 | 2 | 0.19 | 0 | 7 | 0 | 0.05 | 0.8 | 0.26 | 0.11 |
| *1 oz* | | 1.6 | 19.9 | 7.0 | 8.2 | 2.9 | 22 | 35 | 24 | 0.11 | 0.010 | 2.4 | 23 | 0 | 0.02 | 0.05 | 0 | 10006 |
| **salt pork**, raw | 28 | 209 | 3.1 | 0 | 0 | | | 0 | 399 | 2 | 2 | 0.25 | 0.001 | 0 | 0 | 0.06 | 0.5 | 0.08 | 0.06 |
| *1 oz* | | 1.4 | 22.5 | 8.2 | 10.6 | 2.6 | 24 | 18 | 15 | 0.12 | 0.014 | 1.6 | 0 | 0 | 0.02 | 0.02 | 0.3 | 10165 |

| | WT (g) | KCAL / PRO (g) | H₂O / FAT (g) | CHO / SFA (g) | TSUG / MUFA (g) | ASUG / PUFA (g) | DFIB / CHOL | Na / K (mg) | Ca / P (mg) | Mg / Fe (mg) | Zn / Cu (mg) | Mn / Se | A (mcg RAE) / A (IU) | C / E | B-1 / B-2 | NIA / B-6 | B-12 / FOL | PANT / REF |
|---|---|---|---|---|---|---|---|---|---|---|---|---|---|---|---|---|---|---|
| **sea lion fat**, raw | 28 | 238 | 1.3 | 0 | | | | 27 | 0 | | | | 27 | 0 | | | | |
| *1 oz* | | 0.3 | 26.3 | | | | 27 | | | | | | 90 | | | | | 35231 |
| **seal, bearded**, oil | 14 | 126 | 0 | 0 | | | | 0 | 0 | 0 | 0 | 0 | 1 | 0 | 0 | 0 | 0 | 0 |
| *1 T* | | 0.1 | 13.9 | 1.5 | 6.6 | 4.6 | 7 | 0 | 0 | 0 | 0 | 0.5 | 5 | 1.4 | 0 | 0 | | 35057 |
| **seal, spotted**, oil | 14 | 125 | 0 | 0 | 0 | | 0 | 0 | 0 | 0 | 0 | 0 | 146 | 0 | 0 | 0 | 0 | 0 |
| *1 T* | | 0 | 13.9 | 2.1 | 7.6 | 2.5 | | 0 | 0 | 0 | 0 | 0.3 | 487 | 0.9 | 0 | 0 | 0 | 35156 |
| **turkey fat**, raw | 13 | 117 | 0 | 0 | 0 | | 0 | 0 | 0 | 0 | 0 | | 0 | 0 | 0 | 0 | 0 | 0 |
| *1 T* | | 0 | 13.0 | 3.8 | 5.6 | 3.0 | 13 | 0 | 0 | 0 | 0 | | 0 | 0.4 | 0 | 0 | 0 | 4575 |
| **walrus oil** | 14 | 126 | 0 | 0 | | | | | 0 | | | | | 0 | 0 | | | |
| *1 T* | | 0 | 14.0 | | | | 17 | | | | | | 364 | 0 | | | | 35084 |
| **whale, beluga**, oil | 14 | 126 | 0 | 0 | 0 | | | 0 | 0 | 0 | 0 | 0 | 97 | 0 | | 0 | 0 | 0 |
| *1 T* | | 0 | 14.0 | 2.0 | 7.6 | 1.5 | | 0 | 0 | 0 | 0 | 0.4 | 323 | 1.2 | 0 | | | 35014 |
| **whale, bowhead**, oil | 14 | 126 | 0 | 0 | | | | | 0 | | | | | 0 | 0 | | | |
| *1 T* | | 0 | 14.0 | | | | | 0 | 0 | | | | 393 | 0 | | | | 35087 |

## 11.2 FISH OILS

| | WT (g) | KCAL / PRO (g) | H₂O / FAT (g) | CHO / SFA (g) | TSUG / MUFA (g) | ASUG / PUFA (g) | DFIB / CHOL | Na / K (mg) | Ca / P (mg) | Mg / Fe (mg) | Zn / Cu (mg) | Mn / Se | A (mcg RAE) / A (IU) | C / E | B-1 / B-2 | NIA / B-6 | B-12 / FOL | PANT / REF |
|---|---|---|---|---|---|---|---|---|---|---|---|---|---|---|---|---|---|---|
| **cod liver oil** | 14 | 126 | 0 | 0 | | | 0 | 0 | 0 | 0 | 0 | 0 | 4200 | 0 | | 0 | 0 | 0 |
| *1 T* | | 0 | 14.0 | 3.2 | 6.5 | 3.2 | 80 | 0 | 0 | 0 | 0 | 0 | 14000 | | 0 | 0 | 0 | 4589 |
| **herring oil** | 14 | 126 | 0 | 0 | | | 0 | 0 | 0 | 0 | 0 | 0 | 0 | 0 | 0 | 0 | 0 | 0 |
| *1 T* | | 0 | 14.0 | 3.0 | 7.9 | 2.2 | 107 | 0 | 0 | 0 | 0 | 0 | 0 | 0 | 0 | 0 | 0 | 4590 |
| **menhaden oil** | 14 | 126 | 0 | 0 | | | 0 | 0 | 0 | 0 | 0 | 0 | 0 | 0 | 0 | 0 | 0 | 0 |
| *1 T* | | 0 | 14.0 | 4.3 | 3.7 | 4.8 | 73 | 0 | 0 | 0 | 0 | 0 | 0 | 0 | 0 | 0 | 0 | 4591 |
| **menhaden oil**, fully hydrogenated | 13 | 117 | 0 | 0 | | | 0 | 0 | 0 | 0 | 0 | 0 | 0 | 0 | 0 | 0 | 0 | 0 |
| *1 T* | | 0 | 13.0 | 12.4 | 0 | 0 | 65 | 0 | 0 | 0 | 0 | 0 | 0 | 0 | 0 | 0 | 0 | 4592 |
| **salmon oil** | 14 | 126 | 0 | 0 | | | 0 | 0 | 0 | 0 | 0 | 0 | 0 | 0 | 0 | 0 | 0 | 0 |
| *1 T* | | 0 | 14.0 | 2.8 | 4.1 | 5.6 | 68 | 0 | 0 | 0 | 0 | 0 | 0 | 0 | 0 | 0 | 0 | 4593 |
| **sardine oil** | 14 | 126 | 0 | 0 | | | 0 | 0 | 0 | 0 | 0 | 0 | 0 | 0 | 0 | 0 | 0 | 0 |
| *1 T* | | 0 | 14.0 | 4.2 | 4.7 | 4.5 | 99 | 0 | 0 | 0 | 0 | 0 | 0 | 0 | 0 | 0 | 0 | 4594 |

## 11.3 SHORTENINGS

| | WT (g) | KCAL / PRO (g) | H₂O / FAT (g) | CHO / SFA (g) | TSUG / MUFA (g) | ASUG / PUFA (g) | DFIB / CHOL | Na / K (mg) | Ca / P (mg) | Mg / Fe (mg) | Zn / Cu (mg) | Mn / Se | A (mcg RAE) / A (IU) | C / E | B-1 / B-2 | NIA / B-6 | B-12 / FOL | PANT / REF |
|---|---|---|---|---|---|---|---|---|---|---|---|---|---|---|---|---|---|---|
| **shortening**, beef tallow and cottonseed (for frying) - *1 T* | 13 | 117 | 0 | 0 | | | 0 | 0 | 0 | 0 | 0 | | 0 | 0 | 0 | 0 | 0 | 0 |
| | | 0 | 13.0 | 5.8 | 5.0 | 1.1 | 13 | 0 | 0 | 0 | 0 | 0 | 0 | 0.5 | 0 | 0 | 0 | 4550 |
| **shortening**, hydg coconut and palm kernel oils (for confectionery) | 13 | 115 | 0 | 0 | 0 | | 0 | 0 | 0 | 0 | 0 | | 0 | 0 | 0 | 0 | 0 | 0 |
| *1 T* | | 0 | 13.0 | 11.9 | 0.3 | 0.1 | 0 | 0 | 0 | 0 | 0 | 0 | 0 | 0.3 | 0 | 0 | 0 | 4551 |
| **shortening**, lard and veg. oil | 13 | 117 | 0 | 0 | 0 | | 0 | 0 | 0 | 0 | 0 | | 0 | 0 | 0 | 0 | 0 | 0 |
| *1 T* | | 0 | 13.0 | 5.2 | 5.8 | 1.4 | 7 | 0 | 0 | 0 | 0 | 0 | 0 | 0.1 | 0 | 0 | 0 | 4544 |
| **shortening**, palm (for confectionery) | 14 | 124 | 0 | 0 | | | 0 | 0 | 0 | 0 | 0 | | 0 | 0 | 0 | 0 | 0 | 0 |
| *1 T* | | 0 | 14.0 | 9.2 | 4.1 | 0.1 | 0 | 0 | 0 | 0 | 0 | 0 | 0 | 2.7 | 0 | 0 | 0 | 4570 |
| **shortening**, soy (hydg), 30% linoleic acid - *1 T* | 14 | 124 | 0 | 0 | 0 | | 0 | 0 | 0 | 0 | 0 | | 0 | 0 | 0 | 0 | 0 | 0 |
| | | 0 | 14.0 | 2.6 | 6.1 | 4.7 | 0 | 0 | 0 | 0 | 0 | 0 | 0 | 0.1 | 0 | 0 | 0 | 4552 |
| **shortening**, soy (hydg) and cottonseed - *1 T* | 14 | 124 | 0 | 0 | | | 0 | 0 | 0 | 0 | 0 | | 0 | 0 | 0 | 0 | 0 | 0 |
| | | 0 | 14.0 | 2.2 | 8.1 | 3.1 | 0 | 0 | 0 | 0 | 0 | 0 | 0 | 0.1 | 0 | 0 | 0 | 4547 |
| **shortening**, soy (hydg) and cottonseed (household) - *1 T* | 14 | 124 | 0 | 0 | | | 0 | 0 | 0 | 0 | 0 | | 0 | 0 | 0 | 0 | 0 | 0 |
| | | 0 | 14.0 | 3.5 | 6.2 | 3.7 | 0 | 0 | 0 | 0 | 0 | 0 | 0 | 0.1 | 0 | 0 | 0 | 4031 |
| **shortening**, soy (hydg) and palm (household) - *1 T* | 14 | 124 | 0 | 0 | | | 0 | 0 | 0 | 0 | 0 | | 0 | 0 | 0 | 0 | 0 | 0 |
| | | 0 | 14.0 | 3.5 | 6.0 | 3.7 | 0 | 0 | 0 | 0 | 0 | 0 | 0 | | 0 | 0 | 0 | 4559 |
| **shortening**, sunflower oil, hydg | 14 | 124 | 0 | 0 | 0 | | 0 | 0 | 0 | 0 | 0 | | 0 | 0 | 0 | 0 | 0 | 0 |
| *1 T* | | 0 | 14.0 | 1.8 | 6.5 | 5.1 | 0 | 0 | 0 | 0 | 0 | 0 | 0 | 5.8 | 0 | 0 | 0 | 4545 |

## 11.4 SPREADS

| | WT (g) | KCAL / PRO (g) | H₂O / FAT (g) | CHO / SFA (g) | TSUG / MUFA (g) | ASUG / PUFA (g) | DFIB / CHOL | Na / K (mg) | Ca / P (mg) | Mg / Fe (mg) | Zn / Cu (mg) | Mn / Se | A (mcg RAE) / A (IU) | C / E | B-1 / B-2 | NIA / B-6 | B-12 / FOL | PANT / REF |
|---|---|---|---|---|---|---|---|---|---|---|---|---|---|---|---|---|---|---|
| **butter** | 14 | 100 | 2.2 | 0 | 0 | 0 | 0 | 81 | 3 | 0 | 0.01 | 0 | 96 | 0 | 0 | 0 | 0.02 | 0.02 |
| *1 T* | | 0.1 | 11.4 | 7.2 | 2.9 | 0.4 | 30 | 3 | 3 | 0 | 0 | 0.1 | 350 | 0.3 | 0 | 0 | 0.4 | 1001 |
| **butter**, light, stick | 14 | 71 | 5.9 | 0 | 0 | | 0 | 63 | 7 | 1 | 0.04 | | 65 | 0 | 0 | 0 | 0.02 | |
| *1 T* | | 0.5 | 7.7 | 4.8 | 2.2 | 0.3 | 15 | 10 | 5 | 0.15 | 0 | 0.1 | 238 | 0.2 | 0.01 | 0 | 0.1 | 4601 |
| **butter**, sweet (unsalted) | 14 | 100 | 2.5 | 0 | 0 | 0 | 0 | 2 | 3 | 0 | 0.01 | 0.001 | 96 | 0 | 0 | 0 | 0.02 | 0.02 |
| *1 T* | | 0.1 | 11.4 | 7.2 | 2.9 | 0.4 | 30 | 3 | 3 | 0 | 0.002 | 0.1 | 350 | 0.3 | 0 | 0 | 4 | 1145 |
| **butter**, whipped | 9 | 65 | 1.4 | 0 | 0 | 0 | 0 | 74 | 2 | 0 | 0 | 0 | 62 | 0 | 0 | 0 | 0.01 | 0.01 |
| *1 T* | | 0.1 | 7.3 | 4.5 | 2.1 | 0.3 | 20 | 2 | 2 | 0.01 | 0.001 | 0.1 | 225 | 0.2 | 0 | 0 | 0.3 | 1002 |
| **margarine-butter blend** (60% corn oil, 40% butter) - *1 T* | 14 | 100 | 2.4 | 0.1 | 0 | | 0 | 89 | 1 | 0 | 0 | 0.001 | 115 | 0 | 0 | 0 | 0 | 0.01 |
| | | 0 | 11.2 | 2.0 | 4.2 | 3.4 | 2 | 3 | 1 | 0.01 | 0.001 | 0.1 | 501 | 0.5 | 0 | 0 | 0.3 | 4585 |

| | WT (g) | KCAL / PRO (g) | H₂O (g) / FAT (g) | CHO (g) / SFA (g) | TSUG (g) / MUFA (g) | ASUG (g) / PUFA (g) | DFIB (g) / CHOL (mg) | Na (mg) / K (mg) | Ca (mg) / P (mg) | Mg (mg) / Fe (mg) | Zn (mg) / Cu (mg) | Mn (mg) / Se (mcg) | A (mcg RAE) / A (IU) | C (mg) / E (mg ATE) | B-1 (mg) / B-2 (mg) | NIA (mg) / B-6 (mg) | B-12 (mcg) / FOL (mcg DFE) | PANT (mg) / REF |
|---|---|---|---|---|---|---|---|---|---|---|---|---|---|---|---|---|---|---|
| margarine, corn and soy, 80% fat, stick - 1 T | 14 | 100 | 2.3 | 0.1 | | | 0 | 92 | 0 | 0 | 0.02 | | | 0 | 0 | | | 0 |
| | | 0 | 11.3 | 2.1 | 5.4 | 3.4 | 0 | 3 | 1 | 0.02 | | | | 0.7 | 0 | | 0.1 | 4628 |
| margarine, fat-free, tub 1 T | 15 | 7 | 13.6 | 0.7 | 0 | 0 | 0 | 87 | 1 | 0 | 0.01 | 0 | 149 | 0 | 0.15 | 0.1 | 0 | 0.04 |
| | | 0 | 0.5 | 0.3 | 0.1 | 0.1 | 0 | 5 | 0 | 0.01 | 0 | 0 | 496 | 0.1 | 0 | 0 | 0 | 4631 |
| margarine, liquid 1 T | 14 | 101 | 2.2 | 0 | 0 | | 0 | 109 | 9 | 1 | 0 | | 115 | 0 | 0 | 0 | 0.03 | 0.03 |
| | | 0.3 | 11.3 | 1.8 | 3.9 | 5.0 | 0 | 13 | 7 | 0 | 0 | 0 | 501 | 0.6 | 0.01 | 0 | 0.4 | 4105 |
| margarine, soy, 70% fat 1 T | 14 | 87 | 3.7 | 0 | | | 0 | 98 | 1 | 0 | 0.01 | 0.002 | | 0.01 | | | | 0 |
| | | 0 | 9.8 | 1.9 | 4.7 | 2.8 | 0 | 6 | 1 | 0.02 | | | 500 | 0.8 | 0 | 0 | 0.1 | 4629 |
| margarine, stick/tub composite, 60% fat - 1 T | 14 | 74 | 5.4 | 0 | 0 | | 0 | 110 | 3 | 0 | 0 | | 115 | 0 | 0 | 0 | 0.01 | 0 |
| | | 0.1 | 8.3 | 1.4 | 2.8 | 3.5 | 0 | 4 | 2 | 0 | 0 | 0 | 500 | 0.7 | 0 | 0 | 0.1 | 4614 |
| margarine, unspecified oils 1 T | 14 | 100 | 2.3 | 0.1 | 0 | | 0 | 132 | 4 | 0 | 0 | | 115 | 0 | 0 | 0 | 0.01 | 0.01 |
| | | 0 | 11.3 | 2.1 | 5.4 | 3.4 | 0 | 6 | 3 | 0.01 | 0 | 0 | 500 | 1.3 | 0.01 | 0 | 0.1 | 4132 |
| mayonnaise, diet, no cholesterol 1 T | 15 | 58 | 6.0 | 3.6 | 1.0 | 0.9 | 0 | 107 | 2 | 0 | 0.03 | 0.013 | 3 | 0 | 0 | 0 | 0.03 | 0.04 |
| | | 0.1 | 5.0 | 0.8 | 1.3 | 2.7 | 0 | 1 | 4 | 0.03 | 0.002 | 0.2 | 33 | 0.3 | 0 | 0 | 0 | 43599 |
| mayonnaise, fat-free, Kraft 1 T | 16 | 11 | 13.1 | 2.0 | 1.1 | | 0.3 | 120 | 1 | | | | | 0 | | | | |
| | | 0 | 0.4 | 0.1 | | | 2 | 8 | 4 | 0.02 | | | 16 | | | | | 4013 |
| mayonnaise, imitation, soy 1 T | 15 | 35 | 9.4 | 2.4 | 0.9 | 0.9 | 0 | 75 | 0 | 0 | 0.02 | | 0 | 0 | 0 | 0 | 0 | 0 |
| | | 0 | 2.9 | 0.5 | 0.7 | 1.6 | 4 | 2 | 0 | 0 | 0.002 | 0.2 | 0 | 0.3 | 0 | 0 | 0 | 4027 |
| mayonnaise, light, Kraft Mayo Light - 1 T | 15 | 50 | 8.3 | 1.3 | 0.6 | | 0 | 120 | 1 | | | | | 0 | | | | |
| | | 0.1 | 4.9 | 0.8 | | | 5 | 8 | 9 | 0.03 | | | 28 | | | | | 4011 |
| mayonnaise, safflower and soy 1 T | 14 | 100 | 2.1 | 0.4 | 0.1 | | 0 | 80 | 3 | 0 | 0.02 | | 12 | 0 | 0 | 0 | 0.04 | 0.04 |
| | | 0.2 | 11.1 | 1.2 | 1.8 | 7.7 | 8 | 5 | 4 | 0.07 | | 0.2 | 39 | 3.1 | 0 | 0.08 | 1.1 | 4026 |
| mayonnaise, soy 1 T | 14 | 101 | 2.1 | 0.4 | 0.2 | 0.1 | 0 | 80 | 1 | 0 | 0.02 | 0.001 | 11 | 0 | 0 | 0 | 0.05 | 0.03 |
| | | 0.1 | 11.1 | 1.7 | 2.7 | 5.9 | 5 | 2 | 4 | 0.03 | 0.004 | 0.2 | 39 | 0.7 | 0.01 | 0.08 | 0.7 | 4025 |
| Miracle Whip, light, Kraft 1 T | 16 | 37 | 10.1 | 2.3 | 1.6 | | 0 | 131 | 1 | | | | | 0 | | | | |
| | | 0.1 | 3.0 | 0.5 | | | 4 | 4 | 2 | 0.03 | | | 5 | | | | | 4012 |
| Miracle Whip, nonfat, Kraft 1 T | 16 | 13 | 12.6 | 2.5 | 1.6 | | 0.3 | 126 | 1 | | | | | 0 | | | | |
| | | 0 | 0.4 | 0.1 | | | 1 | 8 | 1 | 0.02 | | | 11 | | | | | 4014 |
| sandwich spread (mayo-based) 1 T | 15 | 58 | 6.1 | 3.4 | 2.3 | 2.3 | 0.1 | 150 | 2 | 0 | 0.12 | | 3 | 0 | 0 | 0 | 0.03 | 0 |
| | | 0.1 | 5.1 | 0.8 | 1.1 | 3.0 | 11 | 5 | 4 | 0.03 | 0.002 | 0.2 | 33 | 0.6 | 0 | 0 | 0.9 | 4030 |
| Smart Balance Buttery Spread 1 T | 14 | 85 | 4.3 | 0 | 0 | | 0 | 90 | | | | | | | | | | |
| | | 0 | 9.4 | 2.7 | 3.6 | 2.5 | 0 | 4 | 1 | | | | 535 | 1.6 | | | | 4673 |
| Smart Balance Light Buttery Spread 1 T | 14 | 47 | 8.4 | 0.3 | | | 0 | 81 | 0 | 0 | 0 | 0 | 201 | 0 | 0 | | | |
| | | 0 | 5.1 | 1.4 | 1.9 | 1.4 | 0 | 4 | 0 | 0 | 0 | | 723 | 2.2 | 0 | 0 | | 4674 |
| Smart Balance Omega Plus Spread w/plant sterols and fish oil - 1 T | 14 | 85 | 3.8 | 0 | 0 | | 0 | 102 | | | | | | | | | | |
| | | 0 | 9.4 | 2.7 | 3.5 | 2.5 | 0 | 10 | 3 | | | | 757 | 1.4 | | | | 4677 |
| Smart Beat Super Light Spread 1 T | 14 | 22 | 11.3 | 0 | 0 | | 0 | 106 | | | | | | | | | | |
| | | 0 | 2.4 | 0.3 | 1.1 | 0.6 | 0 | 2 | 0 | | | | 628 | 0.2 | | | | 4675 |
| Smart Squeeze Fat-Free Spread 1 T | 14 | 7 | 12.3 | 1.0 | 0.1 | | 0 | 116 | | | | | | | | | | |
| | | 0 | 0.3 | 0 | 0.1 | 0.2 | 0 | 4 | 0 | | | | 808 | 0 | | | | 4676 |

## 11.5 VEGETABLE OILS AND VEGETABLE OIL SPRAYS

| | WT (g) | KCAL / PRO (g) | H₂O (g) / FAT (g) | CHO (g) / SFA (g) | TSUG (g) / MUFA (g) | ASUG (g) / PUFA (g) | DFIB (g) / CHOL (mg) | Na (mg) / K (mg) | Ca (mg) / P (mg) | Mg (mg) / Fe (mg) | Zn (mg) / Cu (mg) | Mn (mg) / Se (mcg) | A (mcg RAE) / A (IU) | C (mg) / E (mg ATE) | B-1 (mg) / B-2 (mg) | NIA (mg) / B-6 (mg) | B-12 (mcg) / FOL (mcg DFE) | PANT (mg) / REF |
|---|---|---|---|---|---|---|---|---|---|---|---|---|---|---|---|---|---|---|
| almond oil 1 T | 14 | 124 | 0 | 0 | 0 | | 0 | 0 | 0 | 0 | 0 | | 0 | 0 | 0 | 0 | 0 | 0 |
| | | 0 | 14.0 | 1.1 | 9.8 | 2.4 | 0 | 0 | 0 | 0 | 0 | 0 | 0 | 5.5 | 0 | 0 | 0 | 4529 |
| apricot kernel oil 1 T | 14 | 124 | 0 | 0 | 0 | | 0 | 0 | 0 | 0 | 0 | | 0 | 0 | 0 | 0 | 0 | 0 |
| | | 0 | 14.0 | 0.9 | 8.4 | 4.1 | 0 | 0 | 0 | 0 | 0 | 0 | 0 | 0.6 | 0 | 0 | 0 | 4530 |
| avocado oil 1 T | 14 | 124 | 0 | 0 | 0 | | 0 | 0 | 0 | 0 | 0 | | 0 | 0 | 0 | 0 | 0 | 0 |
| | | 0 | 14.0 | 1.6 | 9.9 | 1.9 | 0 | 0 | 0 | 0 | 0 | 0 | 0 | 0 | 0 | 0 | 0 | 4581 |
| babassu oil 1 T | 14 | 124 | 0 | 0 | 0 | | 0 | 0 | 0 | 0 | 0 | | 0 | 0 | 0 | 0 | 0 | 0 |
| | | 0 | 14.0 | 11.4 | 1.6 | 0.2 | 0 | 0 | 0 | 0 | 0 | 0 | 0 | 2.7 | 0 | 0 | 0 | 4534 |
| canola oil 1 T | 14 | 124 | 0 | 0 | 0 | | 0 | 0 | 0 | 0 | 0 | 0 | 0 | 0 | 0 | 0 | 0 | 0 |
| | | 0 | 14.0 | 1.0 | 8.9 | 3.9 | 0 | 0 | 0 | 0 | 0 | 0 | 0 | 2.4 | 0 | 0 | 0 | 4582 |
| canola oil, Natreon 1 T | 14 | 124 | 0 | 0 | 0 | | 0 | | | | | | | 0 | 0 | 0 | | |
| | | 0 | 14.0 | 0.9 | 10.1 | 2.4 | 0 | | | | | | 0 | 3.1 | 0 | | | 4678 |
| cocoa oil (cocoa butter) 1 T | 14 | 124 | 0 | 0 | 0 | | 0 | 0 | 0 | 0 | 0 | 0 | 0 | 0 | 0 | 0 | 0 | 0 |
| | | 0 | 14.0 | 8.4 | 4.6 | 0.4 | 0 | 0 | 0 | 0 | 0 | 0 | 0 | 0.3 | 0 | 0 | 0 | 4501 |
| coconut oil 1 T | 14 | 121 | 0 | 0 | 0 | | 0 | 0 | 0 | 0 | 0 | | 0 | 0 | 0 | 0 | 0 | 0 |
| | | 0 | 14.0 | 12.1 | 0.8 | 0.3 | 0 | 0 | 0 | 0.01 | 0 | 0 | 0 | 0 | 0 | 0 | 0 | 4047 |
| corn and canola oil 1 T | 14 | 124 | 0 | 0 | 0 | | 0 | 0 | 0 | 0 | 0 | | 0 | 0 | 0 | 0 | 0 | 0 |
| | | 0 | 14.0 | 1.1 | 8.2 | 4.1 | 0 | 0 | 0 | 0 | 0 | 0 | 0 | 2.1 | 0 | 0 | 0 | 42289 |

| | WT (g) | KCAL | H₂0 (g) | CHO (g) | TSUG (g) | ASUG (g) | DFIB (g) | Na (mg) | Ca (mg) | Mg (mg) | Zn (mg) | Mn (mg) | A (mcg RAE) | C (mg) | B-1 (mg) | NIA (mg) | B-12 (mcg) | PANT (mg) |
|---|---|---|---|---|---|---|---|---|---|---|---|---|---|---|---|---|---|---|
| | | PRO (g) | FAT (g) | SFA (g) | MUFA (g) | PUFA (g) | CHOL (mg) | K (mg) | P (mg) | Fe (mg) | Cu (mg) | Se (mcg) | A (IU) | E (mg ATE) | B-2 (mg) | B-6 (mg) | FOL (mcg DFE) | REF |
| corn oil | 14 | 124 | 0 | 0 | 0 | | 0 | 0 | 0 | 0 | 0 | | 0 | 0 | 0 | 0 | 0 | 0 |
| 1 T | | 0 | 14.0 | 1.8 | 3.9 | 7.7 | 0 | 0 | 0 | 0 | 0 | 0 | 0 | 2.0 | 0 | 0 | 0 | 4518 |
| cottonseed oil | 14 | 124 | 0 | 0 | 0 | | 0 | 0 | 0 | 0 | 0 | | 0 | 0 | 0 | 0 | 0 | 0 |
| 1 T | | 0 | 14.0 | 3.6 | 2.5 | 7.3 | 0 | 0 | 0 | 0 | 0 | 0 | 0 | 4.9 | 0 | 0 | 0 | 4502 |
| flaxseed oil | 14 | 124 | 0 | 0 | 0 | | 0 | 0 | 0 | 0 | 0 | | 0 | 0 | 0 | 0 | 0 | |
| 1 T | | 0 | 14.0 | 1.3 | 2.8 | 9.2 | 0 | 0 | 0 | 0 | 0 | 0 | 0 | 2.4 | 0 | 0 | 0 | 42231 |
| grapeseed oil | 14 | 124 | 0 | 0 | 0 | | 0 | 0 | 0 | 0 | 0 | 0 | 0 | 0 | 0 | 0 | 0 | 0 |
| 1 T | | 0 | 14.0 | 1.3 | 2.3 | 9.8 | 0 | 0 | 0 | 0 | 0 | 0 | 0 | 4.0 | 0 | 0 | 0 | 4517 |
| hazelnut oil | 14 | 124 | 0 | 0 | 0 | | 0 | 0 | 0 | 0 | 0 | | 0 | 0 | 0 | 0 | 0 | 0 |
| 1 T | | 0 | 14.0 | 1.0 | 10.9 | 1.4 | 0 | 0 | 0 | 0 | 0 | 0 | 0 | 6.6 | 0 | 0 | 0 | 4532 |
| mustard oil | 14 | 124 | 0 | 0 | | | 0 | 0 | 0 | 0 | 0 | 0 | 0 | 0 | 0 | 0 | 0 | 0 |
| 1 T | | 0 | 14.0 | 1.6 | 8.3 | 3.0 | 0 | 0 | 0 | 0 | 0 | 0 | 0 | 0 | 0 | 0 | 0 | 4583 |
| nutmeg oil | 14 | 124 | 0 | 0 | 0 | | 0 | 0 | 0 | 0 | 0 | | 0 | 0 | 0 | 0 | 0 | 0 |
| 1 T | | 0 | 14.0 | 12.6 | 0.7 | 0 | 0 | 0 | 0 | 0 | 0 | 0 | 0 | 0 | 0 | 0 | 0 | 4572 |
| oat oil | 14 | 124 | 0 | 0 | 0 | | 0 | 0 | 0 | 0 | 0 | 0 | 0 | 0 | 0 | 0 | 0 | 0 |
| 1 T | | 0 | 14.0 | 2.7 | 4.9 | 5.7 | 0 | 0 | 0 | 0 | 0 | 0 | 0 | 2.0 | 0 | 0 | 0 | 4588 |
| olive oil | 14 | 124 | 0 | 0 | 0 | | 0 | 0 | 0 | 0 | 0 | 0 | 0 | 0 | 0 | 0 | 0 | 0 |
| 1 T | | 0 | 14.0 | 1.9 | 10.2 | 1.5 | 0 | 0 | 0 | 0.08 | 0 | 0 | 0 | 2.0 | 0 | 0 | 0 | 4053 |
| palm kernel oil | 14 | 121 | 0 | 0 | 0 | | 0 | 0 | 0 | 0 | 0 | 0 | 0 | 0 | 0 | 0 | 0 | 0 |
| 1 T | | 0 | 14.0 | 11.4 | 1.6 | 0.2 | 0 | 0 | 0 | 0 | 0 | 0 | 0 | 0.5 | 0 | 0 | 0 | 4513 |
| palm oil | 14 | 124 | 0 | 0 | 0 | | 0 | 0 | 0 | 0 | 0 | 0 | 0 | 0 | 0 | 0 | 0 | 0 |
| 1 T | | 0 | 14.0 | 6.9 | 5.2 | 1.3 | 0 | 0 | 0 | 0 | 0 | 0 | 0 | 2.2 | 0 | 0 | 0 | 4055 |
| PAM cooking spray, ConAgra | 0.3 | 2 | 0 | 0.1 | 0 | | 0 | 0 | 0 | | | | 0 | | | | | |
| ⅓ sec spray | | 0 | 0.2 | 0 | 0.2 | 0 | 0 | | | 0 | | | 0 | | | | | 4679 |
| peanut oil | 14 | 124 | 0 | 0 | 0 | | 0 | 0 | 0 | 0 | 0 | | 0 | 0 | 0 | 0 | 0 | 0 |
| 1 T | | 0 | 14.0 | 2.4 | 6.5 | 4.5 | 0 | 0 | 0 | 0 | 0 | 0 | 0 | 2.2 | 0 | 0 | 0 | 4042 |
| poppyseed oil | 14 | 124 | 0 | 0 | 0 | | 0 | 0 | 0 | 0 | 0 | | 0 | 0 | 0 | 0 | 0 | 0 |
| 1 T | | 0 | 14.0 | 1.9 | 2.8 | 8.7 | 0 | 0 | 0 | 0 | 0 | 0 | 0 | 1.6 | 0 | 0 | 0 | 4514 |
| rice bran oil | 14 | 124 | 0 | 0 | 0 | | 0 | 0 | 0 | 0 | 0 | | 0 | 0 | 0 | 0 | 0 | 0 |
| 1 T | | 0 | 14.0 | 2.8 | 5.5 | 4.9 | 0 | 0 | 0 | 0.01 | 0 | 0 | 0 | 4.5 | 0 | 0 | 0 | 4037 |
| safflower oil, >70% linoleic acid | 14 | 124 | 0 | 0 | 0 | | 0 | 0 | 0 | 0 | 0 | 0 | 0 | 0 | 0 | 0 | 0 | 0 |
| 1 T | | 0 | 14.0 | 0.9 | 2.0 | 10.4 | 0 | 0 | 0 | 0 | 0 | 0 | 0 | 4.8 | 0 | 0 | 0 | 4510 |
| safflower oil, >70% oleic acid | 14 | 124 | 0 | 0 | 0 | | 0 | 0 | 0 | 0 | 0 | | 0 | 0 | 0 | 0 | 0 | 0 |
| 1 T | | 0 | 14.0 | 0.9 | 10.5 | 2.0 | 0 | 0 | 0 | 0 | 0 | 0 | 0 | 4.8 | 0 | 0 | 0 | 4511 |
| sesame oil | 14 | 124 | 0 | 0 | 0 | | 0 | 0 | 0 | 0 | 0 | | 0 | 0 | 0 | 0 | 0 | 0 |
| 1 T | | 0 | 14.0 | 2.0 | 5.6 | 5.8 | 0 | 0 | 0 | 0 | 0 | 0 | 0 | 0.2 | 0 | 0 | 0 | 4058 |
| sheanut oil (sheanut butter) | 14 | 124 | 0 | 0 | 0 | | 0 | 0 | 0 | 0 | 0 | | 0 | 0 | 0 | 0 | 0 | 0 |
| 1 T | | 0 | 14.0 | 6.5 | 6.2 | 0.7 | 0 | 0 | 0 | 0 | 0 | 0 | 0 | 0 | 0 | 0 | 0 | 4536 |
| soy (hydrogenated) and cottonseed oil - 1 T | 14 | 124 | 0 | 0 | 0 | | 0 | 0 | 0 | 0 | 0 | 0 | 0 | 0 | 0 | 0 | 0 | 0 |
| | | 0 | 14.0 | 2.5 | 4.1 | 6.7 | 0 | 0 | 0 | 0 | 0 | 0 | 0 | 1.7 | 0 | 0 | 0 | 4543 |
| soy (hydrogenated) and cottonseed oil (for bread) - 1 T | 14 | 124 | 0 | 0 | 0 | | 0 | 0 | 0 | 0 | 0 | 0 | 0 | 0 | 0 | 0 | 0 | 0 |
| | | 0 | 14.0 | 3.1 | 4.6 | 5.7 | 0 | 0 | 0 | 0 | 0 | 0 | 0 | 1.1 | 0 | 0 | 0 | 4546 |
| soy lecithin | 14 | 107 | 0 | 0 | 0 | | 0 | 0 | 0 | 0 | 0 | 0 | 0 | 0 | 0 | 0 | 0 | 0 |
| 1 T | | 0 | 14.0 | 2.1 | 1.5 | 6.3 | 0 | 0 | 0 | 0 | 0 | 0 | 0 | 1.1 | 0 | 0 | 0 | 4531 |
| soy oil (hydg) | 14 | 124 | 0 | 0 | 0 | | 0 | 0 | 0 | 0 | 0 | 0 | 0 | 0 | 0 | 0 | 0 | 0 |
| 1 T | | 0 | 14.0 | 2.1 | 6.0 | 5.3 | 0 | 0 | 0 | 0 | 0 | 0 | 0 | 1.1 | 0 | 0 | 0 | 4034 |
| soy oil, salad/cooking | 14 | 124 | 0 | 0 | 0 | | 0 | 0 | 0 | 0 | 0 | 0 | 0 | 0 | 0 | 0 | 0 | 0 |
| 1 T | | 0 | 14.0 | 2.2 | 3.2 | 8.1 | 0 | 0 | 0 | 0.01 | 0 | 0 | 0 | 1.1 | 0 | 0 | 0 | 4044 |
| sunflower oil, <60% linoleic acid | 14 | 124 | 0 | 0 | 0 | | 0 | 0 | 0 | 0 | 0 | 0 | 0 | 0 | 0 | 0 | 0 | 0 |
| 1 T | | 0 | 14.0 | 1.4 | 6.4 | 5.6 | 0 | 0 | 0 | 0 | 0 | 0 | 0 | 5.8 | 0 | 0 | 0 | 4060 |
| sunflower oil, >60% linoleic acid | 14 | 124 | 0 | 0 | 0 | | 0 | 0 | 0 | 0 | 0 | 0 | 0 | 0 | 0 | 0 | 0 | 0 |
| 1 T | | 0 | 14.0 | 1.4 | 2.7 | 9.2 | 0 | 0 | 0 | 0 | 0 | 0 | 0 | 5.8 | 0 | 0 | 0 | 4506 |
| sunflower oil, >70% oleic acid | 14 | 124 | 0 | 0 | 0 | | 0 | 0 | 0 | 0 | 0 | 0 | 0 | 0 | 0 | 0 | 0 | 0 |
| 1 T | | 0 | 14.0 | 1.4 | 11.7 | 0.5 | 0 | 0 | 0 | 0 | 0 | 0 | 0 | 5.8 | 0 | 0 | 0 | 4584 |
| walnut oil | 14 | 124 | 0 | 0 | 0 | | 0 | 0 | 0 | 0 | 0 | 0 | 0 | 0 | 0 | 0 | 0 | 0 |
| 1 T | | 0 | 14.0 | 1.3 | 3.2 | 8.9 | 0 | 0 | 0 | 0 | 0 | 0 | 0 | 0.1 | 0 | 0 | 0 | 4528 |
| wheat germ oil | 14 | 124 | 0 | 0 | 0 | | 0 | 0 | 0 | 0 | 0 | 0 | 0 | 0 | 0 | 0 | 0 | 0 |
| 1 T | | 0 | 14.0 | 2.6 | 2.1 | 8.6 | 0 | 0 | 0 | 0 | 0 | 0 | 0 | 20.9 | 0 | 0 | 0 | 4038 |

| | WT (g) | KCAL | H₂0 (g) | CHO (g) | TSUG (g) | ASUG (g) | DFIB (g) | Na (mg) | Ca (mg) | Mg (mg) | Zn (mg) | Mn (mg) | A (mcg RAE) | C (mg) | B-1 (mg) | NIA (mg) | B-12 (mcg) | PANT (mg) |
|---|---|---|---|---|---|---|---|---|---|---|---|---|---|---|---|---|---|---|
| | | PRO (g) | FAT (g) | SFA (g) | MUFA (g) | PUFA (g) | CHOL (mg) | K (mg) | P (mg) | Fe (mg) | Cu (mg) | Se (mcg) | A (IU) | E (mg ATE) | B-2 (mg) | B-6 (mg) | FOL (mcg DFE) | REF |

## 12. FISH AND SEAFOOD
### 12.1 CRUSTACEA

| Food | WT | KCAL/PRO | H₂O/FAT | CHO/SFA | TSUG/MUFA | ASUG/PUFA | DFIB/CHOL | Na/K | Ca/P | Mg/Fe | Zn/Cu | Mn/Se | A/A(IU) | C/E | B-1/B-2 | NIA/B-6 | B-12/FOL | PANT/REF |
|---|---|---|---|---|---|---|---|---|---|---|---|---|---|---|---|---|---|---|
| **crab, Alaska king**, cooked by moist heat - 3 oz | 85 | 82 | 65.9 | 0 | | | 0 | 911 | 50 | 54 | 6.48 | 0.034 | 8 | 6 | 0.05 | 1.1 | 9.78 | 0.34 |
| | | 16.4 | 1.3 | 0.1 | 0.2 | 0.5 | 45 | 223 | 238 | 0.65 | 1.005 | 34.0 | 25 | | 0.05 | 0.15 | 43.4 | 15137 |
| **crab, Alaska king, imitation**, made from surimi - 3 oz | 85 | 81 | 63.5 | 12.8 | 5.3 | 0 | 0.4 | 715 | 11 | 37 | 0.28 | 0.009 | 0 | 0 | 0.03 | 0.5 | 0.48 | 0 |
| | | 6.5 | 0.4 | 0.1 | 0.2 | 0.2 | 17 | 76 | 240 | 0.33 | 0.027 | 19.0 | 0 | 0.1 | 0.07 | 0.11 | 0 | 15138 |
| **crab, Alaska king**, raw  3 oz | 85 | 71 | 67.6 | 0 | | | 0 | 711 | 39 | 42 | 5.06 | 0.030 | 6 | 6 | 0.04 | 0.9 | 7.65 | 0.30 |
| | | 15.5 | 0.5 | 0.1 | 0.1 | 0.1 | 36 | 173 | 186 | 0.50 | 0.784 | 30.9 | 20 | | 0.04 | 0.13 | 37.4 | 15136 |
| **crab, blue**, canned  3 oz | 85 | 84 | 64.7 | 0 | 0 | | 0 | 283 | 86 | 33 | 3.42 | 0.162 | 2 | 2 | 0.07 | 1.2 | 0.39 | 0.31 |
| | | 17.4 | 1.0 | 0.2 | 0.2 | 0.4 | 76 | 318 | 221 | 0.71 | 0.646 | 27.0 | 6 | 1.6 | 0.07 | 0.13 | 36.6 | 15141 |
| **crab, blue**, cooked by moist heat  3 oz | 85 | 87 | 65.8 | 0 | 0 | | 0 | 237 | 88 | 28 | 3.59 | 0.162 | 2 | 3 | 0.08 | 2.8 | 6.20 | 0.37 |
| | | 17.2 | 1.5 | 0.2 | 0.2 | 0.6 | 85 | 275 | 175 | 0.77 | 0.548 | 34.2 | 6 | 1.6 | 0.04 | 0.15 | 43.4 | 15140 |
| **crab, blue**, raw  3 oz | 85 | 74 | 67.2 | 0 | | | 0 | 249 | 76 | 29 | 3.01 | 0.128 | 2 | 3 | 0.07 | 2.3 | 7.65 | 0.30 |
| | | 15.4 | 0.9 | 0.2 | 0.2 | 0.3 | 66 | 280 | 195 | 0.63 | 0.569 | 31.8 | 4 | | 0.03 | 0.13 | 37.4 | 15139 |
| **crab, dungeness**, ckd by moist heat  3 oz | 85 | 94 | 62.3 | 0.8 | | | 0 | 321 | 50 | 49 | 4.65 | 0.082 | 26 | 3 | 0.05 | 3.1 | 8.82 | 0.34 |
| | | 19.0 | 1.1 | 0.1 | 0.2 | 0.3 | 65 | 347 | 149 | 0.37 | 0.624 | 40.5 | 88 | | 0.17 | 0.15 | 35.7 | 15226 |
| **crab, dungeness**, raw  3 oz | 85 | 73 | 67.3 | 0.6 | | | 0 | 251 | 39 | 38 | 3.63 | 0.068 | 23 | 3 | 0.04 | 2.7 | 7.65 | 0.30 |
| | | 14.8 | 0.8 | 0.1 | 0.1 | 0.3 | 50 | 301 | 155 | 0.31 | 0.573 | 31.5 | 76 | | 0.14 | 0.13 | 37.4 | 15143 |
| **crab, queen**, cooked by moist heat  3 oz | 85 | 98 | 63.8 | 0 | | | 0 | 587 | 28 | 54 | 3.05 | 0.031 | 44 | 6 | 0.08 | 2.5 | 8.82 | 0.34 |
| | | 20.2 | 1.3 | 0.2 | 0.3 | 0.5 | 60 | 170 | 109 | 2.45 | 0.528 | 37.7 | 147 | | 0.21 | 0.15 | 35.7 | 15227 |
| **crab, queen**, raw  3 oz | 85 | 76 | 68.5 | 0 | | | 0 | 458 | 22 | 42 | 2.38 | 0.026 | 38 | 6 | 0.07 | 2.1 | 7.65 | 0.30 |
| | | 15.7 | 1.0 | 0.1 | 0.2 | 0.4 | 47 | 147 | 113 | 2.12 | 0.484 | 29.4 | 128 | | 0.17 | 0.13 | 37.4 | 15144 |
| **crabcake**  2.1 oz cake | 60 | 93 | 42.6 | 0.3 | | | 0 | 198 | 63 | 20 | 2.45 | 0.114 | 34 | 2 | 0.05 | 1.7 | 3.56 | 0.30 |
| | | 12.1 | 4.5 | 0.9 | 1.7 | 1.4 | 90 | 194 | 128 | 0.65 | 0.366 | 24.4 | 151 | | 0.05 | 0.10 | 36.6 | 15142 |
| **crayfish, farmed**, ckd by moist heat  3 oz | 85 | 74 | 68.7 | 0 | | | 0 | 82 | 43 | 28 | 1.26 | 0.184 | 13 | 0 | 0.04 | 1.4 | 2.64 | 0.44 |
| | | 14.9 | 1.1 | 0.2 | 0.2 | 0.4 | 116 | 202 | 205 | 0.94 | 0.493 | 29.1 | 42 | | 0.07 | 0.11 | 9.4 | 15243 |
| **crayfish, farmed**, raw  3 oz | 85 | 61 | 71.4 | 0 | | | 0 | 53 | 21 | 26 | 0.86 | 0.124 | 13 | 0 | 0.04 | 1.6 | 1.78 | 0.48 |
| | | 12.6 | 0.8 | 0.1 | 0.2 | 0.3 | 91 | 222 | 185 | 0.47 | 0.201 | 24.1 | 42 | | 0.03 | 0.06 | 25.5 | 15242 |
| **crayfish, wild**, ckd by moist heat  3 oz | 85 | 70 | 67.5 | 0 | 0 | | 0 | 80 | 51 | 28 | 1.50 | 0.444 | 13 | 1 | 0.04 | 1.9 | 1.83 | 0.49 |
| | | 14.3 | 1.0 | 0.2 | 0.2 | 0.3 | 113 | 252 | 230 | 0.71 | 0.582 | 31.2 | 42 | 1.3 | 0.07 | 0.06 | 37.4 | 15146 |
| **crayfish, wild**, raw  3 oz | 85 | 65 | 69.9 | 0 | 0 | | 0 | 49 | 23 | 23 | 1.10 | 0.192 | 14 | 1 | 0.06 | 1.9 | 1.70 | 0.46 |
| | | 13.6 | 0.8 | 0.1 | 0.1 | 0.2 | 97 | 257 | 218 | 0.71 | 0.356 | 26.9 | 45 | 2.4 | 0.03 | 0.09 | 31.4 | 15145 |
| **lobster, northern**, ckd by moist heat  3 oz | 85 | 83 | 64.6 | 1.1 | 0 | | 0 | 323 | 52 | 30 | 2.48 | 0.052 | 22 | 0 | 0.01 | 0.9 | 2.64 | 0.24 |
| | | 17.4 | 0.5 | 0.1 | 0.1 | 0.1 | 61 | 299 | 157 | 0.33 | 1.649 | 36.3 | 74 | 0.8 | 0.06 | 0.07 | 9.4 | 15148 |
| **lobster, northern**, raw  3 oz | 85 | 76 | 65.2 | 0.4 | 0 | | 0 | 252 | 41 | 23 | 2.57 | 0.047 | 18 | 0 | 0.01 | 1.2 | 0.79 | 1.39 |
| | | 16.0 | 0.8 | 0.2 | 0.2 | 0.1 | 81 | 234 | 122 | 0.26 | 1.414 | 35.2 | 60 | 1.2 | 0.04 | 0.05 | 7.6 | 15147 |
| **shrimp, breaded and fried**  3 oz (11 large) | 85 | 206 | 44.9 | 9.7 | | | 0.3 | 292 | 57 | 34 | 1.17 | 0.085 | | 1 | 0.11 | 2.6 | 1.59 | 0.30 |
| | | 18.2 | 10.4 | 1.8 | 3.2 | 4.3 | 150 | 191 | 185 | 1.07 | 0.233 | 35.4 | 161 | | 0.12 | 0.08 | 20.4 | 15150 |
| **shrimp**, canned  3 oz | 85 | 85 | 64.5 | 0 | 0 | | 0 | 660 | 123 | 28 | 1.67 | 0.337 | 0 | 3 | 0.01 | 0.5 | 0.63 | 0.12 |
| | | 17.4 | 1.2 | 0.2 | 0.1 | 0.6 | 214 | 68 | 166 | 1.81 | 0.223 | 40.4 | 0 | 0.9 | 0.01 | 0.01 | 7.6 | 15152 |
| **shrimp**, cooked by moist heat  3 oz (15½ large) | 85 | 84 | 65.7 | 0 | 0 | | 0 | 190 | 33 | 29 | 1.33 | 0.029 | 58 | 2 | 0.03 | 2.2 | 1.27 | 0.29 |
| | | 17.8 | 0.9 | 0.2 | 0.2 | 0.4 | 166 | 155 | 116 | 2.63 | 0.164 | 33.7 | 191 | 1.2 | 0.03 | 0.11 | 3.4 | 15151 |
| **shrimp, imitation**, made from surimi - 3 oz | 85 | 86 | 63.7 | 7.8 | | | 0 | 599 | 16 | 37 | 0.28 | 0.009 | 17 | 0 | 0.02 | 0.1 | 1.36 | 0.06 |
| | | 10.5 | 1.2 | 0.2 | 0.2 | 0.6 | 31 | 76 | 240 | 0.51 | 0.027 | 19.5 | 56 | | 0.03 | 0.03 | 1.7 | 15153 |
| **shrimp**, raw  3 oz | 85 | 90 | 64.5 | 0.8 | 0 | | 0 | 126 | 44 | 31 | 0.94 | 0.042 | 46 | 2 | 0.02 | 2.2 | 0.99 | 0.23 |
| | | 17.3 | 1.5 | 0.3 | 0.2 | 0.6 | 129 | 157 | 174 | 2.05 | 0.224 | 32.3 | 153 | 0.9 | 0.03 | 0.09 | 2.6 | 15149 |
| **spiny lobster**, cooked by dry heat  3 oz | 85 | 122 | 56.7 | 2.7 | | | 0 | 193 | 54 | 43 | 6.18 | 0.015 | 5 | 2 | 0.01 | 4.2 | 3.43 | 0.34 |
| | | 22.4 | 1.6 | 0.3 | 0.3 | 0.6 | 76 | 177 | 195 | 1.20 | 0.353 | 50.3 | 17 | | 0.05 | 0.15 | 0.8 | 15228 |
| **spiny lobster**, raw  3 oz | 85 | 95 | 63.0 | 2.1 | | | 0 | 150 | 42 | 34 | 4.82 | 0.013 | 4 | 2 | 0.01 | 3.6 | 2.98 | 0.30 |
| | | 17.5 | 1.3 | 0.2 | 0.2 | 0.5 | 60 | 153 | 202 | 1.04 | 0.324 | 39.3 | 14 | | 0.04 | 0.13 | 0.8 | 15154 |

### 12.2 FINFISH

| Food | WT | KCAL/PRO | H₂O/FAT | CHO/SFA | TSUG/MUFA | ASUG/PUFA | DFIB/CHOL | Na/K | Ca/P | Mg/Fe | Zn/Cu | Mn/Se | A/A(IU) | C/E | B-1/B-2 | NIA/B-6 | B-12/FOL | PANT/REF |
|---|---|---|---|---|---|---|---|---|---|---|---|---|---|---|---|---|---|---|
| **anchovies**, canned in olive oil  5 anchovies | 20 | 42 | 10.1 | 0 | 0 | | 0 | 734 | 46 | 14 | 0.49 | 0.020 | 2 | 0 | 0.02 | 4.0 | 0.18 | 0.18 |
| | | 5.8 | 1.9 | 0.4 | 0.8 | 0.5 | 17 | 109 | 50 | 0.93 | 0.068 | 13.6 | 8 | 0.7 | 0.07 | 0.04 | 2.6 | 15002 |
| **anchovies**, raw  3 oz | 85 | 111 | 62.4 | 0 | 0 | | 0 | 88 | 125 | 35 | 1.46 | 0.060 | 13 | 0 | 0.05 | 11.9 | 0.53 | 0.55 |
| | | 17.3 | 4.1 | 1.1 | 1.0 | 1.4 | 51 | 326 | 148 | 2.76 | 0.179 | 31.0 | 42 | 0.5 | 0.22 | 0.12 | 7.6 | 15001 |
| **bass, freshwater**, cooked by dry heat - 3 oz | 85 | 124 | 58.5 | 0 | | | 0 | 76 | 88 | 32 | 0.71 | 0.969 | 30 | 2 | 0.07 | 1.3 | 1.96 | 0.74 |
| | | 20.6 | 4.0 | 0.9 | 1.6 | 1.2 | 74 | 388 | 218 | 1.62 | 0.101 | 13.8 | 98 | | 0.08 | 0.12 | 14.4 | 15187 |
| **bass, freshwater**, raw  3 oz | 85 | 97 | 64.3 | 0 | | | 0 | 60 | 68 | 26 | 0.55 | 0.756 | 26 | 2 | 0.06 | 1.1 | 1.70 | 0.64 |
| | | 16.0 | 3.1 | 0.7 | 1.2 | 0.9 | 58 | 303 | 170 | 1.27 | 0.079 | 10.7 | 85 | | 0.06 | 0.10 | 12.8 | 15003 |

| Food | WT (g) | KCAL / PRO (g) | H₂0 (g) / FAT (g) | CHO (g) / SFA (g) | TSUG (g) / MUFA (g) | ASUG (g) / PUFA (g) | DFIB (g) / CHOL (mg) | Na (mg) / K (mg) | Ca (mg) / P (mg) | Mg (mg) / Fe (mg) | Zn (mg) / Cu (mg) | Mn (mg) / Se (mcg) | A (mcg RAE) / A (IU) | C (mg) / E (mg ATE) | B-1 (mg) / B-2 (mg) | NIA (mg) / B-6 (mg) | B-12 (mcg) / FOL (mcg DFE) | PANT (mg) / REF |
|---|---|---|---|---|---|---|---|---|---|---|---|---|---|---|---|---|---|---|
| **bass, striped**, cooked by dry heat | 85 | 105 | 62.4 | 0 | | | 0 | 75 | 16 | 43 | 0.43 | 0.016 | 26 | 0 | 0.10 | 2.2 | 3.75 | 0.74 |
| *3 oz* | | 19.3 | 2.5 | 0.6 | 0.7 | 0.9 | 88 | 279 | 216 | 0.92 | 0.034 | 39.8 | 88 | | 0.03 | 0.29 | 8.5 | 15188 |
| **bass, striped**, raw | 85 | 82 | 67.3 | 0 | | | 0 | 59 | 13 | 34 | 0.34 | 0.013 | 23 | 0 | 0.08 | 1.8 | 3.25 | 0.64 |
| *3 oz* | | 15.1 | 2.0 | 0.4 | 0.6 | 0.7 | 68 | 218 | 168 | 0.71 | 0.026 | 31.0 | 76 | | 0.03 | 0.26 | 7.6 | 15004 |
| **bluefish**, cooked by dry heat | 85 | 135 | 53.2 | 0 | | | 0 | 65 | 8 | 36 | 0.88 | 0.023 | 117 | 0 | 0.06 | 6.2 | 5.29 | 0.81 |
| *3 oz* | | 21.8 | 4.6 | 1.0 | 2.0 | 1.2 | 65 | 405 | 247 | 0.53 | 0.058 | 39.8 | 390 | | 0.08 | 0.39 | 1.7 | 15189 |
| **bluefish**, raw | 85 | 105 | 60.2 | 0 | | | 0 | 51 | 6 | 28 | 0.69 | 0.018 | 102 | 0 | 0.05 | 5.1 | 4.58 | 0.70 |
| *3 oz* | | 17.0 | 3.6 | 0.8 | 1.5 | 0.9 | 50 | 316 | 193 | 0.41 | 0.045 | 31.0 | 338 | | 0.07 | 0.34 | 1.7 | 15005 |
| **burbot**, cooked by dry heat | 85 | 98 | 62.4 | 0 | | | 0 | 105 | 54 | 35 | 0.82 | 0.762 | 4 | 0 | 0.36 | 1.7 | 0.78 | 0.15 |
| *3 oz* | | 21.0 | 0.9 | 0.2 | 0.1 | 0.3 | 65 | 440 | 218 | 0.98 | 0.218 | 13.8 | 14 | | 0.15 | 0.29 | 0.8 | 15190 |
| **burbot**, raw | 85 | 76 | 67.4 | 0 | | | 0 | 82 | 42 | 27 | 0.65 | 0.595 | 4 | 0 | 0.32 | 1.4 | 0.68 | 0.13 |
| *3 oz* | | 16.4 | 0.7 | 0.1 | 0.1 | 0.3 | 51 | 343 | 170 | 0.76 | 0.170 | 10.7 | 13 | | 0.12 | 0.26 | 0.8 | 15006 |
| **butterfish**, cooked by dry heat | 85 | 159 | 56.8 | 0 | | | 0 | 97 | 24 | 27 | 0.84 | 0.016 | 28 | 0 | 0.12 | 4.9 | 1.56 | 0.74 |
| *3 oz* | | 18.8 | 8.7 | | | | 71 | 409 | 262 | 0.54 | 0.059 | 39.8 | 93 | | 0.16 | 0.29 | 14.4 | 15191 |
| **butterfish**, raw | 85 | 124 | 63.0 | 0 | | | 0 | 76 | 19 | 21 | 0.65 | 0.013 | 26 | 0 | 0.10 | 3.8 | 1.62 | 0.64 |
| *3 oz* | | 14.7 | 6.8 | 2.9 | 2.9 | 0.5 | 55 | 319 | 204 | 0.42 | 0.046 | 31.0 | 85 | | 0.13 | 0.26 | 12.8 | 15007 |
| **carp**, cooked by dry heat | 85 | 138 | 59.2 | 0 | | | 0 | 54 | 44 | 32 | 1.62 | 0.042 | 8 | 1 | 0.12 | 1.8 | 1.25 | 0.74 |
| *3 oz* | | 19.4 | 6.1 | 1.2 | 2.5 | 1.6 | 71 | 363 | 451 | 1.35 | 0.062 | 13.8 | 27 | | 0.06 | 0.19 | 14.4 | 15009 |
| **carp**, raw | 85 | 108 | 64.9 | 0 | 0 | | 0 | 42 | 35 | 25 | 1.26 | 0.036 | 8 | 1 | 0.10 | 1.4 | 1.30 | 0.64 |
| *3 oz* | | 15.2 | 4.8 | 0.9 | 2.0 | 1.2 | 56 | 283 | 353 | 1.05 | 0.048 | 10.7 | 26 | 0.5 | 0.05 | 0.16 | 12.8 | 15008 |
| **catfish, channel**, breaded and fried | 85 | 195 | 50.0 | 6.8 | | | 0.6 | 238 | 37 | 23 | 0.73 | 0.034 | 7 | 0 | 0.06 | 1.9 | 1.62 | 0.62 |
| *3 oz* | | 15.4 | 11.3 | 2.8 | 4.8 | 2.8 | 69 | 289 | 184 | 1.22 | 0.086 | 11.8 | 24 | | 0.11 | 0.16 | 33.2 | 15011 |
| **catfish, channel**, farmed, cooked by dry heat - 3 oz | 85 | 129 | 60.8 | 0 | | | 0 | 68 | 8 | 22 | 0.89 | 0.017 | 13 | 1 | 0.36 | 2.1 | 2.38 | 0.52 |
| | | 15.9 | 6.8 | 1.5 | 3.5 | 1.2 | 54 | 273 | 208 | 0.70 | 0.104 | 12.3 | 42 | | 0.06 | 0.14 | 6.0 | 15235 |
| **catfish, channel**, farmed, raw | 85 | 115 | 64.1 | 0 | 0 | | 0 | 45 | 8 | 20 | 0.63 | 0.015 | 13 | 1 | 0.31 | 2.0 | 2.10 | 0.51 |
| *3 oz* | | 13.2 | 6.5 | 1.5 | 3.0 | 1.3 | 40 | 254 | 172 | 0.42 | 0.086 | 10.7 | 42 | 1.0 | 0.06 | 0.16 | 8.5 | 15234 |
| **catfish, channel**, wild, ckd by dry heat - 3 oz | 85 | 89 | 66.0 | 0 | | | 0 | 42 | 9 | 24 | 0.52 | 0.023 | 13 | 1 | 0.19 | 2.0 | 2.46 | 0.77 |
| | | 15.7 | 2.4 | 0.6 | 0.9 | 0.5 | 61 | 356 | 258 | 0.30 | 0.033 | 12.2 | 42 | | 0.06 | 0.09 | 8.5 | 15233 |
| **catfish, channel**, wild, raw | 85 | 81 | 68.3 | 0 | | | 0 | 37 | 12 | 20 | 0.43 | 0.021 | 13 | 1 | 0.18 | 1.6 | 1.90 | 0.65 |
| *3 oz* | | 13.9 | 2.4 | 0.6 | 0.7 | 0.7 | 49 | 304 | 178 | 0.26 | 0.029 | 10.7 | 42 | | 0.06 | 0.10 | 8.5 | 15010 |
| **cisco**, raw | 85 | 83 | 67.1 | 0 | | | 0 | 47 | 10 | 14 | 0.31 | 0.057 | 26 | 0 | 0.07 | 2.1 | 0.85 | 0.64 |
| *3 oz* | | 16.1 | 1.6 | 0.4 | 0.4 | 0.5 | 42 | 301 | 129 | 0.34 | 0.061 | 10.7 | 85 | | 0.08 | 0.26 | 12.8 | 15013 |
| **cisco**, smoked | 85 | 150 | 59.3 | 0 | 0 | | 0 | 409 | 22 | 14 | 0.26 | 0.018 | 241 | 0 | 0.04 | 2.0 | 3.62 | 0.26 |
| *3 oz* | | 13.9 | 10.1 | 1.5 | 4.7 | 1.9 | 27 | 249 | 128 | 0.42 | 0.183 | 15.4 | 802 | 0.2 | 0.14 | 0.23 | 1.7 | 15014 |
| **cod, Atlantic**, cnd, solids and liquids - 3 oz | 85 | 89 | 64.3 | 0 | 0 | | 0 | 185 | 18 | 35 | 0.49 | 0.017 | 12 | 1 | 0.07 | 2.1 | 0.89 | 0.14 |
| | | 19.3 | 0.7 | 0.1 | 0.1 | 0.2 | 47 | 449 | 221 | 0.42 | 0.031 | 32.4 | 40 | 0.7 | 0.07 | 0.24 | 6.8 | 15017 |
| **cod, Atlantic**, cooked by dry heat | 85 | 89 | 64.5 | 0 | 0 | | 0 | 66 | 12 | 36 | 0.49 | 0.017 | 12 | 1 | 0.07 | 2.1 | 0.89 | 0.15 |
| *3 oz* | | 19.4 | 0.7 | 0.1 | 0.1 | 0.2 | 47 | 207 | 117 | 0.42 | 0.031 | 32.0 | 40 | 0.7 | 0.07 | 0.24 | 6.8 | 15016 |
| **cod, Atlantic**, dried and salted | 85 | 246 | 13.7 | 0 | 0 | | 0 | 5973 | 136 | 113 | 1.35 | 0.042 | 36 | 3 | 0.23 | 6.4 | 8.50 | 1.42 |
| *3 oz* | | 53.4 | 2.0 | 0.4 | 0.3 | 0.7 | 129 | 1239 | 808 | 2.12 | 0.150 | 125.6 | 119 | 2.4 | 0.20 | 0.73 | 21.2 | 15018 |
| **cod, Atlantic**, raw | 85 | 70 | 69.0 | 0 | 0 | | 0 | 46 | 14 | 27 | 0.38 | 0.013 | 10 | 1 | 0.06 | 1.8 | 0.77 | 0.13 |
| *3 oz* | | 15.1 | 0.6 | 0.1 | 0.1 | 0.2 | 37 | 351 | 173 | 0.32 | 0.024 | 28.1 | 34 | 0.5 | 0.06 | 0.21 | 6.0 | 15015 |
| **cod, Pacific**, cooked by dry heat | 85 | 89 | 64.6 | 0 | | | 0 | 77 | 8 | 26 | 0.43 | 0.013 | 8 | 3 | 0.02 | 2.1 | 0.88 | 0.14 |
| *3 oz* | | 19.5 | 0.7 | 0.1 | 0.1 | 0.3 | 40 | 439 | 190 | 0.28 | 0.028 | 39.8 | 27 | | 0.04 | 0.39 | 6.8 | 15192 |
| **cod, Pacific**, raw | 85 | 70 | 69.1 | 0 | 0 | | 0 | 60 | 6 | 20 | 0.34 | 0.010 | 7 | 2 | 0.02 | 1.7 | 0.76 | 0.12 |
| *3 oz* | | 15.2 | 0.6 | 0.1 | 0.1 | 0.2 | 31 | 343 | 148 | 0.22 | 0.022 | 31.0 | 23 | 0.5 | 0.04 | 0.34 | 6.0 | 15019 |
| **croaker, Atlantic**, breaded and fried | 85 | 188 | 50.8 | 6.4 | | | 0.3 | 296 | 27 | 36 | 0.44 | 0.068 | 20 | 0 | 0.08 | 3.7 | 1.78 | 0.63 |
| *3 oz* | | 15.5 | 10.8 | 3.0 | 4.5 | 2.5 | 71 | 289 | 184 | 0.73 | 0.055 | 33.0 | 64 | | 0.11 | 0.22 | 38.2 | 15021 |
| **croaker, Atlantic**, raw | 85 | 88 | 66.3 | 0 | 0 | | 0 | 48 | 13 | 34 | 0.36 | 0.021 | 15 | 0 | 0.06 | 3.6 | 2.12 | 0.64 |
| *3 oz* | | 15.1 | 2.7 | 0.9 | 1.0 | 0.4 | 52 | 293 | 178 | 0.31 | 0.036 | 31.0 | 51 | 0.8 | 0.08 | 0.26 | 12.8 | 15020 |
| **cusk**, cooked by dry heat | 85 | 95 | 59.2 | 0 | | | 0 | 34 | 11 | 34 | 0.42 | 0.016 | 18 | 0 | 0.04 | 2.8 | 1.02 | 0.27 |
| *3 oz* | | 20.7 | 0.7 | | | | 45 | 428 | 223 | 0.90 | 0.020 | 39.8 | 59 | | 0.14 | 0.38 | 1.7 | 15193 |
| **cusk**, raw | 85 | 74 | 64.9 | 0 | | | 0 | 26 | 8 | 26 | 0.32 | 0.013 | 15 | 0 | 0.04 | 2.3 | 0.88 | 0.24 |
| *3 oz* | | 16.1 | 0.6 | 0.1 | 0.1 | 0.2 | 35 | 333 | 173 | 0.71 | 0.015 | 31.0 | 51 | | 0.11 | 0.33 | 1.7 | 15022 |
| **dolphinfish**, cooked by dry heat | 85 | 93 | 60.5 | 0 | | | 0 | 96 | 16 | 32 | 0.50 | 0.016 | 53 | 0 | 0.02 | 6.3 | 0.59 | 0.74 |
| *3 oz* | | 20.2 | 0.8 | 0.2 | 0.1 | 0.2 | 80 | 453 | 156 | 1.23 | 0.045 | 39.8 | 177 | | 0.07 | 0.39 | 5.1 | 15194 |
| **dolphinfish**, raw | 85 | 72 | 65.9 | 0 | | | 0 | 75 | 13 | 26 | 0.39 | 0.013 | 46 | 0 | 0.02 | 5.2 | 0.51 | 0.64 |
| *3 oz* | | 15.7 | 0.6 | 0.2 | 0.1 | 0.1 | 62 | 354 | 122 | 0.96 | 0.035 | 31.0 | 153 | | 0.06 | 0.34 | 4.2 | 15023 |
| **drum, freshwater**, cooked by dry heat - 3 oz | 85 | 130 | 60.3 | 0 | | | 0 | 82 | 65 | 32 | 0.72 | 0.762 | 50 | 1 | 0.07 | 2.4 | 1.96 | 0.74 |
| | | 19.1 | 5.4 | 1.2 | 2.4 | 1.3 | 70 | 300 | 196 | 0.98 | 0.252 | 13.8 | 167 | | 0.18 | 0.29 | 14.4 | 15195 |
| **drum, freshwater**, raw | 85 | 101 | 65.7 | 0 | | | 0 | 64 | 51 | 26 | 0.56 | 0.595 | 43 | 1 | 0.06 | 2.0 | 1.70 | 0.64 |
| *3 oz* | | 14.9 | 4.2 | 1.0 | 1.9 | 1.0 | 54 | 234 | 153 | 0.76 | 0.197 | 10.7 | 144 | | 0.14 | 0.26 | 12.8 | 15024 |

| | WT (g) | KCAL | H₂0 (g) | CHO (g) | TSUG (g) | ASUG (g) | DFIB (g) | Na (mg) | Ca (mg) | Mg (mg) | Zn (mg) | Mn (mg) | A (mcg RAE) | C (mg) | B-1 (mg) | NIA (mg) | B-12 (mcg) | PANT (mg) |
|---|---|---|---|---|---|---|---|---|---|---|---|---|---|---|---|---|---|---|
| | | PRO (g) | FAT (g) | SFA (g) | MUFA (g) | PUFA (g) | CHOL (mg) | K (mg) | P (mg) | Fe (mg) | Cu (mg) | Se (mcg) | A (IU) | E (mg ATE) | B-2 (mg) | B-6 (mg) | FOL (mcg DFE) | REF |
| eel, cooked by dry heat | 85 | 201 | 50.4 | 0 | | | 0 | 55 | 22 | 22 | 1.77 | 0.034 | 966 | 2 | 0.16 | 3.8 | 2.46 | 0.24 |
| 3 oz | | 20.1 | 12.7 | 2.6 | 7.8 | 1.0 | 137 | 297 | 235 | 0.54 | 0.025 | 7.1 | 3219 | | 0.04 | 0.07 | 14.4 | 15026 |
| eel, raw | 85 | 156 | 58.0 | 0 | 0 | | 0 | 43 | 17 | 17 | 1.38 | 0.030 | 887 | 2 | 0.13 | 3.0 | 2.55 | 0.20 |
| 3 oz | | 15.7 | 9.9 | 2.0 | 6.1 | 0.8 | 107 | 231 | 184 | 0.42 | 0.020 | 5.5 | 2955 | 3.4 | 0.03 | 0.06 | 12.8 | 15025 |
| fish fillet, Cajun blackened, frozen, Gorton's - 3.8 oz fillet | 108 | 100 | | 1.0 | 0 | | 0 | 330 | 20 | | | | | 0 | 0.12 | 1.6 | | |
| | | 17.0 | 3.0 | 0.5 | 1.0 | 1.0 | 60 | 360 | | 0.72 | | | 0 | | 0.03 | | | GORT1 |
| fish fillet, garlic butter, frozen, Gorton's - 3.8 oz fillet | 108 | 100 | | 1.0 | 0 | | 0 | 270 | 0 | | | | | 0 | 0.09 | 1.6 | | |
| | | 17.0 | 3.0 | 0.5 | 0.5 | 1.5 | 60 | 350 | | 0.36 | | | 0 | | | | | GORT2 |
| fish sticks/pieces, frozen, reheated | 28 | 70 | 14.9 | 5.9 | 0.7 | 0.5 | 0.4 | 118 | 7 | 8 | 0.13 | 0.059 | 9 | 0 | 0.04 | 0.4 | 0.36 | 0.12 |
| 1 stick (4″ × 1″ × ½″) | | 3.1 | 3.7 | 0.8 | 1.2 | 1.6 | 9 | 60 | 51 | 0.28 | 0.017 | 4.6 | 30 | 0.3 | 0.03 | 0.01 | 13.7 | 15027 |
| flounder/sole (flatfish), ckd by dry heat - 3 oz | 85 | 99 | 62.2 | 0 | 0 | | 0 | 89 | 15 | 49 | 0.54 | 0.017 | 11 | 0 | 0.07 | 1.9 | 2.13 | 0.49 |
| | | 20.5 | 1.3 | 0.3 | 0.2 | 0.5 | 58 | 292 | 246 | 0.29 | 0.022 | 49.5 | 37 | 0.6 | 0.10 | 0.20 | 7.6 | 15029 |
| flounder/sole (flatfish), raw | 85 | 77 | 67.2 | 0 | 0 | | 0 | 69 | 15 | 26 | 0.38 | 0.014 | 8 | 1 | 0.08 | 2.5 | 1.29 | 0.43 |
| 3 oz | | 16.0 | 1.0 | 0.2 | 0.2 | 0.3 | 41 | 307 | 156 | 0.31 | 0.027 | 27.8 | 28 | 0.4 | 0.06 | 0.18 | 6.8 | 15028 |
| gefiltefish with broth, sweet | 42 | 35 | 33.7 | 3.1 | | | 0 | 220 | 10 | 4 | 0.34 | 0.031 | 11 | 0 | 0.03 | 0.4 | 0.35 | 0.08 |
| 1 piece | | 3.8 | 0.7 | 0.2 | 0.3 | 0.1 | 13 | 38 | 31 | 1.04 | 0.082 | 4.4 | 37 | | 0.02 | 0.03 | 1.3 | 15030 |
| grouper, cooked by dry heat | 85 | 100 | 62.4 | 0 | | | 0 | 45 | 18 | 31 | 0.43 | 0.010 | 42 | 0 | 0.07 | 0.3 | 0.59 | 0.74 |
| 3 oz | | 21.1 | 1.1 | 0.3 | 0.2 | 0.3 | 40 | 404 | 122 | 0.97 | 0.038 | 39.8 | 140 | | 0.01 | 0.30 | 8.5 | 15032 |
| grouper, raw | 85 | 78 | 67.3 | 0 | | | 0 | 45 | 23 | 26 | 0.41 | 0.012 | 37 | 0 | 0.06 | 0.3 | 0.51 | 0.64 |
| 3 oz | | 16.5 | 0.9 | 0.2 | 0.2 | 0.3 | 31 | 411 | 138 | 0.76 | 0.017 | 31.0 | 122 | 0 | | 0.26 | 7.6 | 15031 |
| haddock, cooked by dry heat | 85 | 95 | 63.1 | 0 | | | 0 | 74 | 36 | 42 | 0.41 | 0.026 | 16 | 0 | 0.03 | 3.9 | 1.18 | 0.13 |
| 3 oz | | 20.6 | 0.8 | 0.1 | 0.1 | 0.3 | 63 | 339 | 205 | 1.15 | 0.028 | 34.4 | 54 | | 0.04 | 0.29 | 11.0 | 15034 |
| haddock, raw | 85 | 74 | 67.9 | 0 | 0 | | 0 | 58 | 28 | 33 | 0.31 | 0.021 | 14 | 0 | 0.03 | 3.2 | 1.02 | 0.11 |
| 3 oz | | 16.1 | 0.6 | 0.1 | 0.1 | 0.2 | 48 | 264 | 160 | 0.89 | 0.022 | 25.7 | 48 | 0.3 | 0.03 | 0.26 | 10.2 | 15033 |
| haddock, smoked | 85 | 99 | 60.8 | 0 | 0 | | 0 | 649 | 42 | 46 | 0.42 | 0.026 | 19 | 0 | 0.04 | 4.3 | 1.36 | 0.14 |
| 3 oz | | 21.4 | 0.8 | 0.1 | 0.1 | 0.3 | 65 | 353 | 213 | 1.19 | 0.036 | 36.5 | 62 | 0.5 | 0.04 | 0.34 | 12.8 | 15035 |
| halibut, Alaskan, cooked with skin | 85 | 96 | 61.9 | 0 | 0 | | 0 | 73 | 28 | 25 | 0.64 | 0.009 | 41 | | 0.07 | 5.3 | 2.17 | 0.41 |
| 3 oz | | 18.8 | 2.3 | 0.4 | 0.7 | 0.6 | 64 | 426 | 234 | 0.31 | 0.035 | 51.5 | 136 | 0.9 | 0.15 | 0.23 | | 35188 |
| halibut, Atlantic and Pacific, ckd by dry heat - 3 oz | 85 | 119 | 60.9 | 0 | | | 0 | 59 | 51 | 91 | 0.45 | 0.017 | 46 | 0 | 0.06 | 6.1 | 1.16 | 0.32 |
| | | 22.7 | 2.5 | 0.4 | 0.8 | 0.8 | 35 | 490 | 242 | 0.91 | 0.030 | 39.8 | 152 | | 0.08 | 0.34 | 11.9 | 15037 |
| halibut, Atlantic and Pacific, raw | 85 | 94 | 66.2 | 0 | 0 | | 0 | 46 | 40 | 71 | 0.36 | 0.013 | 40 | 0 | 0.05 | 5.0 | 1.00 | 0.28 |
| 3 oz | | 17.7 | 1.9 | 0.3 | 0.6 | 0.6 | 27 | 382 | 189 | 0.71 | 0.023 | 31.0 | 133 | 0.7 | 0.06 | 0.29 | 10.2 | 15036 |
| halibut, Greenland, ckd by dry heat | 85 | 203 | 52.6 | 0 | | | 0 | 88 | 3 | 28 | 0.43 | 0.013 | 15 | 0 | 0.06 | 1.6 | 0.82 | 0.24 |
| 3 oz | | 15.7 | 15.1 | 2.6 | 9.1 | 1.5 | 50 | 292 | 178 | 0.72 | 0.032 | 39.8 | 51 | | 0.09 | 0.41 | 0.8 | 15196 |
| halibut, Greenland, raw | 85 | 158 | 59.7 | 0 | 0 | | 0 | 68 | 3 | 22 | 0.34 | 0.010 | 14 | 0 | 0.05 | 1.3 | 0.85 | 0.21 |
| 3 oz | | 12.2 | 11.8 | 2.1 | 7.1 | 1.2 | 39 | 228 | 139 | 0.56 | 0.026 | 31.0 | 48 | 0.7 | 0.07 | 0.36 | 0.8 | 15038 |
| herring, Atlantic, cooked by dry heat - 3 oz | 85 | 173 | 54.5 | 0 | 0 | | 0 | 98 | 63 | 35 | 1.08 | 0.034 | 31 | 1 | 0.10 | 3.5 | 11.17 | 0.63 |
| | | 19.6 | 9.9 | 2.2 | 4.1 | 2.3 | 65 | 356 | 258 | 1.20 | 0.100 | 39.8 | 102 | 1.2 | 0.25 | 0.30 | 10.2 | 15040 |
| herring, Atlantic, kippered | 40 | 87 | 23.9 | 0 | 0 | | 0 | 367 | 34 | 18 | 0.54 | 0.020 | 16 | 0 | 0.05 | 1.8 | 7.48 | 0.35 |
| 1 piece (5″ × 1¾″ × ¼″) | | 9.8 | 4.9 | 1.1 | 2.0 | 1.2 | 33 | 179 | 130 | 0.60 | 0.054 | 21.0 | 54 | 0.6 | 0.13 | 0.17 | 5.6 | 15042 |
| herring, Atlantic, pickled | 15 | 39 | 8.3 | 1.4 | 1.2 | 1.2 | 0 | 130 | 12 | 1 | 0.08 | 0.006 | 39 | 0 | 0.01 | 0.5 | 0.64 | 0.01 |
| 1 piece (1¾″ × ⅞″ × ½″) | | 2.1 | 2.7 | 0.4 | 1.8 | 0.3 | 2 | 10 | 13 | 0.18 | 0.016 | 8.8 | 129 | 0.3 | 0.02 | 0.03 | 0.3 | 15041 |
| herring, Atlantic, raw | 85 | 134 | 61.2 | 0 | 0 | | 0 | 76 | 48 | 27 | 0.84 | 0.030 | 24 | 1 | 0.08 | 2.7 | 11.62 | 0.49 |
| 3 oz | | 15.3 | 7.7 | 1.7 | 3.2 | 1.8 | 51 | 278 | 201 | 0.94 | 0.078 | 31.0 | 79 | 0.9 | 0.20 | 0.26 | 8.5 | 15039 |
| herring, Pacific, cooked by dry heat | 85 | 212 | 54.0 | 0 | | | 0 | 81 | 90 | 35 | 0.58 | 0.049 | 30 | 0 | 0.06 | 2.4 | 8.18 | 0.98 |
| 3 oz | | 17.9 | 15.1 | 3.5 | 7.5 | 2.6 | 84 | 461 | 248 | 1.22 | 0.085 | 39.8 | 99 | | 0.22 | 0.44 | 5.1 | 15197 |
| herring, Pacific, raw | 85 | 166 | 60.8 | 0 | 0 | | 0 | 63 | 71 | 27 | 0.45 | 0.038 | 27 | 0 | 0.05 | 1.9 | 8.50 | 0.85 |
| 3 oz | | 13.9 | 11.8 | 2.8 | 5.8 | 2.1 | 65 | 360 | 194 | 0.95 | 0.066 | 31.0 | 90 | | 0.17 | 0.38 | 4.2 | 15043 |
| ling, cooked by dry heat | 85 | 94 | 62.8 | 0 | | | 0 | 147 | 37 | 69 | 0.85 | 0.032 | 30 | 0 | 0.11 | 2.4 | 0.55 | 0.31 |
| 3 oz | | 20.7 | 0.7 | | | | 43 | 413 | 216 | 0.71 | 0.120 | 39.8 | 98 | | 0.20 | 0.30 | 6.8 | 15198 |
| ling, raw | 85 | 74 | 67.7 | 0 | | | 0 | 115 | 29 | 54 | 0.66 | 0.026 | 26 | 0 | 0.09 | 2.0 | 0.48 | 0.27 |
| 3 oz | | 16.1 | 0.5 | 0.1 | 0.1 | 0.2 | 34 | 322 | 168 | 0.55 | 0.094 | 31.0 | 85 | | 0.16 | 0.26 | 6.0 | 15044 |
| lingcod, cooked by dry heat | 85 | 93 | 64.3 | 0 | | | 0 | 65 | 15 | 28 | 0.49 | 0.022 | 14 | 0 | 0.03 | 2.0 | 3.53 | 0.74 |
| 3 oz | | 19.2 | 1.2 | 0.2 | 0.4 | 0.3 | 57 | 476 | 219 | 0.35 | 0.030 | 39.8 | 49 | | 0.12 | 0.29 | 8.5 | 15199 |
| lingcod, raw | 85 | 72 | 68.9 | 0 | | | 0 | 50 | 12 | 22 | 0.38 | 0.017 | 13 | 0 | 0.03 | 1.6 | 3.06 | 0.64 |
| 3 oz | | 15.0 | 0.9 | 0.2 | 0.3 | 0.3 | 44 | 371 | 171 | 0.27 | 0.023 | 31.0 | 42 | | 0.10 | 0.26 | 7.6 | 15045 |
| mackerel, Atlantic, ckd by dry heat | 85 | 223 | 45.3 | 0 | | | 0 | 71 | 13 | 82 | 0.80 | 0.017 | 46 | 0 | 0.14 | 5.8 | 16.15 | 0.84 |
| 3 oz | | 20.3 | 15.1 | 3.5 | 6.0 | 3.7 | 64 | 341 | 236 | 1.33 | 0.080 | 43.9 | 153 | | 0.35 | 0.39 | 1.7 | 15047 |
| mackerel, Atlantic, raw | 85 | 174 | 54.0 | 0 | 0 | | 0 | 76 | 10 | 65 | 0.54 | 0.013 | 42 | 0 | 0.15 | 7.7 | 7.40 | 0.73 |
| 3 oz | | 15.8 | 11.8 | 2.8 | 4.6 | 2.8 | 60 | 267 | 184 | 1.39 | 0.062 | 37.5 | 142 | 1.3 | 0.27 | 0.34 | 0.8 | 15046 |
| mackerel, jack, canned, drained | 190 | 296 | 131.4 | 0 | 0 | | 0 | 720 | 458 | 70 | 1.94 | 0.076 | 247 | 2 | 0.08 | 11.7 | 13.19 | 0.58 |
| 1 cup | | 44.1 | 12.0 | 3.5 | 4.2 | 3.1 | 150 | 369 | 572 | 3.88 | 0.279 | 71.6 | 823 | 2.0 | 0.40 | 0.40 | 9.5 | 15048 |

| | WT (g) | KCAL / PRO (g) | H₂0 (g) / FAT (g) | CHO (g) / SFA (g) | TSUG (g) / MUFA (g) | ASUG (g) / PUFA (g) | DFIB (g) / CHOL (mg) | Na (mg) / K (mg) | Ca (mg) / P (mg) | Mg (mg) / Fe (mg) | Zn (mg) / Cu (mg) | Mn (mg) / Se (mcg) | A (mcg RAE) / A (IU) | C (mg) / E (mg ATE) | B-1 (mg) / B-2 (mg) | NIA (mg) / B-6 (mg) | B-12 (mcg) / FOL (mcg DFE) | PANT (mg) / REF |
|---|---|---|---|---|---|---|---|---|---|---|---|---|---|---|---|---|---|---|
| **mackerel, king,** cooked by dry heat | 85 | 114 | 58.7 | 0 | | | 0 | 173 | 34 | 35 | 0.61 | 0.005 | 214 | 1 | 0.10 | 8.9 | 15.30 | 0.82 |
| *3 oz* | | 22.1 | 2.2 | 0.4 | 0.8 | 0.5 | 58 | 474 | 270 | 1.94 | 0.028 | 39.8 | 713 | | 0.49 | 0.43 | 7.6 | 15200 |
| **mackerel, king,** raw | 85 | 89 | 64.5 | 0 | | | 0 | 134 | 26 | 27 | 0.48 | 0.004 | 185 | 1 | 0.08 | 7.3 | 13.26 | 0.71 |
| *3 oz* | | 17.2 | 1.7 | 0.3 | 0.6 | 0.4 | 45 | 370 | 211 | 1.51 | 0.022 | 31.0 | 618 | | 0.40 | 0.38 | 6.8 | 15049 |
| **mackerel, Pacific/jack,** ckd by dry | 85 | 171 | 52.5 | 0 | 0 | | 0 | 94 | 25 | 31 | 0.73 | 0.016 | 14 | 2 | 0.11 | 9.1 | 3.60 | 0.31 |
| heat - *3 oz* | | 21.9 | 8.6 | 2.4 | 2.9 | 2.1 | 51 | 443 | 136 | 1.27 | 0.101 | 39.8 | 46 | 1.1 | 0.46 | 0.32 | 1.7 | 15201 |
| **mackerel, Pacific/jack,** raw | 85 | 134 | 59.6 | 0 | 0 | | 0 | 73 | 20 | 24 | 0.57 | 0.013 | 11 | 2 | 0.09 | 7.1 | 3.74 | 0.27 |
| *3 oz* | | 17.1 | 6.7 | 1.9 | 2.2 | 1.6 | 40 | 345 | 106 | 0.99 | 0.079 | 31.0 | 37 | 0.8 | 0.36 | 0.28 | 1.7 | 15050 |
| **mackerel,** salted | 28 | 85 | 12.0 | 0 | 0 | | 0 | 1246 | 18 | 17 | 0.31 | | 13 | 0 | 0.01 | 0.9 | 3.36 | |
| *1 oz* | | 5.2 | 7.0 | 2.0 | 2.3 | 1.7 | 27 | 146 | 71 | 0.39 | 0.028 | 20.6 | 44 | 0.7 | 0.05 | 0.11 | 4.2 | 83110 |
| **mackerel, Spanish,** ckd by dry heat | 85 | 134 | 58.2 | 0 | | | 0 | 56 | 11 | 32 | 0.53 | 0.010 | 28 | 1 | 0.11 | 4.2 | 5.95 | 0.74 |
| *3 oz* | | 20.1 | 5.4 | 1.5 | 1.8 | 1.5 | 62 | 471 | 230 | 0.63 | 0.055 | 34.5 | 93 | | 0.18 | 0.39 | 0.8 | 15052 |
| **mackerel, Spanish,** raw | 85 | 118 | 60.9 | 0 | 0 | | 0 | 50 | 9 | 28 | 0.42 | 0.012 | 26 | 1 | 0.11 | 2.0 | 2.04 | 0.64 |
| *3 oz* | | 16.4 | 5.4 | 1.6 | 1.3 | 1.5 | 65 | 379 | 174 | 0.37 | 0.047 | 31.0 | 85 | 0.6 | 0.14 | 0.34 | 0.8 | 15051 |
| **milkfish,** cooked by dry heat | 85 | 162 | 53.2 | 0 | | | 0 | 78 | 55 | 32 | 0.89 | 0.022 | 28 | 0 | 0.01 | 7.0 | 2.78 | 0.74 |
| *3 oz* | | 22.4 | 7.3 | | | | 57 | 318 | 177 | 0.35 | 0.037 | 13.8 | 93 | | 0.06 | 0.41 | 15.3 | 15202 |
| **milkfish,** raw | 85 | 126 | 60.2 | 0 | 0 | | 0 | 61 | 43 | 26 | 0.70 | 0.017 | 26 | 0 | 0.01 | 5.5 | 2.89 | 0.64 |
| *3 oz* | | 17.5 | 5.7 | 1.4 | 2.2 | 1.6 | 44 | 248 | 138 | 0.27 | 0.029 | 10.7 | 85 | | 0.05 | 0.36 | 13.6 | 15053 |
| **monkfish,** cooked by dry heat | 85 | 82 | 66.7 | 0 | | | 0 | 20 | 8 | 23 | 0.45 | 0.026 | 12 | 1 | 0.02 | 2.2 | 0.88 | 0.15 |
| *3 oz* | | 15.8 | 1.7 | | | | 27 | 436 | 218 | 0.35 | 0.031 | 39.8 | 39 | | 0.06 | 0.24 | 6.8 | 15203 |
| **monkfish,** raw | 85 | 65 | 70.8 | 0 | | | 0 | 15 | 7 | 18 | 0.35 | 0.020 | 10 | 1 | 0.02 | 1.8 | 0.76 | 0.13 |
| *3 oz* | | 12.3 | 1.3 | 0.3 | 0.2 | 0.5 | 21 | 340 | 170 | 0.27 | 0.024 | 31.0 | 34 | | 0.05 | 0.20 | 6.0 | 15054 |
| **mullet, striped,** cooked by dry heat | 85 | 128 | 59.9 | 0 | | | 0 | 60 | 26 | 28 | 0.75 | 0.019 | 36 | 1 | 0.08 | 5.4 | 0.21 | 0.75 |
| *3 oz* | | 21.1 | 4.1 | 1.2 | 1.2 | 0.8 | 54 | 389 | 207 | 1.20 | 0.120 | 39.8 | 120 | | 0.08 | 0.42 | 8.5 | 15056 |
| **mullet, striped,** raw | 85 | 99 | 65.5 | 0 | 0 | | 0 | 55 | 35 | 25 | 0.44 | 0.014 | 31 | 1 | 0.08 | 4.4 | 0.19 | 0.65 |
| *3 oz* | | 16.4 | 3.2 | 0.9 | 0.9 | 0.6 | 42 | 303 | 188 | 0.87 | 0.043 | 31.0 | 105 | 0.8 | 0.07 | 0.36 | 7.6 | 15055 |
| **ocean perch, Atlantic,** ckd by | 85 | 103 | 61.8 | 0 | | | 0 | 82 | 116 | 33 | 0.52 | 0.017 | 12 | 1 | 0.11 | 2.1 | 0.98 | 0.36 |
| dry heat - *3 oz* | | 20.3 | 1.8 | 0.3 | 0.7 | 0.5 | 46 | 298 | 235 | 1.00 | 0.028 | 47.2 | 39 | | 0.11 | 0.23 | 8.5 | 15058 |
| **ocean perch, Atlantic,** raw | 85 | 80 | 66.9 | 0 | 0 | | 0 | 64 | 91 | 26 | 0.41 | 0.013 | 10 | 1 | 0.09 | 1.7 | 0.85 | 0.31 |
| *3 oz* | | 15.8 | 1.4 | 0.2 | 0.5 | 0.4 | 36 | 232 | 184 | 0.78 | 0.022 | 36.8 | 34 | 1.1 | 0.09 | 0.20 | 7.6 | 15057 |
| **orange roughy,** cooked by dry heat | 85 | 89 | 56.9 | 0 | 0 | | 0 | 59 | 9 | 15 | 0.27 | 0.031 | 20 | 0 | 0.04 | 1.5 | 0.40 | 0.05 |
| *3 oz* | | 19.2 | 0.8 | | 0.4 | 0.2 | 68 | 154 | 87 | 0.96 | 0.064 | 75.1 | 68 | 1.6 | 0.05 | 0.06 | 4.2 | 15232 |
| **orange roughy,** raw | 85 | 65 | 64.3 | 0 | 0 | | 0 | 61 | 8 | 14 | 0.20 | 0.042 | 18 | 0 | 0.03 | 1.3 | 0.32 | 0.04 |
| *3 oz* | | 13.9 | 0.6 | 0 | 0.2 | 0.1 | 51 | 142 | 91 | 0.86 | 0.064 | 56.7 | 60 | 1.0 | 0.04 | 0.04 | 22.1 | 15073 |
| **perch,** cooked by dry heat | 85 | 99 | 62.3 | 0 | | | 0 | 67 | 87 | 32 | 1.22 | 0.765 | 8 | 1 | 0.07 | 1.6 | 1.87 | 0.74 |
| *3 oz* | | 21.1 | 1.0 | 0.2 | 0.2 | 0.4 | 98 | 292 | 218 | 0.99 | 0.163 | 13.7 | 27 | | 0.10 | 0.12 | 5.1 | 15061 |
| **perch,** raw | 85 | 77 | 67.3 | 0 | 0 | | 0 | 53 | 68 | 26 | 0.94 | 0.595 | 8 | 1 | 0.06 | 1.3 | 1.62 | 0.64 |
| *3 oz* | | 16.5 | 0.8 | 0.2 | 0.1 | 0.3 | 76 | 229 | 170 | 0.76 | 0.128 | 10.7 | 26 | 0.2 | 0.08 | 0.10 | 4.2 | 15060 |
| **pike, northern,** cooked by dry heat | 85 | 96 | 62.0 | 0 | | | 0 | 42 | 62 | 34 | 0.73 | 0.264 | 20 | 3 | 0.06 | 2.4 | 1.95 | 0.74 |
| *3 oz* | | 21.0 | 0.7 | 0.1 | 0.2 | 0.2 | 42 | 281 | 240 | 0.60 | 0.055 | 13.8 | 69 | | 0.07 | 0.11 | 14.4 | 15063 |
| **pike, northern,** raw | 85 | 75 | 67.1 | 0 | 0 | | 0 | 33 | 48 | 26 | 0.57 | 0.204 | 18 | 3 | 0.05 | 2.0 | 1.70 | 0.64 |
| *3 oz* | | 16.4 | 0.6 | 0.1 | 0.1 | 0.2 | 33 | 220 | 187 | 0.47 | 0.043 | 10.7 | 60 | 0.2 | 0.05 | 0.10 | 12.8 | 15062 |
| **pike, walleye,** cooked by dry heat | 85 | 101 | 62.4 | 0 | | | 0 | 55 | 120 | 32 | 0.67 | 0.872 | 20 | 0 | 0.27 | 2.4 | 1.96 | 0.74 |
| *3 oz* | | 20.9 | 1.3 | 0.3 | 0.3 | 0.5 | 94 | 424 | 229 | 1.42 | 0.194 | 13.8 | 69 | | 0.17 | 0.12 | 14.4 | 15204 |
| **pike, walleye,** raw | 85 | 79 | 67.4 | 0 | 0 | | 0 | 43 | 94 | 26 | 0.53 | 0.680 | 18 | 0 | 0.23 | 2.0 | 1.70 | 0.64 |
| *3 oz* | | 16.3 | 1.0 | 0.2 | 0.2 | 0.4 | 73 | 331 | 178 | 1.10 | 0.151 | 10.7 | 60 | | 0.14 | 0.10 | 12.8 | 15064 |
| **pollock, Atlantic,** cooked by | 85 | 100 | 61.2 | 0 | | | 0 | 94 | 65 | 73 | 0.51 | 0.016 | 10 | 0 | 0.05 | 3.4 | 3.13 | 0.35 |
| dry heat - *3 oz* | | 21.2 | 1.1 | 0.1 | 0.1 | 0.5 | 77 | 388 | 241 | 0.50 | 0.054 | 39.8 | 34 | | 0.19 | 0.28 | 2.6 | 15205 |
| **pollock, Atlantic,** raw | 85 | 78 | 66.5 | 0 | 0 | | 0 | 73 | 51 | 57 | 0.40 | 0.013 | 9 | 0 | 0.04 | 2.8 | 2.71 | 0.30 |
| *3 oz* | | 16.5 | 0.8 | 0.1 | 0.1 | 0.4 | 60 | 303 | 188 | 0.39 | 0.042 | 31.0 | 31 | 0.2 | 0.16 | 0.24 | 2.6 | 15065 |
| **pollock, walleye,** cooked by | 85 | 96 | 63.0 | 0 | 0 | | 0 | 99 | 5 | 62 | 0.51 | 0.017 | 21 | 0 | 0.06 | 1.4 | 3.57 | 0.14 |
| dry heat - *3 oz* | | 20.0 | 1.0 | 0.2 | 0.1 | 0.4 | 82 | 329 | 410 | 0.24 | 0.047 | 36.9 | 71 | 0.7 | 0.06 | 0.06 | 3.4 | 15067 |
| **pollock, walleye,** raw | 85 | 69 | 69.3 | 0 | 0 | | 0 | 84 | 4 | 48 | 0.37 | 0.013 | 17 | 0 | 0.06 | 1.1 | 2.64 | 0.12 |
| *3 oz* | | 14.6 | 0.7 | 0.1 | 0.1 | 0.4 | 60 | 277 | 320 | 0.20 | 0.037 | 18.6 | 57 | 0.5 | 0.05 | 0.05 | 2.6 | 15066 |
| **pomano, Florida,** cooked by | 85 | 179 | 53.5 | 0 | | | 0 | 65 | 37 | 26 | 0.59 | 0.021 | 31 | 0 | 0.58 | 3.2 | 1.02 | 0.74 |
| dry heat - *3 oz* | | 20.1 | 10.3 | 3.8 | 2.8 | 1.2 | 54 | 541 | 290 | 0.57 | 0.066 | 39.8 | 102 | | 0.13 | 0.20 | 14.4 | 15069 |
| **pomano, Florida,** raw | 85 | 139 | 60.5 | 0 | 0 | | 0 | 55 | 19 | 23 | 0.61 | 0.011 | 28 | 0 | 0.48 | 2.6 | 1.10 | 0.64 |
| *3 oz* | | 15.7 | 8.0 | 3.0 | 2.2 | 1.0 | 42 | 324 | 166 | 0.51 | 0.032 | 31.0 | 94 | 0.2 | 0.10 | 0.17 | 12.8 | 15068 |
| **pout, ocean,** cooked by dry heat | 85 | 87 | 64.7 | 0 | | | 0 | 66 | 11 | 14 | 1.12 | 0.016 | 12 | 0 | 0.08 | 2.2 | 0.88 | 0.15 |
| *3 oz* | | 18.1 | 1.0 | 0.3 | 0.4 | 0 | 57 | 436 | 218 | 0.31 | 0.035 | 39.8 | 39 | | 0.06 | 0.24 | 6.8 | 15206 |
| **pout, ocean,** raw | 85 | 67 | 69.2 | 0 | | | 0 | 52 | 8 | 11 | 0.88 | 0.013 | 10 | 0 | 0.07 | 1.8 | 0.76 | 0.13 |
| *3 oz* | | 14.1 | 0.8 | 0.3 | 0.3 | 0 | 44 | 340 | 170 | 0.24 | 0.027 | 31.0 | 34 | | 0.05 | 0.20 | 6.0 | 15059 |

| | WT (g) | KCAL | H₂O (g) | CHO (g) | TSUG (g) | ASUG (g) | DFIB (g) | Na (mg) | Ca (mg) | Mg (mg) | Zn (mg) | Mn (mg) | A (mcg RAE) | C (mg) | B-1 (mg) | NIA (mg) | B-12 (mcg) | PANT (mg) |
|---|---|---|---|---|---|---|---|---|---|---|---|---|---|---|---|---|---|---|
| | | PRO (g) | FAT (g) | SFA (g) | MUFA (g) | PUFA (g) | CHOL (mg) | K (mg) | P (mg) | Fe (mg) | Cu (mg) | Se (mcg) | A (IU) | E (mg ATE) | B-2 (mg) | B-6 (mg) | FOL (mcg DFE) | REF |
| **rockfish, Pacific**, cooked by | 85 | 103 | 62.4 | 0 | 0 | | 0 | 65 | 10 | 29 | 0.45 | 0.017 | 60 | 0 | 0.04 | 3.3 | 1.02 | 0.74 |
| dry heat - 3 oz | | 20.4 | 1.7 | 0.4 | 0.4 | 0.5 | 37 | 442 | 194 | 0.45 | 0.031 | 39.8 | 202 | 1.3 | 0.07 | 0.23 | 8.5 | 15071 |
| **rockfish, Pacific**, raw | 85 | 80 | 67.4 | 0 | 0 | | 0 | 51 | 8 | 22 | 0.35 | 0.014 | 48 | 0 | 0.03 | 2.7 | 0.85 | 0.64 |
| 3 oz | | 15.9 | 1.3 | 0.3 | 0.3 | 0.4 | 30 | 344 | 151 | 0.35 | 0.025 | 31.0 | 162 | 1.1 | 0.06 | 0.20 | 7.6 | 15070 |
| **sablefish**, cooked by dry heat | 85 | 212 | 53.4 | 0 | | | 0 | 61 | 38 | 60 | 0.35 | 0.016 | 87 | 0 | 0.10 | 4.4 | 1.22 | 0.74 |
| 3 oz | | 14.6 | 16.7 | 3.5 | 8.8 | 2.2 | 54 | 390 | 183 | 1.39 | 0.024 | 39.8 | 287 | | 0.10 | 0.29 | 14.4 | 15208 |
| **sablefish**, raw | 85 | 166 | 60.4 | 0 | | | 0 | 48 | 30 | 47 | 0.27 | 0.013 | 79 | 0 | 0.08 | 3.4 | 1.27 | 0.64 |
| 3 oz | | 11.4 | 13.0 | 2.7 | 6.8 | 1.7 | 42 | 304 | 143 | 1.09 | 0.019 | 31.0 | 264 | | 0.08 | 0.26 | 12.8 | 15074 |
| **sablefish**, smoked | 85 | 218 | 51.1 | 0 | | | 0 | 626 | 42 | 63 | 0.37 | 0.017 | 105 | 0 | 0.11 | 4.5 | 1.70 | 0.84 |
| 3 oz | | 15.0 | 17.1 | 3.6 | 9.0 | 2.3 | 54 | 400 | 189 | 1.44 | 0.031 | 42.7 | 347 | | 0.10 | 0.33 | 17.0 | 15075 |
| **salmon, Atlantic**, farmed, cooked | 85 | 175 | 55.0 | 0 | | | 0 | 52 | 13 | 26 | 0.37 | 0.014 | | 3 | 0.29 | 6.8 | 2.38 | 1.25 |
| by dry heat - 3 oz | | 18.8 | 10.5 | 2.1 | 3.8 | 3.8 | 54 | 326 | 214 | 0.29 | 0.042 | 35.2 | 42 | | 0.11 | 0.55 | 28.9 | 15237 |
| **salmon, Atlantic**, farmed, raw | 85 | 177 | 55.2 | 0 | | | 0 | 50 | 8 | 23 | 0.31 | 0.009 | | 3 | 0.18 | 7.4 | 2.75 | 1.31 |
| 3 oz | | 17.4 | 11.4 | 2.6 | 3.2 | 3.3 | 47 | 309 | 204 | 0.29 | 0.038 | 20.4 | 42 | 3.0 | 0.13 | 0.54 | 22.1 | 15236 |
| **salmon, Atlantic**, wild, ckd by | 85 | 155 | 50.7 | 0 | | | 0 | 48 | 13 | 31 | 0.70 | 0.018 | 11 | 0 | 0.23 | 8.6 | 2.59 | 1.63 |
| dry heat - 3 oz | | 21.6 | 6.9 | 1.1 | 2.3 | 2.8 | 60 | 534 | 218 | 0.88 | 0.273 | 39.8 | 37 | | 0.41 | 0.80 | 24.6 | 15209 |
| **salmon, Atlantic**, wild, raw | 85 | 121 | 58.2 | 0 | | | 0 | 37 | 10 | 25 | 0.54 | 0.014 | 10 | 0 | 0.19 | 6.7 | 2.70 | 1.41 |
| 3 oz | | 16.9 | 5.4 | 0.8 | 1.8 | 2.2 | 47 | 416 | 170 | 0.68 | 0.212 | 31.0 | 34 | | 0.32 | 0.70 | 21.2 | 15076 |
| **salmon, chinook**, cooked by | 85 | 196 | 55.8 | 0 | | | 0 | 51 | 24 | 104 | 0.48 | 0.016 | 127 | 3 | 0.04 | 8.5 | 2.44 | 0.74 |
| dry heat - 3 oz | | 21.9 | 11.4 | 2.7 | 4.9 | 2.3 | 72 | 429 | 315 | 0.77 | 0.045 | 39.8 | 422 | | 0.13 | 0.39 | 29.8 | 15210 |
| **salmon, chinook**, raw | 85 | 152 | 60.9 | 0 | 0 | | 0 | 40 | 22 | 81 | 0.37 | 0.013 | 116 | 3 | 0.05 | 7.2 | 1.10 | 0.64 |
| 3 oz | | 16.9 | 8.9 | 2.6 | 3.7 | 2.4 | 42 | 335 | 246 | 0.21 | 0.035 | 31.0 | 385 | 1.0 | 0.10 | 0.34 | 25.5 | 15078 |
| **salmon, chinook**, smoked (lox) | 85 | 99 | 61.2 | 0 | 0 | | 0 | 666 | 9 | 15 | 0.26 | 0.014 | 22 | 0 | 0.02 | 4.0 | 2.77 | 0.74 |
| 3 oz | | 15.5 | 3.7 | 0.8 | 1.7 | 0.8 | 20 | 149 | 139 | 0.72 | 0.196 | 27.5 | 74 | 1.1 | 0.09 | 0.24 | 1.7 | 15077 |
| **salmon, chum**, cnd w/bone, | 85 | 120 | 60.2 | 0 | 0 | | 0 | 414 | 212 | 26 | 0.85 | 0.017 | 15 | 0 | 0.02 | 6.0 | 3.74 | 0.48 |
| drained - 3 oz | | 18.2 | 4.7 | 1.3 | 1.6 | 1.3 | 33 | 255 | 301 | 0.60 | 0.085 | 36.8 | 51 | 1.4 | 0.14 | 0.32 | 17.0 | 15080 |
| **salmon, chum**, cooked by dry heat | 85 | 131 | 58.2 | 0 | | | 0 | 54 | 12 | 24 | 0.51 | 0.016 | 29 | 0 | 0.08 | 7.2 | 2.94 | 0.74 |
| 3 oz | | 21.9 | 4.1 | 0.9 | 1.7 | 1.0 | 81 | 468 | 309 | 0.60 | 0.060 | 39.8 | 97 | | 0.19 | 0.39 | 4.2 | 15211 |
| **salmon, chum**, raw | 85 | 102 | 64.1 | 0 | | | 0 | 42 | 9 | 19 | 0.40 | 0.013 | 26 | 0 | 0.07 | 6.0 | 2.55 | 0.64 |
| 3 oz | | 17.1 | 3.2 | 0.7 | 1.3 | 0.8 | 63 | 365 | 241 | 0.47 | 0.047 | 31.0 | 84 | 0.9 | 0.15 | 0.34 | 3.4 | 15079 |
| **salmon, coho**, farmed, ckd by | 85 | 151 | 57.0 | 0 | | | 0 | 44 | 10 | 29 | 0.40 | 0.018 | 50 | 1 | 0.08 | 6.3 | 2.69 | 1.08 |
| dry heat - 3 oz | | 20.7 | 7.0 | 1.7 | 3.1 | 1.7 | 54 | 391 | 282 | 0.33 | 0.076 | 12.0 | 167 | | 0.10 | 0.48 | 11.9 | 15239 |
| **salmon, coho**, farmed, raw | 85 | 136 | 59.9 | 0 | | | 0 | 40 | 10 | 26 | 0.37 | 0.010 | 48 | 1 | 0.08 | 5.8 | 2.27 | 0.97 |
| 3 oz | | 18.1 | 6.5 | 1.5 | 2.8 | 1.6 | 43 | 382 | 248 | 0.29 | 0.041 | 10.7 | 160 | | 0.09 | 0.56 | 11.0 | 15238 |
| **salmon, coho**, wild, ckd by dry heat | 85 | 118 | 60.8 | 0 | 0 | | 0 | 49 | 38 | 28 | 0.48 | 0.016 | 32 | 1 | 0.06 | 6.8 | 4.25 | 0.69 |
| 3 oz | | 19.9 | 3.7 | 0.9 | 1.3 | 1.1 | 47 | 369 | 274 | 0.52 | 0.060 | 32.3 | 106 | 0.7 | 0.12 | 0.48 | 11.0 | 15247 |
| **salmon, coho**, wild, ckd by | 85 | 156 | 55.6 | 0 | | | 0 | 45 | 39 | 30 | 0.44 | 0.015 | 27 | 1 | 0.10 | 6.6 | 3.81 | 0.71 |
| moist heat - 3 oz | | 23.3 | 6.4 | 1.4 | 2.3 | 2.1 | 48 | 387 | 253 | 0.60 | 0.055 | 39.3 | 92 | | 0.14 | 0.47 | 7.6 | 15082 |
| **salmon, coho**, wild, raw | 85 | 124 | 61.8 | 0 | 0 | | 0 | 39 | 31 | 26 | 0.35 | 0.012 | 26 | 1 | 0.10 | 6.1 | 3.54 | 0.70 |
| 3 oz | | 18.4 | 5.0 | 1.1 | 1.8 | 1.7 | 38 | 360 | 223 | 0.48 | 0.043 | 31.0 | 85 | 0.6 | 0.12 | 0.47 | 7.6 | 15081 |
| **salmon, pink**, canned with bone | 85 | 118 | 58.5 | 0 | 0 | | 0 | 471 | 181 | 29 | 0.78 | 0.017 | 14 | 0 | 0.02 | 5.6 | 3.74 | 0.47 |
| 3 oz | | 16.8 | 5.1 | 1.3 | 1.5 | 1.7 | 47 | 277 | 280 | 0.71 | 0.087 | 28.2 | 48 | 0.5 | 0.16 | 0.26 | 12.8 | 15084 |
| **salmon, pink**, cooked by dry heat | 85 | 127 | 59.2 | 0 | | | 0 | 73 | 14 | 28 | 0.60 | 0.016 | 35 | 0 | 0.17 | 7.2 | 2.94 | 0.74 |
| 3 oz | | 21.7 | 3.8 | 0.6 | 1.0 | 1.5 | 57 | 352 | 251 | 0.84 | 0.084 | 48.6 | 116 | | 0.06 | 0.20 | 4.2 | 15212 |
| **salmon, pink**, raw | 85 | 99 | 64.9 | 0 | 0 | | 0 | 57 | 11 | 22 | 0.47 | 0.013 | 30 | 0 | 0.14 | 6.0 | 2.55 | 0.64 |
| 3 oz | | 16.9 | 2.9 | 0.5 | 0.8 | 1.2 | 44 | 275 | 196 | 0.65 | 0.065 | 37.9 | 99 | 0.5 | 0.05 | 0.17 | 3.4 | 15083 |
| **salmon, sockeye**, cnd w/bone, | 85 | 141 | 57.4 | 0 | 0 | | 0 | 306 | 188 | 26 | 0.85 | 0.033 | 32 | 0 | 0.03 | 6.5 | 4.68 | 0.45 |
| drained - 3 oz | | 19.8 | 6.2 | 1.3 | 1.7 | 1.7 | 37 | 245 | 268 | 0.59 | 0.127 | 29.2 | 109 | 1.8 | 0.18 | 0.10 | 3.4 | 15087 |
| **salmon, sockeye**, cooked by | 85 | 184 | 52.6 | 0 | 0 | | 0 | 56 | 6 | 26 | 0.43 | 0.017 | 54 | 0 | 0.18 | 5.7 | 4.93 | 0.60 |
| dry heat - 3 oz | | 23.2 | 9.3 | 1.6 | 4.5 | 2.0 | 74 | 319 | 235 | 0.47 | 0.057 | 32.1 | 178 | 0.7 | 0.15 | 0.19 | 4.2 | 15086 |
| **salmon, sockeye**, raw | 85 | 143 | 59.7 | 0 | 0 | | 0 | 40 | 5 | 20 | 0.46 | 0.012 | 49 | 0 | 0.17 | 4.9 | 4.25 | 0.52 |
| 3 oz | | 18.1 | 7.3 | 1.3 | 3.5 | 1.6 | 53 | 332 | 183 | 0.40 | 0.044 | 28.6 | 164 | 0.5 | 0.13 | 0.16 | 3.4 | 15085 |
| **salmon, tipnuk**, fermented | 28 | 45 | 19.3 | 0 | | | | | | | | | | | 0.04 | 0.5 | | |
| 1 oz | | 4.5 | 3.0 | | | | | | 13 | | | | 218 | | 0.04 | | | 35064 |
| **sardines, Atlantic**, cnd in soy oil | 24 | 50 | 14.3 | 0 | 0 | | 0 | 121 | 92 | 9 | 0.31 | 0.026 | 8 | 0 | 0.02 | 1.3 | 2.15 | 0.15 |
| 2 sardines | | 5.9 | 2.7 | 0.4 | 0.9 | 1.2 | 34 | 95 | 118 | 0.70 | 0.045 | 12.6 | 26 | 0.5 | 0.05 | 0.04 | 2.9 | 15088 |
| **sardines, Pacific**, cnd in tom sce | 38 | 71 | 25.3 | 0.3 | 0.2 | 0 | 0 | 157 | 91 | 13 | 0.53 | 0.078 | 13 | 0 | 0.02 | 1.6 | 3.42 | 0.28 |
| 1 sardine | | 7.9 | 4.0 | 1.0 | 1.8 | 0.8 | 23 | 130 | 139 | 0.87 | 0.103 | 15.4 | 54 | 0.5 | 0.09 | 0.05 | 9.1 | 15089 |
| **scup**, cooked by dry heat | 85 | 115 | 58.2 | 0 | | | 0 | 46 | 43 | 25 | 0.53 | 0.038 | 26 | 0 | 0.11 | 4.2 | 1.38 | 0.74 |
| 3 oz | | 20.6 | 3.0 | | | | 57 | 313 | 201 | 0.58 | 0.055 | 39.8 | 88 | | 0.10 | 0.29 | 14.4 | 15213 |
| **scup**, raw | 85 | 89 | 64.1 | 0 | 0 | | 0 | 36 | 34 | 20 | 0.41 | 0.030 | 23 | 0 | 0.09 | 3.5 | 1.19 | 0.64 |
| 3 oz | | 16.0 | 2.3 | 0.5 | 0.5 | 0.9 | 44 | 244 | 157 | 0.45 | 0.043 | 31.0 | 76 | 0.4 | 0.08 | 0.26 | 12.8 | 15090 |

| | WT (g) | KCAL | H₂0 (g) | CHO (g) | TSUG (g) | ASUG (g) | DFIB (g) | Na (mg) | Ca (mg) | Mg (mg) | Zn (mg) | Mn (mg) | A (mcg RAE) | C (mg) | B-1 (mg) | NIA (mg) | B-12 (mcg) | PANT (mg) |
|---|---|---|---|---|---|---|---|---|---|---|---|---|---|---|---|---|---|---|
| | | PRO (g) | FAT (g) | SFA (g) | MUFA (g) | PUFA (g) | CHOL (mg) | K (mg) | P (mg) | Fe (mg) | Cu (mg) | Se (mcg) | A (IU) | E (mg ATE) | B-2 (mg) | B-6 (mg) | FOL (mcg DFE) | REF |
| sea bass, cooked by dry heat | 85 | 105 | 61.3 | 0 | | | 0 | 74 | 11 | 45 | 0.44 | 0.017 | 54 | 0 | 0.11 | 1.6 | 0.26 | 0.74 |
| 3 oz | | 20.1 | 2.2 | 0.6 | 0.5 | 0.8 | 45 | 279 | 211 | 0.31 | 0.020 | 39.8 | 181 | | 0.13 | 0.39 | 5.1 | 15092 |
| sea bass, raw | 85 | 82 | 66.5 | 0 | 0 | | 0 | 58 | 8 | 35 | 0.34 | 0.013 | 47 | 0 | 0.09 | 1.4 | 0.26 | 0.64 |
| 3 oz | | 15.7 | 1.7 | 0.4 | 0.4 | 0.6 | 35 | 218 | 165 | 0.25 | 0.016 | 31.0 | 156 | 0.4 | 0.10 | 0.34 | 4.2 | 15091 |
| seatrout, cooked by dry heat | 85 | 113 | 61.1 | 0 | | | 0 | 63 | 19 | 34 | 0.49 | 0.016 | 30 | 0 | 0.06 | 2.5 | 2.94 | 0.74 |
| 3 oz | | 18.2 | 3.9 | 1.1 | 1.0 | 0.8 | 90 | 371 | 273 | 0.30 | 0.032 | 39.8 | 98 | | 0.18 | 0.39 | 5.1 | 15214 |
| seatrout, raw | 85 | 88 | 66.4 | 0 | | | 0 | 49 | 14 | 26 | 0.38 | 0.013 | 26 | 0 | 0.05 | 2.0 | 2.55 | 0.64 |
| 3 oz | | 14.2 | 3.1 | 0.9 | 0.8 | 0.6 | 71 | 290 | 212 | 0.23 | 0.026 | 31.0 | 85 | | 0.14 | 0.34 | 4.2 | 15093 |
| shad, American, cooked by dry heat - 3 oz | 85 | 214 | 50.3 | 0 | | | 0 | 55 | 51 | 32 | 0.40 | 0.046 | 31 | 0 | 0.16 | 9.2 | 0.12 | 0.74 |
| | | 18.5 | 15.0 | | | | 82 | 418 | 297 | 1.05 | 0.070 | 39.8 | 102 | | 0.26 | 0.39 | 14.4 | 15215 |
| shad, American, raw | 85 | 167 | 58.0 | 0 | 0 | | 0 | 43 | 40 | 26 | 0.31 | 0.036 | 28 | 0 | 0.13 | 7.1 | 0.13 | 0.64 |
| 3 oz | | 14.4 | 11.7 | 2.7 | 4.9 | 2.8 | 64 | 326 | 231 | 0.82 | 0.054 | 31.0 | 94 | 0.8 | 0.20 | 0.34 | 12.8 | 15094 |
| shark, batter-dipped and fried | 85 | 194 | 51.1 | 5.4 | | | 0 | 104 | 42 | 37 | 0.41 | 0.042 | 46 | 0 | 0.06 | 2.4 | 1.03 | 0.53 |
| 3 oz | | 15.8 | 11.7 | 2.7 | 5.0 | 3.1 | 50 | 132 | 165 | 0.94 | 0.036 | 28.9 | 153 | | 0.08 | 0.26 | 18.7 | 15096 |
| shark, raw | 85 | 110 | 62.5 | 0 | 0 | | 0 | 67 | 29 | 42 | 0.37 | 0.013 | 60 | 0 | 0.04 | 2.5 | 1.27 | 0.59 |
| 3 oz | | 17.8 | 3.8 | 0.8 | 1.5 | 1.0 | 43 | 136 | 178 | 0.71 | 0.028 | 31.0 | 198 | 0.8 | 0.05 | 0.34 | 2.6 | 15095 |
| sheefish, dried | 28 | 32 | 20.9 | 0 | 0 | | 0 | 15 | 39 | 7 | 0.17 | 0.010 | 0 | 0 | 0.01 | 0.6 | 1.65 | 0.18 |
| 1 oz | | 6.2 | 0.8 | 0.1 | 0.3 | 0.2 | 16 | 109 | 84 | 0.14 | 0.041 | 11.8 | 0 | 0.1 | 0.04 | 0.05 | 2.5 | 35169 |
| sheepshead, cooked by dry heat | 85 | 107 | 58.7 | 0 | | | 0 | 62 | 31 | 30 | 0.54 | 0.018 | 30 | 0 | 0.01 | 1.5 | 1.95 | 0.74 |
| 3 oz | | 22.1 | 1.4 | 0.3 | 0.3 | 0.3 | 54 | 435 | 298 | 0.57 | 0.104 | 43.6 | 98 | | 0.04 | 0.30 | 14.4 | 15098 |
| sheepshead, raw | 85 | 92 | 66.3 | 0 | | | 0 | 60 | 18 | 27 | 0.33 | 0.011 | 26 | 0 | 0.01 | 1.3 | 1.70 | 0.64 |
| 3 oz | | 17.2 | 2.0 | 0.5 | 0.6 | 0.4 | 42 | 343 | 266 | 0.39 | 0.026 | 31.0 | 85 | | 0.03 | 0.26 | 12.8 | 15097 |
| smelt, dried | 28 | 108 | 4.7 | 0 | 0 | | 0 | 118 | 448 | 25 | 1.88 | 0.202 | 39 | | 0.02 | 1.7 | 5.35 | 0.64 |
| 1 oz | | 15.7 | 5.0 | 1.0 | 1.9 | 0.8 | 70 | 280 | 392 | 1.51 | 0.041 | 54.3 | 130 | 1.3 | 0.07 | 0.05 | | 35184 |
| smelt, rainbow, cooked by dry heat | 85 | 105 | 61.9 | 0 | 0 | | 0 | 65 | 65 | 32 | 1.80 | 0.765 | 14 | 0 | 0.01 | 1.5 | 3.37 | 0.63 |
| 3 oz | | 19.2 | 2.6 | 0.5 | 0.7 | 1.0 | 76 | 316 | 251 | 0.98 | 0.151 | 39.8 | 49 | | 0.12 | 0.14 | 4.2 | 15100 |
| smelt, rainbow, raw | 85 | 82 | 67.0 | 0 | 0 | | 0 | 51 | 51 | 26 | 1.40 | 0.595 | 13 | 0 | 0.01 | 1.2 | 2.92 | 0.54 |
| 3 oz | | 15.0 | 2.1 | 0.4 | 0.5 | 0.8 | 60 | 246 | 196 | 0.76 | 0.118 | 31.0 | 42 | 0.4 | 0.10 | 0.13 | 3.4 | 15099 |
| snapper, cooked by dry heat | 85 | 109 | 59.8 | 0 | | | 0 | 48 | 34 | 31 | 0.37 | 0.014 | 30 | 1 | 0.05 | 0.3 | 2.98 | 0.74 |
| 3 oz | | 22.4 | 1.5 | 0.3 | 0.3 | 0.5 | 40 | 444 | 171 | 0.20 | 0.039 | 41.6 | 98 | 0 | | 0.39 | 5.1 | 15102 |
| snapper, raw | 85 | 85 | 65.3 | 0 | 0 | | 0 | 54 | 27 | 27 | 0.31 | 0.011 | 26 | 1 | 0.04 | 0.2 | 2.55 | 0.64 |
| 3 oz | | 17.4 | 1.1 | 0.2 | 0.2 | 0.4 | 31 | 354 | 168 | 0.15 | 0.024 | 32.5 | 85 | 0.4 | 0 | 0.34 | 4.2 | 15101 |
| spot, cooked by dry heat | 85 | 134 | 58.8 | 0 | | | 0 | 31 | 15 | 46 | 0.55 | 0.038 | 30 | 0 | 0.16 | 7.2 | 2.94 | 0.74 |
| 3 oz | | 20.2 | 5.3 | 1.6 | 1.5 | 1.2 | 65 | 541 | 202 | 0.35 | 0.050 | 39.8 | 98 | | 0.23 | 0.39 | 5.1 | 15216 |
| spot, raw | 85 | 105 | 64.6 | 0 | | | 0 | 25 | 12 | 36 | 0.43 | 0.030 | 26 | 0 | 0.14 | 6.0 | 2.55 | 0.64 |
| 3 oz | | 15.7 | 4.2 | 1.2 | 1.1 | 0.9 | 51 | 422 | 158 | 0.27 | 0.039 | 31.0 | 85 | | 0.19 | 0.34 | 4.2 | 15103 |
| sturgeon, cooked by dry heat | 85 | 115 | 59.4 | 0 | 0 | | 0 | 59 | 14 | 38 | 0.46 | 0.026 | 224 | 0 | 0.07 | 8.6 | 2.12 | 0.74 |
| 3 oz | | 17.6 | 4.4 | 1.0 | 2.1 | 0.8 | 65 | 309 | 230 | 0.76 | 0.045 | 13.8 | 744 | 0.5 | 0.08 | 0.20 | 14.4 | 15105 |
| sturgeon, raw | 85 | 89 | 65.1 | 0 | 0 | | 0 | 46 | 11 | 30 | 0.36 | 0.021 | 178 | 0 | 0.06 | 7.1 | 1.87 | 0.64 |
| 3 oz | | 13.7 | 3.4 | 0.8 | 1.6 | 0.6 | 51 | 241 | 179 | 0.60 | 0.035 | 10.7 | 595 | 0.4 | 0.06 | 0.17 | 12.8 | 15104 |
| sturgeon, smoked | 85 | 147 | 53.1 | 0 | 0 | | 0 | 628 | 14 | 40 | 0.48 | 0.026 | 238 | 0 | 0.08 | 9.4 | 2.46 | 0.85 |
| 3 oz | | 26.5 | 3.7 | 0.9 | 2.0 | 0.4 | 68 | 322 | 239 | 0.79 | 0.042 | 17.1 | 793 | 0.4 | 0.08 | 0.23 | 17.0 | 15106 |
| sucker, white, cooked by dry heat | 85 | 101 | 62.9 | 0 | | | 0 | 43 | 76 | 32 | 0.82 | 0.654 | 50 | | 0.01 | 1.2 | 1.96 | 0.74 |
| 3 oz | | 18.3 | 2.5 | 0.5 | 0.8 | 0.9 | 45 | 414 | 229 | 1.42 | 0.212 | 13.8 | 167 | | 0.07 | 0.20 | 14.4 | 15217 |
| sucker, white, raw | 85 | 78 | 67.8 | 0 | | | 0 | 34 | 60 | 26 | 0.64 | 0.510 | 43 | 0 | 0.01 | 1.0 | 1.70 | 0.64 |
| 3 oz | | 14.2 | 2.0 | 0.4 | 0.6 | 0.7 | 35 | 323 | 178 | 1.10 | 0.166 | 10.7 | 144 | | 0.06 | 0.17 | 12.8 | 15107 |
| sunfish, pumpkinseed, ckd by dry heat - 3 oz | 85 | 97 | 62.7 | 0 | | | 0 | 88 | 88 | 32 | 1.69 | 0.762 | 14 | 1 | 0.08 | 1.2 | 1.96 | 0.74 |
| | | 21.1 | 0.8 | 0.2 | 0.1 | 0.3 | 73 | 382 | 196 | 1.31 | 0.327 | 13.8 | 49 | | 0.07 | 0.12 | 14.4 | 15218 |
| sunfish, pumpkinseed, raw | 85 | 76 | 67.6 | 0 | | | 0 | 68 | 68 | 26 | 1.32 | 0.595 | 13 | 1 | 0.07 | 1.0 | 1.70 | 0.64 |
| 3 oz | | 16.5 | 0.6 | 0.1 | 0.1 | 0.2 | 57 | 298 | 153 | 1.02 | 0.255 | 10.7 | 42 | | 0.06 | 0.10 | 12.8 | 15108 |
| surimi, cooked | 85 | 84 | 64.9 | 5.8 | 0 | | 0 | 122 | 8 | 37 | 0.28 | 0.009 | 17 | 0 | 0.02 | 0.2 | 1.36 | 0.06 |
| 3 oz | | 12.9 | 0.8 | 0.2 | 0.1 | 0.4 | 26 | 95 | 240 | 0.22 | 0.027 | 23.9 | 57 | 0.5 | 0.02 | 0.03 | 1.7 | 15109 |
| swordfish, cooked by dry heat | 85 | 132 | 58.4 | 0 | | | 0 | 98 | 5 | 29 | 1.25 | 0.017 | 35 | 1 | 0.04 | 10.0 | 1.72 | 0.32 |
| 3 oz | | 21.6 | 4.4 | 1.2 | 1.7 | 1.0 | 42 | 314 | 286 | 0.88 | 0.138 | 52.4 | 116 | | 0.10 | 0.32 | 1.7 | 15111 |
| swordfish, raw | 85 | 103 | 64.3 | 0 | | | 0 | 76 | 3 | 23 | 0.98 | 0.016 | 31 | 1 | 0.03 | 8.2 | 1.49 | 0.35 |
| 3 oz | | 16.8 | 3.4 | 0.9 | 1.3 | 0.8 | 33 | 245 | 224 | 0.69 | 0.107 | 40.9 | 102 | 0.4 | 0.08 | 0.28 | 1.7 | 15110 |
| tilapia, cooked by dry heat | 85 | 109 | 60.9 | 0 | 0 | | 0 | 48 | 12 | 29 | 0.35 | 0.031 | 0 | 0 | 0.08 | 4.0 | 1.58 | 0.56 |
| 3 oz | | 22.2 | 2.3 | 0.8 | 0.8 | 0.5 | 48 | 323 | 173 | 0.59 | 0.064 | 46.2 | 0 | 0.7 | 0.06 | 0.10 | 5.1 | 15262 |
| tilefish, cooked by dry heat | 85 | 125 | 59.7 | 0 | | | 0 | 50 | 22 | 28 | 0.45 | 0.013 | 18 | 0 | 0.12 | 3.0 | 2.12 | 0.74 |
| 3 oz | | 20.8 | 4.0 | 0.7 | 1.1 | 1.1 | 54 | 435 | 201 | 0.26 | 0.044 | 43.8 | 59 | | 0.16 | 0.26 | 14.4 | 15113 |
| tilefish, raw | 85 | 82 | 67.1 | 0 | | | 0 | 45 | 22 | 24 | 0.31 | 0.008 | 15 | 0 | 0.10 | 2.5 | 1.87 | 0.64 |
| 3 oz | | 14.9 | 2.0 | 0.4 | 0.5 | 0.5 | 42 | 368 | 159 | 0.21 | 0.035 | 31.0 | 51 | | 0.14 | 0.22 | 12.8 | 15112 |

| | WT (g) | KCAL / PRO (g) | H₂O (g) / FAT (g) | CHO (g) / SFA (g) | TSUG (g) / MUFA (g) | ASUG (g) / PUFA (g) | DFIB (g) / CHOL (mg) | Na (mg) / K (mg) | Ca (mg) / P (mg) | Mg (mg) / Fe (mg) | Zn (mg) / Cu (mg) | Mn (mg) / Se (mcg) | A (mcg RAE) / A (IU) | C (mg) / E (mg ATE) | B-1 (mg) / B-2 (mg) | NIA (mg) / B-6 (mg) | B-12 (mcg) / FOL (mcg DFE) | PANT (mg) / REF |
|---|---|---|---|---|---|---|---|---|---|---|---|---|---|---|---|---|---|---|
| **trout,** cooked by dry heat | 85 | 162 | 53.9 | 0 | | | 0 | 57 | 47 | 24 | 0.72 | 0.927 | 16 | 0 | 0.36 | 4.9 | 6.37 | 1.90 |
| *3 oz* | | 22.6 | 7.2 | 1.3 | 3.5 | 1.6 | 63 | 394 | 267 | 1.63 | 0.205 | 13.8 | 54 | | 0.36 | 0.20 | 12.8 | 15219 |
| **trout, rainbow,** farmed, ckd by dry heat - 3 oz | 85 | 144 | 57.4 | 0 | | | 0 | 36 | 73 | 27 | 0.42 | 0.017 | 73 | 3 | 0.20 | 7.5 | 4.22 | 1.11 |
| | | 20.6 | 6.1 | 1.8 | 1.8 | 2.0 | 58 | 375 | 226 | 0.28 | 0.052 | 12.8 | 244 | | 0.07 | 0.34 | 20.4 | 15241 |
| **trout, rainbow,** farmed, raw | 85 | 117 | 61.8 | 0 | 0 | | 0 | 30 | 57 | 27 | 0.35 | 0.015 | 71 | 2 | 0.17 | 7.0 | 3.20 | 1.22 |
| *3 oz* | | 17.7 | 4.6 | 1.3 | 1.3 | 1.5 | 50 | 383 | 240 | 0.23 | 0.039 | 10.7 | 238 | 0 | 0.06 | 0.53 | 9.4 | 15240 |
| **trout, rainbow,** wild, cooked by dry - 3 oz | 85 | 128 | 59.9 | 0 | | | 0 | 48 | 73 | 26 | 0.43 | 0.018 | 13 | 2 | 0.13 | 4.9 | 5.36 | 0.91 |
| | | 19.5 | 4.9 | 1.4 | 1.5 | 1.6 | 59 | 381 | 229 | 0.32 | 0.049 | 11.2 | 42 | | 0.08 | 0.29 | 16.2 | 15116 |
| **trout, rainbow,** wild, raw | 85 | 101 | 61.1 | 0 | | | 0 | 26 | 57 | 26 | 0.92 | 0.134 | 16 | 2 | 0.10 | 4.6 | 3.78 | 0.79 |
| *3 oz* | | 17.4 | 2.9 | 0.6 | 1.0 | 1.1 | 50 | 409 | 230 | 0.60 | 0.093 | 10.7 | 53 | | 0.09 | 0.35 | 10.2 | 15115 |
| **trout,** raw | 85 | 126 | 60.7 | 0 | 0 | | 0 | 44 | 37 | 19 | 0.56 | 0.723 | 14 | 0 | 0.30 | 3.8 | 6.62 | 1.65 |
| *3 oz* | | 17.7 | 5.6 | 1.0 | 2.8 | 1.3 | 49 | 307 | 208 | 1.27 | 0.160 | 10.7 | 48 | 0.2 | 0.28 | 0.17 | 11.0 | 15114 |
| **trout, steelhead,** boiled, canned | 85 | 135 | 60.0 | 0 | 0 | | 0 | 100 | 26 | 21 | 0.48 | 0.009 | 17 | 0 | | | 4.92 | |
| *3 oz* | | 17.9 | 7.0 | 1.3 | 1.9 | 1.0 | 50 | 310 | 212 | 0.54 | 0.049 | 22.1 | 55 | 1.8 | | | | 35181 |
| **trout, steelhead,** dried | 28 | 107 | 1.8 | 0 | 0 | | 0 | 798 | 24 | 24 | 0.50 | 0.022 | 18 | 0 | | | 6.27 | |
| *1 oz* | | 21.6 | 2.3 | 0.2 | 0.3 | 0.5 | 64 | 482 | 273 | 0.83 | 0.061 | 29.4 | 60 | 0.7 | | | | 35180 |
| **tuna, bluefin,** cooked by dry heat | 85 | 156 | 50.2 | 0 | 0 | | 0 | 42 | 8 | 54 | 0.65 | 0.017 | 643 | 0 | 0.24 | 9.0 | 9.25 | 1.16 |
| *3 oz* | | 25.4 | 5.3 | 1.4 | 1.7 | 1.6 | 42 | 275 | 277 | 1.11 | 0.094 | 39.8 | 2142 | | 0.26 | 0.45 | 1.7 | 15118 |
| **tuna, bluefin,** raw | 85 | 122 | 57.9 | 0 | 0 | | 0 | 33 | 7 | 42 | 0.51 | 0.013 | 557 | 0 | 0.20 | 7.4 | 8.02 | 0.90 |
| *3 oz* | | 19.8 | 4.2 | 1.1 | 1.4 | 1.2 | 32 | 214 | 216 | 0.87 | 0.073 | 31.0 | 1856 | 0.8 | 0.21 | 0.39 | 1.7 | 15117 |
| **tuna, light,** canned in oil | 85 | 168 | 50.9 | 0 | 0 | | 0 | 301 | 11 | 26 | 0.76 | 0.013 | 20 | 0 | 0.03 | 10.5 | 1.87 | 0.31 |
| *3 oz* | | 24.8 | 7.0 | 1.3 | 2.5 | 2.5 | 15 | 176 | 264 | 1.18 | 0.060 | 64.6 | 65 | 0.7 | 0.10 | 0.09 | 4.2 | 15119 |
| **tuna, light,** canned in water | 85 | 99 | 63.3 | 0 | 0 | | 0 | 287 | 9 | 23 | 0.65 | 0.009 | 14 | 0 | 0.03 | 11.3 | 2.54 | 0.18 |
| *3 oz* | | 21.7 | 0.7 | 0.2 | 0.1 | 0.3 | 26 | 201 | 139 | 1.30 | 0.043 | 68.3 | 48 | 0.3 | 0.06 | 0.30 | 3.4 | 15121 |
| **tuna salad,** homemade | 85 | 159 | 53.7 | 8.0 | | | 0 | 342 | 14 | 16 | 0.48 | 0.034 | 20 | 2 | 0.03 | 5.7 | 1.02 | 0.22 |
| *3 oz* | | 13.6 | 7.9 | 1.3 | 2.5 | 3.5 | 11 | 151 | 151 | 0.85 | 0.123 | 35.0 | 82 | | 0.06 | 0.07 | 6.8 | 15128 |
| **tuna, skipjack,** cooked by dry heat | 85 | 112 | 52.9 | 0 | | | 0 | 40 | 31 | 37 | 0.89 | 0.016 | 15 | 1 | 0.03 | 15.9 | 1.86 | 0.41 |
| *3 oz* | | 24.0 | 1.1 | 0.4 | 0.2 | 0.3 | 51 | 444 | 242 | 1.36 | 0.094 | 39.8 | 51 | | 0.10 | 0.83 | 8.5 | 15220 |
| **tuna, skipjack,** raw | 85 | 88 | 60.0 | 0 | | | 0 | 31 | 25 | 29 | 0.70 | 0.013 | 14 | 1 | 0.03 | 13.1 | 1.62 | 0.36 |
| *3 oz* | | 18.7 | 0.9 | 0.3 | 0.2 | 0.3 | 40 | 346 | 189 | 1.06 | 0.073 | 31.0 | 44 | | 0.08 | 0.72 | 7.6 | 15123 |
| **tuna, white,** canned in oil | 85 | 158 | 54.4 | 0 | 0 | | 0 | 337 | 3 | 29 | 0.40 | 0.014 | 4 | 0 | 0.01 | 9.9 | 1.87 | 0.31 |
| *3 oz* | | 22.6 | 6.9 | 1.1 | 2.8 | 2.5 | 26 | 283 | 227 | 0.55 | 0.110 | 51.1 | 14 | 2.0 | 0.07 | 0.37 | 4.2 | 15124 |
| **tuna, white,** canned in water | 85 | 109 | 62.2 | 0 | 0 | | 0 | 320 | 12 | 28 | 0.41 | 0.016 | 5 | 0 | 0.01 | 4.9 | 0.99 | 0.11 |
| *3 oz* | | 20.1 | 2.5 | 0.7 | 0.7 | 0.9 | 36 | 201 | 184 | 0.82 | 0.033 | 55.8 | 17 | 0.7 | 0.04 | 0.18 | 1.7 | 15126 |
| **tuna, yellowfin,** cooked by dry heat - 3 oz | 85 | 118 | 53.4 | 0 | | | 0 | 40 | 18 | 54 | 0.57 | 0.016 | 17 | 1 | 0.43 | 10.1 | 0.51 | 0.74 |
| | | 25.5 | 1.0 | 0.3 | 0.2 | 0.3 | 49 | 484 | 208 | 0.80 | 0.070 | 39.8 | 58 | | 0.05 | 0.88 | 1.7 | 15221 |
| **tuna, yellowfin,** raw | 85 | 92 | 60.3 | 0 | 0 | | 0 | 31 | 14 | 42 | 0.44 | 0.013 | 15 | 1 | 0.37 | 8.3 | 0.44 | 0.64 |
| *3 oz* | | 19.9 | 0.8 | 0.2 | 0.1 | 0.2 | 38 | 377 | 162 | 0.62 | 0.054 | 31.0 | 51 | 0.4 | 0.04 | 0.76 | 1.7 | 15127 |
| **turbot, European,** cooked by dry heat - 3 oz | 85 | 104 | 59.9 | 0 | | | 0 | 163 | 20 | 55 | 0.24 | 0.019 | 10 | 1 | 0.06 | 2.3 | 2.16 | 0.56 |
| | | 17.5 | 3.2 | | | | 53 | 259 | 140 | 0.39 | 0.040 | 39.8 | 34 | | 0.08 | 0.21 | 7.6 | 15222 |
| **turbot, European,** raw | 85 | 81 | 65.4 | 0 | | | 0 | 128 | 15 | 43 | 0.19 | 0.014 | 9 | 1 | 0.06 | 1.9 | 1.87 | 0.48 |
| *3 oz* | | 13.6 | 2.5 | 0.6 | 0.5 | 0.7 | 41 | 202 | 110 | 0.31 | 0.031 | 31.0 | 30 | | 0.07 | 0.18 | 6.8 | 15129 |
| **whitefish,** cooked by dry heat | 85 | 146 | 55.3 | 0 | | | 0 | 55 | 28 | 36 | 1.08 | 0.073 | 33 | 0 | 0.15 | 3.3 | 0.82 | 0.74 |
| *3 oz* | | 20.8 | 6.4 | 1.0 | 2.2 | 2.3 | 65 | 345 | 294 | 0.40 | 0.078 | 13.8 | 111 | | 0.13 | 0.29 | 14.4 | 15223 |
| **whitefish,** dried | 28 | 104 | 5.8 | 0 | 0 | | 0 | 56 | 227 | 24 | 1.40 | 0.064 | 11 | 0 | 0.01 | 3.1 | 5.15 | 0.72 |
| *1 oz* | | 17.5 | 3.8 | 0.8 | 1.2 | 0.6 | 74 | 302 | 291 | 1.15 | 0.050 | 31.6 | 37 | 0.2 | 0.12 | 0.10 | 3.1 | 35165 |
| **whitefish,** raw | 85 | 114 | 61.9 | 0 | 0 | | 0 | 43 | 22 | 28 | 0.84 | 0.057 | 31 | 0 | 0.12 | 2.6 | 0.85 | 0.64 |
| *3 oz* | | 16.2 | 5.0 | 0.8 | 1.7 | 1.8 | 51 | 269 | 230 | 0.31 | 0.061 | 10.7 | 102 | 0.2 | 0.10 | 0.26 | 12.8 | 15130 |
| **whitefish,** smoked | 85 | 92 | 60.2 | 0 | 0 | | 0 | 866 | 15 | 20 | 0.42 | 0.029 | 48 | 0 | 0.03 | 2.0 | 2.77 | 0.09 |
| *3 oz* | | 19.9 | 0.8 | 0.2 | 0.2 | 0.2 | 28 | 360 | 112 | 0.42 | 0.268 | 11.5 | 162 | 0.2 | 0.09 | 0.33 | 6.0 | 15131 |
| **whiting,** cooked by dry heat | 85 | 99 | 63.5 | 0 | 0 | | 0 | 112 | 53 | 23 | 0.45 | 0.110 | 29 | 0 | 0.06 | 1.4 | 2.21 | 0.21 |
| *3 oz* | | 20.0 | 1.4 | 0.3 | 0.4 | 0.5 | 71 | 369 | 242 | 0.36 | 0.034 | 34.9 | 96 | 0.3 | 0.05 | 0.15 | 12.8 | 15133 |
| **whiting,** raw | 85 | 76 | 68.2 | 0 | 0 | | 0 | 61 | 41 | 18 | 0.75 | 0.088 | 26 | 0 | 0.05 | 1.1 | 1.95 | 0.18 |
| *3 oz* | | 15.6 | 1.1 | 0.2 | 0.2 | 0.4 | 57 | 212 | 189 | 0.29 | 0.026 | 27.3 | 85 | 0.3 | 0.04 | 0.13 | 11.0 | 15132 |
| **wolffish, Atlantic,** ckd by dry heat | 85 | 105 | 63.1 | 0 | | | 0 | 93 | 7 | 32 | 0.85 | 0.016 | 110 | 0 | 0.18 | 2.2 | 2.00 | 0.56 |
| *3 oz* | | 19.1 | 2.6 | 0.4 | 0.9 | 0.9 | 50 | 327 | 218 | 0.10 | 0.031 | 39.8 | 368 | | 0.08 | 0.39 | 5.1 | 15224 |
| **wolffish, Atlantic,** raw | 85 | 82 | 67.9 | 0 | | | 0 | 72 | 5 | 26 | 0.66 | 0.013 | 96 | 0 | 0.15 | 1.8 | 1.73 | 0.48 |
| *3 oz* | | 14.9 | 2.0 | 0.3 | 0.7 | 0.7 | 39 | 255 | 170 | 0.08 | 0.025 | 31.0 | 319 | | 0.07 | 0.34 | 4.2 | 15134 |
| **yellowtail,** cooked by dry heat | 85 | 159 | 57.2 | 0 | | | 0 | 42 | 25 | 32 | 0.57 | 0.016 | 26 | 2 | 0.15 | 7.4 | 1.06 | 0.58 |
| *3 oz* | | 25.2 | 5.7 | | | | 60 | 457 | 171 | 0.54 | 0.049 | 39.8 | 88 | | 0.04 | 0.16 | 3.4 | 15225 |
| **yellowtail,** raw | 85 | 124 | 63.3 | 0 | | | 0 | 33 | 20 | 26 | 0.44 | 0.013 | 25 | 2 | 0.12 | 5.8 | 1.10 | 0.50 |
| *3 oz* | | 19.7 | 4.5 | 1.1 | 1.7 | 1.2 | 47 | 357 | 133 | 0.42 | 0.038 | 31.0 | 81 | | 0.03 | 0.14 | 3.4 | 15135 |

| | WT (g) | KCAL / PRO (g) | H2O (g) / FAT (g) | CHO (g) / SFA (g) | TSUG (g) / MUFA (g) | ASUG (g) / PUFA (g) | DFIB (g) / CHOL (mg) | Na (mg) / K (mg) | Ca (mg) / P (mg) | Mg (mg) / Fe (mg) | Zn (mg) / Cu (mg) | Mn (mg) / Se (mcg) | A (mcg RAE) / A (IU) | C (mg) / E (mg ATE) | B-1 (mg) / B-2 (mg) | NIA (mg) / B-6 (mg) | B-12 (mcg) / FOL (mcg DFE) | PANT (mg) / REF |
|---|---|---|---|---|---|---|---|---|---|---|---|---|---|---|---|---|---|---|

## 12.3 FISH EGGS

**caviar, black and red, granular** — 1 T

| WT 16 | 40 | 7.6 | 0.6 | 0 | 0 | 0 | 240 | 44 | 48 | 0.15 | 0.008 | 43 | 0 | 0.03 | 0 | 3.20 | 0.56 |
| | 3.9 | 2.9 | 0.6 | 0.7 | 1.2 | 94 | 29 | 57 | 1.90 | 0.018 | 10.5 | 145 | 0.3 | 0.10 | 0.05 | 8.0 | 15012 |

**roe, mixed species, ckd by dryheat** — 1 oz

| WT 28 | 57 | 16.4 | 0.5 | | | 0 | 33 | 8 | 7 | 0.36 | 0.004 | 25 | 5 | 0.08 | 0.6 | 3.23 | 0.32 |
| | 8.0 | 2.3 | 0.5 | 0.6 | 1.0 | 134 | 79 | 144 | 0.22 | 0.036 | 14.5 | 85 | | 0.27 | 0.05 | 25.8 | 15207 |

**roe, mixed species, raw** — 1 oz

| WT 28 | 40 | 19.0 | 0.4 | 0 | | 0 | 25 | 6 | 6 | 0.28 | 0.003 | 25 | 4 | 0.07 | 0.5 | 2.80 | 0.28 |
| | 6.2 | 1.8 | 0.4 | 0.5 | 0.7 | 105 | 62 | 113 | 0.17 | 0.028 | 11.3 | 84 | 2.0 | 0.21 | 0.04 | 22.4 | 15072 |

**roe, whitefish** — 1 oz

| WT 28 | 29 | 21.3 | 1.4 | 0 | | 0 | 45 | 13 | 8 | 0.59 | 0.062 | 25 | 3 | 0.02 | 0.3 | 15.79 | 0.30 |
| | 4.1 | 0.8 | 0.1 | 0.3 | 0.3 | 123 | 53 | 86 | 1.67 | 0.062 | 26.0 | 85 | 0.8 | 0.11 | 0.04 | 14.8 | 35158 |

## 12.4 MOLLUSKS AND JELLYFISH

**abalone, fried** — 3 oz

| WT 85 | 161 | 51.1 | 9.4 | | | 0 | 502 | 31 | 48 | 0.81 | 0.060 | 2 | 2 | 0.19 | 1.6 | 0.59 | 2.44 |
| | 16.7 | 5.8 | 1.4 | 2.3 | 1.4 | 80 | 241 | 184 | 3.23 | 0.194 | 44.0 | 4 | | 0.11 | 0.13 | 17.0 | 15156 |

**abalone, mixed species, raw** — 3 oz

| WT 85 | 89 | 63.4 | 5.1 | 0 | 0 | 0 | 256 | 26 | 41 | 0.70 | 0.034 | 2 | 2 | 0.16 | 1.3 | 0.62 | 2.55 |
| | 14.5 | 0.6 | 0.1 | 0.1 | 0.1 | 72 | 212 | 162 | 2.71 | 0.167 | 38.1 | 6 | 3.4 | 0.08 | 0.13 | 4.2 | 15155 |

**clam liquid, canned** — 1 cup

| WT 240 | 5 | 234.5 | 0.2 | 0 | 0 | 0 | 516 | 31 | 26 | 0.24 | 0.178 | 22 | 2 | 0.02 | 0.4 | 12.00 | 0.10 |
| | 1.0 | 0 | 0 | 0 | 0 | 7 | 358 | 274 | 0.72 | 0.934 | 9.8 | 72 | 0.7 | 0.05 | 0.02 | 4.8 | 15162 |

**clams, breaded and fried** — 3 oz (9 small)

| WT 85 | 172 | 52.3 | 8.8 | | | | 309 | 54 | 12 | 1.24 | 0.459 | 77 | 8 | 0.08 | 1.8 | 34.23 | 0.37 |
| | 12.1 | 9.5 | 2.3 | 3.9 | 2.4 | 52 | 277 | 160 | 11.82 | 0.303 | 24.6 | 257 | | 0.21 | 0.05 | 40.8 | 15158 |

**clams, canned, drained** — 3 oz

| WT 85 | 126 | 54.1 | 4.4 | 0 | 0 | 0 | 95 | 78 | 15 | 2.32 | 0.850 | 154 | 19 | 0.13 | 2.9 | 84.06 | 0.58 |
| | 21.7 | 1.7 | 0.2 | 0.1 | 0.5 | 57 | 534 | 287 | 23.77 | 0.585 | 41.3 | 513 | 0.5 | 0.36 | 0.09 | 24.6 | 15160 |

**clams, cooked by moist heat** — 3 oz (19 small)

| WT 85 | 126 | 54.1 | 4.4 | | | 0 | 95 | 78 | 15 | 2.32 | 0.850 | 145 | 19 | 0.13 | 2.9 | 84.06 | 0.58 |
| | 21.7 | 1.7 | 0.2 | 0.1 | 0.5 | 57 | 534 | 287 | 23.77 | 0.585 | 54.4 | 484 | | 0.36 | 0.09 | 24.6 | 15159 |

**clams, raw** — 3 oz (4 large or 9 small)

| WT 85 | 63 | 69.5 | 2.2 | 0 | 0 | 0 | 48 | 39 | 8 | 1.16 | 0.425 | 76 | 11 | 0.07 | 1.5 | 42.02 | 0.31 |
| | 10.9 | 0.8 | 0.1 | 0.1 | 0.2 | 29 | 267 | 144 | 11.88 | 0.292 | 20.7 | 255 | 0.3 | 0.18 | 0.05 | 13.6 | 15157 |

**cockles, raw** — 3 oz

| WT 85 | 67 | 67.0 | 4.0 | | | | 26 | | | | | | | 0.01 | 2.7 | | |
| | 11.5 | 0.6 | | | | | | | 13.77 | | | | | 0.17 | | | 35028 |

**conch, baked/broiled** — 3 oz

| WT 85 | 110 | 59.0 | 1.4 | 0 | | 0 | 130 | 83 | 202 | 1.45 | | 6 | 0 | 0.05 | 0.9 | 4.46 | |
| | 22.4 | 1.0 | 0.3 | 0.3 | 0.2 | 55 | 139 | 184 | 1.20 | 0.370 | 34.3 | 20 | 5.4 | 0.07 | 0.05 | 152.2 | 15250 |

**cuttlefish, cooked by moist heat** — 3 oz

| WT 85 | 134 | 52.0 | 1.4 | | | 0 | 632 | 153 | 51 | 2.94 | 0.178 | 173 | 7 | 0.01 | 1.9 | 4.59 | 0.76 |
| | 27.6 | 1.2 | 0.2 | 0.1 | 0.2 | 190 | 541 | 493 | 9.21 | 0.848 | 76.2 | 574 | | 1.47 | 0.23 | 20.4 | 15229 |

**cuttlefish, raw** — 3 oz

| WT 85 | 67 | 68.5 | 0.7 | | | 0 | 316 | 76 | 26 | 1.47 | 0.094 | 96 | 5 | 0.01 | 1.0 | 2.55 | 0.42 |
| | 13.8 | 0.6 | 0.1 | 0.1 | 0.1 | 95 | 301 | 329 | 5.12 | 0.499 | 38.1 | 319 | | 0.77 | 0.13 | 13.6 | 15163 |

**jellyfish, dried, salted** — ½ cup

| WT 29 | 10 | 19.7 | 0 | 0 | | 0 | 2810 | 1 | 1 | 0.12 | | 1 | 0 | 0 | 0.1 | 0.01 | |
| | 1.6 | 0.4 | 0.1 | 0.1 | 0.1 | 1 | 1 | 6 | 0.66 | 0.041 | 12.2 | 2 | 0 | 0 | 0 | 0.3 | 43497 |

**mussels, blue, cooked by moist heat - 3 oz**

| WT 85 | 146 | 52.0 | 6.3 | | | 0 | 314 | 28 | 31 | 2.27 | 5.780 | 77 | 12 | 0.26 | 2.6 | 20.40 | 0.81 |
| | 20.2 | 3.8 | 0.7 | 0.9 | 1.0 | 48 | 228 | 242 | 5.71 | 0.127 | 76.2 | 258 | | 0.36 | 0.08 | 64.6 | 15165 |

**mussels, blue, raw** — 3 oz

| WT 85 | 73 | 68.5 | 3.1 | 0 | 0 | 0 | 243 | 22 | 29 | 1.36 | 2.890 | 41 | 7 | 0.14 | 1.4 | 10.20 | 0.42 |
| | 10.1 | 1.9 | 0.4 | 0.4 | 0.5 | 24 | 272 | 167 | 3.36 | 0.080 | 38.1 | 136 | 0.5 | 0.18 | 0.04 | 35.7 | 15164 |

**octopus, cooked by moist heat** — 3 oz

| WT 85 | 139 | 51.4 | 3.7 | 0 | 0 | 0 | 391 | 90 | 51 | 2.86 | 0.040 | 76 | 7 | 0.05 | 3.2 | 30.60 | 0.76 |
| | 25.3 | 1.8 | 0.4 | 0.3 | 0.4 | 82 | 536 | 237 | 8.11 | 0.628 | 76.2 | 255 | 1.0 | 0.06 | 0.55 | 20.4 | 15230 |

**octopus, raw** — 3 oz

| WT 85 | 70 | 68.2 | 1.9 | 0 | 0 | 0 | 196 | 45 | 26 | 1.43 | 0.021 | 38 | 4 | 0.03 | 1.8 | 17.00 | 0.42 |
| | 12.7 | 0.9 | 0.2 | 0.1 | 0.2 | 41 | 298 | 158 | 4.50 | 0.370 | 38.1 | 128 | 1.0 | 0.03 | 0.31 | 13.6 | 15166 |

**oysters, eastern, breaded and fried** — 6 medium (3 oz)

| WT 88 | 173 | 57.0 | 10.2 | | | | 367 | 55 | 51 | 76.67 | 0.431 | 80 | 3 | 0.13 | 1.5 | 13.75 | 0.24 |
| | 7.7 | 11.1 | 2.8 | 4.1 | 2.9 | 71 | 215 | 140 | 6.12 | 3.779 | 58.5 | 266 | | 0.18 | 0.06 | 37.8 | 15168 |

**oysters, eastern, canned** — 3 oz (~11 oysters)

| WT 85 | 59 | 72.4 | 3.3 | 0 | 0 | 0 | 95 | 38 | 46 | 77.31 | 0.382 | 76 | 4 | 0.13 | 1.1 | 16.26 | 0.15 |
| | 6.0 | 2.1 | 0.5 | 0.2 | 0.6 | 47 | 195 | 118 | 5.70 | 3.792 | 30.4 | 255 | 0.7 | 0.14 | 0.08 | 7.6 | 15170 |

**oysters, eastern, farmed, ckd by dry heat - 6 medium**

| WT 59 | 47 | 48.4 | 4.3 | | | 0 | 96 | 33 | 19 | 26.64 | 0.251 | 11 | 4 | 0.08 | 1.1 | 14.34 | 0.12 |
| | 4.1 | 1.3 | 0.4 | 0.1 | 0.4 | 22 | 90 | 68 | 4.58 | 0.846 | 45.7 | 37 | | 0.03 | 0.04 | 14.2 | 15246 |

**oysters, eastern, farmed, raw** — 6 medium

| WT 84 | 50 | 72.4 | 4.6 | | | 0 | 150 | 37 | 28 | 31.85 | 0.331 | 7 | 4 | 0.09 | 1.1 | 13.61 | 0.13 |
| | 4.4 | 1.3 | 0.4 | 0.1 | 0.5 | 21 | 104 | 78 | 4.86 | 0.620 | 53.5 | 21 | | 0.05 | 0.05 | 15.1 | 15245 |

**oysters, eastern, wild, ckd by dry heat 6 medium**

| WT 59 | 42 | 49.1 | 2.8 | | | 0 | 144 | 27 | 27 | 43.42 | 0.170 | 0 | 2 | 0.05 | 1.0 | 16.40 | 0.13 |
| | 4.9 | 1.1 | 0.3 | 0.1 | 0.5 | 29 | 99 | 80 | 2.55 | 2.038 | 42.3 | 0 | | 0.05 | 0.06 | 10.6 | 15244 |

**oysters, eastern, wild, ckd by moist heat - 6 medium**

| WT 42 | 58 | 29.5 | 3.3 | | | 0 | 177 | 38 | 40 | 76.28 | 0.293 | 23 | 3 | 0.08 | 1.0 | 14.71 | 0.15 |
| | 5.9 | 2.1 | 0.6 | 0.3 | 0.8 | 44 | 118 | 85 | 5.04 | 3.179 | 30.1 | 76 | | 0.08 | 0.05 | 5.9 | 15169 |

**oysters, eastern, wild, raw** — 6 medium

| WT 84 | 57 | 71.5 | 3.3 | 0 | 0 | 0 | 177 | 38 | 39 | 76.28 | 0.308 | 25 | 3 | 0.08 | 1.2 | 16.35 | 0.16 |
| | 5.9 | 2.1 | 0.6 | 0.3 | 0.8 | 45 | 131 | 113 | 5.59 | 3.740 | 53.5 | 84 | 0.7 | 0.08 | 0.05 | 8.4 | 15167 |

**oysters, Pacific, ckd by moist heat** — 3 oz

| WT 85 | 139 | 54.5 | 8.4 | 0 | | 0 | 180 | 14 | 37 | 28.25 | 1.039 | 124 | 11 | 0.11 | 3.1 | 24.48 | 0.76 |
| | 16.1 | 3.9 | 0.9 | 0.7 | 1.5 | 85 | 257 | 207 | 7.82 | 2.277 | 130.9 | 414 | 0.7 | 0.38 | 0.08 | 12.8 | 15231 |

**oysters, Pacific, raw** — 3 oz

| WT 85 | 69 | 69.8 | 4.2 | | | 0 | 90 | 7 | 19 | 14.13 | 0.547 | 69 | 7 | 0.06 | 1.7 | 13.60 | 0.42 |
| | 8.0 | 2.0 | 0.4 | 0.3 | 0.8 | 42 | 143 | 138 | 4.34 | 1.340 | 65.4 | 230 | | 0.20 | 0.04 | 8.5 | 15171 |

| Food | WT (g) | KCAL / PRO (g) | H₂0 (g) / FAT (g) | CHO (g) / SFA (g) | TSUG (g) / MUFA (g) | ASUG (g) / PUFA (g) | DFIB (g) / CHOL (mg) | Na (mg) / K (mg) | Ca (mg) / P (mg) | Mg (mg) / Fe (mg) | Zn (mg) / Cu (mg) | Mn (mg) / Se (mcg) | A (mcg RAE) / A (IU) | C (mg) / E (mg ATE) | B-1 (mg) / B-2 (mg) | NIA (mg) / B-6 (mg) | B-12 (mcg) / FOL (mcg DFE) | PANT (mg) / REF |
|---|---|---|---|---|---|---|---|---|---|---|---|---|---|---|---|---|---|---|
| **scallops**, bay/sea, steamed | 85 | 95 | 62.1 | 0 | 0 |  | 0 | 225 | 98 | 47 | 2.55 |  | 26 | 0 | 0.08 | 1.1 |  | 1.10 |
| 3 oz |  | 19.7 | 1.2 | 0.1 | 0.1 | 0.4 | 45 | 405 | 287 | 2.55 | 0.255 | 23.7 | 85 | 1.3 | 0.05 | 0.08 | 10.2 | 90240 |
| **scallops**, breaded and fried | 31 | 67 | 18.1 | 3.1 |  |  |  | 144 | 13 | 18 | 0.33 | 0.043 | 7 | 1 | 0.01 | 0.5 |  | 0.06 |
| 2 large |  | 5.6 | 3.4 | 0.8 | 1.4 | 0.9 | 19 | 103 | 73 | 0.25 | 0.024 | 8.3 | 23 |  | 0.03 | 0.04 | 15.5 | 15173 |
| **scallops, imitation**, made from surimi - 3 oz | 85 | 84 | 62.7 | 9.0 |  |  | 0 | 676 | 7 | 37 | 0.28 | 0.009 | 17 | 0 | 0.01 | 0.3 |  | 0.06 |
|  |  | 10.9 | 0.3 | 0.1 | 0.1 | 0.2 | 19 | 88 | 240 | 0.26 | 0.027 | 20.1 | 56 |  | 0.01 | 0.03 | 1.7 | 15174 |
| **scallops**, raw | 85 | 75 | 66.8 | 2.0 | 0 | 0 | 0 | 137 | 20 | 48 | 0.81 | 0.076 | 13 | 3 | 0.01 | 1.0 |  | 0.12 |
| 3 oz (6 large) |  | 14.3 | 0.6 | 0.1 | 0 | 0.2 | 28 | 274 | 186 | 0.25 | 0.045 | 18.9 | 42 | 0 | 0.06 | 0.13 | 13.6 | 15172 |
| **snails**, raw | 85 | 76 | 67.3 | 1.7 | 0 | 0 | 0 | 60 | 8 | 212 | 0.85 |  | 26 | 0 | 0.01 | 1.2 |  | 0.42 |
| 3 oz |  | 13.7 | 1.2 | 0.3 | 0.2 | 0.2 | 42 | 325 | 231 | 2.98 | 0.340 | 23.3 | 85 | 4.2 | 0.10 | 0.11 | 5.1 | 90560 |
| **squid**, fried | 85 | 149 | 54.9 | 6.6 |  |  | 0 | 260 | 33 | 32 | 1.48 | 0.060 | 9 | 4 | 0.05 | 2.2 |  | 0.43 |
| 3 oz |  | 15.2 | 6.4 | 1.6 | 2.3 | 1.8 | 221 | 237 | 213 | 0.86 | 1.797 | 44.0 | 30 |  | 0.39 | 0.05 | 17.0 | 15176 |
| **squid**, raw | 85 | 78 | 66.8 | 2.6 | 0 | 0 | 0 | 37 | 27 | 28 | 1.30 | 0.030 | 8 | 4 | 0.02 | 1.8 |  | 0.42 |
| 3 oz |  | 13.2 | 1.2 | 0.3 | 0.1 | 0.4 | 198 | 209 | 188 | 0.58 | 1.607 | 38.1 | 28 | 1.0 | 0.35 | 0.05 | 4.2 | 15175 |
| **whelks**, ckd by moist heat | 85 | 234 | 27.2 | 13.2 |  |  | 0 | 350 | 96 | 146 | 2.77 | 0.756 | 42 | 6 | 0.04 | 1.7 |  | 0.34 |
| 3 oz |  | 40.5 | 0.7 | 0.1 | 0 | 0 | 110 | 590 | 240 | 8.55 | 1.751 | 76.2 | 138 |  | 0.18 | 0.55 | 9.4 | 15178 |
| **whelks**, raw | 85 | 116 | 56.1 | 6.6 | 0 | 0 | 0 | 175 | 48 | 73 | 1.39 | 0.380 | 22 | 3 | 0.02 | 0.9 |  | 0.18 |
| 3 oz |  | 20.3 | 0.3 | 0 | 0 | 0 | 55 | 295 | 120 | 4.28 | 0.876 | 38.1 | 74 | 0.1 | 0.09 | 0.29 | 5.1 | 15177 |

## 13. FLOUR, MEALS, AND GRAIN FRACTIONS

| Food | WT (g) | KCAL / PRO (g) | H₂0 (g) / FAT (g) | CHO (g) / SFA (g) | TSUG (g) / MUFA (g) | ASUG (g) / PUFA (g) | DFIB (g) / CHOL (mg) | Na (mg) / K (mg) | Ca (mg) / P (mg) | Mg (mg) / Fe (mg) | Zn (mg) / Cu (mg) | Mn (mg) / Se (mcg) | A (mcg RAE) / A (IU) | C (mg) / E (mg ATE) | B-1 (mg) / B-2 (mg) | NIA (mg) / B-6 (mg) | B-12 (mcg) / FOL (mcg DFE) | PANT (mg) / REF |
|---|---|---|---|---|---|---|---|---|---|---|---|---|---|---|---|---|---|---|
| **arrowroot flour** | 128 | 457 | 14.6 | 112.8 |  |  | 4.4 | 3 | 51 | 4 | 0.09 | 0.602 | 0 | 0 | 0 | 0 | 0 | 0.17 |
| 1 cup |  | 0.4 | 0.1 | 0 | 0 | 0.1 | 0 | 14 | 6 | 0.42 | 0.051 |  | 0 |  | 0.01 |  | 9.0 | 20003 |
| **barley flour/meal** | 148 | 511 | 17.9 | 110.3 | 1.2 | 0 | 14.9 | 6 | 47 | 142 | 2.96 | 1.530 | 0 | 0 | 0.55 | 9.3 | 0 | 0.21 |
| 1 cup |  | 15.5 | 2.4 | 0.5 | 0.3 | 1.1 | 0 | 457 | 438 | 3.97 | 0.508 | 55.8 | 0 | 0.8 | 0.17 | 0.59 | 11.8 | 20130 |
| **barley malt flour** | 162 | 585 | 13.3 | 126.8 | 1.3 | 0 | 11.5 | 18 | 60 | 157 | 3.34 | 1.933 | 2 | 1 | 0.50 | 9.1 | 0 | 0.93 |
| 1 cup |  | 16.7 | 3.0 | 0.6 | 0.4 | 1.5 | 0 | 363 | 491 | 7.63 | 0.437 | 61.1 | 31 | 0.9 | 0.50 | 1.06 | 61.6 | 20131 |
| **buckwheat flour**, whole groat | 120 | 402 | 13.4 | 84.7 | 3.1 | 0 | 12.0 | 13 | 49 | 301 | 3.74 | 2.436 | 0 | 0 | 0.50 | 7.4 | 0 | 0.53 |
| 1 cup |  | 15.1 | 3.7 | 0.8 | 1.1 | 1.1 | 0 | 692 | 404 | 4.87 | 0.618 | 6.8 | 0 | 0.4 | 0.23 | 0.70 | 64.8 | 20011 |
| **corn bran** | 76 | 170 | 3.6 | 65.1 | 0 | 0 | 60.0 | 5 | 32 | 49 | 1.19 | 0.106 | 3 | 0 | 0.01 | 2.1 | 0 | 0.48 |
| 1 cup |  | 6.4 | 0.7 | 0.1 | 0.2 | 0.3 | 0 | 33 | 55 | 2.12 | 0.188 | 12.5 | 54 | 0.3 | 0.08 | 0.12 | 3.0 | 20015 |
| **corn flour**, yellow, enr | 114 | 416 | 10.3 | 86.9 | 0.7 | 0 | 10.9 | 6 | 161 | 125 | 2.03 | 0.552 | 0 | 0 | 1.63 | 11.2 | 0 | 0.75 |
| 1 cup |  | 10.6 | 4.3 | 0.6 | 1.1 | 2.0 | 0 | 340 | 254 | 8.22 | 0.193 | 17.1 | 3 | 0.2 | 0.86 | 0.42 | 433.2 | 20017 |
| **corn flour**, yellow, whole grain | 117 | 422 | 12.8 | 89.9 | 0.7 | 0 | 8.5 | 6 | 8 | 109 | 2.02 | 0.538 | 13 | 0 | 0.29 | 2.2 | 0 | 0.77 |
| 1 cup |  | 8.1 | 4.5 | 0.6 | 1.2 | 2.1 | 0 | 369 | 318 | 2.78 | 0.269 | 18.0 | 250 | 0.5 | 0.09 | 0.43 | 29.2 | 20016 |
| **cornmeal**, white, bolted, enr, self-rising - 1 cup | 122 | 407 | 15.4 | 85.7 |  |  | 8.2 | 1521 | 440 | 105 | 2.44 |  | 0 | 0 | 0.81 | 6.5 |  | 0.52 |
|  |  | 10.1 | 4.1 | 0.6 | 1.1 | 1.9 | 0 | 311 | 981 | 7.03 | 0.183 |  | 0 |  | 0.49 | 0.66 | 434.3 | 20323 |
| **cornmeal**, white, bolted, enr, self-rising w/wheat flour - 1 cup | 170 | 592 | 17.6 | 124.8 |  |  | 10.7 | 2242 | 508 | 92 | 2.36 |  | 0 | 0 | 1.21 | 8.8 |  | 0.65 |
|  |  | 14.3 | 4.8 | 0.7 | 1.3 | 2.2 | 0 | 352 | 1107 | 8.42 | 0.236 |  | 0 |  | 0.74 | 0.65 | 683.4 | 20324 |
| **cornmeal**, white, degermed, enr, self-rising - 1 cup | 138 | 490 | 14.0 | 103.2 |  |  | 9.8 | 1860 | 483 | 68 | 1.38 |  | 0 | 0 | 0.94 | 6.3 |  | 0.52 |
|  |  | 11.6 | 2.4 | 0.3 | 0.6 | 1.0 | 0 | 235 | 860 | 6.53 | 0.179 |  | 0 |  | 0.53 | 0.54 | 517.5 | 20325 |
| **cornmeal**, white, whole grain | 122 | 442 | 12.5 | 93.8 | 0.8 | 0 | 8.9 | 43 | 7 | 155 | 2.22 | 0.608 | 0 | 0 | 0.47 | 4.4 | 0 | 0.52 |
| 1 cup |  | 9.9 | 4.4 | 0.6 | 1.2 | 2.0 | 0 | 350 | 294 | 4.21 | 0.235 | 18.9 | 4 | 0.5 | 0.25 | 0.37 | 30.5 | 20320 |
| **cornmeal**, yellow, bolted, enr, self-rising - 1 cup | 122 | 407 | 15.4 | 85.7 |  |  | 8.2 | 1521 | 440 | 105 | 2.44 | 0.608 | 28 | 0 | 0.81 | 6.5 |  | 0.52 |
|  |  | 10.1 | 4.1 | 0.6 | 1.1 | 1.9 | 0 | 311 | 981 | 7.03 | 0.183 |  | 572 |  | 0.49 | 0.66 | 434.3 | 20023 |
| **cornmeal**, yellow, bolted, enr, self-rising w/wheat flour - 1 cup | 170 | 592 | 17.6 | 124.8 |  |  | 10.7 | 2242 | 508 | 92 | 2.36 | 0.877 | 24 | 0 | 1.21 | 8.8 |  | 0.65 |
|  |  | 14.3 | 4.8 | 0.7 | 1.3 | 2.2 | 0 | 352 | 1107 | 8.42 | 0.236 |  | 488 |  | 0.74 | 0.65 | 683.4 | 20024 |
| **cornmeal**, yellow, degermed, enr | 138 | 509 | 15.5 | 109.2 | 2.3 | 0 | 5.5 | 10 | 4 | 48 | 0.98 | 0.251 | 15 | 0 | 0.85 | 7.3 | 0 | 0.39 |
| 1 cup |  | 10.0 | 2.5 | 0.3 | 0.5 | 1.0 | 0 | 210 | 145 | 5.96 | 0.105 | 16.0 | 295 | 0.2 | 0.57 | 0.27 | 476.1 | 20022 |
| **cornmeal**, yellow, degermed, enr, self-rising - 1 cup | 138 | 490 | 14.0 | 103.2 |  |  | 9.8 | 1860 | 483 | 68 | 1.38 | 0.145 | 15 | 0 | 0.94 | 6.3 | 0 | 0.43 |
|  |  | 11.6 | 2.4 | 0.3 | 0.6 | 1.0 | 0 | 235 | 860 | 6.53 | 0.179 |  | 295 |  | 0.53 | 0.54 | 516.1 | 20025 |
| **cornmeal**, yellow, whole grain | 122 | 442 | 12.5 | 93.8 | 0.8 | 0 | 8.9 | 43 | 7 | 155 | 2.22 | 0.608 | 13 | 0 | 0.47 | 4.4 | 0 | 0.52 |
| 1 cup |  | 9.9 | 4.4 | 0.6 | 1.2 | 2.0 | 0 | 350 | 294 | 4.21 | 0.235 | 18.9 | 261 | 0.5 | 0.25 | 0.37 | 30.5 | 20020 |
| **cottonseed flour**, lowfat | 94 | 312 | 6.5 | 33.9 |  |  |  | 33 | 446 | 673 | 10.91 | 2.001 | 21 | 2 | 1.96 | 3.8 | 0 | 0.42 |
| 1 cup |  | 46.8 | 1.3 | 0.3 | 0.2 | 0.5 | 0 | 1655 | 1492 | 11.83 | 1.102 |  | 406 |  | 0.37 | 0.72 | 214.3 | 12008 |
| **cottonseed flour**, partially defatted | 80 | 287 | 5.0 | 32.4 |  |  | 2.4 | 28 | 382 | 577 | 9.35 | 1.714 | 18 | 2 | 1.68 | 3.3 | 0 | 0.36 |
| 2.8 oz |  | 32.8 | 5.0 | 1.3 | 0.9 | 2.4 | 0 | 1418 | 1278 | 10.13 | 0.944 | 4.5 | 347 |  | 0.32 | 0.62 | 183.2 | 12007 |
| **cottonseed meal**, partially defatted | 85 | 312 | 1.0 | 32.7 |  |  |  | 31 | 428 | 646 | 10.47 | 1.921 | 20 | 2 | 1.88 | 3.6 | 0 | 0.40 |
| 3 oz |  | 41.7 | 4.1 | 1.0 | 0.7 | 1.9 | 0 | 1589 | 1431 | 11.35 | 0.001 |  | 389 |  | 0.36 | 0.69 | 205.7 | 12011 |
| **oat bran** | 94 | 231 | 6.2 | 62.2 | 1.4 | 0 | 14.5 | 4 | 55 | 221 | 2.92 | 5.292 | 0 | 0 | 1.10 | 0.9 | 0 | 1.40 |
| 1 cup |  | 16.3 | 6.6 | 1.2 | 2.2 | 2.6 | 0 | 532 | 690 | 5.09 | 0.379 | 42.5 | 0 | 0.9 | 0.21 | 0.16 | 48.9 | 20033 |
| **oat flour** | 104 | 420 | 8.9 | 68.3 | 0.8 | 0 | 6.8 | 20 | 57 | 150 | 3.33 | 4.180 | 0 | 0 | 0.72 | 1.5 | 0 | 0.21 |
| 1 cup |  | 15.2 | 9.5 | 1.7 | 3.0 | 3.5 | 0 | 386 | 470 | 4.16 | 0.454 | 35.4 | 0 | 0.7 | 0.13 | 0.13 | 33.3 | 20132 |

| | WT (g) | KCAL | H₂0 (g) | CHO (g) | TSUG (g) | ASUG (g) | DFIB (g) | Na (mg) | Ca (mg) | Mg (mg) | Zn (mg) | Mn (mg) | A (mcg RAE) | C (mg) | B-1 (mg) | NIA (mg) | B-12 (mcg) | PANT (mg) |
|---|---|---|---|---|---|---|---|---|---|---|---|---|---|---|---|---|---|---|
| | | PRO (g) | FAT (g) | SFA (g) | MUFA (g) | PUFA (g) | CHOL (mg) | K (mg) | P (mg) | Fe (mg) | Cu (mg) | Se (mcg) | A (IU) | E (mg ATE) | B-2 (mg) | B-6 (mg) | FOL (mcg DFE) | REF |
| **peanut flour**, defatted | 60 | 196 | 4.7 | 20.8 | 4.9 | 0 | 9.5 | 108 | 84 | 222 | 3.06 | 2.940 | 0 | 0 | 0.42 | 16.2 | 0 | 1.65 |
| *1 cup* | | 31.3 | 0.3 | 0 | 0.1 | 0.1 | 0 | 774 | 456 | 1.26 | 1.080 | 4.3 | 0 | 0 | 0.29 | 0.30 | 148.8 | 16099 |
| **potato flour** | 160 | 571 | 10.4 | 133.0 | 5.6 | 0 | 9.4 | 88 | 104 | 104 | 0.86 | 0.501 | 0 | 6 | 0.36 | 5.6 | 0 | 0.76 |
| *1 cup* | | 11.0 | 0.5 | 0.1 | 0 | 0.2 | 0 | 1602 | 269 | 2.21 | 0.315 | 1.8 | 0 | 0.4 | 0.08 | 1.23 | 40.0 | 11413 |
| **rice bran** | 118 | 373 | 7.2 | 58.6 | 1.1 | 0 | 24.8 | 6 | 67 | 922 | 7.13 | 16.768 | 0 | 0 | 3.25 | 40.1 | 0 | 8.72 |
| *1 cup* | | 15.8 | 24.6 | 4.9 | 8.9 | 8.8 | 0 | 1752 | 1979 | 21.88 | 0.859 | 18.4 | 0 | 5.8 | 0.34 | 4.80 | 74.3 | 20060 |
| **rice flour**, brown | 158 | 574 | 18.9 | 120.8 | 1.3 | 0 | 7.3 | 13 | 17 | 177 | 3.87 | 6.341 | 0 | 0 | 0.70 | 10.0 | 0 | 2.51 |
| *1 cup* | | 11.4 | 4.4 | 0.9 | 1.6 | 1.6 | 0 | 457 | 532 | 3.13 | 0.363 | | 0 | 1.9 | 0.13 | 1.16 | 25.3 | 20090 |
| **rice flour**, white | 158 | 578 | 18.8 | 126.6 | 0.2 | 0 | 3.8 | 0 | 16 | 55 | 1.26 | 1.896 | 0 | 0 | 0.22 | 4.1 | 0 | 1.29 |
| *1 cup* | | 9.4 | 2.2 | 0.6 | 0.7 | 0.6 | 0 | 120 | 155 | 0.55 | 0.205 | 23.9 | 0 | 0.2 | 0.03 | 0.69 | 6.3 | 20061 |
| **rye flour**, dark | 128 | 415 | 14.2 | 88.0 | 1.3 | 0 | 28.9 | 1 | 72 | 317 | 7.19 | 8.614 | 1 | 0 | 0.40 | 5.5 | 0 | 1.86 |
| *1 cup* | | 18.0 | 3.4 | 0.4 | 0.4 | 1.5 | 0 | 934 | 809 | 8.26 | 0.960 | 45.7 | 14 | 1.8 | 0.32 | 0.57 | 76.8 | 20063 |
| **rye flour**, light | 102 | 374 | 9.0 | 81.8 | 1.1 | 0 | 14.9 | 2 | 21 | 71 | 1.78 | 2.009 | 0 | 0 | 0.34 | 0.8 | 0 | 0.68 |
| *1 cup* | | 8.6 | 1.4 | 0.1 | 0.2 | 0.6 | 0 | 238 | 198 | 1.84 | 0.255 | 36.4 | 0 | 0.4 | 0.09 | 0.24 | 22.4 | 20065 |
| **rye flour**, medium | 102 | 361 | 10.0 | 79.0 | 1.1 | 0 | 14.9 | 3 | 24 | 76 | 2.03 | 5.569 | 0 | 0 | 0.29 | 1.8 | 0 | 0.50 |
| *1 cup* | | 9.6 | 1.8 | 0.2 | 0.2 | 0.8 | 0 | 347 | 211 | 2.16 | 0.293 | 36.4 | 0 | 0.8 | 0.12 | 0.27 | 19.4 | 20064 |
| **sesame flour**, high-fat | 85 | 447 | 0.8 | 22.6 | | | | 35 | 135 | 307 | 9.07 | 1.266 | 3 | 0 | 2.28 | 11.4 | 0 | 2.49 |
| *3 oz* | | 26.2 | 31.5 | 4.4 | 11.9 | 13.8 | 0 | 360 | 686 | 12.89 | 1.292 | | 59 | | 0.24 | 0.13 | 26.4 | 12170 |
| **sesame flour**, lowfat | 85 | 283 | 6.0 | 30.2 | | | | 33 | 127 | 287 | 8.50 | 1.187 | 3 | 0 | 2.14 | 10.7 | 0 | 2.33 |
| *3 oz* | | 42.6 | 1.5 | 0.2 | 0.5 | 0.5 | 0 | 337 | 643 | 12.09 | 1.211 | | 54 | | 0.23 | 0.12 | 24.6 | 12033 |
| **sesame flour**, partially defatted | 85 | 325 | 5.6 | 29.9 | | | | 35 | 128 | 308 | 9.09 | 1.193 | 3 | 0 | 2.15 | 10.7 | 0 | 2.35 |
| *3 oz* | | 34.3 | 10.1 | 1.4 | 3.7 | 4.3 | 0 | 361 | 688 | 12.16 | 1.217 | | 59 | | 0.23 | 0.13 | 24.6 | 12032 |
| **sesame meal**, partially defatted | 85 | 482 | 4.2 | 22.1 | | | | 33 | 130 | 294 | 8.70 | 1.213 | 3 | 0 | 2.19 | 10.9 | 0 | 2.39 |
| *3 oz* | | 14.4 | 40.8 | 5.7 | 15.4 | 17.9 | 0 | 345 | 658 | 12.37 | 1.238 | | 56 | | 0.23 | 0.12 | 25.5 | 12034 |
| **soy flour**, defatted | 100 | 330 | 7.2 | 38.4 | 18.9 | 0 | 17.5 | 20 | 241 | 290 | 2.46 | 3.018 | 2 | 0 | 0.70 | 2.6 | 0 | 2.00 |
| *1 cup* | | 47.0 | 1.2 | 0.1 | 0.2 | 0.5 | 0 | 2384 | 674 | 9.24 | 4.065 | 1.7 | 40 | 0.1 | 0.25 | 0.57 | 305.0 | 16117 |
| **soy flour**, full-fat | 84 | 366 | 4.3 | 29.6 | 6.3 | 0 | 8.1 | 11 | 173 | 360 | 3.29 | 1.911 | 5 | 0 | 0.49 | 3.6 | 0 | 1.34 |
| *1 cup* | | 29.0 | 17.3 | 2.5 | 3.8 | 9.8 | 0 | 2113 | 415 | 5.35 | 2.453 | 6.3 | 101 | 1.6 | 0.97 | 0.39 | 289.8 | 16115 |
| **soy flour**, full-fat, roasted | 85 | 375 | 3.2 | 28.6 | 6.5 | 0 | 8.2 | 10 | 160 | 314 | 3.04 | 1.765 | 5 | 0 | 0.35 | 2.8 | 0 | 1.03 |
| *1 cup* | | 29.6 | 18.6 | 2.7 | 4.1 | 10.5 | 0 | 1735 | 405 | 4.95 | 1.888 | 6.4 | 104 | 1.7 | 0.80 | 0.30 | 193.0 | 16116 |
| **soy flour**, lowfat | 88 | 330 | 4.1 | 30.7 | 9.3 | 0 | 14.1 | 8 | 251 | 251 | 3.61 | 2.772 | 2 | 0 | 0.96 | 2.6 | 0 | 1.36 |
| *1 cup* | | 40.0 | 7.8 | 1.1 | 1.3 | 3.7 | 0 | 1839 | 594 | 7.22 | 1.408 | 51.8 | 35 | 0.5 | 0.25 | 0.92 | 254.3 | 16118 |
| **soy meal**, defatted | 122 | 414 | 8.5 | 49.0 | | | | 4 | 298 | 373 | 6.17 | 4.636 | 2 | 0 | 0.84 | 3.2 | 0 | 2.41 |
| *1 cup* | | 54.8 | 2.9 | 0.3 | 0.5 | 1.3 | 0 | 3038 | 855 | 16.71 | 2.440 | 4.0 | 49 | | 0.31 | 0.69 | 369.7 | 16119 |
| **sunflower flour**, partially defatted | 64 | 209 | 4.8 | 22.9 | | | 3.3 | 2 | 73 | 221 | 3.17 | 1.264 | 1 | 1 | 2.04 | 4.7 | 0 | 4.22 |
| *1 cup* | | 30.8 | 1.0 | 0.1 | 0.2 | 0.6 | 0 | 43 | 441 | 4.24 | 1.096 | 37.2 | 31 | | 0.17 | 0.48 | 142.1 | 12041 |
| **triticale flour**, whole grain | 130 | 439 | 13.0 | 95.1 | | | 19.0 | 3 | 46 | 199 | 3.46 | 5.440 | 0 | 0 | 0.49 | 3.7 | 0 | 2.82 |
| *1 cup* | | 17.1 | 2.4 | 0.4 | 0.2 | 1.0 | 0 | 606 | 417 | 3.37 | 0.727 | | 0 | 1.2 | 0.17 | 0.52 | 96.2 | 20070 |
| **wheat bran**, crude | 58 | 125 | 5.7 | 37.4 | 0.2 | 0 | 24.8 | 1 | 42 | 354 | 4.22 | 6.670 | 0 | 0 | 0.30 | 7.9 | 0 | 1.26 |
| *1 cup* | | 9.0 | 2.5 | 0.4 | 0.4 | 1.3 | 0 | 686 | 588 | 6.13 | 0.579 | 45.0 | 5 | 0.9 | 0.33 | 0.76 | 45.8 | 20077 |
| **wheat bran**, toasted, Kretschmer | 28 | 56 | 3.3 | 16.7 | | | 11.6 | 2 | 18 | 170 | 3.14 | 4.866 | 0 | 0 | 0.31 | 5.8 | 0.06 | 0.82 |
| *1 oz* | | 4.9 | 1.4 | 0.2 | 0.2 | 0.8 | 0 | 360 | 368 | 3.89 | 0.305 | | 0 | | 0.13 | 0.19 | 83.7 | 8363 |
| **wheat germ**, honey crunch, Kretschmer - 2 oz | 57 | 212 | 1.9 | 33.1 | 14.2 | | 5.8 | 6 | 28 | 155 | 7.91 | 9.052 | 0 | 0 | 0.76 | 2.7 | 0 | 0.63 |
| | | 15.1 | 4.4 | 0.8 | 0.6 | 2.8 | 0 | 549 | 576 | 4.59 | 0.410 | 33.1 | 0 | 11.5 | 0.39 | 0.28 | 579.1 | 8085 |
| **wheat germ**, Kretschmer | 28 | 102 | 1.3 | 13.8 | | | 3.3 | 2 | 14 | 88 | 4.48 | 5.342 | 0 | 2 | 0.55 | 1.6 | 0.06 | 0.39 |
| *1 oz* | | 8.8 | 2.7 | 0.5 | 0.4 | 1.7 | 0 | 307 | 316 | 2.34 | 0.174 | | 0 | | 0.22 | 0.17 | 249.8 | 8366 |
| **wheat germ**, toasted | 56 | 214 | 3.1 | 27.8 | 4.4 | 0 | 8.5 | 2 | 25 | 179 | 9.34 | 11.175 | 3 | 3 | 0.94 | 3.1 | 0 | 0.78 |
| *½ cup* | | 16.3 | 6.0 | 1.0 | 0.8 | 3.7 | 0 | 530 | 642 | 5.09 | 0.347 | 36.4 | 58 | 9.0 | 0.46 | 0.55 | 197.1 | 8084 |
| **wheat flour**, white, enr, all-purpose | 125 | 455 | 14.9 | 95.4 | 0.3 | 0 | 3.4 | 2 | 19 | 28 | 0.88 | 0.852 | 0 | 0 | 0.98 | 7.4 | 0 | 0.55 |
| *1 cup* | | 12.9 | 1.2 | 0.2 | 0.1 | 0.5 | 0 | 134 | 135 | 5.80 | 0.180 | 42.4 | 0 | 0.1 | 0.62 | 0.05 | 363.8 | 20081 |
| **wheat flour**, white, enriched, bread | 137 | 495 | 18.3 | 99.4 | 0.4 | 0 | 3.3 | 3 | 21 | 34 | 1.16 | 1.085 | 0 | 0 | 1.11 | 10.3 | 0 | 0.60 |
| *1 cup* | | 16.4 | 2.3 | 0.3 | 0.2 | 1.0 | 0 | 137 | 133 | 6.04 | 0.249 | 54.4 | 3 | 0.5 | 0.70 | 0.05 | 394.6 | 20083 |
| **wheat flour**, white, enriched, cake | 137 | 496 | 17.1 | 106.9 | 0.4 | 0 | 2.3 | 3 | 19 | 22 | 0.85 | 0.869 | 0 | 0 | 1.22 | 9.3 | 0 | 0.63 |
| *1 cup* | | 11.2 | 1.2 | 0.2 | 0.1 | 0.5 | 0 | 144 | 116 | 10.03 | 0.190 | 6.7 | 0 | | 0.59 | 0.05 | 386.3 | 20084 |
| **wheat flour**, white, enr, self-rising | 125 | 442 | 13.2 | 92.8 | 0.3 | 0 | 3.4 | 1588 | 422 | 24 | 0.78 | 1.250 | 0 | 0 | 0.84 | 7.3 | 0 | 0.55 |
| *1 cup* | | 12.4 | 1.2 | 0.2 | 0.1 | 0.5 | 0 | 155 | 744 | 5.84 | 0.140 | 43.0 | 0 | 0.1 | 0.52 | 0.06 | 383.8 | 20082 |
| **wheat flour**, white, enr, tortilla mix | 111 | 450 | 11.2 | 74.5 | | | | 751 | 228 | 23 | 0.71 | 0.682 | 0 | 0 | 0.82 | 6.5 | 0 | 0.44 |
| *1 cup* | | 10.7 | 11.8 | 4.6 | 5.0 | 1.7 | 0 | 111 | 233 | 7.83 | 0.111 | | 0 | | 0.55 | 0.04 | 238.7 | 20086 |
| **wheat flour**, whole wheat | 120 | 407 | 12.3 | 87.1 | 0.5 | 0 | 14.6 | 6 | 41 | 166 | 3.52 | 4.559 | 0 | 0 | 0.54 | 7.6 | 0 | 1.21 |
| *1 cup* | | 16.4 | 2.2 | 0.4 | 0.3 | 0.9 | 0 | 486 | 415 | 4.66 | 0.458 | 84.8 | 11 | 1.0 | 0.26 | 0.41 | 52.8 | 20080 |
| **wheat germ**, crude | 57 | 205 | 6.3 | 29.5 | | | 7.5 | 7 | 22 | 136 | 7.01 | 7.582 | 0 | 0 | 1.07 | 3.9 | 0 | 1.29 |
| *½ cup* | | 13.2 | 5.5 | 0.9 | 0.8 | 3.4 | 0 | 508 | 480 | 3.57 | 0.454 | 45.1 | 0 | | 0.28 | 0.74 | 160.2 | 20078 |
| **wheat semolina**, enriched | 167 | 601 | 21.2 | 121.6 | | | 6.5 | 2 | 28 | 78 | 1.75 | 1.034 | 0 | 0 | 1.35 | 10.0 | 0 | 0.97 |
| *1 cup* | | 21.2 | 1.8 | 0.3 | 0.2 | 0.7 | 0 | 311 | 227 | 7.28 | 0.316 | 149.3 | 0 | 0.4 | 0.95 | 0.17 | 435.9 | 20066 |

| | WT (g) | KCAL / PRO (g) | H₂O (g) / FAT (g) | CHO (g) / SFA (g) | TSUG (g) / MUFA (g) | ASUG (g) / PUFA (g) | DFIB (g) / CHOL (mg) | Na (mg) / K (mg) | Ca (mg) / P (mg) | Mg (mg) / Fe (mg) | Zn (mg) / Cu (mg) | Mn (mg) / Se (mcg) | A (mcg RAE) / A (IU) | C (mg) / E (mg ATE) | B-1 (mg) / B-2 (mg) | NIA (mg) / B-6 (mg) | B-12 (mcg) / FOL (mcg DFE) | PANT (mg) / REF |
|---|---|---|---|---|---|---|---|---|---|---|---|---|---|---|---|---|---|---|

## 14. FRUIT AND VEGETABLE JUICES AND JUICE DRINKS

| | WT (g) | KCAL / PRO | H₂O / FAT | CHO / SFA | TSUG / MUFA | ASUG / PUFA | DFIB / CHOL | Na / K | Ca / P | Mg / Fe | Zn / Cu | Mn / Se | A RAE / A IU | C / E | B-1 / B-2 | NIA / B-6 | B-12 / FOL | PANT / REF |
|---|---|---|---|---|---|---|---|---|---|---|---|---|---|---|---|---|---|---|
| **acerola juice**, raw | 242 | 56 | 228.2 | 11.6 | 10.9 | 0 | 0.7 | 7 | 24 | 29 | 0.24 | | 60 | 3872 | 0.05 | 1.0 | 0 | 0.50 |
| *8 fl oz* | | 1.0 | 0.7 | 0.2 | 0.2 | 0.2 | 0 | 235 | 22 | 1.21 | 0.208 | 0.2 | 1232 | 0.4 | 0.15 | 0.01 | 33.9 | 9002 |
| **AntioxiDance jce drink**, btld, Odwalla - *8 fl oz* | 249 | 100 | | 24.0 | 21.0 | | | 10 | | | | | | 180 | | | | |
| | | 0 | 0 | | | | | 55 | | | | | | | | | | ODWA1 |
| **apple juice**, canned/bottled | 248 | 114 | 218.8 | 28.0 | 23.9 | 0 | 0.5 | 10 | 20 | 12 | 0.05 | 0.184 | 0 | 2 | 0.05 | 0.2 | 0 | 0.12 |
| *8 fl oz* | | 0.2 | 0.3 | 0.1 | 0 | 0.1 | 0 | 250 | 17 | 0.30 | 0.030 | 0.2 | 2 | 0 | 0.04 | 0.04 | 0 | 9016 |
| **apple juice**, from frozen conc | 239 | 112 | 210.1 | 27.6 | 26.1 | 0 | 0.2 | 17 | 14 | 12 | 0.10 | 0.151 | 0 | 1 | 0.01 | 0.1 | 0 | 0.15 |
| *8 fl oz* | | 0.3 | 0.2 | 0 | 0 | 0.1 | 0 | 301 | 17 | 0.62 | 0.033 | 0.2 | 0 | 0 | 0.04 | 0.08 | 0 | 9018 |
| **apple juice**, Minute Maid | 208 | 100 | | 23.0 | 21.0 | | | 15 | 100 | 8 | | | | 60 | | | | |
| *6.7 fl oz box* | | 0 | 0 | | | | | | | | | | | | | | | MNTM2 |
| **apple strawberry juice**, Minute Maid - *6.7 fl oz box* | 208 | 100 | | 25.0 | 22.0 | | | 15 | 100 | 8 | | | | 60 | | | | |
| | | 0 | 0 | | | | | 180 | | | | | | | | | | MNTM34 |
| **apricot nectar**, canned/bottled | 251 | 141 | 213.0 | 36.1 | 34.6 | 26.5 | 1.5 | 8 | 18 | 13 | 0.23 | 0.080 | 166 | 2 | 0.02 | 0.7 | 0 | 0.24 |
| *8 fl oz* | | 0.9 | 0.2 | 0 | 0.1 | 0 | 0 | 286 | 23 | 0.95 | 0.183 | 0 | 3303 | 0.8 | 0.04 | 0.06 | 2.5 | 9036 |
| **B Berrier jce drink**, bottled, Odwalla - *8 fl oz* | 249 | 120 | | 29.0 | 27.0 | | | 15 | | | | | | | | | 1.50 | |
| | | 0 | 0 | | | | | 45 | | | | | | | | | 0.50 | ODWA2 |
| **beef broth and tomato juice**, canned - *5.5 fl oz* | 168 | 62 | 151.0 | 14.3 | | | 0.2 | 220 | 18 | 5 | 0.03 | 0.047 | 10 | 2 | 0 | 0.3 | 0.08 | 0.06 |
| | | 1.0 | 0.2 | 0.1 | 0 | 0 | 0 | 161 | 22 | 0.97 | 0.029 | 1.2 | 215 | | 0.05 | 0.04 | 6.7 | 14114 |
| **Berries GoMega jce**, btld, Odwalla | 249 | 160 | | 34.0 | 24.0 | | | 15 | 20 | | | | | | | | | |
| *8 fl oz* | | 2.0 | 2.0 | | | | | 360 | | 1.80 | | | | | | | | ODWA3 |
| **berry juice blend**, Minute Maid | 208 | 5 | | 2.0 | | | | | 100 | | | | | 60 | | | | |
| *6.7 fl oz box* | | 0 | 0 | | | | 4 | | | | | | | | | | | MNTM35 |
| **berry juice**, btld, Odwalla | 249 | 140 | | 35.0 | 27.0 | | | 20 | 40 | | | | | | | | | |
| *8 fl oz* | | 0 | 0 | | | | | 420 | | 0.36 | | | | | | | | ODWA13 |
| **berry punch**, Minute Maid Coolers | 208 | 100 | | 26.0 | 25.0 | | | 15 | 100 | | | | | 60 | | | | |
| *6.7 fl oz pouch* | | 0 | 0 | | | | | | | | | | | | | | | MNTM39 |
| **berry punch**, refrig carton, Minute Maid - *8 fl oz* | 249 | 120 | | 32.0 | 31.0 | | | 15 | | | | | | | | | | |
| | | 0 | 0 | | | | | | | | | | | | | | | MNTM40 |
| **blackberry fruit shake**, btld, Odwalla - *8 fl oz* | 250 | 150 | | 36.0 | 29.0 | | | 10 | 20 | | | | | | | | | |
| | | 2.0 | 0 | | | | | 1060 | | 0.72 | | | | | | | | ODWA4 |
| **blackberry juice**, canned | 249 | 95 | 226.3 | 19.4 | 19.2 | 0 | 0.2 | 2 | 30 | 52 | 1.02 | | 15 | 28 | 0.03 | 1.1 | 0 | |
| *8 fl oz* | | 0.7 | 1.5 | 0 | 0.1 | 0.9 | 0 | 336 | 30 | 1.20 | 0.284 | 0.7 | 306 | 2.2 | 0.04 | 0.05 | 24.9 | 9043 |
| **Blueberry B Monster jce**, btld, Odwalla - *8 fl oz* | 249 | 140 | | 34.0 | 23.0 | | | 10 | | | | | | 15 | 5.40 | 9.0 | 21.60 | 6.00 |
| | | 0 | 0 | | | | | 360 | | | | | | 6.12 | 7.20 | 16.0 | | ODWA5 |
| **carrot juice**, canned | 236 | 94 | 209.7 | 21.9 | 9.2 | 0 | 1.9 | 68 | 57 | 33 | 0.42 | 0.307 | 2256 | 20 | 0.22 | 0.9 | 0 | 0.54 |
| *8 fl oz* | | 2.2 | 0.4 | 0.1 | 0 | 0.2 | 0 | 689 | 99 | 1.09 | 0.109 | 1.4 | 45133 | 2.7 | 0.13 | 0.51 | 9.4 | 11655 |
| **cherry limeade**, cnd, Minute Maid Light - *12 fl oz can* | 372 | 10 | | 3.0 | 1.0 | | | 50 | | | | | | | | | | |
| | | 0 | 0 | | | | | | | | | | | | | | | MNTM41 |
| **cherry limeade**, refrig carton, Minute Maid - *8 fl oz* | 249 | 120 | | 34.0 | 33.0 | | | 15 | | | | | | | | | | |
| | | 0 | 0 | | | | | | | | | | | | | | | MNTM43 |
| **Citrus C Monster jce**, btld, Odwalla - *8 fl oz* | 249 | 150 | | 36.0 | 27.0 | | | 15 | 20 | | | | | 600 | | | | |
| | | 2.0 | 0 | | | | | 640 | | 0.36 | | | | | | | | ODWA7 |
| **citrus fruit jce drink**, from frzn conc - *8 fl oz* | 248 | 114 | 217.8 | 28.3 | 20.2 | | 0.2 | 10 | 22 | 15 | 0.10 | 0.181 | 5 | 67 | 0.03 | 0.2 | 0 | 0.15 |
| | | 0.8 | 0.1 | 0 | 0 | 0 | 0 | 278 | 25 | 2.78 | 0.087 | 0.2 | 92 | 0.1 | 0.02 | 0.05 | 17.4 | 14263 |
| **citrus punch**, refrig carton, Minute Maid - *8 fl oz* | 250 | 110 | | 31.0 | 30.0 | | | 0 | | | | | | | | | | |
| | | 0 | 0 | | | | | | | | | | | | | | | MNTM45 |
| **clam and tomato juice**, canned *5.5 fl oz* | 166 | 80 | 145.1 | 18.2 | 5.5 | | 0.7 | 601 | 13 | 8 | 0.13 | 0.053 | 12 | 8 | 0.03 | 0.4 | 0.05 | 0.14 |
| | | 1.0 | 0.3 | 0 | 0 | 0 | 0 | 148 | 18 | 0.25 | 0.048 | 0.7 | 247 | 0.2 | 0.02 | 0.10 | 13.3 | 14187 |
| **clear cherry jce drink**, Minute Maid Coolers - *6.7 fl oz pouch* | 208 | 100 | | 28.0 | 27.0 | | | 15 | 100 | | | | | 60 | | | | |
| | | 0 | 0 | | | | | | | | | | | | | | | MNTM46 |
| **cranberry apple jce drink**, btld - *8 fl oz* | 245 | 154 | 205.3 | 38.8 | 35.5 | 24.9 | 0 | 5 | 7 | 2 | 0.05 | 0.071 | 0 | 97 | 0 | 0 | 0 | 0 |
| | | 0 | 0.3 | 0 | 0 | 0.1 | 0 | 42 | 5 | 0.17 | 0.024 | 0 | 7 | 0.3 | 0 | 0 | 0 | 14238 |
| **cranberry apple jce drink**, low-cal | 245 | 47 | 233.2 | 11.5 | 11.3 | 0 | 0.2 | 12 | 24 | 7 | 0.05 | 0.034 | 0 | 78 | 0.01 | 0.1 | 0 | 0.03 |
| *8 fl oz* | | 0.2 | 0 | 0 | 0 | 0 | 0 | 110 | 2 | 0.15 | 0.017 | 0.2 | 24 | 0.7 | 0.02 | 0.05 | 0 | 43404 |
| **cranberry apple raspberry jce drink**, Minute Maid - *8 fl oz* | 250 | 120 | | 33.0 | 30.0 | | | 25 | 0 | | | | | 60 | 0 | | | |
| | | 0 | 0 | | | | | 0 | | | | | | | | | | MNTM47 |
| **cranberry apricot jce drink**, btld | 245 | 157 | 204.6 | 39.7 | | | 0.2 | 5 | 22 | 7 | 0.10 | 0.306 | 56 | 0 | 0.01 | 0.3 | 0 | 0.09 |
| *8 fl oz* | | 0.5 | 0 | 0 | 0 | 0 | 0 | 149 | 12 | 0.37 | 0.037 | 0 | 1134 | | 0.02 | 0.05 | 2.4 | 14240 |
| **cranberry grape jce drink**, btld | 245 | 137 | 209.7 | 34.3 | | | 0.2 | 7 | 20 | 7 | 0.10 | 0.387 | 0 | 78 | 0.02 | 0.3 | 0 | 0.13 |
| *8 fl oz* | | 0.5 | 0.2 | 0.1 | 0 | 0.1 | 0 | 59 | 10 | 0.02 | 0.017 | 0 | 12 | | 0.04 | 0.07 | 2.4 | 14241 |

| | WT (g) | KCAL / PRO (g) | H₂0 (g) / FAT (g) | CHO (g) / SFA (g) | TSUG (g) / MUFA (g) | ASUG (g) / PUFA (g) | DFIB (g) / CHOL (mg) | Na (mg) / K (mg) | Ca (mg) / P (mg) | Mg (mg) / Fe (mg) | Zn (mg) / Cu (mg) | Mn (mg) / Se (mcg) | A (mcg RAE) / A (IU) | C (mg) / E (mg ATE) | B-1 (mg) / B-2 (mg) | NIA (mg) / B-6 (mg) | B-12 (mcg) / FOL (mcg DFE) | PANT (mg) / REF |
|---|---|---|---|---|---|---|---|---|---|---|---|---|---|---|---|---|---|---|
| **cranberry grape jce drink**, Minute Maid - *8 fl oz* | 249 | 150 | | 39.0 | 38.0 | | | 20 | 0 | | | | | 60 | 0 | | | |
| | | 0 | 0 | | | | | 0 | | | | | | | | | | MNTM50 |
| **cranberry jce cocktail**, cnd/btld *8 fl oz* | 253 | 137 | 218.0 | 34.2 | 30.0 | 20.6 | 0 | 5 | 8 | 3 | 0.08 | 0.121 | 0 | 107 | 0 | 0.1 | 0 | 0.13 |
| | | 0 | 0.3 | 0 | 0 | 0.1 | 0 | 35 | 3 | 0.25 | 0.025 | 0.5 | 20 | 0.6 | 0 | 0 | 0 | 14242 |
| **cranberry jce cocktail**, from frzn conc - *8 fl oz* | 250 | 118 | 220.2 | 29.5 | 24.4 | | 0 | 10 | 12 | 5 | 0.05 | 0.080 | 0 | 26 | 0.01 | 0 | 0 | 0.28 |
| | | 0 | 0 | 0 | 0 | 0 | 0 | 30 | 2 | 0.18 | 0.030 | 0 | 20 | 0 | 0.02 | 0.03 | 0 | 14431 |
| **cranberry jce cocktail**, low cal, added calcium, btld - *8 fl oz* | 237 | 45 | 225.6 | 10.9 | 10.9 | 1.5 | 0 | 7 | 21 | 5 | 0.05 | 0.014 | 0 | 76 | 0 | 0 | 0 | 0 |
| | | 0 | 0 | 0 | 0 | 0 | 0 | 59 | 2 | 0.09 | 0.024 | 0 | 5 | 0.1 | 0 | 0 | 0 | 14243 |
| **cranberry juice**, unsweetened *4 fl oz* | 126 | 58 | 109.8 | 15.4 | 15.2 | | 0.1 | 3 | 10 | 8 | 0.13 | | 3 | 12 | 0.01 | 0.1 | 0 | |
| | | 0.5 | 0.2 | 0 | 0 | 0.1 | 0 | 97 | 16 | 0.32 | 0.069 | 0.1 | 57 | 1.5 | 0.02 | 0.07 | 1.3 | 43382 |
| **fruit medley jce**, btld, Minute Maid - *10 fl oz* | 310 | 140 | | 36.0 | 32.0 | | | 26 | 16 | | | | | 60 | | | | |
| | | 0 | 0 | | | | | | | | | | | | | | | MNTM51 |
| **fruit punch, 100% jce**, Minute Maid - *6.7 fl oz box* | 208 | 100 | | 24.0 | 21.0 | | | 15 | 100 | 8 | | | | 60 | | | | |
| | | 0 | 0 | | | | | 350 | | | | | | | | | | MNTM53 |
| **fruit punch jce drink**, from frzn conc - *8 fl oz* | 248 | 104 | 221.1 | 25.9 | | | 0 | 12 | 17 | 7 | 0.42 | 0.126 | 0 | 12 | 0 | 0.1 | 0 | 0.06 |
| | | 0.2 | 0.4 | 0.1 | 0.1 | 0.1 | 0 | 164 | 7 | 0.50 | 0.060 | 0 | 12 | 0 | 0.14 | 0.03 | 5.0 | 14406 |
| **fruit punch**, bottled, Minute Maid - *8 fl oz* | 249 | 120 | | 31.0 | 30.0 | | | 35 | 0 | | | | | 60 | 0 | | | |
| | | 0 | 0 | | | | | 20 | | | | | | | | | | MNTM54 |
| **grape jce blend**, Minute Maid *6.7 fl oz box* | 208 | 100 | | 26.0 | 23.0 | | | 15 | 100 | 8 | | | | 60 | | | | |
| | | 0 | 0 | | | | | 160 | | | | | | | | | | MNTM5 |
| **grape jce**, cnd/btld *8 fl oz* | 253 | 152 | 213.8 | 37.4 | 35.9 | 0 | 0.5 | 13 | 28 | 25 | 0.18 | 0.605 | 0 | 0 | 0.04 | 0.3 | 0 | 0.12 |
| | | 0.9 | 0.3 | 0.1 | 0 | 0.1 | 0 | 263 | 35 | 0.63 | 0.046 | 0.2 | 20 | 0 | 0.04 | 0.08 | 0 | 9135 |
| **grape jce cocktail**, from frzn conc *8 fl oz* | 249 | 120 | | 33.0 | 32.0 | | | 5 | 100 | | | | | 72 | | | | |
| | | 0 | 0 | | | | | | | | | | | | | | | MNTM55 |
| **grape jce drink**, cnd/btld *8 fl oz* | 250 | 142 | 213.2 | 36.4 | 35.3 | 9.7 | 0.2 | 22 | 18 | 15 | 0.08 | 0.500 | 0 | 66 | 0.56 | 0.4 | 0 | 0.06 |
| | | 0 | 0 | 0 | 0 | 0 | 0 | 82 | 15 | 0.32 | 0.055 | 0.2 | 10 | 0 | 0.88 | 0.09 | 2.5 | 14282 |
| **grape jce**, swtnd, from frzn conc *8 fl oz* | 250 | 128 | 217.2 | 31.9 | 31.6 | 26.1 | 0.2 | 5 | 10 | 10 | 0.10 | 0.442 | 0 | 60 | 0.04 | 0.3 | 0 | 0.06 |
| | | 0.5 | 0.2 | 0.1 | 0 | 0.1 | 0 | 52 | 10 | 0.25 | 0.032 | 0.2 | 20 | 0 | 0.06 | 0.11 | 2.5 | 9137 |
| **grape punch**, refrig carton, Minute Maid - *8 fl oz* | 249 | 120 | | 32.0 | 31.0 | | | 15 | | | | | | | | | | |
| | | 0 | 0 | | | | | | | | | | | | | | | MNTM56 |
| **grapefruit juice**, canned/bottled *8 fl oz* | 247 | 94 | 222.5 | 22.1 | 21.9 | 0 | 0.2 | 2 | 17 | 25 | 0.22 | 0.049 | 0 | 72 | 0.10 | 0.6 | 0 | 0.32 |
| | | 1.3 | 0.2 | 0 | 0 | 0.1 | 0 | 378 | 27 | 0.49 | 0.094 | 0.2 | 17 | 0.1 | 0.05 | 0.05 | 24.7 | 9123 |
| **grapefruit juice**, from frzn conc *8 fl oz* | 247 | 101 | 220.6 | 24.0 | 23.8 | 0 | 0.2 | 2 | 20 | 27 | 0.12 | 0.049 | 0 | 83 | 0.10 | 0.5 | 0 | 0.47 |
| | | 1.4 | 0.3 | 0 | 0 | 0.1 | 0 | 336 | 35 | 0.35 | 0.082 | 0.2 | 22 | 0.1 | 0.05 | 0.11 | 9.9 | 9126 |
| **grapefruit juice**, pink, raw *8 fl oz* | 247 | 96 | 222.3 | 22.7 | | | | 2 | 22 | 30 | 0.12 | 0.049 | 54 | 94 | 0.10 | 0.5 | 0 | 0.47 |
| | | 1.2 | 0.2 | 0 | 0 | 0.1 | 0 | 400 | 37 | 0.49 | 0.082 | | 1087 | | 0.05 | 0.11 | 24.7 | 9404 |
| **grapefruit juice**, raw *8 fl oz* | 247 | 96 | 222.3 | 22.7 | 22.5 | 0 | 0.2 | 2 | 22 | 30 | 0.12 | 0.049 | 2 | 94 | 0.10 | 0.5 | 0 | 0.47 |
| | | 1.2 | 0.2 | 0 | 0 | 0.1 | 0 | 400 | 37 | 0.49 | 0.082 | 0.2 | 25 | 0.5 | 0.05 | 0.11 | 24.7 | 9128 |
| **grapefruit juice**, swtnd, cnd/btld *8 fl oz* | 250 | 115 | 218.4 | 27.8 | 27.6 | 5.4 | 0.2 | 5 | 20 | 25 | 0.15 | 0.050 | 0 | 67 | 0.10 | 0.8 | 0 | 0.32 |
| | | 1.4 | 0.2 | 0 | 0 | 0.1 | 0 | 405 | 28 | 0.90 | 0.120 | 0.2 | 18 | 0.1 | 0.06 | 0.05 | 25.0 | 9124 |
| **grenadine syrup** (from pomegranate jce) - *1 T* | 20 | 54 | 6.5 | 13.4 | 9.3 | 8.4 | 0 | 5 | 1 | 1 | 0.03 | | 0 | 0 | 0 | 0 | 0 | 0 |
| | | 0 | 0 | 0 | 0 | 0 | 0 | 6 | 1 | 0.01 | 0.005 | 0.1 | 0 | 0 | 0 | 0 | 0 | 42040 |
| **guava citrus jce drink**, light, Minute Maid - *8 fl oz* | 249 | 5 | | 2.0 | 0.5 | | | 80 | 0 | | | | | 0 | 0 | | | |
| | | 0 | 0 | | | | | 19 | | | | | | | | | | MNTM58 |
| **guava nectar**, canned *8 fl oz* | 251 | 143 | 213.1 | 37.3 | 31.0 | | 2.5 | 18 | 28 | 8 | 0.08 | 0.100 | 5 | 49 | 0.01 | 0.5 | | 0.21 |
| | | 0.2 | 0.2 | | | | | 95 | 5 | | 0.043 | | 88 | 0.1 | 0.01 | 0.03 | 7.5 | 9435 |
| **Just 10 Fruit Punch**, Minute Maid *6.7 fl oz pouch* | 208 | 10 | | 2.0 | 2.0 | | | | 100 | | | | | 60 | | | | |
| | | 0 | 0 | | | | 4 | | | | | | | | | | | MNTM59 |
| **lemon juice**, canned/bottled *1 T* | 15 | 3 | 13.9 | 1.0 | 0.4 | 0 | 0.1 | 3 | 2 | 1 | 0.01 | 0.003 | 0 | 4 | 0.01 | 0 | 0 | 0.01 |
| | | 0.1 | 0 | 0 | 0 | 0 | 0 | 15 | 1 | 0.02 | 0.006 | 0 | 2 | 0 | 0 | 0.01 | 1.5 | 9153 |
| **lemon juice**, frzn, single-strength *8 fl oz* | 244 | 54 | 225.4 | 15.9 | 5.9 | 0 | 1.0 | 2 | 20 | 20 | 0.12 | 0.073 | 2 | 77 | 0.14 | 0.3 | 0 | 0.30 |
| | | 1.1 | 0.8 | 0.1 | 0 | 0.2 | 0 | 217 | 20 | 0.29 | 0.073 | 0.2 | 32 | 0.2 | 0.03 | 0.15 | 24.4 | 9154 |
| **lemon juice**, raw *yield from 1 lemon (1.5 fl oz)* | 47 | 12 | 42.6 | 4.1 | 1.1 | 0 | 0.2 | 0 | 3 | 3 | 0.02 | 0.004 | 0 | 22 | 0.01 | 0 | 0 | 0.05 |
| | | 0.2 | 0 | 0 | 0 | 0 | 0 | 58 | 3 | 0.01 | 0.014 | 0 | 9 | 0.1 | 0 | 0.02 | 6.1 | 9152 |
| **lemonade**, bottled, Odwalla *8 fl oz* | 250 | 120 | | 30.0 | 28.0 | | | 10 | | | | | | 12 | | | | |
| | | 0 | 0 | | | | | | | | | | | | | | | ODWA17 |
| **lemonade**, bottled, Simply Lemonade - *8 fl oz* | 249 | 120 | | 30.0 | 28.0 | | | 15 | | | | | | | | | | |
| | | 0 | 0 | | | | | | | | | | | | | | | MNTM62 |
| **lemonade iced tea**, refrig carton, Minute Maid - *8 fl oz* | 249 | 110 | | 29.0 | 28.0 | | | | | | | | | | | | | |
| | | 0 | 0 | | | | | | | | | | | | | | | MNTM60 |
| **lemonade**, light, canned, Minute Maid - *12 fl oz can* | 372 | 5 | | 2.0 | 0 | | | 120 | | | | | | | | | | |
| | | 0 | 0 | | | | | | | | | | | | | | | MNTM63 |

| | WT (g) | KCAL | H₂O (g) | CHO (g) | TSUG (g) | ASUG (g) | DFIB (g) | Na (mg) | Ca (mg) | Mg (mg) | Zn (mg) | Mn (mg) | A (mcg RAE) | C (mg) | B-1 (mg) | NIA (mg) | B-12 (mcg) | PANT (mg) |
|---|---|---|---|---|---|---|---|---|---|---|---|---|---|---|---|---|---|---|
| | | PRO (g) | FAT (g) | SFA (g) | MUFA (g) | PUFA (g) | CHOL (mg) | K (mg) | P (mg) | Fe (mg) | Cu (mg) | Se (mcg) | A (IU) | E (mg ATE) | B-2 (mg) | B-6 (mg) | FOL (mcg DFE) | REF |
| **lemonade**, light, refrig carton, Minute Maid - *8 fl oz* | 249 | 15 | | 4.0 | 2.0 | | | 15 | | | | | | 60 | | | | |
| | | 0 | 0 | | | | | | | | | | | | | | | MNTM64 |
| **lemonade**, pink, canned, Minute Maid - *8 fl oz* | 249 | 100 | | 28.0 | 27.0 | | | 80 | 0 | | | | | 0 | 0 | | | |
| | | 0 | 0 | | | | | 19 | | | | | | | | | | MNTM65 |
| **lemonade**, pink, refrig carton, Minute Maid - *8 fl oz* | 249 | 110 | | 29.0 | 20.0 | | | 15 | | | | | | | | | | |
| | | 0 | 0 | | | | | | | | | | | | | | | MNTM96 |
| **lemonade**, refrig carton, Minute Maid - *8 fl oz* | 249 | 110 | | 31.0 | 29.0 | | | 15 | | | | | | | | | | |
| | | 0 | 0 | | | | | | | | | | | | | | | MNTM66 |
| **lime juice**, canned/bottled *1 fl oz* | 31 | 7 | 28.7 | 2.1 | 0.4 | 0 | 0.1 | 5 | 4 | 2 | 0.02 | 0.002 | 0 | 2 | 0.01 | 0.1 | 0 | 0.02 |
| | | 0.1 | 0.1 | 0 | 0 | 0 | 0 | 23 | 3 | 0.07 | 0.009 | 0 | 5 | 0 | 0 | 0.01 | 2.5 | 9161 |
| **lime juice**, raw *yield from 1 lime (1.2 fl oz)* | 38 | 10 | 34.5 | 3.2 | 0.6 | 0 | 0.2 | 1 | 5 | 3 | 0.03 | 0.007 | 1 | 11 | 0.01 | 0.1 | 0 | 0.05 |
| | | 0.2 | 0 | 0 | 0 | 0 | 0 | 44 | 5 | 0.03 | 0.010 | 0 | 19 | 0.1 | 0.01 | 0.01 | 3.8 | 9160 |
| **limeade**, btld, Odwalla Quencher *8 fl oz* | 249 | 120 | | 29.0 | 27.0 | | | 10 | | | | | | | | | | |
| | | 0 | 0 | | | | | | | | | | | | | | | ODWA24 |
| **limeade**, btld, Simply Limeade *8 fl oz* | 249 | 120 | | 30.0 | 28.0 | | | 15 | | | | | | | | | | |
| | | 0 | 0 | | | | | | | | | | | | | | | MNTM68 |
| **Limonada-Limeade**, light, refrig carton, Minute Maid - *8 fl oz* | 249 | 15 | | 4.0 | 2.0 | | | 15 | | | | | | 60 | | | | |
| | | 0 | 0 | | | | | | | | | | | | | | | MNTM70 |
| **Limonada-Limeade**, refrig carton, Minute Maid - *8 fl oz* | 249 | 120 | | 33.0 | 31.0 | | | 15 | | | | | | | | | | |
| | | 0 | 0 | | | | | | | | | | | | | | | MNTM69 |
| **mango nectar**, canned *8 fl oz* | 251 | 128 | 217.4 | 32.9 | 31.2 | | 0.8 | 13 | 43 | 8 | 0.05 | 0.070 | 88 | 38 | 0.01 | 0.2 | 0 | 0.18 |
| | | 0.3 | 0.2 | 0 | 0.1 | 0 | 0 | 60 | 5 | 0.90 | 0.038 | 1.0 | 1737 | 0.5 | 0.01 | 0.04 | 17.6 | 9436 |
| **Mango Tango juice**, bottled, Odwalla - *8 fl oz* | 250 | 150 | | 34.0 | 30.0 | | | 10 | 20 | | | | | | | | | |
| | | 1.0 | 1.0 | 0.5 | | | | 250 | | 0.36 | | | | | | | | ODWA8 |
| **Micronutrient jce drink**, btld, Odwalla - *8 fl oz* | 250 | 130 | | 30.0 | 25.0 | | | 10 | 20 | | | 0.200 | | 12 | | | | |
| | | 1.0 | 0.5 | | | | | 370 | | 1.44 | | | | | | | | ODWA10 |
| **mixed berry jce blend**, Minute Maid - *6.7 fl oz box* | 208 | 100 | | 25.0 | 23.0 | | | 15 | 100 | 8 | | | | 60 | | | | |
| | | 0 | 0 | | | | | 200 | | | | | | | | | | MNTM8 |
| **mixed berry jce blend**, btld, Minute Maid - *10 fl oz* | 310 | 150 | | 36.0 | 34.0 | | | 25 | | 8 | | | | 60 | | | | |
| | | 0 | 0 | | | | | 430 | | | | | | | | | | MNTM73 |
| **mixed veg and fruit jce drink** *8 fl oz* | 248 | 72 | 229.0 | 18.5 | 5.2 | 4.2 | 0 | 52 | 7 | 2 | 0.02 | 0.030 | 258 | 81 | 0.01 | 0 | 0 | 0.03 |
| | | 0.1 | 0 | 0 | 0 | 0 | 0 | 47 | 5 | 0.10 | 0.022 | 0.2 | 5166 | 4.0 | 0.01 | 0.02 | 0 | 14119 |
| **Mo'Beta juice**, btld, Odwalla *8 fl oz* | 250 | 150 | | 37.0 | 26.0 | | 1.0 | 15 | | 3.00 | | | | 300 | | | | |
| | | 1.0 | 0 | | | | | 270 | | 0.36 | | | 5000 | | | | | ODWA9 |
| **orange apricot juice drink**, canned *8 fl oz* | 250 | 128 | 216.8 | 31.8 | 30.2 | 21.1 | 0.2 | 5 | 12 | 12 | 0.10 | 0.022 | 22 | 50 | 0.05 | 0.5 | 0 | 0.17 |
| | | 0.8 | 0.2 | 0 | 0.1 | 0.1 | 0 | 200 | 20 | 0.25 | 0.080 | 0.2 | 458 | 0.3 | 0.02 | 0.09 | 17.5 | 14327 |
| **orange grapefruit juice**, cnd/btld *8 fl oz* | 247 | 106 | 218.9 | 25.4 | 25.1 | 0 | 0.2 | 7 | 20 | 25 | 0.17 | 0.042 | 15 | 72 | 0.14 | 0.8 | 0 | 0.35 |
| | | 1.5 | 0.2 | 0 | 0 | 0 | 0 | 390 | 35 | 1.14 | 0.188 | 0.2 | 294 | 0.3 | 0.07 | 0.06 | 34.6 | 9217 |
| **orange juice bev**, light, refrig carton - *8 fl oz* | 249 | 50 | | 13.0 | 10.0 | | | 15 | 350 | 24 | | | | 72 | 0.15 | 0.4 | | |
| | | 0 | 0 | | | | | 450 | | | | | | | | 0.08 | 24.0 | MNTM74 |
| **orange juice**, btld, Minute Maid Active - *8 fl oz* | 249 | 120 | | 28.0 | 24.0 | | | 15 | 20 | 24 | | | | 60 | 0.15 | 2.0 | 1.20 | |
| | | 2.0 | 0 | | | | | 450 | | | | | | | | 0.40 | 60.0 | MNTM77 |
| **orange juice**, btld, Minute Maid Heart Wise - *8 fl oz* | 249 | 110 | | 27.0 | 24.0 | | | 20 | 20 | 24 | | | | 60 | 0.15 | 0.4 | 1.20 | |
| | | 2.0 | 0 | | | | | 450 | | | | | | | | 0.40 | 60.0 | MNTM78 |
| **orange juice**, btld, Minute Maid Multi-Vitamin - *8 fl oz* | 249 | 120 | | 27.0 | 24.0 | | | 20 | 350 | 40 | 1.50 | 0.200 | | 60 | 0.15 | 5.0 | 1.50 | 2.50 |
| | | 2.0 | 0 | | | | | 450 | 250 | | 0.200 | 14.0 | 500 | | 0.42 | 0.50 | 60.0 | MNTM79 |
| **orange juice**, btld, Simply Orange Original - *8 fl oz* | 249 | 110 | | 26.0 | 22.0 | | | 0 | 20 | 24 | | | | 84 | 0.15 | 0.4 | | |
| | | 2.0 | 0 | 0 | | | 0 | 450 | | | | | | | | 0.08 | 60.0 | MNTM81 |
| **orange juice**, canned/bottled *8 fl oz* | 249 | 117 | 218.4 | 27.4 | 21.8 | 0 | 0.7 | 10 | 25 | 25 | 0.10 | 0.052 | 22 | 75 | 0.10 | 0.5 | 0 | 0.45 |
| | | 1.7 | 0.4 | 0 | 0.1 | 0.1 | 0 | 458 | 42 | 0.25 | 0.055 | 0.2 | 436 | 0.5 | 0.05 | 0.08 | 59.8 | 9207 |
| **orange juice drink**, canned/bottled *8 fl oz* | 249 | 134 | 214.6 | 33.4 | 23.3 | 3.5 | 0.5 | 5 | 5 | 7 | 0.05 | 0.017 | 5 | 37 | 0.95 | 12.5 | 0 | 0.15 |
| | | 0.5 | 0 | 0 | 0 | 0 | 0 | 105 | 10 | 0.27 | 0.045 | 0 | 110 | 0 | 1.07 | 1.25 | 10.0 | 42270 |
| **orange juice**, from frzn conc *8 fl oz* | 249 | 112 | 219.4 | 26.8 | 20.9 | 0 | 0.5 | 2 | 22 | 25 | 0.12 | 0.035 | 12 | 97 | 0.20 | 0.5 | 0 | 0.39 |
| | | 1.7 | 0.1 | 0 | 0 | 0 | 0 | 473 | 40 | 0.25 | 0.110 | 0.2 | 266 | 0.5 | 0.04 | 0.11 | 109.6 | 9215 |
| **orange juice**, Minute Maid Kids *6.7 fl oz box* | 208 | 100 | | 23.0 | 20.0 | | | 15 | 300 | 16 | | | | 60 | 0.15 | | | |
| | | 1.0 | 0 | | | | | 380 | | | | | 750 | | | | 40.0 | MNTM84 |
| **orange juice**, raw *8 fl oz* | 248 | 112 | 219.0 | 25.8 | 20.8 | 0 | 0.5 | 2 | 27 | 27 | 0.12 | 0.035 | 25 | 124 | 0.22 | 1.0 | 0 | 0.47 |
| | | 1.7 | 0.5 | 0.1 | 0.1 | 0.1 | 0 | 496 | 42 | 0.50 | 0.109 | 0.2 | 496 | 0.1 | 0.07 | 0.10 | 74.4 | 9206 |
| **orange juice**, refrigerated *8 fl oz* | 248 | 109 | 219.2 | 25.3 | | | 0.5 | 2 | 25 | 27 | 0.10 | 0.057 | 10 | 82 | 0.28 | 0.7 | 0 | 0.47 |
| | | 2.0 | 0.3 | 0 | 0.1 | 0.1 | 0 | 471 | 27 | 0.42 | 0.099 | 0.2 | 193 | | 0.05 | 0.13 | 44.6 | 9209 |
| **orange juice**, rfrg crtn, Min Maid Hm Sqzd Plus Ca & Vit D - *8 fl oz* | 249 | 110 | | 27.0 | 24.0 | | | 15 | 350 | 24 | | | | 72 | 0.15 | 0.4 | | |
| | | 2.0 | 0 | | | | | 450 | | | | | | | | 0.08 | 60.0 | MNTM86 |

| Item | WT (g) | KCAL / PRO (g) | H₂O / FAT (g) | CHO / SFA (g) | TSUG / MUFA (g) | ASUG / PUFA (g) | DFIB / CHOL (mg) | Na / K (mg) | Ca / P (mg) | Mg / Fe (mg) | Zn / Cu (mg) | Mn / Se (mg/mcg) | A (mcg RAE) / A (IU) | C / E (mg / mg ATE) | B-1 / B-2 (mg) | NIA / B-6 (mg) | B-12 / FOL (mcg / mcg DFE) | PANT (mg) / REF |
|---|---|---|---|---|---|---|---|---|---|---|---|---|---|---|---|---|---|---|
| orange juice w/calcium and vit D, refrig, Florida's Natural - 8 fl oz | 249 | 110 | | 26.0 | 22.0 | | 0 | 0 | 350 | | | | | 72 | 0.15 | | | |
| | | 2.0 | 0 | 0 | | | 0 | 450 | 0 | | | | 0 | | | | | FLOR1 |
| orange juice w/calcium, btld, Minute Maid Original - 8 fl oz | 249 | 110 | | 27.0 | 24.0 | | | 15 | 350 | 24 | | | | 60 | 0.15 | 0.4 | | |
| | | 2.0 | 0 | | | | | 450 | | | | | | | 0.08 | | 60.0 | MNTM80 |
| orange juice w/calcium, btld, Simply Orange - 8 fl oz | 249 | 110 | | 26.0 | 22.0 | | | 0 | 350 | 24 | | | | 84 | 0.15 | 0.4 | | |
| | | 2.0 | 0 | 0 | | | 0 | 450 | | | | | | | 0.08 | | 60.0 | MNTM82 |
| orange jce w/orange pcs, btld, Simply Orange Grove Made - 8 fl oz | 249 | 110 | | 26.0 | 22.0 | | | 0 | 20 | 24 | | | | 84 | 0.15 | 0.4 | | |
| | | 2.0 | 0 | 0 | | | 0 | 450 | | | | | | | 0.08 | | 60.0 | MNTM75 |
| orange jce w/pulp, btld, Simply Orange Country Stand - 8 fl oz | 249 | 110 | | 26.0 | 22.0 | | | 0 | 350 | 24 | | | | 84 | 0.15 | 0.4 | | |
| | | 2.0 | 0 | 0 | | | 0 | 450 | | | | | | | 0.08 | | 60.0 | MNTM76 |
| orange strawberry banana juice 8 fl oz | 234 | 117 | 203.0 | 28.9 | 22.4 | 0 | 0.5 | 9 | 19 | 23 | 0.16 | | 9 | 58 | 0.06 | 0.4 | 0 | |
| | | 1.0 | 0.4 | 0.1 | 0 | 0.1 | 0 | 342 | 30 | 0.63 | 0.101 | 0.2 | 204 | 0.1 | 0.03 | 0.04 | 39.8 | 42149 |
| orange strawberry juice drink, Min Maid Coolers - 6.7 fl oz pouch | 208 | 100 | | 26.0 | 24.0 | | | 15 | 100 | | | | | 60 | | | | |
| | | 0 | 0 | | | | | | | | | | | | | | | MNTM88 |
| orange tangerine juice, light, refrig carton, Minute Maid - 8 fl oz | 249 | 15 | | 4.0 | 2.0 | | | 15 | | | | | | 60 | | | | |
| | | 0 | 0 | | | | | | | | | | | | | | | MNTM90 |
| orange tangerine juice, refrig carton, Min Maid - 8 fl oz | 249 | 110 | | 27.0 | 24.0 | | | 0 | 350 | | | | | 96 | | | | |
| | | 0 | 0 | | | | | 450 | | | | | | | | | | MNTM89 |
| orange tropical jce blend, cnd, Minute Maid - 11.5 oz can | 357 | 180 | | 46.0 | 43.0 | | | 30 | | 24 | | | | 60 | | | | |
| | | 0 | 0 | | | | | 320 | | | | | | | | | 24.0 | MNTM92 |
| orangeade, canned, Minute Maid 12 fl oz can | 372 | 160 | | 43.0 | 42.0 | | | 110 | | | | | | | | | | |
| | | 0 | 0 | | | | | | | | | | | | | | | MNTM93 |
| orangeade, light, canned, Minute Maid - 12 fl oz can | 372 | 10 | | 2.0 | 1.0 | | | 110 | | | | | | | | | | |
| | | 0 | 0 | | | | | | | | | | | | | | | MNTM94 |
| papaya nectar, canned 8 fl oz | 250 | 142 | 212.6 | 36.3 | 34.8 | 27.5 | 1.5 | 12 | 25 | 8 | 0.38 | 0.032 | 45 | 8 | 0.02 | 0.4 | 0 | 0.14 |
| | | 0.4 | 0.4 | 0.1 | 0.1 | 0.1 | 0 | 78 | 0 | 0.85 | 0.032 | 0.8 | 902 | 0.6 | 0.01 | 0.02 | 5.0 | 9229 |
| passion fruit juice, purple, raw 8 fl oz | 247 | 126 | 211.5 | 33.6 | 33.1 | 0 | 0.5 | 15 | 10 | 42 | 0.12 | | 89 | 74 | 0 | 3.6 | 0 | |
| | | 1.0 | 0.1 | 0 | 0 | 0.1 | 0 | 687 | 32 | 0.59 | 0.131 | 0.2 | 1771 | 0 | 0.32 | 0.12 | 17.3 | 9232 |
| passion fruit juice, yellow, raw 8 fl oz | 247 | 148 | 208.0 | 35.7 | 35.2 | | 0.5 | 15 | 10 | 42 | 0.15 | | 116 | 45 | 0 | 5.5 | 0 | |
| | | 1.7 | 0.4 | 0 | 0.1 | 0.3 | 0 | 687 | 62 | 0.89 | 0.124 | 0.2 | 2329 | 0 | 0.25 | 0.15 | 19.8 | 9233 |
| peach nectar, canned/bottled 8 fl oz | 249 | 134 | 213.2 | 34.7 | 33.2 | 23.7 | 1.5 | 17 | 12 | 10 | 0.20 | 0.047 | 32 | 13 | 0.01 | 0.7 | 0 | 0.17 |
| | | 0.7 | 0 | 0 | 0 | 0 | 0 | 100 | 15 | 0.47 | 0.172 | 0.5 | 642 | 0.7 | 0.03 | 0.02 | 2.5 | 9251 |
| pear nectar, canned/bottled 8 fl oz | 250 | 150 | 210.0 | 39.4 | 37.9 | 28.1 | 1.5 | 10 | 12 | 8 | 0.18 | 0.075 | 0 | 3 | 0 | 0.3 | 0 | 0.05 |
| | | 0.3 | 0 | 0 | 0 | 0 | 0 | 32 | 8 | 0.65 | 0.168 | 0 | 2 | 0.1 | 0.03 | 0.04 | 2.5 | 9262 |
| pineapple grapefruit jce drink, cnd - 8 fl oz | 250 | 118 | 219.8 | 29.0 | 28.8 | 15.2 | 0.2 | 35 | 18 | 15 | 0.15 | 1.032 | 0 | 115 | 0.08 | 0.7 | 0 | 0.13 |
| | | 0.5 | 0.2 | 0 | 0 | 0.1 | 0 | 152 | 15 | 0.78 | 0.112 | 0.2 | 5 | 0 | 0.04 | 0.11 | 22.5 | 14334 |
| pineapple juice, canned/bottled 8 fl oz | 250 | 132 | 215.9 | 32.2 | 25.0 | 0 | 0.5 | 5 | 32 | 30 | 0.28 | 1.260 | 0 | 25 | 0.15 | 0.5 | 0 | 0.14 |
| | | 0.9 | 0.3 | 0 | 0 | 0.1 | 0 | 325 | 20 | 0.78 | 0.173 | 0.2 | 12 | 0 | 0.05 | 0.25 | 45.0 | 9273 |
| pineapple juice, from frzn conc 8 fl oz | 250 | 130 | 216.2 | 31.9 | 31.4 | 0 | 0.5 | 2 | 28 | 22 | 0.28 | 2.475 | 2 | 30 | 0.18 | 0.5 | 0 | 0.31 |
| | | 1.0 | 0.1 | 0 | 0 | 0 | 0 | 340 | 20 | 0.75 | 0.225 | 0.2 | 25 | 0 | 0.05 | 0.18 | 27.5 | 9275 |
| pineapple orange jce drink, cnd/btld - 8 fl oz | 250 | 125 | 217.2 | 29.5 | 29.0 | 7.5 | 0.2 | 8 | 12 | 15 | 0.15 | 0.902 | 2 | 56 | 0.08 | 0.5 | 0 | 0.14 |
| | | 3.2 | 0 | 0 | 0 | 0 | 0 | 115 | 10 | 0.68 | 0.103 | 0.2 | 48 | 0.1 | 0.05 | 0.12 | 22.5 | 14341 |
| PomaGrand Juice, bottled, Odwalla - 8 fl oz | 250 | 160 | | 40.0 | 31.0 | | | 30 | 60 | | | | | | | | | |
| | | 0 | 0 | | | | | 540 | | 0.36 | | | | | | | | ODWA12 |
| pomegranate juice, bottled 8 fl oz | 249 | 134 | 214.0 | 32.7 | 31.5 | | 0.2 | 22 | 27 | 17 | 0.22 | 0.237 | 0 | 0 | 0.04 | 0.6 | 0 | 0.71 |
| | | 0.4 | 0.7 | 0.2 | 0.1 | 0.1 | 0 | 533 | 27 | 0.25 | 0.052 | 0.7 | 0 | 0.9 | 0.04 | 0.10 | 59.8 | 9442 |
| pomegranate lemonade, btld, Odwalla - 8 fl oz | 250 | 110 | | 28.0 | 27.0 | | | 10 | | | | | | | | | | |
| | | 0 | 0 | | | | | | | | | | | | | | | ODWA15 |
| pomegranate limeade, btld, Odwalla - 8 fl oz | 250 | 120 | | 30.0 | 27.0 | | | 10 | | | | | | | | | | |
| | | 0 | 0 | | | | | | | | | | | | | | | ODWA16 |
| prune juice, canned/bottled 8 fl oz | 256 | 182 | 208.0 | 44.7 | 42.1 | 0 | 2.6 | 10 | 31 | 36 | 0.54 | 0.387 | 0 | 10 | 0.04 | 2.0 | 0 | 0.27 |
| | | 1.6 | 0.1 | 0 | 0.1 | 0 | 0 | 707 | 64 | 3.02 | 0.174 | 1.5 | 8 | 0.3 | 0.18 | 0.56 | 0 | 9294 |
| raspberry lemonade, refrig carton, Minute Maid - 8 fl oz | 249 | 120 | | 32.0 | 30.0 | | | 15 | | | | | | | | | | |
| | | 0 | 0 | | | | | | | | | | | | | | | MNTM98 |
| strawberry banana fruit smoothie, btld, Odwalla - 8 fl oz | 248 | 130 | | 31.0 | 26.0 | | 1.0 | 0 | | | | | | | | | | |
| | | 1.0 | 0 | | | | | 430 | | | | | | | | | | ODWA21 |
| Strawberry C Monster frt smoothie, btld, Odwalla - 8 fl oz | 248 | 160 | | 38.0 | 29.0 | | | 20 | 20 | | | | | 600 | | | | |
| | | 2.0 | 0 | | | | | 400 | | 0.72 | | | | | | | | ODWA22 |
| strawberry lemonade, btld, Odwalla Quencher - 8 fl oz | 248 | 110 | | 28.0 | 25.0 | | | 10 | | | | | | | | | | |
| | | 0 | 0 | | | | | | | | | | | | | | | ODWA23 |
| strawberry raspberry jce blend, Minute Maid - 8 fl oz | 249 | 120 | | 33.0 | 31.0 | | | 20 | 0 | | | | | 60 | 0 | | | |
| | | 0 | 0 | | | | | 35 | | | | | | | | | | MNTM103 |

| | WT (g) | KCAL / PRO (g) | H₂O (g) / FAT (g) | CHO (g) / SFA (g) | TSUG (g) / MUFA (g) | ASUG (g) / PUFA (g) | DFIB (g) / CHOL (mg) | Na (mg) / K (mg) | Ca (mg) / P (mg) | Mg (mg) / Fe (mg) | Zn (mg) / Cu (mg) | Mn (mg) / Se (mcg) | A (mcg RAE) / A (IU) | C (mg) / E (mg ATE) | B-1 (mg) / B-2 (mg) | NIA (mg) / B-6 (mg) | B-12 (mcg) / FOL (mcg DFE) | PANT (mg) / REF |
|---|---|---|---|---|---|---|---|---|---|---|---|---|---|---|---|---|---|---|
| **tamarind nectar**, canned | 251 | 143 | 213.3 | 37.0 | 31.9 | | 1.3 | 18 | 25 | 10 | 0.05 | 0.050 | 0 | 18 | 0.01 | 0.2 | 0 | 0.09 |
| *8 fl oz* | | 0.2 | 0.3 | | | | 0 | 68 | 5 | 1.88 | 0.035 | | 0 | 0.3 | 0.01 | 0.02 | 2.5 | 9437 |
| **tangerine juice**, raw | 247 | 106 | 219.6 | 24.9 | 24.5 | 0 | 0.5 | 2 | 44 | 20 | 0.07 | 0.091 | 32 | 77 | 0.15 | 0.2 | 0 | 0.31 |
| *8 fl oz* | | 1.2 | 0.5 | 0.1 | 0.1 | 0.1 | 0 | 440 | 35 | 0.49 | 0.062 | 0.2 | 625 | 0.3 | 0.05 | 0.10 | 12.4 | 9221 |
| **tangerine juice**, swtnd, cnd/btld | 249 | 125 | 216.6 | 29.9 | 29.4 | 4.7 | 0.5 | 2 | 45 | 20 | 0.07 | 0.092 | 32 | 55 | 0.15 | 0.2 | 0 | 0.31 |
| *8 fl oz* | | 1.2 | 0.5 | 0 | 0 | 0.1 | 0 | 443 | 35 | 0.50 | 0.062 | 0.2 | 630 | 0.4 | 0.05 | 0.08 | 12.5 | 9223 |
| **tangerine juice**, swtnd, from frzn conc - *8 fl oz* | 241 | 111 | 212.3 | 26.7 | | | 0.5 | 2 | 19 | 19 | 0.07 | 0.089 | 70 | 58 | 0.13 | 0.2 | 0 | 0.30 |
| | | 1.0 | 0.3 | 0 | 0 | 0 | 0 | 272 | 19 | 0.24 | 0.060 | | 1381 | | 0.05 | 0.10 | 12.0 | 9225 |
| **tangerine juice**, swtnd, frzn conc | 241 | 388 | 140.3 | 93.6 | | | 1.4 | 7 | 65 | 67 | 0.22 | 0.313 | 333 | 205 | 0.44 | 0.8 | 0 | 1.06 |
| *8 fl oz* | | 3.6 | 0.9 | 0.1 | 0.1 | 0.1 | 0 | 957 | 72 | 0.82 | 0.214 | | 6668 | | 0.16 | 0.35 | 38.6 | 9224 |
| **tomato juice**, canned/bottled | 243 | 41 | 228.2 | 10.3 | 8.7 | 0 | 1.0 | 24 | 24 | 27 | 0.36 | 0.170 | 56 | 44 | 0.11 | 1.6 | 0 | 0.61 |
| *8 fl oz* | | 1.8 | 0.1 | 0 | 0 | 0.1 | 0 | 556 | 44 | 1.04 | 0.148 | 0.7 | 1094 | 0.8 | 0.08 | 0.27 | 48.6 | 11886 |
| **tropical punch**, Minute Maid Coolers - *6.7 fl oz pouch* | 208 | 100 | | 26.0 | 25.0 | | | 15 | 100 | | | | | 60 | | | | |
| | | 0 | 0 | | | | | | | | | | | | | | | MNTM108 |
| **tropical punch**, refrig carton, Minute Maid - *8 fl oz* | 249 | 110 | | 30.0 | | | 29.0 | 15 | | | | | | | | | | |
| | | 0 | 0 | | | | | | | | | | | | | | | MNTM109 |
| **V8 Fusion Jce**, acai berry, Campbell's - *8 fl oz* | 246 | 111 | 217.5 | 27.0 | 26.0 | | 0 | 69 | 2 | | | | | 100 | | | | |
| | | 0 | 0 | 0 | 0 | 0 | 0 | 241 | | 1.99 | | | 15 | 4.5 | | | | 14623 |
| **vegetable juice**, canned/bottled | 242 | 46 | 226.3 | 11.0 | 8.0 | 0 | 1.9 | 653 | 27 | 27 | 0.48 | 0.242 | 189 | 67 | 0.10 | 1.8 | 0 | 0.64 |
| *8 fl oz* | | 1.5 | 0.2 | 0 | 0 | 0.1 | 0 | 467 | 41 | 1.02 | 0.484 | 1.2 | 3770 | 0.8 | 0.07 | 0.34 | 50.8 | 11578 |

## 15. FRUITS

| | WT (g) | KCAL / PRO (g) | H₂O (g) / FAT (g) | CHO (g) / SFA (g) | TSUG (g) / MUFA (g) | ASUG (g) / PUFA (g) | DFIB (g) / CHOL (mg) | Na (mg) / K (mg) | Ca (mg) / P (mg) | Mg (mg) / Fe (mg) | Zn (mg) / Cu (mg) | Mn (mg) / Se (mcg) | A (mcg RAE) / A (IU) | C (mg) / E (mg ATE) | B-1 (mg) / B-2 (mg) | NIA (mg) / B-6 (mg) | B-12 (mcg) / FOL (mcg DFE) | PANT (mg) / REF |
|---|---|---|---|---|---|---|---|---|---|---|---|---|---|---|---|---|---|---|
| **abiyuch**, raw | 114 | 79 | 91.1 | 20.1 | 9.7 | | 6.0 | 23 | 9 | 27 | 0.35 | 0.207 | 6 | 62 | | | | |
| *½ cup* | | 1.7 | 0.1 | 0 | | | | 347 | 54 | 1.84 | 0.065 | | 114 | | | | | 9427 |
| **acerola**, raw | 98 | 31 | 89.6 | 7.5 | | | 1.1 | 7 | 12 | 18 | 0.10 | | 37 | 1644 | 0.02 | 0.4 | 0 | 0.30 |
| *1 cup* | | 0.4 | 0.3 | 0.1 | 0.1 | 0.1 | 0 | 143 | 11 | 0.20 | 0.084 | 0.6 | 752 | | 0.06 | 0.01 | 13.7 | 9001 |
| **apple**, dried | 6 | 15 | 1.9 | 4.0 | 3.4 | 0 | 0.5 | 5 | 1 | 1 | 0.01 | 0.005 | 0 | 0 | 0 | 0.1 | 0 | 0.01 |
| *1 ring* | | 0.1 | 0 | | | | 0 | 27 | 2 | 0.08 | 0.011 | 0.1 | 0 | 0 | 0.01 | 0.01 | 0 | 9011 |
| **apple**, dried, cooked | 171 | 97 | 143.9 | 26.2 | 22.8 | 0 | 3.4 | 34 | 5 | 7 | 0.09 | 0.036 | 2 | 2 | 0.01 | 0.2 | 0 | 0.10 |
| *1 cup sliced* | | 0.4 | 0.1 | 0 | 0 | 0 | 0 | 180 | 15 | 0.56 | 0.075 | 0.5 | 29 | 0.2 | 0.03 | 0.09 | 0 | 9012 |
| **apple**, frozen, unsweetened | 171 | 82 | 148.5 | 21.1 | | | 3.2 | 5 | 7 | 5 | 0.09 | 0.289 | 3 | 3 | 0.02 | 0.1 | 0 | 0.09 |
| *1 cup sliced* | | 0.5 | 0.5 | 0.1 | 0 | 0.2 | 0 | 132 | 14 | 0.31 | 0.099 | 0.3 | 58 | | 0.02 | 0.06 | 1.7 | 9014 |
| **apple**, peeled, boiled | 171 | 91 | 146.2 | 23.3 | 18.8 | 0 | 4.1 | 2 | 9 | 5 | 0.07 | 0.202 | 3 | 3 | 0.03 | 0.2 | 0 | 0.08 |
| *1 cup sliced* | | 0.4 | 0.6 | 0.1 | 0 | 0.2 | 0 | 150 | 14 | 0.32 | 0.060 | 0.5 | 75 | 0.1 | 0.02 | 0.08 | 1.7 | 9005 |
| **apple**, peeled, microwaved | 170 | 95 | 143.9 | 24.5 | 19.7 | 0 | 4.8 | 2 | 8 | 5 | 0.07 | 0.241 | 3 | 1 | 0.03 | 0.1 | 0 | 0.08 |
| *1 cup sliced* | | 0.5 | 0.7 | 0.1 | 0 | 0.2 | 0 | 158 | 14 | 0.29 | 0.078 | 0.5 | 68 | 0.1 | 0.02 | 0.08 | 1.7 | 9006 |
| **apple**, peeled, raw | 128 | 61 | 110.9 | 16.3 | 12.9 | 0 | 1.7 | | 6 | 5 | 0.06 | 0.049 | 3 | 5 | 0.02 | 0.1 | 0 | 0.09 |
| *1 medium (2¾" diameter)* | | 0.3 | 0.2 | 0 | 0 | 0 | 0 | 115 | 14 | 0.09 | 0.040 | 0 | 49 | 0.1 | 0.04 | 0.05 | 0 | 9004 |
| **apple**, raw | 138 | 72 | 118.1 | 19.1 | 14.3 | 0 | 3.3 | 1 | 8 | 7 | 0.06 | 0.048 | 4 | 6 | 0.02 | 0.1 | 0 | 0.08 |
| *1 medium (2¾" diameter)* | | 0.4 | 0.2 | 0 | 0 | 0.1 | 0 | 148 | 15 | 0.17 | 0.037 | 0 | 75 | 0.2 | 0.04 | 0.06 | 4.1 | 9003 |
| **apple**, sliced, swtnd, cnd, drained | 204 | 137 | 168.0 | 34.1 | 30.6 | 10.0 | 3.5 | 6 | 8 | 4 | 0.06 | 0.312 | 6 | 1 | 0.02 | 0.1 | 0 | 0.09 |
| *1 cup sliced* | | 0.4 | 1.0 | 0.2 | 0 | 0.3 | 0 | 139 | 10 | 0.47 | 0.108 | 0.6 | 104 | 0.4 | 0.02 | 0.09 | 0 | 9007 |
| **applesauce**, sweetened, cnd/btld | 255 | 173 | 209.0 | 44.6 | 37.4 | 16.3 | 3.1 | 5 | 8 | 8 | 0.08 | 0.076 | 0 | 4 | 0.04 | 0.2 | 0 | 0.11 |
| *1 cup* | | 0.4 | 0.4 | 0.1 | 0 | 0.1 | 0 | 191 | 15 | 0.31 | 0.082 | 0.8 | 15 | 0.5 | 0.06 | 0.07 | 2.6 | 9020 |
| **applesauce**, unsweetened, cnd/btld | 244 | 102 | 215.3 | 27.5 | 22.9 | 0 | 2.7 | 5 | 10 | 7 | 0.07 | 0.061 | 2 | 2 | 0.06 | 0.2 | 0 | 0.10 |
| *1 cup* | | 0.4 | 0.2 | 0 | 0 | 0 | 0 | 181 | 12 | 0.56 | 0.066 | 0.7 | 71 | 0.4 | 0.07 | 0.07 | 7.3 | 9019 |
| **apricot**, canned in heavy syrup | 258 | 214 | 200.1 | 55.0 | 48.1 | 36.6 | 7.0 | 10 | 26 | 18 | 0.28 | | 377 | 8 | 0.05 | 1.0 | 0 | |
| *1 cup whole* | | 1.7 | 0.3 | 0 | 0.1 | 0.1 | 0 | 369 | 34 | 0.77 | 0.250 | 0.3 | 7544 | 2.3 | 0.06 | 0.14 | 5.2 | 9357 |
| **apricot**, canned in juice | 244 | 117 | 211.4 | 30.1 | 26.2 | 0 | 3.9 | 10 | 29 | 24 | 0.27 | 0.127 | 207 | 12 | 0.04 | 0.8 | 0 | 0.22 |
| *1 cup halves* | | 1.5 | 0.1 | 0 | 0 | 0 | 0 | 403 | 49 | 0.73 | 0.132 | 0.2 | 4126 | 1.5 | 0.05 | 0.13 | 4.9 | 9024 |
| **apricot**, canned in light syrup | 253 | 159 | 208.9 | 41.7 | 37.7 | 25.6 | 4.0 | 10 | 28 | 20 | 0.28 | 0.132 | 167 | 7 | 0.04 | 0.8 | 0 | 0.23 |
| *1 cup halves* | | 1.3 | 0.1 | 0 | 0.1 | 0 | 0 | 349 | 33 | 0.99 | 0.200 | 0.3 | 3345 | 1.5 | 0.05 | 0.14 | 5.1 | 9026 |
| **apricot**, canned in water | 227 | 61 | 209.7 | 14.5 | 10.9 | 0 | 3.6 | 7 | 18 | 16 | 0.25 | 0.120 | 222 | 8 | 0.05 | 0.9 | 0 | 0.21 |
| *1 cup whole* | | 1.6 | 0.4 | 0 | 0.2 | 0.1 | 0 | 436 | 30 | 0.73 | 0.186 | 0.2 | 4447 | 1.4 | 0.05 | 0.12 | 4.5 | 9022 |
| **apricot**, dried | 65 | 157 | 20.1 | 40.7 | 34.7 | 0 | 4.7 | 6 | 36 | 21 | 0.25 | 0.153 | 117 | 1 | 0.01 | 1.7 | 0 | 0.34 |
| *½ cup halves* | | 2.2 | 0.3 | 0 | 0 | 0 | 0 | 755 | 46 | 1.73 | 0.223 | 1.4 | 2343 | 2.8 | 0.05 | 0.09 | 6.5 | 9032 |
| **apricot**, peeled, canned in water | 227 | 50 | 212.1 | 12.4 | | | 2.5 | 25 | 18 | 20 | 0.25 | 0.120 | 207 | 4 | 0.05 | 1.0 | 0 | 0.21 |
| *1 cup whole* | | 1.6 | 0.1 | 0 | 0 | 0 | 0 | 350 | 36 | 1.23 | 0.154 | | 4109 | | 0.05 | 0.12 | 4.5 | 9023 |
| **apricot**, peeled, cnd in heavy syrup | 258 | 214 | 200.4 | 55.3 | | | 4.1 | 28 | 23 | 21 | 0.26 | 0.132 | 160 | 7 | 0.05 | 1.1 | 0 | 0.24 |
| *1 cup whole* | | 1.3 | 0.2 | 0 | 0.1 | 0 | 0 | 346 | 34 | 1.11 | 0.168 | | 3199 | | 0.06 | 0.14 | 5.2 | 9028 |
| **apricot**, raw | 105 | 50 | 90.7 | 11.7 | 9.7 | 0 | 2.1 | 1 | 14 | 10 | 0.21 | 0.081 | 101 | 10 | 0.03 | 0.6 | 0 | 0.25 |
| *3 apricots* | | 1.5 | 0.4 | 0 | 0.2 | 0.1 | 0 | 272 | 24 | 0.41 | 0.082 | 0.1 | 2022 | 0.9 | 0.04 | 0.06 | 9.5 | 9021 |

| | WT (g) | Macronutrients | | | | | | Minerals | | | | | Vitamins | | | | | |
|---|---|---|---|---|---|---|---|---|---|---|---|---|---|---|---|---|---|---|
| | | KCAL / PRO (g) | H₂0 (g) / FAT (g) | CHO (g) / SFA (g) | TSUG (g) / MUFA (g) | ASUG (g) / PUFA (g) | DFIB (g) / CHOL (mg) | Na (mg) / K (mg) | Ca (mg) / P (mg) | Mg (mg) / Fe (mg) | Zn (mg) / Cu (mg) | Mn (mg) / Se (mcg) | A (mcg RAE) / A (IU) | C (mg) / E (mg ATE) | B-1 (mg) / B-2 (mg) | NIA (mg) / B-6 (mg) | B-12 (mcg) / FOL (mcg DFE) | PANT (mg) / REF |
| **apricot**, sweetened, frozen | 242 | 237 | 177.4 | 60.7 | | | 5.3 | 10 | 24 | 22 | 0.24 | 0.121 | 203 | 22 | 0.05 | 1.9 | 0 | 0.48 |
| *1 cup* | | 1.7 | 0.2 | 0 | 0.1 | 0 | 0 | 554 | 46 | 2.18 | 0.155 | 1.0 | 4066 | | 0.10 | 0.15 | 4.8 | 9035 |
| **avocado**, California, raw | 173 | 289 | 125.1 | 14.9 | 0.5 | | 11.8 | 14 | 22 | 50 | 1.18 | 0.258 | 12 | 15 | 0.13 | 3.3 | 0 | 2.53 |
| *1 medium (6.1 oz)* | | 3.4 | 26.7 | 3.7 | 17.0 | 3.1 | 0 | 877 | 93 | 1.06 | 0.294 | 0.7 | 254 | 3.4 | 0.25 | 0.50 | 154.0 | 9038 |
| **avocado**, Florida, raw | 304 | 365 | 239.6 | 23.8 | 7.4 | | 17.0 | 6 | 30 | 73 | 1.22 | 0.289 | 21 | 53 | 0.06 | 2.0 | 0 | 2.83 |
| *1 medium (10.7 oz)* | | 6.8 | 30.6 | 6.0 | 16.8 | 5.1 | 0 | 1067 | 122 | 0.52 | 0.945 | | 426 | 8.1 | 0.16 | 0.24 | 106.4 | 9039 |
| **avocado**, raw | 146 | 234 | 106.9 | 12.5 | 1.0 | 0 | 9.8 | 10 | 18 | 42 | 0.93 | 0.207 | 10 | 15 | 0.10 | 2.5 | 0 | 2.03 |
| *1 cup sliced* | | 2.9 | 21.4 | 3.1 | 14.3 | 2.7 | 0 | 708 | 76 | 0.80 | 0.277 | 0.6 | 213 | 3.0 | 0.19 | 0.38 | 118.3 | 9037 |
| **banana chips** | 28 | 145 | 1.2 | 16.4 | 9.9 | 7.2 | 2.2 | 2 | 5 | 21 | 0.21 | 0.437 | 1 | 2 | 0.02 | 0.2 | 0 | 0.17 |
| *1 oz* | | 0.6 | 9.4 | 8.1 | 0.5 | 0.2 | 0 | 150 | 16 | 0.35 | 0.057 | 0.4 | 23 | 0.1 | 0 | 0.07 | 3.9 | 19400 |
| **banana melon**, raw | 100 | 21 | 94.7 | 4.1 | 3.4 | | 0.3 | 11 | 13 | 10 | 0.14 | 0.036 | | 8 | 0.02 | 0.5 | | 0.07 |
| *3.5 oz* | | 0.8 | 0.2 | | | | | 140 | 9 | 0.21 | 0.035 | 0.4 | | | 0.02 | 0.05 | | 35132 |
| **banana**, raw | 118 | 105 | 88.4 | 27.0 | 14.4 | 0 | 3.1 | 1 | 6 | 32 | 0.18 | 0.319 | 4 | 10 | 0.04 | 0.8 | 0 | 0.39 |
| *1 medium (7–8″ long)* | | 1.3 | 0.4 | 0.1 | 0 | 0.1 | 0 | 422 | 26 | 0.31 | 0.092 | 1.2 | 76 | 0.1 | 0.09 | 0.43 | 23.6 | 9040 |
| **blackberries**, canned in heavy syrup - 1 cup | 256 | 236 | 192.2 | 59.1 | 50.4 | 37.9 | 8.7 | 8 | 54 | 44 | 0.46 | 1.784 | 28 | 7 | 0.07 | 0.7 | 0 | 0.39 |
| *syrup - 1 cup* | | 3.4 | 0.4 | 0 | 0 | 0.2 | 0 | 253 | 36 | 1.66 | 0.340 | 0.8 | 561 | 2.0 | 0.10 | 0.09 | 69.1 | 9046 |
| **blackberries**, frozen, unsweetened | 151 | 97 | 124.1 | 23.7 | 16.1 | 0 | 7.6 | 2 | 44 | 33 | 0.38 | 1.847 | 9 | 5 | 0.04 | 1.8 | 0 | 0.23 |
| *1 cup* | | 1.8 | 0.6 | 0 | 0.1 | 0.4 | 0 | 211 | 45 | 1.21 | 0.181 | 0.6 | 172 | 1.8 | 0.07 | 0.09 | 51.3 | 9048 |
| **blackberries**, raw | 144 | 62 | 126.9 | 13.8 | 7.0 | 0 | 7.6 | 1 | 42 | 29 | 0.76 | 0.930 | 16 | 30 | 0.03 | 0.9 | 0 | 0.40 |
| *1 cup* | | 2.0 | 0.7 | 0 | 0.1 | 0.4 | 0 | 233 | 32 | 0.89 | 0.238 | 0.6 | 308 | 1.7 | 0.04 | 0.04 | 36.0 | 9042 |
| **blackberries**, wild, raw | 144 | 75 | 126.8 | 14.2 | 5.3 | | 4.6 | 9 | 7 | 6 | 0.22 | 0.413 | 7 | 7 | 0.09 | 0.5 | 0 | 1.81 |
| *1 cup* | | 1.2 | 1.5 | | | | | 108 | 16 | 0.30 | 0.320 | | 66 | 1.3 | 0.21 | 0.06 | 15.8 | 35015 |
| **blueberries**, canned in heavy syrup | 256 | 225 | 196.6 | 56.5 | 52.4 | 26.9 | 4.1 | 8 | 13 | 10 | 0.18 | 0.520 | 5 | 3 | 0.09 | 0.3 | 0 | 0.23 |
| *1 cup* | | 1.7 | 0.8 | 0.1 | 0.1 | 0.4 | 0 | 102 | 26 | 0.84 | 0.136 | 0.3 | 92 | 1.0 | 0.14 | 0.09 | 5.1 | 9052 |
| **blueberries**, canned in light syrup | 244 | 215 | 184.8 | 55.3 | 42.6 | | 6.3 | 7 | 15 | 10 | 0.22 | 1.074 | | 1 | 0.11 | 0.9 | | 0.10 |
| *1 cup* | | 2.5 | 1.0 | | | | | 132 | 29 | 1.05 | | | | 3.4 | 0.32 | 0.12 | | 9352 |
| **blueberries**, frozen | 155 | 79 | 134.2 | 18.9 | 13.1 | 0 | 4.2 | 2 | 12 | 8 | 0.11 | 0.228 | 3 | 4 | 0.05 | 0.8 | 0 | 0.19 |
| *1 cup* | | 0.7 | 1.0 | 0.1 | 0.1 | 0.4 | 0 | 84 | 17 | 0.28 | 0.051 | 0.2 | 71 | 0.7 | 0.06 | 0.09 | 10.8 | 9054 |
| **blueberries**, frozen, sweetened | 230 | 186 | 178.0 | 50.5 | 45.4 | 25.9 | 5.1 | 2 | 14 | 5 | 0.14 | 0.603 | 5 | 2 | 0.05 | 0.6 | 0 | 0.29 |
| *1 cup* | | 0.9 | 0.3 | 0 | 0 | 0.1 | 0 | 138 | 16 | 0.90 | 0.090 | 0.5 | 113 | 1.2 | 0.12 | 0.14 | 16.1 | 9055 |
| **blueberries**, raw | 145 | 83 | 122.1 | 21.0 | 14.4 | 0 | 3.5 | 1 | 9 | 9 | 0.23 | 0.487 | 4 | 14 | 0.05 | 0.6 | 0 | 0.18 |
| *1 cup* | | 1.1 | 0.5 | 0 | 0.1 | 0.2 | 0 | 112 | 17 | 0.41 | 0.083 | 0.1 | 78 | 0.8 | 0.06 | 0.08 | 8.7 | 9050 |
| **blueberries**, wild, cnd in heavy syrup - 1 cup | 319 | 341 | 225.3 | 90.3 | 61.5 | | 15.6 | 3 | 61 | 19 | 0.38 | 7.337 | | 1 | 0.11 | 1.5 | | 0.13 |
| *syrup - 1 cup* | | 1.8 | 1.1 | | | | | 147 | 45 | 7.02 | | | | | 1.00 | 0.11 | 25.5 | 9353 |
| **blueberries**, wild, Alaska, frozen | 155 | 68 | 137.5 | 16.1 | | | | | | 23 | | | | 3 | | 0.05 | | |
| *1 cup* | | 1.1 | 0 | | | | | | | 1.71 | | | 253 | | 0.16 | | | 35017 |
| **blueberries**, wild, frozen | 140 | 71 | 120.1 | 19.4 | | | 6.2 | 4 | 24 | 10 | 0.94 | 4.018 | 4 | 2 | 0.04 | 0.9 | | |
| *1 cup* | | 0 | 0.2 | 0 | 0 | 0.1 | | 95 | 18 | 0.81 | | | 83 | 0.4 | 0.01 | 0.03 | | 9053 |
| **blueberries**, wild, raw | 148 | 90 | 126.5 | 18.2 | 9.6 | | 3.8 | 9 | 19 | 10 | 0.30 | 2.960 | 9 | 27 | 0.10 | 0.9 | 0 | 0.39 |
| *1 cup* | | 1.8 | 1.1 | | | | | 111 | 43 | 0.55 | 0.044 | | 170 | 2.5 | 0.61 | 0.04 | 48.8 | 35155 |
| **boysenberries**, canned in heavy syrup - 1 cup | 256 | 225 | 195.2 | 57.1 | | | 6.7 | 8 | 46 | 28 | 0.49 | 0.640 | 5 | 16 | 0.07 | 0.6 | 0 | 0.34 |
| *syrup - 1 cup* | | 2.5 | 0.3 | 0 | 0 | 0.2 | 0 | 230 | 26 | 1.10 | 0.179 | 1.0 | 102 | | 0.07 | 0.10 | 87.0 | 9056 |
| **boysenberries**, frozen, unsweetened | 132 | 66 | 113.4 | 16.1 | 9.1 | 0 | 7.0 | 1 | 36 | 21 | 0.29 | 0.722 | 4 | 4 | 0.07 | 1.0 | 0 | 0.33 |
| *1 cup* | | 1.5 | 0.3 | 0 | 0 | 0.2 | 0 | 183 | 36 | 1.12 | 0.106 | 0.3 | 88 | 1.1 | 0.05 | 0.07 | 83.2 | 9057 |
| **candied fruit** | 28 | 90 | 4.7 | 23.2 | 22.6 | 21.8 | 0.4 | 27 | 5 | 1 | 0.01 | 0.031 | 0 | 0 | 0 | 0 | 0 | |
| *1 oz* | | 0.1 | 0 | 0 | 0 | 0 | 0 | 16 | 1 | 0.05 | 0.008 | 0.2 | 5 | 0 | 0 | 0 | 0 | 9426 |
| **cantaloupe**, raw | 177 | 60 | 159.6 | 14.4 | 13.9 | 0 | 1.6 | 28 | 16 | 21 | 0.32 | 0.073 | 299 | 65 | 0.07 | 1.3 | 0 | 0.19 |
| *1 cup pieces* | | 1.5 | 0.3 | 0.1 | 0 | 0.1 | 0 | 473 | 27 | 0.37 | 0.073 | 0.7 | 5986 | 0.1 | 0.03 | 0.13 | 37.2 | 9181 |
| **carambola** (star fruit), raw | 91 | 28 | 83.2 | 6.1 | 3.6 | 0 | 2.5 | 2 | 3 | 9 | 0.11 | 0.034 | 3 | 31 | 0.01 | 0.3 | 0 | 0.36 |
| *1 medium (3⅜″ diameter)* | | 0.9 | 0.3 | 0 | 0 | 0.2 | 0 | 121 | 11 | 0.07 | 0.125 | 0.5 | 56 | 0.1 | 0.01 | 0.02 | 10.9 | 9060 |
| **carissa** (natal plum), raw | 20 | 12 | 16.8 | 2.7 | | | | 1 | 2 | 3 | | | 0 | 8 | 0.01 | 0 | 0 | |
| *1 medium* | | 0.1 | 0.3 | | | | 0 | 52 | 1 | 0.26 | 0.042 | | 8 | | 0.01 | | | 9061 |
| **casaba melon**, raw | 170 | 48 | 156.1 | 11.2 | 9.7 | 0 | 1.5 | 15 | 19 | 19 | 0.12 | 0.060 | 0 | 37 | 0.03 | 0.4 | 0 | 0.14 |
| *1 cup pieces* | | 1.9 | 0.2 | 0 | 0 | 0.1 | 0 | 309 | 8 | 0.58 | 0.102 | 0.7 | 0 | 0.1 | 0.05 | 0.28 | 13.6 | 9183 |
| **cherimoya**, raw | 156 | 115 | 123.8 | 27.6 | | | 3.6 | 6 | 12 | 25 | 0.28 | 0.129 | 0 | 18 | 0.14 | 0.9 | 0 | 0.37 |
| *1 cup diced* | | 2.6 | 1.0 | | | | 0 | 420 | 41 | 0.47 | 0.114 | | 0 | | 0.19 | 0.33 | 28.1 | 9062 |
| **cherries, maraschino**, canned | 10 | 16 | 5.7 | 4.2 | 3.9 | 3.0 | 0.3 | 0 | 5 | 0 | 0.03 | 0.001 | 0 | 0 | 0 | 0 | 0 | 0.01 |
| *2 cherries* | | 0 | 0 | 0 | 0 | 0 | 0 | 2 | 0 | 0.04 | 0.014 | 0 | 4 | 0 | 0 | 0 | 0 | 9328 |
| **cherries, sour**, cnd in heavy syrup | 256 | 233 | 193.7 | 59.6 | 56.8 | 37.3 | 2.8 | 18 | 26 | 15 | 0.15 | 0.184 | 92 | 5 | 0.04 | 0.4 | 0 | 0.27 |
| *1 cup* | | 1.9 | 0.3 | 0.1 | 0.1 | 0.1 | 0 | 238 | 26 | 3.33 | 0.169 | 0 | 1828 | 0.6 | 0.10 | 0.11 | 20.5 | 9066 |
| **cherries, sour**, cnd in light syrup | 252 | 189 | 200.6 | 48.6 | | | 2.0 | 18 | 25 | 15 | 0.18 | 0.184 | 91 | 5 | 0.04 | 0.4 | 0 | 0.26 |
| *1 cup* | | 1.9 | 0.3 | 0.1 | 0.1 | 0.1 | 0 | 239 | 25 | 3.33 | 0.171 | | 1830 | | 0.10 | 0.11 | 20.2 | 9065 |

| | WT (g) | KCAL / PRO (g) | H₂O (g) / FAT (g) | CHO (g) / SFA (g) | TSUG (g) / MUFA (g) | ASUG (g) / PUFA (g) | DFIB (g) / CHOL (mg) | Na (mg) / K (mg) | Ca (mg) / P (mg) | Mg (mg) / Fe (mg) | Zn (mg) / Cu (mg) | Mn (mg) / Se (mcg) | A (mcg RAE) / A (IU) | C (mg) / E (mg ATE) | B-1 (mg) / B-2 (mg) | NIA (mg) / B-6 (mg) | B-12 (mcg) / FOL (mcg DFE) | PANT (mg) / REF |
|---|---|---|---|---|---|---|---|---|---|---|---|---|---|---|---|---|---|---|
| **cherries, sour**, cnd in water | 244 | 88 | 219.4 | 21.8 | 18.5 | 0 | 2.7 | 17 | 27 | 15 | 0.17 | 0.185 | 93 | 5 | 0.04 | 0.4 | 0 | 0.26 |
| *1 cup* | | 1.9 | 0.2 | 0.1 | 0.1 | 0.1 | 0 | 239 | 24 | 3.34 | 0.171 | 0 | 1840 | 0.6 | 0.10 | 0.11 | 19.5 | 9064 |
| **cherries, sour**, frozen | 155 | 71 | 135.2 | 17.1 | 14.0 | 0 | 2.5 | 2 | 20 | 14 | 0.16 | 0.088 | 68 | 3 | 0.07 | 0.2 | 0 | 0.28 |
| *1 cup* | | 1.4 | 0.7 | 0.2 | 0.2 | 0.2 | 0 | 192 | 25 | 0.82 | 0.139 | 0 | 1348 | 0.1 | 0.05 | 0.10 | 7.8 | 9068 |
| **cherries, sour**, raw | 103 | 52 | 88.7 | 12.5 | 8.7 | 0 | 1.6 | 3 | 16 | 9 | 0.10 | 0.115 | 66 | 10 | 0.03 | 0.4 | 0 | 0.15 |
| *1 cup* | | 1.0 | 0.3 | 0.1 | 0.1 | 0.1 | 0 | 178 | 15 | 0.33 | 0.107 | 0 | 1321 | 0.1 | 0.04 | 0.05 | 8.2 | 9063 |
| **cherries, sweet**, cnd in heavy syrup | 179 | 149 | 138.9 | 37.7 | 29.0 | 16.0 | 4.1 | 5 | 18 | 16 | 0.18 | 0.086 | 21 | 6 | 0.04 | 0.7 | 0 | 0.11 |
| *1 cup drained* | | 1.3 | 0.4 | 0.1 | 0.1 | 0.1 | 0 | 265 | 36 | 0.63 | 0.315 | 0 | 424 | 0.3 | 0.08 | 0.04 | 9.0 | 9367 |
| **cherries, sweet**, cnd in juice | 250 | 135 | 212.4 | 34.5 | 30.8 | 0 | 3.8 | 8 | 35 | 30 | 0.25 | 0.152 | 15 | 6 | 0.04 | 1.0 | 0 | 0.32 |
| *1 cup* | | 2.3 | 0 | 0 | 0 | 0 | 0 | 328 | 55 | 1.45 | 0.182 | 0 | 312 | 0.6 | 0.06 | 0.08 | 10.0 | 9072 |
| **cherries, sweet**, cnd in light syrup | 252 | 169 | 205.5 | 43.6 | 39.8 | 13.9 | 3.8 | 8 | 23 | 23 | 0.25 | 0.151 | 20 | 9 | 0.05 | 1.0 | 0 | 0.32 |
| *1 cup* | | 1.5 | 0.4 | 0.1 | 0.1 | 0.1 | 0 | 373 | 45 | 0.91 | 0.365 | 0 | 396 | 0.6 | 0.10 | 0.08 | 10.1 | 9073 |
| **cherries, sweet**, cnd in water | 248 | 114 | 215.9 | 29.2 | 25.4 | 0 | 3.7 | 2 | 27 | 22 | 0.20 | 0.154 | 20 | 5 | 0.05 | 1.0 | 0 | 0.31 |
| *1 cup* | | 1.9 | 0.3 | 0.1 | 0.1 | 0.1 | 0 | 325 | 37 | 0.89 | 0.186 | 0 | 397 | 0.6 | 0.10 | 0.07 | 9.9 | 9071 |
| **cherries, sweet**, raw | 117 | 74 | 96.2 | 18.7 | 15.0 | 0 | 2.5 | 0 | 15 | 13 | 0.08 | 0.082 | 4 | 8 | 0.03 | 0.2 | 0 | 0.23 |
| *1 cup* | | 1.2 | 0.2 | 0 | 0.1 | 0.1 | 0 | 260 | 25 | 0.42 | 0.070 | 0 | 75 | 0.1 | 0.04 | 0.06 | 4.7 | 9070 |
| **cherries, sweet**, sweetened, frozen | 259 | 231 | 195.6 | 57.9 | 52.5 | 19.3 | 5.4 | 3 | 31 | 26 | 0.10 | 0.282 | 23 | 3 | 0.07 | 0.5 | 0 | 0.33 |
| *1 cup* | | 3.0 | 0.3 | 0.1 | 0.1 | 0.1 | 0 | 515 | 41 | 0.91 | 0.062 | 0 | 490 | 0.2 | 0.12 | 0.09 | 10.4 | 9076 |
| **chokecherries**, pitted, raw | 100 | 156 | 61.5 | 33.9 | 14.2 | | 17.0 | 2 | 40 | 21 | 0.19 | 0.192 | 2 | 1 | 0.03 | 0.7 | 0 | 0.33 |
| *3.5 oz* | | 2.9 | 1.0 | | | | | 309 | 45 | 0.40 | 0.068 | 1.7 | 43 | 0.8 | 0.06 | 0.19 | 10.0 | 35179 |
| **clementine**, raw | 74 | 35 | 64.1 | 8.9 | 6.8 | | 1.3 | 1 | 22 | 7 | 0.04 | 0.017 | | 36 | 0.06 | 0.5 | | 0.11 |
| *2.6 oz fruit* | | 0.6 | 0.1 | | | | | 131 | 16 | 0.10 | 0.032 | 0.1 | | 0.1 | 0.02 | 0.06 | 17.8 | 9433 |
| **cloudberries**, raw | 100 | 51 | 87.0 | 8.6 | | | | | 18 | | | | | 158 | 0.05 | 0.9 | | |
| *3.5 oz* | | 2.4 | 0.8 | | | | | | 35 | 0.70 | | | 210 | | 0.07 | | | 35027 |
| **crabapples**, raw | 110 | 84 | 86.8 | 21.9 | | | | 1 | 20 | 8 | | 0.127 | 2 | 9 | 0.03 | 0.1 | 0 | |
| *1 cup sliced* | | 0.4 | 0.3 | 0.1 | 0 | 0.1 | 0 | 213 | 16 | 0.40 | 0.074 | | 44 | | 0.02 | | | 9077 |
| **cranberries**, dried, sweetened | 33 | 102 | 5.3 | 27.2 | 21.4 | 20.7 | 1.9 | 1 | 3 | 2 | 0.04 | 0.087 | 0 | 0 | | 0.3 | 0 | 0.07 |
| *⅓ cup* | | 0 | 0.5 | 0 | 0.1 | 0.2 | 0 | 13 | 3 | 0.17 | 0.026 | 0.2 | 0 | 0.4 | 0.01 | 0.01 | 0 | 9079 |
| **cranberries**, raw | 95 | 44 | 82.8 | 11.6 | 3.8 | 0 | 4.4 | 2 | 8 | 6 | 0.10 | 0.342 | 3 | 13 | 0.01 | 0.1 | 0 | 0.28 |
| *1 cup whole* | | 0.4 | 0.1 | 0 | 0 | 0.1 | 0 | 81 | 12 | 0.24 | 0.058 | 0.1 | 57 | 1.1 | 0.02 | 0.05 | 1.0 | 9078 |
| **cranberries**, wild, raw | 100 | 55 | 86.0 | 12.3 | | | 6.7 | 26 | 20 | | | | | 15 | 0 | 0.9 | | |
| *3.5 oz* | | 1.1 | 0.2 | | | | | 140 | 15 | 1.00 | | | 1060 | | 0.01 | | | 35029 |
| **cranberry orange relish**, canned | 275 | 490 | 146.3 | 127.0 | | | 0 | 88 | 30 | 11 | | | 11 | 50 | 0.08 | 0.3 | 0 | |
| *1 cup* | | 0.8 | 0.3 | 0 | | | 0 | 104 | 22 | 0.55 | 0.110 | | 192 | | 0.06 | | | 9082 |
| **cranberry sauce**, jelled, canned | 57 | 86 | 34.6 | 22.2 | 21.6 | 19.8 | 0.6 | 17 | 2 | 2 | 0.03 | 0.034 | 1 | 1 | 0.01 | 0.1 | 0 | |
| *½" thick slice* | | 0.1 | 0.1 | 0 | 0 | 0 | 0 | 15 | 3 | 0.13 | 0.011 | 0.2 | 24 | 0.5 | 0.01 | 0.01 | 0.6 | 9081 |
| **currants, black**, raw | 112 | 71 | 91.8 | 17.2 | | | | 2 | 62 | 27 | 0.30 | 0.287 | 13 | 203 | 0.06 | 0.3 | 0 | 0.45 |
| *1 cup* | | 1.6 | 0.5 | 0 | 0.1 | 0.2 | 0 | 361 | 66 | 1.72 | 0.096 | | 258 | 1.1 | 0.06 | 0.07 | | 9083 |
| **currants, red/white**, raw | 112 | 63 | 94.0 | 15.5 | 8.3 | 0 | 4.8 | 1 | 37 | 15 | 0.26 | 0.208 | 2 | 46 | 0.04 | 0.1 | 0 | 0.07 |
| *1 cup* | | 1.6 | 0.2 | 0 | 0 | 0.1 | 0 | 308 | 49 | 1.12 | 0.120 | 0.7 | 47 | 0.1 | 0.06 | 0.08 | 9.0 | 9084 |
| **currants, zante**, dried | 72 | 204 | 13.8 | 53.3 | 48.4 | 0 | 4.9 | 6 | 62 | 30 | 0.48 | 0.338 | 3 | 3 | 0.12 | 1.2 | 0 | 0.03 |
| *½ cup* | | 2.9 | 0.2 | 0 | 0 | 0.1 | 0 | 642 | 90 | 2.35 | 0.337 | 0.5 | 53 | 0.1 | 0.10 | 0.21 | 7.2 | 9085 |
| **custard apple** (bullock's heart), raw | 100 | 101 | 71.5 | 25.2 | | | 2.4 | 4 | 30 | 18 | | | 2 | 19 | 0.08 | 0.5 | 0 | 0.14 |
| *3.5 oz* | | 1.7 | 0.6 | 0.2 | | | 0 | 382 | 21 | 0.71 | | | 33 | | 0.10 | 0.22 | | 9086 |
| **date**, dried | 32 | 90 | 6.6 | 24.0 | 20.3 | 0 | 2.6 | 1 | 12 | 14 | 0.09 | 0.084 | 0 | 0 | 0.02 | 0.4 | 0 | 0.19 |
| *4 dates* | | 0.8 | 0.1 | 0 | 0 | 0 | 0 | 210 | 20 | 0.33 | 0.066 | 1.0 | 3 | 0 | 0.02 | 0.05 | 6.1 | 9087 |
| **date, medjool**, dried | 24 | 66 | 5.1 | 18.0 | 16.0 | | 1.6 | 0 | 15 | 13 | 0.11 | 0.071 | 2 | 0 | 0.01 | 0.4 | 0 | 0.19 |
| *1 date* | | 0.4 | 0 | | | | | 167 | 15 | 0.22 | 0.087 | | 36 | | 0.01 | 0.06 | 3.6 | 9421 |
| **durian**, raw/frozen | 243 | 357 | 157.9 | 65.8 | | | 9.2 | 5 | 15 | 73 | 0.68 | 0.790 | 5 | 48 | 0.91 | 2.6 | 0 | 0.56 |
| *1 cup chopped* | | 3.6 | 13.0 | | | | 0 | 1059 | 95 | 1.04 | 0.503 | | 107 | | 0.49 | 0.77 | | 9422 |
| **elderberries**, raw | 145 | 106 | 115.7 | 26.7 | | | 10.2 | 9 | 55 | 7 | 0.16 | | 44 | 52 | 0.10 | 0.7 | 0 | 0.20 |
| *1 cup* | | 1.0 | 0.7 | 0 | 0.1 | 0.4 | 0 | 406 | 57 | 2.32 | 0.088 | 0.9 | 870 | | 0.09 | 0.33 | 8.7 | 9088 |
| **feijoa**, raw | 50 | 24 | 43.3 | 5.3 | | | | 2 | 8 | 4 | 0.02 | 0.042 | 0 | 10 | 0 | 0.1 | 0 | 0.11 |
| *1 medium* | | 0.6 | 0.4 | | | | 0 | 78 | 10 | 0.04 | 0.028 | | 0 | | 0.02 | 0.02 | 19.0 | 9334 |
| **fig**, canned in heavy syrup | 28 | 25 | 21.4 | 6.4 | 5.8 | 2.5 | 0.6 | 0 | 8 | 3 | 0.03 | 0.024 | 1 | 0 | 0.01 | 0.1 | 0 | 0.02 |
| *1 fig with liquid* | | 0.1 | 0 | 0 | 0 | 0 | 0 | 28 | 3 | 0.08 | 0.030 | 0.1 | 10 | 0 | 0.01 | 0.02 | 0.6 | 9092 |
| **fig**, dried | 19 | 47 | 5.7 | 12.1 | 9.1 | 0 | 1.9 | 2 | 31 | 13 | 0.10 | 0.097 | 0 | 0 | 0.02 | 0.1 | 0 | 0.08 |
| *1 fig* | | 0.6 | 0.2 | 0 | 0 | 0.1 | 0 | 129 | 13 | 0.39 | 0.055 | 0.1 | 2 | 0.1 | 0.02 | 0.02 | 1.7 | 9094 |
| **fig**, raw | 50 | 37 | 39.6 | 9.6 | 8.1 | 0 | 1.4 | 0 | 18 | 8 | 0.08 | 0.064 | 4 | 1 | 0.03 | 0.2 | 0 | 0.15 |
| *1 medium (2¼" diameter)* | | 0.4 | 0.2 | 0 | 0 | 0.1 | 0 | 116 | 7 | 0.18 | 0.035 | 0.1 | 71 | 0.1 | 0.02 | 0.06 | 3.0 | 9089 |
| **Fruit by the Foot** (dried fruit), Betty Crocker - .7 oz roll | 21 | 80 | | 17.0 | 10.0 | | | 45 | | | | | | 6 | | | | |
| | | 0 | 1.0 | 0 | | | 0 | | | | | | | | | | | |

| | WT (g) | KCAL | H₂O (g) | CHO (g) | TSUG (g) | ASUG (g) | DFIB (g) | Na (mg) | Ca (mg) | Mg (mg) | Zn (mg) | Mn (mg) | A (mcg RAE) | C (mg) | B-1 (mg) | NIA (mg) | B-12 (mcg) | PANT (mg) |
|---|---|---|---|---|---|---|---|---|---|---|---|---|---|---|---|---|---|---|
| | | PRO (g) | FAT (g) | SFA (g) | MUFA (g) | PUFA (g) | CHOL (mg) | K (mg) | P (mg) | Fe (mg) | Cu (mg) | Se (mcg) | A (IU) | E (mg ATE) | B-2 (mg) | B-6 (mg) | FOL (mcg DFE) | REF |
| **fruit cocktail**, cnd in heavy syrup, drained - *1 cup* | 248 | 174 | 199.4 | 46.6 | 42.5 | 24.7 | 4.2 | 15 | 17 | 12 | 0.20 | | 35 | 5 | 0.05 | 0.9 | 0 | |
| | | 1.2 | 0.2 | 0 | 0 | 0.1 | 0 | 223 | 30 | 0.72 | 0.213 | 1.2 | 677 | 1.5 | 0.05 | 0.13 | 7.4 | 9351 |
| **fruit cocktail**, cnd in heavy syrup, solids and liquid - *1 cup* | 248 | 181 | 199.4 | 46.9 | 44.4 | 25.8 | 2.5 | 15 | 15 | 12 | 0.20 | 0.357 | 25 | 5 | 0.04 | 0.9 | 0 | 0.15 |
| | | 1.0 | 0.2 | 0 | 0 | 0.1 | 0 | 218 | 27 | 0.72 | 0.171 | 1.2 | 508 | 1.0 | 0.05 | 0.12 | 7.4 | 9100 |
| **fruit cocktail**, cnd in juice *1 cup* | 237 | 109 | 207.2 | 28.1 | 25.7 | 0 | 2.4 | 9 | 19 | 17 | 0.21 | 0.346 | 36 | 6 | 0.03 | 1.0 | 0 | 0.15 |
| | | 1.1 | 0 | 0 | 0 | 0 | 0 | 225 | 33 | 0.50 | 0.147 | 1.2 | 723 | 0.9 | 0.04 | 0.12 | 7.1 | 9097 |
| **fruit cocktail**, cnd in water *1 cup* | 237 | 76 | 215.1 | 20.2 | 17.8 | 0 | 2.4 | 9 | 12 | 17 | 0.21 | 0.356 | 31 | 5 | 0.04 | 0.9 | 0 | 0.15 |
| | | 1.0 | 0.1 | 0 | 0 | 0 | 0 | 223 | 26 | 0.59 | 0.168 | 1.2 | 592 | 0.9 | 0.03 | 0.12 | 7.1 | 9096 |
| **Fruit Crisps** (dried fruit), apple, Nature Valley - *.49 oz pouch* | 14 | 50 | | 13.0 | 10.0 | | 1.0 | 75 | | | | | | | | | | |
| | | 0 | 0 | 0 | | | 0 | | | | | | | | | | | GENM400 |
| **Fruit Crisps** (dried fruit), cinn apple, Nature Valley - *.49 oz pouch* | 14 | 50 | | 13.0 | 10.0 | | 1.0 | 75 | | | | | | | | | | |
| | | 0 | 0 | 0 | | | 0 | | | | | | | | | | | GENM401 |
| **Fruit Gushers**, all flavors, Betty Crocker - *.9 oz pouch* | 25 | 90 | | 20.0 | 13.0 | | | 45 | | | | | | 6 | | | | |
| | | 0 | 1.0 | 0 | | | 0 | | | | | | | | | | | GENM207 |
| **fruit roll** (dried fruit) *1 large roll (.74 oz)* | 21 | 78 | 2.1 | 18.0 | 10.3 | 6.4 | 0 | 67 | 7 | 4 | 0.04 | 0.039 | 1 | 25 | 0.02 | 0 | 0 | 0.01 |
| | | 0 | 0.6 | 0.1 | 0.3 | 0.1 | 0 | 62 | 7 | 0.21 | 0.036 | 0.1 | 12 | 0.1 | 0 | 0.06 | 0.4 | 19014 |
| **fruit roll** (dried fruit), berry, Fruit Roll-Ups - *2 rolls* | 28 | 104 | 2.9 | 23.9 | 10.8 | | | 89 | | | | | | 34 | | | | |
| | | 0 | 1.0 | 0.3 | 0.5 | 0 | | | | | | 0.9 | | | | | | 19269 |
| **fruit roll** (dried fruit), cherry, Mariani - *1 roll* | 21 | 70 | | 18.0 | 11.0 | | 2.0 | 10 | 0 | | | | | 15 | | | | |
| | | 0 | 0 | 0 | | | 0 | | 0 | | | | 100 | | | | | MARI1 |
| **fruit roll** (dried fruit), green apple, Mariani - *1 roll* | 21 | 80 | | 19.0 | 12.0 | | 2.0 | 10 | 0 | | | | | 15 | | | | |
| | | 0 | 0 | 0 | | | 0 | | 0 | | | | 0 | | | | | MARI2 |
| **fruit salad**, canned in heavy syrup *1 cup* | 255 | 186 | 204.7 | 48.7 | 46.2 | 27.0 | 2.6 | 15 | 15 | 13 | 0.18 | 0.370 | 64 | 6 | 0.04 | 0.9 | 0 | 0.14 |
| | | 0.9 | 0.2 | 0 | 0 | 0.1 | 0 | 204 | 23 | 0.71 | 0.163 | 1.3 | 1285 | 1.0 | 0.05 | 0.08 | 7.6 | 9105 |
| **fruit salad**, canned in juice *1 cup* | 249 | 125 | 214.5 | 32.5 | | | 2.5 | 12 | 27 | 20 | 0.35 | 0.376 | 75 | 8 | 0.03 | 0.9 | 0 | 0.13 |
| | | 1.3 | 0.1 | 0 | 0 | 0 | 0 | 289 | 35 | 0.62 | 0.125 | | 1494 | | 0.03 | 0.07 | 7.5 | 9103 |
| **fruit salad**, tropical, cnd in heavy syrup - *1 cup* | 257 | 221 | 197.3 | 57.5 | | | 3.3 | 5 | 33 | 33 | 0.28 | | 15 | 45 | 0.14 | 1.4 | 0 | |
| | | 1.1 | 0.3 | 0 | 0 | 0.1 | 0 | 337 | 18 | 1.34 | 0.206 | 1.3 | 326 | | 0.12 | 0.31 | 23.1 | 9325 |
| **Fruit Shapes**, Betty Crocker *.9 oz pouch* | 25 | 80 | | 21.0 | 13.0 | | | 30 | | | | | | 12 | | | | |
| | | 0 | 0 | 0 | | | 0 | | | | | | | | | | | GENM210 |
| **Fruit Snacks**, mixed fruit, Welch's *20 pieces* | 40 | 110 | | 24.0 | 21.0 | | 0 | 20 | 0 | | | | | 60 | | | | |
| | | 1.0 | 0 | | | | 0 | | | | 0.36 | | 1250 | | | | | WLCH1 |
| **Fruit Snacks** with vitamins A, C, and E, Farley - *1 pouch* | 26 | 89 | 3.8 | 21.0 | | | | 9 | | | | | | 23 | | | | |
| | | 1.1 | 0 | | | | | | | | | | 1413 | | | | | 19272 |
| **gooseberries**, canned in light syrup *1 cup* | 252 | 184 | 201.9 | 47.2 | | | 6.0 | 5 | 40 | 15 | 0.28 | 0.446 | 18 | 25 | 0.05 | 0.4 | 0 | 0.35 |
| | | 1.6 | 0.5 | 0 | 0 | 0.3 | 0 | 194 | 18 | 0.83 | 0.547 | 1.0 | 348 | | 0.13 | 0.03 | 7.6 | 9109 |
| **gooseberries**, raw *1 cup* | 150 | 66 | 131.8 | 15.3 | | | 6.4 | 2 | 38 | 15 | 0.18 | 0.216 | 22 | 42 | 0.06 | 0.4 | 0 | 0.43 |
| | | 1.3 | 0.9 | 0.1 | 0.1 | 0.5 | 0 | 297 | 40 | 0.46 | 0.105 | 0.9 | 435 | 0.6 | 0.04 | 0.12 | 9.0 | 9107 |
| **grapefruit**, canned in juice *1 cup* | 249 | 92 | 223.3 | 22.9 | 21.9 | 0 | 1.0 | 17 | 37 | 27 | 0.20 | 0.017 | 0 | 84 | 0.07 | 0.6 | 0 | 0.30 |
| | | 1.7 | 0.2 | 0 | 0 | 0.1 | 0 | 421 | 30 | 0.52 | 0.092 | 2.2 | 0 | 0.2 | 0.04 | 0.05 | 22.4 | 9120 |
| **grapefruit**, canned in light syrup *1 cup* | 254 | 152 | 212.3 | 39.2 | 38.2 | 16.0 | 1.0 | 5 | 36 | 25 | 0.20 | 0.018 | 0 | 54 | 0.10 | 0.6 | 0 | 0.30 |
| | | 1.4 | 0.3 | 0 | 0 | 0.1 | 0 | 328 | 25 | 1.02 | 0.168 | 2.3 | 0 | 0.2 | 0.05 | 0.05 | 22.9 | 9121 |
| **grapefruit**, pink and red, raw *½ medium (3¾" diameter)* | 123 | 52 | 108.3 | 13.1 | 8.5 | 0 | 2.0 | 0 | 27 | 11 | 0.09 | 0.027 | 71 | 38 | 0.05 | 0.3 | 0 | 0.32 |
| | | 0.9 | 0.2 | 0 | 0 | 0 | 0 | 166 | 22 | 0.10 | 0.039 | 0.1 | 1414 | 0.2 | 0.04 | 0.07 | 16.0 | 9112 |
| **grapefruit**, raw *½ medium (3¾" diameter)* | 118 | 38 | 107.3 | 9.5 | 8.2 | 0 | 1.3 | 0 | 14 | 9 | 0.08 | 0.014 | 54 | 41 | 0.04 | 0.3 | 0 | 0.33 |
| | | 0.7 | 0.1 | 0 | 0 | 0 | 0 | 164 | 9 | 0.11 | 0.055 | 0.4 | 1094 | 0.2 | 0.02 | 0.05 | 11.8 | 9111 |
| **grapefruit**, white, raw *½ medium (3¾" diameter)* | 118 | 39 | 106.8 | 9.9 | 8.6 | 0 | 1.3 | 0 | 14 | 11 | 0.08 | 0.015 | 2 | 39 | 0.04 | 0.3 | 0 | 0.33 |
| | | 0.8 | 0.1 | 0 | 0 | 0 | 0 | 175 | 9 | 0.07 | 0.059 | 1.7 | 39 | 0.2 | 0.02 | 0.05 | 11.8 | 9116 |
| **grapes**, American (slip skin), all colors, raw - *1 cup* | 92 | 62 | 74.8 | 15.8 | 15.0 | 0 | 0.8 | 2 | 13 | 5 | 0.04 | 0.661 | 5 | 4 | 0.08 | 0.3 | 0 | 0.02 |
| | | 0.6 | 0.3 | 0.1 | 0 | 0.1 | 0 | 176 | 9 | 0.27 | 0.037 | 0.1 | 92 | 0.2 | 0.05 | 0.10 | 3.7 | 9131 |
| **grapes**, green, canned in water *1 cup* | 245 | 98 | 217.7 | 25.2 | 23.8 | 0 | 1.5 | 15 | 24 | 15 | 0.12 | 0.096 | 5 | 2 | 0.08 | 0.3 | 0 | 0.10 |
| | | 1.2 | 0.3 | 0.1 | 0 | 0.1 | 0 | 262 | 44 | 2.40 | 0.137 | 0.2 | 110 | 0.3 | 0.06 | 0.16 | 7.4 | 9133 |
| **grapes**, green, Thompson seedless, cnd in heavy syrup - *1 cup* | 256 | 195 | 203.6 | 50.3 | 48.8 | 23.9 | 1.5 | 13 | 26 | 15 | 0.13 | 0.097 | 8 | 3 | 0.08 | 0.3 | 0 | 0.10 |
| | | 1.2 | 0.3 | 0.1 | 0 | 0.1 | 0 | 264 | 44 | 2.41 | 0.138 | 0.3 | 164 | 0.3 | 0.06 | 0.17 | 7.7 | 9134 |
| **grapes**, red/green, European, seedless, raw - *1 cup* | 160 | 110 | 128.9 | 29.0 | 24.8 | 0 | 1.4 | 3 | 16 | 11 | 0.11 | 0.114 | 5 | 17 | 0.11 | 0.3 | 0 | 0.08 |
| | | 1.2 | 0.3 | 0.1 | 0 | 0.1 | 0 | 306 | 32 | 0.58 | 0.203 | 0.2 | 106 | 0.3 | 0.11 | 0.14 | 3.2 | 9132 |
| **groundcherries**, raw *1 cup* | 140 | 74 | 119.6 | 15.7 | | | | | 13 | | | | 50 | 15 | 0.15 | 3.9 | 0 | |
| | | 2.7 | 0.1 | | | | 0 | | 56 | 1.40 | | | 1008 | | 0.06 | | | 9138 |
| **guava**, raw *1 medium (3.2 oz)* | 90 | 61 | 72.7 | 12.9 | 8.0 | 0 | 4.9 | 2 | 16 | 20 | 0.21 | 0.135 | 28 | 205 | 0.06 | 1.0 | 0 | 0.41 |
| | | 2.3 | 0.9 | 0.2 | 0.1 | 0.4 | 0 | 375 | 36 | 0.23 | 0.207 | 0.5 | 562 | 0.7 | 0.04 | 0.10 | 44.1 | 9139 |
| **honeydew melon**, raw *1 cup pieces* | 177 | 64 | 159.0 | 16.1 | 14.4 | 0 | 1.4 | 32 | 11 | 18 | 0.16 | 0.048 | 5 | 32 | 0.07 | 0.7 | 0 | 0.27 |
| | | 1.0 | 0.2 | 0.1 | 0 | 0.1 | 0 | 404 | 19 | 0.30 | 0.042 | 1.2 | 88 | 0 | 0.02 | 0.16 | 33.6 | 9184 |

| | WT (g) | KCAL | H₂O (g) | CHO (g) | TSUG (g) | ASUG (g) | DFIB (g) | Na (mg) | Ca (mg) | Mg (mg) | Zn (mg) | Mn (mg) | A (mcg RAE) | C (mg) | B-1 (mg) | NIA (mg) | B-12 (mcg) | PANT (mg) |
|---|---|---|---|---|---|---|---|---|---|---|---|---|---|---|---|---|---|---|
| | | PRO (g) | FAT (g) | SFA (g) | MUFA (g) | PUFA (g) | CHOL (mg) | K (mg) | P (mg) | Fe (mg) | Cu (mg) | Se (mcg) | A (IU) | E (mg ATE) | B-2 (mg) | B-6 (mg) | FOL (mcg DFE) | REF |
| huckleberries, raw | 100 | 37 | 90.7 | 8.7 | | | | 10 | 15 | | | | | | 3 | 0.01 | 0.3 | |
| 3.5 oz | | 0.4 | 0.1 | | | | | | | 0.30 | | | 79 | | 0.03 | | | 35043 |
| jackfruit, canned in syrup | 178 | 164 | 134.0 | 42.6 | | | 1.6 | 20 | 78 | 18 | 0.20 | 0.139 | 0 | 1 | 0.06 | 1.2 | 0 | 0.13 |
| 1 cup | | 0.6 | 0.2 | | | | 0 | 171 | 11 | 0.52 | 0.089 | | 4 | | 0.06 | 0.08 | 24.9 | 9420 |
| jackfruit, raw | 165 | 155 | 120.8 | 39.6 | | | 2.6 | 5 | 56 | 61 | 0.69 | 0.325 | 25 | 11 | 0.05 | 0.7 | 0 | |
| 1 cup sliced | | 2.4 | 0.5 | 0.1 | 0.1 | 0.1 | 0 | 500 | 59 | 0.99 | 0.309 | 1.0 | 490 | | 0.18 | 0.18 | 23.1 | 9144 |
| java plum, raw | 135 | 81 | 112.2 | 21.0 | | | | 19 | 26 | 20 | | | 0 | 19 | 0.01 | 0.4 | 0 | |
| 1 cup | | 1.0 | 0.3 | | | | 0 | 107 | 23 | 0.26 | | | 4 | | 0.02 | 0.05 | | 9145 |
| jujube, dried | 28 | 80 | 5.5 | 20.6 | | | | 3 | 22 | 10 | 0.05 | 0.085 | | 4 | 0.06 | 0.1 | 0 | |
| 1 oz | | 1.0 | 0.3 | | | | 0 | 149 | 28 | 0.50 | 0.074 | | | | 0.10 | | | 9147 |
| jujube, raw | 100 | 79 | 77.9 | 20.2 | | | | 3 | 21 | 10 | 0.05 | 0.084 | 2 | 69 | 0.02 | 0.9 | 0 | |
| 3.5 oz | | 1.2 | 0.2 | | | | 0 | 250 | 23 | 0.48 | 0.073 | | 40 | | 0.04 | 0.08 | | 9146 |
| kiwifruit, raw | 76 | 46 | 63.1 | 11.1 | 6.8 | 0 | 2.3 | 2 | 26 | 13 | 0.11 | 0.074 | 3 | 70 | 0.02 | 0.3 | 0 | 0.14 |
| 1 medium (2.7 oz) | | 0.9 | 0.4 | 0 | 0 | 0.2 | 0 | 237 | 26 | 0.24 | 0.099 | 0.2 | 66 | 1.1 | 0.02 | 0.05 | 19.0 | 9148 |
| kumquat, raw | 19 | 13 | 15.4 | 3.0 | 1.8 | 0 | 1.2 | 2 | 12 | 4 | 0.03 | 0.026 | 3 | 8 | 0.01 | 0.1 | 0 | 0.04 |
| 1 medium | | 0.4 | 0.2 | 0 | 0 | 0 | 0 | 35 | 4 | 0.16 | 0.018 | 0 | 55 | 0 | 0.02 | 0.01 | 3.2 | 9149 |
| lemon peel, raw | 6 | 3 | 4.9 | 1.0 | 0.3 | 0 | 0.6 | 0 | 8 | 1 | 0.02 | | 0 | 8 | 0 | 0 | 0 | 0.02 |
| 1 T | | 0.1 | 0 | 0 | 0 | 0 | 0 | 10 | 1 | 0.05 | 0.006 | 0 | 3 | 0 | 0 | 0.01 | 0.8 | 9156 |
| lemon, raw | 58 | 17 | 51.6 | 5.4 | 1.4 | 0 | 1.6 | 1 | 15 | 5 | 0.03 | 0.017 | 1 | 31 | 0.02 | 0.1 | 0 | 0.11 |
| 1 medium (2⅛" diameter) | | 0.6 | 0.2 | 0 | 0 | 0.1 | 0 | 80 | 9 | 0.35 | 0.021 | 0.2 | 13 | 0.1 | 0.01 | 0.05 | 6.4 | 9150 |
| lime, raw | 67 | 20 | 59.1 | 7.1 | 1.1 | 0 | 1.9 | 1 | 22 | 4 | 0.07 | 0.005 | 1 | 19 | 0.02 | 0.1 | 0 | 0.15 |
| 1 medium (2" diameter) | | 0.5 | 0.1 | 0 | 0 | 0 | 0 | 68 | 12 | 0.40 | 0.044 | 0.3 | 34 | 0.1 | 0.01 | 0.03 | 5.4 | 9159 |
| lingonberries, raw | 100 | 55 | 86.7 | 12.2 | | | | | 26 | | | | | 21 | 0.02 | 0.4 | | |
| 3.5 oz | | 0.4 | 0.5 | | | | | | 21 | 0.40 | | | 90 | | 0.08 | | | 35030 |
| litchee (lychee), dried | 2 | 6 | 0.4 | 1.4 | 1.3 | 0 | 0.1 | 0 | 1 | 1 | 0.01 | 0.005 | 0 | 4 | 0 | 0.1 | 0 | |
| 1 medium | | 0.1 | 0 | 0 | 0 | 0 | 0 | 22 | 4 | 0.03 | 0.013 | 0 | 0 | 0 | 0.01 | 0 | 0.2 | 9165 |
| litchee (lychee), raw | 10 | 7 | 8.2 | 1.7 | 1.5 | 0 | 0.1 | 0 | 0 | 1 | 0.01 | 0.006 | 0 | 7 | 0 | 0.1 | 0 | |
| 1 medium | | 0.1 | 0 | 0 | 0 | 0 | 0 | 17 | 3 | 0.03 | 0.015 | 0.1 | 0 | 0 | 0.01 | 0.01 | 1.4 | 9164 |
| loganberries, frozen | 147 | 81 | 124.4 | 19.1 | 11.3 | 0 | 7.8 | 1 | 38 | 31 | 0.50 | 1.833 | 3 | 22 | 0.07 | 1.2 | 0 | 0.36 |
| 1 cup | | 2.2 | 0.5 | 0 | 0 | 0.3 | 0 | 213 | 38 | 0.94 | 0.172 | 0.3 | 51 | 1.3 | 0.05 | 0.10 | 38.2 | 9167 |
| longan, dried | 28 | 80 | 4.9 | 20.7 | | | | 13 | 13 | 13 | 0.06 | 0.069 | 0 | 8 | 0.01 | 0.3 | 0 | |
| 1 oz | | 1.4 | 0.1 | | | | 0 | 184 | 55 | 1.51 | 0.226 | | 0 | | 0.14 | | | 9173 |
| longan, raw | 3 | 2 | 2.5 | 0.5 | | | | 0 | 0 | 0 | 0 | 0.002 | | 3 | 0 | 0 | 0 | |
| 1 medium | | 0 | 0 | | | | 0 | 8 | 1 | 0 | 0.005 | | | | 0 | | | 9172 |
| loquat, raw | 16 | 8 | 13.9 | 1.9 | | | 0.3 | 0 | 3 | 2 | 0.01 | 0.024 | 12 | 0 | 0 | 0 | 0 | |
| 1 medium | | 0.1 | 0 | 0 | 0 | 0 | 0 | 43 | 4 | 0.04 | 0.006 | 0.1 | 244 | | 0.02 | | 2.2 | 9174 |
| mammy apple (mamey), raw | 846 | 431 | 729.3 | 105.8 | | | 25.4 | 127 | 93 | 135 | 0.85 | | 102 | 118 | 0.17 | 3.4 | 0 | 0.87 |
| 1 medium | | 4.2 | 4.2 | 1.2 | 1.7 | 0.7 | 0 | 398 | 93 | 5.92 | 0.728 | 5.1 | 1946 | | 0.34 | 0.85 | 118.4 | 9175 |
| mandarin oranges, cnd in juice | 249 | 92 | 222.9 | 23.8 | 22.1 | 0 | 1.7 | 12 | 27 | 27 | 1.27 | 0.080 | 107 | 85 | 0.20 | 1.1 | 0 | 0.31 |
| 1 cup | | 1.5 | 0.1 | 0 | 0 | 0 | 0 | 331 | 25 | 0.67 | 0.082 | 1.0 | 2121 | 0.2 | 0.07 | 0.10 | 12.5 | 9219 |
| mandarin oranges, cnd in light syrup - 1 cup | 252 | 154 | 209.3 | 40.8 | 39.0 | 12.4 | 1.8 | 15 | 18 | 20 | 0.60 | 0.081 | 106 | 50 | 0.13 | 1.1 | 0 | 0.32 |
| | | 1.1 | 0.3 | 0 | 0 | 0 | 0 | 197 | 25 | 0.93 | 0.111 | 1.0 | 2117 | 0.3 | 0.11 | 0.11 | 12.6 | 9220 |
| mango, dried, Sunsweet | 40 | 140 | | 34.0 | 28.0 | | 1.0 | 20 | 80 | | | | | 1 | | | | |
| ⅓ cup | | 0 | 0 | 0 | | | 0 | 10 | | 0.36 | | | 500 | 1 | | | | SUNS1 |
| mango, raw | 207 | 135 | 169.1 | 35.2 | 30.6 | 0 | 3.7 | 4 | 21 | 19 | 0.08 | 0.056 | 79 | 57 | 0.12 | 1.2 | 0 | 0.33 |
| 1 medium (7.3 oz) | | 1.1 | 0.6 | 0.1 | 0.2 | 0.1 | 0 | 323 | 23 | 0.27 | 0.228 | 1.2 | 1584 | 2.3 | 0.12 | 0.28 | 29.0 | 9176 |
| mangosteen, canned in syrup | 196 | 143 | 158.6 | 35.1 | | | 3.5 | 14 | 24 | 25 | 0.41 | 0.200 | 4 | 6 | 0.11 | 0.6 | 0 | 0.06 |
| 1 cup | | 0.8 | 1.1 | | | | 0 | 94 | 16 | 0.59 | 0.135 | | 69 | | 0.11 | 0.04 | 60.8 | 9177 |
| melon balls (cantaloupe and honeydew), frzn - 1 cup | 173 | 57 | 156.1 | 13.7 | | | 1.2 | 54 | 17 | 24 | 0.29 | 0.069 | 154 | 11 | 0.29 | 1.1 | 0 | 0.28 |
| | | 1.5 | 0.4 | 0.1 | 0 | 0.2 | 0 | 484 | 21 | 0.50 | 0.104 | | 3069 | | 0.04 | 0.18 | 45.0 | 9185 |
| mixed fruit, canned in heavy syrup | 255 | 184 | 205.4 | 47.8 | | | 2.6 | 10 | 3 | 13 | 0.18 | 0.984 | 26 | 176 | 0.04 | 1.5 | 0 | 0.15 |
| 1 cup | | 0.9 | 0.3 | 0 | 0 | 0.1 | 0 | 214 | 26 | 0.92 | 0.148 | | 495 | | 0.10 | 0.09 | 7.6 | 9187 |
| mixed fruit (prunes, apricots, pears), dried - 11 oz package | 293 | 712 | 91.4 | 187.7 | | | 22.9 | 53 | 111 | 114 | 1.46 | 0.665 | 357 | 11 | 0.13 | 5.6 | 0 | 1.29 |
| | | 7.2 | 1.4 | 0.1 | 0.7 | 0.3 | 0 | 2332 | 226 | 7.94 | 1.128 | | 7155 | | 0.46 | 0.47 | 11.7 | 9188 |
| mixed fruit, sweetened, frozen | 250 | 245 | 184.3 | 60.6 | | | 4.8 | 8 | 18 | 15 | 0.12 | 0.160 | 40 | 188 | 0.04 | 1.0 | 0 | 0.23 |
| 1 cup | | 3.6 | 0.4 | 0.1 | 0.1 | 0.2 | 0 | 328 | 30 | 0.70 | 0.085 | | 805 | | 0.09 | 0.06 | 20.0 | 9189 |
| mulberries, raw | 140 | 60 | 122.8 | 13.7 | 11.3 | 0 | 2.4 | 14 | 55 | 25 | 0.17 | | 1 | 51 | 0.04 | 0.9 | 0 | |
| 1 cup | | 2.0 | 0.5 | 0 | 0.1 | 0.3 | 0 | 272 | 53 | 2.59 | 0.084 | 0.8 | 35 | 1.2 | 0.14 | 0.07 | 8.4 | 9190 |
| nectarine, raw | 136 | 60 | 119.1 | 14.3 | 10.7 | 0 | 2.3 | 0 | 8 | 12 | 0.23 | 0.073 | 23 | 7 | 0.05 | 1.5 | 0 | 0.25 |
| 1 medium (2½" diameter) | | 1.4 | 0.4 | 0 | 0.1 | 0.2 | 0 | 273 | 35 | 0.38 | 0.117 | 0 | 452 | 1.0 | 0.04 | 0.03 | 6.8 | 9191 |
| oheloberries, raw | 140 | 39 | 129.2 | 9.6 | | | | 1 | 10 | 8 | | | 59 | 8 | 0.02 | 0.4 | 0 | |
| 1 cup | | 0.5 | 0.3 | | | | 0 | 53 | 14 | 0.13 | | | 1162 | | 0.05 | | | 9192 |

| | WT | Macronutrients | | | | | | Minerals | | | | | Vitamins | | | | | |
|---|---|---|---|---|---|---|---|---|---|---|---|---|---|---|---|---|---|---|
| | (g) | KCAL | $H_2O$ (g) | CHO (g) | TSUG (g) | ASUG (g) | DFIB (g) | Na (mg) | Ca (mg) | Mg (mg) | Zn (mg) | Mn (mg) | A (mcg RAE) | C (mg) | B-1 (mg) | NIA (mg) | B-12 (mcg) | PANT (mg) |
| | | PRO (g) | FAT (g) | SFA (g) | MUFA (g) | PUFA (g) | CHOL (mg) | K (mg) | P (mg) | Fe (mg) | Cu (mg) | Se (mcg) | A (IU) | E (mg ATE) | B-2 (mg) | B-6 (mg) | FOL (mcg DFE) | REF |
| **orange, all varieties**, raw | 131 | 62 | 113.6 | 15.4 | 12.2 | 0 | 3.1 | 0 | 52 | 13 | 0.09 | 0.033 | 14 | 70 | 0.11 | 0.4 | 0 | 0.33 |
| *1 medium (2⅝" diameter)* | | 1.2 | 0.2 | 0 | 0 | 0 | 0 | 237 | 18 | 0.13 | 0.059 | 0.7 | 295 | 0.2 | 0.05 | 0.08 | 39.3 | 9200 |
| **orange, California navel**, raw | 140 | 69 | 120.4 | 17.6 | 11.9 | | 3.1 | 1 | 60 | 15 | 0.11 | 0.041 | 17 | 83 | 0.10 | 0.6 | 0 | 0.37 |
| *1 medium (2⅞" diameter)* | | 1.3 | 0.2 | 0 | 0 | 0 | 0 | 232 | 32 | 0.18 | 0.055 | 0 | 346 | 0.2 | 0.07 | 0.11 | 47.6 | 9202 |
| **orange, California Valencia**, raw | 121 | 59 | 104.5 | 14.4 | | | 3.0 | 0 | 48 | 12 | 0.07 | 0.028 | 15 | 59 | 0.11 | 0.3 | 0 | 0.30 |
| *1 medium (2⅝" diameter)* | | 1.3 | 0.4 | 0 | 0.1 | 0.1 | 0 | 217 | 21 | 0.11 | 0.045 | | 278 | | 0.05 | 0.08 | 47.2 | 9201 |
| **orange, Florida**, raw | 141 | 65 | 122.9 | 16.3 | 12.9 | 0 | 3.4 | 0 | 61 | 14 | 0.11 | 0.034 | 16 | 63 | 0.14 | 0.6 | 0 | 0.35 |
| *1 medium (2⅝" diameter)* | | 1.0 | 0.3 | 0 | 0.1 | 0.1 | 0 | 238 | 17 | 0.13 | 0.055 | 0.7 | 317 | 0.3 | 0.06 | 0.07 | 24.0 | 9203 |
| **orange peel**, raw | 6 | 6 | 4.4 | 1.5 | | | 0.6 | 0 | 10 | 1 | 0.02 | | 1 | 8 | 0.01 | 0.1 | 0 | 0.03 |
| *1 T* | | 0.1 | 0 | 0 | 0 | 0 | 0 | 13 | 1 | 0.05 | 0.006 | 0.1 | 25 | 0 | 0.01 | 0.01 | 1.8 | 9216 |
| **papaya**, raw - *1 medium* | 304 | 119 | 270.0 | 29.8 | 17.9 | 0 | 5.5 | 9 | 73 | 30 | 0.21 | 0.033 | 167 | 188 | 0.08 | 1.0 | 0 | 0.66 |
| *(5⅛" long × 3" diameter)* | | 1.9 | 0.4 | 0.1 | 0.1 | 0.1 | 0 | 781 | 15 | 0.30 | 0.049 | 1.8 | 3326 | 2.2 | 0.10 | 0.06 | 115.5 | 9226 |
| **passion fruit** (granadilla), purple, | 18 | 17 | 13.1 | 4.2 | 2.0 | 0 | 1.9 | 5 | 2 | 5 | 0.02 | | 12 | 5 | 0 | 0.3 | 0 | |
| raw - *1 medium* | | 0.4 | 0.1 | 0 | 0 | 0.1 | 0 | 63 | 12 | 0.29 | 0.015 | 0.1 | 229 | 0 | 0.02 | 0.02 | 2.5 | 9231 |
| **peach**, canned in heavy syrup, | 262 | 202 | 207.7 | 51.8 | 46.2 | 34.2 | 5.8 | 16 | 8 | 13 | 0.24 | | 100 | 7 | 0.03 | 1.6 | 0 | |
| drained - *1 cup* | | 1.4 | 0.4 | 0 | 0 | 0.1 | 0 | 246 | 31 | 0.71 | 0.165 | 0.8 | 2002 | 1.9 | 0.07 | 0.05 | 7.9 | 9370 |
| **peach**, canned in heavy syrup, | 262 | 194 | 207.7 | 52.2 | 48.8 | 36.2 | 3.4 | 16 | 8 | 13 | 0.24 | 0.118 | 45 | 7 | 0.03 | 1.6 | 0 | 0.13 |
| solids and liquid - *1 cup* | | 1.2 | 0.3 | 0 | 0.1 | 0.1 | 0 | 241 | 29 | 0.71 | 0.134 | 0.8 | 870 | 1.3 | 0.06 | 0.05 | 7.9 | 9241 |
| **peach**, canned in juice | 250 | 110 | 218.7 | 28.9 | 25.7 | 0 | 3.2 | 10 | 15 | 18 | 0.28 | 0.120 | 48 | 9 | 0.02 | 1.5 | 0 | 0.12 |
| *1 cup* | | 1.6 | 0.1 | 0 | 0 | 0 | 0 | 320 | 42 | 0.68 | 0.125 | 0.8 | 952 | 1.2 | 0.04 | 0.05 | 7.5 | 9238 |
| **peach**, canned in light syrup | 251 | 136 | 212.6 | 36.5 | 33.3 | 21.2 | 3.3 | 13 | 8 | 13 | 0.23 | 0.115 | 45 | 6 | 0.02 | 1.5 | 0 | 0.13 |
| *1 cup* | | 1.1 | 0.1 | 0 | 0 | 0 | 0 | 243 | 28 | 0.90 | 0.131 | 0.8 | 889 | 1.2 | 0.06 | 0.05 | 7.5 | 9240 |
| **peach**, canned in water | 244 | 59 | 227.2 | 14.9 | 11.7 | 0 | 3.2 | 7 | 5 | 12 | 0.22 | 0.117 | 66 | 7 | 0.02 | 1.3 | 0 | 0.12 |
| *1 cup* | | 1.1 | 0.1 | 0 | 0.1 | 0.1 | 0 | 242 | 24 | 0.78 | 0.132 | 0.7 | 1298 | 1.2 | 0.05 | 0.05 | 7.3 | 9237 |
| **peach**, dried | 160 | 382 | 50.9 | 98.1 | 66.8 | 0 | 13.1 | 11 | 45 | 67 | 0.91 | 0.488 | 173 | 8 | 0 | 7.0 | 0 | 0.90 |
| *1 cup halves* | | 5.8 | 1.2 | 0.1 | 0.4 | 0.6 | 0 | 1594 | 190 | 6.50 | 0.582 | 0.8 | 3461 | 0.3 | 0.34 | 0.11 | 0 | 9246 |
| **peach**, raw | 98 | 38 | 87.1 | 9.3 | 8.2 | 0 | 1.5 | 0 | 6 | 9 | 0.17 | 0.060 | 16 | 6 | 0.02 | 0.8 | 0 | 0.15 |
| *1 medium (2½" diameter)* | | 0.9 | 0.2 | 0 | 0.1 | 0.1 | 0 | 186 | 20 | 0.24 | 0.067 | 0.1 | 319 | 0.7 | 0.03 | 0.02 | 3.9 | 9236 |
| **peach**, spiced, cnd in heavy syrup | 242 | 182 | 191.7 | 48.6 | 45.4 | 33.8 | 3.1 | 10 | 15 | 17 | 0.19 | | 39 | 13 | 0.03 | 1.3 | 0 | 0.12 |
| *1 cup* | | 1.0 | 0.2 | 0 | 0.1 | 0.1 | 0 | 206 | 22 | 0.68 | 0.237 | 0.7 | 767 | 1.2 | 0.08 | 0.05 | 7.3 | 9243 |
| **peach**, sweetened, frozen | 250 | 235 | 186.8 | 60.0 | 55.4 | 34.5 | 4.5 | 15 | 8 | 12 | 0.12 | 0.073 | 35 | 236 | 0.03 | 1.6 | 0 | 0.33 |
| *1 cup* | | 1.6 | 0.3 | 0 | 0.1 | 0.2 | 0 | 325 | 28 | 0.92 | 0.060 | 1.0 | 710 | 1.6 | 0.09 | 0.04 | 7.5 | 9250 |
| **pear, Asian**, raw | 122 | 51 | 107.7 | 13.0 | 8.6 | 0 | 4.4 | 0 | 5 | 10 | 0.02 | 0.073 | 0 | 5 | 0.01 | 0.3 | 0 | 0.09 |
| *1 pear (2¼" long, 2½" dia)* | | 0.6 | 0.3 | 0 | 0.1 | 0.1 | 0 | 148 | 13 | 0 | 0.061 | 0.1 | 0 | 0.1 | 0.01 | 0.03 | 9.8 | 9340 |
| **pear**, canned in light syrup | 251 | 143 | 212.0 | 38.1 | 30.4 | 15.1 | 4.0 | 13 | 13 | 10 | 0.20 | 0.083 | 0 | 2 | 0.03 | 0.4 | 0 | 0.06 |
| *1 cup halves* | | 0.5 | 0.1 | 0 | 0 | 0 | 0 | 166 | 18 | 0.70 | 0.123 | 0 | 0 | 0.2 | 0.04 | 0.04 | 2.5 | 9256 |
| **pear**, cnd in heavy syrup, drained | 266 | 197 | 213.7 | 50.8 | 43.7 | 26.2 | 7.2 | 13 | 16 | 11 | 0.21 | | 0 | 3 | 0.03 | 0.6 | 0 | |
| *1 cup halves* | | 0.6 | 0.5 | 0 | 0.1 | 0.1 | 0 | 176 | 21 | 0.59 | 0.162 | 0.3 | 21 | 0.3 | 0.06 | 0.04 | 2.7 | 9374 |
| **pear**, cnd in heavy syrup, solids | 266 | 197 | 213.7 | 51.0 | 40.4 | 24.2 | 4.3 | 13 | 13 | 11 | 0.21 | 0.085 | 0 | 3 | 0.03 | 0.6 | 0 | 0.06 |
| and liquid - *1 cup halves* | | 0.5 | 0.3 | 0 | 0.1 | 0.1 | 0 | 173 | 19 | 0.59 | 0.130 | 0 | 0 | 0.2 | 0.06 | 0.04 | 2.7 | 9257 |
| **pear**, cnd in juice | 248 | 124 | 214.4 | 32.1 | 24.1 | 0 | 4.0 | 10 | 22 | 17 | 0.22 | 0.084 | 0 | 4 | 0.03 | 0.5 | 0 | 0.05 |
| *1 cup halves* | | 0.8 | 0.2 | 0 | 0 | 0 | 0 | 238 | 30 | 0.72 | 0.131 | 0 | 15 | 0.2 | 0.03 | 0.03 | 2.5 | 9254 |
| **pear**, cnd in water | 244 | 71 | 224.0 | 19.1 | 14.9 | 0 | 3.9 | 5 | 10 | 10 | 0.22 | 0.083 | 0 | 2 | 0.02 | 0.1 | 0 | 0.05 |
| *1 cup halves* | | 0.5 | 0.1 | 0 | 0 | 0 | 0 | 129 | 17 | 0.51 | 0.124 | 0 | 0 | 0.2 | 0.02 | 0.03 | 2.4 | 9253 |
| **pear**, dried | 175 | 458 | 46.7 | 122.0 | 108.8 | 0 | 13.1 | 10 | 60 | 58 | 0.68 | 0.572 | 0 | 12 | 0.01 | 2.4 | 0 | 0.27 |
| *10 halves* | | 3.3 | 1.1 | 0.1 | 0.2 | 0.3 | 0 | 933 | 103 | 3.68 | 0.649 | 0.4 | 5 | 0.1 | 0.25 | 0.13 | 0 | 9259 |
| **pear**, raw | 166 | 96 | 139.0 | 25.7 | 16.3 | 0 | 5.1 | 2 | 15 | 12 | 0.17 | 0.081 | 2 | 7 | 0.02 | 0.3 | 0 | 0.08 |
| *1 medium (2½" diameter)* | | 0.6 | 0.2 | 0 | 0 | 0 | 0 | 198 | 18 | 0.28 | 0.136 | 0.2 | 38 | 0.2 | 0.04 | 0.05 | 11.6 | 9252 |
| **persimmon, Japanese**, dried | 34 | 93 | 7.8 | 25.0 | | | 4.9 | 1 | 8 | 11 | 0.14 | 0.473 | 13 | 0 | | 0.1 | 0 | |
| *1 medium* | | 0.5 | 0.2 | | | | 0 | 273 | 28 | 0.25 | 0.150 | | 261 | | 0.01 | | | 9264 |
| **persimmon, Japanese**, raw | 168 | 118 | 134.9 | 31.2 | 21.1 | 0 | 6.0 | 2 | 13 | 15 | 0.18 | 0.596 | 136 | 13 | 0.05 | 0.2 | 0 | |
| *1 medium (2½ diameter)* | | 1.0 | 0.3 | 0 | 0.1 | 0.1 | 0 | 270 | 29 | 0.25 | 0.190 | 1.0 | 2733 | 1.2 | 0.03 | 0.17 | 13.4 | 9263 |
| **persimmon**, raw | 25 | 32 | 16.1 | 8.4 | | | | 0 | 7 | | | | | 16 | | | 0 | |
| *1 medium* | | 0.2 | 0.1 | | | | 0 | 78 | 6 | 0.62 | | | | | | | | 9265 |
| **pineapple**, canned in heavy syrup | 254 | 198 | 200.6 | 51.3 | 42.9 | 23.9 | 2.0 | 3 | 36 | 41 | 0.30 | 2.743 | 3 | 19 | 0.23 | 0.7 | 0 | 0.25 |
| *1 cup pieces* | | 0.9 | 0.3 | 0 | 0 | 0.1 | 0 | 264 | 18 | 0.97 | 0.257 | 1.0 | 36 | 0 | 0.06 | 0.19 | 12.7 | 9270 |
| **pineapple**, canned in juice, drained | 249 | 149 | 207.9 | 38.7 | 35.5 | 0 | 3.2 | 2 | 40 | 37 | 0.25 | | 7 | 23 | 0.25 | 0.7 | 0 | |
| *1 cup pieces* | | 1.3 | 0.3 | 0 | 0 | 0.1 | 0 | 309 | 17 | 0.70 | 0.266 | 1.0 | 125 | 0 | 0.05 | 0.19 | 12.5 | 9354 |
| **pineapple**, canned in juice, solids | 249 | 149 | 207.9 | 39.1 | 36.0 | 0 | 2.0 | 2 | 35 | 35 | 0.25 | 2.791 | 5 | 24 | 0.24 | 0.7 | 0 | 0.25 |
| and liquid - *1 cup pieces* | | 1.0 | 0.2 | 0 | 0 | 0.1 | 0 | 304 | 15 | 0.70 | 0.214 | 1.0 | 95 | 0 | 0.05 | 0.18 | 12.5 | 9268 |
| **pineapple**, raw | 155 | 78 | 133.3 | 20.3 | 15.3 | 0 | 2.2 | 2 | 20 | 19 | 0.19 | 1.437 | 5 | 74 | 0.12 | 0.8 | 0 | 0.33 |
| *1 cup pieces* | | 0.8 | 0.2 | 0 | 0 | 0.1 | 0 | 169 | 12 | 0.45 | 0.170 | 0.2 | 90 | 0 | 0.05 | 0.17 | 27.9 | 9266 |

| | WT (g) | KCAL | H₂0 (g) | CHO (g) | TSUG (g) | ASUG (g) | DFIB (g) | Na (mg) | Ca (mg) | Mg (mg) | Zn (mg) | Mn (mg) | A (mcg RAE) | C (mg) | B-1 (mg) | NIA (mg) | B-12 (mcg) | PANT (mg) |
|---|---|---|---|---|---|---|---|---|---|---|---|---|---|---|---|---|---|---|
| | | PRO (g) | FAT (g) | SFA (g) | MUFA (g) | PUFA (g) | CHOL (mg) | K (mg) | P (mg) | Fe (mg) | Cu (mg) | Se (mcg) | A (IU) | E (mg ATE) | B-2 (mg) | B-6 (mg) | FOL (mcg DFE) | REF |
| **pitanga** (surinam cherry), raw | 173 | 57 | 157.1 | 13.0 | | | | 5 | 16 | 21 | | | 130 | 45 | 0.05 | 0.5 | 0 | |
| 1 cup | | 1.4 | 0.7 | | | | 0 | 178 | 19 | 0.35 | | | 2595 | | 0.07 | | | 9276 |
| **plum,** canned in heavy syrup, drained - 1 plum with liquid | 46 | 41 | 35.0 | 10.6 | 9.9 | 5.5 | 0.7 | 9 | 5 | 2 | 0.03 | | 9 | 0 | 0.01 | 0.1 | 0 | |
| | | 0.2 | 0.1 | 0 | 0 | 0 | 0 | 43 | 7 | 0.39 | 0.021 | 0 | 184 | 0.1 | 0.02 | 0.01 | 1.4 | 9379 |
| **plum,** cnd in hvy syrp, solids and lqd - 1 plum with liquid | 46 | 41 | 35.0 | 10.7 | 10.3 | 5.6 | 0.4 | 9 | 4 | 2 | 0.03 | 0.014 | 6 | 0 | 0.01 | 0.1 | 0 | 0.03 |
| | | 0.2 | 0 | 0 | 0 | 0 | 0 | 42 | 6 | 0.39 | 0.017 | 0 | 119 | 0.1 | 0.01 | 0.01 | 1.4 | 9284 |
| **plum,** canned in juice | 46 | 27 | 38.6 | 7.0 | 6.5 | 0 | 0.4 | 0 | 5 | 4 | 0.05 | 0.015 | 23 | 1 | 0.01 | 0.2 | 0 | 0.03 |
| 1 plum with liquid | | 0.2 | 0 | 0 | 0 | 0 | 0 | 71 | 7 | 0.16 | 0.025 | 0 | 464 | 0.1 | 0.03 | 0.01 | 1.4 | 9282 |
| **plum,** raw | 66 | 30 | 57.6 | 7.5 | 6.5 | 0 | 0.9 | 0 | 4 | 5 | 0.07 | 0.034 | 11 | 6 | 0.02 | 0.3 | 0 | 0.09 |
| 1 medium (2⅛" diameter) | | 0.5 | 0.2 | 0 | 0.1 | 0 | 0 | 104 | 11 | 0.11 | 0.038 | 0 | 228 | 0.2 | 0.02 | 0.02 | 3.3 | 9279 |
| **pomegranate,** raw | 154 | 128 | 120.0 | 28.8 | 21.1 | 0 | 6.2 | 5 | 15 | 18 | 0.54 | 0.183 | 0 | 16 | 0.10 | 0.5 | 0 | 0.58 |
| 1 medium (3⅜" diameter) | | 2.6 | 1.8 | 0.2 | 0.1 | 0.1 | 0 | 363 | 55 | 0.46 | 0.243 | 0.8 | 0 | 0.9 | 0.08 | 0.12 | 58.5 | 9286 |
| **prickly pear fruit,** raw | 103 | 42 | 90.2 | 9.9 | | | 3.7 | 5 | 58 | 88 | 0.12 | | 2 | 14 | 0.01 | 0.5 | 0 | |
| 1 medium | | 0.8 | 0.5 | 0.1 | 0.1 | 0.2 | 0 | 227 | 25 | 0.31 | 0.082 | 0.6 | 44 | | 0.06 | 0.06 | 6.2 | 9287 |
| **prune,** canned in heavy syrup | 86 | 90 | 60.8 | 23.9 | | | 3.3 | 3 | 15 | 13 | 0.16 | 0.084 | 34 | 2 | 0.03 | 0.7 | 0 | 0.09 |
| 5 prunes with liquid | | 0.7 | 0.2 | 0 | 0.1 | 0 | 0 | 194 | 22 | 0.35 | 0.101 | | 685 | | 0.10 | 0.17 | 0 | 9288 |
| **prune,** dried | 16 | 38 | 4.9 | 10.2 | 6.1 | 0 | 1.1 | 0 | 7 | 7 | 0.07 | 0.048 | 6 | 0 | 0.01 | 0.3 | 0 | 0.07 |
| 2 prunes | | 0.3 | 0.1 | 0 | 0 | 0 | 0 | 117 | 11 | 0.15 | 0.045 | 0 | 125 | 0.1 | 0.03 | 0.03 | 0.6 | 9291 |
| **prune,** dried, stewed | 248 | 265 | 172.9 | 69.6 | 62.0 | 0 | 7.7 | 2 | 47 | 45 | 0.47 | 0.325 | 42 | 7 | 0.06 | 1.8 | 0 | 0.27 |
| 1 cup pitted | | 2.4 | 0.4 | 0 | 0.2 | 0.1 | 0 | 796 | 74 | 1.02 | 0.305 | 0.2 | 848 | 0.5 | 0.25 | 0.54 | 0 | 9292 |
| **prune puree** | 28 | 72 | 8.4 | 18.2 | 10.9 | | 0.9 | 6 | 9 | | | | 28 | 1 | 0.01 | 0.7 | | 0.12 |
| 1 oz | | 0.6 | 0.1 | 0 | | | 0 | 239 | 20 | 0.78 | | | 560 | | | | | 9423 |
| **pummelo,** raw | 190 | 72 | 169.3 | 18.3 | | | 1.9 | 2 | 8 | 11 | 0.15 | 0.032 | 0 | 116 | 0.06 | 0.4 | 0 | |
| 1 cup pieces | | 1.4 | 0.1 | | | | 0 | 410 | 32 | 0.21 | 0.091 | | 15 | | 0.05 | 0.07 | | 9295 |
| **quince,** raw | 92 | 52 | 77.1 | 14.1 | | | 1.7 | 4 | 10 | 7 | 0.04 | | 2 | 14 | 0.02 | 0.2 | 0 | 0.07 |
| 1 medium | | 0.4 | 0.1 | 0 | 0 | 0 | 0 | 181 | 16 | 0.64 | 0.120 | 0.6 | 37 | | 0.03 | 0.04 | 2.8 | 9296 |
| **raisins,** seeded | 73 | 216 | 12.1 | 57.3 | | | 5.0 | 20 | 20 | 22 | 0.13 | 0.195 | 0 | 4 | 0.08 | 0.8 | 0 | 0.03 |
| ½ cup | | 1.8 | 0.4 | 0.1 | 0 | 0.1 | 0 | 602 | 55 | 1.89 | 0.220 | 0.4 | 0 | | 0.13 | 0.14 | 2.2 | 9299 |
| **raisins,** seedless | 43 | 129 | 6.6 | 34.0 | 25.5 | 0 | 1.6 | 5 | 22 | 14 | 0.09 | 0.129 | 0 | 1 | 0.05 | 0.3 | 0 | 0.04 |
| 1.5 oz box (snack size) | | 1.3 | 0.2 | 0 | 0 | 0 | 0 | 322 | 43 | 0.81 | 0.137 | 0.3 | 0 | 0.1 | 0.05 | 0.07 | 2.2 | 9298 |
| **raisins,** seedless, golden | 73 | 220 | 10.9 | 58.0 | 43.2 | 0 | 2.9 | 9 | 39 | 26 | 0.23 | 0.225 | 0 | 2 | 0.01 | 0.8 | 0 | 0.10 |
| ½ cup | | 2.5 | 0.3 | 0.1 | 0 | 0.1 | 0 | 545 | 84 | 1.31 | 0.265 | 0.5 | 0 | 0.1 | 0.14 | 0.24 | 2.2 | 9297 |
| **rambutan,** canned in syrup | 214 | 175 | 167.0 | 44.7 | | | 1.9 | 24 | 47 | 15 | 0.17 | 0.734 | 0 | 10 | 0.03 | 2.9 | 0 | 0.04 |
| 1 cup | | 1.4 | 0.4 | | | | 0 | 90 | 19 | 0.75 | 0.141 | | 6 | | 0.05 | 0.04 | 17.1 | 9301 |
| **raspberries,** canned in heavy syrup | 256 | 233 | 192.8 | 59.8 | 51.4 | 40.0 | 8.4 | 8 | 28 | 31 | 0.41 | 0.596 | 5 | 22 | 0.05 | 1.1 | 0 | 0.63 |
| 1 cup | | 2.1 | 0.3 | 0 | 0 | 0.2 | 0 | 241 | 23 | 1.08 | 0.146 | 0.3 | 84 | 1.5 | 0.08 | 0.11 | 28.2 | 9304 |
| **raspberries,** raw | 123 | 64 | 105.5 | 14.7 | 5.4 | 0 | 8.0 | 1 | 31 | 27 | 0.52 | 0.824 | 2 | 32 | 0.04 | 0.7 | 0 | 0.40 |
| 1 cup | | 1.5 | 0.8 | 0 | 0.1 | 0.5 | 0 | 186 | 36 | 0.85 | 0.111 | 0.2 | 41 | 1.1 | 0.05 | 0.07 | 25.8 | 9302 |
| **raspberries,** sweetened, frozen | 250 | 258 | 181.9 | 65.4 | 54.4 | 43.4 | 11.0 | 2 | 38 | 32 | 0.45 | 1.625 | 8 | 41 | 0.05 | 0.6 | 0 | 0.38 |
| 1 cup | | 1.8 | 0.4 | 0 | 0 | 0.2 | 0 | 285 | 42 | 1.62 | 0.262 | 0.8 | 150 | 1.8 | 0.11 | 0.08 | 65.0 | 9306 |
| **rose apple,** raw | 100 | 25 | 93.0 | 5.7 | | | | 0 | 29 | 5 | 0.06 | 0.029 | 17 | 22 | 0.02 | 0.8 | 0 | |
| 3.5 oz | | 0.6 | 0.3 | | | | 0 | 123 | 8 | 0.07 | 0.016 | | 339 | | 0.03 | | | 9312 |
| **roselle,** raw | 57 | 28 | 49.4 | 6.4 | | | | 3 | 123 | 29 | | | 8 | 7 | 0.01 | 0.2 | 0 | |
| 1 cup | | 0.5 | 0.4 | | | | 0 | 119 | 21 | 0.84 | | | 164 | | 0.02 | | | 9311 |
| **rowal,** raw | 228 | 253 | 162.8 | 54.5 | 32.1 | | 14.1 | 9 | 34 | 73 | 0.98 | 0.353 | 43 | 59 | | | | |
| 1 cup | | 5.2 | 4.6 | 0.6 | | | | 299 | 119 | 5.02 | 2.417 | | 873 | | | | | 9428 |
| **salmonberries,** raw | 100 | 47 | 88.2 | 10.0 | 3.7 | | 1.9 | 14 | 13 | 15 | 0.28 | 1.100 | 50 | 9 | 0.04 | 0.5 | | 0.17 |
| 3.5 oz | | 0.8 | 0.3 | | | | | 110 | 27 | 0.40 | 0.030 | | 496 | 1.6 | 0.06 | 0.08 | 17.0 | 35154 |
| **sapodilla,** raw | 170 | 141 | 132.6 | 33.9 | | | 9.0 | 20 | 36 | 20 | 0.17 | | 5 | 25 | 0 | 0.3 | 0 | 0.43 |
| 1 medium | | 0.7 | 1.9 | 0.3 | 0.9 | 0 | 0 | 328 | 20 | 1.36 | 0.146 | 1.0 | 102 | | 0.03 | 0.06 | 23.8 | 9313 |
| **sapote,** raw | 225 | 302 | 140.5 | 76.0 | | | 5.9 | 22 | 88 | 68 | | | 47 | 45 | 0.02 | 4.0 | 0 | |
| 1 medium | | 4.8 | 1.3 | | | | 0 | 774 | 63 | 2.25 | | | 922 | | 0.04 | | | 9314 |
| **soursop,** raw | 225 | 148 | 182.6 | 37.9 | 30.5 | 0 | 7.4 | 32 | 32 | 47 | 0.22 | | 0 | 46 | 0.16 | 2.0 | 0 | 0.57 |
| 1 cup | | 2.2 | 0.7 | 0.1 | 0.2 | 0.2 | 0 | 626 | 61 | 1.35 | 0.193 | 1.3 | 4 | 0.2 | 0.11 | 0.13 | 31.5 | 9315 |
| **strawberries,** raw | 144 | 46 | 131.0 | 11.1 | 7.0 | 0 | 2.9 | 1 | 23 | 19 | 0.20 | 0.556 | 1 | 85 | 0.03 | 0.6 | 0 | |
| 1 cup whole | | 1.0 | 0.4 | 0 | 0.1 | 0.2 | 0 | 220 | 35 | 0.59 | 0.069 | 0.6 | 17 | 0.4 | 0.03 | 0.07 | 34.6 | 9316 |
| **strawberries,** swtnd, frzn, thawed | 255 | 199 | 199.0 | 53.6 | 47.5 | 36.8 | 4.8 | 3 | 28 | 15 | 0.13 | 0.635 | 3 | 101 | 0.04 | 0.7 | 0 | 0.28 |
| 1 cup | | 1.3 | 0.4 | 0 | 0 | 0.2 | 0 | 250 | 31 | 1.20 | 0.048 | 1.8 | 69 | 0.6 | 0.20 | 0.07 | 10.2 | 9319 |
| **strawberries,** unswtnd, frzn, thawed | 221 | 77 | 198.8 | 20.2 | 10.1 | 0 | 4.6 | 4 | 35 | 24 | 0.29 | 0.641 | 4 | 91 | 0.05 | 1.0 | 0 | 0.24 |
| 1 cup | | 1.0 | 0.2 | 0 | 0 | 0.1 | 0 | 327 | 29 | 1.66 | 0.108 | 1.5 | 99 | 0.6 | 0.08 | 0.06 | 37.6 | 9318 |
| **strawberry guava,** raw | 244 | 168 | 196.8 | 42.4 | | | 13.2 | 90 | 51 | 41 | | | 12 | 90 | 0.07 | 1.5 | 0 | |
| 1 cup | | 1.4 | 1.5 | 0.4 | 0.1 | 0.6 | 0 | 712 | 66 | 0.54 | | | 220 | | 0.07 | | | 9140 |

| | WT (g) | KCAL | $H_2O$ (g) | CHO (g) | TSUG (g) | ASUG (g) | DFIB (g) | Na (mg) | Ca (mg) | Mg (mg) | Zn (mg) | Mn (mg) | A (mcg RAE) | C (mg) | B-1 (mg) | NIA (mg) | B-12 (mcg) | PANT (mg) |
|---|---|---|---|---|---|---|---|---|---|---|---|---|---|---|---|---|---|---|
| | | PRO (g) | FAT (g) | SFA (g) | MUFA (g) | PUFA (g) | CHOL (mg) | K (mg) | P (mg) | Fe (mg) | Cu (mg) | Se (mcg) | A (IU) | E (mg ATE) | B-2 (mg) | B-6 (mg) | FOL (mcg DFE) | REF |
| **sugar apple**, raw | 155 | 146 | 113.5 | 36.6 | | | 6.8 | 14 | 37 | 33 | 0.16 | | 0 | 56 | 0.17 | 1.4 | 0 | 0.35 |
| *1 medium (2⅞" diameter)* | | 3.2 | 0.4 | 0.1 | 0.2 | 0.1 | 0 | 383 | 50 | 0.93 | 0.133 | 0.9 | 9 | | 0.18 | 0.31 | 21.7 | 9321 |
| **tamarind**, raw | 120 | 287 | 37.7 | 75.0 | 68.9 | 0 | 6.1 | 34 | 89 | 110 | 0.12 | | 2 | 4 | 0.51 | 2.3 | 0 | 0.17 |
| *1 cup* | | 3.4 | 0.7 | 0.3 | 0.2 | 0.1 | 0 | 754 | 136 | 3.36 | 0.103 | 1.6 | 36 | 0.1 | 0.18 | 0.08 | 16.8 | 9322 |
| **tangerine**, raw | 84 | 45 | 71.5 | 11.2 | 8.9 | 0 | 1.5 | 2 | 31 | 10 | 0.06 | 0.033 | 29 | 22 | 0.05 | 0.3 | 0 | 0.18 |
| *1 medium (2⅜" diameter)* | | 0.7 | 0.3 | 0 | 0.1 | 0.1 | 0 | 139 | 17 | 0.13 | 0.035 | 0.1 | 572 | 0.2 | 0.03 | 0.07 | 13.4 | 9218 |
| **watermelon**, raw | 152 | 46 | 139.0 | 11.5 | 9.4 | 0 | 0.6 | 2 | 11 | 15 | 0.15 | 0.058 | 43 | 12 | 0.05 | 0.3 | 0 | 0.34 |
| *1 cup pieces* | | 0.9 | 0.2 | 0 | 0.1 | 0.1 | 0 | 170 | 17 | 0.36 | 0.064 | 0.6 | 865 | 0.1 | 0.03 | 0.07 | 4.6 | 9326 |

## 16. GRAIN- AND VEGETABLE-BASED SNACK FOODS

| | WT (g) | KCAL | $H_2O$ (g) | CHO (g) | TSUG (g) | ASUG (g) | DFIB (g) | Na (mg) | Ca (mg) | Mg (mg) | Zn (mg) | Mn (mg) | A (mcg RAE) | C (mg) | B-1 (mg) | NIA (mg) | B-12 (mcg) | PANT (mg) |
|---|---|---|---|---|---|---|---|---|---|---|---|---|---|---|---|---|---|---|
| | | PRO (g) | FAT (g) | SFA (g) | MUFA (g) | PUFA (g) | CHOL (mg) | K (mg) | P (mg) | Fe (mg) | Cu (mg) | Se (mcg) | A (IU) | E (mg ATE) | B-2 (mg) | B-6 (mg) | FOL (mcg DFE) | REF |
| **Bugles**, Betty Crocker | 30 | 160 | | 18.0 | 1.0 | | 0.5 | 310 | 0 | | | | | 0 | | | | |
| *1⅓ cups (1.06 oz)* | | 1.0 | 9.0 | 8.0 | | | 0 | | | 0 | | | 0 | | | | | GENM213 |
| **cereal bar**, All-Bran brn sugar cinn, | 35 | 130 | | 27.0 | 11.0 | | 5.0 | 180 | 0 | | | | | 0 | 0.15 | 2.0 | 0.60 | |
| Kellogg's - *1.2 oz bar* | | 2.0 | 3.0 | 0.5 | | | 0 | | | 1.80 | | | 500 | | 0.17 | 0.20 | | KELL4 |
| **cereal bar**, All-Bran honey oat, | 35 | 130 | | 27.0 | 11.0 | | 5.0 | 170 | 0 | | 0.60 | | | 0 | 0.15 | 2.0 | 0.60 | |
| Kellogg's - *1.2 oz bar* | | 2.0 | 3.0 | 0.5 | | | 0 | | | 1.80 | | | 500 | | 0.17 | 0.20 | | KELL5 |
| **cereal bar**, All-Bran oatmeal raisin, | 35 | 120 | | 26.0 | 12.0 | | 5.0 | 170 | 0 | | | | | 0 | 0.15 | 2.0 | 0.60 | |
| Kellogg's - *1.2 oz bar* | | 2.0 | 0.5 | 0 | | | 0 | | | 1.80 | | | 500 | | 0.17 | 0.20 | | KELL6 |
| **cereal bar**, cinn, Smart Start Healthy | 40 | 150 | | 30.0 | 12.0 | | 2.0 | 85 | 0 | | | | | 0 | 0.15 | 2.0 | | |
| Heart Bar - *1.4 oz bar* | | 3.0 | 2.5 | 0 | | | 0 | | | 0.72 | | | 500 | | 0.17 | 0.20 | | KELL7 |
| **cereal bar**, fruit, Nutri-Grain | 37 | 139 | 5.4 | 26.8 | 13.0 | | 0.8 | 110 | 200 | 10 | 1.52 | | 225 | 0 | 0.37 | 5.0 | 0 | 0 |
| *1.3 oz bar* | | 1.6 | 2.8 | 0.4 | 1.9 | 0.3 | 0 | 73 | 38 | 1.80 | 0.037 | 3.9 | 750 | 0.2 | 0.41 | 0.52 | 65.5 | 19441 |
| **cereal bar**, mixed berry, Kellogg's | 37 | 137 | 5.4 | 26.9 | 12.4 | | 0.7 | 110 | 14 | 10 | 1.52 | | | 0 | 0.37 | 5.0 | 0 | 0 |
| Nutri-Grain - *1.3 oz bar* | | 1.6 | 2.8 | 0.6 | 1.8 | 0.4 | 0 | 70 | 36 | 1.81 | 0.037 | | 750 | | 0.41 | 0.52 | | 18501 |
| **cereal bar**, multigrain apple cinn, | 37 | 140 | | 28.0 | 14.0 | | 1.0 | 80 | 0 | | | | | 0 | | | | |
| Nature's Choice - *1 bar* | | 2.0 | 2.0 | 0 | | | 0 | | | 0.36 | | | 0 | | | | | BARB9 |
| **cereal bar**, multigrain blueberry, | 37 | 150 | | 29.0 | 15.0 | | 2.0 | 85 | 0 | | | | | 0 | | | | |
| Nature's Choice - *1 bar* | | 2.0 | 2.0 | 0 | | | 0 | | | 0.36 | | | 0 | | | | | BARB10 |
| **cereal bar**, multigrain cherry, | 37 | 150 | | 28.0 | 14.0 | | 1.0 | 80 | 0 | | | | | 0 | | | | |
| Nature's Choice - *1 bar* | | 2.0 | 2.0 | 0 | | | 0 | | | 0.36 | | | 0 | | | | | BARB11 |
| **cereal bar**, multigrain raspberry, | 37 | 150 | | 29.0 | 15.0 | | 2.0 | 85 | 0 | | | | | 0 | | | | |
| Nature's Choice - *1 bar* | | 2.0 | 2.0 | 0 | | | 0 | | | 0.36 | | | 0 | | | | | BARB12 |
| **cereal bar**, multigrain strawberry, | 37 | 150 | | 29.0 | 15.0 | | 2.0 | 85 | 0 | | | | | 0 | | | | |
| Nature's Choice - *1 bar* | | 2.0 | 2.0 | 0 | | | 0 | | | 0.36 | | | 0 | | | | | BARB13 |
| **cereal bar**, multigrain triple berry, | 37 | 150 | | 29.0 | 15.0 | | 2.0 | 85 | 0 | | | | | 0 | | | | |
| Nature's Choice - *1 bar* | | 2.0 | 2.0 | 0 | | | 0 | | | 0.36 | | | 0 | | | | | BARB14 |
| **cereal bar**, whole grain, choc chip, | 28 | 118 | 1.4 | 20.2 | 10.9 | | 0.7 | 69 | 304 | 20 | 0.39 | 0.299 | 4 | 0 | 0.05 | 0.4 | 0.04 | 0.13 |
| Kudos - *1 oz bar* | | 1.3 | 3.6 | 1.3 | 1.3 | 0.8 | 0 | 78 | 58 | 0.39 | 0.087 | | 16 | 3.0 | 0.06 | 0.03 | 3.6 | 19440 |
| **cereal bar**, whole grain, M&M's, | 24 | 100 | 1.9 | 17.5 | 9.1 | | 0.6 | 82 | 226 | | | | | 0 | | | | |
| Kudos - *.85 oz bar* | | 0.9 | 2.9 | 1.6 | | | 1 | | | 0.20 | | | 12 | | | | | 25009 |
| **cereal bar**, whole grain, peanut | 28 | 130 | 2.0 | 18.1 | 12.4 | | 0.7 | 75 | 244 | | | | | 0 | | | | |
| butter, Kudos - *1 oz bar* | | 1.6 | 5.8 | 2.9 | | | 1 | | | 0.25 | | | 20 | | | | | 25007 |
| **Cheese Puff Bakes**, Barbara's | 28 | 160 | | 13.0 | 1.0 | | | 190 | 40 | | | | | 2 | | | | |
| Bakery - *¾ cup* | | 2.0 | 11.0 | 2.0 | | | 0 | | | 0.36 | | | 0 | | | | | BARB15 |
| **Cheese Puff Bakes**, white cheddar, | 28 | 160 | | 13.0 | 1.0 | | | 190 | 40 | | | | | 2 | | | | |
| Barbara's Bakery - *½ cup* | | 2.0 | 11.0 | 2.0 | | | 0 | | | 0.36 | | | 0 | | | | | BARB16 |
| **Cheese Puffs**, Barbara's Bakery | 28 | 150 | | 16.0 | 0 | | | 130 | 20 | | | | | 2 | | | | |
| *¾ cup* | | 2.0 | 10.0 | 1.5 | | | 0 | | | 0 | | | 0 | | | | | BARB17 |
| **Cheese Puffs**, jalapeno, Barbara's | 28 | 150 | | 16.0 | 0 | | | 130 | 20 | | | | | 2 | | | | |
| Bakery - *¾ cup* | | 2.0 | 10.0 | 1.5 | | | 0 | | | 0 | | | 0 | | | | | BARB18 |
| **cheese puffs/twists** | 28 | 158 | 0.5 | 14.7 | 0.8 | 0 | 0.5 | 255 | 16 | 5 | 0.15 | 0.025 | 11 | 0 | 0.04 | 1.3 | 0.13 | 0.27 |
| *1 oz* | | 1.6 | 10.4 | 1.6 | 2.9 | 5.3 | 2 | 53 | 36 | 0.49 | 0.013 | 2.3 | 36 | 1.3 | 0.04 | 0.02 | 24.6 | 19008 |
| **Cheese Twists**, Snyder | 28 | 140 | | 15.0 | 1.0 | | 0 | 230 | 20 | | | | | 0 | | | | |
| *1 oz* | | 2.0 | 8.0 | 1.0 | | | | | | 0 | | | 5 | | | | | SNYD25 |
| **Chewy Nut Bar**, sweet and salty | 45 | 220 | | 22.0 | 8.0 | | 6.0 | 65 | 250 | | | | | 6 | | | | |
| almond, Odwalla - *1.6 oz bar* | | 7.0 | 11.0 | 1.0 | | | 0 | 210 | | 1.44 | | | 500 | | | | | ODWA40 |
| **Chewy Nut Bar**, sweet and salty | 45 | 190 | | 28.0 | 12.0 | | 2.0 | 180 | 250 | | | | | 6 | | | | |
| peanut Odwalla - *1.6 oz bar* | | 5.0 | 6.0 | 1.0 | | | 0 | 160 | | 1.08 | | | 500 | | | | | ODWA41 |
| **Chewy Nut Bar**, trail mix, Odwalla | 45 | 190 | | 27.0 | 11.0 | | 3.0 | 65 | 250 | | | | | 6 | | | | |
| *1.6 oz bar* | | 5.0 | 7.0 | 1.5 | | | 0 | 200 | | 1.44 | | | 500 | | | | | ODWA42 |

| Food | WT (g) | KCAL / PRO (g) | $H_2O$ / FAT (g) | CHO / SFA (g) | TSUG / MUFA (g) | ASUG / PUFA (g) | DFIB (g) / CHOL (mg) | Na / K (mg) | Ca / P (mg) | Mg / Fe (mg) | Zn / Cu (mg) | Mn (mg) / Se (mcg) | A (mcg RAE) / A (IU) | C (mg) / E (mg ATE) | B-1 / B-2 (mg) | NIA / B-6 (mg) | B-12 (mcg) / FOL (mcg DFE) | PANT (mg) / REF |
|---|---|---|---|---|---|---|---|---|---|---|---|---|---|---|---|---|---|---|
| Chex Mix | 28 | 119 | 0.7 | 20.9 | 1.4 |  | 1.1 | 337 | 10 | 11 | 0.30 | 0.231 | 0 |  | 0.10 | 1.2 |  | 0.13 |
| *⅔ cup (1 oz)* |  | 2.5 | 2.8 | 0.4 | 0.8 | 1.3 |  | 55 | 43 | 0.84 | 0.041 | 2.8 | 0 |  | 0.06 | 0.03 | 23.8 | 19033 |
| **Chex Snack Mixes**, Betty Crocker | 49 | 210 |  | 36.0 | 3.0 |  | 2.0 | 620 | 0 |  |  |  |  | 0 |  |  |  |  |
| *1.7 oz pouch* |  | 4.0 | 6.0 | 1.0 |  |  | 0 |  |  | 0.72 |  |  | 0 |  |  |  |  | GENM215 |
| **corn-based cones** | 28 | 143 | 0.6 | 17.6 |  |  | 0.3 | 286 | 1 | 3 | 0.06 | 0.024 | 4 | 0 | 0.09 | 0.4 | 0 | 0.06 |
| *1 oz* |  | 1.6 | 7.5 | 6.4 | 0.5 | 0.2 | 0 | 23 | 12 | 0.71 | 0.011 | 1.1 | 89 |  | 0.07 | 0.01 | 0.8 | 19005 |
| **corn-based cones**, nacho | 28 | 150 | 0.5 | 16.0 |  |  | 0.3 | 267 | 10 | 7 | 0.13 | 0.022 | 7 | 0 | 0.06 | 0.4 | 0 | 0.11 |
| *1 oz* |  | 1.8 | 8.9 | 7.5 | 0.6 | 0.2 | 1 | 34 | 21 | 0.36 | 0.017 | 1.1 | 88 |  | 0.03 | 0.03 | 1.4 | 19006 |
| **corn-based onion flavor snack food** - 1 oz | 28 | 140 | 0.6 | 18.2 | 1.4 | 0.4 | 1.1 | 275 | 8 | 8 | 0.09 | 0.057 | 2 | 1 | 0.06 | 0.9 | 0 | 0.07 |
|  |  | 2.2 | 6.3 | 1.2 | 3.7 | 0.9 | 0 | 40 | 20 | 1.04 | 0.033 | 3.0 | 34 | 0.8 | 0.09 | 0.04 | 49.3 | 19007 |
| **corn chips** | 28 | 145 | 0.1 | 17.6 | 0.3 | 0 | 1.5 | 172 | 46 | 24 | 0.44 | 0.122 | 0 | 0 | 0 | 0.1 | 0 | 0.16 |
| *1 oz* |  | 1.7 | 8.0 | 1.0 | 2.2 | 3.9 | 0 | 38 | 44 | 0.37 | 0.061 | 1.9 | 0 | 0.4 | 0.18 | 0.03 | 3.6 | 19003 |
| **corn chips**, barbecue | 28 | 146 | 0.3 | 15.7 |  |  | 1.5 | 214 | 37 | 22 | 0.30 | 0.217 | 9 | 0 | 0.02 | 0.5 | 0 | 0.04 |
| *1 oz* |  | 2.0 | 9.2 | 1.2 | 2.7 | 4.5 | 0 | 66 | 58 | 0.43 | 0.046 | 1.1 | 171 |  | 0.06 | 0.06 | 10.9 | 19004 |
| **Cracker Jack**, Frito-Lay | 28 | 120 |  | 23.0 | 15.0 |  | 1.0 | 70 | 0 |  |  |  |  | 0 |  |  |  |  |
| *½ cup* |  | 2.0 | 2.0 | 0 |  |  | 0 |  |  | 0.72 |  |  | 0 |  |  |  |  | FRIT1 |
| **crisped rice bar w/choc chips** | 28 | 113 | 0.7 | 20.4 |  |  | 0.6 | 78 | 6 | 13 | 0.24 | 0.280 |  | 2.0 | 0.15 |  | 0 | 0 |
| *1 oz bar* |  | 1.4 | 3.8 | 1.5 | 1.1 | 1.0 | 0 | 47 | 38 | 1.76 | 0.087 | 2.7 | 494 |  | 0.17 | 0.20 | 39.2 | 19010 |
| **Doo Dads**, Nabisco | 28 | 128 | 0.8 | 18.0 |  |  | 1.9 | 356 | 21 | 17 | 0.63 | 0.494 | 12 | 0 | 0.10 | 1.5 | 0 | 0.16 |
| *½ cup (1 oz)* |  | 2.9 | 5.2 | 1.0 |  |  | 0 | 78 | 83 | 0.70 | 0.090 |  | 42 |  | 0.07 | 0.06 | 40.3 | 19032 |
| **fruit & yogurt bar**, apple cinnamon, Barbara's Bakery - 1 bar | 42 | 150 |  | 28.0 | 15.0 |  | 1.0 | 125 | 250 |  | 1.50 |  |  | 6 | 0.15 | 2.0 | 0.60 |  |
|  |  | 3.0 | 3.0 | 0 |  |  | 0 |  |  | 1.80 |  |  | 500 |  | 0.17 | 0.20 |  | BARB28 |
| **fruit & yogurt bar**, blueberry apple, Barbara's Bakery - 1 bar | 42 | 150 |  | 29.0 | 15.0 |  | 1.0 | 125 | 250 |  | 1.50 |  |  | 6 | 0.15 | 2.0 | 0.60 |  |
|  |  | 3.0 | 3.0 | 0 |  |  | 0 |  |  | 1.80 |  |  | 500 |  | 0.17 | 0.20 |  | BARB29 |
| **fruit & yogurt bar**, cherry apple, Barbara's Bakery - 1 bar | 42 | 150 |  | 29.0 | 15.0 |  | 1.0 | 125 | 250 |  | 1.50 |  |  | 6 | 0.15 | 2.0 | 0.60 |  |
|  |  | 3.0 | 3.0 | 0 |  |  | 0 |  |  | 1.80 |  |  | 500 |  | 0.17 | 0.20 |  | BARB30 |
| **fruit & yogurt bar**, strawberry apple, Barbara's Bakery - 1 bar | 42 | 150 |  | 28.0 | 15.0 |  | 1.0 | 125 | 250 |  | 1.50 |  |  | 6 | 0.15 | 2.0 | 0.60 |  |
|  |  | 3.0 | 3.0 | 0 |  |  | 0 |  |  | 1.80 |  |  | 500 |  | 0.17 | 0.20 |  | BARB31 |
| **Gardetto's Snack Mix** | 49 | 240 |  | 33.0 | 2.0 |  | 2.0 | 440 | 0 |  |  |  |  | 0 |  |  |  |  |
| *1.7 oz pouch* |  | 5.0 | 10.0 | 2.0 |  |  | 0 |  |  | 0.36 |  |  | 0 |  |  |  |  | GENM216 |
| **granola bar**, almond, hard | 24 | 119 | 0.7 | 14.9 |  |  | 1.2 | 61 | 8 | 19 | 0.38 | 0.328 | 0 | 0 | 0.07 | 0.1 | 0 | 0.11 |
| *.85 oz bar* |  | 1.8 | 6.1 | 3.0 | 1.9 | 0.9 | 0 | 66 | 55 | 0.60 | 0.030 | 3.6 | 9 |  | 0.02 | 0.01 | 2.9 | 19016 |
| **granola bar**, almond/brn sgr, crnchy, lowfat, Kellogg's - 1 oz bar | 28 | 109 | 1.4 | 21.8 |  |  | 1.7 | 81 | 10 | 24 | 0.62 | 0.503 | 200 | 0 | 0.20 | 2.7 | 0 | 0.19 |
|  |  | 2.2 | 2.1 | 0.3 | 0.5 | 1.3 | 0 | 70 | 69 | 2.41 | 0.196 |  | 667 |  | 0.22 | 0.28 | 0 | 19439 |
| **granola bar**, apl cinn, chewy trail mix, Nature Valley - 1.2 oz bar | 35 | 140 |  | 25.0 | 13.0 |  | 1.0 | 110 |  |  |  |  |  |  |  |  |  |  |
|  |  | 2.0 | 4.0 | 0.5 |  |  | 0 |  |  | 0.36 |  |  |  |  |  |  |  | GENM405 |
| **granola bar**, chocolate chip, hard | 24 | 105 | 0.6 | 17.3 |  |  | 1.1 | 83 | 18 | 17 | 0.46 | 0.362 | 0 | 0 | 0.04 | 0.1 | 0 | 0.12 |
| *.85 oz bar* |  | 1.8 | 3.9 | 2.7 | 0.6 | 0.3 | 0 | 60 | 49 | 0.73 | 0.063 | 3.0 | 10 |  | 0.02 | 0.01 | 3.1 | 19017 |
| **granola bar**, chocolate chip, soft | 28 | 117 | 1.8 | 19.7 | 8.1 |  | 1.1 | 50 | 11 | 18 | 0.36 | 0.354 | 0 | 0 | 0.05 | 0.2 | 0 | 0.10 |
| *1 oz bar* |  | 1.6 | 4.6 | 1.7 | 2.0 | 0.4 | 0 | 66 | 49 | 0.61 | 0.076 | 3.1 | 0 | 0.1 | 0.02 | 0.02 | 4.5 | 19404 |
| **granola bar**, chocolate chip, soft, chocolate-covered - 1 oz bar | 28 | 130 | 1.0 | 17.9 |  |  | 1.0 | 56 | 29 | 18 | 0.36 | 0.260 | 2 | 0 | 0.03 | 0.2 | 0.16 | 0.14 |
|  |  | 1.6 | 7.0 | 4.0 | 2.2 | 0.5 | 1 | 88 | 56 | 0.65 | 0.098 |  | 11 |  | 0.07 | 0.03 | 7.3 | 19024 |
| **granola bar**, chocolate, graham, and marshmallow, soft - 1 oz bar | 28 | 120 | 1.7 | 19.8 |  |  | 1.1 | 88 | 25 | 20 | 0.36 | 0.358 | 1 | 0 | 0.04 | 0.3 | 0 | 0.11 |
|  |  | 1.7 | 4.3 | 2.6 | 0.8 | 0.7 | 0 | 77 | 57 | 0.72 | 0.078 | 4.3 | 13 |  | 0.04 | 0.01 | 5.9 | 19405 |
| **granola bar**, cinn crisp, crunchy, Barbara's Bakery - 2 bars | 42 | 190 |  | 27.0 | 10.0 |  | 3.0 | 60 | 40 |  |  |  |  | 0 |  |  |  |  |
|  |  | 4.0 | 8.0 | 1.0 |  |  | 0 |  |  | 1.44 |  |  | 0 |  |  |  |  | BARB34 |
| **granola bar**, coconut, choc-covered | 28 | 149 | 1.7 | 15.5 | 9.6 | 8.9 | 1.7 | 43 | 12 | 16 | 0.33 |  | 0 | 0 | 0.04 | 0.1 | 0.02 |  |
| *1 oz bar* |  | 1.5 | 9.0 | 6.4 | 1.4 | 0.9 | 0 | 71 | 43 | 0.49 | 0.089 | 4.6 | 0 | 0.1 | 0.02 | 0.03 | 2.5 | 42272 |
| **granola bar**, crunchy, oats and honey, Nature Valley - 2 bars (1.5 oz) | 42 | 180 |  | 29.0 | 11.0 |  | 2.0 | 160 |  |  |  |  |  |  |  |  |  |  |
|  |  | 4.0 | 6.0 | 0.5 |  |  | 0 |  |  | 1.08 |  |  |  |  |  |  |  | GENM217 |
| **granola bar**, fruit & nut, chewy trail mix, Nature Valley - 1.2 oz bar | 35 | 140 |  | 25.0 | 13.0 |  | 1.0 | 80 |  |  |  |  |  |  |  |  |  |  |
|  |  | 3.0 | 4.0 | 0.5 |  |  | 0 |  |  | 0 |  |  |  |  |  |  |  | GENM406 |
| **granola bar**, fruit-filled, nonfat | 28 | 96 | 3.8 | 21.7 | 15.5 |  | 2.1 | 4 | 1 | 14 | 0.40 |  | 7 | 0 | 0.01 | 0.1 | 0.05 |  |
| *1 oz bar* |  | 1.7 | 0.3 | 0.1 | 0.1 | 0.1 | 0 | 62 | 34 | 1.12 | 0.066 | 2.3 | 137 | 0.1 | 0.02 | 0.45 | 146.2 | 19435 |
| **granola bar**, hard | 28 | 132 | 1.1 | 18.0 |  |  | 1.5 | 82 | 17 | 27 | 0.57 | 0.498 | 0 | 0 | 0.07 | 0.4 | 0 | 0.23 |
| *1 oz bar* |  | 2.8 | 5.5 | 0.7 | 1.2 | 3.4 | 0 | 94 | 78 | 0.83 | 0.110 | 4.5 | 42 |  | 0.03 | 0.02 | 6.4 | 19015 |
| **granola bar**, honey nut, chewy, Hlthy Hrt, Nature Valley - 1.4 oz bar | 40 | 160 |  | 28.0 | 13.0 |  | 3.0 | 115 |  |  |  |  |  |  |  |  |  |  |
|  |  | 3.0 | 4.0 | 0.5 |  |  | 0 | 85 |  |  |  |  |  |  |  |  |  | GENM408 |
| **granola bar**, mixed berry, Nature Valley - 1.2 oz bar | 35 | 140 |  | 26.0 | 13.0 |  | 1.0 | 80 |  |  |  |  |  |  |  |  |  |  |
|  |  | 2.0 | 3.5 | 0 |  |  | 0 |  |  | 0 |  |  |  |  |  |  |  | GENM407 |
| **granola bar**, nut and raisin, soft | 28 | 127 | 1.7 | 17.8 |  |  | 1.6 | 71 | 24 | 25 | 0.45 | 0.336 | 1 | 0 | 0.05 | 0.7 | 0.07 | 0.12 |
| *1 oz bar* |  | 2.2 | 5.7 | 2.7 | 1.2 | 1.5 | 0 | 110 | 67 | 0.61 | 0.106 | 4.3 | 11 |  | 0.05 | 0.03 | 8.4 | 19406 |

Column legend (each food occupies two data rows):

Row 1 — KCAL · H₂O (g) · CHO (g) · TSUG (g) · ASUG (g) · DFIB (g) · Na (mg) · Ca (mg) · Mg (mg) · Zn (mg) · Mn (mg) · A (mcg RAE) · C (mg) · B-1 (mg) · NIA (mg) · B-12 (mcg) · PANT (mg)

Row 2 — PRO (g) · FAT (g) · SFA (g) · MUFA (g) · PUFA (g) · CHOL (mg) · K (mg) · P (mg) · Fe (mg) · Cu (mg) · Se (mcg) · A (IU) · E (mg ATE) · B-2 (mg) · B-6 (mg) · FOL (mcg DFE) · REF

| Food | WT (g) | KCAL / PRO | H₂O / FAT | CHO / SFA | TSUG / MUFA | ASUG / PUFA | DFIB / CHOL | Na / K | Ca / P | Mg / Fe | Zn / Cu | Mn / Se | A(RAE) / A(IU) | C / E | B-1 / B-2 | NIA / B-6 | B-12 / FOL | PANT / REF |
|---|---|---|---|---|---|---|---|---|---|---|---|---|---|---|---|---|---|---|
| **granola bar**, oat, fruits, and nut | 28 | 111 | 2.0 | 21.7 | 12.2 | 11.4 | 1.5 | 70 | 10 | 24 | 0.52 | | 8 | 0 | 0.14 | 1.4 | 0 | |
| *1 oz bar* | | 2.2 | 1.8 | 0.2 | 0 | 1.4 | 0 | 67 | 68 | 1.48 | 0.188 | 4.3 | 26 | 0.3 | 0.12 | 0.22 | 44.8 | 19023 |
| **granola bar**, oat raisin, chewy, Hlthy Hrt, Nature Valley - *1.4 oz bar* | 40 | 150 | | 30.0 | 14.0 | | 3.0 | 95 | | | | | | | | | | |
| | | 3.0 | 2.0 | 0.5 | | | 0 | 95 | | | | | | | | | | GENM409 |
| **granola bar**, oats and honey, crunchy, Barbara's Bakery - *2 bars* | 42 | 190 | | 27.0 | 10.0 | | 3.0 | 60 | 40 | | | | | 0 | | | | |
| | | 4.0 | 8.0 | 1.0 | | | 0 | | | 1.44 | | | 0 | | | | | BARB36 |
| **granola bar**, peanut butter and choc chip, soft - *1 oz bar* | 28 | 121 | 1.7 | 17.4 | | | 1.2 | 92 | 22 | 25 | 0.48 | 0.378 | 1 | 0 | 0.03 | 0.9 | 0.13 | 0.15 |
| | | 2.7 | 5.6 | 1.6 | 2.3 | 1.3 | 0 | 106 | 73 | 0.54 | 0.112 | | 3 | | 0.03 | 0.03 | 9.2 | 19027 |
| **granola bar**, pnt butter, crunchy, Barbara's Bakery - *2 bars* | 42 | 200 | | 26.0 | 9.0 | | 3.0 | 55 | 40 | | | | | 0 | | | | |
| | | 4.0 | 9.0 | 1.0 | | | 0 | | | 1.44 | | | 0 | | | | | BARB37 |
| **granola bar**, peanut butter, hard *.85 oz bar* | 24 | 116 | 0.6 | 15.0 | | | 0.7 | 68 | 10 | 13 | 0.30 | 0.221 | 0 | 0 | 0.05 | 0.5 | 0 | 0.09 |
| | | 2.4 | 5.7 | 0.8 | 1.7 | 2.9 | 0 | 70 | 33 | 0.58 | 0.052 | 3.6 | 4 | 0.02 | 0.02 | | 4.3 | 19420 |
| **granola bar**, peanut butter, soft *1 oz bar* | 28 | 119 | 2.0 | 18.0 | | | 1.2 | 115 | 25 | 24 | 0.52 | 0.392 | 1 | 0 | 0.06 | 0.9 | 0.06 | 0.15 |
| | | 2.9 | 4.4 | 1.0 | 1.8 | 1.2 | 0 | 81 | 70 | 0.60 | 0.185 | 5.3 | 4 | | 0.04 | 0.03 | 9.0 | 19021 |
| **granola bar**, peanut butter, soft, choc-covered - *1.3 oz bar* | 37 | 188 | 1.2 | 19.8 | | | 1.0 | 71 | 40 | 25 | 0.54 | 0.500 | 2 | 0 | 0.04 | 1.2 | 0 | 0.20 |
| | | 3.8 | 11.5 | 6.3 | 2.4 | 0.7 | 4 | 125 | 84 | 0.54 | 0.120 | | 9 | | 0.08 | 0.04 | 9.2 | 19026 |
| **granola bar**, peanut, hard *1 oz bar* | 28 | 134 | 0.6 | 17.8 | 9.5 | | 1.2 | 78 | 11 | 31 | 0.59 | 0.394 | 0 | | 0.05 | 0.4 | 0 | 0.17 |
| | | 3.1 | 6.0 | 0.7 | 1.6 | 3.3 | 0 | 85 | 84 | 0.70 | 0.078 | 4.2 | 0 | 1.5 | 0.02 | 0.02 | 9.5 | 19019 |
| **granola bar**, raisin, soft *1 oz bar* | 28 | 125 | 1.8 | 18.6 | | | 1.2 | 79 | 28 | 20 | 0.36 | 0.353 | 0 | | 0.06 | 0.3 | 0.05 | 0.13 |
| | | 2.1 | 5.0 | 2.7 | 0.8 | 0.9 | 0 | 101 | 62 | 0.68 | 0.078 | 4.4 | 0 | | 0.05 | 0.03 | 5.9 | 19022 |
| **granola bar**, soft *1 oz bar* | 28 | 124 | 1.8 | 18.8 | | | 1.3 | 78 | 29 | 21 | 0.42 | 0.428 | 0 | | 0.08 | 0.1 | 0.11 | 0.15 |
| | | 2.1 | 4.8 | 2.0 | 1.1 | 1.5 | 0 | 91 | 64 | 0.72 | 0.076 | 4.5 | 0 | | 0.05 | 0.03 | 6.7 | 19020 |
| **granola bar**, sweet & salty, Nature Valley - *1.2 oz bar* | 35 | 165 | | 20.7 | 11.5 | | 1.5 | 160 | 20 | | | | | | | | | |
| | | 3.0 | 8.0 | 2.2 | | | 0 | | | 0.36 | | | | | | | | GENM403 |
| **granola bar**, toasted almond, crunchy, Barbara's Bakery - *2 bars* | 42 | 200 | | 27.0 | 10.0 | | 3.0 | 60 | 40 | | | | | 0 | | | | |
| | | 4.0 | 8.0 | 1.0 | | | 0 | | | 1.44 | | | 0 | | | | | BARB39 |
| **granola bar**, yogurt-coated, Nature Valley - *1.2 oz bar* | 35 | 140 | | 26.0 | 13.0 | | 1.0 | 110 | 200 | | | | | 0 | | | | |
| | | 2.0 | 3.5 | 2.0 | | | 0 | | | 0.36 | | | 0 | | | | | GENM404 |
| **Milk 'n Cereal Bar**, Cinn Toast Crnch, Gen Mills - *1.6 oz bar* | 45 | 180 | | 32.0 | 15.0 | | 1.0 | 140 | 250 | 16 | 4.50 | | | 9 | 0.45 | 6.0 | 2.10 | |
| | | 3.0 | 4.0 | 2.0 | | | 0 | 115 | 150 | 5.40 | | | 750 | | 0.60 | 0.60 | | GENM219 |
| **Milk 'n Cereal Bar**, Cocoa Puffs, General Mills - *1.4 oz bar* | 40 | 170 | | 29.0 | 14.0 | | 1.0 | 125 | 250 | 8 | 4.50 | | | 9 | 0.45 | 6.0 | 2.10 | |
| | | 3.0 | 4.0 | 2.0 | | | 0 | 50 | 150 | 5.40 | | | 750 | | 0.60 | 0.60 | | GENM220 |
| **Milk 'n Cereal Bar**, Honey Nut Cheerios, Gen Mills - *1.4 oz bar* | 40 | 160 | | 28.0 | 14.0 | | 1.0 | 120 | 250 | 8 | 4.50 | | | 9 | 0.45 | 5.0 | 2.10 | |
| | | 3.0 | 4.0 | 2.0 | | | 0 | 115 | 150 | 5.40 | | | 750 | | 0.60 | 0.50 | | GENM221 |
| **Moose Munch**, dark choc, Harry and David - *½ cup (1.48 oz)* | 42 | 160 | | 24.0 | 20.0 | | 1.0 | 100 | | | | | | | | | | |
| | | 1.0 | 6.0 | 3.0 | | | 5 | | | 0.36 | | | 100 | | | | | HADA10 |
| **Moose Munch**, milk choc, Harry and David - *½ cup (1.41 oz)* | 40 | 170 | | 20.0 | 16.0 | | 1.0 | 120 | 20 | | | | | | | | | |
| | | 2.0 | 8.0 | 3.5 | | | 10 | | | 0.36 | | | 100 | | | | | HADA8 |
| **Munchos Potato Crisps**, Frito-Lay *1.3 oz bag* | 37 | 210 | | 21.0 | | | 1.0 | 300 | 0 | | | | | 0 | | | | |
| | | 1.0 | 13.0 | 1.5 | | | 0 | | 40 | 0 | | | 0 | | | 0.08 | | FRIT2 |
| **Odwalla Bar**, banana nut *2.2 oz bar* | 62 | 240 | | 41.0 | 18.0 | | 5.0 | 115 | 250 | | | | | 12 | | | | |
| | | 4.0 | 6.0 | 1.0 | | | 0 | 200 | | 1.08 | | | 1000 | | | | | ODWA37 |
| **Odwalla Bar**, Berries GoMega *2.2 oz bar* | 62 | 220 | | 41.0 | 20.0 | | 5.0 | 230 | 250 | | | | | 0 | | | | |
| | | 5.0 | 4.5 | 0.5 | 1.0 | 2.5 | 0 | | | 1.44 | | | 2500 | | | | | ODWA31 |
| **Odwalla Bar**, choco-walla *2.2 oz bar* | 62 | 240 | | 42.0 | 20.0 | | 5.0 | 80 | 250 | | | | | 12 | | | | |
| | | 5.0 | 6.0 | 2.0 | | | 0 | 220 | | 2.70 | | | 1250 | | | | | ODWA38 |
| **Odwalla Bar**, peanut crunch *2.2 oz bar* | 62 | 240 | | 37.0 | 14.0 | | 3.0 | 210 | 250 | | | | | 12 | | | | |
| | | 8.0 | 7.0 | 1.5 | | | 0 | | | 1.44 | | | 0 | | | | | ODWA35 |
| **Odwalla Bar**, strawberry pomegranate - *2.2 oz bar* | 62 | 220 | | 44.0 | 20.0 | | 4.0 | 95 | 250 | | | | | 12 | | | | |
| | | 4.0 | 3.0 | 0.5 | | | 0 | 210 | | 1.80 | | | 1250 | | | | | ODWA39 |
| **Odwalla Bar**, Super Protein *2.2 oz bar* | 62 | 230 | | 31.0 | 16.0 | | 4.0 | 160 | 250 | | | | | 12 | 0.38 | 5.0 | 1.50 | 2.50 |
| | | 16.0 | 4.5 | 1.5 | | | 0 | 200 | | 1.80 | | | 2500 | | 0.42 | 0.50 | | ODWA33 |
| **Odwalla Bar**, Superfood *2.2 oz bar* | 62 | 230 | | 43.0 | 20.0 | | 3.0 | 110 | 250 | | | | | 12 | | | | |
| | | 4.0 | 4.0 | 2.0 | | | 0 | 300 | | 2.70 | | | 500 | | | | | ODWA32 |
| **Oriental snack mix**, rice-based *1 oz* | 28 | 142 | 0.7 | 14.5 | 0.8 | 0 | 3.7 | 116 | 15 | 33 | 0.74 | 0.356 | 0 | 0 | 0.09 | 0.9 | 0 | 0.13 |
| | | 4.8 | 7.2 | 1.1 | 2.8 | 3.0 | 0 | 92 | 73 | 0.68 | 0.038 | 2.3 | 0 | 1.6 | 0.04 | 0.02 | 10.6 | 19031 |
| **plantain chips** *1 oz* | 28 | 157 | | 16.0 | | | 1.2 | 109 | 2 | 17 | 0.08 | 0.084 | | | 0.02 | 0.3 | | 0.24 |
| | | 0.5 | 10.1 | 2.6 | 1.6 | 5.1 | | 196 | 18 | 0.22 | 0.008 | | | | 0.03 | 0.13 | | 25027 |
| **popcorn**, 94% fat-free, microwaved *1 oz* | 28 | 113 | 1.2 | 21.3 | 0.2 | | 3.8 | 176 | 4 | 35 | 0.78 | 0.304 | 4 | 0 | 0.02 | 0.6 | 0 | |
| | | 3.0 | 1.7 | 0.3 | 0.8 | 0.6 | 0 | 80 | 85 | 0.80 | 0.073 | 1.9 | 74 | 0.1 | 0.04 | 0.06 | 5.0 | 25000 |
| **popcorn**, air-popped *1 oz (~3.5 cups)* | 28 | 108 | 0.9 | 21.8 | 0.2 | 0 | 4.1 | 2 | 2 | 40 | 0.86 | 0.312 | 3 | 0 | 0.03 | 0.6 | 0 | 0.14 |
| | | 3.6 | 1.3 | 0.2 | 0.3 | 0.5 | 0 | 92 | 100 | 0.89 | 0.073 | 0 | 55 | 0.1 | 0.02 | 0.04 | 8.7 | 19034 |

| | WT (g) | KCAL / PRO | H2O (g) / FAT (g) | CHO (g) / SFA (g) | TSUG (g) / MUFA (g) | ASUG (g) / PUFA (g) | DFIB (g) / CHOL (mg) | Na (mg) / K (mg) | Ca (mg) / P (mg) | Mg (mg) / Fe (mg) | Zn (mg) / Cu (mg) | Mn (mg) / Se (mcg) | A (mcg RAE) / A (IU) | C (mg) / E (mg ATE) | B-1 (mg) / B-2 (mg) | NIA (mg) / B-6 (mg) | B-12 (mcg) / FOL (mcg DFE) | PANT (mg) / REF |
|---|---|---|---|---|---|---|---|---|---|---|---|---|---|---|---|---|---|---|
| popcorn, butter flavored, Snyder .63 oz | 18 | 100 | | 6.0 | 0 | | 1.0 | 150 | 0 | | | | | 0 | | | | |
| | | 1.0 | 8.0 | 0.5 | | | 0 | | 0 | | | | 0 | | | | | SNYD24 |
| popcorn, butter, popped, PopSecret 1 cup | 6 | 40 | | 4.0 | 0 | | 0.5 | 65 | 0 | | | | | 0 | | | | |
| | | 0.5 | 2.5 | 0.5 | | | 0 | | 0 | | | | 0 | | | | | GENM222 |
| popcorn cake .35 oz cake | 10 | 38 | 0.5 | 8.0 | 0.1 | 0.1 | 0.3 | 29 | 1 | 16 | 0.40 | 0.098 | 0 | 0 | 0.01 | 0.6 | 1.8 | 0.04 |
| | | 1.0 | 0.3 | 0 | 0.1 | 0.1 | 0 | 33 | 28 | 0.19 | 0.057 | 1.0 | 7 | 0 | 0.02 | 0.02 | 1.8 | 19036 |
| popcorn, caramel-coated 1 oz | 28 | 121 | 0.8 | 22.1 | 14.9 | 14.8 | 1.5 | 58 | 12 | 10 | 0.16 | 0.062 | 1 | 0 | 0.02 | 0.6 | 0 | 0.02 |
| | | 1.1 | 3.6 | 1.0 | 0.8 | 1.3 | 1 | 31 | 23 | 0.49 | 0.033 | 1.0 | 2 | 0.3 | 0.02 | 0.01 | 1.4 | 19039 |
| popcorn, caramel-coated with peanuts - 1 oz (~⅔ cup) | 28 | 112 | 0.9 | 22.6 | 12.7 | 12.5 | 1.1 | 83 | 18 | 22 | 0.35 | 0.214 | 1 | 0 | 0.01 | 0.6 | 0 | 0.06 |
| | | 1.8 | 2.2 | 0.3 | 0.8 | 0.9 | 0 | 99 | 36 | 1.09 | 0.083 | 1.1 | 22 | 0.2 | 0.04 | 0.05 | 4.5 | 19038 |
| popcorn, cheese 1 oz (~2.6 cups) | 28 | 147 | 0.7 | 14.4 | | | 2.8 | 249 | 32 | 25 | 0.56 | 0.200 | 11 | 0 | 0.03 | 0.4 | 0.15 | 0.13 |
| | | 2.6 | 9.3 | 1.8 | 2.7 | 4.3 | 3 | 73 | 101 | 0.63 | 0.039 | 3.4 | 68 | | 0.07 | 0.07 | 3.1 | 19040 |
| popcorn, extra butter, popped, Pop Secret - 1 cup | 7 | 40 | | 3.0 | 0 | | 0.5 | 60 | 0 | | | | | 0 | | | | |
| | | 0.5 | 3.0 | 0.5 | | | 0 | | 0 | | | | 0 | | | | | GENM223 |
| popcorn, light butter, popped, Pop Secret - 1 cup | 5 | 20 | | 4.0 | 0 | | 0.5 | 55 | 0 | | | | | 0 | | | | |
| | | 0.5 | 1.0 | 0 | | | 0 | | 0 | | | | 0 | | | | | GENM224 |
| popcorn, lowfat, low sodium, microwaved - 1 oz | 28 | 120 | 0.8 | 20.5 | 0.2 | 0 | 4.0 | 137 | 3 | 42 | 1.07 | | 2 | 0 | 0.10 | 0.6 | 0 | |
| | | 3.5 | 2.7 | 0.4 | 1.1 | 1.0 | 0 | 67 | 74 | 0.64 | 0.153 | 2.4 | 41 | 1.4 | 0.03 | 0.05 | 4.8 | 43572 |
| popcorn, oil-popped 1 oz (~2.6 cups) | 28 | 163 | 0.3 | 12.6 | 0.1 | 0 | 2.3 | 296 | 1 | 22 | 0.87 | 0.176 | 2 | 0 | 0.04 | 0.3 | 0 | 0.06 |
| | | 2.0 | 12.2 | 1.9 | 2.7 | 6.5 | 0 | 51 | 56 | 0.55 | 0.045 | 0.6 | 43 | 0.7 | 0.02 | 0.03 | 7.0 | 19035 |
| popcorn, oil-popped, microwaved 1 oz (~2.6 cups) | 28 | 163 | 0.3 | 12.6 | 0.1 | 0 | 2.3 | 296 | 1 | 22 | 0.87 | 0.176 | 2 | 0 | 0.04 | 0.3 | 0 | 0.06 |
| | | 2.0 | 12.2 | 1.9 | 2.7 | 6.5 | 0 | 51 | 56 | 0.55 | 0.045 | 0.6 | 43 | 0.7 | 0.02 | 0.03 | 7.0 | 19035 |
| popcorn, oil-popped, unsalted 1 oz (~2.6 cups) | 28 | 146 | 0.8 | 16.3 | 0.2 | 0 | 2.8 | 1 | 3 | 30 | 0.74 | | 2 | 0 | 0.04 | 0.4 | 0 | |
| | | 2.5 | 7.9 | 1.4 | 2.3 | 3.8 | 0 | 63 | 70 | 0.78 | 0.062 | 2.0 | 43 | 0.7 | 0.04 | 0.06 | 4.8 | 42259 |
| potato chips 1 oz | 28 | 153 | 0.6 | 13.9 | 0.1 | 0 | 1.2 | 147 | 7 | 20 | 0.67 | 0.186 | 0 | 5 | 0.02 | 1.2 | 0 | 1.22 |
| | | 1.8 | 10.5 | 3.1 | 2.8 | 3.4 | 0 | 460 | 43 | 0.45 | 0.111 | 2.3 | 0 | 1.9 | 0.06 | 0.20 | 21.0 | 19411 |
| potato chips, baked 1 oz | 28 | 131 | 0.4 | 20.0 | 1.4 | 0 | 1.3 | 257 | 35 | 12 | 0.13 | | 0 | 0 | 0.10 | 1.1 | 0 | |
| | | 1.4 | 5.1 | 0.7 | 2.8 | 1.2 | 0 | 202 | 77 | 0.22 | 0.029 | 2.3 | 0 | 0.6 | 0.02 | 0.14 | 0 | 42283 |
| potato chips, barbeque 1 oz | 28 | 137 | 0.5 | 14.8 | | | 1.2 | 210 | 14 | 21 | 0.26 | 0.140 | 3 | 9 | 0.06 | 1.3 | 0 | 0.17 |
| | | 2.2 | 9.1 | 2.3 | 1.8 | 4.6 | 0 | 353 | 52 | 0.54 | 0.101 | 2.3 | 61 | | 0.06 | 0.17 | 23.2 | 19042 |
| potato chips, barbeque, Snyder 1 oz | 28 | 150 | | 20.0 | | | 4.0 | 300 | 0 | | | | | 9 | | | | |
| | | 2.0 | 6.0 | 2.0 | | | 0 | | | 0.36 | | | 2 | | | | | SNYD15 |
| potato chips, cheese 1 oz | 28 | 139 | 0.5 | 16.2 | | | 1.5 | 222 | 20 | 21 | 0.25 | 0.125 | 3 | 15 | 0.04 | 1.4 | 0 | 0.22 |
| | | 2.4 | 7.6 | 2.4 | 2.2 | 2.7 | 1 | 428 | 84 | 0.52 | 0.070 | | 9 | | 0.04 | 0.10 | 0 | 19421 |
| potato chips, cheese, from dried potatoes - 1 oz | 28 | 154 | 0.5 | 14.2 | | | 1.0 | 211 | 31 | 15 | 0.18 | 0.016 | 0 | 2 | 0.05 | 0.7 | 0 | 0.09 |
| | | 2.0 | 10.4 | 2.7 | 2.0 | 5.2 | 1 | 107 | 46 | 0.45 | 0.016 | 2.3 | 1 | | 0.03 | 0.15 | 5.0 | 19412 |
| potato chips, fat-free, made w/Olestra - 1 oz | 28 | 77 | 0.6 | 18.2 | 0 | 0 | 1.9 | 155 | 10 | 19 | 0.98 | 0.216 | 0 | 8 | 0.09 | 1.2 | 0 | 0.27 |
| | | 2.2 | 0.2 | 0.1 | 0.1 | 0.1 | 0 | 325 | 49 | 0.67 | 0.123 | 0.3 | 0 | | 0.01 | 0.04 | 23.2 | 19423 |
| potato chips, from dried potatoes 1 oz | 28 | 157 | 0.7 | 14.6 | 0.3 | 0.8 | 0.9 | 109 | | 12 | 0.13 | 0.077 | 0 | 2 | 0.03 | 0.9 | 0 | 0.23 |
| | | 1.2 | 10.8 | 2.7 | 2.0 | 3.8 | 0 | 210 | 35 | 0.23 | 0.034 | 0.6 | 3 | 3.2 | 0 | 0.11 | 2.0 | 19410 |
| potato chips, hot buffalo wing, Snyder - 1 oz | 28 | 150 | | 19.0 | 0 | | 4.0 | 340 | 0 | | | | | 9 | | | | |
| | | 2.0 | 7.0 | 2.0 | | | 0 | | | 0.36 | | | 0 | | | | | SNYD17 |
| potato chips, jalapeno, Snyder 1 oz | 28 | 150 | | 20.0 | | | 4.0 | 330 | 0 | | | | | 9 | | | | |
| | | 2.0 | 6.0 | 2.0 | | | 0 | | | 0.36 | | | 1 | | | | | SNYD18 |
| potato chips, kosher dill, Snyder 1 oz | 28 | 140 | | 20.0 | 1.0 | | 4.0 | 360 | 0 | | | | | 9 | | | | |
| | | 2.0 | 6.0 | 2.0 | | | 0 | | | 0.36 | | | 0 | | | | | SNYD19 |
| potato chips, light 1 oz | 28 | 132 | 0.3 | 18.7 | 0.1 | 0 | 1.7 | 138 | 6 | 25 | 0.02 | 0.123 | 0 | 7 | 0.06 | 2.0 | 0 | 0.08 |
| | | 2.0 | 5.8 | 1.2 | 1.3 | 3.1 | 0 | 488 | 54 | 0.38 | 0.168 | 2.3 | 0 | 1.5 | 0.07 | 0.19 | 7.6 | 19422 |
| potato chips, reduced fat, from dried potatoes - 1 oz | 28 | 141 | 0.6 | 18.2 | 0.2 | 0 | 0.9 | 115 | 8 | 13 | 0.20 | 0.101 | 0 | 3 | 0.06 | 1.0 | 0 | 0.23 |
| | | 1.3 | 7.3 | 1.9 | 1.3 | 3.4 | 0 | 213 | 36 | 0.31 | 0.043 | 0.8 | 0 | 0.6 | 0 | 0.12 | 7.6 | 19045 |
| potato chips, ripple, Snyder 1 oz | 28 | 140 | | 18.0 | 0 | | 4.0 | 100 | 0 | | | | | 9 | | | | |
| | | 2.0 | 6.0 | 2.0 | | | 0 | | | 0.36 | | | 0 | | | | | SNYD20 |
| potato chips, salt and vinegar, Snyder - 1 oz | 28 | 140 | | 19.0 | | | 4.0 | 250 | 0 | | | | | 9 | | | | |
| | | 2.0 | 6.0 | 2.0 | | | 0 | | | 0.36 | | | 0 | | | | | SNYD21 |
| potato chips, Snyder 1 oz | 28 | 150 | | 19.0 | | | 3.0 | 90 | 0 | | | | | 9 | | | | |
| | | 2.0 | 7.0 | 2.0 | | | 0 | | | 0.36 | | | 0 | | | | | SNYD16 |
| potato chips, sour cream and onion, Snyder - 1 oz | 28 | 150 | | 20.0 | 1.0 | | 4.0 | 210 | 0 | | | | | 9 | | | | |
| | | 2.0 | 6.0 | 2.0 | | | 0 | | | 0.36 | | | 0 | | | | | SNYD22 |
| potato chips, sour cream'n onion 1 oz | 28 | 149 | 0.5 | 14.4 | | | 1.5 | 175 | 20 | 21 | 0.27 | 0.113 | 4 | 10 | 0.05 | 1.1 | 0.28 | 0.23 |
| | | 2.3 | 9.5 | 2.5 | 1.7 | 4.9 | 2 | 373 | 49 | 0.45 | 0.084 | 2.3 | 48 | | 0.06 | 0.19 | 17.4 | 19043 |
| potato chips, sour cream'n onion, from dried potatoes - 1 oz | 28 | 153 | 0.6 | 14.4 | | | 0.3 | 202 | 18 | 15 | 0.20 | 0.113 | | 3 | 0.05 | 0.7 | 0 | 0.23 |
| | | 1.8 | 10.4 | 2.7 | 2.0 | 5.3 | 1 | 139 | 47 | 0.39 | 0.018 | | 211 | | 0.03 | 0.13 | 6.4 | 19046 |

| | WT (g) | KCAL / PRO (g) | H2O (g) / FAT (g) | CHO (g) / SFA (g) | TSUG (g) / MUFA (g) | ASUG (g) / PUFA (g) | DFIB (g) / CHOL (mg) | Na (mg) / K (mg) | Ca (mg) / P (mg) | Mg (mg) / Fe (mg) | Zn (mg) / Cu (mg) | Mn (mg) / Se (mcg) | A (mcg RAE) / A (IU) | C (mg) / E (mg ATE) | B-1 (mg) / B-2 (mg) | NIA (mg) / B-6 (mg) | B-12 (mcg) / FOL (mcg DFE) | PANT (mg) / REF |
|---|---|---|---|---|---|---|---|---|---|---|---|---|---|---|---|---|---|---|
| **potato crisps**, jalapeno cheddar, Snyder - *1 oz* | 28 | 120 | | 21.0 | 3.0 | | 2.0 | 380 | 40 | | | | | 0 | | | | |
| | | 2.0 | 2.5 | 0 | | | 5 | | | | 0 | | 0 | | | | | SNYD11 |
| **potato crisps**, zesty ranch, Snyder *1 oz* | 28 | 110 | | 23.0 | 3.0 | | 1.0 | 270 | 0 | | | | | 0 | | | | |
| | | 1.0 | 1.5 | 0 | | | 0 | | | | 0.03 | | 0 | | | | | SNYD9 |
| **potato sticks** *½ cup* | 18 | 94 | 0.4 | 9.6 | 0 | 0 | 0.6 | 45 | 3 | 12 | 0.18 | 0.076 | 0 | 9 | 0.02 | 0.9 | 0 | 0.07 |
| | | 1.2 | 6.2 | 1.6 | 1.1 | 3.2 | 0 | 223 | 31 | 0.41 | 0.057 | 1.5 | 0 | 1.6 | 0.02 | 0.06 | 7.2 | 19415 |
| **pretzel**, chocolate-covered *.39 oz pretzel* | 11 | 50 | 0.3 | 7.8 | | | | 63 | 8 | 5 | 0.10 | 0.062 | 0 | 0 | 0.01 | 0.1 | 0 | 0.08 |
| | | 0.8 | 1.8 | 0.8 | 0.6 | 0.2 | | 25 | 16 | 0.22 | 0.033 | | 1 | | 0.02 | 0.02 | 1.0 | 19048 |
| **pretzel**, hard *10 twists (2.1 oz)* | 60 | 227 | 2.1 | 47.5 | 1.7 | 0.7 | 1.8 | 814 | 11 | 17 | 0.86 | 0.560 | 0 | 0 | 0.30 | 3.1 | 0 | 0.20 |
| | | 6.2 | 1.6 | 0.3 | 0.7 | 0.7 | 0 | 82 | 68 | 3.12 | 0.102 | 3.6 | 0 | 0.2 | 0.19 | 0.03 | 171.6 | 19047 |
| **pretzel**, homestyle, Snyder *1 oz* | 28 | 120 | | 25.0 | | | 1.0 | 230 | 0 | | | | | 0 | | | | |
| | | 3.0 | 1.0 | 0 | | | 0 | | | | 0.36 | | 0 | | | | | SNYD1 |
| **pretzel**, milk chocolate-covered, Snyder - *1 oz* | 28 | 140 | | 19.0 | 11.0 | | | 100 | 40 | | | | | 0 | | | | |
| | | 2.0 | 6.0 | 3.5 | | | | | | | 0.36 | | 0 | | | | | SNYD27 |
| **pretzel**, mini, Snyder *1 oz* | 28 | 110 | | 25.0 | | | | 250 | 0 | | | | | 0 | | | | |
| | | 3.0 | 0 | 0 | | | 0 | | | | 0.36 | | 0 | | | | | SNYD2 |
| **pretzel**, soft *2 oz* | 57 | 193 | 8.5 | 39.6 | 0.1 | 0 | 1.0 | 800 | 13 | 12 | 0.54 | | 0 | 0 | 0.23 | 2.4 | 0 | |
| | | 4.7 | 1.8 | 0.4 | 0.6 | 0.5 | 2 | 50 | 45 | 2.23 | 0.072 | 9.8 | 0 | 0.3 | 0.17 | 0.01 | 13.7 | 43109 |
| **pretzel**, sourdough, Snyder *1 oz* | 28 | 100 | | 22.0 | 0 | | 1.0 | 240 | 0 | | | | | 0 | | | | |
| | | 3.0 | 0 | 0 | | | 0 | | | | 0.36 | | 0 | | | | | SNYD3 |
| **pretzel**, white chocolate-coated, Snyder - *1 oz* | 28 | 140 | | 19.0 | 11.0 | | 0 | 110 | 40 | | | | | 0 | | | | |
| | | 3.0 | 6.0 | 3.0 | | | | | | | 0 | | 0 | | | | | SNYD28 |
| **pretzel**, whole wheat *2 oz* | 57 | 206 | 2.2 | 46.3 | | | 4.4 | 116 | 16 | 17 | 0.35 | 1.517 | 0 | 1 | 0.25 | 3.7 | 0 | 0.46 |
| | | 6.3 | 1.5 | 0.3 | 0.6 | 0.5 | | 245 | 71 | 1.53 | 0.160 | | 0 | | 0.17 | 0.16 | 30.8 | 19050 |
| **rice cake**, brown rice *.32 oz cake* | 9 | 35 | 0.5 | 7.3 | 0.1 | 0 | 0.4 | 29 | 1 | 12 | 0.27 | 0.336 | 0 | 0 | 0.01 | 0.7 | 0 | 0.09 |
| | | 0.7 | 0.3 | 0.1 | 0.1 | 0.1 | 0 | 26 | 32 | 0.13 | 0.040 | 2.2 | 0 | 0.1 | 0.01 | 0.01 | 1.9 | 19051 |
| **rice cake**, brown rice and buckwheat *.32 oz cake* | 9 | 34 | 0.5 | 7.2 | | | 0.3 | 10 | 1 | 14 | 0.22 | 0.556 | 0 | 0 | 0.01 | 0.7 | 0 | 0.10 |
| | | 0.8 | 0.3 | 0.1 | 0.1 | 0.1 | 0 | 27 | 34 | 0.10 | 0.034 | 1.5 | 0 | | 0.01 | 0.01 | 1.9 | 19052 |
| **rice cake**, brown rice and corn *.32 oz cake* | 9 | 35 | 0.5 | 7.3 | | | 0.3 | 26 | 1 | 10 | 0.20 | 0.457 | 0 | 0 | 0.01 | 0.6 | 0 | 0.08 |
| | | 0.8 | 0.3 | 0.1 | 0.1 | 0.1 | 0 | 25 | 29 | 0.11 | 0.038 | | 0 | | 0.01 | 0.01 | 1.7 | 19413 |
| **rice cake**, brown rice and multigrain *.32 oz cake* | 9 | 35 | 0.6 | 7.2 | | | 0.3 | 23 | 2 | 12 | 0.23 | 0.470 | 0 | 0 | 0.01 | 0.6 | 0 | 0.09 |
| | | 0.8 | 0.3 | 0.1 | 0.1 | 0.1 | 0 | 26 | 33 | 0.18 | 0.038 | | 0 | | 0.02 | 0.01 | 1.8 | 19414 |
| **rice cake**, brown rice and rye *.32 oz cake* | 9 | 35 | 0.6 | 7.2 | | | 0.4 | 10 | 2 | 13 | 0.27 | 0.268 | 0 | 0 | 0.01 | 0.6 | 0 | 0.10 |
| | | 0.7 | 0.3 | 0.1 | 0.1 | 0.1 | 0 | 28 | 34 | 0.16 | 0.035 | | 0 | | 0.01 | 0.01 | 0.4 | 19416 |
| **rice cake**, brown rice and sesame seeds - *.32 oz cake* | 9 | 35 | 0.5 | 7.3 | | | 0.5 | 20 | 1 | 12 | 0.27 | 0.387 | 0 | 0 | 0 | 0.6 | 0 | 0.13 |
| | | 0.7 | 0.3 | 0 | 0.1 | 0.1 | 0 | 26 | 34 | 0.14 | 0.035 | 2.2 | 0 | | 0.01 | 0.01 | 1.6 | 19053 |
| **rice cake**, white rice *.32 oz cake* | 9 | 35 | 0.5 | 7.3 | 0.1 | 0 | 0.4 | 6 | 1 | 12 | 0.27 | | 0 | 0 | 0.01 | 0.7 | 0 | |
| | | 0.6 | 0.4 | 0.1 | 0.1 | 0.1 | 0 | 39 | 32 | 0.13 | 0.040 | 2.2 | 0 | 0.1 | 0.01 | 0.01 | 1.9 | 42204 |
| **Rice Krispies Treats**, Kellogg's *1.13 oz bar* | 32 | 132 | 1.9 | 25.8 | | | 0.2 | 112 | 1 | 4 | 0.16 | 0.512 | 104 | 0 | 0.41 | 5.2 | 0 | 0 |
| | | 1.1 | 2.9 | 0.4 | 0.8 | 1.6 | 0 | 12 | 13 | 0.41 | 0.032 | | 346 | | 0.44 | 0.29 | 55.0 | 19438 |
| **sesame sticks**, wheat-based *1 oz* | 28 | 151 | 0.6 | 13.0 | 0.1 | 0 | 0.8 | 417 | 48 | 13 | 0.33 | 0.253 | 0 | 0 | 0.03 | 0.4 | 0 | 0.07 |
| | | 3.1 | 10.3 | 1.8 | 3.1 | 4.9 | 0 | 50 | 39 | 0.21 | 0.114 | 4.8 | 1 | 1.1 | 0.02 | 0.02 | 6.2 | 19418 |
| **Soy Crisps**, parmesan, garlic, olive oil, Snyder - *1 oz* | 28 | 160 | | 11.0 | 0 | | 5.0 | 290 | 0 | | | | | 0 | | | | |
| | | 8.0 | 9.0 | 1.0 | | | 0 | | | | 1.08 | | 0 | | | | | SNYD5 |
| **Soy Crisps**, tomato, romano, olive oil, Snyder - *1 oz* | 28 | 150 | | 11.0 | 0 | | 5.0 | 360 | 0 | | | | | 0 | | | | |
| | | 7.0 | 9.0 | 1.0 | | | 0 | | | | 1.08 | | 0 | | | | | SNYD4 |
| **Sunchips**, Frito Lay *1 oz* | 28 | 137 | 0.6 | 18.8 | 2.0 | | 1.9 | 92 | 6 | 21 | 0.46 | 0.367 | 0 | 0 | 0.04 | 0.6 | 0 | 0.25 |
| | | 2.2 | 5.9 | 0.6 | 3.2 | 1.8 | | 65 | 62 | 0.49 | 0.064 | | 0 | 2.0 | 0.01 | 0.06 | 8.7 | 25013 |
| **Sunchips**, harvest cheddar, Fritolay *1 oz* | 28 | 137 | 0.7 | 18.1 | 2.0 | | 2.3 | 151 | 11 | 17 | 0.38 | | 6 | 0 | 0.05 | 0.6 | 0 | |
| | | 2.3 | 6.2 | 0.8 | 3.5 | 1.9 | 1 | 67 | 69 | 0.39 | | | 62 | | 0.03 | 0.08 | | 25023 |
| **sweet potato chips** *1 oz* | 28 | 139 | 1.1 | 18.2 | 2.0 | | 1.0 | 10 | 20 | 18 | 0.15 | 0.378 | 663 | 0 | 0.02 | 0.6 | 0 | 0.43 |
| | | 1.0 | 6.9 | 0.6 | 2.6 | 3.4 | 0 | 259 | 41 | 0.71 | 0.115 | 0.6 | 6629 | 2.7 | 0.05 | 0.15 | 10.4 | 25012 |
| **sweet potato crisps**, baked, Snyder *1 oz* | 28 | 110 | | 23.0 | 4.0 | | 1.0 | 310 | 40 | | | | | 0 | | | | |
| | | 1.0 | 1.5 | 0 | | | 0 | | | | 0.01 | | 5 | | | | | SNYD10 |
| **taro chips** *10 chips (.8 oz)* | 23 | 115 | 0.5 | 15.7 | 0.9 | 0 | 1.7 | 79 | 14 | 19 | 0.09 | 0 | 2 | 1 | 0.04 | 0.1 | 0 | 0.15 |
| | | 0.5 | 5.7 | 1.5 | 1.0 | 3.0 | 0 | 174 | 30 | 0.28 | 0.064 | 0.4 | 33 | 2.6 | 0.01 | 0.10 | 4.6 | 19524 |
| **tortilla chips**, blue corn, unsalted, Garden of Eatin' - *1 oz (16 chips)* | 28 | 140 | | 18.0 | 0 | | 2.0 | 10 | 20 | | | | | 0 | | | | |
| | | 2.0 | 7.0 | 0.5 | 5.0 | 1.0 | | | | | 0.36 | | 0 | | | | | GARD1 |
| **tortilla chips**, blue corn w/sesame *1 oz (about 14 chips)* | 28 | 140 | | 16.0 | 0 | | 3.0 | 170 | 0 | | | | | 0 | | | | |
| | | 2.0 | 9.0 | 1.5 | | | 0 | | | | 0.36 | | 0 | | | | | ORGA1 |
| **tortilla chips**, light (baked w/less oil) *1 oz* | 28 | 130 | 0.4 | 20.6 | 0.1 | | 1.6 | 281 | 45 | 27 | 0.32 | | 1 | 0 | 0.06 | 0.1 | 0.02 | |
| | | 2.4 | 4.3 | 0.8 | 1.8 | 1.4 | 1 | 76 | 89 | 0.46 | 0.032 | 4.4 | 23 | 1.0 | 0.08 | 0.05 | 4.5 | 43566 |

Each food has two data rows. In every column the upper value corresponds to the first header label and the lower value to the second (e.g. KCAL then PRO, H2O then FAT, etc.).

| Food | WT (g) | KCAL / PRO (g) | H2O (g) / FAT (g) | CHO (g) / SFA (g) | TSUG (g) / MUFA (g) | ASUG (g) / PUFA (g) | DFIB (g) / CHOL (mg) | Na (mg) / K (mg) | Ca (mg) / P (mg) | Mg (mg) / Fe (mg) | Zn (mg) / Cu (mg) | Mn (mg) / Se (mcg) | A (mcg RAE) / A (IU) | C (mg) / E (mg ATE) | B-1 (mg) / B-2 (mg) | NIA (mg) / B-6 (mg) | B-12 (mcg) / FOL (mcg DFE) | PANT (mg) / REF |
|---|---|---|---|---|---|---|---|---|---|---|---|---|---|---|---|---|---|---|
| tortilla chips, lowfat, baked | 28 | 116 | 0.5 | 22.4 | 0.2 | 0 | 1.5 | 117 | 45 | 27 | 0.32 |  | 1 |  | 0.06 | 0.1 |  | 0 |
| *1 oz* |  | 3.1 | 1.6 | 0.2 | 0.5 | 0.8 | 0 | 76 | 89 | 0.45 | 0.031 | 4.4 | 29 | 0.2 | 0.08 | 0.05 | 4.5 | 19433 |
| tortilla chips, lowfat, unsalted | 28 | 116 | 0.5 | 22.4 | 0.2 | 0 | 1.5 | 4 | 45 | 27 | 0.32 |  | 1 | 0 | 0.06 | 0.1 |  | 0 |
| *1 oz* |  | 3.1 | 1.6 | 0.2 | 0.5 | 0.8 | 0 | 76 | 89 | 0.45 | 0.031 | 4.4 | 23 | 1.0 | 0.08 | 0.05 | 4.5 | 19833 |
| tortilla chips, multigrain, Snyder | 28 | 130 |  | 20.0 | 2.0 |  | 3.0 | 110 | 0 |  |  |  |  | 0 |  |  |  |  |
| *1 oz* |  | 2.0 | 5.0 | 0 |  |  | 0 |  |  |  | 0.36 |  | 0 |  |  |  |  | SNYD26 |
| tortilla chips, nacho | 28 | 144 | 0.4 | 17.3 | 1.1 |  | 1.3 | 172 | 41 | 21 | 0.41 | 0.097 | 0 |  | 0.01 | 0.4 |  | 0.20 |
| *1 oz* |  | 2.3 | 7.3 | 1.1 | 2.0 | 3.8 |  | 67 | 72 | 0.31 | 0.029 | 2.2 |  |  | 0.01 | 0.06 |  | 19057 |
| tortilla chips, nacho cheese, lowfat, made w/Olestra - *1 oz* | 28 | 89 | 0.5 | 18.3 | 0.8 | 0 | 1.8 | 169 | 36 | 28 | 0.95 | 0.160 | 3 | 2 | 0.06 | 0.4 | 0.08 | 0.06 |
| *made w/Olestra - 1 oz* |  | 2.4 | 1.0 | 0.3 | 0.4 | 0.3 | 1 | 111 | 69 | 1.34 | 0.039 | 2.6 | 85 | 1.0 | 0.04 | 0.07 | 4.5 | 19444 |
| tortilla chips, nacho, reduced-fat | 28 | 125 | 0.4 | 20.0 |  |  | 1.3 | 281 | 45 | 27 |  | 0.122 | 7 | 0 | 0.06 | 0.1 | 0 |  |
| *1 oz* |  | 2.4 | 4.3 | 0.8 | 2.5 | 0.6 | 1 | 76 | 89 | 0.46 | 0.040 |  | 106 |  | 0.08 | 0.06 | 7.3 | 19424 |
| tortilla chips, ranch | 28 | 140 | 0.9 | 17.6 | 0.8 |  | 1.1 | 145 | 38 | 24 | 0.40 | 0.102 | 0 |  | 0.01 | 0.4 |  | 0.17 |
| *1 oz* |  | 2.0 | 6.9 | 1.0 | 2.0 | 3.8 |  | 73 | 71 | 0.39 | 0.028 | 2.0 |  |  | 0.02 | 0.06 |  | 19058 |
| tortilla chips, taco flavor | 28 | 134 | 0.4 | 17.7 |  |  | 1.5 | 220 | 43 | 25 | 0.36 | 0.124 | 13 | 0 | 0.07 | 0.6 | 0 | 0.08 |
| *1 oz* |  | 2.2 | 6.8 | 1.3 | 4.0 | 0.9 | 1 | 61 | 67 | 0.57 | 0.052 | 1.9 | 253 |  | 0.06 | 0.08 | 5.9 | 19063 |
| tortilla chips, white corn | 28 | 137 | 0.5 | 18.4 | 0.3 | 0 | 1.5 | 118 | 49 | 41 | 0.69 |  | 0 | 0 | 0 | 0.4 | 0.10 | 0.33 |
| *1 oz* |  | 2.2 | 6.5 | 0.8 | 1.9 | 3.4 | 0 | 60 | 56 | 0.65 | 0.146 | 1.9 | 1 | 1.2 | 0.03 | 0.06 | 5.6 | 19056 |
| tortilla chips, white corn, rstrnt-style, Utz - *1 oz (6 chips)* | 28 | 140 |  | 18.0 | 0 |  | 1.0 | 120 | 20 |  |  |  |  | 0 |  |  |  |  |
| *Utz - 1 oz (6 chips)* |  | 2.0 | 7.0 | 1.0 |  |  | 0 |  |  |  | 0.36 |  | 0 |  |  |  |  | UTZQ1 |
| tortilla chips, white corn, unsalted | 28 | 141 | 0.6 | 18.3 | 0.3 | 0 | 1.5 | 4 | 49 | 41 | 0.69 |  | 1 | 0 | 0 | 0.4 | 0.10 | 0.33 |
| *1 oz* |  | 2.2 | 6.5 | 0.7 | 2.7 | 2.8 | 0 | 60 | 56 | 0.65 | 0.146 | 1.9 | 23 | 1.0 | 0.03 | 0.06 | 2.8 | 43364 |
| tortilla chips, yellow corn | 28 | 138 | 0.6 | 18.8 | 0.3 |  | 1.3 | 79 | 26 | 24 | 0.45 | 0.113 |  |  | 0.04 | 0.5 |  | 0.12 |
| *1 oz* |  | 2.0 | 6.0 | 0.7 | 2.9 | 2.0 |  | 62 | 66 | 0.45 | 0.031 | 2.4 |  |  | 0.01 | 0.06 |  | 25028 |
| trail mix bar, fruit 'n nut, Nature Valley - *1.2 oz bar* | 35 | 140 |  | 25.0 | 13.0 |  | 1.0 | 115 |  |  |  |  |  |  |  |  |  |  |
| *Valley - 1.2 oz bar* |  | 3.0 | 4.0 | 0.5 |  |  | 0 |  |  |  |  |  |  |  |  |  |  | GENM225 |
| veggie crisps, cheddar and jalapeno, Snyder - *1 oz* | 28 | 130 |  | 18.0 | 1.0 |  | 2.0 | 430 | 0 |  |  |  |  | 0 |  |  |  |  |
| *jalapeno, Snyder - 1 oz* |  | 1.0 | 7.0 | 0.5 |  |  | 0 |  |  |  | 0.36 |  | 100 |  |  |  |  | SNYD8 |
| veggie crisps, Snyder | 28 | 140 |  | 18.0 | 0 |  | 2.0 | 290 | 0 |  |  |  |  | 0 |  |  |  |  |
| *1 oz* |  | 1.0 | 7.0 | 0.5 |  |  | 0 |  |  |  | 0.36 |  | 0 |  |  |  |  | SNYD6 |
| veggie crisps, sundried tomato and pesto, Snyder - *1 oz* | 28 | 140 |  | 19.0 | 0 |  | 3.0 | 390 | 0 |  |  |  |  | 0 |  |  |  |  |
| *pesto, Snyder - 1 oz* |  | 1.0 | 7.0 | 0.5 |  |  | 0 |  |  |  | 0.36 |  | 100 |  |  |  |  | SNYD7 |

## 17. GRAIN PRODUCTS
### 17.1 BAGELS

| Food | WT (g) | KCAL / PRO (g) | H2O (g) / FAT (g) | CHO (g) / SFA (g) | TSUG (g) / MUFA (g) | ASUG (g) / PUFA (g) | DFIB (g) / CHOL (mg) | Na (mg) / K (mg) | Ca (mg) / P (mg) | Mg (mg) / Fe (mg) | Zn (mg) / Cu (mg) | Mn (mg) / Se (mcg) | A (mcg RAE) / A (IU) | C (mg) / E (mg ATE) | B-1 (mg) / B-2 (mg) | NIA (mg) / B-6 (mg) | B-12 (mcg) / FOL (mcg DFE) | PANT (mg) / REF |
|---|---|---|---|---|---|---|---|---|---|---|---|---|---|---|---|---|---|---|
| bagel, cinnamon raisin | 105 | 287 | 33.6 | 58.0 | 6.3 | 3.8 | 2.4 | 338 | 20 | 29 | 1.19 | 0.920 | 22 | 1 | 0.40 | 3.2 | 0 | 0.53 |
| *3.7 oz bagel (3½" diameter)* |  | 10.3 | 1.8 | 0.3 | 0.2 | 0.7 | 0 | 155 | 105 | 3.99 | 0.171 | 32.6 | 77 | 0.3 | 0.29 | 0.07 | 182.7 | 18005 |
| bagel, egg (egg in bagel dough) | 105 | 292 | 34.3 | 55.6 |  |  | 2.4 | 530 | 14 | 26 | 0.81 | 0.430 | 35 | 1 | 0.56 | 3.6 | 0.17 | 0.70 |
| *3.7 oz bagel (4" diameter)* |  | 11.1 | 2.2 | 0.4 | 0.4 | 0.7 | 25 | 71 | 88 | 4.18 | 0.094 | 32.1 | 114 |  | 0.25 | 0.09 | 140.7 | 18003 |
| bagel, oat bran | 105 | 268 | 34.5 | 56.0 | 1.7 | 1.4 | 3.8 | 532 | 13 | 33 | 0.94 | 0.906 | 1 | 0 | 0.35 | 3.1 | 0 | 0.47 |
| *3.7 oz bagel (4" diameter)* |  | 11.2 | 1.3 | 0.2 | 0.3 | 0.5 | 0 | 121 | 116 | 3.23 | 0.159 | 35.9 | 4 | 0.3 | 0.35 | 0.05 | 140.7 | 18007 |
| bagel, pln/onion/popysd/sesame sd | 105 | 270 | 38.1 | 53.0 | 5.3 | 5.1 | 2.3 | 470 | 93 | 23 | 2.00 | 0.541 | 0 | 1 | 0.63 | 4.2 | 0 | 0.22 |
| *3.7 oz bagel (4" diameter)* |  | 10.5 | 1.7 | 0.4 | 0.5 | 0.7 | 0 | 79 | 91 | 6.35 | 0.136 | 23.9 | 0 | 0.1 | 0.27 | 0.07 | 237.3 | 18001 |

### 17.2 BISCUITS

| Food | WT (g) | KCAL / PRO (g) | H2O (g) / FAT (g) | CHO (g) / SFA (g) | TSUG (g) / MUFA (g) | ASUG (g) / PUFA (g) | DFIB (g) / CHOL (mg) | Na (mg) / K (mg) | Ca (mg) / P (mg) | Mg (mg) / Fe (mg) | Zn (mg) / Cu (mg) | Mn (mg) / Se (mcg) | A (mcg RAE) / A (IU) | C (mg) / E (mg ATE) | B-1 (mg) / B-2 (mg) | NIA (mg) / B-6 (mg) | B-12 (mcg) / FOL (mcg DFE) | PANT (mg) / REF |
|---|---|---|---|---|---|---|---|---|---|---|---|---|---|---|---|---|---|---|
| biscuit, Butter Tastin, from refrig dough, Grands! - *2 oz biscuit* | 58 | 180 |  | 24.0 | 5.0 |  | 0.5 | 590 | 20 |  |  |  |  | 0 |  |  |  |  |
| *dough, Grands! - 2 oz biscuit* |  | 4.0 | 8.0 | 2.5 |  |  | 0 |  |  |  | 1.44 |  | 0 |  |  |  |  | GENM237 |
| biscuit, buttermilk, from refrig dough, Grands! - *2 oz biscuit* | 58 | 190 |  | 24.0 | 4.0 |  | 0.5 | 600 | 20 |  |  |  |  | 0 |  |  |  |  |
| *dough, Grands! - 2 oz biscuit* |  | 4.0 | 8.0 | 3.0 |  |  | 0 |  |  |  | 1.44 |  | 0 |  |  |  |  | GENM231 |
| biscuit, buttermlk, red fat, from refrig dough, Grands! - *2 oz biscuit* | 58 | 170 |  | 26.0 | 5.0 |  | 0.5 | 590 | 20 |  |  |  |  | 0 |  |  |  |  |
| *dough, Grands! - 2 oz biscuit* |  | 4.0 | 6.0 | 3.5 | 1.5 | 0.5 | 0 |  |  |  | 1.44 |  | 0 |  |  |  |  | GENM234 |
| biscuit, country, from refrig dough, Pillsbury - *2.3 oz biscuit* | 64 | 150 |  | 29.0 | 4.0 |  | 1.0 | 570 | 0 |  |  |  |  | 0 |  |  |  |  |
| *Pillsbury - 2.3 oz biscuit* |  | 4.0 | 2.0 | 0 | 0 | 0 | 0 |  |  |  | 1.44 |  | 0 |  |  |  |  | GENM239 |
| biscuit dough, buttermilk, refrig, Pillsbury - *2.3 oz biscuit* | 64 | 150 | 26.0 | 29.0 | 4.0 |  | 1.0 | 570 |  |  |  |  |  |  |  |  |  |  |
| *Pillsbury - 2.3 oz biscuit* |  | 4.0 | 2.0 | 0.3 |  |  | 0 |  |  |  | 1.44 |  |  |  |  |  |  | 18629 |
| biscuit dough, buttermilk, refrig, Pillsbury Grands - *2.2 oz biscuit* | 61 | 193 | 20.4 | 25.2 | 4.2 |  | 0.7 | 631 | 21 |  |  |  |  |  |  |  |  |  |
| *Pillsbury Grands - 2.2 oz biscuit* |  | 4.2 | 8.4 | 3.2 |  |  | 0 |  |  |  | 1.51 |  |  |  |  |  |  | 18633 |
| biscuit dough, btrmlk, refrig, Pillsbury Hungry Jk - *1.2 oz biscuit* | 34 | 104 | 12.1 | 14.0 | 2.0 |  | 0.4 | 360 |  |  |  |  |  |  |  |  |  |  |
| *Hungry Jk - 1.2 oz biscuit* |  | 2.0 | 4.5 | 1.0 |  |  | 0 |  |  |  | 0.72 |  |  |  |  |  |  | 18634 |

| Food | WT (g) | KCAL / PRO (g) | H2O (g) / FAT (g) | CHO (g) / SFA (g) | TSUG (g) / MUFA (g) | ASUG (g) / PUFA (g) | DFIB (g) / CHOL (mg) | Na (mg) / K (mg) | Ca (mg) / P (mg) | Mg (mg) / Fe (mg) | Zn (mg) / Cu (mg) | Mn (mg) / Se (mcg) | A (mcg RAE) / A (IU) | C (mg) / E (mg ATE) | B-1 (mg) / B-2 (mg) | NIA (mg) / B-6 (mg) | B-12 (mcg) / FOL (mcg DFE) | PANT (mg) / REF |
|---|---|---|---|---|---|---|---|---|---|---|---|---|---|---|---|---|---|---|
| biscuit dough, mixed grain, refrig | 44 | 116 | 16.6 | 20.9 | | | | 295 | 7 | 13 | 0.26 | 0.290 | 0 | 0 | 0.17 | 1.5 | 0 | 0.14 |
| *1.6 oz biscuit (2½" diameter)* | | 2.7 | 2.5 | 0.6 | 1.3 | 0.4 | 0 | 201 | 104 | 1.21 | 0.051 | | 0 | | 0.09 | 0.03 | 58.5 | 18017 |
| **biscuit**, extra rich, from refrig dough, Grands! - 2.15 oz biscuit | 61 | 210 | | 26.0 | 6.0 | | 0.5 | 580 | 20 | | | | 0 | 0 | | | | |
| | | 4.0 | 10.0 | 3.0 | | | 0 | | | 1.44 | | | 0 | | | | | GENM240 |
| **biscuit**, flaky, from refrig dough, Grands! - 2.15 oz biscuit | 58 | 190 | | 24.0 | 5.0 | | 0.5 | 550 | 20 | | | | 0 | 0 | | | | |
| | | 4.0 | 9.0 | 2.0 | | | 0 | | | 1.08 | | | 0 | | | | | GENM241 |
| **biscuit**, flaky layer btrmlk, from refrig dough, Pillsbury - 2.3 oz bsct | 64 | 160 | | 28.0 | 4.0 | | 1.0 | 550 | 0 | | | | 0 | 0 | | | | |
| | | 4.0 | 4.0 | 1.0 | | | 0 | | | 1.44 | | | 0 | | | | | GENM249 |
| **biscuit mix**, buttermilk | 35 | 150 | 3.2 | 22.2 | 4.1 | 0 | 0.7 | 447 | 63 | 9 | 0.21 | 0.119 | 1 | 0 | 0.20 | 1.6 | 0.14 | 0.31 |
| *1 biscuit* | | 2.8 | 5.4 | 1.4 | 3.0 | 0.7 | 1 | 57 | 205 | 0.97 | 0.054 | 2.6 | 2 | 0 | 0.15 | 0.03 | 72.4 | 18010 |
| **biscuit**, plain/buttermilk | 51 | 186 | 13.6 | 24.7 | 1.8 | 1.3 | 0.7 | 537 | 25 | 9 | 0.24 | 0.200 | 0 | 0 | 0.22 | 1.7 | 0.07 | 0.15 |
| *1.8 oz medium biscuit* | | 3.2 | 8.4 | 1.3 | 3.5 | 3.2 | 1 | 114 | 219 | 1.68 | 0.042 | 9.6 | 1 | 0.7 | 0.15 | 0.02 | 58.1 | 18009 |
| **biscuit**, plain/buttermilk, from mix | 28 | 94 | 8.1 | 13.6 | | | 0.5 | 267 | 52 | 7 | 0.17 | 0.070 | 7 | 0 | 0.10 | 0.8 | 0.06 | 0.15 |
| *1 oz biscuit* | | 2.0 | 3.4 | 0.8 | 1.2 | 1.2 | 1 | 53 | 132 | 0.57 | 0.032 | 1.7 | 26 | 0 | 0.10 | 0.02 | 23.5 | 18011 |
| **biscuit**, plain/buttermilk, from refrig dough (12–28% fat) - 1 oz biscuit | 27 | 95 | 7.4 | 12.6 | 2.2 | 2.0 | 0.2 | 292 | 15 | 5 | 0.14 | 0.127 | 1 | 0 | 0.11 | 1.0 | 0.02 | 0.11 |
| | | 2.0 | 4.1 | 1.0 | 2.4 | 0.3 | 0 | 48 | 138 | 0.72 | 0.024 | 2.3 | 2 | 0.2 | 0.08 | 0.02 | 18.4 | 18015 |
| **biscuit**, plain/buttermilk, from refrig dough (2–12% fat) - .7 oz biscuit | 21 | 63 | 5.8 | 11.6 | 1.7 | 1.6 | 0.4 | 305 | 4 | 4 | 0.10 | 0.074 | 0 | 0 | 0.09 | 0.7 | 0 | 0.06 |
| | | 1.6 | 1.1 | 0.3 | 0.6 | 0.2 | 0 | 39 | 98 | 0.65 | 0.019 | 3.7 | 0 | 0 | 0.05 | 0.01 | 29.0 | 18013 |
| **biscuit**, plain/buttermilk, homemade | 60 | 212 | 17.3 | 26.8 | 1.3 | 0 | 0.9 | 348 | 141 | 11 | 0.32 | 0.227 | 0 | | 0.21 | 1.8 | 0.05 | 0.17 |
| *2.1 oz biscuit (2½" diameter)* | | 4.2 | 9.8 | 2.6 | 4.2 | 2.5 | 2 | 73 | 98 | 1.74 | 0.049 | 11.7 | 49 | | 0.19 | 0.02 | 57.0 | 18016 |
| **biscuit**, southern style, from refrig dough, Grands! - 2 oz biscuit | 58 | 180 | | 24.0 | 5.0 | | 0.5 | 590 | 20 | | | | 0 | 0 | | | | |
| | | 4.0 | 8.0 | 2.5 | | | 0 | | | 1.44 | | | 0 | | | | | GENM248 |
| **biscuit**, wheat, reduced fat, from refrig dough, Grands! - 2.15 oz biscuit | 61 | 180 | | 28.0 | 6.0 | | 1.0 | 590 | 20 | | | | 0 | 0 | | | | |
| | | 4.0 | 6.0 | 1.5 | | | 0 | | | 1.44 | | | 0 | | | | | GENM250 |

## 17.3 BREADS, QUICK

| Food | WT (g) | KCAL / PRO (g) | H2O (g) / FAT (g) | CHO (g) / SFA (g) | TSUG (g) / MUFA (g) | ASUG (g) / PUFA (g) | DFIB (g) / CHOL (mg) | Na (mg) / K (mg) | Ca (mg) / P (mg) | Mg (mg) / Fe (mg) | Zn (mg) / Cu (mg) | Mn (mg) / Se (mcg) | A (mcg RAE) / A (IU) | C (mg) / E (mg ATE) | B-1 (mg) / B-2 (mg) | NIA (mg) / B-6 (mg) | B-12 (mcg) / FOL (mcg DFE) | PANT (mg) / REF |
|---|---|---|---|---|---|---|---|---|---|---|---|---|---|---|---|---|---|---|
| **banana bread**, homemade w/marg | 60 | 196 | 17.5 | 32.8 | | | 0.7 | 181 | 13 | 8 | 0.21 | 0.125 | 64 | 1 | 0.10 | 0.9 | 0.06 | 0.16 |
| *2.1 oz slice* | | 2.6 | 6.3 | 1.3 | 2.7 | 1.9 | 26 | 80 | 35 | 0.84 | 0.043 | 7.3 | 296 | | 0.12 | 0.09 | 28.8 | 18019 |
| **Boston brown bread**, canned | 45 | 88 | 21.2 | 19.5 | 1.1 | 0.5 | 2.1 | 284 | 32 | 28 | 0.22 | 0.459 | 11 | 0 | 0.01 | 0.5 | 0 | 0.25 |
| *1.6 oz slice* | | 2.3 | 0.7 | 0.1 | 0.1 | 0.3 | 0 | 143 | 50 | 0.94 | 0.036 | 9.9 | 39 | 0.1 | 0.05 | 0.04 | 6.3 | 18021 |
| **cornbread**, from mix | 60 | 188 | 19.1 | 28.9 | | | 1.4 | 467 | 44 | 12 | 0.38 | 0.130 | 26 | 0 | 0.15 | 1.2 | 0.10 | 0.26 |
| *2.1 oz piece* | | 4.3 | 6.0 | 1.6 | 3.1 | 0.7 | 37 | 77 | 226 | 1.14 | 0.037 | 5.9 | 123 | | 0.16 | 0.06 | 51.6 | 18023 |
| **cornbread**, homemade with 2% milk | 65 | 173 | 25.4 | 28.3 | | | | 428 | 162 | 16 | 0.39 | 0.077 | | 0 | 0.19 | 1.5 | 0.10 | 0.22 |
| *2.3 oz piece* | | 4.4 | 4.6 | 1.0 | 1.2 | 2.1 | 26 | 96 | 110 | 1.62 | 0.033 | 6.6 | 180 | | 0.19 | 0.07 | 76.7 | 18024 |
| **hush puppies**, homemade | 22 | 74 | 6.4 | 10.1 | 0.4 | 0 | 0.6 | 147 | 61 | 5 | 0.15 | 0.048 | 9 | 0 | 0.08 | 0.6 | 0.04 | 0.08 |
| *.8 oz hush puppy* | | 1.7 | 3.0 | 0.5 | 0.7 | 1.6 | 10 | 32 | 42 | 0.67 | 0.015 | 3.5 | 41 | 0.3 | 0.07 | 0.02 | 30.1 | 18270 |
| **Irish soda bread**, homemade | 28 | 81 | 8.4 | 15.7 | | | 0.7 | 111 | 23 | 6 | 0.16 | 0.099 | 13 | 0 | 0.08 | 0.7 | 0.01 | 0.07 |
| *1 oz slice* | | 1.8 | 1.4 | 0.3 | 0.6 | 0.4 | 5 | 74 | 32 | 0.75 | 0.036 | 4.5 | 54 | | 0.08 | 0.02 | 20.4 | 18032 |

## 17.4 BREADS, YEAST

| Food | WT (g) | KCAL / PRO (g) | H2O (g) / FAT (g) | CHO (g) / SFA (g) | TSUG (g) / MUFA (g) | ASUG (g) / PUFA (g) | DFIB (g) / CHOL (mg) | Na (mg) / K (mg) | Ca (mg) / P (mg) | Mg (mg) / Fe (mg) | Zn (mg) / Cu (mg) | Mn (mg) / Se (mcg) | A (mcg RAE) / A (IU) | C (mg) / E (mg ATE) | B-1 (mg) / B-2 (mg) | NIA (mg) / B-6 (mg) | B-12 (mcg) / FOL (mcg DFE) | PANT (mg) / REF |
|---|---|---|---|---|---|---|---|---|---|---|---|---|---|---|---|---|---|---|
| **breadcrumbs**, dry, grated | 108 | 427 | 7.0 | 77.7 | 6.7 | 5.6 | 4.9 | 791 | 198 | 46 | 1.57 | 0.993 | 0 | 0 | 1.04 | 7.2 | 0.38 | 0.60 |
| *1 cup* | | 14.4 | 5.7 | 1.3 | 1.1 | 2.2 | 0 | 212 | 178 | 5.22 | 0.275 | 27.2 | 0 | 0.1 | 0.44 | 0.13 | 177.1 | 18079 |
| **breadcrumbs**, dry, grated, seasoned | 120 | 460 | 7.6 | 82.2 | 6.9 | | 5.9 | 2111 | 218 | 55 | 1.72 | 1.181 | 12 | 3 | 1.15 | 7.4 | | 0.75 |
| *1 cup* | | 17.0 | 6.6 | 1.7 | 1.4 | 2.8 | 1 | 277 | 212 | 5.90 | 0.293 | 29.6 | 232 | 0.3 | 0.50 | 0.21 | 225.6 | 18376 |
| **breadcrumbs**, garlic, herb, Progresso | 28 | 110 | | 19.0 | 2.0 | | 1.0 | 520 | 40 | | | | 0 | 0 | | | | |
| *¼ cup (1 oz)* | | 4.0 | 1.5 | 0.5 | | | 0 | | | 1.44 | | | 0 | | | | | GENM391 |
| **breadcrumbs**, Italian style, Progresso | 28 | 110 | | 20.0 | 2.0 | | 1.0 | 450 | 40 | | | | 0 | 0 | | | | |
| *¼ cup (1 oz)* | | 4.0 | 1.5 | 0.5 | | | 0 | | | 1.44 | | | 0 | | | | | GENM392 |
| **breadcrumbs**, Parmesan Progresso | 28 | 100 | | 18.0 | 2.0 | | 1.0 | 850 | 40 | | | | 0 | 0 | | | | |
| *¼ cup (1 oz)* | | 4.0 | 1.5 | 0 | | | 0 | | | 1.08 | | | 0 | | | | | GENM251 |
| **breadcrumbs**, plain, Progresso | 28 | 110 | | 20.0 | 2.0 | | 1.0 | 200 | 40 | | | | 0 | 0 | | | | |
| *¼ cup (1 oz)* | | 4.0 | 1.5 | 0.5 | | | 0 | | | 1.08 | | | 0 | | | | | GENM393 |
| **cracked wheat bread** | 25 | 65 | 9.0 | 12.4 | | | 1.4 | 134 | 11 | 13 | 0.31 | 0.343 | 0 | 0 | 0.09 | 0.9 | 0 | 0.13 |
| *.9 oz slice* | | 2.2 | 1.0 | 0.2 | 0.5 | 0.2 | 0 | 44 | 38 | 0.70 | 0.056 | 6.3 | 0 | | 0.06 | 0.08 | 19.0 | 18025 |
| **croutons** | 30 | 122 | 1.6 | 22.0 | | | 1.5 | 209 | 23 | 9 | 0.27 | 0.150 | 0 | 0 | 0.19 | 1.6 | 0 | 0.13 |
| *1 cup* | | 3.6 | 2.0 | 0.5 | 0.9 | 0.4 | 0 | 37 | 34 | 1.22 | 0.049 | 11.2 | 0 | | 0.08 | 0.01 | 62.7 | 18242 |
| **croutons**, seasoned | 40 | 186 | 1.4 | 25.4 | 1.8 | 0.8 | 2.0 | 495 | 38 | 17 | 0.38 | 0.206 | 3 | 0 | 0.20 | 1.9 | 0.06 | 0.33 |
| *1 cup* | | 4.3 | 7.3 | 2.1 | 3.8 | 0.9 | 3 | 72 | 56 | 1.13 | 0.067 | 11.5 | 13 | 0.2 | 0.17 | 0.03 | 60.4 | 18243 |
| **croutons**, seasoned, classic style, Pepperidge Farm - 1 cup | 7 | 33 | 0.2 | 4.3 | | | | 97 | | | | | | | | | | |
| | | 1.0 | 1.3 | 0.3 | | | | | | | | | | | | | | 18626 |

| | WT (g) | KCAL / PRO (g) | H₂0 (g) / FAT (g) | CHO (g) / SFA (g) | TSUG (g) / MUFA (g) | ASUG (g) / PUFA (g) | DFIB (g) / CHOL (mg) | Na (mg) / K (mg) | Ca (mg) / P (mg) | Mg (mg) / Fe (mg) | Zn (mg) / Cu (mg) | Mn (mg) / Se (mcg) | A (mcg RAE) / A (IU) | C (mg) / E (mg ATE) | B-1 (mg) / B-2 (mg) | NIA (mg) / B-6 (mg) | B-12 (mcg) / FOL (mcg DFE) | PANT (mg) / REF |
|---|---|---|---|---|---|---|---|---|---|---|---|---|---|---|---|---|---|---|
| **egg bread** | 40 | 113 | 13.9 | 19.1 | 0.7 | 0.5 | 0.9 | 197 | 37 | 8 | 0.32 | 0.200 | 25 | 0 | 0.18 | 1.9 | 0.04 | 0.11 |
| *1.4 oz slice (5″ × 3″ × ½″)* | | 3.8 | 2.4 | 0.6 | 0.9 | 0.4 | 20 | 46 | 42 | 1.22 | 0.065 | 12.0 | 84 | 0.1 | 0.17 | 0.03 | 52.0 | 18027 |
| **French bread** | 32 | 92 | 8.9 | 18.1 | 0.8 | 0 | 0.8 | 208 | 14 | 9 | 0.30 | 0.168 | 0 | 0 | 0.14 | 1.5 | 0 | 0.11 |
| *small slice (2″ × 2½″ × 1¾″)* | | 3.8 | 0.6 | 0.2 | 0.1 | 0.3 | 0 | 41 | 36 | 1.16 | 0.044 | 8.7 | 0 | 0.1 | 0.09 | 0.03 | 73.6 | 18029 |
| **French bread dough**, refrigerated, | 62 | 149 | 24.8 | 28.6 | 2.4 | | 1.1 | 358 | | | | | | | | | | |
| Pillsbury - *2.2 oz slice* | | 4.8 | 1.8 | 0.6 | | | 0 | | | 1.72 | | | | | | | | 18631 |
| **French toast**, frozen | 59 | 126 | 31.0 | 18.9 | | | 0.6 | 292 | 63 | 10 | 0.45 | 0.145 | 32 | 0 | 0.16 | 1.6 | 0.99 | 0.55 |
| *2.1 oz piece* | | 4.4 | 3.6 | 0.9 | 1.2 | 0.7 | 48 | 79 | 82 | 1.30 | 0.050 | 9.9 | 110 | | 0.22 | 0.29 | 42.5 | 18268 |
| **French toast**, homemade with 2% | 65 | 149 | 35.6 | 16.2 | | | | 311 | 65 | 11 | 0.44 | 0.122 | 81 | 0 | 0.13 | 1.1 | 0.20 | 0.36 |
| milk - *2.3 oz piece* | | 5.0 | 7.0 | 1.8 | 2.9 | 1.7 | 75 | 87 | 76 | 1.09 | 0.038 | 13.1 | 327 | | 0.21 | 0.05 | 37.1 | 18269 |
| **garlic bread**, Italian, frzn, | 50 | 186 | 14.6 | 20.8 | | | | 200 | | | | | | | | | | |
| Pepperidge Farm - *1.8 oz slice* | | 4.2 | 9.6 | 2.4 | 3.9 | 1.8 | 6 | | | 1.18 | | | | | | | | 18627 |
| **garlic toast**, frozen, Mamma Bella | 38 | 140 | | 16.0 | 0 | | | 220 | 0 | | | | | 0 | | | | |
| *⅞ inch slice* | | 3.0 | 7.0 | 1.5 | | | 0 | | | 0.72 | | | 300 | | | | | MARZ1 |
| **Health Nut bread**, Arnold Hearty | 38 | 110 | | 18.0 | 3.0 | | 2.0 | 200 | 40 | | | | | 0 | | | | |
| Classics - *1.3 oz slice* | | 4.0 | 2.0 | 0 | 1.0 | 0 | 0 | | | 1.44 | | | 0 | | | | | ARNO1 |
| **Italian bread** | 30 | 81 | 10.7 | 15.0 | 0.2 | 0 | 0.8 | 175 | 23 | 8 | 0.26 | 0.139 | 0 | 0 | 0.14 | 1.3 | 0 | 0.11 |
| *1.1 oz slice (4½″ × 3¼″ × ¾″)* | | 2.6 | 1.0 | 0.3 | 0.2 | 0.4 | 0 | 33 | 31 | 0.88 | 0.057 | 8.2 | 0 | 0.1 | 0.09 | 0.01 | 91.2 | 18033 |
| **mixed-/whole-/7-grain bread** | 26 | 69 | 9.6 | 11.3 | 1.7 | 1.7 | 1.9 | 109 | 27 | 20 | 0.44 | 0.526 | 0 | 0 | 0.07 | 1.1 | 0 | 0.09 |
| *.92 oz slice* | | 3.5 | 1.1 | 0.2 | 0.2 | 0.5 | 0 | 60 | 59 | 0.65 | 0.073 | 8.6 | 0 | 0.1 | 0.03 | 0.07 | 19.5 | 18035 |
| **oat bran bread** | 30 | 71 | 13.2 | 11.9 | 2.3 | 2.2 | 1.3 | 122 | 20 | 10 | 0.27 | 0.234 | 1 | 0 | 0.15 | 1.4 | 0 | 0.17 |
| *1.1 oz slice* | | 3.1 | 1.3 | 0.2 | 0.5 | 0.5 | 0 | 44 | 42 | 0.94 | 0.040 | 9.0 | 2 | 0.1 | 0.10 | 0.02 | 36.0 | 18037 |
| **oat bran bread**, reduced calorie | 23 | 46 | 10.6 | 9.5 | 0.8 | 0.5 | 2.8 | 81 | 13 | 13 | 0.24 | 0.253 | 0 | 0 | 0.08 | 0.9 | 0 | 0.11 |
| *.81 oz slice* | | 1.8 | 0.7 | 0.1 | 0.2 | 0.4 | 0 | 23 | 32 | 0.72 | 0.067 | 4.7 | 0 | 0.1 | 0.05 | 0.02 | 26.2 | 18049 |
| **oatmeal bread** | 27 | 73 | 9.9 | 13.1 | 2.2 | 2.1 | 1.1 | 162 | 18 | 10 | 0.28 | 0.254 | 1 | 0 | 0.11 | 0.8 | 0.01 | 0.09 |
| *.95 oz slice* | | 2.3 | 1.2 | 0.2 | 0.4 | 0.5 | 0 | 38 | 34 | 0.73 | 0.056 | 6.6 | 4 | 0.1 | 0.06 | 0.02 | 23.5 | 18039 |
| **oatmeal bread**, reduced calorie | 23 | 48 | 10.1 | 10.0 | | | | 89 | 26 | 6 | 0.19 | 0.124 | 0 | 0 | 0.08 | 0.7 | 0.02 | 0.10 |
| *.81 oz slice* | | 1.7 | 0.8 | 0.1 | 0.2 | 0.3 | 0 | 29 | 23 | 0.53 | 0.023 | 5.3 | 1 | | 0.06 | 0.01 | 16.1 | 18051 |
| **protein/gluten bread** | 19 | 47 | 7.6 | 8.3 | 0.3 | 0 | 0.6 | 104 | 24 | 12 | 0.35 | 0.280 | 0 | 0 | 0.07 | 0.8 | 0 | 0.08 |
| *.67 oz slice* | | 2.3 | 0.4 | 0.1 | 0 | 0.2 | 0 | 61 | 35 | 0.79 | 0.079 | 6.3 | 1 | 0.1 | 0.07 | 0.01 | 32.9 | 18043 |
| **pumpernickel bread** | 26 | 65 | 9.9 | 12.4 | 0.1 | 0 | 1.7 | 174 | 14 | 18 | 0.38 | 0.339 | 0 | 0 | 0.09 | 0.8 | 0 | 0.11 |
| *.92 oz slice* | | 2.3 | 0.8 | 0.1 | 0.2 | 0.3 | 0 | 54 | 46 | 0.75 | 0.075 | 6.4 | 0 | 0.1 | 0.08 | 0.03 | 34.8 | 18044 |
| **raisin bread** | 26 | 71 | 8.7 | 13.6 | 1.5 | 1.3 | 1.1 | 101 | 17 | 7 | 0.19 | 0.130 | 0 | 0 | 0.09 | 0.9 | 0 | 0.10 |
| *.92 oz slice* | | 2.1 | 1.1 | 0.3 | 0.6 | 0.2 | 0 | 59 | 28 | 0.75 | 0.051 | 5.2 | 0 | 0.1 | 0.10 | 0.02 | 40.6 | 18047 |
| **rice bran bread** | 27 | 66 | 11.1 | 11.7 | 1.3 | 1.1 | 1.3 | 119 | 19 | 22 | 0.35 | 0.428 | 0 | 0 | 0.18 | 1.8 | 0 | 0.21 |
| *.95 oz slice* | | 2.4 | 1.2 | 0.2 | 0.4 | 0.5 | 0 | 58 | 48 | 0.97 | 0.050 | 7.7 | 0 | 0.2 | 0.08 | 0.07 | 33.8 | 18059 |
| **rye bread** | 32 | 83 | 11.9 | 15.5 | 1.2 | 1.0 | 1.9 | 211 | 23 | 13 | 0.36 | 0.264 | 0 | 0 | 0.14 | 1.2 | 0 | 0.14 |
| *1.1 oz slice* | | 2.7 | 1.1 | 0.2 | 0.4 | 0.3 | 0 | 53 | 40 | 0.91 | 0.060 | 9.9 | 2 | 0.1 | 0.11 | 0.02 | 48.3 | 18060 |
| **rye bread**, reduced calorie | 23 | 47 | 10.6 | 9.3 | 0.5 | 0.1 | 2.8 | 93 | 17 | 5 | 0.15 | 0.104 | 0 | 0 | 0.08 | 0.6 | 0.01 | 0.07 |
| *.81 oz slice* | | 2.1 | 0.7 | 0.1 | 0.2 | 0.2 | 0 | 23 | 18 | 0.71 | 0.031 | 6.4 | 1 | 0.1 | 0.06 | 0.02 | 19.1 | 18053 |
| **wheat bran bread** | 36 | 89 | 13.6 | 17.2 | 3.5 | 3.4 | 1.4 | 175 | 27 | 29 | 0.49 | 0.600 | 0 | 0 | 0.14 | 1.6 | 0 | 0.19 |
| *1.3 oz slice* | | 3.2 | 1.2 | 0.3 | 0.6 | 0.2 | 0 | 82 | 67 | 1.11 | 0.080 | 11.2 | 0 | 0.1 | 0.10 | 0.06 | 58.0 | 18066 |
| **wheat germ bread** | 28 | 73 | 10.4 | 13.5 | 1.0 | 0.3 | 0.6 | 155 | 25 | 8 | 0.27 | 0.237 | 0 | 0 | 0.10 | 1.3 | 0.02 | 0.15 |
| *1 oz slice* | | 2.7 | 0.8 | 0.2 | 0.4 | 0.2 | 0 | 71 | 34 | 0.97 | 0.057 | 7.6 | 1 | 0.1 | 0.11 | 0.02 | 45.4 | 18068 |
| **wheat/wheat berry bread** | 25 | 66 | 8.9 | 11.9 | 1.4 | 1.0 | 0.9 | 130 | 36 | 12 | 0.30 | 0.281 | 0 | 0 | 0.09 | 1.3 | 0 | 0.09 |
| *.88 oz slice* | | 2.7 | 0.9 | 0.2 | 0.2 | 0.4 | 0 | 46 | 39 | 0.86 | 0.040 | 7.2 | 0 | 0.1 | 0.08 | 0.03 | 24.8 | 18064 |
| **wheat/wheat berry bread**, red cal | 23 | 46 | 9.9 | 10.0 | 0.7 | 0.3 | 2.8 | 118 | 18 | 9 | 0.26 | 0.196 | 0 | 0 | 0.10 | 0.9 | 0 | 0.14 |
| *.81 oz slice* | | 2.1 | 0.5 | 0.1 | 0.1 | 0.2 | 0 | 28 | 23 | 0.68 | 0.032 | 7.0 | 0 | 0.1 | 0.07 | 0.03 | 31.0 | 18055 |
| **white bread** | 25 | 66 | 9.1 | 12.7 | 1.1 | 1.0 | 0.6 | 170 | 38 | 6 | 0.18 | 0.120 | 0 | 0 | 0.11 | 1.1 | 0 | 0.05 |
| *.88 oz slice* | | 1.9 | 0.8 | 0.2 | 0.2 | 0.3 | 0 | 25 | 25 | 0.94 | 0.063 | 4.3 | 0 | 0.1 | 0.08 | 0.02 | 42.8 | 18069 |
| **white bread**, homemade w/2% milk | 42 | 120 | 14.8 | 20.8 | | | 0.8 | 151 | 24 | 8 | 0.27 | 0.175 | 9 | 0 | 0.17 | 1.5 | 0.03 | 0.16 |
| *1.5 oz thick slice* | | 3.3 | 2.4 | 0.5 | 0.5 | 1.2 | 1 | 61 | 48 | 1.25 | 0.048 | 8.9 | 33 | | 0.16 | 0.02 | 52.5 | 18073 |
| **white bread**, homemade w/nonfat | 44 | 121 | 15.3 | 23.6 | | | 0.9 | 148 | 14 | 7 | 0.26 | 0.202 | 5 | 0 | 0.19 | 1.6 | 0.01 | 0.12 |
| milk - *1.6 oz thick slice* | | 3.4 | 1.1 | 0.2 | 0.2 | 0.6 | 0 | 49 | 42 | 1.40 | 0.049 | 10.2 | 18 | | 0.15 | 0.02 | 55.4 | 18071 |
| **white bread**, reduced calorie | 23 | 48 | 9.9 | 10.2 | 1.1 | 0.2 | 2.2 | 104 | 22 | 5 | 0.31 | 0.090 | 0 | 0 | 0.09 | 0.8 | 0.06 | 0.11 |
| *.81 oz slice* | | 2.0 | 0.6 | 0.1 | 0.2 | 0.1 | 0 | 17 | 28 | 0.73 | 0.076 | 5.0 | 1 | | 0.07 | 0.01 | 31.7 | 18057 |
| **white bread**, toasted | 22 | 64 | 6.7 | 12.0 | 1.0 | 1.0 | 0.6 | 130 | 26 | 6 | 0.15 | 0.093 | 0 | 0 | 0.09 | 0.9 | 0 | 0.06 |
| *.78 oz slice* | | 2.0 | 0.9 | 0.1 | 0.2 | 0.5 | 0 | 29 | 23 | 0.73 | 0.030 | 6.8 | 0 | 0.1 | 0.07 | 0.01 | 35.0 | 18070 |
| **whole wheat bread** | 28 | 69 | 10.8 | 11.6 | 1.6 | 1.4 | 1.9 | 132 | 30 | 23 | 0.50 | 0.598 | 0 | 0 | 0.10 | 1.3 | 0 | 0.09 |
| *1 oz slice* | | 3.6 | 0.9 | 0.2 | 0.4 | 0.2 | 0 | 69 | 57 | 0.68 | 0.106 | 11.3 | 1 | 0.1 | 0.06 | 0.06 | 14.0 | 18075 |
| **whole wheat bread**, homemade | 46 | 128 | 15.0 | 23.6 | 1.8 | 1.7 | 2.8 | 159 | 15 | 37 | 0.69 | 0.865 | 0 | 0 | 0.14 | 1.8 | 0 | 0.22 |
| *1.6 oz thick slice* | | 3.9 | 2.5 | 0.4 | 0.5 | 1.4 | 0 | 144 | 86 | 1.43 | 0.116 | 17.8 | 1 | 0.3 | 0.10 | 0.09 | 35.9 | 18077 |

| | WT | Macronutrients | | | | | | Minerals | | | | | Vitamins | | | | | |
|---|---|---|---|---|---|---|---|---|---|---|---|---|---|---|---|---|---|---|
| | (g) | KCAL | $H_2O$ (g) | CHO (g) | TSUG (g) | ASUG (g) | DFIB (g) | Na (mg) | Ca (mg) | Mg (mg) | Zn (mg) | Mn (mg) | A (mcg RAE) | C (mg) | B-1 (mg) | NIA (mg) | B-12 (mcg) | PANT (mg) |
| | | PRO (g) | FAT (g) | SFA (g) | MUFA (g) | PUFA (g) | CHOL (mg) | K (mg) | P (mg) | Fe (mg) | Cu (mg) | Se (mcg) | A (IU) | E (mg ATE) | B-2 (mg) | B-6 (mg) | FOL (mcg DFE) | REF |

## 17.5 BREADSTICKS

| | | | | | | | | | | | | | | | | | | |
|---|---|---|---|---|---|---|---|---|---|---|---|---|---|---|---|---|---|---|
| **breadstick** | 10 | 41 | 0.6 | 6.8 | 0.1 | 0 | 0.3 | 66 | 2 | 3 | 0.09 | 0.056 | 0 | 0 | 0.06 | 0.5 | 0 | 0.05 |
| *.35 oz breadstick (7⅝" × ⅝")* | | 1.2 | 1.0 | 0.1 | 0.4 | 0.4 | 0 | 12 | 12 | 0.43 | 0.019 | 3.8 | 0 | 0.1 | 0.06 | 0.01 | 25.4 | 18080 |
| **breadstick**, Ital Parm garlic, refrig | 60 | 170 | | 24.0 | 3.0 | | | 540 | 0 | | | | | 0 | | | | |
| dough, Pillsbury - *2 pcs (2.1 oz)* | | 5.0 | 6.0 | 1.5 | | | 0 | | | 1.44 | | | 0 | | | | | GENM255 |
| **breadstick**, Italian garlic, herb, refrig | 60 | 170 | | 24.0 | 3.0 | | 0.5 | 560 | 0 | | | | | 0 | | | | |
| dough, Pillsbury - *2 pcs (2.1 oz)* | | 4.0 | 6.0 | 1.0 | | | 0 | | | 1.44 | | | 0 | | | | | GENM254 |
| **breadstick**, soft, from refrig dough, | 52 | 140 | | 25.0 | 3.0 | | 0.5 | 370 | 0 | | | | | 0 | | | | |
| Pillsbury - *2 pieces (1.8 oz)* | | 4.0 | 2.5 | 1.5 | 0.5 | 0.5 | 0 | | | 1.44 | | | 0 | | | | | GENM253 |
| **cornbread breadstick twist**, refrig | 41 | 140 | | 18.0 | 4.0 | | 0 | 340 | 0 | | | | | 0 | | | | |
| dough, Pillsbury - *1.45 oz piece* | | 3.0 | 6.0 | 1.5 | | | 0 | | | 0.72 | | | 0 | | | | | GENM256 |

## 17.6 CRACKERS

| | | | | | | | | | | | | | | | | | | |
|---|---|---|---|---|---|---|---|---|---|---|---|---|---|---|---|---|---|---|
| **cheese cracker** | 14 | 70 | 0.4 | 8.1 | 0 | 0 | 0.3 | 139 | 21 | 5 | 0.16 | 0.088 | 4 | 0 | 0.08 | 0.7 | 0.06 | 0.07 |
| *.5 oz* | | 1.4 | 3.5 | 1.3 | 1.7 | 0.3 | 2 | 20 | 31 | 0.67 | 0.029 | 1.2 | 15 | 0 | 0.06 | 0.08 | 33.7 | 18214 |
| **cheese cracker** w/cheese filling | 39 | 191 | 1.9 | 22.9 | 4.8 | | 0.7 | 342 | 35 | 11 | 0.22 | 0.194 | 4 | 1 | 0.20 | 1.4 | 0.31 | 0.33 |
| *6 cracker sandwiches* | | 3.5 | 9.5 | | | | 2 | 115 | 112 | 0.83 | 0.094 | 3.9 | 15 | 0.8 | 0.18 | 0.04 | 49.9 | 18927 |
| **cheese cracker** w/peanut butter | 7 | 35 | 0.2 | 4.0 | 0.5 | 0.3 | 0.2 | 50 | 4 | 4 | 0.07 | 0.058 | 0 | 0 | 0.04 | 0.4 | 0.02 | 0.03 |
| filling - *2 crackers with filling* | | 0.9 | 1.8 | 0.3 | 0.9 | 0.4 | 0 | 15 | 19 | 0.19 | 0.021 | 0.6 | 0 | 0.2 | 0.02 | 0.01 | 9.9 | 18215 |
| **Cheese Nips**, cheddar, Nabisco | 35 | 170 | | 22.0 | 0 | | 1.0 | 410 | 20 | | | | | 0 | | | | |
| *1.25 oz package* | | 3.0 | 7.0 | 2.0 | | | 0 | | | 1.44 | | | 0 | | | | | NBSC184 |
| **Cheese Nips**, cheddar, reduced fat, | 30 | 130 | | 21.0 | 0 | | 1.0 | 360 | 0 | | | | | 0 | | | | |
| Nabisco - *1.1 oz* | | 3.0 | 3.5 | 1.0 | | | 0 | | | 1.44 | | | 0 | | | | | NBSC186 |
| **Cheese Nips** chips, bold cheddar, | 31 | 150 | | 21.0 | 1.0 | | 1.0 | 390 | 20 | | | | | 0 | | | | |
| Nabisco - *1.1 oz* | | 2.0 | 6.0 | 1.0 | | | 5 | | | 1.08 | | | 0 | | | | | NBSC182 |
| **Cheese Nips**, four cheese, Nabisco | 30 | 150 | | 18.0 | 1.0 | | 1.0 | 310 | 20 | | | | | 0 | | | | |
| *1.1 oz* | | 3.0 | 7.0 | 2.0 | | | 0 | | | 1.08 | | | 0 | | | | | NBSC185 |
| **Cheese Nips**, mini, Nabisco | 30 | 150 | | 19.0 | 0 | | 1.0 | 340 | 20 | | | | | 0 | | | | |
| *53 crackers (1.1 oz)* | | 3.0 | 6.0 | 1.5 | | | 0 | | | 1.08 | | | 0 | | | | | NBSC183 |
| **cracker meal** | 115 | 440 | 8.7 | 93.0 | 0.4 | 0 | 3.0 | 32 | 26 | 28 | 0.79 | 1.086 | 0 | 0 | 0.80 | 6.6 | 0 | 0.54 |
| *1 cup* | | 10.7 | 2.0 | 0.3 | 0.2 | 0.8 | 0 | 132 | 120 | 5.34 | 0.259 | 48.6 | 0 | 0.5 | 0.54 | 0.04 | 248.4 | 18236 |
| **cracker, round** | 14 | 71 | 0.5 | 8.6 | 1.0 | 0.1 | 0.3 | 121 | 13 | 3 | 0.08 | 0.080 | 0 | 0 | 0.06 | 0.6 | 0 | 0.05 |
| *.5 oz (~5 crackers)* | | 0.9 | 3.6 | 0.8 | 0.9 | 1.8 | 0 | 16 | 36 | 0.53 | 0.015 | 0.5 | 0 | 0.5 | 0.03 | 0.01 | 26.0 | 18229 |
| **cracker, round** w/cheese filling | 7 | 33 | 0.3 | 4.3 | 0.2 | 0.1 | 0.1 | 98 | 18 | 3 | 0.04 | 0.020 | 1 | 0 | 0.03 | 0.3 | 0.01 | 0.04 |
| *2 crackers with filling* | | 0.7 | 1.5 | 0.4 | 0.8 | 0.2 | 0 | 30 | 28 | 0.17 | 0.006 | 1.5 | 4 | 0 | 0.05 | 0 | 11.2 | 18230 |
| **cracker, round** w/peanut butter | 7 | 35 | 0.2 | 4.1 | 0.7 | 0.6 | 0.2 | 50 | 6 | 4 | 0.08 | 0.055 | 0 | 0 | 0.03 | 0.4 | 0 | 0.03 |
| filling - *2 crackers w/filling* | | 0.8 | 1.7 | 0.3 | 1.0 | 0.3 | 0 | 15 | 19 | 0.19 | 0.023 | 0.8 | 0 | 0.1 | 0.02 | 0.01 | 8.5 | 18231 |
| **crispbread, rye** | 10 | 37 | 0.6 | 8.2 | 0.1 | 0 | 1.6 | 26 | 3 | 8 | 0.24 | 0.248 | 0 | 0 | 0.02 | 0.1 | 0 | 0.07 |
| *1 crispbread* | | 0.8 | 0.1 | 0 | 0 | 0.1 | 0 | 32 | 27 | 0.24 | 0.026 | 3.7 | 0 | 0.1 | 0.01 | 0.02 | 6.5 | 18216 |
| **melba toast** | 5 | 20 | 0.3 | 3.8 | 0 | 0 | 0.3 | 41 | 5 | 3 | 0.10 | 0.056 | 0 | 0 | 0.02 | 0.2 | 0 | 0.03 |
| *1 toast (3¾" × 1¾" × ⅛")* | | 0.6 | 0.2 | 0 | 0 | 0.1 | 0 | 10 | 10 | 0.19 | 0.014 | 1.7 | 0 | 0 | 0.01 | 0 | 9.6 | 18220 |
| **melba toast**, rye/pumpernickel | 5 | 19 | 0.2 | 3.9 | | | 0.4 | 45 | 4 | 2 | 0.07 | 0.037 | 0 | 0 | 0.02 | 0.2 | 0 | 0.02 |
| *1 toast* | | 0.6 | 0.2 | 0 | 0 | 0.1 | 0 | 10 | 9 | 0.18 | 0.020 | 1.9 | 0 | | 0.01 | 0 | 6.4 | 18221 |
| **melba toast**, wheat | 5 | 19 | 0.3 | 3.8 | | | 0.4 | 42 | 2 | 3 | 0.08 | 0.053 | 0 | 0 | 0.02 | 0.3 | 0 | 0.03 |
| *1 toast* | | 0.6 | 0.1 | 0 | 0 | 0 | 0 | 7 | 8 | 0.22 | 0.013 | 2.8 | 0 | | 0.01 | 0.01 | 10.4 | 18222 |
| **milk cracker** | 11 | 50 | 0.5 | 7.7 | 1.8 | 1.6 | 0.2 | 65 | 19 | 2 | 0.07 | 0.061 | 2 | 0 | 0.06 | 0.5 | 0.01 | 0.04 |
| *1 cracker* | | 0.8 | 1.7 | 0.3 | 0.7 | 0.6 | 1 | 13 | 33 | 0.39 | 0.025 | 1.7 | 6 | 0.1 | 0.05 | 0 | 15.6 | 18223 |
| **Mixers**, cheddar, Nabisco | 28 | 130 | | 19.0 | 1.0 | | 1.0 | 340 | 0 | | | | | 0 | | | | |
| *1 oz* | | 2.0 | 4.5 | 1.0 | | | 0 | | | 1.08 | | | 0 | | | | | NBSC167 |
| **Mixers**, traditional, Nabisco | 30 | 130 | | 21.0 | 2.0 | | 1.0 | 360 | 20 | | | | | 0 | | | | |
| *1.1 oz* | | 2.0 | 5.0 | 1.0 | | | 0 | | | 1.80 | | | 0 | | | | | NBSC168 |
| **Pita Thins toasted chips**, multi-grain, | 28 | 120 | | 20.0 | 3.0 | | 1.0 | 290 | 40 | | | | | 0 | | | | |
| Nabisco - *1 oz* | | 2.0 | 4.0 | 0.5 | | | 0 | | | 1.08 | | | 0 | | | | | NBSC175 |
| **Pita Thins toasted chips**, original, | 28 | 120 | | 19.0 | 1.0 | | 1.0 | 310 | 0 | | | | | 0 | | | | |
| Nabisco - *1 oz* | | 4.0 | 3.0 | 0 | | | 0 | | | 1.08 | | | 0 | | | | | NBSC173 |
| **Pita Thins toasted chips**, roasted | 28 | 120 | | 19.0 | 1.0 | | 1.0 | 330 | 0 | | | | | 0 | | | | |
| garlic, Nabisco - *1 oz* | | 4.0 | 3.0 | 0 | | | 0 | | | 1.44 | | | 0 | | | | | NBSC174 |
| **rice cracker**, sesame, 365 Brand | 30 | 120 | | 25.0 | 0 | | 1.0 | 130 | 0 | | | | | 1 | | | | |
| *15 crackers* | | 3.0 | 1.5 | 0 | | | | | | 0.36 | | | 0 | | | | | THRE1 |

| | WT (g) / PRO (g) | KCAL / FAT (g) | H₂0 (g) / SFA (g) | CHO (g) / MUFA (g) | TSUG (g) / PUFA (g) | ASUG (g) / CHOL (mg) | DFIB (g) / [K (mg)] | Na (mg) / K (mg) | Ca (mg) / P (mg) | Mg (mg) / Fe (mg) | Zn (mg) / Cu (mg) | Mn (mg) / Se (mcg) | A (mcg RAE) / A (IU) | C (mg) / E (mg ATE) | B-1 (mg) / B-2 (mg) | NIA (mg) / B-6 (mg) | B-12 (mcg) / FOL (mcg DFE) | PANT (mg) / REF |
|---|---|---|---|---|---|---|---|---|---|---|---|---|---|---|---|---|---|---|
| Rice Crunch cracker, cheese, | 30 | 120 | | 26.0 | 0 | | 0 | 35 | 0 | | | | 0 | | | | | |
| KA-ME - *about 17 crackers* | 2.0 | 1.0 | 0 | | | 0 | | | 0 | | | 0 | | | | | | KAME1 |
| Rice Crunch cracker, sesame, | 30 | 120 | | 26.0 | 0 | | 0 | 95 | 0 | | | | | 0 | | | | |
| KA-ME - *about 17 crackers* | 2.0 | 1.0 | 0 | | | 0 | | | 0 | | | 0 | | | | | | KAME2 |
| Rite Lite Round, Barbara's Bakery | 15 | 60 | | 11.0 | 1.0 | | | 200 | 0 | | | | | 0 | | | | |
| *5 crackers* | 1.0 | 2.0 | 0 | | | 0 | | | 0 | | | 0 | | | | | | BARB50 |
| Rite Lite Round, savory poppy seed, | 15 | 60 | | 11.0 | 1.0 | | | 200 | 0 | | | | | 0 | | | | |
| Barbara's Bakery - *5 crackers* | 1.0 | 2.0 | 0 | | | 0 | | | 0 | | | 0 | | | | | | BARB51 |
| Rite Lite Round, tamari sesame, | 15 | 70 | | 10.0 | 0.5 | | | 200 | 0 | | | | | 0 | | | | |
| Barbara's Bakery - *5 crackers* | 1.0 | 2.0 | 0 | | | 0 | | | 0 | | | 0 | | | | | | BARB52 |
| Ritz Bits, peanut butter and jelly, | 29 | 140 | | 16.0 | 3.0 | | 1.0 | 230 | 40 | | | | | 0 | | | | |
| Nabisco - *1 oz* | 3.0 | 7.0 | 2.0 | | | 0 | | | 0.72 | | | 0 | | | | | | NBSC196 |
| Ritz Bits w/cheese filling, Nabisco | 29 | 150 | | 16.0 | 4.0 | | 0 | 260 | 40 | | | | | 0 | | | | |
| *12 pieces (1 oz)* | 2.0 | 9.0 | 2.0 | | | 5 | | | 0.72 | | | 0 | | | | | | NBSC194 |
| Ritz Bits w/peanut butter filling, | 29 | 140 | | 16.0 | 3.0 | | 1.0 | 240 | 40 | | | | | 0 | | | | |
| Nabisco - *12 pieces (1 oz)* | 3.0 | 8.0 | 1.5 | | | 0 | | | 0.72 | | | 0 | | | | | | NBSC195 |
| Ritz Cracker, Nabisco | 16 | 79 | 0.5 | 10.2 | 1.3 | | 0.4 | 141 | 25 | 3 | 0.10 | 0.086 | | | 0.07 | 0.8 | | 0.06 |
| *1 cracker* | 1.2 | 3.7 | 0.9 | 1.0 | 1.7 | 0 | 19 | 44 | 0.72 | 0.020 | 0.7 | | 0.6 | 0.04 | 0.01 | 17.8 | 18621 |
| Ritz Cracker, reduced fat, Nabisco | 15 | 70 | | 11.0 | 1.0 | | 0 | 150 | 20 | | | | | 0 | | | | |
| *1 cracker (.53 oz)* | 1.0 | 2.0 | 0 | | | 0 | | | 0.72 | | | 0 | | | | | | NBSC189 |
| Ritz Cracker, whole wheat, Nabisco | 15 | 70 | | 11.0 | 1.0 | | 1.0 | 120 | 20 | | | | | 0 | | | | |
| *1 cracker (.53 oz)* | 1.0 | 2.5 | 0.5 | | | 0 | | | 0.36 | | | 0 | | | | | | NBSC190 |
| Ritz Dinosaur, Nabisco | 30 | 130 | | 22.0 | 3.0 | | 1.0 | 290 | 60 | | | | | 0 | | | | |
| *1.1 oz* | 2.0 | 3.5 | 1.0 | | | 0 | | | 1.08 | | | 0 | | | | | | NBSC193 |
| Ritz Stick, Nabisco | 30 | 150 | | 19.0 | 2.0 | | 1.0 | 280 | 40 | | | | | 0 | | | | |
| *1.1 oz* | 2.0 | 7.0 | 1.5 | | | 0 | | | 1.08 | | | 0 | | | | | | NBSC192 |
| Ritz Toasted Chip, cheddar, | 28 | 130 | | 19.0 | 3.0 | | 0 | 330 | 40 | | | | | 0 | | | | |
| Nabisco - *1 oz* | 2.0 | 6.0 | 1.0 | | | 0 | | | 0.72 | | | 0 | | | | | | NBSC169 |
| Ritz Toasted Chip, original, | 28 | 130 | | 21.0 | 3.0 | | 1.0 | 290 | 40 | | | | | 0 | | | | |
| Nabisco - *1 oz* | 2.0 | 4.5 | 0.5 | | | 0 | | | 1.08 | | | 0 | | | | | | NBSC170 |
| Ritz Toasted Chip, sour cream, | 28 | 130 | | 19.0 | 3.0 | | 0 | 310 | 40 | | | | | 0 | | | | |
| onion, Nabisco - *1 oz* | 2.0 | 6.0 | 1.0 | | | 0 | | | 0.72 | | | 0 | | | | | | NBSC171 |
| Ritz Toasted Chip, south western | 28 | 140 | | 19.0 | 3.0 | | 1.0 | 290 | 40 | | | | | 0 | | | | |
| ranch, Nabisco - *1 oz* | 2.0 | 6.0 | 1.0 | | | 0 | | | 0.72 | | | 0 | | | | | | NBSC172 |
| Ritz, Top'em, Nabisco | 15 | 70 | | 10.0 | 1.0 | | 0 | 130 | 20 | | | | | 0 | | | | |
| *1 cracker (.53 oz)* | 1.0 | 3.0 | 0.5 | | | 0 | | | 0.36 | | | 0 | | | | | | NBSC191 |
| rusk | 10 | 41 | 0.6 | 7.2 | | | | 25 | 3 | 4 | 0.11 | 0.044 | 1 | 0 | 0.04 | 0.5 | 0.02 | 0.06 |
| *1 rusk* | 1.4 | 0.7 | 0.1 | 0.3 | 0.2 | 8 | 24 | 15 | 0.27 | 0.024 | 2.0 | 4 | | 0.04 | 0 | 10.3 | 18224 |
| rye cracker | 25 | 84 | 1.2 | 20.1 | 0.3 | 0 | 5.7 | 198 | 10 | 30 | 0.70 | 1.342 | 0 | | 0.11 | 0.4 | 0 | 0.14 |
| *1 triple cracker* | 2.4 | 0.2 | 0 | 0 | 0.1 | 0 | 124 | 84 | 1.48 | 0.115 | 6.0 | 1 | 0.2 | 0.07 | 0.07 | 11.2 | 18226 |
| rye cracker, seasoned | 22 | 84 | 0.9 | 16.2 | | | 4.6 | 195 | 10 | 23 | 0.56 | 0.522 | 0 | | 0.07 | 0.5 | 0 | 0.12 |
| *1 triple cracker* | 2.0 | 2.0 | 0.3 | 0.7 | 0.8 | | 100 | 68 | 0.67 | 0.109 | 7.2 | 2 | | 0.05 | 0.04 | 11.4 | 18227 |
| rye cracker with cheese filling | 7 | 34 | 0.3 | 4.3 | | | 0.3 | 73 | 16 | 3 | 0.05 | 0.044 | 2 | | 0.04 | 0.2 | 0.01 | 0.04 |
| *2 crackers* | 0.6 | 1.6 | 0.4 | 0.9 | 0.2 | 1 | 24 | 24 | 0.17 | 0.007 | 1.5 | 23 | | 0.03 | 0.01 | 8.9 | 18225 |
| saltine | 14 | 59 | 0.6 | 10.4 | 0.3 | 0 | 0.4 | 156 | 3 | 4 | 0.11 | 0.117 | 0 | 0 | 0.09 | 0.7 | 0 | 0.07 |
| *5 crackers (.49 oz)* | 1.3 | 1.2 | 0.3 | 0.3 | 0.6 | 0 | 22 | 16 | 0.72 | 0.022 | 0.9 | 0 | 0.2 | 0.05 | 0.01 | 30.9 | 18228 |
| saltine, fat-free, low sodium | 30 | 118 | 1.0 | 24.7 | 0.1 | 0 | 0.8 | 191 | 7 | 8 | 0.28 | 0.191 | 0 | 0 | 0.16 | 1.7 | 0 | 0.12 |
| *6 crackers (1.1 oz)* | 3.2 | 0.5 | 0.1 | 0 | 0.2 | 0 | 34 | 34 | 2.32 | 0.044 | 6.4 | 0 | 0 | 0.18 | 0.03 | 60.6 | 18457 |
| saltine, multigrain, Nabisco | 14 | 60 | | 10.0 | 0 | | 0 | 170 | 0 | | | | | 0 | | | | |
| Premium - *.49 oz* | 1.0 | 1.5 | 0 | | | 0 | | | 0.72 | | | 0 | | | | | | NBSC187 |
| saltine, unsalted top | 15 | 65 | 0.6 | 10.7 | | | 0.4 | 115 | 18 | 4 | 0.12 | 0.104 | 0 | 0 | 0.08 | 0.8 | 0 | 0.07 |
| *5 crackers* | 1.4 | 1.8 | 0.4 | 1.0 | 0.3 | 0 | 19 | 16 | 0.81 | 0.030 | | 0 | | 0.07 | 0.01 | 28.4 | 18426 |
| soda cracker | 14 | 59 | 0.6 | 10.4 | 0.3 | 0 | 0.4 | 89 | 17 | 4 | 0.11 | 0.117 | 0 | 0 | 0.09 | 0.7 | 0.01 | 0.07 |
| *5 crackers (.5 oz)* | 1.3 | 1.2 | 0.3 | 0.3 | 0.6 | 0 | 101 | 16 | 0.72 | 0.022 | 0.9 | 0 | 0.2 | 0.05 | 0.01 | 30.9 | 18425 |
| soup and oyster cracker, Nabisco | 15 | 60 | | 11.0 | 0 | | 0 | 170 | | | | | | |
| Premium - *.53 oz* | 1.0 | 1.5 | 0 | | | 0 | | | 0.72 | | | | | | | | | NBSC188 |
| stone ground wheat cracker, | 16 | 80 | | 10.0 | 1.0 | | 1.0 | 180 | | | | | | |
| Wheatsworth - *.56 oz* | 2.0 | 3.5 | 1.0 | | | 0 | | | 0.72 | | | | | | | | | NBSC200 |
| Triscuit, garden herb, Nabisco | 28 | 120 | | 20.0 | 0 | | 3.0 | 125 | 0 | | | | | 0 | | | | |
| *1 oz* | 3.0 | 4.0 | 0.5 | | | 0 | | | 1.44 | | | 100 | | | | | | NBSC197 |
| Triscuit, Nabisco | 28 | 120 | | 19.0 | 0 | | 3.0 | 180 | 0 | | | | | 0 | | | | |
| *1 oz* | 3.0 | 4.5 | 0.5 | | | 0 | | | 1.80 | | | 0 | | | | | | NBSC199 |

| | WT (g) | KCAL / PRO (g) | H₂0 (g) / FAT (g) | CHO (g) / SFA (g) | TSUG (g) / MUFA (g) | ASUG (g) / PUFA (g) | DFIB (g) / CHOL (mg) | Na (mg) / K (mg) | Ca (mg) / P (mg) | Mg (mg) / Fe (mg) | Zn (mg) / Cu (mg) | Mn (mg) / Se (mcg) | A (mcg RAE) / A (IU) | C (mg) / E (mg ATE) | B-1 (mg) / B-2 (mg) | NIA (mg) / B-6 (mg) | B-12 (mcg) / FOL (mcg DFE) | PANT (mg) / REF |
|---|---|---|---|---|---|---|---|---|---|---|---|---|---|---|---|---|---|---|
| **Triscuit**, reduced fat, Nabisco | 29 | 120 | | 21.0 | 0 | | 3.0 | 160 | 0 | | | | | 0 | | | | |
| *1 oz* | | 3.0 | 3.0 | 0 | | | 0 | | | 1.08 | | | 0 | | | | | NBSC198 |
| **wheat cracker** | 14 | 66 | 0.4 | 9.1 | 1.8 | 1.5 | 0.6 | 111 | 7 | 9 | 0.22 | 0.249 | 0 | 0 | 0.07 | 0.7 | 0 | 0.07 |
| *.5 oz (~7 thin squares)* | | 1.2 | 2.9 | 0.7 | 1.6 | 0.4 | 0 | 26 | 31 | 0.62 | 0.045 | 0.9 | 0 | 0.1 | 0.05 | 0.02 | 26.0 | 18232 |
| **wheat cracker** w/cheese filling | 7 | 35 | 0.2 | 4.1 | | | 0.2 | 64 | 14 | 4 | 0.06 | 0.076 | 1 | 0 | 0.03 | 0.2 | 0.01 | 0.04 |
| *2 crackers with filling* | | 0.7 | 1.8 | 0.3 | 0.7 | 0.6 | 0 | 21 | 27 | 0.18 | 0.011 | 1.7 | 5 | | 0.03 | 0.02 | 6.7 | 18233 |
| **wheat cracker** w/peanut butter filling - *2 crackers w/filling* | 7 | 35 | 0.2 | 3.8 | | | 0.3 | 56 | 12 | 3 | 0.06 | 0.049 | 0 | 0 | 0.03 | 0.4 | 0 | 0.04 |
| | | 0.9 | 1.9 | 0.3 | 0.8 | 0.6 | 0 | 21 | 24 | 0.19 | 0.004 | 1.5 | 0 | | 0.02 | 0.01 | 6.5 | 18234 |
| **Wheat Thin**, multigrain, Nabisco | 30 | 130 | | 22.0 | 3.0 | | 2.0 | 230 | 40 | | | | | 0 | | | | |
| *1.1 oz* | | 2.0 | 4.5 | 0.5 | | | 0 | | | 1.08 | | | 0 | | | | | NBSC201 |
| **Wheat Thin**, veggie toasted chips, Nabisco - *1 oz* | 28 | 120 | | 20.0 | 3.0 | | 1.0 | 300 | 40 | | | | | 1 | | | | |
| | | 2.0 | 4.0 | 0.5 | | | 0 | | | 1.08 | | | 0 | | | | | NBSC176 |
| **Wheatines**, Barbara's Bakery | 14 | 60 | | 11.0 | 1.0 | | 0.5 | 80 | 0 | | | | | 0 | | | | |
| *4 crackers* | | 1.0 | 1.0 | 0 | | | 0 | | 0 | | | | 0 | | | | | BARB64 |
| **Wheatines**, cracked pepper, Barbara's Bakery - *4 crackers* | 14 | 50 | | 11.0 | 1.0 | | 1.0 | 120 | 0 | | | | | 0 | | | | |
| | | 1.0 | 1.0 | 0 | | | 0 | | 0 | | | | 0 | | | | | BARB63 |
| **whole wheat cracker** | 14 | 62 | 0.4 | 9.6 | 0.1 | 0 | 1.5 | 92 | 7 | 14 | 0.30 | 0.315 | 0 | 0 | 0.03 | 0.6 | 0 | 0.11 |
| *.5 oz (~3.5 crackers)* | | 1.2 | 2.4 | 0.5 | 0.8 | 0.9 | 0 | 42 | 41 | 0.43 | 0.062 | 2.1 | 0 | 0.1 | 0.01 | 0.03 | 3.9 | 18235 |
| **Zwieback toast**, Nabisco | 8 | 35 | | 6.0 | 1.0 | | 0 | 10 | | | | | | | | | | |
| *.28 oz piece* | | 1.0 | 1.0 | 0 | | | 0 | | | 0.36 | | | | | | | | NBSC202 |

## 17.7 ENGLISH MUFFINS

| | WT (g) | KCAL / PRO (g) | H₂0 (g) / FAT (g) | CHO (g) / SFA (g) | TSUG (g) / MUFA (g) | ASUG (g) / PUFA (g) | DFIB (g) / CHOL (mg) | Na (mg) / K (mg) | Ca (mg) / P (mg) | Mg (mg) / Fe (mg) | Zn (mg) / Cu (mg) | Mn (mg) / Se (mcg) | A (mcg RAE) / A (IU) | C (mg) / E (mg ATE) | B-1 (mg) / B-2 (mg) | NIA (mg) / B-6 (mg) | B-12 (mcg) / FOL (mcg DFE) | PANT (mg) / REF |
|---|---|---|---|---|---|---|---|---|---|---|---|---|---|---|---|---|---|---|
| **English muffin** | 57 | 129 | 24.8 | 25.2 | 2.0 | 1.5 | 2.0 | 242 | 93 | 14 | 0.60 | 0.288 | 0 | 1 | 0.27 | 2.3 | 0.02 | 0.21 |
| *2 oz muffin* | | 5.1 | 1.0 | 0.4 | 0.2 | 0.3 | 0 | 62 | 52 | 2.28 | 0.077 | 12.8 | 0 | 0.2 | 0.14 | 0.03 | 75.2 | 18258 |
| **English muffin**, 100 cal original, Thomas' - *1.8 oz muffin* | 52 | 100 | | 24.0 | 1.0 | | 5.0 | 220 | 40 | | | | | 0 | | | | |
| | | 4.0 | 1.0 | 0 | 0 | 0 | 0 | | | 1.08 | | | 0 | | | | | THOM1 |
| **English muffin**, cherry blossom, Wolferman's - *3.7 oz muffin* | 106 | 240 | | 50.0 | 10.0 | | 2.0 | 470 | 80 | | | | | 0 | | | | |
| | | 8.0 | 1.0 | 0 | 0 | 0 | 0 | | | 2.70 | | | 200 | | | | | WOLF1 |
| **English muffin**, honey wheat, Thomas' - *2 oz muffin* | 57 | 130 | | 27.0 | 3.0 | | 2.0 | 190 | 60 | | | | | 0 | | | | |
| | | 5.0 | 1.0 | 0 | 0 | 0 | 0 | | | 1.44 | | | 0 | | | | | THOM3 |
| **English muffin**, mixed grain/granola - *2.3 oz muffin* | 66 | 155 | 26.5 | 30.6 | 0.5 | 0.4 | 1.8 | 275 | 129 | 27 | 0.92 | 0.399 | 0 | 0 | 0.28 | 2.4 | 0 | 0.27 |
| | | 6.0 | 1.2 | 0.2 | 0.5 | 0.4 | 0 | 103 | 53 | 1.99 | 0.160 | 16.8 | 0 | 0 | 0.21 | 0.03 | 73.9 | 18260 |
| **English muffin**, multi-grain, light, Thomas' - *2 oz muffin* | 57 | 100 | | 24.0 | 1.0 | | 6.0 | 170 | 100 | | | | | 0 | | | | |
| | | 6.0 | 1.5 | 0 | 1.0 | 1.0 | 0 | | | 1.08 | | | 0 | | | | | THOM2 |
| **English muffin**, raisin cinn/apple cinn - *2 oz muffin* | 57 | 137 | 23.1 | 27.4 | 8.4 | 5.6 | 1.5 | 189 | 65 | 13 | 0.55 | 0.328 | 0 | 1 | 0.23 | 2.1 | 0 | 0.12 |
| | | 4.5 | 1.0 | 0.3 | 0.5 | 0.2 | 0 | 99 | 52 | 2.56 | 0.091 | 12.3 | 1 | 0.2 | 0.12 | 0.04 | 63.8 | 18262 |
| **English muffin**, Thomas' | 57 | 132 | 24.3 | 26.2 | | | | 197 | 103 | | | | | 0 | | | | |
| *2 oz muffin* | | 4.6 | 1.0 | 0.2 | 0.2 | 0.5 | | | | 0.80 | | | 0 | | | | | 18639 |
| **English muffin**, wheat | 57 | 127 | 24.1 | 25.5 | 0.9 | 0.5 | 2.6 | 218 | 101 | 21 | 0.61 | 0.571 | 0 | 0 | 0.25 | 1.9 | 0 | 0.25 |
| *2 oz muffin* | | 5.0 | 1.1 | 0.2 | 0.2 | 0.5 | 0 | 106 | 61 | 1.64 | 0.084 | 16.6 | 2 | 0.3 | 0.17 | 0.05 | 46.7 | 18264 |
| **English muffin**, whole wheat | 66 | 134 | 30.2 | 26.7 | 5.3 | 5.1 | 4.4 | 312 | 175 | 47 | 1.06 | 1.181 | 0 | 0 | 0.20 | 2.3 | 0 | 0.46 |
| *2.3 oz muffin* | | 5.8 | 1.4 | 0.2 | 0.3 | 0.6 | 0 | 139 | 186 | 1.62 | 0.140 | 26.6 | 3 | 0.3 | 0.09 | 0.11 | 32.3 | 18266 |

## 17.8 ETHNIC GRAIN PRODUCTS

| | WT (g) | KCAL / PRO (g) | H₂0 (g) / FAT (g) | CHO (g) / SFA (g) | TSUG (g) / MUFA (g) | ASUG (g) / PUFA (g) | DFIB (g) / CHOL (mg) | Na (mg) / K (mg) | Ca (mg) / P (mg) | Mg (mg) / Fe (mg) | Zn (mg) / Cu (mg) | Mn (mg) / Se (mcg) | A (mcg RAE) / A (IU) | C (mg) / E (mg ATE) | B-1 (mg) / B-2 (mg) | NIA (mg) / B-6 (mg) | B-12 (mcg) / FOL (mcg DFE) | PANT (mg) / REF |
|---|---|---|---|---|---|---|---|---|---|---|---|---|---|---|---|---|---|---|
| **chow mein noodles** | 45 | 237 | 0.3 | 25.9 | 0.1 | 0 | 1.8 | 198 | 9 | 23 | 0.63 | 0.611 | 0 | 0 | 0.26 | 2.7 | 0 | 0.24 |
| *1 cup* | | 3.8 | 13.8 | 2.0 | 3.5 | 7.8 | 0 | 54 | 72 | 2.13 | 0.075 | 19.4 | 0 | 1.6 | 0.19 | 0.05 | 62.1 | 20113 |
| **eggroll wrapper** | 32 | 93 | 9.2 | 18.5 | | | 0.6 | 183 | 15 | 6 | 0.23 | 0.204 | 1 | 0 | 0.17 | 1.7 | 0.01 | 0.01 |
| *7" square wrapper* | | 3.1 | 0.5 | 0.1 | 0.1 | 0.2 | 3 | 26 | 26 | 1.08 | 0.047 | 9.0 | 4 | | 0.12 | 0.01 | 42.9 | 18368 |
| **fry bread** made with lard, Apache | 28 | 87 | 9.3 | 12.9 | 0.4 | | 0.5 | 188 | 15 | 5 | 0.13 | 0.113 | | | 0.15 | 1.2 | 0 | |
| *1 oz piece* | | 2.3 | 2.8 | 1.0 | 1.0 | 0.4 | 1 | 21 | 31 | 0.96 | 0.027 | 1.8 | | 0 | 0.07 | 0.02 | 49.6 | 35185 |
| **fry bread** made with lard, Navajo | 28 | 92 | 8.8 | 13.5 | 0.6 | | | 92 | 16 | 5 | 0.10 | 0.083 | | | 0.12 | 1.3 | 0 | 0.05 |
| *1 oz piece* | | 1.9 | 3.4 | 1.3 | 1.2 | 0.3 | 2 | 22 | 34 | 1.13 | 0.025 | 5.2 | | 0 | 0.06 | 0.01 | 54.9 | 35142 |
| **matzo** | 28 | 111 | 1.2 | 23.4 | 0.1 | 0 | 0.8 | 1 | 4 | 7 | 0.19 | 0.182 | 0 | 0 | 0.11 | 1.1 | 0 | 0.12 |
| *1 oz matzo* | | 2.8 | 0.4 | 0.1 | 0.1 | 0.2 | 0 | 31 | 25 | 0.88 | 0.017 | 10.3 | 0 | | 0.08 | 0.03 | 4.8 | 18217 |
| **matzo**, egg (egg in matzo dough) | 28 | 109 | 1.8 | 22.0 | | | 0.8 | 6 | 11 | 7 | 0.20 | 0.168 | 4 | 0 | 0.22 | 1.4 | 0.05 | 0.12 |
| *1 oz matzo* | | 3.4 | 0.6 | 0.2 | 0.2 | 0.1 | 23 | 42 | 41 | 0.76 | 0.043 | 7.8 | 12 | | 0.17 | 0.02 | 6.7 | 18218 |
| **matzo**, egg, onion (egg, onion in matzo dough) - *1 oz matzo* | 28 | 109 | 2.0 | 21.6 | | | 1.4 | 80 | 10 | 8 | 0.20 | 0.230 | 2 | 0 | 0.16 | 1.4 | 0.06 | 0.16 |
| | | 2.8 | 1.1 | 0.3 | 0.3 | 0.3 | 13 | 23 | 25 | 1.22 | 0.022 | 10.2 | 7 | | 0.12 | 0.03 | 3.0 | 18400 |
| **matzo**, whole wheat | 28 | 98 | 1.3 | 22.1 | | | 3.3 | 1 | 6 | 38 | 0.73 | 0.980 | 0 | 0 | 0.10 | 1.5 | 0 | 0.35 |
| *1 oz matzo* | | 3.7 | 0.4 | 0.1 | 0.1 | 0.2 | 0 | 88 | 85 | 1.30 | 0.098 | 21.0 | 0 | | 0.08 | 0.04 | 9.8 | 18219 |
| **Navajo kneel down bread** (Navajo tamales) - *1 oz piece* | 28 | 55 | 14.8 | 11.1 | 1.0 | | | 35 | 1 | 15 | 0.41 | 0.085 | | | 0.03 | 0.7 | | 0.10 |
| | | 1.2 | 0.6 | 0.1 | 0.2 | 0.2 | | 90 | 46 | 0.31 | 0.027 | 3.3 | | 0 | 0.04 | | | 35140 |

| | WT (g) | KCAL / PRO (g) | H₂O (g) / FAT (g) | CHO (g) / SFA (g) | TSUG (g) / MUFA (g) | ASUG (g) / PUFA (g) | DFIB (g) / CHOL (mg) | Na (mg) / K (mg) | Ca (mg) / P (mg) | Mg (mg) / Fe (mg) | Zn (mg) / Cu (mg) | Mn (mg) / Se (mcg) | A (mcg RAE) / A (IU) | C (mg) / E (mg ATE) | B-1 (mg) / B-2 (mg) | NIA (mg) / B-6 (mg) | B-12 (mcg) / FOL (mcg DFE) | PANT (mg) / REF |
|---|---|---|---|---|---|---|---|---|---|---|---|---|---|---|---|---|---|---|
| **phyllo dough** | 19 | 57 | 6.2 | 10.0 | 0 | 0 | 0.4 | 92 | 2 | 3 | 0.09 | 0.090 | 0 | 0 | 0.10 | 0.8 | 0 | 0.06 |
| *1 sheet* | | 1.3 | 1.1 | 0.3 | 0.6 | 0.2 | 0 | 14 | 14 | 0.61 | 0.019 | 4.4 | 0 | 0 | 0.06 | 0.01 | 26.0 | 18338 |
| **pita bread**, white | 60 | 165 | 19.3 | 33.4 | 0.8 | 0.3 | 1.3 | 322 | 52 | 16 | 0.50 | 0.289 | 0 | 0 | 0.36 | 2.8 | 0 | 0.24 |
| *1 large (6½″ diameter)* | | 5.5 | 0.7 | 0.1 | 0.1 | 0.3 | 0 | 72 | 58 | 1.57 | 0.101 | 16.3 | 0 | 0.2 | 0.20 | 0.02 | 99.0 | 18041 |
| **pita bread**, whole wheat | 64 | 170 | 19.6 | 35.2 | 0.5 | 0.4 | 4.7 | 340 | 10 | 44 | 0.97 | 1.114 | 0 | 0 | 0.22 | 1.8 | 0 | 0.53 |
| *1 large (6½″ diameter)* | | 6.3 | 1.7 | 0.3 | 0.2 | 0.7 | 0 | 109 | 115 | 1.96 | 0.186 | 28.2 | 0 | 0.4 | 0.05 | 0.17 | 22.4 | 18042 |
| **pizza crust**, from refrig dough, Pillsbury - ⅙ crust (2.3 oz) | 65 | 160 | | 31.0 | 4.0 | | | 470 | 0 | | | | | 0 | | | | |
| | | 5.0 | 2.0 | 0.5 | | | 0 | | | 1.80 | | | 0 | | | | | GENM257 |
| **pizza crust**, thin, Boboli | 57 | 170 | | 28.0 | 1.0 | | 1.0 | 330 | 80 | | | | | 0 | | | | |
| *⅕ crust (2 oz)* | | 6.0 | 3.5 | 1.5 | | | 0 | | | 1.80 | | | 0 | | | | | BOBO1 |
| **rice noodles**, cellophane, Chinese, | 140 | 491 | 18.8 | 120.5 | 0 | 0 | 0.7 | 14 | 35 | 4 | 0.57 | 0.140 | 0 | 0 | 0.21 | 0.3 | 0 | 0.14 |
| *dry - 1 cup* | | 0.2 | 0.1 | 0 | 0 | 0 | 0 | 14 | 45 | 3.04 | 0.113 | 11.1 | 0 | 0.2 | 0 | 0.07 | 2.8 | 16082 |
| **rice noodles**, cooked | 176 | 192 | 129.9 | 43.8 | | | 1.8 | 33 | 7 | 5 | 0.44 | 0.201 | 0 | 0 | 0.03 | 0.1 | 0 | 0.02 |
| *1 cup* | | 1.6 | 0.4 | 0 | 0 | 0 | 0 | 7 | 35 | 0.25 | 0.067 | 7.9 | 0 | | 0.01 | 0.01 | 5.3 | 20134 |
| **soba** (Japanese noodles), cooked | 114 | 113 | 83.2 | 24.4 | | | | 68 | 5 | 10 | 0.14 | 0.426 | 0 | 0 | 0.11 | 0.6 | 0 | 0.27 |
| *1 cup* | | 5.8 | 0.1 | 0 | 0 | 0 | 0 | 40 | 28 | 0.55 | 0.009 | | 0 | | 0.03 | 0.05 | 8.0 | 20115 |
| **somen** (Japanese noodles), cooked | 176 | 231 | 119.5 | 48.5 | | | | 283 | 14 | 4 | 0.39 | 0.442 | 0 | 0 | 0.04 | 0.2 | 0 | 0.30 |
| *1 cup* | | 7.0 | 0.3 | 0 | 0 | 0 | 0.1 | 51 | 48 | 0.92 | 0.044 | | 0 | | 0.06 | 0.02 | 3.5 | 20117 |
| **taco shell**, from corn tortilla | 13 | 61 | 1.0 | 8.2 | 0.2 | 0 | 0.6 | 51 | 13 | 11 | 0.21 | 0.056 | 0 | 0 | 0.03 | 0.4 | 0 | 0.05 |
| *1 medium (5″ diameter)* | | 0.9 | 2.7 | 0.6 | 1.5 | 0.5 | 0 | 29 | 29 | 0.24 | 0.017 | 0.6 | 2 | 0.1 | 0.01 | 0.03 | 11.0 | 18360 |
| **taco shell**, from corn tortillas, mini, Old El Paso - 6 shells (.9 oz) | 26 | 120 | | 16.0 | 0 | | 1.0 | 0 | 0 | | | | | 0 | | | | |
| | | 2.0 | 6.0 | 1.5 | | | 0 | | | 0.72 | | | 0 | | | | | GENM258 |
| **taco shell**, from corn tortillas, reg, Old El Paso - 3 shells (1.1 oz) | 32 | 150 | | 19.0 | 0 | | 1.0 | 135 | 20 | | | | | 0 | | | | |
| | | 2.0 | 7.0 | 2.0 | | | 0 | | | 0.36 | | | 0 | | | | | GENM259 |
| **taco shell**, fr corn tortillas, super size, Old El Paso - 2 shells (1.3 oz) | 37 | 170 | | 22.0 | 0 | | 1.0 | 150 | 20 | | | | | 0 | | | | |
| | | 2.0 | 8.0 | 2.5 | | | 0 | | | 0 | | | 0 | | | | | GENM260 |
| **taco shell**, from white corn tortilla, reg, Old El Paso - 3 shells (1.1 oz) | 32 | 150 | | 20.0 | 0 | | 1.0 | 140 | 20 | | | | | 0 | | | | |
| | | 2.0 | 7.0 | 2.5 | | | 0 | | | 0 | | | 0 | | | | | GENM261 |
| **tortilla**, corn | 24 | 52 | 11.0 | 10.7 | 0.2 | 0 | 1.5 | 11 | 19 | 17 | 0.31 | 0.078 | 0 | 0 | 0.02 | 0.4 | 0 | 0.03 |
| *1 medium (6″ diameter)* | | 1.4 | 0.7 | 0.1 | 0.2 | 0.3 | 0 | 45 | 75 | 0.30 | 0.037 | 1.5 | 0 | 0.1 | 0.02 | 0.05 | 1.2 | 18363 |
| **tortilla, corn**, Tortilla Maya, Chef Garcia - 2 medium (6″ diameter) | 57 | 130 | | 26.0 | | | 2.0 | 90 | 80 | | | | | 0 | | | | |
| | | 2.0 | 1.5 | 0 | | | 0 | | | 0.72 | | | 100 | | | | | CHEF1 |
| **tortilla**, flour | 46 | 144 | 13.9 | 23.6 | 0.9 | | 1.4 | 293 | 59 | 10 | 0.25 | 0.229 | 0 | 0 | 0.25 | 1.6 | 0 | 0.08 |
| *1 medium (7–8″ diameter)* | | 3.8 | 3.6 | 0.9 | 1.8 | 0.7 | 0 | 71 | 57 | 1.54 | 0.065 | 10.2 | 0 | 0.1 | 0.12 | 0.02 | 77.3 | 18364 |
| **tortilla, flour**, Mission Foods | 51 | 146 | 17.1 | 25.3 | | | | 249 | 97 | | | | | | | | | |
| *1 medium (8″ diameter)* | | 4.4 | 3.1 | 0.4 | 1.4 | 0.5 | | | | 1.01 | | | | | | | | 18616 |
| **tortilla, flour**, Old El Paso | 41 | 130 | | 20.0 | 0.5 | | 0 | 300 | 60 | | | | | 0 | | | | |
| *1 medium (8″ diameter)* | | 3.0 | 4.0 | 1.0 | | | 0 | | | 1.08 | | | 0 | | | | | GENM263 |
| **tortilla, multigrain**, Snyder | 28 | 130 | | 20.0 | 2.0 | | 3.0 | 110 | 0 | | | | | 0 | | | | |
| *1 oz* | | 2.0 | 5.0 | 0 | | | 0 | | | 0 | | | 0 | | | | | SNYD26 |
| **tostada shell**, Old El Paso | 32 | 150 | | 19.0 | 0 | | 1.0 | 135 | 20 | | | | | 0 | | | | |
| *3 shells (1.1 oz)* | | 2.0 | 7.0 | 2.0 | | | 0 | | | 0.36 | | | 0 | | | | | GENM265 |
| **wonton wrapper** | 32 | 93 | 9.2 | 18.5 | | | 0.6 | 183 | 15 | 6 | 0.23 | 0.204 | 1 | 0 | 0.17 | 1.7 | 0.01 | 0.01 |
| *7″ square wrapper* | | 3.1 | 0.5 | 0.1 | 0.1 | 0.2 | 3 | 26 | 26 | 1.08 | 0.047 | 9.0 | 4 | | 0.12 | 0.01 | 42.9 | 18368 |

## 17.9 MUFFINS

| | WT (g) | KCAL / PRO (g) | H₂O (g) / FAT (g) | CHO (g) / SFA (g) | TSUG (g) / MUFA (g) | ASUG (g) / PUFA (g) | DFIB (g) / CHOL (mg) | Na (mg) / K (mg) | Ca (mg) / P (mg) | Mg (mg) / Fe (mg) | Zn (mg) / Cu (mg) | Mn (mg) / Se (mcg) | A (mcg RAE) / A (IU) | C (mg) / E (mg ATE) | B-1 (mg) / B-2 (mg) | NIA (mg) / B-6 (mg) | B-12 (mcg) / FOL (mcg DFE) | PANT (mg) / REF |
|---|---|---|---|---|---|---|---|---|---|---|---|---|---|---|---|---|---|---|
| **banana muffin bar**, Nutri-Grain | 45 | 170 | | 30.0 | 16.0 | | 1.0 | 110 | 0 | | 1.50 | | | 0 | 0.15 | 2.0 | 0.60 | |
| *1.6 oz bar* | | 3.0 | 4.0 | 0.5 | | | 0 | | | 1.80 | | | 500 | | 0.17 | 0.20 | | KELL2 |
| **blueberry muffin bar**, Nutri-Grain | 45 | 170 | | 31.0 | 17.0 | | 1.0 | 100 | 0 | | 1.50 | | | 0 | 0.15 | 2.0 | 0.60 | |
| *1.6 oz bar* | | 2.0 | 4.0 | 0.5 | | | 0 | | | 1.80 | | | 500 | | 0.17 | 0.20 | | KELL3 |
| **blueberry muffin**, homemade | 57 | 162 | 22.5 | 23.2 | | | | 251 | 108 | 9 | 0.31 | 0.178 | 22 | 1 | 0.16 | 1.3 | 0.08 | 0.19 |
| *w/2% milk - 2 oz muffin* | | 3.7 | 6.2 | 1.2 | 1.5 | 3.1 | 21 | 70 | 83 | 1.29 | 0.040 | 9.7 | 80 | | 0.16 | 0.02 | 41.6 | 18278 |
| **corn muffin** | 139 | 424 | 45.3 | 70.8 | 10.4 | 7.6 | 4.7 | 724 | 103 | 44 | 0.75 | 0.493 | 72 | 0 | 0.38 | 2.8 | 0.13 | 0.62 |
| *4.9 oz muffin* | | 8.2 | 11.7 | 1.9 | 2.9 | 4.5 | 36 | 96 | 395 | 3.91 | 0.416 | 21.1 | 289 | 1.1 | 0.45 | 0.12 | 155.7 | 18279 |
| **corn muffin**, from mix | 28 | 90 | 8.5 | 13.7 | | | 0.7 | 223 | 21 | 6 | 0.18 | 0.062 | 11 | 0 | 0.07 | 0.6 | 0.04 | 0.13 |
| *1 oz muffin* | | 2.1 | 2.9 | 0.8 | 1.5 | 0.4 | 17 | 37 | 108 | 0.54 | 0.018 | 4.3 | 59 | | 0.08 | 0.03 | 24.9 | 18280 |
| **corn muffin**, homemade with 2% milk | 57 | 180 | 18.8 | 25.2 | | | | 333 | 148 | 13 | 0.35 | 0.106 | | 0 | 0.17 | 1.4 | 0.09 | 0.20 |
| *2 oz muffin (2¾″ × 2″)* | | 4.0 | 7.0 | 1.3 | 1.7 | 3.5 | 24 | 83 | 101 | 1.49 | 0.034 | 7.6 | 137 | | 0.18 | 0.05 | 65.6 | 18282 |
| **muffin**, homemade with 2% milk | 57 | 169 | 21.5 | 23.6 | | | 1.5 | 266 | 114 | 10 | 0.32 | 0.169 | 23 | 0 | 0.16 | 1.3 | 0.09 | 0.20 |
| *2 oz muffin* | | 3.9 | 6.5 | 1.2 | 1.6 | 3.3 | 22 | 69 | 87 | 1.36 | 0.039 | 10.3 | 80 | | 0.17 | 0.02 | 44.5 | 18273 |
| **oat bran muffin** | 139 | 375 | 48.6 | 67.1 | 11.4 | 10.2 | 6.4 | 546 | 88 | 218 | 2.56 | 3.656 | 0 | 0 | 0.36 | 0.6 | 0.01 | 1.40 |
| *4.9 oz muffin* | | 9.7 | 10.3 | 1.5 | 2.4 | 5.7 | 0 | 705 | 523 | 5.84 | 0.459 | 15.3 | 0 | 0.9 | 0.13 | 0.22 | 193.2 | 18283 |

| | WT (g) | KCAL | H₂0 (g) | CHO (g) | TSUG (g) | ASUG (g) | DFIB (g) | Na (mg) | Ca (mg) | Mg (mg) | Zn (mg) | Mn (mg) | A (mcg RAE) | C (mg) | B-1 (mg) | NIA (mg) | B-12 (mcg) | PANT (mg) |
|---|---|---|---|---|---|---|---|---|---|---|---|---|---|---|---|---|---|---|
| | | PRO (g) | FAT (g) | SFA (g) | MUFA (g) | PUFA (g) | CHOL (mg) | K (mg) | P (mg) | Fe (mg) | Cu (mg) | Se (mcg) | A (IU) | E (mg ATE) | B-2 (mg) | B-6 (mg) | FOL (mcg DFE) | REF |
| **raisin bran muffin**, toasted | 34 | 106 | 9.2 | 18.9 | 7.8 | | 2.8 | 179 | 13 | 7 | 0.15 | 0.147 | 19 | 0 | 0.07 | 0.8 | 0.01 | 0.06 |
| *1 muffin* | | 1.9 | 3.2 | 0.5 | 0.8 | 1.7 | 3 | 60 | 97 | 0.96 | 0.041 | 6.9 | 65 | 0.3 | 0.10 | 0.02 | 15.6 | 18388 |
| **toaster muffin**, blueberry, toasted | 31 | 103 | 8.2 | 17.6 | 4.0 | | 0.6 | 158 | 4 | 5 | 0.15 | 0.146 | 31 | 0 | 0.06 | 0.6 | 0 | 0.06 |
| *1 muffin* | | 1.5 | 3.1 | 0.5 | 0.7 | 1.7 | 2 | 27 | 60 | 0.17 | 0.031 | 5.8 | 106 | 0.3 | 0.09 | 0.01 | 29.1 | 18386 |

## 17.10  PANCAKES

| | WT (g) | KCAL | H₂0 (g) | CHO (g) | TSUG (g) | ASUG (g) | DFIB (g) | Na (mg) | Ca (mg) | Mg (mg) | Zn (mg) | Mn (mg) | A (mcg RAE) | C (mg) | B-1 (mg) | NIA (mg) | B-12 (mcg) | PANT (mg) |
|---|---|---|---|---|---|---|---|---|---|---|---|---|---|---|---|---|---|---|
| | | PRO (g) | FAT (g) | SFA (g) | MUFA (g) | PUFA (g) | CHOL (mg) | K (mg) | P (mg) | Fe (mg) | Cu (mg) | Se (mcg) | A (IU) | E (mg ATE) | B-2 (mg) | B-6 (mg) | FOL (mcg DFE) | REF |
| **pancake**, blueberry, homemade | 38 | 84 | 20.2 | 11.0 | | | | 157 | 78 | 6 | 0.21 | 0.090 | 19 | 1 | 0.07 | 0.6 | 0.08 | 0.15 |
| *4" diameter pancake* | | 2.3 | 3.5 | 0.8 | 0.9 | 1.6 | 21 | 52 | 57 | 0.65 | 0.021 | 5.3 | 76 | | 0.10 | 0.02 | 20.1 | 18294 |
| **pancake**, buttermilk, homemade | 38 | 86 | 20.0 | 10.9 | | | | 198 | 60 | 6 | 0.24 | 0.077 | 11 | 0 | 0.08 | 0.6 | 0.07 | 0.16 |
| *4" diameter pancake* | | 2.6 | 3.5 | 0.7 | 0.9 | 1.7 | 22 | 55 | 53 | 0.65 | 0.020 | 5.7 | 40 | | 0.11 | 0.02 | 21.3 | 18390 |
| **pancake**, buttermilk, Kellogg's Eggo | 116 | 270 | 54.8 | 44.2 | 9.5 | | 1.3 | 615 | 41 | 21 | 0.70 | | | 2 | 0.30 | 4.0 | 1.19 | 0 |
| *3 pancakes* | | 7.0 | 7.8 | 1.7 | 3.4 | 2.5 | 13 | 119 | 396 | 3.60 | 0 | | 1000 | | 0.34 | 0.41 | | 18499 |
| **pancake**, from complete mix | 38 | 74 | 20.1 | 13.9 | | | 0.5 | 239 | 48 | 8 | 0.15 | 0.103 | 4 | 0 | 0.08 | 0.7 | 0.08 | 0.09 |
| *4" diameter pancake* | | 2.0 | 1.0 | 0.2 | 0.3 | 0.3 | 5 | 66 | 127 | 0.59 | 0.036 | 5.1 | 12 | | 0.08 | 0.03 | 21.7 | 18290 |
| **pancake**, from incomplete mix | 38 | 83 | 20.1 | 11.0 | | | 0.7 | 192 | 82 | 8 | 0.29 | 0.053 | 27 | 0 | 0.08 | 0.5 | 0.13 | 0.19 |
| *4" diameter pancake* | | 3.0 | 2.9 | 0.8 | 0.8 | 1.1 | 27 | 76 | 119 | 0.49 | 0.018 | 3.7 | 95 | | 0.12 | 0.04 | 20.5 | 18292 |
| **pancake**, frozen | 41 | 92 | 19.8 | 16.1 | 4.0 | 3.1 | 1.0 | 207 | 29 | 6 | 0.16 | 0.064 | 26 | 0 | 0.14 | 1.2 | 0.04 | 0.06 |
| *4" diameter pancake* | | 2.2 | 2.1 | 0.3 | 0.8 | 0.4 | 7 | 51 | 120 | 0.90 | 0.022 | 2.3 | 89 | 0.1 | 0.21 | 0.06 | 45.5 | 18288 |
| **pancake**, frozen, microwaved | 38 | 91 | 16.6 | 16.5 | 2.7 | 2.1 | 1.0 | 215 | 27 | 6 | 0.17 | 0.054 | 82 | 0 | 0.14 | 1.3 | | 0.07 |
| *4" diameter pancake* | | 2.2 | 1.8 | 0.4 | 1.0 | 0.4 | | 46 | 133 | 0.62 | 0.013 | 2.8 | 273 | 0.1 | 0.13 | 0.11 | 32.7 | 18936 |
| **pancake**, homemade | 38 | 86 | 20.1 | 10.8 | | | | 167 | 83 | 6 | 0.21 | 0.076 | 21 | 0 | 0.08 | 0.6 | 0.08 | 0.15 |
| *4" diameter pancake* | | 2.4 | 3.7 | 0.8 | 0.9 | 1.7 | 22 | 50 | 60 | 0.68 | 0.019 | 5.7 | 74 | | 0.11 | 0.02 | 21.3 | 18293 |
| **pancake**, whl wht from incomplete | 44 | 92 | 23.2 | 12.9 | | | 1.2 | 252 | 110 | 20 | 0.46 | 0.680 | 28 | 0 | 0.09 | 1.0 | 0.13 | 0.23 |
| mix - *4" diameter pancake* | | 3.7 | 2.9 | 0.8 | 0.8 | 1.1 | 27 | 123 | 164 | 1.37 | 0.035 | 8.5 | 99 | | 0.23 | 0.05 | 15.4 | 18300 |

## 17.11  PASTA

| | WT (g) | KCAL | H₂0 (g) | CHO (g) | TSUG (g) | ASUG (g) | DFIB (g) | Na (mg) | Ca (mg) | Mg (mg) | Zn (mg) | Mn (mg) | A (mcg RAE) | C (mg) | B-1 (mg) | NIA (mg) | B-12 (mcg) | PANT (mg) |
|---|---|---|---|---|---|---|---|---|---|---|---|---|---|---|---|---|---|---|
| | | PRO (g) | FAT (g) | SFA (g) | MUFA (g) | PUFA (g) | CHOL (mg) | K (mg) | P (mg) | Fe (mg) | Cu (mg) | Se (mcg) | A (IU) | E (mg ATE) | B-2 (mg) | B-6 (mg) | FOL (mcg DFE) | REF |
| **macaroni**, enriched, boiled | 140 | 221 | 87.0 | 43.2 | 0.8 | 0 | 2.5 | 1 | 10 | 25 | 0.71 | 0.451 | 0 | 0 | 0.38 | 2.4 | 0 | 0.16 |
| *1 cup elbow-shaped* | | 8.1 | 1.3 | 0.2 | 0.2 | 0.4 | 0 | 62 | 81 | 1.79 | 0.140 | 37.0 | 0 | 0.1 | 0.19 | 0.07 | 166.6 | 20100 |
| **macaroni**, pro-fortified, enr, boiled | 140 | 230 | 83.6 | 44.3 | | | | 7 | 14 | 42 | 0.70 | 0.584 | 0 | 0 | 0.42 | 2.6 | 0 | 0.40 |
| *1 cup elbow-shaped* | | 11.3 | 0.3 | 0 | 0 | 0.1 | 0 | 59 | 70 | 1.01 | 0.118 | | 0 | | 0.23 | 0.09 | 184.8 | 20102 |
| **macaroni**, vegetable, enr, boiled | 134 | 172 | 91.6 | 35.7 | 1.5 | 0 | 5.8 | 8 | 15 | 25 | 0.59 | 1.321 | 7 | 0 | 0.15 | 1.4 | 0 | 0.47 |
| *1 cup spiral-shaped* | | 6.1 | 0.1 | 0 | 0 | 0.1 | 0 | 42 | 67 | 0.66 | 0.123 | 26.5 | 123 | 0.3 | 0.08 | 0.03 | 142.0 | 20106 |
| **macaroni**, whole wheat, boiled | 140 | 174 | 94.0 | 37.2 | 1.1 | 0 | 3.9 | 4 | 21 | 42 | 1.13 | 1.931 | 0 | 0 | 0.15 | 1.0 | 0 | 0.59 |
| *1 cup elbow shaped* | | 7.5 | 0.8 | 0.1 | 0.1 | 0.3 | 0 | 62 | 125 | 1.48 | 0.234 | 36.3 | 4 | 0.4 | 0.06 | 0.11 | 7.0 | 20108 |
| **noodles**, egg, enr, boiled (egg in | 160 | 221 | 108.4 | 40.3 | 0.6 | 0 | 1.9 | 8 | 19 | 34 | 1.04 | 0.504 | 10 | 0 | 0.46 | 3.3 | 0.14 | 0.42 |
| dough) - *1 cup* | | 7.3 | 3.3 | 0.7 | 0.9 | 0.9 | 46 | 61 | 122 | 2.35 | 0.157 | 38.2 | 34 | 0.3 | 0.22 | 0.07 | 220.8 | 20110 |
| **noodles**, egg, enr, dry | 57 | 219 | 5.1 | 40.6 | 1.1 | 0 | 1.9 | 12 | 20 | 33 | 1.09 | 0.487 | 10 | 0 | 0.65 | 4.8 | 0.17 | 0.52 |
| (egg in dough) - *2 oz* | | 8.1 | 2.5 | 0.7 | 0.7 | 0.8 | 48 | 139 | 137 | 2.29 | 0.169 | 44.9 | 35 | 0.2 | 0.24 | 0.12 | 210.9 | 20109 |
| **noodles**, egg, homemade, ckd | 112 | 146 | 77.0 | 26.4 | | | | 93 | 11 | 16 | 0.49 | 0.205 | 19 | 0 | 0.19 | 1.4 | 0.11 | 0.26 |
| (egg in dough) - *4 oz* | | 5.9 | 1.9 | 0.5 | 0.6 | 0.6 | 46 | 24 | 58 | 1.30 | 0.063 | | 65 | | 0.19 | 0.04 | 67.2 | 20097 |
| **noodles**, egg, spinach, enr, bld (egg | 160 | 211 | 109.6 | 38.8 | 0.6 | 0 | 3.7 | 19 | 30 | 38 | 1.01 | 0.507 | 16 | 0 | 0.39 | 2.4 | 0.22 | 0.37 |
| & spinach in dough) - *1 cup* | | 8.1 | 2.5 | 0.6 | 0.8 | 0.6 | 53 | 59 | 91 | 1.74 | 0.128 | 34.9 | 165 | 0.9 | 0.20 | 0.18 | 150.4 | 20112 |
| **pasta**, fresh, refrigerated | 128 | 369 | 39.7 | 70.1 | | | | 33 | 19 | 59 | 1.56 | 0.700 | 18 | 0 | 0.90 | 4.3 | 0.40 | 0.68 |
| *4.5 oz* | | 14.5 | 2.9 | 0.4 | 0.3 | 1.2 | 93 | 229 | 209 | 4.29 | 0.292 | | 60 | | 0.56 | 0.12 | 363.5 | 20093 |
| **pasta**, homemade, cooked | 112 | 147 | 76.8 | 27.9 | | | | 7 | 7 | 20 | 0.63 | 0.251 | 7 | 0 | 0.23 | 1.1 | 0.16 | 0.20 |
| *4 oz* | | 5.8 | 1.2 | 0.2 | 0.1 | 0.5 | 37 | 27 | 71 | 1.28 | 0.104 | | 22 | | 0.17 | 0.04 | 116.5 | 20094 |
| **pasta**, homemade without egg, | 112 | 139 | 77.1 | 28.1 | | | | 83 | 7 | 16 | 0.41 | 0.216 | 0 | 0 | 0.20 | 1.5 | 0 | 0.17 |
| cooked - *4 oz* | | 4.9 | 1.1 | 0.2 | 0.2 | 0.6 | 0 | 21 | 45 | 1.27 | 0.067 | | 0 | | 0.17 | 0.03 | 68.3 | 20098 |
| **pasta** made from corn, boiled | 140 | 176 | 95.6 | 39.1 | | | 6.7 | 0 | 1 | 50 | 0.88 | 0.214 | 4 | 0 | 0.07 | 0.8 | 0 | 0.18 |
| *1 cup* | | 3.7 | 1.0 | 0.1 | 0.3 | 0.5 | 0 | 43 | 106 | 0.35 | 0.090 | 3.9 | 80 | | 0.03 | 0.08 | 8.4 | 20092 |
| **pasta**, spinach, fresh, refrigerated | 128 | 370 | 38.5 | 71.3 | | | | 35 | 55 | 81 | 1.79 | 1.000 | 32 | 0 | 0.78 | 4.4 | 0.40 | 0.88 |
| *4.5 oz* | | 14.4 | 2.7 | 0.6 | 0.8 | 0.6 | 93 | 348 | 189 | 4.22 | 0.252 | | 308 | | 0.51 | 0.40 | 335.4 | 20095 |
| **pasta**, spinach, refrig, cooked | 112 | 146 | 76.8 | 28.0 | | | | 7 | 20 | 27 | 0.71 | 0.354 | 11 | 0 | 0.20 | 1.1 | 0.16 | 0.26 |
| *4 oz* | | 5.7 | 1.1 | 0.2 | 0.3 | 0.2 | 37 | 41 | 64 | 1.24 | 0.090 | | 115 | | 0.15 | 0.13 | 107.5 | 20096 |
| **spaghetti**, enriched, boiled | 140 | 221 | 87.0 | 43.2 | 0.8 | 0 | 2.5 | 1 | 10 | 25 | 0.71 | 0.451 | 0 | 0 | 0.38 | 2.4 | 0 | 0.16 |
| *1 cup* | | 8.1 | 1.3 | 0.2 | 0.2 | 0.4 | 0 | 62 | 81 | 1.79 | 0.140 | 37.0 | 0 | 0.1 | 0.19 | 0.07 | 166.6 | 20121 |
| **spaghetti**, enriched, dry | 57 | 211 | 5.6 | 42.6 | 1.5 | 0 | 1.8 | 3 | 12 | 30 | 0.80 | 0.523 | 0 | 0 | 0.51 | 4.1 | 0 | 0.25 |
| *2 oz* | | 7.4 | 0.9 | 0.2 | 0.1 | 0.3 | 0 | 127 | 108 | 1.88 | 0.165 | 36.0 | 0 | 0.1 | 0.23 | 0.08 | 222.9 | 20120 |
| **spaghetti**, pro-fortified, enr, boiled | 140 | 230 | 83.6 | 44.3 | | | 2.4 | 7 | 14 | 42 | 0.70 | 0.584 | 0 | 0 | 0.42 | 2.6 | 0 | 0.40 |
| *1 cup* | | 11.3 | 0.3 | 0 | 0 | 0.1 | 0 | 59 | 70 | 1.01 | 0.118 | 35.3 | 0 | | 0.23 | 0.09 | 184.8 | 20123 |

| | WT (g) | KCAL / PRO (g) | H₂0 (g) / FAT (g) | CHO (g) / SFA (g) | TSUG (g) / MUFA (g) | ASUG (g) / PUFA (g) | DFIB (g) / CHOL (mg) | Na (mg) / K (mg) | Ca (mg) / P (mg) | Mg (mg) / Fe (mg) | Zn (mg) / Cu (mg) | Mn (mg) / Se (mcg) | A (mcg RAE) / A (IU) | C (mg) / E (mg ATE) | B-1 (mg) / B-2 (mg) | NIA (mg) / B-6 (mg) | B-12 (mcg) / FOL (mcg DFE) | PANT (mg) / REF |
|---|---|---|---|---|---|---|---|---|---|---|---|---|---|---|---|---|---|---|
| **spaghetti**, spinach, boiled | 140 | 182 | 95.4 | 36.6 | | | | 20 | 42 | 87 | 1.51 | 2.106 | 11 | 0 | 0.14 | 2.1 | 0 | 0.26 |
| *1 cup* | | 6.4 | 0.9 | 0.1 | 0.1 | 0.4 | 0 | 81 | 151 | 1.46 | 0.287 | 30.9 | 213 | | 0.14 | 0.13 | 16.8 | 20127 |
| **spaghetti**, whole wheat, boiled | 140 | 174 | 94.0 | 37.2 | 1.1 | 0 | 6.3 | 4 | 21 | 42 | 1.13 | 1.931 | 0 | 0 | 0.15 | 1.0 | 0 | 0.59 |
| *1 cup* | | 7.5 | 0.8 | 0.1 | 0.1 | 0.3 | 0 | 62 | 125 | 1.48 | 0.234 | 36.3 | 4 | 0.4 | 0.06 | 0.11 | 7.0 | 20125 |

## 17.12 ROLLS

| | WT (g) | KCAL / PRO (g) | H₂0 (g) / FAT (g) | CHO (g) / SFA (g) | TSUG (g) / MUFA (g) | ASUG (g) / PUFA (g) | DFIB (g) / CHOL (mg) | Na (mg) / K (mg) | Ca (mg) / P (mg) | Mg (mg) / Fe (mg) | Zn (mg) / Cu (mg) | Mn (mg) / Se (mcg) | A (mcg RAE) / A (IU) | C (mg) / E (mg ATE) | B-1 (mg) / B-2 (mg) | NIA (mg) / B-6 (mg) | B-12 (mcg) / FOL (mcg DFE) | PANT (mg) / REF |
|---|---|---|---|---|---|---|---|---|---|---|---|---|---|---|---|---|---|---|
| **crescent roll**, from refrig dough, Pillsbury - *1 oz roll* | 28 | 110 | | 11.0 | 2.0 | | 0 | 220 | 0 | | | | | 0 | | | | |
| | | 2.0 | 6 | 2.0 | | | | | | | 0.7 | | 0 | | | | | GENM269 |
| **dinner roll** | 28 | 87 | 8.0 | 14.6 | 1.6 | 0.5 | 0.6 | 150 | 50 | 7 | 0.28 | 0.163 | 0 | 0 | 0.15 | 1.5 | 0.04 | 0.13 |
| *1 oz roll (2" square, 2" high)* | | 3.0 | 1.8 | 0.4 | 0.5 | 0.7 | 1 | 39 | 34 | 1.04 | 0.038 | 7.5 | 1 | 0.1 | 0.10 | 0.03 | 42.0 | 18342 |
| **dinner roll**, homemade with 2% milk | 35 | 111 | 10.2 | 18.7 | | | 0.7 | 145 | 21 | 7 | 0.24 | 0.140 | 30 | | 0.14 | 1.2 | 0.05 | 0.16 |
| *1.2 oz roll (2½" diameter)* | | 3.0 | 2.6 | 0.6 | 1.0 | 0.7 | 12 | 53 | 44 | 1.04 | 0.040 | 8.0 | 118 | | 0.14 | 0.02 | 43.0 | 18396 |
| **dinner roll** made with egg | 35 | 107 | 10.6 | 18.2 | 1.5 | 1.5 | 1.3 | 191 | 21 | 9 | 0.39 | 0.184 | 2 | 0 | 0.18 | 1.2 | 0.08 | 0.23 |
| *1.2 oz roll (2½" diameter)* | | 3.3 | 2.2 | 0.6 | 1.0 | 0.4 | 18 | 36 | 35 | 1.23 | 0.047 | 10.4 | 7 | 0.1 | 0.18 | 0.02 | 96.6 | 18344 |
| **dinner roll**, wheat | 28 | 76 | 10.4 | 12.9 | 0.5 | 0.4 | 1.1 | 95 | 49 | 10 | 0.25 | 0.286 | 0 | 0 | 0.12 | 1.1 | 0 | 0.10 |
| *1 oz roll* | | 2.4 | 1.8 | 0.4 | 0.9 | 0.3 | 0 | 32 | 29 | 0.99 | 0.042 | 9.2 | 0 | 0.1 | 0.08 | 0.02 | 25.8 | 18347 |
| **dinner roll**, white, from refrig dough, Pillsbury - *1.4 oz roll* | 40 | 110 | | 20.0 | 3.0 | | 0.5 | 280 | 0 | | | | | 0 | | | | |
| | | 3.0 | 2.0 | 1.0 | 0.5 | 0.5 | 0 | | | | 0.72 | | 0 | | | | | GENM272 |
| **dinner roll**, whole wheat | 36 | 96 | 11.9 | 18.4 | 3.0 | 2.7 | 2.7 | 172 | 38 | 31 | 0.72 | 0.827 | 0 | 0 | 0.09 | 1.3 | 0 | 0.18 |
| *1.3 oz roll (2½" diameter)* | | 3.1 | 1.7 | 0.3 | 0.4 | 0.8 | 0 | 98 | 81 | 0.87 | 0.086 | 17.8 | 0 | 0.3 | 0.05 | 0.07 | 10.8 | 18348 |
| **frankfurter roll** | 43 | 120 | 14.9 | 21.3 | 2.7 | 2.6 | 0.9 | 206 | 59 | 9 | 0.28 | 0.117 | 0 | 0 | 0.17 | 1.8 | 0.09 | 0.14 |
| *1.5 oz roll* | | 4.1 | 1.9 | 0.5 | 0.5 | 0.8 | 0 | 40 | 27 | 1.43 | 0.095 | 8.4 | 0 | 0.1 | 0.14 | 0.03 | 73.1 | 18350 |
| **French roll** | 38 | 105 | 13.2 | 19.1 | 0.1 | 0 | 1.2 | 231 | 35 | 8 | 0.34 | 0.212 | 0 | 0 | 0.20 | 1.7 | 0 | 0.17 |
| *1.3 oz roll* | | 3.3 | 1.6 | 0.4 | 0.7 | 0.3 | 0 | 43 | 32 | 1.03 | 0.051 | 10.6 | 0 | 0.1 | 0.11 | 0.01 | 64.2 | 18349 |
| **hamburger roll** | 43 | 120 | 14.9 | 21.3 | 2.7 | 2.6 | 0.9 | 206 | 59 | 9 | 0.28 | 0.117 | 0 | 0 | 0.17 | 1.8 | 0.09 | 0.14 |
| *1.5 oz roll* | | 4.1 | 1.9 | 0.5 | 0.5 | 0.8 | 0 | 40 | 27 | 1.43 | 0.095 | 8.4 | 0 | 0.1 | 0.14 | 0.03 | 73.1 | 18350 |
| **hamburger roll**, mixed grain | 43 | 113 | 16.3 | 19.2 | 2.7 | 2.7 | 1.6 | 197 | 41 | 19 | 0.45 | 0.436 | 0 | 0 | 0.20 | 1.9 | 0 | 0.21 |
| *1.5 oz roll* | | 4.1 | 2.6 | 0.6 | 1.2 | 0.5 | 0 | 69 | 52 | 1.70 | 0.093 | 13.7 | 0 | 0 | 0.13 | 0.04 | 73.5 | 18351 |
| **hamburger roll**, Wonder | 43 | 117 | 14.7 | 21.9 | 4.8 | | 1.1 | 256 | 37 | | | | | | | | | |
| *1.5 oz roll* | | 3.5 | 1.8 | 0.4 | 0.4 | 0.9 | | | | | 0.95 | | | | | | | 18641 |
| **hard/kaiser roll** | 57 | 167 | 17.7 | 30.0 | 1.0 | 0.9 | 1.3 | 310 | 54 | 15 | 0.54 | 0.262 | 0 | 0 | 0.27 | 2.4 | 0 | 0.23 |
| *2 oz roll (3½"diameter)* | | 5.6 | 2.5 | 0.3 | 0.6 | 1.0 | 0 | 62 | 57 | 1.87 | 0.093 | 22.3 | 0 | 0.2 | 0.19 | 0.02 | 86.1 | 18353 |
| **oat bran roll** | 33 | 78 | 14.5 | 13.3 | 2.2 | 2.1 | 1.4 | 136 | 28 | 11 | 0.34 | 0.249 | 0 | 0 | 0.15 | 1.6 | 0 | 0.14 |
| *1.2 oz roll* | | 3.1 | 1.5 | 0.2 | 0.5 | 0.5 | 0 | 40 | 38 | 1.37 | 0.045 | 9.7 | 0 | 0.2 | 0.10 | 0.01 | 46.2 | 18345 |
| **pumpernickel roll** | 36 | 100 | 11.5 | 19.0 | 0.1 | 0 | 1.9 | 205 | 24 | 19 | 0.53 | 0.687 | 0 | 0 | 0.14 | 1.1 | 0 | 0.22 |
| *1.3 oz roll* | | 3.9 | 1.0 | 0.2 | 0.4 | 0.4 | 0 | 75 | 62 | 1.00 | 0.103 | 10.0 | 0 | 0.2 | 0.11 | 0.04 | 45.0 | 43441 |
| **rye roll** | 36 | 103 | 10.8 | 19.1 | 0.4 | 0 | 1.8 | 321 | 11 | 19 | 0.35 | 0.253 | 0 | 0 | 0.14 | 1.4 | 0 | 0.14 |
| *1.3 oz roll* | | 3.7 | 1.2 | 0.2 | 0.4 | 0.3 | 0 | 65 | 57 | 0.97 | 0.072 | 10.0 | 3 | 0.1 | 0.10 | 0.02 | 55.1 | 18346 |

## 17.13 STUFFINGS AND COATINGS

| | WT (g) | KCAL / PRO (g) | H₂0 (g) / FAT (g) | CHO (g) / SFA (g) | TSUG (g) / MUFA (g) | ASUG (g) / PUFA (g) | DFIB (g) / CHOL (mg) | Na (mg) / K (mg) | Ca (mg) / P (mg) | Mg (mg) / Fe (mg) | Zn (mg) / Cu (mg) | Mn (mg) / Se (mcg) | A (mcg RAE) / A (IU) | C (mg) / E (mg ATE) | B-1 (mg) / B-2 (mg) | NIA (mg) / B-6 (mg) | B-12 (mcg) / FOL (mcg DFE) | PANT (mg) / REF |
|---|---|---|---|---|---|---|---|---|---|---|---|---|---|---|---|---|---|---|
| **bread stuffing**, from mix | 100 | 177 | 64.8 | 21.7 | 2.1 | 1.8 | 2.9 | 543 | 32 | 12 | 0.28 | 0.169 | 118 | 0 | 0.14 | 1.5 | 0.01 | 0.08 |
| *½ cup* | | 3.2 | 8.6 | 1.7 | 3.8 | 2.6 | 0 | 74 | 42 | 1.09 | 0.072 | 49.8 | 313 | 1.4 | 0.11 | 0.04 | 54.0 | 18082 |
| **cornbread stuffing**, dry | 28 | 109 | 1.3 | 21.5 | 1.3 | 1.2 | 4.0 | 359 | 22 | 12 | 0.21 | 0.148 | 2 | 1 | 0.14 | 1.4 | 0 | 0.08 |
| *1 oz* | | 2.8 | 1.2 | 0.3 | 0.5 | 0.3 | 0 | 57 | 32 | 0.91 | 0.064 | 8.3 | 44 | | 0.10 | 0.04 | 75.3 | 18084 |
| **cornbread stuffing**, from mix | 100 | 179 | 64.9 | 21.9 | 3.9 | 3.6 | 2.9 | 455 | 26 | 13 | 0.23 | 0.114 | 78 | 1 | 0.12 | 1.2 | 0.01 | 0.06 |
| *½ cup* | | 2.9 | 8.8 | 1.8 | 3.9 | 2.7 | 0 | 62 | 34 | 0.94 | 0.069 | 30.7 | 340 | 0.8 | 0.09 | 0.04 | 159.0 | 18085 |
| **pork coating**, dry, original recipe, Shake 'n Bake - *1 oz* | 28 | 106 | 0.9 | 22.3 | | | | 795 | | | | | | | | | | |
| | | 1.7 | 1.0 | | | | | | | | | | | | | | | 18637 |
| **stuffing mix**, chicken flavor, Stove Top - *amount to make ½ cup* | 28 | 107 | 1.5 | 20.5 | 2.8 | | 0.7 | 429 | 18 | | | | | 1 | 0.11 | 1.1 | | |
| | | 3.5 | 1.1 | 0.2 | | | 1 | 75 | 36 | 1.21 | | | 30 | | 0.08 | | | 18567 |
| **stuffing mix**, sage, onion, Brownberry - *2.4 oz* | 67 | 261 | 2.7 | 48.7 | | | 3.6 | 1126 | | | | | | | | | | |
| | | 8.9 | 3.4 | 0.6 | | | | | | 2.55 | | | | | | | | 18603 |

## 17.14 WAFFLES

| | WT (g) | KCAL / PRO (g) | H₂0 (g) / FAT (g) | CHO (g) / SFA (g) | TSUG (g) / MUFA (g) | ASUG (g) / PUFA (g) | DFIB (g) / CHOL (mg) | Na (mg) / K (mg) | Ca (mg) / P (mg) | Mg (mg) / Fe (mg) | Zn (mg) / Cu (mg) | Mn (mg) / Se (mcg) | A (mcg RAE) / A (IU) | C (mg) / E (mg ATE) | B-1 (mg) / B-2 (mg) | NIA (mg) / B-6 (mg) | B-12 (mcg) / FOL (mcg DFE) | PANT (mg) / REF |
|---|---|---|---|---|---|---|---|---|---|---|---|---|---|---|---|---|---|---|
| **waffle**, banana bread, Kellogg's Eggo - *1 waffle* | 78 | 212 | 32.1 | 32.4 | 5.2 | | 2.0 | 280 | 40 | 14 | 0.47 | | | 1 | 0.31 | 4.0 | 1.17 | 0 |
| | | 5.3 | 7.4 | 1.3 | 4.1 | 2.0 | 0 | 140 | 266 | 3.59 | 0 | | 1000 | | 0.31 | 0.39 | | 18500 |
| **waffle**, blueberry, lowfat, Nutri-Grain | 35 | 73 | 16.1 | 14.9 | 3.1 | | 1.2 | 207 | 21 | 19 | | | | 0 | 0.13 | 1.8 | 0.54 | |
| *1 round waffle (4" diameter)* | | 2.1 | 1.0 | 0.1 | 0.4 | 0.3 | 0 | 24 | 27 | 1.62 | | | 449 | | 0.15 | 0.18 | | 18507 |
| **waffle**, blueberry, wheat-free, Van's | 90 | 201 | | 35.0 | 7.0 | | 1.0 | 390 | 90 | | | | 0 | | | | | |
| *2 waffles (3.17 oz)* | | 4.0 | 5.0 | 0.5 | | | 0 | | | 1.80 | | | 0 | | | | | VANS1 |

| | WT (g) | KCAL / PRO (g) | H₂O (g) / FAT (g) | CHO (g) / SFA (g) | TSUG (g) / MUFA (g) | ASUG (g) / PUFA (g) | DFIB (g) / CHOL (mg) | Na (mg) / K (mg) | Ca (mg) / P (mg) | Mg (mg) / Fe (mg) | Zn (mg) / Cu (mg) | Mn (mg) / Se (mcg) | A (mcg RAE) / A (IU) | C (mg) / E (mg ATE) | B-1 (mg) / B-2 (mg) | NIA (mg) / B-6 (mg) | B-12 (mcg) / FOL (mcg DFE) | PANT (mg) / REF |
|---|---|---|---|---|---|---|---|---|---|---|---|---|---|---|---|---|---|---|
| **waffle**, buttermilk, frozen, microwaved | 33 | 95 | 12.0 | 14.6 | 1.5 | | 0.8 | 219 | 41 | 7 | 0.19 | 0.078 | 142 | 0 | 0.19 | 2.2 | 0.81 | 0.08 |
| *1 waffle (4" square)* | | 2.3 | 3.1 | 0.7 | 1.6 | 0.5 | 5 | 36 | 135 | 2.15 | 0.021 | 3.3 | 472 | 0.2 | 0.23 | 0.36 | 32.7 | 18934 |
| **waffle**, buttermilk, frozen, toasted | 33 | 102 | 10.4 | 16.0 | 1.5 | 1.2 | 0.9 | 234 | 99 | 7 | 0.16 | 0.074 | 144 | 0 | 0.19 | 2.6 | 0.53 | 0.07 |
| *1 waffle (4" square)* | | 2.4 | 3.1 | 0.8 | 1.7 | 0.5 | 4 | 46 | 147 | 2.17 | 0.012 | 3.4 | 483 | 0.2 | 0.21 | 0.37 | 35.3 | 18933 |
| **waffle**, frozen, microwaved | 33 | 98 | 11.5 | 15.0 | 1.7 | | 0.8 | 225 | 65 | 8 | 0.15 | 0.051 | | | 0.18 | 2.6 | 0.72 | 0.11 |
| *1 waffle (4" square)* | | 2.2 | 3.3 | 0.5 | 1.7 | 0.7 | 5 | 49 | 135 | 1.92 | 0.013 | 4.2 | | 0.3 | 0.22 | 0.34 | 35.0 | 18935 |
| **waffle**, frozen, toasted | 33 | 103 | 10.1 | 16.3 | 1.7 | 1.2 | 0.8 | 241 | 101 | 8 | 0.17 | 0.099 | 131 | 0 | 0.17 | 2.9 | 0.96 | 0.11 |
| *1 waffle (4" square)* | | 2.4 | 3.2 | 0.5 | 1.6 | 0.7 | 5 | 48 | 142 | 2.28 | 0.010 | 4.2 | 439 | 0.3 | 0.23 | 0.34 | 39.3 | 18403 |
| **waffle**, homemade | 75 | 218 | 31.5 | 24.7 | | | | 383 | 191 | 14 | 0.51 | 0.199 | 49 | 0 | 0.20 | 1.6 | 0.19 | 0.36 |
| *1 round waffle (7" diameter)* | | 5.9 | 10.6 | 2.1 | 2.6 | 5.1 | 52 | 119 | 142 | 1.73 | 0.046 | 34.7 | 171 | | 0.26 | 0.04 | 51.0 | 18367 |
| **waffle**, homestyle, lowfat, Kellogg's | 35 | 83 | 15.2 | 15.5 | 1.0 | | 0.4 | 155 | 20 | 24 | | | | 0 | 0.31 | 2.6 | 0.55 | |
| Eggo - *1 round waffle (4" dia)* | | 2.5 | 1.2 | 0.3 | 0.4 | 0.4 | 9 | 50 | 28 | 1.95 | | | 506 | | 0.26 | 0.16 | | 18505 |
| **waffle**, lowfat, Nutri-Grain, Kellogg's | 35 | 71 | 16.7 | 14.1 | 2.0 | | 1.3 | 215 | 21 | 20 | | | | 0 | 0.13 | 1.8 | 0.54 | |
| Eggo - *1 round waffle (4" dia)* | | 2.2 | 1.1 | 0.2 | 0.5 | 0.3 | 0 | 25 | 28 | 1.62 | | | 449 | | 0.15 | 0.18 | | 18506 |
| **waffle**, oat, golden, frozen, Kellogg's | 35 | 69 | 17.7 | 13.1 | 1.2 | | 1.2 | 135 | 23 | 15 | | | | 0 | 0.14 | 1.8 | 0.52 | |
| Eggo - *1 round waffle (4" dia)* | | 2.4 | 1.1 | 0.2 | 0.4 | 0.4 | 0 | 67 | 113 | 1.61 | | | 449 | | 0.18 | 0.18 | | 18512 |

## 18. INFANT, JUNIOR, AND TODDLER FOODS
### 18.1 INFANT, JUNIOR, AND TODDLER BAKED PRODUCTS

| | WT (g) | KCAL / PRO (g) | H₂O (g) / FAT (g) | CHO (g) / SFA (g) | TSUG (g) / MUFA (g) | ASUG (g) / PUFA (g) | DFIB (g) / CHOL (mg) | Na (mg) / K (mg) | Ca (mg) / P (mg) | Mg (mg) / Fe (mg) | Zn (mg) / Cu (mg) | Mn (mg) / Se (mcg) | A (mcg RAE) / A (IU) | C (mg) / E (mg ATE) | B-1 (mg) / B-2 (mg) | NIA (mg) / B-6 (mg) | B-12 (mcg) / FOL (mcg DFE) | PANT (mg) / REF |
|---|---|---|---|---|---|---|---|---|---|---|---|---|---|---|---|---|---|---|
| **arrowroot cookie** | 5 | 22 | 0.3 | 3.6 | | | 0 | 18 | 2 | 1 | 0.03 | | | 0 | 0.02 | 0.3 | 0 | 0.03 |
| *.18 oz cookie* | | 0.4 | 0.7 | 0.2 | 0.4 | 0 | 0 | 8 | 6 | 0.15 | 0.004 | 0.9 | 0 | 0 | 0.02 | 0 | 2.7 | 3214 |
| **baby/infant cookie** | 7 | 30 | 0.4 | 4.7 | 1.7 | 1.2 | 0 | 13 | 7 | 3 | 0.08 | | | 0 | 0.10 | 1.1 | 0.32 | 0.04 |
| *.2 oz cookie* | | 0.8 | 0.9 | 0.3 | 0.5 | 0.1 | 0 | 35 | 13 | 0.29 | 0.005 | 1.2 | 2 | 0 | 0.23 | 0.41 | 7.6 | 3213 |
| **baby/infant pretzel** | 6 | 24 | 0.2 | 4.9 | 0.2 | 0.2 | 0.1 | 16 | 2 | 2 | 0.05 | | | 0 | 0.03 | 0.2 | 0 | 0.03 |
| *.2 oz pretzel* | | 0.6 | 0.1 | 0 | 0 | 0 | 0 | 8 | 7 | 0.23 | 0.009 | 0.5 | 0 | 0 | 0.02 | 0 | 7.9 | 3215 |
| **cracker, vegetable** | 3 | 14 | 0.1 | 2.0 | 0.4 | 0.3 | 0.1 | 32 | 1 | 1 | 0.03 | 0.023 | 5 | 2 | 0.01 | 0.1 | 0 | 0.01 |
| *5 crackers* | | 0.3 | 0.6 | 0.1 | 0.2 | 0.3 | 0 | 7 | 6 | 0.13 | 0.004 | 0.4 | 107 | 0.1 | 0.01 | 0 | 4.8 | 3209 |
| **fruit cookie** | 8 | 35 | 0.5 | 5.9 | 1.9 | 1.4 | 0.3 | 1 | 7 | 2 | 0.06 | 0.018 | 9 | 0 | 0.04 | 0.3 | 0.02 | 0.03 |
| *.3 oz cookie* | | 0.5 | 1.0 | 0.2 | 0.4 | 0.3 | 0 | 34 | 15 | 0.23 | 0.003 | 1.6 | 188 | 0.1 | 0.03 | 0.02 | 13.4 | 3206 |
| **teething biscuit** | 11 | 44 | 0.7 | 8.6 | 3.1 | 1.7 | 0.2 | 28 | 11 | 4 | 0.10 | | 3 | 1 | 0.03 | 0.5 | 0.01 | 0.06 |
| *.4 oz biscuit* | | 1.0 | 0.6 | 0.2 | 0.2 | 0.1 | 0 | 36 | 18 | 0.39 | 0.016 | 2.6 | 13 | 0 | 0.06 | 0.01 | 7.6 | 3216 |
| **zwieback toast**, Gerber | 7 | 30 | 0.3 | 5.2 | 0.9 | 0.9 | 0.2 | 16 | 1 | 1 | 0.04 | | 1 | 0 | 0.01 | 0.1 | 0 | 0.04 |
| *.2 oz piece* | | 0.7 | 0.7 | 0.3 | 0.3 | 0.1 | 1 | 21 | 4 | 0.04 | 0.010 | 2.0 | 4 | 0 | 0.02 | 0.01 | 9.4 | 3217 |

### 18.2 INFANT, JUNIOR, AND TODDLER CEREALS

| | WT (g) | KCAL / PRO (g) | H₂O (g) / FAT (g) | CHO (g) / SFA (g) | TSUG (g) / MUFA (g) | ASUG (g) / PUFA (g) | DFIB (g) / CHOL (mg) | Na (mg) / K (mg) | Ca (mg) / P (mg) | Mg (mg) / Fe (mg) | Zn (mg) / Cu (mg) | Mn (mg) / Se (mcg) | A (mcg RAE) / A (IU) | C (mg) / E (mg ATE) | B-1 (mg) / B-2 (mg) | NIA (mg) / B-6 (mg) | B-12 (mcg) / FOL (mcg DFE) | PANT (mg) / REF |
|---|---|---|---|---|---|---|---|---|---|---|---|---|---|---|---|---|---|---|
| **barley infant cereal**, dry | 2.4 | 9 | 0.2 | 1.8 | 0.1 | 0 | 0.2 | 1 | 19 | 3 | 0.08 | | | 0 | 0.07 | 0.9 | 0 | 0.01 |
| *1 T* | | 0.3 | 0.1 | 0 | 0 | 0 | 0 | 9 | 11 | 1.14 | 0.011 | 0.7 | 0 | 0.1 | 0.06 | 0.01 | 0.7 | 3181 |
| **barley infant cereal**, prep | 28 | 31 | 20.9 | 4.6 | | | | 14 | 64 | 8 | 0.23 | | | | 0.13 | 1.7 | 0.08 | 0.10 |
| *w/whole milk - 1 oz* | | 1.3 | 0.9 | | | | | 54 | 42 | 3.46 | 0.024 | | 29 | | 0.16 | 0.03 | 2.5 | 3681 |
| **cereal and egg yolks**, junior | 170 | 88 | 150.8 | 12.1 | | | 1.5 | 56 | 41 | 5 | 0.49 | | 70 | 1 | 0.01 | 0.1 | 0.10 | 1.49 |
| *6 oz jar* | | 3.2 | 3.1 | 1.0 | 1.3 | 0.5 | 107 | 60 | 68 | 0.87 | 0.037 | | 245 | | 0.08 | 0.03 | 5.1 | 3198 |
| **cereal and egg yolks**, strained | 113 | 58 | 100.3 | 7.9 | | | 1.0 | 37 | 27 | 3 | 0.33 | | 45 | 1 | 0.01 | 0.1 | 0.08 | 0.99 |
| *4 oz jar* | | 2.1 | 2.0 | 0.7 | 0.9 | 0.3 | 71 | 44 | 45 | 0.53 | 0.025 | | 159 | | 0.05 | 0.02 | 3.4 | 3197 |
| **cereal and eggs**, strained | 113 | 66 | 98.5 | 9.0 | | | | 43 | 31 | 3 | 0.37 | | | 1 | 0.01 | 0.1 | 0.09 | 1.13 |
| *4 oz jar* | | 2.5 | 1.7 | 0.6 | 0.7 | 0.4 | 58 | 50 | 52 | 0.61 | 0.028 | | 182 | | 0.06 | 0.03 | 10.2 | 3199 |
| **cereal, egg yolks, and bacon**, | 170 | 134 | 146.0 | 10.5 | | | 1.5 | 82 | 48 | 8 | 0.46 | | 48 | 2 | 0.08 | 0.5 | 0.15 | 1.88 |
| junior - *6 oz jar* | | 4.2 | 8.5 | 2.8 | 3.8 | 1.1 | 160 | 60 | 85 | 0.80 | 0.034 | | 160 | | 0.13 | 0.04 | 6.8 | 3201 |
| **high pro infant cereal**, prep | 28 | 31 | 20.9 | 3.2 | | | | 14 | 61 | 13 | 0.29 | | | | 0.13 | 1.6 | 0.08 | 0.13 |
| *w/whole milk - 1 oz* | | 2.4 | 1.1 | | | | | 98 | 50 | 3.40 | 0.061 | | 29 | | 0.16 | 0.03 | 9.8 | 3682 |
| **high pro infant cereal** w/apple | 2 | 7 | 0.1 | 1.2 | | | 0.1 | 2 | 15 | 3 | 0.05 | | 0 | 0 | 0.08 | 0.5 | 0.01 | |
| and orange, dry - *1 T* | | 0.5 | 0.1 | 0 | 0 | 0.1 | 0 | 27 | 11 | 0.95 | 0.019 | 0.6 | 1 | | 0.09 | 0.01 | 3.8 | 3211 |
| **high pro infant cereal** w/apple & | 28 | 31 | 20.8 | 3.8 | | | | 16 | 62 | 10 | 0.21 | | | | 0.18 | 1.1 | 0.10 | |
| orange, prep w/whl mlk - *1 oz* | | 1.9 | 1.1 | | | | | 97 | 46 | 4.04 | 0.046 | | | | 0.24 | 0.03 | 7.8 | 3711 |
| **mixed cereal**, dry, infant | 2.5 | 9 | 0.2 | 1.8 | 0 | 0 | 0.2 | 1 | 18 | 2 | 0.06 | | | 0 | 0.06 | 0.9 | 0 | 0.03 |
| *1 T* | | 0.3 | 0.1 | 0 | 0 | 0 | 0 | 11 | 10 | 1.19 | 0.008 | 0.6 | 0 | 0.1 | 0.07 | 0 | 1.1 | 3185 |
| **mixed cereal**, prep w/whole milk, | 28 | 32 | 20.9 | 4.5 | | | 0.4 | 13 | 62 | 8 | 0.20 | | 7 | 0 | 0.12 | 1.6 | 0.08 | 0.12 |
| infant - *1 oz* | | 1.3 | 1.0 | 0.5 | | | 3 | 56 | 40 | 2.92 | 0.018 | | 29 | | 0.16 | 0.02 | 3.1 | 3685 |
| **mixed cereal** w/applesauce and | 170 | 141 | 135.3 | 31.3 | 13.2 | 0 | 2.0 | 61 | 7 | 12 | 0.37 | | 2 | 15 | 0.48 | 6.9 | 0 | 0.33 |
| bananas, junior - *6 oz jar* | | 2.0 | 0.7 | 0.1 | 0.2 | 0.3 | 0 | 54 | 49 | 9.54 | 0.094 | 4.4 | 32 | 0.1 | 0.61 | 0.24 | 6.8 | 3188 |

| | WT (g) | Macronutrients: KCAL / PRO (g) | H₂0 (g) / FAT (g) | CHO (g) / SFA (g) | TSUG (g) / MUFA (g) | ASUG (g) / PUFA (g) | DFIB (g) / CHOL (mg) | Minerals: Na (mg) / K (mg) | Ca (mg) / P (mg) | Mg (mg) / Fe (mg) | Zn (mg) / Cu (mg) | Mn (mg) / Se (mcg) | Vitamins: A (mcg RAE) / A (IU) | C (mg) / E (mg ATE) | B-1 (mg) / B-2 (mg) | NIA (mg) / B-6 (mg) | B-12 (mcg) / FOL (mcg DFE) | PANT (mg) / REF |
|---|---|---|---|---|---|---|---|---|---|---|---|---|---|---|---|---|---|---|
| **mixed cereal** w/applesauce and | 113 | 93 | 90.4 | 20.2 | 8.8 | 0 | 1.4 | 2 | 7 | 9 | 0.21 | | 1 | 29 | 0.32 | 4.5 | 0 | 0.22 |
| bananas, strained - *4 oz jar* | | 1.4 | 0.6 | 0.1 | 0.2 | 0.2 | 0 | 46 | 26 | 7.48 | 0.061 | 2.9 | 20 | 0 | 0.40 | 0.15 | 4.5 | 3187 |
| **mixed cereal** w/bananas, dry, | 2.5 | 10 | 0.1 | 1.9 | 0.2 | 0 | 0.2 | 3 | 17 | 2 | 0.03 | | 0 | 0 | 0.09 | 0.5 | 0.01 | |
| infant - *1 T* | | 0.3 | 0.1 | 0 | 0 | 0 | 0 | 17 | 9 | 1.19 | 0.006 | 0.5 | 3 | 0 | 0.09 | 0.01 | 0.4 | 3186 |
| **mixed cereal** w/bananas, prep | 28 | 32 | 20.8 | 4.6 | | | 0.4 | 17 | 60 | 7 | 0.15 | | 6 | 0 | 0.18 | 1.0 | 0.10 | |
| w/whole milk, infant - *1 oz* | | 1.3 | 1.0 | 0.6 | | | 3 | 66 | 39 | 3.12 | 0.014 | | 30 | | 0.20 | 0.03 | 2.0 | 3686 |
| **mixed cereal** w/honey, prep | 28 | 32 | 20.8 | 4.5 | | | | 13 | 82 | 8 | 0.20 | | | | 0.13 | 1.8 | 0.08 | 0.12 |
| w/whole milk, infant - *1 oz* | | 1.4 | 1.0 | | | | | 48 | 52 | 3.16 | 0.018 | | | | 0.16 | 0.02 | 3.1 | 3704 |
| **oatmeal**, dry, infant cereal | 2 | 8 | 0.1 | 1.4 | 0.1 | 0 | 0.2 | 0 | 14 | 3 | 0.11 | 0.068 | 0 | 0 | 0.06 | 0.6 | 0 | 0.01 |
| *1 T* | | 0.3 | 0.2 | 0 | 0.1 | 0 | 0 | 8 | 12 | 1.02 | 0.009 | 0.6 | 0 | 0.1 | 0.07 | 0.01 | 0.7 | 3189 |
| **oatmeal**, prep w/whole milk, | 28 | 32 | 20.9 | 4.3 | | | 0.3 | 13 | 62 | 10 | 0.26 | | 6 | 0 | 0.14 | 1.7 | 0.08 | 0.14 |
| infant cereal - *1 oz* | | 1.4 | 1.1 | 0.6 | | | 3 | 57 | 45 | 3.40 | 0.026 | | 29 | | 0.16 | 0.02 | 2.8 | 3689 |
| **oatmeal** w/applesauce and | 170 | 128 | 139.1 | 26.7 | 16.1 | 0 | 1.4 | 53 | 10 | 19 | 12.75 | | 2 | 42 | 0.42 | 9.5 | 0 | 0.39 |
| bananas, junior - *6 oz jar* | | 2.2 | 1.2 | 0.2 | 0.4 | 0.4 | 0 | 82 | 70 | 12.75 | 0.128 | 5.1 | 48 | 0.2 | 0.82 | 0.41 | 6.8 | 3192 |
| **oatmeal** w/applesauce and | 113 | 84 | 92.9 | 17.4 | 11.9 | 0 | 0.9 | 2 | 10 | 12 | 0.40 | | 2 | 25 | 0.47 | 5.7 | 0 | 0.26 |
| bananas, strained - *4 oz jar* | | 1.5 | 0.8 | 0.1 | 0.2 | 0.3 | 0 | 53 | 46 | 6.38 | 0.082 | 3.4 | 34 | 0.2 | 0.41 | 0.23 | 4.5 | 3191 |
| **oatmeal** w/bananas, dry, infant | 2 | 8 | 0.1 | 1.5 | 0.3 | 0 | 0.1 | 2 | 13 | 2 | 0.04 | | 0 | 0 | 0.07 | 0.4 | 0 | |
| cereal - *1 T* | | 0.2 | 0.1 | 0 | 0 | 0 | 0 | 15 | 9 | 0.95 | 0.008 | 0.4 | 1 | 0.1 | 0.07 | 0.01 | 0.4 | 3190 |
| **oatmeal** w/bananas, prep w/whole | 28 | 32 | 20.8 | 4.5 | | | | 17 | 58 | 8 | 0.18 | | 6 | 0 | 0.17 | 0.9 | 0.09 | |
| milk, infant cereal - *1 oz* | | 1.3 | 1.1 | | | | | 69 | 42 | 3.14 | 0.020 | | 28 | | 0.21 | 0.03 | 2.0 | 3690 |
| **oatmeal** w/fruit, dry infant | 5 | 20 | 0.3 | 3.7 | 0.6 | 0 | 0.4 | 10 | 14 | 5 | 0.29 | 0.140 | 0 | 0 | 0.04 | 0.5 | 0 | |
| cereal - *1 T* | | 0.5 | 0.4 | 0.1 | 0.2 | 0.1 | 0 | 17 | 21 | 0.72 | 0.017 | 1.0 | 4 | 0.1 | 0.04 | 0.02 | 0.9 | 3205 |
| **oatmeal** w/honey, dry infant | 2 | 8 | 0.1 | 1.4 | | | | 1 | 23 | 3 | 0.07 | | 0 | 0 | 0.06 | 0.7 | 0 | 0.03 |
| cereal - *1 T* | | 0.3 | 0.1 | | | | | 5 | 15 | 1.34 | 0.011 | 0.7 | 0 | | 0.06 | 0 | 0.7 | 3193 |
| **oatmeal** w/honey, prep w/whole | 28 | 32 | 20.9 | 4.3 | | | | 14 | 81 | 10 | 0.26 | | | | 0.14 | 1.7 | 0.08 | 0.14 |
| milk, infant cereal - *1 oz* | | 1.4 | 1.1 | | | | | 48 | 55 | 3.11 | 0.027 | | | | 0.17 | 0.02 | 2.8 | 3693 |
| **rice, brown cereal**, dry, infant | 4 | 16 | 0 | 3.4 | 0 | 0 | 0.3 | 0 | 2 | 1 | 0 | | 0 | 0 | 0.04 | 0.6 | 0 | |
| *1 T* | | 0.3 | 0.1 | 0 | 0 | 0 | 0 | 15 | 11 | 1.90 | 0.015 | 0.9 | 0 | 0.1 | 0.01 | 0.04 | 0.6 | 42285 |
| **rice cereal**, dry, infant | 2 | 8 | 0.1 | 1.6 | 0 | 0 | 0 | 1 | 17 | 4 | 0.04 | | 0 | 0 | 0.05 | 0.6 | 0 | |
| *1 T* | | 0.1 | 0.1 | 0 | 0 | 0 | 0 | 8 | 12 | 0.95 | 0.007 | 0.2 | 0 | 0.1 | 0.04 | 0.01 | 0.5 | 3194 |
| **rice cereal**, prep w/whole milk, | 28 | 32 | 20.9 | 4.7 | | | 0 | 13 | 67 | 13 | 0.18 | | 6 | 0 | 0.13 | 1.5 | 0.08 | |
| infant - *1 oz* | | 1.1 | 1.0 | 0.7 | | | 3 | 53 | 49 | 3.41 | 0.017 | | 29 | | 0.14 | 0.03 | 2.2 | 3694 |
| **rice cereal** w/aplsce and bananas, | 120 | 96 | 97.2 | 20.5 | 2.7 | 0 | 1.2 | 34 | 20 | 4 | 0.10 | | 1 | 38 | 0.31 | 4.8 | 0 | |
| Gerber 2nd Fds - *4.25 oz jar* | | 1.4 | 0.5 | 0.1 | 0.1 | 0.1 | 0 | 34 | 14 | 8.08 | 0.061 | 2.5 | 25 | 0 | 0.51 | 0.28 | 1.2 | 3195 |
| **rice cereal** w/aplsce and bananas, | 120 | 96 | 97.2 | 20.5 | 2.7 | 0 | 1.2 | 34 | 20 | 4 | 0.10 | | 1 | 38 | 0.31 | 4.8 | 0 | |
| Heinz Str-2 - *4.25 oz jar* | | 1.4 | 0.5 | 0.1 | 0.1 | 0.1 | 0 | 34 | 14 | 8.08 | 0.061 | 2.5 | 25 | 0 | 0.51 | 0.28 | 1.2 | 3195 |
| **rice cereal** w/bananas, dry, | 2 | 8 | 0.1 | 1.6 | 0.3 | 0 | 0 | 2 | 14 | 3 | 0.03 | | 0 | 0 | 0.08 | 0.5 | 0 | |
| infant - *1 T* | | 0.2 | 0.1 | 0 | 0 | 0 | 0 | 15 | 8 | 0.95 | 0.005 | 0.2 | 1 | 0 | 0.08 | 0.01 | 0.2 | 3212 |
| **rice cereal** w/bananas, prep w/ | 28 | 33 | 20.8 | 4.8 | | | 0.1 | 16 | 60 | 10 | 0.16 | | 6 | 0 | 0.19 | 1.1 | 0.09 | |
| whole milk, infant - *1 oz* | | 1.2 | 1.0 | 0.6 | | | 3 | 71 | 41 | 3.09 | 0.014 | | 28 | | 0.21 | 0.04 | 1.7 | 3712 |
| **rice cereal** w/honey, prep w/ | 28 | 32 | 20.8 | 4.8 | | | | 14 | 81 | 13 | 0.18 | | 6 | 0 | 0.13 | 1.7 | 0.08 | |
| whole milk, infant - *1 oz* | | 1.1 | 0.9 | | | | | 39 | 51 | 3.03 | 0.018 | | 30 | | 0.17 | 0.03 | 2.2 | 3696 |
| **rice cereal** w/mixed fruit, | 170 | 139 | 136.7 | 31.1 | 17.8 | 0 | 1.0 | 17 | 27 | 8 | 0.24 | | 2 | 16 | 0.22 | 3.6 | 0.03 | 0.46 |
| Gerber 3rd Foods - *6 oz jar* | | 1.5 | 0.3 | 0.1 | 0.1 | 0.1 | 0 | 85 | 36 | 4.42 | 0.042 | 3.6 | 26 | 0.1 | 0.27 | 0.19 | 1.7 | 3210 |
| **whole wheat cereal** w/apples, dry, | 15 | 60 | 0.3 | 11.6 | 3.3 | 0 | 1.8 | 4 | 90 | 21 | 0.39 | 0.378 | 0 | 9 | 0.22 | 2.0 | 0 | 0.14 |
| infant - *.5 oz* | | 1.9 | 0.7 | 0.1 | 0.2 | 0.3 | 0 | 77 | 75 | 6.75 | 0.093 | 9.7 | 3 | 0.2 | 0.27 | 0.04 | 3.0 | 3184 |

## 18.3 INFANT, JUNIOR, AND TODDLER DESSERTS

| | WT (g) | KCAL / PRO (g) | H₂0 (g) / FAT (g) | CHO (g) / SFA (g) | TSUG (g) / MUFA (g) | ASUG (g) / PUFA (g) | DFIB (g) / CHOL (mg) | Na (mg) / K (mg) | Ca (mg) / P (mg) | Mg (mg) / Fe (mg) | Zn (mg) / Cu (mg) | Mn (mg) / Se (mcg) | A (mcg RAE) / A (IU) | C (mg) / E (mg ATE) | B-1 (mg) / B-2 (mg) | NIA (mg) / B-6 (mg) | B-12 (mcg) / FOL (mcg DFE) | PANT (mg) / REF |
|---|---|---|---|---|---|---|---|---|---|---|---|---|---|---|---|---|---|---|
| **apple yogurt dessert**, strained | 113 | 108 | 88.0 | 22.0 | 13.6 | 3.6 | 0.6 | 23 | 7 | 17 | 0.32 | | 3 | 40 | 1.76 | 0 | 0.56 | |
| *4 oz jar* | | 0.9 | 1.8 | 1.2 | 0.5 | 0 | 7 | 79 | 35 | 0 | 0.056 | 0.8 | 27 | 0 | 0.06 | 0.02 | 10.2 | 42150 |
| **banana apple dessert**, strained | 113 | 77 | 93.9 | 18.4 | 16.6 | 9.2 | 1.1 | 8 | 3 | 9 | 0.06 | | 2 | 14 | 0.02 | 0.1 | 0 | |
| *4 oz jar* | | 0.3 | 0.2 | 0.1 | 0 | 0.1 | 0 | 80 | 10 | 0.11 | 0.034 | 0.7 | 34 | 0 | 0.02 | 0.07 | 4.5 | 43550 |
| **banana pudding**, strained | 113 | 77 | 94.4 | 16.0 | 11.9 | 8.6 | 0.9 | 34 | 12 | 6 | 0.14 | | 1 | 14 | 0.01 | 0.2 | 0.01 | |
| *4 oz jar* | | 1.1 | 0.9 | 0.3 | 0.3 | 0.1 | 33 | 102 | 38 | 0.34 | 0.045 | 1.2 | 21 | 0.1 | 0.07 | 0.15 | 6.8 | 43004 |
| **banana yogurt dessert**, strained | 113 | 89 | 91.2 | 19.7 | 4.5 | 0.3 | 0.6 | 16 | 34 | 11 | 0.29 | | 3 | 16 | 0.01 | 0.2 | 0.15 | |
| *4 oz jar* | | 1.2 | 0.6 | 0.4 | 0.1 | 0 | 1 | 113 | 32 | 0.16 | 0.023 | 1.0 | 23 | 0 | 0.05 | 0.09 | 7.9 | 43539 |
| **bananas, apples, pears**, strained | 113 | 95 | 89.3 | 22.3 | 14.4 | 0 | 1.6 | 8 | 6 | 28 | 0.11 | 0.093 | 3 | 16 | 0.01 | 0.6 | 0 | 0.16 |
| *4 oz jar* | | 1.0 | 0.2 | 0.1 | 0 | 0.1 | 0 | 263 | 21 | 0.34 | 0.090 | 0.7 | 63 | 0.1 | 0.03 | 0.33 | 5.6 | 3163 |
| **blueberry yogurt dessert**, strained | 113 | 87 | 92.0 | 19.3 | 15.4 | 0.3 | 0.5 | 16 | 28 | 15 | 0.16 | | 3 | 14 | 0 | 0.2 | 0.49 | |
| *4 oz jar* | | 0.6 | 0.8 | 0.5 | 0.2 | 0 | 5 | 70 | 123 | 0.23 | 0.034 | 0.9 | 46 | 0.5 | 0.05 | 0.45 | 9.0 | 43537 |
| **cherry cobbler dessert**, junior | 170 | 133 | 135.7 | 32.6 | 17.7 | 14.2 | 0.3 | 73 | 8 | 3 | 0.08 | 0.034 | 3 | 16 | 0.02 | 0.1 | 0 | 0.07 |
| *6 oz jar* | | 0.5 | 0.2 | 0 | 0 | 0.1 | 0 | 76 | 10 | 0.17 | 0.017 | 1.5 | 53 | 0.1 | 0.02 | 0.03 | 3.4 | 3222 |

| | WT (g) | KCAL / PRO (g) | H₂O (g) / FAT (g) | CHO (g) / SFA (g) | TSUG (g) / MUFA (g) | ASUG (g) / PUFA (g) | DFIB (g) / CHOL (mg) | Na (mg) / K (mg) | Ca (mg) / P (mg) | Mg (mg) / Fe (mg) | Zn (mg) / Cu (mg) | Mn (mg) / Se (mcg) | A (mcg RAE) / A (IU) | C (mg) / E (mg ATE) | B-1 (mg) / B-2 (mg) | NIA (mg) / B-6 (mg) | B-12 (mcg) / FOL (mcg DFE) | PANT (mg) / REF |
|---|---|---|---|---|---|---|---|---|---|---|---|---|---|---|---|---|---|---|
| **cherry vanilla pudding, junior** | 170 | 117 | 137.7 | 31.3 | 28.9 | 23.9 | 0.5 | 26 | 8 | 3 | 0.05 | | 31 | 2 | 0.01 | 0.1 | 0.02 | |
| *6 oz jar* | | 0.3 | 0.3 | 0.1 | 0.1 | 0.1 | 17 | 56 | 12 | 0.29 | 0.087 | 1.0 | 444 | 0 | 0.02 | 0.02 | 0 | 3225 |
| **cherry vanilla pudding, strained** | 113 | 77 | 92.1 | 20.1 | 10.3 | 8.4 | 0.3 | 18 | 6 | 2 | 0.05 | | 20 | 1 | 0.01 | 0 | 0.01 | |
| *4 oz jar* | | 0.2 | 0.3 | 0.1 | 0.1 | 0.1 | 11 | 38 | 8 | 0.21 | 0.056 | 0.7 | 295 | 0 | 0.01 | 0.01 | 0 | 3224 |
| **Dutch apple dessert, junior** | 170 | 134 | 136.5 | 32.8 | 30.4 | 16.3 | 2.4 | 5 | 5 | 7 | 0.05 | 0.034 | 2 | 31 | 0.02 | 0.1 | 0 | 0.03 |
| *6 oz jar* | | 0.3 | 0.3 | 0 | 0 | 0 | 0 | 114 | 12 | 0.19 | 0.051 | 0.3 | 31 | 0.1 | 0.02 | 0.03 | 0 | 3221 |
| **Dutch apple dessert, strained** | 113 | 85 | 89.8 | 22.3 | 20.2 | 10.8 | 1.6 | 18 | 6 | 2 | 0.01 | | 2 | 24 | 0.01 | 0.1 | 0 | |
| *4 oz jar* | | 0.2 | 0.5 | 0.2 | 0.1 | 0 | 0 | 37 | 3 | 0.23 | 0.067 | 0.2 | 55 | 0 | 0.01 | 0.01 | 1.1 | 3220 |
| **fruit dessert, Gerber 2nd Foods** | 120 | 71 | 100.1 | 19.2 | 15.1 | 3.7 | 0.7 | 17 | 11 | 6 | 0.05 | | 8 | 3 | 0.02 | 0.2 | 0 | 0.12 |
| *4.25 oz jar* | | 0.4 | 0 | 0 | 0 | 0 | 0 | 113 | 8 | 0.26 | 0.036 | 0.5 | 158 | 0.3 | 0.01 | 0.04 | 3.6 | 3235 |
| **fruit dessert, Gerber 3rd** | 170 | 107 | 139.7 | 29.2 | 20.4 | 8.0 | 1.0 | 22 | 15 | 8 | 0.08 | | 12 | 5 | 0.04 | 0.2 | 0 | 0.17 |
| Foods/Heinz-Jr-3 - *6 oz jar* | | 0.5 | 0 | 0 | 0 | 0 | 0 | 162 | 14 | 0.36 | 0.051 | 0.7 | 224 | 0.5 | 0.02 | 0.06 | 6.8 | 3236 |
| **fruit dessert, Heinz Strained-2** | 120 | 71 | 100.1 | 19.2 | 15.1 | 3.7 | 0.7 | 17 | 11 | 6 | 0.05 | | 8 | 3 | 0.02 | 0.2 | 0 | 0.12 |
| *4.25 oz jar* | | 0.4 | 0 | 0 | 0 | 0 | 0 | 113 | 8 | 0.26 | 0.036 | 0.5 | 158 | 0.3 | 0.01 | 0.04 | 3.6 | 3235 |
| **fruit supreme dessert, infant** | 113 | 82 | 92.2 | 19.4 | 16.8 | 11.3 | 2.3 | 1 | 7 | 8 | 0.09 | | 3 | 14 | 0.01 | 0.3 | 0 | |
| *4 oz jar* | | 0.6 | 0.2 | 0 | 0 | 0.1 | 0 | 146 | 10 | 0.19 | 0.040 | 0.5 | 56 | 0.9 | 0.05 | 0.08 | 6.8 | 43585 |
| **orange pudding, strained** | 113 | 90 | 90.2 | 20.0 | | | 0.7 | 23 | 36 | 6 | 0.19 | | 7 | 10 | 0.05 | 0.1 | 0.01 | 0.28 |
| *4 oz jar* | | 1.2 | 1.0 | 0.6 | 0.3 | 0 | 3 | 97 | 32 | 0.11 | 0.056 | 0.7 | 130 | | 0.06 | 0.03 | 9.0 | 3226 |
| **peach cobbler, Gerber 2nd Foods/** | 113 | 73 | 92.4 | 20.1 | 12.0 | 8.0 | 0.8 | 8 | 5 | 2 | 0.34 | | 8 | 23 | 0.01 | 0.3 | 0 | |
| Heinz Strained-2 - *4 oz jar* | | 0.3 | 0 | 0 | 0 | 0 | 0 | 61 | 6 | 0.11 | 0.215 | 1.1 | 156 | 0.4 | 0.02 | 0.01 | 2.3 | 3227 |
| **peach cobbler, Gerber 3rd Foods** | 170 | 114 | 138.0 | 31.1 | 20.2 | 14.2 | 1.2 | 15 | 7 | 3 | 0.05 | | 12 | 35 | 0.02 | 0.4 | 0 | |
| *6 oz jar* | | 0.5 | 0 | 0 | 0 | 0 | 0 | 95 | 10 | 0.17 | 0.333 | 1.7 | 235 | 0.5 | 0.03 | 0.01 | 6.8 | 3228 |
| **peach yogurt dessert, infant** | 113 | 86 | 91.4 | 19.9 | 7.5 | 5.8 | 0.5 | 16 | 31 | 15 | 0.20 | | 1 | 13 | 0.01 | 0.5 | 0.49 | |
| *4 oz jar* | | 1.0 | 0.2 | 0.1 | 0.1 | 0 | 5 | 115 | 31 | 0.45 | 0.045 | 0.9 | 3 | 0 | 0.06 | 0.02 | 9.0 | 43536 |
| **pineapple pudding,** | 113 | 92 | 87.7 | 22.9 | 11.6 | 7.1 | 0.8 | 21 | 35 | 10 | 0.23 | | 12 | 31 | 0.04 | 0.1 | 0.07 | 0.22 |
| Gerber 2nd Foods - *4 oz jar* | | 1.5 | 0.3 | 0.1 | 0.1 | 0 | 0 | 92 | 35 | 0.20 | 0.026 | 1.4 | 45 | 0 | 0.05 | 0.05 | 5.6 | 3233 |
| **tropical fruit dessert, junior** | 113 | 68 | 94.0 | 18.5 | | | | 8 | 11 | 6 | 0.06 | | 1 | 21 | 0.01 | 0.1 | 0 | 0.11 |
| *4 oz jar* | | 0.2 | 0 | | | | | 66 | 9 | 0.29 | 0.032 | 0.5 | 23 | | 0.04 | 0.04 | 3.4 | 3238 |
| **tutti frutti, junior** | 170 | 117 | 140.9 | 27.2 | 16.0 | 0 | 0.7 | 29 | 24 | 7 | 0.32 | | 17 | 12 | 0.05 | 0.1 | 0.02 | |
| *6 oz jar* | | 0.7 | 0.7 | 0.2 | 0.3 | 0.1 | 26 | 80 | 48 | 0.51 | 0.340 | 0.7 | 338 | 0.3 | 0.03 | 0.03 | 5.1 | 43007 |
| **tutti frutti, strained** | 113 | 75 | 94.4 | 17.5 | 10.5 | 0 | 0.7 | 28 | 17 | 5 | 0.90 | | 8 | 14 | 0.02 | 0.1 | 0.01 | |
| *4 oz jar* | | 0.5 | 0.3 | 0.1 | 0.1 | 0 | 17 | 52 | 19 | 0.23 | 0.023 | 0.5 | 150 | 0.1 | 0.02 | 0.02 | 3.4 | 43006 |
| **van cstrd pddng, Bch-Nut Stg 2/Grbr** | 113 | 96 | 90.3 | 18.1 | 13.0 | 11.0 | 0 | 32 | 62 | 6 | 0.32 | | 20 | 1 | 0.01 | 0 | 0.01 | 0.28 |
| 2nd Fds/Heinz Str-2 - *4 oz jar* | | 1.8 | 2.3 | 1.1 | 0.8 | 0.2 | 9 | 75 | 51 | 0.27 | 0.056 | 2.7 | 72 | 0.3 | 0.09 | 0.02 | 6.8 | 3245 |
| **van cstrd pddng, Bch-Nut Stg 3/Grbr** | 170 | 146 | 134.8 | 29.9 | 20.7 | 15.8 | 0.3 | 44 | 92 | 8 | 0.51 | 0.017 | 22 | 1 | 0.02 | 0.1 | 0.39 | 0.39 |
| 3rd Fds/Heinz Jr-3 - *6 oz jar* | | 3.0 | 1.7 | 0.6 | 0.6 | 0.2 | 65 | 116 | 94 | 0.37 | 0.017 | 4.1 | 80 | 0.2 | 0.09 | 0.05 | 10.2 | 3246 |

## 18.4 INFANT, JUNIOR, AND TODDLER DINNERS

| | WT (g) | KCAL / PRO (g) | H₂O (g) / FAT (g) | CHO (g) / SFA (g) | TSUG (g) / MUFA (g) | ASUG (g) / PUFA (g) | DFIB (g) / CHOL (mg) | Na (mg) / K (mg) | Ca (mg) / P (mg) | Mg (mg) / Fe (mg) | Zn (mg) / Cu (mg) | Mn (mg) / Se (mcg) | A (mcg RAE) / A (IU) | C (mg) / E (mg ATE) | B-1 (mg) / B-2 (mg) | NIA (mg) / B-6 (mg) | B-12 (mcg) / FOL (mcg DFE) | PANT (mg) / REF |
|---|---|---|---|---|---|---|---|---|---|---|---|---|---|---|---|---|---|---|
| **apples, chkn, Bch-Nut Stg 2/Gerber** | 113 | 73 | 96.5 | 12.3 | 8.9 | 0 | 2.0 | 14 | 20 | 7 | 0.41 | 0.034 | 2 | 0 | 0.02 | 0.7 | 0.02 | 0.11 |
| 2nd Fds/Heinz Str-2 - *4 oz jar* | | 2.4 | 1.6 | 0.4 | 0.5 | 0.4 | 6 | 107 | 36 | 0.43 | 0.045 | 2.8 | 34 | 0.1 | 0.06 | 0.09 | 1.1 | 3297 |
| **apples, ham, Gerber 2nd Foods** | 113 | 70 | 96.4 | 12.3 | 9.0 | 0 | 2.0 | 10 | 5 | 8 | 0.45 | 0.023 | 0 | 0 | 0.07 | 0.8 | 0.02 | 0.11 |
| *4 oz jar* | | 2.9 | 1.0 | 0.3 | 0.4 | 0.1 | 9 | 136 | 38 | 0.34 | 0.045 | 5.2 | 7 | 0.1 | 0.07 | 0.08 | 2.3 | 3289 |
| **apples, sweet potatoes** | 113 | 72 | 94.9 | 17.3 | 13.1 | 0 | 1.6 | 2 | 9 | 7 | 0.11 | 0.068 | 116 | 7 | 0.01 | 0.1 | 0 | 0.12 |
| Gerber 2nd Fds - *4 oz jar* | | 0.3 | 0.2 | 0 | 0 | 0.1 | 0 | 168 | 19 | 0.23 | 0.102 | 0.3 | 2316 | 0.2 | 0.02 | 0.06 | 2.3 | 3154 |
| **beef lasagna, toddler** | 170 | 131 | 139.9 | 17.0 | 0 | 0 | | 772 | 31 | 19 | 1.19 | | 99 | 3 | 0.12 | 2.3 | 0.87 | |
| *6 oz jar* | | 7.1 | 3.6 | | | | | 207 | 68 | 1.48 | 0.165 | 14.3 | 1977 | | 0.15 | 0.12 | 10.2 | 3043 |
| **beef ndl, Bch-Nut Stg 2/Gerber** | 113 | 71 | 98.1 | 9.2 | 1.6 | 0 | 1.5 | 17 | 11 | 11 | 0.68 | 0.136 | 41 | 0 | 0.04 | 0.7 | 0.21 | 0.11 |
| 2nd Fds/Heinz Str-2 - *4 oz jar* | | 2.8 | 2.6 | 1.1 | 1.1 | 0.2 | 9 | 98 | 43 | 0.46 | 0.056 | 4.1 | 809 | 0.4 | 0.04 | 0.04 | 12.4 | 3047 |
| **beef ndl, Bch-Nut Stg 3/Gerber 3rd** | 170 | 97 | 149.3 | 12.6 | 2.5 | 0 | 1.9 | 29 | 14 | 12 | 0.68 | | 56 | 2 | 0.05 | 1.0 | 0.17 | 0.39 |
| Fds/Heinz Jr-3 - *6 oz jar* | | 4.2 | 3.2 | 1.3 | 1.4 | 0.2 | 14 | 78 | 51 | 0.73 | 0.054 | 9.7 | 1115 | 0.8 | 0.06 | 0.05 | 28.9 | 3287 |
| **beef, rice, toddler** | 170 | 139 | 139.2 | 15.0 | 0 | 0 | | 607 | 19 | 14 | 1.56 | | 42 | 7 | 0.03 | 2.3 | 0.87 | |
| *6 oz jar* | | 8.5 | 4.9 | | | | | 204 | 60 | 1.17 | 0.092 | 14.3 | 853 | | 0.12 | 0.24 | 10.2 | 3049 |
| **beef stew, Beech-Nut Table Time** | 170 | 87 | 147.7 | 9.4 | 2.4 | 0 | 1.9 | 586 | 15 | 19 | 1.48 | | 139 | 5 | 0.02 | 2.2 | 0.87 | |
| *6 oz jar* | | 8.7 | 2.0 | 1.0 | 0.7 | 0.2 | 22 | 241 | 75 | 1.22 | 0.122 | 7.6 | 2803 | 0.8 | 0.11 | 0.13 | 10.2 | 3052 |
| **beef, vegetables, infant** | 113 | 108 | 95.3 | 7.2 | 2.4 | 0 | 2.0 | 26 | 21 | 17 | 0.40 | 0.007 | 251 | 0 | 0.03 | 0.8 | 0.10 | 0.29 |
| *4 oz jar* | | 2.3 | 7.8 | 3.2 | 3.5 | 1.0 | 14 | 144 | 27 | 0.37 | 0.041 | 2.5 | 5013 | 0.6 | 0.07 | 0.09 | 12.4 | 3055 |
| **beef, vegetables, toddler** | 170 | 116 | 144.9 | 14.8 | 2.0 | 0 | 0.8 | 304 | 19 | 19 | 1.48 | | 97 | 4 | 0.03 | 1.2 | 0.87 | |
| *6 oz jar* | | 6.0 | 3.6 | 1.4 | 1.6 | 0.2 | 20 | 286 | 63 | 0.85 | 0.136 | 3.7 | 1938 | 0.6 | 0.07 | 0.12 | 10.2 | 43417 |
| **broccoli, chkn, Gerber 2nd** | 113 | 70 | 98.2 | 7.2 | 1.6 | 0 | 1.6 | 19 | 42 | 14 | 0.44 | 0.136 | 27 | 20 | 0.02 | 1.1 | 0.37 | 0.31 |
| Fds/Heinz Str-2 - *4 oz jar* | | 4.1 | 2.8 | 0.6 | 0.9 | 0.5 | 15 | 192 | 66 | 0.59 | 0.034 | 2.5 | 536 | 0.7 | 0.11 | 0.06 | 85.9 | 3298 |

| | WT (g) | Macronutrients | | | | | | Minerals | | | | | Vitamins | | | | | |
|---|---|---|---|---|---|---|---|---|---|---|---|---|---|---|---|---|---|---|
| | | KCAL | H₂O (g) | CHO (g) | TSUG (g) | ASUG (g) | DFIB (g) | Na (mg) | Ca (mg) | Mg (mg) | Zn (mg) | Mn (mg) | A (mcg RAE) | C (mg) | B-1 (mg) | NIA (mg) | B-12 (mcg) | PANT (mg) |
| | | PRO (g) | FAT (g) | SFA (g) | MUFA (g) | PUFA (g) | CHOL (mg) | K (mg) | P (mg) | Fe (mg) | Cu (mg) | Se (mcg) | A (IU) | E (mg ATE) | B-2 (mg) | B-6 (mg) | FOL (mcg DFE) | REF |
| carrots, beef, Gerber 2nd Fds | 113 | 67 | 98.6 | 6.4 | 2.3 | 0 | 2.9 | 66 | 25 | 15 | 0.90 | 0.158 | 817 | 1 | 0.02 | 1.1 | 0.34 | |
| *4 oz jar* | | 3.8 | 2.8 | 1.1 | 1.2 | 0.1 | 9 | 255 | 51 | 0.56 | 0.061 | 3.2 | 16331 | 0.7 | 0.07 | 0.11 | 19.2 | 3290 |
| chicken ndl, Bch-Nut Stg 2/Gerber | 113 | 75 | 96.8 | 10.3 | 2.8 | 0 | 2.4 | 26 | 31 | 16 | 0.62 | 0.181 | 124 | 0 | 0.05 | 0.8 | 0.02 | 0.22 |
| 2nd Fds/Heinz - Str-2 - *4 oz jar* | | 3.0 | 2.3 | 0.7 | 1.0 | 0.5 | 18 | 157 | 52 | 0.72 | 0.079 | 4.2 | 2466 | 0.2 | 0.07 | 0.07 | 14.7 | 3068 |
| chicken ndl, Bch-Nut Stg 3/Gerber | 170 | 94 | 148.3 | 14.9 | 1.8 | 0 | 1.5 | 133 | 36 | 12 | 0.68 | 0.170 | 148 | 0 | 0.05 | 1.2 | 0.02 | 0.30 |
| 3rd Fds/Heinz Jr-3 - *6 oz jar* | | 4.0 | 2.0 | 0.6 | 0.8 | 0.5 | 15 | 66 | 134 | 0.65 | 0.051 | 6.3 | 2939 | 0.3 | 0.07 | 0.09 | 13.6 | 3069 |
| chicken, noodles, vegs, infant | 113 | 75 | 96.4 | 10.0 | 0.9 | 0 | 0.7 | 210 | 12 | 11 | 0.46 | | 111 | 2 | 0.05 | 1.4 | 0.16 | |
| *4 oz jar* | | 4.3 | 1.9 | 0.5 | 0.7 | 0.4 | 32 | 107 | 47 | 0.45 | 0.023 | 4.2 | 2204 | 0.2 | 0.06 | 0.07 | 13.6 | 43373 |
| chicken rice, infant | 113 | 58 | 99.4 | 10.4 | 0.6 | 0 | 1.2 | 17 | 20 | 9 | 0.28 | | 66 | 1 | 0.01 | 0.3 | 0.11 | |
| *4 oz jar* | | 1.8 | 1.0 | 0.2 | 0.4 | 0.2 | 11 | 68 | 23 | 0.23 | 0.028 | 3.4 | 1322 | 0.1 | 0.02 | 0.03 | 3.4 | 43008 |
| chicken soup, Bch-Nut Stg 2/ | 113 | 56 | 100.7 | 8.1 | 1.9 | 0 | 1.2 | 18 | 42 | 6 | 0.25 | | 78 | 1 | 0.02 | 0.3 | 0.14 | |
| Heinz Str-2 - *4 oz jar* | | 1.8 | 1.9 | 0.3 | 0.5 | 1.0 | 5 | 75 | 27 | 0.31 | 0.315 | 1.6 | 1564 | 0.6 | 0.04 | 0.04 | 5.6 | 3070 |
| chicken stew, toddler | 170 | 133 | 141.6 | 10.9 | 2.9 | 0 | 1.0 | 340 | 61 | 17 | 0.70 | | 88 | 3 | 0.05 | 2.0 | 0.24 | |
| *6 oz jar* | | 8.8 | 6.3 | 1.9 | 2.9 | 1.3 | 49 | 156 | 87 | 1.12 | 0.034 | 9.4 | 1717 | 0.4 | 0.13 | 0.08 | 45.9 | 3072 |
| macaroni and cheese, junior | 170 | 104 | 147.0 | 13.9 | 2.2 | 0 | 0.5 | 129 | 87 | 12 | 0.54 | | 51 | 2 | 0.10 | 0.9 | 0.05 | |
| *6 oz jar* | | 4.4 | 3.4 | 2.0 | 0.9 | 0.2 | 10 | 75 | 100 | 0.51 | 0.036 | 6.5 | 180 | 0.1 | 0.11 | 0.03 | 30.6 | 3090 |
| macaroni and cheese, strained | 113 | 76 | 96.3 | 10.1 | 1.4 | 0 | 0.8 | 98 | 75 | 9 | 0.45 | 0.102 | 27 | 0 | 0.04 | 0.6 | 0.15 | 0.20 |
| *4 oz jar* | | 3.5 | 2.4 | 1.5 | 0.7 | 0.1 | 8 | 76 | 97 | 0.24 | 0.023 | 4.3 | 97 | 0 | 0.09 | 0.04 | 17.0 | 3089 |
| macaroni and cheese, toddler | 170 | 141 | 138.9 | 19.0 | 1.3 | 0 | 0.8 | 391 | 173 | 15 | 0.73 | | 5 | 0 | 0.07 | 1.3 | 0.10 | |
| *6 oz jar* | | 6.0 | 4.4 | 2.6 | 1.2 | 0.3 | 12 | 31 | 138 | 1.02 | 0.070 | 11.2 | 19 | 0 | 0.15 | 0.08 | 69.7 | 3048 |
| macaroni, beef, tomato sce, | 170 | 138 | 139.1 | 19.6 | 0.6 | 0 | 1.9 | 342 | 20 | 26 | 0.82 | | 5 | 3 | 0.10 | 2.3 | 0.39 | |
| toddler - *6 oz jar* | | 7.4 | 3.2 | 1.2 | 1.3 | 0.2 | 12 | 252 | 83 | 1.36 | 0.034 | 3.1 | 102 | 0.2 | 0.10 | 0.15 | 23.8 | 43432 |
| macaroni, tom, beef, Bch-Nut Stg 3/ | 170 | 100 | 147.4 | 16.0 | 4.1 | 0 | 1.9 | 29 | 24 | 12 | 0.61 | | 60 | 3 | 0.08 | 1.3 | 0.41 | |
| Gerber 3rd Fds - *6 oz jar* | | 4.2 | 1.9 | 0.7 | 0.8 | 0.1 | 7 | 122 | 75 | 0.61 | 0.066 | 14.3 | 1175 | 1.4 | 0.09 | 0.08 | 18.7 | 3045 |
| mac, tom, beef, Bch-Nut Stg 2/Gerber | 113 | 69 | 97.6 | 10.7 | 2.4 | 0 | 1.4 | 43 | 19 | 14 | 0.61 | 0.147 | 50 | 0 | 0.04 | 0.8 | 0.17 | 0.16 |
| 2nd Fds/Heinz Str-2 - *4 oz jar* | | 2.7 | 1.7 | 0.5 | 0.7 | 0.2 | 8 | 127 | 44 | 0.52 | 0.056 | 9.5 | 992 | 3.0 | 0.05 | 0.06 | 13.6 | 3044 |
| mixed vegetable dinner, junior | 170 | 56 | 154.0 | 13.4 | | | | 15 | 29 | 17 | 0.41 | | 207 | 6 | 0.02 | 0.7 | 0 | 0.39 |
| *6 oz jar* | | 1.7 | 0 | | | | | 190 | 37 | 0.53 | 0.061 | 1.2 | 4155 | | 0.04 | 0.13 | 11.9 | 3279 |
| mixed vegetable dinner, strained | 113 | 46 | 100.2 | 10.7 | | | | 9 | 25 | 12 | 0.18 | | 154 | 3 | 0.02 | 0.6 | 0 | 0.31 |
| *4 oz jar* | | 1.4 | 0.1 | | | | | 137 | 27 | 0.37 | 0.050 | 0.8 | 3083 | | 0.04 | 0.08 | 9.0 | 3278 |
| pasta with vegetables, Gerber | 113 | 68 | 98.6 | 9.5 | 1.4 | 0 | 1.7 | 12 | 16 | 27 | 0.45 | 0.441 | 46 | 3 | 0.07 | 0.6 | 0 | 0.20 |
| *4 oz jar* | | 1.9 | 2.4 | 1.4 | 0.7 | 0.2 | 6 | 150 | 56 | 0.56 | 0.124 | 7.2 | 627 | 0.3 | 0.06 | 0.12 | 10.2 | 3077 |
| potatoes w/cheese and ham, | 170 | 133 | 138.5 | 19.6 | 1.4 | 0 | 2.0 | 348 | 90 | 24 | 1.02 | 0.031 | 14 | 0 | 0.08 | 1.8 | 0.17 | 0.59 |
| toddler - *6 oz jar* | | 6.0 | 3.4 | 1.9 | 1.2 | 0.3 | 10 | 243 | 184 | 0.68 | 0.102 | 9.4 | 53 | 0 | 0.17 | 0.27 | 10.2 | 3304 |
| ravioli, cheese, tomato sce, infant | 113 | 112 | 86.4 | 18.4 | 0.7 | 0 | 0.1 | 336 | 61 | | 0.40 | | 58 | 0 | 0.14 | 1.9 | 0.06 | |
| *4 oz jar* | | 4.1 | 2.5 | 1.1 | 0.6 | 0.5 | 8 | 36 | 63 | 0.90 | 0.045 | 15.1 | 558 | 0.5 | 0.16 | 0.10 | 40.7 | 3046 |
| spag, tom, beef, Bch-Nut Stg 3/Gerber | 170 | 116 | 143.1 | 19.4 | 4.6 | 0 | 1.9 | 128 | 26 | 19 | 0.90 | 0.204 | 107 | 0 | 0.08 | 1.6 | 0.05 | 0.15 |
| 3rd Fds/Heinz Jr-3 - *6 oz jar* | | 4.4 | 2.3 | 0.9 | 0.8 | 0.3 | 8 | 207 | 60 | 0.90 | 0.051 | 14.3 | 2134 | 0.1 | 0.12 | 0.11 | 74.8 | 3050 |
| spaghetti, tomato, meat, toddler | 170 | 128 | 138.7 | 18.4 | | | | 609 | 37 | 26 | 0.82 | | 37 | 7 | 0.11 | 2.6 | 0.39 | |
| *6 oz jar* | | 9.0 | 1.7 | | | | | 277 | 76 | 1.53 | 0.034 | 14.3 | 753 | | 0.17 | 0.14 | 85.0 | 3051 |
| sweet potatoes, chicken, Bch-Nut | 113 | 84 | 94.6 | 12.5 | 6.1 | 0 | 1.5 | 25 | 34 | 15 | 0.42 | 0.173 | 244 | 0 | 0.02 | 1.2 | 0.06 | 0.37 |
| Stg 2 - *4 oz jar* | | 2.8 | 2.5 | 0.6 | 1.1 | 0.5 | 12 | 226 | 28 | 0.51 | 0.092 | 1.9 | 4879 | 0.7 | 0.05 | 0.15 | 6.8 | 3303 |
| turkey rice, Bch-Nut Stg 2/Gerber 2nd | 113 | 59 | 99.7 | 9.0 | 1.9 | 0 | 1.0 | 23 | 20 | 9 | 0.45 | 0.147 | 92 | 0 | 0.02 | 0.7 | 0.02 | 0.20 |
| Fds/Heinz Str-2 - *4 oz jar* | | 2.6 | 1.4 | 0.4 | 0.5 | 0.3 | 6 | 103 | 38 | 0.33 | 0.034 | 3.4 | 1833 | 0.2 | 0.05 | 0.06 | 4.5 | 3082 |
| turkey rice, Bch-Nut Stg 3/Gerber | 170 | 95 | 147.3 | 16.3 | 2.1 | 0 | 1.7 | 136 | 41 | 15 | 0.80 | 0.204 | 160 | 1 | 0.06 | 1.2 | 0.03 | 0.34 |
| 3rd Fds/Heinz Jr-3 - *6 oz jar* | | 4.0 | 1.6 | 0.4 | 0.5 | 0.4 | 7 | 146 | 63 | 0.70 | 0.051 | 5.6 | 3206 | 0.5 | 0.07 | 0.09 | 13.6 | 3083 |
| turkey, rice, vegs, toddler | 170 | 100 | 146.7 | 12.8 | 1.1 | 0 | 1.4 | 311 | 19 | 24 | 1.04 | 0.391 | 192 | 1 | 0.12 | 3.6 | 0.17 | 0.45 |
| *6 oz jar* | | 6.5 | 2.7 | 0.8 | 0.9 | 0.5 | 12 | 182 | 107 | 0.68 | 0.170 | 5.6 | 3856 | 0.3 | 0.12 | 0.22 | 5.1 | 3296 |
| vegetables, bacon, Gerber 2nd | 113 | 78 | 96.9 | 10.0 | 2.0 | 0 | 1.9 | 55 | 16 | 11 | 0.34 | 0.158 | 129 | 0 | 0.04 | 0.5 | 0.07 | 0.18 |
| Fds/Heinz Str-2 - *4 oz jar* | | 2.2 | 3.3 | 1.2 | 1.5 | 0.4 | 5 | 131 | 32 | 0.34 | 0.045 | 1.9 | 2581 | 0.6 | 0.04 | 0.07 | 3.4 | 3059 |
| veg, beef, Bch-Nut Stg 2/Gerber 2nd | 113 | 87 | 96.0 | 10.0 | 2.6 | 0 | 1.5 | 24 | 19 | 11 | 0.43 | 0.203 | 278 | 0 | 0.01 | 0.9 | 0.20 | 0.11 |
| Fds/Heinz Str-2 - *4 oz jar* | | 2.5 | 4.1 | 1.5 | 1.5 | 0.3 | 8 | 164 | 37 | 0.40 | 0.034 | 2.5 | 5566 | 0.6 | 0.05 | 0.07 | 7.9 | 3053 |
| veg, beef, Bch-Nut Stg 3/Gerber 3rd | 170 | 131 | 144.4 | 15.0 | 4.0 | 0 | 2.2 | 36 | 29 | 17 | 0.65 | 0.180 | 418 | 0 | 0.01 | 1.3 | 0.56 | 0.17 |
| Fds/Heinz Jr-3 - *6 oz jar* | | 3.8 | 6.1 | 2.3 | 2.2 | 0.5 | 12 | 246 | 56 | 0.60 | 0.051 | 3.7 | 6120 | 0.8 | 0.08 | 0.11 | 11.9 | 3054 |
| vegetables, beef, Earth's Best | 113 | 87 | 96.0 | 10.0 | 2.6 | 0 | 1.5 | 24 | 19 | 11 | 0.43 | 0.203 | 278 | 0 | 0.01 | 0.9 | 0.20 | 0.11 |
| *4 oz jar* | | 2.5 | 4.1 | 1.5 | 1.5 | 0.3 | 8 | 164 | 37 | 0.40 | 0.034 | 2.5 | 5566 | 0.6 | 0.05 | 0.07 | 7.9 | 3053 |
| vegetables, chicken, Bch Nut Stg 3/ | 170 | 90 | 149.2 | 14.7 | 2.5 | 0 | 1.9 | 129 | 46 | 14 | 0.51 | 0.187 | 223 | 0 | 0.04 | 1.1 | 0.03 | 0.22 |
| Gerber 3rd Fds - *6 oz jar* | | 3.5 | 1.9 | 0.5 | 0.7 | 0.5 | 12 | 141 | 54 | 0.56 | 0.034 | 3.6 | 4440 | 0.3 | 0.08 | 0.08 | 5.1 | 3274 |
| vegetables, chicken, strained | 113 | 67 | 98.2 | 9.5 | 1.8 | 0 | 2.4 | 27 | 31 | 16 | 0.54 | 0.169 | 234 | 0 | 0.04 | 0.8 | 0.01 | 0.12 |
| *4 oz jar* | | 2.8 | 2.0 | 0.6 | 0.8 | 0.4 | 12 | 179 | 53 | 0.60 | 0.079 | 3.2 | 4669 | 0.4 | 0.06 | 0.08 | 5.6 | 3073 |
| vegetables, dumplings, beef, | 113 | 54 | 100.5 | 8.7 | 0 | 0 | | 55 | 16 | 7 | 0.45 | | 24 | 1 | 0.06 | 0.6 | 0.10 | 0.24 |
| strained - *4 oz jar* | | 2.3 | 1.0 | | | | | 52 | 32 | 0.44 | 0.033 | 2.4 | 470 | 0.3 | 0.05 | 0.05 | 7.9 | 3041 |

| | WT (g) | KCAL / PRO (g) | $H_2O$ (g) / FAT (g) | CHO (g) / SFA (g) | TSUG (g) / MUFA (g) | ASUG (g) / PUFA (g) | DFIB (g) / CHOL (mg) | Na (mg) / K (mg) | Ca (mg) / P (mg) | Mg (mg) / Fe (mg) | Zn (mg) / Cu (mg) | Mn (mg) / Se (mcg) | A (mcg RAE) / A (IU) | C (mg) / E (mg ATE) | B-1 (mg) / B-2 (mg) | NIA (mg) / B-6 (mg) | B-12 (mcg) / FOL (mcg DFE) | PANT (mg) / REF |
|---|---|---|---|---|---|---|---|---|---|---|---|---|---|---|---|---|---|---|
| | | Macronutrients | | | | | | Minerals | | | | | Vitamins | | | | | |
| **vegetables, dumplings, beef,** | 170 | 82 | 150.6 | 13.6 | 0 | 0 | | 88 | 24 | 12 | 0.56 | | 56 | 1 | 0.07 | 0.8 | 0.15 | 0.36 |
| junior - *6 oz jar* | | 3.6 | 1.4 | | | | | 80 | 49 | 0.80 | 0.051 | 3.6 | 1122 | | 0.06 | 0.08 | 11.9 | 3042 |
| **veg, ham**, Bch-Nut Stg 2/Gerber 2nd | 113 | 67 | 98.8 | 8.8 | 1.5 | 0 | 1.8 | 18 | 18 | 14 | 0.36 | 0.158 | 163 | 2 | 0.04 | 0.8 | 0.07 | 0.17 |
| Fds/Heinz Str-2 - *4 oz jar* | | 2.5 | 2.4 | 0.9 | 1.1 | 0.3 | 6 | 159 | 37 | 0.46 | 0.079 | 2.7 | 3245 | 0.4 | 0.06 | 0.08 | 3.4 | 3061 |
| **vegetables, ham**, Gerber 3rd | 170 | 102 | 147.9 | 14.7 | 1.7 | 0 | 1.7 | 148 | 24 | 14 | 0.51 | 0.119 | 245 | 2 | 0.05 | 0.9 | 0.05 | |
| Fds/Heinz Jr-3 - *6 oz jar* | | 3.4 | 3.2 | 0.8 | 1.4 | 0.8 | 5 | 165 | 56 | 0.41 | 0.051 | 4.1 | 4882 | 0.5 | 0.07 | 0.08 | 13.6 | 3062 |
| **vegetables, lamb**, Bch-Nut Stg | 113 | 59 | 100.1 | 7.8 | 1.1 | 0 | 1.2 | 23 | 14 | 8 | 0.25 | | 113 | 1 | 0.02 | 0.6 | 0.18 | 0.18 |
| Heinz Str-2 - *4 oz jar* | | 2.3 | 2.3 | 0.9 | 0.9 | 0.2 | 7 | 106 | 55 | 0.40 | 0.033 | 2.7 | 2254 | 0.3 | 0.04 | 0.05 | 4.5 | 3066 |
| **vegetables, lamb**, junior | 170 | 87 | 150.6 | 12.1 | 1.6 | 0 | 1.9 | 22 | 22 | 12 | 0.37 | | 235 | 3 | 0.04 | 0.9 | 0.27 | 0.27 |
| *6 oz jar* | | 3.6 | 2.9 | 1.2 | 1.2 | 0.3 | 8 | 162 | 83 | 0.58 | 0.049 | 4.1 | 2521 | 0.4 | 0.05 | 0.07 | 6.8 | 3067 |
| **vegetables, noodles, chicken,** | 113 | 71 | 98.5 | 8.9 | | | 1.2 | 23 | 32 | 11 | 0.28 | | 80 | 1 | 0.04 | 0.5 | 0.09 | 0.21 |
| strained - *4 oz jar* | | 2.3 | 2.8 | | | | | 62 | 35 | 0.40 | 0.061 | 3.6 | 1601 | | 0.06 | 0.02 | 3.4 | 3075 |
| **vegetables, noodles, chicken,** | 170 | 109 | 146.5 | 15.5 | | | 1.9 | 44 | 44 | 19 | 0.54 | | 90 | 1 | 0.07 | 1.1 | 0.15 | 0.35 |
| junior - *6 oz jar* | | 2.9 | 3.7 | | | | | 100 | 56 | 0.83 | 0.099 | 5.4 | 1787 | | 0.06 | 0.04 | 5.1 | 3076 |
| **vegetables, noodles, turkey,** | 170 | 88 | 150.8 | 12.9 | | | 1.9 | 29 | 54 | 15 | 0.51 | | 85 | 1 | 0.04 | 0.5 | 0.20 | 0.37 |
| junior - *6 oz jar* | | 3.1 | 2.6 | | | | | 124 | 49 | 0.44 | 0.044 | 4.8 | 1690 | | 0.07 | 0.03 | 5.1 | 3081 |
| **vegetables, noodles, turkey,** | 113 | 50 | 102.0 | 7.7 | | | 1.2 | 24 | 36 | 9 | 0.31 | | 56 | 1 | 0.02 | 0.3 | 0.11 | 0.21 |
| strained - *4 oz jar* | | 1.4 | 1.4 | | | | | 71 | 28 | 0.21 | 0.025 | 3.2 | 1120 | | 0.05 | 0.02 | 2.3 | 3079 |
| **vegetables, turkey**, Earth's Best | 128 | 61 | 113.7 | 9.8 | 2.0 | 0 | 1.9 | 26 | 35 | 17 | 0.90 | 0.179 | 282 | 1 | 0.03 | 0.6 | 0.03 | 0.29 |
| *4.5 oz jar* | | 3.0 | 1.2 | 0.3 | 0.4 | 0.3 | 5 | 131 | 56 | 0.47 | 0.115 | 2.4 | 5627 | 0.4 | 0.03 | 0.06 | 12.8 | 3084 |
| **vegetables, turkey**, Gerber 2nd Fds | 128 | 61 | 113.7 | 9.8 | 2.0 | 0 | 1.9 | 26 | 35 | 17 | 0.90 | 0.179 | 282 | 1 | 0.03 | 0.6 | 0.03 | 0.29 |
| *4.5 oz jar* | | 3.0 | 1.2 | 0.3 | 0.4 | 0.3 | 5 | 131 | 56 | 0.47 | 0.115 | 2.4 | 5627 | 0.4 | 0.03 | 0.06 | 12.8 | 3084 |
| **vegetables, turkey**, Gerber 3rd Fds | 170 | 90 | 150.4 | 12.8 | 2.3 | 0 | 1.5 | 151 | 27 | 15 | 0.51 | 0.102 | 367 | 1 | 0.04 | 0.9 | 0.02 | 0.28 |
| *6 oz jar* | | 2.9 | 3.0 | 0.8 | 1.2 | 0.7 | 7 | 167 | 54 | 0.61 | 0.034 | 3.2 | 7352 | 0.5 | 0.05 | 0.09 | 11.9 | 3085 |
| **vegetables, turkey**, toddler | 170 | 136 | 139.9 | 13.6 | 0 | 0 | | 568 | 78 | 27 | 0.54 | | 178 | 6 | 0.03 | 1.0 | 0.75 | |
| *6 oz jar* | | 8.2 | 5.8 | | | | | 282 | 97 | 1.02 | 0.071 | 3.2 | 3568 | | 0.15 | 0.10 | 5.1 | 3086 |

## 18.5 INFANT, JUNIOR, AND TODDLER FRUIT JUICES

| | WT (g) | KCAL / PRO (g) | $H_2O$ (g) / FAT (g) | CHO (g) / SFA (g) | TSUG (g) / MUFA (g) | ASUG (g) / PUFA (g) | DFIB (g) / CHOL (mg) | Na (mg) / K (mg) | Ca (mg) / P (mg) | Mg (mg) / Fe (mg) | Zn (mg) / Cu (mg) | Mn (mg) / Se (mcg) | A (mcg RAE) / A (IU) | C (mg) / E (mg ATE) | B-1 (mg) / B-2 (mg) | NIA (mg) / B-6 (mg) | B-12 (mcg) / FOL (mcg DFE) | PANT (mg) / REF |
|---|---|---|---|---|---|---|---|---|---|---|---|---|---|---|---|---|---|---|
| **apl ban jce**, Bch-Nut Stg 2/Gerber | 125 | 64 | 108.9 | 15.4 | 13.8 | 0 | 0.2 | 5 | 9 | 8 | 0.05 | 0.100 | 0 | 35 | 0.01 | 0.2 | 0 | 0.16 |
| 2nd Fds/Heinz Str - *4 fl oz jar* | | 0.2 | 0.1 | 0 | 0 | 0 | 0 | 154 | 10 | 0.25 | 0.025 | 0.4 | 11 | 0 | 0.01 | 0.08 | 1.2 | 3167 |
| **apple banana jce**, Earth's Best | 125 | 64 | 108.9 | 15.4 | 13.8 | 0 | 0.2 | 5 | 9 | 8 | 0.05 | 0.100 | 0 | 35 | 0.01 | 0.2 | 0 | 0.16 |
| *4 fl oz jar* | | 0.2 | 0.1 | 0 | 0 | 0 | 0 | 154 | 10 | 0.25 | 0.025 | 0.4 | 11 | 0 | 0.01 | 0.08 | 1.2 | 3167 |
| **apple cherry jce**, infant | 127 | 60 | 112.0 | 14.2 | 13.3 | 0 | 0.4 | 5 | 9 | 4 | 0.04 | | 1 | 41 | 0.01 | 0.1 | 0 | |
| *4 fl oz jar* | | 0.3 | 0.1 | 0 | 0 | 0 | 0 | 140 | 15 | 0.44 | 0.025 | 0.1 | 23 | 0 | 0.03 | 0.04 | 0 | 43535 |
| **apple cranberry jce**, infant | 124 | 57 | 109.5 | 14.2 | 8.5 | 0 | 0 | 6 | 7 | 4 | 0.06 | 0.198 | 1 | 35 | 0 | 0.1 | 0 | |
| *4 fl oz jar* | | 0 | 0 | 0 | 0 | 0 | 0 | 120 | 9 | 0.27 | 0.012 | 0.1 | 35 | 0.7 | 0.02 | 0.04 | 0 | 3169 |
| **apple grape jce**, Bch-Nut Stg 2/ Gerber 2nd Fds/Heinz Str | 131 | 60 | 115.4 | 14.9 | 14.3 | 0 | 0.1 | 4 | 8 | 8 | 0.05 | | 0 | 41 | 0.01 | 0.1 | 0 | 0.10 |
| *4.2 fl oz jar* | | 0.1 | 0.3 | 0.1 | 0 | 0.1 | 0 | 118 | 7 | 0.51 | 0.102 | 0.1 | 5 | 0 | 0.03 | 0.04 | 1.3 | 3265 |
| **apple grape jce**, Earth's Best | 131 | 60 | 115.4 | 14.9 | 14.3 | 0 | 0.1 | 4 | 8 | 8 | 0.05 | | 0 | 41 | 0.01 | 0.1 | 0 | 0.10 |
| *4.2 fl oz jar* | | 0.1 | 0.3 | 0.1 | 0 | 0.1 | 0 | 118 | 7 | 0.51 | 0.102 | 0.1 | 5 | 0 | 0.03 | 0.04 | 1.3 | 3265 |
| **apple jce**, Bch-Nut Stg 1/Gerber 1st | 127 | 60 | 111.8 | 14.9 | 13.6 | 0 | 0.1 | 4 | 5 | 4 | 0.04 | | 1 | 74 | 0.01 | 0.1 | 0 | 0.15 |
| Fds/Heinz Str - *4 fl oz jar* | | 0 | 0.1 | 0 | 0 | 0 | 0 | 116 | 6 | 0.72 | 0.051 | 0.1 | 23 | 0.8 | 0.02 | 0.04 | 0 | 3166 |
| **apple jce**, Earth's Best | 127 | 60 | 111.8 | 14.9 | 13.6 | 0 | 0.1 | 4 | 5 | 4 | 0.04 | | 1 | 74 | 0.01 | 0.1 | 0 | 0.15 |
| *4 fl oz jar* | | 0 | 0.1 | 0 | 0 | 0 | 0 | 116 | 6 | 0.72 | 0.051 | 0.1 | 23 | 0.8 | 0.02 | 0.04 | 0 | 3166 |
| **apple jce w/calcium**, infant | 127 | 58 | 112.1 | 14.1 | 11.4 | 0 | 0.5 | 4 | 161 | 8 | 0.04 | 0.368 | 0 | 27 | 0.03 | 0.1 | 0 | 0.08 |
| *4 fl oz jar* | | 0.1 | 0.1 | 0 | 0 | 0 | 0 | 117 | 10 | 0.25 | 0.013 | 0.1 | 0 | 0 | 0.03 | 0.04 | 0 | 3269 |
| **apple peach jce**, infant | 127 | 55 | 113.0 | 13.3 | 12.2 | 0 | 0.1 | 1 | 4 | 4 | 0.04 | | 4 | 74 | 0.01 | 0.3 | 0 | 0.10 |
| *4 fl oz jar* | | 0.3 | 0.1 | 0 | 0 | 0 | 0 | 123 | 5 | 0.71 | 0.047 | 0.4 | 80 | 0.2 | 0.01 | 0.03 | 1.3 | 3168 |
| **apple plum jce**, infant | 127 | 62 | 110.9 | 15.6 | 14.7 | 0 | 0.1 | 1 | 6 | 4 | 0.04 | | 3 | 74 | 0.03 | 0.2 | 0 | 0.16 |
| *4 fl oz jar* | | 0.1 | 0 | 0 | 0 | 0 | 0 | 128 | 4 | 0.79 | 0.053 | 0.4 | 55 | 0.1 | 0.02 | 0.04 | 0 | 3170 |
| **apple prune jce**, infant | 127 | 91 | 103.3 | 22.9 | 13.4 | 0 | 0.1 | 6 | 11 | 9 | 0.06 | | 1 | 86 | 0.01 | 0.4 | 0 | 0.23 |
| *4 fl oz jar* | | 0.3 | 0.1 | 0 | 0 | 0 | 0 | 188 | 19 | 1.21 | 0.079 | 0.4 | 20 | 0.1 | 0 | 0.04 | 0 | 3171 |
| **apple sweet potato jce**, infant | 123 | 59 | 108.1 | 14.0 | 11.8 | 0 | 0.6 | 6 | 18 | 9 | 0.10 | | 189 | 42 | 0.01 | 0.1 | 0 | |
| *4 fl oz jar* | | 0.4 | 0.1 | 0 | 0 | 0.1 | 0 | 169 | 17 | 0.37 | 0.039 | 0.1 | 3790 | 0.4 | 0.04 | 0.09 | 3.7 | 42266 |
| **banana jce w/lowfat yogurt,** | 126 | 112 | 98.9 | 22.1 | 16.7 | 0 | 0.5 | 47 | 100 | 13 | 0.18 | | 8 | 43 | 0.04 | 0.3 | 0.54 | |
| infant - *4 fl oz jar* | | 3.2 | 1.0 | 0.7 | 0.3 | 0 | 4 | 202 | 82 | 0.25 | 0.038 | 2.0 | 35 | 0.1 | 0.13 | 0.15 | 7.6 | 42119 |
| **Fruit Juice Snacks**, Gerber Graduates | 28 | 100 | | 24.0 | 17.0 | | 0 | 15 | 0 | | | | | 12 | | | | |
| for Toddlers - *1 oz packet* | | | 0 | 0 | | | 0 | 15 | | 0 | | | 0 | | | | | GERB276 |
| **fruit punch w/calcium**, infant | 124 | 64 | 107.3 | 15.7 | 13.1 | 0 | 0.5 | 5 | 79 | 9 | 0.05 | 0.112 | 0 | 26 | 0.01 | 0.1 | 0 | 0.07 |
| *4 fl oz jar* | | 0.2 | 0.1 | 0 | 0 | 0 | 0 | 107 | 14 | 0.37 | 0.025 | 0.1 | 4 | 0 | 0.02 | 0.06 | 1.2 | 3267 |
| **mixed fruit jce w/lowfat yogurt,** | 126 | 96 | 102.7 | 18.5 | 13.6 | 0 | 0.5 | 45 | 102 | 13 | 0.18 | | 6 | 43 | 0.05 | 0.2 | 0.54 | |
| infant - *4 fl oz jar* | | 3.0 | 1.0 | 0.7 | 0.3 | 0 | 4 | 173 | 76 | 0.25 | 0.038 | 1.6 | 35 | 0 | 0.13 | 0.06 | 7.6 | 42120 |

| | WT (g) | KCAL | H₂0 (g) | CHO (g) | TSUG (g) | ASUG (g) | DFIB (g) | Na (mg) | Ca (mg) | Mg (mg) | Zn (mg) | Mn (mg) | A (mcg RAE) | C (mg) | B-1 (mg) | NIA (mg) | B-12 (mcg) | PANT (mg) |
|---|---|---|---|---|---|---|---|---|---|---|---|---|---|---|---|---|---|---|
| | | PRO (g) | FAT (g) | SFA (g) | MUFA (g) | PUFA (g) | CHOL (mg) | K (mg) | P (mg) | Fe (mg) | Cu (mg) | Se (mcg) | A (IU) | E (mg ATE) | B-2 (mg) | B-6 (mg) | FOL (mcg DFE) | REF |
| **mixed fruit juice, infant** | 127 | 60 | 111.6 | 14.7 | 10.7 | 0 | 0.1 | 5 | 10 | 6 | 0.04 | | 3 | 81 | 0.03 | 0.2 | 0 | 0.15 |
| *4 fl oz jar* | | 0.1 | 0.1 | 0 | 0 | 0 | 0 | 128 | 6 | 0.43 | 0.051 | 0.6 | 53 | 0.1 | 0.02 | 0.05 | 8.9 | 3179 |
| **orange apple banana jce, Heinz Str - 4 fl oz jar** | 127 | 60 | 111.3 | 14.6 | 12.7 | 0 | 0.1 | 5 | 6 | 8 | 0.04 | | 1 | 41 | 0.05 | 0.3 | 0 | 0.17 |
| | | 0.5 | 0.1 | 0 | 0 | 0 | 0 | 170 | 10 | 0.44 | 0.056 | 0.1 | 34 | 0 | 0.03 | 0.08 | 12.7 | 3174 |
| **orange apple juice, infant** | 127 | 55 | 112.9 | 12.8 | | | | 4 | 13 | 6 | 0.04 | | 5 | 98 | 0.05 | 0.2 | 0 | 0.15 |
| *4 fl oz jar* | | 0.5 | 0.3 | | | | | 175 | 9 | 0.25 | 0.051 | 0.1 | 93 | | 0.04 | 0.05 | 15.2 | 3173 |
| **orange apricot juice, infant** | 127 | 58 | 111.5 | 13.8 | | | 0.1 | 8 | 8 | 9 | 0.05 | | 14 | 109 | 0.07 | 0.3 | 0 | 0.12 |
| *4 fl oz jar* | | 1.0 | 0.1 | 0 | 0 | 0 | 0 | 253 | 15 | 0.48 | 0.107 | 0.1 | 274 | 0.8 | 0.04 | 0.07 | 25.4 | 3175 |
| **orange banana juice, infant** | 127 | 64 | 110.4 | 15.1 | | | | 4 | 22 | 18 | 0.11 | | 3 | 43 | 0.06 | 0.2 | 0 | 0.19 |
| *4 fl oz jar* | | 0.9 | 0.1 | | | | | 254 | 17 | 0.14 | 0.053 | 0.1 | 58 | | 0.05 | 0.07 | 30.5 | 3176 |
| **orange carrot juice, infant** | 127 | 55 | 113.2 | 12.6 | 10.7 | 0 | 0.5 | 13 | 20 | 13 | 0.09 | | 119 | 43 | 0.08 | 0.3 | 0 | |
| *4 fl oz jar* | | 0.6 | 0.1 | 0 | 0 | 0 | 0 | 221 | 24 | 0.25 | 0.056 | 0.1 | 2388 | 0.4 | 0.06 | 0.06 | 49.5 | 42267 |
| **orange jce, Bch-Nut Stg 3/Gerber 2nd Fds/Heinz Str - 4 fl oz jar** | 127 | 57 | 112.4 | 13.0 | 10.5 | 0 | 0.1 | 1 | 15 | 11 | 0.08 | | 4 | 79 | 0.06 | 0.3 | 0 | 0.17 |
| | | 0.8 | 0.4 | 0 | 0.1 | 0.1 | 0 | 234 | 14 | 0.22 | 0.058 | 0.1 | 70 | 0.1 | 0.04 | 0.07 | 33.0 | 3172 |
| **orange pineapple juice, infant** | 127 | 61 | 110.9 | 14.9 | | | 0.1 | 3 | 10 | 11 | 0.05 | | 3 | 68 | 0.06 | 0.2 | 0 | 0.07 |
| *4 fl oz jar* | | 0.6 | 0.1 | 0 | 0 | 0 | 0 | 179 | 11 | 0.53 | 0.056 | 0.1 | 39 | 0.8 | 0.03 | 0.08 | 24.1 | 3177 |
| **pear juice, infant** | 127 | 60 | 111.6 | 15.1 | 9.2 | 0 | 0.1 | 0 | 15 | 10 | 0.10 | | 0 | 43 | 0.01 | 0.4 | 0 | |
| *4 fl oz jar* | | 0 | 0 | 0 | 0 | 0 | 0 | 165 | 15 | 0 | 0.083 | 0.5 | 0 | 0.1 | 0.04 | 0.01 | 5.1 | 43408 |
| **prune orange juice, infant** | 127 | 89 | 104.0 | 21.3 | | | | 3 | 15 | 10 | 0.05 | | 9 | 81 | 0.06 | 0.5 | 0 | 0.17 |
| *4 fl oz jar* | | 0.8 | 0.4 | | | | | 230 | 13 | 1.10 | 0.058 | 0.1 | 166 | | 0.15 | 0.08 | 16.5 | 3178 |

## 18.6 INFANT, JUNIOR, AND TODDLER FRUITS

| | WT (g) | KCAL | H₂0 (g) | CHO (g) | TSUG (g) | ASUG (g) | DFIB (g) | Na (mg) | Ca (mg) | Mg (mg) | Zn (mg) | Mn (mg) | A (mcg RAE) | C (mg) | B-1 (mg) | NIA (mg) | B-12 (mcg) | PANT (mg) |
|---|---|---|---|---|---|---|---|---|---|---|---|---|---|---|---|---|---|---|
| | | PRO (g) | FAT (g) | SFA (g) | MUFA (g) | PUFA (g) | CHOL (mg) | K (mg) | P (mg) | Fe (mg) | Cu (mg) | Se (mcg) | A (IU) | E (mg ATE) | B-2 (mg) | B-6 (mg) | FOL (mcg DFE) | REF |
| **apple blueberry, junior** | 170 | 105 | 140.8 | 28.2 | 15.0 | 0 | 3.1 | 22 | 8 | 5 | 0.07 | | 3 | 24 | 0.03 | 0.2 | 0 | 0.28 |
| *6 oz jar* | | 0.3 | 0.3 | 0 | 0 | 0.1 | 0 | 110 | 12 | 0.68 | 0.097 | 0.7 | 70 | 0.5 | 0.07 | 0.07 | 5.1 | 3165 |
| **apple blueberry, strained** | 113 | 69 | 93.9 | 18.4 | 15.7 | 0 | 2.0 | 2 | 5 | 3 | 0.03 | | 1 | 31 | 0.02 | 0.1 | 0 | 0.18 |
| *4 oz jar* | | 0.2 | 0.2 | 0 | 0 | 0.1 | 0 | 78 | 9 | 0.23 | 0.063 | 0.5 | 23 | 0.1 | 0.04 | 0.04 | 4.5 | 3164 |
| **apple raspberry, junior** | 170 | 99 | 142.8 | 26.2 | 22.0 | 0 | 3.6 | 3 | 8 | 7 | 0.05 | | 3 | 49 | 0.02 | 0.2 | 0 | 0.15 |
| *6 oz jar* | | 0.3 | 0.3 | 0.1 | 0 | 0.1 | 0 | 122 | 14 | 0.37 | 0.090 | 0.5 | 58 | 0.1 | 0.05 | 0.06 | 1.7 | 3153 |
| **apple raspberry, strained** | 113 | 66 | 94.7 | 17.6 | 14.6 | 0 | 2.4 | 2 | 6 | 5 | 0.03 | | 1 | 30 | 0.02 | 0.1 | 0 | 0.10 |
| *4 oz jar* | | 0.2 | 0.2 | 0 | 0 | 0.1 | 0 | 90 | 9 | 0.25 | 0.061 | 0.3 | 25 | 0.2 | 0.03 | 0.04 | 1.1 | 3152 |
| **apples, diced, toddler** | 170 | 87 | 148.8 | 20.6 | 18.4 | 0 | 1.5 | 22 | 17 | 10 | 0.07 | 0.068 | 3 | 53 | 0.02 | 0.1 | 0 | 0.07 |
| *6 oz jar* | | 0.3 | 0.2 | 0 | 0 | 0.1 | 0 | 85 | 22 | 0.34 | 0.034 | 0.5 | 53 | 0.4 | 0.03 | 0.08 | 1.7 | 3115 |
| **aplsce & apricots, Bch-Nut Stg 2/Grbr 2nd Fds/Heinz Str-2 - 4 oz jar** | 113 | 50 | 99.1 | 13.2 | 10.5 | 0 | 2.0 | 3 | 7 | 5 | 0.05 | | 19 | 21 | 0.02 | 0.2 | 0 | 0.13 |
| | | 0.2 | 0.2 | 0 | 0 | 0.1 | 0 | 136 | 10 | 0.28 | 0.046 | 0.3 | 383 | 0.2 | 0.03 | 0.03 | 2.3 | 3142 |
| **applesce and apricots, Earth's Best** | 128 | 60 | 111.2 | 15.9 | 11.2 | 0 | 2.3 | 4 | 8 | 5 | 0.04 | | 3 | 23 | 0.02 | 0.2 | 0 | 0.16 |
| *4.5 oz jar* | | 0.3 | 0.3 | 0 | 0 | 0.1 | 0 | 140 | 13 | 0.33 | 0.056 | 0.4 | 42 | 0.1 | 0.04 | 0.04 | 1.3 | 3143 |
| **applesce and apricots, Heinz Jr-3** | 128 | 60 | 111.2 | 15.9 | 11.2 | 0 | 2.3 | 4 | 8 | 5 | 0.04 | | 3 | 23 | 0.02 | 0.2 | 0 | 0.16 |
| *4.5 oz jar* | | 0.3 | 0.3 | 0 | 0 | 0.1 | 0 | 140 | 13 | 0.33 | 0.056 | 0.4 | 42 | 0.1 | 0.04 | 0.04 | 1.3 | 3143 |
| **applesce and banana, Bch-Nut Stg 3 - 6 oz jar** | 170 | 112 | 141.3 | 27.5 | 7.4 | 0 | 2.7 | 5 | 8 | 15 | 0.08 | 0.170 | 0 | 29 | 0.02 | 0.3 | 0 | 0.23 |
| | | 0.6 | 0.2 | 0.1 | 0 | 0.1 | 0 | 223 | 20 | 0.41 | 0.068 | 0.7 | 10 | 0 | 0.05 | 0.17 | 5.1 | 3147 |
| **applesce and cherries, junior** | 170 | 87 | 145.5 | 24.0 | 18.0 | 0 | 1.9 | 2 | 2 | 7 | 0.05 | | 3 | 73 | 0.02 | 0.2 | 0 | 0.22 |
| *6 oz jar* | | 0 | 0 | 0 | 0 | 0 | 0 | 224 | 14 | 0.51 | 0.078 | 0.5 | 76 | 0.1 | 0.05 | 0.07 | | 3145 |
| **applesce and cherries, strained** | 113 | 58 | 96.8 | 15.9 | 12.2 | 0 | 1.2 | 1 | 1 | 5 | 0.03 | | 2 | 48 | 0.01 | 0.2 | 0 | 0.15 |
| *4 oz jar* | | 0 | 0 | 0 | 0 | 0 | 0 | 149 | 9 | 0.34 | 0.051 | 0.3 | 51 | 0.1 | 0.03 | 0.04 | | 3144 |
| **applesce and pineapple, junior** | 170 | 66 | 151.5 | 17.8 | | | 2.6 | 3 | 7 | 7 | 0.05 | | 2 | 46 | 0.04 | 0.1 | 0 | 0.18 |
| *6 oz jar* | | 0.2 | 0.2 | 0 | 0 | 0.1 | 0 | 129 | 10 | 0.17 | 0.061 | 0.5 | 36 | 1.0 | 0.05 | 0.07 | 3.4 | 3151 |
| **applesce and pineapple, strained** | 113 | 42 | 101.1 | 11.4 | | | 1.7 | 2 | 5 | 3 | 0.02 | | 0 | 32 | 0.02 | 0.1 | 0 | 0.11 |
| *4 oz jar* | | 0.1 | 0.1 | 0 | 0 | 0 | 0 | 88 | 7 | 0.11 | 0.040 | 0.3 | 0 | 0.7 | 0.03 | 0.04 | 2.3 | 3150 |
| **applesce, Bch-Nut Baby's 1st/Gerber 1st Fds/Heinz Beg - 2.5 oz jar** | 71 | 29 | 62.9 | 7.7 | 7.0 | 0 | 1.2 | 1 | 3 | 2 | 0.01 | | 1 | 27 | 0.01 | 0 | 0 | 0.08 |
| | | 0.1 | 0.1 | 0 | 0 | 0 | 0 | 50 | 5 | 0.16 | 0.027 | 0.2 | 12 | 0.4 | 0.02 | 0.02 | 1.4 | 3116 |
| **applesce, Bch-Nut Stg 1/Gerber 2nd Fds/Heinz Str-2 - 2.5 oz jar** | 71 | 29 | 62.9 | 7.7 | 7.0 | 0 | 1.2 | 1 | 3 | 2 | 0.01 | | 1 | 27 | 0.01 | 0 | 0 | 0.08 |
| | | 0.1 | 0.1 | 0 | 0 | 0 | 0 | 50 | 5 | 0.16 | 0.027 | 0.2 | 12 | 0.4 | 0.02 | 0.02 | 1.4 | 3116 |
| **applesce, Bch-Nut Stg 3/Gerber 3rd Fds/Heinz Jr-3 - 6 oz jar** | 170 | 63 | 152.2 | 17.5 | 14.4 | 0 | 2.9 | 3 | 8 | 5 | 0.07 | | 0 | 64 | 0.02 | 0.1 | 0 | 0.17 |
| | | 0 | 0 | 0 | 0 | 0 | 0 | 131 | 10 | 0.37 | 0.060 | 0.5 | 15 | 1.0 | 0.05 | 0.05 | 3.4 | 3117 |
| **applesce, Earth's Best** | 71 | 29 | 62.9 | 7.7 | 7.0 | 0 | 1.2 | 1 | 3 | 2 | 0.01 | | 1 | 27 | 0.01 | 0 | 0 | 0.08 |
| *2.5 oz jar* | | 0.1 | 0.1 | 0 | 0 | 0 | 0 | 50 | 5 | 0.16 | 0.027 | 0.2 | 12 | 0.4 | 0.02 | 0.02 | 1.4 | 3116 |
| **apricots w/tapioca, Gerber 2nd Fds** | 113 | 68 | 93.9 | 18.4 | 1.6 | 0 | 1.7 | 9 | 10 | 5 | 0.06 | | 41 | 24 | 0.01 | 0.2 | 0 | 0.15 |
| *4 oz jar* | | 0.3 | 0 | 0 | 0 | 0 | 0 | 137 | 11 | 0.34 | 0.038 | 0.3 | 819 | 0.1 | 0.01 | 0.03 | 2.3 | 3118 |
| **apricots w/tapioca, Gerber 3rd Fds/Heinz Jr-3 - 6 oz jar** | 170 | 107 | 139.6 | 29.4 | 2.4 | 0 | 2.6 | 10 | 14 | 7 | 0.07 | | 61 | 30 | 0.01 | 0.3 | 0 | 0.23 |
| | | 0.5 | 0 | 0 | 0 | 0 | 0 | 212 | 17 | 0.46 | 0.061 | 0.5 | 1229 | 1.0 | 0.02 | 0.05 | 3.4 | 3128 |
| **apricots w/tapioca, Heinz Str-2** | 113 | 68 | 93.9 | 18.4 | 1.6 | 0 | 1.7 | 9 | 10 | 5 | 0.06 | | 41 | 24 | 0.01 | 0.2 | 0 | 0.15 |
| *4 oz jar* | | 0.3 | 0 | 0 | 0 | 0 | 0 | 137 | 11 | 0.34 | 0.038 | 0.3 | 819 | 0.1 | 0.01 | 0.03 | 2.3 | 3118 |

| | WT (g) | KCAL | H₂0 (g) | CHO (g) | TSUG (g) | ASUG (g) | DFIB (g) | Na (mg) | Ca (mg) | Mg (mg) | Zn (mg) | Mn (mg) | A (mcg RAE) | C (mg) | B-1 (mg) | NIA (mg) | B-12 (mcg) | PANT (mg) |
|---|---|---|---|---|---|---|---|---|---|---|---|---|---|---|---|---|---|---|
| | | PRO (g) | FAT (g) | SFA (g) | MUFA (g) | PUFA (g) | CHOL (mg) | K (mg) | P (mg) | Fe (mg) | Cu (mg) | Se (mcg) | A (IU) | E (mg ATE) | B-2 (mg) | B-6 (mg) | FOL (mcg DFE) | REF |
| **bananas**, strained | 113 | 103 | 86.7 | 24.1 | 12.8 | 0 | 1.8 | 3 | 5 | 29 | 0.06 | | 0 | 25 | 0.02 | 0.6 | 0 | |
| *4 oz jar* | | 1.1 | 0.2 | 0.1 | 0 | 0 | 0 | 328 | 23 | 0.34 | 0.045 | 1.2 | 6 | 0.3 | 0.07 | 0.29 | 19.2 | 43546 |
| **bananas w/pineapple and tapioca,** | 120 | 78 | 98.0 | 21.4 | 12.9 | 0 | 1.9 | 7 | 8 | 7 | 0.05 | | 4 | 23 | 0.02 | 0.2 | 0 | 0.17 |
| Gerber 2nd Fds - *4.25 oz jar* | | 0.2 | 0 | 0 | 0 | 0 | 0 | 82 | 6 | 0.28 | 0.047 | 0.7 | 72 | 0.1 | 0.02 | 0.10 | 21.6 | 3157 |
| **ban w/pinaple & tapioca,** Gerber 3rd | 170 | 116 | 137.9 | 31.3 | 14.3 | 0 | 2.7 | 14 | 12 | 10 | 0.05 | | 3 | 36 | 0.03 | 0.3 | 0 | 0.25 |
| Fds/Heinz Jr-3 - *6 oz jar* | | 0.3 | 0.2 | 0.1 | 0 | 0 | 0 | 133 | 8 | 0.22 | 0.068 | 1.0 | 68 | 0 | 0.03 | 0.16 | 10.2 | 3156 |
| **bananas w/pineapple and tapioca,** | 120 | 78 | 98.0 | 21.4 | 12.9 | 0 | 1.9 | 7 | 8 | 7 | 0.05 | | 4 | 23 | 0.02 | 0.2 | 0 | 0.17 |
| Heinz Str-2 - *4.25 oz jar* | | 0.2 | 0 | 0 | 0 | 0 | 0 | 82 | 6 | 0.28 | 0.047 | 0.7 | 72 | 0.1 | 0.02 | 0.10 | 21.6 | 3157 |
| **bananas w/tapioca,** Gerber 2nd | 113 | 63 | 94.9 | 17.3 | 0.4 | 0 | 1.8 | 10 | 6 | 11 | 0.07 | | 2 | 19 | 0.01 | 0.2 | 0 | 0.17 |
| Fds - *4 oz jar* | | 0.5 | 0.1 | 0 | 0 | 0 | 0 | 99 | 8 | 0.23 | 0.045 | 0.7 | 49 | 0.7 | 0.04 | 0.13 | 6.8 | 3129 |
| **bananas w/tapioca,** Gerber 3rd | 170 | 114 | 138.5 | 30.3 | 12.1 | 0 | 2.7 | 15 | 14 | 20 | 0.12 | | 3 | 44 | 0.03 | 0.4 | 0 | 0.29 |
| Fds/Heinz Jr-3 - *6 oz jar* | | 0.7 | 0.3 | 0.1 | 0 | 0.1 | 0 | 184 | 15 | 0.51 | 0.078 | 1.0 | 75 | 1.0 | 0.03 | 0.24 | 10.2 | 3280 |
| **bananas w/tapioca,** Heinz Str-2 | 113 | 63 | 94.9 | 17.3 | 0.4 | 0 | 1.8 | 10 | 6 | 11 | 0.07 | | 2 | 19 | 0.01 | 0.2 | 0 | 0.17 |
| *4 oz jar* | | 0.5 | 0.1 | 0 | 0 | 0 | 0 | 99 | 8 | 0.23 | 0.045 | 0.7 | 49 | 0.7 | 0.04 | 0.13 | 6.8 | 3129 |
| **guava and papaya w/tapioca,** | 113 | 71 | 93.2 | 19.2 | | | | 5 | 8 | 6 | 0.07 | | 10 | 91 | 0.01 | 0.3 | 0 | |
| strained - *4 oz jar* | | 0.2 | 0.1 | | | | | 84 | 7 | 0.23 | | 0.5 | 208 | | 0.02 | 0.02 | 2.3 | 3160 |
| **mango w/tapioca,** Gerber | 113 | 79 | 90.4 | 21.5 | 14.7 | 0 | 1.2 | 5 | 9 | 7 | 0.03 | | 26 | 18 | 0.02 | 0.2 | 0 | 0.11 |
| *4 oz jar* | | 0.3 | 0.2 | 0 | 0.1 | 0 | 0 | 75 | 5 | 0.23 | 0.034 | 0.5 | 508 | 0.7 | 0.02 | 0.09 | 9.0 | 3140 |
| **papaya and applesce w/tapioca,** | 113 | 79 | 91.1 | 21.4 | | | 1.6 | 6 | 8 | 6 | 0.03 | | 5 | 128 | 0.01 | 0.1 | 0 | 0.32 |
| strained - *4 oz jar* | | 0.2 | 0.1 | | | | | 89 | 6 | 0.50 | 0.050 | 0.5 | 86 | | 0.03 | 0.03 | 2.3 | 3162 |
| **peaches,** Bch-Nut Baby's 1st/Gerber | 113 | 73 | 94.5 | 16.4 | 13.0 | 0 | 1.5 | 7 | 5 | 8 | 0.12 | 0.042 | 38 | 52 | 0.02 | 1.9 | 0 | 0.09 |
| 1st Fds/Heinz Beg-1 - *4 oz jar* | | 1.1 | 0.4 | 0 | 0 | 0 | 0 | 220 | 17 | 0.26 | 0.034 | 0.1 | 264 | 2.2 | 0.09 | 0.02 | 23.7 | 3130 |
| **peaches,** Bch-Nut Stg 1/Gerber 2nd | 113 | 73 | 94.5 | 16.4 | 13.0 | 0 | 1.5 | 7 | 5 | 8 | 0.12 | 0.042 | 38 | 52 | 0.02 | 1.9 | 0 | 0.09 |
| Fds/Heinz Str-2 - *4 oz jar* | | 1.1 | 0.4 | 0 | 0 | 0 | 0 | 220 | 17 | 0.26 | 0.034 | 0.1 | 264 | 2.2 | 0.09 | 0.02 | 23.7 | 3130 |
| **peaches,** Bch-Nut Stg 3/Gerber 3rd | 170 | 110 | 142.2 | 24.6 | 19.6 | 0 | 2.2 | 10 | 7 | 12 | 0.19 | 0.063 | 58 | 78 | 0.03 | 2.8 | 0 | 0.14 |
| Fds/Heinz Jr-3 - *6 oz jar* | | 1.6 | 0.6 | 0 | 0 | 0.1 | 0 | 332 | 26 | 0.39 | 0.051 | 0.2 | 1166 | 3.4 | 0.13 | 0.03 | 35.7 | 3131 |
| **peaches,** toddler | 170 | 87 | 148.6 | 20.1 | 16.1 | 0 | 1.4 | 8 | 10 | 14 | 0.20 | 0.085 | 12 | 53 | 0.02 | 0.8 | 0 | 0.29 |
| *6 oz jar* | | 0.8 | 0.3 | 0 | 0.1 | 0.1 | 0 | 141 | 29 | 0.34 | 0.051 | 0.7 | 235 | 1.4 | 0.03 | 0.07 | 8.5 | 3161 |
| **pears & pinaple,** Bch-Nut Stg 2/Grbr | 113 | 46 | 100.0 | 12.3 | 8.8 | 0 | 2.9 | 5 | 11 | 8 | 0.08 | | 1 | 31 | 0.02 | 0.2 | 0 | 0.10 |
| 2nd Fds/Heinz Str-2 - *4 oz jar* | | 0.3 | 0.1 | 0 | 0 | 0 | 0 | 131 | 10 | 0.28 | 0.158 | 0.5 | 33 | 0 | 0.03 | 0.02 | 3.4 | 3158 |
| **pears and pineapple,** Gerber 3rd | 170 | 75 | 149.3 | 19.4 | 12.5 | 0 | 4.4 | 2 | 17 | 12 | 0.22 | | 3 | 29 | 0.04 | 0.3 | 0 | 0.16 |
| Fds *6 oz jar* | | 0.5 | 0.3 | 0 | 0.1 | 0 | 0 | 201 | 17 | 0.36 | 0.178 | 0.7 | 54 | 0.1 | 0.04 | 0.02 | 5.1 | 3159 |
| **pears,** Bch-Nut Baby's 1st/Gerber 1st | 113 | 47 | 99.9 | 12.2 | 7.9 | 0 | 4.1 | 2 | 9 | 9 | 0.09 | | 1 | 28 | 0.01 | 0.2 | 0 | 0.10 |
| Fds/Heinz Beg-1 - *4 oz jar* | | 0.3 | 0.2 | 0 | 0 | 0.1 | 0 | 147 | 14 | 0.27 | 0.073 | 0.5 | 37 | 0.1 | 0.03 | 0.01 | 4.5 | 3132 |
| **pears,** Bch-Nut Stg 1/Gerber 2nd | 113 | 47 | 99.9 | 12.2 | 7.9 | 0 | 4.1 | 2 | 9 | 9 | 0.09 | | 1 | 28 | 0.01 | 0.2 | 0 | 0.10 |
| Fds/Heinz Str-2 - *4 oz jar* | | 0.3 | 0.2 | 0 | 0 | 0.1 | 0 | 147 | 14 | 0.27 | 0.073 | 0.5 | 37 | 0.1 | 0.03 | 0.01 | 4.5 | 3132 |
| **pears,** Bch-Nut Stg 3/Gerber 3rd | 170 | 73 | 149.3 | 19.7 | 12.5 | 0 | 6.1 | 3 | 14 | 15 | 0.14 | | 2 | 37 | 0.02 | 0.3 | 0 | 0.16 |
| Fds/Heinz Jr-3 - *6 oz jar* | | 0.5 | 0.2 | 0 | 0 | 0 | 0 | 196 | 20 | 0.42 | 0.136 | 0.7 | 31 | 1.0 | 0.05 | 0.02 | 6.8 | 3133 |
| **pears,** Earth's Best | 113 | 47 | 99.9 | 12.2 | 7.9 | 0 | 4.1 | 2 | 9 | 9 | 0.09 | | 1 | 28 | 0.01 | 0.2 | 0 | 0.10 |
| *4 oz jar* | | 0.3 | 0.2 | 0 | 0 | 0.1 | 0 | 147 | 14 | 0.27 | 0.073 | 0.5 | 37 | 0.1 | 0.03 | 0.01 | 4.5 | 3132 |
| **pears,** toddler | 170 | 97 | 145.5 | 23.1 | 14.7 | 0 | 2.0 | 10 | 17 | 12 | 0.15 | 0.051 | 2 | 53 | 0.02 | 0.2 | 0 | 0.10 |
| *6 oz jar* | | 0.5 | 0.2 | 0 | 0.1 | 0.1 | 0 | 87 | 22 | 0.34 | 0.068 | 0.7 | 36 | 0.2 | 0.03 | 0.07 | 1.7 | 3141 |
| **plums, bananas, and rice,** | 128 | 73 | 109.6 | 16.3 | 11.9 | 0 | 1.7 | 1 | 4 | 14 | 0.17 | | 9 | 16 | 0.05 | 1.0 | 0 | |
| strained - *4.5 oz jar* | | 1.4 | 0.4 | 0.1 | 0.2 | 0.1 | 0 | 339 | 41 | 0 | 0.069 | 3.1 | 170 | 0.3 | 0.06 | 0.17 | 7.7 | 3293 |
| **plums w/tapioca,** Gerber 2nd | 113 | 80 | 90.4 | 22.3 | 15.1 | 0 | 1.4 | 7 | 7 | 5 | 0.09 | | 8 | 1 | 0.01 | 0.2 | 0 | 0.12 |
| Fds/Heinz Str-2 - *4 oz jar* | | 0.1 | 0.1 | 0 | 0 | 0 | 0 | 96 | 7 | 0.23 | 0.042 | 0.5 | 160 | 0.2 | 0.03 | 0.03 | 2.3 | 3134 |
| **plums w/tapioca,** Gerber 3rd Fds | 170 | 126 | 134.6 | 34.8 | 23.2 | 0 | 2.0 | 14 | 10 | 7 | 0.14 | | 8 | 1 | 0.01 | 0.4 | 0 | 0.19 |
| *6 oz jar* | | 0.2 | 0.2 | 0 | 0 | 0 | 0 | 141 | 10 | 0.37 | 0.065 | 0.7 | 160 | 1.0 | 0.05 | 0.05 | 1.7 | 3135 |
| **prunes,** strained | 128 | 129 | 95.1 | 30.1 | 27.1 | 0 | 3.5 | 8 | 27 | 22 | 0.26 | | 4 | 2 | 0.03 | 0.9 | 0 | |
| *4.5 oz jar* | | 1.3 | 0.3 | 0 | 0.2 | 0.1 | 0 | 392 | 38 | 0.51 | 0.210 | 1.0 | 77 | 0.7 | 0.27 | 0.14 | 1.3 | 3139 |
| **prunes w/tapioca,** Gerber 2nd Fds | 113 | 78 | 90.7 | 20.9 | 12.4 | | 3.1 | 6 | 17 | 11 | 0.10 | | 26 | 1 | 0.02 | 0.6 | 0 | 0.16 |
| *4 oz jar* | | 0.7 | 0.1 | 0 | 0.1 | 0 | 0 | 200 | 17 | 0.40 | 0.069 | 0.6 | 512 | 0.7 | 0.08 | 0.09 | 1.1 | 3136 |
| **prunes w/tapioca,** Heinz Str-2 | 113 | 78 | 90.7 | 20.9 | 12.4 | | 3.1 | 6 | 17 | 11 | 0.10 | | 26 | 1 | 0.02 | 0.6 | 0 | 0.16 |
| *4 oz jar* | | 0.7 | 0.1 | 0 | 0.1 | 0 | 0 | 200 | 17 | 0.40 | 0.069 | 0.6 | 512 | 0.7 | 0.08 | 0.09 | 1.1 | 3136 |
| **prunes w/tapioca,** junior | 170 | 119 | 136.2 | 31.8 | 18.6 | | 4.6 | 3 | 26 | 17 | 0.17 | | 17 | 1 | 0.04 | 0.9 | 0 | 0.24 |
| *6 oz jar* | | 1.0 | 0.2 | 0 | 0.1 | 0 | 0 | 275 | 26 | 0.56 | 0.105 | 0.8 | 354 | 0.2 | 0.14 | 0.15 | 1.7 | 3137 |

## 18.7 INFANT, JUNIOR, AND TODDLER MEATS

| | WT (g) | KCAL | H₂0 | CHO | TSUG | ASUG | DFIB | Na | Ca | Mg | Zn | Mn | A | C | B-1 | NIA | B-12 | PANT |
|---|---|---|---|---|---|---|---|---|---|---|---|---|---|---|---|---|---|---|
| **beef,** strained | 71 | 58 | 58.5 | 1.7 | 0 | | 0 | 33 | 4 | 8 | 1.58 | 0.026 | 0 | 1 | 0.01 | 1.8 | 0.89 | 0.06 |
| *2.5 oz jar* | | 8.5 | 1.8 | 0.8 | 0.7 | 0.1 | 36 | 133 | 66 | 0.70 | 0.105 | 2.1 | 0 | 0.3 | 0.10 | 0.03 | 5.7 | 3002 |
| **beef,** Gerber 3rd Fds/Heinz Jr-3 | 71 | 58 | 58.5 | 1.7 | 0 | | 0 | 33 | 4 | 8 | 1.58 | 0.026 | 0 | 1 | 0.01 | 1.8 | 0.89 | 0.06 |
| *2.5 oz jar* | | 8.5 | 1.8 | 0.8 | 0.7 | 0.1 | 36 | 133 | 66 | 0.70 | 0.105 | 2.1 | 0 | 0.3 | 0.10 | 0.03 | 5.7 | 3003 |

| | WT (g) | KCAL / PRO (g) | H₂O (g) / FAT (g) | CHO (g) / SFA (g) | TSUG (g) / MUFA (g) | ASUG (g) / PUFA (g) | DFIB (g) / CHOL (mg) | Na (mg) / K (mg) | Ca (mg) / P (mg) | Mg (mg) / Fe (mg) | Zn (mg) / Cu (mg) | Mn (mg) / Se (mcg) | A (mcg RAE) / A (IU) | C (mg) / E (mg ATE) | B-1 (mg) / B-2 (mg) | NIA (mg) / B-6 (mg) | B-12 (mcg) / FOL (mcg DFE) | PANT (mg) / REF |
|---|---|---|---|---|---|---|---|---|---|---|---|---|---|---|---|---|---|---|
| **chicken**, Bch-Nut Stg 1/Gerber 2nd Fds/Heinz Str-2 - 2.5 oz jar | 71 | 92 | 55.0 | 0.1 | 0 | | 0 | 33 | 45 | 9 | 0.86 | | 4 | 1 | 0.01 | 2.3 | 0.28 | 0.48 |
| | | 9.7 | 5.6 | 1.4 | 2.5 | 1.4 | 43 | 100 | 69 | 0.99 | 0.032 | 7.8 | 15 | 0.2 | 0.11 | 0.14 | 2.1 | 3012 |
| **chicken**, Gerber 3rd Fds/Heinz Jr-3 2.5 oz jar | 71 | 104 | 54.0 | 0 | 0 | | 0 | 36 | 39 | 8 | 0.72 | | 8 | 1 | 0.01 | 2.4 | 0.28 | 0.52 |
| | | 9.9 | 6.8 | 1.8 | 3.1 | 1.7 | 42 | 87 | 64 | 0.70 | 0.032 | 7.3 | 28 | 0.3 | 0.12 | 0.13 | 7.8 | 3013 |
| **chicken sticks**, Gerber Graduates 2.5 oz jar | 71 | 133 | 48.5 | 1.1 | 1.0 | 0 | 0.1 | 340 | 52 | 10 | 0.72 | | 2 | 1 | 0.01 | 1.4 | 0.28 | 0.52 |
| | | 10.4 | 10.2 | 2.9 | 4.4 | 2.1 | 55 | 75 | 86 | 1.11 | 0.032 | 7.3 | 8 | 0.3 | 0.14 | 0.07 | 7.8 | 3014 |
| **ham**, Gerber 2nd Foods 2.5 oz jar | 71 | 69 | 57.2 | 2.6 | 0 | | 0 | 29 | 4 | 9 | 1.60 | | 1 | 1 | 0.10 | 1.9 | 0.07 | 0.36 |
| | | 8.0 | 2.7 | 0.9 | 1.3 | 0.4 | 17 | 145 | 58 | 0.73 | 0.046 | 10.1 | 4 | 0.1 | 0.11 | 0.18 | 1.4 | 3008 |
| **ham**, junior 2.5 oz jar | 71 | 69 | 57.2 | 2.6 | 0 | | 0 | 48 | 4 | 8 | 1.21 | | 0 | 1 | 0.10 | 2.0 | 0.07 | 0.38 |
| | | 8.0 | 2.7 | 0.9 | 1.3 | 0.4 | 21 | 149 | 63 | 0.72 | 0.048 | 10.6 | 0 | 0.3 | 0.14 | 0.14 | 1.4 | 3009 |
| **lamb**, Bch-Nut Stg 1/Gerber 2nd Fds/Heinz Str-2 - 2.5 oz jar | 71 | 62 | 57.6 | 0.6 | 0 | | 0 | 31 | 5 | 9 | 1.73 | 0.026 | 0 | 1 | 0.01 | 2.1 | 1.35 | 0.08 |
| | | 10.0 | 2.4 | 1.2 | 0.9 | 0.2 | 26 | 137 | 74 | 0.84 | 0.105 | 1.6 | 0 | 0.1 | 0.12 | 0.03 | 0 | 3010 |
| **lamb**, junior 2.5 oz jar | 71 | 80 | 56.5 | 0 | 0 | | 0 | 52 | 5 | 7 | 1.85 | | 6 | 1 | 0.01 | 2.3 | 1.61 | 0.30 |
| | | 10.8 | 3.7 | 1.8 | 1.5 | 0.2 | 27 | 150 | 65 | 1.18 | 0.040 | 5.0 | 19 | 0.3 | 0.14 | 0.13 | 1.4 | 3011 |
| **meat sticks**, Gerber Graduates 2.5 oz jar | 71 | 131 | 49.3 | 0.8 | 0.6 | 0 | 0.1 | 388 | 24 | 8 | 1.35 | | 15 | 2 | 0.04 | 1.1 | 0.21 | 0.34 |
| | | 9.5 | 10.4 | 4.1 | 4.6 | 1.1 | 50 | 81 | 73 | 0.98 | 0.048 | 9.4 | 49 | 0.2 | 0.12 | 0.06 | 2.1 | 3021 |
| **pork**, strained 2.5 oz jar | 71 | 88 | 55.7 | 0 | 0 | | 0 | 30 | 4 | 7 | 1.61 | | 8 | 1 | 0.10 | 1.6 | 0.70 | 0.19 |
| | | 9.9 | 5.0 | 1.7 | 2.5 | 0.6 | 34 | 158 | 67 | 0.71 | 0.051 | 9.2 | 27 | 0.3 | 0.14 | 0.15 | 1.4 | 3007 |
| **turkey**, Bch-Nut Stg 1/Gerber 2nd Fds/Heinz Str-2 - 2.5 oz jar | 71 | 79 | 57.0 | 1.0 | 0 | | 0 | 33 | 29 | 9 | 1.26 | 0.026 | 0 | 2 | 0.01 | 1.9 | 0.79 | 0.29 |
| | | 8.2 | 4.4 | 1.2 | 1.7 | 1.2 | 41 | 96 | 83 | 0.50 | 0.105 | 8.5 | 0 | 0.1 | 0.12 | 0.02 | 5.7 | 3015 |
| **turkey**, Gerber 3rd Foods 2.5 oz jar | 71 | 79 | 57.0 | 1.0 | 0 | | 0 | 33 | 29 | 9 | 1.26 | 0.026 | 0 | 0 | 0.01 | 1.9 | 0.79 | 0.29 |
| | | 8.2 | 4.4 | 1.2 | 1.7 | 1.2 | 41 | 96 | 83 | 0.50 | 0.105 | 8.5 | 0 | 0.1 | 0.12 | 0.02 | 5.7 | 3016 |
| **turkey sticks**, Gerber Graduates 2.5 oz jar | 71 | 129 | 49.6 | 1.0 | 1.0 | 0 | 0.4 | 343 | 51 | 11 | 1.30 | | 4 | 1 | 0.01 | 1.2 | 0.71 | 0.40 |
| | | 9.7 | 10.1 | 2.9 | 3.3 | 2.6 | 46 | 65 | 73 | 0.88 | 0.028 | 7.2 | 13 | 0.3 | 0.11 | 0.05 | 7.8 | 3017 |
| **veal**, Bch-Nut Stg 1/Gerber 2nd Fds/Heinz Str-2 - 2.5 oz jar | 71 | 58 | 58.5 | 1.1 | 0 | | 0 | 28 | 4 | 8 | 1.78 | 0.026 | 0 | 0 | 0.02 | 2.0 | 1.17 | 0.11 |
| | | 9.3 | 1.7 | 0.8 | 0.7 | 0.1 | 23 | 121 | 70 | 0.54 | 0.105 | 2.5 | 0 | 0.2 | 0.08 | 0.03 | 3.6 | 3005 |

## 18.8 INFANT, JUNIOR, AND TODDLER VEGETABLES

| | WT (g) | KCAL / PRO (g) | H₂O (g) / FAT (g) | CHO (g) / SFA (g) | TSUG (g) / MUFA (g) | ASUG (g) / PUFA (g) | DFIB (g) / CHOL (mg) | Na (mg) / K (mg) | Ca (mg) / P (mg) | Mg (mg) / Fe (mg) | Zn (mg) / Cu (mg) | Mn (mg) / Se (mcg) | A (mcg RAE) / A (IU) | C (mg) / E (mg ATE) | B-1 (mg) / B-2 (mg) | NIA (mg) / B-6 (mg) | B-12 (mcg) / FOL (mcg DFE) | PANT (mg) / REF |
|---|---|---|---|---|---|---|---|---|---|---|---|---|---|---|---|---|---|---|
| **beets**, Gerber 2nd Fds/Heinz Str-2 4 oz jar | 113 | 38 | 101.8 | 8.7 | 6.9 | 0 | 2.1 | 94 | 16 | 16 | 0.14 | | 1 | 3 | 0.01 | 0.1 | 0 | 0.11 |
| | | 1.5 | 0.1 | 0 | 0 | 0 | 0 | 206 | 16 | 0.36 | 0.079 | 0.1 | 31 | 0 | 0.05 | 0.03 | 35.0 | 3098 |
| **butternut squash and corn**, Gerber 2nd Foods - 4 oz jar | 113 | 56 | 98.6 | 10.5 | 3.3 | 0 | 2.3 | 6 | 36 | 29 | 0.34 | 0.136 | 158 | 6 | 0.07 | 0.6 | 0 | 0.35 |
| | | 2.3 | 0.7 | 0.1 | 0.2 | 0.3 | 0 | 398 | 40 | 0.45 | 0.113 | 0.7 | 3156 | 0.1 | 0.07 | 0.12 | 26.0 | 3114 |
| **carrots**, Bch-Nut Baby's 1st/Gerber 1st Fds/Heinz Beg-1 - 2.5 oz jar | 71 | 19 | 65.5 | 4.3 | 2.6 | 0 | 1.2 | 26 | 16 | 6 | 0.11 | | 407 | 4 | 0.02 | 0.3 | 0 | 0.17 |
| | | 0.6 | 0.1 | 0 | 0 | 0 | 0 | 139 | 14 | 0.26 | 0.029 | 0.1 | 8137 | 0.4 | 0.03 | 0.05 | 10.6 | 3099 |
| **carrots**, Bch-Nut Stg 1/Gerber 2nd Fds/Heinz Str-2 - 2.5 oz jar | 71 | 19 | 65.5 | 4.3 | 2.6 | 0 | 1.2 | 26 | 16 | 6 | 0.11 | | 407 | 4 | 0.02 | 0.3 | 0 | 0.17 |
| | | 0.6 | 0.1 | 0 | 0 | 0 | 0 | 139 | 14 | 0.26 | 0.029 | 0.1 | 8137 | 0.4 | 0.03 | 0.05 | 10.6 | 3099 |
| **carrots**, Bch-Nut Stg 3/Gerber 3rd Fds/Heinz Jr-3 - 6 oz jar | 170 | 54 | 154.7 | 12.2 | 5.4 | 0 | 2.9 | 83 | 39 | 19 | 0.31 | | 1005 | 9 | 0.04 | 0.8 | 0 | 0.47 |
| | | 1.4 | 0.3 | 0.1 | 0 | 0.2 | 0 | 343 | 34 | 0.66 | 0.080 | 0.3 | 20077 | 0.9 | 0.07 | 0.14 | 28.9 | 3100 |
| **carrots**, Earth's Best 2.5 oz jar | 71 | 19 | 65.5 | 4.3 | 2.6 | 0 | 1.2 | 26 | 16 | 6 | 0.11 | | 407 | 4 | 0.02 | 0.3 | 0 | 0.17 |
| | | 0.6 | 0.1 | 0 | 0 | 0 | 0 | 139 | 14 | 0.26 | 0.029 | 0.1 | 8137 | 0.4 | 0.03 | 0.05 | 10.6 | 3099 |
| **carrots**, toddler 6 oz jar | 170 | 44 | 159.0 | 8.9 | 4.2 | 0 | 3.9 | 44 | 32 | 10 | 0.34 | | 1251 | 1 | 0.03 | 0.4 | 0 | |
| | | 1.0 | 0.5 | 0.1 | 0 | 0.3 | 0 | 219 | 36 | 0.34 | 0.138 | 1.4 | 25007 | 1.0 | 0.05 | 0.08 | 11.9 | 42316 |
| **corn and sweet potatoes**, strained 4.5 oz jar | 128 | 87 | 105.8 | 19.5 | 5.1 | | 2.3 | 42 | 23 | 13 | 0.24 | 0 | 161 | 6 | 0.02 | 0.6 | 0.01 | 0.41 |
| | | 1.6 | 0.4 | 0.1 | 0.1 | 0.2 | 1 | 197 | 37 | 0.40 | 0.065 | 1.4 | 3195 | 0.7 | 0.05 | 0.08 | 17.9 | 3934 |
| **corn, yellow, crmd**, Bch-Nut Stg 2/Grbr 2nd Fds/Heinz Str-2 - 4 oz jar | 113 | 64 | 94.5 | 15.9 | 1.4 | 0 | 2.4 | 49 | 23 | 9 | 0.21 | | 6 | 2 | 0.01 | 0.6 | 0.02 | 0.33 |
| | 1.6 | 0.5 | 0.1 | 0.1 | 0.2 | 1 | 102 | 37 | 0.32 | 0.038 | 1.5 | 78 | 0 | 0.05 | 0.05 | 19.2 | | 3119 |
| **corn, yellow, creamed**, Heinz Jr-3 6 oz jar | 170 | 110 | 138.4 | 27.6 | 2.5 | 0 | 3.6 | 88 | 7 | 14 | 0.39 | | 3 | 4 | 0.02 | 0.9 | 0.03 | 0.56 |
| | | 2.4 | 0.2 | 0.1 | 0.2 | 0.3 | 2 | 138 | 56 | 0.46 | 0.065 | 2.2 | 58 | 0.1 | 0.08 | 0.07 | 34.0 | 3120 |
| **garden vegetables**, strained 4 oz jar | 113 | 36 | 101.7 | 7.7 | 2.9 | 0 | 1.7 | 40 | 32 | 24 | 0.29 | | 342 | 6 | 0.07 | 0.9 | 0 | 0.29 |
| | | 2.6 | 0.2 | 0 | 0 | 0.1 | 0 | 190 | 32 | 0.94 | 0.079 | 0.8 | 6856 | 0.6 | 0.08 | 0.11 | 45.2 | 3283 |
| **green beans and potatoes**, Gerber 2nd Fds - 4 oz jar | 113 | 70 | 97.4 | 10.2 | 2.7 | 0 | 1.6 | 20 | 68 | 23 | 0.34 | 0.316 | 16 | 1 | 0.05 | 0.5 | 0.17 | 0.32 |
| | | 2.5 | 2.1 | 1.3 | 0.6 | 0.1 | 6 | 167 | 69 | 0.56 | 0.045 | 0.8 | 96 | 0.1 | 0.12 | 0.09 | 11.3 | 3096 |
| **green beans**, Bch-Nut Stg 1/Gerber 2nd Fds/Heinz Str-2 - 2.5 oz jar | 71 | 19 | 65.2 | 4.5 | 1.3 | 0 | 1.6 | 4 | 28 | 14 | 0.16 | 0.188 | 13 | 0 | 0.02 | 0.3 | 0 | 0.03 |
| | | 0.9 | 0.1 | 0 | 0 | 0.1 | 0 | 104 | 29 | 0.48 | 0.021 | 0.1 | 252 | 0 | 0.06 | 0.03 | 17.0 | 3091 |
| **green beans**, Beech-Nut Stage 3 6 oz jar | 170 | 41 | 157.2 | 9.7 | 1.8 | 0 | 3.2 | 3 | 110 | 37 | 0.32 | | 41 | 14 | 0.04 | 0.5 | 0 | 0.26 |
| | | 2.0 | 0.2 | 0 | 0 | 0.1 | 0 | 218 | 32 | 1.84 | 0.083 | 0.5 | 736 | 0.5 | 0.17 | 0.06 | 56.1 | 3092 |
| **green beans**, Gerber 1st Fds/Heinz Beginner-1 - 2.5 oz jar | 71 | 19 | 65.2 | 4.5 | 1.3 | 0 | 1.6 | 4 | 28 | 14 | 0.16 | 0.188 | 13 | 0 | 0.02 | 0.3 | 0 | 0.03 |
| | | 0.9 | 0.1 | 0 | 0 | 0.1 | 0 | 104 | 29 | 0.48 | 0.021 | 0.1 | 252 | 0 | 0.06 | 0.03 | 17.0 | 3091 |
| **green beans**, toddler 6 oz jar | 170 | 49 | 157.4 | 9.7 | 1.8 | 0 | 2.2 | 63 | 46 | 32 | 0.17 | 0.136 | 41 | 3 | 0.03 | 0.4 | 0 | 0.09 |
| | | 2.0 | 0.3 | 0.1 | 0 | 0.2 | 0 | 197 | 37 | 0.68 | 0.051 | 0.7 | 818 | 0.5 | 0.07 | 0.05 | 54.4 | 3093 |

| Food | WT (g) | KCAL / PRO (g) | H₂0 (g) / FAT (g) | CHO (g) / SFA (g) | TSUG (g) / MUFA (g) | ASUG (g) / PUFA (g) | DFIB (g) / CHOL (mg) | Na (mg) / K (mg) | Ca (mg) / P (mg) | Mg (mg) / Fe (mg) | Zn (mg) / Cu (mg) | Mn (mg) / Se (mcg) | A (mcg RAE) / A (IU) | C (mg) / E (mg ATE) | B-1 (mg) / B-2 (mg) | NIA (mg) / B-6 (mg) | B-12 (mcg) / FOL (mcg DFE) | PANT (mg) / REF |
|---|---|---|---|---|---|---|---|---|---|---|---|---|---|---|---|---|---|---|
| **green peas**, Bch-Nut Baby's 1st/Gerber 1st Foods - *4 oz jar* | 113 | 56 | 98.9 | 9.4 | 2.3 | 0 | 2.3 | 8 | 20 | 19 | 0.53 | 0.246 | 12 | 1 | 0.10 | 1.3 | 0 | 0.08 |
|  |  | 3.7 | 0.5 | 0.1 | 0.1 | 0.2 | 0 | 120 | 56 | 1.07 | 0.069 | 0.1 | 244 | 0 | 0.07 | 0.02 | 31.6 | 3121 |
| **green peas**, Bch-Nut Stg 1/Gerber 2nd Fds - *4 oz jar* | 113 | 56 | 98.9 | 9.4 | 2.3 | 0 | 2.3 | 8 | 20 | 19 | 0.53 | 0.246 | 12 | 1 | 0.10 | 1.3 | 0 | 0.08 |
|  |  | 3.7 | 0.5 | 0.1 | 0.1 | 0.2 | 0 | 120 | 56 | 1.07 | 0.069 | 0.1 | 244 | 0 | 0.07 | 0.02 | 31.6 | 3121 |
| **green peas**, toddler *6 oz jar* | 170 | 109 | 143.8 | 17.5 | 7.0 | 0 | 6.6 | 82 | 36 | 32 | 0.85 | 0.255 | 26 | 10 | 0.17 | 1.4 | 0 | 0.59 |
|  |  | 6.6 | 1.4 | 0.2 | 0.1 | 0.6 | 0 | 138 | 114 | 1.70 | 0.136 | 0.2 | 517 | 0.8 | 0.10 | 0.10 | 59.5 | 3122 |
| **mixed vegetables**, junior *6 oz jar* | 170 | 61 | 152.0 | 13.9 | 3.0 | 0 | 2.6 | 61 | 19 | 19 | 0.46 |  | 357 | 4 | 0.05 | 1.1 | 0 | 0.44 |
|  |  | 2.4 | 0.7 | 0.1 | 0 | 0.3 | 0 | 289 | 42 | 0.70 | 0.070 | 1.2 | 7132 | 0.9 | 0.05 | 0.14 | 6.8 | 3282 |
| **mixed vegetables**, strained *4 oz jar* | 113 | 41 | 101.5 | 9.1 | 1.8 | 0 | 1.7 | 15 | 15 | 11 | 0.17 |  | 179 | 2 | 0.02 | 0.4 | 0 | 0.28 |
|  |  | 1.4 | 0.6 | 0.1 | 0.1 | 0.2 | 0 | 144 | 25 | 0.36 | 0.045 | 0.8 | 3578 | 0.3 | 0.03 | 0.06 | 4.5 | 3286 |
| **peas and brown rice**, infant *4.5 oz jar* | 128 | 82 | 107.6 | 14.7 | 3.7 | 0 | 3.2 | 8 | 18 | 32 | 0.59 |  | 24 | 4 | 0.13 | 1.8 | 0 |  |
|  |  | 4.4 | 0.6 | 0.1 | 0.2 | 0 | 0 | 119 | 67 | 1.92 | 0.102 | 1.5 | 497 | 0.1 | 0.10 | 0.08 | 20.5 | 42279 |
| **potatoes**, Gerber Graduate *4.5 oz jar* | 128 | 67 | 111.1 | 15.0 | 1.2 | 0 | 1.2 | 73 | 5 | 19 | 0.22 | 0.090 | 0 | 13 | 0.03 | 0.4 | 0 | 0.39 |
|  |  | 1.3 | 0.1 | 0 | 0 | 0 | 0 | 141 | 29 | 0.26 | 0.090 | 1.0 | 0 | 0 | 0.01 | 0.09 | 7.7 | 3112 |
| **spinach, creamed**, Gerber 2nd Fds *4 oz jar* | 113 | 42 | 101.2 | 6.4 | 2.6 | 0 | 2.0 | 55 | 101 | 62 | 0.35 |  | 257 | 10 | 0.02 | 0.2 | 0.07 |  |
|  |  | 2.8 | 1.5 | 0.8 | 0.4 | 0.2 | 6 | 216 | 61 | 0.70 | 0.068 | 2.7 | 4712 | 0.9 | 0.12 | 0.08 | 68.9 | 3127 |
| **sqsh, yelw**, Bch-Nut Baby's 1st/Grbr 1st Fds/Hnz Beg-1 - *4.5 oz jar* | 128 | 36 | 118.6 | 7.3 | 4.3 | 0 | 1.2 | 8 | 31 | 18 | 0.24 | 0.106 | 109 | 0 | 0.04 | 0.9 | 0 | 0.27 |
|  |  | 1.0 | 0.3 | 0 | 0 | 0.1 | 0 | 237 | 27 | 0.41 | 0.038 | 0.3 | 2180 | 0.7 | 0.06 | 0.09 | 10.2 | 3104 |
| **sqsh, yelw**, Bch-Nut Stg 1/Grbr 2nd Fds/Heinz - Str-2 - *4.5 oz jar* | 128 | 36 | 118.6 | 7.3 | 4.3 | 0 | 1.2 | 8 | 31 | 18 | 0.24 | 0.106 | 109 | 0 | 0.04 | 0.9 | 0 | 0.27 |
|  |  | 1.0 | 0.3 | 0 | 0 | 0.1 | 0 | 237 | 27 | 0.41 | 0.038 | 0.3 | 2180 | 0.7 | 0.06 | 0.09 | 10.2 | 3104 |
| **squash, yellow**, Earth's Best *4.5 oz jar* | 128 | 36 | 118.6 | 7.3 | 4.3 | 0 | 1.2 | 8 | 31 | 18 | 0.24 | 0.106 | 109 | 0 | 0.04 | 0.9 | 0 | 0.27 |
|  |  | 1.0 | 0.3 | 0 | 0 | 0.1 | 0 | 237 | 27 | 0.41 | 0.038 | 0.3 | 2180 | 0.7 | 0.06 | 0.09 | 10.2 | 3104 |
| **squash, yellow**, Gerber 3rd Foods *6 oz jar* | 170 | 41 | 157.5 | 9.7 | 5.5 | 0 | 1.5 | 10 | 41 | 24 | 0.32 | 0.141 | 144 | 1 | 0.05 | 1.2 | 0 | 0.36 |
|  |  | 1.4 | 0.3 | 0 | 0 | 0.1 | 0 | 314 | 36 | 0.54 | 0.051 | 0.3 | 2895 | 0.9 | 0.08 | 0.12 | 13.6 | 3105 |
| **swt pot**, Bch-Nut Baby's 1st/Gerber 1st Fds/Hnz Beg-1 - *2.5 oz jar* | 71 | 40 | 60.2 | 9.4 | 2.9 | 0 | 1.1 | 14 | 11 | 9 | 0.15 |  | 229 | 7 | 0.02 | 0.3 | 0 | 0.28 |
|  |  | 0.8 | 0.1 | 0 | 0 | 0 | 0 | 187 | 17 | 0.26 | 0.058 | 0.5 | 4571 | 0.4 | 0.02 | 0.07 | 7.1 | 3108 |
| **swt pot**, Bch-Nut Stg 1/Gerber 2nd Fds/Heinz Str-2 - *2.5 oz jar* | 71 | 40 | 60.2 | 9.4 | 2.9 | 0 | 1.1 | 14 | 11 | 9 | 0.15 |  | 229 | 7 | 0.02 | 0.3 | 0 | 0.28 |
|  |  | 0.8 | 0.1 | 0 | 0 | 0 | 0 | 187 | 17 | 0.26 | 0.058 | 0.5 | 4571 | 0.4 | 0.02 | 0.07 | 7.1 | 3108 |
| **swt pot**, Bch-Nut Stg 3/Gerber 3rd Fds/Heinz Jr-3 - *6 oz jar* | 170 | 102 | 143.0 | 23.6 | 7.2 | 0 | 2.6 | 37 | 27 | 20 | 0.19 |  | 564 | 16 | 0.04 | 0.7 | 0 | 0.69 |
|  |  | 1.9 | 0.2 | 0 | 0 | 0.1 | 0 | 413 | 41 | 0.66 | 0.170 | 1.2 | 11281 | 0.9 | 0.06 | 0.19 | 17.0 | 3109 |
| **sweet potatoes**, Earth's Best *2.5 oz jar* | 71 | 40 | 60.2 | 9.4 | 2.9 | 0 | 1.1 | 14 | 11 | 9 | 0.15 |  | 229 | 7 | 0.02 | 0.3 | 0 | 0.28 |
|  |  | 0.8 | 0.1 | 0 | 0 | 0 | 0 | 187 | 17 | 0.26 | 0.058 | 0.5 | 4571 | 0.4 | 0.02 | 0.07 | 7.1 | 3108 |

# 19. MEATS
## 19.1 BEEF

| Food | WT (g) | KCAL / PRO (g) | H₂0 (g) / FAT (g) | CHO (g) / SFA (g) | TSUG (g) / MUFA (g) | ASUG (g) / PUFA (g) | DFIB (g) / CHOL (mg) | Na (mg) / K (mg) | Ca (mg) / P (mg) | Mg (mg) / Fe (mg) | Zn (mg) / Cu (mg) | Mn (mg) / Se (mcg) | A (mcg RAE) / A (IU) | C (mg) / E (mg ATE) | B-1 (mg) / B-2 (mg) | NIA (mg) / B-6 (mg) | B-12 (mcg) / FOL (mcg DFE) | PANT (mg) / REF |
|---|---|---|---|---|---|---|---|---|---|---|---|---|---|---|---|---|---|---|
| **beef bottom sirloin tri-tip roast,** 0" trim, lean, roasted - *3 oz* | 85 | 155 | 55.0 | 0 | 0 |  | 0 | 47 | 14 | 20 | 4.19 | 0.008 | 0 | 0 | 0.06 | 6.5 | 1.30 | 0.45 |
|  |  | 22.7 | 7.1 | 2.6 | 3.6 | 0.2 | 60 | 289 | 179 | 1.44 | 0.067 | 26.3 | 0 | 0.3 | 0.12 | 0.49 | 7.6 | 13985 |
| **beef bottom sirloin tri-tip steak,** 0" trim, lean and fat, brld - *3 oz* | 85 | 225 | 42.9 | 0 | 0 |  | 0 | 61 | 10 | 22 | 5.99 | 0 | 0 | 0 | 0.11 | 3.6 | 2.41 | 0 |
|  |  | 25.5 | 12.9 | 4.9 | 6.6 | 0.5 | 58 | 371 | 225 | 3.09 | 0.134 | 8.8 | 0 | 0.1 | 0.24 | 0.38 | 8.5 | 23545 |
| **beef bottom sirloin tri-tip steak,** 0" trim, lean, broiled - *3 oz* | 85 | 212 | 43.9 | 0 | 0 |  | 0 | 62 | 10 | 22 | 6.17 |  | 0 | 0 | 0.11 | 3.7 | 2.45 |  |
|  |  | 26.1 | 11.2 | 4.1 | 5.9 | 0.4 | 57 | 382 | 231 | 3.18 | 0.138 | 8.5 | 0 | 0.2 | 0.25 | 0.39 | 8.5 | 13987 |
| **beef brisket, flat half,** 0" trim, lean and fat, braised - *3 oz* | 85 | 181 | 50.1 | 0 | 0 |  | 0 | 46 | 16 | 18 | 6.47 | 0.009 | 0 | 0 | 0.06 | 4.0 | 2.07 | 0.55 |
|  |  | 28.0 | 6.8 | 2.7 | 2.9 | 0.3 | 34 | 224 | 170 | 2.35 | 0.097 | 26.3 | 0 | 0.4 | 0.17 | 0.27 | 8.5 | 13369 |
| **beef brisket, flat half,** 0" trim, lean, braised - *3 oz* | 85 | 174 | 50.6 | 0 | 0 |  | 0 | 46 | 14 | 19 | 6.80 | 0.010 | 0 | 0 | 0.06 | 4.1 | 2.06 | 0.56 |
|  |  | 28.3 | 5.9 | 2.2 | 2.5 | 0.2 | 59 | 227 | 174 | 2.40 | 0.098 | 28.9 | 0 | 0.4 | 0.18 | 0.27 | 9.4 | 13370 |
| **beef brisket, flat half, choice,** ⅛" trim, lean and fat, braised - *3 oz* | 85 | 246 | 44.6 | 0 | 0 |  | 0 | 41 | 14 | 16 | 5.69 | 0.008 | 0 | 0 | 0.05 | 3.5 | 1.80 | 0.48 |
|  |  | 24.5 | 15.7 | 6.2 | 6.7 | 0.6 | 65 | 197 | 149 | 2.07 | 0.085 | 23.0 | 0 | 0.4 | 0.15 | 0.24 | 7.6 | 13806 |
| **beef brisket, flat half, choice,** ⅛" trim, lean, braised - *3 oz* | 85 | 110 | 62.3 | 0 | 0 |  | 0 | 64 | 13 | 20 | 4.70 | 0.013 | 0 | 0 | 0.06 | 4.4 | 1.78 | 0.55 |
|  |  | 18.4 | 3.5 | 1.3 | 1.4 | 0.1 | 37 | 285 | 173 | 1.73 | 0.078 | 21.0 | 0 | 0.2 | 0.14 | 0.41 | 11.0 | 23613 |
| **beef brisket, flat half, select,** ⅛" trim, lean and fat, braised - *3 oz* | 85 | 235 | 50.4 | 0 | 0 |  | 0 | 49 | 14 | 15 | 3.60 | 0.008 | 0 | 0 | 0.06 | 3.4 | 1.17 | 0.43 |
|  |  | 15.1 | 18.9 | 7.6 | 8.1 | 0.7 | 69 | 230 | 139 | 1.27 | 0.064 | 16.5 | 0 | 0.4 | 0.11 | 0.38 | 7.6 | 23659 |
| **beef brisket, flat half, select,** ⅛" trim, lean, braised - *3 oz* | 85 | 105 | 63.1 | 0 | 0 |  | 0 | 65 | 15 | 19 | 4.73 | 0.010 | 0 | 0 | 0.07 | 4.0 | 1.45 | 0.54 |
|  |  | 18.2 | 3.1 | 1.1 | 1.3 | 0.1 | 32 | 283 | 170 | 1.56 | 0.078 | 23.0 | 0 | 0.2 | 0.12 | 0.46 | 11.0 | 23632 |
| **beef brisket, point half,** 0" trim, lean and fat, braised - *3 oz* | 85 | 304 | 39.1 | 0 | 0 |  | 0 | 58 | 7 | 15 | 4.96 | 0.012 | 0 | 0 | 0.05 | 2.6 | 1.98 | 0.25 |
|  |  | 20.0 | 24.2 | 9.6 | 10.8 | 0.8 | 78 | 198 | 159 | 1.99 | 0.082 | 18.6 | 0 |  | 0.16 | 0.20 | 6.0 | 13371 |
| **beef brisket, point half,** 0" trim, lean, braised - *3 oz* | 85 | 207 | 47.3 | 0 | 0 |  | 0 | 65 | 5 | 19 | 6.28 | 0.014 | 0 | 0 | 0.06 | 3.0 | 2.19 | 0.29 |
|  |  | 23.8 | 11.7 | 4.4 | 5.5 | 0.3 | 77 | 232 | 192 | 2.37 | 0.098 | 20.0 | 0 |  | 0.20 | 0.24 | 6.8 | 13372 |
| **beef brisket, whl** (flat & pt, halves), 0" trim, lean & fat braised - *3 oz* | 85 | 247 | 43.8 | 0 | 0 |  | 0 | 55 | 6 | 18 | 5.07 | 0.013 | 0 | 0 | 0.06 | 2.9 | 2.08 | 0.27 |
|  |  | 22.8 | 16.6 | 6.4 | 7.4 | 0.6 | 79 | 220 | 184 | 2.15 | 0.092 | 19.8 | 0 | 0.2 | 0.17 | 0.23 | 6.0 | 13367 |

| | WT (g) | KCAL / PRO (g) | H₂O (g) / FAT (g) | CHO (g) / SFA (g) | TSUG (g) / MUFA (g) | ASUG (g) / PUFA (g) | DFIB (g) / CHOL (mg) | Na (mg) / K (mg) | Ca (mg) / P (mg) | Mg (mg) / Fe (mg) | Zn (mg) / Cu (mg) | Mn (mg) / Se (mcg) | A (mcg RAE) / A (IU) | C (mg) / E (mg ATE) | B-1 (mg) / B-2 (mg) | NIA (mg) / B-6 (mg) | B-12 (mcg) / FOL (mcg DFE) | PANT (mg) / REF |
|---|---|---|---|---|---|---|---|---|---|---|---|---|---|---|---|---|---|---|
| **beef brisket, whl** (flat & pt halves), | 85 | 185 | 49.1 | 0 | 0 | | 0 | 60 | 5 | 20 | 5.86 | 0.014 | 0 | 0 | 0.06 | 3.2 | 2.21 | 0.31 |
| 0″ trim, lean, braised - 3 *oz* | | 25.3 | 8.6 | 3.1 | 4.0 | 0.3 | 79 | 242 | 205 | 2.39 | 0.101 | 20.8 | | 0.1 | 0.19 | 0.25 | 6.8 | 13368 |
| **beef chuck arm pot roast, choice,** | 85 | 180 | 50.0 | 0 | 0 | | 0 | 46 | 12 | 19 | 6.62 | 0.010 | 0 | 0 | 0.06 | 4.3 | 2.20 | 0.56 |
| 0″ trim, lean, braised - 3 *oz* | | 28.4 | 6.5 | 2.5 | 2.8 | 0.2 | 65 | 223 | 172 | 2.46 | 0.105 | 28.0 | | 0.4 | 0.19 | 0.28 | 9.4 | 13377 |
| **beef chuck arm pot rst, choice, ⅛″** | 85 | 212 | 52.5 | 0 | 0 | | 0 | 54 | 14 | 16 | 3.88 | 0.011 | 0 | 0 | 0.05 | 3.7 | 1.52 | 0.48 |
| trim, lean & fat, braised - 3 *oz* | | 16.3 | 15.8 | 6.4 | 6.8 | 0.6 | 58 | 246 | 145 | 1.47 | 0.070 | 16.9 | | 0.3 | 0.12 | 0.36 | 8.5 | 13811 |
| **beef chuck arm pot roast, choice,** | 85 | 118 | 61.6 | 0 | 0 | | 0 | 63 | 13 | 20 | 4.66 | 0.013 | 0 | 0 | 0.07 | 4.4 | 1.79 | 0.56 |
| ⅛″ trim, lean, braised - 3 *oz* | | 18.7 | 4.3 | 1.6 | 1.8 | 0.2 | 46 | 282 | 171 | 1.72 | 0.077 | 20.8 | | 0.2 | 0.14 | 0.42 | 11.0 | 23612 |
| **beef chuck arm pot rst, select, 0″ trim,** | 85 | 241 | 45.4 | 0 | 0 | | 0 | 41 | 14 | 16 | 5.84 | 0.008 | 0 | 0 | 0.05 | 3.6 | 1.64 | 0.49 |
| lean and fat, braised - 3 *oz* | | 24.8 | 14.9 | 5.9 | 6.4 | 0.6 | 74 | 200 | 151 | 2.02 | 0.076 | 23.7 | | 0.4 | 0.14 | 0.24 | 7.6 | 13375 |
| **beef chuck arm pot roast, select,** | 85 | 166 | 52.0 | 0 | 0 | | 0 | 47 | 14 | 19 | 6.88 | 0.010 | 0 | 0 | 0.06 | 4.1 | 1.91 | 0.56 |
| 0″ trim, lean, braised - 3 *oz* | | 28.4 | 4.9 | 1.9 | 2.1 | 0.2 | 48 | 230 | 176 | 2.35 | 0.092 | 32.2 | | 0.3 | 0.17 | 0.26 | 9.4 | 13378 |
| **beef chuck arm pot roast, select, ⅛″** | 85 | 203 | 53.4 | 0 | 0 | | 0 | 53 | 15 | 16 | 3.84 | 0.008 | 0 | 0 | 0.06 | 3.7 | 1.27 | 0.47 |
| trim, lean and fat, braised - 3 *oz* | | 16.4 | 14.8 | 6.0 | 6.3 | 0.6 | 54 | 246 | 150 | 1.37 | 0.068 | 17.7 | | 0.3 | 0.11 | 0.41 | 8.5 | 13813 |
| **beef chuck arm pot roast, select,** | 85 | 106 | 63.0 | 0 | 0 | | 0 | 65 | 15 | 20 | 4.83 | 0.010 | 0 | 0 | 0.07 | 4.2 | 1.50 | 0.56 |
| ⅛″ trim, lean, braised - 3 *oz* | | 18.9 | 2.8 | 1.0 | 1.2 | 0.1 | 30 | 288 | 173 | 1.58 | 0.080 | 23.5 | | 0.2 | 0.12 | 0.47 | 11.0 | 23631 |
| **beef chuck blade rst, choice, 0″ trim,** | 85 | 296 | 39.9 | 0 | 0 | | 0 | 55 | 11 | 17 | 7.22 | 0.014 | 0 | 0 | 0.06 | 2.1 | 1.95 | 0.26 |
| lean and fat, braised - 3 *oz* | | 22.9 | 22.0 | 8.7 | 9.5 | 0.8 | 88 | 199 | 173 | 2.69 | 0.108 | 21.2 | 0 | | 0.21 | 0.22 | 4.2 | 13380 |
| **beef chuck blade roast, choice,** | 85 | 225 | 45.9 | 0 | 0 | | 0 | 60 | 11 | 20 | 8.73 | 0.015 | 0 | 0 | 0.07 | 2.3 | 2.10 | 0.30 |
| 0″ trim, lean, braised - 3 *oz* | | 26.4 | 12.5 | 4.8 | 5.4 | 0.4 | 90 | 224 | 200 | 3.13 | 0.126 | 22.7 | 0 | | 0.24 | 0.25 | 5.1 | 13383 |
| **beef chuck blade rst, choice, ⅛″ trim,** | 85 | 225 | 50.9 | 0 | 0 | | 0 | 57 | 8 | 14 | 4.16 | 0.010 | 0 | 0 | 0.08 | 1.8 | 2.86 | 0.25 |
| lean and fat, braised - 3 *oz* | | 14.4 | 18.1 | 7.3 | 8.0 | 0.7 | 61 | 227 | 136 | 1.71 | 0.061 | 13.8 | 0 | | 0.14 | 0.30 | 4.2 | 13817 |
| **beef chuck blade roast, select,** | 85 | 202 | 47.3 | 0 | 0 | | 0 | 60 | 11 | 20 | 8.73 | 0.015 | 0 | 0 | 0.07 | 2.3 | 2.10 | 0.30 |
| 0″ trim, lean, braised - 3 *oz* | | 26.4 | 9.9 | 3.9 | 4.3 | 0.3 | 90 | 224 | 200 | 3.13 | 0.126 | 22.7 | 0 | | 0.24 | 0.25 | 5.1 | 13384 |
| **beef chuck blade rst, slct, 0″ trim,** | 85 | 266 | 42.0 | 0 | 0 | | 0 | 56 | 11 | 17 | 7.45 | 0.014 | 0 | 0 | 0.06 | 2.1 | 1.98 | 0.27 |
| lean and fat, braised - 3 *oz* | | 23.5 | 18.4 | 7.3 | 8.0 | 0.7 | 88 | 203 | 177 | 2.75 | 0.110 | 21.3 | 0 | | 0.21 | 0.22 | 4.2 | 13381 |
| **beef chuck blade rst, slct, ⅛″ trim,** | 85 | 196 | 53.4 | 0 | 0 | | 0 | 59 | 8 | 14 | 4.31 | 0.011 | 0 | 0 | 0.08 | 1.9 | 2.92 | 0.25 |
| lean and fat, braised - 3 *oz* | | 14.8 | 14.7 | 5.9 | 6.5 | 0.5 | 60 | 235 | 139 | 1.76 | 0.063 | 13.9 | 0 | | 0.14 | 0.31 | 4.2 | 13819 |
| **beef chuck clod rst, choice, 0″ trim,** | 85 | 184 | 51.3 | 0 | 0 | | 0 | 60 | 7 | 17 | 5.06 | 0.001 | 0 | 0 | 0.07 | 2.8 | 2.42 | 0.01 |
| lean and fat, rstd - 3 *oz* | | 20.9 | 10.4 | 3.6 | 5.0 | 0.4 | 57 | 309 | 178 | 2.57 | 0.081 | 24.6 | 0 | 0.1 | 0.20 | 0.22 | 7.6 | 23528 |
| **beef chuck clod roast, choice,** | 85 | 145 | 54.7 | 0 | 0 | | 0 | 63 | 6 | 19 | 5.43 | | 0 | 0 | 0.07 | 2.9 | 2.52 | |
| 0″ trim, lean, roasted - 3 *oz* | | 22.1 | 5.7 | 1.7 | 3.0 | 0.2 | 54 | 328 | 190 | 2.72 | 0.085 | 25.5 | 0 | 0.1 | 0.21 | 0.23 | 7.6 | 13937 |
| **beef chuck clod rst, slct, 0″ trim,** | 85 | 167 | 52.8 | 0 | 0 | | 0 | 61 | 6 | 18 | 5.24 | 0 | 0 | 0 | 0.08 | 3.1 | 2.68 | 0.01 |
| lean and fat, rstd - 3 *oz* | | 23.2 | 7.4 | 2.8 | 3.5 | 0.4 | 62 | 316 | 183 | 2.63 | 0.082 | 25.0 | 0 | 0.1 | 0.22 | 0.24 | 8.5 | 23531 |
| **beef chuck clod roast, select,** | 85 | 146 | 54.6 | 0 | 0 | | 0 | 63 | 6 | 19 | 5.43 | | 0 | 0 | 0.08 | 3.1 | 2.74 | |
| 0″ trim, lean, roasted - 3 *oz* | | 23.9 | 4.9 | 1.8 | 2.5 | 0.3 | 61 | 326 | 189 | 2.71 | 0.085 | 25.5 | 0 | 0.1 | 0.22 | 0.25 | 8.5 | 13940 |
| **beef chuck clod steak, choice, 0″ trim,** | 85 | 196 | 47.8 | 0 | 0 | | 0 | 46 | 7 | 18 | 5.75 | 0.001 | 0 | 0 | 0.07 | 2.3 | 2.38 | 0.01 |
| lean and fat, braised - 3 *oz* | | 23.9 | 10.4 | 3.5 | 4.8 | 0.4 | 76 | 246 | 158 | 3.09 | 0.107 | 24.6 | 0 | 0.2 | 0.20 | 0.18 | 6.0 | 23533 |
| **beef chuck clod steak, choice,** | 85 | 164 | 50.5 | 0 | 0 | | 0 | 47 | 6 | 19 | 6.13 | | 0 | 0 | 0.07 | 2.4 | 2.46 | |
| 0″ trim, lean, braised - 3 *oz* | | 25.1 | 6.3 | 1.8 | 3.0 | 0.2 | 76 | 258 | 166 | 3.26 | 0.113 | 25.5 | 0 | 0.2 | 0.21 | 0.18 | 6.0 | 13943 |
| **beef chuck clod steak, select,** | 85 | 162 | 51.2 | 0 | 0 | | 0 | 54 | 8 | 19 | 7.07 | | 0 | 0 | 0.06 | 2.9 | 2.66 | |
| 0″ trim, lean, braised - 3 *oz* | | 25.8 | 5.8 | 2.1 | 2.7 | 0.3 | 84 | 236 | 219 | 3.26 | 0.134 | 25.5 | 0 | 0.2 | 0.23 | 0.26 | 8.5 | 13946 |
| **beef chuck clod stk, slct, 0″ trim,** | 85 | 174 | 50.3 | 0 | 0 | | 0 | 54 | 8 | 18 | 6.92 | 0 | 0 | 0 | 0.06 | 2.9 | 2.63 | 0 |
| lean and fat, braised - 3 *oz* | | 25.4 | 7.3 | 2.7 | 3.3 | 0.3 | 84 | 232 | 215 | 3.20 | 0.132 | 25.2 | 0 | 0.2 | 0.22 | 0.25 | 8.5 | 23536 |
| **beef chuck shldr medallion, choice,** | 85 | 121 | 61.9 | 0 | 0 | | 0 | 51 | 4 | 21 | 3.72 | 0.015 | 0 | 0 | 0.08 | 4.7 | 4.33 | 0.78 |
| 0″ trim, lean, grilled - 3 *oz* | | 17.8 | 4.9 | 1.7 | 1.7 | 0.3 | 49 | 311 | 186 | 2.03 | 0.110 | 27.0 | 0 | 0.1 | 0.23 | 0.44 | 6.0 | 23036 |
| **beef chuck shldr medallion, select,** | 85 | 150 | 55.8 | 0 | 0 | | 0 | 50 | 4 | 21 | 4.45 | 0.012 | 0 | 0 | 0.07 | 4.4 | 4.39 | 0.73 |
| 0″ trim, lean, grilled - 3 *oz* | | 22.3 | 6.1 | 2.4 | 2.5 | 0.3 | 66 | 303 | 191 | 2.20 | 0.145 | 32.9 | 0 | 0.1 | 0.23 | 0.51 | 6.8 | 23054 |
| **beef chuck shldr top blade stk, choice,** | 85 | 141 | 60.5 | 0 | 0 | | 0 | 64 | 5 | 20 | 6.35 | 0.014 | 0 | 0 | 0.12 | 3.0 | 4.45 | 0.84 |
| 0″ trim, lean & fat, grld - 3 *oz* | | 16.5 | 7.8 | 2.9 | 3.1 | 0.4 | 56 | 275 | 168 | 2.23 | 0.099 | 26.8 | 0 | 0.1 | 0.22 | 0.30 | 2.6 | 23043 |
| **beef chuck shldr top blade stk, slct,** | 85 | 150 | 59.9 | 0 | 0 | | 0 | 63 | 5 | 18 | 5.85 | 0.014 | 0 | 0 | 0.08 | 2.9 | 4.29 | 0.81 |
| 0″ trim, lean & fat, grld - 3 *oz* | | 16.1 | 8.9 | 3.4 | 3.5 | 0.4 | 56 | 263 | 156 | 2.01 | 0.101 | 25.3 | 0 | 0.1 | 0.19 | 0.31 | 2.6 | 23059 |
| **beef chuck shldr top/center stk, slct,** | 85 | 156 | 55.3 | 0 | 0 | | 0 | 50 | 4 | 20 | 5.82 | 0.011 | 0 | 0 | 0.06 | 4.4 | 3.88 | 0.67 |
| 0″ trim, lean & fat, grld - 3 *oz* | | 22.2 | 6.9 | 2.6 | 2.9 | 0.3 | 63 | 291 | 190 | 2.18 | 0.082 | 34.1 | 0 | 0.2 | 0.23 | 0.48 | 9.4 | 23038 |
| **beef chuck shldr top/center steak,** | 85 | 155 | 55.1 | 0 | 0 | | 0 | 51 | 4 | 22 | 6.03 | 0.013 | 0 | 0 | 0.06 | 4.5 | 4.21 | 0.71 |
| select, 0″ trim, lean, grld - 3 *oz* | | 22.4 | 6.5 | 2.4 | 2.6 | 0.3 | 65 | 307 | 197 | 2.37 | 0.076 | 35.3 | 0 | 0.2 | 0.25 | 0.49 | 9.4 | 23058 |
| **beef chuck, tndr stk, choice, 0″ trim,** | 85 | 137 | 55.7 | 0 | 0 | | 0 | 62 | 7 | 20 | 6.66 | 0 | 0 | 0 | 0.09 | 3.1 | 2.86 | 0 |
| lean & fat, brld - 3 *oz* | | 21.9 | 4.9 | 1.5 | 2.3 | 0.3 | 55 | 249 | 199 | 2.57 | 0.103 | 21.4 | 0 | 0.1 | 0.19 | 0.27 | 6.8 | 23519 |
| **beef chuck, tender steak, choice,** | 85 | 137 | 55.8 | 0 | 0 | | 0 | 62 | 7 | 20 | 6.66 | | 0 | 0 | 0.09 | 3.1 | 2.86 | |
| 0″ trim, lean, broiled - 3 *oz* | | 21.9 | 4.8 | 1.5 | 2.3 | 0.3 | 55 | 249 | 199 | 2.57 | 0.103 | 21.4 | 0 | 0.1 | 0.19 | 0.27 | 6.8 | 13961 |
| **beef chuck, tndr stk, slct, 0″ trim,** | 85 | 135 | 57.0 | 0 | 0 | | 0 | 58 | 6 | 20 | 6.64 | 0 | 0 | 0 | 0.10 | 3.1 | 2.91 | 0 |
| lean & fat, brld - 3 *oz* | | 22.2 | 4.5 | 1.8 | 2.2 | 0.3 | 51 | 249 | 184 | 2.38 | 0.095 | 21.5 | 0 | 0.1 | 0.20 | 0.28 | 6.8 | 23521 |

| | WT (g) | KCAL | H₂O (g) | CHO (g) | TSUG (g) | ASUG (g) | DFIB (g) | Na (mg) | Ca (mg) | Mg (mg) | Zn (mg) | Mn (mg) | A (mcg RAE) | C (mg) | B-1 (mg) | NIA (mg) | B-12 (mcg) | PANT (mg) |
|---|---|---|---|---|---|---|---|---|---|---|---|---|---|---|---|---|---|---|
| | | PRO (g) | FAT (g) | SFA (g) | MUFA (g) | PUFA (g) | CHOL (mg) | K (mg) | P (mg) | Fe (mg) | Cu (mg) | Se (mcg) | A (IU) | E (mg ATE) | B-2 (mg) | B-6 (mg) | FOL (mcg DFE) | REF |
| **beef chuck, tender steak, select,** | 85 | 133 | 57.2 | 0 | 0 | | 0 | 58 | 6 | 20 | 6.66 | | 0 | 0 | 0.10 | 3.1 | 2.91 | |
| 0″ trim, lean, broiled - 3 oz | | 22.2 | 4.3 | 1.7 | 2.1 | 0.3 | 50 | 249 | 184 | 2.38 | 0.095 | 21.5 | 0 | 0.1 | 0.20 | 0.28 | 6.8 | 13963 |
| **beef chuck, top blade, choice,** | 85 | 193 | 51.6 | 0 | 0 | | 0 | 58 | 6 | 20 | 7.45 | 0 | 0 | 0 | 0.09 | 3.1 | 2.87 | 0 |
| 0″ trim, lean & fat, brld - 3 oz | | 21.9 | 11.0 | 3.5 | 5.3 | 0.4 | 49 | 255 | 183 | 2.35 | 0.094 | 16.9 | 0 | 0.2 | 0.19 | 0.27 | 6.8 | 23523 |
| **beef chuck, top blade, choice,** | 85 | 184 | 52.4 | 0 | 0 | | 0 | 58 | 6 | 20 | 7.58 | | 0 | 0 | 0.10 | 3.1 | 2.91 | |
| 0″ trim, lean, broiled - 3 oz | | 22.2 | 9.9 | 3.1 | 4.9 | 0.3 | 48 | 258 | 185 | 2.39 | 0.096 | 17.0 | 0 | 0.2 | 0.20 | 0.28 | 6.8 | 13965 |
| **beef chuck, top blade, slct, 0″ trim,** | 85 | 170 | 53.4 | 0 | 0 | | 0 | 57 | 6 | 20 | 7.38 | 0 | 0 | 0 | 0.12 | 3.4 | 3.15 | 0 |
| lean & fat, brld - 3 oz | | 21.8 | 8.5 | 3.0 | 3.6 | 0.3 | 57 | 253 | 180 | 2.33 | 0.094 | 16.9 | 0 | 0.1 | 0.19 | 0.40 | 7.6 | 23525 |
| **beef chuck, top blade, select,** | 85 | 156 | 54.7 | 0 | 0 | | 0 | 58 | 6 | 20 | 7.58 | | 0 | 0 | 0.12 | 3.4 | 3.21 | |
| 0″ trim, lean, broiled - 3 oz | | 22.2 | 6.8 | 2.3 | 2.8 | 0.3 | 56 | 258 | 184 | 2.38 | 0.095 | 17.0 | 0 | 0.1 | 0.19 | 0.41 | 7.6 | 13967 |
| **beef flank, choice,** 0″ trim, lean and | 85 | 172 | 53.8 | 0 | 0 | | 0 | 45 | 15 | 19 | 4.07 | 0.008 | 0 | 0 | 0.06 | 6.4 | 1.55 | 0.46 |
| fat, broiled - 3 oz | | 23.4 | 7.9 | 3.3 | 3.2 | 0.3 | 43 | 277 | 171 | 1.53 | 0.075 | 24.6 | 0 | 0.3 | 0.10 | 0.47 | 7.6 | 13067 |
| **beef flank, choice,** 0″ trim, lean, | 85 | 201 | 48.7 | 0 | 0 | | 0 | 61 | 5 | 20 | 5.14 | 0.016 | 0 | 0 | 0.12 | 3.9 | 2.90 | 0.32 |
| braised - 3 oz | | 23.8 | 11.0 | 4.7 | 4.6 | 0.3 | 60 | 298 | 227 | 2.95 | 0.105 | 26.2 | 0 | 0.1 | 0.16 | 0.31 | 7.6 | 13069 |
| **beef flank, choice,** 0″ trim, lean, | 85 | 165 | 54.5 | 0 | 0 | | 0 | 48 | 13 | 20 | 4.34 | 0.008 | 0 | 0 | 0.06 | 7.0 | 1.48 | 0.46 |
| broiled - 3 oz | | 23.6 | 7.1 | 2.9 | 2.8 | 0.3 | 47 | 287 | 179 | 1.56 | 0.073 | 26.5 | 0 | 0.3 | 0.12 | 0.49 | 7.6 | 13070 |
| **beef flank, select,** 0″ trim, lean and | 85 | 156 | 55.3 | 0 | 0 | | 0 | 49 | 19 | 20 | 4.26 | 0.008 | 0 | 0 | 0.07 | 6.2 | 1.22 | 0.47 |
| fat, broiled - 3 oz | | 23.6 | 6.1 | 2.5 | 2.4 | 0.2 | 33 | 298 | 187 | 1.43 | 0.065 | 25.3 | 0 | 0.3 | 0.12 | 0.52 | 7.6 | 13949 |
| **beef flank, select,** 0″ trim, lean, | 85 | 151 | 55.7 | 0 | 0 | | 0 | 50 | 17 | 20 | 4.33 | 0.008 | 0 | 0 | 0.07 | 6.9 | 1.14 | 0.47 |
| broiled - 3 oz | | 23.8 | 5.5 | 2.3 | 2.2 | 0.2 | 37 | 310 | 192 | 1.45 | 0.065 | 29.5 | 0 | 0.3 | 0.13 | 0.53 | 7.6 | 23655 |
| **beef, ground, 10% fat, crumbles,** | 85 | 196 | 49.8 | 0 | 0 | | 0 | 74 | 14 | 23 | 5.81 | 0.011 | 0 | 0 | 0.04 | 5.8 | 2.30 | 0.69 |
| pan-browned - 3 oz | | 24.2 | 10.2 | 4.0 | 4.3 | 0.4 | 76 | 368 | 212 | 2.62 | 0.084 | 18.1 | 0 | 0.4 | 0.16 | 0.36 | 6.8 | 23565 |
| **beef, ground, 10% fat, loaf,** baked | 85 | 182 | 52.1 | 0 | 0 | | 0 | 52 | 11 | 18 | 5.65 | 0.008 | 0 | 0 | 0.03 | 4.4 | 2.12 | 0.53 |
| 3 oz piece | | 22.6 | 9.4 | 3.7 | 4.0 | 0.3 | 73 | 255 | 164 | 2.46 | 0.066 | 18.4 | 0 | 0.3 | 0.15 | 0.30 | 5.1 | 23566 |
| **beef, ground, 10% fat, patty,** | 85 | 184 | 52.1 | 0 | 0 | | 0 | 58 | 11 | 19 | 5.41 | 0.011 | 0 | 0 | 0.04 | 4.8 | 2.18 | 0.55 |
| broiled - 3 oz patty | | 22.2 | 10.0 | 3.9 | 4.2 | 0.4 | 72 | 283 | 172 | 2.30 | 0.077 | 18.4 | 0 | 0.3 | 0.15 | 0.34 | 6.8 | 23563 |
| **beef, ground, 10% fat, patty,** | 85 | 173 | 53.7 | 0 | 0 | | 0 | 64 | 13 | 20 | 5.38 | 0.009 | 0 | 0 | 0.04 | 5.1 | 2.51 | 0.53 |
| pan-broiled - 3 oz patty | | 21.4 | 9.1 | 3.6 | 3.8 | 0.3 | 70 | 309 | 184 | 2.35 | 0.073 | 17.6 | 0 | 0.3 | 0.15 | 0.32 | 6.8 | 23564 |
| **beef, ground, 15% fat, crumbles,** | 85 | 218 | 47.5 | 0 | 0 | | 0 | 76 | 19 | 21 | 5.63 | 0.010 | 0 | 0 | 0.04 | 5.4 | 2.37 | 0.69 |
| pan-browned - 3 oz | | 23.6 | 13.0 | 4.9 | 5.6 | 0.4 | 76 | 346 | 202 | 2.49 | 0.079 | 18.4 | 0 | 0.4 | 0.16 | 0.36 | 8.5 | 23570 |
| **beef, ground, 15% fat, loaf,** baked | 85 | 204 | 50.1 | 0 | 0 | | 0 | 54 | 15 | 17 | 5.48 | 0.008 | 0 | 0 | 0.03 | 4.2 | 2.12 | 0.51 |
| 3 oz piece | | 22.0 | 12.2 | 4.6 | 5.3 | 0.4 | 77 | 243 | 158 | 2.33 | 0.067 | 17.8 | 0 | 0.4 | 0.15 | 0.29 | 5.1 | 23571 |
| **beef, ground, 15% fat, patty,** | 85 | 212 | 49.3 | 0 | 0 | | 0 | 61 | 15 | 18 | 5.36 | 0.010 | 0 | 0 | 0.04 | 4.6 | 2.24 | 0.56 |
| broiled - 3 oz patty | | 22.0 | 13.2 | 5.0 | 5.7 | 0.4 | 76 | 270 | 168 | 2.21 | 0.072 | 18.4 | 0 | 0.4 | 0.15 | 0.32 | 7.6 | 23568 |
| **beef, ground, 15% fat, patty,** | 85 | 197 | 51.5 | 0 | 0 | | 0 | 67 | 17 | 19 | 5.27 | 0.009 | 0 | 0 | 0.04 | 4.9 | 2.39 | 0.53 |
| pan-broiled - 3 oz patty | | 20.9 | 11.9 | 4.5 | 5.1 | 0.4 | 73 | 297 | 179 | 2.28 | 0.069 | 17.3 | 0 | 0.4 | 0.15 | 0.31 | 6.8 | 23569 |
| **beef, ground, 20% fat, crumbles,** | 85 | 231 | 46.4 | 0 | 0 | | 0 | 77 | 24 | 20 | 5.44 | 0.010 | 0 | 0 | 0.04 | 5.0 | 2.43 | 0.69 |
| pan-browned - 3 oz | | 23.0 | 14.8 | 5.6 | 6.5 | 0.4 | 76 | 323 | 192 | 2.36 | 0.074 | 18.5 | 0 | 0.4 | 0.16 | 0.36 | 9.4 | 23575 |
| **beef, ground, 20% fat, loaf,** baked | 85 | 216 | 49.0 | 0 | 0 | | 0 | 57 | 20 | 16 | 5.30 | 0.008 | 0 | 0 | 0.04 | 3.9 | 2.11 | 0.48 |
| 3 oz piece | | 21.5 | 13.7 | 5.2 | 6.1 | 0.4 | 76 | 230 | 152 | 2.19 | 0.068 | 17.3 | 0 | 0.4 | 0.14 | 0.28 | 6.0 | 23576 |
| **beef, ground, 20% fat, patty,** | 85 | 230 | 47.7 | 0 | 0 | | 0 | 64 | 20 | 17 | 5.31 | 0.009 | 0 | 0 | 0.04 | 4.3 | 2.32 | 0.57 |
| broiled - 3 oz patty | | 21.9 | 15.1 | 5.7 | 6.7 | 0.4 | 77 | 258 | 165 | 2.11 | 0.068 | 18.3 | 0 | 0.4 | 0.15 | 0.31 | 8.5 | 23573 |
| **beef, ground, 20% fat, patty,** | 85 | 209 | 50.2 | 0 | 0 | | 0 | 71 | 22 | 18 | 5.16 | 0.009 | 0 | 0 | 0.04 | 4.7 | 2.26 | 0.53 |
| pan-broiled - 3 oz patty | | 20.4 | 13.5 | 5.1 | 6.0 | 0.4 | 73 | 285 | 174 | 2.20 | 0.065 | 16.9 | 0 | 0.4 | 0.15 | 0.30 | 7.6 | 23574 |
| **beef, ground, 25% fat, crumbles,** | 85 | 235 | 46.3 | 0 | 0 | | 0 | 79 | 29 | 19 | 5.24 | 0.010 | 0 | 0 | 0.04 | 4.5 | 2.50 | 0.68 |
| pan-browned - 3 oz | | 22.3 | 15.5 | 6.0 | 7.1 | 0.4 | 76 | 301 | 182 | 2.24 | 0.068 | 18.7 | 0 | 0.4 | 0.16 | 0.36 | 10.2 | 23580 |
| **beef, ground, 25% fat, loaf,** baked | 85 | 216 | 48.9 | 0 | 0 | | 0 | 60 | 24 | 15 | 5.13 | 0.008 | 0 | 0 | 0.04 | 3.7 | 2.10 | 0.46 |
| 3 oz piece | | 20.9 | 14.0 | 5.4 | 6.4 | 0.4 | 70 | 218 | 146 | 2.07 | 0.068 | 16.7 | 0 | 0.4 | 0.14 | 0.27 | 6.0 | 23581 |
| **beef, ground, 25% fat, patty,** | 85 | 236 | 47.2 | 0 | 0 | | 0 | 66 | 26 | 17 | 5.26 | 0.008 | 0 | 0 | 0.04 | 4.1 | 2.39 | 0.57 |
| broiled - 3 oz patty | | 21.7 | 15.9 | 6.2 | 7.3 | 0.4 | 76 | 246 | 161 | 2.01 | 0.064 | 18.2 | 0 | 0.4 | 0.15 | 0.30 | 9.4 | 23578 |
| **beef, ground, 25% fat, patty,** | 85 | 211 | 49.9 | 0 | 0 | | 0 | 74 | 27 | 17 | 5.06 | 0.009 | 0 | 0 | 0.04 | 4.5 | 2.14 | 0.53 |
| pan-broiled - 3 oz patty | | 19.9 | 14.0 | 5.4 | 6.4 | 0.4 | 71 | 274 | 169 | 2.12 | 0.060 | 16.7 | 0 | 0.4 | 0.15 | 0.29 | 8.5 | 23579 |
| **beef, ground, 30% fat,** broiled | 85 | 232 | 47.8 | 0 | 0 | | 0 | 69 | 30 | 16 | 5.22 | 0.008 | 0 | 0 | 0.04 | 3.9 | 2.46 | 0.58 |
| 3 oz | | 21.6 | 15.5 | 6.2 | 7.5 | 0.4 | 70 | 234 | 157 | 1.91 | 0.059 | 18.2 | 0 | 0.4 | 0.15 | 0.29 | 9.4 | 13497 |
| **beef, ground, 30% fat, crumbles,** | 85 | 230 | 47.4 | 0 | 0 | | 0 | 82 | 35 | 17 | 5.06 | 0.010 | 0 | 0 | 0.04 | 4.1 | 2.56 | 0.68 |
| pan-browned - 3 oz | | 21.7 | 15.2 | 6.1 | 7.4 | 0.4 | 75 | 279 | 172 | 2.11 | 0.063 | 18.9 | 0 | 0.4 | 0.16 | 0.36 | 11.0 | 13494 |
| **beef, ground, 30% fat, loaf,** baked | 85 | 205 | 49.6 | 0 | 0 | | 0 | 62 | 28 | 14 | 4.96 | 0.008 | 0 | 0 | 0.04 | 3.4 | 2.09 | 0.44 |
| 3 oz piece | | 20.3 | 13.1 | 5.3 | 6.3 | 0.4 | 56 | 205 | 141 | 1.93 | 0.069 | 16.2 | 0 | 0.4 | 0.14 | 0.26 | 6.0 | 13495 |
| **beef, ground, 30% fat, patty,** | 85 | 202 | 50.5 | 0 | 0 | | 0 | 78 | 31 | 17 | 4.95 | 0.009 | 0 | 0 | 0.04 | 4.3 | 2.01 | 0.52 |
| pan-broiled - 3 oz patty | | 19.4 | 13.2 | 5.3 | 6.4 | 0.4 | 66 | 262 | 165 | 2.05 | 0.056 | 16.3 | 0 | 0.4 | 0.15 | 0.28 | 8.5 | 13496 |
| **beef, ground, 5% fat, crumbles,** | 85 | 164 | 53.2 | 0 | 0 | | 0 | 72 | 8 | 24 | 6.00 | 0.011 | 0 | 0 | 0.04 | 6.2 | 2.24 | 0.69 |
| pan-browned - 3 oz | | 24.8 | 6.4 | 2.9 | 2.7 | 0.3 | 76 | 390 | 224 | 2.75 | 0.090 | 17.9 | 0 | 0.3 | 0.17 | 0.36 | 6.0 | 23560 |

| | WT(g) / PRO(g) | KCAL / FAT(g) | $H_2O$(g) / SFA(g) | CHO(g) / MUFA(g) | TSUG(g) / PUFA(g) | ASUG(g) / CHOL(mg) | DFIB(g) | Na(mg) / K(mg) | Ca(mg) / P(mg) | Mg(mg) / Fe(mg) | Zn(mg) / Cu(mg) | Mn(mg) / Se(mcg) | A(mcg RAE) / A(IU) | C(mg) / E(mg ATE) | B-1(mg) / B-2(mg) | NIA(mg) / B-6(mg) | B-12(mcg) / FOL(mcg DFE) | PANT(mg) / REF |
|---|---|---|---|---|---|---|---|---|---|---|---|---|---|---|---|---|---|---|
| **beef, ground, 5% fat, loaf**, baked | 85 | 148 | 55.0 | 0 | 0 | | 0 | 49 | 7 | 19 | 5.83 | 0.009 | 0 | 0 | 0.03 | 4.7 | 2.12 | 0.56 |
| *3 oz piece* | | 23.2 | 5.4 | 2.5 | 2.2 | 0.3 | 62 | 268 | 169 | 2.59 | 0.066 | 19.0 | 0 | 0.3 | 0.15 | 0.30 | 5.1 | 23561 |
| **beef, ground, 5% fat, patty**, broiled | 85 | 145 | 56.1 | 0 | 0 | | 0 | 55 | 6 | 19 | 5.47 | 0.012 | 0 | 0 | 0.04 | 5.0 | 2.10 | 0.54 |
| *3 oz patty* | | 22.3 | 5.6 | 2.5 | 2.3 | 0.3 | 65 | 296 | 175 | 2.41 | 0.082 | 18.4 | 0 | 0.3 | 0.15 | 0.35 | 6.0 | 23558 |
| **beef, ground, 5% fat, patty,** pan-broiled - 3 oz patty | 85 | 139 | 56.9 | 0 | 0 | | 0 | 60 | 8 | 20 | 5.48 | 0.009 | 0 | 0 | 0.04 | 5.3 | 2.64 | 0.53 |
| | | 21.9 | 5.0 | 2.3 | 2.1 | 0.3 | 65 | 320 | 189 | 2.42 | 0.077 | 17.9 | 0 | 0.3 | 0.15 | 0.33 | 6.0 | 23559 |
| **beef patty with vegetable protein**, frozen, cooked - 3 oz | 85 | 210 | 49.8 | 6.7 | | | 1.2 | 56 | 33 | 42 | 7.07 | 0.298 | 14 | 0 | 0.22 | 3.3 | 2.44 | 0.99 |
| | | 13.3 | 14.4 | 5.3 | 6.6 | 0.5 | 32 | 276 | 200 | 3.09 | 0.213 | 12.4 | 76 | | 0.18 | 0.22 | 14.4 | 23501 |
| **beef patty with vegetable protein**, frozen, raw - 3 oz | 85 | 191 | 53.8 | 3.3 | | | 1.1 | 47 | 25 | 31 | 4.62 | 0.214 | 14 | 0 | 0.27 | 3.6 | 3.05 | 1.24 |
| | | 12.9 | 14.0 | 5.0 | 6.5 | 0.5 | 28 | 250 | 162 | 2.26 | 0.139 | 9.9 | 82 | | 0.19 | 0.37 | | 23506 |
| **beef ribeye, sml end (ribs 10–12)**, chc, 0" trim, lean & fat, brld - 3 oz | 85 | 233 | 49.3 | 0 | | | 0 | 48 | 8 | 15 | 3.27 | 0.010 | 0 | 0 | 0.07 | 2.7 | 2.64 | 0.25 |
| | | 14.9 | 18.8 | 7.6 | 8.1 | 0.7 | 58 | 259 | 143 | 1.59 | 0.051 | 14.0 | 0 | | 0.11 | 0.31 | 4.2 | 13095 |
| **beef ribeye, small end (ribs 10–12),** choice, 0" trim, lean, brld - 3 oz | 85 | 137 | 58.4 | 0 | | | 0 | 54 | 8 | 19 | 3.96 | 0.012 | 0 | 0 | 0.08 | 3.2 | 3.03 | 0.29 |
| | | 17.1 | 7.1 | 2.7 | 3.0 | 0.2 | 50 | 317 | 167 | 1.85 | 0.057 | 14.5 | 0 | | 0.13 | 0.36 | 5.1 | 13097 |
| **beef ribeye, sml end (ribs 10–12)**, slct, 0" trim, lean & fat, brld - 3 oz | 85 | 210 | 48.9 | 0 | | | 0 | 48 | 17 | 20 | 4.19 | 0.008 | 0 | 0 | 0.06 | 6.2 | 1.36 | 0.46 |
| | | 23.2 | 12.5 | 4.9 | 5.1 | 0.5 | 94 | 289 | 180 | 1.49 | 0.070 | 25.1 | 0 | 0.4 | 0.11 | 0.49 | 6.8 | 13952 |
| **beef ribeye, small end (ribs 10–12),** select, 0" trim, lean, brld - 3 oz | 85 | 155 | 54.3 | 0 | | | 0 | 54 | 18 | 22 | 4.64 | 0.009 | 0 | 0 | 0.07 | 7.4 | 1.22 | 0.50 |
| | | 25.4 | 5.1 | 2.0 | 2.1 | 0.2 | 52 | 333 | 206 | 1.56 | 0.069 | 31.7 | 0 | 0.3 | 0.14 | 0.56 | | 13490 |
| **beef ribs, large end (ribs 6–9)**, choice, 0" trim, lean & fat, rstd - 3 oz | 85 | 316 | 39.2 | 0 | | | 0 | 54 | 8 | 17 | 4.90 | 0.011 | 0 | 0 | 0.06 | 3.1 | 1.98 | 0.31 |
| | | 19.4 | 25.9 | 10.4 | 11.1 | 0.9 | 72 | 246 | 146 | 1.98 | 0.075 | 18.0 | | | 0.16 | 0.20 | 6.0 | 13386 |
| **beef ribs, large end (ribs 6–9)**, choice, 0" trim, lean, rstd - 3 oz | 85 | 215 | 48.3 | 0 | | | 0 | 62 | 7 | 21 | 6.34 | 0.014 | 0 | 0 | 0.08 | 3.8 | 2.22 | 0.38 |
| | | 23.4 | 12.8 | 5.1 | 5.3 | 0.4 | 69 | 303 | 178 | 2.40 | 0.089 | 19.4 | 0 | | 0.19 | 0.22 | 7.6 | 13389 |
| **beef ribs, shortribs**, lean and fat, braised - 3 oz | 85 | 400 | 30.4 | 0 | | | 0 | 42 | 10 | 13 | 4.15 | 0.011 | 0 | 0 | 0.04 | 2.1 | 2.23 | 0.21 |
| | | 18.3 | 35.7 | 15.1 | 16.0 | 1.3 | 80 | 190 | 138 | 1.96 | 0.084 | 17.7 | 0 | 0.2 | 0.13 | 0.19 | 4.2 | 13148 |
| **beef ribs, shortribs**, lean, braised 3 oz | 85 | 251 | 42.6 | 0 | | | 0 | 49 | 9 | 19 | 6.63 | 0.015 | 0 | 0 | 0.06 | 2.7 | 2.94 | 0.29 |
| | | 26.1 | 15.4 | 6.6 | 6.8 | 0.5 | 79 | 266 | 200 | 2.86 | 0.091 | 18.8 | 0 | 0.1 | 0.17 | 0.24 | 6.0 | 13150 |
| **beef ribs, sml end (ribs 10–12)**, chc, 0" trim, lean & fat, brld - 3 oz | 85 | 265 | 43.4 | 0 | | | 0 | 54 | 11 | 20 | 5.04 | 0.012 | 0 | 0 | 0.08 | 3.6 | 2.55 | 0.26 |
| | | 21.0 | 19.4 | 7.9 | 8.3 | 0.7 | 71 | 291 | 156 | 1.94 | 0.076 | 17.8 | 0 | | 0.16 | 0.30 | 6.0 | 13392 |
| **beef ribs, small end (ribs 10–12),** choice, 0" trim, lean, brld - 3 oz | 85 | 191 | 49.9 | 0 | | | 0 | 59 | 11 | 23 | 5.94 | 0.014 | 0 | 0 | 0.08 | 4.1 | 2.82 | 0.29 |
| | | 23.8 | 9.9 | 4.0 | 4.2 | 0.3 | 68 | 335 | 177 | 2.18 | 0.085 | 18.6 | 0 | | 0.19 | 0.34 | 6.8 | 13395 |
| **beef ribs, sml end (ribs 10–12)**, chc, ⅛" trim, lean & fat, brld - 3 oz | 85 | 224 | 51.1 | 0 | | | 0 | 41 | 20 | 16 | 2.87 | 0.010 | 0 | 0 | 0.04 | 5.2 | 0.90 | 0.47 |
| | | 16.2 | 17.1 | 6.9 | 7.3 | 0.7 | 63 | 249 | 146 | 1.17 | 0.054 | 17.6 | 0 | 0.4 | 0.07 | 0.44 | 8.5 | 13853 |
| **beef ribs, small end (ribs 10–12),** choice, ⅛" trim, lean, brld - 3 oz | 85 | 166 | 54.6 | 0 | | | 0 | 53 | 16 | 21 | 4.67 | 0.009 | 0 | 0 | 0.07 | 7.2 | 1.44 | 0.49 |
| | | 25.1 | 6.5 | 2.5 | 2.6 | 0.2 | 60 | 321 | 200 | 1.60 | 0.074 | 29.2 | 0 | 0.3 | 0.13 | 0.54 | 8.5 | 23638 |
| **beef ribs, small end (ribs 10–12)**, slct, 0" trim, lean & fat, brld - 3 oz | 85 | 242 | 44.9 | 0 | | | 0 | 54 | 11 | 20 | 5.08 | 0.012 | 0 | 0 | 0.08 | 3.6 | 2.56 | 0.26 |
| | | 21.2 | 16.8 | 6.8 | 7.2 | 0.6 | 71 | 292 | 156 | 1.95 | 0.076 | 17.9 | 0 | | 0.16 | 0.30 | 6.0 | 13393 |
| **beef ribs, small end (ribs 10–12),** slct, 0" trim, lean, brld - 3 oz | 85 | 168 | 51.3 | 0 | | | 0 | 59 | 11 | 23 | 5.94 | 0.014 | 0 | 0 | 0.08 | 4.1 | 2.82 | 0.29 |
| | | 23.8 | 7.4 | 3.0 | 3.1 | 0.2 | 68 | 335 | 177 | 2.18 | 0.085 | 18.6 | 0 | | 0.19 | 0.34 | 6.8 | 13396 |
| **beef ribs, small end (ribs 10–12)**, slct, ⅛" trim, lean & fat, rstd - 3 oz | 85 | 285 | 45.2 | 0 | | | 0 | 45 | 8 | 14 | 3.08 | 0.010 | 0 | 0 | 0.07 | 2.6 | 2.52 | 0.24 |
| | | 14.2 | 24.8 | 10.3 | 10.9 | 0.9 | 60 | 243 | 136 | 1.50 | 0.048 | 13.9 | 0 | | 0.11 | 0.30 | 4.2 | 13859 |
| **beef ribs, small end (ribs 10–12),** slct, ⅛" trim, lean & fat, rstd - 3 oz | 85 | 301 | 40.3 | 0 | | | 0 | 54 | 11 | 19 | 4.87 | 0.012 | 0 | 0 | 0.08 | 3.5 | 2.50 | 0.26 |
| | | 20.5 | 23.7 | 9.8 | 10.3 | 0.8 | 71 | 282 | 151 | 1.90 | 0.075 | 18.4 | 0 | | 0.16 | 0.29 | 6.0 | 13860 |
| **beef ribs, small end (ribs 10–12),** slct, ⅛" trim, lean, brld - 3 oz | 85 | 126 | 60.6 | 0 | | | 0 | 48 | 24 | 20 | 3.51 | 0.012 | 0 | 0 | 0.05 | 6.4 | 1.02 | 0.56 |
| | | 18.8 | 5.0 | 1.9 | 2.0 | 0.2 | 51 | 290 | 173 | 1.39 | 0.061 | 21.7 | 0 | 0.3 | 0.09 | 0.52 | 11.0 | 23623 |
| **beef ribs, sml end (ribs 20–12)**, chc, ⅛" trim, lean & fat, rstd - 3 oz | 85 | 258 | 45.0 | 0 | | | 0 | 42 | 14 | 17 | 3.71 | 0.008 | 0 | 0 | 0.05 | 5.7 | 1.38 | 0.41 |
| | | 20.9 | 18.8 | 7.4 | 7.8 | 0.7 | 99 | 253 | 156 | 1.39 | 0.068 | 22.4 | 0 | 0.4 | 0.09 | 0.42 | 6.8 | 13854 |
| **beef round, bottom, choice**, 0" trim, lean and fat, braised - 3 oz | 85 | 196 | 48.2 | 0 | | | 0 | 36 | 6 | 18 | 4.60 | 0.009 | 0 | 0 | 0.06 | 5.0 | 1.67 | 0.55 |
| | | 27.8 | 8.5 | 3.1 | 3.6 | 0.3 | 95 | 224 | 169 | 2.30 | 0.060 | 29.3 | 0 | 0.4 | 0.16 | 0.37 | 8.5 | 13401 |
| **beef round, bottom, choice**, 0" trim, lean and fat, roasted - 3 oz | 85 | 169 | 54.0 | 0 | | | 0 | 30 | 5 | 14 | 3.75 | 0.008 | 0 | 0 | 0.05 | 4.1 | 1.37 | 0.45 |
| | | 22.7 | 8.0 | 2.9 | 3.4 | 0.3 | 89 | 183 | 138 | 1.87 | 0.049 | 23.9 | 0 | 0.3 | 0.13 | 0.30 | 6.8 | 13402 |
| **beef round, bottom, choice**, 0" trim, lean, braised - 3 oz | 85 | 190 | 48.8 | 0 | | | 0 | 37 | 6 | 19 | 4.92 | 0.009 | 0 | 0 | 0.06 | 5.4 | 1.66 | 0.55 |
| | | 28.1 | 7.7 | 2.7 | 3.2 | 0.3 | 104 | 230 | 178 | 2.49 | 0.066 | 32.1 | 0 | 0.4 | 0.18 | 0.39 | 9.4 | 13410 |
| **beef round, bottom, choice**, 0" trim, lean, roasted - 3 oz | 85 | 157 | 55.1 | 0 | | | 0 | 31 | 5 | 15 | 4.03 | 0.008 | 0 | 0 | 0.05 | 4.4 | 1.37 | 0.45 |
| | | 23.1 | 6.5 | 2.3 | 2.7 | 0.2 | 88 | 189 | 146 | 2.04 | 0.054 | 26.3 | 0 | 0.3 | 0.14 | 0.32 | 7.6 | 13411 |
| **beef round, bottom, choice**, ⅛" trim, lean and fat, braised - 3 oz | 85 | 168 | 56.4 | 0 | | | 0 | 45 | 14 | 19 | 3.23 | 0.011 | 0 | 0 | 0.07 | 5.3 | 1.50 | 0.51 |
| | | 17.6 | 10.3 | 4.1 | 4.5 | 0.4 | 52 | 271 | 167 | 1.56 | 0.078 | 21.2 | 0 | 0.3 | 0.12 | 0.52 | 9.4 | 13871 |
| **beef round, bottom, choice**, ⅛" trim, lean and fat, roasted - 3 oz | 85 | 216 | 46.1 | 0 | | | 0 | 36 | 6 | 18 | 4.59 | 0.009 | 0 | 0 | 0.06 | 5.0 | 1.67 | 0.55 |
| | | 27.9 | 10.7 | 4.1 | 4.6 | 0.4 | 68 | 224 | 169 | 2.30 | 0.060 | 29.2 | 0 | 0.4 | 0.16 | 0.37 | 8.5 | 13872 |
| **beef round, bottom, choice**, ⅛" trim, lean, braised - 3 oz | 85 | 109 | 61.7 | 0 | | | 0 | 50 | 17 | 20 | 3.59 | 0.012 | 0 | 0 | 0.08 | 5.7 | 1.33 | 0.56 |
| | | 18.9 | 3.7 | 1.3 | 1.5 | 0.2 | 49 | 298 | 182 | 1.63 | 0.084 | 24.0 | 0 | 0.2 | 0.12 | 0.56 | 11.0 | 23594 |

| Food | WT (g) | KCAL / PRO | $H_2O$ / FAT | CHO / SFA | TSUG / MUFA | ASUG / PUFA | DFIB / CHOL | Na / K | Ca / P | Mg / Fe | Zn / Cu | Mn / Se | A (mcg RAE) / A (IU) | C / E | B-1 / B-2 | NIA / B-6 | B-12 / FOL | PANT / REF |
|---|---|---|---|---|---|---|---|---|---|---|---|---|---|---|---|---|---|---|
| beef round, bottom, choice, ⅛" trim, lean, roasted - 3 oz | 85 | 119 | 61.2 | 0 | 0 |  | 0 | 48 | 16 | 20 | 3.54 | 0.012 | 0 | 0 | 0.08 | 5.7 | 1.57 | 0.37 |
|  |  | 18.9 | 4.2 | 1.4 | 1.8 | 0.2 | 57 | 290 | 183 | 1.75 | 0.083 | 23.5 | 0 | 0.3 | 0.14 | 0.56 | 11.0 | 23618 |
| beef round, bottom, select, 0" trim, lean and fat, braised - 3 oz | 85 | 184 | 49.2 | 0 | 0 |  | 0 | 38 | 8 | 19 | 4.91 | 0.010 | 0 | 0 | 0.07 | 4.9 | 1.50 | 0.58 |
|  |  | 29.2 | 6.6 | 2.4 | 2.8 | 0.2 | 73 | 237 | 184 | 2.33 | 0.075 | 28.7 | 0 | 0.4 | 0.15 | 0.38 | 9.4 | 13404 |
| beef round, bottom, select, 0" trim, lean and fat, roasted - 3 oz | 85 | 149 | 55.6 | 0 | 0 |  | 0 | 31 | 6 | 16 | 4.09 | 0.008 | 0 | 0 | 0.06 | 4.0 | 1.22 | 0.47 |
|  |  | 23.9 | 5.2 | 1.9 | 2.2 | 0.2 | 58 | 197 | 152 | 1.94 | 0.062 | 23.9 | 0 | 0.3 | 0.12 | 0.31 | 7.6 | 13405 |
| beef round, bottom, select, 0" trim, lean, braised - 3 oz | 85 | 175 | 50.0 | 0 | 0 |  | 0 | 39 | 6 | 20 | 5.07 | 0.011 | 0 | 0 | 0.07 | 5.1 | 1.53 | 0.58 |
|  |  | 29.7 | 5.4 | 1.9 | 2.3 | 0.2 | 72 | 246 | 189 | 2.42 | 0.082 | 36.8 | 0 | 0.4 | 0.16 | 0.39 | 10.2 | 13413 |
| beef round, bottom, select, 0" trim, lean, roasted - 3 oz | 85 | 144 | 56.0 | 0 | 0 |  | 0 | 32 | 5 | 16 | 4.18 | 0.008 | 0 | 0 | 0.06 | 4.1 | 1.23 | 0.47 |
|  |  | 24.0 | 4.5 | 1.6 | 1.9 | 0.2 | 61 | 202 | 156 | 2.00 | 0.067 | 30.3 | 0 | 0.3 | 0.13 | 0.32 | 7.6 | 13414 |
| beef round, bottom, select, ⅛" trim lean and fat, braised - 3 oz | 85 | 159 | 57.3 | 0 | 0 |  | 0 | 51 | 20 | 19 | 3.27 | 0.011 | 0 | 0 | 0.07 | 5.2 | 1.05 | 0.50 |
|  |  | 17.6 | 9.3 | 3.7 | 4.0 | 0.4 | 47 | 285 | 171 | 1.39 | 0.076 | 21.0 | 0 | 0.3 | 0.09 | 0.52 | 9.4 | 13874 |
| beef round, bottom, select, ⅛" trim lean and fat, roasted - 3 oz | 85 | 204 | 47.3 | 0 | 0 |  | 0 | 37 | 7 | 19 | 4.74 | 0.010 | 0 | 0 | 0.07 | 4.7 | 1.42 | 0.55 |
|  |  | 27.8 | 9.5 | 3.6 | 4.1 | 0.4 | 61 | 229 | 177 | 2.24 | 0.072 | 27.7 | 0 | 0.4 | 0.14 | 0.36 | 8.5 | 13875 |
| beef round, bottom, select, ⅛" trim, lean, braised - 3 oz | 85 | 194 | 48.0 | 0 | 0 |  | 0 | 38 | 6 | 20 | 5.06 | 0.010 | 0 | 0 | 0.06 | 5.6 | 1.72 | 0.57 |
|  |  | 29.1 | 7.7 | 2.6 | 3.2 | 0.3 | 101 | 236 | 183 | 2.56 | 0.068 | 33.0 | 0 | 0.4 | 0.18 | 0.41 | 9.4 | 23622 |
| beef round, bottom, select, ⅛" trim, lean, roasted - 3 oz | 85 | 139 | 56.6 | 0 | 0 |  | 0 | 32 | 5 | 16 | 4.18 | 0.008 | 0 | 0 | 0.06 | 4.2 | 1.24 | 0.48 |
|  |  | 24.2 | 4.0 | 1.4 | 1.7 | 0.2 | 52 | 202 | 156 | 2.00 | 0.067 | 30.3 | 0 | 0.3 | 0.13 | 0.32 | 8.5 | 23590 |
| beef round, eye of, choice, 0" trim, lean and fat, roasted - 3 oz | 85 | 141 | 56.1 | 0 | 0 |  | 0 | 31 | 5 | 15 | 4.03 | 0.008 | 0 | 0 | 0.05 | 4.4 | 1.46 | 0.48 |
|  |  | 24.3 | 4.1 | 1.5 | 1.8 | 0.2 | 46 | 196 | 149 | 2.01 | 0.054 | 25.7 | 0 | 0.3 | 0.14 | 0.32 | 7.6 | 13416 |
| beef round, eye of, choice, 0" trim, lean, roasted - 3 oz | 85 | 138 | 56.5 | 0 | 0 |  | 0 | 32 | 5 | 16 | 4.28 | 0.008 | 0 | 0 | 0.05 | 4.7 | 1.44 | 0.48 |
|  |  | 24.4 | 3.7 | 1.3 | 1.5 | 0.1 | 49 | 201 | 155 | 2.17 | 0.058 | 28.0 | 0 | 0.3 | 0.15 | 0.34 | 8.5 | 13419 |
| beef round, eye of, choice, ⅛" trim, lean and fat, roasted - 3 oz | 85 | 147 | 58.3 | 0 | 0 |  | 0 | 47 | 14 | 20 | 3.37 | 0.011 | 0 | 0 | 0.07 | 5.6 | 1.56 | 0.54 |
|  |  | 18.4 | 7.6 | 3.0 | 3.3 | 0.3 | 37 | 284 | 175 | 1.63 | 0.082 | 22.2 | 0 | 0.3 | 0.13 | 0.54 | 10.2 | 13879 |
| beef round, eye of, choice, ⅛" trim, lean, roasted - 3 oz | 85 | 149 | 55.0 | 0 | 0 |  | 0 | 33 | 5 | 17 | 4.39 | 0.008 | 0 | 0 | 0.05 | 4.9 | 1.50 | 0.50 |
|  |  | 25.4 | 4.5 | 1.6 | 1.9 | 0.2 | 60 | 205 | 159 | 2.22 | 0.059 | 28.6 | 0 | 0.3 | 0.16 | 0.35 | 8.5 | 23620 |
| beef round, eye of, select, 0" trim, lean and fat, roasted - 3 oz | 85 | 144 | 56.0 | 0 | 0 |  | 0 | 33 | 6 | 16 | 4.22 | 0.008 | 0 | 0 | 0.06 | 4.3 | 1.29 | 0.50 |
|  |  | 25.2 | 4.0 | 1.4 | 1.7 | 0.2 | 45 | 203 | 157 | 2.00 | 0.064 | 24.6 | 0 | 0.3 | 0.13 | 0.33 | 7.6 | 13417 |
| beef round, eye of, select, 0" trim, lean, roasted - 3 oz | 85 | 139 | 56.5 | 0 | 0 |  | 0 | 33 | 5 | 17 | 4.32 | 0.009 | 0 | 0 | 0.06 | 4.4 | 1.31 | 0.50 |
|  |  | 25.4 | 3.3 | 1.1 | 1.4 | 0.1 | 44 | 209 | 161 | 2.06 | 0.070 | 31.3 | 0 | 0.3 | 0.14 | 0.34 | 8.5 | 13420 |
| beef round, eye of, select, ⅛" trim, lean and fat, roasted - 3 oz | 85 | 135 | 59.6 | 0 | 0 |  | 0 | 53 | 20 | 20 | 3.38 | 0.011 | 0 | 0 | 0.07 | 5.3 | 1.08 | 0.51 |
|  |  | 18.1 | 6.4 | 2.5 | 2.8 | 0.2 | 32 | 294 | 177 | 1.44 | 0.078 | 21.8 | 0 | 0.3 | 0.10 | 0.54 | 9.4 | 13881 |
| beef round, eye of, select, ⅛" trim, lean, roasted - 3 oz | 85 | 139 | 56.4 | 0 | 0 |  | 0 | 33 | 5 | 17 | 4.30 | 0.009 | 0 | 0 | 0.06 | 4.3 | 1.29 | 0.50 |
|  |  | 25.2 | 3.5 | 1.2 | 1.5 | 0.1 | 46 | 208 | 160 | 2.06 | 0.070 | 31.2 | 0 | 0.3 | 0.14 | 0.33 | 8.5 | 23591 |
| beef round, full cut, choice, ⅛" trim, lean & fat, brld - 3 oz | 85 | 166 | 55.6 | 0 | 0 |  | 0 | 46 | 3 | 19 | 2.75 | 0.011 | 0 | 0 | 0.08 | 3.2 | 2.40 | 0.31 |
|  |  | 17.5 | 10.1 | 3.9 | 4.4 | 0.4 | 53 | 291 | 169 | 1.69 | 0.064 | 16.7 | 0 | 0.2 | 0.14 | 0.40 | 6.8 | 13864 |
| beef round, full cut, select, ⅛" trim, lean and fat, broiled - 3 oz | 85 | 156 | 56.6 | 0 | 0 |  | 0 | 46 | 3 | 19 | 2.75 | 0.011 | 0 | 0 | 0.08 | 3.2 | 2.40 | 0.31 |
|  |  | 17.5 | 9.1 | 3.6 | 3.9 | 0.3 | 53 | 291 | 169 | 1.70 | 0.064 | 16.7 | 0 |  | 0.15 | 0.40 | 6.8 | 13866 |
| beef rnd, knuckle tip cntr stk, choice, 0" trim, lean & fat, grld - 3 oz | 85 | 116 | 61.8 | 0 | 0 |  | 0 | 45 | 4 | 20 | 4.80 | 0.009 | 0 | 0 | 0.06 | 4.5 | 4.58 | 0.66 |
|  |  | 17.8 | 4.4 | 1.6 | 1.7 | 0.3 | 50 | 306 | 184 | 1.71 | 0.058 | 24.5 | 0 | 0.2 | 0.17 | 0.45 | 9.4 | 23047 |
| beef rnd, knuckle tip cntr stk, slct, 0" trim, lean & fat, grld - 3 oz | 85 | 122 | 61.6 | 0 | 0 |  | 0 | 46 | 4 | 20 | 4.52 | 0.009 | 0 | 0 | 0.06 | 4.3 | 3.82 | 0.62 |
|  |  | 17.8 | 5.0 | 1.8 | 2.0 | 0.3 | 50 | 309 | 183 | 1.67 | 0.063 | 25.5 | 0 | 0.2 | 0.16 | 0.45 | 9.4 | 23061 |
| beef rnd, knuckle tip side stk, choice, 0" trim, lean & fat, grld - 3 oz | 85 | 136 | 56.3 | 0 | 0 |  | 0 | 44 | 4 | 23 | 6.85 | 0.016 | 0 | 0 | 0.06 | 5.1 | 3.43 | 0.73 |
|  |  | 24.9 | 3.3 | 1.1 | 1.2 | 0.2 | 66 | 310 | 208 | 2.53 | 0.121 | 34.7 | 0 | 0.2 | 0.18 | 0.45 | 6.8 | 23033 |
| beef rnd, knuckle tip side stk, slct, 0" trim, lean & fat, grld - 3 oz | 85 | 143 | 55.8 | 0 | 0 |  | 0 | 46 | 4 | 22 | 6.16 | 0.012 | 0 | 0 | 0.06 | 5.0 | 3.55 | 0.68 |
|  |  | 24.7 | 4.1 | 1.6 | 1.9 | 0.3 | 68 | 310 | 203 | 2.35 | 0.095 | 35.8 | 0 | 0.2 | 0.17 | 0.48 | 6.8 | 23056 |
| beef rnd, outside bottom stk, choice, 0" trim, lean & fat, grld - 3 oz | 85 | 110 | 62.3 | 0 | 0 |  | 0 | 53 | 4 | 20 | 3.66 | 0.017 | 0 | 0 | 0.08 | 5.4 | 3.07 | 0.65 |
|  |  | 18.8 | 3.3 | 1.2 | 1.4 | 0.3 | 52 | 306 | 184 | 2.47 | 0.112 | 25.8 | 0 | 0.1 | 0.20 | 0.62 | 5.1 | 23051 |
| beef rnd, outside bottom stk, slct, 0" trim, lean & fat, grld - 3 oz | 85 | 121 | 61.4 | 0 | 0 |  | 0 | 53 | 4 | 20 | 3.35 | 0.016 | 0 | 0 | 0.06 | 5.4 | 3.69 | 0.59 |
|  |  | 18.4 | 4.7 | 1.7 | 2.1 | 0.3 | 52 | 293 | 179 | 2.15 | 0.114 | 27.5 | 0 | 0.1 | 0.17 | 0.61 | 5.1 | 23063 |
| beef round, tip, choice, 0" trim, lean and fat, roasted - 3 oz | 85 | 167 | 54.2 | 0 | 0 |  | 0 | 30 | 5 | 14 | 3.77 | 0.008 | 0 | 0 | 0.05 | 4.2 | 1.38 | 0.45 |
|  |  | 23.0 | 7.6 | 2.8 | 3.1 | 0.3 | 86 | 184 | 139 | 1.89 | 0.050 | 24.1 | 0 | 0.3 | 0.13 | 0.30 | 6.8 | 13422 |
| beef round, tip, choice, 0" trim, lean, roasted - 3 oz | 85 | 150 | 55.8 | 0 | 0 |  | 0 | 31 | 5 | 16 | 4.09 | 0.008 | 0 | 0 | 0.05 | 4.5 | 1.39 | 0.46 |
|  |  | 23.5 | 5.5 | 1.9 | 2.2 | 0.2 | 77 | 191 | 148 | 2.07 | 0.055 | 26.7 | 0 | 0.3 | 0.15 | 0.33 | 7.6 | 13425 |
| beef round, tip, choice, ⅛" trim, lean and fat, roasted - 3 oz | 85 | 169 | 55.6 | 0 | 0 |  | 0 | 49 | 4 | 18 | 3.71 | 0.011 | 0 | 0 | 0.09 | 2.7 | 2.55 | 0.28 |
|  |  | 16.6 | 10.9 | 4.3 | 4.7 | 0.4 | 55 | 277 | 163 | 1.69 | 0.065 | 16.7 | 0 |  | 0.15 | 0.35 | 6.0 | 13885 |
| beef round, tip, select, 0" trim, lean and fat, roasted - 3 oz | 85 | 154 | 55.7 | 0 | 0 |  | 0 | 30 | 6 | 15 | 3.85 | 0.008 | 0 | 0 | 0.06 | 3.8 | 1.16 | 0.45 |
|  |  | 22.6 | 6.4 | 2.3 | 2.7 | 0.2 | 73 | 185 | 144 | 1.83 | 0.059 | 22.5 | 0 | 0.3 | 0.11 | 0.30 | 6.8 | 13423 |
| beef round, tip, select, 0" trim, lean, roasted - 3 oz | 85 | 127 | 57.7 | 0 | 0 |  | 0 | 31 | 5 | 15 | 4.04 | 0.008 | 0 | 0 | 0.06 | 4.0 | 1.20 | 0.58 |
|  |  | 23.3 | 3.7 | 1.3 | 1.5 | 0.1 | 53 | 196 | 150 | 1.92 | 0.065 | 29.2 | 0 | 0.3 | 0.13 | 0.31 | 7.6 | 13426 |
| beef round, tip, select, ⅛" trim, lean and fat, roasted - 3 oz | 85 | 151 | 56.8 | 0 | 0 |  | 0 | 49 | 4 | 19 | 3.78 | 0.011 | 0 | 0 | 0.09 | 2.7 | 2.58 | 0.28 |
|  |  | 16.8 | 8.8 | 3.5 | 3.8 | 0.3 | 54 | 282 | 166 | 1.72 | 0.065 | 16.7 | 0 |  | 0.15 | 0.35 | 6.0 | 13887 |

| | WT (g) | KCAL / PRO (g) | H₂O (g) / FAT (g) | CHO (g) / SFA (g) | TSUG (g) / MUFA (g) | ASUG (g) / PUFA (g) | DFIB (g) / CHOL (mg) | Na (mg) / K (mg) | Ca (mg) / P (mg) | Mg (mg) / Fe (mg) | Zn (mg) / Cu (mg) | Mn (mg) / Se (mcg) | A (mcg RAE) / A (IU) | C (mg) / E (mg ATE) | B-1 (mg) / B-2 (mg) | NIA (mg) / B-6 (mg) | B-12 (mcg) / FOL (mcg DFE) | PANT (mg) / REF |
|---|---|---|---|---|---|---|---|---|---|---|---|---|---|---|---|---|---|---|
| beef round, top, **choice**, 0″ trim, | 85 | 184 | 48.7 | 0 | 0 | | 0 | 38 | 3 | 21 | 3.82 | 0.015 | 0 | 0 | 0.06 | 3.2 | 2.28 | 0.31 |
| lean and fat, braised - *3 oz* | | 30.3 | 6.0 | 2.1 | 2.4 | 0.3 | 76 | 280 | 190 | 2.78 | 0.104 | 27.8 | 0 | | 0.21 | 0.24 | 7.6 | 13430 |
| beef round, top, **choice**, 0″ trim, | 85 | 170 | 51.0 | 0 | 0 | | 0 | 36 | 6 | 18 | 4.54 | 0.009 | 0 | 0 | 0.06 | 4.9 | 1.62 | 0.53 |
| lean and fat, broiled - *3 oz* | | 26.8 | 6.1 | 2.2 | 2.6 | 0.2 | 68 | 221 | 167 | 2.27 | 0.060 | 28.9 | 0 | 0.4 | 0.15 | 0.35 | 8.5 | 13968 |
| beef round, top, **choice**, 0″ trim, | 85 | 176 | 49.4 | 0 | 0 | | 0 | 38 | 3 | 22 | 3.88 | 0.015 | 0 | 0 | 0.06 | 3.2 | 2.30 | 0.31 |
| lean, braised - *3 oz* | | 30.7 | 4.9 | 1.7 | 1.9 | 0.2 | 76 | 284 | 192 | 2.82 | 0.105 | 28.0 | 0 | | 0.21 | 0.24 | 7.6 | 13436 |
| beef round, top, **choice**, 0″ trim, | 85 | 167 | 51.2 | 0 | 0 | | 0 | 37 | 6 | 19 | 4.83 | 0.009 | 0 | 0 | 0.06 | 5.2 | 1.59 | 0.53 |
| lean, broiled - *3 oz* | | 26.9 | 5.8 | 2.0 | 2.4 | 0.2 | 78 | 225 | 174 | 2.44 | 0.065 | 31.4 | 0 | 0.4 | 0.17 | 0.38 | | 13492 |
| beef round, top, **choice**, ⅛″ trim, | 85 | 143 | 58.5 | 0 | 0 | | 0 | 48 | 14 | 20 | 3.45 | 0.011 | 0 | 0 | 0.07 | 5.7 | 1.58 | 0.54 |
| lean and fat, braised - *3 oz* | | 18.6 | 7.0 | 2.7 | 3.0 | 0.3 | 35 | 290 | 179 | 1.67 | 0.083 | 22.7 | 0 | 0.3 | 0.13 | 0.55 | 10.2 | 13894 |
| beef round, top, **choice**, ⅛″ trim, | 85 | 212 | 45.8 | 0 | 0 | | 0 | 38 | 4 | 20 | 3.66 | 0.014 | 0 | 0 | 0.06 | 3.1 | 2.22 | 0.30 |
| lean and fat, broiled - *3 oz* | | 29.0 | 9.9 | 3.7 | 4.0 | 0.4 | 76 | 269 | 182 | 2.67 | 0.100 | 27.6 | 0 | | 0.20 | 0.23 | 7.6 | 13895 |
| beef round, top, **choice**, ⅛″ trim, | 85 | 190 | 49.7 | 0 | 0 | | 0 | 34 | 6 | 17 | 4.33 | 0.009 | 0 | 0 | 0.05 | 4.7 | 1.56 | 0.51 |
| lean and fat, panfried - *3 oz* | | 26.1 | 8.7 | 3.3 | 3.7 | 0.3 | 56 | 211 | 159 | 2.16 | 0.057 | 27.5 | 0 | 0.4 | 0.15 | 0.34 | 8.5 | 13896 |
| beef round, top, **choice**, ⅛″ trim, | 85 | 115 | 63.8 | 0 | 0 | | 0 | 52 | 17 | 21 | 3.71 | 0.012 | 0 | 0 | 0.08 | 5.8 | 1.38 | 0.58 |
| lean, broiled - *3 oz* | | 19.5 | 3.5 | 1.2 | 1.5 | 0.1 | 47 | 308 | 189 | 1.69 | 0.087 | 24.8 | 0 | 0.2 | 0.13 | 0.58 | 11.0 | 23609 |
| beef round, top, **select**, 0″ trim, | 85 | 170 | 49.7 | 0 | 0 | | 0 | 38 | 3 | 21 | 3.82 | 0.015 | 0 | 0 | 0.06 | 3.2 | 2.28 | 0.31 |
| lean and fat, braised - *3 oz* | | 30.3 | 4.5 | 1.6 | 1.8 | 0.2 | 76 | 280 | 190 | 2.78 | 0.104 | 27.8 | 0 | | 0.21 | 0.24 | 7.6 | 13432 |
| beef round, top, **select**, 0″ trim, | 85 | 150 | 54.2 | 0 | 0 | | 0 | 36 | 7 | 18 | 4.54 | 0.009 | 0 | 0 | 0.07 | 4.5 | 1.38 | 0.53 |
| lean and fat, broiled - *3 oz* | | 26.9 | 3.9 | 1.4 | 1.7 | 0.1 | 43 | 218 | 169 | 2.15 | 0.069 | 26.5 | 0 | 0.3 | 0.14 | 0.35 | 8.5 | 13969 |
| beef round, top, **select**, 0″ trim, | 85 | 162 | 50.4 | 0 | 0 | | 0 | 38 | 3 | 22 | 3.88 | 0.015 | 0 | 0 | 0.06 | 3.2 | 2.30 | 0.31 |
| lean, braised - *3 oz* | | 30.7 | 3.4 | 1.2 | 1.3 | 0.2 | 76 | 284 | 192 | 2.82 | 0.105 | 28.0 | 0 | | 0.21 | 0.24 | 7.6 | 13438 |
| beef round, top, **select**, 0″ trim, | 85 | 150 | 54.2 | 0 | 0 | | 0 | 36 | 6 | 18 | 4.62 | 0.010 | 0 | 0 | 0.06 | 4.6 | 1.39 | 0.53 |
| lean, broiled - *3 oz* | | 26.9 | 3.8 | 1.3 | 1.6 | 0.1 | 51 | 224 | 172 | 2.20 | 0.075 | 33.5 | 0 | 0.3 | 0.15 | 0.36 | 9.0 | 13493 |
| beef round, top, **select**, ⅛″ trim, | 85 | 171 | 51.6 | 0 | 0 | | 0 | 35 | 7 | 18 | 4.51 | 0.009 | 0 | 0 | 0.07 | 4.4 | 1.33 | 0.51 |
| lean and fat, braised - *3 oz* | | 26.0 | 6.6 | 2.5 | 2.8 | 0.3 | 42 | 218 | 168 | 2.14 | 0.069 | 26.4 | 0 | 0.4 | 0.13 | 0.34 | 8.5 | 13900 |
| beef round, top, **select**, ⅛″ trim, | 85 | 147 | 58.4 | 0 | 0 | | 0 | 43 | 3 | 20 | 2.38 | 0.012 | 0 | 0 | 0.08 | 3.6 | 2.37 | 0.30 |
| lean and fat, broiled - *3 oz* | | 18.9 | 7.4 | 2.8 | 3.1 | 0.3 | 50 | 315 | 181 | 1.73 | 0.068 | 17.4 | 0 | | 0.15 | 0.42 | 7.6 | 13901 |
| beef round, top, **select**, ⅛″ trim, | 85 | 164 | 52.0 | 0 | 0 | | 0 | 36 | 6 | 19 | 4.78 | 0.009 | 0 | 0 | 0.06 | 5.2 | 1.61 | 0.53 |
| lean, broiled - *3 oz* | | 27.2 | 5.3 | 1.8 | 2.2 | 0.2 | 70 | 224 | 173 | 2.41 | 0.064 | 31.1 | 0 | 0.3 | 0.17 | 0.38 | 9.4 | 23621 |
| beef **sndwch steaks**, flaked, chpd, | 56 | 173 | 31.4 | 0 | 0 | | 0 | 38 | 7 | 9 | 2.03 | 0.010 | 0 | 0 | 0.02 | 2.6 | 1.52 | 0.20 |
| formed, thinly slcd - *2 oz steak* | | 9.2 | 15.1 | 6.5 | 6.2 | 0.3 | 40 | 130 | 74 | 1.04 | 0.035 | 7.3 | 0 | 0.1 | 0.09 | 0.14 | 3.9 | 13342 |
| beef **sandwich steaks**, The Philly | 38 | 120 | | 0 | 0 | | | 35 | 0 | | | | 0 | 0 | | | | |
| Steak - *1.3 oz steak* | | 8.0 | 10.0 | 4.0 | | | 30 | | | 0.72 | | | 0 | | | | | PNSS1 |
| beef **short loin porterhse stk**, choice, | 85 | 210 | 52.1 | 0 | 0 | | 0 | 45 | 5 | 16 | 2.71 | 0.011 | 0 | 0 | 0.08 | 3.0 | 2.31 | 0.26 |
| ⅛″ trim, lean and fat - *3 oz* | | 16.0 | 15.7 | 6.3 | 7.0 | 0.6 | 54 | 254 | 144 | 1.67 | 0.065 | 13.9 | 0 | | 0.14 | 0.32 | 5.1 | 23001 |
| beef **short loin porterhse stk**, slct, | 85 | 180 | 51.3 | 0 | 0 | | 0 | 59 | 5 | 21 | 4.30 | 0.014 | 0 | 0 | 0.09 | 3.9 | 1.93 | 0.29 |
| 0″ trim, lean, brld - *3 oz* | | 22.2 | 9.5 | 3.3 | 4.4 | 0.3 | 53 | 279 | 179 | 2.75 | 0.122 | 17.0 | 0 | 0.1 | 0.21 | 0.34 | 6.8 | 13466 |
| beef **short loin porterhse stk**, slct, | 85 | 189 | 54.1 | 0 | 0 | | 0 | 46 | 5 | 17 | 2.79 | 0.011 | 0 | 0 | 0.08 | 3.1 | 2.36 | 0.26 |
| ⅛″ trim, lean & fat, brld - *3 oz* | | 17.6 | 12.6 | 5.1 | 5.5 | 0.5 | 48 | 263 | 148 | 1.71 | 0.067 | 14.0 | 0 | | 0.15 | 0.32 | 5.1 | 23003 |
| beef **short loin, select**, ⅛″ trim, | 85 | 150 | 55.0 | 0 | 0 | | 0 | 53 | 18 | 21 | 4.57 | 0.009 | 0 | 0 | 0.07 | 7.3 | 1.20 | 0.49 |
| lean, broiled - *3 oz* | | 25.0 | 4.9 | 1.9 | 1.9 | 0.2 | 46 | 328 | 203 | 1.54 | 0.068 | 31.2 | 0 | 0.3 | 0.13 | 0.55 | 8.5 | 23589 |
| beef **short loin T-bone steak**, choice, | 85 | 168 | 53.1 | 0 | 0 | | 0 | 60 | 3 | 22 | 4.34 | 0.014 | 0 | 0 | 0.09 | 3.9 | 1.93 | 0.28 |
| 0″ trim, lean, brld - *3 oz* | | 22.1 | 8.2 | 2.8 | 3.9 | 0.3 | 48 | 278 | 183 | 3.11 | 0.122 | 8.5 | 0 | 0.1 | 0.21 | 0.33 | 6.8 | 13481 |
| beef **short loin T-bone stk**, choice, | 85 | 187 | 54.0 | 0 | 0 | | 0 | 46 | 5 | 17 | 2.78 | 0.011 | 0 | 0 | 0.08 | 3.1 | 2.36 | 0.26 |
| ⅛″ trim, lean & fat, brld - *3 oz* | | 16.3 | 13.0 | 5.2 | 5.7 | 0.5 | 48 | 264 | 149 | 1.80 | 0.067 | 14.2 | 0 | | 0.15 | 0.33 | 5.1 | 23005 |
| beef **short loin T-bone stk**, slct, | 85 | 150 | 54.2 | 0 | 0 | | 0 | 60 | 3 | 22 | 4.34 | 0.014 | 0 | 0 | 0.09 | 3.9 | 1.93 | 0.28 |
| 0″ trim, lean, brld - *3 oz* | | 22.1 | 6.3 | 2.4 | 2.8 | 0.3 | 46 | 278 | 183 | 3.11 | 0.122 | 8.5 | 0 | 0.1 | 0.21 | 0.33 | 6.8 | 13484 |
| beef **short loin T-bone stk**, slct, | 85 | 163 | 56.3 | 0 | 0 | | 0 | 47 | 5 | 17 | 2.84 | 0.011 | 0 | 0 | 0.09 | 3.2 | 2.40 | 0.27 |
| ⅛″ trim, lean & fat, brld - *3 oz* | | 16.9 | 10.1 | 4.1 | 4.3 | 0.5 | 38 | 271 | 151 | 1.84 | 0.069 | 14.2 | 0 | | 0.15 | 0.33 | 6.0 | 23007 |
| beef **short loin, top, choice**, 0″ trim, | 85 | 174 | 52.8 | 0 | 0 | | 0 | 48 | 15 | 20 | 4.27 | 0.008 | 0 | 0 | 0.06 | 6.6 | 1.60 | 0.48 |
| lean and fat, broiled - *3 oz* | | 24.2 | 7.8 | 3.0 | 3.2 | 0.3 | 59 | 291 | 178 | 1.61 | 0.078 | 25.8 | 0 | 0.3 | 0.11 | 0.48 | 7.6 | 13446 |
| beef **short loin, top, choice**, 0″ trim, | 85 | 163 | 53.8 | 0 | 0 | | 0 | 50 | 14 | 20 | 4.58 | 0.009 | 0 | 0 | 0.07 | 7.3 | 1.53 | 0.48 |
| lean, broiled - *3 oz* | | 24.6 | 6.5 | 2.5 | 2.6 | 0.2 | 65 | 303 | 189 | 1.65 | 0.077 | 28.0 | 0 | 0.3 | 0.13 | 0.51 | 8.5 | 13449 |
| beef **short loin, top, choice**, ⅛″ trim, | 85 | 197 | 53.5 | 0 | 0 | | 0 | 43 | 21 | 18 | 3.08 | 0.011 | 0 | 0 | 0.05 | 5.7 | 0.98 | 0.51 |
| lean and fat, broiled - *3 oz* | | 17.5 | 13.6 | 5.5 | 5.8 | 0.5 | 49 | 266 | 156 | 1.26 | 0.057 | 18.8 | 0 | 0.3 | 0.07 | 0.47 | 9.4 | 13911 |
| beef **short loin, top, choice**, ⅛″ trim, | 85 | 132 | 59.8 | 0 | 0 | | 0 | 49 | 25 | 20 | 3.59 | 0.013 | 0 | 0 | 0.05 | 6.6 | 1.05 | 0.58 |
| lean, broiled - *3 oz* | | 19.4 | 5.5 | 2.0 | 2.2 | 0.2 | 56 | 296 | 177 | 1.41 | 0.063 | 22.1 | 0 | 0.3 | 0.10 | 0.53 | 11.0 | 23627 |
| beef **short loin, top, select**, 0″ trim, | 85 | 153 | 54.9 | 0 | 0 | | 0 | 52 | 20 | 21 | 4.48 | 0.008 | 0 | 0 | 0.07 | 6.5 | 1.29 | 0.49 |
| lean and fat, broiled - *3 oz* | | 24.9 | 5.2 | 2.0 | 2.1 | 0.2 | 39 | 314 | 197 | 1.50 | 0.068 | 26.7 | 0 | 0.3 | 0.13 | 0.55 | 7.6 | 13447 |
| beef **short loin, top, select**, 0″ trim, | 85 | 146 | 55.5 | 0 | 0 | | 0 | 53 | 18 | 21 | 4.57 | 0.009 | 0 | 0 | 0.07 | 7.4 | 1.20 | 0.50 |
| lean, broiled - *3 oz* | | 25.2 | 4.3 | 1.7 | 1.7 | 0.2 | 43 | 328 | 202 | 1.54 | 0.068 | 31.2 | 0 | 0.3 | 0.13 | 0.56 | 8.5 | 13450 |

| | WT (g) | KCAL / PRO (g) | H₂0 (g) / FAT (g) | CHO (g) / SFA (g) | TSUG (g) / MUFA (g) | ASUG (g) / PUFA (g) | DFIB (g) / CHOL (mg) | Na (mg) / K (mg) | Ca (mg) / P (mg) | Mg (mg) / Fe (mg) | Zn (mg) / Cu (mg) | Mn (mg) / Se (mcg) | A (mcg RAE) / A (IU) | C (mg) / E (mg ATE) | B-1 (mg) / B-2 (mg) | NIA (mg) / B-6 (mg) | B-12 (mcg) / FOL (mcg DFE) | PANT (mg) / REF |
|---|---|---|---|---|---|---|---|---|---|---|---|---|---|---|---|---|---|---|
| **beef short loin, top, select**, ⅛" trim, | 85 | 239 | 49.7 | 0 | 0 | | 0 | 45 | 5 | 15 | 2.67 | 0.010 | 0 | 0 | 0.08 | 3.3 | 2.34 | 0.27 |
| lean and fat, broiled - 3 oz | | 16.2 | 18.8 | 7.7 | 8.3 | 0.7 | 57 | 251 | 139 | 1.34 | 0.059 | 14.7 | 0 | | 0.12 | 0.33 | 5.1 | 13915 |
| **beef skirt steak, inside**, 0" trim, | 85 | 187 | 51.3 | 0 | 0 | | 0 | 64 | 9 | 20 | 6.15 | 0 | 0 | 0 | 0.08 | 3.2 | 3.16 | 0 |
| lean and fat, broiled - 3 oz | | 22.2 | 10.2 | 4.0 | 5.1 | 0.4 | 51 | 246 | 196 | 2.35 | 0.079 | 16.8 | 0 | 0.1 | 0.16 | 0.27 | 6.0 | 23540 |
| **beef skirt steak, inside**, 0" trim, | 85 | 174 | 52.5 | 0 | 0 | | 0 | 65 | 9 | 20 | 6.32 | | 0 | 0 | 0.08 | 3.2 | 3.23 | |
| lean, broiled - 3 oz | | 22.7 | 8.6 | 3.3 | 4.4 | 0.3 | 50 | 251 | 201 | 2.41 | 0.081 | 16.9 | 0 | 0.1 | 0.16 | 0.28 | 6.0 | 13977 |
| **beef skirt steak, outside**, 0" trim, | 85 | 217 | 48.6 | 0 | 0 | | 0 | 78 | 9 | 20 | 4.68 | 0 | 0 | 0 | 0.10 | 3.6 | 3.54 | 0.01 |
| lean and fat, broiled - 3 oz | | 20.0 | 14.6 | 6.0 | 7.2 | 0.6 | 50 | 322 | 182 | 2.19 | 0.074 | 15.8 | 0 | 0.1 | 0.16 | 0.41 | 6.0 | 23541 |
| **beef skirt steak, outside**, 0" trim, | 85 | 198 | 50.3 | 0 | 0 | | 0 | 80 | 8 | 21 | 4.86 | | 0 | 0 | 0.10 | 3.7 | 3.66 | |
| lean, broiled - 3 oz | | 20.6 | 12.2 | 5.1 | 6.3 | 0.5 | 49 | 334 | 188 | 2.26 | 0.076 | 15.9 | 0 | 0.1 | 0.17 | 0.42 | 6.8 | 13979 |
| **beef tenderloin, choice**, 0" trim, | 85 | 196 | 50.5 | 0 | 0 | | 0 | 47 | 15 | 19 | 4.20 | 0.008 | 0 | 0 | 0.06 | 6.4 | 1.57 | 0.47 |
| lean and fat, broiled - 3 oz | | 23.8 | 10.5 | 4.1 | 4.3 | 0.4 | 79 | 286 | 176 | 1.58 | 0.076 | 25.3 | 0 | 0.4 | 0.10 | 0.47 | 7.6 | 13440 |
| **beef tenderloin, choice**, 0" trim, | 85 | 175 | 52.5 | 0 | 0 | | 0 | 50 | 14 | 20 | 4.58 | 0.009 | 0 | 0 | 0.07 | 7.3 | 1.54 | 0.48 |
| lean, broiled - 3 oz | | 24.6 | 7.8 | 3.0 | 3.1 | 0.3 | 78 | 303 | 190 | 1.66 | 0.077 | 28.0 | 0 | 0.3 | 0.13 | 0.51 | 8.5 | 13443 |
| **beef tenderloin, choice**, ⅛" trim, | 85 | 209 | 52.4 | 0 | 0 | | 0 | 42 | 21 | 17 | 2.98 | 0.010 | 0 | 0 | 0.04 | 5.4 | 0.94 | 0.49 |
| lean and fat, broiled - 3 oz | | 16.8 | 15.2 | 6.1 | 6.5 | 0.6 | 55 | 258 | 150 | 1.22 | 0.055 | 18.2 | 0 | 0.3 | 0.07 | 0.45 | 9.4 | 13920 |
| **beef tenderloin, choice**, ⅛" trim, | 85 | 232 | 47.2 | 0 | 0 | | 0 | 44 | 14 | 18 | 3.97 | 0.008 | 0 | 0 | 0.06 | 6.1 | 1.48 | 0.44 |
| lean and fat, roasted - 3 oz | | 22.5 | 15.1 | 6.0 | 6.3 | 0.6 | 79 | 270 | 167 | 1.50 | 0.072 | 24.0 | 0 | 0.4 | 0.10 | 0.45 | 6.8 | 13921 |
| **beef tenderloin, choice**, ⅛" trim, | 85 | 134 | 59.6 | 0 | 0 | | 0 | 48 | 24 | 20 | 3.51 | 0.012 | 0 | 0 | 0.05 | 6.4 | 1.02 | 0.56 |
| lean, broiled - 3 oz | | 18.8 | 6.0 | 2.2 | 2.4 | 0.3 | 61 | 289 | 173 | 1.39 | 0.061 | 21.6 | 0 | 0.3 | 0.09 | 0.52 | 11.0 | 23624 |
| **beef tenderloin, select**, 0" trim, | 85 | 174 | 53.3 | 0 | 0 | | 0 | 49 | 19 | 20 | 4.20 | 0.008 | 0 | 0 | 0.07 | 6.0 | 1.20 | 0.46 |
| lean and fat, broiled - 3 oz | | 23.1 | 8.4 | 3.2 | 3.4 | 0.3 | 63 | 294 | 184 | 1.41 | 0.063 | 25.0 | 0 | 0.3 | 0.12 | 0.51 | 6.8 | 13441 |
| **beef tenderloin, select**, 0" trim, | 85 | 152 | 55.3 | 0 | 0 | | 0 | 50 | 17 | 20 | 4.38 | 0.008 | 0 | 0 | 0.07 | 7.0 | 1.14 | 0.47 |
| lean, broiled - 3 oz | | 23.9 | 5.6 | 2.1 | 2.2 | 0.2 | 56 | 314 | 194 | 1.47 | 0.065 | 29.8 | 0 | 0.3 | 0.13 | 0.53 | 7.6 | 13444 |
| **beef tenderloin, select**, ⅛" trim, | 85 | 212 | 52.1 | 0 | 0 | | 0 | 42 | 19 | 17 | 2.82 | 0.008 | 0 | 0 | 0.06 | 4.4 | 0.78 | 0.47 |
| lean and fat, broiled - 3 oz | | 16.5 | 15.7 | 6.3 | 6.7 | 0.6 | 58 | 255 | 155 | 1.21 | 0.058 | 19.2 | 0 | 0.3 | 0.09 | 0.45 | 8.5 | 13923 |
| **beef tenderloin, select**, ⅛" trim, | 85 | 223 | 48.0 | 0 | 0 | | 0 | 48 | 19 | 20 | 4.12 | 0.008 | 0 | 0 | 0.07 | 5.9 | 1.16 | 0.44 |
| lean and fat, roasted - 3 oz | | 22.5 | 14.1 | 5.5 | 5.9 | 0.5 | 74 | 289 | 182 | 1.39 | 0.062 | 24.6 | 0 | 0.4 | 0.12 | 0.49 | 6.8 | 13924 |
| **beef tenderloin, select**, ⅛" trim, | 85 | 126 | 60.4 | 0 | 0 | | 0 | 47 | 19 | 20 | 3.37 | 0.009 | 0 | 0 | 0.06 | 5.4 | 0.79 | 0.55 |
| lean, broiled - 3 oz | | 18.8 | 5.0 | 1.9 | 2.0 | 0.2 | 52 | 301 | 178 | 1.36 | 0.065 | 25.9 | 0 | 0.3 | 0.10 | 0.53 | 11.0 | 23583 |
| **beef top sirloin, choice**, 0" trim, | 85 | 186 | 50.7 | 0 | 0 | | 0 | 49 | 16 | 20 | 4.43 | 0.008 | 0 | 0 | 0.06 | 6.7 | 1.62 | 0.49 |
| lean and fat, broiled - 3 oz | | 24.7 | 9.0 | 3.5 | 3.7 | 0.3 | 67 | 302 | 185 | 1.67 | 0.081 | 26.8 | 0 | 0.4 | 0.11 | 0.49 | 7.6 | 13452 |
| **beef top sirloin, choice**, 0" trim, | 85 | 160 | 53.0 | 0 | 0 | | 0 | 54 | 14 | 22 | 4.89 | 0.009 | 0 | 0 | 0.07 | 7.6 | 1.61 | 0.51 |
| lean, broiled - 3 oz | | 25.7 | 5.6 | 2.1 | 2.2 | 0.2 | 56 | 323 | 201 | 1.76 | 0.082 | 29.8 | 0 | 0.3 | 0.13 | 0.54 | 8.5 | 13455 |
| **beef top sirloin, choice**, ⅛" trim, | 85 | 182 | 55.1 | 0 | 0 | | 0 | 43 | 21 | 17 | 3.03 | 0.011 | 0 | 0 | 0.05 | 5.5 | 0.94 | 0.49 |
| lean and fat, broiled - 3 oz | | 16.9 | 12.1 | 4.9 | 5.2 | 0.5 | 44 | 263 | 154 | 1.24 | 0.056 | 18.5 | 0 | 0.3 | 0.07 | 0.46 | 9.4 | 13931 |
| **beef top sirloin, choice**, ⅛" trim, | 85 | 218 | 48.3 | 0 | 0 | | 0 | 46 | 15 | 19 | 4.09 | 0.008 | 0 | 0 | 0.06 | 6.2 | 1.50 | 0.45 |
| lean and fat, pan-fried - 3 oz | | 22.8 | 13.4 | 5.3 | 5.6 | 0.5 | 71 | 278 | 171 | 1.54 | 0.075 | 24.6 | 0 | 0.4 | 0.10 | 0.45 | 6.8 | 13932 |
| **beef top sirloin, choice**, ⅛" trim, | 85 | 115 | 61.6 | 0 | 0 | | 0 | 48 | 24 | 20 | 3.52 | 0.012 | 0 | 0 | 0.05 | 6.3 | 1.01 | 0.55 |
| lean, broiled - 3 oz | | 18.6 | 3.9 | 1.5 | 1.6 | 0.2 | 40 | 291 | 174 | 1.39 | 0.062 | 21.7 | 0 | 0.3 | 0.09 | 0.51 | 11.0 | 23625 |
| **beef top sirloin, select**, 0" trim, | 85 | 175 | 51.8 | 0 | 0 | | 0 | 54 | 20 | 22 | 4.62 | 0.008 | 0 | 0 | 0.07 | 6.6 | 1.31 | 0.50 |
| lean and fat, broiled - 3 oz | | 25.2 | 7.5 | 2.9 | 3.1 | 0.3 | 56 | 324 | 203 | 1.56 | 0.070 | 27.5 | 0 | 0.4 | 0.13 | 0.55 | 7.6 | 13453 |
| **beef top sirloin, select**, 0" trim, | 85 | 150 | 54.0 | 0 | 0 | | 0 | 56 | 19 | 23 | 4.84 | 0.009 | 0 | 0 | 0.07 | 7.7 | 1.25 | 0.52 |
| lean, broiled - 3 oz | | 26.2 | 4.3 | 1.6 | 1.7 | 0.2 | 43 | 348 | 215 | 1.63 | 0.072 | 33.1 | 0 | 0.3 | 0.14 | 0.58 | 8.5 | 13456 |
| **beef top sirloin, select**, ⅛" trim, | 85 | 161 | 57.2 | 0 | 0 | | 0 | 45 | 20 | 18 | 3.01 | 0.008 | 0 | 0 | 0.06 | 4.7 | 0.83 | 0.50 |
| lean and fat, broiled - 3 oz | | 17.6 | 9.5 | 3.8 | 4.1 | 0.4 | 35 | 273 | 165 | 1.28 | 0.062 | 20.5 | 0 | 0.3 | 0.10 | 0.49 | 9.4 | 13934 |
| **beef top sirloin, select**, ⅛" trim, | 85 | 108 | 62.3 | 0 | 0 | | 0 | 48 | 19 | 20 | 3.40 | 0.009 | 0 | 0 | 0.06 | 5.5 | 0.80 | 0.56 |
| lean, broiled - 3 oz | | 18.9 | 3.0 | 1.1 | 1.2 | 0.1 | 31 | 303 | 179 | 1.37 | 0.065 | 26.2 | 0 | 0.2 | 0.10 | 0.53 | 11.0 | 23584 |
| **breakfast strips, beef**, cooked | 34 | 153 | 8.9 | 0.5 | 0 | | 0 | 766 | 3 | 9 | 2.17 | 0.006 | 0 | 0 | 0.03 | 2.2 | 1.17 | 0.12 |
| *3 slices (1.2 oz)* | | 10.6 | 11.7 | 4.9 | 5.7 | 0.5 | 40 | 140 | 80 | 1.07 | 0.039 | 9.1 | 0 | 0.1 | 0.09 | 0.11 | 2.7 | 13345 |
| **corned beef** (cured beef brisket), | 85 | 213 | 50.8 | 0.4 | 0 | | 0 | 964 | 7 | 10 | 3.89 | 0.019 | 0 | 0 | 0.02 | 2.6 | 1.39 | 0.36 |
| cooked - 3 oz | | 15.4 | 16.1 | 5.4 | 7.8 | 0.6 | 83 | 123 | 106 | 1.58 | 0.131 | 27.9 | 0 | 0.1 | 0.14 | 0.20 | 5.1 | 13347 |
| **beef sausage** (fresh), pan-fried | 85 | 282 | 43.5 | 0.3 | 0 | | 0 | 554 | 9 | 12 | 3.72 | 0 | 11 | 0 | 0.04 | 3.1 | 1.71 | 0.44 |
| *3 oz* | | 15.5 | 23.8 | 9.3 | 10.7 | 0.6 | 70 | 219 | 120 | 1.33 | 0.059 | 0 | 69 | 0.2 | 0.13 | 0.27 | 2.6 | 7956 |
| **beef tripe**, simmered | 85 | 80 | 69.4 | 1.7 | 0 | | 0 | 58 | 69 | 13 | 1.45 | 0.088 | 0 | 0 | 0 | 0.4 | 0.61 | 0.08 |
| *3 oz* | | 10.0 | 3.4 | 1.2 | 1.4 | 0.2 | 133 | 36 | 56 | 0.56 | 0 | 10.0 | 0 | 0.1 | 0.02 | 0 | 2.6 | 23640 |

## 19.2 GAME AND AMPHIBIANS

| | WT (g) | KCAL / PRO (g) | H₂0 (g) / FAT (g) | CHO (g) / SFA (g) | TSUG (g) / MUFA (g) | ASUG (g) / PUFA (g) | DFIB (g) / CHOL (mg) | Na (mg) / K (mg) | Ca (mg) / P (mg) | Mg (mg) / Fe (mg) | Zn (mg) / Cu (mg) | Mn (mg) / Se (mcg) | A (mcg RAE) / A (IU) | C (mg) / E (mg ATE) | B-1 (mg) / B-2 (mg) | NIA (mg) / B-6 (mg) | B-12 (mcg) / FOL (mcg DFE) | PANT (mg) / REF |
|---|---|---|---|---|---|---|---|---|---|---|---|---|---|---|---|---|---|---|
| **antelope**, roasted | 85 | 128 | 56.0 | 0 | | | 0 | 46 | 3 | 24 | 1.43 | 0.019 | 0 | | 0.22 | | | |
| *3 oz* | | 25.0 | 2.3 | 0.8 | 0.5 | 0.5 | 107 | 316 | 178 | 3.57 | 0.181 | 11.0 | 0 | | 0.62 | | 7.6 | 17145 |
| **bear, polar**, raw | 85 | 110 | 59.8 | 0 | | | | | 14 | | | | | 2 | 0.02 | 3.4 | | |
| *3 oz* | | 21.8 | 2.6 | 0.5 | 1.7 | 0.4 | | 34 | | 5.18 | | | 1190 | | 0.49 | | | 35008 |

| | WT (g) | KCAL | H₂0 (g) | CHO (g) | TSUG (g) | ASUG (g) | DFIB (g) | Na (mg) | Ca (mg) | Mg (mg) | Zn (mg) | Mn (mg) | A (mcg RAE) | C (mg) | B-1 (mg) | NIA (mg) | B-12 (mcg) | PANT (mg) |
|---|---|---|---|---|---|---|---|---|---|---|---|---|---|---|---|---|---|---|
| | | PRO (g) | FAT (g) | SFA (g) | MUFA (g) | PUFA (g) | CHOL (mg) | K (mg) | P (mg) | Fe (mg) | Cu (mg) | Se (mcg) | A (IU) | E (mg ATE) | B-2 (mg) | B-6 (mg) | FOL (mcg DFE) | REF |
| **bear**, simmered | 85 | 220 | 45.5 | 0 | 0 | | 0 | 60 | 4 | 20 | 8.73 | | 0 | 0 | 0.08 | 2.8 | 2.10 | |
| *3 oz* | | 27.6 | 11.4 | 3.0 | 4.8 | 2.0 | 83 | 224 | 144 | 9.12 | 0.126 | 9.5 | 0 | 0.4 | 0.70 | 0.25 | 5.1 | 17147 |
| **beaver**, roasted | 85 | 180 | 49.2 | 0 | 0 | | 0 | 50 | 19 | 25 | 1.93 | | 0 | 3 | 0.04 | 1.9 | 7.06 | 0.79 |
| *3 oz* | | 29.6 | 5.9 | 1.8 | 1.6 | 1.1 | 99 | 343 | 248 | 8.50 | 0.161 | 36.6 | 0 | 0.4 | 0.26 | 0.40 | 9.4 | 17151 |
| **beefalo**, roasted | 85 | 160 | 52.4 | 0 | | | 0 | 70 | 20 | | 5.44 | | 0 | 8 | 0.03 | 4.2 | 2.17 | 0.49 |
| *3 oz* | | 26.1 | 5.4 | 2.3 | 2.3 | 0.2 | 49 | 390 | 212 | 2.59 | | 11.1 | 0 | | 0.09 | | 15.3 | 17153 |
| **bison chuck shoulder clod**, lean, braised - *3 oz* | 85 | 164 | 51.4 | 0 | 0 | | 0 | 48 | 6 | 22 | 7.34 | 0.014 | 0 | 0 | 0.10 | 4.1 | 2.02 | 1.38 |
| | | 28.7 | 4.6 | 2.0 | 1.8 | | 94 | 269 | 203 | 4.13 | 0.177 | 35.4 | 0 | 0.2 | 0.40 | 0.39 | 17.8 | 17333 |
| **bison, ground, grass-fed**, pan-fried | 85 | 152 | 55.3 | 0 | 0 | | 0 | 65 | 12 | 20 | 4.54 | | 0 | 0 | 0.12 | 5.1 | 2.07 | |
| *3 oz* | | 21.6 | 7.3 | 3.0 | 2.8 | 0.3 | 60 | 300 | 181 | 2.71 | 0.128 | 26.4 | 0 | 0.2 | 0.22 | 0.34 | 13.6 | 17148 |
| **bison, ground**, pan-broiled | 85 | 202 | 50.6 | 0 | 0 | | 0 | 62 | 11 | 19 | 4.37 | 0.008 | 0 | 0 | 0.11 | 4.7 | 1.94 | 0.97 |
| *3 oz* | | 20.2 | 12.9 | | | | 71 | 290 | 174 | 2.62 | 0.124 | 25.5 | 0 | 0.2 | 0.21 | 0.32 | 12.8 | 17331 |
| **bison ribeye steak**, lean, broiled | 85 | 150 | 54.8 | 0 | 0 | | 0 | 44 | 6 | 22 | 4.26 | 0.010 | 0 | 0 | 0.12 | 5.7 | 1.10 | 0.86 |
| *3 oz* | | 25.0 | 4.8 | 2.1 | 1.9 | 0.2 | 67 | 315 | 202 | 2.45 | 0.171 | 35.8 | 0 | 0.2 | 0.26 | 0.40 | 15.3 | 17335 |
| **bison top round steak**, lean, broiled - *3 oz* | 85 | 148 | 55.3 | 0 | 0 | | 0 | 35 | 4 | 24 | 3.22 | 0.009 | 0 | 0 | 0.14 | 5.5 | 1.54 | 1.23 |
| | | 25.7 | 4.2 | 1.7 | 1.5 | 0.2 | 72 | 325 | 218 | 2.99 | 0.178 | 34.8 | 0 | 0.2 | 0.31 | 0.56 | 16.2 | 17336 |
| **bison top sirloin steak**, lean, broiled - *3 oz* | 85 | 145 | 55.3 | 0 | 0 | | 0 | 45 | 4 | 23 | 4.34 | 0.011 | 0 | 0 | 0.19 | 4.7 | 2.41 | 1.14 |
| | | 23.8 | 4.8 | 2.1 | 1.9 | 0.2 | 73 | 329 | 215 | 2.95 | 0.179 | 35.0 | 0 | 0.2 | 0.38 | 0.47 | 15.3 | 17332 |
| **boar, wild**, roasted | 85 | 136 | 54.3 | 0 | 0 | | 0 | 51 | 14 | 23 | 2.56 | | 0 | 0 | 0.26 | 3.6 | 0.60 | |
| *3 oz* | | 24.1 | 3.7 | 1.1 | 1.5 | 0.5 | 65 | 337 | 114 | 0.95 | 0.048 | 11.0 | 0 | 0.3 | 0.12 | 0.36 | 5.1 | 17159 |
| **buffalo top round steak**, broiled | 85 | 124 | 54.6 | 0 | 0 | | 0 | 35 | 3 | 24 | 4.30 | 0.009 | | | 0.14 | 6.0 | 1.42 | 0.86 |
| *3 oz* | | 27.6 | 1.5 | 0.5 | 0.5 | 0.1 | 70 | 320 | 209 | 3.20 | 0.161 | 8.9 | | 0.5 | 0.39 | 0.67 | 6.8 | 35176 |
| **caribou**, roasted | 85 | 142 | 53.1 | 0 | 0 | | 0 | 51 | 19 | 23 | 4.47 | 0.074 | 0 | 3 | 0.21 | 4.9 | 5.64 | 2.28 |
| *3 oz* | | 25.3 | 3.8 | 1.4 | 1.1 | 0.5 | 93 | 264 | 198 | 5.24 | 0.224 | 11.6 | 0 | 0.3 | 0.76 | 0.27 | 4.2 | 17163 |
| **caribou shoulder**, dried | 28 | 76 | 9.5 | 0 | 0 | | 0 | 266 | 4 | 17 | 2.63 | 0.031 | 3 | 0 | 0.09 | 4.1 | 4.23 | 1.16 |
| *1 oz* | | 16.6 | 1.0 | 0.4 | 0.3 | 0.1 | 46 | 227 | 154 | 3.08 | 0.218 | 10.3 | 10 | 0 | 0.36 | 0.14 | 2.2 | 35161 |
| **deer, all cuts**, roasted | 85 | 134 | 55.4 | 0 | | | 0 | 46 | 6 | 20 | 2.34 | 0.039 | 0 | 0 | 0.15 | 5.7 | | |
| *3 oz* | | 25.7 | 2.7 | 1.1 | 0.7 | 0.5 | 95 | 285 | 192 | 3.80 | 0.255 | 11.0 | 0 | | 0.51 | | | 17165 |
| **deer, ground**, pan-broiled | 85 | 159 | 54.6 | 0 | 0 | | 0 | 66 | 12 | 20 | 4.42 | 0.011 | 0 | 0 | 0.43 | 7.9 | 1.97 | 0.65 |
| *3 oz* | | 22.5 | 7.0 | 3.4 | 1.6 | 0.4 | 83 | 309 | 194 | 2.85 | 0.085 | 8.8 | 0 | 0.6 | 0.28 | 0.40 | 6.8 | 17344 |
| **deer loin steak**, lean, broiled | 85 | 128 | 57.0 | 0 | 0 | | 0 | 48 | 5 | 26 | 3.09 | 0.025 | 0 | 0 | 0.24 | 9.1 | 1.56 | 0.74 |
| *3 oz* | | 25.7 | 2.0 | 0.7 | 0.3 | 0.1 | 67 | 338 | 235 | 3.48 | 0.193 | 11.3 | 0 | 0.5 | 0.44 | 0.64 | 7.6 | 17345 |
| **deer shoulder clod**, lean, braised | 85 | 162 | 50.8 | 0 | 0 | | 0 | 44 | 5 | 24 | 7.34 | 0.022 | 0 | 0 | 0.13 | 6.3 | 2.60 | 0.87 |
| *3 oz* | | 30.8 | 3.4 | 1.7 | 0.7 | 0.2 | 96 | 266 | 222 | 4.26 | 0.242 | 15.0 | 0 | 0.6 | 0.56 | 0.41 | 9.4 | 17346 |
| **deer tenderloin**, lean, broiled | 85 | 127 | 57.1 | 0 | 0 | | 0 | 48 | 4 | 28 | 3.39 | 0.019 | 0 | 0 | 0.22 | 7.5 | 3.08 | 0.73 |
| *3 oz* | | 25.4 | 2.0 | 1.0 | 0.5 | 0.1 | 75 | 369 | 254 | 3.61 | 0.216 | 9.4 | 0 | 0.5 | 0.48 | 0.52 | 7.6 | 17347 |
| **deer, top round steak**, lean, broiled | 85 | 129 | 56.2 | 0 | 0 | | 0 | 38 | 3 | 26 | 3.12 | 0.015 | 0 | 0 | 0.21 | 7.1 | 1.93 | 0.77 |
| *3 oz* | | 26.7 | 1.6 | 0.9 | 0.4 | 0.1 | 72 | 320 | 231 | 3.60 | 0.231 | 9.6 | 0 | 0.5 | 0.42 | 0.60 | 8.5 | 17348 |
| **elk, eye of round**, cooked | 85 | 126 | 54.9 | 0 | 0 | | 0 | 42 | 3 | 22 | 4.08 | 0.014 | 0 | 0 | 0.14 | 6.8 | 1.66 | 0.76 |
| *3 oz* | | 26.0 | 2.4 | 1.0 | 1.2 | 0.1 | 54 | 314 | 201 | 2.28 | 0.131 | 17.4 | 0 | 0.4 | 0.30 | 0.78 | 0.8 | 35178 |
| **elk, ground**, pan-broiled | 85 | 164 | 54.5 | 0 | 0 | | 0 | 72 | 8 | 20 | 5.58 | 0.009 | 0 | 0 | 0.11 | 4.5 | 2.18 | 0.89 |
| *3 oz* | | 22.6 | 7.4 | 3.4 | 2.3 | | 66 | 301 | 188 | 2.84 | 0.121 | 7.6 | 0 | 0.5 | 0.27 | 0.36 | 6.8 | 17339 |
| **elk, ground patty**, cooked | 85 | 122 | 57.6 | 0 | 0 | | | 48 | 4 | 22 | 6.62 | 0.037 | 0 | 0 | 0.15 | 6.7 | 3.61 | 0.88 |
| *3 oz* | | 25.0 | 2.4 | 1.0 | 0.8 | 0.2 | 60 | 322 | 201 | 7.70 | 0.173 | 20.0 | 0 | 0.7 | 0.42 | 0.66 | 0.8 | 35172 |
| **elk loin**, lean, broiled | 85 | 142 | 54.8 | 0 | 0 | | 0 | 46 | 4 | 24 | 4.34 | 0.010 | 0 | 0 | 0.14 | 7.6 | 0.71 | 1.04 |
| *3 oz* | | 26.4 | 3.3 | 1.3 | 0.9 | 0.2 | 64 | 343 | 218 | 3.37 | 0.147 | 8.9 | 0 | 0.5 | 0.28 | 0.40 | 7.6 | 17340 |
| **elk**, roasted | 85 | 124 | 56.3 | 0 | | | 0 | 52 | 4 | 20 | 2.69 | 0.011 | 0 | | | | | |
| *3 oz* | | 25.7 | 1.6 | 0.6 | 0.4 | 0.3 | 62 | 279 | 153 | 3.09 | 0.121 | 11.0 | 0 | | | | 7.6 | 17167 |
| **elk round**, lean, broiled | 85 | 133 | 55.6 | 0 | 0 | | 0 | 43 | 4 | 24 | 4.79 | 0.013 | 0 | 0 | 0.15 | 6.1 | 1.27 | 1.04 |
| *3 oz* | | 26.3 | 2.2 | 0.9 | 0.6 | 0.1 | 66 | 333 | 226 | 3.47 | 0.188 | 9.0 | 0 | 0.5 | 0.39 | 0.40 | 7.6 | 17341 |
| **elk tenderloin**, lean, broiled | 85 | 138 | 55.2 | 0 | 0 | | 0 | 42 | 4 | 25 | 3.50 | 0.016 | 0 | 0 | 0.12 | 5.2 | 2.52 | 1.03 |
| *3 oz* | | 26.1 | 2.9 | 1.1 | 0.8 | 0.1 | 61 | 333 | 242 | 3.46 | 0.297 | 8.9 | 0 | 0.5 | 0.31 | 0.41 | 7.6 | 17342 |
| **emu fan fillet**, broiled | 85 | 131 | 56.5 | 0 | 0 | | 0 | 45 | 5 | 26 | 2.71 | 0.022 | 0 | 0 | 0.30 | 8.3 | 7.96 | 2.88 |
| *3 oz* | | 26.6 | 2.0 | 0.5 | 0.8 | 0.3 | 70 | 337 | 231 | 3.88 | 0.197 | 39.2 | 0 | 0.2 | 0.51 | 0.78 | 7.6 | 5624 |
| **emu flat fillet**, raw | 85 | 87 | 64.1 | 0 | 0 | | 0 | 128 | 3 | 26 | 2.55 | 0.024 | 0 | 0 | 0.21 | 5.8 | 5.20 | 2.11 |
| *3 oz* | | 18.9 | 0.6 | 0.2 | 0.3 | 0.1 | 60 | 204 | 195 | 4.25 | 0.174 | 26.8 | 0 | 0.2 | 0.35 | 0.49 | 10.2 | 5625 |
| **emu full rump**, broiled | 85 | 143 | 52.7 | 0 | 0 | | 0 | 94 | 6 | 29 | 3.67 | 0.031 | 3 | 0 | 0.37 | 9.0 | 1.87 | 3.10 |
| *3 oz* | | 28.6 | 2.3 | 0.7 | 0.9 | 0.5 | 110 | 275 | 275 | 5.86 | 0.242 | 44.3 | 9 | 0.2 | 0.55 | 0.84 | 8.5 | 5627 |
| **emu, ground**, pan-broiled | 85 | 139 | 56.0 | 0 | 0 | | 0 | 55 | 7 | 25 | 3.88 | 0.026 | 0 | 0 | 0.27 | 7.6 | 7.24 | 2.62 |
| *3 oz patty* | | 24.2 | 4.0 | 1.1 | 1.7 | 0.6 | 74 | 319 | 229 | 4.26 | 0.202 | 37.0 | 0 | 0.2 | 0.46 | 0.71 | 7.6 | 5622 |
| **emu inside drum**, broiled | 85 | 133 | 54.7 | 0 | 0 | | 0 | 100 | 5 | 28 | 4.33 | 0.029 | 3 | 0 | 0.35 | 8.6 | 2.04 | 2.98 |
| *3 oz* | | 27.5 | 1.7 | 0.6 | 0.7 | 0.3 | 77 | 265 | 261 | 6.18 | 0.231 | 42.2 | 8 | 0.2 | 0.53 | 0.81 | 8.5 | 5629 |

| | WT (g) | KCAL / PRO (g) | H₂0 (g) / FAT (g) | CHO (g) / SFA (g) | TSUG (g) / MUFA (g) | ASUG (g) / PUFA (g) | DFIB (g) / CHOL (mg) | Na (mg) / K (mg) | Ca (mg) / P (mg) | Mg (mg) / Fe (mg) | Zn (mg) / Cu (mg) | Mn (mg) / Se (mcg) | A (mcg RAE) / A (IU) | C (mg) / E (mg ATE) | B-1 (mg) / B-2 (mg) | NIA (mg) / B-6 (mg) | B-12 (mcg) / FOL (mcg DFE) | PANT (mg) / REF |
|---|---|---|---|---|---|---|---|---|---|---|---|---|---|---|---|---|---|---|
| emu outside drum, raw | 85 | 88 | 63.6 | 0 | 0 | | 0 | 85 | 3 | 25 | 3.82 | 0.021 | 0 | 0 | 0.22 | 6.2 | 5.88 | 2.12 |
| 3 oz | | 19.6 | 0.4 | 0.1 | 0.2 | 0.1 | 66 | 272 | 191 | 3.82 | 0.169 | 30.9 | 0 | 0.1 | 0.38 | 0.57 | 6.0 | 5630 |
| emu oyster, raw | 85 | 120 | 61.7 | 0 | 0 | | 0 | 128 | 3 | 26 | 5.10 | 0.023 | 0 | 0 | 0.23 | 6.4 | 5.75 | 2.33 |
| 3 oz | | 19.4 | 4.1 | 1.0 | 1.6 | 0.6 | 69 | 212 | 184 | 4.68 | 0.165 | 25.3 | 0 | 0.2 | 0.39 | 0.55 | 11.0 | 5631 |
| emu top loin, broiled | 85 | 129 | 57.3 | 0 | 0 | | 0 | 49 | 8 | 26 | 2.91 | 0.026 | 0 | 0 | 0.28 | 7.8 | 7.40 | 2.68 |
| 3 oz | | 24.7 | 2.7 | 0.7 | 1.1 | 0.4 | 75 | 318 | 233 | 4.31 | 0.238 | 37.0 | 0 | 0.2 | 0.47 | 0.72 | 7.6 | 5632 |
| frog legs, raw | 85 | 62 | 69.6 | 0 | 0 | | 0 | 49 | 15 | 17 | 0.85 | | 13 | 0 | 0.12 | 1.0 | 0.34 | |
| 3 oz | | 13.9 | 0.3 | 0.1 | 0 | 0.1 | 42 | 242 | 125 | 1.27 | 0.212 | 12.0 | 42 | 0.8 | 0.21 | 0.10 | 12.8 | 80200 |
| goat, roasted | 85 | 122 | 58.0 | 0 | 0 | | 0 | 73 | 14 | 0 | 4.48 | 0.036 | 0 | 0 | 0.08 | 3.4 | 1.01 | |
| 3 oz | | 23.0 | 2.6 | 0.8 | 1.2 | 0.2 | 64 | 344 | 171 | 3.17 | 0.258 | 10.0 | 0 | 0.3 | 0.52 | 0 | 4.2 | 17169 |
| horse, roasted | 85 | 149 | 54.4 | 0 | | | 0 | 47 | 7 | 21 | 3.25 | 0.019 | 0 | 2 | 0.08 | 4.1 | 2.69 | |
| 3 oz | | 23.9 | 5.1 | 1.6 | 1.8 | 0.7 | 58 | 322 | 210 | 4.28 | 0.145 | 11.5 | 0 | | 0.10 | 0.28 | | 17171 |
| moose, roasted | 85 | 114 | 57.7 | 0 | 0 | | 0 | 59 | 5 | 20 | 3.13 | 0.008 | 0 | 4 | 0.04 | 4.5 | 5.36 | |
| 3 oz | | 24.9 | 0.8 | 0.2 | 0.2 | 0.3 | 66 | 284 | 150 | 3.59 | 0.067 | 10.9 | 0 | 0.2 | 0.29 | 0.31 | 3.4 | 17173 |
| muskrat, roasted | 85 | 199 | 47.2 | 0 | | | 0 | 81 | 31 | 22 | 1.93 | 0.027 | 0 | 6 | 0.07 | 6.1 | 7.06 | 0.79 |
| 3 oz | | 25.6 | 10.0 | | | | 103 | 272 | 230 | 6.03 | 0.161 | 12.6 | 0 | | 0.60 | 0.40 | 9.4 | 17175 |
| opossum, roasted | 85 | 188 | 49.6 | 0 | 0 | | 0 | 49 | 14 | 29 | 1.94 | | 0 | 0 | 0.08 | 7.2 | 7.06 | |
| 3 oz | | 25.7 | 8.7 | 1.0 | 3.2 | 2.5 | 110 | 372 | 236 | 3.94 | 0.161 | 15.5 | 0 | 0.4 | 0.31 | 0.40 | 8.5 | 17176 |
| ostrich, ground, pan-broiled | 85 | 149 | 57.1 | 0 | 0 | | 0 | 68 | 7 | 20 | 3.68 | 0.014 | 0 | 0 | 0.18 | 5.6 | 4.88 | 1.03 |
| 3 oz | | 22.2 | 6.0 | 1.5 | 1.8 | 0.6 | 71 | 275 | 190 | 2.92 | 0.116 | 28.5 | 0 | 0.2 | 0.23 | 0.43 | 11.9 | 5642 |
| ostrich inside leg, cooked | 85 | 120 | 59.5 | 0 | 0 | | 0 | 71 | 5 | 21 | 4.00 | 0.015 | 0 | 0 | 0.20 | 6.2 | 5.41 | 1.14 |
| 3 oz | | 24.7 | 1.6 | 0.6 | 0.6 | 0.3 | 62 | 299 | 207 | 2.65 | 0.126 | 31.0 | 0 | 0.2 | 0.25 | 0.47 | 13.6 | 5645 |
| ostrich inside strip, cooked | 85 | 139 | 56.6 | 0 | 0 | | 0 | 62 | 4 | 22 | 4.16 | 0.016 | 0 | 0 | 0.20 | 6.3 | 5.47 | 1.16 |
| 3 oz | | 25.0 | 3.6 | 1.5 | 1.5 | 0.6 | 82 | 311 | 215 | 4.08 | 0.130 | 32.2 | 0 | 0.2 | 0.26 | 0.48 | 13.6 | 5647 |
| ostrich outside strip, cooked | 85 | 133 | 56.8 | 0 | 0 | | 0 | 61 | 4 | 22 | 4.17 | 0.016 | 0 | 0 | 0.20 | 6.1 | 5.32 | 1.12 |
| 3 oz | | 24.3 | 3.3 | 1.2 | 1.4 | 0.4 | 79 | 312 | 216 | 3.66 | 0.131 | 32.3 | 0 | 0.2 | 0.25 | 0.46 | 13.6 | 5650 |
| ostrich oyster, cooked | 85 | 135 | 57.4 | 0 | 0 | | 0 | 69 | 5 | 25 | 4.20 | 0.020 | 0 | 0 | 0.20 | 6.1 | 5.37 | 1.13 |
| 3 oz | | 24.5 | 3.4 | 1.4 | 1.2 | 0.4 | 76 | 348 | 239 | 4.16 | 0.153 | 39.5 | 0 | 0.2 | 0.25 | 0.47 | 13.6 | 5652 |
| ostrich tip, trimmed, cooked | 85 | 123 | 58.2 | 0 | 0 | | 0 | 68 | 5 | 21 | 4.12 | 0.016 | 0 | 0 | 0.20 | 6.1 | 5.31 | 1.12 |
| 3 oz | | 24.2 | 2.2 | 0.8 | 0.8 | 0.4 | 72 | 308 | 213 | 2.37 | 0.129 | 31.9 | 0 | 0.2 | 0.25 | 0.46 | 12.8 | 5656 |
| ostrich top loin, cooked | 85 | 132 | 57.8 | 0 | 0 | | 0 | 65 | 5 | 21 | 4.01 | 0.015 | 0 | 0 | 0.19 | 6.0 | 5.24 | 1.11 |
| 3 oz | | 23.9 | 3.3 | 1.1 | 1.1 | 0.3 | 79 | 300 | 208 | 2.81 | 0.126 | 31.1 | 0 | 0.2 | 0.25 | 0.46 | 12.8 | 5658 |
| rabbit, domesticated, raw | 85 | 116 | 61.9 | 0 | | | 0 | 35 | 11 | 16 | 1.33 | 0.022 | 0 | 0 | 0.08 | 6.2 | 6.09 | 0.68 |
| 3 oz | | 17.0 | 4.7 | 1.4 | 1.3 | 0.9 | 48 | 280 | 181 | 1.33 | 0.123 | 20.1 | 0 | | 0.13 | 0.42 | 6.8 | 17177 |
| rabbit, domesticated, roasted | 85 | 167 | 51.5 | 0 | | | 0 | 40 | 16 | 18 | 1.93 | 0.027 | 0 | 0 | 0.08 | 7.2 | 7.06 | 0.79 |
| 3 oz | | 24.7 | 6.8 | 2.0 | 1.8 | 1.3 | 70 | 326 | 224 | 1.93 | 0.161 | 32.7 | 0 | | 0.18 | 0.40 | 9.4 | 17178 |
| rabbit, domesticated, stewed | 85 | 175 | 50.0 | 0 | 0 | | 0 | 31 | 17 | 17 | 2.01 | 0.027 | 0 | 0 | 0.05 | 6.1 | 5.53 | 0.57 |
| 3 oz | | 25.8 | 7.1 | 2.1 | 1.9 | 1.4 | 73 | 255 | 192 | 2.01 | 0.150 | 32.7 | 0 | 0.4 | 0.14 | 0.29 | 7.6 | 17179 |
| rabbit, wild hare, raw | 85 | 97 | 63.0 | 0 | | | 0 | 42 | 10 | 25 | | | 0 | 0 | 0.03 | 5.5 | | |
| 3 oz | | 18.5 | 2.0 | 0.6 | 0.5 | 0.4 | 69 | 321 | 192 | 2.72 | | 8.0 | 0 | | 0.05 | | | 17180 |
| rabbit, wild hare, stewed | 85 | 147 | 52.2 | 0 | 0 | | 0 | 38 | 15 | 26 | 2.02 | | 0 | 0 | 0.02 | 5.4 | 5.53 | |
| 3 oz | | 28.1 | 3.0 | 0.9 | 0.8 | 0.6 | 105 | 292 | 204 | 4.12 | 0.150 | 12.9 | 0 | 0.3 | 0.06 | 0.29 | 6.8 | 17181 |
| raccoon, roasted | 85 | 217 | 46.2 | 0 | 0 | | 0 | 67 | 12 | 26 | 1.93 | | 0 | 0 | 0.50 | 4.0 | 7.06 | |
| 3 oz | | 24.8 | 12.3 | 3.5 | 4.4 | 1.8 | 82 | 338 | 222 | 6.03 | 0.161 | 15.3 | 0 | 0.4 | 0.44 | 0.40 | 9.4 | 17182 |
| sea lion, raw | 85 | 102 | 60.5 | 0 | | | | 53 | 5 | 19 | 2.82 | 0.014 | | 0 | | | | |
| 3 oz | | 22.0 | 1.6 | | 0.1 | | 54 | 345 | 215 | 9.76 | 0.448 | 95.0 | | | | | | 35229 |
| seal, bearded, dried | 28 | 98 | 3.2 | 0 | 0 | | 0 | | | | | | 110 | | 0.04 | | | |
| 1 oz | | 23.1 | 0.6 | 0.2 | 0.4 | 0.1 | | | 220 | 13.89 | | | 367 | | 0.18 | | | 35055 |
| seal, bearded, dried in oil | 28 | 103 | 9.9 | 0 | 0 | | 0 | 34 | 2 | 8 | 0.87 | 0.010 | | 0 | 0 | 1.8 | 1.64 | 0.20 |
| 1 oz | | 9.9 | 7.0 | 1.1 | 3.1 | 0.3 | 18 | 112 | 67 | 4.76 | 0.076 | 25.4 | 545 | 0.2 | 0.10 | 0.03 | 3.1 | 35164 |
| squirrel, roasted | 85 | 147 | 52.8 | 0 | 0 | | 0 | 101 | 3 | 24 | 1.51 | 0.027 | 0 | 0 | 0.05 | 3.9 | 5.53 | 0.79 |
| 3 oz | | 26.2 | 4.0 | 0.7 | 1.1 | 1.2 | 103 | 299 | 179 | 5.79 | 0.126 | 12.8 | 0 | 0.3 | 0.25 | 0.31 | 7.6 | 17184 |
| turtle, green, raw | 85 | 76 | 66.7 | 0 | 0 | | 0 | 58 | 100 | 17 | 0.85 | | 26 | 0 | 0.10 | 0.9 | 0.85 | |
| 3 oz | | 16.8 | 0.4 | 0.1 | 0.1 | 0.1 | 42 | 196 | 153 | 1.19 | 0.212 | 14.3 | 85 | 0.4 | 0.13 | 0.10 | 12.8 | 93600 |
| walrus, dried | 85 | 213 | 33.0 | 0 | | | | | | | | | | | 0.18 | 8.6 | | |
| 3 oz | | 48.4 | 2.2 | | | | | | 353 | 36.55 | | | 348 | | 0.67 | | | 35079 |
| water buffalo, roasted | 85 | 111 | 58.5 | 0 | | | 0 | 48 | 13 | 28 | 2.16 | | 0 | 0 | 0.03 | 5.3 | 1.49 | 0.14 |
| 3 oz | | 22.8 | 1.5 | 0.5 | 0.5 | 0.3 | 52 | 266 | 187 | 1.80 | 0.151 | 10.2 | 0 | | 0.21 | 0.39 | 7.6 | 17161 |
| whale, beluga, dried | 85 | 94 | 61.6 | 0 | 0 | | 0 | 66 | 6 | 19 | 2.35 | 0.039 | 87 | 0 | 0.01 | 4.6 | 2.20 | 0.51 |
| 3 oz | | 22.5 | 0.4 | 0.1 | 0.3 | 0 | 68 | 241 | 203 | 22.01 | 0.096 | 31.0 | 289 | | 0.16 | 0.04 | 3.4 | 35011 |

### 19.3 LAMB, DOMESTIC US

| | WT (g) | KCAL / PRO (g) | $H_2O$ (g) / FAT (g) | CHO (g) / SFA (g) | TSUG (g) / MUFA (g) | ASUG (g) / PUFA (g) | DFIB (g) / CHOL (mg) | Na (mg) / K (mg) | Ca (mg) / P (mg) | Mg (mg) / Fe (mg) | Zn (mg) / Cu (mg) | Mn (mg) / Se (mcg) | A (mcg RAE) / A (IU) | C (mg) / E (mg ATE) | B-1 (mg) / B-2 (mg) | NIA (mg) / B-6 (mg) | B-12 (mcg) / FOL (mcg DFE) | PANT (mg) / REF |
|---|---|---|---|---|---|---|---|---|---|---|---|---|---|---|---|---|---|---|
| **lamb foreshank, choice**, ¼" trim, lean and fat, braised - *3 oz* | 85 | 207 | 48.3 | 0 | 0 | | 0 | 61 | 17 | 19 | 6.54 | 0.021 | 0 | 0 | 0.04 | 4.6 | 1.94 | 0.54 |
| | | 24.1 | 11.4 | 4.8 | 4.8 | 0.8 | 90 | 218 | 141 | 1.82 | 0.105 | 26.0 | 0 | 0.2 | 0.16 | 0.08 | 14.4 | 17008 |
| **lamb foreshank, choice**, ¼" trim, lean, braised - *3 oz* | 85 | 159 | 52.5 | 0 | | | 0 | 63 | 17 | 20 | 7.36 | 0.024 | 0 | 0 | 0.03 | 4.3 | 1.92 | 0.54 |
| | | 26.4 | 5.1 | 1.8 | 2.2 | 0.3 | 88 | 227 | 149 | 1.93 | 0.110 | 30.0 | 0 | 0.2 | 0.16 | 0.09 | 16.2 | 17010 |
| **lamb, ground**, broiled *3 oz* | 85 | 241 | 46.8 | 0 | 0 | | 0 | 69 | 19 | 20 | 3.97 | 0.020 | 0 | 0 | 0.08 | 5.7 | 2.22 | 0.56 |
| | | 21.0 | 16.7 | 6.9 | 7.1 | 1.2 | 82 | 288 | 171 | 1.52 | 0.109 | 23.5 | 0 | 0.1 | 0.21 | 0.12 | 16.2 | 17225 |
| **lamb leg and shoulder**, cubed, lean, braised - *3 oz* | 85 | 190 | 47.8 | 0 | 0 | | 0 | 60 | 13 | 24 | 5.59 | 0.027 | 0 | 0 | 0.06 | 5.1 | 2.32 | 0.50 |
| | | 28.6 | 7.5 | 2.7 | 3.0 | 0.7 | 92 | 221 | 174 | 2.38 | 0.120 | 32.4 | 0 | 0.2 | 0.20 | 0.10 | 17.8 | 17060 |
| **lamb leg and shoulder**, cubed, lean, broiled - *3 oz* | 85 | 158 | 54.0 | 0 | 0 | | 0 | 65 | 11 | 26 | 4.90 | 0.025 | 0 | 0 | 0.09 | 5.6 | 2.58 | 0.59 |
| | | 23.9 | 6.2 | 2.2 | 2.5 | 0.6 | 76 | 285 | 190 | 1.99 | 0.128 | 26.9 | 0 | 0.2 | 0.26 | 0.12 | 19.6 | 17061 |
| **lamb leg, shank half, choice**, ¼" trim, lean & fat, rstd - *3 oz* | 85 | 191 | 51.6 | 0 | | | 0 | 55 | 8 | 21 | 3.96 | 0.021 | 0 | 0 | 0.08 | 5.6 | 2.27 | 0.60 |
| | | 22.4 | 10.6 | 4.3 | 4.5 | 0.7 | 76 | 277 | 168 | 1.68 | 0.099 | 25.0 | 0 | 0.1 | 0.23 | 0.14 | 18.7 | 17016 |
| **lamb leg, shank half, choice**, ¼" trim, lean, roasted - *3 oz* | 85 | 153 | 55.2 | 0 | | | 0 | 56 | 7 | 22 | 4.27 | 0.024 | 0 | 0 | 0.09 | 5.4 | 2.30 | 0.60 |
| | | 23.9 | 5.7 | 2.0 | 2.5 | 0.4 | 74 | 291 | 177 | 1.75 | 0.103 | 26.9 | 0 | 0.2 | 0.24 | 0.14 | 20.4 | 17018 |
| **lamb leg, sirloin half, choice**, ¼" trim, lean & fat, rstd - *3 oz* | 85 | 248 | 46.0 | 0 | | | 0 | 58 | 9 | 19 | 3.51 | 0.019 | 0 | 0 | 0.09 | 5.6 | 2.15 | 0.57 |
| | | 20.9 | 17.6 | 7.4 | 7.4 | 1.3 | 82 | 256 | 156 | 1.70 | 0.095 | 21.7 | 0 | 0.1 | 0.24 | 0.12 | 14.4 | 17020 |
| **lamb leg, sirloin half, choice**, ¼" trim, lean, roasted - *3 oz* | 85 | 173 | 53.1 | 0 | 0 | | 0 | 60 | 7 | 21 | 4.12 | 0.024 | 0 | 0 | 0.10 | 5.3 | 2.19 | 0.60 |
| | | 24.1 | 7.8 | 2.8 | 3.4 | 0.5 | 78 | 283 | 173 | 1.87 | 0.101 | 26.2 | 0 | 0.1 | 0.26 | 0.14 | 17.8 | 17022 |
| **lamb leg, whole, choice**, ¼" trim, lean & fat, rstd - *3 oz* | 85 | 219 | 48.9 | 0 | 0 | | 0 | 56 | 9 | 20 | 3.74 | 0.020 | 0 | 0 | 0.08 | 5.6 | 2.20 | 0.58 |
| | | 21.7 | 14.0 | 5.9 | 5.9 | 1.0 | 79 | 266 | 162 | 1.68 | 0.098 | 23.1 | 0 | 0.1 | 0.23 | 0.13 | 17.0 | 17012 |
| **lamb leg, whole, choice**, ¼" trim, lean, roasted - *3 oz* | 85 | 162 | 54.3 | 0 | 0 | | 0 | 58 | 7 | 22 | 4.20 | 0.024 | 0 | 0 | 0.09 | 5.4 | 2.24 | 0.60 |
| | | 24.1 | 6.6 | 2.3 | 2.9 | 0.4 | 76 | 287 | 175 | 1.80 | 0.102 | 25.6 | 0 | 0.2 | 0.25 | 0.14 | 19.6 | 17014 |
| **lamb loin, choice**, ¼" trim, lean and fat, broiled - *3 oz* | 85 | 269 | 43.8 | 0 | 0 | | 0 | 65 | 17 | 20 | 2.96 | 0.019 | 0 | 0 | 0.08 | 6.0 | 2.10 | 0.54 |
| | | 21.4 | 19.6 | 8.4 | 8.2 | 1.4 | 85 | 278 | 167 | 1.54 | 0.110 | 23.3 | 0 | 0.1 | 0.21 | 0.11 | 15.3 | 17024 |
| **lamb loin, choice**, ¼" trim, lean, and fat, broiled - *3 oz* | 85 | 184 | 51.8 | 0 | 0 | | 0 | 71 | 16 | 24 | 3.51 | 0.024 | 0 | 0 | 0.09 | 5.8 | 2.14 | 0.56 |
| | | 25.5 | 8.3 | 3.0 | 3.6 | 0.5 | 81 | 320 | 192 | 1.70 | 0.123 | 27.9 | 0 | 0.1 | 0.24 | 0.14 | 20.4 | 17027 |
| **lamb loin, choice**, ¼" trim, lean and fat, roasted - *3 oz* | 85 | 263 | 44.6 | 0 | 0 | | 0 | 54 | 15 | 20 | 2.90 | 0.017 | 0 | 0 | 0.08 | 6.0 | 1.88 | 0.55 |
| | | 19.2 | 20.1 | 8.7 | 8.2 | 1.6 | 81 | 209 | 153 | 1.80 | 0.101 | 20.9 | 0 | 0.1 | 0.20 | 0.09 | 16.2 | 17025 |
| **lamb loin, choice**, ¼" trim, lean, roasted - *3 oz* | 85 | 172 | 53.3 | 0 | 0 | | 0 | 56 | 14 | 23 | 3.45 | 0.022 | 0 | 0 | 0.08 | 5.8 | 1.84 | 0.58 |
| | | 22.6 | 8.3 | 3.2 | 3.4 | 0.7 | 74 | 227 | 175 | 2.07 | 0.112 | 25.8 | 0 | 0.1 | 0.23 | 0.14 | 21.2 | 17028 |
| **lamb rib, choice**, ¼" trim, lean and fat, broiled - *3 oz* | 85 | 305 | 40.7 | 0 | | | 0 | 62 | 19 | 17 | 2.97 | 0.016 | 0 | 0 | 0.08 | 5.7 | 1.90 | 0.54 |
| | | 18.0 | 25.3 | 10.9 | 10.6 | 1.8 | 82 | 230 | 141 | 1.36 | 0.098 | 18.5 | 0 | 0.1 | 0.18 | 0.09 | 12.8 | 17031 |
| **lamb rib, choice**, ¼" trim, lean and fat, roasted - *3 oz* | 85 | 316 | 43.2 | 0 | | | 0 | 48 | 13 | 15 | 2.30 | 0.014 | 0 | 0 | 0.08 | 5.2 | 1.78 | 0.53 |
| | | 12.3 | 29.2 | 12.9 | 12.0 | 2.3 | 65 | 162 | 116 | 1.18 | 0.076 | 14.3 | 0 | 0.2 | 0.16 | 0.09 | 11.9 | 17029 |
| **lamb rib, choice**, ¼" trim, lean, broiled - *3 oz* | 85 | 289 | 41.7 | 0 | | | 0 | 65 | 15 | 20 | 3.58 | 0.018 | 0 | 0 | 0.08 | 5.9 | 2.18 | 0.52 |
| | | 19.6 | 22.8 | 9.7 | 9.3 | 1.8 | 83 | 235 | 156 | 1.64 | 0.105 | 21.0 | 0 | | 0.20 | 0.09 | 12.8 | 17240 |
| **lamb rib, choice**, ¼" trim, lean, roasted - *3 oz* | 85 | 290 | 42.2 | 0 | | | 0 | 63 | 16 | 17 | 3.08 | 0.018 | 0 | 0 | 0.08 | 5.7 | 1.89 | 0.54 |
| | | 18.5 | 23.4 | 9.9 | 9.9 | 1.7 | 82 | 235 | 144 | 1.38 | 0.099 | 19.0 | 0 | | 0.18 | 0.10 | 13.6 | 17241 |
| **lamb shoulder, arm, choice**, ¼" trim, lean and fat, braised - *3 oz* | 85 | 294 | 37.6 | 0 | | | 0 | 61 | 21 | 22 | 5.17 | 0.020 | 0 | 0 | 0.06 | 5.7 | 2.19 | 0.52 |
| | | 25.8 | 20.4 | 8.4 | 8.7 | 1.5 | 102 | 260 | 175 | 2.03 | 0.118 | 31.6 | 0 | 0.1 | 0.21 | 0.09 | 15.3 | 17044 |
| **lamb shoulder, arm, choice**, ¼ trim, lean and fat, broiled - *3 oz* | 85 | 239 | 46.5 | 0 | | | 0 | 65 | 15 | 22 | 4.16 | 0.020 | 0 | 0 | 0.08 | 6.0 | 2.43 | 0.58 |
| | | 20.8 | 16.6 | 7.1 | 6.8 | 1.3 | 82 | 263 | 167 | 1.78 | 0.113 | 23.5 | 0 | 0.1 | 0.23 | 0.10 | 15.3 | 17045 |
| **lamb shoulder, arm, choice**, ¼" trim, lean and fat, roasted - *3 oz* | 85 | 237 | 47.5 | 0 | | | 0 | 55 | 15 | 20 | 3.81 | 0.018 | 0 | 0 | 0.08 | 5.7 | 2.17 | 0.60 |
| | | 19.2 | 17.2 | 7.4 | 7.1 | 1.4 | 78 | 220 | 156 | 1.73 | 0.096 | 21.6 | 0 | 0.1 | 0.21 | 0.10 | 17.0 | 17046 |
| **lamb shoulder, arm, choice**, ¼" trim, lean, braised - *3 oz* | 85 | 237 | 41.9 | 0 | | | 0 | 65 | 22 | 25 | 6.20 | 0.024 | 0 | 0 | 0.06 | 5.4 | 2.25 | 0.53 |
| | | 30.2 | 12.0 | 4.3 | 5.2 | 0.8 | 103 | 287 | 197 | 2.30 | 0.131 | 32.1 | 0 | 0.2 | 0.23 | 0.11 | 18.7 | 17048 |
| **lamb shoulder, arm, choice**, ¼" trim, lean, broiled - *3 oz* | 85 | 170 | 52.9 | 0 | | | 0 | 70 | 14 | 26 | 4.87 | 0.024 | 0 | 0 | 0.08 | 5.8 | 2.55 | 0.60 |
| | | 23.6 | 7.7 | 2.9 | 3.1 | 0.7 | 78 | 289 | 186 | 1.96 | 0.123 | 26.8 | 0 | 0.2 | 0.25 | 0.12 | 19.6 | 17049 |
| **lamb shoulder, arm, choice**, ¼" trim, lean, roasted - *3 oz* | 85 | 163 | 54.7 | 0 | | | 0 | 57 | 14 | 22 | 4.46 | 0.022 | 0 | 0 | 0.08 | 5.4 | 2.22 | 0.63 |
| | | 21.6 | 7.9 | 3.1 | 3.2 | 0.7 | 73 | 235 | 172 | 1.90 | 0.102 | 24.7 | 0 | 0.1 | 0.23 | 0.12 | 21.2 | 17050 |
| **lamb shldr, blade, choice**, ¼" trim, lean & fat, braised - *3 oz* | 85 | 293 | 38.4 | 0 | | | 0 | 64 | 23 | 20 | 5.83 | 0.023 | 0 | 0 | 0.05 | 5.1 | 2.41 | 0.52 |
| | | 24.2 | 21.0 | 8.7 | 8.6 | 1.7 | 99 | 207 | 157 | 2.00 | 0.103 | 28.1 | 0 | 0.1 | 0.18 | 0.09 | 15.3 | 17052 |
| **lamb shldr, blade, choice**, ¼" trim, lean & fat, braised - *3 oz* | 85 | 236 | 47.5 | 0 | 0 | | 0 | 70 | 20 | 20 | 4.78 | 0.020 | 0 | 0 | 0.08 | 5.4 | 2.32 | 0.57 |
| | | 19.6 | 16.9 | 7.0 | 7.2 | 1.2 | 81 | 286 | 168 | 1.46 | 0.104 | 23.3 | 0 | 0.1 | 0.21 | 0.13 | 15.3 | 17053 |
| **lamb shldr, blade, choice**, ¼" trim, lean & fat, rstd - *3 oz* | 85 | 239 | 47.5 | 0 | | | 0 | 56 | 18 | 19 | 4.74 | 0.019 | 0 | 0 | 0.08 | 5.0 | 2.27 | 0.59 |
| | | 18.9 | 17.5 | 7.3 | 7.2 | 1.4 | 78 | 209 | 156 | 1.63 | 0.090 | 21.4 | 0 | 0.1 | 0.20 | 0.09 | 17.8 | 17054 |
| **lamb shoulder, blade, choice**, ¼" trim, lean, braised - *3 oz* | 85 | 245 | 42.2 | 0 | | | 0 | 67 | 24 | 22 | 6.85 | 0.027 | 0 | 0 | 0.05 | 4.8 | 2.50 | 0.52 |
| | | 27.5 | 14.1 | 5.4 | 5.7 | 1.2 | 99 | 216 | 172 | 2.21 | 0.109 | 31.1 | 0 | 0.2 | 0.19 | 0.10 | 17.8 | 17056 |
| **lamb shoulder, blade, choice**, ¼" trim, lean, broiled - *3 oz* | 85 | 179 | 53.1 | 0 | | | 0 | 75 | 20 | 22 | 5.51 | 0.024 | 0 | 0 | 0.08 | 5.2 | 2.39 | 0.59 |
| | | 21.7 | 9.6 | 3.4 | 4.2 | 0.6 | 77 | 313 | 184 | 1.54 | 0.110 | 26.3 | 0 | 0.1 | 0.22 | 0.14 | 17.8 | 17057 |

| | WT (g) | KCAL / PRO (g) | H₂0 (g) / FAT (g) | CHO (g) / SFA (g) | TSUG (g) / MUFA (g) | ASUG (g) / PUFA (g) | DFIB (g) / CHOL (mg) | Na (mg) / K (mg) | Ca (mg) / P (mg) | Mg (mg) / Fe (mg) | Zn (mg) / Cu (mg) | Mn (mg) / Se (mcg) | A (mcg RAE) / A (IU) | C (mg) / E (mg ATE) | B-1 (mg) / B-2 (mg) | NIA (mg) / B-6 (mg) | B-12 (mcg) / FOL (mcg DFE) | PANT (mg) / REF |
|---|---|---|---|---|---|---|---|---|---|---|---|---|---|---|---|---|---|---|
| **lamb shoulder, blade, choice,** ¼″ trim, lean, roasted - *3 oz* | 85 | 178 / 20.9 | 53.4 / 9.8 | 0 / 3.7 | / 4.0 | / 0.9 | 0 / 74 | 58 / 219 | 18 / 169 | 21 / 1.76 | 5.51 / 0.094 | 0.022 / 23.9 | 0 / 0 | 0 / 0.1 | 0.08 / 0.21 | 4.6 / 0.13 | 2.33 / 21.2 | 0.61 / 17058 |
| **lamb shldr, whl, choice,** ¼″ trim, lean & fat, braised - *3 oz* | 85 | 292 / 24.4 | 38.4 / 20.9 | 0 / 8.8 | / 8.5 | / 1.7 | 0 / 99 | 64 / 211 | 21 / 158 | 20 / 2.04 | 5.41 / 0.105 | 0.022 / 28.0 | 0 / 0 | 0 / 0.1 | 0.06 / 0.19 | 5.4 / 0.08 | 2.38 / 14.4 | 0.52 / 17036 |
| **lamb shldr, whl, choice,** ¼″ trim, lean & fat, braised - *3 oz* | 85 | 236 / 20.8 | 46.8 / 16.4 | 0 / 6.8 | / 6.7 | / 1.3 | 0 / 82 | 66 / 256 | 18 / 168 | 22 / 1.73 | 4.86 / 0.109 | 0.020 / 23.3 | 0 / 0 | 0 / 0.1 | 0.08 / 0.22 | 5.5 / 0.10 | 2.52 / 16.2 | 0.57 / 17037 |
| **lamb shldr, whl, choice,** ¼″ trim, lean & fat, rstd - *3 oz* | 85 | 235 / 19.1 | 47.8 / 17.0 | 0 / 7.2 | 0 / 6.9 | / 1.4 | 0 / 78 | 56 / 213 | 17 / 156 | 20 / 1.67 | 4.45 / 0.092 | 0.019 / 22.3 | 0 / 0 | 0 / 0.1 | 0.08 / 0.20 | 5.2 / 0.11 | 2.24 / 17.8 | 0.60 / 17038 |
| **lamb shoulder, whole, choice,** ¼″ trim, lean, braised - *3 oz* | 85 | 241 / 27.9 | 42.5 / 13.5 | 0 / 5.2 | / 5.5 | / 1.2 | 0 / 99 | 67 / 222 | 22 / 173 | 23 / 2.27 | 6.39 / 0.112 | 0.027 / 31.4 | 0 / 0 | 0 / 0.2 | 0.05 / 0.20 | 5.1 / 0.10 | 2.47 / 17.8 | 0.53 / 17040 |
| **lamb shoulder, whole, choice,** ¼″ trim, lean, broiled - *3 oz* | 85 | 178 / 23.1 | 52.2 / 8.9 | 0 / 3.3 | 0 / 3.6 | / 0.8 | 0 / 79 | 71 / 275 | 18 / 184 | 25 / 1.86 | 5.61 / 0.116 | 0.024 / 26.6 | 0 / 0 | 0 / 0.2 | 0.08 / 0.24 | 5.2 / 0.12 | 2.64 / 19.6 | 0.59 / 17041 |
| **lamb shoulder, whole, choice,** ¼″ trim, lean, roasted - *3 oz* | 85 | 173 / 21.2 | 53.8 / 9.2 | 0 / 3.5 | 0 / 3.7 | / 0.8 | 0 / 74 | 58 / 225 | 16 / 170 | 21 / 1.81 | 5.13 / 0.096 | 0.022 / 24.2 | 0 / 0 | 0 / 0.2 | 0.08 / 0.22 | 4.9 / 0.13 | 2.30 / 21.2 | 0.62 / 17042 |
| **mutton,** roasted *3 oz* | 85 | 199 / 28.4 | 45.9 / 9.4 | 0.1 / 4.4 | / 3.8 | / 0.7 | / 93 | 115 / 348 | 8 / 231 | 26 / 4.05 | 5.04 / 0.053 | 0.028 / 32.3 | | / 0.7 | 0.05 / 0.26 | 5.5 / 0.32 | 3.77 / | 0.76 / 35141 |

## 19.4 LAMB, IMPORTED FROM AUSTRALIA

| | WT (g) | KCAL / PRO (g) | H₂0 (g) / FAT (g) | CHO (g) / SFA (g) | TSUG (g) / MUFA (g) | ASUG (g) / PUFA (g) | DFIB (g) / CHOL (mg) | Na (mg) / K (mg) | Ca (mg) / P (mg) | Mg (mg) / Fe (mg) | Zn (mg) / Cu (mg) | Mn (mg) / Se (mcg) | A / A | C / E | B-1 / B-2 | NIA / B-6 | B-12 / FOL | PANT / REF |
|---|---|---|---|---|---|---|---|---|---|---|---|---|---|---|---|---|---|---|
| **lamb foreshank,** ⅛″ trim, lean and fat, braised - *3 oz* | 85 | 201 / 21.1 | 51.4 / 12.3 | 0 / 5.8 | / 5.1 | / 0.5 | / 77 | 79 / 207 | 14 / 142 | 18 / 1.52 | 5.92 / 0.099 | 0.009 / 7.1 | | | 0.07 / 0.22 | 4.3 / 0.21 | 2.55 / | 0.53 / 17287 |
| **lamb foreshank,** ⅛″ trim, lean, braised - *3 oz* | 85 | 140 / 23.4 | 56.9 / 4.4 | 0 / 1.6 | / 2.0 | / 0.2 | / 78 | 85 / 217 | 12 / 150 | 19 / 1.62 | 6.74 / 0.106 | 0.009 / 7.6 | | | 0.08 / 0.24 | 4.6 / 0.22 | 2.72 / | 0.56 / 17289 |
| **lamb leg, whole,** ⅛″ trim, lean and fat, roasted - *3 oz* | 85 | 207 / 21.4 | 50.7 / 12.9 | 0 / 6.0 | / 5.2 | / 0.5 | / 75 | 60 / 263 | 9 / 172 | 20 / 1.73 | 3.77 / 0.125 | 0.012 / 4.8 | | | 0.11 / 0.33 | 4.6 / 0.36 | 2.58 / | 0.78 / 17291 |
| **lamb leg, whole,** ⅛″ trim, lean, roasted - *3 oz* | 85 | 162 / 23.2 | 54.9 / 6.9 | 0 / 2.8 | / 2.8 | / 0.3 | / 76 | 61 / 277 | 8 / 182 | 21 / 1.83 | 4.11 / 0.134 | 0.012 / 5.0 | | | 0.11 / 0.36 | 4.9 / 0.39 | 2.71 / | 0.84 / 17293 |
| **lamb loin,** ⅛″ trim, lean and fat, broiled - *3 oz* | 85 | 186 / 21.7 | 52.7 / 10.4 | 0 / 4.7 | / 4.2 | / 0.4 | / 70 | 66 / 281 | 18 / 182 | 21 / 1.80 | 2.86 / 0.128 | 0.011 / 8.2 | | | 0.15 / 0.27 | 6.7 / 0.42 | 1.70 / | 0.69 / 17311 |
| **lamb loin,** ⅛″ trim, lean, broiled *3 oz* | 85 | 163 / 22.6 | 54.8 / 7.4 | 0 / 3.1 | / 3.0 | / 0.3 | / 69 | 68 / 289 | 18 / 187 | 22 / 1.85 | 2.96 / 0.133 | 0.012 / 8.8 | | | 0.15 / 0.28 | 6.9 / 0.44 | 1.71 / | 0.71 / 17313 |
| **lamb retail cuts,** ⅛″ trim, lean and fat, cooked - *3 oz* | 85 | 218 / 20.8 | 49.9 / 14.3 | 0 / 6.7 | / 5.7 | / 0.6 | / 74 | 65 / 256 | 14 / 166 | 19 / 1.64 | 3.98 / 0.121 | 0.011 / 8.6 | | | 0.10 / 0.28 | 4.6 / 0.31 | 2.44 / | 0.69 / 17281 |
| **lamb retail cuts,** ⅛″ trim, lean, cooked - *3 oz* | 85 | 171 / 22.7 | 54.2 / 8.2 | 0 / 3.4 | / 3.3 | / 0.4 | / 74 | 68 / 270 | 14 / 176 | 20 / 1.74 | 4.37 / 0.130 | 0.012 / 9.4 | | | 0.11 / 0.31 | 4.9 / 0.33 | 2.56 / | 0.74 / 17283 |
| **lamb rib,** ⅛″ trim, lean and fat, roasted - *3 oz* | 85 | 235 / 18.9 | 48.9 / 17.2 | 0 / 8.3 | / 6.7 | / 0.6 | / 68 | 65 / 240 | 14 / 155 | 18 / 1.42 | 2.85 / 0.111 | 0.010 / 7.7 | | | 0.11 / 0.23 | 4.7 / 0.32 | 1.65 / | 0.55 / 17315 |
| **lamb rib,** ⅛″ trim, lean, roasted *3 oz* | 85 | 178 / 20.9 | 54.2 / 9.9 | 0 / 4.3 | / 3.8 | / 0.4 | / 68 | 70 / 257 | 13 / 166 | 20 / 1.51 | 3.14 / 0.122 | 0.011 / 8.2 | | | 0.12 / 0.25 | 5.1 / 0.36 | 1.67 / | 0.59 / 17317 |
| **lamb shoulder, whole,** lean and fat, braised - *3 oz* | 85 | 252 / 20.0 | 47.0 / 18.4 | 0 / 8.8 | / 7.3 | / 0.7 | / 76 | 72 / 245 | 24 / 156 | 18 / 1.51 | 4.97 / 0.116 | 0.012 / 3.8 | | | 0.08 / 0.23 | 3.8 / 0.17 | 2.80 / | 0.61 / 17319 |
| **lamb shoulder, whole,** lean, braised - *3 oz* | 85 | 132 / 16.5 | 61.5 / 6.8 | 0 / 2.9 | / 2.7 | / 0.3 | / 54 | 75 / 260 | 15 / 151 | 18 / 1.21 | 4.14 / 0.110 | 0.011 / 3.3 | | | 0.10 / 0.20 | 3.9 / 0.25 | 2.56 / | 0.67 / 17320 |

## 19.5 LAMB, IMPORTED FROM NEW ZEALAND

| | WT (g) | KCAL / PRO (g) | H₂0 (g) / FAT (g) | CHO (g) / SFA (g) | TSUG (g) / MUFA (g) | ASUG (g) / PUFA (g) | DFIB (g) / CHOL (mg) | Na (mg) / K (mg) | Ca (mg) / P (mg) | Mg (mg) / Fe (mg) | Zn (mg) / Cu (mg) | Mn (mg) / Se (mcg) | A / A | C / E | B-1 / B-2 | NIA / B-6 | B-12 / FOL | PANT / REF |
|---|---|---|---|---|---|---|---|---|---|---|---|---|---|---|---|---|---|---|
| **lamb foreshank,** lean and fat, braised - *3 oz* | 85 | 219 / 22.9 | 48.2 / 13.5 | 0 / 6.6 | / 5.2 | / 0.6 | 0 / 87 | 40 / 100 | 12 / 149 | 13 / 1.76 | 4.08 / 0.087 | 0.020 / 4.5 | 0 / 0 | 0 / 0.2 | 0.06 / 0.28 | 5.2 / 0.07 | 2.07 / 0.8 | 0.35 / 17069 |
| **lamb foreshank,** lean, braised *3 oz* | 85 | 158 / 26.1 | 54.0 / 5.1 | 0 / 2.2 | / 2.0 | / 0.3 | 0 / 86 | 42 / 106 | 8 / 156 | 14 / 1.89 | 4.76 / 0.095 | 0.024 / 5.2 | 0 / 0 | 0 / 0.2 | 0.06 / 0.31 | 4.8 / 0.08 | 2.08 / 0.8 | 0.31 / 17071 |
| **lamb leg, whole,** lean and fat, roasted - *3 oz* | 85 | 209 / 21.1 | 49.2 / 13.2 | 0 / 6.5 | / 5.1 | / 0.6 | 0 / 86 | 37 / 142 | 8 / 185 | 17 / 1.78 | 3.04 / 0.088 | 0.020 / 3.4 | 0 / 0 | 0 / 0.1 | 0.10 / 0.38 | 6.5 / 0.11 | 2.21 / 0.8 | 0.47 / 17073 |
| **lamb leg, whole,** lean, roasted *3 oz* | 85 | 154 / 23.5 | 54.3 / 6.0 | 0 / 2.6 | / 2.3 | / 0.3 | 0 / 85 | 38 / 156 | 6 / 199 | 18 / 1.90 | 3.43 / 0.094 | 0.023 / 3.6 | 0 / 0 | 0 / 0.2 | 0.10 / 0.42 | 6.4 / 0.12 | 2.24 / 0 | 0.46 / 17075 |
| **lamb loin,** lean and fat, broiled *3 oz* | 85 | 268 / 19.9 | 42.9 / 20.3 | 0 / 10.2 | 0 / 7.8 | / 0.9 | 0 / 95 | 42 / 135 | 20 / 177 | 16 / 1.74 | 2.25 / 0.093 | 0.018 / 1.7 | 0 / 0 | 0 / 0.1 | 0.10 / 0.31 | 6.7 / 0.09 | 2.15 / 0.8 | 0.42 / 17077 |
| **lamb loin,** lean, broiled *3 oz* | 85 | 169 / 24.9 | 51.7 / 7.0 | 0 / 3.0 | / 2.7 | / 0.4 | 0 / 97 | 47 / 161 | 18 / 204 | 19 / 1.99 | 2.80 / 0.110 | 0.024 / 1.7 | 0 / 0 | 0 / 0.1 | 0.11 / 0.37 | 6.7 / 0.12 | 2.19 / 0 | 0.39 / 17079 |
| **lamb retail cuts,** lean and fat, cooked *3 oz* | 85 | 259 / 20.8 | 43.5 / 18.9 | 0 / 9.4 | / 7.3 | / 0.9 | 0 / 93 | 39 / 138 | 14 / 184 | 16 / 1.78 | 2.97 / 0.085 | 0.020 / 1.7 | 0 / 0 | 0 / 0.1 | 0.10 / 0.35 | 6.6 / 0.10 | 2.39 / 0.8 | 0.49 / 17063 |
| **lamb retail cuts,** lean, cooked *3 oz* | 85 | 175 / 25.2 | 51.0 / 7.5 | 0 / 3.3 | / 3.0 | / 0.4 | 0 / 93 | 42 / 160 | 11 / 209 | 19 / 2.00 | 3.66 / 0.097 | 0.025 / 1.7 | 0 / 0 | 0 / 0.2 | 0.11 / 0.42 | 6.5 / 0.12 | 2.51 / 0 | 0.49 / 17065 |
| **lamb rib,** lean and fat, roasted *3 oz* | 85 | 289 / 16.1 | 42.7 / 24.4 | 0 / 12.3 | 0 / 9.4 | / 1.1 | 0 / 85 | 37 / 105 | 16 / 144 | 12 / 1.45 | 2.21 / 0.060 | 0.014 / 1.5 | 0 / 0 | 0 / 0.1 | 0.08 / 0.23 | 5.8 / 0.07 | 1.98 / 0.8 | 0.43 / 17081 |

| | WT (g) | KCAL | H₂0 (g) | CHO (g) | TSUG (g) | ASUG (g) | DFIB (g) | Na (mg) | Ca (mg) | Mg (mg) | Zn (mg) | Mn (mg) | A (mcg RAE) | C (mg) | B-1 (mg) | NIA (mg) | B-12 (mcg) | PANT (mg) |
|---|---|---|---|---|---|---|---|---|---|---|---|---|---|---|---|---|---|---|
| | | PRO (g) | FAT (g) | SFA (g) | MUFA (g) | PUFA (g) | CHOL (mg) | K (mg) | P (mg) | Fe (mg) | Cu (mg) | Se (mcg) | A (IU) | E (mg ATE) | B-2 (mg) | B-6 (mg) | FOL (mcg DFE) | REF |
| **lamb rib**, lean, roasted | 85 | 167 | 54.7 | 0 | 0 | | 0 | 41 | 12 | 14 | 2.92 | 0.020 | 0 | 0 | 0.09 | 5.2 | 1.94 | 0.38 |
| *3 oz* | | 20.8 | 8.6 | 3.8 | 3.4 | 0.5 | 80 | 124 | 162 | 1.61 | 0.065 | 1.4 | 0 | 0.1 | 0.28 | 0.09 | 0 | 17083 |
| **lamb shoulder, whole**, lean and fat, braised - *3 oz* | 85 | 303 | 36.2 | 0 | | | 0 | 43 | 23 | 15 | 3.85 | 0.021 | 0 | 0 | 0.07 | 5.4 | 2.89 | 0.44 |
| | | 24.0 | 22.3 | 10.8 | 8.7 | 1.1 | 105 | 125 | 167 | 1.79 | 0.088 | 3.8 | 0 | | 0.27 | 0.06 | 0.8 | 17085 |
| **lamb shoulder, whole**, lean, braised - *3 oz* | 85 | 242 | 40.7 | 0 | | | 0 | 48 | 23 | 17 | 4.76 | 0.027 | 0 | 0 | 0.07 | 5.0 | 3.15 | 0.42 |
| | | 29.0 | 13.2 | 5.8 | 5.2 | 0.8 | 108 | 141 | 183 | 1.99 | 0.099 | 4.5 | 0 | | 0.31 | 0.07 | | 17087 |

## 19.6 PORK

| | WT (g) | KCAL | H₂0 (g) | CHO (g) | TSUG (g) | ASUG (g) | DFIB (g) | Na (mg) | Ca (mg) | Mg (mg) | Zn (mg) | Mn (mg) | A (mcg RAE) | C (mg) | B-1 (mg) | NIA (mg) | B-12 (mcg) | PANT (mg) |
|---|---|---|---|---|---|---|---|---|---|---|---|---|---|---|---|---|---|---|
| | | PRO (g) | FAT (g) | SFA (g) | MUFA (g) | PUFA (g) | CHOL (mg) | K (mg) | P (mg) | Fe (mg) | Cu (mg) | Se (mcg) | A (IU) | E (mg ATE) | B-2 (mg) | B-6 (mg) | FOL (mcg DFE) | REF |
| **Canadian bacon** (cured pork), grilled - *2 slices* | 47 | 87 | 29.0 | 0.6 | 0 | | 0 | 727 | 5 | 10 | 0.80 | 0.013 | 0 | 0 | 0.39 | 3.3 | 0.37 | 0.24 |
| | | 11.4 | 4.0 | 1.3 | 1.9 | 0.4 | 27 | 183 | 139 | 0.39 | 0.025 | 11.6 | 0 | 0.2 | 0.09 | 0.21 | 1.9 | 10131 |
| **Canadian bacon** (cured pork), unheated - *2 slices* | 57 | 89 | 38.2 | 1.0 | 0 | | 0 | 803 | 5 | 10 | 0.79 | 0.013 | 0 | 0 | 0.43 | 3.6 | 0.38 | 0.30 |
| | | 11.8 | 4.0 | 1.3 | 1.8 | 0.4 | 28 | 196 | 139 | 0.39 | 0.026 | 14.2 | 0 | 0.1 | 0.10 | 0.22 | 2.3 | 10130 |
| **Canadian bacon** (cured pork), unheated, Hormel - *2 oz patty* | 56 | 68 | 40.9 | 1.0 | 0.8 | | | 569 | 3 | 11 | 1.01 | | | 1 | | | | |
| | | 9.5 | 2.8 | 1.0 | 1.4 | 0.3 | 27 | 156 | | 0.50 | 0.056 | | 0 | | | | | 10857 |
| **pork bacon**, cured, broiled/pan-fried *3 medium slices* | 19 | 103 | 2.3 | 0.3 | 0 | | 0 | 439 | 2 | 6 | 0.66 | 0.004 | 2 | 0 | 0.08 | 2.1 | 0.23 | 0.22 |
| | | 7.0 | 7.9 | 2.6 | 3.5 | 0.9 | 21 | 107 | 101 | 0.27 | 0.031 | 11.8 | 7 | 0.1 | 0.05 | 0.07 | 0.4 | 10124 |
| **pork bacon**, cured, raw *3 medium slices* | 68 | 311 | 27.3 | 0.4 | 0 | | 0 | 566 | 4 | 8 | 0.80 | 0.015 | 7 | 0 | 0.19 | 2.6 | 0.47 | 0.35 |
| | | 7.9 | 30.6 | 10.2 | 13.6 | 3.4 | 46 | 141 | 128 | 0.33 | 0.048 | 13.7 | 25 | 0.2 | 0.08 | 0.14 | 1.4 | 10123 |
| **ham, cured** (purchased fully ckd), lean (4% fat), canned - *3 oz* | 85 | 102 | 62.5 | 0 | 0 | | 0 | 1067 | 5 | 14 | 1.64 | 0.021 | 0 | 0 | 0.71 | 4.5 | 0.70 | 0.42 |
| | | 15.7 | 3.9 | 1.3 | 1.9 | 0.3 | 32 | 309 | 190 | 0.80 | 0.071 | 12.3 | 0 | 0.1 | 0.20 | 0.38 | 5.1 | 10137 |
| **ham, cured** (purchased fully ckd), lean (4% fat), canned, roasted - *3 oz* | 85 | 116 | 59.0 | 0 | 0 | | 0 | 965 | 5 | 18 | 1.90 | 0.020 | 0 | 0 | 0.88 | 4.2 | 0.60 | 0.48 |
| | | 18.0 | 4.1 | 1.4 | 2.1 | 0.4 | 26 | 296 | 178 | 0.78 | 0.042 | 14.8 | 0 | | 0.21 | 0.38 | 4.2 | 10138 |
| **ham, cured** (purchased fully ckd) lean (5% fat), roasted - *3 oz* | 85 | 123 | 57.5 | 1.3 | 0 | | 0 | 1023 | 7 | 12 | 2.45 | 0.046 | 0 | 0 | 0.64 | 3.4 | 0.55 | 0.34 |
| | | 17.8 | 4.7 | 1.5 | 2.2 | 0.5 | 45 | 244 | 167 | 1.26 | 0.067 | 16.6 | 0 | 0.2 | 0.17 | 0.34 | 2.6 | 10134 |
| **ham, cured** (purchased fully ckd), reg (11% fat), roasted - *3 oz* | 85 | 151 | 54.9 | 0 | 0 | | 0 | 1275 | 7 | 19 | 2.10 | 0.035 | 0 | 0 | 0.62 | 5.2 | 0.60 | 0.61 |
| | | 19.2 | 7.7 | 2.7 | 3.8 | 1.2 | 50 | 348 | 239 | 1.14 | 0.123 | 16.8 | 0 | 0.3 | 0.28 | 0.26 | 2.6 | 10136 |
| **ham, cured** (purchased fully ckd), reg (13% fat), canned - *3 oz* | 85 | 162 | 56.6 | 0 | 0 | | 0 | 1054 | 5 | 12 | 1.41 | 0.020 | 0 | 0 | 0.82 | 2.7 | 0.66 | 0.33 |
| | | 14.4 | 11.0 | 3.6 | 5.3 | 1.2 | 33 | 269 | 149 | 0.71 | 0.057 | 25.3 | 0 | 0.2 | 0.20 | 0.41 | 4.2 | 10139 |
| **ham, cured** (purchased fully ckd), reg (13% fat), canned, roasted - *3 oz* | 85 | 192 | 51.8 | 0.4 | 0 | | 0 | 800 | 7 | 14 | 2.12 | 0.025 | 0 | 12 | 0.70 | 4.5 | 0.90 | 0.62 |
| | | 17.5 | 12.9 | 4.3 | 6.0 | 1.5 | 53 | 303 | 207 | 1.16 | 0.110 | 30.5 | 0 | | 0.22 | 0.26 | 4.2 | 10140 |
| **ham, cured** (purchased fully ckd), reg, cntr slice, lean & fat, unheated - *3 oz* | 85 | 173 | 53.9 | 0 | | | | 1178 | 6 | 14 | 1.60 | 0.026 | 0 | 0 | 0.72 | 4.1 | 0.68 | 0.42 |
| | | 17.1 | 11.0 | 3.9 | 5.2 | 1.2 | 46 | 286 | 183 | 0.64 | 0.063 | 19.2 | 0 | | 0.17 | 0.40 | 3.4 | 10142 |
| **ham, cured** (purchased fully ckd), whole, lean and fat, roasted - *3 oz* | 85 | 207 | 49.6 | 0 | 0 | | 0 | 1009 | 6 | 16 | 1.97 | 0.012 | 0 | 0 | 0.51 | 3.8 | 0.54 | 0.39 |
| | | 18.3 | 14.3 | 5.1 | 6.7 | 1.5 | 53 | 243 | 182 | 0.74 | 0.071 | 19.3 | 0 | 0.3 | 0.19 | 0.32 | 2.6 | 10151 |
| **ham, cured** (purchased fully ckd), whole, lean and fat, unheated - *3 oz* | 85 | 209 | 50.8 | 0.1 | 0 | | 0 | 1091 | 6 | 13 | 1.50 | 0.024 | 0 | 30 | 0.66 | 3.8 | 0.63 | 0.40 |
| | | 15.7 | 15.7 | 5.6 | 7.4 | 1.4 | 48 | 264 | 171 | 0.60 | 0.060 | 13.0 | 0 | 0.2 | 0.16 | 0.35 | 0.8 | 10150 |
| **ham, cured** (purchased fully ckd), whole, lean, roasted - *3 oz* | 85 | 133 | 55.9 | 0 | 0 | | 0 | 1128 | 6 | 19 | 2.18 | 0.014 | 0 | 0 | 0.58 | 4.3 | 0.60 | 0.42 |
| | | 21.3 | 4.7 | 1.6 | 2.2 | 0.5 | 47 | 269 | 193 | 0.80 | 0.074 | 21.6 | 0 | 0.2 | 0.22 | 0.40 | 3.4 | 10153 |
| **ham, cured** (purchased fully ckd), whole, lean, unheated - *3 oz* | 85 | 125 | 58.0 | 0 | 0 | | 0 | 1289 | 6 | 15 | 1.73 | 0.030 | 0 | 0 | 0.79 | 4.5 | 0.74 | 0.46 |
| | | 19.0 | 4.9 | 1.6 | 2.2 | 0.6 | 44 | 315 | 197 | 0.69 | 0.067 | 16.0 | 0 | 0.2 | 0.19 | 0.45 | 3.4 | 10152 |
| **ham patties**, cured, grilled *2 oz patty* | 60 | 205 | 30.8 | 1.0 | 0 | | 0 | 638 | 5 | 6 | 1.14 | 0.013 | 0 | 0 | 0.21 | 1.9 | 0.42 | 0.16 |
| | | 8.0 | 18.5 | 6.7 | 8.8 | 2.0 | 43 | 146 | 61 | 0.97 | 0.060 | 12.7 | 0 | 0.3 | 0.11 | 0.10 | 1.8 | 10147 |
| **ham patties**, cured, unheated *2.3 oz patty* | 65 | 205 | 35.4 | 1.1 | | | 0 | 707 | 5 | 6 | 1.02 | 0.015 | 0 | 0 | 0.30 | 2.0 | 0.70 | 0.20 |
| | | 8.3 | 18.3 | 6.6 | 8.6 | 2.0 | 46 | 155 | 97 | 0.68 | 0.046 | 10.3 | 0 | | 0.10 | 0.10 | 2.0 | 10146 |
| **ham steak**, extra lean, cured, unheated - *3 oz* | 85 | 104 | 61.4 | 0 | | | 0 | 1079 | 3 | 16 | 1.72 | 0.031 | 0 | 27 | 0.68 | 4.3 | 0.67 | 0.53 |
| | | 16.6 | 3.6 | 1.2 | 1.7 | 0.4 | 38 | 276 | 221 | 0.85 | 0.068 | 13.2 | 0 | | 0.17 | 0.31 | 3.4 | 10149 |
| **pork arm, picnic, cured**, lean and fat, roasted - *3 oz* | 85 | 238 | 46.5 | 0 | 0 | | 0 | 911 | 8 | 12 | 2.13 | 0.020 | 0 | 0 | 0.52 | 3.5 | 0.79 | 0.48 |
| | | 17.4 | 18.1 | 6.5 | 8.6 | 2.0 | 49 | 219 | 188 | 0.81 | 0.096 | 28.6 | 0 | 0.2 | 0.16 | 0.24 | 2.6 | 10168 |
| **pork arm, picnic, cured**, lean, roasted - *3 oz* | 85 | 144 | 54.3 | 0 | 0 | | 0 | 1046 | 9 | 14 | 2.50 | 0.026 | 0 | 0 | 0.62 | 4.1 | 0.94 | 0.56 |
| | | 21.2 | 6.0 | 2.0 | 2.7 | 0.7 | 41 | 248 | 207 | 0.92 | 0.109 | 35.1 | 0 | 0.2 | 0.19 | 0.31 | 3.4 | 10169 |
| **pork arm, picnic**, lean and fat, braised - *3 oz* | 85 | 280 | 40.5 | 0 | 0 | | 0 | 75 | 15 | 16 | 3.55 | 0.012 | 3 | 0 | 0.46 | 4.4 | 0.55 | 0.51 |
| | | 23.8 | 19.7 | 7.2 | 8.8 | 1.9 | 93 | 314 | 180 | 1.37 | 0.117 | 27.7 | 8 | 0.3 | 0.26 | 0.30 | 3.4 | 10075 |
| **pork arm, picnic**, lean and fat, roasted - *3 oz* | 85 | 269 | 44.2 | 0 | 0 | | 0 | 60 | 16 | 14 | 2.93 | 0.028 | 2 | 0 | 0.44 | 3.3 | 0.60 | 0.45 |
| | | 19.9 | 20.4 | 7.5 | 9.1 | 2.0 | 80 | 276 | 194 | 1.00 | 0.094 | 28.6 | 7 | | 0.26 | 0.30 | 3.4 | 10076 |
| **pork arm, picnic**, lean, braised - *3 oz* | 85 | 211 | 46.1 | 0 | 0 | | 0 | 87 | 7 | 19 | 4.22 | 0.014 | 2 | 0 | 0.51 | 5.0 | 0.60 | 0.57 |
| | | 27.4 | 10.4 | 3.5 | 4.9 | 1.0 | 97 | 344 | 192 | 1.66 | 0.137 | 31.4 | 7 | 0.2 | 0.31 | 0.35 | 4.2 | 10078 |
| **pork arm, picnic**, lean, roasted - *3 oz* | 85 | 194 | 51.2 | 0 | 0 | | 0 | 68 | 8 | 17 | 3.46 | 0.035 | 2 | 0 | 0.49 | 3.7 | 0.66 | 0.50 |
| | | 22.7 | 10.7 | 3.7 | 5.1 | 1.0 | 81 | 298 | 210 | 1.21 | 0.109 | 32.7 | 6 | | 0.30 | 0.35 | 4.2 | 10079 |

| | WT (g) | KCAL / PRO (g) | H₂O (g) / FAT (g) | CHO (g) / SFA (g) | TSUG (g) / MUFA (g) | ASUG (g) / PUFA (g) | DFIB (g) / CHOL (mg) | Na (mg) / K (mg) | Ca (mg) / P (mg) | Mg (mg) / Fe (mg) | Zn (mg) / Cu (mg) | Mn (mg) / Se (mcg) | A (mcg RAE) / A (IU) | C (mg) / E (mg ATE) | B-1 (mg) / B-2 (mg) | NIA (mg) / B-6 (mg) | B-12 (mcg) / FOL (mcg DFE) | PANT (mg) / REF |
|---|---|---|---|---|---|---|---|---|---|---|---|---|---|---|---|---|---|---|
| **pork backribs**, lean and fat, roasted | 85 | 314 | 38.6 | 0 | | | 0 | 86 | 38 | 18 | 2.86 | 0.008 | 3 | 0 | 0.36 | 3.0 | 0.54 | 0.49 |
| *3 oz* | | 20.6 | 25.1 | 9.3 | 11.4 | 2.0 | 100 | 268 | 166 | 1.17 | 0.069 | 33.4 | 8 | | 0.17 | 0.26 | 2.6 | 10193 |
| **pork blade roll, cured**, lean and fat, roasted - *3 oz* | 85 | 244 | 47.8 | 0.3 | | | 0 | 827 | 6 | 11 | 2.08 | 0.020 | 0 | 3 | 0.39 | 2.0 | 0.89 | 0.65 |
| | | 14.7 | 20.0 | 7.1 | 9.4 | 2.1 | 57 | 165 | 133 | 0.76 | 0.065 | 24.3 | 0 | | 0.24 | 0.18 | 2.6 | 10171 |
| **pork Boston blade**, lean and fat, braised - *3 oz* | 85 | 227 | 46.7 | 0 | 0 | | 0 | 49 | 22 | 20 | 4.11 | 0.010 | 2 | 0 | 0.43 | 3.3 | 0.79 | 1.10 |
| | | 21.3 | 15.0 | 5.6 | 6.8 | 1.8 | 83 | 259 | 177 | 1.49 | 0.110 | 36.0 | 7 | 0.1 | 0.31 | 0.38 | 0 | 10081 |
| **pork Boston blade**, lean and fat, broiled - *3 oz* | 85 | 220 | 48.7 | 0 | 0 | | 0 | 59 | 31 | 18 | 3.83 | 0.003 | 3 | 0 | 0.59 | 3.5 | 0.90 | 0.62 |
| | | 21.7 | 14.1 | 5.1 | 6.3 | 1.2 | 81 | 277 | 178 | 1.19 | 0.049 | 30.9 | 8 | 0.2 | 0.34 | 0.24 | 3.4 | 10082 |
| **pork Boston blade**, lean and fat, roasted - *3 oz* | 85 | 229 | 48.8 | 0 | 0 | | 0 | 57 | 24 | 15 | 3.37 | 0.010 | 2 | 1 | 0.54 | 3.5 | 0.75 | 0.57 |
| | | 19.6 | 16.0 | 5.9 | 7.0 | 1.5 | 73 | 282 | 167 | 1.23 | 0.097 | 29.2 | 6 | 0.2 | 0.30 | 0.20 | 4.2 | 10083 |
| **pork Boston blade**, lean, braised *3 oz* | 85 | 198 | 49.3 | 0 | 0 | | 0 | 51 | 21 | 20 | 4.42 | 0.011 | 0 | 0 | 0.45 | 3.3 | 0.76 | 1.16 |
| | | 22.6 | 11.2 | 4.3 | 5.3 | 1.2 | 85 | 270 | 184 | 1.57 | 0.116 | 38.2 | 0 | 0.1 | 0.33 | 0.40 | 0 | 10085 |
| **pork Boston blade**, lean, broiled *3 oz* | 85 | 193 | 51.1 | 0 | 0 | | 0 | 63 | 28 | 20 | 4.27 | 0.008 | 2 | 0 | 0.64 | 3.7 | 0.96 | 0.69 |
| | | 22.7 | 10.7 | 3.8 | 4.8 | 0.9 | 80 | 292 | 187 | 1.33 | 0.050 | 33.4 | 7 | 0.2 | 0.37 | 0.26 | 4.2 | 10086 |
| **pork Boston blade**, lean, roasted *3 oz* | 85 | 197 | 51.8 | 0 | 0 | | 0 | 75 | 23 | 22 | 3.60 | 0.013 | 3 | 1 | 0.95 | 4.2 | 0.99 | 0.92 |
| | | 20.6 | 12.2 | 4.4 | 5.4 | 1.1 | 72 | 363 | 200 | 1.33 | 0.103 | 30.7 | 8 | 0.2 | 0.34 | 0.37 | 6.8 | 10087 |
| **pork breakfast strips**, cured, cooked *3 slices (1.2 oz)* | 34 | 156 | 9.2 | 0.4 | 0 | | 0 | 714 | 5 | 9 | 1.25 | 0.015 | 0 | 0 | 0.25 | 2.6 | 0.60 | 0.31 |
| | | 9.8 | 12.5 | 4.3 | 5.6 | 1.9 | 36 | 158 | 90 | 0.67 | 0.052 | 8.4 | 0 | 0.1 | 0.13 | 0.12 | 1.4 | 10129 |
| **pork breakfast strips**, cured, raw *3 slices (2.4 oz)* | 68 | 264 | 32.2 | 0.5 | 0 | | 0 | 671 | 5 | 8 | 1.13 | 0.020 | 0 | 18 | 0.32 | 2.5 | 0.67 | 0.32 |
| | | 8.0 | 25.3 | 8.8 | 11.4 | 3.8 | 47 | 139 | 93 | 0.64 | 0.043 | 17.0 | 0 | | 0.12 | 0.14 | 2.0 | 10128 |
| **pork breast**, lean and fat, broiled *3 oz* | 85 | 138 | 57.2 | 0 | 0 | | 0 | 46 | 6 | 22 | 2.07 | 0.010 | 0 | 0 | 0.46 | 8.9 | 0.52 | 0.61 |
| | | 24.2 | 3.8 | 1.1 | 1.5 | 0.5 | 66 | 309 | 204 | 0.78 | 0.060 | 28.6 | 0 | 0.1 | 0.37 | 0.46 | 1.7 | 10959 |
| **pork center loin (chops)** w/bone, lean and fat, braised - *3 oz* | 85 | 210 | 48.8 | 0 | 0 | | 0 | 50 | 22 | 16 | 1.84 | 0.013 | 2 | 1 | 0.65 | 3.9 | 0.42 | 0.60 |
| | | 23.7 | 12.0 | 4.5 | 5.3 | 1.1 | 73 | 300 | 152 | 0.89 | 0.062 | 34.8 | 7 | | 0.18 | 0.32 | 2.6 | 10037 |
| **pork center loin (chops)** w/bone, lean and fat, broiled - *3 oz* | 85 | 178 | 52.9 | 0 | 0 | | 0 | 47 | 20 | 21 | 1.82 | 0.008 | 2 | 0 | 0.51 | 6.9 | 0.50 | 0.56 |
| | | 21.8 | 9.4 | 3.0 | 3.6 | 1.2 | 71 | 292 | 187 | 0.67 | 0.066 | 37.1 | 5 | 0.1 | 0.20 | 0.57 | 0 | 10038 |
| **pork center loin (chops)** w/bone, lean and fat, pan-fried - *3 oz* | 85 | 235 | 45.0 | 0 | 0 | | 0 | 68 | 23 | 25 | 1.96 | 0.009 | 2 | 1 | 0.97 | 4.8 | 0.62 | 0.78 |
| | | 25.4 | 14.1 | 5.1 | 6.0 | 1.6 | 78 | 361 | 220 | 0.77 | 0.064 | 33.2 | 7 | 0.2 | 0.26 | 0.40 | 5.1 | 10179 |
| **pork center loin (chops)** w/bone, lean, braised - *3 oz* | 85 | 172 | 52.2 | 0 | 0 | | 0 | 53 | 20 | 17 | 1.92 | 0.014 | 2 | 1 | 0.70 | 4.1 | 0.43 | 0.64 |
| | | 25.3 | 7.1 | 2.6 | 3.2 | 0.5 | 72 | 312 | 154 | 0.96 | 0.065 | 37.3 | 6 | 0.2 | 0.19 | 0.34 | 2.6 | 10041 |
| **pork center loin (chops)** w/bone, lean, broiled - *3 oz* | 85 | 153 | 55.3 | 0 | 0 | | 0 | 48 | 20 | 22 | 1.89 | 0.008 | 0 | 0 | 0.53 | 7.2 | 0.46 | 0.57 |
| | | 22.7 | 6.2 | 1.8 | 2.2 | 0.7 | 71 | 303 | 194 | 0.68 | 0.069 | 38.8 | 0 | 0.1 | 0.21 | 0.60 | 0 | 10042 |
| **pork center loin (chops)** w/bone, lean, pan-fried - *3 oz* | 85 | 197 | 48.3 | 0 | 0 | | 0 | 73 | 20 | 27 | 2.07 | 0.010 | 2 | 1 | 1.06 | 5.1 | 0.65 | 0.85 |
| | | 27.4 | 8.9 | 3.1 | 3.8 | 1.1 | 78 | 382 | 230 | 0.83 | 0.066 | 40.6 | 7 | 0.2 | 0.28 | 0.44 | 5.1 | 10176 |
| **pork center loin (roasts)**, lean and fat, roasted - *3 oz* | 85 | 199 | 50.8 | 0 | 0 | | 0 | 54 | 23 | 17 | 1.72 | 0.013 | 2 | 1 | 0.73 | 4.4 | 0.48 | 0.56 |
| | | 22.4 | 11.4 | 4.3 | 5.0 | 1.0 | 68 | 299 | 183 | 0.84 | 0.058 | 34.8 | 6 | | 0.22 | 0.30 | 3.4 | 10039 |
| **pork center loin (roasts)**, lean, roasted - *3 oz* | 85 | 169 | 53.5 | 0 | 0 | | 0 | 56 | 21 | 19 | 1.78 | 0.014 | 2 | 1 | 0.78 | 4.6 | 0.49 | 0.59 |
| | | 23.4 | 7.7 | 2.8 | 3.4 | 0.6 | 67 | 308 | 186 | 0.88 | 0.060 | 36.7 | 6 | | 0.23 | 0.32 | 3.4 | 10043 |
| **pork center rib (chops)** w/bone, lean and fat, braised - *3 oz* | 85 | 212 | 48.4 | 0 | 0 | | 0 | 34 | 21 | 15 | 1.71 | 0.008 | 2 | 0 | 0.50 | 4.2 | 0.45 | 0.44 |
| | | 22.7 | 12.8 | 5.0 | 5.8 | 1.1 | 62 | 329 | 150 | 0.77 | 0.061 | 34.8 | 6 | | 0.20 | 0.27 | 1.7 | 10045 |
| **pork center rib (chops)** w/bone, lean and fat, broiled - *3 oz* | 85 | 189 | 52.4 | 0 | 0 | | 0 | 47 | 24 | 20 | 1.83 | 0.005 | 2 | 0 | 0.46 | 6.4 | 0.49 | 0.54 |
| | | 20.8 | 11.1 | 3.8 | 4.6 | 1.4 | 57 | 280 | 178 | 0.58 | 0.071 | 36.4 | 7 | 0.1 | 0.18 | 0.54 | 0 | 10046 |
| **pork center rib (chops)** w/bone, lean, braised - *3 oz* | 85 | 175 | 51.8 | 0 | 0 | | 0 | 35 | 19 | 16 | 1.78 | 0.008 | 2 | 0 | 0.53 | 4.4 | 0.46 | 0.46 |
| | | 24.1 | 8.0 | 3.1 | 3.8 | 0.6 | 60 | 344 | 152 | 0.82 | 0.064 | 37.3 | 5 | 0.2 | 0.21 | 0.29 | 1.7 | 10049 |
| **pork center rib (chops)** w/bone, lean, broiled - *3 oz* | 85 | 158 | 55.4 | 0 | 0 | | 0 | 48 | 22 | 21 | 1.91 | 0.006 | 0 | 0 | 0.48 | 6.7 | 0.44 | 0.55 |
| | | 21.9 | 7.1 | 2.4 | 3.0 | 0.8 | 56 | 292 | 185 | 0.58 | 0.075 | 38.6 | 0 | 0.1 | 0.19 | 0.57 | 0 | 10050 |
| **pork center rib (chops)** w/bone, lean, panfried - *3 oz* | 85 | 232 | 47.9 | 0 | 0 | | 0 | 42 | 9 | 20 | 1.73 | 0.006 | 2 | 0 | 0.60 | 4.1 | 0.50 | 0.61 |
| | | 21.9 | 15.3 | 5.7 | 6.8 | 1.8 | 62 | 364 | 194 | 0.62 | 0.057 | 35.6 | 6 | 0.2 | 0.27 | 0.30 | 6.0 | 10197 |
| **pork center rib (roasts)**, lean and fat, roasted - *3 oz* | 85 | 217 | 47.6 | 0 | 0 | | 0 | 39 | 24 | 18 | 1.75 | 0.008 | 2 | 0 | 0.62 | 5.2 | 0.56 | 0.45 |
| | | 23.3 | 13.0 | 5.0 | 5.9 | 1.1 | 62 | 358 | 196 | 0.80 | 0.063 | 34.8 | 5 | | 0.26 | 0.28 | 2.6 | 10047 |
| **pork center rib (roasts)**, lean, roasted - *3 oz* | 85 | 190 | 50.0 | 0 | 0 | | 0 | 40 | 22 | 19 | 1.81 | 0.009 | 2 | 0 | 0.64 | 5.5 | 0.58 | 0.46 |
| | | 24.4 | 9.5 | 3.7 | 4.5 | 0.7 | 60 | 371 | 201 | 0.83 | 0.065 | 36.7 | 5 | | 0.27 | 0.29 | 2.6 | 10051 |
| **pork, ground**, cooked *3 oz* | 85 | 252 | 44.8 | 0 | 0 | | 0 | 62 | 19 | 20 | 2.73 | 0.009 | 2 | 1 | 0.60 | 3.6 | 0.46 | 0.44 |
| | | 21.8 | 17.7 | 6.6 | 7.9 | 1.6 | 80 | 308 | 192 | 1.10 | 0.037 | 30.1 | 7 | 0.2 | 0.19 | 0.33 | 5.1 | 10220 |
| **pork leg (rump and shank half)**, lean and fat, roasted - *3 oz* | 85 | 232 | 46.8 | 0 | 0 | | 0 | 51 | 12 | 19 | 2.52 | 0.027 | 3 | 0 | 0.54 | 3.9 | 0.58 | 0.52 |
| | | 22.8 | 15.0 | 5.5 | 6.7 | 1.4 | 80 | 299 | 224 | 0.86 | 0.085 | 38.5 | 8 | 0.2 | 0.27 | 0.34 | 8.5 | 10009 |
| **pork leg (rump and shank half)**, lean roasted - *3 oz* | 85 | 179 | 51.6 | 0 | 0 | | 0 | 54 | 6 | 21 | 2.77 | 0.031 | 3 | 0 | 0.59 | 4.2 | 0.61 | 0.57 |
| | | 25.0 | 8.0 | 2.8 | 3.8 | 0.7 | 80 | 317 | 239 | 0.95 | 0.092 | 42.4 | 8 | 0.2 | 0.30 | 0.38 | 10.2 | 10011 |
| **pork loin blade (chops)** w/bone, lean and fat, braised - *3 oz* | 85 | 275 | 44.1 | 0 | 0 | | 0 | 47 | 26 | 13 | 2.78 | 0.009 | 2 | 1 | 0.40 | 3.1 | 0.55 | 0.48 |
| | | 18.6 | 21.6 | 8.1 | 9.3 | 2.0 | 72 | 258 | 138 | 0.94 | 0.072 | 30.6 | 7 | 0.2 | 0.20 | 0.25 | 1.7 | 10029 |
| **pork loin blade (chops)** w/bone, lean and fat, broiled - *3 oz* | 85 | 272 | 44.1 | 0 | 0 | | 0 | 60 | 25 | 19 | 2.86 | 0.007 | 2 | 1 | 0.55 | 3.5 | 0.71 | 0.52 |
| | | 19.1 | 21.1 | 7.9 | 9.1 | 1.9 | 73 | 292 | 180 | 0.79 | 0.071 | 31.5 | 7 | | 0.25 | 0.32 | 3.4 | 10030 |

| | WT (g) | KCAL / PRO (g) | H₂O (g) / FAT (g) | CHO (g) / SFA (g) | TSUG (g) / MUFA (g) | ASUG (g) / PUFA (g) | DFIB (g) / CHOL (mg) | Na (mg) / K (mg) | Ca (mg) / P (mg) | Mg (mg) / Fe (mg) | Zn (mg) / Cu (mg) | Mn (mg) / Se (mcg) | A (mcg RAE) / A (IU) | C (mg) / E (mg ATE) | B-1 (mg) / B-2 (mg) | NIA (mg) / B-6 (mg) | B-12 (mcg) / FOL (mcg DFE) | PANT (mg) / REF |
|---|---|---|---|---|---|---|---|---|---|---|---|---|---|---|---|---|---|---|
| **pork loin blade (chops)** w/bone, lean and fat, panfried - 3 oz | 85 | 291 | 42.5 | 0 | 0 | | 0 | 57 | 26 | 18 | 2.71 | 0.007 | 2 | 1 | 0.53 | 3.4 | 0.71 | 0.56 |
| | | 18.3 | 23.6 | 8.6 | 10.0 | 2.6 | 72 | 282 | 175 | 0.75 | 0.068 | 29.7 | 7 | 0.2 | 0.25 | 0.29 | 3.4 | 10178 |
| **pork loin blade (chops)** w/bone, lean, braised - 3 oz | 85 | 191 | 51.9 | 0 | 0 | | 0 | 53 | 20 | 15 | 3.32 | 0.012 | 2 | 1 | 0.45 | 3.3 | 0.60 | 0.54 |
| | | 21.3 | 11.1 | 4.0 | 4.8 | 0.9 | 71 | 277 | 137 | 1.15 | 0.082 | 36.0 | 6 | 0.2 | 0.23 | 0.30 | 2.6 | 10033 |
| **pork loin blade (chops)** w/bone, lean, broiled - 3 oz | 85 | 199 | 50.9 | 0 | 0 | | 0 | 68 | 20 | 22 | 3.37 | 0.008 | 2 | 1 | 0.63 | 3.9 | 0.80 | 0.59 |
| | | 21.6 | 11.8 | 4.3 | 5.1 | 0.9 | 71 | 318 | 192 | 0.93 | 0.078 | 36.5 | 6 | | 0.30 | 0.38 | 3.4 | 10034 |
| **pork loin blade (chops)** w/bone, lean, panfried - 3 oz | 85 | 205 | 50.4 | 0 | 0 | | 0 | 66 | 19 | 22 | 3.29 | 0.008 | 2 | 1 | 0.62 | 3.8 | 0.82 | 0.66 |
| | | 21.0 | 12.8 | 4.4 | 5.3 | 1.7 | 70 | 310 | 188 | 0.91 | 0.076 | 36.0 | 6 | 0.2 | 0.30 | 0.35 | 3.4 | 10120 |
| **pork loin blade (roasts)**, lean and fat, roasted - 3 oz | 85 | 275 | 43.5 | 0 | 0 | | 0 | 26 | 29 | 17 | 2.80 | 0.009 | 3 | 1 | 0.45 | 3.6 | 0.62 | 0.41 |
| | | 20.2 | 20.9 | 7.8 | 9.0 | 1.8 | 79 | 277 | 178 | 0.94 | 0.067 | 31.5 | 8 | 0.2 | 0.25 | 0.32 | 3.4 | 10031 |
| **pork loin blade (roasts)**, lean, roasted - 3 oz | 85 | 210 | 49.5 | 0 | 0 | | 0 | 25 | 25 | 20 | 3.24 | 0.011 | 2 | 1 | 0.49 | 4.0 | 0.68 | 0.45 |
| | | 22.6 | 12.6 | 4.5 | 5.5 | 0.9 | 79 | 297 | 188 | 1.10 | 0.073 | 36.0 | 7 | | 0.29 | 0.37 | 4.2 | 10035 |
| **pork loin, whole,** lean and fat, braised - 3 oz | 85 | 203 | 49.5 | 0 | 0 | | 0 | 41 | 18 | 16 | 2.02 | 0.010 | 2 | 1 | 0.54 | 3.8 | 0.46 | 0.55 |
| | | 23.1 | 11.6 | 4.3 | 5.2 | 1.0 | 68 | 318 | 154 | 0.91 | 0.065 | 38.5 | 6 | 0.2 | 0.22 | 0.31 | 2.6 | 10021 |
| **pork loin, whole,** lean and fat, broiled - 3 oz | 85 | 206 | 49.2 | 0 | 0 | | 0 | 53 | 16 | 24 | 2.03 | 0.008 | 2 | 1 | 0.75 | 4.3 | 0.60 | 0.59 |
| | | 23.2 | 11.8 | 4.4 | 5.3 | 1.0 | 68 | 360 | 209 | 0.74 | 0.062 | 38.5 | 6 | 0.2 | 0.27 | 0.39 | 4.2 | 10022 |
| **pork loin, whole,** lean and fat, roasted - 3 oz | 85 | 211 | 48.9 | 0 | 0 | | 0 | 50 | 16 | 22 | 1.97 | 0.009 | 3 | 1 | 0.84 | 4.7 | 0.60 | 0.65 |
| | | 23.0 | 12.5 | 4.6 | 5.5 | 1.0 | 70 | 347 | 206 | 0.84 | 0.048 | 28.4 | 8 | 0.2 | 0.27 | 0.44 | 5.1 | 10023 |
| **pork loin, whole,** lean, braised 3 oz | 85 | 173 | 52.2 | 0 | 0 | | 0 | 42 | 15 | 17 | 2.11 | 0.011 | 2 | 1 | 0.56 | 3.9 | 0.47 | 0.58 |
| | | 24.3 | 7.8 | 2.9 | 3.5 | 0.6 | 67 | 329 | 156 | 0.96 | 0.067 | 41.0 | 6 | 0.2 | 0.23 | 0.33 | 3.4 | 10025 |
| **pork loin, whole,** lean, broiled 3 oz | 85 | 178 | 51.6 | 0 | 0 | | 0 | 54 | 14 | 25 | 2.11 | 0.008 | 2 | 1 | 0.78 | 4.5 | 0.61 | 0.62 |
| | | 24.3 | 8.3 | 3.1 | 3.8 | 0.7 | 67 | 372 | 215 | 0.77 | 0.064 | 41.0 | 6 | 0.2 | 0.29 | 0.42 | 5.1 | 10026 |
| **pork loin, whole,** lean, roasted 3 oz | 85 | 178 | 51.9 | 0 | 0 | | 0 | 49 | 15 | 24 | 2.15 | 0.014 | 2 | 1 | 0.86 | 5.0 | 0.62 | 0.66 |
| | | 24.3 | 8.2 | 3.0 | 3.7 | 0.6 | 69 | 361 | 212 | 0.93 | 0.050 | 29.8 | 7 | 0.2 | 0.28 | 0.47 | 0.8 | 10027 |
| **pork petite tender,** lean and fat, broiled - 3 oz | 85 | 132 | 58.4 | 0 | 0 | | 0 | 45 | 7 | 23 | 2.33 | 0.010 | 0 | 0 | 0.62 | 5.4 | 0.65 | 0.83 |
| | | 23.3 | 3.6 | 1.1 | 1.5 | 0.5 | 70 | 353 | 216 | 1.06 | 0.084 | 23.0 | 0 | 0.1 | 0.40 | 0.50 | 0.8 | 10960 |
| **pork, raw** 3 oz | 85 | 193 | 54.6 | 0 | 0 | | 0 | 46 | 13 | 17 | 1.79 | 0.013 | 2 | 1 | 0.68 | 3.8 | 0.57 | 0.61 |
| | | 15.5 | 14.0 | 4.9 | 6.2 | 1.5 | 59 | 275 | 167 | 0.76 | 0.058 | 24.2 | 6 | 0.2 | 0.21 | 0.35 | 5.1 | 10003 |
| **pork rump,** lean and fat, roasted 3 oz | 85 | 214 | 48.3 | 0 | 0 | | 0 | 53 | 10 | 23 | 2.40 | 0.020 | 3 | 0 | 0.64 | 4.0 | 0.61 | 0.53 |
| | | 24.5 | 12.1 | 4.5 | 5.4 | 1.2 | 82 | 318 | 231 | 0.89 | 0.088 | 39.8 | 8 | 0.2 | 0.28 | 0.27 | 2.6 | 10013 |
| **pork rump,** lean, roasted 3 oz | 85 | 175 | 51.8 | 0 | | | 0 | 55 | 6 | 25 | 2.56 | 0.022 | 3 | 0 | 0.68 | 4.2 | 0.64 | 0.56 |
| | | 26.3 | 6.9 | 2.4 | 3.2 | 0.6 | 82 | 332 | 242 | 0.97 | 0.093 | 41.8 | 8 | 0.2 | 0.30 | 0.29 | 2.6 | 10015 |
| **pork sausage (fresh),** maple, cooked, Jimmy Dean - 3 links (2.4 oz) | 68 | 280 | | 2.0 | 3.0 | | 0 | 250 | | | | | | 1 | | | | |
| | | 8.0 | 27.0 | 9.0 | | | 50 | | | 0.36 | | | 0 | | | | | JIMM1 |
| **pork sausage (fresh),** Oscar Mayer, pan-fried - 2 links (1.7 oz) | 48 | 165 | 23.8 | 0.5 | 0.4 | | 0 | 401 | 8 | 9 | 1.25 | | | 0 | | | | |
| | | 7.8 | 14.6 | 5.1 | 7.1 | 1.8 | 37 | 114 | 76 | 0.83 | 0.154 | | 0 | | | | | 7225 |
| **pork sausage (fresh),** pan-fried 1.1 oz patty (3⅛" diameter) | 27 | 92 | 13.4 | 0 | 0 | | 0 | 202 | 4 | 5 | 0.56 | 0.001 | 3 | 0 | 0.08 | 1.7 | 0.32 | 0.20 |
| | | 5.2 | 7.7 | 2.5 | 3.3 | 1.0 | 23 | 79 | 44 | 0.37 | 0.023 | 0 | 11 | 0.1 | 0.05 | 0.09 | 0.8 | 7064 |
| **pork sausage (fresh),** raw 3 oz | 85 | 258 | 47.8 | 0 | 0 | | 0 | 541 | 8 | 12 | 1.84 | 0.004 | 11 | 1 | 0.23 | 4.0 | 0.72 | 0.57 |
| | | 12.8 | 22.6 | 7.5 | 10.0 | 3.0 | 61 | 211 | 115 | 0.94 | 0.056 | 0 | 64 | 0.2 | 0.10 | 0.26 | 0.8 | 7063 |
| **pork shank,** lean and fat, roasted 3 oz | 85 | 246 | 45.7 | 0 | 0 | | 0 | 50 | 13 | 19 | 2.60 | 0.024 | 3 | 0 | 0.49 | 3.8 | 0.56 | 0.53 |
| | | 21.5 | 17.1 | 6.3 | 7.7 | 1.6 | 78 | 287 | 218 | 0.83 | 0.083 | 36.8 | 8 | | 0.26 | 0.34 | 4.2 | 10017 |
| **pork shank,** lean, roasted 3 oz | 85 | 183 | 51.4 | 0 | | | 0 | 54 | 6 | 21 | 2.93 | 0.029 | 2 | 0 | 0.54 | 4.1 | 0.60 | 0.58 |
| | | 24.0 | 8.9 | 3.1 | 4.3 | 0.8 | 78 | 306 | 236 | 0.94 | 0.092 | 42.3 | 7 | 0.2 | 0.29 | 0.39 | 5.1 | 10019 |
| **pork shoulder, whole,** lean and fat, roasted - 3 oz | 85 | 248 | 46.6 | 0 | 0 | | 0 | 58 | 20 | 15 | 3.15 | 0.019 | 2 | 0 | 0.49 | 3.4 | 0.68 | 0.51 |
| | | 19.8 | 18.2 | 6.7 | 8.0 | 1.7 | 76 | 280 | 180 | 1.12 | 0.096 | 28.4 | 7 | 0.2 | 0.28 | 0.24 | 4.2 | 10071 |
| **pork shoulder, whole,** lean, roasted 3 oz | 85 | 196 | 51.5 | 0 | 0 | | 0 | 64 | 15 | 17 | 3.54 | 0.022 | 2 | 1 | 0.53 | 3.6 | 0.73 | 0.55 |
| | | 21.5 | 11.5 | 4.1 | 5.2 | 1.1 | 76 | 294 | 188 | 1.27 | 0.105 | 31.8 | 6 | 0.2 | 0.31 | 0.27 | 4.2 | 10073 |
| **pork sirloin (chops)** with bone, lean and fat, braised - 3 oz | 85 | 208 | 49.9 | 0 | 0 | | 0 | 43 | 15 | 16 | 2.08 | 0.011 | 2 | 1 | 0.56 | 3.2 | 0.48 | 0.55 |
| | | 21.6 | 12.8 | 4.7 | 5.6 | 1.2 | 70 | 276 | 148 | 0.99 | 0.049 | 34.4 | 6 | | 0.22 | 0.35 | 2.6 | 10053 |
| **pork sirloin (chops)** with bone, lean and fat, broiled - 3 oz | 85 | 220 | 47.9 | 0 | 0 | | 0 | 58 | 14 | 25 | 2.18 | 0.008 | 2 | 1 | 0.81 | 3.8 | 0.64 | 0.62 |
| | | 22.7 | 13.7 | 5.0 | 5.9 | 1.3 | 73 | 326 | 209 | 0.84 | 0.049 | 40.5 | 7 | 0.3 | 0.29 | 0.46 | 4.2 | 10054 |
| **pork sirloin (chops)** with bone, lean, braised - 3 oz | 85 | 167 | 53.7 | 0 | 0 | | 0 | 45 | 11 | 17 | 2.21 | 0.012 | 2 | 1 | 0.59 | 3.4 | 0.48 | 0.59 |
| | | 23.0 | 7.7 | 2.7 | 3.4 | 0.7 | 69 | 286 | 150 | 1.08 | 0.050 | 36.2 | 6 | | 0.24 | 0.38 | 2.6 | 10057 |
| **pork sirloin (chops)** with bone, lean, broiled - 3 oz | 85 | 181 | 51.5 | 0 | 0 | | 0 | 61 | 11 | 26 | 2.33 | 0.008 | 2 | 1 | 0.87 | 4.0 | 0.67 | 0.67 |
| | | 24.2 | 8.6 | 3.1 | 3.8 | 0.8 | 72 | 341 | 218 | 0.91 | 0.050 | 43.9 | 6 | 0.2 | 0.32 | 0.51 | 0.8 | 10058 |
| **pork sirloin (roasts),** lean and fat, roasted - 3 oz | 85 | 196 | 50.4 | 0 | 0 | | 0 | 48 | 13 | 21 | 2.14 | 0.008 | 2 | 0 | 0.54 | 6.7 | 0.54 | 0.88 |
| | | 22.6 | 10.9 | 3.5 | 4.3 | 1.3 | 76 | 289 | 194 | 0.80 | 0.099 | 37.7 | 5 | 0.1 | 0.31 | 0.64 | 0 | 10055 |
| **pork sirloin (roasts),** lean, roasted 3 oz | 85 | 173 | 52.5 | 0 | 0 | | 0 | 50 | 11 | 22 | 2.23 | 0.008 | 0 | 0 | 0.57 | 6.9 | 0.52 | 0.91 |
| | | 23.6 | 8.0 | 2.4 | 3.1 | 0.8 | 76 | 299 | 200 | 0.82 | 0.103 | 39.4 | 0 | 0.1 | 0.32 | 0.67 | 0 | 10059 |
| **pork sirloin tip roast,** lean and fat, braised - 3 oz | 85 | 133 | 56.9 | 0 | 0 | | 0 | 37 | 4 | 21 | 2.43 | 0.008 | 0 | 0 | 0.51 | 6.5 | 0.49 | 0.68 |
| | | 26.4 | 2.2 | 0.7 | 0.9 | 0.4 | 71 | 309 | 201 | 0.90 | 0.058 | 32.0 | 0 | 0.1 | 0.43 | 0.42 | 0.8 | 10962 |

| Food | WT (g) | KCAL / PRO (g) | $H_2O$ (g) / FAT (g) | CHO (g) / SFA (g) | TSUG (g) / MUFA (g) | ASUG (g) / PUFA (g) | DFIB (g) / CHOL (mg) | Na (mg) / K (mg) | Ca (mg) / P (mg) | Mg (mg) / Fe (mg) | Zn (mg) / Cu (mg) | Mn (mg) / Se (mcg) | A (mcg RAE) / A (IU) | C (mg) / E (mg ATE) | B-1 (mg) / B-2 (mg) | NIA (mg) / B-6 (mg) | B-12 (mcg) / FOL (mcg DFE) | PANT (mg) / REF |
|---|---|---|---|---|---|---|---|---|---|---|---|---|---|---|---|---|---|---|
| **pork spareribs**, lean and fat, braised 3 oz | 85 | 337 | 34.4 | 0 | 0 | | 0 | 79 | 40 | 20 | 3.91 | 0.012 | 3 | 0 | 0.35 | 4.7 | 0.92 | 0.64 |
| | | 24.7 | 25.8 | 9.5 | 11.5 | 2.3 | 103 | 272 | 222 | 1.57 | 0.121 | 31.8 | 8 | 0.3 | 0.32 | 0.30 | 3.4 | 10089 |
| **pork tenderloin**, lean and fat, broiled - 3 oz | 85 | 171 | 51.9 | 0 | 0 | | 0 | 54 | 4 | 30 | 2.46 | 0.010 | 2 | 1 | 0.82 | 4.3 | 0.83 | 0.76 |
| | | 25.4 | 6.9 | 2.5 | 2.8 | 0.6 | 80 | 377 | 246 | 1.18 | 0.057 | 40.5 | 6 | | 0.32 | 0.44 | 5.1 | 10221 |
| **pork tenderloin**, lean and fat, roasted - 3 oz | 85 | 125 | 58.7 | 0 | 0 | | 0 | 48 | 5 | 25 | 2.05 | 0.011 | 0 | 0 | 0.80 | 6.3 | 0.48 | 0.86 |
| | | 22.1 | 3.4 | 1.2 | 1.3 | 0.5 | 62 | 356 | 225 | 0.98 | 0.094 | 32.3 | 1 | 0.1 | 0.33 | 0.62 | 0 | 10222 |
| **pork tenderloin**, lean, broiled 3 oz | 85 | 159 | 53.0 | 0 | 0 | | 0 | 55 | 4 | 31 | 2.51 | 0.010 | 2 | 1 | 0.84 | 4.4 | 0.85 | 0.78 |
| | | 25.9 | 5.4 | 1.9 | 2.2 | 0.5 | 80 | 383 | 251 | 1.22 | 0.058 | 43.9 | 6 | | 0.33 | 0.45 | 5.1 | 10223 |
| **pork tenderloin**, lean, roasted 3 oz | 85 | 122 | 59.0 | 0 | 0 | | 0 | 48 | 5 | 25 | 2.06 | 0.011 | 0 | 0 | 0.81 | 6.3 | 0.48 | 0.86 |
| | | 22.2 | 3.0 | 1.0 | 1.1 | 0.4 | 62 | 358 | 227 | 0.98 | 0.094 | 32.5 | 0 | 0.1 | 0.33 | 0.63 | 0 | 10061 |
| **pork top loin (chops)**, lean and fat, braised - 3 oz | 85 | 198 | 49.5 | 0 | 0 | | 0 | 36 | 18 | 16 | 1.79 | 0.008 | 2 | 0 | 0.47 | 3.9 | 0.39 | 0.54 |
| | | 23.6 | 10.8 | 4.0 | 4.8 | 0.9 | 64 | 346 | 157 | 0.82 | 0.065 | 35.1 | 6 | 0.2 | 0.22 | 0.28 | 3.4 | 10063 |
| **pork top loin (chops)**, lean and fat, broiled - 3 oz | 85 | 167 | 53.4 | 0 | 0 | | 0 | 37 | 6 | 22 | 1.78 | 0.006 | 1 | 0 | 0.54 | 7.0 | 0.50 | 0.58 |
| | | 22.6 | 7.8 | 2.7 | 3.4 | 0.9 | 62 | 303 | 196 | 0.54 | 0.069 | 37.1 | 4 | 0.1 | 0.16 | 0.59 | 0 | 10064 |
| **pork top loin (chops)**, lean and fat, pan-fried - 3 oz | 85 | 218 | 46.6 | 0 | 0 | | 0 | 47 | 18 | 24 | 1.87 | 0.006 | 2 | 0 | 0.68 | 4.6 | 0.55 | 0.69 |
| | | 24.6 | 12.6 | 4.5 | 5.5 | 1.4 | 66 | 407 | 223 | 0.69 | 0.064 | 39.0 | 6 | 0.2 | 0.30 | 0.34 | 6.8 | 10186 |
| **pork top loin (chops)**, lean, braised 3 oz | 85 | 172 | 51.9 | 0 | 0 | | 0 | 36 | 20 | 17 | 1.85 | 0.009 | 2 | 0 | 0.49 | 4.0 | 0.39 | 0.56 |
| | | 24.7 | 7.3 | 2.7 | 3.4 | 0.5 | 62 | 358 | 158 | 0.86 | 0.066 | 36.8 | 5 | 0.2 | 0.23 | 0.29 | 4.2 | 10067 |
| **pork top loin (chops)**, lean, broiled 3 oz | 85 | 147 | 55.3 | 0 | 0 | | 0 | 38 | 4 | 23 | 1.83 | 0.006 | 0 | 0 | 0.56 | 7.2 | 0.48 | 0.59 |
| | | 23.4 | 5.2 | 1.8 | 2.3 | 0.5 | 61 | 312 | 201 | 0.54 | 0.071 | 38.5 | 0 | 0.1 | 0.17 | 0.61 | 0 | 10068 |
| **pork top loin (chops)**, lean, pan-fried 3 oz | 85 | 191 | 49.0 | 0 | 0 | | 0 | 48 | 19 | 26 | 1.95 | 0.007 | 2 | 0 | 0.71 | 4.8 | 0.57 | 0.73 |
| | | 25.9 | 8.9 | 3.1 | 3.9 | 1.1 | 65 | 425 | 230 | 0.72 | 0.065 | 38.9 | 5 | 0.2 | 0.32 | 0.36 | 6.8 | 10181 |
| **pork top loin (roasts)**, lean and fat, roasted - 3 oz | 85 | 163 | 54.2 | 0 | 0 | | 0 | 39 | 6 | 21 | 1.79 | 0.006 | 1 | 0 | 0.46 | 6.0 | 0.49 | 0.57 |
| | | 22.5 | 7.5 | 2.4 | 3.0 | 0.8 | 68 | 297 | 190 | 0.54 | 0.065 | 29.7 | 3 | 0.1 | 0.20 | 0.59 | 0 | 10065 |
| **pork top loin (roasts)**, lean, roasted 3 oz | 85 | 147 | 55.8 | 0 | 0 | | 0 | 40 | 5 | 22 | 1.84 | 0.006 | 0 | 0 | 0.48 | 6.2 | 0.47 | 0.58 |
| | | 23.1 | 5.3 | 1.6 | 2.1 | 0.5 | 67 | 303 | 193 | 0.54 | 0.067 | 30.4 | 0 | 0.1 | 0.20 | 0.61 | 0 | 10069 |
| **pork w/beef sausage** (fresh), pan-fried 1 oz patty (3⅞" dia, ¼" thick) | 27 | 107 | 12.0 | 0.7 | 0 | 0 | 0 | 217 | 3 | 3 | 0.50 | 0.010 | 0 | 0 | 0.10 | 0.9 | 0.12 | 0.13 |
| | | 3.7 | 9.8 | 3.5 | 4.6 | 1.1 | 19 | 51 | 29 | 0.31 | 0.011 | 3.9 | 0 | 0.1 | 0.04 | 0.01 | 0.5 | 7065 |

## 19.7 VEAL

| Food | WT (g) | KCAL / PRO (g) | $H_2O$ (g) / FAT (g) | CHO (g) / SFA (g) | TSUG (g) / MUFA (g) | ASUG (g) / PUFA (g) | DFIB (g) / CHOL (mg) | Na (mg) / K (mg) | Ca (mg) / P (mg) | Mg (mg) / Fe (mg) | Zn (mg) / Cu (mg) | Mn (mg) / Se (mcg) | A (mcg RAE) / A (IU) | C (mg) / E (mg ATE) | B-1 (mg) / B-2 (mg) | NIA (mg) / B-6 (mg) | B-12 (mcg) / FOL (mcg DFE) | PANT (mg) / REF |
|---|---|---|---|---|---|---|---|---|---|---|---|---|---|---|---|---|---|---|
| **veal breast, plate half**, bone out, lean and fat, braised - 3 oz | 85 | 240 | 46.6 | 0 | | | | 54 | 7 | 16 | 2.95 | 0.007 | | | 0.05 | 6.7 | 1.13 | 0.88 |
| | | 22.0 | 16.1 | 6.3 | 7.7 | 1.0 | 95 | 226 | 158 | 0.64 | 0.059 | 9.0 | | | 0.25 | 0.22 | 11.0 | 17273 |
| **veal breast, point half**, bone out, lean and fat, braised - 3 oz | 85 | 211 | 48.8 | 0 | | | | 56 | 8 | 18 | 3.27 | 0.007 | | | 0.05 | 7.1 | 1.18 | 0.91 |
| | | 24.0 | 12.0 | 4.7 | 5.7 | 0.8 | 97 | 236 | 167 | 0.67 | 0.062 | 9.8 | | | 0.26 | 0.23 | 11.9 | 17274 |
| **veal breast, whole**, bone out, lean and fat, braised - 3 oz | 85 | 226 | 47.6 | 0 | | | | 55 | 8 | 17 | 3.09 | 0.007 | | | 0.05 | 6.8 | 1.13 | 0.88 |
| | | 22.9 | 14.3 | 5.6 | 6.8 | 1.0 | 96 | 231 | 162 | 0.65 | 0.060 | 9.4 | | | 0.25 | 0.22 | 11.0 | 17272 |
| **veal breast, whole**, bone out, lean, braised - 3 oz | 85 | 185 | 50.8 | 0 | | | | 58 | 8 | 19 | 3.56 | 0.007 | | | 0.05 | 7.6 | 1.26 | 0.97 |
| | | 25.8 | 8.3 | 3.2 | 3.8 | 0.7 | 99 | 246 | 177 | 0.71 | 0.065 | 10.6 | | | 0.28 | 0.25 | 12.8 | 17275 |
| **veal, ground**, broiled 3 oz | 85 | 146 | 56.7 | 0 | 0 | | 0 | 71 | 14 | 20 | 3.29 | 0.030 | 0 | 0 | 0.06 | 6.8 | 1.08 | 0.99 |
| | | 20.7 | 6.4 | 2.6 | 2.4 | 0.5 | 88 | 286 | 184 | 0.84 | 0.088 | 11.6 | 0 | 0.1 | 0.23 | 0.33 | 9.4 | 17143 |
| **veal leg (top round)**, lean and fat, braised - 3 oz | 85 | 179 | 47.2 | 0 | 0 | | 0 | 57 | 7 | 25 | 3.37 | 0.033 | 0 | 0 | 0.05 | 9.0 | 0.99 | 0.87 |
| | | 30.7 | 5.4 | 2.2 | 2.0 | 0.4 | 114 | 326 | 212 | 1.12 | 0.119 | 13.1 | 0 | 0.4 | 0.30 | 0.31 | 15.3 | 17095 |
| **veal leg (top round)**, lean and fat, breaded, pan-fried - 3 oz | 85 | 202 | 43.6 | 8.4 | 0.5 | | 0.3 | 386 | 33 | 26 | 2.34 | 0.115 | 8 | 0 | 0.14 | 8.8 | 1.05 | 0.91 |
| | | 23.2 | 7.8 | 2.6 | 2.9 | 1.3 | 95 | 315 | 212 | 1.39 | 0.062 | 14.0 | 29 | 0.5 | 0.30 | 0.34 | 28.0 | 17096 |
| **veal leg (top round)**, lean and fat, pan-fried - 3 oz | 85 | 179 | 49.6 | 0 | 0 | | 0 | 65 | 5 | 26 | 2.75 | 0.026 | 0 | 0 | 0.06 | 10.2 | 1.23 | 0.99 |
| | | 27.0 | 7.1 | 2.7 | 2.7 | 0.5 | 89 | 361 | 237 | 0.75 | 0.053 | 11.4 | 0 | 0.4 | 0.30 | 0.42 | 12.8 | 17097 |
| **veal leg (top round)**, lean and fat, roasted - 3 oz | 85 | 136 | 56.2 | 0 | 0 | | 0 | 58 | 5 | 24 | 2.58 | 0.026 | 0 | 0 | 0.05 | 8.4 | 0.99 | 0.84 |
| | | 23.5 | 4.0 | 1.6 | 1.5 | 0.3 | 88 | 331 | 199 | 0.77 | 0.110 | 9.5 | 0 | 0.4 | 0.27 | 0.26 | 13.6 | 17098 |
| **veal leg (top round)**, lean, braised 3 oz | 85 | 173 | 47.8 | 0 | 0 | | 0 | 57 | 8 | 26 | 3.43 | 0.034 | 0 | 0 | 0.05 | 9.1 | 1.01 | 0.88 |
| | | 31.2 | 4.3 | 1.6 | 1.6 | 0.3 | 115 | 329 | 214 | 1.12 | 0.121 | 13.3 | 0 | 0.4 | 0.31 | 0.31 | 15.3 | 17100 |
| **veal leg (top round)**, lean, breaded, pan-fried - 3 oz | 85 | 184 | 45.2 | 8.4 | 0.5 | | 0.2 | 387 | 33 | 27 | 2.44 | 0.116 | 8 | 0 | 0.14 | 9.2 | 1.09 | 0.94 |
| | | 24.1 | 5.3 | 1.4 | 1.8 | 1.1 | 96 | 326 | 219 | 1.39 | 0.063 | 11.5 | 29 | 0.5 | 0.31 | 0.36 | 28.9 | 17101 |
| **veal leg (top round)**, lean, pan-fried 3 oz | 85 | 156 | 51.6 | 0 | 0 | | 0 | 65 | 6 | 27 | 2.87 | 0.027 | 0 | 0 | 0.06 | 10.7 | 1.28 | 1.04 |
| | | 28.2 | 3.9 | 1.1 | 1.4 | 0.3 | 91 | 376 | 246 | 0.74 | 0.054 | 8.8 | 0 | 0.4 | 0.31 | 0.43 | 13.6 | 17102 |
| **veal leg (top round)**, lean, roasted 3 oz | 85 | 128 | 57.0 | 0 | 0 | | 0 | 58 | 5 | 24 | 2.62 | 0.026 | 0 | 0 | 0.05 | 8.6 | 1.00 | 0.85 |
| | | 23.9 | 2.9 | 1.0 | 1.0 | 0.2 | 88 | 334 | 201 | 0.76 | 0.110 | 10.1 | 0 | 0.5 | 0.28 | 0.26 | 13.6 | 17103 |
| **veal leg and shoulder**, cubed for stew, lean, braised - 3 oz | 85 | 160 | 50.4 | 0 | | | 0 | 79 | 25 | 24 | 5.11 | 0.034 | 0 | 0 | 0.06 | 7.1 | 1.42 | 1.01 |
| | | 29.7 | 3.7 | 1.1 | 1.2 | 0.4 | 123 | 291 | 203 | 1.22 | 0.130 | 12.9 | 0 | 0.4 | 0.34 | 0.32 | 13.6 | 17141 |
| **veal loin**, lean and fat, braised 3 oz | 85 | 241 | 44.2 | 0 | 0 | | 0 | 68 | 24 | 20 | 3.09 | 0.029 | 0 | 0 | 0.03 | 7.7 | 1.03 | 0.67 |
| | | 25.7 | 14.6 | 5.7 | 5.7 | 1.0 | 100 | 238 | 187 | 0.93 | 0.077 | 11.2 | 0 | 0.3 | 0.26 | 0.24 | 11.9 | 17105 |
| **veal loin**, lean and fat, roasted 3 oz | 85 | 184 | 51.6 | 0 | 0 | | 0 | 79 | 16 | 21 | 2.58 | 0.025 | 0 | 0 | 0.04 | 7.5 | 1.05 | 1.02 |
| | | 21.1 | 10.5 | 4.5 | 4.1 | 0.7 | 88 | 276 | 180 | 0.74 | 0.094 | 9.4 | 0 | 0.4 | 0.24 | 0.29 | 12.8 | 17106 |

| | WT (g) | KCAL / PRO (g) | H₂O (g) / FAT (g) | CHO (g) / SFA (g) | TSUG (g) / MUFA (g) | ASUG (g) / PUFA (g) | DFIB (g) / CHOL (mg) | Na (mg) / K (mg) | Ca (mg) / P (mg) | Mg (mg) / Fe (mg) | Zn (mg) / Cu (mg) | Mn (mg) / Se (mcg) | A (mcg RAE) / A (IU) | C (mg) / E (mg ATE) | B-1 (mg) / B-2 (mg) | NIA (mg) / B-6 (mg) | B-12 (mcg) / FOL (mcg DFE) | PANT (mg) / REF |
|---|---|---|---|---|---|---|---|---|---|---|---|---|---|---|---|---|---|---|
| **veal loin, lean, braised** | 85 | 192 | 48.4 | 0 | 0 | | 0 | 71 | 27 | 23 | 3.48 | 0.032 | 0 | 0 | 0.04 | 8.5 | 1.12 | 0.72 |
| 3 oz | | 28.5 | 7.8 | 2.2 | 2.8 | 0.7 | 106 | 252 | 201 | 0.94 | 0.084 | 12.2 | 0 | 0.4 | 0.29 | 0.24 | 12.8 | 17108 |
| **veal loin, lean, roasted** | 85 | 149 | 54.9 | 0 | 0 | | 0 | 82 | 18 | 22 | 2.75 | 0.026 | 0 | 0 | 0.05 | 8.0 | 1.11 | 1.08 |
| 3 oz | | 22.4 | 5.9 | 2.2 | 2.1 | 0.5 | 90 | 289 | 189 | 0.72 | 0.099 | 9.9 | 0 | 0.4 | 0.26 | 0.31 | 13.6 | 17109 |
| **veal ribs, lean and fat, braised** | 85 | 213 | 45.3 | 0 | 0 | | 0 | 81 | 19 | 21 | 4.73 | 0.032 | 0 | 0 | 0.04 | 6.4 | 1.23 | 0.91 |
| 3 oz | | 27.6 | 10.7 | 4.2 | 4.0 | 0.8 | 118 | 260 | 178 | 1.20 | 0.112 | 11.8 | 0 | 0.3 | 0.25 | 0.27 | 13.6 | 17111 |
| **veal ribs, lean and fat, roasted** | 85 | 194 | 50.9 | 0 | 0 | | 0 | 78 | 9 | 19 | 3.48 | 0.026 | 0 | 0 | 0.04 | 5.9 | 1.24 | 1.09 |
| 3 oz | | 20.4 | 11.9 | 4.6 | 4.6 | 0.8 | 94 | 251 | 167 | 0.82 | 0.084 | 8.9 | 0 | 0.3 | 0.23 | 0.21 | 11.0 | 17112 |
| **veal ribs, lean, braised** | 85 | 185 | 47.7 | 0 | 0 | | 0 | 84 | 20 | 22 | 5.08 | 0.034 | 0 | 0 | 0.05 | 6.7 | 1.30 | 0.96 |
| 3 oz | | 29.3 | 6.6 | 2.2 | 2.2 | 0.6 | 122 | 270 | 185 | 1.23 | 0.119 | 12.4 | 0 | 0.3 | 0.26 | 0.29 | 13.6 | 17114 |
| **veal ribs, lean, roasted** | 85 | 150 | 54.9 | 0 | | | 0 | 82 | 10 | 20 | 3.82 | 0.027 | 0 | 0 | 0.05 | 6.4 | 1.34 | 1.17 |
| 3 oz | | 21.9 | 6.3 | 1.8 | 2.3 | 0.6 | 98 | 264 | 176 | 0.82 | 0.090 | 9.4 | 0 | 0.3 | 0.25 | 0.23 | 11.9 | 17115 |
| **veal shank (fore and hind), lean and fat, braised - 3 oz** | 85 | 162 | 52.5 | 0 | | | 0 | 79 | 28 | 21 | 5.64 | 0.013 | | | 0.04 | 8.0 | 1.37 | 1.04 |
| | | 26.8 | 5.3 | 1.8 | 2.0 | 0.5 | 105 | 259 | 191 | 1.06 | 0.094 | 13.0 | | | 0.25 | 0.23 | 14.4 | 17277 |
| **veal shank (fore and hind), lean braised - 3 oz** | 85 | 150 | 53.5 | 0 | | | 0 | 80 | 29 | 21 | 5.79 | 0.013 | 0 | | 0.04 | 8.2 | 1.39 | 1.06 |
| | | 27.4 | 3.7 | 1.0 | 1.3 | 0.4 | 107 | 263 | 194 | 1.07 | 0.096 | 11.6 | 0 | | 0.26 | 0.23 | 14.4 | 17279 |
| **veal shoulder, arm, lean and fat, braised - 3 oz** | 85 | 201 | 47.0 | 0 | | | 0 | 74 | 24 | 25 | 4.94 | 0.031 | 0 | 0 | 0.05 | 8.6 | 1.46 | 1.11 |
| | | 28.6 | 8.7 | 3.4 | 3.4 | 0.6 | 126 | 283 | 224 | 1.17 | 0.109 | 12.3 | 0 | 0.4 | 0.26 | 0.25 | 15.3 | 17123 |
| **veal shoulder, arm, lean and fat, roasted - 3 oz** | 85 | 156 | 55.0 | 0 | | | 0 | 76 | 22 | 22 | 3.55 | 0.026 | 0 | 0 | 0.05 | 6.8 | 1.30 | 0.99 |
| | | 21.6 | 7.0 | 3.0 | 2.7 | 0.5 | 92 | 296 | 188 | 0.98 | 0.120 | 9.4 | 0 | 0.4 | 0.27 | 0.25 | 14.4 | 17124 |
| **veal shoulder, arm, lean, braised** | 85 | 171 | 49.5 | 0 | | | 0 | 76 | 26 | 26 | 5.30 | 0.032 | 0 | 0 | 0.05 | 9.1 | 1.55 | 1.18 |
| 3 oz | | 30.4 | 4.5 | 1.3 | 1.6 | 0.4 | 132 | 295 | 235 | 1.20 | 0.119 | 13.0 | 0 | 0.4 | 0.28 | 0.26 | 16.2 | 17126 |
| **veal shoulder, arm, lean, roasted** | 85 | 139 | 56.5 | 0 | | | 0 | 77 | 23 | 23 | 3.67 | 0.026 | 0 | 0 | 0.06 | 7.0 | 1.33 | 1.01 |
| 3 oz | | 22.2 | 4.9 | 2.0 | 1.8 | 0.4 | 93 | 303 | 192 | 0.99 | 0.124 | 9.6 | 0 | 0.4 | 0.28 | 0.26 | 14.4 | 17127 |
| **veal shoulder, blade, lean and fat, braised - 3 oz** | 85 | 191 | 48.4 | 0 | 0 | | 0 | 83 | 32 | 22 | 5.95 | 0.031 | 0 | 0 | 0.05 | 4.7 | 1.64 | 1.29 |
| | | 26.6 | 8.6 | 3.1 | 3.3 | 0.6 | 130 | 252 | 207 | 1.22 | 0.139 | 11.9 | 0 | 0.4 | 0.30 | 0.20 | 12.8 | 17129 |
| **veal shoulder, blade, lean and fat, roasted - 3 oz** | 85 | 158 | 55.7 | 0 | | | 0 | 85 | 24 | 20 | 4.74 | 0.026 | 0 | 0 | 0.06 | 4.9 | 1.71 | 1.17 |
| | | 21.4 | 7.4 | 2.9 | 2.8 | 0.5 | 99 | 260 | 180 | 0.85 | 0.117 | 9.0 | 0 | 0.4 | 0.30 | 0.20 | 9.4 | 17130 |
| **veal shoulder, blade, lean, braised** | 85 | 168 | 50.4 | 0 | 0 | | 0 | 86 | 34 | 24 | 6.28 | 0.032 | 0 | 0 | 0.05 | 4.8 | 1.71 | 1.35 |
| 3 oz | | 27.8 | 5.5 | 1.5 | 2.0 | 0.5 | 134 | 259 | 214 | 1.25 | 0.145 | 12.3 | 0 | 0.4 | 0.31 | 0.21 | 12.8 | 17132 |
| **veal shoulder, blade, lean, roasted** | 85 | 145 | 56.9 | 0 | | | 0 | 87 | 24 | 20 | 4.86 | 0.026 | 0 | 0 | 0.06 | 4.9 | 1.75 | 1.20 |
| 3 oz | | 21.8 | 5.8 | 2.2 | 2.1 | 0.5 | 101 | 264 | 183 | 0.85 | 0.120 | 9.1 | 0 | 0.4 | 0.31 | 0.20 | 9.4 | 17133 |
| **veal shoulder, whole, lean and fat, braised - 3 oz** | 85 | 194 | 47.9 | 0 | 0 | | 0 | 81 | 30 | 23 | 5.60 | 0.031 | 0 | 0 | 0.05 | 5.5 | 1.56 | 1.30 |
| | | 27.3 | 8.6 | 3.2 | 3.3 | 0.6 | 107 | 263 | 212 | 1.21 | 0.128 | 12.1 | 0 | 0.4 | 0.29 | 0.21 | 12.8 | 17117 |
| **veal shoulder, whole, lean and fat, roasted - 3 oz** | 85 | 156 | 55.5 | 0 | 0 | | 0 | 82 | 23 | 21 | 4.35 | 0.026 | 0 | 0 | 0.06 | 5.4 | 1.55 | 1.10 |
| | | 21.5 | 7.2 | 2.9 | 2.7 | 0.5 | 96 | 274 | 183 | 0.88 | 0.118 | 9.1 | 0 | 0.4 | 0.29 | 0.22 | 10.2 | 17118 |
| **veal shoulder, whole, lean, braised** | 85 | 169 | 50.0 | 0 | | | 0 | 82 | 31 | 24 | 5.95 | 0.032 | 0 | 0 | 0.05 | 5.7 | 1.65 | 1.37 |
| 3 oz | | 28.6 | 5.2 | 1.4 | 1.9 | 0.5 | 110 | 271 | 221 | 1.23 | 0.135 | 12.5 | 0 | 0.4 | 0.30 | 0.22 | 13.6 | 17120 |
| **veal shoulder, whole, lean, roasted** | 85 | 144 | 56.7 | 0 | | | 0 | 82 | 23 | 21 | 4.46 | 0.026 | 0 | C | 0.06 | 5.5 | 1.58 | 1.12 |
| 3 oz | | 21.9 | 5.6 | 2.1 | 2.0 | 0.5 | 97 | 278 | 185 | 0.88 | 0.121 | 9.3 | 0 | 0.4 | 0.29 | 0.22 | 11.0 | 17121 |
| **veal sirloin, lean and fat, braised** | 85 | 214 | 46.3 | 0 | | | 0 | 67 | 14 | 23 | 3.67 | 0.030 | 0 | 0 | 0.04 | 5.6 | 1.26 | 0.86 |
| 3 oz | | 26.6 | 11.2 | 4.4 | 4.4 | 0.7 | 92 | 273 | 207 | 1.02 | 0.109 | 11.9 | 0 | 0.3 | 0.30 | 0.30 | 12.8 | 17135 |
| **veal sirloin, lean and fat, roasted** | 85 | 172 | 53.3 | 0 | 0 | | 0 | 71 | 11 | 22 | 2.85 | 0.025 | 0 | 0 | 0.05 | 7.5 | 1.21 | 1.07 |
| 3 oz | | 21.4 | 8.9 | 3.8 | 3.5 | 0.6 | 87 | 298 | 190 | 0.78 | 0.110 | 9.4 | 0 | 0.4 | 0.30 | 0.27 | 12.8 | 17136 |
| **veal sirloin, lean, braised** | 85 | 173 | 49.8 | 0 | | | 0 | 69 | 16 | 25 | 4.04 | 0.032 | 0 | 0 | 0.05 | 6.0 | 1.35 | 0.92 |
| 3 oz | | 28.9 | 5.5 | 1.5 | 2.0 | 0.5 | 96 | 288 | 220 | 1.05 | 0.117 | 12.8 | 0 | 0.4 | 0.32 | 0.32 | 13.6 | 17138 |
| **veal sirloin, lean, roasted** | 85 | 143 | 55.9 | 0 | | | 0 | 72 | 12 | 23 | 3.01 | 0.026 | 0 | 0 | 0.05 | 7.9 | 1.27 | 1.12 |
| 3 oz | | 22.4 | 5.3 | 2.0 | 1.9 | 0.4 | 88 | 310 | 196 | 0.77 | 0.116 | 9.8 | 0 | 0.4 | 0.31 | 0.29 | 13.6 | 17139 |

## 19.8 INTERNAL ORGANS AND OTHER PARTS

| | WT (g) | KCAL / PRO | H₂O / FAT | CHO / SFA | TSUG / MUFA | ASUG / PUFA | DFIB / CHOL | Na / K | Ca / P | Mg / Fe | Zn / Cu | Mn / Se | A RAE / A IU | C / E | B-1 / B-2 | NIA / B-6 | B-12 / FOL | PANT / REF |
|---|---|---|---|---|---|---|---|---|---|---|---|---|---|---|---|---|---|---|
| **beef brain, pan-fried** | 85 | 167 | 60.1 | 0 | | | 0 | 134 | 8 | 13 | 1.15 | 0.027 | 0 | 3 | 0.11 | 3.2 | 12.92 | 0.48 |
| 3 oz | | 10.7 | 13.5 | 3.2 | 3.4 | 2.0 | 1696 | 301 | 328 | 1.89 | 0.187 | 22.1 | 0 | | 0.22 | 0.33 | 5.1 | 13319 |
| **beef brain, raw** | 85 | 122 | 64.8 | 0.9 | 0 | | 0 | 107 | 37 | 11 | 0.87 | 0.022 | 6 | 9 | 0.08 | 3.0 | 8.08 | 1.71 |
| 3 oz | | 9.2 | 8.8 | 2.0 | 1.6 | 1.3 | 2558 | 233 | 308 | 2.17 | 0.244 | 18.1 | 125 | 0.8 | 0.17 | 0.19 | 2.6 | 13318 |
| **beef brain, simmered** | 85 | 128 | 63.6 | 1.3 | 0 | | 0 | 92 | 8 | 10 | 0.93 | 0.024 | 5 | 9 | 0.06 | 3.1 | 8.58 | 1.03 |
| 3 oz | | 9.9 | 9.0 | 2.0 | 1.6 | 1.4 | 2635 | 207 | 285 | 1.95 | 0.196 | 18.5 | 99 | 1.4 | 0.18 | 0.12 | 4.2 | 13320 |
| **beef heart, raw** | 85 | 95 | 65.5 | 0.1 | 0 | | 0 | 83 | 6 | 18 | 1.44 | 0.030 | 0 | 2 | 0.20 | 6.4 | 7.27 | 1.52 |
| 3 oz | | 15.1 | 3.3 | 1.2 | 1.0 | 0.5 | 105 | 244 | 180 | 3.66 | 0.337 | 18.5 | 0 | 0.2 | 0.77 | 0.24 | 2.6 | 13321 |
| **beef heart, simmered** | 85 | 140 | 55.8 | 0.1 | 0 | | 0 | 50 | 4 | 18 | 2.44 | 0.028 | 0 | 0 | 0.09 | 5.7 | 9.18 | 1.36 |
| 3 oz | | 24.2 | 4.0 | 1.2 | 0.9 | 0.8 | 180 | 186 | 216 | 5.42 | 0.475 | 33.1 | 0 | 0.2 | 1.03 | 0.21 | 4.2 | 13322 |

| | WT (g) | KCAL / PRO (g) | H₂0 (g) / FAT (g) | CHO (g) / SFA (g) | TSUG (g) / MUFA (g) | ASUG (g) / PUFA (g) | DFIB (g) / CHOL (mg) | Na (mg) / K (mg) | Ca (mg) / P (mg) | Mg (mg) / Fe (mg) | Zn (mg) / Cu (mg) | Mn (mg) / Se (mcg) | A (mcg RAE) / A (IU) | C (mg) / E (mg ATE) | B-1 (mg) / B-2 (mg) | NIA (mg) / B-6 (mg) | B-12 (mcg) / FOL (mcg DFE) | PANT (mg) / REF |
|---|---|---|---|---|---|---|---|---|---|---|---|---|---|---|---|---|---|---|
| **beef kidney**, raw | 85 | 88 | 66.2 | 0.2 | 0 | | 0 | 155 | 11 | 14 | 1.63 | 0.121 | 356 | 8 | 0.30 | 6.8 | 23.38 | 3.37 |
| *3 oz* | | 14.8 | 2.6 | 0.7 | 0.5 | 0.5 | 349 | 223 | 218 | 3.91 | 0.362 | 119.8 | 1187 | 0.2 | 2.41 | 0.57 | 83.3 | 13323 |
| **beef kidney**, simmered | 85 | 134 | 56.8 | 0 | 0 | | 0 | 80 | 16 | 10 | 2.41 | 0.157 | 0 | 0 | 0.14 | 3.3 | 21.16 | 1.33 |
| *3 oz* | | 23.2 | 4.0 | 0.9 | 0.6 | 0.7 | 609 | 115 | 258 | 4.93 | 0.479 | 142.8 | 0 | 0.1 | 2.52 | 0.33 | 70.6 | 13324 |
| **beef liver**, braised | 85 | 162 | 50.0 | 4.4 | 0 | 0 | 0 | 67 | 5 | 18 | 4.50 | 0.303 | 8026 | 2 | 0.16 | 14.9 | 59.99 | 6.04 |
| *3 oz* | | 24.7 | 4.5 | 1.4 | 0.5 | 0.5 | 337 | 299 | 422 | 5.56 | 12.141 | 30.7 | 26957 | 0.4 | 2.91 | 0.86 | 215.0 | 13326 |
| **beef liver**, pan-fried | 85 | 149 | 52.7 | 4.4 | 0 | 0 | 0 | 65 | 5 | 19 | 4.45 | 0.303 | 6582 | 1 | 0.15 | 14.9 | 70.66 | 5.90 |
| *3 oz* | | 22.5 | 4.0 | 1.3 | 0.6 | 0.5 | 324 | 298 | 412 | 5.24 | 12.400 | 27.9 | 22175 | 0.4 | 2.91 | 0.87 | 221.0 | 13327 |
| **beef liver**, raw | 85 | 115 | 60.2 | 3.3 | 0 | | 0 | 59 | 4 | 15 | 3.40 | 0.264 | 4223 | 1 | 0.16 | 11.2 | 50.40 | 6.10 |
| *3 oz* | | 17.3 | 3.1 | 1.0 | 0.4 | 0.4 | 234 | 266 | 329 | 4.16 | 8.292 | 33.7 | 14363 | 0.3 | 2.34 | 0.92 | 246.5 | 13325 |
| **beef lungs**, braised | 85 | 102 | 64.9 | 0 | | | 0 | 86 | 9 | 8 | 1.39 | 0.013 | 10 | 28 | 0.03 | 2.1 | 2.20 | 0.53 |
| *3 oz* | | 17.3 | 3.1 | 1.1 | 0.8 | 0.4 | 235 | 147 | 151 | 4.59 | 0.188 | 42.8 | 33 | | 0.12 | 0.02 | 6.8 | 13329 |
| **beef pancreas** (sweetbread), braised | 85 | 230 | 47.3 | 0 | | | 0 | 51 | 14 | 18 | 3.91 | 0.177 | 0 | 17 | 0.15 | 3.4 | 14.11 | 3.61 |
| *3 oz* | | 23.0 | 14.6 | 5.0 | 5.0 | 2.7 | 223 | 209 | 385 | 2.22 | 0.076 | 41.2 | 0 | | 0.41 | 0.15 | 2.6 | 13332 |
| **beef spleen**, braised | 85 | 123 | 59.5 | 0 | | | 0 | 48 | 10 | 16 | 2.37 | 0.064 | 0 | 43 | 0.04 | 4.7 | 4.27 | 0.74 |
| *3 oz* | | 21.3 | 3.6 | 1.2 | 1.0 | 0.3 | 295 | 241 | 259 | 33.46 | 0.785 | 77.7 | 0 | | 0.26 | 0.03 | 3.4 | 13334 |
| **beef thymus** (sweetbread), braised | 85 | 271 | 44.9 | 0 | | | 0 | 99 | 8 | 8 | 1.87 | 0.084 | 0 | 26 | 0.07 | 1.6 | 1.28 | 1.68 |
| *3 oz* | | 18.6 | 21.2 | 7.3 | 7.3 | 4.0 | 250 | 368 | 309 | 1.27 | 0.037 | 18.4 | 0 | | 0.19 | 0.07 | 2.6 | 13338 |
| **beef tongue**, simmered | 85 | 241 | 49.2 | 0 | 0 | | 0 | 55 | 4 | 13 | 3.48 | 0.015 | 0 | 1 | 0.02 | 3.0 | 2.66 | 0.63 |
| *3 oz* | | 16.4 | 19.0 | 6.9 | 8.6 | 0.6 | 112 | 156 | 123 | 2.22 | 0.126 | 11.2 | 0 | 0.3 | 0.25 | 0.13 | 6.0 | 13340 |
| **calf brain**, raw | 85 | 100 | 67.8 | 0 | | | 0 | 108 | 8 | 12 | 0.94 | 0.031 | 0 | 12 | 0.11 | 3.7 | 10.37 | 2.31 |
| *3 oz* | | 8.8 | 7.0 | 1.6 | 1.4 | 0.8 | 1352 | 268 | 233 | 1.81 | 0.187 | 8.5 | 0 | | 0.22 | 0.24 | 2.6 | 17188 |
| **calf heart**, raw | 85 | 94 | 66.0 | 0.1 | | | 0 | 65 | 4 | 15 | 1.25 | 0.031 | 0 | 7 | 0.44 | 5.4 | 11.70 | 2.36 |
| *3 oz* | | 14.6 | 3.4 | 0.9 | 0.7 | 0.9 | 88 | 222 | 179 | 3.60 | 0.289 | 28.3 | 0 | | 0.85 | 0.37 | 1.7 | 17193 |
| **calf kidney**, raw | 85 | 84 | 67.2 | 0.7 | | | 0 | 151 | 9 | 14 | 1.67 | 0.068 | 78 | 4 | 0.27 | 5.9 | 23.97 | 2.80 |
| *3 oz* | | 13.4 | 2.7 | 0.8 | 0.6 | 0.5 | 309 | 231 | 205 | 2.86 | 0.420 | 68.0 | 262 | | 1.62 | 0.31 | 17.8 | 17197 |
| **calf liver**, raw | 85 | 119 | 60.3 | 2.5 | 0 | | 0 | 65 | 4 | 17 | 10.22 | 0.217 | 9951 | 1 | 0.15 | 9.0 | 50.87 | 5.16 |
| *3 oz* | | 16.9 | 4.1 | 1.3 | 0.8 | 0.7 | 284 | 262 | 322 | 5.44 | 10.085 | 19.3 | 33198 | 0.3 | 2.07 | 0.81 | 106.2 | 17202 |
| **calf lung**, raw | 85 | 76 | 68.4 | 0 | | | 0 | 92 | 6 | 10 | 0.99 | 0.015 | 0 | 33 | 0.04 | 3.4 | 3.26 | |
| *3 oz* | | 13.9 | 2.0 | 0.7 | 0.6 | 0.3 | 195 | 233 | 245 | 4.45 | 0.205 | 14.6 | 0 | | 0.20 | 0.09 | 9.4 | 17207 |
| **calf neck**, raw | 85 | 86 | 67.3 | 0 | 0 | | 0 | 57 | 3 | 20 | 1.32 | 0.015 | 0 | 42 | 0.06 | 4.1 | 2.83 | 1.05 |
| *3 oz* | | 14.6 | 2.6 | 0.7 | 0.7 | 0.2 | 212 | 415 | 453 | 0.89 | 0.067 | 13.7 | 0 | 0.1 | 0.16 | 0.03 | 18.7 | 17218 |
| **calf spleen**, raw | 85 | 83 | 66.4 | 0 | | | 0 | 82 | 5 | 14 | 1.37 | 0.061 | 0 | 35 | 0.04 | 6.7 | 4.54 | |
| *3 oz* | | 15.6 | 1.9 | 0.6 | 0.5 | 0.1 | 289 | 308 | 288 | 7.92 | 0.142 | 52.4 | 0 | | 0.30 | 0.09 | 3.4 | 17216 |
| **calf tongue**, raw | 85 | 111 | 63.4 | 1.6 | | | 0 | 70 | 6 | 14 | 2.24 | 0.020 | 0 | 4 | 0.14 | 1.9 | 5.18 | 1.02 |
| *3 oz* | | 14.6 | 4.7 | 2.0 | 2.1 | 0.3 | 53 | 230 | 135 | 2.31 | 0.170 | 6.0 | 1 | | 0.35 | 0.16 | 4.2 | 17222 |
| **lamb brain**, braised | 85 | 123 | 64.4 | 0 | | | 0 | 114 | 10 | 12 | 1.16 | 0.050 | 0 | 10 | 0.09 | 2.1 | 7.86 | 0.84 |
| *3 oz* | | 10.7 | 8.6 | 2.2 | 1.6 | 0.9 | 1737 | 174 | 286 | 1.43 | 0.178 | 10.2 | 0 | | 0.20 | 0.09 | 4.2 | 17186 |
| **lamb brain**, pan-fried | 85 | 232 | 51.6 | 0 | | | 0 | 133 | 18 | 19 | 1.70 | 0.057 | 0 | 20 | 0.14 | 3.9 | 20.48 | 1.33 |
| *3 oz* | | 14.4 | 18.9 | 4.8 | 3.4 | 1.9 | 2128 | 304 | 421 | 1.73 | 0.408 | 10.2 | 0 | | 0.31 | 0.20 | 6.0 | 17187 |
| **lamb heart**, braised | 85 | 157 | 54.6 | 1.6 | | | 0 | 54 | 12 | 20 | 3.13 | 0.047 | 0 | 6 | 0.14 | 3.7 | 9.52 | 1.16 |
| *3 oz* | | 21.2 | 6.7 | 2.7 | 1.9 | 1.0 | 212 | 160 | 216 | 4.69 | 0.518 | 39.9 | 0 | | 1.01 | 0.26 | 1.7 | 17192 |
| **lamb heart**, raw | 85 | 104 | 65.2 | 0.2 | | | 0 | 76 | 5 | 14 | 1.59 | 0.039 | 0 | 4 | 0.31 | 5.2 | 8.71 | 2.24 |
| *3 oz* | | 14.0 | 4.8 | 1.9 | 1.4 | 0.5 | 115 | 269 | 149 | 3.91 | 0.337 | 27.2 | 0 | | 0.84 | 0.33 | 1.7 | 17191 |
| **lamb kidney**, braised | 85 | 116 | 59.9 | 0.8 | | | 0 | 128 | 15 | 17 | 3.23 | 0.122 | 116 | 10 | 0.30 | 5.1 | 67.06 | 1.73 |
| *3 oz* | | 20.1 | 3.1 | 1.0 | 0.7 | 0.6 | 480 | 151 | 246 | 10.54 | 0.314 | 186.0 | 387 | | 1.76 | 0.10 | 68.8 | 17196 |
| **lamb liver**, braised | 85 | 187 | 48.2 | 2.2 | | | 0 | 48 | 7 | 19 | 6.71 | 0.442 | 6367 | 3 | 0.20 | 10.3 | 65.02 | 3.37 |
| *3 oz* | | 26.0 | 7.5 | 2.9 | 1.6 | 1.1 | 426 | 188 | 357 | 7.04 | 6.013 | 94.7 | 21203 | | 3.43 | 0.42 | 62.0 | 17200 |
| **lamb liver**, pan-fried | 85 | 202 | 47.8 | 3.2 | | | 0 | 105 | 8 | 20 | 4.79 | 0.505 | 6615 | 11 | 0.30 | 14.2 | 72.84 | 5.38 |
| *3 oz* | | 21.7 | 10.8 | 4.2 | 2.2 | 1.6 | 419 | 299 | 363 | 8.67 | 8.356 | 98.7 | 22098 | | 3.90 | 0.81 | 340.0 | 17201 |
| **lamb liver**, raw | 85 | 118 | 60.7 | 1.5 | | | 0 | 60 | 6 | 16 | 3.96 | 0.156 | 6282 | 3 | 0.29 | 13.7 | 76.54 | 5.21 |
| *3 oz* | | 17.3 | 4.3 | 1.6 | 0.9 | 0.6 | 315 | 266 | 309 | 6.26 | 5.932 | 70.0 | 20920 | | 3.09 | 0.76 | 195.5 | 17199 |
| **lamb lung**, braised | 85 | 96 | 64.5 | 0 | | | 0 | 71 | 10 | 9 | 1.64 | 0.014 | 27 | 24 | 0.03 | 2.1 | 2.14 | |
| *3 oz* | | 16.9 | 2.6 | 0.9 | 0.7 | 0.4 | 241 | 108 | 160 | 3.88 | 0.199 | 17.9 | 90 | | 0.12 | 0.05 | 6.8 | 17206 |
| **lamb pancreas** (sweetbread), braised - 3 oz | 85 | 199 | 50.7 | 0 | | | 0 | 44 | 10 | 16 | 2.28 | 0.037 | 0 | 17 | 0.02 | 2.2 | 4.71 | 0.72 |
| *3 oz* | | 19.4 | 12.0 | 5.8 | 4.6 | 0.6 | 340 | 247 | 366 | 1.80 | 0.071 | 55.1 | 0 | | 0.18 | 0.04 | 11.0 | 17211 |
| **lamb spleen**, braised | 85 | 133 | 56.4 | 0 | | | 0 | 49 | 11 | 14 | 3.35 | 0.053 | 0 | 22 | 0.04 | 5.0 | 4.50 | |
| *3 oz* | | 22.5 | 4.1 | 1.3 | 1.1 | 0.3 | 327 | 211 | 290 | 32.87 | 0.118 | 42.3 | 0 | | 0.27 | 0.07 | 3.4 | 17215 |
| **lamb tongue**, braised | 85 | 234 | 49.2 | 0 | | | 0 | 57 | 8 | 14 | 2.54 | 0.028 | 0 | 6 | 0.07 | 3.1 | 5.36 | 0.29 |
| *3 oz* | | 18.3 | 17.2 | 6.7 | 8.5 | 1.1 | 161 | 134 | 114 | 2.24 | 0.178 | 23.8 | 0 | | 0.36 | 0.14 | 2.6 | 17221 |
| **pork belly**, raw | 85 | 440 | 31.2 | 0 | 0 | | 0 | 27 | 4 | 3 | 0.87 | 0.005 | 3 | 0 | 0.34 | 3.9 | 0.71 | 0.22 |
| *3 oz* | | 7.9 | 45.1 | 16.4 | 21.0 | 4.8 | 61 | 157 | 92 | 0.44 | 0.044 | 6.8 | 8 | 0.3 | 0.21 | 0.11 | 0.8 | 10005 |

| | WT (g) / PRO (g) | KCAL / FAT (g) | H₂0 (g) / SFA (g) | CHO (g) / MUFA (g) | TSUG (g) / PUFA (g) | ASUG (g) / CHOL (mg) | DFIB (g) | Na (mg) / K (mg) | Ca (mg) / P (mg) | Mg (mg) / Fe (mg) | Zn (mg) / Cu (mg) | Mn (mg) / Se (mcg) | A (mcg RAE) / A (IU) | C (mg) / E (mg ATE) | B-1 (mg) / B-2 (mg) | NIA (mg) / B-6 (mg) | B-12 (mcg) / FOL (mcg DFE) | PANT (mg) / REF |
|---|---|---|---|---|---|---|---|---|---|---|---|---|---|---|---|---|---|---|
| **pork brain**, braised | 85 | 117 | 64.5 | 0 | | | 0 | 77 | 8 | 10 | 1.26 | 0.072 | 0 | 12 | 0.07 | 2.8 | 1.21 | 1.55 |
| *3 oz* | 10.3 | 8.1 | 1.8 | 1.5 | 1.2 | 2169 | | 166 | 187 | 1.55 | 0.224 | 15.7 | 0 | | 0.19 | 0.12 | 3.4 | 10097 |
| **pork brain**, raw | 85 | 108 | 66.6 | 0 | | | 0 | 102 | 8 | 12 | 1.08 | 0.080 | 0 | 11 | 0.13 | 3.6 | 1.86 | 2.38 |
| *3 oz* | 8.7 | 7.8 | 1.8 | 1.4 | 1.2 | 1866 | | 219 | 240 | 1.36 | 0.204 | 13.5 | 0 | | 0.23 | 0.16 | 5.1 | 10096 |
| **pork chitterlings**, simmered | 85 | 198 | 57.7 | 0 | 0 | | 0 | 15 | 21 | 8 | 1.57 | 0.076 | 0 | 0 | 0.01 | 0.1 | 0.36 | 0.07 |
| *3 oz* | 10.6 | 17.3 | 8.1 | 6.0 | 1.0 | 235 | | 12 | 56 | 1.25 | 0.039 | 23.0 | 0 | 0.2 | 0.04 | 0 | 0.8 | 10099 |
| **pork ears**, simmered | 111 | 184 | 80.6 | 0.2 | | | 0 | 185 | 20 | 8 | 0.22 | 0.011 | 0 | 0 | 0.02 | 0.6 | 0.04 | 0.04 |
| *1 ear (3.9 oz)* | 17.7 | 12.0 | 4.3 | 5.5 | 1.3 | 100 | | 44 | 27 | 1.66 | 0.007 | 4.9 | 0 | | 0.08 | 0.01 | 0 | 10101 |
| **pork heart**, braised | 129 | 191 | 87.8 | 0.5 | | | 0 | 45 | 9 | 31 | 3.99 | 0.094 | 9 | 3 | 0.72 | 7.8 | 4.89 | 3.19 |
| *1 heart (4.6 oz)* | 30.4 | 6.5 | 1.7 | 1.5 | 1.7 | 285 | | 266 | 230 | 7.52 | 0.655 | 23.6 | 28 | | 2.20 | 0.50 | 5.2 | 10104 |
| **pork heart**, raw | 85 | 100 | 64.8 | 1.1 | 0 | | 0 | 48 | 4 | 16 | 2.38 | 0.054 | 7 | 5 | 0.52 | 5.8 | 3.22 | 2.14 |
| *3 oz* | 14.7 | 3.7 | 1.0 | 0.9 | 1.0 | 111 | | 250 | 144 | 3.98 | 0.347 | 8.8 | 21 | 0.5 | 1.01 | 0.33 | 3.4 | 10103 |
| **pork jowl**, raw | 85 | 557 | 18.9 | 0 | 0 | | 0 | 21 | 3 | 3 | 0.71 | 0.004 | 3 | 0 | 0.33 | 3.9 | 0.70 | 0.21 |
| *3 oz* | 5.4 | 59.2 | 21.5 | 28.0 | 6.9 | 76 | | 126 | 73 | 0.36 | 0.034 | 1.3 | 8 | 0.2 | 0.20 | 0.08 | 0.8 | 10105 |
| **pork kidney**, braised | 85 | 128 | 58.4 | 0 | | | 0 | 68 | 11 | 15 | 3.53 | 0.127 | 66 | 9 | 0.34 | 4.9 | 6.62 | 2.44 |
| *3 oz* | 21.6 | 4.0 | 1.3 | 1.3 | 0.3 | 408 | | 122 | 204 | 4.50 | 0.581 | 264.8 | 221 | | 1.35 | 0.39 | 34.8 | 10107 |
| **pork kidney**, raw | 85 | 85 | 68.1 | 0 | | | 0 | 103 | 8 | 14 | 2.34 | 0.105 | 50 | 11 | 0.29 | 7.0 | 7.22 | 2.66 |
| *3 oz* | 14.0 | 2.8 | 0.9 | 0.9 | 0.2 | 271 | | 195 | 173 | 4.16 | 0.529 | 161.5 | 168 | | 1.44 | 0.37 | 35.7 | 10106 |
| **pork liver**, braised | 85 | 140 | 54.7 | 3.2 | | | 0 | 42 | 8 | 12 | 5.71 | 0.255 | 4594 | 20 | 0.22 | 7.2 | 15.87 | 4.06 |
| *3 oz* | 22.1 | 3.7 | 1.2 | 0.5 | 0.9 | 302 | | 128 | 205 | 15.23 | 0.539 | 57.4 | 15297 | | 1.87 | 0.48 | 138.5 | 10111 |
| **pork liver**, raw | 85 | 114 | 60.4 | 2.1 | | | 0 | 74 | 8 | 15 | 4.90 | 0.292 | 5527 | 22 | 0.24 | 13.0 | 22.10 | 5.65 |
| *3 oz* | 18.2 | 3.1 | 1.0 | 0.4 | 0.7 | 256 | | 232 | 245 | 19.80 | 0.575 | 44.8 | 18402 | | 2.55 | 0.59 | 180.2 | 10110 |
| **pork lung**, braised | 85 | 84 | 68.0 | 0 | | | 0 | 69 | 7 | 10 | 2.08 | 0.013 | 0 | 7 | 0.07 | 1.2 | 1.73 | 0.56 |
| *3 oz* | 14.1 | 2.6 | 0.9 | 0.6 | 0.3 | 329 | | 128 | 158 | 13.95 | 0.068 | 19.9 | 0 | | 0.27 | 0.07 | 1.7 | 10113 |
| **pork lung**, raw | 85 | 72 | 67.6 | 0 | | | 0 | 130 | 6 | 12 | 1.73 | 0.014 | 0 | 10 | 0.07 | 2.8 | 2.34 | 0.76 |
| *3 oz* | 12.0 | 2.3 | 0.8 | 0.5 | 0.3 | 272 | | 258 | 167 | 16.06 | 0.071 | 15.1 | 0 | | 0.37 | 0.08 | 2.6 | 10112 |
| **pork pancreas** (sweetbread), braised | 85 | 186 | 51.3 | 0 | | | 0 | 36 | 14 | 20 | 3.65 | 0.168 | 0 | 5 | 0.08 | 2.7 | 14.51 | 4.03 |
| *3 oz* | 24.2 | 9.2 | 3.2 | 3.2 | 1.7 | 268 | | 143 | 247 | 2.29 | 0.094 | 61.9 | 0 | | 0.56 | 0.37 | 4.2 | 10116 |
| **pork (pig) feet**, cured, pickled | 85 | 119 | 63.8 | 0 | 0 | 0 | 0 | 476 | 27 | 9 | 0.17 | 0.019 | 9 | 0 | 0.01 | 0.2 | 0.18 | 0.22 |
| *3 oz* | 9.9 | 8.5 | 2.5 | 4.8 | 0.7 | 71 | | 11 | 74 | 0.26 | 0.031 | 13.4 | 31 | 0.2 | 0.01 | 0.01 | 0.8 | 10132 |
| **pork (pig) feet**, simmered | 85 | 197 | 53.4 | 0 | 0 | | 0 | 62 | 0 | 4 | 0.89 | 0.015 | 0 | 0 | 0.01 | 0.5 | 0.35 | 0.20 |
| *3 oz* | 18.6 | 13.6 | 3.7 | 6.8 | 1.3 | 91 | | 28 | 70 | 0.83 | 0.053 | 19.6 | 0 | 0.1 | 0.05 | 0.03 | 1.7 | 10173 |
| **pork spleen**, braised | 85 | 127 | 56.7 | 0 | | | 0 | 91 | 11 | 13 | 3.01 | 0.038 | 0 | 10 | 0.12 | 5.0 | 2.35 | 0.76 |
| *3 oz* | 24.0 | 2.7 | 0.9 | 0.7 | 0.2 | 428 | | 193 | 241 | 18.90 | 0.113 | 42.2 | 0 | | 0.22 | 0.05 | 3.4 | 10118 |
| **pork spleen**, raw | 85 | 85 | 66.7 | 0 | | | 0 | 83 | 8 | 11 | 2.16 | 0.061 | 0 | 24 | 0.11 | 5.0 | 2.77 | 0.90 |
| *3 oz* | 15.2 | 2.2 | 0.7 | 0.6 | 0.2 | 309 | | 337 | 221 | 18.97 | 0.111 | 27.9 | 0 | | 0.26 | 0.05 | 3.4 | 10117 |
| **pork stomach**, raw | 85 | 135 | 62.5 | 0 | 0 | | 0 | 64 | 9 | 9 | 1.57 | 0.032 | 0 | 0 | 0.04 | 2.1 | 0.26 | 1.04 |
| *3 oz* | 14.3 | 8.6 | 3.4 | 3.1 | 0.8 | 190 | | 119 | 110 | 0.86 | 0.144 | 26.4 | 0 | 0 | 0.17 | 0.03 | 2.6 | 10119 |
| **pork tail**, simmered | 85 | 337 | 39.7 | 0 | | | 0 | 21 | 12 | 6 | 1.39 | 0.005 | 0 | 0 | 0.06 | 1.0 | 0.47 | 0.36 |
| *3 oz* | 14.4 | 30.4 | 10.6 | 14.4 | 3.3 | 110 | | 133 | 40 | 0.67 | 0.057 | 2.6 | 0 | | 0.06 | 0.23 | 3.4 | 10175 |
| **pork tongue**, braised | 85 | 230 | 48.4 | 0 | | | 0 | 93 | 16 | 17 | 3.85 | 0.008 | 0 | 1 | 0.27 | 4.5 | 2.03 | 0.43 |
| *3 oz* | 20.5 | 15.8 | 5.5 | 7.4 | 1.6 | 124 | | 201 | 148 | 4.24 | 0.094 | 13.2 | 0 | | 0.43 | 0.20 | 3.4 | 10122 |
| **pork tongue**, raw | 85 | 191 | 56.0 | 0 | 0 | | 0 | 94 | 14 | 15 | 2.56 | 0.009 | 0 | 4 | 0.42 | 4.5 | 2.41 | 0.54 |
| *3 oz* | 13.9 | 14.6 | 5.1 | 6.9 | 1.5 | 86 | | 207 | 164 | 2.85 | 0.060 | 8.8 | 0 | | 0.41 | 0.20 | 3.4 | 10121 |
| **sea lion heart**, raw | 85 | 87 | 64.8 | 0.8 | | | | 98 | 4 | 19 | 1.90 | 0.031 | | | | | | |
| *3 oz* | 14.4 | 2.8 | | | | | | 271 | 224 | 5.70 | 0.260 | 103.7 | | | | | | 35228 |
| **sea lion kidney**, raw | 85 | 79 | 65.8 | 1.2 | | | | 196 | 8 | 14 | 2.46 | 0.111 | | 0 | | | | |
| *3 oz* | 15.4 | 1.4 | 0.3 | 0.3 | 0.3 | 332 | | 215 | 256 | 5.95 | 0.744 | 232.9 | 0 | 0 | | | | 35227 |
| **sea lion liver**, raw | 85 | 116 | 60.6 | 0 | | | | 75 | 5 | 19 | 3.48 | 0.595 | | | | | | |
| *3 oz* | 19.5 | 4.2 | 1.1 | 0.8 | 0.2 | 305 | | 247 | 337 | 7.65 | 1.606 | 589.0 | | | | | | 35226 |
| **sheep spleen**, raw | 85 | 86 | 66.4 | 0 | | | 0 | 71 | 8 | 18 | 2.41 | 0.043 | 0 | 20 | 0.04 | 6.7 | 4.54 | |
| *3 oz* | 14.6 | 2.6 | 0.9 | 0.7 | 0.2 | 212 | | 304 | 238 | 35.61 | 0.103 | 27.5 | 0 | | 0.30 | 0.09 | 3.4 | 17214 |
| **veal brain**, braised | 85 | 116 | 65.4 | 0 | | | 0 | 133 | 14 | 14 | 1.37 | 0.032 | 0 | 11 | 0.07 | 2.1 | 8.20 | 0.85 |
| *3 oz* | 9.8 | 8.2 | 1.9 | 1.5 | 1.3 | 2635 | | 182 | 327 | 1.42 | 0.221 | 9.4 | 0 | | 0.17 | 0.14 | 2.6 | 17189 |
| **veal brain**, pan-fried | 85 | 181 | 58.3 | 0 | | | 0 | 150 | 8 | 15 | 1.55 | 0.037 | 0 | 13 | 0.13 | 4.8 | 18.10 | 0.96 |
| *3 oz* | 12.3 | 14.2 | 3.4 | 3.6 | 2.1 | 1802 | | 401 | 369 | 0.91 | 0.255 | 10.2 | 0 | | 0.31 | 0.28 | 5.1 | 17190 |
| **veal heart**, braised | 85 | 158 | 52.9 | 0.1 | | | 0 | 49 | 7 | 15 | 1.90 | 0.052 | 0 | 8 | 0.30 | 4.1 | 12.29 | 1.40 |
| *3 oz* | 24.8 | 5.7 | 1.5 | 1.2 | 1.5 | 150 | | 169 | 212 | 3.67 | 0.367 | 44.5 | 0 | | 0.79 | 0.18 | 1.7 | 17194 |
| **veal kidney**, braised | 85 | 139 | 57.5 | 0 | | | 0 | 94 | 25 | 20 | 3.61 | 0.108 | 171 | 7 | 0.16 | 3.9 | 31.36 | 0.73 |
| *3 oz* | 22.4 | 4.8 | 1.5 | 1.1 | 1.0 | 672 | | 135 | 316 | 2.58 | 0.306 | 85.0 | 569 | | 1.69 | 0.15 | 17.8 | 17198 |
| **veal liver**, braised | 85 | 163 | 50.9 | 3.2 | 0 | | 0 | 66 | 5 | 17 | 9.55 | 0.230 | 17973 | 1 | 0.15 | 11.2 | 71.91 | 5.57 |
| *3 oz* | 24.2 | 5.3 | 1.7 | 1.0 | 0.9 | 434 | | 280 | 391 | 4.34 | 12.699 | 16.4 | 59979 | 0.6 | 2.43 | 0.78 | 281.3 | 17203 |

| | WT (g) | KCAL | H₂O (g) | CHO (g) | TSUG (g) | ASUG (g) | DFIB (g) | Na (mg) | Ca (mg) | Mg (mg) | Zn (mg) | Mn (mg) | A (mcg RAE) | C (mg) | B-1 (mg) | NIA (mg) | B-12 (mcg) | PANT (mg) |
|---|---|---|---|---|---|---|---|---|---|---|---|---|---|---|---|---|---|---|
| | | PRO (g) | FAT (g) | SFA (g) | MUFA (g) | PUFA (g) | CHOL (mg) | K (mg) | P (mg) | Fe (mg) | Cu (mg) | Se (mcg) | A (IU) | E (mg ATE) | B-2 (mg) | B-6 (mg) | FOL (mcg DFE) | REF |
| **veal liver**, pan-fried | 85 | 164 | 50.9 | 3.8 | 0 | | 0 | 72 | 6 | 20 | 10.12 | 0.257 | 17063 | 1 | 0.15 | 12.2 | 61.62 | 6.01 |
| *3 oz* | | 23.3 | 5.5 | 1.8 | 1.0 | 1.0 | 412 | 300 | 411 | 5.08 | 12.792 | 21.2 | 56941 | 0.5 | 2.60 | 0.76 | 297.5 | 17204 |
| **veal lung**, braised | 85 | 88 | 66.0 | 0 | | | 0 | 48 | 6 | 7 | 1.02 | 0.013 | 0 | 29 | 0.03 | 1.9 | 2.02 | |
| *3 oz* | | 15.9 | 2.2 | 0.8 | 0.6 | 0.3 | 224 | 121 | 197 | 3.07 | 0.188 | 16.8 | 0 | | 0.11 | 0.05 | 6.8 | 17208 |
| **veal pancreas** (sweetbread), braised | 85 | 218 | 47.3 | 0 | | | 0 | 58 | 15 | 20 | 4.42 | 0.200 | 0 | 5 | 0.16 | 3.5 | 14.73 | |
| *3 oz* | | 24.7 | 12.4 | 4.3 | 4.3 | 2.3 | | 236 | 435 | 2.02 | 0.086 | 33.2 | 0 | | 0.43 | 0.16 | 2.6 | 17213 |
| **veal spleen**, braised | 85 | 110 | 60.6 | 0 | | | 0 | 49 | 6 | 12 | 1.62 | 0.064 | 0 | 34 | 0.04 | 4.5 | 4.10 | |
| *3 oz* | | 20.5 | 2.5 | 0.8 | 0.7 | 0.2 | 380 | 183 | 265 | 6.26 | 0.786 | 69.0 | 0 | | 0.24 | 0.06 | 3.4 | 17217 |
| **veal thymus** (sweetbread), braised | 85 | 106 | 62.6 | 0 | | | 0 | 50 | 3 | 20 | 1.81 | 0.018 | 0 | 33 | 0.05 | 2.9 | 2.42 | 0.92 |
| *3 oz* | | 19.3 | 2.6 | 0.8 | 0.8 | 0.3 | 298 | 370 | 533 | 1.05 | 0.061 | 18.3 | 0 | 0.1 | 0.08 | 0.02 | 17.0 | 17219 |
| **veal tongue**, braised | 85 | 172 | 54.5 | 0 | | | 0 | 54 | 8 | 15 | 3.83 | 0.040 | 0 | 5 | 0.06 | 1.2 | 4.50 | 0.63 |
| *3 oz* | | 22.0 | 8.6 | 3.7 | 3.9 | 0.3 | 202 | 138 | 141 | 1.78 | 0.178 | 9.4 | 0 | | 0.30 | 0.13 | 7.6 | 17223 |

## 20. MEATS, LUNCHEON AND SNACK
### 20.1 FRANKFURTERS AND OTHER LUNCHEON-TYPE SAUSAGES

| | WT (g) | KCAL | H₂O (g) | CHO (g) | TSUG (g) | ASUG (g) | DFIB (g) | Na (mg) | Ca (mg) | Mg (mg) | Zn (mg) | Mn (mg) | A (mcg RAE) | C (mg) | B-1 (mg) | NIA (mg) | B-12 (mcg) | PANT (mg) |
|---|---|---|---|---|---|---|---|---|---|---|---|---|---|---|---|---|---|---|
| | | PRO (g) | FAT (g) | SFA (g) | MUFA (g) | PUFA (g) | CHOL (mg) | K (mg) | P (mg) | Fe (mg) | Cu (mg) | Se (mcg) | A (IU) | E (mg ATE) | B-2 (mg) | B-6 (mg) | FOL (mcg DFE) | REF |
| **beef sausage**, smoked, pan-fried | 43 | 134 | 23.0 | 1.0 | | | 0 | 486 | 3 | 6 | 1.20 | 0.004 | 0 | 0 | 0.02 | 1.4 | 0.80 | 0.08 |
| *1.5 oz sausage* | | 6.1 | 11.6 | 4.9 | 5.6 | 0.5 | 29 | 76 | 45 | 0.76 | 0.031 | 6.3 | 0 | | 0.06 | 0.05 | 1.7 | 13357 |
| **blood sausage** (blood/black pudding, blutwurst) - .9 oz slice | 25 | 95 | 11.8 | 0.3 | 0.3 | 0.3 | 0 | 170 | 2 | 2 | 0.32 | 0.002 | 0 | 0 | 0.02 | 0.3 | 0.25 | 0.15 |
| | | 3.6 | 8.6 | 3.4 | 4.0 | 0.9 | 30 | 10 | 6 | 1.60 | 0.010 | 3.9 | 0 | 0 | 0.03 | 0.01 | 1.2 | 7005 |
| **bockwurst** (pork, veal, milk, eggs), raw - 3.2 oz sausage | 91 | 274 | 49.6 | 2.7 | 1.2 | | 0.9 | 452 | 37 | 24 | 1.88 | 0.156 | 70 | 3 | 0.18 | 5.1 | 0.78 | 0.81 |
| | | 12.8 | 23.5 | 9.3 | 12.0 | 2.1 | 85 | 246 | 154 | 1.05 | 0.091 | 10.3 | 233 | 0.3 | 0.21 | 0.34 | 15.5 | 7006 |
| **bratwurst**, beef and pork, smoked - 2.3 oz | 66 | 196 | 37.4 | 1.3 | 0 | | 0 | 560 | 5 | 10 | 1.63 | 0.027 | 0 | 0 | 0.25 | 2.1 | 1.76 | 0.46 |
| | | 8.1 | 17.4 | 4.0 | 5.3 | 1.0 | 51 | 187 | 86 | 0.66 | 0.053 | 9.3 | 0 | | 0.14 | 0.13 | 2.6 | 7922 |
| **bratwurst**, chicken, cooked | 84 | 148 | 59.0 | 0 | 0 | | 0 | 60 | 9 | 19 | 1.20 | | 25 | 2 | 0.06 | 6.3 | 0.29 | 0.81 |
| *3 oz* | | 16.3 | 8.7 | | | | 60 | 177 | 134 | 0.73 | 0.042 | | 85 | | 0.11 | 0.32 | 5.0 | 7923 |
| **bratwurst**, pork, beef, and turkey, lite, smoked - 2.3 oz | 66 | 123 | 43.5 | 1.1 | 1.0 | | 0 | 648 | 9 | 9 | 1.77 | 0.010 | 0 | 0 | 0.06 | 1.2 | 1.06 | 0.27 |
| | | 9.5 | 8.9 | | 4.7 | 0.6 | 37 | 162 | 87 | 0.62 | 0.042 | 13.3 | 1 | | 0.11 | 0.14 | 3.3 | 7924 |
| **bratwurst**, pork, cooked | 85 | 283 | 43.7 | 2.4 | 0 | 0 | 0 | 719 | 24 | 18 | 2.76 | 0.012 | 2 | 0 | 0.39 | 4.1 | 0.62 | 0.57 |
| *3 oz* | | 11.7 | 24.8 | 8.5 | 12.5 | 2.2 | 63 | 296 | 177 | 0.45 | 0.088 | 33.7 | 5 | 0.2 | 0.26 | 0.28 | 2.6 | 7013 |
| **bratwurst**, veal, cooked | 85 | 290 | 45.5 | 0 | | | 0 | 51 | 9 | 14 | 1.74 | 0.042 | 0 | 0 | 0.05 | 4.6 | 0.83 | 0.81 |
| *3 oz* | | 11.9 | 26.9 | 12.7 | 11.0 | 1.4 | 67 | 196 | 128 | 0.63 | 0.069 | 16.3 | 0 | | 0.16 | 0.26 | 7.6 | 7910 |
| **brotwurst**, pork and beef w/nonfat dry milk - 2.5 oz link (7/lb) | 70 | 226 | 35.9 | 2.1 | 2.1 | 2.1 | 0 | 778 | 34 | 11 | 1.47 | 0.028 | 0 | 0 | 0.18 | 2.3 | 1.43 | 0.04 |
| | | 10.0 | 19.5 | 7.0 | 9.3 | 2.0 | 44 | 197 | 94 | 0.72 | 0.056 | 11.9 | 0 | 0.2 | 0.16 | 0.09 | 3.5 | 7015 |
| **chicken and beef sausage**, smoked - 2 oz | 56 | 166 | 31.1 | 0 | 0 | | 0 | 571 | 6 | 8 | 0.97 | | 17 | 0 | 0.02 | 2.3 | 0.21 | |
| | | 10.4 | 13.4 | 4.0 | 5.7 | 2.6 | 39 | 78 | 62 | 0.60 | 0.029 | 8.1 | 60 | 0.3 | 0.07 | 0.10 | 2.2 | 42262 |
| **chicken, beef, and pork sausage**, skinless, smoked - 1 link | 84 | 181 | 50.8 | 6.8 | 1.6 | | 0 | 869 | 84 | 12 | 2.25 | 0.013 | 0 | 0 | 0.08 | 1.6 | 1.34 | 0.35 |
| | | 11.4 | 12.0 | 4.0 | 6.0 | 0.7 | 101 | 207 | 111 | 4.03 | 0.053 | 17.0 | 0 | | 0.14 | 0.18 | 5.0 | 7928 |
| **chorizo**, pork and beef 2.1 oz link (4" long) | 60 | 273 | 19.1 | 1.1 | 0 | | 0 | 741 | 5 | 11 | 2.05 | 0.024 | 0 | 0 | 0.38 | 3.1 | 1.20 | 0.67 |
| | | 14.5 | 23.0 | 8.6 | 11.0 | 2.1 | 53 | 239 | 90 | 0.95 | 0.048 | 12.7 | 0 | 0.1 | 0.18 | 0.32 | 1.2 | 7019 |
| **frankfurter** | 52 | 151 | 29.3 | 2.2 | | | 0 | 567 | 51 | 8 | 0.62 | 0.023 | 0 | 0 | 0.03 | 1.4 | 0.82 | 0.16 |
| *1.8 oz frankfurter* | | 5.3 | 13.4 | | | | 40 | 79 | 107 | 0.57 | 0.050 | 6.5 | 0 | 0.1 | 0.06 | 0.09 | 3.1 | 7950 |
| **frankfurter**, beef | 43 | 142 | 22.4 | 1.7 | 1.5 | 0 | 0 | 490 | 6 | 6 | 1.06 | 0.035 | 0 | 0 | 0.02 | 1.0 | 0.74 | 0.10 |
| *1.5 oz frankfurter* | | 4.8 | 12.7 | 5.0 | 6.2 | 0.5 | 23 | 67 | 69 | 0.65 | 0.079 | 3.5 | 0 | 0.1 | 0.06 | 0.04 | 2.2 | 7022 |
| **frankfurter**, beef and pork | 45 | 137 | 25.2 | 0.8 | 0 | | 0 | 504 | 5 | 4 | 0.83 | 0.014 | 8 | 0 | 0.09 | 1.2 | 0.59 | 0.16 |
| *1.6 oz frankfurter* | | 5.2 | 12.4 | 4.8 | 6.2 | 1.2 | 22 | 75 | 39 | 0.52 | 0.036 | 6.2 | 26 | 0.1 | 0.05 | 0.06 | 1.8 | 7023 |
| **frankfurter**, beef and pork, lowfat | 57 | 88 | 40.6 | 2.5 | 0 | 0 | 0 | 716 | 6 | 6 | 1.12 | | 0 | 0 | 0.10 | 1.4 | 0.74 | |
| *2 oz frankfurter* | | 6.3 | 5.7 | 2.1 | 2.7 | 0.5 | 25 | 85 | 80 | 0.68 | 0.043 | 8.6 | 0 | 0 | 0.06 | 0.06 | 2.3 | 42188 |
| **frankfurter**, beef, bun length, Oscar Mayer - 2 oz frankfurter | 57 | 185 | 30.3 | 1.5 | 1.0 | | 0 | 584 | 7 | 9 | 1.28 | | 0 | 0 | | | | |
| | | 6.3 | 17.2 | 7.1 | 8.3 | 0.5 | 34 | 90 | 60 | 0.89 | 0.085 | | 0 | | | | 6.3 | 7242 |
| **frankfurter**, beef, fat-free, Oscar Mayer - 1.8 oz frankfurter | 50 | 39 | 39.0 | 2.6 | 1.9 | | 0 | 464 | 10 | 10 | 1.20 | | 0 | 0 | | | | |
| | | 6.6 | 0.2 | 0.1 | 0.1 | 0 | 15 | 234 | 64 | 0.98 | 0.080 | | 0 | | | | | 7243 |
| **frankfurter**, beef, heated | 52 | 170 | 27.1 | 2.0 | 1.8 | | 0 | 600 | 6 | 7 | 1.22 | 0.040 | 0 | 0 | 0.02 | 1.2 | 0.86 | 0.13 |
| *1.8 oz frankfurter* | | 6.0 | 15.3 | 5.9 | 7.4 | 0.6 | 29 | 76 | 89 | 0.81 | 0.080 | 6.3 | 0 | 0.1 | 0.07 | 0.05 | 3.6 | 7945 |
| **frankfurter**, beef, Hormel Wrangler | 56 | 162 | 31.7 | 1.2 | 0.9 | | 0 | 557 | 8 | 8 | 1.29 | | 2 | 11 | | | | |
| *2 oz frankfurter* | | 7.0 | 14.4 | 5.9 | 7.3 | 0.5 | 38 | 96 | | 1.01 | 0.056 | | 7 | | | | 6.2 | 7279 |
| **frankfurter**, beef, light, Oscar Mayer - 2 oz frankfurter | 57 | 110 | 38.1 | 2.3 | 1.2 | | 0 | 615 | 12 | 10 | 1.20 | | 0 | 0 | | | | |
| | | 6.1 | 8.5 | 3.6 | 4.3 | 0.6 | 28 | 229 | 93 | 0.89 | 0.120 | | 0 | | | | | 7244 |
| **frankfurter**, beef, lowfat | 57 | 133 | 36.4 | 0.9 | 0 | | 0 | 593 | 5 | 6 | 1.12 | | 0 | 1 | 0.03 | 1.3 | 0.80 | |
| *2 oz frankfurter* | | 6.8 | 11.1 | 4.6 | 5.6 | 0.3 | 23 | 74 | 109 | 0.66 | 0.037 | 7.9 | 0 | 0.1 | 0.06 | 0.06 | 2.3 | 42179 |
| **frankfurter**, beef, Oscar Mayer | 45 | 147 | 23.9 | 1.1 | 0.7 | | 0 | 461 | 4 | 6 | 0.99 | 0.009 | 0 | 0 | 0.02 | 1.0 | 0.73 | 0.10 |
| *1.6 oz frankfurter* | | 5.1 | 13.6 | 5.6 | 6.6 | 0.6 | 25 | 58 | 63 | 0.60 | 0.063 | 5.2 | 0 | | 0.05 | 0.03 | 2.7 | 7241 |

| | WT (g) | KCAL / PRO (g) | H₂O (g) / FAT (g) | CHO (g) / SFA (g) | TSUG (g) / MUFA (g) | ASUG (g) / PUFA (g) | DFIB (g) / CHOL (mg) | Na (mg) / K (mg) | Ca (mg) / P (mg) | Mg (mg) / Fe (mg) | Zn (mg) / Cu (mg) | Mn (mg) / Se (mcg) | A (mcg RAE) / A (IU) | C (mg) / E (mg ATE) | B-1 (mg) / B-2 (mg) | NIA (mg) / B-6 (mg) | B-12 (mcg) / FOL (mcg DFE) | PANT (mg) / REF |
|---|---|---|---|---|---|---|---|---|---|---|---|---|---|---|---|---|---|---|
| frankfurter, beef, pork, and turkey, fat-free - 2 oz frankfurter | 57 | 62 | 40.8 | 6.4 | 0 | 0 | 0 | 455 | 31 | 8 | 1.66 | | 0 | 14 | 0.09 | 2.0 | 0.60 | |
| | | 7.1 | 0.9 | 0.3 | 0.4 | 0.2 | 23 | 125 | 75 | 1.01 | 0.067 | 10.7 | 0 | 0 | 0.09 | 0.10 | 3.4 | 7905 |
| frankfurter, cheese w/turkey, Oscar Mayer - 1.6 oz frankfurter | 45 | 143 | 23.8 | 1.3 | 0.8 | | 0 | 514 | 74 | 11 | 0.83 | | | 0 | | | | |
| | | 5.4 | 12.9 | 4.5 | 5.9 | 1.7 | 33 | 59 | 97 | 0.67 | 0.081 | | 0 | | | | | 7245 |
| frankfurter, chicken - 1.6 oz frankfurter | 45 | 100 | 28.1 | 1.2 | 0.2 | 0 | 0.2 | 380 | 33 | 9 | 0.50 | 0.027 | 0 | 0 | 0.03 | 2.1 | 0.24 | 0.48 |
| | | 7.0 | 7.3 | 1.7 | 2.7 | 1.7 | 43 | 91 | 73 | 0.53 | 0.035 | 10.4 | 0 | 0.1 | 0.12 | 0.15 | 5.0 | 7024 |
| frankfurter, fat-free, Oscar Mayer - 1.8 oz frankfurter | 50 | 36 | 39.4 | 2.2 | 1.0 | | 0 | 487 | 8 | 10 | 0.60 | | | 0 | | | | |
| | | 6.3 | 0.3 | 0.1 | 0.1 | 0.1 | 14 | 236 | 81 | 0.46 | 0.110 | | 0 | | | | | 7246 |
| frankfurter, heated - 1.8 oz frankfurter | 52 | 145 | 30.1 | 2.5 | | | 0 | 527 | 51 | 8 | 0.56 | 0.027 | 0 | 0 | 0.03 | 1.4 | 0.82 | 0.16 |
| | | 5.1 | 12.6 | | | | 38 | 73 | 110 | 0.63 | 0.079 | 6.5 | 0 | 0.1 | 0.06 | 0.09 | 3.1 | 7949 |
| frankfurter, pork - 2.7 oz frankfurter | 76 | 204 | 45.5 | 0.2 | 0 | | 0.1 | 620 | 203 | 11 | 1.59 | 0.012 | 60 | 2 | 0.45 | 2.1 | 0.37 | 0.39 |
| | | 9.7 | 18.0 | 6.6 | 8.3 | 1.7 | 50 | 201 | 130 | 2.81 | 0.056 | 21.1 | 200 | | 0.14 | 0.24 | 2.3 | 7939 |
| frankfurter, pork and turkey, Oscar Mayer - 1.6 oz frankfurter | 45 | 147 | 24.0 | 1.2 | 0.8 | | 0 | 445 | 27 | 8 | 0.77 | | 0 | 0 | | | | |
| | | 4.9 | 13.5 | 4.3 | 6.2 | 1.9 | 32 | 73 | 62 | 0.52 | 0.117 | | 0 | | | | | 7240 |
| frankfurter, pork & turkey, sml, Oscar Mayer - 6 sml frnks (2 oz) | 57 | 177 | 31.4 | 1.3 | 0.9 | | 0 | 592 | 7 | 7 | 1.05 | | | 0 | | | | |
| | | 6.2 | 16.4 | 6.4 | 8.2 | 1.5 | 31 | 91 | 55 | 0.58 | 0.063 | | 0 | | | | | 7248 |
| frankfurter, pork, beef, (cheesefurter) Am chs - 1.5 oz frankfurter | 43 | 141 | 22.6 | 0.6 | 0.6 | 0 | 0 | 465 | 25 | 6 | 0.97 | 0.013 | 20 | 0 | 0.11 | 1.2 | 0.74 | 0.33 |
| | | 6.1 | 12.5 | 4.5 | 5.9 | 1.3 | 29 | 89 | 77 | 0.46 | 0.030 | 6.8 | 68 | 0.1 | 0.07 | 0.06 | 1.3 | 7016 |
| frankfurter, pork, turkey, beef, light, Oscar Mayer - 2 oz frankfurter | 57 | 111 | 38.0 | 1.6 | 0.9 | | 0 | 591 | 22 | 10 | 1.01 | | | 0 | | | | |
| | | 6.9 | 8.5 | 3.0 | 3.9 | 1.2 | 35 | 226 | 96 | 0.73 | 0.114 | | 0 | | | | | 7247 |
| frankfurter, turkey - 1.6 oz frankfurter | 45 | 100 | 28.3 | 1.7 | 0.5 | | 0 | 485 | 67 | 6 | 0.83 | 0.015 | 0 | 0 | 0.02 | 1.7 | 0.37 | 0.20 |
| | | 5.5 | 7.8 | 1.8 | 2.6 | 1.8 | 35 | 176 | 77 | 0.66 | 0.032 | 6.8 | 0 | 0.3 | 0.08 | 0.06 | 4.5 | 7025 |
| frankfurter, turkey and chicken, Louis Rich - 1.6 oz frankfurter | 45 | 85 | 30.1 | 2.4 | 0.7 | | 0 | 511 | 59 | 10 | 0.84 | | | 0 | | | | |
| | | 5.0 | 6.1 | 1.7 | 2.5 | 1.4 | 41 | 72 | 66 | 0.98 | 0.099 | | 0 | | | | | 7253 |
| frankfurter, turkey, Butcher Boy Meats - 2 oz frankfurter | 56 | 134 | 33.1 | 2.6 | 1.4 | | 0.1 | 651 | 83 | 8 | 1.61 | | 8 | 0 | 0.03 | 1.2 | 0.14 | 0.37 |
| | | 7.5 | 10.2 | 3.3 | 3.1 | 2.8 | 58 | 106 | 138 | 1.02 | 0.055 | | 166 | | 0.08 | 0.12 | 3.9 | 7269 |
| frankfurter, turkey, chicken, cheese, Louis Rich - 1.6 oz frankfurter | 45 | 90 | 28.8 | 2.3 | 0.8 | | 0 | 482 | 109 | 10 | 0.81 | | | 0 | | | | |
| | | 5.7 | 6.5 | 2.3 | 2.8 | 1.3 | 42 | 71 | 92 | 0.95 | 0.090 | | 0 | | | | | 7252 |
| Italian sausage, pork, cooked - 2.4 oz link | 67 | 230 | 31.6 | 2.9 | 0.6 | 0 | 0.1 | 809 | 14 | 12 | 1.60 | | 7 | 0 | 0.42 | 2.8 | 0.87 | |
| | | 12.8 | 18.3 | 6.4 | 8.0 | 2.2 | 38 | 204 | 114 | 0.96 | 0.054 | 14.7 | 21 | 0.2 | 0.16 | 0.22 | 3.4 | 7089 |
| Italian sausage, sweet, cooked - 3 oz link | 84 | 125 | 60.1 | 1.8 | 0 | | 0 | 479 | 21 | 10 | 1.28 | 0.006 | 0 | 0 | 0.14 | 1.5 | 0.87 | 0.23 |
| | | 13.5 | 7.1 | 2.7 | 3.0 | 0.4 | 25 | 163 | 87 | 1.00 | 0.034 | 9.1 | 2 | | 0.10 | 0.16 | 3.4 | 7914 |
| Italian sausage, turkey, smoked - 2 oz | 56 | 88 | 38.4 | 2.6 | 1.8 | | 0.5 | 520 | 12 | 14 | 1.19 | 0.037 | 24 | 17 | 0.04 | 2.1 | 0.24 | 0.45 |
| | | 8.4 | 4.9 | | | | 30 | 110 | 104 | 5.38 | 0.062 | 12.4 | 81 | | 0.10 | 0.21 | 4.5 | 7927 |
| kielbasa, Polish, turkey and beef, smoked - 2 oz | 56 | 127 | 34.7 | 2.2 | 0 | | 0 | 672 | | | | | 0 | 8 | | | | |
| | | 7.3 | 9.9 | 3.5 | 4.6 | 1.3 | 39 | | | 0.69 | | | 0 | | | | | 7934 |
| kielbasa (pork, beef w/nonfat dry milk) cooked - .9 oz slice | 26 | 80 | 14.2 | 0.7 | 0.4 | 0 | 0 | 235 | 4 | 3 | 0.41 | 0.012 | 0 | 0 | 0.05 | 0.9 | 0.19 | 0.17 |
| | | 3.2 | 7.1 | 2.4 | 3.1 | 1.0 | 17 | 78 | 44 | 0.21 | 0.096 | 5.0 | 0 | 0.1 | 0.05 | 0.05 | 0.3 | 7037 |
| knockwurst/knackwurst, pork, beef - 2.5 oz sausage | 72 | 221 | 39.8 | 2.3 | 0 | 0 | 0 | 670 | 8 | 8 | 1.20 | 0.015 | 0 | 0 | 0.25 | 2.0 | 0.85 | 0.23 |
| | | 8.0 | 19.9 | 7.4 | 9.2 | 2.1 | 43 | 143 | 71 | 0.48 | 0.043 | 9.7 | 0 | 0.4 | 0.10 | 0.12 | 1.4 | 7038 |
| Polish sausage, beef with chicken, hot, cooked - 5 pieces | 55 | 142 | 30.4 | 2.0 | 0 | | 0 | 847 | 7 | 8 | 1.06 | 0.027 | 0 | 0 | 0.28 | 1.9 | 0.54 | 0.25 |
| | | 9.7 | 10.7 | 4.4 | 5.3 | 0.4 | 36 | 130 | 75 | 0.48 | 0.050 | 9.7 | 0 | | 0.08 | 0.10 | 1.1 | 7915 |
| Polish sausage, pork and beef, smoked - 2.7 oz | 76 | 229 | 43.0 | 1.5 | 0 | | 0 | 644 | 5 | 9 | 1.60 | 0.028 | 0 | 0 | 0.20 | 2.5 | 1.15 | 0.33 |
| | | 9.2 | 20.2 | 7.0 | 9.3 | 2.1 | 54 | 144 | 81 | 0.76 | 0.046 | 10.0 | 0 | | 0.13 | 0.13 | 3.0 | 7916 |
| Polish sauge, pork, ckd - 8 oz sausage (10" long, 1¼" diameter) | 227 | 740 | 120.7 | 3.7 | | | 0 | 1989 | 27 | 32 | 4.38 | 0.111 | 0 | 2 | 1.14 | 7.8 | 2.22 | 1.02 |
| | | 32.0 | 65.2 | 23.4 | 30.7 | 7.0 | 159 | 538 | 309 | 3.27 | 0.204 | 40.2 | 0 | | 0.34 | 0.43 | 4.5 | 7059 |
| pork and beef sausage w/cheddar cheese, smoked - 2.7 oz | 77 | 228 | 43.2 | 1.6 | 0.1 | | 0 | 653 | 44 | 10 | 1.73 | 0.025 | 0 | 0 | 0.19 | 2.2 | 1.33 | 0.59 |
| | | 9.9 | 19.9 | 7.3 | 9.5 | 2.1 | 49 | 159 | 137 | 0.56 | 0.054 | 5.8 | 0 | | 0.12 | 0.10 | 2.3 | 7917 |
| Smokie (smkd sausg), beef, Oscar Mayer - 1.5 oz link | 43 | 127 | 24.2 | 0.8 | 0.6 | | 0 | 416 | 5 | 6 | 1.27 | | 0 | 0 | | | | |
| | | 5.3 | 11.5 | 4.8 | 5.5 | 0.4 | 27 | 74 | 99 | 0.75 | 0.086 | | 0 | | | | 4.7 | 7233 |
| Smokie (smkd sausg), pork - 2.4 oz link (4" long) | 68 | 209 | 38.4 | 0.6 | 0.6 | 0 | 0 | 562 | 7 | 7 | 0.89 | 0.007 | 0 | 0 | 0.14 | 1.9 | 0.45 | 0.36 |
| | | 8.1 | 19.2 | 6.3 | 7.6 | 2.5 | 41 | 328 | 107 | 0.40 | 0.120 | 12.4 | 0 | 0.2 | 0.12 | 0.12 | 0.7 | 7074 |
| Smokie (smkd sausg), pork & beef - 2.4 oz link (4" long) | 68 | 218 | 36.7 | 1.6 | 0 | 0 | 0 | 619 | 8 | 9 | 0.86 | 0.033 | 9 | 0 | 0.13 | 2.0 | 0.39 | 0.36 |
| | | 8.2 | 19.5 | 6.6 | 8.3 | 2.7 | 39 | 122 | 82 | 0.51 | 0.052 | 0 | 50 | 0.1 | 0.07 | 0.11 | 1.4 | 7075 |
| Smokie (smkd sausg), pork, beef w/flr & nfdm - 2.4 oz link (4" long) | 68 | 182 | 39.0 | 2.7 | 2.0 | | 0 | 865 | 45 | 9 | 1.36 | 0.035 | 0 | 2 | 0.16 | 1.8 | 0.90 | 0.41 |
| | | 9.5 | 14.6 | 5.3 | 6.8 | 1.5 | 44 | 105 | 75 | 0.98 | 0.061 | 10.8 | 0 | 0.1 | 0.12 | 0.09 | 1.4 | 7076 |
| Smokie (smkd sausg), pork, beef w/nfdm - 2.4 oz link (4" long) | 68 | 213 | 36.7 | 1.3 | | | 0 | 798 | 28 | 11 | 1.33 | 0.026 | 0 | 0 | 0.13 | 1.9 | 1.07 | 0.41 |
| | | 9.0 | 18.8 | 6.6 | 8.6 | 2.1 | 44 | 194 | 93 | 1.00 | 0.061 | 9.5 | 0 | | 0.15 | 0.12 | 1.4 | 7077 |
| Smokie (smkd sausg), pork, turkey, Little Smokies - 6 links (2 oz) | 57 | 172 | 31.6 | 1.0 | 0.8 | | 0 | 583 | 6 | 10 | 1.12 | | | 0 | | | | |
| | | 7.1 | 15.4 | 5.4 | 7.3 | 1.6 | 36 | 99 | 121 | 0.67 | 0.114 | | 0 | | | | | 7235 |

| Food | WT (g) | KCAL / PRO (g) | H₂0 (g) / FAT (g) | CHO (g) / SFA (g) | TSUG (g) / MUFA (g) | ASUG (g) / PUFA (g) | DFIB (g) / CHOL (mg) | Na (mg) / K (mg) | Ca (mg) / P (mg) | Mg (mg) / Fe (mg) | Zn (mg) / Cu (mg) | Mn (mg) / Se (mcg) | A (mcg RAE) / A (IU) | C (mg) / E (mg ATE) | B-1 (mg) / B-2 (mg) | NIA (mg) / B-6 (mg) | B-12 (mcg) / FOL (mcg DFE) | PANT (mg) / REF |
|---|---|---|---|---|---|---|---|---|---|---|---|---|---|---|---|---|---|---|
| **Smokie** (smkd sausg), prk, trky w/chs, Little Smokies - 6 links (2 oz) | 57 | 180 | 30.3 | 1.0 | 0.2 |  | 0 | 591 | 38 | 12 | 1.16 |  |  | 0 |  |  |  |  |
|  |  | 7.7 | 16.1 | 6.4 | 7.5 | 1.6 | 38 | 87 | 141 | 0.71 | 0.171 |  | 0 |  |  |  |  | 7236 |
| **Smokie** (smkd sausg), Smokie Links, Oscar Mayer - 1.5 oz link | 43 | 130 | 23.9 | 0.7 | 0.7 |  | 0 | 433 | 4 | 7 | 0.90 |  |  | 0 |  |  |  |  |
|  |  | 5.3 | 11.7 | 4.0 | 5.7 | 1.2 | 27 | 77 | 103 | 0.50 | 0.108 |  | 0 |  |  |  |  | 7232 |
| **Smokie** (smkd sausg), turkey, Louis Rich - 2 oz link | 56 | 90 | 38.7 | 1.8 | 1.6 |  | 0 | 530 | 15 | 12 | 1.20 |  | 0 | 0 |  |  |  |  |
|  |  | 8.3 | 5.5 | 1.5 | 2.0 | 1.5 | 37 | 113 | 114 | 0.77 | 0.095 |  | 0 |  |  |  | 3.4 | 7268 |
| **Smokie** (smkd sausg) w/cheese, Oscar Mayer - 1.5 oz link | 43 | 130 | 23.6 | 0.8 | 0.6 |  | 0 | 450 | 19 | 7 | 0.84 |  |  |  |  |  |  |  |
|  |  | 5.5 | 11.7 | 4.4 | 5.6 | 1.2 | 30 | 78 | 124 | 0.46 | 0.086 |  | 69 |  |  |  |  | 7234 |
| **turkey sausage**, hot, smoked 2 oz | 56 | 88 | 38.4 | 2.6 | 1.8 |  | 0.5 | 520 | 12 | 14 | 1.19 |  | 24 | 17 | 0.04 | 2.1 | 0.24 |  |
|  |  | 8.4 | 4.9 | 1.9 | 1.3 | 0.9 | 30 | 110 | 104 | 5.38 | 0.062 | 12.4 | 81 | 0.1 | 0.10 | 0.21 | 4.5 | 7929 |
| **turkey, pork and beef sausage**, lowfat, smoked - 2 oz | 56 | 57 | 42.7 | 6.4 | 0 | 0 | 0.3 | 446 | 6 | 9 | 0.67 |  | 0 | 1 | 0.07 | 0.9 | 0.16 | 0.09 |
|  |  | 4.5 | 1.4 | 0.5 | 0.6 | 0.2 | 12 | 136 | 41 | 1.23 | 0.075 | 13.8 | 0 | 0.1 | 0.04 | 0.06 | 3.4 | 7900 |
| **turkey, pork, and beef sausage**, reduced fat, smoked - 2 oz | 56 | 134 | 33.2 | 1.5 | 0 | 0 | 0 | 536 | 10 | 10 | 1.22 |  | 1 | 0 | 0.10 | 1.8 | 0.25 |  |
|  |  | 10.4 | 9.4 | 3.4 | 3.9 | 1.3 | 36 | 114 | 80 | 0.63 | 0.034 | 15.6 | 1 | 0.1 | 0.08 | 0.15 | 2.2 | 42241 |
| **Vienna sausage**, beef and pork, cnd .6 oz sausage (2" long, ⅞" dia) | 16 | 37 | 10.4 | 0.4 | 0 | 0 | 0 | 155 | 2 | 1 | 0.26 |  | 0 | 0 | 0.01 | 0.3 | 0.16 | 0.06 |
|  |  | 1.7 | 3.1 | 1.1 | 1.5 | 0.2 | 14 | 16 | 8 | 0.14 | 0.005 | 2.7 | 0 | 0 | 0.02 | 0.02 | 0.6 | 7083 |

## 20.2 LUNCH MEATS AND SPREADS

| Food | WT (g) | KCAL / PRO (g) | H₂0 (g) / FAT (g) | CHO (g) / SFA (g) | TSUG (g) / MUFA (g) | ASUG (g) / PUFA (g) | DFIB (g) / CHOL (mg) | Na (mg) / K (mg) | Ca (mg) / P (mg) | Mg (mg) / Fe (mg) | Zn (mg) / Cu (mg) | Mn (mg) / Se (mcg) | A (mcg RAE) / A (IU) | C (mg) / E (mg ATE) | B-1 (mg) / B-2 (mg) | NIA (mg) / B-6 (mg) | B-12 (mcg) / FOL (mcg DFE) | PANT (mg) / REF |
|---|---|---|---|---|---|---|---|---|---|---|---|---|---|---|---|---|---|---|
| **barbeque loaf lunch meat** .8 oz slice | 23 | 40 | 14.9 | 1.5 |  |  | 0 | 307 | 13 | 4 | 0.57 | 0.009 | 1 | 0 | 0.08 | 0.5 | 0.39 | 0.36 |
|  |  | 3.6 | 2.0 | 0.7 | 1.0 | 0.2 | 9 | 76 | 30 | 0.27 | 0.016 | 4.9 | 16 |  | 0.06 | 0.06 | 2.1 | 7001 |
| **beef, chopped, smoked** 1 oz slice | 28 | 37 | 19.3 | 0.5 |  |  | 0 | 352 | 2 | 6 | 1.10 | 0.008 | 0 | 0 | 0.02 | 1.3 | 0.48 | 0.17 |
|  |  | 5.7 | 1.2 | 0.5 | 0.5 | 0.1 | 13 | 106 | 51 | 0.80 | 0.007 | 5.5 | 0 |  | 0.05 | 0.10 | 2.2 | 13358 |
| **beef loaf lunch meat** 1 oz slice | 28 | 86 | 14.7 | 0.8 | 0 | 0 | 0 | 372 | 3 | 4 | 0.71 | 0.013 | 0 | 0 | 0.03 | 1.0 | 1.09 | 0.15 |
|  |  | 4.0 | 7.3 | 3.1 | 3.4 | 0.2 | 18 | 58 | 33 | 0.65 | 0.034 | 6.2 | 0 | 0.1 | 0.06 | 0.05 | 1.4 | 7042 |
| **beef lunch meat, jellied** 1 oz slice | 28 | 31 | 20.9 | 0 |  |  | 0 | 370 | 3 | 5 | 0.99 | 0.015 | 0 |  | 0.04 | 1.4 | 1.44 | 0.19 |
|  |  | 5.3 | 0.9 | 0.4 | 0.4 | 0 | 10 | 113 | 39 | 0.97 | 0.034 | 4.6 | 0 |  | 0.08 | 0.07 | 2.0 | 13353 |
| **beef, smoked**, sliced lunch meat, Carl Buddig - 2 oz | 57 | 79 | 39.6 | 0.3 |  |  | 0 | 816 | 8 |  |  |  |  |  | 0.05 | 2.2 |  |  |
|  |  | 11.0 | 3.7 | 1.5 |  | 0.2 | 38 | 192 |  | 1.29 |  |  |  |  | 0.14 |  |  | 7272 |
| **beef, thin sliced lunch meat** 5 slices (.7 oz) | 21 | 25 | 15.2 | 0.5 | 0 |  | 0 | 235 | 1 | 4 | 0.70 | 0.003 | 0 | 0 | 0.01 | 1.0 | 0.41 | 0.09 |
|  |  | 3.8 | 0.7 | 0.2 | 0.3 | 0 | 10 | 65 | 53 | 0.43 | 0.038 | 3.0 | 0 | 0 | 0.06 | 0.08 | 0.6 | 7043 |
| **beerwurst, pork and beef** 1 oz slice | 28 | 77 | 15.9 | 1.2 | 0 |  | 0.3 | 205 | 8 | 5 | 0.62 | 0.043 | 1 | 0 | 0.07 | 0.8 | 0.32 | 0.08 |
|  |  | 3.9 | 6.3 | 2.4 | 2.8 | 0.6 | 17 | 68 | 38 | 0.48 | 0.029 | 4.9 | 3 |  | 0.05 | 0.06 | 1.4 | 7931 |
| **berliner, pork and beef** .8 oz slice | 23 | 53 | 14.0 | 0.6 | 0.5 |  | 0 | 298 | 3 | 3 | 0.57 | 0.009 | 0 | 0 | 0.09 | 0.7 | 0.61 | 0.16 |
|  |  | 3.5 | 4.0 | 1.4 | 1.8 | 0.4 | 11 | 65 | 30 | 0.26 | 0.018 | 3.2 | 0 |  | 0.05 | 0.05 | 1.2 | 7004 |
| **bologna, beef** 1 oz slice | 28 | 87 | 15.2 | 1.1 | 0 | 0 | 0 | 302 | 9 | 4 | 2.55 | 0.012 | 4 | 4 | 0.01 | 0.7 | 0.36 | 0.11 |
|  |  | 2.9 | 7.9 | 3.1 | 3.4 | 0.2 | 16 | 48 | 48 | 0.31 | 0.019 | 0 | 20 | 0.1 | 0.03 | 0.05 | 2.5 | 7007 |
| **bologna, beef and pork** 1 oz slice | 28 | 86 | 14.5 | 1.5 | 1.2 | 1.2 | 0 | 206 | 24 | 5 | 0.64 | 0.005 | 7 | 0 | 0.06 | 0.7 | 0.51 | 0.12 |
|  |  | 4.3 | 6.9 | 2.6 | 2.9 | 0.3 | 17 | 88 | 46 | 0.34 | 0.015 | 6.9 | 24 | 0 | 0.05 | 0.08 | 1.7 | 7008 |
| **bologna, beef, light, Oscar Mayer** 1 oz slice | 28 | 56 | 18.2 | 1.6 | 0.6 |  | 0 | 322 | 4 | 4 | 0.53 |  | 0 |  |  |  |  |  |
|  |  | 3.3 | 4.1 | 1.6 | 2.0 | 0.1 | 12 | 44 | 50 | 0.34 | 0.059 |  | 0 |  |  |  | 3.6 | 7202 |
| **bologna, beef, Oscar Mayer** 1 oz slice | 28 | 88 | 15.2 | 0.7 | 0.4 |  | 0 | 330 | 3 | 4 | 0.57 |  | 0 | 0 | 0.01 | 0.7 | 0.40 | 0.08 |
|  |  | 3.1 | 8.1 | 3.6 | 4.3 | 0.3 | 18 | 47 | 31 | 0.38 | 0.031 |  | 0 |  | 0.03 | 0.05 | 3.6 | 7201 |
| **bologna, chicken, pork, and beef,** Oscar Mayer - 1 oz slice | 28 | 89 | 15.0 | 0.7 | 0.4 |  | 0 | 289 | 19 | 6 | 0.40 |  | 0 | 0 |  |  |  |  |
|  |  | 3.1 | 8.2 | 2.9 | 4.1 | 1.1 | 29 | 43 | 56 | 0.50 | 0.056 |  | 0 |  |  |  |  | 7200 |
| **bologna, fat-free, Oscar Mayer** 1 oz slice | 28 | 22 | 21.8 | 1.7 | 0.6 |  | 0 | 274 | 4 | 6 | 0.32 |  | 0 | 0 |  |  |  |  |
|  |  | 3.5 | 0.2 | 0.1 | 0.1 | 0 | 7 | 44 | 43 | 0.26 | 0.056 |  | 0 |  |  |  |  | 7203 |
| **bologna, pork** 1 oz slice | 28 | 69 | 17.0 | 0.2 | 0 |  | 0 | 332 | 3 | 4 | 0.57 |  | 0 | 0 | 0.15 | 1.1 | 0.26 | 0.20 |
|  |  | 4.3 | 5.6 | 1.9 | 2.7 | 0.6 | 17 | 79 | 39 | 0.22 | 0.022 | 3.6 | 0 | 0.1 | 0.04 | 0.08 | 1.4 | 7010 |
| **bologna, pork and turkey, lite** 1 oz slice | 28 | 59 | 18.2 | 1.0 | 0 |  | 0 | 200 | 13 | 5 | 0.20 | 0.043 | 0 | 0 | 0.04 | 0.9 | 0.08 | 0.10 |
|  |  | 3.7 | 4.5 | 1.5 | 2.1 | 0.9 | 22 | 39 | 26 | 0.32 | 0.023 | 1.6 | 1 |  | 0.03 | 0.05 | 5.0 | 7936 |
| **bologna, pork, chicken, and beef,** light, Oscar Mayer - 1 oz slice | 28 | 57 | 18.1 | 1.6 | 0.7 |  | 0 | 313 | 14 | 6 | 0.45 | 0.043 | 0 | 0 | 0.04 | 0.9 | 0.08 | 0.10 |
|  |  | 3.2 | 4.1 | 1.6 | 2.0 | 0.4 | 16 | 46 | 52 | 0.39 | 0.056 | 1.6 | 0 |  | 0.03 | 0.05 | 5.0 | 7205 |
| **bologna, pork, turkey, beef** 1 oz slice | 28 | 94 | 12.7 | 1.9 | 0.4 |  | 0 | 295 | 9 | 4 | 0.62 | 0.074 | 0 | 3 | 0.04 | 0.9 | 0.30 | 0.10 |
|  |  | 3.2 | 8.2 | 3.3 | 3.6 | 0.7 | 21 | 62 | 36 | 0.34 | 0.026 | 3.5 | 0 | 0 | 0.04 | 0.11 | 1.1 | 7937 |
| **bologna, turkey** 1 oz slice | 28 | 59 | 18.1 | 1.3 | 0.8 | 0 | 0.1 | 351 | 34 | 4 | 0.36 | 0.014 | 3 | 4 | 0.01 | 0.7 | 0.06 | 0.13 |
|  |  | 3.2 | 4.5 | 1.2 | 1.9 | 1.1 | 21 | 38 | 32 | 0.84 | 0.020 | 4.3 | 9 | 0.1 | 0.03 | 0.07 | 2.5 | 7011 |
| **bologna, turkey, Louis Rich** 1 oz slice | 28 | 52 | 18.9 | 1.4 | 0.3 |  | 0 | 302 | 35 | 6 | 0.52 |  | 0 | 0 |  |  |  |  |
|  |  | 3.2 | 3.7 | 1.1 | 1.5 | 1.0 | 19 | 43 | 55 | 0.46 | 0.050 |  | 0 |  |  |  | 1.7 | 7255 |
| **bologna, Wisconsin ring, Oscar Mayer** - 1 oz slice | 28 | 88 | 15.3 | 0.7 | 0.6 |  | 0 | 232 | 4 | 4 | 0.52 | 0.014 | 0 | 0 | 0.08 | 0.7 | 0.35 |  |
|  |  | 3.3 | 8.0 | 3.1 | 3.9 | 0.6 | 17 | 39 | 30 | 0.32 | 0.036 |  | 0 |  | 0.04 | 0.04 |  | 7206 |
| **braunschweiger** (pork liver sausage) .6 oz slice (2½" dia, ¼" thick) | 18 | 59 | 9.1 | 0.6 | 0 | 0 | 0 | 209 | 2 | 2 | 0.51 | 0.028 | 760 | 0 | 0.04 | 1.5 | 3.62 | 0.61 |
|  |  | 2.6 | 5.1 | 1.7 | 2.3 | 0.6 | 32 | 36 | 30 | 2.02 | 0.043 | 10.4 | 2529 | 0.1 | 0.27 | 0.06 | 7.9 | 7014 |

| | WT (g) | KCAL / PRO (g) | H₂0 (g) / FAT (g) | CHO (g) / SFA (g) | TSUG (g) / MUFA (g) | ASUG (g) / PUFA (g) | DFIB (g) / CHOL (mg) | Na (mg) / K (mg) | Ca (mg) / P (mg) | Mg (mg) / Fe (mg) | Zn (mg) / Cu (mg) | Mn (mg) / Se (mcg) | A (mcg RAE) / A (IU) | C (mg) / E (mg ATE) | B-1 (mg) / B-2 (mg) | NIA (mg) / B-6 (mg) | B-12 (mcg) / FOL (mcg DFE) | PANT (mg) / REF |
|---|---|---|---|---|---|---|---|---|---|---|---|---|---|---|---|---|---|---|
| braunschweiger (pork liver sausage), saren tube, Oscar Mayer - 2 oz | 56 | 191 | 27.8 | 1.3 | 0.4 | | 0.1 | 626 | 5 | 7 | 1.77 | 0.050 | | 5 | 0.13 | 4.6 | 10.37 | 1.61 |
| | | 8.0 | 17.1 | 6.1 | 8.7 | 2.1 | 90 | 103 | 109 | 5.45 | 0.224 | | 9335 | | 0.87 | 0.19 | 34.2 | 7208 |
| braunschweiger (pork liver sausage), sliced, Oscar Mayer - 1 oz | 28 | 93 | 14.1 | 0.7 | 0.3 | | 0.1 | 325 | 3 | 4 | 0.95 | 0.041 | 1322 | 3 | 0.06 | 2.6 | 5.26 | 0.97 |
| | | 4.0 | 8.2 | 3.1 | 4.3 | 1.0 | 50 | 57 | 56 | 2.94 | 0.140 | 4404 | | 0.45 | 0.09 | 13.2 | 7207 |
| chicken breast, baked/grilled, Louis Rich - 2 slices (1.6 oz) | 45 | 44 | 32.8 | 1.7 | 0.3 | | 0 | 514 | 4 | 14 | 0.40 | | | 0 | | | | |
| | | 8.9 | 0.2 | 0.1 | 0.1 | 0 | 23 | 131 | 127 | 0.58 | 0.108 | | 0 | | | | | 7249 |
| chicken breast, fat-free, mesquite flavor, sliced - 2 slices | 42 | 34 | 32.2 | 0.9 | 0.1 | | 0 | 437 | 2 | 15 | 0.25 | 0.014 | 0 | 0 | 0.01 | 1.2 | 0.03 | 0.08 |
| | | 7.1 | 0.2 | 0.1 | 0.1 | 0 | 15 | 133 | 108 | 0.13 | 0.097 | 2.6 | 0 | | 0.01 | 0.05 | 0.4 | 7932 |
| chicken breast, fat-free, oven-roasted, sliced - 2 slices | 42 | 33 | 32.2 | 0.9 | 0 | | 0 | 457 | 3 | 4 | 0.13 | 0.018 | 0 | 0 | 0.01 | 1.4 | 0.04 | 0.10 |
| | | 7.1 | 0.2 | 0.1 | 0.1 | 0 | 15 | 28 | 25 | 0.13 | 0.014 | 3.2 | 0 | | 0.01 | 0.06 | 0.4 | 7933 |
| chicken breast, honey glazed, Oscar Mayer - 4 slices (1.8 oz) | 52 | 57 | 36.6 | 2.1 | 2.2 | | 0 | 748 | 5 | 19 | 0.36 | | 0 | 0 | | | | |
| | | 10.3 | 0.8 | 0.2 | 0.3 | 0.1 | 28 | 171 | 150 | 0.59 | 0.088 | | 0 | | | | 2.1 | 7209 |
| chicken breast, roasted, fat-free, Oscar Mayer - 4 slices (1.8 oz) | 52 | 44 | 39.4 | 0.9 | 0.5 | | 0 | 646 | 6 | 19 | 0.31 | | | 0 | | | | |
| | | 9.5 | 0.3 | 0.1 | 0.1 | 0 | 23 | 164 | 133 | 0.69 | 0.120 | | 0 | | | | | 7210 |
| chicken breast, roasted, Louis Rich - 1 oz | 28 | 28 | 20.6 | 0.7 | 0.4 | | 0 | 333 | 2 | 7 | 0.20 | | | 0 | | | | |
| | | 5.1 | 0.6 | 0.2 | 0.2 | 0.1 | 14 | 74 | 74 | 0.32 | 0.064 | | 0 | | | | | 7250 |
| chicken breast roll, oven-roasted - 2 oz | 56 | 75 | 40.9 | 1.0 | 0.2 | | 0 | 494 | 3 | 10 | 0.36 | 0.010 | 0 | 0 | 0.02 | 3.7 | 0.13 | 0.32 |
| | | 8.2 | 4.3 | 1.4 | 1.6 | 0.8 | 22 | 181 | 68 | 0.18 | 0.039 | 6.6 | 0 | 0 | 0.03 | 0.17 | 1.7 | 7935 |
| chicken, light and dark, smoked, Carl Buddig - 2 oz | 57 | 94 | 38.9 | 0.4 | | | 0 | 544 | 71 | | | | | | 0.04 | 3.8 | | |
| | | 10.2 | 5.8 | 1.5 | | 1.2 | 30 | 146 | | 0.89 | | | | | 0.14 | | | 7271 |
| chicken roll, light meat 2 slices (2 oz) | 57 | 63 | 41.3 | 2.7 | 0.3 | 0 | 0 | 604 | 9 | 14 | 0.34 | 0.010 | 14 | 0 | 0.02 | 4.6 | 0.21 | 0.63 |
| | | 9.5 | 1.6 | 0.4 | 0.5 | 0.2 | 26 | 250 | 169 | 0.23 | 0.050 | 8.3 | 47 | 0.2 | 0.09 | 0.21 | 3.4 | 7017 |
| chicken spread, canned 1 oz | 28 | 44 | 16.1 | 1.1 | 0.1 | | 0.1 | 202 | 4 | 3 | 0.32 | 0.003 | 8 | 0 | | 0.8 | 0.04 | 0.12 |
| | | 5.0 | 4.9 | 0.9 | 1.3 | 0.7 | 16 | 30 | 25 | 0.24 | 0.011 | 3.0 | 28 | | 0.03 | 0.04 | 0.8 | 7018 |
| chicken, white, roasted, Louis Rich - 1 oz | 28 | 36 | 20.0 | 0.6 | 0.3 | | 0 | 335 | 5 | 7 | 0.32 | | | 0 | | | | |
| | | 4.8 | 1.6 | 0.4 | 0.7 | 0.3 | 17 | 85 | 69 | 0.44 | 0.064 | | 0 | | | | | 7251 |
| chicken/turkey salad spread 1 oz (~2T) | 28 | 56 | 18.5 | 2.1 | 0 | 0 | 0 | 106 | 3 | 3 | 0.29 | 0.003 | 12 | 0 | 0.01 | 0.5 | 0.11 | 0.08 |
| | | 3.3 | 3.8 | 1.0 | 0.9 | 1.7 | 8 | 51 | 9 | 0.17 | 0.008 | 3.1 | 39 | 0.6 | 0.02 | 0.03 | 1.4 | 7067 |
| corned beef, canned .7 oz slice | 21 | 52 | 12.1 | 0 | 0 | | 0 | 211 | 3 | 3 | 0.75 | 0.003 | 0 | 0 | 0 | 0.5 | 0.34 | 0.13 |
| | | 5.7 | 3.1 | 1.3 | 1.3 | 0.1 | 18 | 29 | 23 | 0.44 | 0.013 | 9.0 | 0 | 0 | 0.03 | 0.03 | 1.9 | 13348 |
| corned beef, chopped, pressed, Carl Buddig) - 2 oz | 57 | 81 | 39.4 | 0.6 | | | 0 | 765 | 10 | | | | | | 0.05 | 2.4 | | |
| | | 11.0 | 3.9 | 1.6 | | 0.2 | 37 | 201 | | 1.37 | | | | | 0.14 | | | 7270 |
| corned beef, jellied loaf 1 oz slice | 28 | 43 | 19.3 | 0 | | | 0 | 267 | 3 | 3 | 1.15 | 0.009 | 0 | 0 | 0 | 0.5 | 0.36 | 0.05 |
| | | 6.4 | 1.7 | 0.7 | 0.8 | 0.1 | 13 | 28 | 20 | 0.57 | 0.017 | 4.8 | 0 | 0 | 0.03 | 0.03 | 2.2 | 7020 |
| ham and cheese loaf 1 oz slice | 28 | 67 | 16.9 | 1.1 | 0 | 0 | 0 | 302 | 16 | 4 | 0.56 | | 0 | 0 | 0.17 | 1.0 | 0.23 | 0.15 |
| | | 3.8 | 5.2 | 2.0 | 2.4 | 0.6 | 16 | 82 | 71 | 0.25 | 0.022 | 9.7 | 0 | 0.1 | 0.05 | 0.07 | 0.8 | 7032 |
| ham and cheese loaf, Oscar Mayer - 1 oz slice | 28 | 66 | 16.9 | 1.0 | 0.9 | | 0 | 327 | 19 | 5 | 0.51 | 0.005 | 0 | 0 | 0.16 | 1.0 | 0.21 | 0.12 |
| | | 3.9 | 5.1 | 1.8 | 2.3 | 0.5 | 17 | 74 | 76 | 0.24 | 0.034 | | 0 | | 0.05 | 0.07 | 0.8 | 7211 |
| ham and cheese spread 1 oz (about 2 T) | 28 | 69 | 16.6 | 0.6 | | | 0 | 335 | 61 | 5 | 0.63 | 0.010 | 25 | 0 | 0.09 | 0.6 | 0.20 | 0.17 |
| | | 4.5 | 5.2 | 2.4 | 2.0 | 0.4 | 17 | 45 | 139 | 0.21 | 0.025 | 9.4 | 85 | | 0.06 | 0.04 | 0.8 | 7033 |
| ham, baked, 96% fat free, water added, Oscar Mayer - .7 oz slice | 21 | 22 | 15.6 | 0.4 | 0.2 | | 0 | 261 | 2 | 7 | 0.38 | | 0 | 0 | | | | |
| | | 3.4 | 0.7 | 0.2 | 0.2 | 0.3 | 10 | 56 | 49 | 0.27 | 0.050 | | 0 | | | | 0.8 | 7213 |
| ham, boiled, water added, Oscar Mayer - .7 oz slice | 21 | 22 | 15.7 | 0.3 | 0.1 | | 0 | 283 | 2 | 7 | 0.39 | | | 0 | | | | |
| | | 3.5 | 0.8 | 0.3 | 0.4 | 0.1 | 10 | 59 | 50 | 0.31 | 0.050 | | 0 | | | | | 7214 |
| ham, chopped, canned .7 oz slice | 21 | 50 | 12.8 | 0.1 | 0 | | 0 | 287 | 1 | 3 | 0.38 | 0.005 | 0 | 0 | 0.11 | 0.7 | 0.15 | 0.06 |
| | | 3.4 | 4.0 | 1.3 | 1.9 | 0.4 | 10 | 60 | 29 | 0.20 | 0.010 | 3.9 | 0 | 0.1 | 0.03 | 0.07 | 0.2 | 7026 |
| ham, chopped, Oscar Mayer 1 oz | 28 | 50 | 18.3 | 1.0 | 0.6 | | 0 | 350 | 3 | 6 | 0.63 | | 0 | 0 | | | | |
| | | 4.6 | 3.1 | 1.1 | 1.6 | 0.4 | 17 | 73 | 61 | 0.36 | 0.067 | | 0 | | | | 0.8 | 7212 |
| ham, chopped, packaged 1 oz slice | 28 | 50 | 18.3 | 1.2 | 0 | 0 | 0 | 372 | 2 | 4 | 0.54 | | 0 | 0 | 0.18 | 1.1 | 0.26 | |
| | | 4.6 | 2.9 | 1.0 | 1.4 | 0.4 | 17 | 89 | 43 | 0.23 | 0.017 | 4.9 | 0 | 0.1 | 0.06 | 0.10 | 0.3 | 7027 |
| ham, honey, water added, Oscar Mayer - .7 oz slice | 21 | 23 | 15.3 | 0.7 | 0.7 | | 0 | 262 | 2 | 7 | 0.44 | | | 0 | | | | |
| | | 3.5 | 0.7 | 0.2 | 0.4 | 0.1 | 9 | 59 | 54 | 0.28 | 0.048 | | 0 | | | | | 7215 |
| ham, minced .7 oz slice | 21 | 55 | 12.0 | 0.4 | 0 | | 0 | 261 | 2 | 3 | 0.40 | 0.007 | 0 | 0 | 0.15 | 0.9 | 0.20 | 0.04 |
| | | 3.4 | 4.3 | 1.5 | 2.0 | 0.5 | 15 | 65 | 33 | 0.17 | 0.017 | 4.2 | 0 | 0.1 | 0.04 | 0.05 | 0.2 | 7030 |
| ham salad spread 1 oz (about 2 T) | 28 | 60 | 17.5 | 3.0 | 0 | 0 | 0 | 255 | 2 | 3 | 0.31 | 0.004 | 0 | 0 | 0.12 | 0.6 | 0.21 | 0.09 |
| | | 2.4 | 4.3 | 1.4 | 2.0 | 0.8 | 10 | 42 | 34 | 0.17 | 0.020 | 5.0 | 0 | 0.5 | 0.03 | 0.04 | 0.3 | 7031 |
| ham, sliced, lean (5% fat) 1 oz slice | 28 | 30 | 20.7 | 0.2 | 0 | 0 | 0 | 297 | 2 | 6 | 0.52 | 0.006 | 0 | 0 | 0.09 | 1.6 | 0.10 | 0.20 |
| | | 5.3 | 0.7 | 0.2 | 0.3 | 0.1 | 13 | 182 | 81 | 0.20 | 0.136 | 8.8 | 0 | 0.1 | 0.07 | 0.11 | 0 | 7028 |
| ham, sliced, regular (11% fat) 1 oz slice | 28 | 46 | 18.8 | 1.1 | 0 | | 0.4 | 365 | 7 | 6 | 0.38 | 0.156 | 0 | 0 | 0.18 | 0.8 | 0.12 | 0.12 |
| | | 4.6 | 2.4 | 0.8 | 1.2 | 0.2 | 16 | 80 | 43 | 0.29 | 0.025 | 5.8 | 0 | 1 | 0.05 | 0.09 | 2.0 | 7029 |
| ham, smoked, fat free, 40% water, Oscar Mayer - 3 slices (1.7 oz) | 47 | 34 | 37.2 | 0.9 | 0.5 | | 0 | 509 | 5 | 13 | 0.74 | | | 0 | | | | |
| | | 6.9 | 0.3 | 0.1 | 0.1 | 0.1 | 18 | 110 | 93 | 0.43 | 0.094 | | 0 | | | | | 7217 |

| | WT (g) | KCAL | H2O (g) | CHO (g) | TSUG (g) | ASUG (g) | DFIB (g) | Na (mg) | Ca (mg) | Mg (mg) | Zn (mg) | Mn (mg) | A (mcg RAE) | C (mg) | B-1 (mg) | NIA (mg) | B-12 (mcg) | PANT (mg) |
|---|---|---|---|---|---|---|---|---|---|---|---|---|---|---|---|---|---|---|
| | | PRO (g) | FAT (g) | SFA (g) | MUFA (g) | PUFA (g) | CHOL (mg) | K (mg) | P (mg) | Fe (mg) | Cu (mg) | Se (mcg) | A (IU) | E (mg ATE) | B-2 (mg) | B-6 (mg) | FOL (mcg DFE) | REF |
| **ham**, smoked, sliced, Carl Buddig | 57 | 93 | 38.2 | 0.6 | | | 0 | 787 | 9 | | | | | | 0.43 | 2.9 | | |
| *2 oz* | | 10.5 | 5.3 | 1.8 | | 0.6 | 31 | 194 | | 1.16 | | | | | 0.20 | | | 7275 |
| **ham**, smoked, water added, | 21 | 21 | 15.9 | 0 | 0 | | 0 | 255 | 2 | 7 | 0.38 | | | 0 | | | | |
| *Oscar Mayer - .7 oz slice* | | 3.5 | 0.8 | 0.3 | 0.4 | 0.1 | 10 | 56 | 49 | 0.27 | 0.050 | | 0 | | | | | 7216 |
| **headcheese**, pork | 28 | 44 | 20.7 | 0 | 0 | | 0 | 232 | 4 | 3 | 0.27 | | 0 | 0 | 0.01 | 0.1 | 0.29 | |
| *1 oz slice* | | 3.9 | 3.1 | 1.0 | 1.6 | 0.3 | 19 | 9 | 16 | 0.42 | 0.034 | 0 | 0 | 0.1 | 0.03 | 0.05 | 0.6 | 7034 |
| **headcheese**, pork, Oscar Mayer | 28 | 52 | 18.9 | 0 | 0 | | 0 | 300 | 6 | 3 | 0.33 | | | 0 | 0.01 | 0.3 | 0.27 | 0.06 |
| *1 oz slice* | | 4.4 | 3.8 | 1.2 | 1.9 | 0.4 | 25 | 8 | 18 | 0.46 | 0.056 | | 28 | | 0.05 | 0.04 | 0.3 | 7218 |
| **honey loaf**, pork and beef | 28 | 35 | 19.7 | 2.8 | 0 | 0 | 0.2 | 370 | 5 | 5 | 0.68 | 0.008 | 1 | 0 | 0.13 | 0.9 | 0.30 | 0.18 |
| *1 oz slice* | | 3.1 | 1.3 | 0.4 | 0.6 | 0.1 | 10 | 96 | 40 | 0.38 | 0.017 | 7.9 | 3 | 0 | 0.07 | 0.09 | 2.2 | 7035 |
| **honey roll sausage**, beef | 23 | 42 | 14.9 | 0.5 | | | 0 | 304 | 2 | 4 | 0.75 | 0.009 | 0 | 0 | 0.02 | 1.0 | 0.54 | 0.11 |
| *.8 oz slice* | | 4.3 | 2.4 | 0.9 | 1.1 | 0.1 | 12 | 67 | 32 | 0.51 | 0.023 | 3.6 | 0 | | 0.04 | 0.06 | 0.9 | 7088 |
| **Lebanon bologna**, beef | 23 | 40 | 15.1 | 0.1 | 0 | | 0 | 316 | 5 | 5 | 0.88 | 0.005 | 3 | 0 | 0.02 | 0.7 | 0.67 | 0.07 |
| *.8 oz slice* | | 4.4 | 2.4 | 0.6 | 1.0 | 0.1 | 13 | 76 | 44 | 0.49 | 0.017 | 3.6 | 9 | 0.1 | 0.04 | 0.09 | 1.4 | 7039 |
| **liver cheese**, pork | 38 | 116 | 20.4 | 0.8 | | | 0 | 466 | 3 | 5 | 1.41 | 0.076 | 1996 | 1 | 0.08 | 4.5 | 9.33 | 1.34 |
| *1.3 oz slice* | | 5.8 | 9.7 | 3.4 | 4.7 | 1.3 | 66 | 86 | 79 | 4.12 | 0.146 | 13.9 | 6646 | | 0.85 | 0.18 | 39.5 | 7040 |
| **liver cheese**, pork, Oscar Mayer | 38 | 119 | 19.8 | 1.0 | 0.5 | | 0 | 420 | 3 | 6 | 1.46 | 0.074 | 2711 | 1 | 0.08 | 4.6 | 9.23 | 1.42 |
| *1.3 oz slice* | | 5.8 | 10.0 | 3.5 | 5.0 | 1.6 | 80 | 81 | 89 | 4.52 | 0.222 | | 9036 | | 0.84 | 0.17 | 42.9 | 7220 |
| **liver pate**, canned | 28 | 89 | 15.1 | 0.4 | | | 0 | 195 | 20 | 4 | 0.80 | 0.034 | 277 | 1 | 0.01 | 0.9 | 0.90 | 0.34 |
| *1 oz (~2 T)* | | 4.0 | 7.8 | 2.7 | 3.5 | 0.9 | 71 | 39 | 56 | 1.54 | 0.112 | 11.6 | 924 | | 0.17 | 0.02 | 16.8 | 7055 |
| **liver pate**, chicken, canned | 28 | 56 | 18.4 | 1.8 | 0 | 0 | 0 | 108 | 3 | 4 | 0.60 | 0.045 | 61 | 3 | 0.01 | 2.1 | 2.26 | 0.73 |
| *1 oz (2 T)* | | 3.8 | 3.7 | 1.1 | 1.5 | 0.7 | 109 | 27 | 49 | 2.57 | 0.050 | 12.9 | 203 | 0.3 | 0.39 | 0.07 | 89.9 | 7053 |
| **liver pate**, goose, smoked, canned | 28 | 129 | 10.4 | 1.3 | | | 0 | 195 | 20 | 4 | 0.26 | 0.034 | 280 | 0 | 0.02 | 0.7 | 2.63 | 0.34 |
| *1 oz (~2 T)* | | 3.2 | 12.3 | 4.0 | 7.2 | 0.2 | 42 | 39 | 56 | 1.54 | 0.112 | 12.3 | 933 | | 0.08 | 0.02 | 16.8 | 7054 |
| **liver pate**, truffle flavor | 56 | 183 | 29.0 | 3.5 | | | | 452 | 39 | 7 | 1.60 | 0.067 | 2523 | 1 | 0.02 | 1.8 | 1.79 | 0.67 |
| *2 oz* | | 6.3 | 16.0 | 5.7 | 7.6 | 1.9 | 59 | 77 | 112 | 2.21 | 0.224 | 23.3 | 8400 | | 0.34 | 0.03 | 33.6 | 7942 |
| **liverwurst**, pork | 28 | 91 | 14.6 | 0.6 | | | 0 | 241 | 7 | 3 | 0.64 | 0.043 | 2326 | 0 | 0.08 | 1.2 | 3.77 | 0.83 |
| *1 oz* | | 3.9 | 8.0 | 3.0 | 3.7 | 0.7 | 44 | 48 | 64 | 1.79 | 0.067 | 16.2 | 7747 | | 0.29 | 0.05 | 8.4 | 7041 |
| **liverwurst spread** | 55 | 168 | 29.4 | 3.2 | 0.9 | | 1.4 | 385 | 12 | 7 | 1.26 | 0.085 | 2250 | 2 | 0.15 | 2.4 | 7.40 | 1.62 |
| *4 T* | | 6.8 | 14.0 | 5.5 | 6.8 | 1.3 | 65 | 94 | 127 | 4.87 | 0.132 | 31.9 | 7500 | | 0.57 | 0.10 | 16.5 | 7911 |
| **luncheon loaf**, spiced, | 28 | 66 | 16.4 | 2.0 | 1.3 | | 0 | 343 | 31 | 7 | 0.55 | | | 0 | | | | |
| *Oscar Mayer - 1 oz slice* | | 3.8 | 4.7 | 1.5 | 2.1 | 0.8 | 19 | 76 | 55 | 0.38 | 0.647 | | 0 | | | | | 7221 |
| **luxury loaf**, pork | 28 | 39 | 19.1 | 1.4 | | | 0 | 343 | 10 | 6 | 0.85 | 0.011 | 0 | 0 | 0.20 | 1.0 | 0.38 | 0.14 |
| *1 oz slice* | | 5.2 | 1.3 | 0.4 | 0.7 | 0.1 | 10 | 106 | 52 | 0.29 | 0.028 | 6.0 | 0 | | 0.08 | 0.09 | 0.6 | 7060 |
| **macaroni and cheese loaf**, chicken, | 38 | 87 | 21.9 | 4.4 | 0 | | 0 | 1 | 46 | 10 | 0.57 | 0.105 | 0 | 6 | 0.09 | 1.1 | 0.26 | 0.20 |
| pork, and beef - *1 slice* | | 4.5 | 5.7 | 2.1 | 2.9 | 0.6 | 17 | 119 | 66 | 0.46 | 0.042 | 8.7 | 0 | | 0.09 | 0.13 | 12.5 | 7940 |
| **mortadella**, beef and pork | 15 | 47 | 7.8 | 0.5 | 0 | 0 | 0 | 187 | 3 | 2 | 0.32 | 0.004 | 0 | 0 | 0.02 | 0.4 | 0.22 | 0.07 |
| *.5 oz slice* | | 2.5 | 3.8 | 1.4 | 1.7 | 0.5 | 8 | 24 | 15 | 0.21 | 0.009 | 3.4 | 0 | | 0.02 | 0.02 | 0.4 | 7050 |
| **mother's loaf**, pork | 21 | 59 | 11.5 | 1.6 | | | 0 | 237 | 9 | 3 | 0.30 | 0.014 | 0 | 0 | 0.12 | 0.7 | 0.22 | 0.10 |
| *.7 oz slice* | | 2.5 | 4.7 | 1.7 | 2.2 | 0.5 | 9 | 47 | 27 | 0.28 | 0.019 | 7.4 | 0 | | 0.04 | 0.04 | 1.7 | 7061 |
| **old fashioned loaf**, Oscar Mayer | 28 | 65 | 16.5 | 2.2 | 1.3 | | 0 | 332 | 32 | 6 | 0.52 | | | 0 | | | | |
| *1 oz slice* | | 3.7 | 4.6 | 1.6 | 2.2 | 0.7 | 17 | 82 | 58 | 0.37 | 0.039 | | 0 | | | | | 7222 |
| **olive loaf**, chicken, pork, and turkey, | 28 | 74 | 16.1 | 1.9 | 0.9 | | 0 | 369 | 31 | 8 | 0.29 | | | 0 | | | | |
| *Oscar Mayer - 1 oz slice* | | 2.8 | 6.1 | 2.0 | 3.1 | 0.7 | 20 | 52 | 37 | 0.49 | 0.062 | | 0 | | | | | 7223 |
| **olive loaf**, pork | 28 | 66 | 16.3 | 2.6 | 0 | 0 | 0 | 416 | 31 | 5 | 0.39 | 0.010 | 17 | 0 | 0.08 | 0.5 | 0.35 | 0.22 |
| *1 oz slice* | | 3.3 | 4.6 | 1.6 | 2.2 | 0.5 | 11 | 83 | 36 | 0.15 | 0.014 | 4.6 | 56 | 0.1 | 0.07 | 0.06 | 0.6 | 7051 |
| **pastrami**, beef | 28 | 41 | 19.5 | 0 | 0 | | 0 | 248 | 3 | 5 | 1.39 | 0.008 | 1 | 0 | 0.01 | 1.2 | 0.52 | 0.07 |
| *1 oz slice* | | 6.1 | 1.6 | 0.8 | 0.6 | 0 | 19 | 59 | 49 | 0.62 | 0.025 | 5.0 | 12 | 0 | 0.05 | 0.06 | 1.7 | 13355 |
| **pastrami**, beef, 98% fat-free | 57 | 54 | 42.4 | 0.9 | 0 | | 0 | 576 | 5 | 10 | 2.43 | 0.007 | 0 | 20 | 0.05 | 2.9 | 1.00 | 0.17 |
| *6 slices* | | 11.2 | 0.7 | 0 | 0.3 | 0 | 27 | 130 | 85 | 1.58 | 0.045 | 5.9 | 0 | | 0.10 | 0.10 | 4.0 | 7925 |
| **pastrami**, beef, smoked, | 57 | 80 | 39.8 | 0.6 | | | 0 | 602 | 10 | | | | | | 0.05 | 2.3 | | |
| Carl Buddig - *2 oz* | | 11.2 | 3.7 | 1.7 | | 0.2 | 37 | 208 | | 1.40 | | | | | 0.13 | | | 7274 |
| **pastrami**, Healthy Choice | 52 | 60 | | 2.0 | 0 | | 0 | 450 | 0 | | | | | 0 | | | | |
| *4 slices* | | 10.0 | 1.5 | 0.5 | | | 25 | | | 0.72 | | | 0 | | | | | HLCH14 |
| **pastrami**, turkey | 57 | 76 | 40.9 | 1.9 | 1.9 | 0 | 0.1 | 559 | 6 | 8 | 1.23 | 0.007 | 2 | 5 | 0.03 | 2.0 | 0.14 | 0.33 |
| *2 slices* | | 9.3 | 3.5 | 1.0 | 1.2 | 0.9 | 39 | 197 | 114 | 2.39 | 0.028 | 9.2 | 14 | 0.1 | 0.14 | 0.15 | 2.8 | 7052 |
| **peppered loaf**, pork and beef | 28 | 42 | 18.9 | 1.3 | 1.3 | | 0 | 426 | 15 | 6 | 0.90 | 0.017 | 0 | 0 | 0.11 | 0.9 | 0.55 | 0.15 |
| *1 oz slice* | | 4.8 | 1.8 | 0.6 | 0.8 | 0.1 | 13 | 110 | 48 | 0.30 | 0.034 | 3.2 | 0 | 0.1 | 0.08 | 0.08 | 0.6 | 7056 |
| **pepperoni**, pork and beef | 6 | 30 | 1.8 | 0 | 0 | 0 | 0 | 99 | 1 | 1 | 0.15 | 0.036 | 0 | 0 | 0.02 | 0.3 | 0.10 | 0.07 |
| *.2 oz slice (1⅜" dia, ⅛" thick)* | | 1.4 | 2.6 | 0.9 | 1.0 | 0.2 | 6 | 17 | 11 | 0.10 | 0.007 | 2.1 | 0 | 0 | 0.02 | 0.02 | 0.3 | 7057 |
| **pepperoni**, turkey, Hormel | 30 | 73 | 14.4 | 1.1 | 0 | | 0 | 557 | 8 | 12 | 1.29 | | 4 | 0 | | | | |
| Pillow Pak *~1 oz* | | 9.3 | 3.5 | 1.1 | 1.5 | 1.0 | 37 | 135 | | 0.81 | 0.060 | | 15 | | | | 1.2 | 7278 |

| | WT (g) | KCAL / PRO (g) | H₂0 (g) / FAT (g) | CHO (g) / SFA (g) | TSUG (g) / MUFA (g) | ASUG (g) / PUFA (g) | DFIB (g) / CHOL (mg) | Na (mg) / K (mg) | Ca (mg) / P (mg) | Mg (mg) / Fe (mg) | Zn (mg) / Cu (mg) | Mn (mg) / Se (mcg) | A (mcg RAE) / A (IU) | C (mg) / E (mg ATE) | B-1 (mg) / B-2 (mg) | NIA (mg) / B-6 (mg) | B-12 (mcg) / FOL (mcg DFE) | PANT (mg) / REF |
|---|---|---|---|---|---|---|---|---|---|---|---|---|---|---|---|---|---|---|
| **pickle and pimento loaf**, chicken, Oscar Mayer - *1 oz slice* | 28 | 75 | 15.6 | 2.5 | 1.9 | | 0 | 357 | 31 | 8 | 0.33 | | | 0 | | | | |
| | | 2.7 | 6.0 | 2.0 | 2.9 | 0.8 | 22 | 49 | 42 | 0.61 | 0.078 | | 0 | | | | | 7224 |
| **pickle and pimento loaf**, pork *1 oz slice* | 28 | 63 | 16.9 | 2.4 | 2.4 | 0.9 | 0.4 | 365 | 31 | 10 | 0.47 | 0.031 | 22 | 2 | 0.11 | 0.7 | 0.15 | 0.12 |
| | | 3.1 | 4.5 | 1.5 | 2.0 | 0.8 | 16 | 104 | 43 | 0.37 | 0.029 | 2.2 | 73 | 0.1 | 0.03 | 0.12 | 10.4 | 7058 |
| **picnic loaf**, pork and beef *1 oz slice* | 28 | 65 | 16.9 | 1.3 | | | 0 | 326 | 13 | 4 | 0.61 | 0.008 | 0 | 0 | 0.10 | 0.6 | 0.42 | 0.19 |
| | | 4.2 | 4.7 | 1.7 | 2.2 | 0.5 | 11 | 75 | 35 | 0.29 | 0.020 | 10.0 | 0 | | 0.07 | 0.08 | 0.6 | 7062 |
| **pork and beef loaf**, Dutch Brand *1.3 oz slice* | 38 | 104 | 22.1 | 1.5 | 0.3 | 0 | 0.1 | 401 | 3 | 6 | 0.96 | 0.015 | 13 | 1 | 0.05 | 1.3 | 0.34 | 0.19 |
| | | 4.6 | 8.7 | 3.4 | 4.3 | 1.2 | 23 | 80 | 45 | 0.06 | 0.026 | 7.0 | 42 | 0.1 | 0.05 | 0.09 | 4.2 | 7021 |
| **pork and beef lunch meat** *2 oz slice* | 57 | 201 | 28.1 | 1.3 | 0 | 0 | 0 | 737 | 5 | 8 | 0.95 | 0.017 | 0 | 0 | 0.18 | 1.6 | 0.73 | 0.36 |
| | | 7.2 | 18.3 | 6.6 | 8.6 | 2.1 | 31 | 115 | 49 | 0.49 | 0.023 | 16.3 | 0 | 0.1 | 0.09 | 0.11 | 3.4 | 7047 |
| **pork and beef luncheon sausage** *.8 oz slice (4" dia, ⅛" thick)* | 23 | 60 | 13.5 | 0.4 | | | 0 | 272 | 3 | 3 | 0.56 | 0.010 | 0 | 0 | 0.05 | 0.8 | 0.45 | 0.09 |
| | | 3.5 | 4.8 | 1.8 | 2.3 | 0.5 | 15 | 56 | 28 | 0.33 | 0.018 | 3.5 | 0 | | 0.04 | 0.05 | 0.7 | 7090 |
| **pork and beef sausage,** New England Brand *.8 oz slice (4" dia, ⅛" thick)* | 23 | 37 | 15.4 | 1.1 | | | 0 | 281 | 2 | 4 | 0.62 | 0.008 | 0 | 0 | 0.15 | 0.8 | 0.31 | 0.16 |
| | | 4.0 | 1.7 | 0.6 | 0.8 | 0.2 | 11 | 74 | 31 | 0.22 | 0.023 | 4.4 | 0 | | 0.06 | 0.08 | 1.6 | 7091 |
| **pork lunch meat**, canned *.7 oz slice* | 21 | 70 | 10.8 | 0.4 | 0 | 0 | 0 | 271 | 1 | 2 | 0.31 | 0.005 | 0 | 0 | 0.08 | 0.7 | 0.19 | 0.10 |
| | | 2.6 | 6.4 | 2.3 | 3.0 | 0.7 | 13 | 45 | 17 | 0.15 | 0.008 | 5.9 | 0 | 0.1 | 0.04 | 0.04 | 1.3 | 7045 |
| **roast beef spread** *4 T* | 57 | 127 | 35.2 | 2.1 | 0.4 | | 0.1 | 413 | 13 | 14 | 3.47 | | 0 | 0 | 0.01 | 2.4 | 1.36 | |
| | | 8.7 | 9.3 | 3.6 | 3.2 | 0.2 | 40 | 148 | 66 | 1.17 | 0.058 | 12.9 | 1 | | 0.13 | 0.09 | 4.6 | 7912 |
| **salami**, beef *2 slices (1.6 oz)* | 46 | 120 | 27.6 | 0.9 | 0.7 | 0 | 0 | 524 | 3 | 6 | 0.81 | 0.021 | 0 | 0 | 0.05 | 1.5 | 1.41 | 0.44 |
| | | 5.8 | 10.2 | 4.5 | 4.9 | 0.5 | 33 | 86 | 94 | 1.01 | 0.087 | 6.7 | 0 | 0.1 | 0.09 | 0.08 | 0.9 | 7068 |
| **salami**, beef and pork *2 slices (1.6 oz)* | 46 | 155 | 20.8 | 1.1 | 0.4 | 0 | 0 | 667 | 7 | 9 | 1.35 | 0.450 | 0 | 0 | 0.17 | 2.8 | 0.70 | 0.55 |
| | | 10.1 | 11.9 | 4.3 | 5.1 | 1.2 | 41 | 145 | 88 | 0.72 | 0.164 | 14.4 | 0 | 0.1 | 0.16 | 0.21 | 1.4 | 7069 |
| **salami**, beef and pork, less sodium - *1 oz* | 28 | 111 | 9.4 | 4.3 | 1.7 | | 0.1 | 174 | 26 | 9 | 0.86 | 0.016 | 1 | 0 | 0.21 | 1.3 | 0.49 | 0.24 |
| | | 4.2 | 8.5 | 3.0 | 3.7 | 0.9 | 25 | 384 | 76 | 0.43 | 0.025 | 4.1 | 3 | | 0.09 | 0.14 | 2.2 | 7913 |
| **salami**, beef cotto, Oscar Mayer *2 slices (1.6 oz)* | 46 | 95 | 29.7 | 0.9 | 0.5 | | 0 | 602 | 3 | 8 | 0.96 | | 0 | 0 | | | | |
| | | 6.5 | 7.2 | 3.1 | 3.2 | 0.4 | 38 | 95 | 103 | 1.25 | 0.106 | | 0 | | | | | 7226 |
| **salami**, beerwurst, Oscar Mayer *2 slices (1.6 oz)* | 46 | 104 | 28.9 | 0.9 | 0.5 | | 0 | 566 | 4 | 8 | 0.94 | | 0 | | | | | |
| | | 6.2 | 8.4 | 2.9 | 4.1 | 0.9 | 32 | 98 | 106 | 0.54 | 0.110 | | 0 | | | | | 7228 |
| **salami**, beerwurst, pork *2 slices (1.6 oz)* | 46 | 109 | 28.3 | 0.9 | | | 0 | 570 | 4 | 6 | 0.79 | 0.015 | 0 | 0 | 0.25 | 1.5 | 0.40 | 0.23 |
| | | 6.6 | 8.6 | 2.9 | 4.1 | 1.1 | 27 | 116 | 47 | 0.35 | 0.023 | 9.6 | 0 | | 0.09 | 0.16 | 1.4 | 7003 |
| **salami**, beerwurst, pork and beef *2 slices (1.6 oz)* | 46 | 127 | 26.1 | 1.7 | 0 | 0 | 0.4 | 337 | 12 | 9 | 1.02 | 0.071 | 1 | 0 | 0.11 | 1.4 | 0.53 | 0.14 |
| | | 6.4 | 10.4 | 3.9 | 4.6 | 1.0 | 29 | 112 | 62 | 0.80 | 0.047 | 8.0 | 5 | 0.1 | 0.08 | 0.11 | 2.3 | 7002 |
| **salami**, cotto, beef, pork, chicken, Oscar Mayer - *2 slices (1.6 oz)* | 46 | 113 | 27.9 | 1.0 | 0.7 | | 0 | 504 | 34 | 13 | 0.91 | | 0 | 0 | | | | |
| | | 6.2 | 9.3 | 3.9 | 4.7 | 0.8 | 37 | 100 | 114 | 1.33 | 0.193 | | 0 | | | | | 7227 |
| **salami**, cotto, turkey, Louis Rich *1 oz* | 28 | 42 | 20.0 | 0.3 | 0.1 | | 0 | 285 | 9 | 6 | 0.66 | | 0 | | | | | |
| | | 4.2 | 2.7 | 0.8 | 1.1 | 0.7 | 22 | 62 | 76 | 0.46 | 0.101 | | | | | | | 7267 |
| **salami**, dry/hard, beef and pork *3 slices (1 oz)* | 27 | 104 | 10.0 | 1.0 | 0 | 0 | 0 | 543 | 2 | 5 | 0.87 | | 0 | 0 | 0.16 | 1.3 | 0.51 | |
| | | 6.3 | 8.1 | 2.9 | 4.0 | 0.8 | 27 | 102 | 38 | 0.41 | 0.022 | 7.0 | 0 | 0.1 | 0.08 | 0.14 | 0.5 | 7072 |
| **salami**, dry/hard, beef and pork, Oscar Mayer - *3 slices (1 oz)* | 27 | 99 | 10.3 | 0.4 | 0.1 | | 0 | 534 | 3 | 6 | 0.85 | 0.011 | 1 | 0 | 0.15 | 1.4 | 0.51 | 0.29 |
| | | 7.0 | 7.7 | 3.0 | 4.1 | 0.8 | 26 | 96 | 49 | 0.49 | 0.051 | | 12 | | 0.07 | 0.12 | 0.8 | 7230 |
| **salami**, dry/hard, Italian, pork, beef, 50% less Na - *3 slices (1 oz)* | 28 | 98 | 11.3 | 1.8 | 0 | | 0 | 262 | 2 | 5 | 0.90 | 0.011 | 0 | 0 | 0.17 | 1.4 | 0.53 | 0.30 |
| | | 6.1 | 7.4 | 2.7 | 3.7 | 0.6 | 25 | 106 | 40 | 0.42 | 0.022 | 7.3 | 0 | | 0.08 | 0.14 | 0.6 | 7941 |
| **salami**, dry/hard, pork *3 slices (1 oz)* | 27 | 110 | 9.8 | 0.4 | | | 0 | 610 | 4 | 6 | 1.13 | 0.019 | 0 | 0 | 0.25 | 1.5 | 0.76 | 0.29 |
| | | 6.1 | 9.1 | 3.2 | 4.3 | 1.0 | 21 | 102 | 62 | 0.35 | 0.043 | 6.9 | 0 | | 0.09 | 0.15 | 0.5 | 7071 |
| **salami**, Genoa, Oscar Mayer *3 slices (1 oz)* | 27 | 105 | 10.6 | 0.3 | 0.1 | | 0 | 493 | 5 | 6 | 0.91 | 0.012 | 0 | 0 | 0.17 | 1.2 | 0.36 | |
| | | 5.6 | 9.0 | 3.3 | 4.5 | 0.7 | 28 | 90 | 55 | 0.50 | 0.068 | | 0 | | 0.08 | 0.09 | | 7229 |
| **salami**, Italian, pork *1 oz* | 28 | 119 | 9.7 | 0.3 | 0.3 | | 0 | 529 | 3 | 6 | 1.18 | 0.020 | 0 | 0 | 0.26 | 1.6 | 0.78 | 0.30 |
| | | 6.1 | 10.4 | 3.7 | 5.1 | 1.0 | 22 | 95 | 64 | 0.43 | 0.045 | 7.1 | 0 | | 0.09 | 0.15 | 0.6 | 7926 |
| **salami**, turkey *2 slices (2 oz)* | 57 | 96 | 39.3 | 0.4 | 0.6 | 0 | 0.1 | 572 | 23 | 13 | 1.32 | 0.011 | 1 | 0 | 0.24 | 2.3 | 0.56 | 0.61 |
| | | 11.0 | 5.2 | 1.6 | 1.8 | 1.4 | 43 | 123 | 152 | 0.71 | 0.108 | 15.0 | 5 | 0.1 | 0.17 | 0.24 | 5.7 | 7070 |
| **salami**, turkey, Louis Rich *1 oz* | 28 | 41 | 20.1 | 0.1 | 0.1 | | 0 | 281 | 11 | 6 | 0.65 | | 0 | | | | | |
| | | 4.3 | 2.6 | 0.8 | 0.9 | 0.7 | 21 | 60 | 74 | 0.35 | 0.053 | | 0 | | | | | 7266 |
| **sandwich spread**, pork and beef *1 oz (~2T)* | 28 | 66 | 16.9 | 3.3 | 0 | 0 | 0.1 | 284 | 3 | 2 | 0.29 | 0.007 | 7 | 0 | 0.05 | 0.5 | 0.31 | 0.12 |
| | | 2.1 | 4.9 | 1.7 | 2.1 | 0.7 | 11 | 31 | 17 | 0.22 | 0.036 | 2.7 | 24 | 0.5 | 0.04 | 0.03 | 0.6 | 7073 |
| **sandwich spread**, pork, chicken, beef, Oscar Mayer - *1 oz* | 30 | 71 | 17.8 | 4.6 | 2.4 | | 0.1 | 246 | 8 | 4 | 0.26 | | 0 | 0 | | | | |
| | | 2.0 | 5.0 | 1.7 | 2.2 | 0.7 | 14 | 35 | 21 | 0.24 | 0.054 | | 30 | | | | | 7231 |
| **Spam**, pork and chicken, lite, cnd, Hormel - *2 oz* | 56 | 107 | 36.8 | 0.8 | 0.7 | | 0 | 578 | 22 | 10 | 1.23 | | 0 | 22 | | | | |
| | | 8.5 | 7.8 | 2.5 | 3.9 | 0.8 | 42 | 258 | | 0.78 | 0.056 | | 0 | | | | 1.7 | 7277 |

| | WT (g) | KCAL | H₂O (g) | CHO (g) | TSUG (g) | ASUG (g) | DFIB (g) | Na (mg) | Ca (mg) | Mg (mg) | Zn (mg) | Mn (mg) | A (mcg RAE) | C (mg) | B-1 (mg) | NIA (mg) | B-12 (mcg) | PANT (mg) |
|---|---|---|---|---|---|---|---|---|---|---|---|---|---|---|---|---|---|---|
| | | PRO (g) | FAT (g) | SFA (g) | MUFA (g) | PUFA (g) | CHOL (mg) | K (mg) | P (mg) | Fe (mg) | Cu (mg) | Se (mcg) | A (IU) | E (mg ATE) | B-2 (mg) | B-6 (mg) | FOL (mcg DFE) | REF |
| **Spam**, pork and ham, cnd, | 56 | 174 | 29.5 | 1.7 | | | 0 | 767 | 8 | 8 | 1.01 | | 0 | 1 | | | | 1.7 |
| Hormel - *2 oz* | | 7.4 | 15.3 | 5.5 | 7.7 | 1.7 | 39 | 128 | | 0.50 | 0.056 | | 0 | | | | 1.7 | 7276 |
| **Swisswurst**, pork, beef, Swiss | 77 | 236 | 42.6 | 1.2 | 0 | | 0 | 637 | 57 | 10 | 1.73 | 0.025 | 77 | 0 | 0.19 | 2.2 | 1.33 | 0.59 |
| cheese, smoked - *2.7 oz* | | 9.8 | 21.1 | | 10.5 | 2.3 | 47 | 159 | 137 | 0.55 | 0.054 | 5.8 | 257 | | 0.12 | 0.10 | 2.3 | 7920 |
| **thuringer**, beef and pork | 46 | 167 | 20.8 | 1.5 | 0.4 | 0 | 0 | 598 | 4 | 6 | 1.18 | | 0 | 8 | 0.07 | 2.0 | 2.53 | |
| *2 slices (1.6 oz)* | | 8.0 | 14.0 | 5.3 | 6.0 | 0.6 | 34 | 120 | 51 | 0.94 | 0.069 | 9.3 | 0 | 0.1 | 0.15 | 0.12 | 0.9 | 7078 |
| **thuringer**, beef, Oscar Mayer | 46 | 142 | 24.2 | 0.9 | 0.5 | | 0 | 655 | 4 | 7 | 1.08 | 0.015 | | 0 | 0.07 | 2.0 | 2.53 | |
| *2 slices (1.6 oz)* | | 6.7 | 12.4 | 5.4 | 5.9 | 0.5 | 37 | 107 | 56 | 1.15 | 0.087 | | | | 0.15 | 0.12 | 2.3 | 7237 |
| **thuringer**, Oscar Mayer | 46 | 140 | 24.5 | 0.4 | 0.2 | | 0 | 658 | 4 | 7 | 0.98 | 0.014 | | 0 | 0.11 | 2.0 | 1.73 | 0.25 |
| *2 slices (1.6 oz)* | | 6.9 | 12.3 | 4.9 | 5.6 | 1.0 | 39 | 105 | 60 | 1.03 | 0.078 | | | | 0.13 | 0.14 | 2.3 | 7238 |
| **turkey breast** lunch meat | 21 | 22 | 15.6 | 0.9 | 0.7 | 0 | 0.1 | 213 | 2 | 4 | 0.28 | 0.004 | 2 | 1 | 0.03 | 0 | 0.02 | 0.03 |
| *.7 oz slice (3½" square)* | | 3.6 | 0.3 | 0.1 | 0.1 | 0.1 | 9 | 63 | 34 | 0.30 | 0.012 | 4.8 | 7 | 0 | 0.07 | 0.03 | 0.8 | 7079 |
| **turkey breast** lunch meat, roasted, | 28 | 24 | 21.4 | 1.3 | 0.5 | | 0 | 334 | 3 | 8 | 0.24 | | | 0 | | | | |
| fat-free, Louis Rich - *1 oz* | | 4.2 | 0.2 | 0.1 | 0.1 | 0 | 9 | 57 | 65 | 0.31 | 0.070 | | 0 | | | | | 7259 |
| **turkey breast** lunch meat, smoked, | 56 | 52 | 41.4 | 1.2 | 0.3 | | 0 | 721 | 9 | 15 | 0.49 | | | 0 | | | | |
| fat-free, Louis Rich - *2 oz* | | 10.8 | 0.4 | 0.1 | 0.1 | 0.1 | 23 | 161 | 169 | 0.63 | 0.112 | | 0 | | | | | 7262 |
| **turkey breast** lnch meat, smkd, fat-free, | 52 | 42 | 40.3 | 1.9 | 0.6 | | 0 | 569 | 5 | 16 | 0.44 | | | 0 | | | | |
| Oscar Mayer - *4 slices (1.8 oz)* | | 7.7 | 0.3 | 0.1 | 0.1 | 0.1 | 16 | 113 | 126 | 0.40 | 0.135 | | 0 | | | | | 7239 |
| **turkey breast** lunch meat, smkd, lmn | 28 | 27 | 20.6 | 0.4 | 0 | | 0 | 325 | | | | | | | | | | |
| pepr, 97% fat-free - *1 slice* | | 5.9 | 0.2 | 0.1 | 0.1 | 0.1 | 13 | | | | | | 0 | | | | | 7943 |
| **turkey breast** lunch meat, smoked, | 45 | 42 | 33.4 | 0.7 | 0.1 | | 0 | 540 | 7 | 14 | 0.43 | | | 0 | | | | |
| Louis Rich - *2 slices (1.6 oz)* | | 8.9 | 0.4 | 0.1 | 0.1 | 0.1 | 19 | 140 | 143 | 0.66 | 0.077 | | 0 | | | | | 7261 |
| **turkey ham** (cured thigh meat) | 57 | 72 | 41.0 | 1.2 | 0.8 | 0 | 0.1 | 635 | 5 | 13 | 1.48 | 0.011 | 4 | 5 | 0.02 | 1.2 | 0.13 | 0.43 |
| lunch meat - *2 slices* | | 10.0 | 2.8 | 0.9 | 1.1 | 0.8 | 41 | 164 | 168 | 1.33 | 0.142 | 18.4 | 14 | 0.4 | 0.08 | 0.12 | 4.0 | 7080 |
| **turkey ham**, extra lean, sliced, | 56 | 69 | 40.3 | 1.6 | 0 | | 0 | 581 | 3 | 11 | 1.32 | | 0 | 0 | 0.03 | 2.0 | 0.15 | |
| packaged/deli-sliced - *2 oz* | | 11.0 | 2.1 | 0.6 | 0.5 | 0.6 | 38 | 167 | 170 | 0.76 | 0.062 | 20.7 | 0 | 0.2 | 0.14 | 0.13 | 3.4 | 42128 |
| **turkey ham** lunch meat, 10% water | 28 | 32 | 20.5 | 0.3 | 0.3 | | 0 | 316 | 1 | 6 | 0.73 | | | 0 | | | | |
| added, Louis Rich - *1 oz* | | 5.1 | 1.3 | 0.3 | 0.3 | 0.2 | 19 | 81 | 82 | 0.36 | 0.070 | | 0 | | | | | 7264 |
| **turkey lunch meat**, honey roasted, | 56 | 57 | 40.3 | 2.5 | 2.2 | | 0 | 661 | 8 | 16 | 0.56 | | | 0 | | | | |
| fat-free, Louis Rich - *2 oz* | | 10.8 | 0.4 | 0.1 | 0.1 | 0.1 | 22 | 147 | 155 | 0.62 | 0.123 | | 0 | | | | | 7258 |
| **turkey lunch meat**, smoked, sliced, | 57 | 91 | 38.9 | 1.0 | | | 0 | 625 | 34 | | | | | | 0.10 | 3.3 | | |
| Carl Buddig - *2 oz* | | 10.0 | 5.2 | 1.8 | | 1.5 | 32 | 188 | | 1.05 | | | | | 0.18 | | | 7273 |
| **turkey roll**, light and dark meat | 57 | 85 | 40.0 | 1.2 | 0 | 0 | 0 | 334 | 18 | 10 | 1.14 | 0.007 | 0 | 0 | 0.05 | 2.7 | 0.13 | 0.32 |
| *2 slices* | | 10.3 | 4.0 | 1.2 | 1.3 | 1.0 | 31 | 154 | 96 | 0.77 | 0.040 | 16.6 | 0 | 0.2 | 0.16 | 0.15 | 2.8 | 7082 |
| **turkey roll**, light meat | 57 | 56 | 42.7 | 2.9 | 0 | 0 | 0 | 594 | 4 | 11 | 0.51 | 0.007 | 0 | 0 | 0.01 | 4.1 | 0.21 | 0.19 |
| *2 slices* | | 8.4 | 0.9 | 0.2 | 0.2 | 0.1 | 19 | 243 | 146 | 0.21 | 0.197 | 7.4 | 0 | 0.1 | 0.08 | 0.23 | 2.3 | 7081 |
| **yachtwurst** (sausage w/pistachio | 56 | 150 | 32.6 | 0.8 | 0 | | 0 | 524 | 11 | | | | 0 | 0 | | | | |
| nuts), cooked - *2 oz* | | 8.3 | 12.7 | 4.4 | | | 36 | | | 0.56 | | | 0 | | | | | 7930 |

## 20.3  MEAT-BASED SNACKS

| | WT (g) | KCAL | H₂O (g) | CHO (g) | TSUG (g) | ASUG (g) | DFIB (g) | Na (mg) | Ca (mg) | Mg (mg) | Zn (mg) | Mn (mg) | A (mcg RAE) | C (mg) | B-1 (mg) | NIA (mg) | B-12 (mcg) | PANT (mg) |
|---|---|---|---|---|---|---|---|---|---|---|---|---|---|---|---|---|---|---|
| | | PRO (g) | FAT (g) | SFA (g) | MUFA (g) | PUFA (g) | CHOL (mg) | K (mg) | P (mg) | Fe (mg) | Cu (mg) | Se (mcg) | A (IU) | E (mg ATE) | B-2 (mg) | B-6 (mg) | FOL (mcg DFE) | REF |
| **bacon and beef sticks** | 28 | 145 | 6.0 | 0.2 | 0.2 | | 0 | 398 | 4 | 5 | 0.90 | 0.011 | 0 | 0 | 0.17 | 1.4 | 0.53 | 0.30 |
| *1 oz* | | 8.1 | 12.4 | 4.5 | 6.1 | 1.2 | 29 | 108 | 40 | 0.52 | 0.022 | 7.3 | 0 | | 0.08 | 0.14 | 0.6 | 7921 |
| **beef, dried** | 21 | 32 | 11.3 | 0.6 | 0.6 | 0.5 | 0 | 586 | 2 | 4 | 1.04 | 0.004 | 0 | 0 | 0.01 | 1.1 | 0.33 | 0.12 |
| *5 slices (.7 oz)* | | 6.5 | 0.4 | 0.2 | 0.2 | 0 | 17 | 49 | 38 | 0.51 | 0.016 | 6.8 | 0 | 0.1 | 0.03 | 0.08 | 2.1 | 13350 |
| **beef jerky**, Bridgford | 28 | 70 | | 3.0 | 3.0 | | 0 | 450 | 0 | | | | | 0 | | | | |
| *1 oz* | | 12.0 | 1.0 | 0 | | | 20 | | | 1.08 | | | 0 | | | | | BRID1 |
| **beef jerky**, chopped and formed | 20 | 82 | 4.7 | 2.2 | 1.8 | 0 | 0.4 | 443 | 4 | 10 | 1.62 | 0.022 | 0 | 0 | 0.03 | 0.3 | 0.20 | 0.03 |
| *1 large piece (.7 oz)* | | 6.6 | 5.1 | 2.2 | 2.3 | 0.2 | 10 | 119 | 81 | 1.08 | 0.045 | 2.1 | 0 | 0.1 | 0.03 | 0.04 | 26.8 | 19002 |
| **beef sticks**, smoked | 20 | 110 | 3.8 | 1.1 | | | 0 | 296 | 14 | 4 | 0.48 | 0.017 | 3 | 1 | 0.03 | 0.9 | 0.20 | 0.07 |
| *.7 oz stick* | | 4.3 | 9.9 | 4.2 | 4.1 | 0.9 | 27 | 51 | 36 | 0.68 | 0.026 | | 50 | | 0.09 | 0.04 | 0 | 19407 |
| **pork skins** | 28 | 152 | 0.5 | 0 | 0 | | 0 | 515 | 8 | 3 | 0.16 | 0.019 | 3 | 0 | 0.03 | 0.4 | 0.18 | 0.12 |
| *1 oz* | | 17.2 | 8.8 | 3.2 | 4.1 | 1.0 | 27 | 36 | 24 | 0.25 | 0.026 | 11.5 | 11 | 0.1 | 0.08 | 0.01 | 0 | 19041 |
| **pork skins**, barbecue | 28 | 151 | 0.6 | 0.4 | | | 0 | 747 | 12 | 0 | 0.20 | 0.021 | 18 | 0 | 0.02 | 0.9 | 0.04 | 0.12 |
| *1 oz* | | 16.2 | 8.9 | 3.2 | 4.2 | 1.0 | 32 | 50 | 62 | 0.29 | 0.098 | | 187 | | 0.12 | 0.04 | 8.7 | 19408 |
| **summer sausage sticks**, pork, beef, | 28 | 119 | 10.1 | 0.5 | 0 | | 0.1 | 415 | 23 | 4 | 0.63 | 0.009 | 63 | 0 | 0.07 | 0.8 | 0.48 | 0.21 |
| cheddar cheese - *1 oz* | | 5.4 | 10.6 | 2.9 | 3.8 | 0.8 | 25 | 58 | 50 | 0.63 | 0.020 | 2.1 | 210 | | 0.04 | 0.04 | 2.0 | 7918 |

# 21. MEAT SUBSTITUTES, TOFU, AND RELATED SOY PRODUCTS
## 21.1 MEAT SUBSTITUTES

Each food item occupies two rows. The first row uses the headers: WT (g), KCAL, H₂O (g), CHO (g), TSUG (g), ASUG (g), DFIB (g), Na (mg), Ca (mg), Mg (mg), Zn (mg), Mn (mg), A (mcg RAE), C (mg), B-1 (mg), NIA (mg), B-12 (mcg), PANT (mg). The second row uses: PRO (g), FAT (g), SFA (g), MUFA (g), PUFA (g), CHOL (mg), K (mg), P (mg), Fe (mg), Cu (mg), Se (mcg), A (IU), E (mg ATE), B-2 (mg), B-6 (mg), FOL (mcg DFE), REF.

| Food | WT / PRO | KCAL / FAT | H₂O / SFA | CHO / MUFA | TSUG / PUFA | ASUG / CHOL | DFIB / K | Na / P | Ca / Fe | Mg / Cu | Zn / Se | Mn / A(IU) | A(RAE) / E | C / B-2 | B-1 / B-6 | NIA / FOL | B-12 / REF | PANT |
|---|---|---|---|---|---|---|---|---|---|---|---|---|---|---|---|---|---|---|
| Asian Veggie Patty, Morningstar Farms - 1 patty | 67 | 104 | 43.4 | 10.0 | 3.3 | | 2.0 | 486 | 34 | | | | | 2 | 0.03 | 1.3 | 0 | |
| | 7.3 | 4.2 | 0.5 | 1.1 | 2.5 | 0 | 263 | 60 | 1.01 | | | 1283 | | 0.13 | | | 16551 | |
| bacon bits, simulated meat product - 1 T | 7 | 5 | 5.9 | 0.8 | 0.2 | 0 | 0.1 | 1 | 1 | 1 | 0.02 | | 1 | 0 | 0 | 0.1 | 0 | |
| | 0.1 | 0.1 | 0 | 0.1 | 0 | 0 | 9 | 2 | 0.03 | 0.006 | 0.1 | 11 | 0 | 0 | 0 | 1.1 | 42278 | |
| bacon, simulated meat product 3 strips (.6 oz) | 16 | 50 | 7.8 | 1.0 | 0 | 0 | 0.4 | 234 | 4 | 3 | 0.07 | 0.033 | 1 | 0 | 0.70 | 1.2 | 0 | 0.02 |
| | 1.7 | 4.7 | 0.7 | 1.1 | 2.5 | 0 | 27 | 11 | 0.39 | 0.017 | 1.2 | 14 | 1.1 | 0.08 | 0.08 | 6.7 | 16104 | |
| Better 'n Burger, frzn, Morningstar Farms - 3 oz patty | 85 | 112 | 58.0 | 7.7 | 0.3 | | 4.4 | 336 | 31 | | 0.68 | | | 0 | 0 | | | |
| | 13.9 | 2.9 | 0.4 | 1.0 | 1.4 | 0 | 423 | 188 | 2.46 | | | 0 | | 0.08 | | | 22121 | |
| Big Franks, cnd, Loma Linda/Worthington Fds - 1.8 oz frank | 51 | 111 | 30.1 | 2.9 | 0.2 | | 1.8 | 217 | 9 | | 1.17 | | | 0 | 0.30 | 7.6 | 6.69 | 1.61 |
| | 10.9 | 6.1 | 0.8 | 1.6 | 3.8 | 0 | 59 | 73 | 1.29 | | | 0 | | 0.50 | 0.73 | | 22126 | |
| Big Franks, lowfat, canned Loma Linda - 1 link | 51 | 79 | 33.5 | 2.5 | 0.2 | | 2.1 | 245 | 9 | | 1.27 | | | 0 | 0.31 | 7.7 | 0 | |
| | 11.8 | 2.4 | 0.3 | 0.6 | 1.6 | 0 | 51 | 70 | 1.17 | | | 0 | | 0.67 | 0 | | 16502 | |
| Breakfast Patty, frzn, Morningstar Farms - 1.3 oz patty | 38 | 80 | 20.7 | 3.3 | 0.6 | | 1.6 | 255 | 17 | | 0.53 | | | 0 | 4.18 | 2.3 | 1.41 | |
| | 9.8 | 3.0 | 0.4 | 0.7 | 1.9 | 1 | 125 | 116 | 1.71 | | | 0 | | 0.11 | 0.19 | | 22122 | |
| Burger Crumbles, frzn, Morningstar Farms - ½ cup (~2 oz) | 55 | 72 | 36.2 | 4.2 | 0.3 | | 2.6 | 235 | 18 | | 0.55 | | | 0 | 0.66 | 6.4 | 4.46 | |
| | 9.8 | 2.4 | 0.3 | 0.5 | 1.6 | 0 | 104 | 111 | 2.53 | | | 0 | | 0.11 | 0.38 | | 22120 | |
| Cheddar Burger, frzn, Morningstar Farms - 1 patty | 64 | 142 | 32.3 | 10.3 | 1.2 | | 3.2 | 458 | 153 | | | | | 14 | | | | |
| | 12.6 | 6.7 | 1.8 | 1.7 | 2.7 | 8 | 264 | | 1.54 | | | 65 | | | | | 16547 | |
| Chic-Ketts, frozen, Worthington 1 slice | 55 | 112 | 31.9 | 2.5 | 0.5 | | 2.0 | 405 | 12 | | 0.73 | | | 0 | 0 | 0.27 | 4.0 | 0 |
| | 14.3 | 5.0 | 0.8 | 1.2 | 3.0 | 0 | 43 | 72 | 1.88 | | | 0 | | 0.14 | 0 | | 16525 | |
| Chik Patty, frozen, Morningstar Farms - 1 patty | 71 | 140 | 38.3 | 16.3 | 1.4 | | 2.1 | 593 | 29 | | 0.36 | | | 0 | 0.21 | 3.0 | 1.21 | |
| | 8.4 | 5.0 | 0.6 | 1.0 | 3.3 | 0 | 278 | 89 | 1.78 | | | 18 | | 0.07 | 0.14 | | 16557 | |
| Chik'n Nuggets, frozen, Morningstar Farms - 4 pieces | 86 | 187 | 45.6 | 17.9 | 1.1 | | 2.0 | 565 | 32 | | 0.71 | | | 0 | 1.35 | 4.7 | 2.17 | |
| | 12.2 | 7.5 | 1.0 | 2.0 | 3.6 | 1 | 282 | | 2.43 | | | 0 | | 0.28 | 0.28 | | 16556 | |
| Chik'n Tenders, frozen, Morningstar Farms - 2 pieces | 81 | 189 | 40.8 | 20.4 | 0.5 | | 2.9 | 578 | 42 | | | | | 0 | | | | |
| | 11.9 | 6.6 | 0.9 | 1.9 | 3.7 | 0 | 200 | | 2.59 | | | 24 | | | | | 16559 | |
| Chili, canned, Worthington 1 cup | 230 | 283 | 167.4 | 25.0 | 3.0 | | 7.8 | 1042 | 41 | | 1.84 | | 9 | 0 | 0.53 | 0 | 3.75 | 0.16 |
| | 23.9 | 9.7 | 1.6 | 2.0 | 6.6 | 0 | 373 | 177 | 7.29 | | | 193 | | 0.25 | 0.85 | | 16510 | |
| Choplets, canned, Worthington 2 slices | 92 | 95 | 68.2 | 3.7 | 0.4 | | 2.6 | 420 | 7 | | 0.96 | | 0 | 0 | 0.02 | 0 | 0 | |
| | 17.8 | 0.9 | 0.1 | 0.1 | 0.5 | 0 | 36 | 70 | 1.39 | | | 0 | | 0.05 | 0 | | 16511 | |
| Deli Franks, frzn, Morningstar Farms - 1.6 oz frankfurter | 45 | 59 | 29.2 | 5.5 | 1.8 | | 1.6 | 481 | 10 | | 0.45 | | | 0 | 0.14 | 0 | 0 | |
| | 8.9 | 0.6 | 0.1 | 0.1 | 0.4 | 0 | 54 | 58 | 0.68 | | | 0 | | 0.09 | 0.03 | | 22119 | |
| Diced Chik, canned, Worthington ¼ cup | 55 | 44 | 43.4 | 2.1 | 0.1 | | 0.8 | 189 | 30 | | 0.38 | | | 0 | 0.09 | 1.7 | 1.19 | |
| | 8.1 | 0.4 | 0 | 0 | 0 | 1 | 119 | 0 | 1.04 | | | 0 | | 0.13 | 0.06 | | 16512 | |
| Dinner Cuts, canned, Loma Linda 2 slices | 92 | 96 | 67.8 | 3.8 | 0.4 | | 2.2 | 456 | 9 | | 0.95 | | | 0 | 0.02 | 0.5 | | |
| | 17.9 | 1.0 | 0.2 | 0.1 | 0.6 | 1 | 36 | 68 | 1.29 | | | 0 | | 0.06 | | | 16503 | |
| Dinner Roast, frozen, Worthington 1 slice | 85 | 181 | 52.4 | 5.8 | 0.8 | | 2.6 | 570 | 39 | | 0.78 | | | 0 | 2.58 | 13.0 | 0 | |
| | 13.6 | 11.5 | 2.0 | 4.6 | 4.8 | 1 | 128 | 111 | 3.81 | | | 0 | | 0.31 | 0 | | 16528 | |
| frankfurter, simulated meat product - 2.5 oz frankfurter | 70 | 163 | 40.6 | 5.4 | 0 | 0 | 2.7 | 330 | 23 | 13 | 0.84 | | 0 | 0 | 0.31 | 2.2 | 1.64 | 0.55 |
| | 13.7 | 9.6 | 1.4 | 2.7 | 5.5 | 0 | 69 | 241 | 0.99 | 0.494 | 5.2 | 0 | 1.3 | 0.58 | 0.05 | 54.6 | 43130 | |
| FriChik, canned, Worthington 2 pieces | 90 | 144 | 64.0 | 3.0 | 0.1 | | 1.4 | 361 | 31 | | 0.63 | | | 0 | 0 | 0.22 | 3.4 | 2.92 |
| | 12.1 | 9.3 | 1.3 | 2.1 | 4.9 | 1 | 139 | 0 | 2.37 | | | 0 | | 0.18 | 0.21 | | 16513 | |
| FriChik, lowfat, canned, Worthington - 2 pieces | 85 | 87 | 64.9 | 4.2 | 0 | | 0.8 | 354 | 30 | | 0.65 | | | 0 | 0 | 0.19 | 4.1 | 3.13 |
| | 12.2 | 2.3 | 0.3 | 0.6 | 0.9 | 1 | 144 | 105 | 2.76 | | | 0 | | 0.20 | 0.23 | | 16514 | |
| Fried Chik'n with Gravy, canned, Loma Linda - 2 pieces | 80 | 145 | 54.6 | 4.2 | 0.4 | | 2.2 | 358 | 9 | | 0.42 | | | 0 | 1.13 | 5.0 | 6.71 | |
| | 10.5 | 9.5 | 1.5 | 2.4 | 5.7 | 1 | 46 | 99 | 1.31 | | | 0 | | 0.49 | 0.35 | | 16501 | |
| FriPats, frozen, Worthigton 1 patty | 64 | 134 | 36.3 | 5.1 | 0.9 | | 1.8 | 331 | 62 | | 0.77 | | | 0 | 6.73 | 7.8 | 0 | |
| | 15.2 | 5.8 | 0.9 | 1.4 | 3.3 | 1 | 118 | 120 | 3.64 | | | 0 | | 0.34 | 0 | | 16529 | |
| Garden Veg Patties, frzn, Morningstar Frms - 2.4 oz patty | 67 | 118 | 40.1 | 9.2 | 1.2 | | 3.0 | 352 | 40 | | 0.67 | | | 1 | 7.50 | 0.9 | | |
| | 11.9 | 3.8 | 0.5 | 1.0 | 2.1 | 1 | 141 | 110 | 1.47 | | | 250 | | 0.20 | 0.60 | | 22118 | |
| Grillers Original, frozen, Morningstar Farms - 1 patty | 64 | 136 | 35.6 | 5.4 | 0.8 | | 2.8 | 270 | 39 | | 0.77 | | | 0 | 1.79 | 4.1 | 2.88 | |
| | 15.3 | 6.0 | 1.1 | 1.7 | 3.2 | 2 | 116 | 118 | 2.69 | | | 0 | | 0.22 | 0.38 | | 16548 | |
| Grillers Prime, frozen, Morningstar Farms - 1 patty | 71 | 169 | 38.6 | 4.2 | 0.2 | | 1.8 | 356 | 41 | | 0.85 | | | 0 | 0.21 | | | |
| | 17.0 | 9.4 | 1.1 | 4.0 | 4.3 | 1 | 159 | | 1.99 | | | 0 | | 0.14 | | | 16549 | |
| Harvest Burger, frzn, Green Giant 3.2 oz patty | 90 | 138 | 58.5 | 7.0 | | | 5.7 | 411 | 102 | 70 | 8.07 | | | 0 | 0.32 | 6.3 | 0 | |
| | 18.0 | 4.1 | 1.0 | 2.1 | 0.3 | 0 | 432 | 225 | 3.85 | 0.441 | 9.0 | 0 | | 0.20 | 0.39 | 21.6 | 22125 | |

| Food | WT (g) | KCAL / PRO (g) | H₂0 (g) / FAT (g) | CHO (g) / SFA (g) | TSUG (g) / MUFA (g) | ASUG (g) / PUFA (g) | DFIB (g) / CHOL (mg) | Na (mg) / K (mg) | Ca (mg) / P (mg) | Mg (mg) / Fe (mg) | Zn (mg) / Cu (mg) | Mn (mg) / Se (mcg) | A (mcg RAE) / A (IU) | C (mg) / E (mg ATE) | B-1 (mg) / B-2 (mg) | NIA (mg) / B-6 (mg) | B-12 (mcg) / FOL (mcg DFE) | PANT (mg) / REF |
|---|---|---|---|---|---|---|---|---|---|---|---|---|---|---|---|---|---|---|
| **Italian Herb Chik Patty**, frozen, Morningstar Farms - 1 patty | 71 | 168 | 33.3 | 22.1 | 1.1 |  | 2.4 | 484 | 36 |  |  |  |  | 0 | 0.28 | 4.0 | 1.49 |  |
|  |  | 9.7 | 5.0 | 0.6 | 0.9 | 3.4 | 0 | 343 | 99 | 2.70 |  |  | 33 |  | 0.07 | 0.21 |  | 16558 |
| **Linketts**, canned, Loma Linda 1 link | 35 | 73 | 21.4 | 1.5 | 0.1 |  | 1.0 | 140 | 4 |  | 0.52 |  |  | 0 | 0.14 | 3.3 | 1.02 | 0.71 |
|  |  | 7.5 | 4.1 | 0.5 | 1.0 | 2.5 | 0 | 22 | 40 | 0.61 |  |  | 0 |  | 0.27 | 0.16 |  | 16509 |
| **Little Links**, canned, Loma Linda 2 links | 46 | 102 | 27.6 | 2.5 | 0.4 |  | 1.9 | 217 | 9 |  | 0.69 |  |  | 0 | 0.45 | 7.2 |  |  |
|  |  | 8.9 | 6.2 | 0.9 | 1.6 | 3.5 | 0 | 26 | 47 | 1.51 |  |  | 0 |  | 0.63 |  |  | 16500 |
| **Meal Starters Chik'n Strips**, frozen, Moringstar Farms - 12 strips | 85 | 139 | 51.3 | 5.7 | 1.0 |  | 1.2 | 507 | 38 | 27 | 3.82 |  |  | 0 | 0.38 | 6.0 | 1.53 | 0.68 |
|  |  | 22.8 | 3.3 | 0.5 | 1.3 | 1.4 | 0 | 105 |  | 4.59 |  |  | 0 |  | 0.42 | 0.34 |  | 16563 |
| **Meal Starters Steak Strips**, frozen, Morningstar Farms - 12 strips | 85 | 147 | 49.7 | 7.6 | 1.0 |  | 0.9 | 530 | 40 | 27 | 3.82 |  |  | 0 | 0.38 | 6.0 | 1.53 | 0.68 |
|  |  | 22.2 | 3.5 | 0.5 | 1.5 | 1.4 | 0 | 182 |  | 7.06 |  |  | 0 |  | 0.42 | 0.26 |  | 16564 |
| **meat extender**, simulated meat product - 1 oz | 28 | 88 | 2.1 | 10.7 |  |  | 4.9 | 3 | 57 | 60 | 0.62 | 0.076 | 1 | 0 | 0.20 | 6.2 | 1.68 | 0.42 |
|  |  | 10.7 | 0.8 | 0.1 | 0.2 | 0.5 | 0 | 533 | 179 | 3.36 | 0.085 | 2.1 | 9 |  | 0.25 | 0.37 | 55.4 | 16106 |
| **Meat-Free Buffalo Wings**, frozen, Morningstar Farms - 5 pieces | 85 | 196 | 42.8 | 19.8 | 1.7 |  | 3.1 | 658 | 43 |  |  |  |  | 1 | 0.42 | 4.0 | 1.53 |  |
|  |  | 12.3 | 8.0 | 1.0 | 1.7 | 5.2 | 0 | 419 | 126 | 2.72 |  |  | 108 |  | 0.17 | 0.17 |  | 16555 |
| **Meatless Chicken**, frzn, Worthington - 1 slice | 55 | 84 | 37.4 | 2.4 | 0.4 |  | 1.3 | 249 | 150 |  | 0.39 |  |  | 0 | 0.38 | 4.1 | 2.02 |  |
|  |  | 8.8 | 4.4 | 0.7 | 1.0 | 2.5 | 1 | 227 | 0 | 2.07 |  |  | 0 |  | 0.13 | 0.28 |  | 16526 |
| **Meatless Corn Dog**, frzn, Morningstar Farms - 1 corn dog | 71 | 162 | 34.6 | 22.5 | 5.3 |  | 3.0 | 466 | 9 |  | 0.50 |  |  | 2 | 0.19 | 6.1 | 0 |  |
|  |  | 8.1 | 4.4 | 0.7 | 1.4 | 2.5 | 0 | 62 | 111 | 1.31 |  |  | 45 |  | 0.23 | 0.04 |  | 16560 |
| **Meatless Corned Beef**, frozen, Worthington - 3 slices | 57 | 139 | 30.8 | 5.6 | 1.2 |  | 2.7 | 432 | 14 |  | 0.44 |  |  | 0 | 11.72 | 7.8 | 3.37 |  |
|  |  | 10.6 | 8.2 | 1.3 | 2.0 | 4.9 | 1 | 123 | 80 | 2.66 |  |  | 0 |  | 0.23 | 0.46 |  | 16527 |
| **Meatless Mini Corn Dogs**, frozen, Morningstar Farms 4 corn dogs | 76 | 174 | 36.8 | 22.3 | 2.7 |  | 3.2 | 515 | 15 |  | 0.59 |  |  | 1 | 0.22 |  |  |  |
|  |  | 10.2 | 4.9 | 0.5 | 1.9 | 1.3 | 1 | 83 | 135 | 1.32 |  |  | 12 |  | 0.14 |  |  | 16561 |
| **Multigrain Cutlets**, cnd, Worthington - 2 slices | 92 | 99 | 67.5 | 5.5 | 0.6 |  | 2.9 | 288 | 9 |  | 1.10 |  |  | 0 |  |  |  |  |
|  |  | 16.7 | 1.2 | 0.5 | 0.2 | 0.6 | 0 | 29 | 78 | 1.38 |  |  | 0 |  |  |  |  | 16516 |
| **Mushroom Lover's Burger**, frozen, Morningstar Farms - 1 patty | 64 | 108 | 42.3 | 7.6 | 1.0 |  | 0.8 | 221 | 0 |  |  |  |  | 0 |  |  |  |  |
|  |  | 7.4 | 5.6 | 0.8 | 1.6 | 3.1 | 0 |  |  | 0.70 |  |  | 0 |  |  |  |  | 16552 |
| **Okara Patty**, frzn, Morningstar Farms - 1 patty | 64 | 114 | 39.6 | 6.1 | 0.8 |  | 2.9 | 304 | 24 |  | 0.83 |  |  | 0 |  |  |  |  |
|  |  | 11.9 | 4.6 | 0.5 | 2.5 | 1.4 | 1 | 244 |  | 1.54 |  |  | 0 |  |  |  |  | 16539 |
| **Philly Cheesesteak Burger**, frozen, Morningstar Farms - 1 patty | 64 | 119 | 40.1 | 6.7 | 0.5 |  | 2.0 | 384 | 38 |  | 0.70 |  |  | 0 | 8 |  |  |  |
|  |  | 9.3 | 6.1 | 1.5 | 1.5 | 2.2 | 0 | 140 | 115 | 1.14 |  |  | 0 |  |  |  |  | 16550 |
| **Prime Stakes**, canned, Worthington - 1 piece | 92 | 124 | 67.6 | 6.9 | 0.3 |  | 1.3 | 442 | 14 |  | 0.57 |  |  | 0 | 0.29 | 6.8 | 3.52 |  |
|  |  | 9.3 | 6.6 | 0.9 | 1.6 | 3.3 | 1 | 93 | 0 | 3.10 |  |  | 0 |  | 0.21 | 0.40 |  | 16517 |
| **Prosage Links**, frozen, Worthington - 2 links | 45 | 64 | 30.4 | 2.3 | 0.3 |  | 1.3 | 369 | 12 |  | 0.45 |  |  | 0 | 1.80 | 7.1 | 0 |  |
|  |  | 9.1 | 2.1 | 0.4 | 0.8 | 0.9 | 1 | 51 | 62 | 2.74 |  |  | 0 |  | 0.22 | 0 |  | 16531 |
| **Prosage Roll**, frozen, Worthington 1 slice | 55 | 144 | 29.9 | 3.3 | 0.1 |  | 1.9 | 367 | 15 |  | 0.42 |  |  | 0 | 0.68 |  | 0 |  |
|  |  | 10.8 | 9.7 | 1.9 | 3.2 | 4.6 | 1 | 76 | 51 | 2.00 |  |  | 0 |  | 0.20 | 0 |  | 16532 |
| **Redi-Burger**, canned, Loma Linda 1 slice | 85 | 127 | 55.1 | 6.9 | 1.0 |  | 3.7 | 432 | 14 |  | 1.45 |  |  | 0 | 0.23 | 4.3 | 1.39 |  |
|  |  | 18.6 | 2.7 | 0.5 | 0.5 | 1.5 | 0 | 144 | 135 | 1.70 |  |  | 0 |  | 0.41 | 0.45 |  | 16507 |
| **Roasted Herb Chik'n**, frozen, Morningstar Farms - 1 patty | 64 | 107 | 38.8 | 8.7 | 0.9 |  | 1.7 | 340 | 19 |  | 0.77 |  |  | 0 |  |  |  |  |
|  |  | 12.1 | 2.6 | 0.3 | 1.2 | 1.1 | 1 | 179 |  | 1.66 |  |  | 0 |  |  |  |  | 16540 |
| **Saucettes**, canned, Worthington 1 link | 38 | 83 | 23.7 | 2.1 | 0.1 |  | 1.1 | 202 | 15 |  | 0.34 |  |  | 0 | 0.70 | 2.5 | 0 |  |
|  |  | 5.7 | 5.8 | 0 | 0 | 0 | 1 | 26 | 59 | 1.94 |  |  | 0 |  | 0.11 | 0 |  | 16518 |
| **sausage meat substitute**, pan-fried .9 oz link | 25 | 64 | 12.6 | 2.5 | 0 | 0 | 0.7 | 222 | 16 | 9 | 0.36 | 0.181 | 0 | 0.59 | 2.8 | 0 | 0.08 |
|  |  | 4.6 | 4.5 | 0.7 | 1.1 | 2.3 | 0 | 58 | 56 | 0.93 | 0.062 | 1.8 | 0 | 0.5 | 0.10 | 0.21 | 6.5 | 16107 |
| **Sausage Style Crumbles**, frozen, Morningstar Farms - ⅔ cup | 55 | 90 | 33.8 | 7.5 | 0.6 |  | 1.1 | 445 | 53 |  |  |  |  | 0 | 0.74 | 11.0 | 6.38 |  |
|  |  | 9.8 | 2.3 | 0.3 | 0.6 | 1.3 | 0 | 116 | 76 | 3.80 |  |  | 0 |  | 0.33 | 0.66 |  | 16565 |
| **Smoked Turkey**, frozen, Worthington - 1 slice | 55 | 138 | 29.5 | 4.4 | 1.3 |  | 0.6 | 472 | 81 |  | 0.42 |  |  | 0 |  | 5.9 | 3.38 |  |
|  |  | 10.2 | 8.9 | 1.3 | 2.1 | 4.9 | 0 | 54 | 0 | 2.97 |  |  | 0 |  | 0 | 0.45 |  | 16533 |
| **Spicy Black Bean burger**, frzn, Mrngstr Frms - 2.8 oz patty | 78 | 133 | 44.1 | 15.4 | 2.2 |  | 5.3 | 406 | 80 | 40 | 0.78 | 0.546 | 1 |  | 1.4 | 0 |  |  |
|  |  | 12.6 | 4.4 | 0.6 | 1.2 | 2.6 | 1 | 296 | 147 | 1.72 | 0.156 |  | 78 |  | 0.23 | 0.12 |  | 22123 |
| **Stakelets**, frozen, Worthington 1 piece | 71 | 150 | 40.8 | 6.8 | 0.8 |  | 2.0 | 462 | 52 |  | 0.87 |  |  | 0 | 1.61 | 7.6 | 0 |  |
|  |  | 14.0 | 7.4 | 1.3 | 2.5 | 3.6 | 1 | 136 | 149 | 2.49 |  |  | 0 |  | 0.28 | 0 |  | 16534 |
| **Stripples**, frozen, Worthington 2 strips | 16 | 55 | 6.7 | 2.3 | 0.1 |  | 0.8 | 234 | 7 |  | 0.10 |  |  | 0 | 1.62 | 1.4 | 0.54 |  |
|  |  | 2.0 | 4.3 | 0.7 | 1.0 | 2.6 | 0 | 16 | 46 | 0.58 |  |  | 0 |  | 0.06 | 0.08 |  | 16535 |
| **Super Links**, canned, Worthington 1 link | 48 | 105 | 29.8 | 2.6 | 0.3 |  | 0.9 | 340 | 16 |  | 0.45 |  |  | 0 | 0.15 | 1.9 | 2.65 |  |
|  |  | 6.9 | 7.4 | 1.0 | 1.5 | 4.0 | 0 | 37 | 45 | 2.05 |  |  | 0 |  | 0.15 | 0.24 |  | 16519 |
| **Swiss Stake with Gravy**, cnd, Loma Linda - 1 piece | 92 | 130 | 65.2 | 9.5 | 0.8 |  | 2.9 | 433 | 32 |  | 0.62 |  |  | 0 | 1.17 | 14.1 | 6.73 |  |
|  |  | 9.4 | 6.0 | 0.8 | 1.5 | 3.4 | 1 | 208 | 129 | 1.63 |  |  | 0 |  | 0.81 | 1.02 |  | 16505 |
| **Tender Bits**, canned, Loma Linda 6 pieces | 85 | 115 | 59.5 | 7.0 | 0.5 |  | 3.7 | 521 | 14 |  | 0.81 |  |  | 0 | 0.42 | 6.4 | 0 |  |
|  |  | 12.9 | 3.9 | 0.6 | 0.9 | 2.2 | 0 | 55 | 75 | 1.39 |  |  | 0 |  | 0.51 | 0 |  | 16508 |
| **Tender Rounds with Gravy**, canned, Loma Linda - 6 pieces | 80 | 116 | 55.3 | 5.9 | 0.8 |  | 2.8 | 354 | 11 |  | 0.69 |  |  | 0 | 0.80 | 0.4 | 1.73 |  |
|  |  | 13.0 | 4.5 | 0.6 | 1.1 | 1.8 | 1 | 76 | 82 | 1.21 |  |  | 0 |  | 0.40 | 0.18 |  | 16504 |

| | WT (g) | Macronutrients | | | | | | Minerals | | | | | Vitamins | | | | | |
|---|---|---|---|---|---|---|---|---|---|---|---|---|---|---|---|---|---|---|
| | | KCAL | H₂0 (g) | CHO (g) | TSUG (g) | ASUG (g) | DFIB (g) | Na (mg) | Ca (mg) | Mg (mg) | Zn (mg) | Mn (mg) | A (mcg RAE) | C (mg) | B-1 (mg) | NIA (mg) | B-12 (mcg) | PANT (mg) |
| | | PRO (g) | FAT (g) | SFA (g) | MUFA (g) | PUFA (g) | CHOL (mg) | K (mg) | P (mg) | Fe (mg) | Cu (mg) | Se (mcg) | A (IU) | E (mg ATE) | B-2 (mg) | B-6 (mg) | FOL (mcg DFE) | REF |
| **Tomato and Basil Pizza Burger**, frzn, Morningstar Farms - *1 patty* | 67 | 121 | 42.1 | 7.4 | 1.6 | | 2.5 | 261 | 32 | | | | | 15 | 0.07 | | | |
| | | 10.4 | 5.6 | 1.5 | 1.4 | 2.6 | 7 | 159 | 93 | 1.21 | | | 285 | | 0.20 | | | 16554 |
| **Turkee Slices**, canned, Worthington *3 slices* | 94 | 190 | 59.7 | 5.3 | 1.2 | | 0 | 531 | 141 | | 0.60 | | 0 | 0 | 3.09 | 5.6 | 4.55 | |
| | | 13.6 | 12.7 | 1.9 | 3.9 | 7.8 | 1 | 55 | 0 | 3.87 | | | 0 | | 0.24 | 0.29 | | 16520 |
| **Vega-Links**, canned, Worthington *1 link* | 31 | 48 | 21.8 | 1.3 | 0.1 | | 1.0 | 164 | 7 | | 0.16 | | 0 | 0 | 0.10 | 1.6 | 1.51 | |
| | | 4.5 | 2.8 | 0.4 | 0.6 | 1.4 | 1 | 17 | 31 | 1.05 | | | 0 | | 0.10 | 0.11 | | 16524 |
| **Vegan Burger**, frozen, Natural Touch - *3 oz patty* | 85 | 117 | 55.1 | 9.1 | 1.8 | | 4.8 | 547 | 26 | | 0.42 | | 0 | | | | | |
| | | 16.1 | 1.9 | 0.3 | 0.7 | 0.9 | 0 | 297 | | 2.38 | | | 0 | | | | | 22128 |
| **Vege-Burger**, canned, Loma Linda *¼ cup* | 55 | 63 | 39.6 | 2.0 | 0.5 | | 1.4 | 122 | 9 | | 0.72 | | | 0 | 0.13 | 5.5 | 3.66 | 0.32 |
| | | 12.2 | 0.7 | 0.1 | 0.1 | 0.4 | 0 | 41 | 44 | 0.94 | | | 0 | | 0.25 | 0.34 | | 16506 |
| **Vegetable Skallops**, cnd, Worthington - *½ cup* | 85 | 93 | 62.0 | 3.9 | 0.3 | | 2.9 | 391 | 6 | | 0.88 | | | 0 | 0.03 | 0 | 0 | |
| | | 16.9 | 1.0 | 0.1 | 0.1 | 0.4 | 0 | 14 | 44 | 1.18 | | | 0 | | 0.03 | 0 | | 16521 |
| **Vegetable Steaks**, cnd, Worthington *2 slices* | 72 | 81 | 51.7 | 3.6 | 0.4 | | 1.6 | 300 | 4 | | 0.79 | | | 0 | 0.84 | 5.7 | 0 | |
| | | 14.9 | 0.8 | 0 | 0 | 0 | 0 | 23 | 55 | 4.17 | | | 0 | | 0.27 | 0 | | 16522 |
| **Vegetarian Burger**, cnd, Worthington - *¼ cup* | 55 | 69 | 38.9 | 3.4 | 0.3 | | 1.5 | 248 | 4 | | 0.64 | | | 0 | 0.20 | 4.7 | 3.05 | |
| | | 10.3 | 1.6 | 0.3 | 0.3 | 1.0 | 0 | 24 | 54 | 2.15 | | | 0 | | 0.13 | 0.21 | | 16523 |
| **Veggie Bacon Strips**, frzn, Morningstar Farms - *2 strips* | 16 | 55 | 6.7 | 2.3 | 0.1 | | 0.8 | 234 | 7 | | 0.10 | | | 0 | 1.62 | 1.4 | 0.54 | |
| | | 2.0 | 4.3 | 0.7 | 1.0 | 2.6 | 1 | 16 | 46 | 0.58 | | | 0 | | 0.06 | 0.08 | | 16542 |
| **Veggie Bites**, broccoli cheddar, frzn, Morningstar Farms - *3 pieces* | 85 | 178 | 50.0 | 14.8 | 2.9 | | 1.3 | 545 | 74 | | | | | 6 | 0.94 | 8.9 | 5.78 | |
| | | 8.4 | 9.9 | 2.4 | 2.6 | 4.7 | 7 | 139 | 128 | 3.23 | | | 268 | | 0.26 | 0.51 | | 16566 |
| **Veggie Bites** Country Scramble, frzn, Morningstar Farms - *3 pieces* | 85 | 184 | 46.8 | 16.8 | 1.8 | | 2.0 | 544 | 68 | | | | | 6 | 1.44 | 6.9 | 3.91 | |
| | | 11.0 | 8.0 | 1.9 | 2.1 | 3.9 | 11 | 94 | 59 | 2.98 | | | 144 | | 0.42 | 0.34 | | 16544 |
| **Veggie Bites** Eggs Florentine, frzn, Morningstar Farms - *3 pieces* | 85 | 175 | 45.3 | 17.1 | 2.8 | | 1.9 | 558 | 97 | 15 | 0.60 | | | 1 | 0.60 | 6.0 | 3.48 | 0.68 |
| | | 9.9 | 7.4 | 1.7 | 1.3 | 4.4 | 12 | 142 | 76 | 2.80 | | | 1016 | | 0.42 | 0.34 | | 16545 |
| **Veggie Bites**, spinach artichoke, frzn, Morningstar Farms - *3 pieces* | 85 | 188 | 47.6 | 16.0 | 4.0 | | 1.8 | 570 | 91 | | | | | 4 | 0.76 | 7.3 | 4.25 | |
| | | 9.4 | 10.1 | 2.6 | 2.7 | 4.6 | 7 | 149 | 135 | 2.80 | | | 931 | | 0.34 | 0.44 | | 16567 |
| **Veggie Cake**, ginger teriyaki, frzn, Morningstar Farms - *1 cake* | 68 | 111 | 41.2 | 19.0 | 1.8 | | 1.8 | 323 | 22 | 2 | 1.50 | 0.476 | | 4 | 0.75 | 10.0 | 2.99 | |
| | | 5.6 | 1.6 | 0.3 | 0.3 | 1.0 | 0 | 171 | 78 | 3.60 | | | 1217 | | 0.20 | 0.48 | | 16568 |
| **Veggie Cake**, southwestern style, frzn, Mrngstr Frms - *1 cake* | 68 | 134 | 35.6 | 20.9 | 0.3 | | 2.2 | 340 | 56 | 2 | 0.68 | 0.408 | | 2 | 0.75 | 10.0 | 2.99 | |
| | | 6.5 | 3.1 | 1.2 | 0.4 | 2.0 | 5 | 141 | 99 | 3.60 | | | 117 | | 0.20 | 0.48 | | 16569 |
| **Veggie Corn Dog**, frzn, Morningstar Farms - *1 corn dog* | 71 | 164 | 34.4 | 21.9 | 5.8 | | 1.6 | 522 | 9 | | 0.50 | | | 0 | | | | |
| | | 8.2 | 4.8 | 0.8 | 1.2 | 2.8 | 0 | 62 | | 1.70 | | | 0 | | | 0.51 | | 16537 |
| **Veggie Sausage Links**, frozen, Morninngstar Farms - *1 link* | 45 | 72 | 28.8 | 3.1 | 0.4 | | 1.8 | 302 | 12 | | | | | 0 | 0.86 | 7.6 | 3.33 | |
| | | 8.6 | 2.7 | 0.3 | 0.8 | 1.6 | 1 | 49 | | 2.66 | | | 0 | | 0.27 | 0.50 | | 16546 |
| **Veja-Links**, lowfat, cnd, Worthington - *1 link* | 31 | 38 | 22.6 | 1.3 | 0.2 | | 0.4 | 190 | 7 | | 0.20 | | | 0 | 0.07 | 2.1 | 1.47 | |
| | | 4.9 | 1.5 | 0.2 | 0.3 | 0.8 | 1 | 22 | 23 | 1.77 | | | 0 | | 0.11 | 0.13 | | 16515 |
| **Wham**, frozen, Worthington *1 slice* | 55 | 108 | 34.2 | 3.1 | 1.8 | | 0 | 394 | 25 | | 0.45 | | | 0 | 0 | 6.5 | 3.21 | |
| | | 9.8 | 6.2 | 0.9 | 1.4 | 3.2 | 0 | 107 | 0 | 2.71 | | | 0 | | 0 | 0.51 | | 16536 |

## 21.2 TOFU AND RELATED SOY PRODUCTS

| | WT (g) | KCAL / PRO | H₂0 / FAT | CHO / SFA | TSUG / MUFA | ASUG / PUFA | DFIB / CHOL | Na / K | Ca / P | Mg / Fe | Zn / Cu | Mn / Se | A(RAE) / A(IU) | C / E | B-1 / B-2 | NIA / B-6 | B-12 / FOL | PANT / REF |
|---|---|---|---|---|---|---|---|---|---|---|---|---|---|---|---|---|---|---|
| **fuyu** (salted, fermented tofu), prep w/calcium sulfate - *.4 oz block* | 11 | 13 | 7.7 | 0.6 | | | | 316 | 135 | 6 | 0.17 | 0.129 | 0 | 0 | 0.02 | 0 | 0 | 0.01 |
| | | 0.9 | 0.9 | 0.1 | 0.2 | 0.5 | 0 | 8 | 8 | 0.22 | 0.041 | 1.9 | 0 | | 0.01 | 0.01 | 3.2 | 16432 |
| **miso** (soybean paste) *1 oz* | 28 | 56 | 12.0 | 7.4 | 1.7 | 0 | 1.5 | 1044 | 16 | 13 | 0.72 | 0.241 | 1 | 0 | 0.03 | 0.3 | 0.02 | 0.09 |
| | | 3.3 | 1.7 | 0.3 | 0.3 | 0.9 | 0 | 59 | 45 | 0.70 | 0.118 | 2.0 | 24 | 0 | 0.07 | 0.06 | 5.3 | 16112 |
| **natto** (boiled, fermented soybeans) *1 cup (6.2 oz)* | 175 | 371 | 96.3 | 25.1 | 8.6 | 0 | 9.5 | 12 | 380 | 201 | 5.30 | 2.674 | 0 | 23 | 0.28 | 0 | 0 | 0.38 |
| | | 31.0 | 19.2 | 2.8 | 4.3 | 10.9 | 0 | 1276 | 304 | 15.05 | 1.167 | 15.4 | 0 | 0 | 0.33 | 0.23 | 14.0 | 16113 |
| **okara** (soybean pulp) *1 cup (4.3 oz)* | 122 | 94 | 99.6 | 15.3 | | | | 11 | 98 | 32 | 0.68 | 0.493 | 0 | 0 | 0.02 | 0 | 0 | 0.11 |
| | | 3.9 | 2.1 | 0.2 | 0.4 | 0.9 | 0 | 260 | 73 | 1.59 | 0.244 | 12.9 | 0 | | 0.02 | 0.14 | 31.7 | 16130 |
| **tempeh**, cooked *3.5 oz* | 100 | 196 | 59.6 | 9.4 | | | | 14 | 96 | 77 | 1.57 | 1.285 | | | 0.05 | 2.1 | 0.14 | 0.45 |
| | | 18.2 | 11.4 | 3.4 | 3.7 | 2.6 | | 401 | 253 | 2.13 | 0.540 | 0 | | | 0.36 | 0.20 | 21.0 | 16174 |
| **tempeh**, uncooked *1 cup (5.9 oz)* | 166 | 320 | 99.0 | 15.6 | | | | 15 | 184 | 134 | 1.89 | 2.158 | 0 | 0 | 0.13 | 4.4 | 0.13 | 0.46 |
| | | 30.8 | 17.9 | 3.7 | 5.0 | 6.4 | 0 | 684 | 442 | 4.48 | 0.930 | 0 | 0 | | 0.59 | 0.36 | 39.8 | 16114 |
| **tofu**, extra firm, prep w/nigari (MgCl) - *3 oz* | 85 | 77 | 69.1 | 1.7 | 0.4 | | 0.3 | 7 | 149 | 45 | 0.94 | 0.645 | 0 | 0 | 0.04 | 0.2 | 0 | 0.39 |
| | | 8.4 | 5.0 | 0.5 | 3.7 | 0.5 | 0 | 112 | 116 | 1.56 | 0.162 | 11.0 | 0 | | 0.04 | 0.05 | 14.4 | 16159 |
| **tofu**, extra firm, silken, lite, Mori-Nu *3 oz* | 85 | 32 | 77.3 | 0.8 | 0.4 | | 0 | 83 | 37 | 8 | 0.22 | | 0 | 0 | 0.03 | 0.1 | 0 | |
| | | 6.0 | 0.6 | 0.1 | 0.1 | 0.3 | 0 | 48 | 71 | 0.67 | 0.110 | | 0 | | 0.02 | 0 | | 16165 |
| **tofu**, extra firm, silken, Mori-Nu *3 oz* | 85 | 47 | 74.9 | 1.7 | 0.8 | | 0.1 | 54 | 26 | 23 | 0.51 | | 0 | 0 | 0.07 | 0.2 | 0 | |
| | | 6.3 | 1.6 | 0.3 | 0.3 | 0.9 | 0 | 131 | 85 | 1.01 | 0.170 | | 0 | | 0.03 | 0.01 | | 16163 |
| **tofu**, firm, prep w/calcium sulfate *3 oz* | 85 | 123 | 59.4 | 3.6 | | | 2.0 | 12 | 581 | 49 | 1.33 | 1.004 | | 0 | 0.13 | 0.3 | 0 | 0.11 |
| | | 13.4 | 7.4 | 1.1 | 1.6 | 4.2 | 0 | 201 | 162 | 2.26 | 0.321 | 14.8 | 141 | | 0.09 | 0.08 | 24.6 | 16426 |
| **tofu**, firm, prep w/calcium sulfate and nigari (MgCl) - *3 oz* | 85 | 60 | 72.2 | 1.4 | 0.5 | | 0.8 | 10 | 171 | 31 | 0.71 | 0.531 | 0 | 0 | 0.05 | 0.1 | 0 | 0.09 |
| | | 7.0 | 3.5 | 0.7 | 1.0 | 1.5 | 0 | 126 | 103 | 1.37 | 0.181 | 8.4 | 0 | | 0.05 | 0.06 | 16.2 | 16126 |

| | WT (g) | KCAL / PRO (g) | H₂O (g) / FAT (g) | CHO (g) / SFA (g) | TSUG (g) / MUFA (g) | ASUG (g) / PUFA (g) | DFIB (g) / CHOL (mg) | Na (mg) / K (mg) | Ca (mg) / P (mg) | Mg (mg) / Fe (mg) | Zn (mg) / Cu (mg) | Mn (mg) / Se (mcg) | A (mcg RAE) / A (IU) | C (mg) / E (mg ATE) | B-1 (mg) / B-2 (mg) | NIA (mg) / B-6 (mg) | B-12 (mcg) / FOL (mcg DFE) | PANT (mg) / REF |
|---|---|---|---|---|---|---|---|---|---|---|---|---|---|---|---|---|---|---|
| **tofu**, firm, prep w/nigari (MgCl) | 85 | 124 | 60.5 | 3.7 | | | 0.5 | 2 | 293 | 45 | 1.41 | 0.894 | | | 0.04 | 0.5 | 0 | 0.03 |
| *3 oz* | | 10.8 | 8.5 | 1.2 | 1.9 | 4.8 | 0 | 124 | 196 | 2.34 | 0.279 | 14.3 | | | 0.07 | 0.03 | 18.7 | 16160 |
| **tofu**, firm, silken, lite, Mori-Nu | 85 | 31 | 77.7 | 0.9 | 0.4 | | 0 | 72 | 31 | 8 | 0.28 | | 0 | 0 | 0.03 | 0.1 | 0 | |
| *3 oz* | | 5.4 | 0.7 | 0.1 | 0.1 | 0.4 | 0 | 54 | 69 | 0.64 | 0.103 | | 0 | | 0.02 | 0 | | 16164 |
| **tofu**, firm, silken, Mori-Nu | 85 | 53 | 74.3 | 2.0 | 1.1 | | 0.1 | 31 | 27 | 23 | 0.52 | | 0 | 0 | 0.09 | 0.2 | 0 | |
| *3 oz* | | 5.9 | 2.3 | 0.3 | 0.5 | 1.3 | 0 | 165 | 76 | 0.88 | 0.173 | | 0 | | 0.03 | 0.01 | | 16162 |
| **tofu**, fried | 13 | 35 | 6.6 | 1.4 | 0.4 | 0 | 0.5 | 2 | 48 | 8 | 0.26 | 0.194 | 0 | 0 | 0.02 | 0 | 0 | 0.02 |
| *.5 oz piece* | | 2.2 | 2.6 | 0.4 | 0.6 | 1.5 | 0 | 19 | 37 | 0.63 | 0.052 | 3.7 | 4 | 0 | 0.01 | 0.01 | 3.5 | 16129 |
| **tofu**, frozen, dried (koyadofu, kori tofu, tung tou-fu) | 17 | 82 | 1.0 | 2.5 | | | 1.2 | 1 | 62 | 10 | 0.83 | 0.627 | 4 | 0 | 0.08 | 0.2 | 0 | 0.07 |
| *1 piece* | | 8.1 | 5.2 | 0.7 | 1.1 | 2.9 | 0 | 3 | 82 | 1.65 | 0.200 | 9.2 | 88 | | 0.05 | 0.05 | 15.6 | 16128 |
| **tofu**, frozen, dried, prep w/calcium sulfate | 17 | 80 | 1.0 | 2.2 | | | 0.2 | 1 | 363 | 31 | 0.83 | 0.627 | 0 | 0 | 0.08 | 0.2 | 0 | 0.07 |
| *.6 oz piece* | | 8.1 | 5.2 | 0.7 | 1.1 | 2.9 | 0 | 3 | 82 | 1.65 | 0.200 | 9.2 | 0 | | 0.05 | 0.05 | 15.6 | 16428 |
| **tofu**, prep w/calcium sulfate, fried | 13 | 35 | 6.6 | 1.4 | | | 0.5 | 2 | 125 | 12 | 0.26 | 0.194 | 0 | 0 | 0.02 | 0 | 0 | 0.02 |
| *.5 oz piece* | | 2.2 | 2.6 | 0.4 | 0.6 | 1.5 | 0 | 19 | 37 | 0.63 | 0.052 | 3.7 | 0 | | 0.01 | 0.01 | 3.5 | 16429 |
| **tofu**, regular, prep w/calcium sulfate | 85 | 65 | 71.9 | 1.6 | | | 0.3 | 6 | 298 | 26 | 0.68 | 0.514 | 3 | 0 | 0.07 | 0.2 | 0 | 0.06 |
| *3 oz* | | 6.9 | 4.1 | 0.6 | 0.9 | 2.3 | 0 | 103 | 82 | 4.56 | 0.164 | 7.6 | 72 | | 0.04 | 0.04 | 12.8 | 16427 |
| **tofu**, soft, prep w/calcium sulfate and nigari (MgCl) | 85 | 52 | 74.2 | 1.5 | 0.6 | 0 | 0.2 | 7 | 94 | 23 | 0.54 | 0.331 | 0 | 0 | 0.04 | 0.5 | 0 | 0.04 |
| *3 oz* | | 5.6 | 3.1 | 0.5 | 0.7 | 1.8 | 0 | 102 | 78 | 0.94 | 0.133 | 7.6 | 6 | 0 | 0.03 | 0.04 | 37.4 | 16127 |
| **tofu**, soft, silken, Mori-Nu | 85 | 47 | 75.6 | 2.5 | 1.1 | | 0.1 | 4 | 26 | 25 | 0.44 | | 0 | 0 | 0.08 | 0.3 | 0 | |
| *3 oz* | | 4.1 | 2.3 | 0.3 | 0.4 | 1.3 | 0 | 153 | 53 | 0.70 | 0.176 | | 0 | | 0.03 | 0.01 | | 16161 |
| **yufu** (salted, fermented tofu) | 11 | 13 | 7.7 | 0.6 | | | | 316 | 5 | 6 | 0.17 | 0.129 | 0 | 0 | 0.02 | 0 | 0 | 0.01 |
| *.4 oz block* | | 0.9 | 0.9 | 0.1 | 0.2 | 0.5 | 0 | 8 | 8 | 0.22 | 0.041 | 1.9 | 0 | | 0.01 | 0.01 | 3.2 | 16132 |

## 22. MILKS, MILK BEVERAGES, AND YOGURT
### 22.1 COW MILK

| | WT (g) | KCAL / PRO (g) | H₂O (g) / FAT (g) | CHO (g) / SFA (g) | TSUG (g) / MUFA (g) | ASUG (g) / PUFA (g) | DFIB (g) / CHOL (mg) | Na (mg) / K (mg) | Ca (mg) / P (mg) | Mg (mg) / Fe (mg) | Zn (mg) / Cu (mg) | Mn (mg) / Se (mcg) | A (mcg RAE) / A (IU) | C (mg) / E (mg ATE) | B-1 (mg) / B-2 (mg) | NIA (mg) / B-6 (mg) | B-12 (mcg) / FOL (mcg DFE) | PANT (mg) / REF |
|---|---|---|---|---|---|---|---|---|---|---|---|---|---|---|---|---|---|---|
| **buttermilk**, cultured, lowfat | 245 | 98 | 220.8 | 11.7 | 11.7 | 0 | 0 | 257 | 284 | 27 | 1.03 | 0.005 | 17 | 2 | 0.08 | 0.1 | 0.54 | 0.67 |
| *8 fl oz* | | 8.1 | 2.2 | 1.3 | 0.6 | 0.1 | 10 | 370 | 218 | 0.12 | 0.027 | 4.9 | 64 | 0.1 | 0.38 | 0.08 | 12.2 | 1088 |
| **buttermilk**, cultured, reduced fat | 245 | 137 | 214.9 | 13.0 | 13.0 | 0 | 0 | 211 | 350 | 32 | 0.59 | | 39 | 4 | 0.12 | 0.2 | 0.91 | |
| *8 fl oz* | | 10.0 | 4.9 | 3.0 | 1.4 | 0.2 | 20 | 441 | 201 | 0.15 | 0.020 | 5.6 | 142 | 0.3 | 0.51 | 0.07 | 14.7 | 42189 |
| **buttermilk**, dry | 7 | 27 | 0.2 | 3.4 | 3.4 | 0 | 0 | 36 | 83 | 8 | 0.28 | 0.002 | 3 | 0 | 0.03 | 0.1 | 0.27 | 0.22 |
| *1 T* | | 2.4 | 0.4 | 0.3 | 0.1 | 0 | 5 | 111 | 65 | 0.02 | 0.008 | 1.4 | 12 | 0 | 0.11 | 0.02 | 3.3 | 1094 |
| **condensed milk**, sweetened, canned | 38 | 122 | 10.3 | 20.7 | 20.7 | 18.3 | 0 | 48 | 108 | 10 | 0.36 | 0.002 | 28 | 1 | 0.03 | 0.1 | 0.17 | 0.29 |
| *1 fl oz* | | 3.0 | 3.3 | 2.1 | 0.9 | 0.1 | 13 | 141 | 96 | 0.07 | 0.006 | 5.6 | 101 | 0.1 | 0.16 | 0.02 | 4.2 | 1095 |
| **evaporated milk**, nonfat, canned | 32 | 25 | 25.4 | 3.6 | 3.6 | 0 | 0 | 37 | 93 | 9 | 0.29 | 0.002 | 38 | 0 | 0.01 | 0.1 | 0.08 | 0.24 |
| *1 fl oz* | | 2.4 | 0.1 | 0 | 0 | 0 | 1 | 106 | 62 | 0.09 | 0.005 | 0.8 | 126 | 0 | 0.10 | 0.02 | 2.9 | 1097 |
| **evaporated milk**, whole, canned | 32 | 43 | 23.7 | 3.2 | 3.2 | 0 | 0 | 34 | 84 | 8 | 0.25 | 0.002 | 21 | 1 | 0.02 | 0.1 | 0.05 | 0.20 |
| *1 fl oz* | | 2.2 | 2.4 | 1.5 | 0.7 | 0.1 | 9 | 97 | 65 | 0.06 | 0.005 | 0.7 | 75 | 0.1 | 0.10 | 0.02 | 2.6 | 1096 |
| **milk**, lowfat, 1% fat | 244 | 102 | 219.4 | 12.2 | 12.7 | 0 | 0 | 107 | 290 | 27 | 1.02 | 0.007 | 142 | 0 | 0.05 | 0.2 | 1.07 | 0.88 |
| *8 fl oz* | | 8.2 | 2.4 | 1.5 | 0.7 | 0.1 | 12 | 366 | 232 | 0.07 | 0.024 | 8.1 | 478 | 0 | 0.45 | 0.09 | 12.2 | 1082 |
| **milk**, lowfat, 1% fat, pro-fortified | 246 | 118 | 218.3 | 13.6 | | | 0 | 143 | 349 | 39 | 1.11 | 0.005 | 150 | 3 | 0.11 | 0.2 | 1.06 | 0.92 |
| *8 fl oz* | | 9.7 | 2.9 | 1.8 | 0.8 | 0.1 | 10 | 443 | 273 | 0.15 | 0.025 | 6.2 | 499 | | 0.47 | 0.12 | 14.8 | 1084 |
| **milk**, lowfat, 1% fat w/ndms | 245 | 105 | 220.0 | 12.2 | | | 0 | 127 | 314 | 34 | 0.98 | 0.005 | 145 | 2 | 0.10 | 0.2 | 0.93 | 0.83 |
| *8 fl oz* | | 8.5 | 2.4 | 1.5 | 0.7 | 0.1 | 10 | 397 | 245 | 0.12 | 0.024 | 5.6 | 500 | | 0.42 | 0.11 | 12.2 | 1083 |
| **milk**, nonfat | 245 | 83 | 222.6 | 12.2 | 12.5 | 0 | 0 | 103 | 306 | 27 | 1.03 | 0.007 | 149 | 0 | 0.11 | 0.2 | 1.30 | 0.87 |
| *8 fl oz* | | 8.3 | 0.2 | 0.1 | 0.1 | 0 | 5 | 382 | 247 | 0.07 | 0.032 | 7.6 | 500 | 0 | 0.45 | 0.09 | 12.2 | 1085 |
| **milk**, nonfat, pro-fortified | 246 | 101 | 219.8 | 13.7 | | | 0 | 145 | 352 | 39 | 1.11 | 0.005 | 150 | 3 | 0.11 | 0.2 | 1.06 | 0.92 |
| *8 fl oz* | | 9.7 | 0.6 | 0.4 | 0.2 | 0 | 5 | 448 | 276 | 0.15 | 0.027 | 5.9 | 499 | | 0.48 | 0.12 | 14.8 | 1087 |
| **milk**, nonfat w/ndms | 245 | 91 | 221.4 | 12.3 | 12.3 | 0 | 0 | 130 | 316 | 37 | 1.00 | 0.005 | 149 | 2 | 0.10 | 0.2 | 0.96 | 0.83 |
| *8 fl oz* | | 8.7 | 0.6 | 0.4 | 0.2 | 0 | 5 | 419 | 255 | 0.12 | 0.027 | 5.4 | 497 | 0 | 0.43 | 0.11 | 12.2 | 1086 |
| **milk powder**, nonfat, calcium-reduced | 28 | 99 | 1.4 | 14.5 | | | 0 | 638 | 78 | 17 | 1.13 | 0.002 | 1 | 2 | 0.05 | 0.2 | 1.11 | 0.93 |
| *1 oz* | | 9.9 | 0.1 | 0 | 0 | 0 | 1 | 190 | 283 | 0.09 | 0.004 | 7.6 | 2 | | 0.46 | 0.08 | 14.0 | 1093 |
| **milk powder**, nonfat, instant w/vit A | 91 | 326 | 3.6 | 47.5 | 47.5 | 0 | 0 | 500 | 1120 | 106 | 4.01 | 0.018 | 645 | 5 | 0.38 | 0.8 | 3.63 | 2.94 |
| *1⅓ cups (3.2 oz pkt)* | | 31.9 | 0.7 | 0.4 | 0.2 | 0 | 16 | 1552 | 896 | 0.28 | 0.037 | 24.8 | 2152 | 0 | 1.59 | 0.31 | 45.5 | 1092 |
| **milk powder**, nonfat, regular w/o vit A | 30 | 109 | 0.9 | 15.6 | 15.6 | 0 | 0 | 160 | 377 | 33 | 1.22 | 0.006 | 2 | 2 | 0.12 | 0.3 | 1.21 | 1.07 |
| *¼ cup* | | 10.8 | 0.2 | 0.1 | 0.1 | 0 | 6 | 538 | 290 | 0.10 | 0.012 | 8.2 | 7 | | 0.46 | 0.11 | 15.0 | 1091 |
| **milk powder**, whole | 32 | 159 | 0.8 | 12.3 | 12.3 | 0 | 0 | 119 | 292 | 27 | 1.07 | 0.013 | 82 | 3 | 0.09 | 0.2 | 1.04 | 0.73 |
| *¼ cup* | | 8.4 | 8.5 | 5.4 | 2.5 | 0.2 | 31 | 426 | 248 | 0.15 | 0.026 | 5.2 | 293 | 0.2 | 0.39 | 0.11 | 11.8 | 1090 |
| **milk, reduced fat**, 2% fat | 244 | 122 | 218.0 | 11.4 | 12.3 | 0 | 0 | 100 | 285 | 27 | 1.05 | 0.007 | 134 | 0 | 0.10 | 0.2 | 1.12 | 0.87 |
| *8 fl oz* | | 8.1 | 4.8 | 3.1 | 1.4 | 0.2 | 20 | 366 | 229 | 0.07 | 0.029 | 6.1 | 461 | 0.1 | 0.45 | 0.09 | 12.2 | 1079 |
| **milk, reduced fat**, 2% fat, pro-fortified | 246 | 138 | 215.8 | 13.5 | 12.9 | | 0 | 145 | 352 | 39 | 1.11 | 0.005 | 0 | 3 | 0.11 | 0.2 | 1.06 | 0.92 |
| *8 fl oz* | | 9.7 | 4.9 | 3.0 | 1.4 | 0.2 | 20 | 448 | 276 | 0.15 | 0.020 | 6.4 | 12 | 0.1 | 0.48 | 0.13 | 14.8 | 1081 |

| | WT (g) | KCAL | H₂0 (g) | CHO (g) | TSUG (g) | ASUG (g) | DFIB (g) | Na (mg) | Ca (mg) | Mg (mg) | Zn (mg) | Mn (mg) | A (mcg RAE) | C (mg) | B-1 (mg) | NIA (mg) | B-12 (mcg) | PANT (mg) |
|---|---|---|---|---|---|---|---|---|---|---|---|---|---|---|---|---|---|---|
| | | PRO (g) | FAT (g) | SFA (g) | MUFA (g) | PUFA (g) | CHOL (mg) | K (mg) | P (mg) | Fe (mg) | Cu (mg) | Se (mcg) | A (IU) | E (mg ATE) | B-2 (mg) | B-6 (mg) | FOL (mcg DFE) | REF |
| **milk, reduced fat, 2% fat w/ndms** | 245 | 125 | 217.7 | 12.2 | | | 0 | 127 | 314 | 34 | 0.98 | 0.005 | 137 | 2 | 0.10 | 0.2 | 0.93 | 0.82 |
| *8 fl oz* | | 8.5 | 4.7 | 2.9 | 1.4 | 0.2 | 20 | 397 | 245 | 0.12 | 0.020 | 5.6 | 500 | | 0.42 | 0.11 | 12.2 | 1080 |
| **milk, whole, 3.25% fat** | 244 | 146 | 215.5 | 11.0 | 12.8 | 0 | 0 | 98 | 276 | 24 | 0.98 | 0.007 | 68 | 0 | 0.11 | 0.3 | 1.07 | 0.88 |
| *8 fl oz* | | 7.9 | 7.9 | 4.6 | 2.0 | 0.5 | 24 | 349 | 222 | 0.07 | 0.027 | 9.0 | 249 | 0.1 | 0.45 | 0.09 | 12.2 | 1077 |
| **milk, whole, 3.7% fat** | 244 | 156 | 214.0 | 11.3 | | | 0 | 120 | 290 | 32 | 0.93 | 0.010 | 81 | 4 | 0.09 | 0.2 | 0.88 | 0.76 |
| *8 fl oz* | | 8.0 | 8.9 | 5.6 | 2.6 | 0.3 | 34 | 368 | 227 | 0.12 | 0.024 | 4.9 | 337 | | 0.39 | 0.10 | 12.2 | 1078 |
| **milk, whole, low sodium** | 244 | 149 | 215.2 | 10.9 | 10.9 | 0 | 0 | 7 | 246 | 12 | 0.93 | 0.010 | 68 | 2 | 0.05 | 0.1 | 0.88 | 0.74 |
| *8 fl oz* | | 7.6 | 8.4 | 5.3 | 2.4 | 0.3 | 34 | 617 | 210 | 0.12 | 0.024 | 4.9 | 251 | 0.1 | 0.26 | 0.08 | 12.2 | 1089 |

## 22.2 COW MILK BEVERAGES

| | WT (g) | KCAL | H₂0 (g) | CHO (g) | TSUG (g) | ASUG (g) | DFIB (g) | Na (mg) | Ca (mg) | Mg (mg) | Zn (mg) | Mn (mg) | A (mcg RAE) | C (mg) | B-1 (mg) | NIA (mg) | B-12 (mcg) | PANT (mg) |
|---|---|---|---|---|---|---|---|---|---|---|---|---|---|---|---|---|---|---|
| | | PRO | FAT | SFA | MUFA | PUFA | CHOL | K | P | Fe | Cu | Se | A (IU) | E | B-2 | B-6 | FOL | REF |
| **carob-flavored milk,** from carob mix in whole milk - *8 fl oz* | 256 | 192 | 215.9 | 22.2 | | | 1.0 | 118 | 251 | 26 | 0.95 | 0.015 | 69 | 0 | 0.11 | 0.4 | 1.08 | 0.89 |
| | | 8.1 | 8.0 | 4.6 | 2.0 | 0.5 | 26 | 335 | 205 | 0.64 | 0.064 | 9.2 | 248 | | 0.45 | 0.10 | 12.8 | 14169 |
| **chocolate malted milk,** whole milk - *8 fl oz* | 265 | 225 | 215.6 | 29.7 | 17.7 | | 1.3 | 159 | 260 | 40 | 1.09 | 0.212 | 69 | 0 | 0.14 | 0.7 | 1.11 | 0.94 |
| | | 8.9 | 8.7 | 5.0 | 2.2 | 0.6 | 26 | 456 | 241 | 0.56 | 0.098 | 14.3 | 252 | 0.2 | 0.49 | 0.12 | 23.8 | 14318 |
| **chocolate malted milk,** whole milk with added nutrients - *8 fl oz* | 265 | 223 | 215.8 | 28.9 | 27.8 | | 1.1 | 231 | 339 | 45 | 1.17 | 0.140 | 904 | 32 | 0.76 | 11.1 | 1.14 | 1.03 |
| | | 8.9 | 8.6 | 5.0 | 2.2 | 0.5 | 26 | 578 | 289 | 3.76 | 0.191 | 12.5 | 3032 | 0.2 | 1.32 | 1.01 | 18.6 | 14316 |
| **chocolate milk,** 1% milk - *8 fl oz* | 250 | 158 | 211.2 | 26.1 | 24.8 | 11.9 | 1.2 | 152 | 288 | 32 | 1.02 | 0.192 | 145 | 2 | 0.10 | 0.3 | 0.85 | 0.76 |
| | | 8.1 | 2.5 | 1.5 | 0.8 | 0.1 | 8 | 425 | 258 | 0.60 | 0.162 | 4.8 | 490 | 0 | 0.42 | 0.10 | 12.5 | 1104 |
| **chocolate milk,** from instant mix with aspartame - *6 fl oz* | 204 | 59 | 188.2 | 9.2 | 5.9 | | 1.6 | 124 | 259 | 39 | 0.65 | 0.131 | 37 | 1 | 0.02 | 0.2 | 0.37 | 0.38 |
| | | 4.5 | 0.5 | 0.3 | 0.1 | 0 | 4 | 402 | 159 | 1.39 | 0.161 | 3.9 | 124 | 0 | 0.35 | 0.02 | 6.1 | 14423 |
| **chocolate milk,** reduced fat - *8 fl oz* | 250 | 190 | 205.4 | 30.3 | 23.9 | 14.3 | 1.8 | 165 | 272 | 35 | 0.98 | 0.155 | 160 | 0 | 0.11 | 0.4 | 0.82 | 1.35 |
| | | 7.5 | 4.8 | 2.9 | 1.1 | 0.2 | 20 | 422 | 255 | 0.60 | 0.188 | 8.5 | 568 | 0.1 | 0.46 | 0.06 | 5.0 | 1103 |
| **chocolate milk,** whole milk - *8 fl oz* | 250 | 208 | 205.8 | 25.8 | 23.8 | 10.7 | 2.0 | 150 | 280 | 32 | 1.02 | 0.192 | 65 | 2 | 0.09 | 0.3 | 0.82 | 0.74 |
| | | 7.9 | 8.5 | 5.3 | 2.5 | 0.3 | 30 | 418 | 252 | 0.60 | 0.162 | 4.8 | 238 | 0.2 | 0.40 | 0.10 | 12.5 | 1102 |
| **chocolate milk,** whole milk with chocolate syrup - *8 fl oz* | 282 | 254 | 227.0 | 36.0 | 31.9 | | 0.8 | 133 | 251 | 51 | 1.21 | 0.155 | 70 | 0 | 0.11 | 0.4 | 1.07 | 0.89 |
| | | 8.7 | 8.3 | 4.7 | 2.1 | 0.5 | 25 | 409 | 254 | 0.90 | 0.254 | 9.6 | 248 | 0.1 | 0.47 | 0.09 | 14.1 | 14182 |
| **chocolate milk,** whole milk with instant mix - *8 fl oz* | 266 | 226 | 214.9 | 31.7 | | | 1.1 | 154 | 253 | 48 | 1.28 | 0.170 | 69 | 0 | 0.11 | 0.4 | 1.06 | 0.89 |
| | | 8.6 | 8.6 | 4.9 | 2.2 | 0.5 | 24 | 458 | 234 | 0.80 | 0.218 | 9.6 | 250 | 0.2 | 0.48 | 0.09 | 13.3 | 14177 |
| **eggnog,** from mix w/whole milk nonalcoholic - *8 fl oz* | 272 | 258 | 215.3 | 38.6 | 34.4 | | 0 | 150 | 250 | 27 | 0.95 | 0.019 | 71 | 0 | 0.11 | 0.3 | 1.06 | 0.90 |
| | | 8.0 | 8.2 | 4.6 | 2.1 | 0.5 | 30 | 329 | 209 | 0.33 | 0.060 | 9.2 | 256 | 0.2 | 0.45 | 0.09 | 13.6 | 14245 |
| **eggnog,** nonalcoholic - *8 fl oz* | 254 | 343 | 188.9 | 34.4 | 21.4 | 13.4 | 0 | 137 | 330 | 48 | 1.17 | 0.013 | 117 | 4 | 0.09 | 0.3 | 1.14 | 1.06 |
| | | 9.7 | 19.0 | 11.3 | 5.7 | 0.9 | 150 | 419 | 277 | 0.51 | 0.033 | 10.7 | 409 | 0.5 | 0.48 | 0.13 | 2.5 | 1057 |
| **hot chocolate,** from mix, prep w/ water - *1 oz pkt in 6 fl oz water* | 206 | 113 | 177.9 | 23.8 | 18.6 | | 1.0 | 150 | 43 | 25 | 0.43 | 0.076 | 0 | 0 | 0.03 | 0.2 | 0.10 | 0.25 |
| | | 1.9 | 1.1 | 0.7 | 0.4 | 0 | 0 | 204 | 89 | 0.35 | 0.099 | 1.4 | 2 | 0.1 | 0.16 | 0.03 | 2.1 | 14194 |
| **hot chocolate,** from mix w/aspartame, prep w/wtr - *1 pkt in 6 fl oz wtr* | 192 | 56 | 177.4 | 10.8 | 5.6 | | 1.2 | 138 | 92 | 33 | 0.52 | 0.100 | 0 | 0 | 0.04 | 0.2 | 0.17 | 0.57 |
| | | 2.3 | 0.4 | 0.3 | 0.1 | 0 | 0 | 405 | 134 | 0.75 | 0.127 | 2.5 | 2 | 0 | 0.21 | 0.05 | 1.9 | 14390 |
| **hot chocolate,** homemade w/ 2% milk - *8 fl oz* | 250 | 192 | 206.4 | 26.6 | 24.2 | | 2.5 | 110 | 262 | 58 | 1.58 | 0.032 | 128 | 0 | 0.10 | 0.3 | 1.05 | 0.82 |
| | | 8.8 | 5.8 | 3.6 | 1.7 | 0.1 | 20 | 492 | 262 | 1.20 | 0.258 | 6.8 | 438 | 0.1 | 0.45 | 0.10 | 12.5 | 1105 |
| **malted milk,** whole milk - *8 fl oz* | 265 | 233 | 215.7 | 27.1 | 25.3 | | 0.3 | 209 | 310 | 45 | 1.14 | 0.056 | 87 | 1 | 0.21 | 1.4 | 1.22 | 1.07 |
| | | 10.2 | 9.6 | 5.4 | 2.4 | 0.7 | 32 | 485 | 281 | 0.24 | 0.098 | 13.8 | 310 | | 0.64 | 0.17 | 21.2 | 14312 |
| **malted milk,** whole milk w/added nutrients - *8 fl oz* | 265 | 228 | 215.9 | 28.3 | 22.2 | | 0 | 191 | 326 | 40 | 1.09 | 0.098 | 745 | 28 | 0.73 | 10.6 | 1.06 | 0.94 |
| | | 9.7 | 8.5 | 4.8 | 2.1 | 0.6 | 29 | 530 | 284 | 3.60 | 0.117 | 11.1 | 2496 | | 1.21 | 0.86 | 15.9 | 14310 |
| **strawberry flavored mix** in whole milk - *8 fl oz* | 266 | 234 | 215.2 | 32.7 | | | 0 | 128 | 293 | 32 | 0.93 | 0.005 | 69 | 2 | 0.09 | 0.2 | 0.88 | 0.77 |
| | | 8.0 | 8.2 | 5.1 | 2.4 | 0.3 | 32 | 370 | 229 | 0.21 | 0.024 | 4.8 | 309 | | 0.42 | 0.10 | 13.3 | 14351 |

## 22.3 COW MILK MIXES

| | WT (g) | KCAL | H₂0 (g) | CHO (g) | TSUG (g) | ASUG (g) | DFIB (g) | Na (mg) | Ca (mg) | Mg (mg) | Zn (mg) | Mn (mg) | A (mcg RAE) | C (mg) | B-1 (mg) | NIA (mg) | B-12 (mcg) | PANT (mg) |
|---|---|---|---|---|---|---|---|---|---|---|---|---|---|---|---|---|---|---|
| | | PRO | FAT | SFA | MUFA | PUFA | CHOL | K | P | Fe | Cu | Se | A (IU) | E | B-2 | B-6 | FOL | REF |
| **carob mix** - *1 T* | 12 | 45 | 0.3 | 11.2 | | | 1.0 | 12 | 4 | 1 | 0.01 | 0.008 | 0 | 0 | 0 | 0.1 | 0 | 0 |
| | | 0.2 | 0 | 0 | 0 | 0 | 0 | 12 | 1 | 0.55 | 0.007 | 0.2 | 0 | 0 | 0.01 | 0 | | 14168 |
| **chocolate malted mix** - *3 heaping t (.7 oz)* | 21 | 86 | 0.3 | 18.3 | 14.0 | 14.5 | 1.0 | 40 | 13 | 15 | 0.17 | | 7 | 0 | 0.04 | 0.4 | 0.09 | 0.07 |
| | | 1.1 | 1.0 | 0.5 | 0.2 | 0.1 | 0 | 130 | 37 | 0.48 | 0.042 | 1.4 | 25 | 0 | 0.04 | 0.03 | 10.5 | 14317 |
| **chocolate mix** - *2 T* | 21 | 85 | 0.2 | 19.1 | 17.6 | 16.8 | 1.0 | 44 | 8 | 21 | 0.33 | 0.148 | 0 | 0 | 0.01 | 0.1 | 0 | 0.01 |
| | | 0.7 | 0.7 | 0.4 | 0.2 | 0 | 0 | 124 | 27 | 0.66 | 0.148 | 0.5 | 0 | 0.1 | 0.03 | 0 | 1.0 | 14175 |
| **chocolate mix, Nestle** NesQuik - *.6 oz* | 16 | 60 | | 14.0 | 13.0 | | | 30 | | 8 | 1.50 | | 0 | 6 | | 0.6 | | |
| | | | 0.5 | 0 | | | 0 | | 0 | | | | 0 | | | | | NTEA31 |
| **chocolate mix w/aspartame** - *.75 oz packet* | 21 | 69 | 2.7 | 10.8 | 6.9 | 0 | 2.0 | 138 | 297 | 44 | 0.76 | 0.153 | 44 | 1 | 0.02 | 0.3 | 0.43 | 0.45 |
| | | 5.2 | 0.5 | 0.4 | 0.1 | 0 | 5 | 470 | 188 | 1.62 | 0.168 | 4.5 | 147 | 0 | 0.41 | 0.02 | 6.9 | 14422 |
| **cocoa mix** - *1 oz packet (3–4 heaping t)* | 28 | 111 | 0.4 | 23.4 | 18.4 | 17.0 | 1.0 | 141 | 37 | 23 | 0.41 | 0.075 | 0 | 0 | 0.03 | 0.2 | 0.10 | 0.25 |
| | | 1.9 | 1.1 | 0.7 | 0.4 | 0 | 0 | 199 | 88 | 0.33 | 0.080 | 1.4 | 1 | 0.1 | 0.16 | 0.03 | 1.7 | 14192 |
| **cocoa mix, rich chocolate,** Carnation - *1 oz packet* | 28 | 112 | 1.0 | 21.0 | 16.8 | | 1.1 | 238 | 28 | | | | | 0 | | | | |
| | | 0.8 | 4.2 | 2.8 | | | 0 | 0 | | 0.50 | | | 3 | | | | | 14197 |

| | WT (g) | KCAL / PRO (g) | H₂O (g) / FAT (g) | CHO (g) / SFA (g) | TSUG (g) / MUFA (g) | ASUG (g) / PUFA (g) | DFIB (g) / CHOL (mg) | Na (mg) / K (mg) | Ca (mg) / P (mg) | Mg (mg) / Fe (mg) | Zn (mg) / Cu (mg) | Mn (mg) / Se (mcg) | A (mcg RAE) / A (IU) | C (mg) / E (mg ATE) | B-1 (mg) / B-2 (mg) | NIA (mg) / B-6 (mg) | B-12 (mcg) / FOL (mcg DFE) | PANT (mg) / REF |
|---|---|---|---|---|---|---|---|---|---|---|---|---|---|---|---|---|---|---|
| cocoa mix w/marshmallows, | 28 | 112 | 1.2 | 21.0 | 18.2 | | 1.0 | 224 | 22 | | | | | 0 | | | | |
| Carnation - *1 oz packet* | | 0.8 | 4.2 | 4.2 | | | 0 | | | 0.50 | | | 3 | | | | | 14195 |
| **Instant Breakfast mix**, chocolate | 37 | 132 | 2.7 | 24.5 | 24.3 | 9.9 | 0.1 | 142 | 105 | 84 | 3.16 | | 554 | 28 | 0.31 | 5.3 | 0.63 | |
| *1 packet* | | 7.4 | 0.5 | 0.2 | 0.1 | 0.1 | 4 | 350 | 158 | 4.74 | 0.527 | 4.5 | 1845 | 3.5 | 0.07 | 0.42 | 179.4 | 43205 |
| **Instant Breakfast mix** w/low cal | 20 | 72 | 1.5 | 8.2 | 7.8 | 0 | 0.4 | 143 | 100 | 82 | 3.08 | | 537 | 28 | 0.30 | 5.1 | 0.62 | |
| sweetener, choc - *1 pkt* | | 7.2 | 1.0 | 0.4 | 0.2 | 0.2 | 9 | 341 | 100 | 0.46 | 0.520 | 4.4 | 1792 | 3.4 | 0.07 | 0.40 | 170.0 | 43260 |
| **malted milk mix** | 21 | 90 | 0.4 | 15.0 | 10.0 | 0 | 0 | 85 | 63 | 20 | 0.21 | 0.050 | 13 | 1 | 0.11 | 1.1 | 0.17 | 0.13 |
| *3 heaping t (.7 oz)* | | 3.0 | 2.0 | 1.0 | 0.5 | 0.3 | 5 | 159 | 75 | 0.15 | 0.042 | 3.4 | 47 | 0.1 | 0.19 | 0.09 | 9.7 | 14311 |
| **malted milk mix** w/added | 21 | 78 | 0.7 | 17.6 | 13.3 | 9.8 | 0.4 | 54 | 79 | 13 | 0.15 | 0.068 | 666 | 27 | 0.89 | 8.9 | 0.10 | 0.20 |
| nutrients *4–5 heaping t (.7 oz)* | | 2.0 | 0.3 | 0.1 | 0.1 | 0 | 0 | 124 | 79 | 2.67 | 0.144 | 1.5 | 2222 | 0 | 0.76 | 0.89 | 9.0 | 14309 |
| **strawberry flavored mix** | 22 | 86 | 0.1 | 21.8 | 21.0 | 20.8 | 0 | 8 | 1 | 0 | 0 | 0 | 0 | 0 | 0 | 0 | 0 | 0 |
| *2–3 heaping t (.8 oz)* | | 0 | 0 | 0 | 0 | 0 | 0 | 1 | 1 | 0.10 | 0 | 0.1 | 0 | 0 | 0.02 | 0 | 0 | 14350 |

## 22.4  COW MILK YOGURT

| | WT (g) | KCAL / PRO (g) | H₂O (g) / FAT (g) | CHO (g) / SFA (g) | TSUG (g) / MUFA (g) | ASUG (g) / PUFA (g) | DFIB (g) / CHOL (mg) | Na (mg) / K (mg) | Ca (mg) / P (mg) | Mg (mg) / Fe (mg) | Zn (mg) / Cu (mg) | Mn (mg) / Se (mcg) | A (mcg RAE) / A (IU) | C (mg) / E (mg ATE) | B-1 (mg) / B-2 (mg) | NIA (mg) / B-6 (mg) | B-12 (mcg) / FOL (mcg DFE) | PANT (mg) / REF |
|---|---|---|---|---|---|---|---|---|---|---|---|---|---|---|---|---|---|---|
| **yogurt**, fruit flavors with Trix, | 113 | 100 | | 20.0 | 16.0 | | 0 | 50 | 100 | | | | | | | | | |
| Yoplait - *4 oz container* | | 4.0 | 0.5 | 0.5 | | | 2 | 160 | 80 | | | | 500 | | | | | GENM276 |
| **yogurt**, fruit flavors, Yoplait | 64 | 70 | | 13.0 | 10.0 | | 0 | 30 | 100 | | | | | 0 | | | | |
| Go-Gurt - *2.3 oz tube* | | 2.0 | 0.5 | 0 | | | 2 | 95 | 60 | 0 | | | 300 | | 0.07 | | | GENM278 |
| **yogurt**, light, fruit flavors, Yoplalt | 170 | 100 | | 19.0 | 14.0 | | 0 | 85 | 200 | | | | | 0 | | | | |
| *6 oz container* | | 5.0 | 0 | 0 | | | 2 | 250 | 150 | 0 | | | 750 | | | | | GENM280 |
| **yogurt**, lowfat (1%), strawberry, | 227 | 218 | 173.7 | 41.3 | 39.5 | | 0.5 | 118 | 284 | | | | | 0 | | | 1.20 | |
| Breyers - *8 oz container* | | 8.6 | 1.8 | 1.1 | | | 20 | 436 | 202 | 0.23 | | | 77 | | 0.43 | | | 1195 |
| **yogurt**, lowfat (1%), strawbry, | 125 | 135 | 91.6 | 27.4 | 24.5 | | 0.2 | 56 | 114 | | | | | 0 | | | 0.58 | |
| Breyers Lght N' Lively - *4.4 oz* | | 4.0 | 1.0 | 0.6 | | | 11 | 189 | 84 | 0.14 | | | 38 | | 0.18 | | | 1196 |
| **yogurt**, lowfat (1%), strawbry, | 227 | 232 | 169.8 | 45.2 | 39.0 | | 0.7 | 125 | 245 | | | | | 0 | | | 1.18 | |
| Breyers Smooth & Crmy - *8 oz* | | 8.6 | 2.0 | 1.1 | | | 20 | 402 | 177 | 0.30 | | | 70 | | 0.41 | | | 1197 |
| **yogurt**, lowfat, fruit | 227 | 232 | 169.1 | 43.2 | 43.2 | 25.9 | 0 | 132 | 345 | 34 | 1.68 | 0.148 | 23 | 2 | 0.08 | 0.2 | 1.07 | 1.11 |
| *8 oz container* | | 9.9 | 2.5 | 1.6 | 0.7 | 0.1 | 9 | 443 | 270 | 0.16 | 0.182 | 7.0 | 82 | 0 | 0.40 | 0.09 | 20.4 | 1121 |
| **yogurt**, lowfat, fruit w/low-cal | 227 | 238 | 168.2 | 42.2 | 6.6 | 0 | 0 | 132 | 345 | 36 | 1.86 | 0.148 | 297 | 2 | 0.09 | 0.2 | 1.18 | 1.23 |
| sweetener - *8 oz container* | | 11.0 | 3.2 | 2.1 | 0.9 | 0.1 | 14 | 440 | 302 | 0.16 | 0.182 | 7.0 | 1001 | 0.1 | 0.41 | 0.10 | 22.7 | 1203 |
| **yogurt**, lowfat, plain | 227 | 143 | 193.1 | 16.0 | 16.0 | 0 | 0 | 159 | 415 | 39 | 2.02 | 0.009 | 32 | 2 | 0.10 | 0.3 | 1.27 | 1.34 |
| *8 oz container* | | 11.9 | 3.5 | 2.3 | 1.0 | 0.1 | 14 | 531 | 327 | 0.18 | 0.030 | 7.5 | 116 | 0.1 | 0.49 | 0.11 | 25.0 | 1117 |
| **yogurt**, lowfat, plain, Colombo | 227 | 220 | | 42.0 | 34.0 | | 0 | 130 | 250 | | | | | 0 | | | | |
| *8 oz container* | | 8.0 | 2.5 | 1.5 | | | 15 | 390 | 200 | 0 | | | 1000 | | 0.17 | | | GENM285 |
| **yogurt**, lowfat, strawberry | 227 | 225 | 170.9 | 42.3 | 42.3 | 25.0 | 0 | 120 | 313 | 30 | 1.52 | 0.145 | 25 | 1 | 0.08 | 0.2 | 0.98 | 1.01 |
| *8 oz container* | | 9.0 | 2.6 | 1.7 | 0.7 | 0.1 | 11 | 402 | 247 | 0.14 | 0.179 | 6.4 | 91 | 0 | 0.37 | 0.08 | 20.4 | 1120 |
| **yogurt**, lowfat, vanilla | 227 | 193 | 179.3 | 31.3 | 31.3 | 19.0 | 0 | 150 | 388 | 36 | 1.88 | 0.009 | 27 | 2 | 0.10 | 0.2 | 1.20 | 1.25 |
| *8 oz container* | | 11.2 | 2.8 | 1.8 | 0.8 | 0.1 | 11 | 497 | 306 | 0.16 | 0.030 | 11.1 | 98 | 0 | 0.46 | 0.10 | 25.0 | 1119 |
| **yogurt**, nonfat, chocolate | 227 | 245 | 162.5 | 53.4 | 34.0 | 21.6 | 2.7 | 306 | 200 | 91 | 2.57 | | 0 | 0 | 0.11 | 0.5 | 1.14 | |
| *8 oz container* | | 8.0 | 0 | 0 | 0 | 0 | 2 | 770 | 377 | 0.95 | 0.474 | 15.9 | 0 | 0 | 0.49 | 0.11 | 27.2 | 1187 |
| **yogurt**, nonfat, fruit | 227 | 216 | 171.2 | 43.1 | 43.1 | 25.8 | 0 | 132 | 345 | 34 | 1.68 | 0.079 | 5 | 2 | 0.09 | 0.2 | 1.07 | |
| *8 oz container* | | 10.0 | 0.5 | 0.3 | 0.1 | 0 | 5 | 440 | 270 | 0.16 | 0.025 | 13.6 | 27 | 0.1 | 0.41 | 0.09 | 20.4 | 43261 |
| **yogurt**, nonfat, plain | 227 | 127 | 193.5 | 17.4 | 17.4 | 0 | 0 | 175 | 452 | 43 | 2.20 | 0.011 | 5 | 2 | 0.11 | 0.3 | 1.38 | 1.46 |
| *8 oz container* | | 13.0 | 0.4 | 0.3 | 0.1 | 0 | 5 | 579 | 356 | 0.20 | 0.034 | 8.2 | 16 | 0.1 | 0.53 | 0.12 | 27.2 | 1118 |
| **yogurt**, nonfat, plain, Colombo | 227 | 100 | | 16.0 | 10.0 | | 0 | 160 | 300 | 32 | | | | 0 | | | | |
| *8 oz container* | | 10.0 | 0 | 0 | | | 10 | 440 | 250 | 0 | | | 0 | | 0.42 | | | GENM287 |
| **yogurt**, nonfat, strawberry w/ | 227 | 125 | 195.2 | 22.5 | 17.5 | | 0 | 102 | 216 | | | | | 1 | | | 0.93 | |
| aspartame, Breyers Light - *8 oz* | | 7.7 | 0.5 | 0.3 | | | 11 | 331 | 154 | 0.25 | | | 9 | | 0.32 | | | 1198 |
| **yogurt**, nonfat, vanilla, Colombo | 227 | 160 | | 32.0 | 26.0 | | 0 | 140 | 250 | 24 | | | | 0 | | | | |
| *8 oz container* | | 8.0 | 0 | 0 | | | 5 | 410 | 200 | 0 | | | 0 | | 0.34 | | | GENM288 |
| **yogurt**, nonfat, vanilla/lemon w/low- | 227 | 107 | 198.5 | 17.0 | 17.0 | 0 | 0 | 134 | 325 | 30 | 1.52 | | 0 | 2 | 0.08 | 0.2 | 0.98 | |
| cal sweetener - *8 oz container* | | 8.8 | 0.4 | 0.3 | 0.1 | 0 | 5 | 402 | 247 | 0.27 | 0.179 | 7.0 | 0 | 0 | 0.37 | 0.08 | 18.2 | 1184 |
| **yogurt**, whole, plain | 227 | 138 | 199.5 | 10.6 | 10.6 | 0 | 0 | 104 | 275 | 27 | 1.34 | 0.009 | 61 | 1 | 0.07 | 0.2 | 0.84 | 0.88 |
| *8 oz container* | | 7.9 | 7.4 | 4.8 | 2.0 | 0.2 | 30 | 352 | 216 | 0.11 | 0.020 | 5.0 | 225 | 0.1 | 0.32 | 0.07 | 15.9 | 1116 |

## 22.5  OTHER MAMMAL MILKS

| | WT (g) | KCAL / PRO (g) | H₂O (g) / FAT (g) | CHO (g) / SFA (g) | TSUG (g) / MUFA (g) | ASUG (g) / PUFA (g) | DFIB (g) / CHOL (mg) | Na (mg) / K (mg) | Ca (mg) / P (mg) | Mg (mg) / Fe (mg) | Zn (mg) / Cu (mg) | Mn (mg) / Se (mcg) | A (mcg RAE) / A (IU) | C (mg) / E (mg ATE) | B-1 (mg) / B-2 (mg) | NIA (mg) / B-6 (mg) | B-12 (mcg) / FOL (mcg DFE) | PANT (mg) / REF |
|---|---|---|---|---|---|---|---|---|---|---|---|---|---|---|---|---|---|---|
| **ewe (sheep) milk** | 245 | 265 | 197.7 | 13.1 | | | 0 | 108 | 473 | 44 | 1.32 | 0.044 | 108 | 10 | 0.16 | 1.0 | 1.74 | 1.00 |
| *8 fl oz* | | 14.7 | 17.2 | 11.3 | 4.2 | 0.8 | 66 | 336 | 387 | 0.25 | 0.113 | 4.2 | 360 | | 0.87 | 0.15 | 17.2 | 1109 |
| **goat milk** | 244 | 168 | 212.4 | 10.9 | 10.9 | 0 | 0 | 122 | 327 | 34 | 0.73 | 0.044 | 139 | 3 | 0.12 | 0.7 | 0.17 | 0.76 |
| *8 fl oz* | | 8.7 | 10.1 | 6.5 | 2.7 | 0.4 | 27 | 498 | 271 | 0.12 | 0.112 | 3.4 | 483 | 0.2 | 0.34 | 0.11 | 2.4 | 1106 |

| | WT (g) | KCAL / PRO | H₂0 / FAT | CHO / SFA | TSUG / MUFA | ASUG / PUFA | DFIB / CHOL | Na / K | Ca / P | Mg / Fe | Zn / Cu | Mn / Se | A (RAE) / A (IU) | C / E | B-1 / B-2 | NIA / B-6 | B-12 / FOL | PANT / REF |
|---|---|---|---|---|---|---|---|---|---|---|---|---|---|---|---|---|---|---|
| human milk | 31 | 22 | 27.1 | 2.1 | 2.1 | 0 | 0 | 5 | 10 | 1 | 0.05 | 0.008 | 19 | 2 | 0 | 0.1 | 0.02 | 0.07 |
| *1 fl oz* | | 0.3 | 1.4 | 0.6 | 0.5 | 0.2 | 4 | 16 | 4 | 0.01 | 0.016 | 0.6 | 66 | 0 | 0.01 | 0 | 1.6 | 1107 |
| Indian buffalo milk | 244 | 237 | 203.5 | 12.6 | | | 0 | 127 | 412 | 76 | 0.54 | 0.044 | 129 | 6 | 0.13 | 0.2 | 0.88 | 0.47 |
| *8 fl oz* | | 9.2 | 16.8 | 11.2 | 4.4 | 0.4 | 46 | 434 | 285 | 0.29 | 0.112 | | 434 | | 0.33 | 0.06 | 14.6 | 1108 |

## 22.6 NON-DAIRY MILK-LIKE BEVERAGES AND YOGURTS

| | WT (g) | KCAL / PRO | H₂0 / FAT | CHO / SFA | TSUG / MUFA | ASUG / PUFA | DFIB / CHOL | Na / K | Ca / P | Mg / Fe | Zn / Cu | Mn / Se | A (RAE) / A (IU) | C / E | B-1 / B-2 | NIA / B-6 | B-12 / FOL | PANT / REF |
|---|---|---|---|---|---|---|---|---|---|---|---|---|---|---|---|---|---|---|
| soy yogurt | 262 | 246 | 203.0 | 41.8 | 3.2 | 3.1 | 0.5 | 92 | 309 | 105 | 0.81 | | 5 | 7 | 0.16 | 0.6 | 0 | |
| *1 cup* | | 9.2 | 4.7 | 0.7 | 1.0 | 2.7 | 0 | 123 | 100 | 2.78 | 0.196 | 34.1 | 86 | 0.8 | 0.05 | 0.05 | 15.7 | 43476 |
| soy yogurt, black cherry, Silk | 170 | 150 | 132.9 | 29.0 | 20.0 | | 1.0 | 20 | 299 | | | | | 30 | | | | |
| *1 container* | | 4.0 | 2.0 | 0 | | | 0 | | | 1.09 | | | 0 | | | | | 16256 |
| soy yogurt, blueberry, Silk | 170 | 150 | 132.9 | 29.0 | 21.0 | | 1.0 | 26 | 299 | | | | | 30 | | | | |
| *1 container* | | 4.0 | 2.0 | 0 | | | 0 | | | 1.09 | | | 0 | | | | | 16257 |
| soy yogurt, peach, Silk | 170 | 160 | 129.9 | 32.0 | 25.0 | | 1.0 | 26 | 299 | | | | | 30 | | | | |
| *1 container* | | 4.0 | 2.0 | 0 | | | 0 | | | 1.09 | | | 0 | | | | | 16255 |
| soy yogurt, raspberry, Silk | 170 | 150 | 131.9 | 30.0 | 22.0 | | 1.0 | 26 | 299 | | | | | 30 | | | | |
| *1 container* | | 4.0 | 2.0 | 0 | | | 0 | | | 1.09 | | | 0 | | | | | 16254 |
| soy yogurt, Silk | 227 | 150 | 192.2 | 22.0 | 12.0 | | 0.9 | 30 | 300 | | | | | 30 | | | | |
| *1 container* | | 6.0 | 4.0 | 0.5 | | | 0 | | | | | | 0 | | | | | 16252 |
| soy yogurt, strawberry, Silk | 170 | 160 | 130.9 | 31.0 | 22.0 | | 1.0 | 26 | 299 | | | | | 30 | | | | |
| *1 container* | | 4.0 | 2.0 | 0 | | | 0 | | | 1.09 | | | 0 | | | | | 16253 |
| soy yogurt, vanilla, Silk | 170 | 150 | 134.9 | 25.0 | 18.0 | | 1.0 | 20 | 299 | | | | | 30 | | | | |
| *1 container* | | 5.0 | 3.0 | 0 | | | 0 | | | 1.44 | | | 0 | | | | | 16251 |
| soymilk | 245 | 132 | 215.7 | 15.4 | 9.8 | 0 | 1.5 | 125 | 61 | 61 | 0.29 | 0.546 | 0 | 0 | 0.15 | 1.3 | 0 | 0.91 |
| *8 fl oz* | | 8.0 | 4.3 | 0.5 | 1.0 | 2.4 | 0 | 289 | 127 | 1.57 | 0.314 | 11.8 | 7 | 0.3 | 0.17 | 0.19 | 44.1 | 16120 |
| soymilk, chai, Odwalla Soy Smart | 245 | 150 | | 22.0 | 20.0 | | | 30 | 300 | 40 | | 0.600 | | | | | | |
| *8 fl oz* | | 6.0 | 4.0 | 0.5 | 0.5 | 2.5 | | 410 | 150 | 0.72 | | | | | | 0.12 | | ODWA18 |
| soymilk, chai, Silk | 243 | 129 | 212.9 | 19.0 | 14.0 | | 0 | 100 | 299 | | 0.90 | | | 0 | | | | 0.90 |
| *8 fl oz* | | 6.0 | 3.5 | 0.5 | | | 0 | 299 | | 1.07 | | 0 | 299 | | 0.34 | | | 16247 |
| soymilk, chocolate, Odwalla Super Protein | 245 | 170 | | 24.0 | 20.0 | | | 240 | 350 | 60 | 3.00 | 0.700 | | | | | | 6.00 |
| *8 fl oz* | | 10.0 | 3.5 | 0.5 | | | | 470 | 300 | 2.70 | 0.400 | | | | | 2.00 | | ODWA28 |
| soymilk, chocolate, Silk | 243 | 141 | 209.9 | 23.0 | 19.0 | | 1.9 | 100 | 299 | 39 | 0.61 | | | 0 | | | | 2.99 |
| *8 fl oz* | | 5.0 | 3.5 | 0.5 | | | 0 | 350 | | 1.43 | | 4.1 | 501 | | 0.51 | | | 16237 |
| soymilk, chocolate, unfortified | 243 | 153 | 208.0 | 24.2 | 19.1 | 9.8 | 1.0 | 129 | 61 | 36 | 0.83 | | 0 | 4 | 0.05 | 1.2 | 1.70 | 0.22 |
| *8 fl oz* | | 5.5 | 3.7 | 0.6 | 0.9 | 2.0 | 0 | 347 | 124 | 1.17 | 0.501 | 11.7 | 7 | 0 | 0.64 | 0.19 | 26.7 | 16166 |
| soymilk, mocha, Silk | 243 | 141 | 210.9 | 22.0 | 18.0 | | 0 | 100 | 299 | 0 | 0.90 | | | 0 | | | | 0.90 |
| *8 fl oz* | | 5.0 | 3.5 | 0.5 | | | 0 | 299 | | 1.07 | | 0 | 299 | | 0.34 | | | 16248 |
| soymilk, Odwalla Super Protein | 245 | 190 | | 35.0 | 29.0 | | 1.0 | 180 | 350 | 40 | 3.00 | | | | | | | |
| *8 fl oz* | | 10.0 | 1.0 | | | | | 420 | | 1.80 | | | | | | 3.00 | | ODWA26 |
| soymilk, pumpkin, Odwalla Super Protein - 8 fl oz | 245 | 160 | | 22.0 | 17.0 | | | 115 | 350 | 40 | 3.00 | 0.400 | | | | | | 6.00 |
| | | 10.0 | 3.5 | 0.5 | | | | 390 | 150 | 1.44 | 0.200 | | | | | 2.00 | | ODWA27 |
| soymilk, Silk | 243 | 100 | 222.4 | 8.0 | 6.0 | | 1.0 | 119 | 299 | 39 | 0.61 | | | 0 | | | | 2.99 |
| *8 fl oz* | | 7.0 | 4.0 | 0.5 | | | 0 | 299 | | 1.07 | | 5.6 | 501 | | 0.51 | | | 16235 |
| soymilk, vanilla al'mondo, Odwalla Super Protein - 8 fl oz | 245 | 190 | | 25.0 | 19.0 | | | 80 | 350 | 40 | 3.00 | | | | | | | 6.00 |
| | | 10.0 | 6.0 | 1.0 | | | | 390 | | 1.08 | | | | | | 2.00 | | ODWA29 |
| soymilk, vanilla, Silk | 243 | 100 | 221.9 | 10.0 | 7.0 | | 1.0 | 95 | 299 | 39 | 0.61 | | | 0 | | | | 2.99 |
| *8 fl oz* | | 6.0 | 3.5 | 0.5 | | | 0 | 299 | | 1.07 | | 5.6 | 501 | | 0.51 | | | 16236 |

## 23. NUTS AND SEEDS
### 23.1 NUTS, NUT PRODUCTS, AND NUT-LIKE PRODUCTS

| | WT (g) | KCAL / PRO | H₂0 / FAT | CHO / SFA | TSUG / MUFA | ASUG / PUFA | DFIB / CHOL | Na / K | Ca / P | Mg / Fe | Zn / Cu | Mn / Se | A (RAE) / A (IU) | C / E | B-1 / B-2 | NIA / B-6 | B-12 / FOL | PANT / REF |
|---|---|---|---|---|---|---|---|---|---|---|---|---|---|---|---|---|---|---|
| acorn flour, full-fat | 100 | 501 | 6.0 | 54.6 | | | | 0 | 43 | 110 | 0.64 | 1.743 | 3 | 0 | 0.15 | 2.4 | 0 | 0.93 |
| *3.5 oz* | | 7.5 | 30.2 | 3.9 | 19.1 | 5.8 | 0 | 712 | 103 | 1.21 | 0.611 | | 51 | | 0.15 | 0.69 | 114.0 | 12060 |
| acorns, dried | 28 | 143 | 1.4 | 15.0 | | | | 0 | 15 | 23 | 0.19 | 0.382 | 0 | 0 | 0.04 | 0.7 | 0 | 0.26 |
| *1 oz* | | 2.3 | 8.8 | 1.1 | 5.6 | 1.7 | 0 | 199 | 29 | 0.29 | 0.229 | | 0 | | 0.04 | 0.19 | 32.2 | 12059 |
| acorns, raw | 28 | 108 | 7.8 | 11.4 | | | | 0 | 11 | 17 | 0.14 | 0.374 | 1 | 0 | 0.03 | 0.5 | 0 | 0.20 |
| *1 oz* | | 1.7 | 6.7 | 0.9 | 4.2 | 1.3 | 0 | 151 | 22 | 0.22 | 0.174 | | 11 | | 0.03 | 0.15 | 24.4 | 12058 |
| almond butter | 16 | 101 | 0.2 | 3.4 | | | 0.6 | 2 | 43 | 48 | 0.49 | 0.377 | 0 | 0 | 0.02 | 0.5 | 0 | 0.04 |
| *1 T* | | 2.4 | 9.5 | 0.9 | 6.1 | 2.0 | 0 | 121 | 84 | 0.59 | 0.144 | | 0 | | 0.10 | 0.01 | 10.4 | 12195 |
| almond paste | 28 | 128 | 3.9 | 13.4 | 10.2 | 9.4 | 1.3 | 3 | 48 | 36 | 0.41 | 0.240 | 0 | 0 | 0.02 | 0.4 | 0 | 0.03 |
| *1 oz* | | 2.5 | 7.8 | 0.7 | 5.0 | 1.6 | 0 | 88 | 72 | 0.45 | 0.127 | 1.2 | 0 | 3.8 | 0.12 | 0.01 | 20.4 | 12071 |
| almonds, dry-roasted | 28 | 167 | 0.7 | 5.4 | 1.4 | 0 | 3.3 | 0 | 74 | 80 | 0.99 | 0.734 | 0 | 0 | 0.02 | 1.1 | 0 | 0.06 |
| *1 oz (~22 nuts)* | | 6.2 | 14.8 | 1.1 | 9.4 | 3.5 | 0 | 209 | 137 | 1.26 | 0.328 | 0.8 | 0 | 7.3 | 0.24 | 0.04 | 9.2 | 12063 |

| | WT (g) | Macronutrients | | | | | | Minerals | | | | | Vitamins | | | | | |
|---|---|---|---|---|---|---|---|---|---|---|---|---|---|---|---|---|---|---|
| | | KCAL | H₂0 (g) | CHO (g) | TSUG (g) | ASUG (g) | DFIB (g) | Na (mg) | Ca (mg) | Mg (mg) | Zn (mg) | Mn (mg) | A (mcg RAE) | C (mg) | B-1 (mg) | NIA (mg) | B-12 (mcg) | PANT (mg) |
| | | PRO (g) | FAT (g) | SFA (g) | MUFA (g) | PUFA (g) | CHOL (mg) | K (mg) | P (mg) | Fe (mg) | Cu (mg) | Se (mcg) | A (IU) | E (mg ATE) | B-2 (mg) | B-6 (mg) | FOL (mcg DFE) | REF |
| **almonds**, honey-roasted | 28 | 166 | 0.5 | 7.8 | | | 3.8 | 36 | 74 | 67 | 0.73 | 0.561 | 0 | 0 | 0.03 | 0.8 | 0 | 0.07 |
| *1 oz (~22 nuts)* | | 5.1 | 14.0 | 1.3 | 9.1 | 2.9 | 0 | 157 | 112 | 0.79 | 0.272 | | 0 | | 0.27 | 0.02 | 9.0 | 12206 |
| **almonds**, oil-roasted | 28 | 170 | 0.8 | 5.0 | 1.3 | 0 | 2.9 | 0 | 81 | 77 | 0.86 | 0.689 | 0 | 0 | 0.03 | 1.0 | 0 | 0.06 |
| *1 oz (22 nuts)* | | 5.9 | 15.4 | 1.2 | 9.7 | 3.8 | 0 | 196 | 130 | 1.03 | 0.267 | 0.8 | 0 | 7.3 | 0.22 | 0.03 | 7.6 | 12065 |
| **almonds**, raw | 28 | 161 | 1.3 | 6.1 | 1.1 | 0 | 3.4 | 0 | 74 | 75 | 0.86 | 0.640 | 0 | 0 | 0.06 | 0.9 | 0 | 0.13 |
| *1 oz* | | 5.9 | 13.8 | 1.0 | 8.6 | 3.4 | 0 | 197 | 136 | 1.04 | 0.279 | 0.7 | 0 | 7.3 | 0.28 | 0.04 | 14.0 | 12061 |
| **almonds**, sugar-coated | 3.5 | 17 | 0.1 | 2.4 | 2.2 | 1.7 | 0.1 | 0 | 4 | 5 | 0.05 | 0.039 | 0 | 0 | 0 | 0 | 0 | 0.01 |
| *1 piece* | | 0.4 | 0.6 | 0.1 | 0.4 | 0.1 | 0 | 9 | 6 | 0.07 | 0.021 | 0.1 | 0 | 0.4 | 0.01 | 0 | 0.5 | 19858 |
| **beechnuts**, dried | 28 | 161 | 1.8 | 9.4 | | | | 11 | 0 | 0 | 0.10 | 0.375 | 0 | 4 | 0.09 | 0.2 | 0 | 0.26 |
| *1 oz* | | 1.7 | 14.0 | 1.6 | 6.1 | 5.6 | 0 | 285 | 0 | 0.69 | 0.188 | | 0 | | 0.10 | 0.19 | 31.6 | 12077 |
| **brazilnuts**, raw | 28 | 184 | 1.0 | 3.4 | 0.7 | 0 | 2.1 | 1 | 45 | 105 | 1.14 | 0.342 | 0 | 0 | 0.17 | 0.1 | 0 | 0.05 |
| *1 oz (6–8 nuts)* | | 4.0 | 18.6 | 4.2 | 6.9 | 5.8 | 0 | 185 | 203 | 0.68 | 0.488 | 536.8 | 0 | 1.6 | 0.01 | 0.03 | 6.2 | 12078 |
| **butternuts**, dried | 28 | 171 | 0.9 | 3.4 | | | 1.3 | 0 | 15 | 66 | 0.88 | 1.837 | 2 | 1 | 0.11 | 0.3 | 0 | 0.18 |
| *1 oz (about 9 nuts)* | | 7.0 | 16.0 | 0.4 | 2.9 | 12.0 | 0 | 118 | 125 | 1.13 | 0.126 | 4.8 | 35 | | 0.04 | 0.16 | 18.5 | 12084 |
| **cashew butter** | 16 | 94 | 0.5 | 4.4 | | | 0.3 | 2 | 7 | 41 | 0.83 | 0.130 | 0 | 0 | 0.05 | 0.3 | 0 | 0.19 |
| *1 T* | | 2.8 | 7.9 | 1.6 | 4.7 | 1.3 | 0 | 87 | 73 | 0.80 | 0.350 | 1.8 | 0 | | 0.03 | 0.04 | 10.9 | 12088 |
| **cashews**, dry-roasted | 28 | 161 | 0.5 | 9.2 | 1.4 | 0 | 0.8 | 4 | 13 | 73 | 1.57 | 0.231 | 0 | 0 | 0.06 | 0.4 | 0 | 0.34 |
| *1 oz* | | 4.3 | 13.0 | 2.6 | 7.6 | 2.2 | 0 | 158 | 137 | 1.68 | 0.622 | 3.3 | 0 | 0.3 | 0.06 | 0.07 | 19.3 | 12085 |
| **cashews**, oil-roasted | 28 | 162 | 1.0 | 8.4 | 1.4 | 0 | 0.9 | 4 | 12 | 76 | 1.50 | 0.467 | 0 | 0 | 0.10 | 0.5 | 0 | 0.25 |
| *1 oz (18 nuts)* | | 4.7 | 13.4 | 2.4 | 7.3 | 2.4 | 0 | 177 | 149 | 1.69 | 0.572 | 5.7 | 0 | 0.3 | 0.06 | 0.09 | 7.0 | 12086 |
| **cashews**, raw | 28 | 155 | 1.5 | 8.5 | 1.7 | 0 | 0.9 | 4 | 10 | 82 | 1.62 | 0.463 | 0 | 0 | 0.12 | 0.3 | 0 | 0.24 |
| *1 oz* | | 5.1 | 12.3 | 2.2 | 6.7 | 2.2 | 0 | 185 | 166 | 1.87 | 0.615 | 5.6 | 0 | 0.3 | 0.02 | 0.12 | 7.0 | 12087 |
| **chestnuts, Chinese**, boiled, steamed | 28 | 43 | 17.2 | 9.4 | | | | 1 | 3 | 16 | 0.17 | 0.307 | 2 | 7 | 0.03 | 0.2 | 0 | 0.11 |
| *1 oz* | | 0.8 | 0.2 | 0 | 0.1 | 0.1 | 0 | 86 | 18 | 0.27 | 0.070 | | 39 | | 0.03 | 0.08 | 12.9 | 12095 |
| **chestnuts, Chinese**, dried | 28 | 102 | 2.5 | 22.3 | | | | 1 | 8 | 38 | 0.39 | 0.728 | 4 | 16 | 0.07 | 0.4 | 0 | 0.25 |
| *1 oz* | | 1.9 | 0.5 | 0.1 | 0.3 | 0.1 | 0 | 203 | 43 | 0.64 | 0.165 | | 92 | | 0.08 | 0.19 | 30.8 | 12094 |
| **chestnuts, Chinese**, raw | 28 | 63 | 12.3 | 13.7 | | | | 1 | 5 | 24 | 0.24 | 0.448 | 3 | 10 | 0.04 | 0.2 | 0 | 0.16 |
| *1 oz* | | 1.2 | 0.3 | 0 | 0.2 | 0.1 | 0 | 125 | 27 | 0.39 | 0.102 | | 57 | | 0.05 | 0.11 | 19.0 | 12093 |
| **chestnuts, Chinese**, roasted | 28 | 67 | 11.3 | 14.7 | | | | 1 | 5 | 25 | 0.26 | 0.478 | 0 | 11 | 0.04 | 0.4 | 0 | 0.17 |
| *1 oz* | | 1.3 | 0.3 | 0 | 0.2 | 0.1 | 0 | 134 | 29 | 0.42 | 0.108 | | 1 | | 0.03 | 0.12 | 20.2 | 12096 |
| **chestnuts, European**, boiled, steamed | 28 | 37 | 19.1 | 7.8 | | | | 8 | 13 | 15 | 0.07 | 0.239 | 0 | 7 | 0.04 | 0.2 | 0 | 0.09 |
| *1 oz* | | 0.6 | 0.4 | 0.1 | 0.1 | 0.2 | 0 | 200 | 28 | 0.48 | 0.132 | | 5 | | 0.03 | 0.07 | 10.6 | 12101 |
| **chestnuts, European**, dried | 28 | 105 | 2.6 | 21.6 | | | 3.3 | 10 | 19 | 21 | 0.10 | 0.364 | 0 | 4 | 0.08 | 0.2 | 0 | 0.25 |
| *1 oz* | | 1.8 | 1.2 | 0.2 | 0.4 | 0.5 | 0 | 276 | 49 | 0.67 | 0.182 | 0.5 | 0 | | 0.10 | 0.19 | 30.5 | 12099 |
| **chestnuts, European**, raw | 28 | 60 | 13.6 | 12.8 | | | 2.3 | 1 | 8 | 9 | 0.15 | 0.267 | 0 | 12 | 0.07 | 0.3 | 0 | 0.14 |
| *1 oz* | | 0.7 | 0.6 | 0.1 | 0.2 | 0.3 | 0 | 145 | 26 | 0.28 | 0.125 | | 8 | | 0.05 | 0.11 | 17.4 | 12097 |
| **chestnuts, European**, roasted | 28 | 69 | 11.3 | 14.8 | 3.0 | 0 | 1.4 | 1 | 8 | 9 | 0.16 | 0.330 | 0 | 7 | 0.07 | 0.4 | 0 | 0.16 |
| *1 oz (3 nuts)* | | 0.9 | 0.6 | 0.1 | 0.2 | 0.2 | 0 | 166 | 30 | 0.25 | 0.142 | 0.3 | 7 | 0.1 | 0.05 | 0.14 | 19.6 | 12167 |
| **chestnuts, Japanese**, boiled, steamed | 28 | 16 | 24.1 | 3.5 | | | | 1 | 3 | 5 | 0.11 | 0.161 | 0 | 3 | 0.04 | 0.2 | 0 | 0.02 |
| *1 oz* | | 0.2 | 0.1 | 0 | 0 | 0 | 0 | 33 | 7 | 0.15 | 0.057 | | 4 | | 0.02 | 0.03 | 4.8 | 12203 |
| **chestnuts, Japanese**, dried | 28 | 101 | 2.8 | 22.8 | | | | 10 | 20 | 32 | 0.72 | 1.039 | 1 | 17 | 0.22 | 1.0 | 0 | 0.13 |
| *1 oz* | | 1.5 | 0.3 | 0.1 | 0.2 | 0.1 | 0 | 215 | 47 | 0.95 | 0.367 | | 24 | | 0.11 | 0.18 | 30.5 | 12175 |
| **chestnuts, Japanese**, raw | 28 | 43 | 17.2 | 9.8 | | | | 4 | 9 | 14 | 0.31 | 0.445 | 1 | 7 | 0.10 | 0.4 | 0 | 0.06 |
| *1 oz* | | 0.6 | 0.1 | 0 | 0.1 | 0 | 0 | 92 | 20 | 0.41 | 0.157 | | 10 | | 0.05 | 0.08 | 13.2 | 12202 |
| **chestnuts, Japanese**, roasted | 28 | 56 | 14.0 | 12.6 | | | | 5 | 10 | 18 | 0.40 | 0.578 | 1 | 8 | 0.13 | 0.2 | 0 | 0.13 |
| *1 oz* | | 0.8 | 0.2 | 0 | 0.1 | 0.1 | 0 | 120 | 26 | 0.59 | 0.204 | | 21 | | 0.12 | 0.12 | 16.5 | 12204 |
| **coconut cream**, raw | 240 | 792 | 129.4 | 16.0 | | | 5.3 | 10 | 26 | 67 | 2.30 | 3.130 | 0 | 7 | 0.07 | 2.1 | 0 | 0.63 |
| *8 fl oz* | | 8.7 | 83.2 | 73.8 | 3.5 | 0.9 | 0 | 780 | 293 | 5.47 | 0.907 | | 0 | 0 | 0.11 | | 55.2 | 12115 |
| **coconut cream**, sweetened, canned | 296 | 1057 | 85.8 | 157.5 | 152.4 | 0 | 0.6 | 107 | 12 | 50 | 1.78 | 2.412 | 0 | 0 | 0.07 | 0.1 | 0 | 0.48 |
| *8 fl oz* | | 3.5 | 48.3 | 45.8 | 2.0 | 0.5 | 0 | 299 | 65 | 0.38 | 0.699 | 16.3 | 0 | 0.4 | 0.12 | 0.09 | 41.4 | 12116 |
| **coconut**, dried | 28 | 185 | 0.8 | 6.6 | 2.1 | 0 | 4.6 | 10 | 7 | 25 | 0.56 | 0.769 | 0 | 0 | 0.02 | 0.2 | 0 | 0.22 |
| *1 oz* | | 1.9 | 18.1 | 16.0 | 0.8 | 0.2 | 0 | 152 | 58 | 0.93 | 0.223 | 5.2 | 0 | 0.1 | 0.03 | 0.08 | 2.5 | 12108 |
| **coconut**, dried, creamed | 28 | 192 | 0.5 | 6.0 | | | | 10 | 7 | 26 | 0.57 | 0.779 | 0 | 0 | 0.02 | 0.2 | 0 | 0.23 |
| *1 oz* | | 1.5 | 19.3 | 17.2 | 0.8 | 0.2 | 0 | 154 | 59 | 0.94 | 0.226 | | 0 | | 0.03 | 0.09 | 2.5 | 12177 |
| **coconut**, dried, sweetened, flaked, canned - *1 oz* | 28 | 124 | 6.5 | 11.5 | | | 1.3 | 6 | 4 | 14 | 0.45 | 0.608 | 0 | 0 | 0.01 | 0.1 | 0 | 0.18 |
| | | 0.9 | 8.9 | 7.9 | 0.4 | 0.1 | 0 | 91 | 29 | 0.52 | 0.086 | | 0 | | 0.01 | 0.07 | 2.0 | 12110 |
| **coconut**, dried, sweetened, flaked, packaged - *1 oz* | 28 | 128 | 4.3 | 14.5 | 10.3 | 10.1 | 2.8 | 80 | 3 | 14 | 0.20 | 0.269 | 0 | 0 | 0 | 0.2 | 0 | 0.04 |
| | | 0.9 | 7.8 | 7.4 | 0.4 | 0.1 | 0 | 101 | 28 | 0.42 | 0.083 | 4.5 | 0 | 0 | 0 | 0.01 | 0.8 | 12109 |
| **coconut**, dried, sweetened, shredded | 28 | 140 | 3.5 | 13.3 | 12.1 | 10.0 | 1.3 | 73 | 4 | 14 | 0.51 | 0.693 | 0 | 0 | 0.01 | 0.1 | 0 | 0.20 |
| *1 oz* | | 0.8 | 9.9 | 8.8 | 0.4 | 0.1 | 0 | 94 | 30 | 0.54 | 0.088 | 4.7 | 0 | 0.1 | 0.01 | 0.08 | 2.2 | 12179 |
| **coconut**, dried, toasted | 28 | 166 | 0.3 | 12.4 | | | | 10 | 8 | 26 | 0.57 | 0.784 | 0 | 0 | 0.02 | 0.2 | 0 | 0.23 |
| *1 oz* | | 1.5 | 13.2 | 11.7 | 0.6 | 0.1 | 0 | 155 | 59 | 0.95 | 0.227 | | 0 | | 0.03 | 0.09 | 2.5 | 12114 |

| | WT (g) | KCAL | H₂0 (g) | CHO (g) | TSUG (g) | ASUG (g) | DFIB (g) | Na (mg) | Ca (mg) | Mg (mg) | Zn (mg) | Mn (mg) | A (mcg RAE) | C (mg) | B-1 (mg) | NIA (mg) | B-12 (mcg) | PANT (mg) |
|---|---|---|---|---|---|---|---|---|---|---|---|---|---|---|---|---|---|---|
| | | PRO (g) | FAT (g) | SFA (g) | MUFA (g) | PUFA (g) | CHOL (mg) | K (mg) | P (mg) | Fe (mg) | Cu (mg) | Se (mcg) | A (IU) | E (mg ATE) | B-2 (mg) | B-6 (mg) | FOL (mcg DFE) | REF |
| **coconut milk**, canned | 226 | 445 | 164.7 | 6.4 | | | | 29 | 41 | 104 | 1.27 | 1.736 | 0 | 2 | 0.05 | 1.4 | 0 | 0.35 |
| *8 fl oz* | | 4.6 | 48.2 | 42.7 | 2.0 | 0.5 | 0 | 497 | 217 | 7.46 | 0.504 | | 0 | 0 | 0.06 | | 31.6 | 12118 |
| **coconut milk**, frozen | 240 | 485 | 171.4 | 13.4 | | | | 29 | 10 | 77 | 1.42 | 1.942 | 0 | 3 | 0.06 | 1.6 | 0 | 0.39 |
| *8 fl oz* | | 3.9 | 49.9 | 44.3 | 2.1 | 0.5 | 0 | 557 | 142 | 1.94 | 0.564 | | 0 | 0 | 0.07 | | 33.6 | 12176 |
| coconut milk, raw | 240 | 552 | 162.3 | 13.3 | 8.0 | 0 | 5.3 | 36 | 38 | 89 | 1.61 | 2.198 | 0 | 7 | 0.06 | 1.8 | 0 | 0.44 |
| *8 fl oz* | | 5.5 | 57.2 | 50.7 | 2.4 | 0.6 | 0 | 631 | 240 | 3.94 | 0.638 | 14.9 | 0 | 0.4 | 0 | 0.08 | 38.4 | 12117 |
| coconut, raw | 45 | 159 | 21.1 | 6.9 | 2.8 | 0 | 4.0 | 9 | 6 | 14 | 0.50 | 0.675 | 0 | 1 | 0.03 | 0.2 | 0 | 0.14 |
| *1.6 oz piece (2"×2"×½")* | | 1.5 | 15.1 | 13.4 | 0.6 | 0.2 | 0 | 160 | 51 | 1.09 | 0.196 | 4.5 | 0 | 0.1 | 0.01 | 0.02 | 11.7 | 12104 |
| coconut water | 240 | 46 | 228.0 | 8.9 | 6.3 | 0 | 2.6 | 252 | 58 | 60 | 0.24 | 0.341 | 0 | 6 | 0.07 | 0.2 | 0 | 0.10 |
| *8 fl oz* | | 1.7 | 0.5 | 0.4 | 0 | 0 | 0 | 600 | 48 | 0.70 | 0.096 | 2.4 | 0 | 0 | 0.14 | 0.08 | 7.2 | 12119 |
| **CornNuts** | 28 | 125 | 0.4 | 20.1 | 0.2 | | 1.9 | 154 | 3 | 32 | 0.50 | 0.127 | 0 | 0 | 0.01 | 0.5 | 0 | 0.10 |
| *1 oz* | | 2.4 | 4.4 | 0.7 | 2.6 | 0.9 | 0 | 78 | 77 | 0.47 | 0.032 | 4.1 | 0 | 0.6 | 0.04 | 0.06 | 0 | 19009 |
| **CornNuts**, barbeque | 28 | 122 | 0.4 | 20.1 | | | 2.4 | 273 | 5 | 31 | 0.53 | 0.136 | 5 | 0 | 0.10 | 0.4 | 0 | 0.10 |
| *1 oz* | | 2.5 | 4.0 | 0.7 | 2.1 | 0.9 | 0 | 80 | 79 | 0.48 | 0.038 | | 95 | | 0.04 | 0.05 | 0 | 19401 |
| **CornNuts**, nacho | 28 | 123 | 0.6 | 20.0 | | | 2.2 | 178 | 10 | 31 | 0.50 | 0.115 | 1 | 4 | 0.10 | 0.3 | 0 | 0.15 |
| *1 oz* | | 2.6 | 4.0 | 0.7 | 2.0 | 0.9 | 1 | 87 | 87 | 0.47 | 0.043 | | 11 | | 0.02 | 0.06 | 4.2 | 19402 |
| **filbert (hazelnut) spread**, chocolate | 37 | 200 | 0.4 | 23.0 | 20.0 | 18.8 | 2.0 | 15 | 40 | 24 | 0.39 | 0.321 | 0 | 0 | 0.03 | 0.2 | 0.10 | 0.13 |
| *2 T* | | 2.0 | 11.0 | 10.5 | 0 | 0 | 0 | 151 | 56 | 1.62 | 0.174 | 1.3 | 1 | 1.8 | 0.06 | 0.03 | 5.2 | 19125 |
| **filberts (hazelnuts)**, dried | 28 | 176 | 1.5 | 4.7 | 1.2 | 0 | 2.7 | 0 | 32 | 46 | 0.69 | 1.729 | 0 | 2 | 0.18 | 0.5 | 0 | 0.26 |
| *1 oz (20 nuts)* | | 4.2 | 17.0 | 1.2 | 12.8 | 2.2 | 0 | 190 | 81 | 1.32 | 0.483 | 0.7 | 6 | 4.2 | 0.03 | 0.16 | 31.6 | 12120 |
| **filberts (hazelnuts)**, dry-roasted | 28 | 181 | 0.7 | 4.9 | 1.4 | | 2.6 | 0 | 34 | 48 | 0.70 | 1.554 | 1 | 1 | 0.09 | 0.6 | 0 | 0.26 |
| *1 oz* | | 4.2 | 17.5 | 1.3 | 13.1 | 2.4 | 0 | 211 | 87 | 1.23 | 0.490 | 1.1 | 17 | 4.3 | 0.03 | 0.17 | 24.6 | 12122 |
| **ginkgo nuts**, canned | 28 | 31 | 20.4 | 6.2 | | | 2.6 | 86 | 1 | 4 | 0.06 | 0.019 | 5 | 3 | 0.04 | 1.0 | 0 | 0.03 |
| *1 oz (14 nuts)* | | 0.6 | 0.5 | 0.1 | 0.2 | 0.2 | 0 | 50 | 15 | 0.08 | 0.046 | 0.1 | 94 | | 0.02 | 0.06 | 9.2 | 12129 |
| **ginkgo nuts**, dried | 28 | 97 | 3.5 | 20.3 | | | | 4 | 6 | 15 | 0.19 | 0.062 | 15 | 8 | 0.12 | 3.3 | 0 | 0.38 |
| *1 oz* | | 2.9 | 0.6 | 0.1 | 0.2 | 0.2 | 0 | 279 | 75 | 0.45 | 0.150 | | 305 | | 0.05 | 0.18 | 29.7 | 12128 |
| **ginkgo nuts**, raw | 28 | 51 | 15.5 | 10.5 | | | | 2 | 1 | 8 | 0.10 | 0.032 | 8 | 4 | 0.06 | 1.7 | 0 | 0.04 |
| *1 oz* | | 1.2 | 0.5 | 0.1 | 0.2 | 0.2 | 0 | 143 | 35 | 0.28 | 0.077 | | 156 | | 0.03 | 0.09 | 15.1 | 12127 |
| **hickorynuts**, dried | 28 | 184 | 0.7 | 5.1 | | | 1.8 | 0 | 17 | 48 | 1.21 | 1.291 | 2 | 1 | 0.24 | 0.3 | 0 | 0.49 |
| *1 oz (~9–10 nuts)* | | 3.6 | 18.0 | 2.0 | 9.1 | 6.1 | 0 | 122 | 94 | 0.59 | 0.207 | 2.3 | 37 | | 0.04 | 0.05 | 11.2 | 12130 |
| **macadamia nuts**, butter candy-glazed, Mauna Loa - ¼ cup (1 oz) | 28 | 190 | | 10.0 | 6.0 | | 1.0 | 55 | | | | | | | | | | |
| | | 2.0 | 15.0 | 2.5 | | | | | | | | | | | | | | MAUN10 |
| **macadamia nuts**, dry-roasted | 28 | 201 | 0.5 | 3.7 | 1.2 | | 2.2 | 1 | 20 | 33 | 0.36 | 0.850 | 0 | 0 | 0.20 | 0.6 | 0 | 0.17 |
| *1 oz (10–12 nuts)* | | 2.2 | 21.3 | 3.3 | 16.6 | 0.4 | 0 | 102 | 55 | 0.74 | 0.160 | 3.3 | 0 | 0.2 | 0.02 | 0.10 | 2.8 | 12132 |
| **macadamia nuts**, honey-roasted, Mauna Loa - ¼ cup (1 oz) | 28 | 210 | | 6.0 | 4.0 | | 2.0 | 35 | | | | | | | | | | |
| | | 2.0 | 21.0 | 2.5 | | | 0 | | | | | | | | | | | MAUN8 |
| **macadamia nuts**, kona coffee-glazed, Mauna Loa - ¼ cup (1 oz) | 28 | 190 | | 10.0 | 6.0 | | 1.0 | 55 | | | | | | | | | | |
| | | 2.0 | 15.0 | 2.5 | | | | | | | | | | | | | | MAUN9 |
| **macadamia nuts**, raw | 28 | 201 | 0.4 | 3.9 | 1.3 | | 2.4 | 1 | 24 | 36 | 0.36 | 1.157 | 0 | 0 | 0.33 | 0.7 | 0 | 0.21 |
| *1 oz (10–12 nuts)* | | 2.2 | 21.2 | 3.4 | 16.5 | 0.4 | 0 | 103 | 53 | 1.03 | 0.212 | 1.0 | 0 | 0.2 | 0.05 | 0.08 | 3.1 | 12131 |
| **mixed nuts**, dry-roasted | 28 | 166 | 0.5 | 7.1 | | | 2.5 | 3 | 20 | 63 | 1.06 | 0.542 | 0 | 0 | 0.06 | 1.3 | 0 | 0.34 |
| *1 oz* | | 4.8 | 14.4 | 1.9 | 8.8 | 3.0 | 0 | 167 | 122 | 1.04 | 0.358 | | 4 | | 0.06 | 0.08 | 14.0 | 12135 |
| **mixed nuts**, oil-roasted | 28 | 173 | 0.6 | 6.0 | | | 2.8 | 3 | 30 | 66 | 1.42 | 0.530 | 0 | 0 | 0.14 | 1.4 | 0 | 0.35 |
| *1 oz* | | 4.7 | 15.8 | 2.4 | 8.9 | 3.7 | 0 | 163 | 130 | 0.90 | 0.465 | | 5 | | 0.06 | 0.07 | 23.2 | 12137 |
| **mixed nuts** w/o peanuts, oil-roasted | 28 | 172 | 0.9 | 6.2 | | | 1.5 | 3 | 30 | 70 | 1.30 | 0.433 | 0 | 0 | 0.14 | 0.5 | 0 | 0.27 |
| *1 oz* | | 4.3 | 15.7 | 2.5 | 9.3 | 3.2 | 0 | 152 | 126 | 0.72 | 0.503 | | 6 | | 0.14 | 0.05 | 15.7 | 12138 |
| **peanut butter**, chunk style/crunchy | 32 | 188 | 0.4 | 6.9 | 2.7 | | 2.6 | 156 | 14 | 51 | 0.89 | 0.576 | 0 | 0 | 0.03 | 4.4 | 0 | 0.36 |
| *2 T* | | 7.7 | 16.0 | 2.6 | 7.9 | 4.7 | 0 | 238 | 102 | 0.61 | 0.185 | 2.6 | 0 | 2.0 | 0.04 | 0.13 | 29.4 | 16097 |
| **peanut butter**, smooth | 32 | 188 | 0.6 | 6.3 | 3.0 | 1.0 | 1.9 | 147 | 14 | 49 | 0.93 | 0.469 | 0 | 0 | 0.02 | 4.3 | 0 | 0.34 |
| *2 T* | | 8.0 | 16.1 | 3.4 | 7.7 | 4.5 | 0 | 208 | 115 | 0.60 | 0.151 | 1.8 | 0 | 2.9 | 0.03 | 0.17 | 23.7 | 16098 |
| **peanut flour**, lowfat | 60 | 257 | 4.7 | 18.8 | | | 9.5 | 1 | 78 | 29 | 3.59 | 2.539 | 0 | 0 | 0.27 | 6.9 | 0 | 0.93 |
| *1 cup* | | 20.3 | 13.1 | 1.8 | 6.5 | 4.2 | 0 | 815 | 305 | 2.84 | 1.223 | 4.3 | 0 | | 0.10 | 0.18 | 79.8 | 16100 |
| **peanuts**, all types, boiled | 28 | 89 | 11.7 | 6.0 | 0.7 | 0 | 2.5 | 210 | 15 | 29 | 0.51 | 0.286 | 0 | 0 | 0.07 | 1.5 | 0 | 0.23 |
| *½ cup (33 nuts)* | | 3.8 | 6.2 | 0.9 | 3.1 | 1.9 | 0 | 50 | 55 | 0.28 | 0.140 | 1.2 | 0 | 1.1 | 0.02 | 0.04 | 21.0 | 16088 |
| **peanuts**, all types, dry-roasted, salted | 28 | 164 | 0.4 | 6.0 | 1.2 | 0 | 2.2 | 228 | 15 | 49 | 0.93 | 0.583 | 0 | 0 | 0.12 | 3.8 | 0 | 0.39 |
| *1 oz (28 nuts)* | | 6.6 | 13.9 | 1.9 | 6.9 | 4.4 | 0 | 184 | 100 | 0.63 | 0.188 | 2.1 | 0 | 2.2 | 0.03 | 0.07 | 40.6 | 16090 |
| **peanuts**, all types, oil-roasted | 28 | 168 | 0.4 | 4.3 | 1.2 | 0 | 2.6 | 90 | 17 | 49 | 0.92 | 0.517 | 0 | 0 | 0.02 | 3.9 | 0 | 0.39 |
| *1 oz* | | 7.8 | 14.7 | 2.4 | 7.3 | 4.3 | 0 | 203 | 111 | 0.43 | 0.149 | 0.9 | 0 | 1.9 | 0.02 | 0.13 | 33.6 | 16089 |
| **peanuts**, all types, raw | 28 | 159 | 1.8 | 4.5 | 1.1 | 0 | 2.4 | 5 | 26 | 47 | 0.92 | 0.542 | 0 | 0 | 0.18 | 3.4 | 0 | 0.49 |
| *1 oz* | | 7.2 | 13.8 | 1.9 | 6.8 | 4.4 | 0 | 197 | 105 | 1.28 | 0.320 | 2.0 | 0 | 2.3 | 0.04 | 0.10 | 67.2 | 16087 |
| **peanuts**, Spanish, oil-roasted | 28 | 162 | 0.5 | 4.9 | | | 2.5 | 121 | 28 | 47 | 0.56 | 0.659 | 0 | 0 | 0.09 | 4.2 | 0 | 0.39 |
| *1 oz* | | 7.8 | 13.7 | 2.1 | 6.2 | 4.8 | 0 | 217 | 108 | 0.64 | 0.185 | 2.1 | 0 | | 0.02 | 0.07 | 35.3 | 16092 |

| | WT (g) | KCAL | $H_2O$ (g) | CHO (g) | TSUG (g) | ASUG (g) | DFIB (g) | Na (mg) | Ca (mg) | Mg (mg) | Zn (mg) | Mn (mg) | A (mcg RAE) | C (mg) | B-1 (mg) | NIA (mg) | B-12 (mcg) | PANT (mg) |
|---|---|---|---|---|---|---|---|---|---|---|---|---|---|---|---|---|---|---|
| | | PRO (g) | FAT (g) | SFA (g) | MUFA (g) | PUFA (g) | CHOL (mg) | K (mg) | P (mg) | Fe (mg) | Cu (mg) | Se (mcg) | A (IU) | E (mg ATE) | B-2 (mg) | B-6 (mg) | FOL (mcg DFE) | REF |
| **peanuts, Spanish**, raw | 28 | 160 | 1.8 | 4.4 | | | 2.7 | 6 | 30 | 53 | 0.59 | 0.739 | 0 | 0 | 0.19 | 4.5 | 0 | 0.50 |
| *1 oz* | | 7.3 | 13.9 | 2.1 | 6.3 | 4.8 | 0 | 208 | 109 | 1.09 | 0.252 | 2.0 | 0 | | 0.04 | 0.10 | 67.2 | 16091 |
| **peanuts, Valencia**, oil-roasted | 28 | 165 | 0.6 | 4.6 | | | 2.5 | 216 | 15 | 45 | 0.86 | 0.482 | 0 | 0 | 0.03 | 4.0 | 0 | 0.39 |
| *1 oz* | | 7.6 | 14.3 | 2.2 | 6.5 | 5.0 | 0 | 171 | 89 | 0.46 | 0.235 | 2.1 | 0 | | 0.04 | 0.07 | 35.3 | 16094 |
| **peanuts, Valencia**, raw | 28 | 160 | 1.2 | 5.9 | | | 2.4 | 0 | 17 | 52 | 0.94 | 0.554 | 0 | 0 | 0.18 | 3.6 | 0 | 0.51 |
| *1 oz* | | 7.0 | 13.3 | 2.1 | 6.0 | 4.6 | 0 | 93 | 94 | 0.59 | 0.328 | 2.0 | 0 | | 0.08 | 0.10 | 68.9 | 16093 |
| **peanuts, Virginia**, oil-roasted | 28 | 162 | 0.6 | 5.6 | | | 2.5 | 121 | 24 | 53 | 1.85 | 0.562 | 0 | 0 | 0.08 | 4.1 | 0 | 0.39 |
| *1 oz* | | 7.2 | 13.6 | 1.8 | 7.1 | 4.1 | 0 | 183 | 142 | 0.47 | 0.356 | 2.1 | 0 | | 0.03 | 0.07 | 35.0 | 16096 |
| **peanuts, Virginia**, raw | 28 | 158 | 1.9 | 4.6 | 1.1 | | 2.4 | 3 | 25 | 48 | 1.24 | 0.475 | 0 | 0 | 0.18 | 3.5 | 0 | 0.49 |
| *1 oz* | | 7.1 | 13.7 | 1.8 | 7.1 | 4.1 | 0 | 193 | 106 | 0.71 | 0.311 | 2.0 | 0 | 1.8 | 0.04 | 0.10 | 66.9 | 16095 |
| **pecans**, dried | 28 | 193 | 1.0 | 3.9 | 1.1 | 0 | 2.7 | 0 | 20 | 34 | 1.27 | 1.260 | 1 | 0 | 0.18 | 0.3 | 0 | 0.24 |
| *1 oz (20 halves)* | | 2.6 | 20.2 | 1.7 | 11.4 | 6.1 | 0 | 115 | 78 | 0.71 | 0.336 | 1.1 | 16 | 0.4 | 0.04 | 0.06 | 6.2 | 12142 |
| **pecans**, dry-roasted without salt | 28 | 199 | 0.3 | 3.8 | 1.1 | 0 | 2.6 | 0 | 20 | 37 | 1.42 | 1.101 | 2 | 0 | 0.13 | 0.3 | 0 | 0.20 |
| *1 oz (20 halves)* | | 2.7 | 20.8 | 1.8 | 12.3 | 5.8 | 0 | 119 | 82 | 0.78 | 0.327 | 1.1 | 39 | 0.4 | 0.03 | 0.05 | 4.5 | 12143 |
| **pecans**, oil-roasted | 28 | 200 | 0.3 | 3.6 | 1.1 | | 2.7 | 0 | 19 | 34 | 1.25 | 1.036 | 1 | 0 | 0.13 | 0.3 | 0 | 0.21 |
| *1 oz (15 halves)* | | 2.6 | 21.1 | 2.0 | 11.5 | 6.6 | 0 | 110 | 74 | 0.69 | 0.336 | 1.7 | 29 | 0.7 | 0.03 | 0.05 | 4.2 | 12144 |
| **pilinuts**, dried | 28 | 201 | 0.8 | 1.1 | | | | 1 | 41 | 85 | 0.83 | 0.648 | 1 | 0 | 0.26 | 0.1 | 0 | 0.13 |
| *1 oz (15 nuts)* | | 3.0 | 22.3 | 8.7 | 10.4 | 2.1 | 0 | 142 | 161 | 0.99 | 0.268 | | 11 | | 0.03 | 0.03 | 16.8 | 12145 |
| **pine nuts, pignolia**, dried | 28 | 188 | 0.6 | 3.7 | 1.0 | 0 | 1.0 | 1 | 4 | 70 | 1.81 | 2.465 | 0 | 0 | 0.10 | 1.2 | 0 | 0.09 |
| *1 oz (15–16 nuts)* | | 3.8 | 19.1 | 1.4 | 5.3 | 9.5 | 0 | 167 | 161 | 1.55 | 0.371 | 0.2 | 8 | 2.6 | 0.06 | 0.03 | 9.5 | 12147 |
| **pine nuts, pinyon**, dried | 28 | 176 | 1.7 | 5.4 | | | 3.0 | 20 | 2 | 66 | 1.20 | 1.213 | 0 | 1 | 0.35 | 1.2 | 0 | 0.06 |
| *1 oz* | | 3.2 | 17.1 | 2.6 | 6.4 | 7.2 | 0 | 176 | 10 | 0.86 | 0.290 | | 8 | | 0.06 | 0.03 | 16.2 | 12149 |
| **pistachios**, dried | 28 | 156 | 1.1 | 7.8 | 2.1 | | 2.9 | 0 | 30 | 34 | 0.62 | 0.336 | 8 | 1 | 0.24 | 0.4 | 0 | 0.15 |
| *1 oz (47 nuts)* | | 5.8 | 12.4 | 1.5 | 6.5 | 3.8 | 0 | 287 | 137 | 1.16 | 0.364 | 2.0 | 155 | 0.6 | 0.04 | 0.48 | 14.3 | 12151 |
| **pistachios**, dry-roasted | 28 | 160 | 0.6 | 7.7 | 2.2 | 0 | 2.9 | 3 | 31 | 34 | 0.64 | 0.357 | 4 | 1 | 0.24 | 0.4 | 0 | 0.14 |
| *1 oz (47 nuts)* | | 6.0 | 12.9 | 1.6 | 6.8 | 3.9 | 0 | 292 | 136 | 1.18 | 0.371 | 2.6 | 73 | 0.5 | 0.04 | 0.36 | 14.0 | 12152 |
| **soy nuts**, chocolate-covered, GeniSoy | 28 | 140 | | 15.0 | 12.0 | | 2.0 | 25 | 70 | | | | | 3 | | | | |
| *1 oz* | | 4.0 | 7.5 | 4.5 | | | | | | 0.90 | | | 150 | | | | | GENI3 |
| **soy nuts**, dry-roasted | 28 | 126 | 0.2 | 9.2 | | | 2.3 | 1 | 39 | 64 | 1.34 | 0.612 | 0 | 1 | 0.12 | 0.3 | 0 | 0.13 |
| *1 oz* | | 11.1 | 6.1 | 0.9 | 1.3 | 3.4 | 0 | 382 | 182 | 1.11 | 0.302 | 5.4 | 0 | | 0.21 | 0.06 | 57.4 | 16111 |
| **soy nuts**, roasted | 172 | 810 | 3.4 | 57.7 | 7.2 | 0 | 30.4 | 280 | 237 | 249 | 5.40 | 3.712 | 17 | 4 | 0.17 | 2.4 | 0 | 0.78 |
| *1 cup* | | 60.6 | 43.7 | 6.3 | 9.6 | 24.7 | 0 | 2528 | 624 | 6.71 | 1.424 | 32.9 | 344 | 1.6 | 0.25 | 0.36 | 362.9 | 16110 |
| **trail mix** | 28 | 129 | 2.6 | 12.6 | | | | 64 | 22 | 44 | 0.90 | 0.290 | 0 | 0 | 0.13 | 1.3 | 0 | 0.25 |
| *1 oz* | | 3.9 | 8.2 | 1.6 | 3.5 | 2.7 | 0 | 192 | | 0.85 | 0.276 | | 5 | | 0.06 | 0.08 | 19.9 | 19059 |
| **trail mix**, tropical | 28 | 114 | 2.5 | 18.4 | | | | 3 | 16 | 27 | 0.33 | 0.270 | 1 | 2 | 0.13 | 0.4 | 0 | 0.34 |
| *1 oz* | | 1.8 | 4.8 | 2.4 | 0.7 | 1.4 | 0 | 199 | 52 | 0.74 | 0.148 | | 14 | | 0.03 | 0.09 | 11.8 | 19061 |
| **trail mix**, unsalted | 28 | 129 | 2.6 | 12.6 | | | | 3 | 22 | 44 | 0.90 | 0.290 | 0 | 0 | 0.13 | 1.3 | 0 | 0.25 |
| *1 oz* | | 3.9 | 8.2 | 1.6 | 3.5 | 2.7 | 0 | 192 | 97 | 0.85 | 0.276 | | 5 | | 0.06 | 0.08 | 19.9 | 19821 |
| **trail mix** with chocolate chips | 28 | 136 | 1.8 | 12.6 | | | | 34 | 31 | 45 | 0.88 | 0.297 | 1 | 0 | 0.12 | 1.2 | 0 | 0.27 |
| *1 oz* | | 4.0 | 8.9 | 1.7 | 3.8 | 3.2 | 1 | 181 | 108 | 0.95 | 0.236 | | 12 | | 0.06 | 0.07 | 18.2 | 19062 |
| **trail mix** with chocolate chips, | 28 | 136 | 1.8 | 12.6 | | | | 8 | 31 | 45 | 0.88 | 0.297 | 1 | 0 | 0.12 | 1.2 | 0 | 0.27 |
| unsalted - *1 oz* | | 4.0 | 8.9 | 1.7 | 3.8 | 3.2 | 1 | 181 | 108 | 0.95 | 0.236 | | 12 | | 0.06 | 0.07 | 18.2 | 19822 |
| **walnuts, black**, dried | 28 | 173 | 1.3 | 2.8 | 0.3 | 0 | 1.9 | 1 | 17 | 56 | 0.94 | 1.091 | 1 | 0 | 0.02 | 0.1 | 0 | 0.46 |
| *1 oz* | | 6.7 | 16.5 | 0.9 | 4.2 | 9.8 | 0 | 146 | 144 | 0.87 | 0.381 | 4.8 | 11 | 0.5 | 0.04 | 0.16 | 8.7 | 12154 |
| **walnuts, English/Persian**, dried | 28 | 183 | 1.1 | 3.8 | 0.7 | 0 | 1.9 | 1 | 27 | 44 | 0.87 | 0.956 | 0 | 0 | 0.10 | 0.3 | 0 | 0.16 |
| *1 oz (14 halves)* | | 4.3 | 18.3 | 1.7 | 2.5 | 13.2 | 0 | 123 | 97 | 0.81 | 0.444 | 1.4 | 6 | 0.2 | 0.04 | 0.15 | 27.4 | 12155 |
| **wheat-base formulated nuts**, | 28 | 181 | 0.6 | 5.8 | | | 1.5 | 25 | 6 | 17 | 0.83 | 1.946 | 0 | 0 | 0.11 | 0.4 | 0 | 0.09 |
| flavored - *1 oz* | | 3.7 | 17.4 | 2.6 | 7.2 | 6.8 | 0 | 90 | 102 | 0.73 | 0.051 | | 0 | | 0.08 | 0.10 | 35.0 | 12200 |
| **wheat-base formulated nuts**, | 28 | 173 | 0.9 | 7.8 | | | 1.5 | 13 | 6 | 16 | 0.82 | 1.443 | 0 | 0 | 0.06 | 0.3 | 0 | 0.09 |
| macadamia-flavored - *1 oz* | | 3.1 | 15.8 | 2.4 | 6.6 | 6.1 | 0 | 73 | 84 | 0.56 | 0.050 | | 0 | | 0.06 | 0.07 | 26.3 | 12199 |
| **wheat-base formulated nuts**, | 28 | 174 | 0.7 | 6.6 | | | 1.5 | 141 | 7 | 16 | 0.82 | 2.217 | 0 | 0 | 0.08 | 0.4 | 0 | 0.09 |
| unflavored - *1 oz* | | 3.9 | 16.2 | 2.4 | 6.6 | 6.4 | 0 | 89 | 104 | 0.67 | 0.050 | | 0 | | 0.08 | 0.11 | 39.8 | 12140 |

## 23.2 SEEDS AND SEED PRODUCTS

| | WT (g) | KCAL | $H_2O$ (g) | CHO (g) | TSUG (g) | ASUG (g) | DFIB (g) | Na (mg) | Ca (mg) | Mg (mg) | Zn (mg) | Mn (mg) | A (mcg RAE) | C (mg) | B-1 (mg) | NIA (mg) | B-12 (mcg) | PANT (mg) |
|---|---|---|---|---|---|---|---|---|---|---|---|---|---|---|---|---|---|---|
| | | PRO (g) | FAT (g) | SFA (g) | MUFA (g) | PUFA (g) | CHOL (mg) | K (mg) | P (mg) | Fe (mg) | Cu (mg) | Se (mcg) | A (IU) | E (mg ATE) | B-2 (mg) | B-6 (mg) | FOL (mcg DFE) | REF |
| **breadfruit seeds**, boiled | 28 | 47 | 16.6 | 9.0 | | | 1.3 | 6 | 17 | 14 | 0.23 | 0.037 | 3 | 2 | 0.08 | 1.5 | 0 | 0.23 |
| *1 oz* | | 1.5 | 0.6 | 0.2 | 0.1 | 0.3 | 0 | 245 | 35 | 0.17 | 0.299 | | 67 | | 0.05 | 0.08 | 13.7 | 12003 |
| **breadfruit seeds**, raw | 28 | 53 | 15.8 | 8.2 | | | 1.5 | 7 | 10 | 15 | 0.25 | 0.040 | 4 | 2 | 0.13 | 0.1 | 0 | 0.25 |
| *1 oz* | | 2.1 | 1.6 | 0.4 | 0.2 | 0.8 | 0 | 263 | 49 | 1.03 | 0.321 | | 72 | | 0.08 | 0.09 | 14.8 | 12001 |
| **breadfruit seeds**, roasted | 28 | 58 | 13.9 | 11.2 | | | 1.7 | 8 | 24 | 17 | 0.29 | 0.046 | 4 | 2 | 0.11 | 2.1 | 0 | 0.28 |
| *1 oz* | | 1.7 | 0.8 | 0.2 | 0.1 | 0.4 | 0 | 303 | 49 | 0.25 | 0.370 | | 82 | | 0.07 | 0.12 | 16.5 | 12158 |
| **cottonseed kernels**, roasted | 10 | 51 | 0.5 | 2.2 | | | 0.6 | 2 | 10 | 44 | 0.60 | 0.218 | 2 | 1 | 0.08 | 0.3 | 0 | 0.05 |
| *1 T* | | 3.3 | 3.6 | 1.0 | 0.7 | 1.8 | 0 | 135 | 80 | 0.54 | 0.120 | | 44 | | 0.03 | 0.08 | 23.3 | 12160 |

| | WT (g) | KCAL | H₂0 (g) | CHO (g) | TSUG (g) | ASUG (g) | DFIB (g) | Na (mg) | Ca (mg) | Mg (mg) | Zn (mg) | Mn (mg) | A (mcg RAE) | C (mg) | B-1 (mg) | NIA (mg) | B-12 (mcg) | PANT (mg) |
|---|---|---|---|---|---|---|---|---|---|---|---|---|---|---|---|---|---|---|
| | | PRO (g) | FAT (g) | SFA (g) | MUFA (g) | PUFA (g) | CHOL (mg) | K (mg) | P (mg) | Fe (mg) | Cu (mg) | Se (mcg) | A (IU) | E (mg ATE) | B-2 (mg) | B-6 (mg) | FOL (mcg DFE) | REF |
| **flaxseeds** | 12 | 64 | 0.8 | 3.5 | 0.2 | 0 | 3.3 | 4 | 31 | 47 | 0.52 | 0.298 | 0 | 0 | 0.20 | 0.4 | 0 | 0.12 |
| *1 T* | | 2.2 | 5.1 | 0.4 | 0.9 | 3.4 | 0 | 98 | 77 | 0.69 | 0.146 | 3.0 | 0 | 0 | 0.02 | 0.06 | 10.4 | 12220 |
| **lotus seeds**, dried | 28 | 93 | 4.0 | 18.1 | | | | 1 | 46 | 59 | 0.29 | 0.649 | 1 | 0 | 0.18 | 0.4 | 0 | 0.24 |
| *1 oz (42 seeds)* | | 4.3 | 0.6 | 0.1 | 0.1 | 0.3 | 0 | 383 | 175 | 0.99 | 0.098 | | 14 | | 0.04 | 0.18 | 29.1 | 12013 |
| **lotus seeds**, raw | 28 | 25 | 21.6 | 4.8 | | | | 0 | 12 | 16 | 0.08 | 0.174 | 0 | 0 | 0.05 | 0.1 | 0 | 0.06 |
| *1 oz* | | 1.2 | 0.1 | 0 | 0 | 0.1 | 0 | 103 | 47 | 0.27 | 0.026 | | 4 | | 0.01 | 0.05 | 7.8 | 12205 |
| **pumpkin and squash seed kernels,** dried - *1 oz (142 seeds)* | 28 | 151 | 1.9 | 5.0 | 0.3 | 0 | 1.1 | 5 | 12 | 150 | 2.09 | 0.846 | 5 | 1 | 0.06 | 0.5 | 0 | 0.09 |
| | | 6.9 | 12.8 | 2.4 | 4.0 | 5.9 | 0 | 226 | 329 | 4.19 | 0.388 | 1.6 | 106 | 0 | 0.09 | 0.06 | 16.2 | 12014 |
| **pumpkin and squash seed kernels,** roasted - *1 oz* | 28 | 146 | 2.0 | 3.8 | 0.3 | 0 | 1.1 | 5 | 12 | 150 | 2.08 | 0.844 | 5 | 1 | 0.06 | 0.5 | 0 | 0.09 |
| | | 9.2 | 11.8 | 2.2 | 3.7 | 5.4 | 0 | 226 | 328 | 4.18 | 0.388 | 1.6 | 106 | 0 | 0.09 | 0.03 | 16.0 | 12016 |
| **safflower seed kernels**, dried | 28 | 145 | 1.6 | 9.6 | | | | 1 | 22 | 99 | 1.41 | 0.564 | 1 | 0 | 0.33 | 0.6 | 0 | 1.13 |
| *1 oz* | | 4.5 | | | 1.4 | 7.9 | 0 | 192 | 180 | 1.37 | 0.489 | | 14 | | 0.12 | 0.33 | 44.8 | 12021 |
| **safflower seed meal**, partially defatted - *1 oz* | 28 | 96 | 1.8 | 13.6 | | | | 1 | 22 | 98 | 1.40 | 0.559 | 1 | 0 | 0.32 | 0.6 | 0 | 1.12 |
| | | 10.0 | 0.7 | 0.1 | 0.1 | 0.4 | 0 | 19 | 179 | 1.36 | 0.485 | | 14 | | 0.12 | 0.33 | 44.5 | 12022 |
| **sesame butter** (tahini), from roasted, toasted kernels - *1 T* | 15 | 89 | 0.5 | 3.2 | 0.1 | 0 | 1.4 | 17 | 64 | 14 | 0.69 | 0.218 | 0 | 0 | 0.18 | 0.8 | 0 | 0.10 |
| | | 2.6 | 8.1 | 1.1 | 3.0 | 3.5 | 0 | 62 | 110 | 1.34 | 0.242 | 0.3 | 10 | 0 | 0.07 | 0.02 | 14.7 | 12166 |
| **sesame butter** (tahini), from unroasted kernels - *1 T* | 14 | 85 | 0.4 | 2.5 | | | 1.3 | 0 | 20 | 49 | 1.46 | 0.204 | 0 | 0 | 0.22 | 0.8 | 0 | 0.10 |
| | | 2.5 | 7.9 | 1.1 | 3.0 | 3.5 | 0 | 64 | 111 | 0.89 | 0.208 | | 9 | | 0.02 | 0.02 | 13.7 | 12171 |
| **sesame butter paste** | 16 | 94 | 0.3 | 3.8 | | | 0.9 | 2 | 154 | 58 | 1.17 | 0.406 | 0 | 0 | 0.04 | 1.1 | 0 | 0.01 |
| *1 T* | | 2.9 | 8.1 | 1.1 | 3.1 | 3.6 | 0 | 93 | 105 | 3.07 | 0.674 | 0.9 | 8 | | 0.03 | 0.13 | 16.0 | 12169 |
| **sesame seed kernels**, dried | 8 | 50 | 0.3 | 0.9 | 0 | 0 | 0.9 | 4 | 5 | 28 | 0.54 | 0.115 | 0 | 0 | 0.06 | 0.5 | 0 | 0.02 |
| *1 T* | | 1.6 | 4.9 | 0.7 | 1.9 | 2.0 | 0 | 30 | 53 | 0.51 | 0.112 | 7.8 | 5 | 0.1 | 0.01 | 0.03 | 9.2 | 12201 |
| **sesame seed kernels**, toasted | 28 | 159 | 1.4 | 7.3 | 0.1 | 0 | 4.7 | 11 | 37 | 97 | 2.86 | 0.400 | 1 | 0 | 0.34 | 1.5 | 0 | 0.19 |
| *1 oz* | | 4.7 | 13.4 | 1.9 | 5.1 | 5.9 | 0 | 114 | 217 | 2.18 | 0.408 | 0.5 | 18 | 0.1 | 0.13 | 0.04 | 26.9 | 12029 |
| **sesame seeds, whole**, dried | 9 | 52 | 0.4 | 2.1 | 0 | 0 | 1.1 | 1 | 88 | 32 | 0.70 | 0.221 | 0 | 0 | 0.07 | 0.4 | 0 | 0 |
| *1 T* | | 1.6 | 4.5 | 0.6 | 1.7 | 2.0 | 0 | 42 | 57 | 1.31 | 0.367 | 0.5 | 1 | 0 | 0.02 | 0.07 | 8.7 | 12023 |
| **sesame seeds, whole**, roasted, toasted - *1 oz* | 28 | 158 | 0.9 | 7.2 | | | 3.9 | 3 | 277 | 100 | 2.00 | 0.699 | 0 | 0 | 0.22 | 1.3 | 0 | 0.01 |
| | | 4.7 | 13.4 | 1.9 | 5.1 | 5.9 | 0 | 133 | 179 | 4.13 | 0.692 | 1.6 | 3 | | 0.07 | 0.22 | 27.4 | 12024 |
| **sunflower seed butter** | 16 | 93 | 0.2 | 4.4 | | | | 0 | 20 | 59 | 0.85 | 0.338 | 0 | 0 | 0.05 | 0.9 | 0 | 1.13 |
| *1 T* | | 3.1 | 7.6 | 0.8 | 1.5 | 5.0 | 0 | 12 | 118 | 0.76 | 0.293 | | 8 | | 0.05 | 0.13 | 37.9 | 12040 |
| **sunflower seed kernels**, dried | 144 | 841 | 6.8 | 28.8 | 3.8 | 0 | 12.4 | 13 | 112 | 468 | 7.20 | 2.808 | 4 | 2 | 2.13 | 12.0 | 0 | 1.63 |
| *1 cup without hulls* | | 29.9 | 74.1 | 6.4 | 26.7 | 33.3 | 0 | 929 | 950 | 7.56 | 2.592 | 76.3 | 72 | 47.9 | 0.51 | 1.94 | 326.9 | 12036 |
| **sunflower seed kernels**, dry-roasted | 28 | 163 | 0.3 | 6.7 | 0.8 | 0 | 3.1 | 1 | 20 | 36 | 1.48 | 0.591 | 0 | 0 | 0.03 | 2.0 | 0 | 1.97 |
| *1 oz* | | 5.4 | 13.9 | 1.5 | 2.7 | 9.2 | 0 | 238 | 323 | 1.06 | 0.512 | 22.2 | 3 | 7.3 | 0.07 | 0.23 | 66.4 | 12037 |
| **sunflower seed kernels**, oil-roasted without salt - *1 oz* | 28 | 166 | 0.4 | 6.4 | 0.9 | 0 | 3.0 | 1 | 24 | 36 | 1.46 | 0.582 | 0 | 0 | 0.09 | 1.2 | 0 | 1.94 |
| | | 5.6 | 14.4 | 2.0 | 2.3 | 9.6 | 0 | 135 | 319 | 1.20 | 0.505 | 21.9 | 3 | 10.2 | 0.08 | 0.22 | 65.5 | 12038 |
| **sunflower seed kernels**, toasted | 28 | 173 | 0.3 | 5.8 | | | 3.2 | 1 | 16 | 36 | 1.48 | 0.592 | 0 | 0 | 0.09 | 1.2 | 0 | 1.98 |
| *1 oz* | | 4.8 | 15.9 | 1.7 | 3.0 | 10.5 | 0 | 137 | 324 | 1.91 | 0.514 | | 0 | | 0.08 | 0.23 | 66.6 | 12039 |
| **watermelon seeds**, dried | 28 | 156 | 1.4 | 4.3 | | | | 28 | 15 | 144 | 2.87 | 0.452 | 0 | 0 | 0.05 | 1.0 | 0 | 0.10 |
| *1 oz (95 large seeds)* | | 7.9 | 13.3 | 2.7 | 2.1 | 7.9 | 0 | 181 | 211 | 2.04 | 0.192 | | 0 | | 0.04 | 0.02 | 16.2 | 12174 |

## 24. POULTRY
### 24.1 CHICKEN, BROILER/FRYER PARTS

| | WT (g) | KCAL | H₂0 (g) | CHO (g) | TSUG (g) | ASUG (g) | DFIB (g) | Na (mg) | Ca (mg) | Mg (mg) | Zn (mg) | Mn (mg) | A (mcg RAE) | C (mg) | B-1 (mg) | NIA (mg) | B-12 (mcg) | PANT (mg) |
|---|---|---|---|---|---|---|---|---|---|---|---|---|---|---|---|---|---|---|
| | | PRO (g) | FAT (g) | SFA (g) | MUFA (g) | PUFA (g) | CHOL (mg) | K (mg) | P (mg) | Fe (mg) | Cu (mg) | Se (mcg) | A (IU) | E (mg ATE) | B-2 (mg) | B-6 (mg) | FOL (mcg DFE) | REF |
| **Chckn (brlr/fryer) back** w/skin, flour-coated, fried - *½ back (2.5 oz)* | 72 | 238 | 31.7 | 4.7 | | | | 65 | 17 | 17 | 1.78 | 0.036 | 27 | 0 | 0.08 | 5.3 | 0.20 | 0.79 |
| | | 20.0 | 14.9 | 4.0 | 5.9 | 3.5 | 64 | 163 | 120 | 1.17 | 0.066 | 17.1 | 89 | | 0.17 | 0.22 | 14.4 | 5050 |
| **Chckn (brlr/fryer) back** w/skin, stewed - *¼ cup (1.4 oz)* | 40 | 103 | 24.4 | 0 | 0 | | | 26 | 7 | 6 | 0.77 | 0.008 | 35 | 0 | 0.02 | 1.7 | 0.07 | 0.28 |
| | | 8.9 | 7.3 | 2.0 | 2.9 | 1.6 | 31 | 58 | 48 | 0.49 | 0.025 | 8.0 | 123 | 0.1 | 0.06 | 0.06 | 2.0 | 5052 |
| **Chckn (brlr/fryer) breast** w/skin, rotisseried - *3 oz* | 85 | 156 | 54.0 | 0 | 0 | | 0 | 295 | 13 | 22 | 0.78 | 0.014 | 10 | 0 | 0.07 | 8.0 | 0.27 | 1.20 |
| | | 23.4 | 7.0 | 1.8 | 3.0 | 1.0 | 82 | 246 | 217 | 0.47 | 0.037 | 26.0 | 35 | 0.2 | 0.11 | 0.25 | 9.4 | 5348 |
| **Chckn (brlr/fryer) breast** w/skin, battered, fried - *½ breast (4.9 oz)* | 140 | 364 | 72.3 | 12.6 | 0 | | 0.4 | 385 | 28 | 34 | 1.33 | 0.076 | 28 | 0 | 0.16 | 14.7 | 0.42 | 1.15 |
| | | 34.8 | 18.5 | 4.9 | 7.6 | 4.3 | 119 | 281 | 259 | 1.75 | 0.084 | 39.2 | 94 | 1.5 | 0.20 | 0.60 | 29.4 | 5058 |
| **Chckn (brlr/fryer) breast** w/skn, flour-coated, fried - *½ breast (3.5 oz)* | 98 | 218 | 55.5 | 1.6 | | | 0.1 | 74 | 16 | 29 | 1.08 | 0.025 | 15 | 0 | 0.08 | 13.5 | 0.33 | 0.98 |
| | | 31.2 | 8.7 | 2.4 | 3.4 | 1.9 | 87 | 254 | 228 | 1.17 | 0.056 | 23.4 | 49 | | 0.13 | 0.57 | 6.9 | 5059 |
| **Chckn (brlr/fryer) breast** w/skin, roasted - *½ breast (3.5 oz)* | 98 | 193 | 61.2 | 0 | 0 | | 0 | 70 | 14 | 26 | 1.00 | 0.018 | 27 | 0 | 0.06 | 12.5 | 0.31 | 0.92 |
| | | 29.2 | 7.6 | 2.1 | 3.0 | 1.6 | 82 | 240 | 210 | 1.05 | 0.049 | 24.2 | 91 | 0.3 | 0.12 | 0.55 | 3.9 | 5060 |
| **Chckn (brlr/fryer) breast** w/skin, stewed - *½ breast (3.9 oz)* | 110 | 202 | 72.8 | 0 | 0 | | 0 | 68 | 14 | 24 | 1.07 | 0.020 | 28 | 0 | 0.05 | 8.6 | 0.23 | 0.60 |
| | | 30.1 | 8.2 | 2.3 | 3.2 | 1.7 | 82 | 196 | 172 | 1.01 | 0.048 | 24.0 | 90 | 0.3 | 0.13 | 0.32 | 3.3 | 5061 |
| **Chckn (brlr/fryr) breast** w/o skn, flour-coated, fried - *½ breast (3 oz)* | 86 | 161 | 51.8 | 0.4 | 0 | | 0 | 68 | 14 | 27 | 0.93 | 0.018 | 6 | 0 | 0.07 | 12.7 | 0.32 | 0.89 |
| | | 28.8 | 4.1 | 1.1 | 1.5 | 0.9 | 78 | 237 | 212 | 0.98 | 0.046 | 22.5 | 20 | 0.4 | 0.11 | 0.55 | 3.4 | 5063 |
| **Chckn (brlr/fryr) breast** w/o skin, roasted - *½ breast (3 oz)* | 86 | 142 | 56.1 | 0 | 0 | | 0 | 64 | 13 | 25 | 0.86 | 0.015 | 5 | 0 | 0.06 | 11.8 | 0.29 | 0.83 |
| | | 26.7 | 3.1 | 0.9 | 1.1 | 0.7 | 73 | 220 | 196 | 0.89 | 0.042 | 23.7 | 18 | 0.2 | 0.10 | 0.52 | 3.4 | 5064 |

| Food | WT (g) / — | KCAL / PRO (g) | H₂O (g) / FAT (g) | CHO (g) / SFA (g) | TSUG (g) / MUFA (g) | ASUG (g) / PUFA (g) | DFIB (g) / CHOL (mg) | Na (mg) / K (mg) | Ca (mg) / P (mg) | Mg (mg) / Fe (mg) | Zn (mg) / Cu (mg) | Mn (mg) / Se (mcg) | A (mcg RAE) / A (IU) | C (mg) / E (mg ATE) | B-1 (mg) / B-2 (mg) | NIA (mg) / B-6 (mg) | B-12 (mcg) / FOL (mcg DFE) | PANT (mg) / REF |
|---|---|---|---|---|---|---|---|---|---|---|---|---|---|---|---|---|---|---|
| Chckn (brlr/fryer) breast w/o skin, | 95 | 143 | 64.9 | 0 | 0 |  | 0 | 60 | 12 | 23 | 0.92 | 0.017 | 6 | 0 | 0.04 | 8.0 | 0.22 | 0.54 |
| stewed - ½ breast (3.4 oz) |  | 27.5 | 2.9 | 0.8 | 1.0 | 0.6 | 73 | 178 | 157 | 0.84 | 0.041 | 21.2 | 18 | 0.3 | 0.11 | 0.31 | 2.8 | 5065 |
| Chckn (brlr/fryer) drumstick w/skn, | 72 | 193 | 38.0 | 6.0 |  |  | 0.2 | 194 | 12 | 14 | 1.68 | 0.037 | 19 | 0 | 0.08 | 3.7 | 0.20 | 0.73 |
| battered, fried - 2.5 oz drmstck |  | 15.8 | 11.3 | 3.0 | 4.6 | 2.7 | 62 | 134 | 106 | 0.97 | 0.055 | 15.8 | 62 |  | 0.15 | 0.19 | 17.3 | 5067 |
| Chckn (brlr/fryr) drmstk w/skn, flour- | 49 | 120 | 27.8 | 0.8 |  |  | 0 | 44 | 6 | 11 | 1.42 | 0.014 | 12 | 0 | 0.04 | 3.0 | 0.16 | 0.60 |
| coated, fried - 1.7 oz drmstk |  | 13.2 | 6.7 | 1.8 | 2.7 | 1.6 | 44 | 112 | 86 | 0.66 | 0.039 | 9.0 | 41 |  | 0.11 | 0.17 | 5.4 | 5068 |
| Chckn (brlr/fryer) drumstick w/skn, | 52 | 112 | 32.6 | 0 | 0 |  | 0 | 47 | 6 | 12 | 1.49 | 0.011 | 16 | 0 | 0.04 | 3.1 | 0.17 | 0.63 |
| roasted - 1.8 oz drumstick |  | 14.1 | 5.8 | 1.6 | 2.2 | 1.3 | 47 | 119 | 91 | 0.69 | 0.040 | 9.7 | 52 | 0.1 | 0.11 | 0.18 | 4.2 | 5069 |
| Chckn (brlr/fryer) drumstick w/skn, | 52 | 112 | 31.1 | 0 | 0 |  | 0 | 214 | 11 | 13 | 1.37 | 0.012 | 9 | 0 | 0.03 | 3.1 | 0.27 | 0.68 |
| rotisseried - 1.8 oz drumstick |  | 14.0 | 6.2 | 1.6 | 2.7 | 0.9 | 81 | 151 | 133 | 0.56 | 0.044 | 18.1 | 31 | 0.2 | 0.11 | 0.09 | 5.7 | 5349 |
| Chckn (brlr/fryer) drumstick w/skn, | 57 | 116 | 37.1 | 0 | 0 |  | 0 | 43 | 6 | 11 | 1.51 | 0.011 | 15 | 0 | 0.03 | 2.4 | 0.13 | 0.49 |
| stewed - 2 oz drumstick |  | 14.4 | 6.1 | 1.7 | 2.3 | 1.4 | 47 | 105 | 80 | 0.76 | 0.040 | 9.7 | 52 | 0.2 | 0.11 | 0.11 | 4.0 | 5070 |
| Chicken (brlr/fryer) drumstick w/o | 44 | 76 | 29.4 | 0 | 0 |  | 0 | 42 | 5 | 11 | 1.40 | 0.009 | 8 | 0 | 0.03 | 2.7 | 0.15 | 0.57 |
| skin, roasted - 1.6 oz drumstick |  | 12.4 | 2.5 | 0.7 | 0.8 | 0.6 | 41 | 108 | 81 | 0.57 | 0.035 | 8.4 | 26 | 0.1 | 0.10 | 0.17 | 4.0 | 5073 |
| Chicken (broiler/fryer) leg w/skin, | 112 | 284 | 61.9 | 2.8 |  |  | 0.1 | 99 | 15 | 27 | 3.00 | 0.036 | 31 | 0 | 0.10 | 7.3 | 0.35 | 1.34 |
| flour-coated, fried - 4 oz leg |  | 30.1 | 16.2 | 4.4 | 6.4 | 3.7 | 105 | 261 | 204 | 1.60 | 0.095 | 23.3 | 103 |  | 0.26 | 0.38 | 14.6 | 5077 |
| Chicken (broiler/fryer) leg w/skin, | 114 | 264 | 69.4 | 0 | 0 |  | 0 | 99 | 14 | 26 | 2.96 | 0.024 | 47 | 0 | 0.08 | 7.1 | 0.34 | 1.32 |
| roasted - 4 oz leg |  | 29.6 | 15.3 | 4.2 | 6.0 | 3.4 | 105 | 256 | 198 | 1.52 | 0.088 | 23.6 | 154 | 0.3 | 0.24 | 0.38 | 8.0 | 5078 |
| Chicken (broiler/fryer) leg w/skin, | 125 | 275 | 80.0 | 0 | 0 |  | 0 | 91 | 14 | 25 | 3.04 | 0.024 | 46 | 0 | 0.07 | 5.7 | 0.25 | 1.02 |
| stewed - 4.4 oz leg |  | 30.2 | 16.2 | 4.5 | 6.3 | 3.6 | 105 | 220 | 174 | 1.69 | 0.089 | 23.6 | 155 | 0.3 | 0.24 | 0.22 | 7.5 | 5079 |
| Chicken (broiler/fryer) leg w/o skin, | 101 | 187 | 67.1 | 0 | 0 |  | 0 | 79 | 11 | 21 | 2.81 | 0.019 | 18 | 0 | 0.06 | 4.8 | 0.23 | 0.92 |
| stewed - 3.6 oz leg |  | 26.5 | 8.1 | 2.2 | 3.0 | 1.9 | 90 | 192 | 150 | 1.41 | 0.078 | 26.8 | 61 | 0.3 | 0.22 | 0.21 | 8.1 | 5083 |
| Chicken (broiler/fryer) neck w/skin, | 43 | 142 | 20.2 | 3.7 |  |  |  | 119 | 13 | 7 | 1.08 | 0.028 | 22 | 0 | 0.04 | 1.9 | 0.10 | 0.36 |
| battered, fried - 1.5 oz neck |  | 8.5 | 10.1 | 2.7 | 4.2 | 2.4 | 39 | 65 | 49 | 0.92 | 0.049 | 9.2 | 73 |  | 0.10 | 0.09 | 9.0 | 5085 |
| Chicken (broiler/fryer) neck w/skin, | 36 | 120 | 17.1 | 1.5 |  |  |  | 30 | 11 | 7 | 1.11 | 0.019 | 21 | 0 | 0.03 | 1.9 | 0.09 | 0.35 |
| flour-coated, fried - 1.3 oz neck |  | 8.6 | 8.5 | 2.3 | 3.5 | 2.0 | 34 | 65 | 48 | 0.87 | 0.047 | 6.7 | 68 |  | 0.09 | 0.09 | 5.4 | 5086 |
| Chicken (broiler/fryer) neck w/skin, | 38 | 94 | 23.5 | 0 | 0 |  | 0 | 20 | 10 | 5 | 1.03 | 0.017 | 18 | 0 | 0.02 | 1.3 | 0.05 | 0.20 |
| simmered - 1.3 oz neck |  | 7.5 | 6.9 | 1.9 | 2.7 | 1.5 | 27 | 41 | 46 | 0.87 | 0.037 | 6.6 | 61 | 0.1 | 0.09 | 0.04 | 1.1 | 5087 |
| Chckn (brlr/fryer) neck w/o skin, | 18 | 32 | 12.1 | 0 |  |  | 0 | 12 | 8 | 3 | 0.68 | 0.009 | 6 | 0 | 0.01 | 0.7 | 0.03 | 0.12 |
| simmered - .63 oz neck |  | 4.4 | 1.5 | 0.4 | 0.5 | 0.4 | 14 | 25 | 23 | 0.47 | 0.023 | 3.7 | 22 |  | 0.05 | 0.03 | 1.1 | 5090 |
| Chckn (brlr/fryer) thigh w/skn, flour- | 62 | 162 | 33.6 | 2.0 |  |  | 0.1 | 55 | 9 | 16 | 1.56 | 0.022 | 18 | 0 | 0.06 | 4.3 | 0.19 | 0.73 |
| coated, fried - 2.2 oz thigh |  | 16.6 | 9.3 | 2.5 | 3.6 | 2.1 | 60 | 147 | 116 | 0.92 | 0.055 | 12.3 | 61 |  | 0.15 | 0.20 | 9.3 | 5093 |
| Chicken (broiler/fryer) thigh w/skin, | 62 | 153 | 36.8 | 0 | 0 |  | 0 | 52 | 7 | 14 | 1.46 | 0.013 | 31 | 0 | 0.04 | 3.9 | 0.18 | 0.69 |
| roasted - 2.2 oz thigh |  | 15.5 | 9.6 | 2.7 | 3.8 | 2.1 | 58 | 138 | 108 | 0.83 | 0.048 | 12.1 | 102 | 0.2 | 0.13 | 0.19 | 4.3 | 5094 |
| Chicken (broiler/fryer) thigh w/skin, | 85 | 198 | 51.3 | 0 | 0 |  | 0 | 293 | 13 | 19 | 1.56 | 0.017 | 18 | 0 | 0.04 | 4.7 | 0.40 | 1.06 |
| rotisseried - 3 oz |  | 19.5 | 13.3 | 3.5 | 5.9 | 2.0 | 112 | 221 | 189 | 0.82 | 0.065 | 21.7 | 60 | 0.2 | 0.18 | 0.14 | 10.2 | 5351 |
| Chicken (broiler/fryer) thigh w/skin, | 68 | 158 | 42.9 | 0 | 0 |  | 0 | 48 | 7 | 13 | 1.53 | 0.013 | 31 | 0 | 0.04 | 3.3 | 0.13 | 0.53 |
| stewed - 2.4 oz thigh |  | 15.8 | 10.0 | 2.8 | 4.0 | 2.2 | 57 | 116 | 95 | 0.93 | 0.048 | 12.2 | 103 | 0.2 | 0.13 | 0.12 | 4.1 | 5095 |
| Chckn (brlr/fryer) thigh w/o skin, | 52 | 109 | 32.7 | 0 | 0 |  | 0 | 46 | 6 | 12 | 1.34 | 0.011 | 10 | 0 | 0.04 | 3.4 | 0.16 | 0.62 |
| roasted - 1.8 oz thigh |  | 13.5 | 5.7 | 1.6 | 2.2 | 1.3 | 49 | 124 | 95 | 0.68 | 0.042 | 15.1 | 34 | 0.1 | 0.12 | 0.18 | 4.2 | 5098 |
| Chicken (broiler/fryer) wing w/skin, | 49 | 159 | 22.6 | 5.4 |  |  | 0.1 | 157 | 10 | 8 | 0.68 | 0.029 | 17 | 0 | 0.05 | 2.6 | 0.12 | 0.35 |
| battered, fried - 1.7 oz wing |  | 9.7 | 10.7 | 2.9 | 4.4 | 2.5 | 39 | 68 | 59 | 0.63 | 0.031 | 12.6 | 55 |  | 0.07 | 0.15 | 12.7 | 5101 |
| Chckn (brlr/fryer) wing w/skn, flour- | 32 | 103 | 15.6 | 0.8 |  |  | 0 | 25 | 5 | 6 | 0.56 | 0.009 | 12 | 0 | 0.02 | 2.1 | 0.09 | 0.28 |
| coated, fried - 1.1 oz wing |  | 8.4 | 7.1 | 1.9 | 2.8 | 1.6 | 26 | 57 | 48 | 0.40 | 0.020 | 6.8 | 40 |  | 0.04 | 0.13 | 2.6 | 5102 |
| Chicken (broiler/fryer) wing w/skin, | 34 | 99 | 18.7 | 0 | 0 |  | 0 | 28 | 5 | 6 | 0.62 | 0.006 | 16 | 0 | 0.01 | 2.3 | 0.10 | 0.30 |
| roasted - 1.2 oz wing |  | 9.1 | 6.6 | 1.9 | 2.6 | 1.4 | 29 | 63 | 51 | 0.43 | 0.019 | 7.5 | 54 | 0.1 | 0.04 | 0.14 | 1.0 | 5103 |
| Chicken (broiler/fryer) wing w/skin, | 85 | 226 | 47.0 | 0 | 0 |  | 0 | 518 | 25 | 20 | 1.45 | 0.021 | 22 | 0 | 0.06 | 5.9 | 0.38 | 1.08 |
| rotisseried - 3 oz |  | 20.7 | 16.0 | 4.1 | 6.9 | 2.3 | 119 | 252 | 219 | 0.82 | 0.050 | 34.2 | 74 | 0.3 | 0.11 | 0.14 | 6.8 | 5352 |
| Chicken (broiler/fryer) wing w/skin, | 40 | 100 | 24.9 | 0 | 0 |  | 0 | 27 | 5 | 6 | 0.65 | 0.007 | 16 | 0 | 0.02 | 1.8 | 0.07 | 0.20 |
| stewed - 1.4 oz wing |  | 9.1 | 6.7 | 1.9 | 2.6 | 1.4 | 28 | 56 | 48 | 0.45 | 0.018 | 7.4 | 53 | 0.1 | 0.04 | 0.09 | 1.2 | 5104 |

## 24.2 CHICKEN, BROILERS/FRYERS

| Food | WT (g) / — | KCAL / PRO (g) | H₂O (g) / FAT (g) | CHO (g) / SFA (g) | TSUG (g) / MUFA (g) | ASUG (g) / PUFA (g) | DFIB (g) / CHOL (mg) | Na (mg) / K (mg) | Ca (mg) / P (mg) | Mg (mg) / Fe (mg) | Zn (mg) / Cu (mg) | Mn (mg) / Se (mcg) | A (mcg RAE) / A (IU) | C (mg) / E (mg ATE) | B-1 (mg) / B-2 (mg) | NIA (mg) / B-6 (mg) | B-12 (mcg) / FOL (mcg DFE) | PANT (mg) / REF |
|---|---|---|---|---|---|---|---|---|---|---|---|---|---|---|---|---|---|---|
| Chicken (broiler/fryer) dark meat | 85 | 215 | 49.8 | 0 |  |  | 0 | 74 | 13 | 19 | 2.12 | 0.018 | 51 | 0 | 0.06 | 5.4 | 0.25 | 0.94 |
| w/skin, roasted - 3 oz |  | 22.1 | 13.4 | 3.7 | 5.3 | 3.0 | 77 | 187 | 143 | 1.16 | 0.065 | 17.2 | 171 |  | 0.18 | 0.26 | 6.0 | 5037 |
| Chicken (broiler/fryer) dark meat | 85 | 198 | 53.5 | 0 |  |  | 0 | 60 | 12 | 15 | 1.92 | 0.016 | 48 | 0 | 0.04 | 3.8 | 0.17 | 0.66 |
| w/skin, stewed - 3 oz |  | 20.0 | 12.5 | 3.5 | 4.9 | 2.8 | 70 | 141 | 113 | 1.11 | 0.058 | 15.6 | 158 |  | 0.15 | 0.14 | 5.1 | 5038 |
| Chicken (broiler/fryer) dark meat | 85 | 203 | 47.3 | 2.2 |  |  | 0 | 82 | 15 | 21 | 2.47 | 0.028 | 20 | 0 | 0.08 | 6.0 | 0.28 | 1.07 |
| w/o skin, fried - 3 oz |  | 24.6 | 9.9 | 2.7 | 3.7 | 2.4 | 82 | 215 | 159 | 1.27 | 0.076 | 17.4 | 67 |  | 0.21 | 0.31 | 7.6 | 5044 |
| Chicken (broiler/fryer) dark meat | 85 | 174 | 53.6 | 0 | 0 |  | 0 | 79 | 13 | 20 | 2.38 | 0.018 | 19 | 0 | 0.06 | 5.6 | 0.27 | 1.03 |
| w/o skin, roasted - 3 oz |  | 23.3 | 8.3 | 2.3 | 3.0 | 1.9 | 79 | 204 | 152 | 1.13 | 0.068 | 15.3 | 61 | 0.2 | 0.19 | 0.31 | 6.8 | 5045 |
| Chicken (broiler/fryer) dark meat | 85 | 163 | 56.0 | 0 | 0 |  | 0 | 63 | 12 | 17 | 2.26 | 0.017 | 18 | 0 | 0.05 | 4.0 | 0.19 | 0.76 |
| w/o skin, stewed - 3 oz |  | 22.1 | 7.6 | 2.1 | 2.8 | 1.8 | 75 | 154 | 122 | 1.16 | 0.064 | 14.7 | 59 | 0.2 | 0.17 | 0.18 | 6.0 | 5046 |

| | WT (g) | KCAL / PRO (g) | H₂O (g) / FAT (g) | CHO (g) / SFA (g) | TSUG (g) / MUFA (g) | ASUG (g) / PUFA (g) | DFIB (g) / CHOL (mg) | Na (mg) / K (mg) | Ca (mg) / P (mg) | Mg (mg) / Fe (mg) | Zn (mg) / Cu (mg) | Mn (mg) / Se (mcg) | A (mcg RAE) / A (IU) | C (mg) / E (mg ATE) | B-1 (mg) / B-2 (mg) | NIA (mg) / B-6 (mg) | B-12 (mcg) / FOL (mcg DFE) | PANT (mg) / REF |
|---|---|---|---|---|---|---|---|---|---|---|---|---|---|---|---|---|---|---|
| Chckn (brlr/fryr) light & dark meat | 85 | 246 | 42.0 | 8.0 | 0 | | 0.3 | 248 | 18 | 18 | 1.42 | 0.048 | 24 | 0 | 0.10 | 6.0 | 0.24 | 0.76 |
| w/skin, battered, fried - 3 oz | | 19.2 | 14.7 | 3.9 | 6.0 | 3.5 | 74 | 157 | 132 | 1.16 | 0.061 | 21.7 | 79 | 1.1 | 0.16 | 0.26 | 21.2 | 5007 |
| Chckn (brlr/fryr) light & dark meat | 85 | 229 | 44.5 | 2.7 | 0 | | 0.1 | 71 | 14 | 21 | 1.73 | 0.029 | 23 | 0 | 0.07 | 7.6 | 0.26 | 0.92 |
| w/skn, flour-coated, fried - 3 oz | | 24.3 | 12.7 | 3.5 | 5.0 | 2.9 | 76 | 199 | 162 | 1.17 | 0.064 | 18.4 | 76 | 0.5 | 0.16 | 0.35 | 9.4 | 5008 |
| Chckn (brlr/fryr) light & dark meat | 85 | 203 | 50.5 | 0 | 0 | | 0 | 70 | 13 | 20 | 1.65 | 0.017 | 41 | 0 | 0.05 | 7.2 | 0.26 | 0.88 |
| with skin, roasted - 3 oz | | 23.2 | 11.6 | 3.2 | 4.5 | 2.5 | 75 | 190 | 155 | 1.07 | 0.056 | 20.3 | 137 | 0.2 | 0.14 | 0.34 | 4.2 | 5009 |
| Chckn (brlr/fryr) light & dark meat | 85 | 186 | 54.3 | 0 | 0 | | 0 | 57 | 11 | 16 | 1.50 | 0.016 | 37 | 0 | 0.04 | 4.8 | 0.17 | 0.57 |
| with skin, stewed - 3 oz | | 21.0 | 10.7 | 3.0 | 4.2 | 2.3 | 66 | 141 | 118 | 0.99 | 0.048 | 15.3 | 124 | 0.2 | 0.13 | 0.19 | 4.2 | 5010 |
| Chckn (brlr/fryr) light & dark meat w/o | 85 | 186 | 48.9 | 1.4 | 0 | | 0.1 | 77 | 14 | 23 | 1.90 | 0.024 | 15 | 0 | 0.07 | 8.2 | 0.29 | 0.99 |
| skn, flour-coated, fried - 3 oz | | 26.0 | 7.8 | 2.1 | 2.8 | 1.8 | 80 | 218 | 174 | 1.15 | 0.064 | 20.8 | 50 | 0.4 | 0.17 | 0.41 | 6.0 | 5012 |
| Chckn (brlr/fryr) light & dark meat | 85 | 162 | 54.2 | 0 | 0 | | 0 | 73 | 13 | 21 | 1.78 | 0.016 | 14 | 0 | 0.06 | 7.8 | 0.28 | 0.94 |
| w/o skin, roasted - 3 oz | | 24.6 | 6.3 | 1.7 | 2.3 | 1.4 | 76 | 207 | 166 | 1.03 | 0.057 | 18.7 | 45 | 0.2 | 0.15 | 0.40 | 5.1 | 5013 |
| Chckn (brlr/fryr) light & dark meat | 85 | 150 | 56.8 | 0 | 0 | | 0 | 60 | 12 | 18 | 1.69 | 0.016 | 13 | 0 | 0.04 | 5.2 | 0.19 | 0.63 |
| w/o skin, stewed - 3 oz | | 23.2 | 5.7 | 1.6 | 2.0 | 1.3 | 71 | 153 | 128 | 0.99 | 0.052 | 17.8 | 42 | 0.2 | 0.14 | 0.22 | 5.1 | 5014 |
| Chckn (brlr/fryr) light meat w/skin, | 85 | 209 | 46.5 | 1.5 | 0 | | 0.1 | 65 | 14 | 23 | 1.07 | 0.022 | 17 | 0 | 0.06 | 10.2 | 0.28 | 0.82 |
| flour-coated, fried - 3 oz | | 25.9 | 10.3 | 2.8 | 4.1 | 2.3 | 74 | 203 | 181 | 1.03 | 0.049 | 24.7 | 58 | 0.5 | 0.11 | 0.46 | 7.6 | 5031 |
| Chckn (brlr/fryr) light meat w/skin, | 85 | 189 | 51.4 | 0 | | | 0 | 64 | 13 | 21 | 1.05 | 0.015 | 28 | 0 | 0.05 | 9.5 | 0.27 | 0.79 |
| roasted - 3 oz | | 24.7 | 9.2 | 2.6 | 3.6 | 2.0 | 71 | 193 | 170 | 0.97 | 0.045 | 20.5 | 94 | | 0.10 | 0.44 | 2.6 | 5032 |
| Chckn (brlr/fryr) light meat w/skin, | 85 | 171 | 55.4 | 0 | | | 0 | 54 | 11 | 17 | 0.97 | 0.015 | 25 | 0 | 0.03 | 5.9 | 0.17 | 0.45 |
| stewed - 3 oz | | 22.2 | 8.5 | 2.4 | 3.3 | 1.8 | 63 | 142 | 124 | 0.83 | 0.037 | 18.0 | 82 | | 0.10 | 0.23 | 2.6 | 5033 |
| Chicken (broiler/fryer) light meat | 85 | 163 | 51.1 | 0.4 | | | 0 | 69 | 14 | 25 | 1.08 | 0.017 | 8 | 0 | 0.06 | 11.4 | 0.31 | 0.88 |
| w/o skin, fried - 3 oz | | 27.9 | 4.7 | 1.3 | 1.7 | 1.1 | 76 | 224 | 196 | 0.97 | 0.046 | 22.3 | 26 | | 0.11 | 0.54 | 3.4 | 5040 |
| Chicken (broiler/fryer) light meat | 85 | 147 | 55.0 | 0 | 0 | | 0 | 65 | 13 | 23 | 1.05 | 0.014 | 8 | 0 | 0.06 | 10.6 | 0.29 | 0.83 |
| w/o skin, roasted - 3 oz | | 26.3 | 3.8 | 1.1 | 1.3 | 0.8 | 72 | 210 | 184 | 0.90 | 0.042 | 20.7 | 25 | 0.2 | 0.10 | 0.51 | 3.4 | 5041 |
| Chicken (broiler/fryer) light meat | 85 | 135 | 57.8 | 0 | 0 | | 0 | 55 | 11 | 19 | 1.01 | 0.015 | 7 | 0 | 0.04 | 6.6 | 0.20 | 0.49 |
| w/o skin, stewed - 3 oz | | 24.5 | 3.4 | 1.0 | 1.1 | 0.7 | 65 | 153 | 135 | 0.79 | 0.037 | 19.0 | 23 | 0.2 | 0.10 | 0.28 | 2.6 | 5042 |

## 24.3 CHICKEN, ROASTERS

| | WT (g) | KCAL / PRO (g) | H₂O (g) / FAT (g) | CHO (g) / SFA (g) | TSUG (g) / MUFA (g) | ASUG (g) / PUFA (g) | DFIB (g) / CHOL (mg) | Na (mg) / K (mg) | Ca (mg) / P (mg) | Mg (mg) / Fe (mg) | Zn (mg) / Cu (mg) | Mn (mg) / Se (mcg) | A (mcg RAE) / A (IU) | C (mg) / E (mg ATE) | B-1 (mg) / B-2 (mg) | NIA (mg) / B-6 (mg) | B-12 (mcg) / FOL (mcg DFE) | PANT (mg) / REF |
|---|---|---|---|---|---|---|---|---|---|---|---|---|---|---|---|---|---|---|
| chicken (roaster) dark meat w/o | 85 | 151 | 57.0 | 0 | | | 0 | 81 | 9 | 17 | 1.81 | 0.016 | 14 | 0 | 0.05 | 4.9 | 0.23 | 0.87 |
| skin, roasted - 3 oz | | 19.8 | 7.4 | 2.1 | 2.8 | 1.7 | 64 | 190 | 145 | 1.13 | 0.060 | 16.7 | 46 | | 0.16 | 0.26 | 6.0 | 5120 |
| chicken (roaster) light and dark | 85 | 190 | 52.8 | 0 | | | 0 | 62 | 10 | 17 | 1.23 | 0.015 | | 0 | 0.05 | 6.3 | 0.23 | 0.78 |
| meat with skin, roasted - 3 oz | | 20.4 | 11.4 | 3.2 | 4.6 | 2.5 | 65 | 179 | 152 | 1.07 | 0.049 | 20.1 | 71 | | 0.12 | 0.30 | 4.2 | 5112 |
| chicken (roaster) light and dark | 85 | 142 | 57.3 | 0 | | | 0 | 64 | 10 | 18 | 1.29 | 0.014 | 10 | 0 | 0.05 | 6.7 | 0.25 | 0.83 |
| meat w/o skin, roasted - 3 oz | | 21.3 | 5.6 | 1.5 | 2.1 | 1.3 | 64 | 195 | 163 | 1.03 | 0.048 | 20.9 | 35 | | 0.12 | 0.35 | 4.2 | 5114 |
| chicken (roaster) light meat w/o | 85 | 130 | 57.7 | 0 | 0 | | 0 | 43 | 11 | 20 | 0.66 | 0.013 | 7 | 0 | 0.05 | 8.9 | 0.26 | 0.77 |
| skin, roasted - 3 oz | | 23.1 | 3.5 | 0.9 | 1.3 | 0.8 | 64 | 201 | 184 | 0.92 | 0.036 | 21.9 | 21 | 0.2 | 0.08 | 0.46 | 2.6 | 5118 |

## 24.4 CHICKEN, STEWERS

| | WT (g) | KCAL / PRO (g) | H₂O (g) / FAT (g) | CHO (g) / SFA (g) | TSUG (g) / MUFA (g) | ASUG (g) / PUFA (g) | DFIB (g) / CHOL (mg) | Na (mg) / K (mg) | Ca (mg) / P (mg) | Mg (mg) / Fe (mg) | Zn (mg) / Cu (mg) | Mn (mg) / Se (mcg) | A (mcg RAE) / A (IU) | C (mg) / E (mg ATE) | B-1 (mg) / B-2 (mg) | NIA (mg) / B-6 (mg) | B-12 (mcg) / FOL (mcg DFE) | PANT (mg) / REF |
|---|---|---|---|---|---|---|---|---|---|---|---|---|---|---|---|---|---|---|
| chicken (stewer) dark meat w/o | 85 | 219 | 46.8 | 0 | | | 0 | 81 | 10 | 19 | 2.65 | 0.020 | 37 | 0 | 0.11 | 3.9 | 0.21 | 0.86 |
| skin, stewed - 3 oz | | 23.9 | 13.0 | 3.5 | 4.5 | 3.1 | 81 | 173 | 159 | 1.39 | 0.122 | 18.5 | 123 | | 0.29 | 0.20 | 6.8 | 5132 |
| chicken (stewer) light and dark | 85 | 242 | 45.1 | 0 | | | 0 | 62 | 11 | 17 | 1.50 | 0.018 | 33 | 0 | 0.08 | 4.9 | 0.20 | 0.64 |
| meat with skin, stewed - 3 oz | | 22.8 | 16.0 | 4.3 | 6.1 | 3.6 | 67 | 155 | 153 | 1.16 | 0.085 | 16.7 | 111 | | 0.20 | 0.21 | 4.2 | 5124 |
| chicken (stewer) light and dark | 85 | 201 | 47.9 | 0 | 0 | | 0 | 66 | 11 | 19 | 1.75 | 0.009 | 29 | 0 | 0.10 | 5.4 | 0.22 | 0.73 |
| meat w/o skin, stewed - 3 oz | | 25.9 | 10.1 | 2.6 | 3.4 | 2.4 | 71 | 172 | 173 | 1.22 | 0.099 | 21.4 | 95 | 0.3 | 0.24 | 0.26 | 5.1 | 5126 |
| chicken (stewer) light meat w/o | 85 | 181 | 49.1 | 0 | 0 | | 0 | 49 | 12 | 20 | 0.71 | 0.017 | 19 | 0 | 0.08 | 7.3 | 0.23 | 0.59 |
| skin, stewed - 3 oz | | 28.1 | 6.8 | 1.7 | 2.3 | 1.6 | 60 | 169 | 191 | 1.01 | 0.072 | 24.4 | 62 | | 0.17 | 0.33 | 3.4 | 5130 |

## 24.5 CHICKEN, UNSPECIFIED TYPES

| | WT (g) | KCAL / PRO (g) | H₂O (g) / FAT (g) | CHO (g) / SFA (g) | TSUG (g) / MUFA (g) | ASUG (g) / PUFA (g) | DFIB (g) / CHOL (mg) | Na (mg) / K (mg) | Ca (mg) / P (mg) | Mg (mg) / Fe (mg) | Zn (mg) / Cu (mg) | Mn (mg) / Se (mcg) | A (mcg RAE) / A (IU) | C (mg) / E (mg ATE) | B-1 (mg) / B-2 (mg) | NIA (mg) / B-6 (mg) | B-12 (mcg) / FOL (mcg DFE) | PANT (mg) / REF |
|---|---|---|---|---|---|---|---|---|---|---|---|---|---|---|---|---|---|---|
| chicken breast, oven roasted, | 52 | 60 | | 3.0 | 0 | | 0 | 450 | 0 | | | | | 0 | | | | 0 |
| Healthy Choice - 4 slices | | 10.0 | 1.5 | 0.5 | | | 25 | | 0 | | | | 0 | | | | | HLCH12 |
| chicken, canned with broth | 142 | 234 | 97.5 | 0 | 0 | | 0 | 714 | 20 | 17 | 2.00 | 0.021 | 48 | 3 | 0.02 | 9.0 | 0.41 | 1.21 |
| 5 oz can | | 30.9 | 11.3 | 3.1 | 4.5 | 2.5 | 88 | 196 | 158 | 2.24 | 0.065 | 22.4 | 166 | 0.4 | 0.18 | 0.50 | 5.7 | 5277 |
| chicken, raw | 85 | 101 | 64.1 | 0 | 0 | | 0 | 65 | 10 | 21 | 1.31 | 0.016 | 14 | 2 | 0.06 | 7.0 | 0.31 | 0.90 |
| 3 oz | | 18.2 | 2.6 | 0.7 | 0.8 | 0.6 | 60 | 195 | 147 | 0.76 | 0.045 | 13.3 | 44 | 0.2 | 0.12 | 0.37 | 6.0 | 5011 |

## 24.6 TURKEY, ROASTERS

| | WT (g) | KCAL / PRO (g) | H₂O (g) / FAT (g) | CHO (g) / SFA (g) | TSUG (g) / MUFA (g) | ASUG (g) / PUFA (g) | DFIB (g) / CHOL (mg) | Na (mg) / K (mg) | Ca (mg) / P (mg) | Mg (mg) / Fe (mg) | Zn (mg) / Cu (mg) | Mn (mg) / Se (mcg) | A (mcg RAE) / A (IU) | C (mg) / E (mg ATE) | B-1 (mg) / B-2 (mg) | NIA (mg) / B-6 (mg) | B-12 (mcg) / FOL (mcg DFE) | PANT (mg) / REF |
|---|---|---|---|---|---|---|---|---|---|---|---|---|---|---|---|---|---|---|
| turkey (roaster) back w/skin, | 85 | 173 | 53.8 | 0 | | | 0 | 60 | 31 | 17 | 2.84 | 0.020 | 0 | 0 | 0.03 | 3.0 | 0.31 | 0.96 |
| roasted - 3 oz | | 22.2 | 8.7 | 2.5 | 3.0 | 2.2 | 92 | 177 | 144 | 1.57 | 0.141 | 32.0 | 0 | | 0.16 | 0.26 | 7.6 | 5214 |
| turkey (roaster) back w/o skin, | 99 | 168 | 65.3 | 0 | | | 0 | 72 | 36 | 22 | 3.76 | 0.025 | 0 | 0 | 0.04 | 3.8 | 0.41 | 1.41 |
| roasted - ½ back (3.5 oz) | | 27.7 | 5.6 | 1.9 | 1.3 | 1.7 | 94 | 215 | 175 | 1.83 | 0.177 | 40.5 | 0 | | 0.20 | 0.40 | 9.9 | 5216 |

| | WT (g) | KCAL / PRO (g) | H₂O (g) / FAT (g) | CHO (g) / SFA (g) | TSUG (g) / MUFA (g) | ASUG (g) / PUFA (g) | DFIB (g) / CHOL (mg) | Na (mg) / K (mg) | Ca (mg) / P (mg) | Mg (mg) / Fe (mg) | Zn (mg) / Cu (mg) | Mn (mg) / Se (mcg) | A (mcg RAE) / A (IU) | C (mg) / E (mg ATE) | B-1 (mg) / B-2 (mg) | NIA (mg) / B-6 (mg) | B-12 (mcg) / FOL (mcg DFE) | PANT (mg) / REF |
|---|---|---|---|---|---|---|---|---|---|---|---|---|---|---|---|---|---|---|
| **turkey (roaster) breast** w/skin, | 85 | 130 | 57.5 | 0 | | | 0 | 45 | 13 | 24 | 1.50 | 0.020 | 0 | 0 | 0.03 | 5.9 | 0.31 | 0.56 |
| roasted - *3 oz* | | 24.7 | 2.7 | 0.7 | 1.0 | 0.6 | 76 | 237 | 184 | 1.33 | 0.065 | 25.9 | 0 | | 0.11 | 0.43 | 5.1 | 5218 |
| **turkey (roaster) breast** w/o skin, | 85 | 115 | 58.1 | 0 | 0 | | 0 | 44 | 10 | 25 | 1.48 | 0.020 | 0 | 0 | 0.04 | 6.4 | 0.33 | 0.60 |
| roasted - *3 oz* | | 25.6 | 0.6 | 0.2 | 0.1 | 0.2 | 71 | 248 | 190 | 1.30 | 0.060 | 27.3 | 0 | 0.1 | 0.11 | 0.48 | 5.1 | 5220 |
| **turkey (roaster) dark meat** w/skin, | 85 | 155 | 55.1 | 0 | | | 0 | 65 | 23 | 20 | 3.26 | 0.020 | 0 | 0 | 0.04 | 2.8 | 0.31 | 1.02 |
| roasted - *3 oz* | | 23.5 | 6.0 | 1.8 | 1.9 | 1.6 | 99 | 201 | 162 | 1.98 | 0.178 | 33.2 | 0 | | 0.20 | 0.28 | 7.6 | 5208 |
| **turkey (roaster) dark meat** w/o | 85 | 138 | 56.4 | 0 | | | 0 | 67 | 22 | 20 | 3.51 | 0.021 | 0 | 0 | 0.04 | 3.0 | 0.33 | 1.15 |
| skin, roasted - *3 oz* | | 24.5 | 3.7 | 1.2 | 0.8 | 1.1 | 95 | 209 | 167 | 2.05 | 0.190 | 34.8 | 0 | | 0.21 | 0.32 | 8.5 | 5212 |
| **turkey (roaster) leg** w/skin, | 245 | 417 | 160.8 | 0 | | | 0 | 196 | 56 | 59 | 10.02 | 0.061 | 0 | 0 | 0.13 | 8.0 | 0.91 | 3.03 |
| roasted - *8.6 oz leg* | | 69.8 | 13.3 | 4.1 | 3.9 | 3.6 | 172 | 617 | 490 | 6.35 | 0.571 | 97.3 | 0 | | 0.63 | 0.83 | 22.0 | 5222 |
| **turkey (roaster) leg** w/o skin, | 224 | 356 | 149.0 | 0 | | | 0 | 181 | 49 | 56 | 9.59 | 0.058 | 0 | 0 | 0.12 | 7.4 | 0.85 | 2.97 |
| roasted - *7.9 oz leg* | | 65.4 | 8.4 | 2.8 | 1.9 | 2.5 | 267 | 578 | 457 | 5.96 | 0.542 | 91.6 | 0 | | 0.60 | 0.83 | 22.4 | 5224 |
| **turkey (roaster) light meat** w/skin, | 85 | 139 | 56.6 | 0 | | | 0 | 48 | 15 | 22 | 1.77 | 0.020 | 0 | 0 | 0.03 | 5.3 | 0.31 | 0.55 |
| roasted - *3 oz* | | 24.5 | 3.9 | 1.1 | 1.4 | 0.9 | 81 | 223 | 174 | 1.37 | 0.078 | 25.4 | 0 | | 0.12 | 0.42 | 5.1 | 5206 |
| **turkey (roaster) light meat** w/o | 85 | 119 | 58.3 | 0 | | | 0 | 48 | 13 | 24 | 1.77 | 0.021 | 0 | 0 | 0.03 | 5.9 | 0.33 | 0.61 |
| skin, roasted - *3 oz* | | 25.7 | 1.0 | 0.3 | 0.2 | 0.3 | 73 | 235 | 184 | 1.33 | 0.073 | 27.3 | 0 | | 0.12 | 0.48 | 5.1 | 5210 |
| **turkey (roaster) skin, roasted** | 34 | 102 | 18.9 | 0 | | | 0 | 21 | 12 | 6 | 0.70 | 0.007 | 0 | 0 | 0.01 | 0.9 | 0.07 | 0.09 |
| *1.2 oz (yield from 1 lb of turkey)* | | 7.1 | 7.9 | 2.1 | 3.4 | 1.8 | 49 | 62 | 51 | 0.63 | 0.044 | 52.1 | 0 | | 0.05 | 0.02 | 1.4 | 5204 |
| **turkey (roaster) wing** w/skin, | 90 | 186 | 56.1 | 0 | | | 0 | 66 | 26 | 18 | 2.92 | 0.022 | 0 | 0 | 0.03 | 3.3 | 0.32 | 0.54 |
| roasted - *3.2 oz wing* | | 24.9 | 8.9 | 2.4 | 3.3 | 2.1 | 104 | 176 | 149 | 1.63 | 0.139 | 25.3 | 0 | | 0.14 | 0.38 | 5.4 | 5226 |
| **turkey (roaster) wing** w/o skin, | 60 | 98 | 39.4 | 0 | 0 | | 0 | 47 | 16 | 13 | 2.30 | 0.016 | 0 | 0 | 0.02 | 2.5 | 0.25 | 0.45 |
| roasted - *2.1 oz wing* | | 18.5 | 2.1 | 0.7 | 0.4 | 0.6 | 61 | 122 | 104 | 1.07 | 0.100 | 19.3 | 0 | 0.1 | 0.10 | 0.35 | 4.2 | 5228 |

## 24.7  TURKEY, YOUNG HEN

| | WT (g) | KCAL / PRO (g) | H₂O (g) / FAT (g) | CHO (g) / SFA (g) | TSUG (g) / MUFA (g) | ASUG (g) / PUFA (g) | DFIB (g) / CHOL (mg) | Na (mg) / K (mg) | Ca (mg) / P (mg) | Mg (mg) / Fe (mg) | Zn (mg) / Cu (mg) | Mn (mg) / Se (mcg) | A (mcg RAE) / A (IU) | C (mg) / E (mg ATE) | B-1 (mg) / B-2 (mg) | NIA (mg) / B-6 (mg) | B-12 (mcg) / FOL (mcg DFE) | PANT (mg) / REF |
|---|---|---|---|---|---|---|---|---|---|---|---|---|---|---|---|---|---|---|
| **turkey (young hen) back** w/skin, | 85 | 216 | 48.4 | 0 | | | 0 | 59 | 26 | 20 | 3.31 | 0.020 | A | 0 | 0.04 | 3.0 | 0.28 | 0.88 |
| roasted - *3 oz* | | 22.4 | 13.3 | 3.9 | 4.6 | 3.4 | 72 | 224 | 161 | 1.89 | 0.113 | 29.2 | 0 | | 0.18 | 0.25 | 6.8 | 5246 |
| **turkey (young hen) breast** w/skin, | 85 | 165 | 53.3 | 0 | | | 0 | 49 | 19 | 22 | 1.67 | 0.018 | A | 0 | 0.05 | 5.7 | 0.30 | 0.53 |
| roasted - *3 oz* | | 24.5 | 6.7 | 1.9 | 2.1 | 1.6 | 61 | 246 | 178 | 1.16 | 0.037 | 23.7 | 0 | | 0.11 | 0.40 | 5.1 | 5248 |
| **turkey (young hen) dark meat** | 85 | 197 | 50.7 | 0 | | | 0 | 61 | 26 | 20 | 3.48 | 0.020 | A | 0 | 0.05 | 3.1 | 0.29 | 0.95 |
| w/skin, roasted - *3 oz* | | 23.3 | 10.9 | 3.3 | 3.5 | 2.9 | 71 | 235 | 167 | 1.94 | 0.118 | 31.6 | 0 | | 0.19 | 0.26 | 6.8 | 5240 |
| **turkey (young hen) dark meat** w/o | 85 | 163 | 53.3 | 0 | | | 0 | 64 | 26 | 21 | 3.73 | 0.020 | A | 0 | 0.05 | 3.2 | 0.31 | 1.05 |
| skin, roasted - *3 oz* | | 24.2 | 6.6 | 2.2 | 1.5 | 2.0 | 68 | 248 | 173 | 1.98 | 0.126 | 34.8 | 0 | | 0.20 | 0.29 | 7.6 | 5244 |
| **turkey (young hen) leg** w/skin, | 85 | 181 | 51.6 | 0 | | | 0 | 62 | 26 | 20 | 3.59 | 0.020 | A | 0 | 0.05 | 3.1 | 0.30 | 0.99 |
| roasted - *3 oz* | | 23.6 | 8.9 | 2.8 | 2.6 | 2.5 | 70 | 240 | 168 | 1.95 | 0.122 | 32.8 | 0 | | 0.19 | 0.27 | 7.6 | 5250 |
| **turkey (young hen) light and dark** | 85 | 185 | 51.9 | 0 | | | 0 | 54 | 22 | 21 | 2.46 | 0.019 | | 0 | 0.05 | 4.5 | 0.29 | 0.71 |
| **meat** w/skin, roasted - *3 oz* | | 23.9 | 9.2 | 2.7 | 3.0 | 2.4 | 66 | 240 | 173 | 1.51 | 0.073 | 26.7 | 0 | | 0.14 | 0.34 | 6.0 | 5232 |
| **turkey (young hen) light and dark** | 85 | 149 | 54.8 | 0 | | | 0 | 57 | 21 | 22 | 2.58 | 0.019 | A | 0 | 0.05 | 4.8 | 0.31 | 0.77 |
| **meat** w/o skin, roasted - *3 oz* | | 24.9 | 4.7 | 1.5 | 1.0 | 1.3 | 62 | 254 | 180 | 1.50 | 0.074 | 29.2 | 0 | | 0.15 | 0.37 | 6.0 | 5234 |
| **turkey (young hen) light meat** | 85 | 176 | 52.8 | 0 | | | 0 | 49 | 20 | 22 | 1.68 | 0.018 | A | 0 | 0.04 | 5.6 | 0.29 | 0.52 |
| w/skin, roasted - *3 oz* | | 24.3 | 8.0 | 2.3 | 2.7 | 1.9 | 63 | 243 | 177 | 1.18 | 0.037 | 24.2 | 0 | | 0.11 | 0.39 | 5.1 | 5238 |
| **turkey (young hen) light meat** | 85 | 137 | 55.9 | 0 | | | 0 | 51 | 18 | 24 | 1.67 | 0.017 | A | 0 | 0.05 | 6.0 | 0.31 | 0.56 |
| w/o skin, roasted - *3 oz* | | 25.4 | 3.2 | 1.0 | 0.6 | 0.8 | 58 | 258 | 185 | 1.11 | 0.033 | 27.3 | 0 | | 0.11 | 0.44 | 5.1 | 5242 |
| **turkey (young hen) wing** w/skin, | 85 | 202 | 49.8 | 0 | | | 0 | 48 | 20 | 21 | 1.69 | 0.018 | A | 0 | 0.04 | 5.2 | 0.28 | 0.48 |
| roasted - *3 oz* | | 23.2 | 11.4 | 3.1 | 4.3 | 2.7 | 65 | 228 | 168 | 1.22 | 0.042 | 23.5 | 0 | | 0.11 | 0.35 | 4.2 | 5252 |

## 24.8  TURKEY, YOUNG TOM

| | WT (g) | KCAL / PRO (g) | H₂O (g) / FAT (g) | CHO (g) / SFA (g) | TSUG (g) / MUFA (g) | ASUG (g) / PUFA (g) | DFIB (g) / CHOL (mg) | Na (mg) / K (mg) | Ca (mg) / P (mg) | Mg (mg) / Fe (mg) | Zn (mg) / Cu (mg) | Mn (mg) / Se (mcg) | A (mcg RAE) / A (IU) | C (mg) / E (mg ATE) | B-1 (mg) / B-2 (mg) | NIA (mg) / B-6 (mg) | B-12 (mcg) / FOL (mcg DFE) | PANT (mg) / REF |
|---|---|---|---|---|---|---|---|---|---|---|---|---|---|---|---|---|---|---|
| **turkey (young tom) back with skin,** | 85 | 202 | 49.6 | 0 | | | 0 | 65 | 30 | 19 | 3.41 | 0.019 | A | 0 | 0.05 | 2.8 | 0.30 | 0.94 |
| roasted - *3 oz* | | 22.8 | 11.6 | 3.4 | 4.0 | 3.0 | 80 | 224 | 162 | 1.88 | 0.125 | 32.3 | 0 | | 0.20 | 0.26 | 6.8 | 5270 |
| **turkey (young tom) breast** w/skin, | 85 | 161 | 53.8 | 0 | | | 0 | 57 | 18 | 23 | 1.78 | 0.016 | A | 0 | 0.05 | 5.1 | 0.31 | 0.55 |
| roasted - *3 oz* | | 24.3 | 6.3 | 1.8 | 2.1 | 1.5 | 64 | 246 | 178 | 1.20 | 0.041 | 25.7 | 0 | | 0.11 | 0.42 | 5.1 | 5272 |
| **turkey (young tom) dark meat** | 85 | 157 | 53.6 | 0 | | | 0 | 70 | 30 | 20 | 3.88 | 0.019 | A | 0 | 0.06 | 3.0 | 0.32 | 1.13 |
| w/skin, roasted - *3 oz* | | 24.4 | 5.9 | 2.0 | 1.3 | 1.8 | 75 | 249 | 174 | 1.98 | 0.139 | 34.8 | 0 | | 0.22 | 0.31 | 8.5 | 5268 |
| **turkey (young tom) dark meat** | 85 | 184 | 51.3 | 0 | | | 0 | 68 | 30 | 20 | 3.61 | 0.019 | A | 0 | 0.05 | 2.9 | 0.31 | 1.02 |
| w/o skin, roasted - *3 oz* | | 23.4 | 9.2 | 2.8 | 2.9 | 2.5 | 77 | 235 | 167 | 1.92 | 0.131 | 33.7 | 0 | | 0.21 | 0.28 | 7.6 | 5264 |
| **turkey (young tom) leg** w/skin, | 85 | 175 | 52.0 | 0 | | | 0 | 68 | 30 | 20 | 3.69 | 0.019 | A | 0 | 0.05 | 3.0 | 0.31 | 1.05 |
| roasted - *3 oz* | | 23.7 | 8.2 | 2.5 | 2.4 | 2.3 | 76 | 239 | 170 | 1.94 | 0.133 | 34.9 | 0 | | 0.21 | 0.29 | 7.6 | 5274 |
| **turkey (young tom) light and dark** | 85 | 172 | 52.6 | 0 | | | 0 | 61 | 23 | 21 | 2.57 | 0.017 | | 0 | 0.05 | 4.2 | 0.31 | 0.75 |
| **meat** w/skin, roasted - *3 oz* | | 23.9 | 7.7 | 2.2 | 2.5 | 2.0 | 70 | 240 | 173 | 1.51 | 0.080 | 29.3 | 0 | | 0.16 | 0.36 | 6.0 | 5256 |
| **turkey (young tom) light and dark** | 85 | 143 | 55.3 | 0 | | | 0 | 63 | 21 | 22 | 2.69 | 0.017 | A | 0 | 0.06 | 4.5 | 0.32 | 0.82 |
| **meat** w/o skin, roasted - *3 oz* | | 25.0 | 4.0 | 1.3 | 0.8 | 1.1 | 65 | 256 | 182 | 1.51 | 0.081 | 31.3 | 0 | | 0.16 | 0.40 | 6.8 | 5258 |
| **turkey (young tom) light meat** | 85 | 162 | 53.7 | 0 | | | 0 | 57 | 18 | 23 | 1.78 | 0.016 | A | 0 | 0.05 | 5.1 | 0.31 | 0.54 |
| w/skin, roasted - *3 oz* | | 24.2 | 6.5 | 1.8 | 2.3 | 1.6 | 64 | 244 | 178 | 1.20 | 0.041 | 26.1 | 0 | | 0.11 | 0.41 | 5.1 | 5262 |

| | WT (g) | KCAL / PRO (g) | H₂0 (g) / FAT (g) | CHO (g) / SFA (g) | TSUG (g) / MUFA (g) | ASUG (g) / PUFA (g) | DFIB (g) / CHOL (mg) | Na (mg) / K (mg) | Ca (mg) / P (mg) | Mg (mg) / Fe (mg) | Zn (mg) / Cu (mg) | Mn (mg) / Se (mcg) | A (mcg RAE) / A (IU) | C (mg) / E (mg ATE) | B-1 (mg) / B-2 (mg) | NIA (mg) / B-6 (mg) | B-12 (mcg) / FOL (mcg DFE) | PANT (mg) / REF |
|---|---|---|---|---|---|---|---|---|---|---|---|---|---|---|---|---|---|---|
| turkey (young tom) light meat w/o skin, roasted - 3 oz | 85 | 131 | 56.6 | 0 | | | 0 | 58 | 15 | 24 | 1.78 | 0.016 | 0 | 0 | 0.06 | 5.6 | 0.32 | 0.59 |
| | | 25.4 | 2.5 | 0.8 | 0.4 | 0.7 | 59 | 262 | 187 | 1.16 | 0.036 | 27.3 | 0 | | 0.11 | 0.47 | 5.1 | 5266 |
| turkey (young tom) wing w/skin, roasted - 3 oz | 85 | 188 | 51.3 | 0 | | | 0 | 56 | 20 | 21 | 1.78 | 0.017 | 0 | 0 | 0.05 | 4.7 | 0.30 | 0.51 |
| | | 23.3 | 9.8 | 2.7 | 3.7 | 2.3 | 69 | 230 | 170 | 1.24 | 0.045 | 25.7 | 0 | | 0.12 | 0.37 | 5.1 | 5276 |

## 24.9 TURKEY, UNSPECIFIED TYPES

| | WT (g) | KCAL / PRO | H₂0 / FAT | CHO / SFA | TSUG / MUFA | ASUG / PUFA | DFIB / CHOL | Na / K | Ca / P | Mg / Fe | Zn / Cu | Mn / Se | A RAE / A IU | C / E | B-1 / B-2 | NIA / B-6 | B-12 / FOL | PANT / REF |
|---|---|---|---|---|---|---|---|---|---|---|---|---|---|---|---|---|---|---|
| turkey and pork sausage (fresh), patty/link, pan-fried - 2 oz | 56 | 172 | 28.5 | 0.4 | 0 | | 0 | 492 | 18 | 11 | 1.78 | | 0 | 1 | 0.29 | 2.4 | 0.71 | |
| | | 12.7 | 12.9 | 4.5 | 5.4 | 1.8 | 47 | 189 | 107 | 0.91 | 0.083 | 11.8 | 0 | 0.2 | 0.14 | 0.19 | 2.2 | 42173 |
| turkey bacon, Louis Rich .5 oz | 14 | 35 | 8.3 | 0.2 | 0.2 | | 0 | 170 | 6 | 3 | 0.35 | | 0 | 0 | | | | |
| | | 2.1 | 2.8 | 0.7 | 1.1 | 0.7 | 13 | 29 | 28 | 0.20 | 0.035 | | 0 | | | | 1.1 | 7254 |
| turkey bacon, pan-fried 1 oz | 28 | 107 | 9.1 | 0.9 | 0 | 0 | 0 | 640 | 3 | 8 | 0.85 | | 0 | 0 | 0.02 | 1.0 | 0.10 | |
| | | 8.3 | 7.8 | 2.3 | 3.1 | 1.9 | 27 | 111 | 129 | 0.59 | 0.042 | 7.2 | 0 | 0.3 | 0.07 | 0.09 | 2.5 | 42130 |
| turkey breast, honey rstd & smoked, Hlthy Chc - 4 slices | 52 | 60 | | 3.0 | 2.0 | | 0 | 450 | 0 | | | | 0 | 0 | | | | |
| | | 9.0 | 1.5 | 0.5 | | | 25 | | 0 | | | | 0 | | | | | HLCH16 |
| turkey breast, raw 3 oz | 85 | 133 | 59.5 | 0 | | | 0 | 50 | 11 | 20 | 1.33 | 0.015 | 2 | 0 | 0.05 | 4.4 | 0.36 | 0.53 |
| | | 18.6 | 6.0 | 1.6 | 2.3 | 1.4 | 55 | 234 | 158 | 1.02 | 0.063 | 19.0 | 5 | | 0.10 | 0.41 | 6.0 | 5191 |
| turkey breast w/skin, prebasted, roasted - 3 oz | 85 | 107 | 60.3 | 0 | | | 0 | 337 | 8 | 18 | 1.30 | 0.013 | 0 | 0 | 0.05 | 7.7 | 0.27 | 0.42 |
| | | 18.8 | 2.9 | 0.8 | 1.0 | 0.7 | 36 | 211 | 182 | 0.56 | 0.035 | 21.8 | 0 | | 0.11 | 0.27 | 4.2 | 5293 |
| turkey, canned with broth 5 oz can | 142 | 231 | 93.8 | 0 | 0 | | 0 | 663 | 17 | 28 | 3.37 | 0.024 | 0 | 3 | 0.02 | 9.4 | 0.40 | 0.97 |
| | | 33.6 | 9.7 | 2.8 | 3.2 | 2.5 | 94 | 318 | 230 | 2.64 | 0.105 | 36.8 | 0 | 0.4 | 0.24 | 0.47 | 8.5 | 5284 |
| turkey, diced, seasoned 1 oz | 28 | 39 | 20.1 | 0.3 | | | 0 | 238 | 0 | 5 | 0.57 | 0.004 | 0 | 0 | 0.01 | 1.3 | 0.07 | 0.16 |
| | | 5.2 | 1.7 | 0.5 | 0.6 | 0.4 | 15 | 87 | 67 | 0.50 | 0.018 | 7.3 | 0 | | 0.03 | 0.08 | 1.4 | 5285 |
| turkey drumstick w/skin, bone out, smoked, cooked - 3 oz | 85 | 177 | 52.0 | 0 | 0 | | 0 | 847 | 27 | 20 | 3.63 | | 0 | 0 | 0.05 | 3.0 | 0.31 | |
| | | 23.7 | 8.3 | 2.6 | 2.4 | 2.3 | 72 | 238 | 169 | 1.95 | 0.131 | 32.6 | 0 | 0.5 | 0.20 | 0.28 | 7.6 | 43367 |
| turkey, ground, cooked 2.9 oz patty | 82 | 193 | 48.7 | 0 | 0 | | 0 | 88 | 20 | 20 | 2.35 | 0.016 | 0 | 0 | 0.04 | 4.0 | 0.27 | 0.67 |
| | | 22.4 | 10.8 | 2.8 | 4.0 | 2.6 | 84 | 221 | 161 | 1.58 | 0.074 | 30.5 | 0 | 0.3 | 0.14 | 0.32 | 5.7 | 5306 |
| turkey, lght/dark meat w/skin, bone out, smkd, rstd - 3 oz | 85 | 177 | 52.4 | 0 | 0 | | 0 | 847 | 22 | 21 | 2.52 | | 0 | 0 | 0.05 | 4.3 | 0.30 | |
| | | 23.9 | 8.2 | 2.4 | 2.7 | 2.1 | 70 | 238 | 173 | 1.52 | 0.079 | 25.8 | 0 | 0.3 | 0.15 | 0.35 | 6.0 | 43390 |
| turkey nuggets/sticks, breaded, Louis Rich - 3 pieces (3 oz) | 85 | 235 | 43.1 | 13.1 | 0 | | 0.4 | 577 | 8 | 18 | 1.56 | | 0 | | | | | |
| | | 12.2 | 14.9 | 2.9 | 7.0 | 4.7 | 34 | 150 | 167 | 0.74 | 0.246 | | 0 | | | | | 7265 |
| turkey patty, breaded/battered, fried - 3.3 oz patty | 94 | 266 | 46.7 | 14.8 | 0.3 | | 0.5 | 752 | 13 | 14 | 1.35 | 0.072 | 9 | 0 | 0.09 | 2.2 | 0.22 | 0.49 |
| | | 13.2 | 16.9 | 4.4 | 7.0 | 4.4 | 70 | 258 | 254 | 2.07 | 0.087 | 20.8 | 34 | 0.9 | 0.18 | 0.19 | 57.3 | 5292 |
| turkey, raw 3 oz | 85 | 101 | 63.0 | 0 | 0 | | 0 | 60 | 12 | 21 | 2.01 | 0.018 | 0 | 0 | 0.06 | 3.9 | 0.37 | 0.77 |
| | | 18.5 | 2.4 | 0.8 | 0.5 | 0.7 | 55 | 252 | 166 | 1.23 | 0.093 | 22.5 | 0 | 0.3 | 0.14 | 0.40 | 7.6 | 5167 |
| turkey roast, boneless, frozen, seasoned, roasted - 3 oz | 85 | 132 | 57.7 | 2.6 | 0 | 0 | 0 | 578 | 4 | 19 | 2.16 | 0.013 | 0 | 0 | 0.04 | 5.3 | 1.29 | 0.69 |
| | | 18.1 | 4.9 | 1.6 | 1.0 | 1.4 | 45 | 253 | 207 | 1.39 | 0.051 | 31.0 | 0 | 0.3 | 0.14 | 0.23 | 4.2 | 5296 |
| turkey sausage (fresh), breakfast, mild - 2 links (2 oz) | 56 | 129 | 35.3 | 0.9 | 0 | | 0 | 328 | 18 | 9 | 1.67 | | 0 | 0 | 0.03 | 2.1 | 0.44 | |
| | | 8.6 | 10.1 | 2.1 | 2.9 | 2.6 | 90 | 128 | 87 | 0.60 | 0.062 | 0 | 0 | 0.1 | 0.09 | 0.12 | 2.2 | 7919 |
| turkey sausage (fresh), pan-fried 2 oz | 56 | 110 | 36.4 | 0 | 0 | | 0 | 372 | 12 | 12 | 2.17 | 0.013 | 7 | 0 | 0.05 | 3.2 | 0.69 | 0.60 |
| | | 13.4 | 5.8 | 1.3 | 1.7 | 1.5 | 52 | 167 | 113 | 0.83 | 0.081 | | 42 | 0.1 | 0.14 | 0.18 | 3.4 | 7958 |
| turkey sausage (fresh), red fat brown and serve, ckd - 2 oz | 56 | 112 | 33.4 | 6.0 | | | 0.2 | 346 | 17 | 12 | 1.29 | 0.124 | 1 | 0 | 0.04 | 1.2 | 0.16 | 0.40 |
| | | 9.5 | 5.8 | 1.6 | 2.2 | 1.4 | 32 | 116 | 92 | 1.01 | 0.083 | 11.6 | 4 | 0 | 0.08 | 0.13 | 12.9 | 7066 |
| turkey skin 1 oz | 28 | 108 | 13.9 | 0 | | | 0 | 10 | 5 | 2 | 0.36 | 0.003 | 3 | 0 | 0.01 | 0.4 | 0.07 | 0.07 |
| | | 3.6 | 10.3 | 2.7 | 4.4 | 2.4 | 25 | 29 | 23 | 0.38 | 0.021 | 3.5 | 11 | | 0.02 | 0.02 | 1.1 | 5169 |
| turkey sticks, breaded/battered, fried - 2.3 oz stick | 64 | 179 | 31.6 | 10.9 | | | | 536 | 9 | 10 | 0.93 | 0.053 | 8 | 0 | 0.06 | 1.3 | 0.15 | 0.34 |
| | | 9.1 | 10.8 | 2.8 | 4.4 | 2.8 | 41 | 166 | 150 | 1.41 | 0.047 | 13.2 | 26 | | 0.12 | 0.13 | 27.5 | 5300 |
| turkey thigh w/skin, prebasted, roasted - 3 oz | 85 | 133 | 60.0 | 0 | | | 0 | 371 | 7 | 14 | 3.50 | 0.013 | 0 | 0 | 0.07 | 2.0 | 0.20 | 0.69 |
| | | 16.0 | 7.3 | 2.3 | 2.2 | 2.0 | 53 | 205 | 145 | 1.28 | 0.118 | 23.7 | 0 | | 0.22 | 0.20 | 5.1 | 5294 |
| turkey wing w/skin, bone out, smoked, cooked - 3 oz | 85 | 195 | 50.6 | 0 | 0 | | 0 | 847 | 20 | 21 | 1.78 | | 0 | 0 | 0.04 | 4.9 | 0.29 | |
| | | 23.3 | 10.5 | 2.9 | 4.0 | 2.5 | 69 | 226 | 167 | 1.24 | 0.048 | 22.1 | 0 | 0.1 | 0.11 | 0.36 | 5.1 | 43366 |

## 24.10 OTHER POULTRY

| | WT (g) | KCAL / PRO | H₂0 / FAT | CHO / SFA | TSUG / MUFA | ASUG / PUFA | DFIB / CHOL | Na / K | Ca / P | Mg / Fe | Zn / Cu | Mn / Se | A RAE / A IU | C / E | B-1 / B-2 | NIA / B-6 | B-12 / FOL | PANT / REF |
|---|---|---|---|---|---|---|---|---|---|---|---|---|---|---|---|---|---|---|
| Cornish game hen w/skin, roasted 3 oz | 85 | 221 | 49.9 | 0 | 0 | | 0 | 54 | 11 | 15 | 1.27 | 0.013 | 27 | 0 | 0.06 | 5.0 | 0.24 | 0.50 |
| | | 18.9 | 15.5 | 4.3 | 6.8 | 3.1 | 111 | 208 | 124 | 0.77 | 0.052 | 13.2 | 90 | 0.3 | 0.17 | 0.26 | 1.7 | 5308 |
| Cornish game hen w/o skin, roasted - 3 oz | 85 | 114 | 61.1 | 0 | 0 | | 0 | 54 | 11 | 16 | 1.30 | 0.013 | 17 | 1 | 0.06 | 5.3 | 0.26 | 0.47 |
| | | 19.8 | 3.3 | 0.8 | 1.1 | 0.8 | 90 | 212 | 127 | 0.65 | 0.050 | 17.7 | 55 | 0.2 | 0.19 | 0.30 | 1.7 | 5310 |
| duck w/skin, roasted 3 oz | 85 | 286 | 44.1 | 0 | 0 | | 0 | 50 | 9 | 14 | 1.58 | 0.016 | 54 | 0 | 0.15 | 4.1 | 0.26 | 0.93 |
| | | 16.1 | 24.1 | 8.2 | 11.0 | 3.1 | 71 | 173 | 133 | 2.30 | 0.193 | 17.0 | 178 | 0.6 | 0.23 | 0.15 | 5.1 | 5140 |
| duck w/o skin, roasted 3 oz | 85 | 171 | 54.6 | 0 | 0 | | 0 | 55 | 10 | 17 | 2.21 | 0.016 | 20 | 0 | 0.22 | 4.3 | 0.34 | 1.27 |
| | | 20.0 | 9.5 | 3.5 | 3.1 | 1.2 | 76 | 214 | 173 | 2.30 | 0.196 | 19.0 | 65 | 0.6 | 0.40 | 0.21 | 8.5 | 5142 |

| | WT (g) | KCAL | H₂0 (g) | CHO (g) | TSUG (g) | ASUG (g) | DFIB (g) | Na (mg) | Ca (mg) | Mg (mg) | Zn (mg) | Mn (mg) | A (mcg RAE) | C (mg) | B-1 (mg) | NIA (mg) | B-12 (mcg) | PANT (mg) |
|---|---|---|---|---|---|---|---|---|---|---|---|---|---|---|---|---|---|---|
| | | PRO (g) | FAT (g) | SFA (g) | MUFA (g) | PUFA (g) | CHOL (mg) | K (mg) | P (mg) | Fe (mg) | Cu (mg) | Se (mcg) | A (IU) | E (mg ATE) | B-2 (mg) | B-6 (mg) | FOL (mcg DFE) | REF |
| **duckling, white pekin breast w/** skin, boneless, roasted - *3 oz* | 85 | 172 | 53.8 | 0 | | | | 71 | 7 | | | | | 2 | | 6.7 | | |
| | | 20.8 | 9.2 | 2.5 | 4.6 | 1.4 | 116 | | | 2.77 | | 22.4 | | | | | | 5315 |
| **duckling, white pekin breast w/o** skin, boneless, broiled - *3 oz* | 85 | 119 | 58.0 | 0 | | | | 89 | 8 | | | | | 3 | | 8.8 | | |
| | | 23.5 | 2.1 | 0.5 | 0.7 | 0.3 | 122 | | | 3.82 | | 24.6 | | | | | | 5316 |
| **duckling, white pekin leg w/skin,** bone in, roasted - *3 oz* | 85 | 184 | 51.8 | 0 | | | | 94 | 8 | | | | | 1 | | 4.9 | | |
| | | 22.7 | 9.7 | 2.5 | 4.8 | 1.6 | 97 | | | 1.77 | | 18.5 | | | | | | 5317 |
| **duckling, white pekin leg w/o** skin, bone in, braised - *3 oz* | 85 | 151 | 54.9 | 0 | | | | 92 | 8 | | | | | 2 | | 4.5 | | |
| | | 24.7 | 5.1 | 1.1 | 2.2 | 0.8 | 89 | | | 1.98 | | 18.4 | | | | | | 5318 |
| **goose** w/skin, roasted | 85 | 259 | 44.2 | 0 | 0 | | 0 | 60 | 11 | 19 | 2.23 | 0.020 | 18 | 0 | 0.07 | 3.5 | 0.35 | 1.30 |
| *3 oz* | | 21.4 | 18.6 | 5.8 | 8.7 | 2.1 | 77 | 280 | 230 | 2.41 | 0.224 | 18.5 | 60 | 1.5 | 0.27 | 0.31 | 1.7 | 5147 |
| **goose** w/o skin, roasted | 85 | 202 | 48.6 | 0 | | | 0 | 65 | 12 | 21 | 2.69 | 0.020 | 10 | 0 | 0.08 | 3.5 | 0.42 | 1.56 |
| *3 oz* | | 24.6 | 10.8 | 3.9 | 3.7 | 1.3 | 82 | 330 | 263 | 2.44 | 0.235 | 21.7 | 34 | | 0.33 | 0.40 | 10.2 | 5149 |
| **Guinea hen** w/o skin, raw | 85 | 94 | 63.3 | 0 | | | 0 | 59 | 9 | 20 | 1.02 | 0.015 | 10 | 1 | 0.06 | 7.5 | 0.31 | 0.80 |
| *3 oz* | | 17.5 | 2.1 | 0.5 | 0.6 | 0.5 | 54 | 187 | 144 | 0.65 | 0.037 | 14.9 | 35 | | 0.10 | 0.40 | 5.1 | 5152 |
| **owl, horned,** raw | 85 | 116 | 60.6 | 0 | | | | | 14 | | | | | | | | | |
| *3 oz* | | 19.3 | 4.2 | | | | | | 185 | 4.08 | | | 298 | | | | | 35059 |
| **pheasant** w/skin, raw | 85 | 154 | 57.6 | 0 | | | 0 | 34 | 10 | 17 | 0.82 | 0.014 | 45 | 5 | 0.06 | 5.5 | 0.65 | 0.79 |
| *3 oz* | | 19.3 | 7.9 | 2.3 | 3.7 | 1.0 | 60 | 207 | 182 | 0.98 | 0.055 | 13.3 | 150 | | 0.12 | 0.56 | 5.1 | 5153 |
| **pheasant** w/o skin, raw | 85 | 113 | 61.9 | 0 | | | 0 | 31 | 11 | 17 | 0.82 | 0.014 | 42 | 5 | 0.07 | 5.7 | 0.71 | 0.82 |
| *3 oz* | | 20.0 | 3.1 | 1.1 | 1.0 | 0.5 | 56 | 223 | 196 | 0.98 | 0.059 | 13.8 | 140 | | 0.13 | 0.63 | 5.1 | 5154 |
| **quail,** edible portion, cooked | 85 | 199 | 51.0 | 0 | 0 | | 0 | 44 | 13 | 19 | 2.64 | | 60 | 2 | 0.19 | 6.7 | 0.31 | |
| *3 oz* | | 21.3 | 12.0 | 3.4 | 4.2 | 3.0 | 73 | 184 | 237 | 3.77 | 0.503 | 18.5 | 199 | 0.6 | 0.26 | 0.53 | 5.1 | 43282 |
| **squab** (pigeon), cooked | 85 | 186 | 52.7 | 0 | 0 | | 0 | 48 | 14 | 22 | 3.26 | | 24 | 2 | 0.24 | 6.5 | 0.35 | |
| *3 oz* | | 20.3 | 11.0 | 3.2 | 4.6 | 2.3 | 99 | 218 | 282 | 5.02 | 0.649 | 17.1 | 81 | 0.1 | 0.30 | 0.48 | 5.1 | 43287 |
| **squab** (pigeon), w/o skin, raw | 85 | 121 | 61.9 | 0 | | | 0 | 43 | 11 | 21 | 2.30 | 0.016 | 24 | 6 | 0.24 | 5.8 | 0.40 | 0.67 |
| *3 oz* | | 14.9 | 6.4 | 1.7 | 2.3 | 1.4 | 76 | 201 | 261 | 3.83 | 0.505 | 11.5 | 80 | | 0.24 | 0.45 | 6.0 | 5161 |

## 24.11  POULTRY INTERNAL ORGANS AND OTHER PARTS

| | WT (g) | KCAL | H₂0 (g) | CHO (g) | TSUG (g) | ASUG (g) | DFIB (g) | Na (mg) | Ca (mg) | Mg (mg) | Zn (mg) | Mn (mg) | A (mcg RAE) | C (mg) | B-1 (mg) | NIA (mg) | B-12 (mcg) | PANT (mg) |
|---|---|---|---|---|---|---|---|---|---|---|---|---|---|---|---|---|---|---|
| | | PRO (g) | FAT (g) | SFA (g) | MUFA (g) | PUFA (g) | CHOL (mg) | K (mg) | P (mg) | Fe (mg) | Cu (mg) | Se (mcg) | A (IU) | E (mg ATE) | B-2 (mg) | B-6 (mg) | FOL (mcg DFE) | REF |
| **chicken feet,** boiled | 85 | 183 | 55.9 | 0.2 | 0 | | 0 | 57 | 75 | 4 | 0.59 | | 26 | 0 | 0.05 | 0.3 | 0.40 | |
| *3 oz* | | 16.5 | 12.4 | 3.3 | 4.7 | 2.5 | 71 | 26 | 71 | 0.77 | 0.087 | 3.1 | 85 | 0.2 | 0.17 | 0.01 | 73.1 | 5335 |
| **chicken giblets,** fried | 85 | 235 | 40.7 | 3.7 | | | 0 | 96 | 15 | 21 | 5.33 | 0.189 | 3045 | 7 | 0.08 | 9.3 | 11.31 | 3.79 |
| *3 oz* | | 27.7 | 11.4 | 3.2 | 3.8 | 2.9 | 379 | 280 | 243 | 8.77 | 0.359 | 88.6 | 10140 | | 1.30 | 0.52 | 322.2 | 5021 |
| **chicken giblets,** simmered | 85 | 134 | 57.6 | 0.4 | | | 0 | 57 | 12 | 12 | 3.60 | 0.169 | 1490 | 11 | 0.12 | 5.6 | 8.02 | 2.78 |
| *3 oz* | | 23.1 | 3.8 | 1.1 | 0.8 | 0.7 | 376 | 190 | 246 | 5.98 | 0.281 | 50.7 | 4989 | 0.4 | 0.89 | 0.34 | 218.4 | 5022 |
| **chicken gizzard,** simmered | 85 | 131 | 57.7 | 0 | | | 0 | 48 | 14 | 3 | 3.76 | 0.063 | 0 | 0 | 0.02 | 2.7 | 0.88 | 0.40 |
| *3 oz* | | 25.8 | 2.3 | 0.6 | 0.4 | 0.3 | 314 | 152 | 161 | 2.71 | 0.137 | 34.9 | 0 | 0.2 | 0.18 | 0.06 | 4.2 | 5024 |
| **chicken heart,** simmered | 85 | 157 | 55.1 | 0.1 | | | 0 | 41 | 16 | 17 | 6.20 | 0.091 | 7 | 2 | 0.06 | 2.4 | 6.20 | 2.26 |
| *3 oz* | | 22.4 | 6.7 | 1.9 | 1.7 | 2.0 | 206 | 112 | 169 | 7.68 | 0.427 | 6.8 | 24 | | 0.63 | 0.27 | 68.0 | 5026 |
| **chicken liver,** raw | 85 | 99 | 65.0 | 0 | | | 0 | 60 | 7 | 16 | 2.27 | 0.217 | 2802 | 15 | 0.26 | 8.3 | 14.09 | 5.30 |
| *3 oz* | | 14.4 | 4.1 | 1.3 | 1.1 | 1.1 | 293 | 196 | 252 | 7.64 | 0.418 | 46.4 | 9416 | 0.6 | 1.51 | 0.73 | 499.8 | 5027 |
| **chicken liver,** simmered | 85 | 142 | 56.8 | 0.7 | | | 0 | 65 | 9 | 21 | 3.38 | 0.305 | 3384 | 24 | 0.25 | 9.4 | 14.32 | 5.67 |
| *3 oz* | | 20.8 | 5.5 | 1.8 | 1.2 | 1.7 | 479 | 224 | 344 | 9.89 | 0.422 | 70.0 | 11329 | 0.7 | 1.69 | 0.64 | 491.3 | 5028 |
| **duck liver,** raw | 85 | 116 | 61.0 | 3.0 | | | 0 | 119 | 9 | 20 | 2.61 | 0.219 | 10186 | 4 | 0.48 | 5.5 | 45.90 | 5.26 |
| *3 oz* | | 15.9 | 3.9 | 1.2 | 0.6 | 0.5 | 438 | 196 | 229 | 25.95 | 5.068 | 57.0 | 33921 | | 0.76 | 0.65 | 627.3 | 5143 |
| **goose liver pate** (pate de foie gras), smoked, canned - *2 T* | 26 | 120 | 9.6 | 1.2 | | | 0 | 181 | 18 | 3 | 0.24 | 0.031 | 260 | 1 | 0.02 | 0.7 | 2.44 | 0.31 |
| | | 3.0 | 11.4 | 3.8 | 6.7 | 0.2 | 39 | 36 | 52 | 1.43 | 0.104 | 11.4 | 867 | | 0.08 | 0.02 | 15.6 | 5282 |
| **goose liver,** raw | 85 | 113 | 61.0 | 5.4 | | | 0 | 119 | 37 | 20 | 2.61 | 0 | 7913 | 4 | 0.48 | 5.5 | 45.90 | 5.26 |
| *3 oz* | | 13.9 | 3.6 | 1.4 | 0.7 | 0.2 | 438 | 196 | 222 | 25.95 | 6.394 | 57.9 | 26348 | | 0.76 | 0.65 | 627.3 | 5150 |
| **turkey giblets,** simmered | 85 | 169 | 55.5 | 0.7 | | | 0 | 54 | 5 | 15 | 2.65 | 0.135 | 9126 | 12 | 0.02 | 5.9 | 28.26 | 2.08 |
| *3 oz* | | 17.8 | 10.1 | 3.3 | 4.2 | 1.1 | 246 | 230 | 196 | 6.55 | 0.229 | 49.2 | 30422 | 0.1 | 1.28 | 0.49 | 284.8 | 5172 |
| **turkey gizzard,** simmered | 85 | 110 | 62.0 | 0.3 | | | 0 | 57 | 6 | 14 | 2.86 | 0.046 | 0 | 5 | 0.01 | 3.6 | 6.87 | 0.45 |
| *3 oz* | | 18.5 | 3.3 | 1.0 | 1.0 | 0.4 | 173 | 282 | 131 | 4.21 | 0.107 | 28.4 | 0 | 0 | 0.18 | 0.09 | 11.0 | 5174 |
| **turkey heart,** simmered | 85 | 116 | 61.2 | 0.6 | | | 0 | 76 | 6 | 22 | 3.78 | 0.055 | 16 | 2 | 0.03 | 2.9 | 18.44 | 1.34 |
| *3 oz* | | 18.2 | 3.9 | 1.1 | 1.0 | 1.0 | 156 | 247 | 220 | 4.42 | 0.418 | 38.7 | 54 | 0 | 0.88 | 0.36 | 6.8 | 5176 |
| **turkey liver,** simmered | 85 | 232 | 48.4 | 1.0 | | | 0 | 48 | 4 | 14 | 2.23 | 0.232 | 19210 | 19 | 0.03 | 8.7 | 49.47 | 3.70 |
| *3 oz* | | 17.0 | 17.5 | 5.9 | 7.7 | 1.7 | 330 | 179 | 250 | 9.09 | 0.297 | 70.1 | 64033 | 0.1 | 2.35 | 0.88 | 587.4 | 5178 |

| | WT (g) | KCAL | H$_2$O (g) | CHO (g) | TSUG (g) | ASUG (g) | DFIB (g) | Na (mg) | Ca (mg) | Mg (mg) | Zn (mg) | Mn (mg) | A (mcg RAE) | C (mg) | B-1 (mg) | NIA (mg) | B-12 (mcg) | PANT (mg) |
|---|---|---|---|---|---|---|---|---|---|---|---|---|---|---|---|---|---|---|
| | | PRO (g) | FAT (g) | SFA (g) | MUFA (g) | PUFA (g) | CHOL (mg) | K (mg) | P (mg) | Fe (mg) | Cu (mg) | Se (mcg) | A (IU) | E (mg ATE) | B-2 (mg) | B-6 (mg) | FOL (mcg DFE) | REF |

## 25. SALAD DRESSINGS
### 25.1 LOW AND REDUCED CALORIE SALAD DRESSINGS

| | WT | KCAL/PRO | H₂O/FAT | CHO/SFA | TSUG/MUFA | ASUG/PUFA | DFIB/CHOL | Na/K | Ca/P | Mg/Fe | Zn/Cu | Mn/Se | A(RAE)/A(IU) | C/E | B-1/B-2 | NIA/B-6 | B-12/FOL | PANT/REF |
|---|---|---|---|---|---|---|---|---|---|---|---|---|---|---|---|---|---|---|
| **balsamic vinaigrette salad dressing**, Newman's Own Lighten Up – 2 T | 30 | 45 | | 2.0 | 1.0 | | 0 | 470 | 0 | | | | | 0 | | | | |
| | | 0 | 4.0 | 0.5 | | | 0 | | 0 | | | | 0 | | | | | NEWM1 |
| **blue cheese salad dressing**, fat-free – 1 T | 17 | 20 | 11.6 | 4.4 | 1.3 | 1.3 | 0.3 | 138 | 9 | 3 | 0.04 | 0.002 | 1 | 0 | 0.01 | 0 | 0.04 | 0.07 |
| | | 0.3 | 0.2 | 0.1 | 0.1 | 0 | 0 | 33 | 18 | 0.02 | 0.003 | 0.3 | 3 | 0 | 0.03 | 0.01 | 0.3 | 42192 |
| **blue cheese salad dressing**, low cal – 1 T | 15 | 15 | 11.9 | 0.4 | 0.4 | 0.4 | 0 | 180 | 13 | 1 | 0.04 | | 0 | 0 | 0 | 0 | 0.03 | |
| | | 0.8 | 1.1 | 0.4 | 0.3 | 0.4 | 0 | 1 | 12 | 0.08 | 0.002 | 0.2 | 0 | 0 | 0.02 | 0 | 0.4 | 43020 |
| **blue cheese salad dressing**, reduced calorie – 1 T | 16 | 14 | 12.4 | 2.1 | 0.6 | 0.1 | 0 | 258 | 11 | 1 | 0.05 | | 11 | 0 | 0 | 0 | 0.02 | |
| | | 0.3 | 0.4 | 0.1 | 0.2 | 0.1 | 2 | 8 | 8 | 0.02 | 0.002 | 0.3 | 41 | 0.1 | 0.01 | 0 | 4.5 | 42153 |
| **buttermilk salad dressing**, lite – 1 T | 15 | 30 | 9.3 | 3.2 | 0.6 | 0.5 | 0.2 | 136 | 6 | 1 | 0.09 | 0.008 | 3 | 0 | 0 | 0 | 0.13 | |
| | | 0.2 | 1.9 | 0.2 | 0.4 | 0.6 | 2 | 20 | 29 | 0.10 | 0.024 | 0.4 | 10 | 0.2 | 0 | 0 | 0.6 | 43215 |
| **Caesar salad dressing**, low calorie – 1 T | 15 | 16 | 11.0 | 2.8 | 2.4 | 2.4 | 0 | 162 | 4 | 0 | 0.02 | 0.007 | 0 | 0 | 0 | 0 | 0 | 0 |
| | | 0 | 0.7 | 0.1 | 0.2 | 0.4 | 0 | 4 | 3 | 0.03 | 0.002 | 0.2 | 1 | 0.1 | 0 | 0 | 0.3 | 43021 |
| **Caesar salad dressing**, Newman's Own Lighten Up – 2 T | 30 | 70 | | 3.0 | 1.0 | | 0 | 520 | 40 | | | | | 0 | | | | |
| | | 2.0 | 6.0 | 1.0 | | | 5 | | 0 | | | | 0 | | | | | NEWM2 |
| **coleslaw salad dressing**, reduced fat – 1 T | 17 | 56 | 6.3 | 6.8 | 6.6 | 6.5 | 0.1 | 272 | 6 | 1 | 0.03 | 0.001 | 0 | 0 | 0 | 0 | 0.02 | 0 |
| | | 0 | 3.4 | 0.5 | 1.5 | 1.3 | 4 | 8 | 5 | 0.04 | 0 | 0.3 | 0 | 0.3 | 0 | 0 | 0 | 42230 |
| **dried tomato salad dressing**, Newman's Own Lighten Up – 2 T | 30 | 60 | | 5.0 | 3.0 | | 0 | 380 | 0 | | | | | 2 | | | | |
| | | 0 | 4.0 | 0.5 | | | 0 | | 0 | | | | 0 | | | | | NEWM3 |
| **French salad dressing**, low/red calorie – 1 T | 16 | 36 | 8.7 | 5.0 | 2.7 | 2.2 | 0.2 | 126 | 2 | 1 | 0.03 | 0.018 | 4 | 1 | 0 | 0.1 | 0 | 0 |
| | | 0.1 | 1.8 | 0.1 | 0.7 | 0.6 | 0 | 17 | 3 | 0.12 | 0.026 | 0.3 | 87 | 0.2 | 0.01 | 0.01 | 0.3 | 4020 |
| **French salad dressing**, red cal – 1 T | 16 | 32 | 9.4 | 4.3 | 4.1 | 3.6 | 0 | 160 | 2 | 0 | 0.03 | 0.011 | 2 | 0 | 0 | 0 | 0 | 0 |
| | | 0.1 | 2.1 | 0.3 | 0.5 | 1.2 | 0 | 13 | 2 | 0.06 | 0.002 | 0.3 | 33 | 0.5 | 0 | 0 | 0.3 | 42171 |
| **honey mustard salad dressing**, Newman's Own Lighten Up – 2 T | 30 | 70 | | 7.0 | 5.0 | | 0 | 290 | 40 | | | | | 0 | | | | |
| | | 0 | 4.0 | 0.5 | | | 0 | | 0 | | | | 0 | | | | | NEWM4 |
| **Italian salad dressing**, fat-free, Kraft Free – 2 T | 33 | 20 | 26.9 | 3.6 | 2.2 | | 0.2 | 430 | 14 | | | | | 0 | | | | |
| | | 0.5 | 0.3 | 0.2 | | | 1 | 38 | 68 | 0.08 | | | 52 | | | | | 4121 |
| **Italian salad dressing**, low/reduced calorie – 1 T | 15 | 11 | 12.7 | 0.7 | 0.7 | 0.4 | 0 | 205 | 1 | 1 | 0.03 | 0 | 0 | 0 | 0 | 0 | 0 | 0 |
| | | 0.1 | 1.0 | 0.1 | 0.3 | 0.3 | 1 | 13 | 2 | 0.10 | 0 | 1.2 | 2 | 0 | 0 | 0.01 | 0 | 4021 |
| **Italian salad dressing**, low/red cal, Light Done Right, Kraft – 2 T | 31 | 53 | 22.6 | 2.5 | 1.5 | | 0.4 | 228 | 9 | | | | | 1 | | | | |
| | | 0.3 | 4.5 | 0.4 | | | 0 | 28 | 8 | 0.10 | | | 55 | | | | | 4118 |
| **Italian salad dressing**, red cal – 1 T | 14 | 28 | 9.8 | 0.9 | 0.3 | 0.2 | 0 | 199 | 1 | 0 | 0.01 | 0.003 | 0 | 0 | 0 | 0 | 0.01 | 0 |
| | | 0 | 2.8 | 0.4 | 0.7 | 1.6 | 0 | 5 | 1 | 0.02 | 0.001 | 0.2 | 0 | 0.1 | 0 | 0 | 0.4 | 42140 |
| **ranch salad dressing**, fat-free, Kraft Free – 2 T | 35 | 48 | 22.3 | 10.7 | 2.1 | | 0.2 | 354 | 9 | | | | | 0 | | | | |
| | | 0.2 | 0.4 | 0.1 | | | 0 | 31 | 28 | 0.02 | | | 3 | | | | | 4119 |
| **ranch salad dressing**, low/red cal, Light Done Right, Kraft – 2 T | 30 | 77 | 18.4 | 3.2 | 1.3 | | 0.2 | 303 | 8 | | | | | 0 | | | | |
| | | 0.4 | 6.8 | 0.6 | | | 8 | 40 | 46 | 0.06 | | | 12 | | | | | 4117 |
| **raspberry & walnut salad dressing**, Newman's Own Lighten Up – 2 T | 30 | 70 | | 7.0 | 5.0 | | 0 | 120 | 0 | | | | | 0 | | | | |
| | | 0 | 5.0 | 0.5 | | | 0 | | 0 | | | | 0 | | | | | NEWM5 |
| **Russian salad dressing**, low/red calorie – 2 T | 32 | 45 | 20.8 | 8.8 | 7.0 | 6.9 | 0.1 | 278 | 6 | 0 | 0.03 | | 1 | 2 | 0 | 0 | 0.04 | 0.04 |
| | | 0.2 | 1.3 | 0.2 | 0.3 | 0.7 | 2 | 50 | 12 | 0.19 | 0.003 | 0.5 | 11 | 0.1 | 0 | 0 | 1.0 | 4022 |
| **mayo type salad dressing**, fat-free – 1 T | 16 | 13 | 12.6 | 2.5 | 1.6 | 1.6 | 0.3 | 126 | 1 | 0 | 0.01 | 0.004 | 0 | 0 | 0 | 0 | 0 | 0 |
| | | 0 | 0.4 | 0.1 | 0.3 | 0 | 1 | 8 | 1 | 0.02 | 0.003 | 0 | 0 | 0 | 0 | 0 | 0 | 42193 |
| **mayo type salad dressing**, low cal – 1 T | 15 | 39 | 8.1 | 3.6 | 0.7 | 0.6 | 0 | 104 | 2 | 0 | 0.03 | | 3 | 0 | 0 | 0 | 0.03 | 0.01 |
| | | 0.1 | 2.8 | 0.4 | 0.7 | 1.6 | 4 | 4 | 4 | 0.04 | 0 | 0.2 | 33 | 0.5 | 0 | 0 | 0.9 | 43329 |
| **sesame ginger salad drsng**, Newman's Own Lighten Up – 2 T | 30 | 35 | | 5.0 | 4.0 | | 0 | 5 | 0 | | | | | 0 | | | | |
| | | 0 | 1.5 | 0 | | | 0 | 390 | | 0.36 | | | 0 | | | | | NEWM6 |
| **thousand island salad dressing**, low/reduced calorie – 1 T | 15 | 29 | 9.1 | 3.6 | 2.6 | 2.3 | 0.2 | 125 | 4 | 1 | 0.03 | 0.018 | 2 | 0 | 0.01 | 0.1 | 0 | 0 |
| | | 0.1 | 1.7 | 0.1 | 1.0 | 0.4 | 2 | 30 | 2 | 0.14 | 0 | 0 | 47 | 0.2 | 0.01 | 0 | 0 | 4023 |

### 25.2 REGULAR SALAD DRESSINGS

| | WT | KCAL/PRO | H₂O/FAT | CHO/SFA | TSUG/MUFA | ASUG/PUFA | DFIB/CHOL | Na/K | Ca/P | Mg/Fe | Zn/Cu | Mn/Se | A(RAE)/A(IU) | C/E | B-1/B-2 | NIA/B-6 | B-12/FOL | PANT/REF |
|---|---|---|---|---|---|---|---|---|---|---|---|---|---|---|---|---|---|---|
| **bacon and tomato salad dressing** – 1 T | 15 | 49 | 8.8 | 0.3 | 0.3 | 0.3 | 0 | 163 | 1 | 1 | 0.03 | | 2 | 1 | 0.01 | 0.1 | 0.01 | |
| | | 0.3 | 5.2 | 0.8 | 1.3 | 2.9 | 1 | 16 | 4 | 0.04 | 0.004 | 0.2 | 32 | 0.6 | 0 | 0.01 | 0 | 43331 |
| **blue cheese salad dressing** – 1 T | 15 | 71 | 6.0 | 0.7 | 0.5 | 0.4 | 0.1 | 140 | 6 | 1 | 0.03 | 0.001 | 3 | 0 | 0 | 0 | 0.02 | 0.06 |
| | | 0.2 | 7.7 | 1.2 | 2.0 | 4.1 | 5 | 13 | 11 | 0.01 | 0.001 | 0.2 | 11 | 0.6 | 0.02 | 0.01 | 1.2 | 4539 |

| | WT (g) | KCAL | H₂O (g) | CHO (g) | TSUG (g) | ASUG (g) | DFIB (g) | Na (mg) | Ca (mg) | Mg (mg) | Zn (mg) | Mn (mg) | A (mcg RAE) | C (mg) | B-1 (mg) | NIA (mg) | B-12 (mcg) | PANT (mg) |
|---|---|---|---|---|---|---|---|---|---|---|---|---|---|---|---|---|---|---|
| | | PRO (g) | FAT (g) | SFA (g) | MUFA (g) | PUFA (g) | CHOL (mg) | K (mg) | P (mg) | Fe (mg) | Cu (mg) | Se (mcg) | A (IU) | E (mg ATE) | B-2 (mg) | B-6 (mg) | FOL (mcg DFE) | REF |
| **Caesar salad dressing** | 15 | 81 | 5.1 | 0.5 | 0.4 | 0.1 | 0.1 | 162 | 7 | 0 | 0.02 | 0.006 | 1 | 0 | 0 | 0 | 0 | 0.01 |
| *1 T* | | 0.3 | 8.7 | 1.3 | 2.0 | 4.9 | 6 | 4 | 3 | 0.16 | 0.002 | 0.2 | 5 | 0.7 | 0 | 0 | 0.3 | 43015 |
| **Caesar salad dressing**, Newman's Own - *2 T* | 31 | 150 | | 1.0 | 1.0 | | 0 | 420 | 20 | | | | | 0 | | | | |
| | | 1.0 | 16.0 | 1.5 | | | 0 | | 0 | | | | 0 | | | | | NEWM7 |
| **coleslaw salad dressing** | 15 | 58 | 6.0 | 3.6 | 3.0 | 2.8 | | 106 | 2 | 0 | 0.03 | 0.016 | 3 | 0 | 0 | 0 | 0.03 | 0.02 |
| *1 T* | | 0.1 | 5.0 | 0.7 | 1.3 | 2.7 | 4 | 1 | 4 | 0.03 | 0.002 | 0.2 | 9 | 0.5 | 0 | 0 | 2.1 | 43016 |
| **creamy Italian salad dressing**, Newman's Own - *2 T* | 30 | 140 | | 2.0 | 1.0 | | 0 | 270 | 20 | | | | | 0 | | | | |
| | | 1.0 | 14.0 | 2.5 | | | 10 | | 0 | | | | 0 | | | | | NEWM8 |
| **French salad dressing** | 16 | 73 | 5.8 | 2.5 | 2.6 | 2.4 | 0 | 134 | 4 | 1 | 0.05 | 0.003 | 4 | 1 | 0 | 0 | 0.02 | 0 |
| *1 T* | | 0.1 | 7.2 | 0.9 | 1.3 | 3.4 | 0 | 11 | 3 | 0.13 | 0 | 0 | 74 | 0.8 | 0.01 | 0 | 0 | 4120 |
| **French salad dressing**, homemade | 14 | 88 | 3.4 | 0.5 | | | 0 | 92 | 1 | 0 | 0 | | 4 | 0 | 0 | 0 | 0 | 0 |
| *1 T* | | 0 | 9.8 | 1.8 | 2.9 | 4.7 | 0 | 3 | 0 | 0.03 | | 0.2 | 72 | 1.1 | 0 | 0 | 0 | 4133 |
| **Green Goddess salad dressing** | 15 | 64 | 6.8 | 1.1 | 1.0 | 1.0 | 0 | 130 | 5 | 1 | 0.04 | | 2 | 0 | 0 | 0 | 0.04 | |
| *1 T* | | 0.3 | 6.5 | 0.9 | 1.4 | 3.5 | 6 | 9 | 5 | 0.05 | 0.002 | 0.2 | 6 | 0.7 | 0.01 | 0 | 0.6 | 43017 |
| **homemade salad dressing**, cooked | 16 | 25 | 11.1 | 2.4 | 1.5 | 1.0 | 0 | 117 | 13 | 1 | 0.06 | | 8 | 0 | 0.01 | 0 | 0.06 | 0 |
| *1 T* | | 0.7 | 1.5 | 0.5 | 0.6 | 0.3 | 9 | 19 | 14 | 0.08 | 0.002 | 0.3 | 27 | 0.1 | 0.02 | 0 | 3.5 | 4134 |
| **Italian salad dressing** | 15 | 44 | 8.5 | 1.6 | 1.2 | 0.9 | 0 | 248 | 1 | 0 | 0.02 | 0.003 | 0 | 0 | 0 | 0 | 0 | 0 |
| *1 T* | | 0.1 | 4.3 | 0.7 | 0.9 | 1.9 | 0 | 7 | 1 | 0.09 | 0 | 0.3 | 5 | 0.8 | 0 | 0.01 | 0 | 4114 |
| **Italian salad dressing**, zesty, Kraft | 31 | 109 | 16.3 | 1.8 | 1.3 | | 0.2 | 505 | 1 | | | | 11 | 0 | | | | |
| *2 T* | | 0.1 | 11.1 | 1.2 | | | 0 | 9 | 4 | 0.05 | | | 11 | | | | | 4116 |
| **mayonnaise type salad dressing** | 15 | 58 | 6.0 | 3.6 | 1.0 | 0.9 | 0 | 107 | 2 | 0 | 0.03 | 0.013 | 3 | 0 | 0 | 0 | 0.03 | 0.04 |
| *2 T* | | 0.1 | 5.0 | 0.7 | 1.3 | 2.7 | 4 | 1 | 4 | 0.03 | 0.002 | 0.2 | 33 | 0.3 | 0 | 0 | 0.9 | 4018 |
| **peppercorn salad dressing** | 13 | 73 | 4.1 | 0.5 | 0.3 | 0.2 | 0 | 138 | 3 | 0 | 0.02 | | 1 | 0 | 0 | 0 | 0.02 | |
| *1 T* | | 0.2 | 8.0 | 1.4 | 1.9 | 4.3 | 6 | 23 | 3 | 0.05 | 0.001 | 0.2 | 5 | 0.6 | 0 | 0.01 | 0.5 | 42137 |
| **ranch salad dressing** | 30 | 145 | 11.5 | 2.0 | 0.7 | | 0.2 | 245 | 9 | 2 | 0.12 | 0.013 | 3 | 1 | 0.03 | 0 | 0.10 | 0.24 |
| *2 T* | | 0.3 | 15.4 | 2.4 | 3.4 | 8.5 | 10 | 19 | 48 | 0.19 | 0.013 | 0.7 | 11 | 1.4 | 0.02 | 0.01 | 1.2 | 4639 |
| **ranch salad dressing**, Kraft | 29 | 148 | 10.7 | 1.3 | 1.2 | | 0.1 | 287 | 8 | | | | 11 | 0 | | | | |
| *2 T* | | 0.4 | 15.6 | 2.4 | | | 8 | 14 | 26 | 0.05 | | | 11 | | | | | 4115 |
| **Russian salad dressing** | 30 | 106 | 11.6 | 9.6 | 5.3 | 5.8 | 0.2 | 298 | 4 | 3 | 0.07 | 0.019 | 9 | 2 | 0.01 | 0.2 | 0 | 0.12 |
| *2 T* | | 0.2 | 7.9 | 0.7 | 1.8 | 4.4 | 0 | 52 | 6 | 0.18 | 0.017 | 0.5 | 173 | 1.0 | 0.01 | 0.03 | 1.5 | 4015 |
| **sesame seed salad dressing** | 15 | 66 | 5.9 | 1.3 | 1.2 | 1.2 | 0.2 | 150 | 1 | 0 | 0.02 | | 0 | 0 | 0 | 0 | 0 | 0 |
| *1 T* | | 0.5 | 6.8 | 0.9 | 1.8 | 3.8 | 0 | 24 | 6 | 0.09 | 0 | 0.2 | 5 | 0.8 | 0 | 0 | 0 | 4016 |
| **sweet and sour salad dressing** | 16 | 2 | 15.3 | 0.6 | 0.6 | 0.6 | 0 | 33 | 1 | 0 | 0 | 0.010 | 0 | 1 | 0 | 0 | 0 | 0 |
| *1 T* | | 0 | 0 | 0 | 0 | 0 | 0 | 5 | 0 | 0.01 | 0.002 | 0.3 | 0 | 0.4 | 0 | 0 | 0.3 | 43019 |
| **thousand island salad dressing** | 16 | 59 | 7.4 | 2.3 | 2.4 | 2.3 | 0.1 | 138 | 3 | 1 | 0.04 | 0.006 | 2 | 0 | 0.23 | 0.1 | 0 | 0 |
| *1 T* | | 0.2 | 5.6 | 0.8 | 1.3 | 2.9 | 4 | 17 | 4 | 0.19 | 0 | 0.2 | 34 | 0.6 | 0.01 | 0 | 0 | 4017 |
| **three cheese balsamic viniagrette** salad dressing, Newman's Own - *2 T* | 30 | 100 | | 2.0 | 1.0 | | 0 | 380 | 20 | | | | | 1 | | | | |
| | | 0 | 11.0 | 1.5 | | | 0 | | 0 | | | | 0 | | | | | NEWM9 |
| **Tuscan Italian salad dressing**, Newman's Own - *2 T* | 30 | 100 | | 1.0 | 1.0 | | 0 | 380 | 20 | | | | | 0 | | | | |
| | | 0 | 11.0 | 1.5 | | | 0 | | 0 | | | | 0 | | | | | NEWM10 |
| **vinegar and oil salad dressing**, homemade - *1 T* | 16 | 72 | 7.6 | 0.4 | 0.4 | 0 | 0 | 0 | 0 | 0 | 0 | 0 | 0 | 0 | 0 | 0 | 0 | 0 |
| | | 0 | 8.0 | 1.5 | 2.4 | 3.9 | 0 | 1 | 0 | 0 | 0 | 0.3 | 0 | 0.7 | 0 | 0 | 0 | 4135 |

## 26. SAUCES, GRAVIES, CONDIMENTS
### 26.1 CONDIMENT SAUCES

| | WT (g) | KCAL | H₂O (g) | CHO (g) | TSUG (g) | ASUG (g) | DFIB (g) | Na (mg) | Ca (mg) | Mg (mg) | Zn (mg) | Mn (mg) | A (mcg RAE) | C (mg) | B-1 (mg) | NIA (mg) | B-12 (mcg) | PANT (mg) |
|---|---|---|---|---|---|---|---|---|---|---|---|---|---|---|---|---|---|---|
| | | PRO (g) | FAT (g) | SFA (g) | MUFA (g) | PUFA (g) | CHOL (mg) | K (mg) | P (mg) | Fe (mg) | Cu (mg) | Se (mcg) | A (IU) | E (mg ATE) | B-2 (mg) | B-6 (mg) | FOL (mcg DFE) | REF |
| **barbeque sauce** | 9 | 14 | 5.4 | 3.3 | 2.3 | 0.3 | 0.1 | 101 | 1 | 1 | 0.01 | 0.020 | 1 | 0 | 0 | 0 | 0 | 0 |
| *1 packet* | | 0 | 0 | 0 | 0 | 0 | 0 | 19 | 2 | 0.02 | 0.007 | 0.1 | 21 | 0.1 | 0 | 0 | 0.2 | 6150 |
| **catsup (ketchup)** | 15 | 15 | 10.4 | 3.8 | 3.4 | 2.5 | 0 | 167 | 3 | 3 | 0.04 | 0.019 | 7 | 2 | 0 | 0.2 | 0 | 0.01 |
| *1 T* | | 0.3 | 0 | 0 | 0 | 0 | 0 | 57 | 5 | 0.08 | 0.027 | 0 | 140 | 0.2 | 0.02 | 0.02 | 1.5 | 11935 |
| **catsup (ketchup)**, low sodium | 15 | 15 | 10.4 | 3.8 | 3.4 | 2.5 | 0 | 3 | 3 | 3 | 0.04 | 0.019 | 7 | 2 | 0 | 0.2 | 0 | 0.01 |
| *1 T* | | 0.3 | 0 | 0 | 0 | 0 | 0 | 57 | 5 | 0.08 | 0.027 | 0 | 140 | 0.2 | 0.02 | 0.02 | 1.5 | 11949 |
| **hoisin sauce** | 16 | 35 | 7.1 | 7.1 | 4.4 | 4.1 | 0.4 | 258 | 5 | 4 | 0.05 | 0.041 | 0 | 0 | 0 | 0.2 | 0 | 0.01 |
| *1 T* | | 0.5 | 0.5 | 0.1 | 0.2 | 0.3 | 0 | 19 | 6 | 0.16 | 0.020 | 0.3 | 1 | 0 | 0.03 | 0.01 | 3.7 | 6175 |
| **horseradish sauce** | 15 | 7 | 12.8 | 1.7 | 1.2 | 0 | 0.5 | 47 | 8 | 4 | 0.12 | 0.019 | 0 | 4 | 0 | 0.1 | 0 | 0.01 |
| *1 T* | | 0.2 | 0.1 | 0 | 0 | 0.1 | 0 | 37 | 5 | 0.06 | 0.009 | 0.4 | 0 | 0 | 0 | 0.01 | 8.5 | 2055 |
| **hot pepper sauce** | 4.7 | 1 | 4.2 | 0.1 | 0.1 | | 0 | 124 | 0 | 0 | 0.01 | 0.002 | 0 | 4 | 0 | 0 | 0 | 0.01 |
| *1 t* | | 0 | 0 | 0 | 0 | 0 | 0 | 7 | 1 | 0.02 | 0.001 | 0 | 8 | 0 | 0 | 0.01 | 0.3 | 6168 |
| **mustard** | 5 | 3 | 4.1 | 0.3 | 0 | 0 | 0.2 | 57 | 3 | 2 | 0.03 | 0.021 | 0 | 0 | 0.02 | 0 | 0 | 0.02 |
| *1 t* | | 0.2 | 0.2 | 0 | 0.1 | 0 | 0 | 7 | 5 | 0.08 | 0.004 | 1.6 | 4 | 0 | 0 | 0 | 0.4 | 2046 |

| | WT (g) | Macronutrients | | | | | | Minerals | | | | | Vitamins | | | | | |
| --- | --- | --- | --- | --- | --- | --- | --- | --- | --- | --- | --- | --- | --- | --- | --- | --- | --- | --- |
| | | KCAL | H₂O (g) | CHO (g) | TSUG (g) | ASUG (g) | DFIB (g) | Na (mg) | Ca (mg) | Mg (mg) | Zn (mg) | Mn (mg) | A (mcg RAE) | C (mg) | B-1 (mg) | NIA (mg) | B-12 (mcg) | PANT (mg) |
| | | PRO (g) | FAT (g) | SFA (g) | MUFA (g) | PUFA (g) | CHOL (mg) | K (mg) | P (mg) | Fe (mg) | Cu (mg) | Se (mcg) | A (IU) | E (mg ATE) | B-2 (mg) | B-6 (mg) | FOL (mcg DFE) | REF |
| **pico de gallo**, Pace | 32 | 10 | 28.2 | 3.0 | 2.0 | | | 150 | 0 | | | | | 1 | | | | |
| 2 T | | 0 | 0 | 0 | | | 0 | | 0 | | | | 100 | | | | | 27027 |
| **plum sauce** | 19 | 35 | 10.2 | 8.1 | | | 0.1 | 102 | 2 | 2 | 0.04 | 0.022 | 0 | 0 | 0 | 0.2 | 0 | 0.01 |
| 1 T | | 0.2 | 0.2 | 0 | 0 | 0.1 | 0 | 49 | 4 | 0.27 | 0.015 | 0.1 | 8 | | 0.02 | 0.01 | 1.1 | 6151 |
| **salsa** | 32 | 9 | 28.8 | 2.0 | 1.0 | | 0.5 | 192 | 9 | 5 | 0.12 | 0.039 | 5 | 1 | 0.01 | 0 | | |
| 2 T | | 0.5 | 0.1 | 0 | 0 | 0 | 0 | 95 | 10 | 0.15 | 0.042 | 0.3 | 93 | 0.4 | 0.01 | 0.06 | 1.3 | 6164 |
| **salsa**, bandito peach, Newman's Own - 2 T | 32 | 25 | | 6.0 | 5.0 | | | 90 | 0 | | | | | 0 | | | | |
| | | 0 | 0 | 0 | | | 0 | | 0 | | | | 750 | | | | | NEWM11 |
| **salsa**, bandito tequila lime, Newman's Own - 2 T | 31 | 15 | | 3.0 | 2.0 | | | 170 | 20 | | | | | 0 | | | | |
| | | 0 | 0 | 0 | | | 0 | | 0.36 | | | | 200 | | | | | NEWM12 |
| **salsa**, black bean and corn, Newman's Own - 2 T | 32 | 20 | | 5.0 | 1.0 | | 2.0 | 140 | 20 | | | | | 0 | | | | |
| | | 1.0 | 0 | 0 | | | 0 | | 0.36 | | | | 100 | | | | | NEWM13 |
| **salsa con queso**, Snyder | 32 | 35 | | 4.0 | 1.0 | | 0 | 160 | 20 | | | | | 0 | | | | |
| 2 T | | 0 | 2.0 | 0 | | | 0 | | 0 | | | | 1 | | | | | SNYD13 |
| **salsa**, garden style sweet, Snyder | 32 | 20 | | 5.0 | 4.0 | | 0 | 95 | 20 | | | | | 0 | | | | |
| 2 T | | 0 | 0 | 0 | | | 0 | | 0 | | | | 2 | | | | | SNYD12 |
| **salsa**, mango, Newman's Own | 32 | 20 | | 5.0 | 1.0 | | 2.0 | 140 | 20 | | | | | 0 | | | | |
| 2 T | | 1.0 | 0 | 0 | | | 0 | | 0.36 | | | | 100 | | | | | NEWM14 |
| **salsa**, tequila lime, Pace | 32 | 15 | 28.4 | 3.0 | 2.0 | | 0 | 190 | 0 | | | | | 2 | | | | |
| 2 T | | 0 | 0 | 0 | | | 0 | 100 | 0 | | | | 200 | | | | | 27029 |
| **salsa**, thick 'n chunky, medium, Old El Paso - 2 T | 30 | 10 | | 2.0 | 1.0 | | 0 | 230 | 0 | | | | | 0 | | | | |
| | | 0 | 0 | 0 | | | 0 | | 0 | | | | 200 | | | | | GENM293 |
| **salsa**, triple pepper, Pace | 32 | 15 | 27.6 | 3.0 | 2.0 | | 1.0 | 190 | | | | | | 2 | | | | |
| 2 T | | 1.0 | 0 | 0 | | | 0 | | | | | | 200 | | | | | 27030 |
| **salsa verde**, Pace | 32 | 15 | 28.2 | 2.0 | 2.0 | | 0 | 230 | 0 | | | | | 1 | | | | |
| 2 T | | 0 | 0.5 | 0 | | | 0 | 65 | 0 | | | | 200 | | | | | 27028 |
| **soy sauce** made w/hydrolyzed veg pro - 1 T | 18 | 7 | 13.6 | 1.4 | 0.3 | 0 | 0.1 | 1024 | 1 | 1 | 0.06 | 0.064 | 0 | 0 | 0.01 | 0.5 | 0 | 0.05 |
| | | 0.4 | 0 | 0 | 0 | 0 | 0 | 27 | 17 | 0.27 | 0.017 | 0.1 | 0 | 0 | 0.02 | 0.03 | 2.3 | 16125 |
| **soy sauce** made w/soy and wheat (shoyu) - 1 T | 16 | 8 | 11.3 | 1.2 | 0.3 | 0 | 0.1 | 902 | 3 | 7 | 0.08 | 0.068 | 0 | 0 | 0.01 | 0.4 | 0 | 0.05 |
| | | 1.0 | 0 | 0 | 0 | 0 | 0 | 35 | 20 | 0.31 | 0.017 | 0.1 | 0 | 0 | 0.03 | 0.02 | 2.2 | 16123 |
| **soy sauce** made w/soy (tamari) | 18 | 11 | 11.9 | 1.0 | 0.3 | 0 | 0.1 | 1005 | 4 | 7 | 0.08 | 0.090 | 0 | 0 | 0.01 | 0.7 | 0 | 0.07 |
| 1 T | | 1.9 | 0 | 0 | 0 | 0 | 0 | 38 | 23 | 0.43 | 0.024 | 0.1 | 0 | 0 | 0.03 | 0.04 | 3.2 | 16124 |
| **tabasco Sauce**, McIlhenny | 4.7 | 1 | 4.5 | 0 | 0 | 0 | 0 | 30 | 1 | 1 | 0.01 | 0.005 | 4 | 0 | 0 | 0 | 0 | 0.01 |
| 1 t | | 0.1 | 0 | 0 | 0 | 0 | 0 | 6 | 1 | 0.05 | 0.004 | 0 | 77 | 0 | 0 | 0.01 | 0.1 | 6169 |
| **taco sauce**, medium, Old El Paso | 15 | 5 | | 1.0 | 0 | | 0 | 90 | 0 | | | | | 0 | | | | |
| 1 T | | 0 | 0 | 0 | | | 0 | | 0 | | | | 0 | | | | | GENM294 |
| **teriyaki sauce** | 18 | 16 | 12.2 | 2.8 | 2.5 | 2.1 | 0 | 690 | 4 | 11 | 0.02 | 0 | 0 | 0 | 0.01 | 0.2 | 0 | 0.04 |
| 1 T | | 1.1 | 0 | 0 | 0 | 0 | 0 | 40 | 28 | 0.31 | 0.018 | 0.2 | 0 | 0 | 0.01 | 0.02 | 1.4 | 6112 |
| **Worcestershire sauce** | 17 | 13 | 13.4 | 3.3 | 1.7 | 1.7 | 0 | 167 | 18 | 2 | 0.03 | | 1 | 2 | 0.01 | 0.1 | 0 | |
| 1 T | | 0 | 0 | 0 | 0 | 0 | 0 | 136 | 10 | 0.90 | 0.034 | 0.1 | 13 | 0 | 0.02 | | 1.4 | 6971 |

## 26.2 ENTRÉE SAUCES

| | WT (g) | | | | | | | | | | | | | | | | | |
| --- | --- | --- | --- | --- | --- | --- | --- | --- | --- | --- | --- | --- | --- | --- | --- | --- | --- | --- |
| **enchilada sauce**, green chili, Old El Paso - ¼ cup | 60 | 30 | | 4.0 | 1.0 | | 0 | 300 | 0 | | | | | 0 | | | | |
| | | 0 | 1.5 | 0 | | | 0 | | 0 | | | | 100 | | | | | GENM295 |
| **enchilada sauce**, mild/medium/hot, Old El Paso - ¼ cup | 60 | 25 | | 3.0 | 1.0 | | 0 | 270 | 0 | | | | | 0 | | | | |
| | | 0 | 1.0 | 0 | | | 0 | | 0 | | | | 100 | | | | | GENM296 |
| **fish sauce** | 28 | 10 | 19.9 | 1.0 | 1.0 | 1.0 | 0 | 2162 | 12 | 49 | 0.06 | 0.065 | 1 | 0 | 0 | 0.6 | 0.13 | 0.03 |
| 1 fl oz (1.5 T) | | 1.4 | 0 | 0 | 0 | 0 | 0 | 81 | 2 | 0.22 | 0.014 | 2.5 | 3 | 0 | 0.02 | 0.11 | 14.3 | 6179 |
| **guava sauce** | 238 | 86 | 213.2 | 22.6 | 14.0 | 0 | 8.6 | 10 | 17 | 17 | 0.40 | 0.257 | 33 | 348 | 0.06 | 1.0 | 0 | |
| 1 cup | | 0.8 | 0.3 | 0.1 | 0 | 0.1 | 0 | 536 | 26 | 0.43 | 0.183 | 1.2 | 674 | 1.3 | 0.03 | 0.21 | 11.9 | 9143 |
| **mole poblano sauce mix** | 125 | 714 | 5.2 | 52.1 | | | 12.6 | 1455 | 378 | 159 | 3.12 | 1.421 | 1 | 0 | 0.17 | 3.2 | | 0.29 |
| ½ cup | | 9.4 | 52.0 | | | | | 752 | 318 | 7.14 | 0.855 | | 19 | | 0.72 | 0.94 | 92.5 | 6137 |
| **oyster sauce** | 18 | 9 | 14.4 | 2.0 | 0 | 0 | 0.1 | 492 | 6 | 1 | 0.02 | 0.010 | 0 | 0 | 0 | 0.3 | 0.07 | 0 |
| 1 T | | 0.2 | 0 | 0 | 0 | 0 | 0 | 10 | 4 | 0.03 | 0.026 | 0.8 | 0 | 0 | 0.02 | 0 | 2.7 | 6176 |
| **pesto and tomato sauce**, Newman's Own - ½ cup | 124 | 80 | | 10.0 | 9.0 | | | 640 | 80 | | | | | 0 | | | | |
| | | 2.0 | 4.0 | 0.5 | | | 0 | | 1.44 | | | | 1000 | | | | | NEWM15 |
| **pizza sauce**, canned | 126 | 68 | 109.3 | 10.9 | 2.2 | | 2.5 | 233 | 68 | 26 | 0.32 | 0.278 | | 14 | 0.08 | 1.8 | 0.03 | 0.47 |
| ½ cup | | 2.7 | 1.4 | 0.6 | 0.6 | 0.1 | 4 | 446 | 63 | 1.13 | 0.173 | | 840 | | 0.07 | 0.17 | | 6152 |
| **sofrito sauce**, homemade | 103 | 244 | 61.4 | 5.6 | | | 1.8 | 1179 | 21 | 26 | 1.45 | 0.197 | | 21 | 0.29 | 3.0 | | 0.61 |
| ½ cup | | 13.2 | 18.7 | | | | | 413 | 143 | 0.97 | 0.170 | | | | 0.22 | 0.37 | 44.3 | 6142 |
| **sweet and sour sauce**, homemade | 18 | 14 | 14.1 | 3.0 | 1.9 | | 0.1 | 62 | 3 | 2 | 0.03 | 0.044 | 1 | 1 | 0.01 | 0.2 | 0 | 0.01 |
| 1 T | | 0.3 | 0.1 | 0 | 0 | 0 | 0 | 35 | 5 | 0.12 | 0.018 | 0.3 | 20 | 0.1 | 0.01 | 0.02 | 1.8 | 6285 |

| Food | WT (g) | KCAL / PRO (g) | H2O (g) / FAT (g) | CHO (g) / SFA (g) | TSUG (g) / MUFA (g) | ASUG (g) / PUFA (g) | DFIB (g) / CHOL (mg) | Na (mg) / K (mg) | Ca (mg) / P (mg) | Mg (mg) / Fe (mg) | Zn (mg) / Cu (mg) | Mn (mg) / Se (mcg) | A (mcg RAE) / A (IU) | C (mg) / E (mg ATE) | B-1 (mg) / B-2 (mg) | NIA (mg) / B-6 (mg) | B-12 (mcg) / FOL (mcg DFE) | PANT (mg) / REF |
|---|---|---|---|---|---|---|---|---|---|---|---|---|---|---|---|---|---|---|
| tomato basil sauce, Newman's Own | 124 | 90 | | 12.0 | 11.0 | | | 650 | 40 | | | | | 0 | | | | |
| ½ cup | | 2.0 | 4.5 | 0.5 | | | 0 | | | 1.44 | | | 1000 | | | | | NEWM16 |
| tomato sauce, bottled | 122 | 29 | 111.2 | 6.6 | 5.2 | 0 | 1.8 | 639 | 16 | 20 | 0.24 | 0.131 | 27 | 9 | 0.03 | 1.2 | 0 | 0.38 |
| ½ cup | | 1.6 | 0.2 | 0 | 0 | 0.1 | 0 | 404 | 32 | 1.24 | 0.143 | 0.2 | 528 | 1.7 | 0.08 | 0.12 | 13.4 | 11549 |
| tomato sauce, marinara, bottled | 122 | 106 | 97.6 | 16.8 | 10.8 | 0.5 | 3.2 | 500 | 27 | 26 | 0.66 | 0.195 | 46 | 2 | 0.03 | 4.8 | 0 | 0.09 |
| ½ cup | | 2.2 | 3.3 | 0.9 | 0.7 | 1.4 | 2 | 386 | 44 | 0.88 | 0.229 | 1.7 | 917 | 2.9 | 0.07 | 0.21 | 15.9 | 6931 |
| tomato sauce, marinara w/mshrms, Newman's Own - ½ cup | 124 | 70 | | 12.0 | 11.0 | | | 520 | 40 | | | | | 0 | | | | |
| | | 2.0 | 2.0 | 0 | | | 0 | | | 1.80 | | | 1250 | | | | | NEWM17 |
| tomato sauce, Spanish style, bottled - ½ cup | 122 | 40 | 108.7 | 8.8 | | | 1.7 | 576 | 21 | 23 | 0.41 | 0.264 | 60 | 10 | 0.09 | 1.6 | 0 | 0.34 |
| | | 1.8 | 0.3 | 0 | | 0.1 | 0 | 450 | 59 | 4.25 | 0.195 | 0.7 | 1202 | | 0.08 | 0.22 | 17.1 | 11649 |
| tomato sauce, traditional 100% natural, bottled, Prego - ½ cup | 125 | 78 | 98.7 | 12.5 | 10.6 | | 2.9 | 558 | 19 | | | | | 2 | | | | |
| | | 1.9 | 2.9 | 1.0 | | | 0 | 365 | | 0.69 | | | 481 | | | | | 6932 |
| tomato sauce w/five cheeses, Newman's Own - ½ cup | 124 | 80 | | 10.0 | 0 | | | 610 | 0 | | | | | 0 | | | | |
| | | 3.0 | 3.0 | 1.5 | | | 5 | | | 0.72 | | | 0 | | | | | NEWM18 |
| tomato sauce w/herbs and cheese, bottled - ½ cup | 122 | 72 | 101.8 | 12.5 | | | 2.7 | 662 | 45 | 23 | 0.44 | 0.229 | 60 | 12 | 0.09 | 1.5 | | 0.34 |
| | | 2.6 | 2.4 | 0.8 | 0.5 | 1.0 | 4 | 434 | 66 | 1.06 | 0.212 | 1.1 | 1204 | | 0.15 | 0.02 | 9.8 | 11555 |
| tomato sauce w/mushrooms, bottled - ½ cup | 122 | 43 | 107.3 | 10.3 | 7.0 | 0 | 1.8 | 551 | 16 | 23 | 0.26 | 0.229 | 59 | 15 | 0.09 | 1.5 | | 0.45 |
| | | 1.8 | 0.2 | 0 | | 0.1 | 0 | 464 | 39 | 1.09 | 0.243 | 0.2 | 1165 | 2.3 | 0.13 | 0.16 | 11.0 | 11551 |
| tomato sauce w/onions, bottled | 122 | 51 | 105.0 | 12.1 | | | 2.2 | 672 | 21 | 23 | 0.28 | 0.367 | 54 | 15 | 0.09 | 1.5 | | 0.45 |
| ½ cup | | 1.9 | 0.2 | 0 | 0 | 0.1 | 0 | 504 | 48 | 1.13 | 0.221 | 1.0 | 1037 | | 0.16 | 0.33 | 26.8 | 11553 |
| tomato sauce w/onions, grn pepper, celery, bottled - ½ cup | 125 | 51 | 110.4 | 11.0 | 9.2 | 3.6 | 1.8 | 682 | 16 | 26 | 0.35 | 0.305 | 51 | 16 | 0.08 | 1.4 | | 0.28 |
| | | 1.2 | 0.9 | 0.2 | 0.1 | 0.4 | 0 | 498 | 48 | 0.95 | 0.248 | 0.8 | 1012 | 1.5 | 0.15 | 0.24 | 17.5 | 11557 |
| tomato sauce w/tomato pieces, bottled - ½ cup | 122 | 39 | 108.7 | 8.6 | | | 1.7 | 18 | 12 | 24 | 0.23 | 0.268 | 49 | 26 | 0.09 | 1.4 | 0 | 0.27 |
| | | 1.6 | 0.5 | 0.1 | 0.1 | 0.2 | 0 | 455 | 51 | 0.83 | 0.017 | 0.7 | 977 | | 0.12 | 0.19 | 11.0 | 11559 |
| white sauce, medium, homemade | 125 | 184 | 93.6 | 11.5 | 5.4 | 0 | 0.2 | 442 | 148 | 18 | 0.51 | 0.054 | 112 | 1 | 0.09 | 0.5 | 0.35 | 0.41 |
| ½ cup | | 4.8 | 13.3 | 3.6 | 5.5 | 3.6 | 9 | 195 | 122 | 0.41 | 0.020 | 5.1 | 409 | 0.4 | 0.23 | 0.05 | 12.5 | 6166 |
| white sauce, thick, homemade | 125 | 232 | 86.4 | 14.5 | 5.0 | 0 | 0.4 | 466 | 139 | 18 | 0.50 | 0.084 | 146 | 1 | 0.11 | 0.7 | 0.32 | 0.39 |
| ½ cup | | 5.0 | 17.3 | 4.3 | 7.3 | 4.9 | 8 | 186 | 120 | 0.62 | 0.026 | 6.5 | 530 | 0.5 | 0.24 | 0.05 | 18.8 | 6167 |
| white sauce, thin, homemade | 125 | 131 | 100.8 | 9.2 | 6.0 | 0 | 0.1 | 410 | 158 | 19 | 0.52 | 0.030 | 71 | 1 | 0.07 | 0.3 | 0.38 | 0.42 |
| ½ cup | | 4.7 | 8.4 | 2.7 | 3.3 | 2.0 | 10 | 204 | 126 | 0.26 | 0.016 | 4.1 | 260 | 0.2 | 0.23 | 0.05 | 21.2 | 6165 |
| white sauce, thin, homemade w/butter - ½ cup | 125 | 90 | 105.0 | 10.4 | 6.6 | | 0.1 | 230 | 164 | 15 | 0.59 | 0.039 | 105 | 0 | 0.08 | 0.4 | 0.69 | 0.49 |
| | | 4.9 | 3.2 | 2.0 | 0.8 | 0.1 | 10 | 209 | 138 | 0.28 | 0.024 | 5.9 | 358 | 0.1 | 0.26 | 0.05 | 16.2 | 6264 |

## 26.3 GRAVIES

| Food | WT (g) | KCAL / PRO (g) | H2O (g) / FAT (g) | CHO (g) / SFA (g) | TSUG (g) / MUFA (g) | ASUG (g) / PUFA (g) | DFIB (g) / CHOL (mg) | Na (mg) / K (mg) | Ca (mg) / P (mg) | Mg (mg) / Fe (mg) | Zn (mg) / Cu (mg) | Mn (mg) / Se (mcg) | A (mcg RAE) / A (IU) | C (mg) / E (mg ATE) | B-1 (mg) / B-2 (mg) | NIA (mg) / B-6 (mg) | B-12 (mcg) / FOL (mcg DFE) | PANT (mg) / REF |
|---|---|---|---|---|---|---|---|---|---|---|---|---|---|---|---|---|---|---|
| au jus gravy, canned | 298 | 48 | 281.6 | 7.4 | | | 0 | 149 | 12 | 6 | 2.98 | 0.596 | 0 | 3 | 0.06 | 2.7 | 0.30 | 0.06 |
| 10.5 oz can | | 3.6 | 0.6 | 0.3 | 0.2 | 0 | 0 | 241 | 89 | 1.79 | 0.298 | 1.2 | 0 | | 0.18 | 0.03 | 6.0 | 6114 |
| au jus gravy mix | 3 | 9 | 0.1 | 1.4 | | | | 348 | 4 | 2 | 0.02 | 0.008 | 0 | 0 | 0.01 | 0.1 | 0.01 | 0 |
| 1 t | | 0.3 | 0.3 | 0.1 | 0.1 | 0 | 0 | 8 | 5 | 0.28 | 0.004 | 0.2 | 0 | | 0.01 | 0.01 | 2.4 | 6115 |
| beef gravy, canned | 291 | 154 | 254.6 | 14.0 | 0.6 | 0 | 1.2 | 1630 | 17 | 6 | 2.91 | 0.582 | 3 | 0 | 0.09 | 1.9 | 0.29 | 0.06 |
| 10.3 oz can | | 10.9 | 6.9 | 3.4 | 2.8 | 0.2 | 9 | 236 | 87 | 2.04 | 0.291 | 2.9 | 9 | 0.1 | 0.10 | 0.03 | 5.8 | 6116 |
| beef gravy, Heinz Home Style | 114 | 44 | 102.6 | 7.1 | 0.6 | | 0.8 | 669 | 7 | 3 | 0.17 | 0.031 | | 0 | 0.01 | 0.2 | 0.10 | 0.10 |
| ½ cup | | 1.2 | 1.3 | 0.5 | 0.5 | 0.1 | 2 | 25 | 11 | 0.15 | 0.022 | 2.5 | | | 0.03 | 0.02 | | 6985 |
| brown gravy mix | 6 | 22 | 0.3 | 3.6 | | | 0.1 | 291 | 8 | 2 | 0.07 | 0.025 | 0 | 0 | 0.01 | 0.2 | 0.04 | 0.01 |
| 1 T | | 0.6 | 0.6 | 0.2 | 0.3 | 0 | 0 | 16 | 12 | 0.10 | 0.011 | 0.4 | 2 | | 0.02 | 0.01 | 2.6 | 6118 |
| chicken gravy, canned | 119 | 94 | 101.6 | 6.4 | 0.9 | 0.4 | 0.5 | 687 | 24 | 2 | 0.95 | 0.238 | 1 | 0 | 0.02 | 0.5 | 0.12 | 0.02 |
| ½ cup | | 2.3 | 6.8 | 1.7 | 3.0 | 1.8 | 2 | 130 | 35 | 0.56 | 0.119 | 1.0 | 4 | 0.2 | 0.05 | 0.01 | 2.4 | 6119 |
| chicken gravy mix | 8 | 30 | 0.3 | 5.0 | | | | 332 | 12 | 3 | 0.11 | 0.018 | 3 | 0 | 0.02 | 0.3 | 0.04 | 0.10 |
| 1 T (amount for 1 serving) | | 0.9 | 0.8 | 0.2 | 0.4 | 0.2 | 2 | 32 | 20 | 0.11 | 0.009 | 0.4 | 25 | | 0.05 | 0.02 | 10.9 | 6120 |
| mushroom gravy, canned | 298 | 149 | 265.2 | 16.3 | | | 1.2 | 1699 | 21 | 6 | 2.09 | 0.894 | 0 | 0 | 0.10 | 2.0 | 0 | 3.28 |
| 10.5 oz can | | 3.8 | 8.1 | 1.2 | 3.5 | 3.0 | 0 | 316 | 45 | 1.97 | 0.298 | 5.7 | 0 | | 0.19 | 0.06 | 35.8 | 6121 |
| pork gravy mix | 7 | 26 | 0.3 | 4.4 | 1.7 | 0.6 | 0.2 | 375 | 10 | 2 | 0.07 | 0.022 | 2 | 0 | 0.01 | 0.2 | 0.04 | 0.02 |
| amount to make 1 serving | | 0.6 | 0.6 | 0.3 | 0.3 | 0 | 1 | 16 | 13 | 0.28 | 0.011 | 0.4 | 8 | 0 | 0.02 | 0.01 | 2.9 | 6124 |
| turkey gravy, canned | 15 | 8 | 13.3 | 0.8 | 0 | 0 | 0.1 | 87 | 1 | 0 | 0.12 | 0.030 | 0 | 0 | 0 | 0.2 | 0.02 | 0 |
| 1 T | | 0.4 | 0.3 | 0.1 | 0.1 | 0 | 0 | 16 | 4 | 0.10 | 0.015 | 0.1 | 0 | | 0.01 | 0 | 0.3 | 6125 |
| turkey gravy mix | 7 | 26 | 0.3 | 4.6 | | | | 307 | 10 | 3 | 0.09 | 0.015 | 1 | 0 | 0.01 | 0.2 | 0.04 | 0.07 |
| amount to make 1 serving | | 0.7 | 0.5 | 0.1 | 0.2 | 0.2 | 1 | 30 | 18 | 0.23 | 0.009 | 0.4 | 2 | | 0.03 | 0.01 | 6.5 | 6126 |

## 26.4 OLIVES

| Food | WT (g) | KCAL / PRO (g) | H2O (g) / FAT (g) | CHO (g) / SFA (g) | TSUG (g) / MUFA (g) | ASUG (g) / PUFA (g) | DFIB (g) / CHOL (mg) | Na (mg) / K (mg) | Ca (mg) / P (mg) | Mg (mg) / Fe (mg) | Zn (mg) / Cu (mg) | Mn (mg) / Se (mcg) | A (mcg RAE) / A (IU) | C (mg) / E (mg ATE) | B-1 (mg) / B-2 (mg) | NIA (mg) / B-6 (mg) | B-12 (mcg) / FOL (mcg DFE) | PANT (mg) / REF |
|---|---|---|---|---|---|---|---|---|---|---|---|---|---|---|---|---|---|---|
| olives, black, canned/bottled | 8.3 | 7 | 7.0 | 0.5 | 0 | 0 | 0.2 | 75 | 8 | 0 | 0.02 | 0.002 | 1 | 0 | 0 | 0 | 0 | 0 |
| 1 jumbo | | 0.1 | 0.6 | 0.1 | 0.4 | 0 | 0 | 1 | 0 | 0.28 | 0.019 | 0.1 | 29 | 0.1 | 0 | 0 | | 9194 |
| olives, green, canned/bottled | 15 | 22 | 11.3 | 0.6 | 0.1 | 0 | 0.5 | 233 | 8 | 2 | 0.01 | | 3 | 0 | 0 | 0 | 0 | 0 |
| 5 olives | | 0.2 | 2.3 | 0.3 | 1.7 | 0.2 | 0 | 6 | 1 | 0.07 | 0.018 | 0.1 | 59 | 0.6 | 0 | 0 | 0.4 | 9195 |

| | WT (g) | KCAL / PRO (g) | H₂O (g) / FAT (g) | CHO (g) / SFA (g) | TSUG (g) / MUFA (g) | ASUG (g) / PUFA (g) | DFIB (g) / CHOL (mg) | Na (mg) / K (mg) | Ca (mg) / P (mg) | Mg (mg) / Fe (mg) | Zn (mg) / Cu (mg) | Mn (mg) / Se (mcg) | A (mcg RAE) / A (IU) | C (mg) / E (mg ATE) | B-1 (mg) / B-2 (mg) | NIA (mg) / B-6 (mg) | B-12 (mcg) / FOL (mcg DFE) | PANT (mg) / REF |
|---|---|---|---|---|---|---|---|---|---|---|---|---|---|---|---|---|---|---|
| **26.5 PICKLES** | | | | | | | | | | | | | | | | | | |
| **dill pickle** | 30 | 4 | 28.3 | 0.8 | 0.4 | 0 | 0.3 | 262 | 13 | 2 | 0.03 | 0.014 | 3 | 0 | 0.01 | 0 | 0 | 0.02 |
| *1 spear* | | 0.2 | 0 | 0 | 0 | 0 | 0 | 28 | 4 | 0.11 | 0.010 | 0 | 55 | 0 | 0.01 | 0.01 | 0.3 | 11937 |
| **pickle relish**, hamburger | 122 | 157 | 74.6 | 42.1 | | | 3.9 | 1337 | 5 | 9 | 0.13 | 0.018 | 16 | 3 | 0.02 | 0.8 | 0 | 0.01 |
| *½ cup* | | 0.8 | 0.7 | 0.1 | 0.3 | 0.2 | 0 | 93 | 21 | 1.39 | 0.101 | 0 | 326 | | 0.05 | 0.02 | 1.2 | 11958 |
| **pickle relish**, hot dog | 122 | 111 | 87.4 | 28.5 | | | 1.8 | 1331 | 6 | 23 | 0.26 | 0.018 | 10 | 1 | 0.05 | 0.6 | 0 | 0.01 |
| *½ cup* | | 1.8 | 0.6 | 0.1 | 0.3 | 0.1 | 0 | 95 | 49 | 1.52 | 0.100 | 0 | 204 | | 0.05 | 0.02 | 1.2 | 11944 |
| **pickle relish**, sweet | 15 | 20 | 9.3 | 5.3 | 4.4 | 0.5 | 0.2 | 122 | 0 | 1 | 0.02 | 0.002 | 9 | 0 | 0 | 0 | 0 | 0.01 |
| *1 T* | | 0.1 | 0.1 | 0 | 0 | 0 | 0 | 4 | 2 | 0.13 | 0.013 | 0 | 183 | 0.1 | 0 | 0 | 0.2 | 11945 |
| **pickled cabbage**, Japanese style | 75 | 22 | 68.6 | 4.3 | 1.0 | 0.1 | 2.3 | 208 | 36 | 9 | 0.15 | 0.178 | 7 | 1 | 0 | 0.1 | 0 | 0.15 |
| *½ cup* | | 1.2 | 0.1 | 0 | 0 | 0 | 0 | 640 | 32 | 0.37 | 0.019 | 0.8 | 142 | 0.1 | 0.03 | 0.08 | 31.5 | 43143 |
| **pickled eggplant** | 68 | 33 | 59.1 | 6.6 | 3.3 | 2.6 | 1.7 | 1138 | 17 | 4 | 0.16 | | 2 | 0 | 0.03 | 0.4 | 0 | |
| *½ cup* | | 0.6 | 0.5 | 0.1 | 0 | 0.2 | 0 | 8 | 6 | 0.52 | 0.118 | 0.4 | 34 | 0 | 0.05 | 0.10 | 13.6 | 43146 |
| **pickled radishes**, Hawaiian style | 75 | 21 | 68.6 | 3.9 | 1.5 | 0 | 1.6 | 592 | 21 | 6 | 0.16 | 0.043 | 0 | 0 | 0.02 | 0.2 | 0 | 0.15 |
| *½ cup* | | 0.8 | 0.2 | 0.1 | 0 | 0.1 | 0 | 250 | 23 | 0.17 | 0.128 | 0.5 | 0 | 0 | 0.02 | 0.08 | 6.8 | 43142 |
| **sour pickle** | 65 | 7 | 61.2 | 1.5 | 0.7 | 0 | 0.8 | 785 | 0 | 3 | 0.01 | 0.007 | 6 | 1 | 0 | 0 | 0 | 0.02 |
| *1 medium (3¾" long)* | | 0.2 | 0.1 | 0 | 0 | 0.1 | 0 | 15 | 9 | 0.26 | 0.055 | 0 | 124 | 0.1 | 0.01 | 0.01 | 0.6 | 11941 |
| **sweet gherkin pickle** | 15 | 14 | 11.4 | 3.2 | 2.7 | 0.5 | 0.2 | 69 | 1 | | 0.02 | 0.010 | 6 | 0 | 0 | 0 | 0 | 0.01 |
| *1 small (2½" long)* | | 0.1 | 0.1 | 0 | 0 | 0 | 0 | 15 | 3 | 0.04 | 0.004 | 0 | 115 | 0.1 | 0 | 0 | 0.2 | 11940 |

## 27. SOUPS
### 27.1 CONDENSED SOUPS

| | WT (g) | KCAL / PRO (g) | H₂O (g) / FAT (g) | CHO (g) / SFA (g) | TSUG (g) / MUFA (g) | ASUG (g) / PUFA (g) | DFIB (g) / CHOL (mg) | Na (mg) / K (mg) | Ca (mg) / P (mg) | Mg (mg) / Fe (mg) | Zn (mg) / Cu (mg) | Mn (mg) / Se (mcg) | A (mcg RAE) / A (IU) | C (mg) / E (mg ATE) | B-1 (mg) / B-2 (mg) | NIA (mg) / B-6 (mg) | B-12 (mcg) / FOL (mcg DFE) | PANT (mg) / REF |
|---|---|---|---|---|---|---|---|---|---|---|---|---|---|---|---|---|---|---|
| **beef broth/bouillon**, cond, cnd | 298 | 39 | 282.4 | 2.5 | 0.3 | 0.3 | 0 | 1946 | 21 | 12 | 0.03 | 0.057 | 0 | 2 | 0.05 | 1.7 | 0.42 | 0.12 |
| *10.5 oz can* | | 7.5 | 0 | 0 | 0 | 0 | 0 | 372 | 77 | 1.28 | 0.006 | 4.2 | 0 | 0 | 0.07 | 0.06 | 14.9 | 6032 |
| **celery soup, cream of**, cond, cnd | 305 | 220 | 259.1 | 21.4 | 4.1 | 0 | 1.8 | 2089 | 98 | 15 | 0.37 | 0.610 | 67 | 1 | 0.07 | 0.8 | 0.12 | 2.81 |
| *10.8 oz can* | | 4.0 | 13.6 | 3.4 | 3.1 | 6.1 | 34 | 299 | 92 | 1.52 | 0.345 | 5.5 | 860 | 4.2 | 0.12 | 0.03 | 6.1 | 6010 |
| **cheddar cheese soup**, cond, Campbell's - ⅛ cup | 124 | 100 | 103.2 | 11.0 | 2.0 | | 1.0 | 890 | 40 | | | | 0 | | | | | |
| | | 2.0 | 5.0 | 2.0 | 1.0 | 1.5 | 5 | 20 | | 0 | | | 500 | | | | | 27012 |
| **cheese soup**, cond, cnd | 312 | 378 | 240.7 | 25.6 | 1.9 | 0 | 2.5 | 2162 | 346 | 9 | 1.56 | 0.624 | 228 | 0 | 0.04 | 1.0 | 0 | 0.22 |
| *11 oz can* | | 13.2 | 25.4 | 16.2 | 7.2 | 0.7 | 72 | 374 | 331 | 1.81 | 0.312 | 11.2 | 927 | 1.7 | 0.33 | 0.06 | 9.4 | 6011 |
| **chicken noodle soup**, cond, cnd | 246 | 128 | 215.2 | 14.8 | 1.3 | 0.5 | 0.7 | 1323 | 22 | 20 | 0.79 | 0.256 | 54 | 0 | 0.28 | 2.7 | 0.10 | 0.37 |
| *1 cup (8 fl oz)* | | 6.4 | 4.8 | 1.3 | 2.1 | 1.3 | 27 | 108 | 86 | 3.32 | 0.298 | 24.4 | 1009 | 0.1 | 0.23 | 0.10 | 61.5 | 6019 |
| **chicken soup, cream of**, cond, cnd | 305 | 274 | 252.4 | 21.8 | 1.6 | 0.7 | 0 | 1998 | 43 | 12 | 0.88 | 0.207 | 131 | 0 | 0.04 | 1.2 | 0 | 0.59 |
| *10.8 oz can* | | 7.3 | 17.6 | 4.9 | 6.2 | 3.2 | 24 | 149 | 95 | 3.23 | 0.390 | 5.8 | 555 | 1.6 | 0.14 | 0 | 6.1 | 6016 |
| **minestrone soup**, cond, cnd | 123 | 84 | 102.0 | 11.3 | 1.8 | 0 | 1.0 | 915 | 34 | 7 | 0.74 | 0.369 | 105 | 1 | 0.05 | 0.9 | 0 | 0.34 |
| *½ cup* | | 4.3 | 2.5 | 0.5 | 0.7 | 1.1 | 1 | 314 | 57 | 0.92 | 0.123 | 3.4 | 2101 | 0.6 | 0.04 | 0.10 | 49.2 | 6040 |
| **mushroom soup, cream of**, cond, cnd - 10.8 oz can | 305 | 259 | 255.7 | 20.5 | 4.5 | 0 | 0 | 1967 | 37 | 12 | 0.61 | 0.250 | 24 | 0 | 0.13 | 1.3 | 0 | 0.71 |
| | | 4.9 | 18.0 | 4.2 | 3.4 | 4.4 | 0 | 189 | 74 | 3.39 | 0.467 | 7.3 | 88 | 2.5 | 0.14 | 0 | 6.1 | 6043 |
| **tomato soup**, cond, cnd | 305 | 183 | 251.6 | 40.9 | 24.7 | 4.7 | 3.7 | 1681 | 40 | 43 | 0.76 | 0.363 | 61 | 39 | 0.12 | 3.1 | 0 | 0.16 |
| *10.8 oz can* | | 4.9 | 1.7 | 0.5 | 0.5 | 0.6 | 0 | 698 | 88 | 3.39 | 0.485 | 15.6 | 1196 | 1.0 | 0.19 | 0.26 | 0 | 6159 |
| **vegetable beef soup**, cond, cnd | 125 | 79 | 104.6 | 10.1 | 1.1 | 0.1 | 2.0 | 789 | 16 | 6 | 1.54 | 0.312 | 194 | 2 | 0.04 | 1.0 | 0.31 | 0.35 |
| *½ cup (4 fl oz)* | | 5.6 | 1.9 | 0.8 | 0.8 | 0.1 | 5 | 172 | 40 | 1.11 | 0.181 | 2.8 | 3880 | 0.6 | 0.05 | 0.08 | 10.0 | 6071 |
| **vegetarian vegetable soup**, cond, cnd - ½ cup (4 fl oz) | 123 | 73 | 104.4 | 12.0 | 3.8 | 0 | 0.6 | 827 | 21 | 7 | 0.47 | 0.461 | 175 | 1 | 0.05 | 0.9 | 0 | 0.34 |
| | | 2.1 | 1.9 | 0.3 | 0.8 | 0.7 | 0 | 210 | 34 | 1.08 | 0.123 | 4.3 | 3496 | 1.4 | 0.05 | 0.06 | 11.1 | 6068 |

### 27.2 CONDENSED SOUPS, PREPARED WITH MILK

| | WT (g) | KCAL / PRO (g) | H₂O (g) / FAT (g) | CHO (g) / SFA (g) | TSUG (g) / MUFA (g) | ASUG (g) / PUFA (g) | DFIB (g) / CHOL (mg) | Na (mg) / K (mg) | Ca (mg) / P (mg) | Mg (mg) / Fe (mg) | Zn (mg) / Cu (mg) | Mn (mg) / Se (mcg) | A (mcg RAE) / A (IU) | C (mg) / E (mg ATE) | B-1 (mg) / B-2 (mg) | NIA (mg) / B-6 (mg) | B-12 (mcg) / FOL (mcg DFE) | PANT (mg) / REF |
|---|---|---|---|---|---|---|---|---|---|---|---|---|---|---|---|---|---|---|
| **asparagus soup, cream of**, cond, prep w/milk - 1 cup (8 fl oz) | 248 | 161 | 213.3 | 16.4 | | | 0.7 | 1042 | 174 | 20 | 0.92 | 0.379 | 62 | 4 | 0.10 | 0.9 | 0.50 | 0.52 |
| | | 6.3 | 8.2 | 3.3 | 2.1 | 2.2 | 22 | 360 | 154 | 0.87 | 0.139 | | 600 | | 0.28 | 0.06 | 29.8 | 6201 |
| **celery soup, cream of**, cond, cnd, prep w/milk - 1 cup (8 fl oz) | 248 | 164 | 214.4 | 14.5 | | | 0.7 | 1009 | 186 | 22 | 0.20 | 0.253 | 114 | 1 | 0.07 | 0.4 | 0.50 | 1.51 |
| | | 5.7 | 9.7 | 3.9 | 2.5 | 2.7 | 32 | 310 | 151 | 0.69 | 0.154 | 4.7 | 461 | | 0.25 | 0.06 | 7.4 | 6210 |
| **cheese soup**, cond, cnd, prep w/milk - 1 cup (8 fl oz) | 251 | 231 | 206.9 | 16.2 | | | 1.0 | 1019 | 289 | 20 | 0.68 | 0.259 | 359 | 1 | 0.06 | 0.5 | 0.43 | 0.48 |
| | | 9.5 | 14.6 | 9.1 | 4.1 | 0.5 | 48 | 341 | 251 | 0.80 | 0.141 | 7.0 | 1242 | | 0.33 | 0.08 | 10.0 | 6211 |
| **chicken soup, cream of**, cond, prep w/milk - 1 cup (8 fl oz) | 248 | 191 | 210.4 | 15.0 | | | 0.2 | 1047 | 181 | 17 | 0.67 | 0.379 | 179 | 1 | 0.07 | 0.9 | 0.55 | 0.57 |
| | | 7.5 | 11.5 | 4.6 | 4.5 | 1.6 | 27 | 273 | 151 | 0.67 | 0.139 | | 714 | | 0.26 | 0.07 | 7.4 | 6216 |
| **clam chowder, New England**, cond, cnd, prep w/milk - 1 cup (8 fl oz) | 248 | 151 | 212.2 | 18.4 | 7.0 | 0.2 | 0.7 | 888 | 169 | 30 | 0.99 | 0.201 | 92 | 5 | 0.20 | 2.0 | 11.90 | 0.73 |
| | | 8.0 | 5.0 | 2.1 | 0.7 | 0.6 | 17 | 456 | 432 | 3.00 | 0.300 | 10.9 | 312 | 0.5 | 0.44 | 0.17 | 22.3 | 6230 |
| **green pea soup**, cond, cnd, prep w/milk - 1 cup (8 fl oz) | 254 | 239 | 197.9 | 32.2 | | | 2.8 | 970 | 173 | 56 | 1.75 | 0.660 | 66 | 3 | 0.15 | 1.3 | 0.43 | 0.56 |
| | | 12.6 | 7.0 | 4.0 | 2.2 | 0.5 | 18 | 376 | 239 | 2.01 | 0.391 | | 356 | | 0.27 | 0.10 | 7.6 | 6249 |
| **mshrm soup, cream of**, cond, cnd, prep w/milk - 1 cup (8 fl oz) | 248 | 166 | 215.0 | 14.0 | 8.3 | 0 | 0 | 823 | 164 | 20 | 0.79 | 0.102 | 82 | 0 | 0.10 | 0.6 | 0.60 | 0.74 |
| | | 6.2 | 9.6 | 3.3 | 2.0 | 1.8 | 10 | 268 | 154 | 1.36 | 0.198 | 6.0 | 278 | 1.0 | 0.29 | 0.05 | 7.4 | 6243 |

| | WT (g) | KCAL | H₂0 (g) | CHO (g) | TSUG (g) | ASUG (g) | DFIB (g) | Na (mg) | Ca (mg) | Mg (mg) | Zn (mg) | Mn (mg) | A (mcg RAE) | C (mg) | B-1 (mg) | NIA (mg) | B-12 (mcg) | PANT (mg) |
|---|---|---|---|---|---|---|---|---|---|---|---|---|---|---|---|---|---|---|
| | | PRO (g) | FAT (g) | SFA (g) | MUFA (g) | PUFA (g) | CHOL (mg) | K (mg) | P (mg) | Fe (mg) | Cu (mg) | Se (mcg) | A (IU) | E (mg ATE) | B-2 (mg) | B-6 (mg) | FOL (mcg DFE) | REF |
| **onion soup, cream of**, cond, cnd, | 248 | 186 | 209.6 | 18.4 | | | 0.7 | 1004 | 179 | 22 | 0.62 | 0.248 | 52 | 2 | 0.10 | 0.6 | 0.50 | 0.69 |
| prep w/milk - *1 cup (8 fl oz)* | | 6.8 | 9.4 | 4.0 | 3.3 | 1.6 | 32 | 310 | 154 | 0.69 | 0.149 | | 451 | | 0.27 | 0.07 | 22.3 | 6246 |
| **oyster stew**, cond, cnd, prep | 245 | 135 | 217.9 | 9.8 | | | 0 | 1041 | 167 | 20 | 10.34 | 0.370 | 56 | 4 | 0.07 | 0.3 | 2.62 | 0.49 |
| w/milk - *1 cup (8 fl oz)* | | 6.1 | 7.9 | 5.0 | 2.1 | 0.3 | 32 | 235 | 162 | 1.05 | 1.605 | | 225 | | 0.23 | 0.06 | 9.8 | 6248 |
| **potato soup, cream of**, cond, cnd, | 248 | 149 | 214.9 | 17.2 | | | 0.5 | 1061 | 166 | 17 | 0.67 | 0.379 | 52 | 1 | 0.08 | 0.6 | 0.50 | 1.69 |
| prep w/milk - *1 cup (8 fl oz)* | | 5.8 | 6.4 | 3.8 | 1.7 | 0.6 | 22 | 322 | 161 | 0.55 | 0.263 | | 444 | | 0.24 | 0.09 | 9.9 | 6253 |
| **shrimp soup, cream of**, cond, cnd, | 248 | 149 | 216.2 | 13.8 | 6.5 | 0 | 0.2 | 982 | 166 | 22 | 1.26 | 0.362 | 109 | 0 | 0.07 | 0.5 | 1.14 | 0.59 |
| prep w/milk - *1 cup (8 fl oz)* | | 6.9 | 7.5 | 4.7 | 2.1 | 0.3 | 25 | 250 | 151 | 0.55 | 0.134 | 8.7 | 392 | 0 | 0.27 | 0.08 | 9.9 | 6256 |
| **tomato bisque**, cond, cnd, prep | 251 | 198 | 204.6 | 29.4 | | | 0.5 | 1109 | 186 | 25 | 0.63 | 0.259 | 63 | 7 | 0.11 | 1.3 | 0.43 | 0.50 |
| w/milk - *1 cup (8 fl oz)* | | 6.3 | 6.6 | 3.1 | 1.9 | 1.2 | 23 | 605 | 173 | 0.88 | 0.141 | | 878 | | 0.27 | 0.14 | 22.6 | 6358 |
| **tomato soup**, cond, cnd, prep | 248 | 136 | 213.4 | 22.0 | 16.2 | 3.4 | 1.5 | 712 | 166 | 30 | 0.84 | 0.146 | 94 | 16 | 0.10 | 1.4 | 0.60 | 0.52 |
| w/milk - *1 cup (8 fl oz)* | | 6.2 | 3.2 | 1.8 | 0.9 | 0.3 | 10 | 466 | 156 | 1.36 | 0.203 | 9.2 | 709 | 0.4 | 0.31 | 0.15 | 5.0 | 6359 |

## 27.3 CONDENSED SOUPS, PREPARED WITH WATER

| | WT (g) | KCAL | H₂0 (g) | CHO (g) | TSUG (g) | ASUG (g) | DFIB (g) | Na (mg) | Ca (mg) | Mg (mg) | Zn (mg) | Mn (mg) | A (mcg RAE) | C (mg) | B-1 (mg) | NIA (mg) | B-12 (mcg) | PANT (mg) |
|---|---|---|---|---|---|---|---|---|---|---|---|---|---|---|---|---|---|---|
| | | PRO (g) | FAT (g) | SFA (g) | MUFA (g) | PUFA (g) | CHOL (mg) | K (mg) | P (mg) | Fe (mg) | Cu (mg) | Se (mcg) | A (IU) | E (mg ATE) | B-2 (mg) | B-6 (mg) | FOL (mcg DFE) | REF |
| **asparagus soup, crm of**, cond, cnd, | 244 | 85 | 224.0 | 10.7 | | | 0.5 | 981 | 29 | 5 | 0.88 | 0.376 | 37 | 3 | 0.05 | 0.8 | 0.05 | 0.12 |
| prep w/wtr - *1 cup (8 fl oz)* | | 2.3 | 4.1 | 1.0 | 1.0 | 1.9 | 5 | 173 | 39 | 0.81 | 0.124 | | 444 | | 0.08 | 0.01 | 22.0 | 6401 |
| **bean with frankurters soup**, cond, | 250 | 188 | 207.6 | 22.0 | | | | 1092 | 88 | 48 | 1.17 | 0.788 | 42 | 1 | 0.11 | 1.0 | 0.08 | 0.10 |
| cnd, prep w/wtr - *1 cup (8 fl oz)* | | 10.0 | 7.0 | 2.1 | 2.7 | 1.6 | 12 | 478 | 165 | 2.35 | 0.395 | 8.5 | 870 | | 0.06 | 0.13 | 30.0 | 6406 |
| **bean with pork soup**, cond, cnd, | 253 | 159 | 215.9 | 21.0 | 3.7 | 0.9 | 7.3 | 883 | 78 | 43 | 0.96 | 0.620 | 43 | 2 | 0.08 | 0.5 | 0.03 | 0.09 |
| prep w/wtr - *1 cup (8 fl oz)* | | 7.3 | 5.5 | 1.4 | 2.0 | 1.7 | 3 | 372 | 121 | 1.90 | 0.385 | 7.8 | 820 | 1.1 | 0.03 | 0.04 | 30.4 | 6404 |
| **beef broth/bouillon**, cond, cnd, prep | 241 | 29 | 231.9 | 1.8 | | | 0 | 636 | 10 | 0 | 0.36 | 0.366 | 0 | 1 | 0.02 | 0.7 | 0 | 0.05 |
| w/water - *1 cup (8 fl oz)* | | 5.4 | 0 | 0 | 0 | 0 | 0 | 154 | 31 | 0.53 | 0.246 | | 0 | | 0.03 | 0.02 | 2.4 | 6432 |
| **beef mushroom soup**, cond, cnd, | 244 | 73 | 225.9 | 6.3 | | | 0.2 | 942 | 5 | 10 | 1.46 | 0.488 | 0 | 5 | 0.04 | 1.0 | 0.20 | 0.22 |
| prep w/water - *1 cup (8 fl oz)* | | 5.8 | 3.0 | 1.5 | 1.2 | 0.1 | 7 | 154 | 34 | 0.88 | 0.244 | | 0 | | 0.06 | 0.05 | 9.8 | 6547 |
| **beef noodle soup**, cond, cnd, prep | 244 | 83 | 224.9 | 8.7 | 2.5 | 0.6 | 0.7 | 930 | 20 | 7 | 1.51 | 0.266 | 12 | 0 | 0.07 | 1.0 | 0.20 | 0.20 |
| w/water - *1 cup (8 fl oz)* | | 4.7 | 3.0 | 1.1 | 1.2 | 0.5 | 5 | 98 | 46 | 1.07 | 0.146 | 7.3 | 246 | 1.2 | 0.06 | 0.04 | 29.3 | 6409 |
| **black bean soup**, cond, cnd, prep | 247 | 114 | 216.4 | 19.0 | 3.1 | 2.8 | 8.4 | 1203 | 47 | 42 | 1.36 | 0.618 | 27 | 0 | 0.05 | 0.5 | 0 | 0.20 |
| w/water - *1 cup (8 fl oz)* | | 6.0 | 1.6 | 0.4 | 0.6 | 0.5 | 0 | 309 | 94 | 1.85 | 0.383 | 0 | 548 | 0.4 | 0.05 | 0.09 | 81.5 | 6402 |
| **cheese soup**, cond, cnd, prep | 247 | 156 | 217.7 | 10.5 | | | 1.0 | 958 | 141 | 5 | 0.64 | 0.257 | 296 | 0 | 0.02 | 0.4 | 0 | 0.10 |
| w/water - *1 cup (8 fl oz)* | | 5.4 | 10.5 | 6.7 | 3.0 | 0.3 | 30 | 153 | 136 | 0.74 | 0.128 | 4.4 | 1087 | | 0.14 | 0.02 | 4.9 | 6411 |
| **chicken and dumplings soup**, cond, | 241 | 96 | 221.2 | 6.0 | 0.8 | 0 | 0.5 | 860 | 14 | 5 | 0.36 | 0.489 | 46 | 0 | 0.02 | 1.8 | 0.17 | 0.14 |
| cnd, prep w/wtr - *1 cup (8 fl oz)* | | 5.6 | 5.5 | 1.3 | 2.5 | 1.3 | 34 | 116 | 60 | 0.63 | 0.123 | 11.8 | 525 | 0.6 | 0.07 | 0.04 | 2.4 | 6412 |
| **chicken broth**, cond, cnd, prep | 240 | 38 | 230.3 | 0.9 | 0.7 | 0.7 | 0 | 763 | 10 | 2 | 0.24 | 0.245 | 0 | 0 | 0.01 | 3.3 | 0.24 | 0.05 |
| w/water - *1 cup (8 fl oz)* | | 4.8 | 1.4 | 0.4 | 0.6 | 0.3 | 0 | 206 | 72 | 0.50 | 0.122 | 0 | 0 | 0 | 0.07 | 0.02 | 4.8 | 6413 |
| **chicken gumbo**, cond, cnd, prep | 244 | 56 | 229.0 | 8.4 | 2.5 | 1.2 | 2.0 | 954 | 24 | 5 | 0.37 | 0.251 | 7 | 5 | 0.02 | 0.7 | 0.02 | 0.20 |
| w/water - *1 cup (8 fl oz)* | | 2.6 | 1.4 | 0.3 | 0.7 | 0.3 | 5 | 76 | 24 | 0.90 | 0.124 | 8.1 | 134 | 0.4 | 0.05 | 0.06 | 4.9 | 6417 |
| **chicken mushroom soup**, cond, cnd, | 244 | 132 | 219.6 | 9.3 | | | 0.2 | 942 | 29 | 10 | 0.98 | 0.244 | 56 | 0 | 0.02 | 1.6 | 0.05 | 0.24 |
| prep w/water - *1 cup (8 fl oz)* | | 4.4 | 9.2 | 2.4 | 4.0 | 2.3 | 10 | 154 | 27 | 0.88 | 0.244 | | 1135 | | 0.11 | 0.05 | 0 | 6549 |
| **chicken noodle soup**, cond, cnd, | 241 | 60 | 226.1 | 7.1 | 0.7 | 0 | 0.5 | 639 | 14 | 10 | 0.39 | 0.123 | 27 | 0 | 0.13 | 1.3 | 0.05 | 0.18 |
| prep w/water - *1 cup (8 fl oz)* | | 3.1 | 2.3 | 0.6 | 1.0 | 0.6 | 12 | 53 | 41 | 1.59 | 0.154 | 11.6 | 484 | 0.1 | 0.11 | 0.05 | 28.9 | 6419 |
| **chicken rice soup**, cond, cnd, prep | 241 | 58 | 226.2 | 7.0 | 0.2 | 0 | 0.7 | 805 | 22 | 0 | 0.27 | 0.362 | 22 | 0 | 0.02 | 1.1 | 0.17 | 0.17 |
| w/water - *1 cup (8 fl oz)* | | 3.5 | 1.9 | 0.4 | 0.9 | 0.4 | 7 | 99 | 22 | 0.75 | 0.128 | 5.1 | 422 | 0.1 | 0.02 | 0.02 | 0 | 6423 |
| **chicken soup, cream of**, cond, cnd, | 244 | 117 | 221.1 | 9.3 | | | 0.2 | 986 | 34 | 2 | 0.63 | 0.376 | 163 | 0 | 0.03 | 0.8 | 0.10 | 0.20 |
| prep w/water - *1 cup (8 fl oz)* | | 3.4 | 7.4 | 2.1 | 3.3 | 1.5 | 10 | 88 | 37 | 0.61 | 0.124 | | 561 | | 0.06 | 0.02 | 2.4 | 6416 |
| **chicken vegetable soup**, cond, cnd, | 241 | 75 | 223.3 | 8.6 | 1.3 | 0.1 | 1.0 | 945 | 17 | 7 | 0.36 | 0.366 | 101 | 1 | 0.04 | 1.2 | 0.10 | 0.17 |
| prep w/water - *1 cup (8 fl oz)* | | 3.6 | 2.8 | 0.8 | 1.3 | 0.6 | 10 | 154 | 41 | 0.87 | 0.123 | 5.3 | 1851 | 0.4 | 0.06 | 0.05 | 4.8 | 6425 |
| **chili beef soup**, cond, cnd, prep | 250 | 142 | 214.2 | 23.1 | 6.2 | 6.1 | 3.0 | 970 | 45 | 25 | 1.92 | 0.980 | 70 | 4 | 0.05 | 1.0 | 0.38 | 0.27 |
| w/water - *1 cup (8 fl oz)* | | 6.2 | 3.1 | 1.5 | 1.2 | 0.1 | 12 | 490 | 138 | 1.98 | 0.380 | 6.0 | 1408 | 1.3 | 0.07 | 0.15 | 10.0 | 6426 |
| **clam chowder, Manhattan**, cond, cnd, | 244 | 73 | 225.1 | 11.6 | 3.2 | 0 | 1.5 | 551 | 27 | 10 | 0.88 | 0.359 | 49 | 4 | 0.03 | 0.8 | 3.86 | 0.18 |
| prep w/wtr - *1 cup (8 fl oz)* | | 2.1 | 2.1 | 0.4 | 0.4 | 1.2 | 2 | 181 | 39 | 1.56 | 0.132 | 9.0 | 910 | 1.2 | 0.04 | 0.10 | 9.8 | 6428 |
| **clam chowder, New England**, cond, | 244 | 85 | 221.8 | 12.3 | 0.5 | 0.1 | 0.7 | 839 | 22 | 17 | 0.44 | 0.198 | 20 | 5 | 0.15 | 1.9 | 11.30 | 0.28 |
| cnd, prep w/wtr - *1 cup (8 fl oz)* | | 3.8 | 2.5 | 1.1 | 0 | 1.1 | 7 | 264 | 310 | 2.98 | 0.298 | 7.6 | 71 | 0.5 | 0.20 | 0.12 | 17.1 | 6430 |
| **green pea soup**, cond, cnd, prep | 250 | 152 | 211.4 | 24.7 | 8.0 | 5.7 | 4.8 | 860 | 30 | 38 | 1.60 | 0.612 | 8 | 2 | 0.10 | 1.2 | 0 | 0.12 |
| w/water - *1 cup (8 fl oz)* | | 8.0 | 2.7 | 1.3 | 0.9 | 0.4 | 0 | 178 | 118 | 1.82 | 0.365 | 9.0 | 30 | 0.2 | 0.06 | 0.05 | 2.5 | 6449 |
| **minestrone soup**, cond, cnd, prep | 241 | 82 | 220.1 | 11.2 | | | 1.0 | 911 | 34 | 7 | 0.75 | 0.366 | 118 | 1 | 0.05 | 0.9 | 0 | 0.34 |
| w/water - *1 cup (8 fl oz)* | | 4.3 | 2.5 | 0.6 | 0.7 | 1.1 | 2 | 313 | 55 | 0.92 | 0.123 | | 2338 | | 0.04 | 0.10 | 50.6 | 6440 |
| **mushroom barley soup**, cond, cnd, | 244 | 73 | 225.5 | 11.7 | | | 0.7 | 891 | 12 | 10 | 0.49 | 0.122 | 10 | 0 | 0.02 | 0.9 | 0 | 0.12 |
| prep w/water - *1 cup (8 fl oz)* | | 1.9 | 2.3 | 0.4 | 1.0 | 0.7 | 0 | 93 | 61 | 0.51 | 0.244 | | 198 | | 0.09 | 0.17 | 4.9 | 6442 |
| **mshrm soup, cream of**, cond, cnd, | 244 | 102 | 224.6 | 8.0 | 1.8 | 0 | 0 | 776 | 17 | 5 | 0.24 | 0.098 | 10 | 0 | 0.05 | 0.5 | 0 | 0.28 |
| prep w/wtr - *1 cup (8 fl oz)* | | 1.9 | 7.0 | 1.6 | 1.3 | 1.7 | 0 | 73 | 32 | 1.32 | 0.195 | 2.9 | 34 | 1.0 | 0.05 | 0 | 2.4 | 6443 |
| **onion soup**, cond, cnd, prep | 241 | 55 | 224.8 | 7.9 | 3.2 | 0.8 | 0.7 | 1019 | 29 | 2 | 0.60 | 0.236 | 2 | 1 | 0.03 | 0.6 | 0 | 0 |
| w/water - *1 cup (8 fl oz)* | | 3.6 | 1.7 | 0.2 | 0.7 | 0.6 | 0 | 67 | 10 | 0.65 | 0.130 | 4.1 | 12 | 0.3 | 0.02 | 0.05 | 14.5 | 6445 |

| | WT (g) | Macronutrients | | | | | | Minerals | | | | | Vitamins | | | | | |
|---|---|---|---|---|---|---|---|---|---|---|---|---|---|---|---|---|---|---|
| | | KCAL | H₂O (g) | CHO (g) | TSUG (g) | ASUG (g) | DFIB (g) | Na (mg) | Ca (mg) | Mg (mg) | Zn (mg) | Mn (mg) | A (mcg RAE) | C (mg) | B-1 (mg) | NIA (mg) | B-12 (mcg) | PANT (mg) |
| | | PRO (g) | FAT (g) | SFA (g) | MUFA (g) | PUFA (g) | CHOL (mg) | K (mg) | P (mg) | Fe (mg) | Cu (mg) | Se (mcg) | A (IU) | E (mg ATE) | B-2 (mg) | B-6 (mg) | FOL (mcg DFE) | REF |
| onion soup, cream of, cond, cnd, prep w/water - 1 cup (8 fl oz) | 244 | 107 | 220.8 | 12.7 | | | 1.0 | 927 | 34 | 5 | 0.15 | 0.244 | 15 | 1 | 0.05 | 0.5 | 0.05 | 0.29 |
| | | 2.8 | 5.3 | 1.5 | 2.1 | 1.5 | 15 | 120 | 37 | 0.63 | 0.146 | | 295 | | 0.08 | 0.02 | 7.3 | 6446 |
| oyster stew, cond, cnd, prep w/water - 1 cup (8 fl oz) | 241 | 58 | 228.6 | 4.1 | | | | 981 | 22 | 5 | 10.29 | 0.366 | 19 | 3 | 0.02 | 0.2 | 2.19 | 0.12 |
| | | 2.1 | 3.8 | 2.5 | 0.9 | 0.2 | 14 | 48 | 48 | 0.99 | 1.593 | | 70 | | 0.04 | 0.01 | 2.4 | 6448 |
| pepperpot soup, cond, cnd, prep w/water - 1 cup (8 fl oz) | 241 | 99 | 218.0 | 9.0 | 1.1 | 0.3 | 0.5 | 940 | 27 | 5 | 1.18 | 0.590 | 46 | 1 | 0.05 | 1.2 | 0.17 | 0.33 |
| | | 6.1 | 4.5 | 2.0 | 1.9 | 0.3 | 10 | 147 | 41 | 0.87 | 0.130 | 0 | 834 | 0.1 | 0.05 | 0.06 | 9.6 | 6452 |
| potato soup, cream of, cond, cnd, prep w/water - 1 cup (8 fl oz) | 244 | 73 | 225.7 | 11.5 | | | 0.5 | 1000 | 20 | 2 | 0.63 | 0.376 | 71 | 0 | 0.03 | 0.5 | 0.05 | 0.83 |
| | | 1.8 | 2.4 | 1.2 | 0.6 | 0.4 | 5 | 137 | 46 | 0.49 | 0.251 | | 288 | | 0.04 | 0.04 | 2.4 | 6453 |
| Scotch broth, cond, cnd, prep w/water - 1 cup (8 fl oz) | 241 | 80 | 221.3 | 9.3 | 0.6 | 0 | 1.2 | 1000 | 19 | 5 | 1.57 | 0.362 | 0 | 1 | 0.02 | 1.1 | 0.27 | 0.34 |
| | | 4.9 | 2.6 | 1.1 | 0.8 | 0.5 | 5 | 157 | 55 | 0.82 | 0.253 | 2.7 | 0 | 0.1 | 0.05 | 0.07 | 9.6 | 6455 |
| shrimp soup, cream of, cond, cnd, prep w/water - 1 cup (8 fl oz) | 244 | 88 | 225.4 | 8.0 | 0.6 | 0 | 0.2 | 954 | 22 | 10 | 0.73 | 0.366 | 39 | 0 | 0.02 | 0.4 | 0.59 | 0.13 |
| | | 2.7 | 5.1 | 3.1 | 1.5 | 0.2 | 17 | 59 | 32 | 0.51 | 0.134 | 5.6 | 154 | 0 | 0.03 | 0.04 | 4.9 | 6456 |
| split pea w/ham soup, cond, cnd, prep w/wtr - 1 cup (8 fl oz) | 253 | 190 | 206.9 | 28.0 | | | 2.3 | 1007 | 23 | 48 | 1.32 | 0.670 | 23 | 2 | 0.15 | 1.5 | 0.25 | 0.25 |
| | | 10.3 | 4.4 | 1.8 | 1.8 | 0.6 | 8 | 400 | 213 | 2.28 | 0.369 | | 445 | | 0.08 | 0.07 | 2.5 | 6451 |
| stockpot soup, cond, cnd, prep w/water - 1 cup (8 fl oz) | 247 | 99 | 223.7 | 11.5 | | | | 1047 | 22 | 5 | 1.16 | 0.257 | 200 | 2 | 0.04 | 1.2 | 0 | 0.35 |
| | | 4.9 | 3.9 | 0.9 | 1.0 | 1.8 | 5 | 237 | 54 | 0.86 | 0.128 | | 3979 | | 0.05 | 0.09 | 9.9 | 6460 |
| tom beef w/ndls soup, cond, cnd, prep w/wtr - 1 cup (8 fl oz) | 244 | 137 | 212.3 | 20.6 | 1.8 | 0 | 1.5 | 895 | 22 | 7 | 0.73 | 0.244 | 29 | | 0.08 | 1.8 | 0.20 | 0.18 |
| | | 4.3 | 4.2 | 1.5 | 1.7 | 0.7 | 5 | 215 | 56 | 1.10 | 0.134 | 4.9 | 534 | 0.8 | 0.09 | 0.09 | 26.8 | 6461 |
| tomato bisque, cond, cnd, prep w/water - 1 cup (8 fl oz) | 247 | 124 | 215.3 | 23.7 | | | 0.5 | 1047 | 40 | 10 | 0.59 | 0.257 | 44 | 6 | 0.07 | 1.1 | 0 | 0.12 |
| | | 2.3 | 2.5 | 0.5 | 0.7 | 1.1 | 5 | 417 | 59 | 0.82 | 0.128 | | 721 | | 0.07 | 0.09 | 14.8 | 6558 |
| tomato rice soup, cond, cnd, prep w/water - 1 cup (8 fl oz) | 247 | 116 | 218.6 | 21.1 | 7.3 | 2.9 | 1.7 | 788 | 27 | 5 | 0.49 | 0.370 | 30 | 14 | 0.06 | 1.0 | 0 | 0.12 |
| | | 2.0 | 2.6 | 0.5 | 0.6 | 1.3 | 2 | 319 | 32 | 0.77 | 0.136 | 2.2 | 519 | 2.1 | 0.05 | 0.07 | 14.8 | 6463 |
| tomato soup, cond, cnd, prep w/water - 1 cup (8 fl oz) | 244 | 73 | 223.0 | 16.0 | 9.7 | 4.4 | 1.5 | 664 | 20 | 17 | 0.29 | 0.142 | 24 | 15 | 0.05 | 1.2 | 0 | 0.06 |
| | | 1.9 | 0.7 | 0.2 | 0.2 | 0.2 | 0 | 273 | 34 | 1.32 | 0.203 | 6.1 | 468 | 0.4 | 0.08 | 0.10 | 0 | 6559 |
| turkey noodle soup, cond, cnd, prep w/water - 1 cup (8 fl oz) | 244 | 68 | 226.9 | 8.6 | | | 0.7 | 815 | 12 | 5 | 0.59 | 0.251 | 15 | 0 | 0.07 | 1.4 | 0.15 | 0.17 |
| | | 3.9 | 2.0 | 0.6 | 0.8 | 0.5 | 5 | 76 | 49 | 0.95 | 0.124 | 10.7 | 293 | | 0.06 | 0.04 | 31.7 | 6465 |
| turkey vegetable soup, cond, cnd, prep w/water - 1 cup (8 fl oz) | 241 | 72 | 223.9 | 8.6 | | | 0.5 | 906 | 17 | 5 | 0.60 | 0.246 | 123 | 0 | 0.03 | 1.0 | 0.17 | 0.48 |
| | | 3.1 | 3.0 | 0.9 | 1.3 | 0.7 | 2 | 176 | 41 | 0.77 | 0.123 | | 2444 | | 0.04 | 0.05 | 4.8 | 6466 |
| vegetable beef soup, cond, cnd, prep w/water - 1 cup (8 fl oz) | 244 | 76 | 224.0 | 9.9 | 1.1 | 0.3 | 2.0 | 773 | 20 | 7 | 1.51 | 0.305 | 190 | 2 | 0.04 | 1.0 | 0.32 | 0.34 |
| | | 5.4 | 1.9 | 0.8 | 0.8 | 0.1 | 5 | 168 | 39 | 1.10 | 0.188 | 2.7 | 3787 | 0.6 | 0.05 | 0.07 | 9.8 | 6471 |
| veg vegetarian soup, cond, cnd, prep w/wtr - 1 cup (8 fl oz) | 241 | 67 | 222.7 | 11.8 | 3.8 | 0.5 | 0.7 | 815 | 24 | 7 | 0.46 | 0.453 | 171 | 1 | 0.05 | 0.9 | 0 | 0.34 |
| | | 2.1 | 1.9 | 0.3 | 0.8 | 0.7 | 0 | 207 | 34 | 1.06 | 0.133 | 4.3 | 3425 | 1.4 | 0.05 | 0.06 | 9.6 | 6468 |
| veg w/beef broth, cond, cnd, prep w/wtr - 1 cup (8 fl oz) | 241 | 80 | 220.7 | 12.9 | 2.0 | 1.5 | 1.7 | 800 | 22 | 7 | 0.80 | 0.333 | 104 | 2 | 0.05 | 1.0 | 0 | 0.34 |
| | | 2.9 | 1.9 | 0.4 | 0.5 | 0.8 | 2 | 190 | 39 | 0.96 | 0.161 | 2.7 | 2056 | 0.1 | 0.05 | 0.06 | 9.6 | 6472 |

## 27.4 DEHYDRATED SOUPS

| | WT (g) | KCAL/PRO | H₂O/FAT | CHO/SFA | TSUG/MUFA | ASUG/PUFA | DFIB/CHOL | Na/K | Ca/P | Mg/Fe | Zn/Cu | Mn/Se | A/A | C/E | B-1/B-2 | NIA/B-6 | B-12/FOL | PANT/REF |
|---|---|---|---|---|---|---|---|---|---|---|---|---|---|---|---|---|---|---|
| beef broth/bouillon cube - 1 cube (amount for 6 fl oz) | 3.6 | 6 | 0.1 | 0.6 | 0.5 | 0.5 | 0 | 864 | 2 | 2 | 0.01 | 0.014 | 0 | 0 | 0.01 | 0.1 | 0.04 | 0.01 |
| | | 0.6 | 0.1 | 0.1 | 0.1 | 0 | 0 | 15 | 8 | 0.08 | 0 | 1.0 | 0 | 0 | 0.01 | 0.01 | 1.2 | 6076 |
| beef noodle soup, dehydrated - 1 packet | 9 | 29 | 0.4 | 4.4 | 0.5 | 0 | 0.2 | 757 | 4 | 7 | 0.07 | 0.063 | 9 | 0 | 0.09 | 0.5 | 0 | 0 |
| | | 1.6 | 0.6 | 0.2 | 0.2 | 0.1 | 1 | 59 | 29 | 0.24 | 0.027 | 3.2 | 179 | 0.1 | 0.04 | 0.02 | 17.9 | 6077 |
| chicken broth cube - 1 cube (amount for 6 fl oz) | 4.8 | 10 | 0.1 | 1.1 | 0 | | 0 | 1152 | 9 | 3 | 0.01 | 0.018 | 0 | 0 | 0.01 | 0.2 | 0.01 | 0.03 |
| | | 0.7 | 0.2 | 0.1 | 0.1 | 0.1 | 1 | 18 | 9 | 0.09 | 0 | 1.3 | 0 | 0 | 0.02 | 0 | 1.5 | 6081 |
| chicken noodle soup, dehydrated - amount for 1 serving | 11 | 41 | 0.5 | 6.9 | 0.2 | 0 | 0.4 | 401 | 6 | 4 | 0.18 | 0.051 | 1 | 0 | 0.06 | 0.5 | 0.08 | 0.10 |
| | | 1.7 | 0.7 | 0.2 | 0.2 | 0.2 | 8 | 34 | 21 | 0.27 | 0.031 | 3.6 | 5 | 0 | 0.04 | 0.03 | 12.6 | 6128 |
| onion soup, dehydrated - 1 packet (amount of 6 fl oz) | 7 | 21 | 0.3 | 4.6 | 0.3 | 0.2 | 0.5 | 562 | 10 | 4 | 0.08 | 0.047 | 0 | 0 | 0.02 | 0.1 | 0 | 0.06 |
| | | 0.5 | 0 | 0 | 0 | 0 | 0 | 50 | 15 | 0.09 | 0.025 | 0.4 | 1 | 0 | 0.02 | 0.04 | 0 | 6094 |
| ramen noodle soup, all flavors, dehydrated - amt for 1 serving | 43 | 195 | 2.0 | 28.2 | 0.3 | 0 | 1.0 | 499 | 7 | 10 | 0.27 | | 0 | 0 | 0.28 | 2.3 | 0 | |
| | | 4.0 | 7.4 | 3.3 | 2.8 | 1.1 | 0 | 52 | 46 | 1.84 | 0.060 | 12.1 | 5 | 0.9 | 0.19 | 0.03 | 99.3 | 6583 |
| ramen noodle soup, beef flavor, dehydrated - amt for 1 serving | 43 | 187 | 2.4 | 27.2 | 0.8 | | 0.9 | 861 | 13 | 10 | 0.46 | 0.228 | 0 | 0 | 0.64 | 1.8 | 0.08 | 0.13 |
| | | 4.4 | 6.8 | 3.4 | 2.9 | 0.7 | | 80 | 52 | 1.77 | 0.064 | 4.6 | 0 | 0.7 | 0.11 | 0.04 | 72.2 | 6982 |
| ramen noodle soup, chicken flavor, dehydrated - amt for 1 serving | 43 | 188 | 1.8 | 27.3 | 0.6 | | 1.0 | 891 | 12 | 9 | 0.26 | 0.204 | 0 | 0 | 0.24 | 1.7 | 0.13 | 0.11 |
| | | 4.6 | 6.7 | 3.1 | 2.6 | 0.6 | | 74 | 51 | 1.69 | 0.085 | 4.0 | 0 | 0.6 | 0.11 | 0.04 | 75.7 | 6983 |

## 27.5 DEHYDRATED SOUPS, RECONSTITUTED

| | WT (g) | KCAL/PRO | H₂O/FAT | CHO/SFA | TSUG/MUFA | ASUG/PUFA | DFIB/CHOL | Na/K | Ca/P | Mg/Fe | Zn/Cu | Mn/Se | A/A | C/E | B-1/B-2 | NIA/B-6 | B-12/FOL | PANT/REF |
|---|---|---|---|---|---|---|---|---|---|---|---|---|---|---|---|---|---|---|
| bean with bacon soup, dehydrated, reconstituted - 1 cup (8 fl oz) | 265 | 106 | 237.8 | 16.4 | 0.6 | 0 | 9.0 | 928 | 56 | 29 | 0.69 | 0.530 | 3 | 1 | 0.05 | 0.4 | 0.03 | 0.05 |
| | | 5.5 | 2.1 | 1.0 | 0.9 | 0.2 | 3 | 326 | 90 | 1.32 | 0.265 | 5.8 | 53 | 0.6 | 0.26 | 0.03 | 8.0 | 6474 |
| beef broth/bouillon, dehydrated, reconstituted - ¾ cup (6 fl oz) | 181 | 5 | 178.6 | 0.5 | 0.4 | 0.3 | 0 | 471 | 7 | 4 | 0.02 | 0.011 | 0 | 0 | 0 | 0.1 | 0.02 | 0.01 |
| | | 0.4 | 0.1 | 0.1 | 0.1 | 0 | 0 | 11 | 5 | 0.04 | 0.018 | 0.5 | 0 | 0 | 0.01 | 0.01 | 0 | 6476 |
| chicken broth/bouillon, dehydrated, reconstituted - ¾ cup (6 fl oz) | 182 | 9 | 177.3 | 1.1 | | | | 593 | 9 | 2 | 0.02 | 0.018 | 2 | 0 | 0.01 | 0.2 | 0.02 | 0.04 |
| | | 0.7 | 0.2 | 0.1 | 0.1 | 0.1 | 0 | 18 | 9 | 0.09 | 0 | | 13 | | 0.02 | 0 | 1.8 | 6481 |
| chicken noodle soup, dehydrated, reconstituted - 1 cup (8 fl oz) | 252 | 58 | 237.3 | 9.2 | 0.8 | 0.6 | 0.3 | 577 | 5 | 8 | 0.20 | 0.081 | 3 | 0 | 0.20 | 1.1 | 0.05 | 0.11 |
| | | 2.1 | 1.4 | 0.3 | 0.5 | 0.4 | 10 | 33 | 30 | 0.50 | 0.035 | 9.6 | 28 | 0.1 | 0.08 | 0.03 | 27.7 | 6528 |

| | WT (g) | KCAL / PRO (g) | H₂O / FAT (g) | CHO / SFA (g) | TSUG / MUFA (g) | ASUG / PUFA (g) | DFIB / CHOL (g/mg) | Na / K (mg) | Ca / P (mg) | Mg / Fe (mg) | Zn / Cu (mg) | Mn / Se (mg/mcg) | A (mcg RAE) / A (IU) | C / E (mg/ATE) | B-1 / B-2 (mg) | NIA / B-6 (mg) | B-12 / FOL (mcg/DFE) | PANT / REF (mg) |
|---|---|---|---|---|---|---|---|---|---|---|---|---|---|---|---|---|---|---|
| **chicken rice soup**, dehydrated, | 240 | 58 | 225.2 | 8.8 | 0.7 | 0.3 | 0.7 | 931 | 7 | 0 | 0.12 | 0.192 | 0 | 0 | 0 | 0.3 | 0.07 | 0.07 |
| reconstituted - *1 cup (8 fl oz)* | | 2.3 | 1.4 | 0.3 | 0.6 | 0.4 | 2 | 10 | 10 | 0 | 0.048 | 5.0 | 5 | 0 | 0 | 0.02 | 0 | 6485 |
| **chicken soup, cream of**, dehydrated, | 261 | 107 | 237.4 | 13.3 | 4.1 | 1.1 | 0.3 | 1185 | 76 | 5 | 1.57 | 0.783 | 21 | 1 | 0.10 | 2.6 | 0.26 | 0.78 |
| reconstituted - *1 cup (8 fl oz)* | | 1.8 | 5.3 | 3.4 | 1.2 | 0.4 | 3 | 214 | 97 | 0.26 | 0.261 | 8.1 | 407 | 0.6 | 0.20 | 0.05 | 5.2 | 6483 |
| **consommé with gelatin**, dehydrated, | 249 | 17 | 235.9 | 1.9 | 1.1 | 1.0 | 0 | 3299 | 12 | 7 | 0.05 | 0.030 | 0 | 0 | 0.12 | 1.3 | 0.05 | 0.02 |
| reconstituted - *1 cup (8 fl oz)* | | 2.2 | 0.2 | 0 | 0 | 0 | 0 | 57 | 15 | 0.22 | 0.055 | 2.0 | 7 | 0 | 0.17 | 0.03 | 12.5 | 6489 |
| **mushroom soup**, dehydrated, | 253 | 83 | 233.7 | 11.1 | 0.5 | 0 | 0.5 | 1020 | 13 | 8 | 0.13 | 0.068 | 0 | 1 | 0.02 | 0.6 | 0.05 | 0.19 |
| reconstituted - *1 cup (8 fl oz)* | | 1.7 | 4.6 | 0.8 | 2.3 | 1.5 | 0 | 96 | 23 | 0.46 | 0.078 | 3.3 | 99 | 0.6 | 0.03 | 0.02 | 5.1 | 6493 |
| **onion soup**, dehydrated, | 246 | 30 | 235.7 | 6.8 | 0.5 | 0.2 | 0.7 | 851 | 22 | 10 | 0.12 | 0.071 | 0 | 0 | 0.03 | 0.2 | 0 | 0.09 |
| reconsituted - *1 cup (8 fl oz)* | | 0.8 | 0 | 0 | 0 | 0 | 0 | 76 | 22 | 0.12 | 0.062 | 0.5 | 2 | 0 | 0.03 | 0.06 | 0 | 6494 |
| **oxtail soup**, dehydrated, | 253 | 71 | 235.2 | 9.0 | 2.5 | 1.8 | 0.3 | 1202 | 20 | 8 | 0.18 | 0.083 | 0 | 0 | 0.02 | 0.2 | 0.03 | 0.03 |
| reconstitued - *1 cup (8 fl oz)* | | 2.8 | 2.6 | 1.3 | 1.1 | 0.1 | 0 | 33 | 35 | 0.48 | 0.073 | 2.0 | 10 | 0.3 | 0.01 | 0.03 | 7.6 | 6495 |
| **tomato soup**, dehydrated, | 265 | 101 | 238.2 | 19.0 | 10.3 | 3.4 | 1.1 | 943 | 77 | 26 | 0.34 | 0.095 | 53 | 5 | 0.28 | 2.5 | 0.16 | 0.48 |
| reconstitued - *1 cup (8 fl oz)* | | 2.5 | 1.6 | 0.8 | 0.6 | 0.2 | 5 | 294 | 87 | 0.48 | 0.090 | 2.9 | 832 | 0.6 | 0.46 | 0.15 | 29.2 | 6498 |
| **tomato vegetable soup**, dehydrated, | 253 | 56 | 238.4 | 10.2 | 2.5 | 0.9 | 0.8 | 334 | 20 | 10 | 0.20 | 0.116 | 10 | 3 | 0.06 | 1.3 | 0.05 | 0.12 |
| reconstituted - *1 cup (8 fl oz)* | | 2.0 | 0.9 | 0.4 | 0.3 | 0.1 | 0 | 170 | 35 | 0.61 | 0.114 | 2.0 | 190 | 0.4 | 0.10 | 0.07 | 12.6 | 6499 |
| **vegetable beef soup**, dehydrated, | 253 | 53 | 238.3 | 8.0 | 0.9 | 0.2 | 0.8 | 789 | 15 | 13 | 0.28 | 0.076 | 13 | 2 | 0.16 | 1.8 | 0.08 | 0.15 |
| reconstituted - *1 cup (8 fl oz)* | | 2.9 | 1.1 | 0.6 | 0.5 | 0.1 | 0 | 182 | 35 | 0.53 | 0.089 | 1.8 | 238 | 0.2 | 0.20 | 0.11 | 20.2 | 6500 |

## 27.6 READY-TO-SERVE SOUPS

| | WT (g) | KCAL / PRO (g) | H₂O / FAT (g) | CHO / SFA (g) | TSUG / MUFA (g) | ASUG / PUFA (g) | DFIB / CHOL (g/mg) | Na / K (mg) | Ca / P (mg) | Mg / Fe (mg) | Zn / Cu (mg) | Mn / Se (mg/mcg) | A (mcg RAE) / A (IU) | C / E (mg/ATE) | B-1 / B-2 (mg) | NIA / B-6 (mg) | B-12 / FOL (mcg/DFE) | PANT / REF (mg) |
|---|---|---|---|---|---|---|---|---|---|---|---|---|---|---|---|---|---|---|
| **bean with ham soup**, chunky, | 243 | 231 | 191.1 | 27.1 | | | 11.2 | 972 | 78 | 46 | 1.07 | 0.705 | 197 | 4 | 0.15 | 1.7 | 0.07 | 0.10 |
| cnd, rts - *1 cup (8 fl oz)* | | 12.6 | 8.5 | 3.3 | 3.8 | 0.9 | 22 | 425 | 143 | 3.23 | 0.389 | 16.8 | 3951 | | 0.15 | 0.12 | 29.2 | 6007 |
| **beef and baked potato soup**, cnd, | 236 | 100 | | 15.0 | 2.0 | | 1.0 | 930 | 20 | | | | | 0 | | | | |
| rts Progresso - *1 cup (8 fl oz)* | | 6.0 | 2.5 | 1.0 | 0.5 | 0 | 15 | | | 0.72 | | | 750 | | | | | GENM302 |
| **beef barley soup**, cnd, rts | 242 | 140 | | 18.0 | 3.0 | | 2.0 | 650 | 20 | | | | | 0 | | | | |
| Progresso - *1 cup (8 fl oz)* | | 9.0 | 3.5 | 1.5 | 0 | 0 | 15 | | | 1.08 | | | 750 | | | | | GENM305 |
| **beef broth/bouillon**, cnd, rts, | 240 | 17 | 234.1 | 0.1 | 0 | | 0 | 782 | 14 | 5 | 0 | 0.024 | 0 | 0 | 0 | 1.9 | 0.17 | 0.05 |
| *1 cup (8 fl oz)* | | 2.7 | 0.5 | 0.3 | 0.2 | 0 | 0 | 130 | 31 | 0.41 | 0 | 1.7 | 0 | 0 | 0.05 | 0.02 | 4.8 | 6008 |
| **beef broth/stock**, homemade | 240 | 31 | 230.1 | 2.9 | 1.3 | 0 | 0 | 475 | 19 | 17 | 0.41 | | 0 | 0 | 0.08 | 2.1 | 0 | |
| *1 cup (8 fl oz)* | | 4.7 | 0.2 | 0.1 | 0.1 | 0 | 0 | 444 | 74 | 0.65 | 0.120 | 2.9 | 0 | 0 | 0.22 | 0.13 | 4.8 | 6170 |
| **beef soup**, chunky, cnd, rts | 240 | 158 | 200.0 | 24.2 | 1.6 | 0 | 1.4 | 862 | 31 | 5 | 2.64 | 0.240 | 130 | 7 | 0.06 | 2.7 | 0.62 | 0.43 |
| *1 cup (8 fl oz)* | | 9.5 | 2.7 | 1.3 | 1.1 | 0.1 | 14 | 336 | 120 | 2.33 | 0.240 | 6.0 | 2611 | 0.7 | 0.15 | 0.13 | 14.4 | 6070 |
| **beef stroganoff soup**, chunky, cnd, | 240 | 235 | 191.8 | 21.6 | 4.0 | 0 | 1.4 | 1044 | 48 | 5 | 2.64 | | 202 | 0 | 0.10 | 0.2 | 0.62 | |
| rts - *1 cup (8 fl oz)* | | 12.2 | 11.0 | 5.6 | 3.7 | 0.6 | 50 | 336 | 120 | 2.11 | 0.240 | 18.2 | 1968 | 1.0 | 0.22 | 0.14 | 177.6 | 6980 |
| **beef vegetable soup**, cnd, rts, | 236 | 100 | | 17.0 | 4.0 | | 2.0 | 850 | 40 | | | | | 4 | | | | |
| Progresso - *1 cup (8 fl oz)* | | 7.0 | 1.0 | 0 | 0 | 0 | 15 | | | 1.08 | | | 1000 | | | | | GENM304 |
| **beef w/country vegs soup**, chunky, | 243 | 151 | 207.3 | 20.8 | | | | 892 | | | | | 219 | | | | | |
| cnd, rts - *1 cup (8 fl oz)* | | 9.9 | 3.0 | 1.5 | 1.1 | 1.2 | 24 | | | 2.16 | | | 4374 | | | | | 6749 |
| **black bean soup**, cnd, rts, | 242 | 160 | | 29.0 | 3.0 | | 8.0 | 760 | 60 | | | | | 0 | | | | |
| Progresso - *1 cup (8 fl oz)* | | 8.0 | 1.0 | 0.5 | 0 | 0.5 | 2 | | | 3.60 | | | 300 | | | | | GENM306 |
| **Chickarina w/meatballs soup**, cnd, | 237 | 120 | | 12.0 | 1.0 | | 2.0 | 950 | 20 | | | | | 1 | | | | |
| rts, Progresso - *1 cup (8 fl oz)* | | 8.0 | 5.0 | 2.0 | 2.5 | 0 | 20 | | | 1.08 | | | 500 | | | | | GENM310 |
| **chicken and rice soup**, cnd, rts, | 240 | 89 | 216.7 | 13.7 | 0.9 | | 1.9 | 434 | 36 | | | | | 2 | | | | |
| Healthy Choice - *1 cup (8 fl oz)* | | 6.1 | 1.3 | 0.4 | 0.6 | 0.3 | 17 | | | 0.22 | | | 802 | | | | | 6315 |
| **chicken and rotini soup**, cnd, rts, | 235 | 100 | | 13.0 | 1.0 | | 1.0 | 960 | 20 | | | | | 0 | | | | |
| Progresso - *1 cup (8 fl oz)* | | 7.0 | 2.0 | 0.5 | 0.5 | 0.5 | 15 | | | 0.36 | | | 750 | | | | | GENM308 |
| **chicken and wild rice soup**, cnd, | 239 | 100 | | 15.0 | 1.0 | | 1.0 | 870 | 20 | | | | | 0 | | | | |
| rts, Progresso - *1 cup (8 fl oz)* | | 6.0 | 1.5 | 0.5 | 0.5 | 0 | 15 | | | 0.36 | | | 1000 | | | | | GENM309 |
| **chicken barley soup**, cnd, rts, | 241 | 100 | | 16.0 | 2.0 | | 3.0 | 900 | 0 | | | | | 0 | | | | |
| Progresso - *1 cup (8 fl oz)* | | 6.0 | 2.5 | 0.5 | 0.5 | 0.5 | 15 | | | 0.72 | | | 1250 | | | | | GENM311 |
| **chkn broth**, 99% fat-free, cnd/carton, | 227 | 9 | 222.7 | 0.3 | 0.3 | | 0 | 928 | 9 | 2 | 0.05 | 0.025 | 0 | | 0.02 | 1.3 | 0.45 | 0.27 |
| Swanson - *1 cup (8 fl oz)* | | 1.2 | 0.4 | 0 | 0 | 0 | 0 | 68 | 25 | 0.32 | 0.043 | 5.0 | | | 0.05 | 0.03 | | 6984 |
| **chicken broth**, cnd, rts, Campbell | 248 | 17 | 242.5 | 1.0 | 0 | | 1.0 | 392 | 15 | 2 | 0.17 | 0.114 | 0 | 17 | 0 | 1.3 | 0.10 | 0.02 |
| Hlthy Request - *1 cup (8 fl oz)* | | 2.5 | 0.2 | 0.1 | 0.1 | 0.1 | 0 | 198 | 32 | 0.50 | 0.067 | 0 | 0 | 0 | 0.02 | 0.01 | 0 | 6194 |
| **chicken broth/stock**, homemade | 240 | 86 | 221.2 | 8.5 | 3.8 | 0 | 0 | 343 | 7 | 10 | 0.34 | | 2 | 0 | 0.08 | 3.8 | 0 | |
| *1 cup (8 fl oz)* | | 6.0 | 2.9 | 0.8 | 1.4 | 0.5 | 7 | 252 | 65 | 0.50 | 0.130 | 5.3 | 7 | 0.1 | 0.20 | 0.15 | 12.0 | 6172 |
| **chicken corn chowder**, cnd, rts | 240 | 238 | 197.0 | 18.0 | | | 2.2 | 718 | | | | | 139 | | | | | |
| *1 cup (8 fl oz)* | | 7.4 | 15.1 | 4.2 | 3.0 | 4.6 | 26 | | | | | | 2760 | | | | | 6725 |
| **chicken mshrm chowder**, chunky, | 240 | 192 | 202.1 | 17.0 | | | 3.4 | 814 | | | | | | 5 | | | | |
| cnd, rts - *1 cup (8 fl oz)* | | 7.2 | 10.6 | 2.8 | 2.0 | 4.2 | 14 | | | 1.15 | | | 0 | | | | | 6726 |
| **chicken noodle soup**, cnd, rts, | 243 | 100 | 218.0 | 12.6 | 1.4 | | 1.9 | 474 | 19 | | | | | 0 | | | | |
| Hlthy Chc - *1 cup (8 fl oz)* | | 9.0 | 1.5 | 1.0 | 0 | 0.4 | 12 | | | 0 | | | 1380 | | | | | 6314 |

| Food | WT (g) | KCAL<br>PRO (g) | H₂O (g)<br>FAT (g) | CHO (g)<br>SFA (g) | TSUG (g)<br>MUFA (g) | ASUG (g)<br>PUFA (g) | DFIB (g)<br>CHOL (mg) | Na (mg)<br>K (mg) | Ca (mg)<br>P (mg) | Mg (mg)<br>Fe (mg) | Zn (mg)<br>Cu (mg) | Mn (mg)<br>Se (mcg) | A (mcg RAE)<br>A (IU) | C (mg)<br>E (mg ATE) | B-1 (mg)<br>B-2 (mg) | NIA (mg)<br>B-6 (mg) | B-12 (mcg)<br>FOL (mcg DFE) | PANT (mg)<br>REF |
|---|---|---|---|---|---|---|---|---|---|---|---|---|---|---|---|---|---|---|
| chicken noodle soup, cnd, rts, | 237 | 100 | | 12.0 | 1.0 | | 1.0 | 950 | 20 | | | | | 0 | | | | |
| Progresso - 1 cup (8 fl oz) | | 7.0 | 2.5 | 0.5 | 1.0 | 0.5 | 25 | | | 0.72 | | | 1000 | | | | | GENM313 |
| chicken noodle soup, chunky, cnd, | 240 | 89 | 217.6 | 9.6 | 1.8 | 0.8 | 1.0 | 823 | 19 | 12 | 0.46 | 0.266 | 149 | 1 | 0.11 | 4.3 | 0.19 | 0.23 |
| rts - 1 cup (8 fl oz) | | 7.8 | 2.2 | 1.0 | 0.5 | 0.3 | 12 | 240 | 151 | 0.79 | 0.118 | 6.7 | 2938 | 0.3 | 0.15 | 0.12 | 26.4 | 6018 |
| chicken rice soup, chunky, cnd, rts | 240 | 127 | 208.3 | 13.0 | 1.4 | 0 | 1.0 | 888 | 34 | 10 | 0.96 | 0.240 | 293 | 4 | 0.02 | 4.1 | 0.31 | 0.36 |
| 1 cup (8 fl oz) | | 12.3 | 3.2 | 1.0 | 1.4 | 0.7 | 12 | 108 | 72 | 1.87 | 0.240 | 10.8 | 5803 | 0.6 | 0.10 | 0.05 | 4.8 | 6022 |
| chicken rice soup w/veg, cnd, rts, | 238 | 100 | | 16.0 | 1.0 | | 0.5 | 870 | 20 | | | | | 0 | | | | |
| Progresso - 1 cup (8 fl oz) | | 5.0 | 1.0 | 0.5 | 0 | 0 | 15 | | | 0.36 | | | 1000 | | | | | GENM314 |
| chicken (roasted) rotini soup, cnd, | 230 | 80 | | 11.0 | 1.0 | | 0.5 | 980 | 0 | | | | | 0 | | | | |
| rts, Progresso - 1 cup (8 fl oz) | | 6.0 | 2.5 | 0.5 | 0.5 | 0.5 | 10 | | | 0.36 | | | 750 | | | | | GENM336 |
| chicken soup, chunky, cnd, rts | 240 | 170 | 201.9 | 16.5 | 2.1 | 0.4 | 1.4 | 850 | 24 | 7 | 0.96 | 0.240 | 65 | 1 | 0.08 | 4.2 | 0.24 | 0.38 |
| 1 cup (8 fl oz) | | 12.1 | 6.3 | 1.9 | 2.8 | 1.3 | 29 | 168 | 108 | 1.66 | 0.240 | 6.0 | 1226 | 0.3 | 0.17 | 0.05 | 4.8 | 6015 |
| chicken veg w/pot & chs soup, | 240 | 156 | 211.0 | 12.5 | 1.5 | 0.5 | 0.7 | 998 | 36 | 12 | 0.38 | | 46 | 10 | 0.04 | 0.8 | 0.05 | |
| chunky, cnd, rts - 1 cup (8 fl oz) | | 2.8 | 10.7 | 3.9 | 3.9 | 2.3 | 17 | 175 | 46 | 0.38 | 0.096 | 8.9 | 900 | 0.1 | 0.04 | 0.10 | 21.6 | 6208 |
| chkn veg soup, chunky, red fat, red | 240 | 96 | 214.8 | 15.1 | | | | 461 | | | | | | | | | | |
| sdm, cnd, rts - 1 cup (8 fl oz) | | 6.5 | 1.2 | 0.3 | 0.4 | 0.3 | 10 | | | | | | 3079 | | | | | 6740 |
| chicken vegetable soup, chunky, | 240 | 166 | 200.3 | 18.9 | | | | 833 | 26 | 10 | 2.16 | 0.240 | | 6 | 0.04 | 3.3 | 0.24 | 0.34 |
| cnd, rts - 1 cup (8 fl oz) | | 12.3 | 4.8 | 1.4 | 2.2 | 1.0 | 17 | 367 | 106 | 1.46 | 0.240 | 12.2 | 5990 | | 0.17 | 0.10 | 12.0 | 6024 |
| clam chowder, Manhattan, chunky, | 240 | 134 | 206.5 | 18.8 | 4.0 | 0.3 | 2.9 | 1001 | 67 | 19 | 1.68 | 0.240 | 168 | 12 | 0.06 | 1.8 | 7.92 | 0.24 |
| cnd, rts - 1 cup (8 fl oz) | | 7.2 | 3.4 | 2.1 | 1.0 | 0.1 | 14 | 384 | 84 | 2.64 | 0.240 | 16.1 | 3216 | 1.6 | 0.06 | 0.26 | 9.6 | 6027 |
| clam chowder, Manhattan, cnd, rts | 239 | 100 | | 17.0 | 4.0 | | 2.0 | 970 | 20 | | | | | 0 | | | | |
| Progresso - 1 cup (8 fl oz) | | 3.0 | 2.0 | 0 | 0 | 1.0 | 10 | | | 1.08 | | | 1500 | | | | | GENM319 |
| clam chowder, New England, cnd, | 240 | 190 | | 20.0 | 2.0 | | 2.0 | 900 | 20 | | | | | 0 | | | | |
| rts, Progresso - 1 cup (8 fl oz) | | 5.0 | 10.0 | 2.5 | 2.0 | 4.5 | 30 | | | 1.08 | | | 100 | | | | | GENM320 |
| crab soup, rts | 244 | 76 | 223.3 | 10.3 | | | 0.7 | 1235 | 66 | 15 | 1.46 | 0.488 | 24 | 0 | 0.20 | 1.3 | 0.20 | 0.29 |
| 1 cup (8 fl oz) | | 5.5 | 1.5 | 0.4 | 0.7 | 0.4 | 10 | 327 | 88 | 1.22 | 0.488 | 6.3 | 505 | | 0.07 | 0.12 | 14.6 | 6034 |
| escarole (chickory) soup, cnd, rts | 248 | 27 | 240.3 | 1.8 | | | | 3864 | 32 | 5 | 2.23 | 1.240 | 109 | 4 | 0.07 | 2.3 | 0.50 | 0.17 |
| 1 cup (8 fl oz) | | 1.5 | 1.8 | 0.5 | 0.8 | 0.4 | 2 | 265 | 79 | 0.74 | 0.372 | | 2170 | | 0.05 | 0.22 | 34.7 | 6035 |
| fish soup, homemade | 233 | 168 | 195.7 | 13.0 | | | | 70 | 82 | 2 | | 0.023 | | 1 | 0.16 | 6.2 | | 0.02 |
| 1 cup (8 fl oz) | | 17.2 | 5.1 | 1.2 | | | 28 | 298 | 261 | 1.16 | | | 93 | | 0.05 | 0.02 | | 35073 |
| fish stock, homemade | 233 | 40 | 225.9 | 0 | 0 | | 0 | 363 | 7 | 16 | 0.14 | 0.121 | 5 | 0 | 0.08 | 2.8 | 1.61 | 0.77 |
| 1 cup (8 fl oz) | | 5.3 | 1.9 | 0.5 | 0.5 | 0.3 | 2 | 336 | 130 | 0.02 | 0.135 | 2.3 | 14 | 0.4 | 0.18 | 0.09 | 4.7 | 6174 |
| French onion soup, cnd, rts | 230 | 50 | | 8.0 | 3.0 | | 0.5 | 850 | 20 | | | | | | | | | |
| 1 cup (8 fl oz) | | 1.0 | 1.5 | 0.5 | 0 | 0 | 2 | | | | | | 100 | | | | | GENM324 |
| garden vegetable soup, cnd, rts, | 246 | 125 | 213.6 | 24.7 | 5.2 | | 4.7 | 480 | 39 | | | | | 2 | | | | |
| Hlthy Chc - 1 cup (8 fl oz) | | 5.2 | 0.5 | 0.1 | 0.2 | 0.2 | 2 | | | 0 | | | 1520 | | | | | 6316 |
| gazpacho, cnd, rts | 244 | 46 | 228.8 | 4.4 | 1.4 | 0.5 | 0.5 | 739 | 24 | 7 | 0.24 | 0.732 | 15 | 7 | 0.05 | 0.9 | 0 | 0.17 |
| 1 cup (8 fl oz) | | 7.1 | 0.2 | 0 | 0 | 0.1 | 0 | 224 | 37 | 0.98 | 0.146 | 3.7 | 298 | 0.4 | 0.02 | 0.15 | 19.5 | 6036 |
| lentil soup, cnd, rts, Progresso | 241 | 150 | | 28.0 | 1.0 | | 5.0 | 870 | 40 | | | | | 0 | | | | |
| 1 cup (8 fl oz) | | 9.0 | 2.0 | 0 | 0 | 0 | 0 | | | 2.70 | | | 300 | | | | | GENM327 |
| lentil soup with ham, cnd, rts | 248 | 139 | 212.7 | 20.2 | | | | 1319 | 42 | 22 | 0.74 | 0.298 | 17 | 4 | 0.17 | 1.4 | 0.30 | 0.35 |
| 1 cup (8 fl oz) | | 9.3 | 2.8 | 1.1 | 1.3 | 0.3 | 7 | 357 | 184 | 2.65 | 0.174 | 0.7 | 360 | | 0.11 | 0.22 | 49.6 | 6037 |
| macaroni and bean soup, cnd, rts, | 246 | 160 | | 25.0 | 1.0 | | 6.0 | 890 | 40 | | | | | 0 | | | | |
| Progresso - 1 cup (8 fl oz) | | 7.0 | 3.5 | 1.0 | 0.5 | 1.5 | 0 | | | 1.80 | | | 200 | | | | | GENM328 |
| minestrone soup, chunky, cnd, rts | 240 | 127 | 208.1 | 20.7 | 5.2 | 0.2 | 5.8 | 864 | 60 | 14 | 1.44 | 0.720 | 214 | 5 | 0.06 | 1.2 | 0 | 0.72 |
| 1 cup (8 fl oz) | | 5.1 | 2.8 | 1.5 | 0.9 | 0.3 | 5 | 612 | 110 | 1.78 | 0.240 | 5.3 | 4279 | 1.6 | 0.12 | 0.24 | 67.2 | 6039 |
| minestrone soup, cnd, rts, Progresso | 240 | 100 | | 18.0 | 2.0 | | 4.0 | 980 | 40 | | | | | 0 | | | | |
| 1 cup (8 fl oz) | | 4.0 | 2.0 | 0.5 | 0 | 1.0 | 0 | | | 1.44 | | | 1000 | | | | | GENM329 |
| pot, broc, chs chowder, cnd, rts, | 252 | 180 | | 18.0 | 2.0 | | 2.0 | 920 | 60 | | | | | 0 | | | | |
| Progresso - 1 cup (8 fl oz) | | 5.0 | 10.0 | 3.0 | 2.0 | 3.5 | 10 | | | 0.72 | | | 200 | | | | | GENM332 |
| potato ham chowder, cnd, rts | 240 | 192 | 204.7 | 13.4 | | | 1.4 | 874 | | | | | | 0 | | | | |
| 1 cup (8 fl oz) | | 6.5 | 12.5 | 3.9 | 5.9 | 0.8 | 22 | | | 1.68 | | | 0 | | | | | 6728 |
| shark fin soup, from restaurant | 216 | 99 | 194.7 | 8.2 | | | 0 | 1082 | 22 | 15 | 1.77 | 0.052 | 0 | 0 | 0.06 | 1.1 | 0.41 | 0.28 |
| 1 cup (8 fl oz) | | 6.9 | 4.3 | 1.1 | 1.3 | 0.7 | 4 | 114 | 45 | 2.03 | 0.233 | | 0 | | 0.08 | 0.06 | 19.4 | 6180 |
| sirloin burger w/vegetables soup, | 240 | 185 | 201.8 | 16.3 | | | 5.5 | 866 | | | | | | 0 | | | | |
| cnd, rts - 1 cup (8 fl oz) | | 10.1 | 8.9 | 3.2 | 3.2 | 1.3 | 26 | | | 2.09 | | | 3000 | | | | | 6729 |
| split pea soup, cnd, Progresso | 253 | 180 | 208.5 | 29.9 | 12.8 | | 4.8 | 420 | 43 | 35 | 1.01 | 0.506 | 71 | 0 | 0.18 | 1.2 | 0.03 | 0.60 |
| Healthy Classics - 1 cup (8 fl oz) | | 9.7 | 2.3 | 0.8 | 0.9 | 0.4 | 5 | 463 | 137 | 1.95 | 0.278 | 0.8 | 1397 | 0.5 | 0.07 | 0.18 | 50.6 | 6192 |
| splt pea w/ham soup, cnd, rts, Cmpbl's | 245 | 167 | 202.9 | 27.9 | 3.8 | | 4.7 | 480 | 39 | 34 | 1.20 | 0.485 | 51 | 2 | 0.20 | 1.7 | 0.07 | 0.61 |
| Hlthy Rqst - 1 cup (8 fl oz) | | 9.8 | 1.7 | 0.7 | 0.7 | 0.3 | 7 | 500 | 132 | 1.72 | 0.245 | 0.7 | 1017 | 0.1 | 0.09 | 0.12 | 71.1 | 6193 |

| | WT (g) | KCAL / PRO (g) | H₂0 (g) / FAT (g) | CHO (g) / SFA (g) | TSUG (g) / MUFA (g) | ASUG (g) / PUFA (g) | DFIB (g) / CHOL (mg) | Na (mg) / K (mg) | Ca (mg) / P (mg) | Mg (mg) / Fe (mg) | Zn (mg) / Cu (mg) | Mn (mg) / Se (mcg) | A (mcg RAE) / A (IU) | C (mg) / E (mg ATE) | B-1 (mg) / B-2 (mg) | NIA (mg) / B-6 (mg) | B-12 (mcg) / FOL (mcg DFE) | PANT (mg) / REF |
|---|---|---|---|---|---|---|---|---|---|---|---|---|---|---|---|---|---|---|
| **split pea with ham soup**, cnd, rts, | 243 | 140 | | 26.0 | 4.0 | | 4.0 | 790 | 20 | | | | | 0 | | | | |
| Progresso - *1 cup (8 fl oz)* | | 9.0 | 1.0 | 0 | 0 | 0 | 5 | | | 1.08 | | | 750 | | | | | GENM340 |
| **split pea with ham soup**, chunky, | 240 | 185 | 194.3 | 26.8 | 4.6 | 1.5 | 4.1 | 965 | 34 | 38 | 3.12 | 0.600 | 245 | 7 | 0.12 | 2.5 | 0.24 | 0.48 |
| cnd, rts - *1 cup (8 fl oz)* | | 11.1 | 4.0 | 1.6 | 1.6 | 0.6 | 7 | 305 | 178 | 2.14 | 0.240 | 9.8 | 4872 | 0.5 | 0.09 | 0.22 | 4.8 | 6050 |
| **tomato basil soup**, cnd, rts, | 244 | 160 | | 30.0 | 16.0 | | 1.0 | 960 | 20 | | | | | 6 | | | | |
| Progresso - *1 cup (8 fl oz)* | | 2.0 | 3.0 | 0.5 | 0.5 | 1.5 | 0 | | | 1.08 | | | 1000 | | | | | GENM341 |
| **tomato, roasted red pepper soup**, | 245 | 100 | | 16.0 | 10.0 | | 1.0 | 750 | 150 | | | | | 2 | | | | |
| Trader Joe's, rts - *1 cup (8 fl oz)* | | 5.0 | 2.0 | 1.5 | | | 10 | | | 0.36 | | | 500 | | | | | TRAD6 |
| **tomato rotini soup**, cnd, rts, | 243 | 140 | | 29.0 | 12.0 | | 3.0 | 950 | 20 | | | | | 5 | | | | |
| Progresso - *1 cup (8 fl oz)* | | 4.0 | 1.0 | 0 | 0 | 0 | 0 | | | 1.44 | | | 1000 | | | | | GENM342 |
| **tomato veg Italiano soup**, cnd, rts, | 241 | 100 | | 19.0 | 9.0 | | 3.0 | 990 | 20 | | | | 0 | | | | | |
| Progresso - *1 cup (8 fl oz)* | | 3.0 | 2.0 | 0.5 | 0 | 1.0 | 0 | | | 0.36 | | | 1000 | | | | | GENM343 |
| **turkey noodle soup**, cnd, rts, | 238 | 80 | | 12.0 | 1.0 | | 1.0 | 930 | 0 | | | | 0 | | | | | |
| Progresso - *1 cup (8 fl oz)* | | 5.0 | 1.5 | 0 | 0 | 0.5 | 15 | | | 0.72 | | | 1000 | | | | | GENM345 |
| **turkey soup**, chunky, cnd, rts | 236 | 135 | 203.8 | 14.1 | | | | 923 | 50 | 24 | 2.12 | 0.236 | 359 | 6 | 0.04 | 3.6 | 2.12 | 0.92 |
| *1 cup (8 fl oz)* | | 10.2 | 4.4 | 1.2 | 1.8 | 1.1 | 9 | 361 | 104 | 1.91 | 0.236 | | 7156 | | 0.11 | 0.31 | 11.8 | 6064 |
| **vegetable beef soup**, microwave | 292 | 128 | 258.7 | 9.6 | | | 4.4 | 1098 | | | | | 96 | | | | | |
| container - *9.7 fl oz container* | | 18.1 | 2.0 | 0.6 | 0.7 | 0.3 | 9 | | | | | | 1898 | | | | | 6742 |
| **vegetable soup**, chunky, cnd, rts | 240 | 122 | 210.2 | 19.0 | 4.4 | 0.6 | 1.2 | 862 | 55 | 7 | 3.12 | 0.480 | 293 | 6 | 0.07 | 1.2 | 0 | 0.34 |
| *1 cup (8 fl oz)* | | 3.5 | 3.7 | 0.6 | 1.6 | 1.4 | 0 | 396 | 72 | 1.63 | 0.240 | 7.0 | 5878 | 1.3 | 0.06 | 0.19 | 16.8 | 6067 |
| **vegetable soup**, cnd, rts, | 238 | 80 | | 16.0 | 4.0 | | 3.0 | 880 | 20 | | | | 0 | | | | | |
| Progresso - *1 cup (8 fl oz)* | | 3.0 | 0.5 | 0 | 0 | 0 | 0 | | | 0.72 | | | 1250 | | | | | GENM347 |
| **vegetarian veg w/barley soup**, cnd, | 242 | 100 | | 20.0 | 5.0 | | 4.0 | 980 | 20 | | | | 0 | | | | | |
| rts, Progresso - *1 cup (8 fl oz)* | | 3.0 | 0.5 | 0 | 0 | 0 | 0 | | | 1.08 | | | 1500 | | | | | GENM348 |

## 28. SPICES, HERBS, AND FLAVORINGS

| | WT (g) | KCAL / PRO (g) | H₂0 (g) / FAT (g) | CHO (g) / SFA (g) | TSUG (g) / MUFA (g) | ASUG (g) / PUFA (g) | DFIB (g) / CHOL (mg) | Na (mg) / K (mg) | Ca (mg) / P (mg) | Mg (mg) / Fe (mg) | Zn (mg) / Cu (mg) | Mn (mg) / Se (mcg) | A (mcg RAE) / A (IU) | C (mg) / E (mg ATE) | B-1 (mg) / B-2 (mg) | NIA (mg) / B-6 (mg) | B-12 (mcg) / FOL (mcg DFE) | PANT (mg) / REF |
|---|---|---|---|---|---|---|---|---|---|---|---|---|---|---|---|---|---|---|
| **allspice**, ground | 6 | 16 | 0.5 | 4.3 | | | 1.3 | 5 | 40 | 8 | 0.06 | 0.177 | 2 | 2 | 0.01 | 0.2 | 0 | |
| *1 T* | | 0.4 | 0.5 | 0.2 | 0 | 0.1 | 0 | 63 | 7 | 0.42 | 0.033 | 0.2 | 32 | | 0.01 | | 2.2 | 2001 |
| **anise seeds** | 7 | 24 | 0.7 | 3.5 | | | 1.0 | 1 | 45 | 12 | 0.37 | 0.161 | 1 | 1 | 0.02 | 0.2 | 0 | 0.06 |
| *1 T* | | 1.2 | 1.1 | 0 | 0.7 | 0.2 | 0 | 101 | 31 | 2.59 | 0.064 | 0.4 | 22 | | 0.02 | 0.05 | 0.7 | 2002 |
| **basil**, dried | 5 | 11 | 0.3 | 2.7 | 0.1 | 0 | 1.8 | 2 | 95 | 19 | 0.26 | 0.143 | 21 | 3 | 0.01 | 0.3 | 0 | |
| *1 T* | | 0.6 | 0.2 | 0 | 0 | 0.1 | 0 | 154 | 22 | 1.89 | 0.062 | 0.1 | 422 | 0.3 | 0.01 | 0.10 | 12.3 | 2003 |
| **basil**, raw | 5 | 1 | 4.6 | 0.1 | 0 | | 0.1 | 0 | 9 | 3 | 0.04 | 0.057 | 13 | 1 | 0 | 0 | 0 | 0.01 |
| *1 T* | | 0.2 | 0 | 0 | 0 | 0 | 0 | 15 | 3 | 0.16 | 0.019 | 0 | 264 | 0 | 0 | 0.01 | 3.4 | 2044 |
| **bay leaves**, dried | 2 | 6 | 0.1 | 1.3 | | | 0.5 | 0 | 15 | 2 | 0.07 | 0.147 | 6 | 1 | 0 | 0 | 0 | |
| *1 T* | | 0.1 | 0.2 | 0 | 0 | 0 | 0 | 10 | 2 | 0.77 | 0.007 | 0.1 | 111 | | 0.01 | 0.03 | 3.2 | 2004 |
| **black pepper** | 6 | 15 | 0.6 | 3.9 | 0 | | 1.6 | 3 | 26 | 12 | 0.09 | 0.337 | 1 | 1 | 0.01 | 0.1 | 0 | |
| *1 T* | | 0.7 | 0.2 | 0.1 | 0.1 | 0.1 | 0 | 76 | 10 | 1.73 | 0.068 | 0.2 | 18 | 0 | 0.01 | 0.02 | 0.6 | 2030 |
| **capers**, canned | 9 | 2 | 7.5 | 0.4 | 0 | | 0.3 | 267 | 4 | 3 | 0.03 | 0.007 | 1 | 0 | | 0.1 | 0 | 0 |
| *1 T* | | 0.2 | 0.1 | 0 | 0 | 0 | 0 | 4 | 1 | 0.15 | 0.034 | 0.1 | 12 | 0.1 | 0.01 | 0 | 2.1 | 2054 |
| **caraway seeds** | 7 | 23 | 0.7 | 3.5 | | 0 | 2.7 | 1 | 48 | 18 | 0.38 | 0.091 | 1 | 1 | 0.03 | 0.3 | 0 | |
| *1 T* | | 1.4 | 1.0 | 0 | 0.5 | 0.2 | 0 | 95 | 40 | 1.14 | 0.064 | 0.8 | 25 | 0.2 | 0.03 | 0.03 | 0.7 | 2005 |
| **cardamon** (cardamom) | 6 | 19 | 0.5 | 4.1 | | | 1.7 | 1 | 23 | 14 | 0.45 | 1.680 | 0 | 1 | 0.01 | 0.1 | 0 | |
| *1 T* | | 0.6 | 0.4 | 0 | 0.1 | 0 | 0 | 67 | 11 | 0.84 | 0.023 | | | | 0.01 | 0.01 | | 2006 |
| **celery seeds** | 7 | 27 | 0.4 | 2.9 | | 0 | 0.8 | 11 | 124 | 31 | 0.49 | 0.530 | 0 | 1 | 0.02 | 0.2 | 0 | |
| *1 T* | | 1.3 | 1.8 | 0.2 | 1.1 | 0.3 | 0 | 98 | 38 | 3.14 | 0.096 | 0.8 | 4 | 0.1 | 0.02 | 0.06 | 0.7 | 2007 |
| **chili powder** | 8 | 25 | 0.6 | 4.4 | 0.6 | 0 | 2.7 | 81 | 22 | 14 | 0.22 | 0.173 | 119 | 5 | 0.03 | 0.6 | 0 | |
| *1 T* | | 1.0 | 1.3 | 0.2 | 0.3 | 0.6 | 0 | 153 | 24 | 1.14 | 0.034 | 0.5 | 2372 | 2.3 | 0.06 | 0.29 | 8.0 | 2009 |
| **chives**, freeze-dried | 1 | 2 | 0 | 0.5 | | | 0.2 | 1 | 7 | 5 | 0.04 | 0.011 | 27 | 5 | 0.01 | 0 | 0 | 0.02 |
| *¼ cup* | | 0.2 | 0 | 0 | 0 | 0 | 0 | 24 | 4 | 0.16 | 0.005 | 0.1 | 546 | | 0.01 | 0.02 | 0.9 | 11615 |
| **chives**, raw | 3 | 1 | 2.7 | 0.1 | 0.1 | 0 | 0.1 | 0 | 3 | 1 | 0.02 | 0.011 | 7 | 2 | 0 | 0 | 0 | 0.01 |
| *1 T chopped* | | 0.1 | 0 | 0 | 0 | 0 | 0 | 9 | 2 | 0.05 | 0.005 | 0 | 131 | 0 | 0 | 0 | 3.2 | 11156 |
| **cilantro**, dried | 2 | 5 | 0.1 | 0.9 | 0.1 | 0 | 0.2 | 4 | 22 | 12 | 0.08 | 0.114 | 5 | 10 | 0.02 | 0.2 | 0 | |
| *1 T* | | 0.4 | 0.1 | 0 | 0 | 0 | 0 | 80 | 9 | 0.76 | 0.032 | 0.5 | 105 | 0 | 0.03 | 0.01 | 4.9 | 2012 |
| **cinnamon**, ground | 7 | 17 | 0.7 | 5.6 | 0.2 | 0 | 3.7 | 1 | 70 | 4 | 0.13 | 1.223 | 1 | 0 | 0 | 0.1 | 0 | 0.03 |
| *1 T* | | 0.3 | 0.1 | 0 | 0 | 0 | 0 | 30 | 4 | 0.58 | 0.024 | 0.2 | 21 | 0.2 | 0 | 0.01 | 0.4 | 2010 |
| **cloves**, ground | 7 | 23 | 0.5 | 4.3 | 0.2 | 0 | 2.4 | 17 | 45 | 18 | 0.08 | 2.102 | 2 | 6 | 0.01 | 0.1 | 0 | |
| *1 T* | | 0.4 | 1.4 | 0.4 | 0.1 | 0.5 | 0 | 77 | 7 | 0.61 | 0.024 | 0.4 | 37 | 0.6 | 0.02 | 0.04 | 6.5 | 2011 |
| **coriander seeds** | 5 | 15 | 0.4 | 2.7 | | | 2.1 | 2 | 35 | 16 | 0.24 | 0.095 | 0 | 1 | 0.01 | 0.1 | 0 | |
| *1 T* | | 0.6 | 0.9 | 0 | 0.7 | 0.1 | 0 | 63 | 20 | 0.82 | 0.049 | 1.3 | 0 | | 0.01 | | 0 | 2013 |

| | WT (g) | KCAL / PRO (g) | H₂O (g) / FAT (g) | CHO (g) / SFA (g) | TSUG (g) / MUFA (g) | ASUG (g) / PUFA (g) | DFIB (g) / CHOL (mg) | Na (mg) / K (mg) | Ca (mg) / P (mg) | Mg (mg) / Fe (mg) | Zn (mg) / Cu (mg) | Mn (mg) / Se (mcg) | A (mcg RAE) / A (IU) | C (mg) / E (mg ATE) | B-1 (mg) / B-2 (mg) | NIA (mg) / B-6 (mg) | B-12 (mcg) / FOL (mcg DFE) | PANT (mg) / REF |
|---|---|---|---|---|---|---|---|---|---|---|---|---|---|---|---|---|---|---|
| cumin | 6 | 22 | 0.5 | 2.7 | 0.1 | 0 | 0.6 | 10 | 56 | 22 | 0.29 | 0.200 | 4 | | 0.04 | 0.3 | 0 | |
| *1 T* | | 1.1 | 1.3 | 0.1 | 0.8 | 0.2 | 0 | 107 | 30 | 3.98 | 0.052 | 0.3 | 76 | 0.2 | 0.02 | 0.03 | 0.6 | 2014 |
| curry powder | 6 | 20 | 0.6 | 3.5 | 0.2 | 0 | 2.0 | 3 | 29 | 15 | 0.24 | 0.257 | 3 | 1 | 0.02 | 0.2 | 0 | |
| *1 T* | | 0.8 | 0.8 | 0.1 | 0.3 | 0.2 | 0 | 93 | 21 | 1.78 | 0.049 | 1.0 | 59 | 1.3 | 0.02 | 0.07 | 9.2 | 2015 |
| dill seeds | 7 | 21 | 0.5 | 3.9 | | | 1.5 | 1 | 106 | 18 | 0.36 | 0.128 | 0 | 1 | 0.03 | 0.2 | 0 | |
| *1 T* | | 1.1 | 1.0 | 0.1 | 0.7 | 0.1 | 0 | 83 | 19 | 1.14 | 0.055 | 0.8 | 4 | | 0.02 | 0.02 | 0.7 | 2016 |
| dill weed, dried | 3 | 8 | 0.2 | 1.7 | | | 0.4 | 6 | 55 | 14 | 0.10 | 0.122 | 9 | 2 | 0.01 | 0.1 | 0 | |
| *1 T* | | 0.6 | 0.1 | 0 | | | 0 | 103 | 17 | 1.51 | 0.015 | | 181 | | 0.01 | 0.05 | | 2017 |
| dill weed, raw | 9 | 4 | 7.7 | 0.6 | | | 0.2 | 5 | 19 | 5 | 0.08 | 0.114 | 35 | 8 | 0.01 | 0.1 | 0 | 0.04 |
| *1 cup sprigs* | | 0.3 | 0.1 | 0 | 0.1 | 0 | 0 | 66 | 6 | 0.59 | 0.013 | | 695 | | 0.03 | 0.02 | 13.5 | 2045 |
| epazote sprig, raw | 2 | 1 | 1.8 | 0.1 | | | 0.1 | 1 | 6 | 2 | 0.02 | 0.062 | 0 | 0 | 0 | 0 | 0 | 0 |
| *1 sprig* | | 0 | 0 | | | | 0 | 13 | 2 | 0.04 | 0.004 | 0 | 1 | | 0.01 | 0 | 4.3 | 11984 |
| fennel seeds | 6 | 21 | 0.5 | 3.1 | | | 2.4 | 5 | 72 | 23 | 0.22 | 0.392 | 0 | 1 | 0.02 | 0.4 | 0 | |
| *1 T* | | 0.9 | 0.9 | 0 | 0.6 | 0.1 | 0 | 102 | 29 | 1.11 | 0.064 | | 8 | | 0.02 | 0.03 | | 2018 |
| fenugreek seeds | 11 | 36 | 1.0 | 6.4 | | | 2.7 | 7 | 19 | 21 | 0.28 | 0.135 | 0 | 0 | 0.04 | 0.2 | 0 | |
| *1 T* | | 2.5 | 0.7 | 0.2 | | | 0 | 85 | 33 | 3.69 | 0.122 | 0.7 | 7 | | 0.04 | 0.07 | 6.3 | 2019 |
| garlic powder | 8 | 27 | 0.5 | 5.8 | 1.9 | 0 | 0.8 | 2 | 6 | 5 | 0.21 | 0.044 | 0 | 1 | 0.04 | 0.1 | 0 | |
| *1 T* | | 1.3 | 0.1 | 0 | 0 | 0 | 0 | 88 | 33 | 0.22 | 0.012 | 3.0 | 0 | 0.1 | 0 | 0.24 | 0.2 | 2020 |
| ginger, ground | 5 | 17 | 0.5 | 3.5 | 0.2 | 0 | 0.6 | 2 | 6 | 9 | 0.24 | 1.325 | 0 | 0 | 0 | 0.3 | 0 | |
| *1 T* | | 0.5 | 0.3 | 0.1 | 0.1 | 0.1 | 0 | 67 | 7 | 0.58 | 0.024 | 1.9 | 7 | 0.9 | 0.01 | 0.04 | 2.0 | 2021 |
| ginger root, raw | 5 | 4 | 3.9 | 0.9 | 0.1 | 0 | 0.1 | 1 | 1 | 2 | 0.02 | 0.011 | 0 | 0 | 0 | 0 | 0 | 0.01 |
| *1 T* | | 0.1 | 0 | 0 | 0 | 0 | 0 | 21 | 2 | 0.03 | 0.011 | 0 | 0 | | 0 | 0.01 | 0.6 | 11216 |
| lemon grass (citronella), raw | 5 | 5 | 3.4 | 1.2 | | | | 0 | 3 | 3 | 0.11 | 0.251 | 0 | 0 | 0 | 0.1 | 0 | 0 |
| *1 T* | | 0.1 | 0 | 0 | 0 | 0 | 0 | 35 | 5 | 0.39 | 0.013 | 0 | | | 0.01 | 0 | 3.6 | 11972 |
| mace, ground | 5 | 24 | 0.4 | 2.5 | | | 1.0 | 4 | 13 | 8 | 0.12 | 0.075 | 2 | 1 | 0.02 | 0.1 | 0 | |
| *1 T* | | 0.3 | 1.6 | 0.5 | 0.6 | 0.2 | 0 | 23 | 6 | 0.70 | 0.123 | 0.1 | 40 | | 0.02 | 0.01 | 3.8 | 2022 |
| marjoram, dried | 2 | 5 | 0.1 | 1.0 | 0.1 | 0 | 0.7 | 1 | 34 | 6 | 0.06 | 0.092 | 7 | 1 | 0 | 0.1 | 0 | |
| *1 T* | | 0.2 | 0.1 | 0 | 0 | 0.1 | 0 | 26 | 5 | 1.41 | 0.019 | 0.1 | 137 | 0 | 0.01 | 0.02 | 4.7 | 2023 |
| mustard seeds, yellow | 11 | 52 | 0.8 | 3.8 | 0.7 | 0 | 1.6 | 1 | 57 | 33 | 0.63 | 0.194 | 0 | 0 | 0.06 | 0.9 | 0 | |
| *1 T* | | 2.7 | 3.2 | 0.2 | 2.2 | 0.6 | 0 | 75 | 93 | 1.10 | 0.045 | 14.7 | 7 | 0.3 | 0.04 | 0.05 | 8.4 | 2024 |
| nutmeg, ground | 7 | 37 | 0.4 | 3.5 | 2.0 | 0 | 1.5 | 1 | 13 | 13 | 0.15 | 0.203 | 0 | 0 | 0.02 | 0.1 | 0 | |
| *1 T* | | 0.4 | 2.5 | 1.8 | 0.2 | 0 | 0 | 25 | 15 | 0.21 | 0.072 | 0.1 | 7 | 0 | 0 | 0.01 | 5.3 | 2025 |
| onion flakes, dehydrated | 14 | 49 | 0.6 | 11.7 | 5.2 | 0 | 1.3 | 3 | 36 | 13 | 0.26 | 0.194 | 0 | 11 | 0.07 | 0.1 | 0 | 0.19 |
| *¼ cup* | | 1.3 | 0.1 | 0 | 0 | 0 | 0 | 227 | 42 | 0.22 | 0.058 | 0.7 | 3 | 0 | 0.01 | 0.22 | 23.2 | 11284 |
| onion powder | 7 | 24 | 0.4 | 5.6 | 2.5 | 0 | 0.4 | 4 | 25 | 9 | 0.16 | 0.026 | 0 | 1 | 0.03 | 0 | 0 | |
| *1 T* | | 0.7 | 0.1 | 0 | 0 | 0 | 0 | 66 | 24 | 0.18 | 0.012 | 0.1 | 0 | 0 | 0 | 0.09 | 11.6 | 2026 |
| oregano, dried, ground | 5 | 14 | 0.3 | 2.9 | 0.2 | 0 | 1.9 | 1 | 71 | 12 | 0.20 | 0.210 | 16 | 2 | 0.02 | 0.3 | 0 | |
| *1 T* | | 0.5 | 0.5 | 0.1 | 0 | 0.2 | 0 | 75 | 9 | 1.98 | 0.042 | 0.3 | 311 | 0.8 | 0.01 | 0.05 | 12.3 | 2027 |
| paprika | 7 | 20 | 0.7 | 3.9 | 0.7 | 0 | 2.6 | 2 | 12 | 13 | 0.28 | 0.059 | 185 | 5 | 0.05 | 1.1 | 0 | 0.12 |
| *1 T* | | 1.0 | 0.9 | 0.1 | 0.1 | 0.6 | 0 | 164 | 24 | 1.65 | 0.042 | 0.3 | 3691 | 2.1 | 0.12 | 0.28 | 7.4 | 2028 |
| parsley, dried | 1 | 4 | 0.1 | 0.7 | 0.1 | 0 | 0.4 | 6 | 19 | 3 | 0.06 | 0.136 | 7 | 2 | 0 | 0.1 | 0 | |
| *1 T* | | 0.3 | 0.1 | 0 | 0 | 0 | 0 | 49 | 5 | 1.27 | 0.008 | 0.4 | 132 | 0.1 | 0.02 | 0.01 | 2.3 | 2029 |
| peppermint, raw | 3 | 2 | 2.5 | 0.5 | | | 0.3 | 1 | 8 | 3 | 0.04 | 0.038 | 7 | 1 | 0 | 0.1 | 0 | 0.01 |
| *2 T* | | 0.1 | 0 | 0 | 0 | 0 | 0 | 18 | 2 | 0.16 | 0.011 | | 136 | | 0.01 | 0 | 3.6 | 2064 |
| poppy seeds | 9 | 47 | 0.5 | 2.5 | 0.3 | 0 | 1.8 | 2 | 129 | 31 | 0.71 | 0.604 | 0 | 0 | 0.08 | 0.1 | 0 | 0.03 |
| *1 T* | | 1.6 | 3.7 | 0.4 | 0.5 | 2.6 | 0 | 65 | 78 | 0.88 | 0.146 | 1.2 | 0 | 0.2 | 0.01 | 0.02 | 7.4 | 2033 |
| poultry seasoning | 4 | 11 | 0.3 | 2.4 | 0.1 | 0 | 0.4 | 1 | 37 | 8 | 0.12 | 0.254 | 5 | 0 | 0.01 | 0.1 | 0 | |
| *1 T* | | 0.4 | 0.3 | 0.1 | 0 | 0.1 | 0 | 25 | 6 | 1.31 | 0.031 | 0.3 | 97 | 0 | 0.01 | 0.05 | 5.1 | 2034 |
| pumpkin pie spice | 6 | 21 | 0.5 | 4.2 | 0.5 | 0 | 0.9 | 3 | 41 | 8 | 0.14 | 0.951 | 1 | 0 | 0.01 | 0.1 | 0 | |
| *1 T* | | 0.3 | 0.8 | 0.4 | 0.1 | 0 | 0 | 40 | 7 | 1.18 | 0.029 | 0.6 | 16 | 0 | 0.01 | 0.02 | 3.1 | 2035 |
| red/cayenne pepper | 5 | 16 | 0.4 | 2.8 | 0.5 | 0 | 1.4 | 2 | 7 | 8 | 0.12 | 0.100 | 104 | 4 | 0.02 | 0.4 | 0 | |
| *1 T* | | 0.6 | 0.9 | 0.2 | 0.1 | 0.4 | 0 | 101 | 15 | 0.39 | 0.019 | 0.4 | 2080 | 1.5 | 0.05 | 0.12 | 5.3 | 2031 |
| rosemary, raw | 2 | 2 | 1.2 | 0.4 | | | 0.2 | 0 | 5 | 2 | 0.02 | 0.016 | 2 | 0 | 0 | 0 | 0 | 0.01 |
| *1 T* | | 0.1 | 0.1 | 0 | 0 | 0 | 0 | 11 | 1 | 0.11 | 0.005 | | 50 | | 0.01 | 0 | 1.9 | 2063 |
| saffron, ground | 2 | 7 | 0.2 | 1.4 | | | 0.1 | 3 | 2 | 6 | 0.02 | 0.597 | 1 | 2 | 0 | 0 | 0 | |
| *1 T* | | 0.2 | 0.1 | 0 | 0 | 0 | 0 | 36 | 5 | 0.23 | 0.007 | 0.1 | 11 | | 0.01 | 0.02 | 2.0 | 2037 |
| sage, ground | 2 | 6 | 0.2 | 1.2 | | | 0.8 | 0 | 33 | 9 | 0.09 | 0.063 | 6 | 1 | 0.02 | 0.1 | 0 | |
| *1 T* | | 0.2 | 0.3 | 0.1 | 0 | 0 | 0 | 21 | 2 | 0.56 | 0.015 | 0.1 | 118 | 0.1 | 0.01 | 0.05 | 5.5 | 2038 |
| salt | 18 | 0 | 0 | 0 | 0 | 0 | 0 | 6976 | 4 | 0 | 0.02 | 0.018 | 0 | 0 | 0 | 0 | 0 | 0 |
| *1 T* | | 0 | 0 | 0 | 0 | 0 | 0 | 1 | 0 | 0.06 | 0.005 | 0 | 0 | 0 | 0 | 0 | 0 | 2047 |
| savory, ground | 4 | 12 | 0.4 | 3.0 | | | 2.0 | 1 | 94 | 17 | 0.19 | 0.268 | 11 | 2 | 0.02 | 0.2 | 0 | |
| *1 T* | | 0.3 | 0.3 | 0.1 | | | 0 | 46 | 6 | 1.67 | 0.037 | 0.2 | 226 | | | 0.08 | | 2039 |

| | WT (g) | KCAL | H₂O (g) | CHO (g) | TSUG (g) | ASUG (g) | DFIB (g) | Na (mg) | Ca (mg) | Mg (mg) | Zn (mg) | Mn (mg) | A (mcg RAE) | C (mg) | B-1 (mg) | NIA (mg) | B-12 (mcg) | PANT (mg) |
|---|---|---|---|---|---|---|---|---|---|---|---|---|---|---|---|---|---|---|
| | | PRO (g) | FAT (g) | SFA (g) | MUFA (g) | PUFA (g) | CHOL (mg) | K (mg) | P (mg) | Fe (mg) | Cu (mg) | Se (mcg) | A (IU) | E (mg ATE) | B-2 (mg) | B-6 (mg) | FOL (mcg DFE) | REF |
| **shallots**, freeze-dried | 4 | 13 | 0.1 | 2.9 | | | | 2 | 7 | 4 | 0.07 | 0.051 | 101 | 1 | 0.01 | 0 | 0 | 0.05 |
| ¼ cup | | 0.4 | 0 | 0 | 0 | 0 | 0 | 59 | 11 | 0.22 | 0.015 | 0.2 | 2020 | | 0 | 0.06 | 4.2 | 11640 |
| **spearmint**, dried | 2 | 5 | 0.2 | 0.8 | | | 0.5 | 6 | 24 | 10 | 0.04 | 0.184 | 8 | 0 | 0 | 0.1 | 0 | 0.02 |
| 1 T | | 0.3 | 0.1 | 0 | 0 | 0.1 | 0 | 31 | 4 | 1.40 | 0.025 | | 169 | | 0.02 | 0.04 | 8.5 | 2066 |
| **spearmint**, raw | 11 | 5 | 9.4 | 0.9 | | | 0.7 | 3 | 22 | 7 | 0.12 | 0.123 | 22 | 1 | 0.01 | 0.1 | 0 | 0.03 |
| 2 T | | 0.4 | 0.1 | 0 | 0 | 0 | 0 | 50 | 7 | 1.31 | 0.026 | | 446 | | 0.02 | 0.02 | 11.6 | 2065 |
| **tarragon**, ground | 5 | 14 | 0.4 | 2.4 | | | 0.4 | 3 | 55 | 17 | 0.19 | 0.382 | 10 | 2 | 0.01 | 0.4 | 0 | |
| 1 T | | 1.1 | 0.3 | 0.1 | 0 | 0.2 | 0 | 145 | 15 | 1.55 | 0.032 | 0.2 | 202 | | 0.06 | 0.12 | 13.2 | 2041 |
| **thyme**, ground | 4 | 12 | 0.3 | 2.7 | 0.1 | | 1.6 | 2 | 81 | 9 | 0.27 | 0.338 | 8 | 2 | 0.02 | 0.2 | 0 | |
| 1 T | | 0.4 | 0.3 | 0.1 | 0 | 0.1 | 0 | 35 | 9 | 5.31 | 0.037 | 0.2 | 163 | 0.3 | 0.02 | 0.02 | 11.8 | 2042 |
| **thyme**, raw | 2 | 2 | 1.6 | 0.6 | | | 0.3 | 0 | 10 | 4 | 0.04 | 0.041 | 6 | 4 | 0 | 0 | 0 | 0.01 |
| 1 T | | 0.1 | 0 | 0 | 0 | 0 | 0 | 15 | 3 | 0.42 | 0.013 | | 114 | | 0.01 | 0.01 | 1.1 | 2049 |
| **turmeric**, ground | 7 | 25 | 0.8 | 4.5 | 0.2 | 0 | 1.5 | 3 | 13 | 14 | 0.30 | 0.548 | 0 | 2 | 0.01 | 0.4 | 0 | |
| 1 T | | 0.5 | 0.7 | 0.2 | 0.1 | 0.2 | 0 | 177 | 19 | 2.90 | 0.042 | 0.3 | 0 | 0.2 | 0.02 | 0.13 | 2.7 | 2043 |
| **vanilla extract** | 13 | 37 | 6.8 | 1.6 | 1.6 | 0 | 0 | 1 | 1 | 2 | 0.01 | 0.030 | 0 | 0 | 0 | 0.1 | 0 | 0 |
| 1 T | | 0 | 0 | 0 | 0 | 0 | 0 | 19 | 1 | 0.02 | 0.009 | 0 | 0 | 0 | 0.01 | 0 | 0 | 2050 |
| **vanilla extract**, imitation w/ | 13 | 31 | 8.4 | 0.3 | | | 0 | 1 | 0 | 1 | 0.01 | 0.063 | 0 | 0 | 0 | 0 | 0 | 0 |
| alcohol - 1 T | | 0 | 0 | | | | 0 | 13 | 3 | 0.02 | 0.003 | | 0 | | 0.01 | 0 | 0 | 2051 |
| **vanilla extract**, imitation w/o | 13 | 7 | 11.1 | 1.9 | 1.9 | 0 | 0 | 0 | 0 | 0 | 0 | 0 | 0 | 0 | 0 | 0 | 0 | 0 |
| alcohol - 1 T | | 0 | 0 | 0 | 0 | 0 | 0 | 0 | 0 | 0.01 | 0 | 0 | 0 | 0 | 0 | 0 | 0 | 2052 |
| **white pepper** | 7 | 21 | 0.8 | 4.8 | | | 1.8 | 0 | 19 | 6 | 0.08 | 0.301 | 0 | 1 | 0 | 0 | 0 | |
| 1 T | | 0.7 | 0.1 | 0.1 | 0 | 0 | 0 | 5 | 12 | 1.00 | 0.064 | 0.2 | 0 | | 0.01 | 0.01 | 0.7 | 2032 |

## 29. SUGARS, SYRUPS, AND OTHER SWEETENERS

| | WT (g) | KCAL | H₂O (g) | CHO (g) | TSUG (g) | ASUG (g) | DFIB (g) | Na (mg) | Ca (mg) | Mg (mg) | Zn (mg) | Mn (mg) | A (mcg RAE) | C (mg) | B-1 (mg) | NIA (mg) | B-12 (mcg) | PANT (mg) |
|---|---|---|---|---|---|---|---|---|---|---|---|---|---|---|---|---|---|---|
| | | PRO (g) | FAT (g) | SFA (g) | MUFA (g) | PUFA (g) | CHOL (mg) | K (mg) | P (mg) | Fe (mg) | Cu (mg) | Se (mcg) | A (IU) | E (mg ATE) | B-2 (mg) | B-6 (mg) | FOL (mcg DFE) | REF |
| **apple butter** | 17 | 29 | 9.6 | 7.2 | 6.0 | 4.3 | 0.3 | 3 | 2 | 1 | 0.01 | 0.054 | 0 | 0 | 0 | 0 | 0 | 0.01 |
| 1 T | | 0.1 | 0.1 | 0 | 0 | 0 | 0 | 15 | 1 | 0.05 | 0.014 | 0.1 | 4 | 0 | 0 | 0.01 | 0.2 | 19294 |
| **corn syrup**, dark | 40 | 114 | 8.8 | 31.0 | 10.7 | 0 | 0 | 62 | 7 | 3 | 0.02 | 0.040 | 0 | 0 | 0 | 0 | 0 | 0.01 |
| 2 T | | 0 | 0 | 0 | 0 | 0 | 0 | 18 | 4 | 0.15 | 0.021 | 1.2 | 0 | 0 | 0 | 0 | 0 | 19349 |
| **corn syrup**, high fructose | 38 | 107 | 9.1 | 28.9 | 10.0 | 0 | 0 | 1 | 0 | 0 | 0.01 | 0.036 | 0 | 0 | 0 | 0 | 0 | 0 |
| 2 T | | 0 | 0 | 0 | 0 | 0 | 0 | 0 | 0 | 0.01 | 0.011 | 0.3 | 0 | 0 | 0.01 | 0 | 0 | 19351 |
| **corn syrup**, light (in color) | 40 | 113 | 9.1 | 30.7 | 10.7 | 0 | 0 | 25 | 5 | 0 | 0.18 | 0 | 0 | 0 | 0.02 | 0 | 0 | 0 |
| 2 T | | 0.1 | 0 | 0 | 0 | 0 | 0 | 0 | 0 | 0 | 0 | 0.3 | 0 | 0 | 0 | 0 | 0 | 19350 |
| **corn syrup with sugar cane syrup** | 20 | 64 | 3.1 | 16.8 | | | 0 | 14 | 5 | 2 | 0.01 | 0.018 | 0 | 0 | 0 | 0 | 0 | 0.01 |
| 1 T | | 0 | 0 | 0 | | | 0 | 13 | 2 | 0.15 | 0.012 | 0.2 | 0 | | 0.01 | 0 | 0.6 | 19362 |
| **honey** | 21 | 64 | 3.6 | 17.3 | 17.2 | 0 | 0 | 1 | 1 | 0 | 0.05 | 0.017 | 0 | 0 | 0 | 0 | 0 | 0.01 |
| 1 T | | 0.1 | 0 | 0 | 0 | 0 | 0 | 11 | 1 | 0.09 | 0.008 | 0.2 | 0 | 0 | 0.01 | 0.01 | 0.4 | 19296 |
| **jam/preserves** | 20 | 56 | 6.1 | 13.8 | 9.7 | 8.6 | 0.2 | 6 | 4 | 1 | 0.01 | 0.008 | 0 | 2 | 0 | 0 | 0 | 0 |
| 1 T | | 0.1 | 0 | 0 | 0 | 0 | 0 | 15 | 4 | 0.10 | 0.020 | 0.4 | 0 | 0 | 0.02 | 0 | 2.2 | 19297 |
| **jam/preserves**, apricot | 20 | 48 | 6.9 | 12.9 | 8.7 | 7.1 | 0.1 | 8 | 4 | 1 | 0.01 | 0.008 | 3 | 2 | 0 | 0 | 0 | 0 |
| 1 T | | 0.1 | 0 | 0 | 0 | 0 | 0 | 15 | 1 | 0.10 | 0.020 | 0.4 | 41 | 0 | 0 | 0 | 0.2 | 19719 |
| **jelly** | 19 | 51 | 5.7 | 13.3 | 9.7 | 8.0 | 0.2 | 6 | 1 | 1 | 0.01 | 0.025 | 0 | 0 | 0 | 0 | 0 | 0.04 |
| 1 T | | 0 | 0 | 0 | 0 | 0 | 0 | 10 | 1 | 0.04 | 0.002 | 0.1 | 1 | 0 | 0 | 0 | 0.4 | 19300 |
| **malt syrup** | 24 | 76 | 5.1 | 17.1 | 17.1 | 0 | 0 | 8 | 15 | 17 | 0.03 | 0.024 | 0 | 0 | 0 | 1.9 | 0 | 0.04 |
| 1 T | | 1.5 | 0 | 0 | 0 | 0 | 0 | 77 | 57 | 0.23 | 0.048 | 3.0 | 0 | | 0.09 | 0.12 | 2.9 | 19352 |
| **maple sugar** | 28 | 99 | 2.2 | 25.5 | 23.8 | 0 | 0 | 3 | 25 | 5 | 1.70 | 1.238 | 0 | 0 | 0 | 0 | 0 | 0.01 |
| 1 oz (~3.2 t) | | 0 | 0.1 | 0 | 0 | 0 | 0 | 77 | 1 | 0.45 | 0.028 | 0.2 | 0 | 0 | 0 | 0 | 0 | 19340 |
| **maple syrup** | 40 | 104 | 12.8 | 26.8 | 23.8 | 0 | 0 | 4 | 27 | 6 | 1.66 | 1.319 | 0 | 0 | 0 | 0 | 0 | 0.01 |
| 2 T | | 0 | 0.1 | 0 | 0 | 0 | 0 | 82 | 1 | 0.48 | 0.030 | 0.2 | 0 | 0 | 0 | 0 | 0 | 19353 |
| **marmalade**, orange | 20 | 49 | 6.6 | 13.3 | 12.0 | 11.3 | 0.1 | 11 | 8 | 0 | 0.01 | 0.004 | 1 | 1 | 0 | 0 | 0 | 0 |
| 1 T | | 0.1 | 0 | 0 | 0 | 0 | 0 | 7 | 1 | 0.03 | 0.018 | 0.1 | 12 | 0 | 0.01 | 0 | 1.8 | 19303 |
| **molasses** | 40 | 116 | 8.7 | 29.9 | 22.2 | 0 | 0 | 15 | 82 | 97 | 0.12 | 0.612 | 0 | 0 | 0.02 | 0.4 | 0 | 0.32 |
| 2 T | | 0 | 0 | 0 | 0 | 0 | 0 | 586 | 12 | 1.89 | 0.195 | 7.1 | 0 | 0 | 0 | 0.27 | 0 | 19304 |
| **pancake/waffle syrup** | 20 | 47 | 7.6 | 12.3 | 6.6 | 6.6 | 0 | 16 | 1 | 0 | 0.02 | 0.014 | 0 | 0 | 0 | 0 | 0 | 0 |
| 1 T | | 0 | 0 | 0 | 0 | 0 | 0 | 3 | 2 | 0.01 | 0 | 0 | 0 | 0 | 0 | 0 | 0 | 19129 |
| **pancake/waffle syrup**, red cal | 15 | 25 | 8.2 | 6.7 | 4.9 | 2.3 | 0 | 27 | 2 | 0 | 0.03 | 0.003 | 0 | 0 | 0 | 0 | 0 | 0 |
| 1 T | | 0 | 0 | 0 | 0 | 0 | 0 | 0 | 6 | 0 | 0.003 | 0.1 | 0 | 0 | 0 | 0 | 0 | 19128 |
| **pancake/waffle syrup** w/15% | 20 | 56 | 6.0 | 13.9 | 13.6 | 13.6 | 0 | 21 | 2 | 0 | 0.13 | 0.099 | 0 | 0 | 0 | 0 | 0 | 0 |
| maple syrup - 1 T | | 0 | 0 | 0 | 0 | 0 | 0 | 11 | 0 | 0.04 | 0.003 | 0.1 | 0 | 0 | 0 | 0 | 0 | 19361 |
| **pancake/waffle syrup** w/2% maple | 20 | 53 | 6.0 | 13.9 | 8.4 | 8.4 | 0 | 12 | 1 | 0 | 0.05 | 0.037 | 0 | 0 | 0 | 0 | 0 | 0 |
| syrup - 1 T | | 0 | 0 | 0 | 0 | 0 | 0 | 1 | 2 | 0.01 | 0.009 | 0.1 | 0 | 0 | 0 | 0 | 0 | 19360 |

| | WT | Macronutrients | | | | | | Minerals | | | | | Vitamins | | | | | |
|---|---|---|---|---|---|---|---|---|---|---|---|---|---|---|---|---|---|---|
| | (g) | KCAL | $H_2O$ (g) | CHO (g) | TSUG (g) | ASUG (g) | DFIB (g) | Na (mg) | Ca (mg) | Mg (mg) | Zn (mg) | Mn (mg) | A (mcg RAE) | C (mg) | B-1 (mg) | NIA (mg) | B-12 (mcg) | PANT (mg) |
| | | PRO (g) | FAT (g) | SFA (g) | MUFA (g) | PUFA (g) | CHOL (mg) | K (mg) | P (mg) | Fe (mg) | Cu (mg) | Se (mcg) | A (IU) | E (mg ATE) | B-2 (mg) | B-6 (mg) | FOL (mcg DFE) | REF |
| **pancake/waffle syrup** w/butter | 20 | 59 | 4.8 | 14.8 | | | 0 | 20 | 0 | 0 | 0.01 | 0.017 | 3 | 0 | 0 | 0 | 0 | 0.01 |
| *1 T* | | 0 | 0.3 | 0.2 | 0.1 | 0 | 1 | 1 | 2 | 0.02 | 0.042 | 0.1 | 12 | | 0 | 0 | 0 | 19113 |
| **sorghum syrup** | 21 | 61 | 4.8 | 15.7 | 15.7 | 0 | 0 | 2 | 32 | 21 | 0.09 | 0.321 | 0 | 0 | 0.02 | 0 | 0 | 0.17 |
| *1 T* | | 0 | 0 | 0 | 0 | 0 | 0 | 210 | 12 | 0.80 | 0.027 | 0.4 | 0 | 0 | 0.03 | 0.14 | 0 | 19355 |
| **sugar, brown** | 14 | 53 | 0.2 | 13.7 | 13.6 | 0 | 0 | 4 | 12 | 1 | 0 | 0.009 | 0 | 0 | 0 | 0 | 0 | 0.02 |
| *1T* | | 0 | 0 | 0 | 0 | 0 | 0 | 19 | 1 | 0.10 | 0.007 | 0.2 | 0 | 0 | 0 | 0.01 | 0.1 | 19334 |
| **sugar substitute**, Equal, Nutrasweet | 1 | 4 | 0.1 | 0.9 | 0.8 | | 0 | 0 | 0 | 0 | 0 | 0 | 0 | 0 | 0 | 0 | 0 | 0 |
| *1 packet* | | 0 | 0 | 0 | 0 | 0 | 0 | 0 | 0 | 0 | 0 | 0 | 0 | 0 | 0 | 0 | 0 | 19337 |
| **sugar substitute**, fructose liquid | 5 | 14 | 1.2 | 3.8 | 3.8 | | 0 | 0 | 0 | 0 | 0 | | 0 | 0 | 0 | 0 | 0 | |
| *1 tsp* | | 0 | 0 | 0 | 0 | 0 | 0 | 0 | 0 | 0.01 | 0.002 | 0 | 0 | 0 | 0 | 0 | 0 | 44018 |
| **sugar substitute**, fructose powder | 3 | 11 | 0 | 3.0 | 2.8 | | 0 | 0 | 0 | 0 | 0 | | 0 | 0 | 0 | 0 | 0 | |
| *1 packet* | | 0 | 0 | 0 | 0 | 0 | 0 | 0 | 0 | 0 | 0.007 | 0 | 0 | 0 | 0 | 0 | 0 | 43216 |
| **sugar substitute**, saccharin powder | 1 | 4 | 0.1 | 0.9 | 0.9 | | 0 | 4 | 0 | 0 | 0 | 0 | 0 | 0 | 0 | 0 | 0 | 0 |
| *1 packet* | | 0 | 0 | 0 | 0 | 0 | 0 | 0 | 0 | 0 | 0 | 0 | 0 | 0 | 0 | 0 | 0 | 43158 |
| **sugar substitute**, sucralose powder, | 1 | 3 | 0.1 | 0.9 | 0.8 | | 0 | 0 | 0 | 0 | 0 | 0 | 0 | 0 | 0 | 0 | 0 | 0 |
| Splenda - *1 packet* | | 0 | 0 | 0 | 0 | 0 | 0 | 0 | 0 | 0 | 0 | 0 | 0 | 0 | 0 | 0 | 0 | 19868 |
| **sugar, white**, granulated | 12 | 46 | 0 | 12.0 | 12.0 | 0 | 0 | 0 | 0 | 0 | 0 | 0 | 0 | 0 | 0 | 0 | 0 | 0 |
| *1 T* | | 0 | 0 | 0 | 0 | 0 | 0 | 0 | 0 | 0 | 0 | 0.1 | 0 | 0 | 0 | 0 | 0 | 19335 |
| **sugar, white**, powdered | 8 | 31 | 0 | 8.0 | 7.8 | 0 | 0 | 0 | 0 | 0 | 0 | 0 | 0 | 0 | 0 | 0 | 0 | 0 |
| *1 T* | | 0 | 0 | 0 | 0 | 0 | 0 | 0 | 0 | 0 | 0 | 0 | 0 | 0 | 0 | 0 | 0 | 19336 |

# 30. VEGETABLES AND VEGETABLE DISHES

## 30.1 FLOWER, STEM, AND STALK VEGETABLES

| | | | | | | | | | | | | | | | | | | |
|---|---|---|---|---|---|---|---|---|---|---|---|---|---|---|---|---|---|---|
| **artichoke**, boiled, drained | 120 | 64 | 100.9 | 14.3 | 1.2 | 0 | 10.3 | 72 | 25 | 50 | 0.48 | 0.270 | 1 | 9 | 0.06 | 1.3 | 0 | 0.29 |
| *4.2 oz artichoke* | | 3.5 | 0.4 | 0.1 | 0 | 0.2 | 0 | 343 | 88 | 0.73 | 0.152 | 0.2 | 16 | 0.2 | 0.11 | 0.10 | 106.8 | 11008 |
| **artichoke**, frozen | 80 | 30 | 70.9 | 6.2 | | | 3.1 | 38 | 15 | 22 | 0.26 | 0.194 | 6 | 4 | 0.05 | 0.7 | 0 | 0.15 |
| *2.8 oz (⅓ of 9 oz package)* | | 2.1 | 0.3 | 0.1 | 0 | 0.1 | 0 | 198 | 46 | 0.40 | 0.043 | 0.2 | 123 | | 0.11 | 0.07 | 100.8 | 11009 |
| **artichoke**, frozen, boiled, drained | 80 | 36 | 69.2 | 7.3 | 0.7 | 0 | 3.7 | 42 | 17 | 25 | 0.29 | 0.218 | 1 | 4 | 0.05 | 0.7 | 0 | 0.16 |
| *2.8 oz (⅓ of 9 oz package)* | | 2.5 | 0.4 | 0.1 | 0 | 0.2 | 0 | 211 | 49 | 0.45 | 0.049 | 0.2 | 9 | 0.1 | 0.13 | 0.07 | 95.2 | 11010 |
| **artichoke**, raw | 120 | 56 | 101.9 | 12.6 | 1.2 | | 6.5 | 113 | 53 | 72 | 0.59 | 0.307 | 1 | 14 | 0.09 | 1.3 | 0 | 0.41 |
| *4.2 oz artichoke* | | 3.9 | 0.2 | 0 | 0 | 0.1 | 0 | 444 | 108 | 1.54 | 0.277 | 0.2 | 16 | 0.2 | 0.08 | 0.14 | 81.6 | 11007 |
| **asparagus**, boiled, drained | 180 | 40 | 166.7 | 7.4 | 2.3 | 0 | 3.6 | 25 | 41 | 25 | 1.08 | 0.277 | 90 | 14 | 0.29 | 2.0 | 0 | 0.40 |
| *1 cup (12 spears)* | | 4.3 | 0.4 | 0.1 | 0 | 0.2 | 0 | 403 | 97 | 1.64 | 0.297 | 11.0 | 1811 | 2.7 | 0.25 | 0.14 | 268.2 | 11012 |
| **asparagus**, canned, drained | 242 | 46 | 227.4 | 6.0 | 2.6 | 0 | 3.9 | 695 | 39 | 24 | 0.97 | 0.411 | 99 | 45 | 0.15 | 2.3 | 0 | 0.34 |
| *1 cup* | | 5.2 | 1.6 | 0.4 | 0.1 | 0.7 | 0 | 416 | 104 | 4.43 | 0.232 | 4.1 | 1989 | 3.0 | 0.24 | 0.27 | 232.3 | 11015 |
| **asparagus**, frozen | 180 | 43 | 165.3 | 7.4 | | | 3.4 | 14 | 45 | 25 | 1.06 | 0.365 | 85 | 57 | 0.22 | 2.2 | 0 | 0.33 |
| *1 cup* | | 5.8 | 0.4 | 0.1 | 0 | 0.2 | 0 | 455 | 115 | 1.31 | 0.247 | 3.1 | 1706 | | 0.24 | 0.20 | 343.8 | 11018 |
| **asparagus**, frozen, boiled, drained | 180 | 32 | 169.4 | 3.5 | 0.6 | 0 | 2.9 | 5 | 32 | 18 | 0.74 | 0.252 | 72 | 44 | 0.12 | 1.9 | 0 | 0.28 |
| *1 cup* | | 5.3 | 0.8 | 0.2 | 0 | 0.3 | 0 | 310 | 88 | 1.01 | 0.189 | 7.0 | 1451 | 2.2 | 0.19 | 0.04 | 243.0 | 11019 |
| **asparagus**, raw | 134 | 27 | 124.9 | 5.2 | 2.5 | 0 | 2.8 | 3 | 32 | 19 | 0.72 | 0.212 | 51 | 8 | 0.19 | 1.3 | 0 | 0.37 |
| *1 cup* | | 2.9 | 0.2 | 0.1 | 0 | 0.1 | 0 | 271 | 70 | 2.87 | 0.253 | 3.1 | 1013 | 1.5 | 0.19 | 0.12 | 69.7 | 11011 |
| **broccoflower**, boiled | 90 | 29 | 80.5 | 5.7 | | | 3.0 | 21 | 29 | 17 | 0.57 | 0.218 | 6 | 65 | 0.06 | 0.6 | 0 | 0.61 |
| *⅕ head* | | 2.7 | 0.3 | 0 | 0 | 0.1 | 0 | 250 | 51 | 0.65 | 0.036 | 0.7 | 127 | | 0.09 | 0.19 | 36.9 | 11967 |
| **broccoflower**, raw | 64 | 20 | 57.5 | 3.9 | 1.9 | 0 | 2.0 | 15 | 21 | 13 | 0.41 | 0.158 | 5 | 56 | 0.05 | 0.5 | 0 | 0.45 |
| *1 cup pieces* | | 1.9 | 0.2 | 0 | 0 | 0.1 | 0 | 192 | 40 | 0.47 | 0.026 | 0.4 | 99 | 0 | 0.07 | 0.14 | 36.5 | 11965 |
| **broccoli**, boiled, drained | 180 | 63 | 160.6 | 12.9 | 2.5 | 0 | 5.9 | 74 | 72 | 38 | 0.81 | 0.349 | 139 | 117 | 0.11 | 1.0 | 0 | 1.11 |
| *1 medium stalk* | | 4.3 | 0.7 | 0.1 | 0.1 | 0.3 | 0 | 527 | 121 | 1.21 | 0.110 | 2.9 | 2786 | 2.6 | 0.22 | 0.36 | 194.4 | 11091 |
| **broccoli**, chopped, frozen | 156 | 41 | 142.7 | 7.5 | 2.1 | 0 | 4.7 | 37 | 87 | 28 | 0.75 | 0.459 | 81 | 88 | 0.08 | 0.7 | 0 | 0.44 |
| *1 cup* | | 4.4 | 0.5 | 0.1 | 0 | 0.2 | 0 | 331 | 78 | 1.26 | 0.059 | 4.4 | 1613 | 1.9 | 0.15 | 0.20 | 104.5 | 11092 |
| **broccoli**, chopped, frozen, boiled, | 184 | 52 | 166.9 | 9.8 | 2.7 | 0 | 5.5 | 20 | 61 | 24 | 0.52 | 0.410 | 94 | 74 | 0.10 | 0.8 | 0 | 0.50 |
| drained - *1 cup* | | 5.7 | 0.2 | 0 | 0 | 0.1 | 0 | 261 | 90 | 1.12 | 0.063 | 1.3 | 1860 | 2.4 | 0.15 | 0.24 | 103.0 | 11093 |
| **broccoli**, chopped, raw | 91 | 31 | 81.3 | 6.0 | 1.5 | 0 | 2.4 | 30 | 43 | 19 | 0.37 | 0.191 | 28 | 81 | 0.06 | 0.6 | 0 | 0.52 |
| *1 cup* | | 2.6 | 0.3 | 0 | 0 | 0 | 0 | 288 | 60 | 0.66 | 0.045 | 2.3 | 567 | 0.7 | 0.11 | 0.16 | 57.3 | 11090 |
| **broccoli** florets, raw | 71 | 20 | 64.4 | 3.7 | | | | 19 | 34 | 18 | 0.28 | 0.163 | 106 | 66 | 0.05 | 0.5 | 0 | 0.38 |
| *1 cup* | | 2.1 | 0.2 | 0 | 0 | 0.1 | 0 | 231 | 47 | 0.62 | 0.032 | 2.1 | 2130 | | 0.08 | 0.11 | 50.4 | 11740 |
| **broccoli** spears, frozen, boiled, | 184 | 52 | 166.9 | 9.9 | 2.7 | 0 | 5.5 | 44 | 94 | 37 | 0.55 | 0.598 | 94 | 74 | 0.10 | 0.8 | 0 | 0.50 |
| drained - *1 cup* | | 5.7 | 0.2 | 0 | 0 | 0.1 | 0 | 331 | 101 | 1.12 | 0.079 | 3.5 | 1860 | 2.4 | 0.15 | 0.24 | 55.2 | 11095 |
| **broccoli** with cheese sauce, frozen, | 168 | 113 | 142.0 | 15.0 | | | | 806 | | | | | | 59 | | | | |
| Green Giant - *1 cup* | | 3.9 | 4.2 | 0.8 | 1.7 | 0.4 | | | | | | | 2268 | | | | | 22600 |
| **cardoon**, boiled, drained | 100 | 22 | 93.5 | 5.3 | | | 1.7 | 176 | 72 | 43 | 0.18 | 0.133 | 6 | 2 | 0.02 | 0.3 | 0 | 0.10 |
| *3.5 oz* | | 0.8 | 0.1 | 0 | 0 | 0 | 0 | 392 | 23 | 0.73 | | 1.0 | 118 | | 0.03 | 0.04 | 22.0 | 11123 |

| | WT (g) | KCAL / PRO (g) | H₂O (g) / FAT (g) | CHO (g) / SFA (g) | TSUG (g) / MUFA (g) | ASUG (g) / PUFA (g) | DFIB (g) / CHOL (mg) | Na (mg) / K (mg) | Ca (mg) / P (mg) | Mg (mg) / Fe (mg) | Zn (mg) / Cu (mg) | Mn (mg) / Se (mcg) | A (mcg RAE) / A (IU) | C (mg) / E (mg ATE) | B-1 (mg) / B-2 (mg) | NIA (mg) / B-6 (mg) | B-12 (mcg) / FOL (mcg DFE) | PANT (mg) / REF |
|---|---|---|---|---|---|---|---|---|---|---|---|---|---|---|---|---|---|---|
| **cardoon**, raw | 89 | 15 | 83.7 | 3.6 | | | 1.4 | 151 | 62 | 37 | 0.15 | 0.228 | 0 | 2 | 0.02 | 0.3 | 0 | 0.30 |
| ½ cup shredded | | 0.6 | 0.1 | 0 | 0 | 0 | 0 | 356 | 20 | 0.62 | 0.206 | 0.2 | 0 | | 0.03 | 0.10 | 60.5 | 11122 |
| **cauliflower**, boiled, drained | 124 | 29 | 115.3 | 5.1 | 2.6 | 0 | 2.9 | 19 | 20 | 11 | 0.21 | 0.164 | 1 | 55 | 0.05 | 0.5 | 0 | 0.63 |
| 1 cup pieces | | 2.3 | 0.6 | 0.1 | 0 | 0.3 | 0 | 176 | 40 | 0.40 | 0.022 | 0.7 | 15 | 0.1 | 0.06 | 0.21 | 54.6 | 11136 |
| **cauliflower**, frozen | 180 | 43 | 166.5 | 8.4 | 4.0 | 0 | 4.1 | 43 | 40 | 22 | 0.31 | 0.355 | 2 | 88 | 0.09 | 0.8 | 0 | 0.24 |
| 1 cup pieces | | 3.6 | 0.5 | 0.1 | 0 | 0.2 | 0 | 347 | 63 | 0.97 | 0.056 | 1.4 | 22 | 0.1 | 0.13 | 0.22 | 115.2 | 11137 |
| **cauliflower**, frozen, boiled, drained | 180 | 34 | 169.2 | 6.8 | 1.9 | 0 | 4.9 | 32 | 31 | 16 | 0.23 | 0.270 | 1 | 56 | 0.07 | 0.6 | 0 | 0.18 |
| 1 cup pieces | | 2.9 | 0.4 | 0.1 | 0 | 0.2 | 0 | 250 | 43 | 0.74 | 0.043 | 1.1 | 18 | 0.1 | 0.10 | 0.16 | 73.8 | 11138 |
| **cauliflower**, raw | 100 | 25 | 91.9 | 5.3 | 2.4 | 0 | 2.5 | 30 | 22 | 15 | 0.28 | 0.156 | 1 | 46 | 0.06 | 0.5 | 0 | 0.65 |
| 1 cup pieces | | 2.0 | 0.1 | 0 | 0 | 0 | 0 | 303 | 44 | 0.44 | 0.042 | 0.6 | 13 | 0.1 | 0.06 | 0.22 | 57.0 | 11135 |
| **cauliflower** with cheese sauce, frozen, Green Giant - ½ cup | 98 | 50 | | 6.0 | 2.0 | | 1.0 | 410 | 40 | | | | | 15 | | | | |
| | | 2.0 | 2.5 | 1.0 | 0.5 | 0 | 0 | | 0.36 | | | | 100 | | | | | GENM353 |
| **celery**, boiled, drained | 150 | 27 | 141.2 | 6.0 | 3.6 | 0 | 2.4 | 136 | 63 | 18 | 0.21 | 0.159 | 39 | 9 | 0.06 | 0.5 | 0 | 0.29 |
| 1 cup diced | | 1.2 | 0.2 | 0.1 | 0 | 0.1 | 0 | 426 | 38 | 0.63 | 0.054 | 1.5 | 782 | 0.5 | 0.07 | 0.13 | 33.0 | 11144 |
| **celery**, raw | 40 | 6 | 38.2 | 1.2 | 0.7 | 0 | 0.6 | 32 | 16 | 4 | 0.05 | 0.041 | 9 | 1 | 0.01 | 0.1 | 0 | 0.10 |
| 1 medium stalk (7.5" long) | | 0.3 | 0.1 | 0 | 0 | 0 | 0 | 104 | 10 | 0.08 | 0.014 | 0.2 | 180 | 0.1 | 0.02 | 0.03 | 14.4 | 11143 |
| **Chinese broccoli** (Chinese kale), boiled - 3.5 oz | 100 | 22 | 93.5 | 3.8 | 0.8 | 0 | 2.5 | 7 | 100 | 18 | 0.39 | 0.264 | 82 | 28 | 0.10 | 0.4 | 0 | 0.16 |
| | | 1.1 | 0.7 | 0.1 | 0 | 0.3 | 0 | 261 | 41 | 0.56 | 0.061 | 1.3 | 1638 | 0.5 | 0.15 | 0.07 | 99.0 | 11969 |
| **hearts of palm** (heart palm), canned - 1 cup | 146 | 41 | 131.7 | 6.7 | | | 3.5 | 622 | 85 | 55 | 1.68 | 2.035 | 0 | 12 | 0.02 | 0.6 | 0 | 0.18 |
| | | 3.7 | 0.9 | 0.2 | 0.2 | 0.3 | 0 | 258 | 95 | 4.57 | 0.194 | 1.0 | 0 | 0.08 | | 56.9 | | 11961 |
| **kohlrabi**, boiled, drained | 165 | 48 | 149.0 | 11.0 | 4.6 | 0 | 1.8 | 35 | 41 | 31 | 0.51 | 0.234 | 3 | 89 | 0.06 | 0.6 | 0 | 0.26 |
| 1 cup slices | | 3.0 | 0.2 | 0 | 0 | 0.1 | 0 | 561 | 74 | 0.66 | 0.218 | 1.3 | 58 | 0.9 | 0.03 | 0.25 | 19.8 | 11242 |
| **kohlrabi**, raw | 135 | 36 | 122.8 | 8.4 | 3.5 | 0 | 4.9 | 27 | 32 | 26 | 0.04 | 0.188 | 3 | 84 | 0.07 | 0.5 | 0 | 0.22 |
| 1 cup slices | | 2.3 | 0.1 | 0 | 0 | 0.1 | 0 | 473 | 62 | 0.54 | 0.174 | 0.9 | 49 | 0.6 | 0.03 | 0.20 | 21.6 | 11241 |
| **leek**, boiled, drained | 124 | 38 | 112.6 | 9.4 | 2.6 | | 1.2 | 12 | 37 | 17 | 0.07 | 0.306 | 51 | 5 | 0.03 | 0.2 | 0 | 0.09 |
| 1 leek | | 1.0 | 0.2 | 0 | 0 | 0.1 | 0 | 108 | 21 | 1.36 | 0.077 | 0.6 | 1007 | 0.6 | 0.02 | 0.14 | 29.8 | 11247 |
| **leek**, raw | 89 | 54 | 73.9 | 12.6 | 3.5 | 0 | 1.6 | 18 | 53 | 25 | 0.11 | 0.428 | 74 | 11 | 0.05 | 0.4 | 0 | 0.12 |
| 1 leek (~ 1 cup) | | 1.3 | 0.3 | 0 | 0 | 0.1 | 0 | 160 | 31 | 1.87 | 0.107 | 0.9 | 1484 | 0.8 | 0.03 | 0.21 | 57.0 | 11246 |
| **pumpkin flowers**, boiled, drained | 134 | 20 | 127.6 | 4.4 | 3.2 | 0 | 1.2 | 8 | 50 | 34 | 0.13 | | 117 | 7 | 0.02 | 0.4 | 0 | |
| 1 cup | | 1.5 | 0.1 | 0.1 | 0 | 0 | 0 | 142 | 46 | 1.18 | 0.134 | 0.9 | 2324 | 0.1 | 0.04 | 0.07 | 54.9 | 11417 |
| **pumpkin flowers**, raw | 33 | 5 | 31.4 | 1.1 | | | | 2 | 13 | 8 | | | 32 | 9 | 0.01 | 0.2 | 0 | |
| 1 cup | | 0.3 | 0 | 0 | 0 | 0 | 0 | 57 | 16 | 0.23 | | 0.2 | 643 | | 0.02 | | 19.5 | 11416 |
| **rhubarb**, cooked, sweetened, frozen - 1 cup | 240 | 278 | 162.7 | 74.9 | 68.9 | 67.0 | 4.8 | 2 | 348 | 29 | 0.19 | 0.175 | 10 | 8 | 0.04 | 0.5 | 0 | 0.12 |
| frozen - 1 cup | | 0.9 | 0.1 | 0 | 0 | 0.1 | 0 | 230 | 19 | 0.50 | 0.065 | 2.2 | 175 | 0.5 | 0.06 | 0.05 | 12.0 | 9310 |
| **rhubarb**, frozen | 137 | 29 | 128.1 | 7.0 | 1.5 | 0 | 2.5 | 3 | 266 | 25 | 0.14 | 0.133 | 7 | 7 | 0.04 | 0.3 | 0 | 0.09 |
| 1 cup | | 0.8 | 0.2 | 0 | 0 | 0.1 | 0 | 148 | 16 | 0.40 | 0.032 | 1.5 | 147 | 0.4 | 0.04 | 0.03 | 11.0 | 9309 |
| **rhubarb**, raw | 122 | 26 | 114.2 | 5.5 | 1.3 | 0 | 2.2 | 5 | 105 | 15 | 0.12 | 0.239 | 6 | 10 | 0.02 | 0.4 | 0 | 0.10 |
| 1 cup | | 1.1 | 0.2 | 0.1 | 0 | 0.1 | 0 | 351 | 17 | 0.27 | 0.026 | 1.3 | 124 | 0.3 | 0.04 | 0.03 | 8.5 | 9307 |
| **scallions** (green/spring onions), raw - 1 cup chopped | 100 | 32 | 89.8 | 7.3 | 2.3 | 0 | 2.6 | 16 | 72 | 20 | 0.39 | 0.160 | 50 | 19 | 0.06 | 0.5 | 0 | 0.08 |
| | | 1.8 | 0.2 | 0 | 0 | 0.1 | 0 | 276 | 37 | 1.48 | 0.083 | 0.6 | 997 | 0.6 | 0.08 | 0.06 | 64.0 | 11291 |
| **sesbania flower**, steamed | 104 | 23 | 97.0 | 5.4 | | | | 11 | 23 | 12 | | | 0 | 38 | 0.05 | 0.3 | 0 | |
| 1 cup | | 1.2 | 0.1 | | | | 0 | 111 | 22 | 0.58 | | 0.7 | 0 | | 0.04 | | 59.3 | 11448 |

## 30.2 FRUIT (SEED-CONTAINING) VEGETABLES

| | WT (g) | KCAL / PRO (g) | H₂O (g) / FAT (g) | CHO (g) / SFA (g) | TSUG (g) / MUFA (g) | ASUG (g) / PUFA (g) | DFIB (g) / CHOL (mg) | Na (mg) / K (mg) | Ca (mg) / P (mg) | Mg (mg) / Fe (mg) | Zn (mg) / Cu (mg) | Mn (mg) / Se (mcg) | A (mcg RAE) / A (IU) | C (mg) / E (mg ATE) | B-1 (mg) / B-2 (mg) | NIA (mg) / B-6 (mg) | B-12 (mcg) / FOL (mcg DFE) | PANT (mg) / REF |
|---|---|---|---|---|---|---|---|---|---|---|---|---|---|---|---|---|---|---|
| **acorn winter squash**, baked | 205 | 115 | 169.9 | 29.9 | | | 9.0 | 8 | 90 | 88 | 0.35 | 0.496 | 43 | 22 | 0.34 | 1.8 | 0 | 1.03 |
| 1 cup cubed | | 2.3 | 0.3 | 0.1 | 0 | 0.1 | 0 | 896 | 92 | 1.91 | 0.176 | 1.4 | 877 | | 0.03 | 0.40 | 38.9 | 11483 |
| **acorn winter squash**, boiled | 245 | 83 | 219.8 | 21.5 | | | 6.4 | 7 | 64 | 64 | 0.27 | 0.358 | 100 | 16 | 0.25 | 1.3 | 0 | 0.74 |
| 1 cup mashed | | 1.6 | 0.2 | 0.1 | 0 | 0.1 | 0 | 644 | 66 | 1.37 | 0.127 | 1.0 | 2002 | | 0.02 | 0.29 | 27.0 | 11484 |
| **acorn winter squash**, raw | 140 | 56 | 122.9 | 14.6 | | | 2.1 | 4 | 46 | 45 | 0.18 | 0.234 | 25 | 15 | 0.20 | 1.0 | 0 | 0.56 |
| 1 cup cubed | | 1.1 | 0.1 | 0 | 0 | 0.1 | 0 | 486 | 50 | 0.98 | 0.091 | 0.7 | 514 | | 0.01 | 0.22 | 23.8 | 11482 |
| **ancho pepper**, dried | 17 | 48 | 3.8 | 8.7 | | | 3.7 | 7 | 10 | 19 | 0.24 | 0.217 | 174 | 0 | 0.03 | 1.1 | 0 | 0.34 |
| 1 pepper | | 2.0 | 1.4 | 0.1 | 0.1 | 0.8 | 0 | 410 | 34 | 1.86 | 0.086 | 0.5 | 3474 | | 0.38 | 0.60 | 11.7 | 11978 |
| **balsam pear pods**, boiled, drained | 124 | 24 | 116.5 | 5.4 | 2.4 | 0 | 2.5 | 7 | 11 | 20 | 0.95 | 0.107 | 7 | 41 | 0.06 | 0.3 | 0 | 0.24 |
| 1 cup pieces | | 1.0 | 0.2 | 0 | 0 | 0.1 | 0 | 396 | 45 | 0.47 | 0.041 | 0.2 | 140 | 0.2 | 0.07 | 0.05 | 63.2 | 11025 |
| **balsam pear pods**, raw | 93 | 16 | 87.4 | 3.4 | | | 2.6 | 5 | 18 | 16 | 0.74 | 0.083 | 22 | 78 | 0.04 | 0.4 | 0 | 0.20 |
| 1 cup (½" pieces) | | 0.9 | 0.2 | | | | 0 | 275 | 29 | 0.40 | 0.032 | 0.2 | 438 | | 0.04 | 0.04 | 67.0 | 11024 |
| **banana pepper**, raw | 46 | 12 | 42.2 | 2.5 | 0.9 | 0 | 1.6 | 6 | 6 | 8 | 0.12 | 0.046 | 8 | 38 | 0.04 | 0.6 | 0 | 0.12 |
| 1 medium (4½" long) | | 0.8 | 0.2 | 0 | 0 | 0.1 | 0 | 118 | 15 | 0.21 | 0.043 | 0.1 | 156 | 0.3 | 0.02 | 0.16 | 13.3 | 11976 |
| **breadfruit**, raw | 96 | 99 | 67.8 | 26.0 | 10.6 | 0 | 4.7 | 2 | 16 | 24 | 0.12 | 0.058 | 0 | 28 | 0.11 | 0.9 | 0 | 0.44 |
| ¼ small | | 1.0 | 0.2 | 0 | 0 | 0.1 | 0 | 470 | 29 | 0.52 | 0.081 | 0.6 | 0 | 0.1 | 0.03 | 0.10 | 13.4 | 9059 |
| **butternut winter squash**, baked | 205 | 82 | 180.0 | 21.5 | 4.0 | | | 8 | 84 | 59 | 0.27 | 0.353 | 1144 | 31 | 0.15 | 2.0 | 0 | 0.74 |
| 1 cup cubed | | 1.8 | 0.2 | 0 | 0 | 0.1 | 0 | 582 | 55 | 1.23 | 0.133 | 1.0 | 22868 | 2.6 | 0.03 | 0.25 | 38.9 | 11486 |

| | WT (g) | KCAL / PRO (g) | H₂0 (g) / FAT (g) | CHO (g) / SFA (g) | TSUG (g) / MUFA (g) | ASUG (g) / PUFA (g) | DFIB (g) / CHOL (mg) | Na (mg) / K (mg) | Ca (mg) / P (mg) | Mg (mg) / Fe (mg) | Zn (mg) / Cu (mg) | Mn (mg) / Se (mcg) | A (mcg RAE) / A (IU) | C (mg) / E (mg ATE) | B-1 (mg) / B-2 (mg) | NIA (mg) / B-6 (mg) | B-12 (mcg) / FOL (mcg DFE) | PANT (mg) / REF |
|---|---|---|---|---|---|---|---|---|---|---|---|---|---|---|---|---|---|---|
| butternut winter squash, cooked | 140 | 56 | 122.9 | 14.7 | 2.8 | 0 | | 336 | 57 | 41 | 0.18 | 0.241 | 781 | 21 | 0.10 | 1.4 | 0 | 0.50 |
| *1 cup cubed* | | 1.3 | 0.1 | 0 | 0 | 0.1 | 0 | 398 | 38 | 0.84 | 0.091 | 0.7 | 15617 | 1.8 | 0.02 | 0.17 | 26.6 | 11866 |
| **butternut winter squash, frzn,** | 240 | 94 | 210.7 | 24.1 | | | | 5 | 46 | 22 | 0.29 | 0.415 | 401 | 8 | 0.12 | 1.1 | 0 | 0.37 |
| **boiled** - *1 cup mashed* | | 3.0 | 0.2 | 0 | 0 | 0.1 | 0 | 319 | 34 | 1.39 | 0.086 | 1.2 | 8014 | | 0.09 | 0.17 | 38.4 | 11488 |
| butternut winter squash, raw | 140 | 63 | 121.0 | 16.4 | 3.1 | | 2.8 | 6 | 67 | 48 | 0.21 | 0.283 | 745 | 29 | 0.14 | 1.7 | 0 | 0.56 |
| *1 cup cubed* | | 1.4 | 0.1 | 0 | 0 | 0.1 | 0 | 493 | 46 | 0.98 | 0.101 | 0.7 | 14882 | 2.0 | 0.03 | 0.22 | 37.8 | 11485 |
| **calabash gourd, white-flowered,** | 146 | 22 | 139.2 | 5.4 | | | | 3 | 35 | 16 | 1.02 | 0.096 | 0 | 12 | 0.04 | 0.6 | 0 | 0.21 |
| **boiled, drained** - *1 cup cubed* | | 0.9 | 0 | 0 | 0 | 0 | 0 | 248 | 19 | 0.36 | 0.038 | 0.3 | 0 | | 0.03 | 0.06 | 5.8 | 11219 |
| chayote, boiled, drained | 160 | 38 | 149.5 | 8.1 | | | 4.5 | 2 | 21 | 19 | 0.50 | 0.270 | 3 | 13 | 0.04 | 0.7 | 0 | 0.65 |
| *1 cup pieces* | | 1.0 | 0.8 | 0.1 | | | 0 | 277 | 46 | 0.35 | 0.176 | 0.5 | 75 | | 0.06 | 0.19 | 28.8 | 11150 |
| **chayote, raw** | 132 | 25 | 124.4 | 6.0 | 2.2 | 0 | 2.2 | 3 | 22 | 16 | 0.98 | 0.249 | 0 | 10 | 0.03 | 0.6 | 0 | 0.33 |
| *1 cup pieces* | | 1.1 | 0.2 | 0 | 0 | 0.1 | 0 | 165 | 24 | 0.45 | 0.162 | 0.3 | 0 | 0.2 | 0.04 | 0.10 | 122.8 | 11149 |
| chili pepper, green, canned | 139 | 29 | 129.6 | 6.4 | | | 2.4 | 552 | 50 | 6 | 0.13 | | 8 | 48 | 0.01 | 0.9 | 0 | 0.12 |
| *1 cup* | | 1.0 | 0.4 | 0 | 0 | 0.2 | 0 | 157 | 15 | 1.85 | | 0.4 | 175 | | 0.04 | 0.17 | 75.1 | 11980 |
| **chili pepper, green, cnd,** | 30 | 5 | | 1.0 | 0 | | 0.5 | 110 | 20 | | | | 0 | 6 | | | | |
| **Old El Paso** - *2 T chopped* | | 0 | 0 | 0 | | | 0 | | 0 | | | | 0 | | | | | GENM354 |
| chili pepper, green, hot, cnd, | 73 | 15 | 67.5 | 3.7 | 2.3 | 0 | 0.9 | 856 | 5 | 10 | 0.12 | 0.101 | 26 | 50 | 0.01 | 0.6 | 0 | 0.02 |
| solids and liquid - *1 pepper* | | 0.7 | 0.1 | 0 | 0 | 0 | 0 | 137 | 12 | 0.36 | 0.074 | 0.2 | 526 | 0.5 | 0.04 | 0.11 | 7.3 | 11329 |
| **chili pepper, green, hot, raw** | 45 | 18 | 39.5 | 4.3 | 2.3 | 0 | 0.7 | 3 | 8 | 11 | 0.14 | 0.107 | 27 | 109 | 0.04 | 0.4 | 0 | 0.03 |
| *1 pepper* | | 0.9 | 0.1 | 0 | 0 | 0 | 0 | 153 | 21 | 0.54 | 0.078 | 0.2 | 531 | 0.3 | 0.04 | 0.13 | 10.4 | 11670 |
| chili pepper, green, whole, canned, | 35 | 10 | | 2.0 | 0 | | 0 | 230 | 0 | | | | | 9 | | | | |
| Old El Paso - *1.2 oz pepper* | | 0 | 0 | 0 | | | 0 | | 0 | | | | 100 | | | | | GENM355 |
| **chili pepper, red, hot, canned,** | 73 | 15 | 67.5 | 3.7 | 2.4 | 0 | 0.9 | 856 | 5 | 10 | 0.12 | 0.101 | 434 | 50 | 0.01 | 0.6 | 0 | 0.02 |
| **solids and liquid** - *1 pepper* | | 0.7 | 0.1 | 0 | 0 | 0 | 0 | 137 | 12 | 0.36 | 0.074 | 0.2 | 8681 | 0.5 | 0.04 | 0.11 | 7.3 | 11820 |
| chili pepper, red, hot, raw | 45 | 18 | 39.6 | 4.0 | 2.4 | 0 | 0.7 | 4 | 6 | 10 | 0.12 | 0.084 | 22 | 65 | 0.03 | 0.6 | 0 | 0.09 |
| *1 pepper* | | 0.8 | 0.2 | 0 | 0 | 0.1 | 0 | 145 | 19 | 0.46 | 0.058 | 0.2 | 428 | 0.3 | 0.04 | 0.23 | 10.4 | 11819 |
| **chili pepper, red, hot, sun-dried** | 0.5 | 2 | 0 | 0.3 | 0.2 | 0 | 0.1 | 0 | 0 | 0 | 0.01 | 0.004 | 7 | 0 | 0 | 0 | 0 | 0 |
| *1 pepper* | | 0.1 | 0 | 0 | 0 | 0 | 0 | 9 | 1 | 0.03 | 0.001 | 0 | 132 | 0 | 0.01 | 0 | 0.3 | 11962 |
| crook/straightneck summer squash, | 180 | 36 | 168.7 | 7.8 | 3.4 | 0 | 2.5 | 0 | 40 | 27 | 0.40 | 0.279 | 14 | 10 | 0.09 | 0.9 | 0 | 0.25 |
| boiled, drained - *1 cup sliced* | | 1.6 | 0.6 | 0.1 | 0 | 0.2 | 0 | 306 | 52 | 0.67 | 0.113 | 0.4 | 293 | 0.2 | 0.09 | 0.17 | 36.0 | 11468 |
| **crook/straightneck summer squash,** | 216 | 28 | 207.4 | 6.4 | 2.6 | 0 | 3.0 | 11 | 26 | 28 | 0.63 | 0.210 | 11 | 6 | 0.03 | 0.9 | 0 | 0.10 |
| **canned, drained** - *1 cup sliced* | | 1.3 | 0.2 | 0 | 0 | 0.1 | 0 | 207 | 45 | 1.53 | 0.173 | 0.4 | 220 | 0.3 | 0.06 | 0.09 | 21.6 | 11471 |
| crook/straightneck summer squash, | 192 | 48 | 177.1 | 10.6 | 4.5 | 0 | 2.7 | 12 | 38 | 52 | 0.65 | 0.505 | 19 | 13 | 0.07 | 0.8 | 0 | 0.20 |
| frzn, bld, drnd - *1 cup sliced* | | 2.5 | 0.4 | 0.1 | 0 | 0.2 | 0 | 486 | 79 | 1.00 | 0.140 | 0.6 | 386 | 0.3 | 0.09 | 0.19 | 25.0 | 11474 |
| **crook/straightneck summer** | 130 | 25 | 122.5 | 5.3 | | | 2.5 | 3 | 27 | 27 | 0.38 | 0.204 | 10 | 11 | 0.07 | 0.6 | 0 | 0.13 |
| **squash, raw** - *1 cup sliced* | | 1.2 | 0.3 | 0.1 | 0 | 0.1 | 0 | 276 | 42 | 0.62 | 0.133 | 0.3 | 195 | | 0.06 | 0.14 | 29.9 | 11467 |
| cucumber, raw | 301 | 45 | 286.6 | 10.9 | 5.0 | 0 | 1.5 | 6 | 48 | 39 | 0.60 | 0.238 | 15 | 8 | 0.08 | 0.3 | 0 | 0.78 |
| *1 large (8¼" long)* | | 2.0 | 0.3 | 0.1 | 0 | 0.1 | 0 | 442 | 72 | 0.84 | 0.123 | 0.9 | 316 | 0.1 | 0.10 | 0.12 | 21.1 | 11205 |
| **cucumber, raw, peeled** | 201 | 24 | 194.4 | 4.3 | 2.8 | 0 | 1.4 | 4 | 28 | 24 | 0.34 | 0.147 | 8 | 6 | 0.06 | 0.1 | 0 | 0.48 |
| *1 medium* | | 1.2 | 0.3 | 0 | 0 | 0 | 0 | 273 | 42 | 0.44 | 0.143 | 0.2 | 145 | 0.1 | 0.05 | 0.10 | 28.1 | 11206 |
| dishcloth (towel) gourd, boiled | 95 | 19 | 89.2 | 4.1 | | | | 3 | 19 | 13 | 0.07 | 0.087 | 20 | 11 | 0.05 | 0.4 | 0 | 0.21 |
| *1 cup sliced* | | 1.1 | 0.2 | 0 | | | 0 | 132 | 30 | 0.34 | 0.033 | 0.2 | 390 | | 0.06 | 0.04 | 6.6 | 11220 |
| **dishcloth (towel) gourd, boiled** | 178 | 100 | 150.0 | 25.5 | | | | 37 | 16 | 36 | 0.30 | 0.397 | 23 | 10 | 0.08 | 0.5 | 0 | 0.89 |
| **drained** - *1 cup sliced* | | 1.2 | 0.6 | 0 | 0.1 | 0.3 | 0 | 806 | 55 | 0.64 | 0.151 | 0.4 | 463 | | 0.07 | 0.18 | 21.4 | 11221 |
| dishcloth (towel) gourd, raw | 95 | 19 | 89.2 | 4.1 | | | | 3 | 19 | 13 | 0.07 | 0.087 | 20 | 11 | 0.05 | 0.4 | 0 | 0.21 |
| *1 cup sliced* | | 1.1 | 0.2 | 0 | 0 | 0.1 | 0 | 132 | 30 | 0.34 | 0.033 | 0.2 | 390 | | 0.06 | 0.04 | 6.6 | 11220 |
| **eggplant (aubergine), boiled,** | 99 | 35 | 88.8 | 8.6 | 3.2 | 0 | 2.5 | 1 | 6 | 11 | 0.12 | 0.112 | 2 | 1 | 0.08 | 0.6 | 0 | 0.07 |
| **drained** - *1 cup* | | 0.8 | 0.2 | 0 | 0 | 0.1 | 0 | 122 | 15 | 0.25 | 0.058 | 0.1 | 37 | 0.4 | 0.02 | 0.09 | 13.9 | 11210 |
| eggplant (aubergine), raw | 82 | 20 | 75.8 | 4.7 | 1.9 | 0 | 2.8 | 2 | 7 | 11 | 0.13 | 0.205 | 1 | 2 | 0.03 | 0.5 | 0 | 0.23 |
| *1 cup* | | 0.8 | 0.2 | 0 | 0 | 0.1 | 0 | 189 | 20 | 0.20 | 0.067 | 0.2 | 22 | 0.2 | 0.03 | 0.07 | 18.0 | 11209 |
| **green snap beans, boiled,** | 125 | 44 | 111.5 | 9.8 | 1.9 | 0 | 4.0 | 1 | 55 | 22 | 0.31 | 0.356 | 44 | 12 | 0.09 | 0.8 | 0 | 0.09 |
| **drained, no salt** - *1 cup* | | 2.4 | 0.4 | 0.1 | 0 | 0.2 | 0 | 182 | 36 | 0.81 | 0.071 | 0.2 | 875 | 0.6 | 0.12 | 0.07 | 41.2 | 11053 |
| green snap beans, canned, drained | 135 | 31 | 125.9 | 6.0 | 1.1 | 0 | 3.1 | 354 | 38 | 18 | 0.38 | 0.275 | 24 | 6 | 0.02 | 0.3 | 0 | 0.05 |
| *1 cup* | | 1.6 | 0.1 | 0 | 0 | 0.1 | 0 | 150 | 27 | 1.17 | 0.053 | 0.5 | 477 | 0 | 0.08 | 0.04 | 43.2 | 11056 |
| **green snap beans, frozen** | 124 | 48 | 111.5 | 9.3 | 2.7 | 0 | 3.2 | 4 | 52 | 27 | 0.32 | 0.458 | 33 | 16 | 0.12 | 0.6 | 0 | 0.13 |
| *1 cup* | | 2.2 | 0.3 | 0.1 | 0 | 0.1 | 0 | 231 | 40 | 1.05 | 0.061 | 0.7 | 678 | 0.5 | 0.11 | 0.05 | 18.6 | 11060 |
| green snap beans, frozen, boiled, | 135 | 38 | 123.4 | 8.7 | 1.7 | 0 | 4.1 | 1 | 57 | 26 | 0.32 | 0.389 | 38 | 6 | 0.05 | 0.5 | 0 | 0.07 |
| drained - *1 cup* | | 2.0 | 0.2 | 0.1 | 0 | 0.1 | 0 | 215 | 39 | 0.89 | 0.080 | 0.5 | 752 | 0.1 | 0.12 | 0.08 | 31.0 | 11061 |
| **green snap beans, frzn,** | 111 | 44 | 99.8 | 7.7 | 2.9 | 0 | 3.8 | 3 | 68 | 32 | 0.34 | 0.366 | 29 | 12 | 0.08 | 0.5 | | 0.19 |
| **microwaved** - *1 cup* | | 2.2 | 0.5 | 0.1 | 0 | 0.1 | | 263 | 47 | 0.89 | 0.073 | 1.1 | 576 | 0.5 | 0.11 | 0.07 | | 11062 |
| green snap beans, raw | 110 | 34 | 99.3 | 7.8 | 1.5 | 0 | 3.7 | 7 | 41 | 28 | 0.26 | 0.235 | 38 | 18 | 0.09 | 0.8 | 0 | 0.10 |
| *1 cup* | | 2.0 | 0.1 | 0 | 0 | 0.1 | 0 | 230 | 42 | 1.14 | 0.076 | 0.7 | 759 | 0.5 | 0.12 | 0.08 | 40.7 | 11052 |

| | WT (g) | KCAL | H₂O (g) | CHO (g) | TSUG (g) | ASUG (g) | DFIB (g) | Na (mg) | Ca (mg) | Mg (mg) | Zn (mg) | Mn (mg) | A (mcg RAE) | C (mg) | B-1 (mg) | NIA (mg) | B-12 (mcg) | PANT (mg) |
|---|---|---|---|---|---|---|---|---|---|---|---|---|---|---|---|---|---|---|
| | | PRO (g) | FAT (g) | SFA (g) | MUFA (g) | PUFA (g) | CHOL (mg) | K (mg) | P (mg) | Fe (mg) | Cu (mg) | Se (mcg) | A (IU) | E (mg ATE) | B-2 (mg) | B-6 (mg) | FOL (mcg DFE) | REF |
| **horseradish tree pods**, boiled, | 118 | 42 | 104.3 | 9.7 | | | 5.0 | 51 | 24 | 50 | 0.50 | 0.284 | 5 | 114 | 0.05 | 0.7 | 0 | 0.83 |
| drained - *1 cup sliced* | | 2.5 | 0.2 | 0 | 0.1 | 0 | 0 | 539 | 58 | 0.53 | 0.092 | 0.8 | 83 | | 0.08 | 0.13 | 35.4 | 11621 |
| **hubbard winter squash**, baked | 205 | 102 | 174.5 | 22.2 | | | | 16 | 35 | 45 | 0.31 | 0.348 | 619 | 19 | 0.15 | 1.1 | 0 | 0.92 |
| *1 cup cubed* | | 5.1 | 1.3 | 0.3 | 0.1 | 0.5 | 0 | 734 | 47 | 0.96 | 0.092 | 1.2 | 12372 | | 0.10 | 0.35 | 32.8 | 11490 |
| **hubbard winter squash**, boiled | 236 | 71 | 215.0 | 15.2 | 6.9 | 0 | 6.8 | 12 | 24 | 31 | 0.24 | 0.297 | 472 | 15 | 0.10 | 0.8 | 0 | 0.70 |
| *1 cup mashed* | | 3.5 | 0.9 | 0.2 | 0.1 | 0.4 | 0 | 505 | 33 | 0.66 | 0.111 | 0.7 | 9452 | 0.3 | 0.07 | 0.24 | 23.6 | 11491 |
| **hubbard winter squash**, raw | 116 | 46 | 102.1 | 10.1 | | | | 8 | 16 | 22 | 0.15 | 0.208 | 79 | 13 | 0.08 | 0.6 | 0 | 0.46 |
| *1 cup cubed* | | 2.3 | 0.6 | 0.1 | 0 | 0.2 | 0 | 371 | 24 | 0.46 | 0.074 | 0.6 | 1586 | | 0.05 | 0.18 | 18.6 | 11489 |
| **Hungarian pepper**, raw | 27 | 8 | 24.7 | 1.8 | | | | 0 | 3 | 4 | 0.08 | 0.055 | 2 | 25 | 0.02 | 0.3 | 0 | 0.06 |
| *1 pepper* | | 0.2 | 0.1 | 0 | 0 | 0.1 | 0 | 55 | 8 | 0.12 | 0.031 | 0.1 | 38 | | 0.01 | 0.14 | 14.3 | 11981 |
| **jalapeno pepper**, cnd, solids and | 22 | 6 | 19.6 | 1.0 | 0.5 | | 0.6 | 368 | 5 | 3 | 0.07 | 0.025 | 19 | 2 | 0.01 | 0.1 | 0 | 0.09 |
| liquid - *1 pepper* | | 0.2 | 0.2 | 0 | 0.1 | | 0 | 42 | 4 | 0.41 | 0.032 | 0.1 | 374 | 0.2 | 0.01 | 0.04 | 3.1 | 11632 |
| **jalapeno pepper**, pickled, sliced, | 31 | 5 | | 1.0 | 0 | | 0.5 | 190 | 0 | | | | | 0 | | | | |
| cnd, Old El Paso - *2 T* | | 0 | 0 | 0 | | | 0 | | 0 | | | | 0 | | | | | GENM356 |
| **jalapeno pepper**, raw | 14 | 4 | 12.8 | 0.8 | 0.5 | 0 | 0.4 | 0 | 1 | 3 | 0.03 | 0.035 | 6 | 6 | 0.02 | 0.2 | 0 | 0.03 |
| *1 pepper* | | 0.2 | 0.1 | 0 | 0 | 0 | 0 | 30 | 4 | 0.10 | 0.019 | 0 | 112 | 0.1 | 0.01 | 0.07 | 6.6 | 11979 |
| **kanpyo** (dried gourd strips) | 27 | 70 | 5.4 | 17.6 | | | | 4 | 76 | 34 | 1.58 | 0.307 | 0 | 0 | 0 | 0.8 | 0 | 0.69 |
| *½ cup* | | 2.3 | 0.2 | 0 | 0 | 0.1 | 0 | 427 | 51 | 1.38 | 0.117 | 0.7 | 0 | | 0.01 | 0.14 | 16.5 | 11237 |
| **okra**, boiled, drained | 85 | 19 | 78.7 | 3.8 | 2.0 | 0 | 2.1 | 5 | 65 | 31 | 0.37 | 0.250 | 12 | 14 | 0.11 | 0.7 | 0 | 0.18 |
| *8 pods (3" long)* | | 1.6 | 0.2 | 0 | 0 | 0 | 0 | 115 | 27 | 0.24 | 0.072 | 0.3 | 241 | 0.2 | 0.05 | 0.16 | 39.1 | 11279 |
| **okra**, frozen, cooked, drained | 184 | 52 | 167.7 | 10.6 | 5.3 | 0 | 5.2 | 6 | 177 | 94 | 1.14 | 1.879 | 31 | 22 | 0.18 | 1.4 | 0 | 0.44 |
| *1 cup sliced* | | 3.8 | 0.6 | 0.1 | 0.1 | 0.1 | 0 | 431 | 85 | 1.23 | 0.178 | 1.1 | 624 | 0.6 | 0.23 | 0.09 | 268.6 | 11281 |
| **okra**, raw | 100 | 31 | 90.2 | 7.0 | 1.2 | 0 | 3.2 | 8 | 81 | 57 | 0.60 | 0.990 | 19 | 21 | 0.20 | 1.0 | 0 | 0.24 |
| *1 cup sliced* | | 2.0 | 0.1 | 0 | 0 | 0 | 0 | 303 | 63 | 0.80 | 0.094 | 0.7 | 375 | 0.4 | 0.06 | 0.22 | 88.0 | 11278 |
| **pasilla pepper**, dried | 7 | 24 | 1.0 | 3.6 | | | 1.9 | 6 | 7 | 9 | 0.10 | 0.111 | 125 | 0 | 0.01 | 0.5 | 0 | 0.11 |
| *1 pepper* | | 0.9 | 1.1 | | | | 0 | 156 | 19 | 0.69 | 0.030 | 0.2 | 2503 | | 0.22 | 0.30 | 11.9 | 11982 |
| **pimiento pepper**, canned | 12 | 3 | 11.2 | 0.6 | 0.3 | 0 | 0.2 | 2 | 1 | 1 | 0.02 | 0.011 | 16 | 10 | 0 | 0.1 | 0 | 0 |
| *1 T* | | 0.1 | 0 | 0 | 0 | 0 | 0 | 19 | 2 | 0.20 | 0.006 | 0 | 319 | 0.1 | 0.01 | 0.03 | 0.7 | 11943 |
| **plantain**, cooked | 154 | 179 | 103.6 | 48.0 | 21.6 | 0 | 3.5 | 8 | 3 | 49 | 0.20 | | 69 | 17 | 0.07 | 1.2 | 0 | 0.36 |
| *1 cup sliced* | | 1.2 | 0.3 | 0.1 | 0 | 0.1 | 0 | 716 | 43 | 0.89 | 0.102 | 2.2 | 1400 | 0.2 | 0.08 | 0.37 | 40.0 | 9278 |
| **pumpkin winter squash**, boiled, | 245 | 49 | 229.5 | 12.0 | 2.5 | 0 | 2.7 | 2 | 37 | 22 | 0.56 | 0.218 | 612 | 12 | 0.08 | 1.0 | 0 | 0.49 |
| drained - *1 cup mashed* | | 1.8 | 0.2 | 0.1 | 0 | 0 | 0 | 564 | 74 | 1.40 | 0.223 | 0.5 | 12230 | 2.0 | 0.19 | 0.11 | 22.0 | 11423 |
| **pumpkin winter squash**, canned | 245 | 83 | 220.4 | 19.8 | 8.1 | 0 | 7.1 | 12 | 64 | 56 | 0.42 | 0.365 | 1906 | 10 | 0.06 | 0.9 | 0 | 0.98 |
| *1 cup mashed* | | 2.7 | 0.7 | 0.4 | 0.1 | 0 | 0 | 505 | 86 | 3.41 | 0.262 | 1.0 | 38129 | 2.6 | 0.13 | 0.14 | 29.4 | 11424 |
| **pumpkin winter squash**, raw | 116 | 30 | 106.3 | 7.5 | 1.6 | 0 | 0.6 | 1 | 24 | 14 | 0.37 | 0.145 | 428 | 10 | 0.06 | 0.7 | 0 | 0.35 |
| *1 cup cubed* | | 1.2 | 0.1 | 0.1 | 0 | 0 | 0 | 394 | 51 | 0.93 | 0.147 | 0.3 | 8565 | 1.2 | 0.13 | 0.07 | 18.6 | 11422 |
| **scallop summer squash**, boiled, | 180 | 29 | 171.0 | 5.9 | 2.7 | 0 | 3.4 | 2 | 27 | 34 | 0.43 | 0.230 | 7 | 19 | 0.09 | 0.8 | 0 | 0.14 |
| drained - *1 cup sliced* | | 1.9 | 0.3 | 0.1 | 0 | 0.1 | 0 | 252 | 50 | 0.59 | 0.149 | 0.4 | 153 | 0.2 | 0.05 | 0.15 | 37.8 | 11476 |
| **scallop summer squash**, raw | 130 | 23 | 122.4 | 5.0 | | | | 1 | 25 | 30 | 0.38 | 0.204 | 8 | 23 | 0.09 | 0.8 | 0 | 0.13 |
| *1 cup sliced* | | 1.6 | 0.3 | 0.1 | 0 | 0.1 | 0 | 237 | 47 | 0.52 | 0.133 | 0.3 | 143 | | 0.04 | 0.14 | 39.0 | 11475 |
| **serrano pepper**, raw | 6 | 2 | 5.4 | 0.4 | 0.2 | 0 | 0.2 | 1 | 1 | 1 | 0.02 | 0.011 | 3 | 3 | 0 | 0.1 | 0 | 0.01 |
| *1 pepper* | | 0.1 | 0 | 0 | 0 | 0 | 0 | 18 | 2 | 0.05 | 0.008 | 0 | 56 | 0 | 0 | 0.03 | 1.4 | 11977 |
| **snow peas**, boiled, drained | 160 | 67 | 142.3 | 11.3 | 6.4 | 0 | 4.5 | 6 | 67 | 42 | 0.59 | 0.269 | 83 | 77 | 0.20 | 0.9 | 0 | 1.08 |
| *1 cup* | | 5.2 | 0.4 | 0.1 | 0 | 0.2 | 0 | 384 | 88 | 3.15 | 0.123 | 1.1 | 1648 | 0.6 | 0.12 | 0.23 | 46.4 | 11301 |
| **snow peas**, frozen, boiled, drained | 160 | 83 | 138.6 | 14.4 | 7.7 | 0 | 5.0 | 8 | 94 | 45 | 0.78 | 0.448 | 106 | 35 | 0.10 | 0.9 | 0 | 1.37 |
| *1 cup* | | 5.6 | 0.6 | 0.1 | 0.1 | 0.3 | 0 | 347 | 93 | 3.84 | 0.144 | 1.3 | 2098 | 0.8 | 0.19 | 0.28 | 56.0 | 11303 |
| **snow peas**, raw | 63 | 26 | 56.0 | 4.8 | 2.5 | 0 | 1.6 | 3 | 27 | 15 | 0.17 | 0.154 | 34 | 38 | 0.09 | 0.4 | 0 | 0.47 |
| *1 cup whole* | | 1.8 | 0.1 | 0 | 0 | 0.1 | 0 | 126 | 33 | 1.31 | 0.050 | 0.4 | 685 | 0.2 | 0.05 | 0.10 | 26.5 | 11300 |
| **spaghetti winter squash**, boiled/ | 155 | 42 | 143.1 | 10.0 | 3.9 | 0 | 2.2 | 28 | 33 | 17 | 0.31 | 0.169 | 9 | 5 | 0.06 | 1.3 | 0 | 0.55 |
| baked - *1 cup* | | 1.0 | 0.4 | 0.1 | 0 | 0.2 | 0 | 181 | 22 | 0.53 | 0.054 | 0.5 | 170 | 0.2 | 0.03 | 0.15 | 12.4 | 11493 |
| **summer squash**, all varieties, boiled, | 180 | 36 | 168.7 | 7.8 | 4.7 | 0 | 2.5 | 2 | 49 | 43 | 0.70 | 0.383 | 20 | 10 | 0.08 | 0.9 | 0 | 0.25 |
| drained - *1 cup sliced* | | 1.6 | 0.6 | 0.1 | 0 | 0.2 | 0 | 346 | 70 | 0.65 | 0.185 | 0.4 | 382 | 0.3 | 0.07 | 0.12 | 36.0 | 11642 |
| **summer squash**, all varieties, raw | 113 | 18 | 106.9 | 3.8 | 2.5 | 0 | 1.2 | 2 | 17 | 19 | 0.33 | 0.198 | 11 | 19 | 0.05 | 0.6 | 0 | 0.18 |
| *1 cup sliced* | | 1.4 | 0.2 | 0 | 0 | 0.1 | 0 | 296 | 43 | 0.40 | 0.058 | 0.2 | 226 | 0.1 | 0.16 | 0.25 | 32.8 | 11641 |
| **sweet pepper**, green, boiled, | 135 | 38 | 124.0 | 9.0 | 4.3 | 0 | 1.6 | 3 | 12 | 14 | 0.16 | 0.155 | 31 | 100 | 0.08 | 0.6 | 0 | 0.11 |
| drained - *1 cup* | | 1.2 | 0.3 | 0 | 0 | 0.1 | 0 | 224 | 24 | 0.62 | 0.088 | 0.4 | 632 | 0.7 | 0.04 | 0.31 | 21.6 | 11334 |
| **sweet pepper**, green, cnd, solids | 140 | 25 | 127.7 | 5.5 | | | 1.7 | 1917 | 57 | 15 | 0.25 | 0.224 | 11 | 65 | 0.03 | 0.8 | 0 | 0.05 |
| and liquid - *1 cup halves* | | 1.1 | 0.4 | 0.1 | 0 | 0.2 | 0 | 204 | 28 | 1.12 | 0.182 | 0.4 | 217 | | 0.04 | 0.25 | 22.4 | 11335 |
| **sweet pepper**, green, frozen | 100 | 20 | 94.0 | 4.4 | | | 1.6 | 5 | 9 | 8 | 0.06 | 0.117 | 18 | 59 | 0.07 | 1.4 | 0 | 0.03 |
| *3.5 oz* | | 1.1 | 0.2 | 0 | 0 | 0.1 | 0 | 91 | 17 | 0.62 | 0.053 | 0.2 | 367 | | 0.04 | 0.14 | 14.0 | 11337 |
| **sweet pepper**, green, frzn, boiled, | 135 | 24 | 127.8 | 5.3 | | | 1.2 | 5 | 11 | 9 | 0.07 | 0.131 | 20 | 56 | 0.07 | 1.5 | 0 | 0.03 |
| drained - *1 cup chopped* | | 1.3 | 0.2 | 0 | 0 | 0.1 | 0 | 97 | 18 | 0.70 | 0.059 | 0.3 | 392 | | 0.04 | 0.15 | 13.5 | 11338 |

| | WT (g) | KCAL | H₂O (g) | CHO (g) | TSUG (g) | ASUG (g) | DFIB (g) | Na (mg) | Ca (mg) | Mg (mg) | Zn (mg) | Mn (mg) | A (mcg RAE) | C (mg) | B-1 (mg) | NIA (mg) | B-12 (mcg) | PANT (mg) |
|---|---|---|---|---|---|---|---|---|---|---|---|---|---|---|---|---|---|---|
| | | PRO (g) | FAT (g) | SFA (g) | MUFA (g) | PUFA (g) | CHOL (mg) | K (mg) | P (mg) | Fe (mg) | Cu (mg) | Se (mcg) | A (IU) | E (mg ATE) | B-2 (mg) | B-6 (mg) | FOL (mcg DFE) | REF |
| sweet pepper, green, raw | 119 | 24 | 111.7 | 5.5 | 2.9 | 0 | 2.0 | 4 | 12 | 12 | 0.15 | 0.145 | 21 | 96 | 0.07 | 0.6 | 0 | 0.12 |
| 1 medium (2¾" long) | | 1.0 | 0.2 | 0.1 | 0 | 0.1 | 0 | 208 | 24 | 0.40 | 0.079 | 0 | 440 | 0.4 | 0.03 | 0.27 | 11.9 | 11333 |
| sweet pepper, red, boiled, drained | 135 | 38 | 124.0 | 9.0 | 5.9 | 0 | 1.6 | 3 | 12 | 14 | 0.16 | 0.155 | 198 | 231 | 0.08 | 0.6 | 0 | 0.11 |
| 1 cup | | 1.2 | 0.3 | 0 | 0 | 0.1 | 0 | 224 | 24 | 0.62 | 0.088 | 0.4 | 3970 | 2.2 | 0.04 | 0.31 | 21.6 | 11823 |
| sweet pepper, red, frozen, boiled, drained - 1 cup chopped | 135 | 22 | 127.8 | 4.5 | 3.9 | | | 5 | 11 | 9 | 0.07 | 0.131 | 242 | 56 | 0.07 | 1.5 | 0 | 0.03 |
| | | 1.3 | 0.2 | 0 | 0 | 0.1 | 0 | 97 | 18 | 0.70 | 0.059 | 0.3 | 4837 | 1.5 | 0.04 | 0.15 | 13.5 | 11918 |
| sweet pepper, red, raw | 119 | 37 | 109.7 | 7.2 | 5.0 | 0 | 2.5 | 5 | 8 | 14 | 0.30 | 0.133 | 187 | 152 | 0.06 | 1.2 | 0 | 0.38 |
| 1 medium (2¾" long) | | 1.2 | 0.4 | 0 | 0 | 0.1 | 0 | 251 | 31 | 0.51 | 0.020 | 0.1 | 3726 | 1.9 | 0.10 | 0.35 | 54.7 | 11821 |
| sweet pepper, yellow, raw | 186 | 50 | 171.2 | 11.8 | | | 1.7 | 4 | 20 | 22 | 0.32 | 0.218 | 19 | 341 | 0.05 | 1.7 | 0 | 0.31 |
| 1 large (3¾" long) | | 1.9 | 0.4 | 0.1 | | | 0 | 394 | 45 | 0.86 | 0.199 | 0.6 | 372 | | 0.05 | 0.31 | 48.4 | 11951 |
| tomatillo, raw | 34 | 11 | 31.2 | 2.0 | 1.3 | 0 | 0.6 | 0 | 2 | 7 | 0.07 | 0.052 | 2 | 4 | 0.01 | 0.6 | 0 | 0.05 |
| 1 medium | | 0.3 | 0.3 | 0 | 0.1 | 0.1 | 0 | 91 | 13 | 0.21 | 0.027 | 0.2 | 39 | 0.1 | 0.01 | 0.02 | 2.4 | 11954 |
| tomato, green, raw | 123 | 28 | 114.4 | 6.3 | 4.9 | 0 | 1.4 | 16 | 16 | 12 | 0.09 | 0.123 | 39 | 29 | 0.07 | 0.6 | 0 | 0.62 |
| 1 medium (2⅗" diameter) | | 1.5 | 0.2 | 0 | 0 | 0.1 | 0 | 251 | 34 | 0.63 | 0.111 | 0.5 | 790 | 0.5 | 0.05 | 0.10 | 11.1 | 11527 |
| tomato, orange, raw | 111 | 18 | 105.2 | 3.5 | | | 1.0 | 47 | 6 | 9 | 0.16 | 0.098 | 83 | 18 | 0.05 | 0.7 | 0 | 0.21 |
| 1 tomato | | 1.3 | 0.2 | 0 | 0 | 0.1 | 0 | 235 | 32 | 0.52 | 0.069 | 0.4 | 1661 | | 0.04 | 0.07 | 32.2 | 11695 |
| tomato paste, canned | 170 | 139 | 125.0 | 32.1 | 20.7 | 0 | 7.0 | 167 | 61 | 71 | 1.07 | 0.513 | 129 | 37 | 0.10 | 5.2 | 0 | 0.24 |
| 6 oz can | | 7.3 | 0.8 | 0.2 | 0.1 | 0.3 | 0 | 1724 | 141 | 5.07 | 0.620 | 9.0 | 2592 | 7.3 | 0.26 | 0.37 | 20.4 | 11546 |
| tomato puree, canned | 125 | 48 | 109.8 | 11.2 | 6.0 | 0 | 2.4 | 35 | 22 | 29 | 0.45 | 0.211 | 32 | 13 | 0.03 | 1.8 | 0 | 0.55 |
| ½ cup | | 2.1 | 0.3 | 0 | 0 | 0.1 | 0 | 549 | 50 | 2.22 | 0.359 | 0.9 | 638 | 2.5 | 0.10 | 0.16 | 13.8 | 11547 |
| tomato, red, boiled | 240 | 43 | 226.4 | 9.6 | 6.0 | 0 | 1.7 | 26 | 26 | 22 | 0.34 | 0.252 | 58 | 55 | 0.09 | 1.3 | 0 | 0.31 |
| 1 cup | | 2.3 | 0.3 | 0 | 0 | 0.1 | 0 | 523 | 67 | 1.63 | 0.180 | 1.2 | 1174 | 1.3 | 0.05 | 0.19 | 31.2 | 11530 |
| tomato, red, canned | 240 | 41 | 226.3 | 9.6 | 5.7 | 0 | 2.4 | 343 | 74 | 26 | 0.34 | 0.185 | 14 | 22 | 0.11 | 1.7 | 0 | 0.28 |
| 1 cup | | 1.9 | 0.3 | 0 | 0.1 | 0.1 | 0 | 451 | 46 | 2.33 | 0.166 | 0.2 | 281 | 1.6 | 0.13 | 0.27 | 19.2 | 11531 |
| tomato, red, cherry, raw | 62 | 11 | 58.6 | 2.4 | 1.6 | 0 | 0.7 | 3 | 6 | 7 | 0.11 | 0.071 | 26 | 8 | 0.02 | 0.4 | 0 | 0.06 |
| 1 tomato | | 0.5 | 0.1 | 0 | 0 | 0.1 | 0 | 147 | 15 | 0.17 | 0.037 | 0 | 516 | 0.3 | 0.01 | 0.05 | 9.3 | 11529 |
| tomato, red, Italian, raw | 62 | 11 | 58.6 | 2.4 | 1.6 | 0 | 0.7 | 3 | 6 | 7 | 0.11 | 0.071 | 26 | 8 | 0.02 | 0.4 | 0 | 0.06 |
| 1 tomato | | 0.5 | 0.1 | 0 | 0 | 0.1 | 0 | 147 | 15 | 0.17 | 0.037 | 0 | 516 | 0.3 | 0.01 | 0.05 | 9.3 | 11529 |
| tomato, red, plum, raw | 62 | 11 | 58.6 | 2.4 | 1.6 | 0 | 0.7 | 3 | 6 | 7 | 0.11 | 0.071 | 26 | 8 | 0.02 | 0.4 | 0 | 0.06 |
| 1 tomato | | 0.5 | 0.1 | 0 | 0 | 0.1 | 0 | 147 | 15 | 0.17 | 0.037 | 0 | 516 | 0.3 | 0.01 | 0.05 | 9.3 | 11529 |
| tomato, red, raw | 62 | 11 | 58.6 | 2.4 | 1.6 | 0 | 0.7 | 3 | 6 | 7 | 0.11 | 0.071 | 26 | 8 | 0.02 | 0.4 | 0 | 0.06 |
| 1 tomato | | 0.5 | 0.1 | 0 | 0 | 0.1 | 0 | 147 | 15 | 0.17 | 0.037 | 0 | 516 | 0.3 | 0.01 | 0.05 | 9.3 | 11529 |
| tomato, red, stewed | 255 | 201 | 205.6 | 33.3 | | | 4.3 | 1160 | 66 | 38 | 0.46 | 0.492 | 84 | 46 | 0.28 | 2.8 | 0 | 0.65 |
| 1 cup | | 5.0 | 6.8 | 1.3 | 2.7 | 2.2 | 0 | 630 | 97 | 2.70 | 0.242 | 3.1 | 1698 | | 0.20 | 0.22 | 28.0 | 11660 |
| tomato, red, stewed, canned | 255 | 66 | 233.4 | 15.8 | 9.0 | 3.6 | 2.6 | 564 | 87 | 31 | 0.43 | 0.150 | 23 | 20 | 0.12 | 1.8 | 0 | 0.29 |
| 1 cup | | 2.3 | 0.5 | 0.1 | 0.1 | 0.2 | 0 | 528 | 51 | 3.39 | 0.286 | 1.5 | 439 | 2.1 | 0.09 | 0.04 | 12.8 | 11533 |
| tom, red, stewed w/onions, clry, grn peprs, cnd, Del Monte - ½ cup | 126 | 35 | | 9.0 | 7.0 | | 2.0 | 360 | 20 | | | | | 9 | | | | |
| | | 1.0 | 0 | 0 | | | 0 | | | 0.36 | | | 500 | | | | | DELM1 |
| tomato, red, sun-dried | 54 | 139 | 7.9 | 30.1 | 20.3 | 0 | 6.6 | 1131 | 59 | 105 | 1.07 | 0.997 | 24 | 21 | 0.29 | 4.9 | 0 | 1.13 |
| 1 cup | | 7.6 | 1.6 | 0.2 | 0.3 | 0.6 | 0 | 1851 | 192 | 4.91 | 0.768 | 3.0 | 472 | 0 | 0.26 | 0.18 | 36.7 | 11955 |
| tomato, red, sun-dried, canned in oil, drained - 1 cup | 110 | 234 | 59.2 | 25.7 | | | 6.4 | 293 | 52 | 89 | 0.86 | 0.513 | 70 | 112 | 0.21 | 4.0 | 0 | 0.53 |
| | | 5.6 | 15.5 | 2.1 | 9.5 | 2.3 | 0 | 1722 | 153 | 2.95 | 0.520 | 3.3 | 1415 | | 0.42 | 0.35 | 25.3 | 11956 |
| tomato, red with green chili, cnd | 241 | 36 | 227.1 | 8.7 | | | | 966 | 48 | 27 | 0.31 | 0.318 | 48 | 15 | 0.08 | 1.5 | 0 | 0.36 |
| 1 cup | | 1.7 | 0.2 | 0 | 0 | 0.1 | 0 | 258 | 34 | 0.63 | 0.217 | 1.0 | 940 | | 0.05 | 0.25 | 21.7 | 11537 |
| tomato, yellow, raw | 212 | 32 | 202.0 | 6.3 | | | 1.5 | 49 | 23 | 25 | 0.59 | 0.254 | 0 | 19 | 0.09 | 2.5 | 0 | 0.23 |
| 1 tomato | | 2.1 | 0.6 | 0.1 | 0.1 | 0.2 | 0 | 547 | 76 | 1.04 | 0.214 | 0.8 | 0 | | 0.10 | 0.12 | 63.6 | 11696 |
| waxgourd (Chinese preserving melon), boiled, drained - 1 cup cubed | 175 | 24 | 168.1 | 5.3 | 2.1 | 0 | 1.8 | 187 | 32 | 18 | 1.03 | 0.098 | 0 | 18 | 0.06 | 0.7 | 0 | 0.21 |
| | | 0.7 | 0.4 | 0 | 0.1 | 0.2 | 0 | 9 | 30 | 0.66 | 0.038 | 0.4 | 0 | 0.1 | 0 | 0.06 | 7.0 | 11594 |
| waxgourd (Chinese preserving melon), raw - 1 cup cubed | 132 | 17 | 126.9 | 4.0 | | | 3.8 | 147 | 25 | 13 | 0.81 | 0.077 | 0 | 17 | 0.05 | 0.5 | 0 | 0.18 |
| | | 0.5 | 0.3 | 0 | 0 | 0.1 | 0 | 8 | 25 | 0.53 | 0.030 | 0.3 | 0 | | 0.15 | 0.05 | 6.6 | 11593 |
| winter squash, all varieties, baked | 205 | 76 | 182.9 | 18.1 | 6.8 | 0 | 5.7 | 2 | 45 | 27 | 0.45 | 0.383 | 535 | 20 | 0.03 | 1.0 | 0 | 0.48 |
| 1 cup cubed | | 1.8 | 0.7 | 0.1 | 0.1 | 0.3 | 0 | 494 | 39 | 0.90 | 0.168 | 0.8 | 10707 | 0.2 | 0.14 | 0.33 | 41.0 | 11644 |
| winter squash, raw | 116 | 39 | 104.1 | 10.0 | 2.6 | 0 | 1.7 | 5 | 32 | 16 | 0.24 | 0.189 | 79 | 14 | 0.03 | 0.6 | 0 | 0.22 |
| 1 cup cubed | | 1.1 | 0.2 | 0 | 0 | 0.1 | 0 | 406 | 27 | 0.67 | 0.082 | 0.5 | 1586 | 0.1 | 0.07 | 0.18 | 27.8 | 11643 |
| yellow snap beans, boiled, drained | 125 | 44 | 111.5 | 9.8 | 1.9 | 0 | 4.1 | 4 | 58 | 31 | 0.45 | 0.368 | 5 | 12 | 0.09 | 0.8 | 0 | 0.09 |
| 1 cup | | 2.4 | 0.4 | 0.1 | 0 | 0.2 | 0 | 374 | 49 | 1.60 | 0.129 | 0.5 | 101 | 0.6 | 0.12 | 0.07 | 41.2 | 11724 |
| yellow snap beans, canned, drained | 135 | 27 | 126.0 | 6.1 | 1.3 | 0 | 1.8 | 339 | 35 | 18 | 0.39 | 0.270 | 7 | 6 | 0.02 | 0.3 | 0 | 0.17 |
| 1 cup | | 1.6 | 0.1 | 0 | 0 | 0.1 | 0 | 147 | 26 | 1.22 | 0.051 | 0.5 | 142 | 0.4 | 0.08 | 0.05 | 43.2 | 11932 |
| yellow snap beans, frozen, drained | 135 | 38 | 123.4 | 8.7 | 1.7 | 0 | 4.1 | 12 | 66 | 32 | 0.65 | 0.436 | 8 | 6 | 0.05 | 0.5 | 0 | 0.07 |
| 1 cup | | 2.0 | 0.2 | 0.1 | 0 | 0.1 | 0 | 170 | 42 | 1.19 | 0.082 | 0.5 | 151 | 0.1 | 0.12 | 0.08 | 31.0 | 11732 |
| zucchini summer squash, baby, raw - 1 medium | 11 | 2 | 10.2 | 0.3 | | | 0.1 | 0 | 2 | 4 | 0.09 | 0.022 | 3 | 4 | 0 | 0.1 | 0 | 0.04 |
| | | 0.3 | 0 | 0 | 0 | 0 | 0 | 50 | 10 | 0.09 | 0.011 | 0 | 54 | | 0.02 | | 2.2 | 11953 |

| | WT (g) | KCAL | H₂O (g) | CHO (g) | TSUG (g) | ASUG (g) | DFIB (g) | Na (mg) | Ca (mg) | Mg (mg) | Zn (mg) | Mn (mg) | A (mcg RAE) | C (mg) | B-1 (mg) | NIA (mg) | B-12 (mcg) | PANT (mg) |
|---|---|---|---|---|---|---|---|---|---|---|---|---|---|---|---|---|---|---|
| | | PRO (g) | FAT (g) | SFA (g) | MUFA (g) | PUFA (g) | CHOL (mg) | K (mg) | P (mg) | Fe (mg) | Cu (mg) | Se (mcg) | A (IU) | E (mg ATE) | B-2 (mg) | B-6 (mg) | FOL (mcg DFE) | REF |
| **zucchini summer squash**, boiled, | 180 | 29 | 170.5 | 7.1 | 3.0 | 0 | 2.5 | 5 | 23 | 40 | 0.32 | 0.320 | 101 | 8 | 0.07 | 0.8 | 0 | 0.21 |
| drained - *1 cup sliced* | | 1.2 | 0.1 | 0 | 0 | 0 | 0 | 455 | 72 | 0.63 | 0.155 | 0.4 | 2011 | 0.2 | 0.07 | 0.14 | 30.6 | 11478 |
| **zucchini summer squash**, frozen, | 223 | 38 | 211.3 | 7.9 | 3.8 | 0 | 2.9 | 4 | 38 | 29 | 0.45 | 0.513 | 20 | 8 | 0.09 | 0.9 | 0 | 0.59 |
| boiled, drained - *1 cup sliced* | | 2.6 | 0.3 | 0.1 | 0 | 0.1 | 0 | 433 | 56 | 1.07 | 0.105 | 0.4 | 395 | 0.3 | 0.09 | 0.10 | 17.8 | 11480 |
| **zucchini summer squash**, Italian | 227 | 66 | 205.7 | 15.5 | | | | 849 | 39 | 32 | 0.59 | 0.545 | 61 | 5 | 0.10 | 1.2 | 0 | 0.62 |
| style, cnd - *1 cup* | | 2.3 | 0.2 | 0.1 | 0 | 0.1 | 0 | 622 | 66 | 1.54 | 0.222 | 0.9 | 1224 | | 0.09 | 0.35 | 68.1 | 11481 |
| **zucchini summer squash**, raw | 113 | 18 | 106.9 | 3.8 | 2.0 | 0 | 1.2 | 11 | 17 | 19 | 0.33 | 0.198 | 11 | 19 | 0.05 | 0.6 | 0 | 0.18 |
| *1 cup sliced* | | 1.4 | 0.2 | 0 | 0 | 0.1 | 0 | 296 | 43 | 0.40 | 0.058 | 0.2 | 226 | 0.1 | 0.16 | 0.25 | 32.8 | 11477 |

## 30.3 LEAFY VEGETABLES

| | WT (g) | KCAL | H₂O (g) | CHO (g) | TSUG (g) | ASUG (g) | DFIB (g) | Na (mg) | Ca (mg) | Mg (mg) | Zn (mg) | Mn (mg) | A (mcg RAE) | C (mg) | B-1 (mg) | NIA (mg) | B-12 (mcg) | PANT (mg) |
|---|---|---|---|---|---|---|---|---|---|---|---|---|---|---|---|---|---|---|
| | | PRO (g) | FAT (g) | SFA (g) | MUFA (g) | PUFA (g) | CHOL (mg) | K (mg) | P (mg) | Fe (mg) | Cu (mg) | Se (mcg) | A (IU) | E (mg ATE) | B-2 (mg) | B-6 (mg) | FOL (mcg DFE) | REF |
| **agave**, boiled | 100 | 135 | 65.4 | 32.0 | 20.9 | | 10.6 | 13 | 460 | 39 | 0.25 | 0.142 | 6 | 0 | 0.01 | 0.2 | 0 | 0.04 |
| *3.5 oz* | | 1.0 | 0.3 | | | | 0 | 59 | 9 | 3.55 | 0.112 | 0.2 | 113 | 0.4 | 0.10 | 0.09 | 3.0 | 35193 |
| **agave**, dried | 28 | 95 | 3.3 | 23.0 | 14.2 | | 4.4 | 4 | 216 | 58 | 3.39 | 0.094 | 0 | 0 | 0.01 | 0.2 | 0 | 0.04 |
| *1 oz* | | 0.5 | 0.2 | | | | 0 | 215 | 10 | 1.02 | 0.053 | 0.2 | 5 | 0.2 | 0.18 | 0.06 | 2.0 | 35194 |
| **agave**, raw | 100 | 68 | 81.8 | 16.2 | 2.6 | | 6.6 | 14 | 417 | 55 | 0.15 | 0.094 | 2 | 4 | 0.03 | 0.2 | 0 | 0.04 |
| *3.5 oz* | | 0.5 | 0.2 | | | | 0 | 127 | 7 | 1.80 | 0.138 | 0.4 | 37 | 0.2 | 0.04 | 0.06 | 7.0 | 35192 |
| **amaranth leaves**, boiled, drained | 132 | 28 | 120.8 | 5.4 | | | | 28 | 276 | 73 | 1.16 | 1.137 | 183 | 54 | 0.03 | 0.7 | 0 | 0.08 |
| *1 cup* | | 2.8 | 0.2 | 0.1 | 0.1 | 0.1 | 0 | 846 | 95 | 2.98 | 0.209 | 1.2 | 3656 | | 0.18 | 0.23 | 75.2 | 11004 |
| **amaranth leaves**, raw | 28 | 6 | 25.7 | 1.1 | | | | 6 | 60 | 15 | 0.25 | 0.248 | 41 | 12 | 0.01 | 0.2 | 0 | 0.02 |
| *1 cup* | | 0.7 | 0.1 | 0 | 0 | 0 | 0 | 171 | 14 | 0.65 | 0.045 | 0.3 | 817 | | 0.04 | 0.05 | 23.8 | 11003 |
| **arugula**, raw | 20 | 5 | 18.3 | 0.7 | 0.4 | 0 | 0.3 | 5 | 32 | 9 | 0.09 | 0.064 | 24 | 3 | 0.01 | 0.1 | 0 | 0.09 |
| *1 cup leaves* | | 0.5 | 0.1 | 0 | 0 | 0.1 | 0 | 74 | 10 | 0.29 | 0.015 | 0.1 | 475 | 0.1 | 0.02 | 0.01 | 19.4 | 11959 |
| **balsam pear leafy tips**, boiled, | 58 | 20 | 51.4 | 3.9 | 0.6 | | 1.1 | 8 | 24 | 55 | 0.17 | 0.311 | 70 | 32 | 0.09 | 0.6 | 0 | 0.03 |
| drained - *1 cup* | | 2.1 | 0.1 | 0 | 0 | 0 | 0 | 349 | 45 | 0.59 | 0.117 | 0.5 | 1401 | 0.8 | 0.16 | 0.44 | 51.0 | 11023 |
| **balsam pear leafy tips**, raw | 48 | 14 | 42.8 | 1.6 | | | | 5 | 40 | 41 | 0.14 | 0.257 | 42 | 42 | 0.09 | 0.5 | 0 | 0.03 |
| *1 cup* | | 2.5 | 0.3 | | | | 0 | 292 | 48 | 0.98 | 0.096 | 0.4 | 832 | | 0.17 | 0.39 | 61.4 | 11022 |
| **beet greens**, boiled, drained | 144 | 39 | 128.3 | 7.9 | 0.9 | 0 | 4.2 | 347 | 164 | 98 | 0.72 | 0.740 | 552 | 36 | 0.17 | 0.7 | 0 | 0.47 |
| *1 cup* | | 3.7 | 0.3 | 0 | 0.1 | 0.1 | 0 | 1309 | 59 | 2.74 | 0.361 | 1.3 | 11022 | 2.6 | 0.42 | 0.19 | 20.2 | 11087 |
| **beet greens**, raw | 38 | 8 | 34.6 | 1.6 | 0.2 | 0 | 1.4 | 86 | 44 | 27 | 0.14 | 0.149 | 120 | 11 | 0.04 | 0.2 | 0 | 0.10 |
| *1 cup* | | 0.8 | 0 | 0 | 0 | 0 | 0 | 290 | 16 | 0.98 | 0.073 | 0.3 | 2404 | 0.6 | 0.08 | 0.04 | 5.7 | 11086 |
| **borage**, boiled, drained | 100 | 25 | 91.9 | 3.6 | | | | 88 | 102 | 57 | 0.22 | 0.385 | 219 | 32 | 0.06 | 0.9 | 0 | 0.04 |
| *3.5 oz* | | 2.1 | 0.8 | 0.2 | 0.2 | 0.1 | 0 | 491 | 55 | 3.64 | 0.143 | 0.9 | 4385 | | 0.16 | 0.09 | 10.0 | 11614 |
| **borage**, raw | 88 | 18 | 81.8 | 2.7 | | | | 70 | 82 | 46 | 0.18 | 0.307 | 185 | 31 | 0.05 | 0.8 | 0 | 0.04 |
| *1 cup* | | 1.6 | 0.6 | 0.1 | 0.2 | 0.1 | 0 | 414 | 47 | 2.90 | 0.114 | 0.8 | 3696 | | 0.13 | 0.07 | 11.4 | 11613 |
| **broccoli raab** (rapini), boiled | 100 | 33 | 91.4 | 3.1 | 0.6 | | 2.8 | 56 | 118 | 27 | 0.54 | 0.380 | 227 | 37 | 0.17 | 2.0 | | 0.45 |
| *3.5 oz* | | 3.8 | 0.5 | 0.1 | 0 | 0.2 | | 343 | 82 | 1.27 | 0.075 | 1.3 | 4533 | 2.5 | 0.14 | 0.22 | | 11097 |
| **broccoli raab** (rapini), raw | 40 | 13 | 37.0 | 1.1 | 0.2 | | 1.1 | 13 | 43 | 9 | 0.31 | 0.158 | 52 | 8 | 0.06 | 0.5 | | 0.13 |
| *1 cup chopped* | | 1.3 | 0.2 | 0 | 0 | 0.1 | | 78 | 29 | 0.86 | 0.017 | 0.4 | 1049 | 0.6 | 0.05 | 0.07 | | 11096 |
| **Brussels sprouts**, boiled, drained | 156 | 56 | 138.7 | 11.1 | 2.7 | 0 | 4.1 | 33 | 56 | 31 | 0.51 | 0.354 | 61 | 97 | 0.17 | 0.9 | 0 | 0.39 |
| *1 cup* | | 4.0 | 0.8 | 0.2 | 0.1 | 0.4 | 0 | 495 | 87 | 1.87 | 0.129 | 2.3 | 1209 | 0.7 | 0.12 | 0.28 | 93.6 | 11099 |
| **Brussels sprouts**, frozen | 155 | 64 | 135.0 | 12.2 | | | 5.9 | 16 | 40 | 31 | 0.48 | 0.482 | 48 | 115 | 0.16 | 1.0 | 0 | 0.44 |
| *1 cup* | | 5.9 | 0.6 | 0.1 | 0 | 0.3 | 0 | 574 | 96 | 1.44 | 0.051 | 2.3 | 956 | | 0.19 | 0.31 | 190.6 | 11100 |
| **Brussels sprouts**, frzn, boiled, | 155 | 65 | 134.4 | 12.9 | 3.2 | 0 | 6.4 | 23 | 40 | 28 | 0.37 | 0.319 | 71 | 71 | 0.16 | 0.8 | 0 | 0.53 |
| drained - *1 cup* | | 5.6 | 0.6 | 0.1 | 0 | 0.3 | 0 | 450 | 87 | 0.74 | 0.053 | 0.9 | 1435 | 0.8 | 0.18 | 0.45 | 156.6 | 11101 |
| **Brussels sprouts**, raw | 88 | 38 | 75.7 | 7.9 | 1.9 | 0 | 3.3 | 22 | 37 | 20 | 0.37 | 0.297 | 33 | 75 | 0.12 | 0.7 | 0 | 0.27 |
| *1 cup* | | 3.0 | 0.3 | 0.1 | 0 | 0.1 | 0 | 342 | 61 | 1.23 | 0.062 | 1.4 | 664 | 0.8 | 0.08 | 0.19 | 53.7 | 11098 |
| **cabbage**, green/white, boiled, | 150 | 34 | 138.9 | 8.3 | 4.2 | 0 | 2.8 | 12 | 72 | 22 | 0.30 | 0.308 | 6 | 56 | 0.09 | 0.4 | 0 | 0.26 |
| drained - *1 cup shredded* | | 1.9 | 0.1 | 0 | 0 | 0 | 0 | 294 | 50 | 0.26 | 0.026 | 0.9 | 120 | 0.2 | 0.06 | 0.17 | 45.0 | 11110 |
| **cabbage**, green/white, raw | 70 | 18 | 64.5 | 4.1 | 2.2 | 0 | 1.8 | 13 | 28 | 8 | 0.13 | 0.112 | 4 | 26 | 0.04 | 0.2 | 0 | 0.15 |
| *1 cup shredded* | | 0.9 | 0.1 | 0 | 0 | 0 | 0 | 119 | 18 | 0.33 | 0.013 | 0.2 | 69 | 0.1 | 0.03 | 0.09 | 30.1 | 11109 |
| **cabbage**, napa, boiled | 109 | 13 | 105.0 | 2.4 | | | | 12 | 32 | 9 | 0.15 | 0.221 | 14 | 3 | 0.01 | 0.5 | 0 | 0.09 |
| *1 cup* | | 1.2 | 0.2 | | | | 0 | 95 | 21 | 0.81 | 0.105 | 0.4 | 287 | | 0.03 | 0.04 | 46.9 | 11970 |
| **cabbage**, red/purple, boiled, | 150 | 44 | 136.3 | 10.4 | 5.0 | 0 | 3.9 | 42 | 63 | 26 | 0.38 | 0.334 | 3 | 52 | 0.11 | 0.6 | 0 | 0.23 |
| drained - *1 cup shredded* | | 2.3 | 0.1 | 0 | 0 | 0.1 | 0 | 393 | 50 | 0.99 | 0.081 | 3.4 | 50 | 0.2 | 0.09 | 0.34 | 36.0 | 11113 |
| **cabbage**, red/purple, raw | 70 | 22 | 63.3 | 5.2 | 2.7 | 0 | 1.5 | 19 | 31 | 11 | 0.15 | 0.170 | 39 | 40 | 0.04 | 0.3 | 0 | 0.10 |
| *1 cup shredded* | | 1.0 | 0.1 | 0 | 0 | 0.1 | 0 | 170 | 21 | 0.56 | 0.012 | 0.4 | 781 | 0.1 | 0.05 | 0.15 | 12.6 | 11112 |
| **cabbage**, savoy, boiled, drained | 145 | 35 | 133.4 | 7.8 | | | 4.1 | 35 | 44 | 35 | 0.33 | 0.220 | 64 | 25 | 0.07 | 0 | 0 | 0.23 |
| *1 cup shredded* | | 2.6 | 0.1 | 0 | 0 | 0.1 | 0 | 267 | 48 | 0.55 | 0.075 | 1.0 | 1289 | | 0.03 | 0.22 | 66.7 | 11115 |
| **cabbage**, savoy, raw | 70 | 19 | 63.7 | 4.3 | 1.6 | 0 | 2.2 | 20 | 24 | 20 | 0.19 | 0.126 | 35 | 22 | 0.05 | 0.2 | 0 | 0.13 |
| *1 cup shredded* | | 1.4 | 0.1 | 0 | 0 | 0 | 0 | 161 | 29 | 0.28 | 0.043 | 0.6 | 700 | 0.1 | 0.02 | 0.13 | 56.0 | 11114 |
| **cabbage**, swamp (skunk cabbage), | 98 | 20 | 91.1 | 3.6 | | | 1.9 | 120 | 53 | 29 | 0.16 | 0.140 | 255 | 16 | 0.05 | 0.5 | 0 | 0.12 |
| boiled, drained - *1 cup* | | 2.0 | 0.2 | 0 | 0 | 0.1 | 0 | 278 | 41 | 1.29 | 0.021 | 0.9 | 5096 | | 0.08 | 0.08 | 34.3 | 11504 |

| | WT (g) | KCAL | H₂O (g) | CHO (g) | TSUG (g) | ASUG (g) | DFIB (g) | Na (mg) | Ca (mg) | Mg (mg) | Zn (mg) | Mn (mg) | A (mcg RAE) | C (mg) | B-1 (mg) | NIA (mg) | B-12 (mcg) | PANT (mg) |
|---|---|---|---|---|---|---|---|---|---|---|---|---|---|---|---|---|---|---|
| | | PRO (g) | FAT (g) | SFA (g) | MUFA (g) | PUFA (g) | CHOL (mg) | K (mg) | P (mg) | Fe (mg) | Cu (mg) | Se (mcg) | A (IU) | E (mg ATE) | B-2 (mg) | B-6 (mg) | FOL (mcg DFE) | REF |
| **cabbage,** swamp (skunk cabbage), raw - *1 cup* | 56 | 11 | 51.8 | 1.8 | | | 1.2 | 63 | 43 | 40 | 0.10 | 0.090 | 176 | 31 | 0.02 | 0.5 | 0 | 0.08 |
| | | 1.5 | 0.1 | | | | 0 | 175 | 22 | 0.94 | 0.013 | 0.5 | 3528 | | 0.06 | 0.05 | 31.9 | 11503 |
| **celtuce leaves,** raw *12 leaves* | 100 | 18 | 94.5 | 3.6 | | | 1.7 | 11 | 39 | 28 | 0.27 | 0.688 | 175 | 20 | 0.06 | 0.6 | 0 | 0.18 |
| | | 0.8 | 0.3 | | | | 0 | 330 | 39 | 0.55 | 0.040 | 0.9 | 3500 | | 0.07 | 0.05 | 46.0 | 11145 |
| **chicory greens,** raw *1 cup chopped* | 180 | 41 | 165.6 | 8.5 | 1.3 | 0 | 7.2 | 81 | 180 | 54 | 0.76 | 0.772 | 515 | 43 | 0.11 | 0.9 | 0 | 2.09 |
| | | 3.1 | 0.5 | 0.1 | 0 | 0.2 | 0 | 756 | 85 | 1.62 | 0.531 | 0.5 | 10291 | 4.1 | 0.18 | 0.19 | 198.0 | 11152 |
| **chicory, witloof,** raw *1 cup* | 90 | 15 | 85.1 | 3.6 | | | 2.8 | 2 | 17 | 9 | 0.14 | 0.090 | 1 | 3 | 0.06 | 0.1 | 0 | 0.13 |
| | | 0.8 | 0.1 | 0 | 0 | 0 | 0 | 190 | 23 | 0.22 | 0.046 | 0.2 | 26 | | 0.02 | 0.04 | 33.3 | 11151 |
| **Chinese cabbage,** pak-choi, boiled, drained - *1 cup shredded* | 170 | 20 | 162.4 | 3.0 | 1.4 | 0 | 1.7 | 58 | 158 | 19 | 0.29 | 0.245 | 360 | 44 | 0.05 | 0.7 | 0 | 0.13 |
| | | 2.7 | 0.3 | 0 | 0 | 0.1 | 0 | 631 | 49 | 1.77 | 0.032 | 0.7 | 7223 | 0.2 | 0.11 | 0.28 | 69.7 | 11117 |
| **Chinese cabbage,** pak-choi, raw *1 cup shredded* | 70 | 9 | 66.7 | 1.5 | 0.8 | 0 | 0.7 | 46 | 74 | 13 | 0.13 | 0.111 | 156 | 31 | 0.03 | 0.4 | 0 | 0.06 |
| | | 1.0 | 0.1 | 0 | 0 | 0.1 | 0 | 176 | 26 | 0.56 | 0.015 | 0.4 | 3128 | 0.1 | 0.05 | 0.14 | 46.2 | 11116 |
| **Chinese cabbage,** pe-tsai, boiled, drained - *1 cup shredded* | 119 | 17 | 113.3 | 2.9 | | | 2.0 | 11 | 38 | 12 | 0.21 | 0.182 | 57 | 19 | 0.05 | 0.6 | 0 | 0.10 |
| | | 1.8 | 0.2 | 0 | 0 | 0.1 | 0 | 268 | 46 | 0.36 | 0.035 | 0.5 | 1151 | | 0.05 | 0.21 | 63.1 | 11120 |
| **Chinese cabbage,** pe-tsai, raw *1 cup shredded* | 76 | 12 | 71.7 | 2.5 | 1.1 | 0 | 0.9 | 7 | 59 | 10 | 0.17 | 0.144 | 12 | 21 | 0.03 | 0.3 | 0 | 0.08 |
| | | 0.9 | 0.2 | 0 | 0 | 0.1 | 0 | 181 | 22 | 0.24 | 0.027 | 0.5 | 242 | 0.1 | 0.04 | 0.18 | 60.0 | 11119 |
| **chrysanthemum leaves,** raw *1 cup chopped* | 51 | 12 | 46.6 | 1.5 | | | 1.5 | 60 | 60 | 16 | 0.36 | 0.481 | 48 | 1 | 0.07 | 0.3 | 0 | 0.11 |
| | | 1.7 | 0.3 | | | | 0 | 289 | 28 | 1.17 | 0.070 | 0.2 | 954 | | 0.07 | 0.09 | 90.3 | 11698 |
| **cilantro,** raw *9 pieces* | 20 | 5 | 18.4 | 0.7 | 0.2 | | 0.6 | 9 | 13 | 5 | 0.10 | 0.085 | 67 | 5 | 0.01 | 0.2 | 0 | 0.11 |
| | | 0.4 | 0.1 | | 0.1 | 0 | 0 | 104 | 10 | 0.35 | 0.045 | 0.2 | 1350 | 0.5 | 0.03 | 0.03 | 12.4 | 11165 |
| **coleslaw,** homemade *½ cup* | 60 | 47 | 48.9 | 7.4 | | | 0.9 | 14 | 27 | 6 | 0.12 | 0.058 | 32 | 20 | 0.04 | 0.2 | 0 | 0.08 |
| | | 0.8 | 1.6 | 0.2 | 0.4 | 0.8 | | 109 | 19 | 0.35 | 0.014 | 0.4 | 220 | | 0.04 | 0.08 | 16.2 | 11159 |
| **collards,** boiled, drained *1 cup chopped* | 190 | 49 | 174.5 | 9.3 | 0.8 | 0 | 5.3 | 30 | 266 | 38 | 0.44 | 0.828 | 771 | 35 | 0.08 | 1.1 | 0 | 0.41 |
| | | 4.0 | 0.7 | 0.1 | 0 | 0.3 | 0 | 220 | 57 | 2.20 | 0.072 | 1.0 | 15417 | 1.7 | 0.20 | 0.24 | 176.7 | 11162 |
| **collards,** frozen *1 cup chopped* | 170 | 56 | 152.2 | 11.0 | | | 6.1 | 82 | 342 | 49 | 0.44 | 1.076 | 780 | 68 | 0.08 | 1.1 | 0 | 0.19 |
| | | 4.6 | 0.6 | 0.1 | 0 | 0.3 | 0 | 430 | 46 | 1.82 | 0.090 | 2.4 | 15611 | | 0.19 | 0.20 | 124.1 | 11163 |
| **collards,** frozen, boiled, drained *1 cup chopped* | 170 | 61 | 150.4 | 12.1 | 1.0 | 0 | 4.8 | 85 | 357 | 51 | 0.46 | 1.127 | 978 | 45 | 0.08 | 1.1 | 0 | 0.20 |
| | | 5.0 | 0.7 | 0.1 | 0 | 0.4 | 0 | 427 | 46 | 1.90 | 0.094 | 2.6 | 19538 | 2.1 | 0.20 | 0.19 | 129.2 | 11164 |
| **collards,** raw *1 cup chopped* | 36 | 11 | 32.6 | 2.0 | 0.2 | 0 | 1.3 | 7 | 52 | 3 | 0.05 | 0.099 | 120 | 13 | 0.02 | 0.3 | 0 | 0.10 |
| | | 0.9 | 0.2 | 0 | 0 | 0.1 | 0 | 61 | 4 | 0.07 | 0.014 | 0.5 | 2400 | 0.8 | 0.05 | 0.06 | 59.8 | 11161 |
| **cornsalad** (lamb's lettuce), raw *1 cup* | 56 | 12 | 52.0 | 2.0 | | | | 2 | 21 | 7 | 0.33 | 0.201 | 199 | 21 | 0.04 | 0.2 | 0 | 0.02 |
| | | 1.1 | 0.2 | | | | 0 | 257 | 30 | 1.22 | 0.075 | 0.5 | 3972 | | 0.05 | 0.15 | 7.8 | 11190 |
| **cowpea plant leafy tips,** boiled, drained - *1 cup chopped* | 53 | 12 | 48.4 | 1.5 | | | | 3 | 37 | 33 | 0.13 | 0.218 | 15 | 10 | 0.14 | 0.5 | 0 | 0.02 |
| | | 2.5 | 0.1 | 0 | 0 | 0 | 0 | 186 | 22 | 0.58 | 0.082 | 0.5 | 305 | | 0.08 | 0.07 | 31.8 | 11202 |
| **dandelion greens,** boiled, drained *1 cup* | 105 | 35 | 94.3 | 6.7 | 0.5 | 0 | 3.0 | 46 | 147 | 25 | 0.29 | 0.242 | 359 | 19 | 0.14 | 0.5 | 0 | 0.06 |
| | | 2.1 | 0.6 | 0.2 | 0 | 0.3 | 0 | 244 | 44 | 1.89 | 0.121 | 0.3 | 7179 | 2.6 | 0.18 | 0.17 | 13.6 | 11208 |
| **dandelion greens,** raw *1 cup chopped* | 55 | 25 | 47.1 | 5.1 | 0.4 | 0 | 1.9 | 42 | 103 | 20 | 0.23 | 0.188 | 279 | 19 | 0.10 | 0.4 | 0 | 0.05 |
| | | 1.5 | 0.4 | 0.1 | 0 | 0.2 | 0 | 218 | 36 | 1.71 | 0.094 | 0.3 | 5589 | 1.9 | 0.14 | 0.14 | 14.8 | 11207 |
| **endive,** raw *1 cup chopped* | 50 | 8 | 46.9 | 1.7 | 0.1 | 0 | 1.6 | 11 | 26 | 8 | 0.40 | 0.210 | 54 | 3 | 0.04 | 0.2 | 0 | 0.45 |
| | | 0.6 | 0.1 | 0 | 0 | 0 | 0 | 157 | 14 | 0.42 | 0.050 | 0.1 | 1084 | 0.2 | 0.04 | 0.01 | 71.0 | 11213 |
| **eppaw,** raw *1 cup* | 100 | 150 | 60.0 | 31.7 | | | | 12 | 110 | 32 | 1.15 | 1.094 | 0 | 13 | 0.11 | 0.3 | 0 | 1.17 |
| | | 4.6 | 1.8 | | | | 0 | 340 | 165 | 1.15 | 0.234 | 0.9 | 0 | | 0.12 | 0.18 | 24.0 | 11618 |
| **fiddlehead ferns,** frozen *3.5 oz* | 100 | 34 | 88.9 | 5.7 | | | | 0 | 24 | 19 | 0.71 | 0.940 | 168 | 18 | 0.01 | 3.3 | 0 | |
| | | 4.3 | 0.4 | | | | 0 | 129 | 58 | 0.73 | 0.220 | | 3350 | | 0.13 | | | 11996 |
| **fiddlehead ferns,** raw *1 cup chopped* | 23 | 8 | 20.4 | 1.3 | | | | 0 | 7 | 8 | 0.19 | 0.117 | 42 | 6 | 0 | 1.1 | 0 | |
| | | 1.0 | 0.1 | | | | 0 | 85 | 23 | 0.30 | 0.074 | | 832 | | 0.05 | | | 11995 |
| **fireweed leaves,** raw *1 cup chopped* | 23 | 24 | 16.3 | 4.4 | | | 2.4 | 8 | 99 | 36 | 0.61 | 1.542 | 41 | 1 | 0.01 | 1.1 | 0 | 0.31 |
| | | 1.1 | 0.6 | | | | 0 | 114 | 25 | 0.55 | 0.074 | 0.2 | 828 | | 0.03 | 0.15 | 25.8 | 11985 |
| **garden cress,** boiled, drained *1 cup* | 135 | 31 | 124.9 | 5.1 | 4.2 | 0 | 0.9 | 11 | 82 | 35 | 0.20 | 0.502 | 313 | 31 | 0.08 | 1.1 | 0 | 0.22 |
| | | 2.6 | 0.8 | 0 | 0.3 | 0.3 | 0 | 477 | 65 | 1.08 | 0.154 | 1.2 | 6276 | 0.7 | 0.22 | 0.21 | 50.0 | 11204 |
| **garden cress,** raw *1 cup* | 50 | 16 | 44.7 | 2.8 | 2.2 | 0 | 0.6 | 7 | 40 | 19 | 0.12 | 0.276 | 173 | 34 | 0.04 | 0.5 | 0 | 0.12 |
| | | 1.3 | 0.4 | 0 | 0.1 | 0.1 | 0 | 303 | 38 | 0.65 | 0.085 | 0.4 | 3458 | 0.4 | 0.13 | 0.12 | 40.0 | 11203 |
| **garland chrysanthemum,** boiled, drained - *1 cup pieces* | 100 | 20 | 92.5 | 4.3 | 2.0 | 0 | 2.3 | 53 | 69 | 18 | 0.20 | 0.355 | 129 | 24 | 0.02 | 0.7 | 0 | 0.04 |
| | | 1.6 | 0.1 | 0 | 0 | 0 | 0 | 569 | 43 | 3.74 | 0.133 | 0.3 | 2572 | 2.5 | 0.16 | 0.12 | 50.0 | 11158 |
| **garland chrysanthemum,** raw *1 cup pieces* | 25 | 6 | 22.8 | 0.8 | | | 0.8 | 30 | 29 | 8 | 0.18 | 0.236 | 29 | 0 | 0.03 | 0.1 | 0 | 0.06 |
| | | 0.8 | 0.1 | | | | 0 | 142 | 14 | 0.57 | 0.034 | | 580 | | 0.04 | 0.04 | 44.2 | 11157 |
| **grape leaves,** canned *5 leaves* | 20 | 14 | 15.2 | 2.3 | | | | 571 | 58 | 3 | 0.08 | 0.058 | 53 | 2 | 0.01 | 0.9 | 0 | 0.85 |
| | | 0.9 | 0.4 | 0.1 | 0 | 0.2 | 0 | 6 | 7 | 0.60 | 0.368 | 0.2 | 1051 | | 0.07 | 0.03 | 15.6 | 11975 |
| **grape leaves,** raw *1 cup* | 14 | 13 | 10.3 | 2.4 | 0.9 | 0 | 1.5 | 1 | 51 | 13 | 0.09 | 0.400 | 193 | 2 | 0.01 | 0.3 | 0 | 0.03 |
| | | 0.8 | 0.3 | 0 | 0 | 0.1 | 0 | 38 | 13 | 0.37 | 0.058 | 0.1 | 3853 | 0.3 | 0.05 | 0.06 | 11.6 | 11974 |
| **horseradish tree leafy tips,** chopped, boiled, drained - *1 cup* | 42 | 25 | 34.3 | 4.7 | 0.4 | 0 | 0.8 | 4 | 63 | 63 | 0.21 | 0.365 | 147 | 13 | 0.09 | 0.8 | 0 | 0.04 |
| | | 2.2 | 0.4 | 0.1 | 0.2 | 0 | 0 | 144 | 28 | 0.97 | 0.036 | 0.4 | 2945 | 0 | 0.21 | 0.39 | 9.7 | 11223 |

| Food | WT (g) | KCAL / PRO (g) | H₂O (g) / FAT (g) | CHO (g) / SFA (g) | TSUG (g) / MUFA (g) | ASUG (g) / PUFA (g) | DFIB (g) / CHOL (mg) | Na (mg) / K (mg) | Ca (mg) / P (mg) | Mg (mg) / Fe (mg) | Zn (mg) / Cu (mg) | Mn (mg) / Se (mcg) | A (mcg RAE) / A (IU) | C (mg) / E (mg ATE) | B-1 (mg) / B-2 (mg) | NIA (mg) / B-6 (mg) | B-12 (mcg) / FOL (mcg DFE) | PANT (mg) / REF |
|---|---|---|---|---|---|---|---|---|---|---|---|---|---|---|---|---|---|---|
| **jute** (potherb), boiled, drained | 87 | 32 | 75.8 | 6.3 | 0.9 | 0 | 1.7 | 10 | 184 | 54 | 0.69 | 0.107 | 225 | 29 | 0.08 | 0.8 | 0 | 0.06 |
| *1 cup* | | 3.2 | 0.2 | 0 | 0 | 0.1 | 0 | 478 | 63 | 2.73 | 0.222 | 0.8 | 4511 | 0.6 | 0.17 | 0.50 | 90.5 | 11232 |
| **jute** (potherb), raw | 28 | 10 | 24.6 | 1.6 | | | | 2 | 58 | 18 | 0.22 | 0.034 | 78 | 10 | 0.04 | 0.4 | 0 | 0.02 |
| *1 cup* | | 1.3 | 0.1 | 0 | 0 | 0 | 0 | 157 | 23 | 1.33 | 0.071 | 0.3 | 1557 | | 0.15 | 0.17 | 34.4 | 11231 |
| **kale**, boiled, drained | 130 | 36 | 118.6 | 7.3 | 1.6 | 0 | 2.6 | 30 | 94 | 23 | 0.31 | 0.541 | 885 | 53 | 0.07 | 0.6 | 0 | 0.06 |
| *1 cup chopped* | | 2.5 | 0.5 | 0.1 | 0 | 0.3 | 0 | 296 | 36 | 1.17 | 0.203 | 1.2 | 17707 | 1.1 | 0.09 | 0.18 | 16.9 | 11234 |
| **kale**, frozen, boiled, drained | 130 | 39 | 117.6 | 6.8 | 1.7 | 0 | 2.6 | 20 | 179 | 23 | 0.23 | 0.585 | 956 | 33 | 0.06 | 0.9 | 0 | 0.07 |
| *1 cup chopped* | | 3.7 | 0.6 | 0.1 | 0 | 0.3 | 0 | 417 | 36 | 1.22 | 0.061 | 1.2 | 19115 | 1.2 | 0.15 | 0.11 | 18.2 | 11236 |
| **kale**, raw | 67 | 34 | 56.6 | 6.7 | | | 1.3 | 29 | 90 | 23 | 0.29 | 0.519 | 515 | 80 | 0.07 | 0.7 | 0 | 0.06 |
| *1 cup chopped* | | 2.2 | 0.5 | 0.1 | 0 | 0.2 | 0 | 299 | 38 | 1.14 | 0.194 | 0.6 | 10302 | | 0.09 | 0.18 | 19.4 | 11233 |
| **kale, Scotch** (curly leaves), boiled, drained - *1 cup chopped* | 130 | 36 | 118.6 | 7.3 | | | 1.6 | 58 | 172 | 74 | 0.31 | 0.542 | 130 | 69 | 0.05 | 1.0 | 0 | 0.06 |
| | | 2.5 | 0.5 | 0.1 | 0 | 0.3 | 0 | 356 | 49 | 2.51 | 0.203 | 1.2 | 2592 | | 0.05 | 0.18 | 16.9 | 11623 |
| **lambsquarters**, boiled, drained - *1 cup* | 180 | 58 | 160.0 | 9.0 | 1.1 | 0 | 3.8 | 52 | 464 | 41 | 0.54 | 0.945 | 704 | 67 | 0.18 | 1.6 | 0 | 0.11 |
| | | 5.8 | 1.3 | 0.1 | 0.2 | 0.6 | 0 | 518 | 81 | 1.26 | 0.355 | 1.6 | 14069 | 3.3 | 0.47 | 0.31 | 25.2 | 11245 |
| **lettuce**, butterhead, raw | 55 | 7 | 52.6 | 1.2 | 0.5 | 0 | 0.6 | 3 | 19 | 7 | 0.11 | 0.098 | 91 | 2 | 0.03 | 0.2 | 0 | 0.08 |
| *1 cup* | | 0.7 | 0.1 | 0 | 0 | 0.1 | 0 | 131 | 18 | 0.68 | 0.009 | 0.3 | 1822 | 0.1 | 0.03 | 0.05 | 40.2 | 11250 |
| **lettuce**, iceberg, raw | 55 | 8 | 52.6 | 1.6 | 1.1 | 0 | 0.7 | 6 | 10 | 4 | 0.08 | 0.069 | 14 | 2 | 0.02 | 0.1 | 0 | 0.05 |
| *1 cup* | | 0.5 | 0.1 | 0 | 0 | 0 | 0 | 78 | 11 | 0.23 | 0.014 | 0.1 | 276 | 0.1 | 0.01 | 0.02 | 16.0 | 11252 |
| **lettuce**, looseleaf (leaf), raw | 56 | 8 | 53.2 | 1.6 | 0.4 | 0 | 0.7 | 16 | 20 | 7 | 0.10 | 0.140 | 207 | 10 | 0.04 | 0.2 | 0 | 0.06 |
| *1 cup* | | 0.8 | 0.1 | 0 | 0 | 0 | 0 | 109 | 16 | 0.48 | 0.016 | 0.3 | 4147 | 0.2 | 0.04 | 0.05 | 21.3 | 11253 |
| **malabar spinach**, boiled | 100 | 23 | 92.5 | 2.7 | | | 2.1 | 55 | 124 | 48 | 0.30 | 0.255 | 58 | 6 | 0.11 | 0.8 | 0 | 0.14 |
| *3.5 oz* | | 3.0 | 0.8 | | | | 0 | 256 | 36 | 1.48 | 0.111 | 0.9 | 1158 | | 0.13 | 0.09 | 114.0 | 11986 |
| **mustard greens**, boiled, drained | 140 | 21 | 132.2 | 2.9 | 0.1 | 0 | 2.8 | 22 | 104 | 21 | 0.15 | 0.384 | 442 | 35 | 0.06 | 0.6 | 0 | 0.17 |
| *1 cup chopped* | | 3.2 | 0.3 | 0 | 0.2 | 0.1 | 0 | 283 | 57 | 0.98 | 0.118 | 0.8 | 8852 | 1.7 | 0.09 | 0.14 | 102.2 | 11271 |
| **mustard greens**, frozen | 146 | 29 | 136.1 | 5.0 | | | 4.8 | 42 | 169 | 22 | 0.34 | 0.495 | 377 | 37 | 0.07 | 0.5 | 0 | 0.03 |
| *1 cup chopped* | | 3.6 | 0.4 | 0 | 0.2 | 0.1 | 0 | 248 | 44 | 1.88 | 0.098 | 1.0 | 7526 | | 0.09 | 0.19 | 201.5 | 11272 |
| **mustard greens**, frozen, boiled, drained - *1 cup chopped* | 150 | 28 | 140.7 | 4.7 | 0.5 | 0 | 4.2 | 38 | 152 | 20 | 0.30 | 0.441 | 531 | 21 | 0.06 | 0.4 | 0 | 0.02 |
| | | 3.4 | 0.4 | 0 | 0.2 | 0.1 | 0 | 208 | 36 | 1.68 | 0.087 | 0.9 | 10614 | 2.0 | 0.08 | 0.16 | 105.0 | 11273 |
| **mustard greens**, raw | 56 | 15 | 50.8 | 2.7 | 0.9 | 0 | 1.8 | 14 | 58 | 18 | 0.11 | 0.269 | 294 | 39 | 0.04 | 0.4 | 0 | 0.12 |
| *1 cup chopped* | | 1.5 | 0.1 | 0 | 0.1 | 0 | 0 | 198 | 24 | 0.82 | 0.082 | 0.5 | 5880 | 1.1 | 0.06 | 0.10 | 104.7 | 11270 |
| **mustard spinach** (tendergreen), boiled, drained - *1 cup chopped* | 180 | 29 | 170.1 | 5.0 | | | 3.6 | 25 | 284 | 13 | 0.20 | 0.486 | 738 | 117 | 0.07 | 0.8 | 0 | 0.21 |
| | | 3.1 | 0.4 | | | | 0 | 513 | 32 | 1.44 | 0.090 | 1.1 | 14760 | | 0.11 | 0.17 | 131.4 | 11275 |
| **mustard spinach** (tendergreen), raw - *1 cup chopped* | 150 | 33 | 138.3 | 5.8 | | | 4.2 | 32 | 315 | 16 | 0.26 | 0.610 | 742 | 195 | 0.10 | 1.0 | 0 | 0.27 |
| | | 3.3 | 0.4 | 0 | 0.2 | 0.1 | 0 | 674 | 42 | 2.25 | 0.112 | 1.2 | 14850 | | 0.14 | 0.23 | 238.5 | 11274 |
| **New Zealand spinach**, boiled, drained - *1 cup chopped* | 180 | 22 | 170.6 | 4.0 | | | | 193 | 86 | 58 | 0.56 | 0.947 | 326 | 29 | 0.05 | 0.7 | 0 | 0.46 |
| | | 2.3 | 0.3 | 0 | 0 | 0.1 | 0 | 184 | 40 | 1.19 | 0.139 | 1.6 | 6520 | | 0.19 | 0.43 | 14.4 | 11277 |
| **New Zealand spinach**, raw | 56 | 8 | 52.6 | 1.4 | | | | 73 | 32 | 22 | 0.21 | 0.358 | 123 | 17 | 0.02 | 0.3 | 0 | 0.17 |
| *1 cup chopped* | | 0.8 | 0.1 | 0 | 0 | 0 | 0 | 73 | 16 | 0.45 | 0.052 | 0.4 | 2464 | | 0.07 | 0.17 | 8.4 | 11276 |
| **parsley**, raw | 10 | 4 | 8.8 | 0.6 | 0.1 | 0 | 0.3 | 6 | 14 | 5 | 0.11 | 0.016 | 42 | 13 | 0.01 | 0.1 | 0 | 0.04 |
| *10 sprigs* | | 0.3 | 0.1 | 0 | 0 | 0 | 0 | 55 | 6 | 0.62 | 0.015 | 0 | 842 | 0.1 | 0.01 | 0.01 | 15.2 | 11297 |
| **pumpkin leaves**, boiled, drained | 71 | 15 | 65.7 | 2.4 | 0.5 | 0 | 1.9 | 6 | 31 | 27 | 0.14 | 0.252 | 57 | 1 | 0.05 | 0.6 | 0 | 0.03 |
| *1 cup* | | 1.9 | 0.2 | 0.1 | 0 | 0 | 0 | 311 | 56 | 2.27 | 0.094 | 0.6 | 1136 | 0.7 | 0.10 | 0.14 | 17.8 | 11419 |
| **purslane**, boiled, drained | 115 | 21 | 107.5 | 4.1 | | | | 51 | 90 | 77 | 0.20 | 0.353 | 107 | 12 | 0.04 | 0.5 | 0 | 0.04 |
| *1 cup* | | 1.7 | 0.2 | | | | 0 | 561 | 43 | 0.89 | 0.131 | 1.0 | 2130 | | 0.10 | 0.08 | 10.4 | 11428 |
| **purslane**, raw | 43 | 7 | 40.4 | 1.5 | | | | 19 | 28 | 29 | 0.07 | 0.130 | 28 | 9 | 0.02 | 0.2 | 0 | 0.02 |
| *1 cup* | | 0.6 | 0 | | | | 0 | 212 | 19 | 0.86 | 0.049 | 0.4 | 568 | | 0.05 | 0.03 | 5.2 | 11427 |
| **radicchio**, raw | 40 | 9 | 37.3 | 1.8 | 0.2 | 0 | 0.4 | 9 | 8 | 5 | 0.25 | 0.055 | 0 | 3 | 0.01 | 0.1 | 0 | 0.11 |
| *1 cup shredded* | | 0.6 | 0.1 | 0 | 0 | 0 | 0 | 121 | 16 | 0.23 | 0.136 | 0.4 | 11 | 0.9 | 0.01 | 0.02 | 24.0 | 11952 |
| **romaine** (cos lettuce), raw | 56 | 10 | 53.0 | 1.8 | 0.7 | 0 | 1.2 | 4 | 18 | 8 | 0.13 | 0.087 | 244 | 13 | 0.04 | 0.2 | 0 | 0.08 |
| *1 cup* | | 0.7 | 0.2 | 0 | 0 | 0.1 | 0 | 138 | 17 | 0.54 | 0.027 | 0.2 | 4878 | 0.1 | 0.04 | 0.04 | 76.2 | 11251 |
| **salsify, black** (viper's grass), raw | 134 | 110 | 103.2 | 24.9 | | | 4.4 | 27 | 80 | 31 | 0.51 | 0.359 | 0 | 11 | 0.11 | 0.7 | 0 | 0.50 |
| *1 cup* | | 4.4 | 0.3 | | | | 0 | 509 | 100 | 0.94 | 0.119 | 1.1 | 0 | | 0.29 | 0.37 | 34.8 | 11437 |
| **salsify** (oyster plant/veg oyster), boiled, drained - *1 cup sliced* | 135 | 92 | 109.4 | 20.7 | 3.9 | 0 | 4.2 | 22 | 63 | 24 | 0.40 | 0.284 | 0 | 6 | 0.08 | 0.5 | 0 | 0.37 |
| | | 3.7 | 0.2 | 0.1 | 0 | 0.1 | 0 | 382 | 76 | 0.74 | 0.095 | 0.8 | 0 | 0.3 | 0.23 | 0.29 | 20.2 | 11438 |
| **sauerkraut**, canned, solids and liquid - *1 cup* | 142 | 27 | 131.4 | 6.1 | 2.5 | 0 | 4.1 | 939 | 43 | 18 | 0.27 | 0.214 | 1 | 21 | 0.03 | 0.2 | 0 | 0.13 |
| | | 1.3 | 0.2 | 0 | 0 | 0.1 | 0 | 241 | 28 | 2.09 | 0.136 | 0.9 | 26 | 0.2 | 0.03 | 0.18 | 34.1 | 11439 |
| **sorrel** (dock), boiled, drained | 133 | 27 | 124.5 | 3.9 | | | 3.5 | 4 | 51 | 118 | 0.23 | 0.403 | 231 | 35 | 0.05 | 0.5 | 0 | 0.05 |
| *1 cup chopped* | | 2.4 | 0.9 | | | | 0 | 427 | 69 | 2.77 | 0.152 | 1.2 | 4620 | | 0.11 | 0.13 | 10.6 | 11617 |
| **sorrel** (dock), raw | 133 | 29 | 123.7 | 4.3 | | | 3.9 | 5 | 59 | 137 | 0.27 | 0.464 | 266 | 64 | 0.05 | 0.7 | 0 | 0.05 |
| *1 cup chopped* | | 2.7 | 0.9 | | | | 0 | 519 | 84 | 3.19 | 0.174 | 1.2 | 5320 | | 0.13 | 0.16 | 17.3 | 11616 |
| **spinach au gratin**, frozen, Budget Gourmet - *5.5 oz package* | 155 | 222 | 116.4 | 11.5 | | | 2.3 | 654 | 243 | | | | | 27 | | | | |
| | | 6.7 | 16.6 | 7.6 | | | 42 | | | 1.95 | | | 7079 | | | | | 22603 |

| | WT (g) | KCAL / PRO (g) | H₂O (g) / FAT (g) | CHO (g) / SFA (g) | TSUG (g) / MUFA (g) | ASUG (g) / PUFA (g) | DFIB (g) / CHOL (mg) | Na (mg) / K (mg) | Ca (mg) / P (mg) | Mg (mg) / Fe (mg) | Zn (mg) / Cu (mg) | Mn (mg) / Se (mcg) | A (mcg RAE) / A (IU) | C (mg) / E (mg ATE) | B-1 (mg) / B-2 (mg) | NIA (mg) / B-6 (mg) | B-12 (mcg) / FOL (mcg DFE) | PANT (mg) / REF |
|---|---|---|---|---|---|---|---|---|---|---|---|---|---|---|---|---|---|---|
| spinach, boiled, drained | 180 | 41 | 164.2 | 6.8 | 0.8 | 0 | 4.3 | 126 | 245 | 157 | 1.37 | 1.683 | 943 | 18 | 0.17 | 0.9 | 0 | 0.26 |
| 1 cup | | 5.3 | 0.5 | 0.1 | 0 | 0.2 | 0 | 839 | 101 | 6.43 | 0.313 | 2.7 | 18866 | 3.7 | 0.42 | 0.44 | 262.8 | 11458 |
| spinach, canned, drained | 214 | 49 | 196.4 | 7.3 | 0.9 | 0 | 5.1 | 58 | 272 | 163 | 0.98 | 1.278 | 1049 | 31 | 0.03 | 0.8 | 0 | 0.10 |
| 1 cup | | 6.0 | 1.1 | 0.2 | 0 | 0.5 | 0 | 740 | 94 | 4.92 | 0.385 | 3.0 | 20974 | 4.2 | 0.30 | 0.21 | 209.7 | 11461 |
| spinach, creamed, frzn, Green | 109 | 70 | | 9.0 | 4.0 | | 1.0 | 510 | 100 | | | | | 4 | | | | |
| Giant ½ cup | | 3.0 | 2.5 | 1.5 | | | 0 | | | 0.72 | | | 2250 | | | | | GENM358 |
| spinach, frozen | 156 | 45 | 140.7 | 6.6 | 1.0 | 0 | 4.5 | 115 | 201 | 117 | 0.87 | 1.098 | 914 | 9 | 0.15 | 0.8 | 0 | 0.15 |
| 1 cup | | 5.7 | 0.9 | 0.1 | 0 | 0.1 | 0 | 540 | 76 | 2.95 | 0.225 | 9.4 | 18293 | 4.5 | 0.35 | 0.27 | 226.2 | 11463 |
| spinach, frozen, boiled, drained | 190 | 65 | 169.0 | 9.1 | 1.0 | 0 | 7.0 | 184 | 291 | 156 | 0.93 | 1.362 | 1146 | 4 | 0.15 | 0.8 | 0 | 0.14 |
| 1 cup | | 7.6 | 1.7 | 0.3 | 0 | 0.7 | 0 | 574 | 95 | 3.72 | 0.306 | 10.4 | 22916 | 6.7 | 0.33 | 0.26 | 229.9 | 11464 |
| spinach, raw | 30 | 7 | 27.4 | 1.1 | 0.1 | 0 | 0.7 | 24 | 30 | 24 | 0.16 | 0.269 | 141 | 8 | 0.02 | 0.2 | 0 | 0.02 |
| 1 cup | | 0.9 | 0.1 | 0 | 0 | 0 | 0 | 167 | 15 | 0.81 | 0.039 | 0.3 | 2813 | 0.6 | 0.06 | 0.06 | 58.2 | 11457 |
| spinach souffle, homemade | 136 | 233 | 96.3 | 7.9 | 2.5 | 0 | 1.0 | 770 | 224 | 41 | 1.17 | 0.366 | 325 | 10 | 0.11 | 0.7 | 0.53 | 0.59 |
| 1 cup | | 10.8 | 17.6 | 8.3 | 4.1 | 0.8 | 160 | 318 | 192 | 1.62 | 0.075 | 15.1 | 3909 | 1.3 | 0.36 | 0.13 | 104.7 | 11658 |
| sweet potato leaves, raw | 35 | 12 | 30.8 | 2.2 | | | 0.7 | 3 | 13 | 21 | 0.10 | 0.090 | 18 | 4 | 0.05 | 0.4 | 0 | 0.08 |
| 1 cup chopped | | 1.4 | 0.1 | 0 | 0 | 0 | 0 | 181 | 33 | 0.35 | 0.013 | 0.3 | 360 | | 0.12 | 0.07 | 28.0 | 11505 |
| sweet potato leaves, steamed | 64 | 22 | 56.8 | 4.7 | 3.5 | 0 | 1.2 | 8 | 15 | 39 | 0.17 | 0.147 | 29 | 1 | 0.07 | 0.6 | 0 | 0.13 |
| 1 cup | | 1.5 | 0.2 | 0 | 0 | 0.1 | 0 | 305 | 38 | 0.38 | 0.021 | 0.6 | 586 | 0.6 | 0.17 | 0.10 | 31.4 | 11506 |
| Swiss chard, boiled, drained | 175 | 35 | 162.1 | 7.2 | 1.9 | 0 | 3.7 | 313 | 102 | 150 | 0.58 | 0.584 | 536 | 32 | 0.06 | 0.6 | 0 | 0.29 |
| 1 cup chopped | | 3.3 | 0.1 | 0 | 0 | 0 | 0 | 961 | 58 | 3.95 | 0.285 | 1.6 | 10717 | 3.3 | 0.15 | 0.15 | 15.8 | 11148 |
| Swiss chard, raw | 36 | 7 | 33.4 | 1.3 | 0.4 | 0 | 0.6 | 77 | 18 | 29 | 0.13 | 0.132 | 110 | 11 | 0.01 | 0.1 | 0 | 0.06 |
| 1 cup | | 0.6 | 0.1 | 0 | 0 | 0 | 0 | 136 | 17 | 0.65 | 0.064 | 0.3 | 2202 | 0.7 | 0.03 | 0.04 | 5.0 | 11147 |
| taro leaves, steamed | 145 | 35 | 133.6 | 5.8 | | | 2.9 | 3 | 125 | 29 | 0.30 | 0.538 | 307 | 51 | 0.20 | 1.8 | 0 | 0.06 |
| 1 cup | | 3.9 | 0.6 | 0.1 | 0 | 0.2 | 0 | 667 | 39 | 1.71 | 0.203 | 1.3 | 6145 | | 0.55 | 0.10 | 69.6 | 11521 |
| turnip greens and root, frozen, boiled, drained - 1 cup | 163 | 57 | 148.4 | 7.9 | 1.7 | 0 | 5.1 | 31 | 209 | 39 | 0.60 | 0.652 | 703 | 30 | 0.08 | 0.8 | 0 | 0.14 |
| | | 4.9 | 0.6 | 0.1 | 0 | 0.3 | 0 | 352 | 52 | 2.85 | 0.217 | 1.8 | 14038 | 3.5 | 0.11 | 0.11 | 53.8 | 11577 |
| turnip greens, boiled, drained | 144 | 29 | 134.2 | 6.3 | 0.8 | 0 | 5.0 | 42 | 197 | 32 | 0.20 | 0.485 | 549 | 39 | 0.06 | 0.6 | 0 | 0.39 |
| 1 cup | | 1.6 | 0.3 | 0.1 | 0 | 0.1 | 0 | 292 | 42 | 1.15 | 0.364 | 1.3 | 10980 | 2.7 | 0.10 | 0.26 | 169.9 | 11569 |
| turnip greens, cnd, solids and liquid - 1 cup | 234 | 33 | 221.6 | 5.7 | | | 4.0 | 648 | 276 | 47 | 0.54 | 0.648 | 419 | 36 | 0.03 | 0.8 | 0 | 0.09 |
| | | 3.2 | 0.7 | 0.2 | 0 | 0.3 | 0 | 330 | 49 | 3.53 | 0.194 | 1.6 | 8391 | | 0.15 | 0.09 | 95.9 | 11570 |
| turnip greens, frozen | 164 | 36 | 152.4 | 6.0 | | | 4.1 | 20 | 194 | 44 | 0.28 | 0.605 | 507 | 44 | 0.07 | 0.6 | 0 | 0.23 |
| 1 cup | | 4.1 | 0.5 | 0.1 | 0 | 0.2 | 0 | 302 | 44 | 2.48 | 0.093 | 1.5 | 10142 | | 0.15 | 0.16 | 121.4 | 11574 |
| turnip greens, frzn, boiled, drained | 164 | 48 | 148.3 | 8.2 | 1.2 | 0 | 5.6 | 25 | 249 | 43 | 0.67 | 0.779 | 882 | 36 | 0.09 | 0.8 | 0 | 0.11 |
| 1 cup chopped | | 5.5 | 0.7 | 0.2 | 0 | 0.3 | 0 | 367 | 56 | 3.18 | 0.246 | 2.0 | 17655 | 4.4 | 0.12 | 0.11 | 64.0 | 11575 |
| turnip greens, raw | 55 | 18 | 49.3 | 3.9 | 0.4 | | 1.8 | 22 | 105 | 17 | 0.10 | 0.256 | 318 | 33 | 0.04 | 0.3 | 0 | 0.21 |
| 1 cup | | 0.8 | 0.2 | 0 | 0 | 0.1 | 0 | 163 | 23 | 0.61 | 0.192 | 0.7 | 6373 | 1.6 | 0.06 | 0.14 | 106.7 | 11568 |
| vinespinach, raw | 100 | 19 | 93.1 | 3.4 | | | | 24 | 109 | 65 | 0.43 | 0.735 | 400 | 102 | 0.05 | 0.5 | 0 | 0.05 |
| 3.5 oz | | 1.8 | 0.3 | | | | 0 | 510 | 52 | 1.20 | 0.107 | 0.8 | 8000 | | 0.16 | 0.24 | 140.0 | 11587 |
| watercress, raw | 34 | 4 | 32.3 | 0.4 | 0.1 | 0 | 0.2 | 14 | 41 | 7 | 0.04 | 0.083 | 54 | 15 | 0.03 | 0.1 | 0 | 0.11 |
| 1 cup | | 0.8 | 0 | 0 | 0 | 0 | 0 | 112 | 20 | 0.07 | 0.026 | 0.3 | 1085 | 0.3 | 0.04 | 0.04 | 3.1 | 11591 |
| winged bean leaves, raw | 100 | 74 | 76.8 | 14.1 | | | | 9 | 224 | 8 | 1.28 | 1.367 | 405 | 45 | 0.83 | 3.5 | 0 | 0.14 |
| 3.5 oz | | 5.8 | 1.1 | 0.3 | 0.3 | 0.2 | 0 | 176 | 63 | 4.00 | 0.456 | 0.9 | 8090 | | 0.60 | 0.23 | 16.0 | 11597 |

## 30.4 LEGUMES (BEANS AND PEAS)

| | WT (g) | KCAL / PRO (g) | H₂O (g) / FAT (g) | CHO (g) / SFA (g) | TSUG (g) / MUFA (g) | ASUG (g) / PUFA (g) | DFIB (g) / CHOL (mg) | Na (mg) / K (mg) | Ca (mg) / P (mg) | Mg (mg) / Fe (mg) | Zn (mg) / Cu (mg) | Mn (mg) / Se (mcg) | A (mcg RAE) / A (IU) | C (mg) / E (mg ATE) | B-1 (mg) / B-2 (mg) | NIA (mg) / B-6 (mg) | B-12 (mcg) / FOL (mcg DFE) | PANT (mg) / REF |
|---|---|---|---|---|---|---|---|---|---|---|---|---|---|---|---|---|---|---|
| adzuki beans, mature, boiled | 230 | 294 | 152.5 | 57.0 | | | 16.8 | 18 | 64 | 120 | 4.07 | 1.318 | 0 | 0 | 0.26 | 1.6 | 0 | 0.99 |
| 1 cup | | 17.3 | 0.2 | 0.1 | | | 0 | 1224 | 386 | 4.60 | 0.685 | 2.8 | 14 | | 0.15 | 0.22 | 278.3 | 16002 |
| adzuki beans, mature, dry | 99 | 326 | 13.3 | 62.3 | | | 12.6 | 5 | 65 | 126 | 4.99 | 1.713 | 1 | 0 | 0.45 | 2.6 | 0 | 1.46 |
| ½ cup | | 19.7 | 0.5 | 0.2 | | | 0 | 1241 | 377 | 4.93 | 1.083 | 3.1 | 17 | | 0.22 | 0.35 | 615.8 | 16001 |
| adzuki beans, mature, sweetened (yokan) - 1 slice | 14 | 36 | 5.0 | 8.5 | | | | 12 | 4 | 3 | 0.01 | 0.020 | 0 | 0 | 0 | 0 | 0 | 0.01 |
| | | 0.5 | 0 | 0 | | | 0 | 6 | 6 | 0.16 | 0.004 | 0.1 | 0 | | 0 | 0 | 1.1 | 16004 |
| adzuki beans, mature, sweetened (yokan), canned - 1 cup | 296 | 702 | 120.1 | 162.8 | | | | 645 | 65 | 92 | 4.62 | 1.492 | 0 | 0 | 0.30 | 1.9 | 0 | 1.12 |
| | | 11.2 | 0.1 | 0 | | | 0 | 352 | 219 | 3.34 | 0.784 | 9.5 | 15 | | 0.17 | 0.25 | 316.7 | 16003 |
| baked beans, homemade | 253 | 392 | 164.9 | 54.7 | | | 13.9 | 1068 | 154 | 109 | 1.85 | 0.645 | 0 | 3 | 0.34 | 1.0 | 0 | 0.39 |
| 1 cup | | 14.0 | 13.0 | 4.9 | 5.4 | 1.9 | 13 | 906 | 276 | 5.03 | 0.402 | 14.4 | 0 | | 0.12 | 0.23 | 121.4 | 16005 |
| baked beans, vegetarian, canned | 254 | 239 | 182.9 | 53.7 | 20.2 | 15.4 | 10.4 | 871 | 86 | 69 | 5.79 | 0.277 | 13 | 0 | 0.24 | 1.1 | 0 | 0.55 |
| 1 cup | | 12.1 | 0.9 | 0.2 | 0.2 | 0.3 | 0 | 569 | 188 | 3.02 | 0.368 | 12.7 | 274 | 0.4 | 0.10 | 0.21 | 30.5 | 16006 |
| baked beans with pork, canned | 253 | 268 | 180.8 | 50.6 | | | 13.9 | 1047 | 134 | 86 | 3.69 | 0.913 | 0 | 5 | 0.13 | 1.1 | 0 | 0.25 |
| 1 cup | | 13.1 | 3.9 | 1.5 | 1.7 | 0.5 | 18 | 782 | 273 | 4.30 | 0.544 | 11.9 | 0 | | 0.10 | 0.16 | 91.1 | 16009 |
| baked beans w/pork in sweet sce, cnd - 1 cup | 253 | 283 | 178.6 | 53.4 | 21.7 | 21.0 | 10.6 | 845 | 149 | 83 | 3.47 | 0.215 | 0 | 7 | 0.12 | 0.9 | 0 | 0.50 |
| | | 13.4 | 3.6 | 1.2 | 1.3 | 1.0 | 18 | 653 | 258 | 4.17 | 0.352 | 12.6 | 20 | 0.1 | 0.15 | 0.14 | 20.2 | 16010 |
| baked beans w/pork in tomato sce, cnd - 1 cup | 253 | 238 | 186.0 | 47.3 | 14.3 | 11.4 | 10.1 | 1106 | 142 | 86 | 13.86 | 0.764 | 10 | 8 | 0.13 | 1.2 | 0 | 0.99 |
| | | 13.0 | 2.4 | 0.7 | 0.7 | 0.4 | 18 | 746 | 293 | 8.20 | 0.539 | 11.9 | 213 | 0.3 | 0.12 | 0.16 | 37.9 | 16011 |

| Food | WT (g) | KCAL / PRO (g) | H₂O (g) / FAT (g) | CHO (g) / SFA (g) | TSUG (g) / MUFA (g) | ASUG (g) / PUFA (g) | DFIB (g) / CHOL (mg) | Na (mg) / K (mg) | Ca (mg) / P (mg) | Mg (mg) / Fe (mg) | Zn (mg) / Cu (mg) | Mn (mg) / Se (mcg) | A (mcg RAE) / A (IU) | C (mg) / E (mg ATE) | B-1 (mg) / B-2 (mg) | NIA (mg) / B-6 (mg) | B-12 (mcg) / FOL (mcg DFE) | PANT (mg) / REF |
|---|---|---|---|---|---|---|---|---|---|---|---|---|---|---|---|---|---|---|
| **bean dip**, Tres, Snyder | 30 | 25 | | 5.0 | 1.0 | | 1.0 | 150 | 0 | | | | 1 | 0 | | | | 0.42 |
| 2 T | | 1.0 | 0 | 0 | | | 0 | | | 0 | | | 1 | 0 | | | | SNYD14 |
| **black beans**, mature, boiled | 172 | 227 | 113.1 | 40.8 | | | 15.0 | 2 | 46 | 120 | 1.93 | 0.764 | 0 | 0 | 0.42 | 0.9 | 0 | 0.42 |
| 1 cup | | 15.2 | 0.9 | 0.2 | 0.1 | 0.4 | 0 | 611 | 241 | 3.61 | 0.359 | 2.1 | 10 | | 0.10 | 0.12 | 256.3 | 16015 |
| **black beans**, mature, dry | 97 | 331 | 10.7 | 60.5 | 2.1 | 0 | 14.7 | 5 | 119 | 166 | 3.54 | 1.028 | 0 | 0 | 0.87 | 1.9 | 0 | 0.87 |
| ½ cup | | 21.0 | 1.4 | 0.4 | 0.1 | 0.6 | 0 | 1439 | 341 | 4.87 | 0.816 | 3.1 | 0 | 0.2 | 0.19 | 0.28 | 430.7 | 16014 |
| **black turtle beans**, mature, boiled | 185 | 240 | 121.6 | 45.0 | 0.6 | 0 | 9.8 | 6 | 102 | 91 | 1.41 | 0.605 | 0 | 0 | 0.42 | 1.0 | 0 | 0.48 |
| 1 cup | | 15.1 | 0.6 | 0.2 | 0.1 | 0.3 | 0 | 801 | 281 | 5.27 | 0.498 | 2.2 | 0 | 1.6 | 0.10 | 0.14 | 159.1 | 16017 |
| **black turtle beans**, mature, canned - 1 cup | 240 | 218 | 181.5 | 39.7 | | | 16.6 | 922 | 84 | 84 | 1.30 | 0.559 | 0 | 6 | 0.34 | 1.5 | 0 | 0.44 |
| | | 14.5 | 0.7 | 0.2 | 0.1 | 0.3 | 0 | 739 | 259 | 4.56 | 0.461 | 3.1 | 10 | | 0.29 | 0.13 | 146.4 | 16018 |
| **broadbeans** (fava beans), immature, boiled, drained - 1 cup | 170 | 105 | 142.3 | 17.2 | | | 6.1 | 70 | 31 | 53 | 0.80 | 0.444 | 24 | 34 | 0.22 | 2.0 | 0 | 0.11 |
| | | 8.2 | 0.8 | 0.2 | | 0.5 | 0 | 328 | 124 | 2.55 | 0.102 | 1.7 | 459 | | 0.15 | 0.05 | 98.6 | 11089 |
| **broadbeans** (fava beans), immature, raw - 1 cup | 109 | 78 | 88.3 | 12.8 | | | 4.6 | 55 | 24 | 41 | 0.63 | 0.349 | 20 | 36 | 0.19 | 1.6 | 0 | 0.09 |
| | | 6.1 | 0.7 | 0.2 | | 0.3 | 0 | 272 | 104 | 2.07 | 0.081 | 1.3 | 382 | | 0.12 | 0.04 | 104.6 | 11088 |
| **broadbeans** (fava beans) in pod, immature, raw - 1 cup | 109 | 96 | 79.1 | 19.2 | | | | 27 | 40 | 36 | 1.09 | 0.720 | 19 | 4 | 0.14 | 2.5 | 0 | 0.25 |
| | | 8.6 | 0.8 | 0.1 | 0.1 | 0.4 | 0 | 362 | 141 | 1.69 | 0.438 | 0.9 | 363 | | 0.32 | 0.11 | 161.3 | 11973 |
| **broadbeans** (fava beans), mature, boiled - 1 cup | 170 | 187 | 121.6 | 33.4 | 3.1 | 0 | 9.2 | 8 | 61 | 73 | 1.72 | 0.716 | 2 | 1 | 0.16 | 1.2 | 0 | 0.27 |
| | | 12.9 | 0.7 | 0.1 | 0.1 | 0.3 | 0 | 456 | 212 | 2.55 | 0.440 | 4.4 | 26 | 0 | 0.15 | 0.12 | 176.8 | 16053 |
| **broadbeans** (fava beans), mature, canned - 1 cup | 256 | 182 | 205.6 | 31.8 | | | 9.5 | 1160 | 67 | 82 | 1.59 | 0.737 | 3 | 5 | 0.05 | 2.5 | 0 | 0.30 |
| | | 14.0 | 0.6 | 0.1 | 0.1 | 0.2 | 0 | 620 | 202 | 2.56 | 0.279 | 4.6 | 26 | | 0.13 | 0.12 | 84.5 | 16054 |
| **broadbeans** (fava beans), mature, dry - ½ cup | 75 | 256 | 8.2 | 43.7 | 4.3 | 0 | 18.8 | 10 | 77 | 144 | 2.36 | 1.220 | 2 | 1 | 0.42 | 2.1 | 0 | 0.73 |
| | | 19.6 | 1.1 | 0.2 | 0.2 | 0.5 | 0 | 796 | 316 | 5.03 | 0.618 | 6.1 | 40 | 0 | 0.25 | 0.27 | 317.2 | 16052 |
| **cannelloni beans**, canned, Goya | 122 | 80 | | 18.0 | 0 | | 7.0 | 390 | 40 | | | | | 0 | | | | |
| ½ cup | | 6.0 | 0 | 0 | | | 0 | | | 1.80 | | | 0 | | | | | GOYA1 |
| **chickpeas** (garbanzo beans), mature, boiled - 1 cup | 164 | 269 | 98.7 | 45.0 | 7.9 | 0 | 12.5 | 11 | 80 | 79 | 2.51 | 1.689 | 2 | 2 | 0.19 | 0.9 | 0 | 0.47 |
| | | 14.5 | 4.2 | 0.4 | 1.0 | 1.9 | 0 | 477 | 276 | 4.74 | 0.577 | 6.1 | 44 | 0.6 | 0.10 | 0.23 | 282.1 | 16057 |
| **chickpeas** (garbanzo beans), mature, canned - 1 cup | 240 | 286 | 167.3 | 54.3 | | | 10.6 | 718 | 77 | 70 | 2.54 | 1.450 | 2 | 9 | 0.07 | 0.3 | 0 | 0.72 |
| | | 11.9 | 2.7 | 0.3 | 0.6 | 1.2 | 0 | 413 | 216 | 3.24 | 0.418 | 6.7 | 50 | | 0.08 | 1.14 | 160.8 | 16058 |
| **chickpeas** (garbanzo beans), mature, dry - ½ cup | 100 | 364 | 11.5 | 60.6 | 10.7 | 0 | 17.4 | 24 | 105 | 115 | 3.43 | 2.204 | 3 | 4 | 0.48 | 1.5 | 0 | 1.59 |
| | | 19.3 | 6.0 | 0.6 | 1.4 | 2.7 | 0 | 875 | 366 | 6.24 | 0.847 | 8.2 | 67 | 0.8 | 0.21 | 0.54 | 557.0 | 16056 |
| **chili beans**, barbecue ranch style | 253 | 245 | 191.0 | 42.8 | 13.3 | 9.3 | 10.6 | 1834 | 78 | 114 | 5.06 | | 3 | 4 | 0.10 | 0.9 | | 0.03 |
| 1 cup | | 12.6 | 2.5 | 0.4 | 0.2 | 1.4 | 0 | 1138 | 390 | 4.71 | 0.638 | 3.3 | 30 | 0.5 | 0.38 | 0.68 | 65.8 | 43112 |
| **cowpeas** (blackeyed peas), immature, boiled, drained - 1 cup | 165 | 160 | 124.5 | 33.5 | 5.3 | 0 | 8.2 | 7 | 211 | 86 | 1.70 | 0.944 | 66 | 4 | 0.17 | 2.3 | 0 | 0.25 |
| | | 5.2 | 0.6 | 0.2 | 0.1 | 0.3 | 0 | 690 | 84 | 1.85 | 0.219 | 4.1 | 1305 | 0.4 | 0.24 | 0.11 | 209.6 | 11192 |
| **cowpeas** (blackeyed peas), immature, frozen - 1 cup | 160 | 222 | 102.6 | 40.2 | | | 8.0 | 10 | 42 | 88 | 2.53 | 1.410 | 6 | 6 | 0.39 | 1.3 | 0 | 0.38 |
| | | 14.4 | 1.1 | 0.3 | 0.1 | 0.5 | 0 | 706 | 195 | 3.76 | 0.328 | 5.8 | 134 | | 0.11 | 0.17 | 299.2 | 11195 |
| **cowpeas** (blackeyed peas), immature, frzn, boiled, drained - 1 cup | 170 | 224 | 112.4 | 40.4 | 7.6 | 0 | 10.9 | 8 | 39 | 85 | 2.41 | 1.345 | 7 | 4 | 0.44 | 1.2 | 0 | 0.36 |
| | | 14.4 | 1.1 | 0.3 | 0.1 | 0.5 | 0 | 638 | 207 | 3.60 | 0.313 | 5.8 | 128 | 0.5 | 0.11 | 0.16 | 239.7 | 11196 |
| **cowpeas** (blackeyed peas), immature, raw - 1 cup | 168 | 151 | 129.7 | 31.6 | 5.0 | 0 | 8.4 | 7 | 212 | 86 | 1.70 | 0.941 | 69 | 4 | 0.18 | 2.4 | 0 | 0.25 |
| | | 5.0 | 0.6 | 0.2 | 0.1 | 0.3 | 0 | 724 | 89 | 1.85 | 0.218 | 3.9 | 1373 | | 0.24 | 0.11 | 282.2 | 11191 |
| **cowpeas** (blackeyed peas), mature, boiled - 1 cup | 172 | 200 | 120.5 | 35.7 | 5.7 | 0 | 11.2 | 7 | 41 | 91 | 2.22 | 0.817 | 2 | 1 | 0.35 | 0.9 | 0 | 0.71 |
| | | 13.3 | 0.9 | 0.2 | 0.1 | 0.4 | 0 | 478 | 268 | 4.32 | 0.461 | 4.3 | 26 | 0.5 | 0.09 | 0.17 | 357.8 | 16063 |
| **cowpeas** (blackeyed peas), mature, canned - 1 cup | 240 | 185 | 191.1 | 32.7 | | | 7.9 | 718 | 48 | 67 | 1.68 | 0.679 | 2 | 6 | 0.18 | 0.8 | 0 | 0.46 |
| | | 11.4 | 1.3 | 0.3 | 0.1 | 0.6 | 0 | 413 | 168 | 2.33 | 0.281 | 5.5 | 31 | | 0.18 | 0.11 | 122.4 | 16064 |
| **cowpeas** (blackeyed peas), mature, dry - ½ cup | 84 | 282 | 10.0 | 50.4 | 5.8 | 0 | 8.9 | 13 | 92 | 155 | 2.83 | 1.284 | 3 | 1 | 0.72 | 1.7 | 0 | 1.26 |
| | | 19.8 | 1.1 | 0.3 | 0.1 | 0.5 | 0 | 934 | 356 | 6.95 | 0.710 | 7.6 | 42 | 0.3 | 0.19 | 0.30 | 531.7 | 16062 |
| **cowpeas** (blackeyed peas) with pork, canned - 1 cup | 240 | 199 | 186.2 | 39.7 | | | 7.9 | 840 | 41 | 103 | 2.50 | 0.941 | 0 | 0 | 0.15 | 1.0 | 0 | 0.46 |
| | | 6.6 | 3.8 | 1.5 | 1.6 | 0.5 | 17 | 427 | 230 | 3.41 | 0.408 | 5.5 | 0 | | 0.12 | 0.11 | 122.4 | 16065 |
| **cowpeas** (blackeyed peas), young pods/seeds, boiled, drained 1 cup | 95 | 32 | 85.0 | 6.6 | | | | 3 | 52 | 39 | 0.23 | 0.208 | 66 | 16 | 0.09 | 0.8 | 0 | 0.61 |
| | | 2.5 | 0.3 | 0.1 | 0 | 0.1 | 0 | 186 | 47 | 0.66 | 0.067 | 0.7 | 1330 | | 0.09 | 0.12 | 24.7 | 11198 |
| **cowpeas, catjang**, mature, boiled | 171 | 200 | 119.2 | 34.7 | | | 6.2 | 32 | 44 | 164 | 3.20 | 0.809 | 2 | 1 | 0.28 | 1.2 | 0 | 0.66 |
| 1 cup | | 13.9 | 1.2 | 0.3 | 0.1 | 0.6 | 0 | 641 | 243 | 5.22 | 0.463 | 4.3 | 17 | | 0.08 | 0.16 | 242.8 | 16061 |
| **cranberry beans** (Roman beans), mature, boiled - 1 cup | 177 | 241 | 114.4 | 43.3 | | | 17.7 | 2 | 88 | 88 | 2.02 | 0.655 | 0 | 0 | 0.37 | 0.9 | 0 | 0.42 |
| | | 16.5 | 0.8 | 0.2 | 0.1 | 0.4 | 0 | 685 | 239 | 3.70 | 0.409 | 2.3 | 0 | | 0.12 | 0.14 | 366.4 | 16020 |
| **cranberry beans** (Roman beans), mature, canned - 1 cup | 260 | 216 | 201.7 | 39.3 | | | 16.4 | 863 | 88 | 83 | 2.18 | 0.520 | 0 | 2 | 0.10 | 1.3 | 0 | 0.37 |
| | | 14.4 | 0.7 | 0.2 | 0.1 | 0.3 | 0 | 676 | 224 | 4.03 | 0.369 | 8.1 | 0 | | 0.10 | 0.14 | 200.2 | 16021 |
| **falafel**, from mature broadbeans, homemade - .6 oz patty (2¼" dia) | 17 | 57 | 5.9 | 5.4 | | | | 50 | 9 | 14 | 0.26 | 0.117 | 0 | 0 | 0.02 | 0.2 | 0 | 0.05 |
| | | 2.3 | 3.0 | 0.4 | 1.7 | 0.7 | 0 | 99 | 33 | 0.58 | 0.044 | 0.2 | 2 | | 0.03 | 0.02 | 17.7 | 16138 |
| **French beans**, mature, boiled | 177 | 228 | 117.8 | 42.5 | | | 16.6 | 11 | 112 | 99 | 1.13 | 0.676 | 0 | 2 | 0.23 | 1.0 | 0 | 0.39 |
| 1 cup | | 12.5 | 1.3 | 0.1 | 0.1 | 0.8 | 0 | 655 | 181 | 1.91 | 0.204 | 2.1 | 5 | | 0.11 | 0.19 | 132.8 | 16023 |

| | WT (g) | KCAL | H₂0 (g) | CHO (g) | TSUG (g) | ASUG (g) | DFIB (g) | Na (mg) | Ca (mg) | Mg (mg) | Zn (mg) | Mn (mg) | A (mcg RAE) | C (mg) | B-1 (mg) | NIA (mg) | B-12 (mcg) | PANT (mg) |
|---|---|---|---|---|---|---|---|---|---|---|---|---|---|---|---|---|---|---|
| | | PRO (g) | FAT (g) | SFA (g) | MUFA (g) | PUFA (g) | CHOL (mg) | K (mg) | P (mg) | Fe (mg) | Cu (mg) | Se (mcg) | A (IU) | E (mg ATE) | B-2 (mg) | B-6 (mg) | FOL (mcg DFE) | REF |
| **great northern beans**, mature, | 177 | 209 | 122.1 | 37.3 | | | 12.4 | 4 | 120 | 88 | 1.56 | 0.917 | 0 | 2 | 0.28 | 1.2 | 0 | 0.47 |
| boiled - *1 cup* | | 14.7 | 0.8 | 0.2 | 0 | 0.3 | 0 | 692 | 292 | 3.77 | 0.437 | 7.3 | 2 | | 0.10 | 0.21 | 180.5 | 16025 |
| **great northern beans**, mature, cnd | 262 | 299 | 183.1 | 55.1 | | | 12.8 | 10 | 139 | 134 | 1.70 | 1.069 | 0 | 3 | 0.37 | 1.2 | 0 | 0.73 |
| *1 cup* | | 19.3 | 1.0 | 0.3 | 0 | 0.4 | 0 | 920 | 356 | 4.11 | 0.419 | 10.7 | 0 | | 0.16 | 0.28 | 212.2 | 16026 |
| **great northern beans**, mature, dry | 92 | 312 | 9.8 | 57.4 | 2.1 | | 18.6 | 13 | 161 | 174 | 2.13 | 1.309 | 0 | 5 | 0.60 | 1.8 | 0 | 1.01 |
| *½ cup* | | 20.1 | 1.0 | 0.3 | 0 | 0.4 | 0 | 1276 | 411 | 5.03 | 0.770 | 11.9 | 0 | 0.2 | 0.22 | 0.41 | 443.4 | 16024 |
| **green peas**, boiled, drained | 160 | 134 | 124.6 | 25.0 | 9.5 | 0 | 8.8 | 5 | 43 | 62 | 1.90 | 0.840 | 64 | 23 | 0.41 | 3.2 | 0 | 0.24 |
| *1 cup* | | 8.6 | 0.4 | 0.1 | 0 | 0.2 | 0 | 434 | 187 | 2.46 | 0.277 | 3.0 | 1282 | 0.2 | 0.24 | 0.35 | 100.8 | 11305 |
| **green peas**, canned, drained | 170 | 117 | 140.1 | 19.3 | 5.1 | 0 | 8.3 | 495 | 39 | 31 | 1.07 | 0.362 | 73 | 16 | 0.22 | 1.7 | 0 | 0.41 |
| *1 cup* | | 7.6 | 1.1 | 0.1 | 0.1 | 0.3 | 0 | 175 | 117 | 2.07 | 0.178 | 2.9 | 1470 | 0.6 | 0.11 | 0.10 | 57.8 | 11308 |
| **green peas**, frozen | 144 | 111 | 115.2 | 19.6 | 7.2 | 0 | 6.5 | 156 | 32 | 37 | 1.18 | 0.484 | 148 | 26 | 0.37 | 2.5 | 0 | 0.79 |
| *1 cup* | | 7.5 | 0.6 | 0.1 | 0 | 0.3 | 0 | 220 | 118 | 2.20 | 0.179 | 2.7 | 2964 | 0 | 0.14 | 0.12 | 76.3 | 11312 |
| **green peas**, frozen, boiled, drained | 160 | 125 | 127.2 | 22.8 | 7.4 | 0 | 8.8 | 115 | 38 | 35 | 1.07 | 0.446 | 168 | 16 | 0.45 | 2.4 | 0 | 0.23 |
| *1 cup* | | 8.2 | 0.4 | 0.1 | 0 | 0.2 | 0 | 176 | 123 | 2.43 | 0.168 | 1.6 | 3360 | 0 | 0.16 | 0.18 | 94.4 | 11313 |
| **green peas**, raw | 145 | 117 | 114.3 | 21.0 | 8.2 | 0 | 7.4 | 7 | 36 | 48 | 1.80 | 0.594 | 55 | 58 | 0.39 | 3.0 | 0 | 0.15 |
| *1 cup* | | 7.9 | 0.6 | 0.1 | 0.1 | 0.3 | 0 | 354 | 157 | 2.13 | 0.255 | 2.6 | 1109 | 0.2 | 0.19 | 0.25 | 94.2 | 11304 |
| **green peas** w/onions, red peppers, garlic, cnd, solids & liquid | 228 | 114 | 197.2 | 21.1 | | | 4.6 | 579 | 34 | 34 | 1.48 | 0.611 | 50 | 26 | 0.22 | 1.6 | 0 | 0.20 |
| *1 cup* | | 7.0 | 0.6 | 0.1 | 0.1 | 0.3 | 0 | 278 | 123 | 2.74 | 0.226 | 3.0 | 987 | | 0.16 | 0.22 | 66.1 | 11310 |
| **hummus** from chickpeas | 14 | 23 | 9.3 | 2.0 | | | 0.8 | 53 | 5 | 10 | 0.26 | 0.108 | | 0 | 0.03 | 0.1 | 0 | 0.02 |
| *1 T* | | 1.1 | 1.3 | 0.2 | 0.6 | 0.5 | 0 | 32 | 25 | 0.34 | 0.074 | 0.4 | 4 | | 0.01 | 0.03 | 11.6 | 16158 |
| **hummus** from chickpeas, homemade - *1 T* | 15 | 27 | 9.7 | 3.0 | 0 | 0 | 0.6 | 36 | 7 | 4 | 0.16 | 0.085 | 0 | 1 | 0.01 | 0.1 | 0 | 0.04 |
| | | 0.7 | 1.3 | 0.2 | 0.7 | 0.3 | 0 | 26 | 16 | 0.23 | 0.034 | 0.4 | 1 | 0.1 | 0.01 | 0.06 | 8.8 | 16137 |
| **hyacinth beans**, immature, boiled, drained - *1 cup* | 87 | 44 | 75.6 | 8.0 | | | 0 | 2 | 36 | 37 | 0.33 | 0.183 | 6 | 4 | 0.05 | 0.4 | 0 | 0.05 |
| | | 2.6 | 0.2 | 0.1 | 0.1 | 0 | 0 | 228 | 43 | 0.66 | 0.042 | 1.4 | 124 | | 0.08 | 0.02 | 40.9 | 11225 |
| **hyacinth beans**, mature, boiled | 194 | 227 | 134.1 | 40.2 | | | | 14 | 78 | 159 | 5.53 | 0.935 | 0 | 0 | 0.52 | 0.8 | 0 | 0.61 |
| *1 cup* | | 15.8 | 1.1 | 0.2 | | | 0 | 654 | 233 | 8.89 | 0.662 | 5.4 | 0 | | 0.07 | 0.07 | 7.8 | 16068 |
| **kidney beans**, all types, mature, boiled - *1 cup* | 176 | 224 | 117.8 | 40.1 | 0.6 | 0 | 11.3 | 2 | 62 | 74 | 1.76 | 0.757 | 0 | 2 | 0.28 | 1.0 | 0 | 0.39 |
| | | 15.3 | 0.9 | 0.1 | 0.1 | 0.5 | 0 | 713 | 243 | 3.91 | 0.380 | 1.9 | 0 | 0.1 | 0.10 | 0.21 | 228.8 | 16028 |
| **kidney beans**, all types, mature, cnd - *1 cup* | 256 | 215 | 199.8 | 37.1 | 4.7 | 0 | 13.6 | 758 | 87 | 69 | 1.18 | 0.430 | 0 | 3 | 0.30 | 1.1 | 0 | 0.35 |
| | | 13.4 | 1.5 | 0.4 | 1.0 | 0.7 | 0 | 607 | 230 | 3.00 | 0.346 | 2.3 | 0 | 0.1 | 0.13 | 0.19 | 92.2 | 16029 |
| **kidney beans**, all types, mature, dry - *½ cup* | 92 | 306 | 10.8 | 55.2 | 2.1 | 0 | 22.9 | 22 | 132 | 129 | 2.57 | 0.939 | 0 | 4 | 0.49 | 1.9 | 0 | 0.72 |
| | | 21.7 | 0.8 | 0.1 | 0.1 | 0.4 | 0 | 1294 | 374 | 7.54 | 0.881 | 2.9 | 0 | 0.2 | 0.20 | 0.37 | 362.5 | 16027 |
| **kidney beans**, California red, mature, boiled - *1 cup* | 256 | 317 | 171.3 | 57.4 | | | 23.8 | 10 | 169 | 123 | 2.20 | 0.814 | 0 | 3 | 0.33 | 1.4 | 0 | 0.56 |
| | | 23.4 | 0.2 | 0 | 0 | 0.1 | 0 | 1073 | 351 | 7.63 | 0.740 | 3.1 | 8 | | 0.16 | 0.27 | 189.4 | 16031 |
| **kidney beans**, red, mature, boiled | 177 | 225 | 118.5 | 40.4 | 0.6 | 0 | 13.1 | 4 | 50 | 80 | 1.89 | 0.844 | 0 | 2 | 0.28 | 1.0 | 0 | 0.39 |
| *1 cup* | | 15.3 | 0.9 | 0.1 | 0.1 | 0.5 | 0 | 713 | 251 | 5.20 | 0.428 | 2.1 | 0 | 0.1 | 0.10 | 0.21 | 230.1 | 16033 |
| **kidney beans**, red, mature, canned | 256 | 215 | 198.1 | 39.8 | 4.8 | 0 | 13.8 | 660 | 64 | 72 | 4.20 | 0.397 | 0 | 3 | 0.27 | 1.1 | 0 | 0.35 |
| *1 cup* | | 13.5 | 0.9 | 0.2 | 0.4 | 0.4 | 0 | 655 | 233 | 3.25 | 0.358 | 1.3 | 0 | 0.1 | 0.22 | 0.20 | 51.2 | 16034 |
| **kidney beans**, red, mature, dry | 92 | 310 | 10.8 | 56.4 | 1.9 | 0 | 14.0 | 11 | 76 | 127 | 2.57 | 1.022 | 0 | 4 | 0.56 | 1.9 | 0 | 0.72 |
| *½ cup* | | 20.7 | 1.0 | 0.1 | 0.1 | 0.5 | 0 | 1250 | 374 | 6.15 | 0.643 | 2.9 | 0 | 0.2 | 0.20 | 0.37 | 362.5 | 16032 |
| **kidney beans**, royal red, mature, boiled - *1 cup* | 177 | 218 | 118.6 | 38.7 | | | 16.5 | 9 | 78 | 74 | 1.59 | 0.451 | 0 | 2 | 0.17 | 1.0 | 0 | 0.39 |
| | | 16.8 | 0.3 | 0 | 0 | 0.2 | 0 | 669 | 251 | 4.90 | 0.464 | 2.1 | 5 | | 0.12 | 0.18 | 131.0 | 16036 |
| **lentils**, mature, boiled | 198 | 230 | 137.9 | 39.9 | 3.6 | 0 | 15.6 | 4 | 38 | 71 | 2.51 | 0.978 | 0 | 3 | 0.33 | 2.1 | 0 | 1.26 |
| *1 cup* | | 17.9 | 0.8 | 0.1 | 0.1 | 0.3 | 0 | 731 | 356 | 6.59 | 0.497 | 5.5 | 16 | 0.2 | 0.14 | 0.35 | 358.4 | 16070 |
| **lentils**, mature, dry | 96 | 339 | 10.0 | 57.7 | 1.9 | 0 | 29.3 | 6 | 54 | 117 | 4.59 | 1.277 | 2 | 4 | 0.84 | 2.5 | 0 | 2.05 |
| *½ cup* | | 24.8 | 1.0 | 0.1 | 0.2 | 0.5 | 0 | 917 | 433 | 7.24 | 0.498 | 8.0 | 37 | 0.5 | 0.20 | 0.52 | 459.8 | 16069 |
| **lentils**, pink, mature, dry | 96 | 331 | 11.3 | 56.8 | | | 10.4 | 7 | 39 | 69 | 3.74 | 1.360 | 3 | 2 | 0.49 | 1.4 | 0 | 0.33 |
| *½ cup* | | 24.0 | 2.1 | 0.4 | 0.5 | 1.1 | 0 | 555 | 282 | 7.26 | 1.251 | 7.9 | 56 | | 0.10 | 0.39 | 195.8 | 16144 |
| **lima beans**, immature, baby, frozen, boiled, drained - *1 cup* | 180 | 189 | 130.2 | 35.0 | 2.5 | 0 | 10.8 | 52 | 50 | 101 | 0.99 | 1.463 | 14 | 10 | 0.13 | 1.4 | 0 | 0.32 |
| | | 12.0 | 0.5 | 0.1 | 0 | 0.3 | 0 | 740 | 202 | 3.53 | 0.355 | 3.1 | 301 | 1.2 | 0.10 | 0.21 | 28.8 | 11040 |
| **lima beans**, immature, baby green, frzn - *1 cup* | 164 | 216 | 107.4 | 41.2 | | | 9.8 | 85 | 57 | 82 | 1.03 | 1.151 | 15 | 14 | 0.19 | 1.7 | 0 | 0.31 |
| | | 12.4 | 0.7 | 0.2 | 0 | 0.4 | 0 | 741 | 171 | 3.62 | 0.210 | 3.4 | 310 | | 0.12 | 0.26 | 45.9 | 11039 |
| **lima beans**, immature, boiled, drained - *1 cup* | 170 | 209 | 114.2 | 40.2 | 2.8 | 0 | 9.0 | 29 | 54 | 126 | 1.34 | 2.128 | 26 | 17 | 0.24 | 1.8 | 0 | 0.44 |
| | | 11.6 | 0.5 | 0.1 | 0 | 0.3 | 0 | 969 | 221 | 4.16 | 0.518 | 3.4 | 515 | 0.4 | 0.10 | 0.33 | 44.2 | 11032 |
| **lima beans**, immature, green, cnd, solids and liquid - *1 cup* | 248 | 176 | 201.3 | 33.1 | 2.3 | 0 | 8.9 | 10 | 69 | 84 | 1.59 | 1.736 | 20 | 22 | 0.07 | 1.3 | 0 | 0.24 |
| | | 10.1 | 0.7 | 0.2 | 0 | 0.3 | 0 | 707 | 176 | 3.99 | 0.402 | 2.7 | 372 | 0.7 | 0.11 | 0.15 | 39.7 | 11715 |
| **lima beans**, immature, green Fordhook, frozen, boiled, drained - *1 cup* | 170 | 175 | 124.1 | 32.8 | 2.3 | 0 | 9.9 | 117 | 51 | 71 | 1.26 | 1.102 | 17 | 22 | 0.13 | 1.8 | 0 | 0.28 |
| | | 10.3 | 0.6 | 0.1 | 0 | 0.3 | 0 | 517 | 165 | 3.09 | 0.289 | 1.0 | 323 | 0.5 | 0.10 | 0.21 | 35.7 | 11038 |
| **lima beans**, mature, baby, boiled | 182 | 229 | 122.2 | 42.4 | | | 14.0 | 5 | 53 | 96 | 1.87 | 1.065 | 0 | 0 | 0.29 | 1.2 | 0 | 0.86 |
| *1 cup* | | 14.6 | 0.7 | 0.2 | 0.1 | 0.3 | 0 | 730 | 231 | 4.37 | 0.391 | 8.9 | 0 | | 0.10 | 0.14 | 273.0 | 16075 |

In each food entry the first data row carries the top header labels (KCAL, $H_2O$, CHO, TSUG, ASUG, DFIB, Na, Ca, Mg, Zn, Mn, A (mcg RAE), C, B-1, NIA, B-12, PANT) and the second row carries the lower header labels (PRO, FAT, SFA, MUFA, PUFA, CHOL, K, P, Fe, Cu, Se, A (IU), E (mg ATE), B-2, B-6, FOL, REF).

| Food | WT (g) | KCAL / PRO | $H_2O$ / FAT | CHO / SFA | TSUG / MUFA | ASUG / PUFA | DFIB / CHOL | Na / K | Ca / P | Mg / Fe | Zn / Cu | Mn / Se | A RAE / A IU | C / E | B-1 / B-2 | NIA / B-6 | B-12 / FOL | PANT / REF |
|---|---|---|---|---|---|---|---|---|---|---|---|---|---|---|---|---|---|---|
| **lima beans**, mature, baby, dry | 101 | 338 | 12.2 | 63.5 | 8.4 |  | 20.8 | 13 | 82 | 190 | 2.63 | 1.703 | 0 | 0 | 0.58 | 1.7 | 0 | 1.28 |
| ½ cup |  | 20.8 | 0.9 | 0.2 | 0.1 | 0.4 | 0 | 1417 | 374 | 6.25 | 0.672 | 7.1 | 0 | 0.7 | 0.22 | 0.33 | 404.0 | 16074 |
| **lima beans**, mature, large, boiled | 184 | 212 | 128.4 | 38.4 | 5.3 | 0 | 12.9 | 4 | 31 | 79 | 1.75 | 0.949 | 0 | 0 | 0.30 | 0.8 | 0 | 0.78 |
| 1 cup |  | 14.4 | 0.7 | 0.2 | 0.1 | 0.3 | 0 | 935 | 204 | 4.40 | 0.432 | 8.3 | 0 | 0.3 | 0.10 | 0.30 | 152.7 | 16072 |
| **lima beans**, mature, large, canned | 241 | 190 | 185.8 | 35.9 |  |  | 11.6 | 810 | 51 | 94 | 1.57 | 0.875 | 0 | 0 | 0.13 | 0.6 | 0 | 0.62 |
| 1 cup |  | 11.9 | 0.4 | 0.1 | 0 | 0.2 | 0 | 530 | 178 | 4.36 | 0.434 | 10.8 | 0 |  | 0.08 | 0.22 | 120.5 | 16073 |
| **lima beans**, mature, large, dry | 89 | 301 | 9.1 | 56.4 | 7.6 | 0 | 16.9 | 16 | 72 | 199 | 2.52 | 1.488 | 0 | 0 | 0.45 | 1.4 | 0 | 1.21 |
| ½ cup |  | 19.1 | 0.6 | 0.1 | 0.1 | 0.3 | 0 | 1534 | 343 | 6.68 | 0.659 | 6.4 | 0 | 0.6 | 0.18 | 0.46 | 351.6 | 16071 |
| **lupins**, mature, boiled | 166 | 198 | 118.0 | 16.4 |  |  | 4.6 | 7 | 85 | 90 | 2.29 | 1.122 | 0 | 2 | 0.22 | 0.8 | 0 | 0.31 |
| 1 cup |  | 25.8 | 4.8 | 0.6 | 2.0 | 1.2 | 0 | 407 | 212 | 1.99 | 0.383 | 4.3 | 12 |  | 0.09 | 0.01 | 97.9 | 16077 |
| **lupins**, mature, dry | 83 | 308 | 8.7 | 33.5 |  |  |  | 12 | 146 | 164 | 3.94 | 1.977 | 1 | 4 | 0.53 | 1.8 | 0 | 0.62 |
| ½ cup |  | 30.0 | 8.1 | 1.0 | 3.3 | 2.0 | 0 | 841 | 365 | 3.62 | 0.848 | 6.8 | 19 |  | 0.18 | 0.30 | 294.6 | 16076 |
| **mothbeans**, mature, boiled | 177 | 207 | 122.5 | 37.1 |  |  |  | 18 | 5 | 184 | 1.04 | 0.933 | 2 | 2 | 0.22 | 1.2 | 0 | 0.69 |
| 1 cup |  | 13.8 | 1.0 | 0.2 | 0.1 | 0.5 | 0 | 538 | 266 | 5.56 | 0.290 | 5.0 | 18 |  | 0.04 | 0.16 | 253.1 | 16079 |
| **mung beans**, mature, boiled | 202 | 212 | 146.8 | 38.7 | 4.0 | 0 | 15.4 | 4 | 55 | 97 | 1.70 | 0.602 |  |  | 0.33 | 1.2 | 0 | 0.83 |
| 1 cup |  | 14.2 | 0.8 | 0.2 | 0.1 | 0.3 | 0 | 537 | 200 | 2.83 | 0.315 | 5.0 | 48 | 0.3 | 0.12 | 0.14 | 321.2 | 16081 |
| **mung beans**, mature, dry | 103 | 357 | 9.3 | 64.5 | 6.8 | 0 | 16.8 | 15 | 136 | 195 | 2.76 | 1.066 | 6 | 5 | 0.64 | 2.3 | 0 | 1.97 |
| ½ cup |  | 24.6 | 1.2 | 0.4 | 0.2 | 0.4 | 0 | 1283 | 378 | 6.94 | 0.969 | 8.4 | 117 | 0.5 | 0.24 | 0.39 | 643.8 | 16080 |
| **mungo beans**, mature, boiled | 180 | 189 | 130.5 | 33.0 | 3.6 | 0 | 11.5 | 13 | 95 | 113 | 1.49 | 0.742 | 4 | 2 | 0.27 | 2.7 | 0 | 0.78 |
| 1 cup |  | 13.6 | 1.0 | 0.1 | 0.1 | 0.6 | 0 | 416 | 281 | 3.15 | 0.250 | 4.5 | 56 | 0.3 | 0.14 | 0.10 | 169.2 | 16084 |
| **mungo beans**, mature, dry | 103 | 351 | 11.1 | 60.8 |  |  | 18.8 | 39 | 142 | 275 | 3.45 | 1.573 | 1 | 0 | 0.28 | 1.5 | 0 | 0.93 |
| ½ cup |  | 26.0 | 1.7 | 0.1 | 0.1 | 1.1 | 0 | 1012 | 390 | 7.80 | 1.010 | 8.4 | 24 |  | 0.26 | 0.29 | 222.5 | 16083 |
| **navy beans**, mature, boiled | 182 | 255 | 116.1 | 47.4 | 0.7 |  | 19.1 | 0 | 126 | 96 | 1.87 | 0.959 | 0 | 2 | 0.43 | 1.2 | 0 | 0.48 |
| 1 cup |  | 15.0 | 1.1 | 0.2 | 0.3 | 0.9 |  | 708 | 262 | 4.30 | 0.382 | 5.3 | 0 | 0 | 0.12 | 0.25 | 254.8 | 16038 |
| **navy beans**, mature, canned | 262 | 296 | 184.6 | 53.6 | 0.7 | 0 | 13.4 | 1174 | 123 | 123 | 2.02 | 0.982 | 0 | 2 | 0.37 | 1.3 | 0 | 0.45 |
| 1 cup |  | 19.7 | 1.1 | 0.3 | 0.1 | 0.5 | 0 | 755 | 351 | 4.85 | 0.545 | 15.2 | 0 | 2.0 | 0.14 | 0.27 | 162.4 | 16039 |
| **navy beans**, mature, dry | 104 | 350 | 12.6 | 63.2 | 4.0 | 0 | 25.4 | 5 | 153 | 182 | 3.80 | 1.475 | 0 | 0 | 0.81 | 2.3 | 0 | 0.77 |
| ½ cup |  | 23.2 | 1.6 | 0.3 | 0.3 | 1.5 | 0 | 1232 | 423 | 5.71 | 0.867 | 11.4 | 0 | 0 | 0.17 | 0.45 | 378.6 | 16037 |
| **peas, split**, mature, boiled | 196 | 231 | 136.2 | 41.4 | 5.7 | 0 | 16.3 | 4 | 27 | 71 | 1.96 | 0.776 | 0 | 1 | 0.37 | 1.7 | 0 | 1.17 |
| 1 cup |  | 16.3 | 0.8 | 0.1 | 0.2 | 0.3 | 0 | 710 | 194 | 2.53 | 0.355 | 1.2 | 14 | 0.1 | 0.11 | 0.09 | 127.4 | 16086 |
| **peas, split**, yellow and green, | 98 | 334 | 11.0 | 59.2 | 7.8 | 0 | 25.0 | 15 | 54 | 113 | 2.95 | 1.363 | 7 | 2 | 0.71 | 2.8 | 0 | 1.72 |
| mature, dry - ½ cup |  | 24.1 | 1.1 | 0.2 | 0.2 | 0.5 | 0 | 961 | 359 | 4.34 | 0.849 | 1.6 | 146 | 0.1 | 0.21 | 0.17 | 268.5 | 16085 |
| **pigeon peas**, immature, boiled, | 153 | 170 | 109.9 | 29.8 | 3.8 | 0 | 9.5 | 8 | 63 | 61 | 1.25 | 0.690 | 3 | 43 | 0.54 | 3.3 | 0 | 0.96 |
| drained - 1 cup |  | 9.1 | 2.1 | 0.2 | 0 | 1.8 | 0 | 698 | 181 | 2.40 | 0.161 | 1.8 | 76 | 0.5 | 0.25 | 0.08 | 153.0 | 11345 |
| **pigeon peas**, mature, boiled | 168 | 203 | 115.2 | 39.1 |  |  | 11.3 | 8 | 72 | 77 | 1.51 | 0.842 | 0 | 0 | 0.25 | 1.3 | 0 | 0.54 |
| 1 cup |  | 11.4 | 0.6 | 0.1 | 0 | 0.3 | 0 | 645 | 200 | 1.86 | 0.452 | 4.9 | 5 |  | 0.10 | 0.08 | 186.5 | 16102 |
| **pigeon peas**, mature, dry | 103 | 353 | 10.9 | 64.7 |  |  | 15.4 | 18 | 134 | 188 | 2.84 | 1.845 | 1 | 0 | 0.66 | 3.1 | 0 | 1.30 |
| ½ cup |  | 22.4 | 1.5 | 0.3 | 0 | 0.8 | 0 | 1434 | 378 | 5.39 | 1.089 | 8.4 | 29 |  | 0.19 | 0.29 | 469.7 | 16101 |
| **pink beans**, mature, boiled | 169 | 252 | 103.4 | 47.2 | 0.6 | 0 | 9.0 | 3 | 88 | 110 | 1.62 | 0.926 | 0 | 0 | 0.43 | 1.0 | 0 | 0.51 |
| 1 cup |  | 15.3 | 0.8 | 0.2 | 0.1 | 0.4 | 0 | 859 | 279 | 3.89 | 0.458 | 2.4 | 0 | 1.7 | 0.11 | 0.30 | 283.9 | 16041 |
| **pink beans**, mature, dry | 105 | 360 | 10.6 | 67.4 | 2.2 | 0 | 13.3 | 8 | 136 | 191 | 2.68 | 1.445 | 0 | 0 | 0.81 | 2.0 | 0 | 1.05 |
| ½ cup |  | 22.0 | 1.2 | 0.1 | 0.1 | 0.5 | 0 | 1537 | 436 | 7.11 | 0.851 | 13.6 | 0 | 0.2 | 0.20 | 0.55 | 486.2 | 16040 |
| **pinto beans**, mature, boiled | 171 | 245 | 107.6 | 44.8 | 0.6 | 0 | 15.4 | 2 | 79 | 86 | 1.68 | 0.775 | 0 | 1 | 0.33 | 0.5 | 0 | 0.36 |
| 1 cup |  | 15.4 | 1.1 | 0.2 | 0.2 | 0.4 | 0 | 746 | 251 | 3.57 | 0.374 | 10.6 | 0 | 1.6 | 0.11 | 0.39 | 294.1 | 16043 |
| **pinto beans**, mature, canned | 240 | 206 | 186.1 | 36.6 | 0.5 |  | 11.0 | 706 | 103 | 65 | 1.66 | 0.550 | 0 | 2 | 0.24 | 0.7 | 0 | 0.33 |
| 1 cup |  | 11.7 | 1.9 | 0.4 | 0.4 | 0.7 | 0 | 583 | 221 | 3.50 | 0.336 | 17.0 | 0 | 1.4 | 0.15 | 0.18 | 144.0 | 16044 |
| **pinto beans**, mature, dry | 96 | 333 | 10.9 | 60.0 | 2.0 | 0 | 14.9 | 12 | 108 | 169 | 2.19 | 1.102 | 0 | 6 | 0.68 | 1.1 | 0 | 0.75 |
| ½ cup |  | 20.6 | 1.2 | 0.2 | 0.2 | 0.4 | 0 | 1337 | 395 | 4.87 | 0.857 | 26.8 | 0 | 0.2 | 0.20 | 0.46 | 504.0 | 16042 |
| **refried beans**, canned | 252 | 229 | 191.9 | 38.5 | 1.2 | 0 | 12.9 | 1131 | 83 | 96 | 1.64 | 0.832 | 0 | 15 | 0.09 | 1.1 | 0 | 0.54 |
| 1 cup |  | 13.6 | 2.9 | 1.0 | 1.0 | 0.8 | 0 | 847 | 280 | 4.21 | 0.418 | 16.4 | 0 | 0.1 | 0.04 | 0.28 | 27.7 | 16103 |
| **refried beans**, canned, Old El Paso | 240 | 90 |  | 16.0 | 0 |  | 5.0 | 560 | 20 |  |  |  | 0 |  |  |  |  |  |
| 1 cup |  | 6.0 | 0.5 | 0 |  |  | 0 |  |  | 1.08 |  |  | 0 |  |  |  |  | GENM360 |
| **refried beans**, fat-free, canned, | 248 | 90 |  | 17.0 | 0 |  | 5.0 | 580 | 20 |  |  |  | 0 |  |  |  |  |  |
| Old El Paso - 1 cup |  | 6.0 | 0 | 0 |  |  | 0 |  |  | 1.08 |  |  | 0 | 0 |  |  |  | GENM361 |
| **refried beans**, vegetarian, canned | 242 | 201 | 189.7 | 32.7 | 1.4 | 0 | 11.4 | 1041 | 85 | 92 | 1.79 | 0.803 |  |  | 0.10 | 0.9 |  | 0.42 |
| 1 cup |  | 12.8 | 2.1 | 0.3 | 0.5 | 1.1 | 0 | 832 | 276 | 4.11 | 0.414 | 13.6 |  | 0.2 | 0.04 | 0.26 |  | 16171 |
| **refried beans**, vegetarian, canned, | 236 | 90 |  | 16.0 | 0 |  | 5.0 | 550 | 20 |  |  |  | 0 |  |  |  |  |  |
| Old El Paso - 1 cup |  | 5.0 | 0.5 | 0 |  |  | 0 |  |  | 1.08 |  |  | 0 |  |  |  |  | GENM362 |
| **refried beans** with green chilies, | 244 | 90 |  | 16.0 | 1.0 |  | 5.0 | 570 | 20 |  |  |  | 0 |  |  |  |  |  |
| canned, Old El Paso - 1 cup |  | 5.0 | 0.5 | 0 |  |  | 0 |  |  | 1.08 |  |  | 0 |  |  |  |  | GENM364 |
| **shellie (shell) beans**, canned, | 245 | 74 | 222.2 | 15.2 | 1.5 | 0 | 8.3 | 818 | 71 | 37 | 0.66 | 0.936 | 27 | 8 | 0.08 | 0.5 | 0 | 0.33 |
| solids and liquid - 1 cup |  | 4.3 | 0.5 | 0.1 | 0 | 0.3 | 0 | 267 | 74 | 2.43 | 0.196 | 5.1 | 559 | 0.1 | 0.13 | 0.12 | 44.1 | 11050 |

| | WT (g) | KCAL / PRO (g) | H₂O (g) / FAT (g) | CHO (g) / SFA (g) | TSUG (g) / MUFA (g) | ASUG (g) / PUFA (g) | DFIB (g) / CHOL (mg) | Na (mg) / K (mg) | Ca (mg) / P (mg) | Mg (mg) / Fe (mg) | Zn (mg) / Cu (mg) | Mn (mg) / Se (mcg) | A (mcg RAE) / A (IU) | C (mg) / E (mg ATE) | B-1 (mg) / B-2 (mg) | NIA (mg) / B-6 (mg) | B-12 (mcg) / FOL (mcg DFE) | PANT (mg) / REF |
|---|---|---|---|---|---|---|---|---|---|---|---|---|---|---|---|---|---|---|
| **soybeans**, grn/immature (edamame), boiled, drnd - *1 cup* | 180 | 254 | 123.5 | 19.9 | | | 7.6 | 25 | 261 | 108 | 1.64 | 0.904 | 14 | 31 | 0.47 | 2.2 | 0 | 0.23 |
| | | 22.2 | 11.5 | 1.3 | 2.2 | 5.4 | 0 | 970 | 284 | 4.50 | 0.211 | 2.5 | 281 | | 0.28 | 0.11 | 199.8 | 11451 |
| **soybeans**, grn/immature (edamame), frzn, heated - *1 cup* | 155 | 189 | 112.8 | 15.4 | 3.4 | | 8.1 | 9 | 98 | 99 | 2.12 | 1.587 | | 9 | 0.31 | 1.4 | | 0.61 |
| | | 16.9 | 8.1 | 1.0 | 2.0 | 3.3 | | 676 | 262 | 3.52 | 0.535 | | | 1.1 | 0.24 | 0.16 | 482.0 | 11212 |
| **soybeans**, green/immature (edamame), raw - *1 cup* | 256 | 376 | 172.8 | 28.3 | | | 10.8 | 38 | 504 | 166 | 2.53 | 1.400 | 23 | 74 | 1.11 | 4.2 | 0 | 0.38 |
| | | 33.2 | 17.4 | 2.0 | 3.3 | 8.2 | 0 | 1587 | 497 | 9.09 | 0.328 | 3.8 | 461 | | 0.45 | 0.17 | 422.4 | 11450 |
| **soybeans**, mature, boiled *1 cup* | 172 | 298 | 107.6 | 17.1 | 5.2 | 0 | 10.3 | 2 | 175 | 148 | 1.98 | 1.417 | 0 | 3 | 0.27 | 0.7 | 0 | 0.31 |
| | | 28.6 | 15.4 | 2.2 | 3.4 | 8.7 | 0 | 886 | 421 | 8.84 | 0.700 | 12.6 | 15 | 0.6 | 0.49 | 0.40 | 92.9 | 16109 |
| **soybeans**, mature, dry *½ cup* | 93 | 415 | 7.9 | 28.0 | 6.8 | | 8.6 | 2 | 258 | 260 | 4.55 | 2.341 | 1 | 6 | 0.81 | 1.5 | 0 | 0.74 |
| | | 33.9 | 18.5 | 2.7 | 4.1 | 10.5 | 0 | 1671 | 655 | 14.60 | 1.542 | 16.6 | 20 | 0.8 | 0.81 | 0.35 | 348.8 | 16108 |
| **white beans**, mature, boiled *1 cup* | 179 | 249 | 112.9 | 44.9 | 0.6 | 0 | 11.3 | 11 | 161 | 113 | 2.47 | 1.138 | 0 | 0 | 0.21 | 0.3 | 0 | 0.41 |
| | | 17.4 | 0.6 | 0.2 | 0.1 | 0.3 | 0 | 1004 | 202 | 6.62 | 0.514 | 2.3 | 0 | 1.7 | 0.08 | 0.17 | 145.0 | 16050 |
| **white beans**, mature, canned *1 cup* | 262 | 299 | 183.7 | 55.5 | 0.8 | | 12.6 | 13 | 191 | 134 | 2.93 | 1.349 | 0 | 0 | 0.25 | 0.3 | 0 | 0.48 |
| | | 19.0 | 0.8 | 0.2 | 0.1 | 0.3 | 0 | 1189 | 238 | 7.83 | 0.608 | 4.2 | 0 | 2.1 | 0.10 | 0.20 | 170.3 | 16051 |
| **white beans**, mature, dry *½ cup* | 101 | 336 | 11.4 | 60.9 | 2.1 | 0 | 15.4 | 16 | 242 | 192 | 3.71 | 1.814 | 0 | 0 | 0.44 | 0.5 | 0 | 0.74 |
| | | 23.6 | 0.9 | 0.2 | 0.1 | 0.4 | 0 | 1813 | 304 | 10.54 | 0.994 | 12.9 | 0 | 0.2 | 0.15 | 0.32 | 391.9 | 16049 |
| **white beans**, small, mature, boiled *1 cup* | 179 | 254 | 113.2 | 46.2 | | | 18.6 | 4 | 131 | 122 | 1.95 | 0.913 | 0 | 0 | 0.42 | 0.5 | 0 | 0.45 |
| | | 16.1 | 1.1 | 0.3 | 0.1 | 0.5 | 0 | 829 | 303 | 5.08 | 0.267 | 2.3 | 0 | | 0.11 | 0.23 | 245.2 | 16046 |
| **white beans**, small, mature, dry *½ cup* | 107 | 360 | 12.5 | 66.6 | | | 26.6 | 13 | 185 | 196 | 3.01 | 1.367 | 0 | 0 | 0.80 | 1.4 | 0 | 0.78 |
| | | 22.6 | 1.3 | 0.3 | 0.1 | 0.5 | 0 | 1650 | 476 | 8.27 | 0.679 | 13.7 | 0 | | 0.22 | 0.47 | 413.0 | 16045 |
| **winged beans**, immature, boiled, drained - *1 cup* | 62 | 24 | 55.9 | 2.0 | | | | 2 | 38 | 19 | 0.17 | 0.098 | 2 | 6 | 0.05 | 0.4 | 0 | 0.03 |
| | | 3.3 | 0.4 | 0.1 | 0.1 | 0.1 | 0 | 170 | 16 | 0.68 | 0.023 | 0.7 | 55 | | 0.04 | 0.05 | 21.7 | 11596 |
| **winged beans**, mature, boiled *1 cup* | 172 | 253 | 115.6 | 25.7 | | | | 22 | 244 | 93 | 2.48 | 2.062 | 0 | 0 | 0.51 | 1.4 | 0 | 0.27 |
| | | 18.3 | 10.0 | 1.4 | 3.7 | 2.7 | 0 | 482 | 263 | 7.45 | 1.330 | 5.0 | 0 | | 0.22 | 0.08 | 17.2 | 16136 |
| **winged beans**, mature, dry *½ cup* | 90 | 368 | 7.5 | 37.5 | | | | 34 | 396 | 161 | 4.03 | 3.349 | 0 | 0 | 0.93 | 2.8 | 0 | 0.72 |
| | | 26.7 | 14.7 | 2.1 | 5.4 | 3.9 | 0 | 879 | 406 | 12.10 | 2.592 | 7.4 | 0 | | 0.40 | 0.16 | 40.5 | 16135 |
| **yardlong bean**, immature, boiled, drained - *1 cup sliced* | 104 | 49 | 91.0 | 9.5 | | | | 4 | 46 | 44 | 0.37 | 0.209 | 24 | 17 | 0.09 | 0.7 | 0 | 0.05 |
| | | 2.6 | 0.1 | 0 | 0 | 0 | 0 | 302 | 59 | 1.02 | 0.049 | 1.6 | 468 | | 0.10 | 0.02 | 46.8 | 11200 |
| **yardlong bean**, mature, boiled *1 cup sliced* | 171 | 202 | 117.6 | 36.1 | | | 6.5 | 9 | 72 | 168 | 1.85 | 0.833 | 0 | 1 | 0.36 | 0.9 | 0 | 0.68 |
| | | 14.2 | 0.8 | 0.2 | 0.1 | 0.3 | 0 | 539 | 310 | 4.51 | 0.385 | 4.8 | 0 | | 0.11 | 0.16 | 249.7 | 16134 |
| **yellow beans**, mature, boiled *1 cup* | 177 | 255 | 111.5 | 44.7 | | | 18.4 | 9 | 110 | 131 | 1.88 | 0.805 | 0 | 3 | 0.33 | 1.3 | 0 | 0.41 |
| | | 16.2 | 1.9 | 0.5 | 0.2 | 0.8 | 0 | 575 | 324 | 4.39 | 0.329 | 2.3 | 4 | | 0.18 | 0.23 | 143.4 | 16048 |
| **yellow snap beans**, raw *1 cup* | 110 | 34 | 99.3 | 7.9 | | | 3.7 | 7 | 41 | 28 | 0.26 | 0.235 | 6 | 18 | 0.09 | 0.8 | 0 | 0.10 |
| | | 2.0 | 0.1 | 0 | 0 | 0.1 | 0 | 230 | 42 | 1.14 | 0.076 | 0.7 | 119 | | 0.12 | 0.08 | 40.7 | 11722 |

## 30.5 SPROUT AND SHOOT VEGETABLES

| | WT (g) | KCAL / PRO (g) | H₂O (g) / FAT (g) | CHO (g) / SFA (g) | TSUG (g) / MUFA (g) | ASUG (g) / PUFA (g) | DFIB (g) / CHOL (mg) | Na (mg) / K (mg) | Ca (mg) / P (mg) | Mg (mg) / Fe (mg) | Zn (mg) / Cu (mg) | Mn (mg) / Se (mcg) | A (mcg RAE) / A (IU) | C (mg) / E (mg ATE) | B-1 (mg) / B-2 (mg) | NIA (mg) / B-6 (mg) | B-12 (mcg) / FOL (mcg DFE) | PANT (mg) / REF |
|---|---|---|---|---|---|---|---|---|---|---|---|---|---|---|---|---|---|---|
| **alfalfa sprouts**, raw *1 cup* | 33 | 8 | 30.6 | 0.7 | 0.1 | 0 | 0.6 | 2 | 11 | 9 | 0.30 | 0.062 | 3 | 3 | 0.03 | 0.2 | 0 | 0.19 |
| | | 1.3 | 0.2 | 0 | 0 | 0.1 | 0 | 26 | 23 | 0.32 | 0.052 | 0.2 | 51 | 0 | 0.04 | 0.01 | 11.9 | 11001 |
| **bamboo shoots**, boiled, drained *1 cup* | 120 | 14 | 115.1 | 2.3 | | | 1.2 | 5 | 14 | 4 | 0.56 | 0.136 | 0 | 0 | 0.02 | 0.4 | 0 | 0.08 |
| | | 1.8 | 0.3 | 0.1 | 0 | 0.1 | 0 | 640 | 24 | 0.29 | 0.098 | 0.5 | 0 | | 0.06 | 0.12 | 2.4 | 11027 |
| **bamboo shoots**, canned, drained *1 cup* | 131 | 25 | 123.6 | 4.2 | 2.5 | 0 | 1.8 | 9 | 10 | 5 | 0.85 | 0.206 | 1 | 1 | 0.03 | 0.2 | 0 | 0.12 |
| | | 2.3 | 0.5 | 0.1 | 0 | 0.2 | 0 | 105 | 33 | 0.42 | 0.149 | 0.7 | 17 | 0.8 | 0.03 | 0.18 | 3.9 | 11028 |
| **bamboo shoots**, raw *1 cup* | 151 | 41 | 137.4 | 7.9 | 4.5 | 0 | 3.3 | 6 | 20 | 5 | 1.66 | 0.396 | 2 | 6 | 0.23 | 0.9 | 0 | 0.24 |
| | | 3.9 | 0.5 | 0.1 | 0 | 0.2 | 0 | 805 | 89 | 0.76 | 0.287 | 1.2 | 30 | 1.5 | 0.11 | 0.36 | 10.6 | 11026 |
| **kidney bean sprouts**, boiled, drained - *1 cup* | 125 | 41 | 111.6 | 5.9 | | | | 9 | 24 | 29 | 0.55 | 0.249 | 0 | 44 | 0.45 | 3.8 | 0 | 0.48 |
| | | 6.0 | 0.7 | 0.1 | 0.1 | 0.4 | 0 | 242 | 48 | 1.11 | 0.217 | 0.8 | 2 | | 0.34 | 0.12 | 58.8 | 11030 |
| **lentil sprouts**, stir-fried *1 cup* | 125 | 126 | 85.9 | 26.6 | | | | 12 | 18 | 44 | 2.00 | 0.628 | 2 | 16 | 0.28 | 1.5 | 0 | 0.71 |
| | | 11.0 | 0.6 | 0.1 | 0.1 | 0.3 | 0 | 355 | 191 | 3.88 | 0.421 | 0.8 | 51 | | 0.11 | 0.20 | 83.8 | 11249 |
| **mung bean sprouts**, boiled, drained *1 cup* | 124 | 26 | 115.8 | 5.2 | 3.5 | 0 | 1.0 | 12 | 15 | 17 | 0.58 | 0.174 | 1 | 14 | 0.06 | 1.0 | 0 | 0.30 |
| | | 2.5 | 0.1 | 0 | 0 | 0 | 0 | 125 | 35 | 0.81 | 0.151 | 0.7 | 16 | 0.1 | 0.13 | 0.07 | 36.0 | 11044 |
| **mung bean sprouts**, canned, drained *1 cup* | 125 | 15 | 120.1 | 2.7 | 1.7 | 0 | 1.0 | 175 | 18 | 11 | 0.35 | 0.091 | 0 | 0 | 0.04 | 0.3 | 0 | 0.18 |
| | | 1.8 | 0.1 | 0 | 0 | 0 | 0 | 34 | 40 | 0.54 | 0.196 | 0.8 | 10 | 0 | 0.09 | 0.04 | 12.5 | 11626 |
| **mung bean sprouts**, raw *1 cup* | 104 | 31 | 94.0 | 6.2 | 4.3 | 0 | 1.9 | 6 | 14 | 22 | 0.43 | 0.196 | 1 | 14 | 0.09 | 0.8 | 0 | 0.40 |
| | | 3.2 | 0.2 | 0 | 0 | 0.1 | 0 | 155 | 56 | 0.95 | 0.171 | 0.6 | 22 | 0.1 | 0.13 | 0.09 | 63.4 | 11043 |
| **mung bean sprouts**, stir-fried *1 cup* | 124 | 62 | 104.5 | 13.1 | | | 2.4 | 11 | 16 | 41 | 1.12 | 0.362 | 2 | 20 | 0.17 | 1.5 | 0 | 0.69 |
| | | 5.3 | 0.3 | 0 | 0.1 | 0.1 | 0 | 272 | 98 | 2.36 | 0.316 | 0.7 | 38 | | 0.22 | 0.16 | 86.8 | 11045 |
| **navy bean sprouts**, boiled, drained *1 cup* | 125 | 98 | 95.0 | 18.8 | | | | 18 | 20 | 139 | 1.21 | 0.558 | 0 | 22 | 0.48 | 1.6 | 0 | 1.07 |
| | | 8.8 | 1.0 | 0.1 | 0.1 | 0.6 | 0 | 396 | 129 | 2.64 | 0.486 | 0.8 | 5 | | 0.29 | 0.25 | 132.5 | 11047 |
| **pea sprouts**, boiled, drained *1 cup* | 125 | 122 | 93.0 | 21.3 | | | | 4 | 32 | 51 | 0.98 | 0.406 | 6 | 8 | 0.27 | 1.3 | 0 | 0.85 |
| | | 8.8 | 0.6 | 0.1 | 0.1 | 0.3 | 0 | 335 | 30 | 2.09 | 0.025 | 0.8 | 134 | | 0.36 | 0.16 | 45.0 | 11317 |
| **pokeberry shoots** (poke), boiled, drained - *1 cup* | 165 | 33 | 153.3 | 5.1 | 2.6 | 0 | 2.5 | 30 | 87 | 23 | 0.31 | 0.554 | 718 | 135 | 0.12 | 1.8 | 0 | 0.06 |
| | | 3.8 | 0.7 | 0.1 | 0 | 0.3 | 0 | 304 | 54 | 1.98 | 0.208 | 1.5 | 14355 | 1.4 | 0.41 | 0.18 | 14.8 | 11351 |

| Food | WT (g) | KCAL / PRO (g) | H₂0 (g) / FAT (g) | CHO (g) / SFA (g) | TSUG (g) / MUFA (g) | ASUG (g) / PUFA (g) | DFIB (g) / CHOL (mg) | Na (mg) / K (mg) | Ca (mg) / P (mg) | Mg (mg) / Fe (mg) | Zn (mg) / Cu (mg) | Mn (mg) / Se (mcg) | A (mcg RAE) / A (IU) | C (mg) / E (mg ATE) | B-1 (mg) / B-2 (mg) | NIA (mg) / B-6 (mg) | B-12 (mcg) / FOL (mcg DFE) | PANT (mg) / REF |
|---|---|---|---|---|---|---|---|---|---|---|---|---|---|---|---|---|---|---|
| radish seed sprouts, raw | 38 | 16 | 34.2 | 1.4 | | | | 2 | 19 | 17 | 0.21 | 0.099 | 8 | 11 | 0.04 | 1.1 | 0 | 0.28 |
| 1 cup | | 1.4 | 1.0 | 0.3 | 0.2 | 0.4 | 0 | 33 | 43 | 0.33 | 0.046 | 0.2 | 149 | | 0.04 | 0.11 | 36.1 | 11676 |
| soybean sprouts, raw | 70 | 85 | 48.3 | 6.7 | | | 0.8 | 10 | 47 | 50 | 0.82 | 0.491 | 1 | 11 | 0.24 | 0.8 | 0 | 0.65 |
| 1 cup | | 9.2 | 4.7 | 0.7 | 1.1 | 2.6 | 0 | 339 | 115 | 1.47 | 0.299 | 0.4 | 8 | | 0.08 | 0.12 | 120.4 | 11452 |
| soybean sprouts, steamed | 94 | 76 | 74.7 | 6.1 | 0.5 | 0 | 0.8 | 9 | 55 | 56 | 0.98 | 0.667 | 2 | 8 | 0.19 | 1.0 | 0 | 0.70 |
| 1 cup | | 8.0 | 4.2 | 0.6 | 0.9 | 2.4 | 0 | 334 | 127 | 1.23 | 0.310 | 0.6 | 38 | 0.2 | 0.05 | 0.10 | 75.2 | 11453 |
| soybean sprouts, stir-fried | 125 | 156 | 84.0 | 11.8 | | | 1.0 | 18 | 102 | 120 | 2.62 | 1.416 | 1 | 15 | 0.52 | 1.4 | 0 | 1.48 |
| 1 cup | | 16.4 | 8.9 | 1.2 | 2.0 | 5.0 | 0 | 709 | 270 | 0.50 | 0.659 | 0.8 | 21 | | 0.24 | 0.21 | 158.8 | 11454 |
| taro shoots, cooked | 140 | 20 | 133.4 | 4.5 | | | | 3 | 20 | 11 | 0.76 | 0.182 | 4 | 26 | 0.05 | 1.1 | 0 | 0.11 |
| 1 cup sliced | | 1.0 | 0.1 | 0 | 0 | 0 | 0 | 482 | 36 | 0.57 | 0.132 | 1.4 | 71 | | 0.07 | 0.16 | 4.2 | 11523 |

## 30.6  TUBER AND ROOT VEGETABLES

| Food | WT (g) | KCAL / PRO (g) | H₂0 (g) / FAT (g) | CHO (g) / SFA (g) | TSUG (g) / MUFA (g) | ASUG (g) / PUFA (g) | DFIB (g) / CHOL (mg) | Na (mg) / K (mg) | Ca (mg) / P (mg) | Mg (mg) / Fe (mg) | Zn (mg) / Cu (mg) | Mn (mg) / Se (mcg) | A (mcg RAE) / A (IU) | C (mg) / E (mg ATE) | B-1 (mg) / B-2 (mg) | NIA (mg) / B-6 (mg) | B-12 (mcg) / FOL (mcg DFE) | PANT (mg) / REF |
|---|---|---|---|---|---|---|---|---|---|---|---|---|---|---|---|---|---|---|
| arrowhead tuber/root, boiled, drained | 12 | 9 | 9.2 | 1.9 | | | | 2 | 1 | 6 | 0.03 | 0.034 | 0 | 0 | 0.02 | 0.1 | 0 | 0.05 |
| drained - 1 medium | | 0.5 | 0 | | | | 0 | 106 | 24 | 0.15 | 0.016 | 0.1 | 0 | | 0.01 | 0.02 | 1.1 | 11006 |
| arrowroot tuber/root, raw | 120 | 78 | 96.9 | 16.1 | | | 1.6 | 31 | 7 | 30 | 0.76 | 0.209 | 1 | 2 | 0.17 | 2.0 | 0 | 0.35 |
| 1 cup sliced | | 5.1 | 0.2 | 0 | 0 | 0.1 | 0 | 545 | 118 | 2.66 | 0.145 | 0.8 | 23 | | 0.07 | 0.32 | 405.6 | 11697 |
| beet, boiled, drained | 85 | 37 | 74.0 | 8.5 | 6.8 | 0 | 1.7 | 65 | 14 | 20 | 0.30 | 0.277 | 2 | 3 | 0.02 | 0.3 | 0 | 0.12 |
| ½ cup sliced | | 1.4 | 0.2 | 0 | 0 | 0.1 | 0 | 259 | 32 | 0.67 | 0.063 | 0.6 | 30 | 0 | 0.03 | 0.06 | 68.0 | 11081 |
| beet, canned, drained | 170 | 53 | 154.6 | 12.3 | 9.4 | 0 | 3.1 | 330 | 26 | 29 | 0.36 | 0.488 | 2 | 7 | 0.02 | 0.3 | 0 | 0.27 |
| 1 cup | | 1.5 | 0.2 | 0 | 0 | 0.1 | 0 | 252 | 29 | 3.09 | 0.100 | 0.8 | 41 | 0.1 | 0.07 | 0.10 | 51.0 | 11084 |
| beet, Harvard, canned, solids and | 246 | 180 | 197.2 | 44.7 | | | 6.2 | 399 | 27 | 47 | 0.57 | 0.593 | 2 | 6 | 0.02 | 0.2 | 0 | 0.37 |
| liquid - 1 cup | | 2.1 | 0.1 | 0 | 0 | 0 | 0 | 403 | 42 | 0.89 | 0.239 | 2.7 | 27 | | 0.12 | 0.14 | 71.3 | 11605 |
| beet, pickled, canned, solids and | 227 | 148 | 185.9 | 37.0 | | | 5.9 | 599 | 25 | 34 | 0.59 | 0.499 | 2 | 5 | 0.02 | 0.6 | 0 | 0.31 |
| liquid - 1 cup | | 1.8 | 0.2 | 0 | 0 | 0.1 | 0 | 336 | 39 | 0.93 | 0.263 | 2.3 | 25 | | 0.11 | 0.11 | 61.3 | 11609 |
| beet, raw | 68 | 29 | 59.6 | 6.5 | 4.6 | 0 | 1.9 | 53 | 11 | 16 | 0.24 | 0.224 | 1 | 3 | 0.02 | 0.2 | 0 | 0.11 |
| ½ cup sliced | | 1.1 | 0.1 | 0 | 0 | 0 | 0 | 221 | 27 | 0.54 | 0.051 | 0.5 | 22 | 0 | 0.03 | 0.05 | 74.1 | 11080 |
| burdock root, boiled, drained | 125 | 110 | 94.6 | 26.4 | 4.4 | 0 | 2.2 | 5 | 61 | 49 | 0.48 | 0.338 | 0 | 3 | 0.05 | 0.4 | 0 | 0.44 |
| 1 cup pieces | | 2.6 | 0.2 | 0 | 0 | 0.1 | 0 | 450 | 116 | 0.96 | 0.111 | 1.1 | 0 | 0.6 | 0.07 | 0.35 | 25.0 | 11105 |
| butterbur (fuki), boiled, | 100 | 8 | 96.7 | 2.2 | | | | 4 | 59 | 8 | 0.09 | 0.156 | 1 | 19 | 0.01 | 0.1 | 0 | 0.02 |
| drained - 3.5 oz | | 0.2 | 0 | | | | 0 | 354 | 7 | 0.10 | 0.059 | 0.9 | 27 | | 0.01 | 0.05 | 4.0 | 11107 |
| carrot, baby, raw | 10 | 4 | 9.0 | 0.8 | 0.5 | | 0.3 | 8 | 3 | 1 | 0.02 | 0.015 | 69 | 0 | 0 | 0.1 | 0 | 0.04 |
| 1 medium | | 0.1 | 0 | 0 | 0 | 0 | 0 | 24 | 3 | 0.09 | 0.010 | 0.1 | 1379 | | 0 | 0.01 | 2.7 | 11960 |
| carrot, boiled, drained | 78 | 27 | 70.3 | 6.4 | 2.7 | 0 | 2.3 | 45 | 23 | 8 | 0.16 | 0.121 | 665 | 3 | 0.05 | 0.5 | 0 | 0.18 |
| ½ cup sliced | | 0.6 | 0.1 | 0 | 0 | 0.1 | 0 | 183 | 23 | 0.27 | 0.013 | 0.5 | 13286 | 0.8 | 0.03 | 0.12 | 10.9 | 11125 |
| carrot, canned, drained | 146 | 36 | 135.7 | 8.1 | 3.6 | 0 | 2.2 | 353 | 36 | 12 | 0.38 | 0.657 | 815 | 4 | 0.03 | 0.8 | 0 | 0.20 |
| 1 cup sliced | | 0.9 | 0.3 | 0.1 | 0 | 0.1 | 0 | 261 | 35 | 0.93 | 0.152 | 0.6 | 16308 | 1.1 | 0.04 | 0.16 | 13.1 | 11128 |
| carrot, frozen, boiled, drained | 146 | 54 | 131.9 | 11.3 | 6.0 | 0 | 4.8 | 86 | 51 | 16 | 0.51 | 0.244 | 1235 | 3 | 0.04 | 0.6 | 0 | 0.25 |
| 1 cup sliced | | 0.8 | 1.0 | 0.2 | 0 | 0.5 | 0 | 280 | 45 | 0.77 | 0.120 | 0.9 | 24715 | 1.5 | 0.05 | 0.12 | 16.1 | 11131 |
| carrot, raw | 72 | 30 | 63.6 | 6.9 | 3.4 | 0 | 2.0 | 50 | 24 | 9 | 0.17 | 0.103 | 601 | 4 | 0.05 | 0.7 | 0 | 0.20 |
| 1 carrot (7½" long) | | 0.7 | 0.2 | 0 | 0 | 0.1 | 0 | 230 | 25 | 0.22 | 0.032 | 0.1 | 12028 | 0.5 | 0.04 | 0.10 | 13.7 | 11124 |
| cassava, raw | 206 | 330 | 122.9 | 78.4 | 3.5 | 0 | 3.7 | 29 | 33 | 43 | 0.70 | 0.791 | 2 | 42 | 0.18 | 1.8 | 0 | 0.22 |
| 1 cup | | 2.8 | 0.6 | 0.2 | 0.2 | 0.1 | 0 | 558 | 56 | 0.56 | 0.206 | 1.4 | 27 | 0.4 | 0.10 | 0.18 | 55.6 | 11134 |
| celeriac (celery root), boiled, drained | 155 | 42 | 143.1 | 9.1 | | | 1.9 | 95 | 40 | 19 | 0.31 | 0.149 | 0 | 6 | 0.04 | 0.7 | 0 | 0.31 |
| 1 cup pieces | | 1.5 | 0.3 | | | | 0 | 268 | 102 | 0.67 | 0.067 | 0.6 | 0 | | 0.06 | 0.16 | 4.6 | 11142 |
| celeriac (celery root), raw | 156 | 66 | 137.3 | 14.4 | 2.5 | 0 | 2.8 | 156 | 67 | 31 | 0.51 | 0.246 | 0 | 12 | 0.08 | 1.1 | 0 | 0.55 |
| 1 cup pieces | | 2.3 | 0.5 | 0.1 | 0.1 | 0.2 | 0 | 468 | 179 | 1.09 | 0.109 | 1.1 | 0 | 0.6 | 0.09 | 0.26 | 12.5 | 11141 |
| chicory root, raw | 90 | 66 | 72.0 | 15.8 | | | | 45 | 37 | 20 | 0.30 | 0.210 | 0 | 4 | 0.04 | 0.4 | 0 | 0.29 |
| 1 cup chopped | | 1.3 | 0.2 | 0 | 0 | 0.1 | 0 | 261 | 55 | 0.72 | 0.069 | 0.6 | 5 | | 0.03 | 0.22 | 20.7 | 11154 |
| fennel bulb, raw | 87 | 27 | 78.5 | 6.3 | | | 2.7 | 45 | 43 | 15 | 0.17 | 0.166 | 6 | 10 | 0.01 | 0.6 | 0 | 0.20 |
| 1 cup sliced | | 1.1 | 0.2 | | | | 0 | 360 | 44 | 0.64 | 0.057 | 0.6 | 117 | | 0.03 | 0.04 | 23.5 | 11957 |
| garlic, raw | 9 | 13 | 5.3 | 3.0 | 0.1 | 0 | 0.2 | 2 | 16 | 2 | 0.10 | 0.150 | 0 | 3 | 0.02 | 0.1 | 0 | 0.05 |
| 3 cloves | | 0.6 | 0 | 0 | 0 | 0 | 0 | 36 | 14 | 0.15 | 0.027 | 1.3 | 1 | 0 | 0.01 | 0.11 | 0.3 | 11215 |
| Jerusalem artichoke (sunchoke), raw | 150 | 110 | 117.0 | 26.2 | 14.4 | 0 | 2.4 | 6 | 21 | 26 | 0.18 | 0.090 | 2 | 6 | 0.30 | 2.0 | 0 | 0.60 |
| 1 cup sliced | | 3.0 | 0 | 0 | 0 | 0 | 0 | 644 | 117 | 5.10 | 0.210 | 1.0 | 30 | 0.3 | 0.09 | 0.12 | 19.5 | 11226 |
| jicama (yambean), boiled, drained | 100 | 38 | 90.1 | 8.8 | | | | 4 | 11 | 11 | 0.15 | 0.057 | 1 | 14 | 0.02 | 0.2 | 0 | 0.12 |
| 3.5 oz | | 0.7 | 0.1 | | | | 0 | 135 | 16 | 0.57 | 0.046 | 0.7 | 19 | | 0.03 | 0.04 | 8.0 | 11604 |
| jicama (yambean), raw | 120 | 46 | 108.1 | 10.6 | 2.2 | 0 | 5.9 | 5 | 14 | 14 | 0.19 | 0.072 | 1 | 24 | 0.02 | 0.2 | 0 | 0.16 |
| 1 cup sliced | | 0.9 | 0.1 | 0 | 0 | 0.1 | 0 | 180 | 22 | 0.72 | 0.058 | 0.8 | 25 | 0.6 | 0.03 | 0.05 | 14.4 | 11603 |
| lotus root, boiled, drained | 89 | 59 | 72.5 | 14.3 | 0.4 | 0 | 2.8 | 40 | 23 | 20 | 0.29 | 0.196 | 0 | 24 | 0.11 | 0.3 | 0 | 0.27 |
| 10 slices (2½" diameter) | | 1.4 | 0.1 | 0 | 0 | 0 | 0 | 323 | 69 | 0.80 | 0.193 | 0.5 | 0 | 0 | 0.01 | 0.19 | 7.1 | 11255 |
| lotus root, raw | 81 | 60 | 64.1 | 14.0 | | | 4.0 | 32 | 36 | 19 | 0.32 | 0.211 | 0 | 36 | 0.13 | 0.3 | 0 | 0.31 |
| 10 slices (2½" diameter) | | 2.1 | 0.1 | 0 | 0 | 0 | 0 | 450 | 81 | 0.94 | 0.208 | 0.6 | 0 | | 0.18 | 0.21 | 10.5 | 11254 |

| Food | WT (g) | KCAL / PRO (g) | H$_2$O (g) / FAT (g) | CHO (g) / SFA (g) | TSUG (g) / MUFA (g) | ASUG (g) / PUFA (g) | DFIB (g) / CHOL (mg) | Na (mg) / K (mg) | Ca (mg) / P (mg) | Mg (mg) / Fe (mg) | Zn (mg) / Cu (mg) | Mn (mg) / Se (mcg) | A (mcg RAE) / A (IU) | C (mg) / E (mg ATE) | B-1 (mg) / B-2 (mg) | NIA (mg) / B-6 (mg) | B-12 (mcg) / FOL (mcg DFE) | PANT (mg) / REF |
|---|---|---|---|---|---|---|---|---|---|---|---|---|---|---|---|---|---|---|
| mountain yam, Hawaiian, steamed | 145 | 119 | 111.9 | 29.0 | | | | 17 | 12 | 14 | 0.46 | 0.410 | 0 | 0 | 0.12 | 0.2 | 0 | 0.70 |
| 1 cup cubed | | 2.5 | 0.1 | 0 | 0 | 0.1 | 0 | 718 | 58 | 0.62 | 0.187 | 1.3 | 0 | | 0.02 | 0.30 | 17.4 | 11259 |
| onion rings, breaded, parfried, frzn, heated - 10 med rings (2-3" dia) | 60 | 244 | 17.1 | 22.9 | | | 0.8 | 225 | 19 | 11 | 0.25 | 0.252 | 7 | 1 | 0.17 | 2.2 | 0 | 0.14 |
| | | 3.2 | 16.0 | 5.2 | 6.5 | 3.1 | 0 | 77 | 49 | 1.01 | 0.048 | 2.1 | 135 | | 0.08 | 0.05 | 61.8 | 11296 |
| onion, white, boiled, drained | 210 | 92 | 184.5 | 21.3 | 9.9 | 0 | 2.9 | 6 | 46 | 23 | 0.44 | 0.321 | 0 | 11 | 0.09 | 0.3 | 0 | 0.24 |
| 1 cup chopped | | 2.9 | 0.4 | 0.1 | 0.1 | 0.2 | 0 | 349 | 74 | 0.50 | 0.141 | 1.3 | 4 | 0 | 0.05 | 0.27 | 31.5 | 11283 |
| onion, white, canned, solids and liquid - 1 cup chopped | 224 | 43 | 210.8 | 9.0 | 4.9 | 0 | 2.7 | 831 | 101 | 13 | 0.65 | 0.228 | 0 | 10 | 0.07 | 0.1 | 0 | 0.22 |
| | | 1.9 | 0.2 | 0 | 0 | 0.1 | 0 | 249 | 63 | 0.29 | 0.123 | 0.7 | 2 | 0.2 | 0.01 | 0.31 | 22.4 | 11285 |
| onion, white, frozen, boiled, drained | 210 | 59 | 193.7 | 13.8 | 6.1 | 0 | 3.8 | 25 | 34 | 13 | 0.15 | 0.149 | 0 | 5 | 0.05 | 0.3 | 0 | 0.21 |
| 1 cup chopped | | 1.6 | 0.2 | 0 | 0 | 0.1 | 0 | 227 | 40 | 0.63 | 0.040 | 0.8 | 4 | 0 | 0.05 | 0.14 | 27.3 | 11288 |
| onion, white, raw | 160 | 64 | 142.6 | 14.9 | 6.8 | 0 | 2.7 | 6 | 37 | 16 | 0.27 | 0.206 | 0 | 12 | 0.07 | 0.2 | 0 | 0.20 |
| 1 cup chopped | | 1.8 | 0.2 | 0.1 | 0 | 0 | 0 | 234 | 46 | 0.34 | 0.062 | 0.8 | 3 | 0 | 0.04 | 0.19 | 30.4 | 11282 |
| onion, Welsh, raw | 160 | 54 | 144.8 | 10.4 | | | | 27 | 29 | 37 | 0.83 | 0.219 | 93 | 43 | 0.08 | 0.6 | 0 | 0.27 |
| 1 cup chopped | | 3.0 | 0.6 | 0.1 | 0.1 | 0.2 | 0 | 339 | 78 | 1.95 | 0.112 | 1.0 | 1856 | | 0.14 | 0.12 | 25.6 | 11293 |
| parsnip, boiled, drained | 160 | 114 | 128.4 | 27.2 | 7.7 | 0 | 5.8 | 16 | 59 | 46 | 0.42 | 0.470 | 0 | 21 | 0.13 | 1.2 | 0 | 0.94 |
| 1 parsnip (9" long) | | 2.1 | 0.5 | 0.1 | 0.2 | 0.1 | 0 | 587 | 110 | 0.93 | 0.221 | 2.7 | 0 | 1.6 | 0.08 | 0.15 | 92.8 | 11299 |
| parsnip, raw | 67 | 50 | 53.3 | 12.1 | 3.2 | 0 | 3.3 | 7 | 24 | 19 | 0.40 | 0.375 | 0 | 11 | 0.06 | 0.5 | 0 | 0.40 |
| ½ cup | | 0.8 | 0.2 | 0 | 0.1 | 0 | 0 | 251 | 48 | 0.40 | 0.080 | 1.2 | 0 | 1.0 | 0.03 | 0.06 | 44.9 | 11298 |
| poi | 240 | 269 | 171.9 | 65.4 | 0.9 | 0 | 1.0 | 29 | 38 | 58 | 0.53 | 0.888 | 7 | 10 | 0.31 | 2.6 | 0 | 0.70 |
| 1 cup | | 0.9 | 0.3 | 0.1 | 0 | 0.1 | 0 | 439 | 94 | 2.11 | 0.398 | 1.7 | 158 | 5.5 | 0.10 | 0.66 | 50.4 | 11349 |
| potato, baked | 173 | 161 | 129.6 | 36.6 | 2.0 | 0 | 3.8 | 17 | 26 | 48 | 0.62 | 0.379 | 2 | 17 | 0.11 | 2.4 | 0 | 0.65 |
| 1 medium (2¼" diameter) | | 4.3 | 0.2 | 0.1 | 0 | 0.1 | 0 | 926 | 121 | 1.87 | 0.204 | 0.7 | 17 | 0.1 | 0.08 | 0.54 | 48.4 | 11674 |
| potato, baked, peeled | 156 | 145 | 117.7 | 33.6 | 2.7 | 0 | 2.3 | 8 | 8 | 39 | 0.45 | 0.251 | 0 | 20 | 0.16 | 2.2 | 0 | 0.87 |
| 1 potato (2⅓" × 4¾") | | 3.1 | 0.2 | 0 | 0 | 0.1 | 0 | 610 | 78 | 0.55 | 0.335 | 0.5 | 0 | 0.1 | 0.03 | 0.47 | 14.0 | 11363 |
| potato, cheesy scalloped, from mix, Betty Crocker - ½ cup prep | 143 | 120 | | 22.0 | 2.0 | | 1.0 | 590 | 40 | | | | | | | 0.8 | | |
| | | 3.0 | 3.0 | 1.0 | | | 0 | 300 | | 0.36 | | | 100 | | 0.07 | | | GENM368 |
| potato, cottage fries, frzn, heated | 50 | 109 | 26.4 | 17.0 | | | 1.6 | 22 | 5 | 11 | 0.20 | 0.152 | 0 | 5 | 0.06 | 1.2 | 0 | 0.34 |
| 10 pieces | | 1.7 | 4.1 | 1.9 | 1.7 | 0.3 | 0 | 240 | 32 | 0.74 | 0.100 | 0.2 | 0 | | 0.02 | 0.12 | 8.5 | 11407 |
| potato, French fries, extruded, frzn, heated - 10 pieces | 50 | 166 | 17.7 | 19.8 | | | 1.6 | 306 | 6 | 12 | 0.20 | 0.142 | 0 | 3 | 0.04 | 1.3 | 0 | 0.30 |
| | | 1.8 | 9.4 | 3.0 | 5.7 | 0.7 | 0 | 270 | 48 | 0.83 | 0.020 | 0.3 | 0 | | 0.02 | 0.11 | 11.0 | 11409 |
| potato, French fries, frozen | 50 | 74 | 33.3 | 12.4 | 0.1 | 0 | 1.0 | 166 | 4 | 10 | 0.18 | 0.079 | 0 | 9 | 0.05 | 1.0 | 0 | 0.24 |
| 10 pieces | | 1.1 | 2.3 | 0.5 | 1.6 | 0.2 | 0 | 204 | 42 | 0.31 | 0.046 | | 2 | 0 | 0.02 | 0.09 | 17.5 | 11402 |
| potato, French fries, frozen, baked | 50 | 67 | 31.2 | 13.9 | 0.1 | 0 | 1.4 | 194 | 6 | 13 | 0.19 | 0.105 | 0 | 7 | 0.06 | 1.1 | 0 | 0.26 |
| 10 pieces | | 1.3 | 2.6 | 0.5 | 1.6 | 0.2 | 0 | 226 | 48 | 0.37 | 0.068 | 0.1 | 2 | 0.1 | 0.02 | 0.09 | 14.0 | 11403 |
| potato, hashed brown, frzn, prep | 156 | 340 | 87.5 | 43.8 | 2.4 | 0 | 3.1 | 53 | 23 | 27 | 0.50 | 0.348 | 0 | 10 | 0.17 | 3.8 | 0 | 0.70 |
| 1 cup | | 4.9 | 17.9 | 7.0 | 8.0 | 2.1 | 0 | 680 | 112 | 2.36 | 0.237 | 0.5 | 0 | 0.3 | 0.03 | 0.20 | 10.9 | 11391 |
| potato, hashed brown, homemade | 156 | 413 | 73.7 | 54.8 | 2.3 | 0 | 5.0 | 534 | 22 | 55 | 0.73 | 0.385 | 0 | 20 | 0.27 | 3.6 | 0 | 1.39 |
| 1 cup | | 4.7 | 19.5 | 2.9 | 8.3 | 7.4 | 0 | 899 | 109 | 0.86 | 0.457 | 0.8 | 8 | 0 | 0.05 | 0.74 | 25.0 | 11370 |
| potato, hashed brown w/butter sce, frozen, prepared - 1 cup | 152 | 271 | 96.8 | 36.7 | | | 5.8 | 154 | 50 | 23 | 0.50 | 0.371 | 40 | 6 | 0.08 | 2.2 | 0 | 0.56 |
| | | 3.7 | 13.4 | 5.1 | 4.8 | 2.8 | 35 | 497 | 58 | 1.50 | 0.155 | 0.5 | 169 | | 0.05 | 0.40 | 19.8 | 11393 |
| potato, mashed | 240 | 199 | 188.4 | 42.1 | 3.6 | 0 | 3.6 | 725 | 58 | 43 | 0.70 | 0.286 | 10 | 15 | 0.21 | 2.7 | 0.17 | 1.16 |
| 1 cup | | 4.6 | 1.4 | 0.6 | 0.2 | 0.1 | 5 | 715 | 113 | 0.65 | 0.343 | 1.9 | 43 | 0 | 0.10 | 0.56 | 19.2 | 11657 |
| potato, mashed, four cheese, from mix, Bty Crkr - ½ cup prep | 105 | 170 | | 22.0 | 4.0 | | 1.0 | 490 | 100 | | | | | | | 0.8 | | |
| | | 4.0 | 7.0 | 2.0 | | | 5 | 440 | | 0.36 | | | 300 | | 0.14 | | | GENM370 |
| potato, mashed, from flakes w/o milk - 1 cup | 210 | 204 | 170.6 | 22.7 | 3.4 | 0 | 1.7 | 344 | 67 | 23 | 0.38 | 0.044 | 90 | 20 | 0.27 | 1.6 | 0.23 | 0.71 |
| | | 3.8 | 10.8 | 6.7 | 2.8 | 0.5 | 29 | 349 | 86 | 0.34 | 0.059 | 5.2 | 332 | 0.3 | 0.12 | 0.21 | 14.7 | 11379 |
| potato, mashed, from granules w/milk - 1 cup | 210 | 244 | 159.6 | 33.8 | 3.7 | 0 | 2.7 | 359 | 71 | 42 | 0.52 | 0.418 | 99 | 14 | 0.19 | 1.8 | 0.21 | 0.30 |
| | | 4.6 | 10.1 | 2.5 | 4.1 | 2.8 | 4 | 330 | 134 | 0.42 | 0.050 | 11.8 | 424 | 1.1 | 0.18 | 0.34 | 16.8 | 11383 |
| potato, mashed, from mix, Potato Buds - ½ cup prepared | 105 | 160 | | 19.0 | 2.0 | | 1.0 | 460 | 20 | | | | | | | 1.2 | | |
| | | 3.0 | 8.0 | 1.5 | | | 5 | 370 | | 0.36 | | | 300 | | | | | GENM371 |
| potato, mashed, homemade w/ whole milk and butter - 1 cup | 210 | 237 | 158.1 | 35.5 | 3.0 | 0 | 3.2 | 699 | 46 | 40 | 0.63 | 0.235 | 86 | 22 | 0.19 | 2.5 | 0.15 | 1.00 |
| | | 4.1 | 8.8 | 2.0 | 3.9 | 2.4 | 2 | 689 | 103 | 0.55 | 0.321 | 1.7 | 376 | 0.9 | 0.09 | 0.52 | 18.9 | 11371 |
| potato, mashed, roasted garlic, from mix, Betty Crocker - ½ cup prep | 105 | 170 | | 22.0 | 4.0 | | 1.0 | 350 | 80 | | | | | | | 0.8 | | |
| | | 4.0 | 7.0 | 2.0 | | | 5 | 400 | | 0.36 | | | 300 | | 0.14 | | | GENM372 |
| potato, mashed, sour crm and chives, from mix, Bty Crkr - ½ cup prep | 105 | 170 | | 22.0 | 5.0 | | 1.0 | 460 | 100 | | | | | | | 0.8 | | |
| | | 4.0 | 7.0 | 2.0 | | | 5 | 410 | | 0.36 | | | 300 | | 0.14 | | | GENM373 |
| potato, microwaved | 202 | 212 | 145.5 | 49.0 | | | 4.6 | 16 | 22 | 55 | 0.73 | 0.590 | 0 | 31 | 0.24 | 3.5 | 0 | 0.92 |
| 1 potato (2½" diameter) | | 4.9 | 0.2 | 0.1 | 0 | 0.1 | 0 | 903 | 212 | 2.50 | 0.675 | 0.8 | 0 | | 0.06 | 0.69 | 24.2 | 11675 |
| potato pancake, homemade | 76 | 204 | 36.2 | 21.2 | 1.4 | 0 | 2.4 | 581 | 24 | 27 | 0.53 | 0.198 | 24 | 21 | 0.12 | 1.3 | 0.22 | 0.58 |
| 1 pancake | | 4.6 | 11.2 | 1.9 | 2.8 | 5.7 | 72 | 473 | 97 | 1.27 | 0.137 | 6.8 | 86 | 0.2 | 0.13 | 0.34 | 34.2 | 11672 |

| | WT (g) | Macronutrients KCAL | H₂0 (g) | CHO (g) | TSUG (g) | ASUG (g) | DFIB (g) | Minerals Na (mg) | Ca (mg) | Mg (mg) | Zn (mg) | Mn (mg) | Vitamins A (mcg RAE) | C (mg) | B-1 (mg) | NIA (mg) | B-12 (mcg) | PANT (mg) |
|---|---|---|---|---|---|---|---|---|---|---|---|---|---|---|---|---|---|---|
| | | PRO (g) | FAT (g) | SFA (g) | MUFA (g) | PUFA (g) | CHOL (mg) | K (mg) | P (mg) | Fe (mg) | Cu (mg) | Se (mcg) | A (IU) | E (mg ATE) | B-2 (mg) | B-6 (mg) | FOL (mcg DFE) | REF |
| **potato peel**, baked | 58 | 115 | 27.4 | 26.7 | 0.8 | 0 | 4.6 | 12 | 20 | 25 | 0.28 | 0.357 | 1 | 8 | 0.07 | 1.8 | 0 | 0.50 |
| *2 oz peel* | | 2.5 | 0.1 | 0 | 0 | 0 | 0 | 332 | 59 | 4.08 | 0.474 | 0.4 | 6 | 0 | 0.06 | 0.36 | 12.8 | 11364 |
| **potato**, peeled, boiled | 167 | 144 | 129.4 | 33.4 | 1.4 | 0 | 3.0 | 8 | 13 | 33 | 0.45 | 0.234 | 0 | 12 | 0.16 | 2.2 | 0 | 0.85 |
| *1 medium (2¼–3¼″ diameter)* | | 2.9 | 0.2 | 0 | 0 | 0.1 | 0 | 548 | 67 | 0.52 | 0.279 | 0.5 | 5 | 0 | 0.03 | 0.45 | 15.0 | 11367 |
| **potato**, peeled, canned, drained | 180 | 108 | 151.7 | 24.5 | | | 4.1 | 394 | 9 | 25 | 0.50 | 0.175 | 0 | 9 | 0.12 | 1.6 | 0 | 0.64 |
| *1 cup* | | 2.5 | 0.4 | 0.1 | 0 | 0.2 | 0 | 412 | 50 | 2.27 | 0.103 | 1.6 | 0 | | 0.02 | 0.34 | 10.8 | 11376 |
| **potato**, peeled, microwaved | 156 | 156 | 114.7 | 36.3 | | | 2.5 | 11 | 8 | 39 | 0.51 | 0.265 | 0 | 24 | 0.20 | 2.5 | 0 | 0.93 |
| *1 potato (2⅓″ × 4¾″)* | | 3.3 | 0.2 | 0 | 0 | 0.1 | 0 | 641 | 170 | 0.64 | 0.370 | 0.6 | 0 | | 0.04 | 0.50 | 18.7 | 11368 |
| **potato puffs**, frozen, heated | 128 | 243 | 76.4 | 35.5 | 0.3 | 0 | 3.2 | 614 | 18 | 22 | 0.41 | 0.163 | 0 | 8 | 0.17 | 1.9 | 0 | 0.38 |
| *1 cup (18 puffs)* | | 2.6 | 11.0 | 2.3 | 7.7 | 0.6 | 0 | 399 | 132 | 0.82 | 0.090 | 0.8 | 6 | 0.3 | 0.04 | 0.16 | 17.9 | 11399 |
| **potato**, raw | 213 | 164 | 169.0 | 37.2 | 1.7 | 0 | 4.7 | 13 | 26 | 49 | 0.62 | 0.326 | 0 | 42 | 0.17 | 2.2 | 0 | 0.63 |
| *1 medium (2¼–3¼″ diameter)* | | 4.3 | 0.2 | 0.1 | 0 | 0.1 | 0 | 897 | 121 | 1.66 | 0.230 | 0.6 | 4 | 0 | 0.07 | 0.63 | 34.1 | 11352 |
| **potato**, red-skinned, baked | 138 | 123 | 105.8 | 27.0 | 2.0 | | 2.5 | 17 | 12 | 39 | 0.55 | 0.239 | 1 | 17 | 0.10 | 2.2 | 0 | 0.47 |
| *1 small (1¾–2½″ diameter)* | | 3.2 | 0.2 | 0 | 0 | 0.1 | 0 | 752 | 99 | 0.97 | 0.240 | 1.1 | 14 | 0.1 | 0.07 | 0.29 | 37.3 | 11358 |
| **potato**, red-skinned, raw | 213 | 149 | 172.4 | 33.9 | 2.1 | | 3.6 | 13 | 21 | 47 | 0.70 | 0.300 | 0 | 18 | 0.17 | 2.4 | 0 | 0.59 |
| *1 medium (2¼–3¼″ diameter)* | | 4.0 | 0.3 | 0.1 | 0 | 0.1 | 0 | 969 | 130 | 1.55 | 0.285 | 1.1 | 15 | 0 | 0.07 | 0.36 | 38.3 | 11355 |
| **potato**, russet, baked | 138 | 134 | 102.7 | 29.6 | 1.5 | | 3.2 | 19 | 25 | 41 | 0.48 | 0.315 | 1 | 18 | 0.09 | 1.9 | 0 | 0.52 |
| *1 small (1¾–2½″ diameter)* | | 3.6 | 0.2 | 0 | 0 | 0.1 | 0 | 759 | 98 | 1.48 | 0.148 | 0.7 | 14 | 0.1 | 0.07 | 0.49 | 35.9 | 11356 |
| **potato**, russet, raw | 213 | 168 | 167.4 | 38.5 | 1.3 | | 2.8 | 11 | 28 | 49 | 0.62 | 0.334 | 0 | 12 | 0.17 | 2.2 | 0 | 0.64 |
| *1 medium (2¼–3¼″ diameter)* | | 4.6 | 0.2 | 0 | 0 | 0.1 | 0 | 888 | 117 | 1.83 | 0.219 | 0.9 | 2 | 0 | 0.07 | 0.73 | 29.8 | 11353 |
| **potato salad**, homemade | 250 | 358 | 190.0 | 27.9 | | | 3.2 | 1322 | 48 | 38 | 0.78 | 0.252 | 80 | 25 | 0.19 | 2.2 | 0 | 1.34 |
| *1 cup* | | 6.7 | 20.5 | 3.6 | 6.2 | 9.3 | 170 | 635 | 130 | 1.62 | 0.295 | 10.2 | 392 | | 0.15 | 0.35 | 17.5 | 11414 |
| **potato**, scalloped, from mix | 137 | 127 | 108.5 | 17.5 | | | 1.5 | 467 | 49 | 19 | 0.34 | 0.248 | 48 | 5 | 0.03 | 1.4 | 0 | 0.45 |
| *⅙ of 5.5 oz package* | | 2.9 | 5.9 | 3.6 | 1.7 | 0.3 | 15 | 278 | 77 | 0.52 | 0.067 | 2.2 | 203 | | 0.08 | 0.06 | 13.7 | 11387 |
| **potato**, scalloped, homemade | 245 | 216 | 198.3 | 26.4 | | | 4.7 | 821 | 140 | 47 | 0.98 | 0.407 | | 26 | 0.17 | 2.6 | 0 | 1.26 |
| *1 cup* | | 7.0 | 9.0 | 5.5 | 2.5 | 0.4 | 29 | 926 | 154 | 1.40 | 0.399 | 3.9 | 331 | | 0.23 | 0.44 | 31.8 | 11372 |
| **potato**, sour crm 'n chive, from mix, | 139 | 120 | | 21.0 | 2.0 | | 1.0 | 680 | 20 | | | | | | | 1.2 | | |
| Betty Crocker - *½ cup prep* | | 2.0 | 3.5 | 1.0 | | | 0 | 250 | | 0.36 | | | 100 | | 0.03 | | | GENM376 |
| **potato**, white-skinned, baked | 138 | 130 | 104.1 | 29.1 | 1.9 | | 2.9 | 10 | 14 | 37 | 0.48 | 0.261 | 1 | 17 | 0.07 | 2.1 | 0 | 0.53 |
| *1 small (1¾–2½″ diameter)* | | 2.9 | 0.2 | 0 | 0 | 0 | 0 | 751 | 103 | 0.88 | 0.175 | 0.7 | 14 | 0.1 | 0.06 | 0.29 | 52.4 | 11357 |
| **potato**, white-skinned, raw | 213 | 147 | 173.8 | 33.5 | 2.4 | | 5.1 | 13 | 19 | 45 | 0.62 | 0.309 | 0 | 42 | 0.15 | 2.3 | 0 | 0.60 |
| *1 medium (2¼–3¼″ diameter)* | | 3.6 | 0.2 | 0.1 | 0 | 0.1 | 0 | 867 | 132 | 1.11 | 0.247 | 0.6 | 17 | 0 | 0.07 | 0.43 | 38.3 | 11354 |
| **potatoes** au gratin, from mix | 137 | 127 | 108.2 | 17.6 | | | 1.2 | 601 | 114 | 21 | 0.33 | 0.178 | 71 | 4 | 0.03 | 1.3 | 0 | 0.33 |
| *⅙ of 5.5 oz package* | | 3.2 | 5.6 | 3.5 | 1.6 | 0.2 | 21 | 300 | 130 | 0.44 | 0.063 | 3.7 | 292 | | 0.11 | 0.05 | 9.6 | 11385 |
| **potatoes** au gratin, from mix, Betty | 141 | 140 | | 21.0 | 3.0 | | 1.0 | 600 | 40 | | | | | | | 1.2 | | |
| Crocker - *½ cup prep* | | 3.0 | 5.0 | 1.5 | | | 2 | 250 | | 0.36 | | | 200 | | 0.07 | | | GENM367 |
| **potatoes** au gratin, homemade | 245 | 323 | 181.3 | 27.6 | | | 4.4 | 1061 | 292 | 49 | 1.69 | 0.394 | 157 | 24 | 0.16 | 2.4 | 0 | 0.95 |
| *1 cup* | | 12.4 | 18.6 | 11.6 | 5.3 | 0.7 | 56 | 970 | 277 | 1.57 | 0.392 | 6.6 | 647 | | 0.28 | 0.43 | 31.8 | 11373 |
| **potatoes** O'Brien, frozen, prepared | 85 | 173 | 52.7 | 18.6 | | | 1.4 | 37 | 17 | 29 | 0.47 | 0.192 | 8 | 9 | 0.04 | 1.2 | 0 | 0.62 |
| *⅔ cup* | | 1.9 | 11.2 | 2.8 | 5.0 | 3.0 | 0 | 402 | 79 | 0.82 | 0.205 | 1.0 | 160 | | 0.11 | 0.32 | 10.2 | 11397 |
| **potatoes** O'Brien, homemade | 194 | 157 | 154.4 | 30.0 | | | | 421 | 70 | 35 | 0.58 | 0.235 | | 32 | 0.15 | 2.0 | 0 | 0.85 |
| *1 cup* | | 4.6 | 2.5 | 1.5 | 0.7 | 0.1 | 8 | 516 | 97 | 0.91 | 0.250 | 2.3 | 933 | | 0.11 | 0.41 | 15.5 | 11671 |
| **radish**, Oriental, boiled, drained | 147 | 25 | 139.7 | 5.0 | 2.7 | 0 | 2.4 | 19 | 25 | 13 | 0.19 | 0.049 | 0 | 22 | 0 | 0.2 | 0 | 0.17 |
| *1 cup sliced* | | 1.0 | 0.4 | 0.1 | 0.1 | 0.2 | 0 | 419 | 35 | 0.22 | 0.148 | 1.0 | 0 | 0 | 0.03 | 0.06 | 25.0 | 11431 |
| **radish**, Oriental, dried | 116 | 314 | 22.8 | 73.5 | | | | 322 | 730 | 197 | 2.47 | 0.625 | 0 | 0 | 0.31 | 3.9 | 0 | 2.15 |
| *1 cup* | | 9.2 | 0.8 | 0.3 | 0.1 | 0.4 | 0 | 4053 | 237 | 7.81 | 1.892 | 0.8 | 0 | | 0.79 | 0.72 | 342.2 | 11432 |
| **radish**, Oriental, raw | 338 | 61 | 319.8 | 13.9 | 8.4 | 0 | 5.4 | 71 | 91 | 54 | 0.51 | 0.128 | 0 | 74 | 0.07 | 0.7 | 0 | 0.47 |
| *1 radish 7″ long* | | 2.0 | 0.3 | 0.1 | 0.1 | 0.2 | 0 | 767 | 78 | 1.35 | 0.389 | 2.4 | 0 | 0 | 0.07 | 0.16 | 94.6 | 11430 |
| **radish**, red, raw | 58 | 9 | 55.3 | 2.0 | 1.1 | 0 | 0.9 | 23 | 14 | 6 | 0.16 | 0.040 | 0 | 9 | 0.01 | 0.1 | 0 | 0.10 |
| *½ cup sliced* | | 0.4 | 0.1 | 0 | 0 | 0 | 0 | 135 | 12 | 0.20 | 0.029 | 0.3 | 4 | 0 | 0.02 | 0.04 | 14.5 | 11429 |
| **radish**, white icicle, raw | 50 | 7 | 47.7 | 1.3 | | | 0.7 | 8 | 14 | 4 | 0.06 | 0.016 | 0 | 14 | 0.02 | 0.2 | 0 | 0.09 |
| *½ cup sliced* | | 0.6 | 0 | 0 | 0 | 0 | 0 | 140 | 14 | 0.40 | 0.050 | 0.4 | 0 | | 0.01 | 0.04 | 7.0 | 11637 |
| **rutabaga** (swede), boiled, drained | 170 | 66 | 151.1 | 14.9 | 10.2 | 0 | 3.1 | 34 | 82 | 39 | 0.60 | 0.296 | 0 | 32 | 0.14 | 1.2 | 0 | 0.26 |
| *1 cup cubed* | | 2.2 | 0.4 | 0 | 0 | 0.2 | 0 | 554 | 95 | 0.90 | 0.070 | 1.2 | 3 | 0.5 | 0.07 | 0.17 | 25.5 | 11436 |
| **rutabaga** (swede), raw | 140 | 50 | 125.5 | 11.4 | 7.8 | 0 | 3.5 | 28 | 66 | 32 | 0.48 | 0.238 | 0 | 35 | 0.13 | 1.0 | 0 | 0.22 |
| *1 cup cubed* | | 1.7 | 0.3 | 0 | 0 | 0.1 | 0 | 472 | 81 | 0.73 | 0.056 | 1.0 | 3 | 0.4 | 0.06 | 0.14 | 29.4 | 11435 |
| **shallots**, raw | 40 | 29 | 31.9 | 6.7 | | | | 5 | 15 | 8 | 0.16 | 0.117 | 24 | 3 | 0.02 | 0.1 | | 0.12 |
| *4 T chopped* | | 1.0 | 0 | 0 | 0 | 0 | 0 | 134 | 24 | 0.48 | 0.035 | 0.5 | 476 | | 0.01 | 0.14 | 13.6 | 11677 |
| **sweet potato**, baked - *1 medium* | 114 | 103 | 86.4 | 23.6 | 7.4 | 0 | 3.8 | 41 | 43 | 31 | 0.36 | 0.567 | 1096 | 22 | 0.12 | 1.7 | 0 | 1.01 |
| *(2″ diameter, 5″ long)* | | 2.3 | 0.2 | 0 | 0 | 0.1 | 0 | 542 | 62 | 0.79 | 0.184 | 0.2 | 21909 | 0.8 | 0.12 | 0.33 | 6.8 | 11508 |
| **sweet potato**, candied, frzn, Green | 137 | 240 | | 41.0 | 20.0 | | 3.0 | 430 | 20 | | | | | 12 | | | | |
| Giant - *¾ cup* | | 2.0 | 7.0 | 1.0 | | | 0 | | | 0.72 | | | 13500 | | | | | GENM378 |

| Food | WT (g) | KCAL / PRO | H₂0 / FAT | CHO / SFA | TSUG / MUFA | ASUG / PUFA | DFIB / CHOL | Na / K | Ca / P | Mg / Fe | Zn / Cu | Mn / Se | A (mcg RAE) / A (IU) | C / E | B-1 / B-2 | NIA / B-6 | B-12 / FOL | PANT / REF |
|---|---|---|---|---|---|---|---|---|---|---|---|---|---|---|---|---|---|---|
| **sweet potato, candied, homemade** | 105 | 151 | 70.3 | 29.3 | | | 2.5 | 74 | 27 | 12 | 0.16 | 0.448 | 0 | 7 | 0.02 | 0.4 | 0 | 0.28 |
| *1 piece (2" diameter, 2½" long)* | | 0.9 | 3.4 | 1.4 | 0.7 | 0.2 | 8 | 198 | 27 | 1.19 | 0.107 | 0.8 | 0 | | 0.04 | 0.04 | 11.6 | 11659 |
| **sweet potato, canned in light syrup, drained** - *1 cup* | 196 | 212 | 142.0 | 49.7 | 11.3 | | 5.9 | 76 | 33 | 24 | 0.31 | 1.205 | 898 | 21 | 0.05 | 0.7 | 0 | 0.79 |
| | | 2.5 | 0.6 | 0.1 | 0 | 0.3 | 0 | 378 | 49 | 1.86 | 0.327 | 1.6 | 17971 | 2.3 | 0.07 | 0.12 | 15.7 | 11647 |
| **sweet potato, canned, mashed** | 255 | 258 | 188.4 | 59.1 | 13.9 | | 4.3 | 191 | 76 | 61 | 0.54 | 2.519 | 1109 | 13 | 0.07 | 2.4 | 0 | 1.31 |
| *1 cup* | | 5.0 | 0.5 | 0.1 | 0 | 0.2 | 0 | 536 | 133 | 3.39 | 0.709 | 2.0 | 22182 | 2.8 | 0.23 | 0.60 | 28.0 | 11514 |
| **sweet potato, canned, vacuum pack** | 200 | 182 | 152.1 | 42.2 | 10.0 | 0 | 3.6 | 106 | 44 | 44 | 0.36 | 0.910 | 798 | 53 | 0.07 | 1.5 | 0 | 1.05 |
| *1 cup pieces* | | 3.3 | 0.4 | 0.1 | 0 | 0.2 | 0 | 624 | 98 | 1.78 | 0.278 | 1.4 | 15966 | 2.0 | 0.11 | 0.38 | 34.0 | 11512 |
| **sweet potato, frozen** | 176 | 169 | 131.8 | 39.1 | | | 3.0 | 11 | 65 | 39 | 0.55 | 1.170 | 912 | 23 | 0.12 | 1.1 | 0 | 0.91 |
| *1 cup cubed* | | 3.0 | 0.3 | 0.1 | | 0.1 | 0 | 642 | 79 | 0.93 | 0.312 | 1.1 | 18246 | | 0.09 | 0.31 | 37.0 | 11516 |
| **sweet potato, frozen, baked** | 176 | 176 | 129.7 | 41.2 | 16.1 | | 3.2 | 14 | 62 | 37 | 0.53 | 1.170 | 1836 | 16 | 0.12 | 1.0 | 0 | 0.99 |
| *1 cup cubed* | | 3.0 | 0.2 | 0 | | 0.1 | 0 | 664 | 77 | 0.95 | 0.322 | 1.1 | 36731 | 1.4 | 0.10 | 0.33 | 38.7 | 11517 |
| **sweet potato, peeled, boiled** | 328 | 249 | 262.8 | 58.1 | 18.8 | 0 | 8.2 | 89 | 89 | 59 | 0.66 | 0.872 | 2581 | 42 | 0.18 | 1.8 | 0 | 1.91 |
| *1 cup mashed* | | 4.5 | 0.5 | 0.1 | 0 | 0.2 | 0 | 754 | 105 | 2.36 | 0.308 | 0.7 | 51627 | 3.1 | 0.15 | 0.54 | 19.7 | 11510 |
| **sweet potato, raw** | 130 | 112 | 100.5 | 26.2 | 5.4 | 0 | 3.9 | 72 | 39 | 32 | 0.39 | 0.335 | 922 | 3 | 0.10 | 0.7 | 0 | 1.04 |
| *1 medium (5" long)* | | 2.0 | 0.1 | 0 | 0 | 0 | 0 | 438 | 61 | 0.79 | 0.196 | 0.8 | 18443 | 0.3 | 0.08 | 0.27 | 14.3 | 11507 |
| **taro, cooked** | 132 | 187 | 84.2 | 45.7 | 0.6 | 0 | 6.7 | 20 | 24 | 40 | 0.36 | 0.593 | 5 | 7 | 0.14 | 0.7 | 0 | 0.44 |
| *1 cup sliced* | | 0.7 | 0.1 | 0 | 0 | 0.1 | 0 | 639 | 100 | 0.95 | 0.265 | 1.2 | 111 | 3.9 | 0.04 | 0.44 | 25.1 | 11519 |
| **taro, raw** | 104 | 116 | 73.5 | 27.5 | 0.4 | 0 | 4.3 | 11 | 45 | 34 | 0.24 | 0.398 | 4 | 5 | 0.10 | 0.6 | 0 | 0.32 |
| *1 cup* | | 1.6 | 0.2 | 0 | 0 | 0.1 | 0 | 615 | 87 | 0.57 | 0.179 | 0.7 | 79 | 2.5 | 0.03 | 0.29 | 22.9 | 11518 |
| **taro, Tahitian, cooked** | 137 | 60 | 118.5 | 9.4 | | | | 74 | 204 | 70 | 0.14 | 0.230 | 121 | 52 | 0.06 | 0.7 | 0 | 0.17 |
| *1 cup sliced* | | 5.7 | 0.9 | 0.2 | 0.1 | 0.4 | 0 | 854 | 92 | 2.14 | 0.104 | 1.1 | 2417 | | 0.27 | 0.16 | 9.6 | 11526 |
| **turnip, boiled, drained** | 156 | 34 | 146.0 | 7.9 | 4.7 | 0 | 3.1 | 25 | 51 | 14 | 0.19 | 0.111 | 0 | 18 | 0.04 | 0.5 | 0 | 0.22 |
| *1 cup cubed* | | 1.1 | 0.1 | 0 | 0 | 0.1 | 0 | 276 | 41 | 0.28 | 0.003 | 0.3 | 0 | 0 | 0.04 | 0.10 | 14.0 | 11565 |
| **turnip, frozen, boiled, drained** | 156 | 36 | 146.0 | 6.8 | 3.7 | 0 | 3.1 | 56 | 50 | 22 | 0.31 | 0.156 | 0 | 6 | 0.05 | 0.9 | 0 | 0.22 |
| *1 cup* | | 2.4 | 0.4 | 0 | 0 | 0.2 | 0 | 284 | 41 | 1.53 | 0.098 | 0.9 | 0 | 0 | 0.04 | 0.10 | 12.5 | 11567 |
| **turnip, raw** | 130 | 36 | 119.4 | 8.4 | 4.9 | 0 | 2.3 | 87 | 39 | 14 | 0.35 | 0.174 | 0 | 27 | 0.05 | 0.5 | 0 | 0.26 |
| *1 cup cubed* | | 1.2 | 0.1 | 0 | 0 | 0.1 | 0 | 248 | 35 | 0.39 | 0.111 | 0.9 | 0 | 0 | 0.04 | 0.12 | 19.5 | 11564 |
| **wasabi root, raw** | 130 | 142 | 89.8 | 30.6 | | | 10.1 | 22 | 166 | 90 | 2.11 | 0.508 | 3 | 54 | 0.17 | 1.0 | 0 | 0.26 |
| *1 cup sliced* | | 6.2 | 0.8 | | | | 0 | 738 | 104 | 1.34 | 0.202 | | 46 | | 0.15 | 0.36 | 23.4 | 11990 |
| **yam, baked/boiled, drained** | 136 | 158 | 95.4 | 37.4 | 0.7 | 0 | 5.3 | 11 | 19 | 24 | 0.27 | 0.505 | 8 | 16 | 0.13 | 0.8 | 0 | 0.42 |
| *1 cup cubed* | | 2.0 | 0.2 | 0 | 0 | 0.1 | 0 | 911 | 67 | 0.71 | 0.207 | 1.0 | 166 | 0.5 | 0.04 | 0.31 | 21.8 | 11602 |
| **yautia (tannier), raw** | 135 | 132 | 98.6 | 31.9 | | | 2.0 | 28 | 12 | 32 | 0.68 | 0.251 | 0 | 7 | 0.13 | 0.9 | 0 | 0.28 |
| *1 cup sliced* | | 2.0 | 0.5 | 0.1 | | | 0 | 807 | 69 | 1.32 | 0.347 | 0.9 | 11 | | 0.05 | 0.32 | 23.0 | 11991 |

## 30.7 VEGETABLE COMBINATIONS

| Food | WT (g) | KCAL / PRO | H₂0 / FAT | CHO / SFA | TSUG / MUFA | ASUG / PUFA | DFIB / CHOL | Na / K | Ca / P | Mg / Fe | Zn / Cu | Mn / Se | A (mcg RAE) / A (IU) | C / E | B-1 / B-2 | NIA / B-6 | B-12 / FOL | PANT / REF |
|---|---|---|---|---|---|---|---|---|---|---|---|---|---|---|---|---|---|---|
| **broc, cauliflower, carrots in chs sce,** | 120 | 60 | | 8.0 | 3.0 | | 2.0 | 460 | 40 | | | | | 18 | | | | |
| frzn, Green Giant - *⅔ cup* | | 2.0 | 2.5 | 1.0 | 0.5 | 0 | 0 | | | 0.36 | | | 1000 | | | | | GENM381 |
| **corn, yellow w/red and green** | 227 | 170 | 175.9 | 41.2 | | | | 788 | 11 | 57 | 0.84 | 0.098 | 27 | 20 | 0.05 | 2.2 | 0 | 1.01 |
| peprs, cnd, slds & lqu - *1 cup* | | 5.3 | 1.2 | 0.2 | 0.4 | 0.6 | 0 | 347 | 141 | 1.79 | 0.136 | 1.4 | 527 | | 0.18 | 0.22 | 77.2 | 11184 |
| **edamame, mshrms, green beans,** | 85 | 50 | | 5.0 | 1.0 | | 2.0 | 10 | 40 | | | | | 5 | | | | |
| frzn, Petite Blends - *⅔ cup* | | 3.0 | 1.5 | 0 | | | 0 | | | 0.72 | | | 200 | | | | | SAFE44 |
| **green peas and carrots, cnd, solids** | 255 | 97 | 224.8 | 21.6 | | | 5.1 | 663 | 59 | 36 | 1.48 | 0.910 | 737 | 17 | 0.19 | 1.5 | 0 | 0.31 |
| and liquid - *1 cup* | | 5.5 | 0.7 | 0.1 | 0.1 | 0.3 | 0 | 255 | 117 | 1.91 | 0.263 | 2.3 | 14713 | | 0.14 | 0.22 | 45.9 | 11318 |
| **green peas and carrots, frzn,** | 80 | 38 | 68.6 | 8.1 | 3.5 | 0 | 2.5 | 54 | 18 | 13 | 0.36 | 0.162 | 381 | 6 | 0.18 | 0.9 | 0 | 0.13 |
| drained - *½ cup* | | 2.5 | 0.3 | 0.1 | 0 | 0.2 | 0 | 126 | 39 | 0.75 | 0.061 | 0.9 | 7611 | 0.4 | 0.05 | 0.07 | 20.8 | 11323 |
| **green peas and onions, cnd, solids** | 120 | 61 | 103.7 | 10.3 | | | 2.8 | 530 | 20 | 19 | 0.70 | 0.306 | 10 | 4 | 0.12 | 1.5 | 0 | 0.19 |
| and liquid - *1 cup* | | 3.9 | 0.5 | 0.1 | 0 | 0.2 | 0 | 115 | 61 | 1.04 | 0.120 | 0.5 | 193 | | 0.08 | 0.23 | 32.4 | 11324 |
| **green peas and onions, frzn, boiled,** | 180 | 61 | 158.7 | 15.5 | 6.8 | 0 | 4.0 | 67 | 25 | 23 | 0.52 | 0.299 | 95 | 12 | 0.27 | 1.9 | 0 | 0.16 |
| drained - *1 cup* | | 4.6 | 0.4 | 0.1 | 0 | 0.2 | 0 | 211 | 61 | 1.69 | 0.113 | 0.7 | 1892 | | 0.12 | 0.16 | 36.0 | 11327 |
| **mixed vegetables, cnd, drained** | 163 | 80 | 141.8 | 15.1 | 3.9 | 0 | 4.9 | 243 | 44 | 26 | 0.67 | 0.926 | 950 | 8 | 0.07 | 0.9 | 0 | 0.23 |
| *1 cup* | | 4.2 | 0.4 | 0.1 | 0 | 0.2 | 0 | 474 | 68 | 1.71 | 0.119 | 0.5 | 18991 | 0.5 | 0.08 | 0.13 | 39.1 | 11581 |
| **mixed vegetables, frozen** | 182 | 116 | 149.4 | 24.5 | | | 7.3 | 86 | 46 | 44 | 0.82 | 0.444 | 462 | 19 | 0.22 | 2.3 | 0 | 0.30 |
| *1 cup* | | 6.1 | 0.9 | 0.2 | 0.1 | 0.4 | 0 | 386 | 107 | 1.73 | 0.169 | 0.7 | 9242 | | 0.15 | 0.17 | 52.8 | 11583 |
| **mixed vegetables, frzn, boiled,** | 182 | 118 | 151.5 | 23.8 | 5.7 | 0 | 8.0 | 64 | 46 | 40 | 0.89 | 0.690 | 389 | 6 | 0.13 | 1.5 | 0 | 0.27 |
| drained - *1 cup* | | 5.2 | 0.3 | 0.1 | 0 | 0.1 | 0 | 308 | 93 | 1.49 | 0.151 | 0.5 | 7784 | 0.7 | 0.22 | 0.13 | 34.6 | 11584 |
| **mixed vegetables, frzn, drained** | 182 | 118 | 151.5 | 23.8 | 5.7 | 0 | 8.0 | 64 | 46 | 40 | 0.89 | 0.690 | 389 | 6 | 0.13 | 1.5 | 0 | 0.27 |
| *1 cup* | | 5.2 | 0.3 | 0.1 | 0 | 0.1 | 0 | 308 | 93 | 1.49 | 0.151 | 0.5 | 7784 | 0.7 | 0.22 | 0.13 | 34.6 | 11584 |
| **succotash (corn and lima beans),** | 192 | 221 | 131.3 | 46.8 | | | 8.6 | 33 | 33 | 102 | 1.21 | 1.476 | 29 | 16 | 0.32 | 2.5 | 0 | 1.09 |
| boiled, drained - *1 cup* | | 9.7 | 1.5 | 0.3 | 0.3 | 0.7 | 0 | 787 | 225 | 2.92 | 0.344 | 1.2 | 564 | | 0.18 | 0.22 | 63.4 | 11496 |

| | WT (g) | KCAL | H₂0 (g) | CHO (g) | TSUG (g) | ASUG (g) | DFIB (g) | Na (mg) | Ca (mg) | Mg (mg) | Zn (mg) | Mn (mg) | A (mcg RAE) | C (mg) | B-1 (mg) | NIA (mg) | B-12 (mcg) | PANT (mg) |
|---|---|---|---|---|---|---|---|---|---|---|---|---|---|---|---|---|---|---|
| | | PRO (g) | FAT (g) | SFA (g) | MUFA (g) | PUFA (g) | CHOL (mg) | K (mg) | P (mg) | Fe (mg) | Cu (mg) | Se (mcg) | A (IU) | E (mg ATE) | B-2 (mg) | B-6 (mg) | FOL (mcg DFE) | REF |
| **succotash** (corn and lima beans), cnd, solids and liquid - *1 cup* | 255 | 161 | 209.0 | 35.6 | | | 6.6 | 564 | 28 | 48 | 1.27 | 0.933 | 18 | 12 | 0.07 | 1.6 | 0 | 0.79 |
| | | 6.6 | 1.2 | 0.2 | 0.2 | 0.6 | 0 | 416 | 140 | 1.35 | 0.278 | 1.5 | 372 | | 0.15 | 0.12 | 81.6 | 11499 |
| **succotash** (corn and lima beans), frzn, boiled, drained - *1 cup* | 170 | 158 | 126.0 | 33.9 | 3.8 | 0 | 7.0 | 76 | 26 | 39 | 0.76 | 0.476 | 17 | 10 | 0.13 | 2.2 | 0 | 0.39 |
| | | 7.3 | 1.5 | 0.3 | 0.3 | 0.7 | 0 | 450 | 119 | 1.51 | 0.102 | 1.0 | 330 | 0.3 | 0.12 | 0.16 | 56.1 | 11502 |
| **succotash** (corn and lima beans) w/ cream style corn, cnd - *1 cup* | 266 | 205 | 207.9 | 46.8 | | | 8.0 | 652 | 29 | 3 | 1.14 | 1.716 | 19 | 17 | 0.07 | 1.6 | 0 | 0.58 |
| | | 7.0 | 1.4 | 0.3 | 0.3 | 0.7 | 0 | 487 | 157 | 1.46 | 0.473 | 1.6 | 375 | | 0.17 | 0.34 | 117.0 | 11497 |

## 30.8 OTHER VEGETABLES

| | WT (g) | KCAL | H₂0 (g) | CHO (g) | TSUG (g) | ASUG (g) | DFIB (g) | Na (mg) | Ca (mg) | Mg (mg) | Zn (mg) | Mn (mg) | A (mcg RAE) | C (mg) | B-1 (mg) | NIA (mg) | B-12 (mcg) | PANT (mg) |
|---|---|---|---|---|---|---|---|---|---|---|---|---|---|---|---|---|---|---|
| | | PRO (g) | FAT (g) | SFA (g) | MUFA (g) | PUFA (g) | CHOL (mg) | K (mg) | P (mg) | Fe (mg) | Cu (mg) | Se (mcg) | A (IU) | E (mg ATE) | B-2 (mg) | B-6 (mg) | FOL (mcg DFE) | REF |
| **agar**, dried (seaweed) - *1 oz* | 28 | 86 | 2.4 | 22.6 | 0.8 | 0 | 2.2 | 29 | 175 | 216 | 1.62 | 1.204 | 0 | 0 | 0 | 0.1 | 0 | 0.85 |
| | | 1.7 | 0.1 | 0 | 0 | 0 | 0 | 315 | 15 | 5.99 | 0.171 | 2.1 | 0 | 1.4 | 0.06 | 0.08 | 162.4 | 11663 |
| **agar**, raw (seaweed) - *2 T* | 10 | 3 | 9.1 | 0.7 | 0 | 0 | | 1 | 5 | 7 | 0.06 | 0.037 | 0 | 0 | 0 | 0 | 0 | 0.03 |
| | | 0.1 | 0 | 0 | 0 | 0 | 0 | 23 | 0 | 0.19 | 0.006 | 0.1 | 0 | 0.1 | 0 | 0 | 8.5 | 11442 |
| **corn pudding**, homemade - *1 cup* | 250 | 328 | 180.8 | 42.5 | 17.4 | 9.4 | 3.5 | 702 | 100 | 38 | 1.30 | 0.200 | 140 | 9 | 0.17 | 2.6 | 0.68 | 1.19 |
| | | 10.9 | 12.7 | 6.1 | 3.8 | 1.4 | 185 | 440 | 232 | 1.35 | 0.080 | 15.0 | 750 | 0.3 | 0.39 | 0.34 | 82.5 | 11656 |
| **corn, white**, steamed (Navajo) - *1 cup* | 164 | 633 | 13.3 | 123.3 | 10.6 | | 27.2 | 7 | 23 | 202 | 5.17 | 1.519 | | 0 | 0.13 | 5.4 | | 0.49 |
| | | 15.9 | 8.5 | 1.4 | 2.4 | 3.1 | | 872 | 512 | 3.76 | 0.379 | | 0 | | 0.11 | 0.47 | | 35135 |
| **corn, yellow**, boiled, drained - *1 baby ear* | 8 | 9 | 5.6 | 2.0 | 0.3 | 0 | 0.2 | 0 | 0 | 2 | 0.05 | 0.013 | 1 | 0 | 0.02 | 0.1 | 0 | 0.07 |
| | | 0.3 | 0.1 | 0 | 0 | 0 | 0 | 17 | 6 | 0.04 | 0.004 | 0 | 21 | 0 | 0.01 | 0 | 3.7 | 11168 |
| **corn, yellow**, canned, drained - *1 cup* | 164 | 133 | 125.8 | 30.8 | 5.0 | 0 | 3.1 | 489 | 8 | 25 | 0.61 | 0.231 | 3 | 1 | 0.03 | 0.6 | 0 | 0.58 |
| | | 4.3 | 1.5 | 0.3 | 0.4 | 0.8 | 0 | 221 | 79 | 1.18 | 0.087 | 1.1 | 74 | 0.1 | 0.08 | 0.11 | 70.5 | 11172 |
| **corn, yellow**, canned, vacuum pack - *1 cup* | 210 | 166 | 160.8 | 40.8 | 7.5 | 0 | 4.2 | 571 | 10 | 48 | 0.97 | 0.141 | 8 | 17 | 0.09 | 2.5 | 0 | 1.42 |
| | | 5.1 | 1.0 | 0.2 | 0.3 | 0.5 | 0 | 391 | 134 | 0.88 | 0.101 | 1.5 | 170 | 0.1 | 0.15 | 0.12 | 102.9 | 11176 |
| **corn, yellow**, creamed, canned - *1 cup* | 256 | 184 | 201.5 | 46.4 | 8.3 | 6.1 | 3.1 | 730 | 8 | 44 | 1.36 | 0.174 | 10 | 12 | 0.06 | 2.5 | 0 | 0.46 |
| | | 4.5 | 1.2 | 0.2 | 0.3 | 0.5 | 0 | 343 | 131 | 0.97 | 0.133 | 1.0 | 189 | 0.2 | 0.14 | 0.16 | 115.2 | 11174 |
| **corn, yellow**, frozen - *1 cup* | 164 | 144 | 123.0 | 34.0 | 4.1 | 0 | 3.4 | 5 | 7 | 30 | 0.62 | 0.202 | 16 | 10 | 0.14 | 2.9 | 0 | 0.59 |
| | | 5.0 | 1.3 | 0.2 | 0.4 | 0.6 | 0 | 349 | 115 | 0.69 | 0.059 | 1.1 | 320 | 0.1 | 0.11 | 0.28 | 59.0 | 11178 |
| **corn, yellow**, frzn, boiled, drained - *1 cup* | 164 | 133 | 126.3 | 31.7 | 5.0 | 0 | 3.9 | 2 | 5 | 46 | 1.03 | 0.254 | 16 | 6 | 0.05 | 2.2 | 0 | 0.25 |
| | | 4.2 | 1.1 | 0.2 | 0.3 | 0.5 | 0 | 382 | 130 | 0.77 | 0.079 | 1.1 | 326 | 0.1 | 0.10 | 0.16 | 57.4 | 11179 |
| **corn, yellow**, frozen, microwaved - *1 cup* | 141 | 185 | 96.4 | 36.5 | 4.7 | | 3.7 | 6 | 7 | 35 | 0.75 | 0.182 | 17 | | 0.12 | 2.9 | 0 | 0.90 |
| | | 5.1 | 2.0 | 0.2 | 0.4 | 0.7 | 0 | 389 | 134 | 0.55 | 0.076 | | 330 | 0.1 | 0.07 | 0.17 | | 11182 |
| **corn, yellow**, raw - *1 cup* | 154 | 132 | 117.0 | 29.3 | 5.0 | 0 | 4.2 | 23 | 3 | 57 | 0.69 | 0.248 | 14 | 10 | 0.31 | 2.6 | 0 | 1.17 |
| | | 5.0 | 1.8 | 0.3 | 0.5 | 0.9 | 0 | 416 | 137 | 0.80 | 0.083 | 0.9 | 288 | 0.1 | 0.09 | 0.08 | 70.8 | 11167 |
| **hominy, white**, canned - *1 cup* | 165 | 119 | 136.2 | 23.5 | 3.0 | 0 | 4.1 | 346 | 16 | 26 | 1.73 | 0.116 | 0 | 0 | 0 | 0.1 | 0 | 0.25 |
| | | 2.4 | 1.5 | 0.2 | 0.4 | 0.7 | 0 | 15 | 58 | 1.02 | 0.049 | 4.9 | 2 | 0.1 | 0.01 | 0.01 | 1.6 | 20030 |
| **hominy, yellow**, canned - *1 cup* | 160 | 115 | 132.0 | 22.8 | | | 4.0 | 336 | 16 | 26 | 1.68 | 0.112 | 10 | 0 | 0 | 0.1 | 0 | 0.25 |
| | | 2.4 | 1.4 | 0.2 | 0.4 | 0.6 | 0 | 14 | 56 | 0.99 | 0.048 | 4.8 | 176 | | 0.01 | 0.01 | 1.6 | 20330 |
| **Irish moss**, raw (seaweed) - *2 T* | 10 | 5 | 8.1 | 1.2 | 0.1 | 0 | 0.1 | 7 | 7 | 14 | 0.20 | 0.037 | 1 | 0 | 0 | 0.1 | 0 | 0.02 |
| | | 0.2 | 0 | 0 | 0 | 0 | 0 | 6 | 16 | 0.89 | 0.015 | 0.1 | 12 | 0.1 | 0.05 | 0.01 | 18.2 | 11444 |
| **kelp** (kombu/tangle), raw (seaweed) - *2 T* | 10 | 4 | 8.2 | 1.0 | 0.1 | 0 | 0.1 | 23 | 17 | 12 | 0.12 | 0.020 | 1 | 0 | 0 | 0 | 0 | 0.06 |
| | | 0.2 | 0.1 | 0 | 0 | 0 | 0 | 9 | 4 | 0.29 | 0.013 | 0.1 | 12 | 0.1 | 0.02 | 0 | 18.0 | 11445 |
| **laver** (nori), raw (seaweed) - *2 T (~4 sheets)* | 10 | 4 | 8.5 | 0.5 | 0 | 0 | 0 | 5 | 7 | 0 | 0.11 | 0.099 | 26 | 4 | 0.01 | 0.1 | 0 | 0.05 |
| | | 0.6 | 0 | 0 | 0 | 0 | 0 | 36 | 6 | 0.18 | 0.026 | 0.1 | 520 | 0.1 | 0.04 | 0.02 | 14.6 | 11446 |
| **mushrooms, cloud ears**, dried - *1 cup pieces* | 28 | 80 | 4.1 | 20.4 | | | 19.6 | 10 | 45 | 23 | 0.37 | 0.546 | 0 | 0 | 0 | 1.8 | 0 | 0.13 |
| | | 2.6 | 0.2 | | | | 0 | 211 | 52 | 1.65 | 0.051 | 12.2 | 0 | | 0.24 | 0.03 | 10.6 | 11988 |
| **mushrooms, common white**, boiled, drained - *1 cup pieces* | 156 | 44 | 142.1 | 8.3 | 3.0 | 0 | 3.4 | 3 | 9 | 19 | 1.36 | 0.179 | 0 | 6 | 0.11 | 7.0 | 0 | 3.37 |
| | | 3.4 | 0.7 | 0.1 | 0 | 0.3 | 0 | 555 | 136 | 2.71 | 0.786 | 18.6 | 0 | | 0.47 | 0.15 | 28.1 | 11261 |
| **mushrooms, common white**, canned, drained - *1 cup pieces* | 156 | 39 | 142.1 | 7.9 | 3.0 | 0 | 3.7 | 663 | 17 | 23 | 1.12 | 0.134 | 0 | 0 | 0.13 | 2.5 | 0 | 1.27 |
| | | 2.9 | 0.5 | 0 | 0 | 0.2 | 0 | 201 | 103 | 1.23 | 0.367 | 6.4 | 0 | | 0.03 | 0.10 | 18.7 | 11264 |
| **mushrooms, common white**, raw - *1 cup pieces* | 70 | 15 | 64.7 | 2.3 | 1.2 | 0 | 0.7 | 4 | 2 | 6 | 0.36 | 0.033 | 0 | 1 | 0.06 | 2.5 | 0 | 1.05 |
| | | 2.2 | 0.2 | 0 | 0 | 0.1 | 0 | 223 | 60 | 0.35 | 0.223 | 6.5 | 0 | | 0.28 | 0.07 | 11.2 | 11260 |
| **mushrooms, crimini, italian**, brown, raw - *1 piece* | 14 | 4 | 12.9 | 0.6 | 0.2 | 0 | 0.1 | 1 | 3 | 1 | 0.15 | 0.020 | 0 | 0 | 0.01 | 0.5 | 0.01 | 0.21 |
| | | 0.4 | 0 | 0 | 0 | 0 | 0 | 63 | 17 | 0.06 | 0.070 | 3.6 | 0 | 0 | 0.07 | 0.02 | 2.0 | 11266 |
| **mushrooms, enoki**, raw - *1 large* | 5 | 2 | 4.4 | 0.4 | 0 | | 0.1 | 0 | 0 | 1 | 0.03 | 0.004 | 0 | 0 | 0.01 | 0.3 | 0 | 0.05 |
| | | 0.1 | 0 | | | | 0 | 18 | 5 | 0.05 | 0.005 | 0.1 | 0 | 0 | 0.01 | 0 | 2.6 | 11950 |
| **mushrooms, oyster**, raw - *1 large* | 148 | 64 | 131.4 | 9.6 | 1.6 | 0 | 3.4 | 27 | 4 | 27 | 1.14 | 0.167 | 3 | 0 | 0.18 | 7.3 | 0 | 1.92 |
| | | 4.9 | 0.6 | 0 | 0 | 0.1 | 0 | 622 | 178 | 1.97 | 0.361 | 3.8 | 71 | 0 | 0.52 | 0.16 | 40.0 | 11987 |
| **mushrooms, portabella**, raw - *1 medium (3.9 oz)* | 110 | 29 | 100.3 | 5.6 | 2.0 | 0 | 1.6 | 7 | 9 | 12 | 0.66 | 0.156 | 0 | 0 | 0.08 | 5.0 | 0.06 | 1.65 |
| | | 2.8 | 0.2 | 0 | 0 | 0.1 | 0 | 532 | 143 | 0.66 | 0.440 | 12.1 | 0 | | 0.53 | 0.11 | 24.2 | 11265 |
| **mushrooms, shitake**, cooked - *4 mushrooms* | 72 | 40 | 60.1 | 10.4 | 2.6 | 0 | 1.5 | 3 | 2 | 10 | 0.96 | 0.147 | 0 | 0 | 0.03 | 1.1 | 0 | 2.59 |
| | | 1.1 | 0.2 | 0 | 0.1 | 0 | 0 | 84 | 21 | 0.32 | 0.645 | 17.9 | 0 | | 0.12 | 0.11 | 15.1 | 11269 |
| **mushrooms, shitake**, dried - *4 mushrooms* | 15 | 44 | 1.4 | 11.3 | 0.3 | 0 | 1.7 | 2 | 2 | 20 | 1.15 | 0.176 | 0 | 1 | 0.04 | 2.1 | 0 | 3.28 |
| | | 1.4 | 0.1 | 0 | 0 | 0 | 0 | 230 | 44 | 0.26 | 0.775 | 6.9 | 0 | | 0.19 | 0.14 | 24.4 | 11268 |

| | WT (g) | KCAL | H₂O (g) | CHO (g) | TSUG (g) | ASUG (g) | DFIB (g) | Na (mg) | Ca (mg) | Mg (mg) | Zn (mg) | Mn (mg) | A (mcg RAE) | C (mg) | B-1 (mg) | NIA (mg) | B-12 (mcg) | PANT (mg) |
|---|---|---|---|---|---|---|---|---|---|---|---|---|---|---|---|---|---|---|
| | | PRO (g) | FAT (g) | SFA (g) | MUFA (g) | PUFA (g) | CHOL (mg) | K (mg) | P (mg) | Fe (mg) | Cu (mg) | Se (mcg) | A (IU) | E (mg ATE) | B-2 (mg) | B-6 (mg) | FOL (mcg DFE) | REF |
| mushrooms, straw, canned, drained | 182 | 58 | 163.6 | 8.4 | | | 4.6 | 699 | 18 | 13 | 1.22 | 0.178 | 0 | 0 | 0.02 | 0.4 | 0 | 0.75 |
| *1 cup pieces* | | 7.0 | 1.2 | 0.2 | 0 | 0.5 | 0 | 142 | 111 | 2.60 | 0.242 | 27.7 | 0 | | 0.13 | 0.03 | 69.2 | 11989 |
| nopales (prickly pear), cooked | 149 | 22 | 140.5 | 4.9 | 1.7 | 0 | 3.0 | 30 | 244 | 70 | 0.31 | 0.608 | 33 | 8 | 0.02 | 0.4 | 0 | 0.22 |
| *1 cup sliced* | | 2.0 | 0.1 | 0 | 0 | 0 | 0 | 291 | 24 | 0.74 | 0.073 | 1.0 | 660 | 0 | 0.06 | 0.10 | 4.5 | 11964 |
| nopales (prickly pear), raw | 86 | 14 | 80.9 | 2.9 | 1.0 | 0 | 1.9 | 18 | 141 | 45 | 0.22 | 0.393 | 20 | 8 | 0.01 | 0.4 | 0 | 0.14 |
| *1 cup sliced* | | 1.1 | 0.1 | 0 | 0 | 0 | 0 | 221 | 14 | 0.51 | 0.045 | 0.2 | 393 | 0 | 0.04 | 0.06 | 2.6 | 11963 |
| pepeao, dried | 24 | 72 | 2.7 | 19.4 | | | | 17 | 27 | 35 | 1.80 | 0.276 | 0 | 0 | 0.20 | 0.7 | 0 | 5.15 |
| *1 cup pieces* | | 1.2 | 0.1 | | | | 0 | 170 | 28 | 1.47 | 1.217 | 10.9 | 0 | | 0.08 | 0.23 | 38.4 | 11230 |
| pepeao, raw | 99 | 25 | 91.7 | 6.7 | | | | 9 | 16 | 25 | 0.65 | 0.100 | 0 | 1 | 0.08 | 0.1 | 0 | 1.97 |
| *1 cup sliced* | | 0.5 | 0 | | | | 0 | 43 | 14 | 0.55 | 0.441 | 11.0 | 0 | | 0.20 | 0.09 | 18.8 | 11228 |
| spirulina (seaweed), dried | 15 | 44 | 0.7 | 3.6 | 0.5 | 0 | 0.5 | 157 | 18 | 29 | 0.30 | 0.285 | 4 | 2 | 0.36 | 1.9 | 0 | 0.52 |
| *1 cup* | | 8.6 | 1.2 | 0.4 | 0.1 | 0.3 | 0 | 204 | 18 | 4.27 | 0.915 | 1.1 | 86 | 0.8 | 0.55 | 0.05 | 14.1 | 11667 |
| spirulina (seaweed), raw | 28 | 7 | 25.4 | 0.7 | | | | 27 | 3 | 5 | 0.06 | 0.052 | 1 | 0 | 0.06 | 0.3 | 0 | 0.09 |
| *1 oz* | | 1.7 | 0.1 | 0 | 0 | 0 | 0 | 36 | 3 | 0.78 | 0.167 | 0.2 | 16 | | 0.10 | 0.01 | 2.5 | 11666 |
| tree fern, chopped, cooked | 142 | 57 | 125.8 | 15.6 | | | 5.3 | 7 | 11 | 7 | 0.44 | 0.765 | 14 | 43 | 0 | 5.0 | 0 | 0.09 |
| *1 cup* | | 0.4 | 0.1 | 0 | 0 | 0 | 0 | 7 | 6 | 0.23 | 0.287 | 1.3 | 284 | | 0.43 | 0.25 | 21.3 | 11563 |
| wakame (seaweed), raw | 10 | 4 | 8.0 | 0.9 | 0.1 | 0 | 0 | 87 | 15 | 11 | 0.04 | 0.140 | 2 | 0 | 0.01 | 0.2 | 0 | 0.07 |
| *2 T* | | 0.3 | 0.1 | 0 | 0 | 0 | 0 | 5 | 8 | 0.22 | 0.028 | 0.1 | 36 | 0.1 | 0.02 | 0.11 | 19.6 | 11669 |
| water chestnuts, Chinese (matai), cnd, | 70 | 35 | 60.5 | 8.6 | 1.7 | 0 | 1.8 | 6 | 3 | 4 | 0.27 | 0.113 | 0 | 1 | 0.01 | 0.3 | 0 | 0.15 |
| solids and liquid - ½ *cup sliced* | | 0.6 | 0 | 0 | 0 | 0 | 0 | 83 | 13 | 0.61 | 0.070 | 0.5 | 0 | 0.4 | 0.02 | 0.11 | 4.2 | 11590 |
| water chestnuts, Chinese (matai), | 62 | 60 | 45.5 | 14.8 | 3.0 | 0 | 1.9 | 9 | 7 | 14 | 0.31 | 0.205 | 0 | 2 | 0.09 | 0.6 | 0 | 0.30 |
| raw - ½ *cup sliced* | | 0.9 | 0.1 | 0 | 0 | 0 | 0 | 362 | 39 | 0.04 | 0.202 | 0.4 | 0 | 0.7 | 0.12 | 0.20 | 9.9 | 11588 |

# 31. MISCELLANEOUS FOOD INGREDIENTS

| | WT (g) | KCAL | H₂O (g) | CHO (g) | TSUG (g) | ASUG (g) | DFIB (g) | Na (mg) | Ca (mg) | Mg (mg) | Zn (mg) | Mn (mg) | A (mcg RAE) | C (mg) | B-1 (mg) | NIA (mg) | B-12 (mcg) | PANT (mg) |
|---|---|---|---|---|---|---|---|---|---|---|---|---|---|---|---|---|---|---|
| | | PRO (g) | FAT (g) | SFA (g) | MUFA (g) | PUFA (g) | CHOL (mg) | K (mg) | P (mg) | Fe (mg) | Cu (mg) | Se (mcg) | A (IU) | E (mg ATE) | B-2 (mg) | B-6 (mg) | FOL (mcg DFE) | REF |
| baking chocolate (unsweetened) | 28 | 140 | 0.4 | 8.4 | 0.3 | 0 | 4.6 | 7 | 28 | 92 | 2.70 | 1.167 | 0 | 0 | 0.04 | 0.4 | 0 | 0.05 |
| *1 oz* | | 3.6 | 14.6 | 9.1 | 4.5 | 0.4 | 0 | 232 | 112 | 4.87 | 0.905 | 2.3 | 0 | 0.1 | 0.03 | 0.01 | 7.8 | 19078 |
| baking chocolate (unsweetened) | 28 | 132 | 0.3 | 9.5 | 0 | 0 | 5.1 | 3 | 15 | 74 | 1.03 | 0.462 | 0 | 0 | 0.01 | 0.6 | 0 | 0.04 |
| liquid - *1 oz packet* | | 3.4 | 13.4 | 7.1 | 2.6 | 3.0 | 0 | 326 | 95 | 1.16 | 0.535 | 2.2 | 3 | | 0.08 | 0.02 | 5.3 | 19077 |
| baking soda (sodium bicarbonate) | 5 | 0 | 0 | 0 | 0 | | 0 | 1368 | 0 | 0 | 0 | 0 | 0 | 0 | 0 | 0 | 0 | 0 |
| *1 t* | | 0 | 0 | 0 | 0 | 0 | 0 | 0 | 0 | 0 | 0 | 0 | 0 | 0 | 0 | 0 | 0 | 18372 |
| carob powder | 103 | 229 | 3.7 | 91.5 | 50.6 | 0 | 41.0 | 36 | 358 | 56 | 0.95 | 0.523 | 1 | 0 | 0.05 | 2.0 | 0 | 0.05 |
| *1 cup* | | 4.8 | 0.7 | 0.1 | 0.2 | 0.2 | 0 | 852 | 81 | 3.03 | 0.588 | 5.5 | 14 | 0.6 | 0.47 | 0.38 | 29.9 | 16055 |
| cocoa powder, unsweetened | 5.4 | 12 | 0.2 | 3.1 | 0.1 | 0 | 1.8 | 1 | 7 | 27 | 0.37 | 0.207 | 0 | 0 | 0 | 0.1 | 0 | 0.01 |
| *1 T* | | 1.1 | 0.7 | 0.4 | 0.2 | 0 | 0 | 82 | 40 | 0.75 | 0.205 | 0.8 | 0 | | 0.01 | 0.01 | 1.7 | 19165 |
| cocoa powder, unsweetened, European style, Hershey - *1 T* | 5.4 | 22 | | 3.2 | 0 | | 1.1 | 0 | 0 | | | | | 0 | | 0 | | |
| | | 1.1 | 0.5 | 0 | | | 0 | | | 1.94 | | | 0 | | | | | 19171 |
| cocoa pwdr, unsweetened, processed w/alkali - *1 T* | 5.4 | 12 | 0.1 | 3.1 | 0.1 | 0 | 1.6 | 1 | 6 | 26 | 0.34 | 0.202 | 0 | 0 | 0.01 | 0.1 | 0 | 0.01 |
| | | 1.0 | 0.7 | 0.4 | 0.2 | 0 | 0 | 135 | 39 | 0.84 | 0.195 | 0.7 | 0 | 0 | 0.02 | 0.01 | 1.7 | 19166 |
| cornstarch | 32 | 122 | 2.7 | 29.2 | 0 | 0 | 0.3 | 3 | 1 | 1 | 0.02 | 0.017 | 0 | 0 | 0 | 0 | 0 | 0 |
| *¼ cup* | | 0.1 | 0 | 0 | 0 | 0 | 0 | 1 | 4 | 0.15 | 0.016 | 0.9 | 0 | 0 | 0 | 0 | 0 | 20027 |
| cream of tartar (potassium acid tartrate) - *1 t* | 3 | 8 | 0.1 | 1.8 | 0 | 0 | 0 | 2 | 0 | 0 | 0.01 | 0.006 | 0 | 0 | 0 | 0 | 0 | 0 |
| | | 0 | 0 | 0 | 0 | 0 | 0 | 495 | 0 | 0.11 | 0.006 | 0 | 0 | 0 | 0 | 0 | 0 | 18373 |
| gelatin, dry, unsweetened | 28 | 94 | 3.6 | 0 | 0 | | 0 | 55 | 15 | 6 | 0.04 | 0.029 | 0 | 0 | 0.01 | 0 | 0 | 0.04 |
| *1 oz packet (4 T)* | | 24.0 | 0 | 0 | 0 | 0 | 0 | 4 | 11 | 0.31 | 0.605 | 11.1 | 0 | | 0.06 | 0 | 8.4 | 19177 |
| pectin, dry, unsweetened | 50 | 162 | 4.4 | 45.2 | | | 4.3 | 100 | 4 | 0 | 0.24 | 0.035 | 0 | 0 | 0 | 0 | 0 | 0.06 |
| *1.75 oz packet* | | 0.2 | 0.2 | 0 | | | 0 | 4 | 1 | 1.36 | 0.210 | 0 | 2 | | 0.03 | 0 | 0.5 | 19310 |
| rennin, unsweetened | 10 | 8 | 0.6 | 2.0 | | | 0 | 2605 | 373 | 2 | 0.64 | 0.090 | 0 | 0 | 0 | 0 | 0 | 0 |
| *.35 oz packet* | | 0.1 | 0 | 0 | 0 | 0 | 0 | 29 | 34 | 0.71 | 0.020 | 0 | 0 | | | | | 19225 |
| soy pro concentrate, acid wash | 28 | 93 | 1.6 | 8.7 | 5.6 | | 1.5 | 252 | 102 | 39 | 1.23 | 1.173 | 0 | 0 | 0.09 | 0.2 | 0 | 0.02 |
| *1 oz* | | 16.3 | 0.1 | 0 | 0 | 0.1 | 0 | 126 | 235 | 3.02 | 0.273 | 0.2 | 0 | | 0.04 | 0.04 | 95.2 | 16420 |
| soy pro concentrate, alcohol extraction - *1 oz* | 28 | 93 | 1.6 | 8.7 | 5.6 | 0 | 1.5 | 1 | 102 | 88 | 1.23 | 1.173 | 0 | 0 | 0.09 | 0.2 | 0 | 0.02 |
| | | 16.3 | 0.1 | 0 | 0 | 0.1 | 0 | 617 | 235 | 3.02 | 0.273 | 0.2 | 0 | | 0.04 | 0.04 | 95.2 | 16121 |
| soy protein isolate | 28 | 95 | 1.4 | 2.1 | 0 | 0 | 1.6 | 281 | 50 | 11 | 1.13 | 0.418 | 0 | 0 | 0.05 | 0.4 | 0 | 0.02 |
| *1 oz* | | 22.6 | 0.9 | 0.1 | 0.2 | 0.5 | 0 | 23 | 217 | 4.06 | 0.448 | 0.2 | 0 | 0 | 0.03 | 0.03 | 49.3 | 16122 |
| soy protein isolate, potassium type | 28 | 91 | 1.4 | 2.9 | 0 | | 1.6 | 14 | 50 | 11 | 1.13 | 0.418 | 0 | 0 | 0.05 | 0.4 | 0 | 0.02 |
| *1 oz* | | 22.6 | 0.1 | 0 | 0 | 0.1 | 0 | 445 | 217 | 4.06 | 0.448 | 0.2 | 0 | 0 | 0.03 | 0.03 | 49.3 | 16422 |
| soy protein isolate, ProPlus, Protein Tech International - *1 oz* | 28 | 106 | 1.4 | 0 | | | | 11 | 56 | | 16.80 | | 157 | 0 | 0.73 | 10.1 | 2.80 | 2.52 |
| Tech International - *1 oz* | | 24.1 | 1.1 | 0.1 | 0.2 | 0.5 | 0 | 448 | 224 | 5.04 | 0.840 | | 521 | | 0.28 | 0.73 | 56.0 | 16176 |
| soy protein isolate, Supro, Protein Tech International - *1 oz* | 28 | 109 | 1.2 | 0 | | | | 333 | 56 | 11 | 1.12 | | 0 | 0 | 0.06 | 0.1 | 0 | 0.06 |
| Tech International - *1 oz* | | 24.6 | 1.1 | 0.2 | 0.2 | 0.5 | 0 | 28 | 241 | 4.48 | 0.392 | | 0 | | 0.03 | | 56.0 | 16175 |

| | WT (g) | KCAL | H$_2$0 (g) | CHO (g) | TSUG (g) | ASUG (g) | DFIB (g) | Na (mg) | Ca (mg) | Mg (mg) | Zn (mg) | Mn (mg) | A (mcg RAE) | C (mg) | B-1 (mg) | NIA (mg) | B-12 (mcg) | PANT (mg) |
|---|---|---|---|---|---|---|---|---|---|---|---|---|---|---|---|---|---|---|
| | | PRO (g) | FAT (g) | SFA (g) | MUFA (g) | PUFA (g) | CHOL (mg) | K (mg) | P (mg) | Fe (mg) | Cu (mg) | Se (mcg) | A (IU) | E (mg ATE) | B-2 (mg) | B-6 (mg) | FOL (mcg DFE) | REF |
| **tapioca**, pearl, dry | 152 | 544 | 16.7 | 134.8 | 5.1 | 0 | 1.4 | 2 | 30 | 2 | 0.18 | 0.167 | 0 | 0 | 0.01 | 0 | 0 | 0.21 |
| *1 cup* | | 0.3 | 0 | 0 | 0 | 0 | 0 | 17 | 11 | 2.40 | 0.030 | 1.2 | 0 | 0 | 0 | 0.01 | 6.1 | 20068 |
| **vinegar**, balsamic | 15 | 13 | 11.5 | 2.6 | 2.2 | | | 3 | 4 | 2 | 0.01 | 0.020 | 0 | 0 | | | | |
| *1 T* | | 0.1 | 0 | 0 | | | | 17 | 3 | 0.11 | 0.004 | | 0 | | | | | 2069 |
| **vinegar**, balsamic, Progresso | 15 | 10 | | 2.0 | | | | 0 | | | | | | | | | | |
| *1 T* | | 0 | 0 | | | | | | | | | | | | | | | GENM390 |
| **vinegar**, cider | 15 | 3 | 14.1 | 0.1 | 0.1 | 0 | 0 | 1 | 1 | 1 | 0.01 | 0.037 | 0 | 0 | 0 | 0 | 0 | 0 |
| *1 T* | | 0 | 0 | 0 | 0 | 0 | 0 | 11 | 1 | 0.03 | 0.001 | 0 | 0 | 0 | 0 | 0 | 0 | 2048 |
| **vinegar**, red wine | 15 | 3 | 14.2 | 0 | 0 | | 0 | 1 | 1 | 1 | 0 | 0.007 | 0 | 0 | | | | |
| *1 T* | | 0 | 0 | 0 | | | | 6 | 1 | 0.07 | 0.002 | | 0 | | | | | 2068 |
| **whey, acid**, dry | 57 | 193 | 2.0 | 41.9 | 41.9 | 0 | 0 | 552 | 1171 | 113 | 3.60 | 0.009 | 10 | 1 | 0.35 | 0.7 | 1.42 | 3.21 |
| *1 cup* | | 6.7 | 0.3 | 0.2 | 0.1 | 0 | 2 | 1305 | 769 | 0.71 | 0.028 | 15.6 | 34 | 0 | 1.17 | 0.35 | 18.8 | 1113 |
| **whey, acid**, fluid | 246 | 59 | 229.8 | 12.6 | 12.6 | 0 | | 118 | 253 | 25 | 1.06 | 0.005 | 5 | 0 | 0.10 | 0.2 | 0.44 | 0.94 |
| *1 cup* | | 1.9 | 0.2 | 0.1 | 0.1 | 0 | 2 | 352 | 192 | 0.20 | 0.007 | 4.4 | 17 | 0 | 0.34 | 0.10 | 4.9 | 1112 |
| **whey, sweet**, dry | 145 | 512 | 4.6 | 108.0 | 108.0 | 0 | 0 | 1565 | 1154 | 255 | 2.86 | 0.013 | 12 | 2 | 0.75 | 1.8 | 3.44 | 8.15 |
| *1 cup* | | 18.7 | 1.6 | 1.0 | 0.4 | 0 | 9 | 3016 | 1351 | 1.28 | 0.102 | 39.4 | 44 | 0 | 3.20 | 0.85 | 17.4 | 1115 |
| **whey, sweet**, fluid | 246 | 66 | 229.1 | 12.6 | 12.6 | 0 | 0 | 133 | 116 | 20 | 0.32 | 0.002 | 7 | 0 | 0.09 | 0.2 | 0.69 | 0.94 |
| *1 cup* | | 2.1 | 0.9 | 0.6 | 0.2 | 0 | 5 | 396 | 113 | 0.15 | 0.010 | 4.7 | 30 | 0 | 0.39 | 0.08 | 2.5 | 1114 |
| **yeast, baker's**, active dry | 7 | 21 | 0.5 | 2.7 | 0 | 0 | 1.5 | 4 | 4 | 7 | 0.45 | 0.039 | 0 | 0 | 0.17 | 2.8 | 0 | 0.79 |
| *.25 oz package* | | 2.7 | 0.3 | 0 | 0.2 | 0 | 0 | 140 | 90 | 1.16 | 0.035 | 1.7 | 0 | 0 | 0.38 | 0.11 | 163.8 | 18375 |
| **yeast, baker's**, compressed | 17 | 18 | 11.7 | 3.1 | 0 | 0 | 1.4 | 5 | 3 | 7 | 1.69 | 0.034 | 0 | 0 | 0.32 | 2.1 | 0 | 0.83 |
| *.6 oz cake* | | 1.4 | 0.3 | 0 | 0.2 | 0 | 0 | 102 | 57 | 0.55 | 0.025 | 1.4 | 0 | 0 | 0.19 | 0.07 | 133.5 | 18374 |

| | WT (g) | Macronutrients and Amino Acids | | | | | | | Minerals | | | | | Vitamins | | | | |
|---|---|---|---|---|---|---|---|---|---|---|---|---|---|---|---|---|---|---|
| | | KCAL | H₂O (g) | CHO (g) | TSUG (g) | ASUG (g) | DFIB (g) | | Na (mg) | Ca (mg) | Mg (mg) | Zn (mg) | Mn (mg) | A (mcg RAE) | C (mg) | B-1 (mg) | NIA (mg) | B-12 (mcg) |
| | | PRO (g) | FAT (g) | SFA (g) | MUFA (g) | PUFA (g) | CHOL (mg) | | K (mg) | P (mg) | Fe (mg) | Cu (mg) | Se (mcg) | A (IU) | E (mg ATE) | B-2 (mg) | B-6 (mg) | FOL (mcg DFE) |
| | | HIS (mg) | ISO (mg) | LEU (mg) | LYS (mg) | MET (mg) | CYS (mg) | TAU (mg) | Cl (mg) | I (mcg) | Mo (mcg) | Cr (mcg) | | PANT (mg) | E (IU) | D (IU) | K (mcg) | |
| | | PHE (mg) | TYR (mg) | THR (mg) | TRY (mg) | VAL (mg) | ARG (mg) | CAR (mg) | | | | | | BIO (mcg) | CHLN (mg) | INOS (mg) | | REF |

## 32. SPECIAL DIETARY FOODS
### 32.1 FORMULAS AND MEDICAL FOODS FOR INFANTS AND CHILDREN

**Acerflex, powder (iso-, leu-, & val-free), Nutricia (child formula) - ¼ cup**

| WT | KCAL | H₂O | CHO | TSUG | ASUG | DFIB | — | Na | Ca | Mg | Zn | Mn | A(RAE) | C | B-1 | NIA | B-12 |
|---|---|---|---|---|---|---|---|---|---|---|---|---|---|---|---|---|---|
| 30 | 118 | | 12.2 | | | | | 90 | 255 | 33 | 3.60 | 0.480 | 146 | 14 | 0.24 | | 0.33 |
| | 6.0 | 5.1 | 0.6 | 3.2 | 1.0 | | | 336 | 255 | 3.60 | 0.480 | 6.9 | 484 | 2.3 | 0.28 | 0.33 | 43.4 |
| | 378 | 0 | 0 | 681 | 159 | 243 | 42 | 150 | 26 | 16 | 15.0 | | 1.0 | 3 | 132 | 6.30 | |
| | 444 | 444 | 492 | 195 | 0 | 660 | 6 | | | | | | 9 | 24 | 9 | | NTRI1 |

**Alimentum, Abbott (medical formula) - 1 fl oz**

| 31 | 20 | 27.1 | 2.1 | 1.4 | | 0 | | 9 | 21 | 2 | 0.15 | 0.002 | 18 | 2 | 0.01 | 0.3 | 0.09 |
|---|---|---|---|---|---|---|---|---|---|---|---|---|---|---|---|---|---|
| | 0.6 | 1.1 | 0.6 | 0.1 | 0.3 | 0 | | 24 | 15 | 0.37 | 0.015 | 0.4 | 61 | 0.4 | 0.02 | 0.01 | 5.3 |
| | | | | | | | | | | | | | 0.2 | | | | 3846 |

**E028 Splash (amino acid-based), Nutricia (child formula) 237 mL drink box (8 fl oz)**

| 248 | 237 | | 34.6 | | | | | 47 | 147 | 21 | 1.80 | 0.240 | 83 | 7 | 0.13 | 2.1 | 0.17 |
|---|---|---|---|---|---|---|---|---|---|---|---|---|---|---|---|---|---|
| | 5.9 | 8.3 | | | | | | 220 | 147 | 1.80 | 0.240 | 3.7 | 277 | 1.3 | 0.15 | 0.19 | 24.1 |
| | | | | | | | | 83 | 14 | 8 | 7.1 | | 0.6 | | 74 | 3.60 | NTRI3 |

**Enfamil AR LIPIL, 20 cal/fl oz, Mead Johnson - 1 fl oz**

| 31 | 21 | | 2.3 | | | | | 8 | 16 | 2 | 0.21 | 0.003 | | 3 | 0.02 | 0.2 | 0.06 |
|---|---|---|---|---|---|---|---|---|---|---|---|---|---|---|---|---|---|
| | 0.5 | 1.1 | | | | | | 23 | 11 | 0.38 | 0.016 | 0.6 | 62 | | 0.03 | 0.01 | 5.7 |
| | | | | | | | 1 | 16 | 2 | | | | 0.1 | 0 | 13 | 1.67 | |
| | | | | | | | 0 | | | | | | 1 | 3 | 1 | | MDJN21 |

**Enfamil EnfaCare LIPIL, 22 cal/fl oz, Mead Johnson 1 fl oz**

| 31 | 23 | | 2.4 | | | | | 8 | 28 | 2 | 0.29 | 0.003 | | 4 | 0.05 | 0.5 | 0.07 |
|---|---|---|---|---|---|---|---|---|---|---|---|---|---|---|---|---|---|
| | 0.7 | 1.2 | | | | | | 24 | 15 | 0.41 | 0.028 | 0.7 | 102 | | 0.05 | 0.02 | 10.1 |
| | | | | | | | 1 | 18 | 5 | | | | 0.2 | 1 | 18 | 1.83 | |
| | | | | | | | 0 | | | | | | 1 | 6 | 7 | | MDJN19 |

**Enfamil Gentlease LIPIL, 20 cal/fl oz, Mead Johnson 1 fl oz**

| 31 | 21 | | 2.3 | | | | | 7 | 17 | 2 | 0.21 | 0.003 | | 3 | 0.02 | 0.2 | 0.06 |
|---|---|---|---|---|---|---|---|---|---|---|---|---|---|---|---|---|---|
| | 0.5 | 1.1 | | | | | | 23 | 10 | 0.38 | 0.016 | 0.6 | 62 | | 0.03 | 0.01 | 5.7 |
| | | | | | | | 1 | 13 | 2 | | | | 0.1 | 0 | 13 | 1.67 | |
| | | | | | | | 0 | | | | | | 1 | 5 | 1 | | MDJN51 |

**Enfamil Human Milk Fortifier, powder, Mead Johnson 4 pckts**

| 3 | 14 | | 0.4 | | | | | 16 | 90 | 1 | 0.72 | 0.010 | | 12 | 0.15 | 3.0 | 0.18 |
|---|---|---|---|---|---|---|---|---|---|---|---|---|---|---|---|---|---|
| | 1.1 | 1.0 | | | | | | 29 | 50 | 1.44 | 0.044 | | 950 | | 0.22 | 0.12 | 42.5 |
| | | | | | | | | 13 | | | | | 0.7 | 5 | 150 | 4.40 | |
| | | | | | | | | | | | | | 3 | | | | MDJN22 |

**Enfamil Lacto-Free LIPIL, 20 cal/fl oz, Mead Johnson 1 fl oz**

| 31 | 21 | | 2.3 | | | | | 6 | 17 | 2 | 0.21 | 0.003 | | 3 | 0.02 | 0.2 | 0.06 |
|---|---|---|---|---|---|---|---|---|---|---|---|---|---|---|---|---|---|
| | 0.4 | 1.1 | | | | | | 23 | 10 | 0.38 | 0.016 | 0.6 | 62 | | 0.03 | 0.01 | 5.7 |
| | | | | | | | 1 | 14 | 3 | | | | 0.1 | 0 | 13 | 1.67 | |
| | | | | | | | 0 | | | | | | 1 | 5 | 1 | | MDJN59 |

**Enfamil LIPIL with iron, 20 cal/fl oz, - 1 fl oz**

| 31 | 21 | | 2.3 | | | | | 6 | 16 | 2 | 0.21 | 0.003 | | 3 | 0.02 | 0.2 | 0.06 |
|---|---|---|---|---|---|---|---|---|---|---|---|---|---|---|---|---|---|
| | 0.4 | 1.1 | | | | | | 23 | 9 | 0.38 | 0.016 | 0.6 | 62 | | 0.03 | 0.01 | 5.7 |
| | | | | | | | 1 | 13 | 2 | | | | 0.1 | 0 | 13 | 1.67 | |
| | | | | | | | 0 | | | | | | 1 | 5 | 1 | | MDJN55 |

**Enfamil LIPIL with iron, 24 cal/fl oz, Mead Johnson 1 fl oz**

| 31 | 25 | | 2.7 | | | | | 7 | 20 | 2 | 0.25 | 0.004 | | 3 | 0.02 | 0.3 | 0.07 |
|---|---|---|---|---|---|---|---|---|---|---|---|---|---|---|---|---|---|
| | 0.5 | 1.3 | | | | | | 27 | 11 | 0.45 | 0.019 | 0.7 | 74 | | 0.04 | 0.02 | 6.9 |
| | | | | | | | 2 | 16 | 3 | | | | 0.1 | 1 | 15 | 2.02 | |
| | | | | | | | 1 | | | | | | 1 | 6 | 2 | | MDJN52 |

**Enfamil Premature LIPIL low iron, 20 cal/fl oz, Mead Johnson 1 fl oz**

| 31 | 21 | | 2.3 | | | | | 12 | 35 | 2 | 0.31 | 0.001 | | 4 | 0.04 | 0.8 | 0.05 |
|---|---|---|---|---|---|---|---|---|---|---|---|---|---|---|---|---|---|
| | 0.6 | 1.1 | | | | | | 20 | 17 | 0.11 | 0.025 | 0.6 | 264 | | 0.06 | 0.03 | 14.2 |
| | | | | | | | 1 | 19 | 5 | 0 | 0 | | 0.3 | 1 | 50 | 1.67 | |
| | | | | | | | 1 | | | | | | 1 | 4 | 9 | | MDJN54 |

**Enfamil Premature LIPIL low iron, 24 cal/fl oz, Mead Johnson 1 fl oz**

| 31 | 25 | | 2.8 | | | | | 15 | 42 | 2 | 0.38 | 0.002 | | 5 | 0.05 | 1.0 | 0.06 |
|---|---|---|---|---|---|---|---|---|---|---|---|---|---|---|---|---|---|
| | 0.7 | 1.3 | | | | | | 25 | 21 | 0.13 | 0.030 | 0.7 | 313 | | 0.07 | 0.04 | 16.9 |
| | | | | | | | 2 | 23 | 6 | 0 | 0 | | 0.3 | 2 | 60 | 2.02 | |
| | | | | | | | 1 | | | | | | 1 | 5 | 11 | | MDJN53 |

**Enfamil Premature LIPIL with iron, 20 cal/fl oz, Mead Johnson 1 fl oz**

| 31 | 21 | | 2.3 | | | | | 12 | 35 | 2 | 0.31 | 0.001 | | 4 | 0.04 | 0.8 | 0.05 |
|---|---|---|---|---|---|---|---|---|---|---|---|---|---|---|---|---|---|
| | 0.6 | 1.1 | | | | | | 20 | 17 | 0.38 | 0.025 | 0.6 | 264 | | 0.06 | 0.03 | 14.2 |
| | | | | | | | 1 | 19 | 5 | 0 | 0 | | 0.3 | 1 | 50 | 1.67 | |
| | | | | | | | 1 | | | | | | 1 | 4 | 9 | | MDJN23 |

**Enfamil Premature LIPIL with iron, 24 cal/fl oz, Mead Johnson 1 fl oz**

| 31 | 25 | | 2.8 | | | | | 15 | 42 | 2 | 0.38 | 0.002 | | 5 | 0.05 | 1.0 | 0.06 |
|---|---|---|---|---|---|---|---|---|---|---|---|---|---|---|---|---|---|
| | 0.7 | 1.3 | | | | | | 25 | 21 | 0.45 | 0.030 | 0.7 | 313 | | 0.07 | 0.04 | 16.9 |
| | | | | | | | 2 | 23 | 6 | 0 | 0 | | 0.3 | 2 | 60 | 2.02 | |
| | | | | | | | 1 | | | | | | 1 | 5 | 11 | | MDJN24 |

Column key (each nutrient column cycles through four label rows, shown separated by `/`):

| Item | WT (g) | KCAL / PRO(g) / HIS(mg) / PHE(mg) | H₂O(g) / FAT(g) / ISO(mg) / TYR(mg) | CHO(g) / SFA(g) / LEU(mg) / THR(mg) | TSUG(g) / MUFA(g) / LYS(mg) / TRY(mg) | ASUG(g) / PUFA(g) / MET(mg) / VAL(mg) | DFIB(g) / CHOL(mg) / CYS(mg) / ARG(mg) | TAU(mg) / CAR(mg) | Na(mg) / K(mg) / Cl(mg) | Ca(mg) / P(mg) / I(mcg) | Mg(mg) / Fe(mg) / Mo(mcg) | Zn(mg) / Cu(mg) / Cr(mcg) | Mn(mg) / Se(mcg) | A(mcg RAE) / A(IU) / PANT(mg) / BIO(mcg) | C(mg) / E(mg ATE) / E(IU) / CHLN(mg) | B-1(mg) / B-2(mg) / D(IU) / INOS(mg) | NIA(mg) / B-6(mg) / K(mcg) | B-12(mcg) / FOL(mcg DFE) / REF |
|---|---|---|---|---|---|---|---|---|---|---|---|---|---|---|---|---|---|---|
| **Enfamil ProSobee LIPIL, 20 cal/fl oz, Mead Johnson** - *1 fl oz* | 31 | 21 |  | 2.2 |  |  |  |  | 7 | 22 | 2 | 0.25 | 0.005 |  | 3 | 0.02 | 0.2 | 0.06 |
|  |  | 0.5 | 1.1 |  |  |  |  |  | 25 | 15 | 0.38 | 0.016 | 0.6 | 62 |  | 0.02 | 0.01 | 5.7 |
|  |  |  |  |  |  |  |  | 1 | 17 | 3 |  |  |  | 0.1 | 0 | 13 | 1.67 |  |
|  |  |  |  |  |  |  |  | 0 |  |  |  |  |  | 1 | 5 | 1 |  | MDJN58 |
| **Follow-Up with iron, Carnation (medical formula)** - *1 fl oz* | 31 | 20 | 26.8 | 2.6 | 1.9 |  | 0 |  | 8 | 24 | 2 | 0.16 |  | 15 | 2 | 0.02 | 0.2 | 0.05 |
|  |  | 0.5 | 0.8 | 0.4 | 0.3 | 0.2 | 0 |  | 27 | 16 | 0.37 | 0.017 | 0.4 | 51 | 0.3 | 0.03 | 0.01 | 5.3 |
|  |  |  |  |  |  |  |  |  |  |  |  |  |  |  |  | 13 |  |  |
|  |  |  |  |  |  |  |  |  |  |  |  |  |  |  |  |  |  | 3900 |
| **Follow-Up with iron, liquid concentrate, Carnation (medical formula)** - *1 fl oz* | 31 | 39 | 23.0 | 5.1 | 3.7 |  | 0 |  | 15 | 46 | 3 | 0.31 |  | 30 | 3 | 0.03 | 0.4 | 0.10 |
|  |  | 1.0 | 1.6 | 0.7 | 0.5 | 0.4 | 1 |  | 52 | 31 | 0.70 | 0.033 | 0.8 | 97 | 0.5 | 0.05 | 0.03 | 9.9 |
|  |  |  |  |  |  |  |  |  |  |  |  |  |  |  |  | 25 |  |  |
|  |  |  |  |  |  |  |  |  |  |  |  |  |  |  |  |  |  | 3901 |
| **Follow-Up with iron, powder, Carnation (medical formula)** *1 scoop* | 9 | 42 | 0.2 | 5.6 | 4.0 |  | 0 |  | 17 | 51 | 3 | 0.36 |  | 32 | 4 | 0.03 | 0.4 | 0.11 |
|  |  | 1.1 | 1.7 | 0.8 | 0.6 | 0.4 | 1 |  | 57 | 34 | 0.76 | 0.036 | 0.8 | 106 | 0.6 | 0.06 | 0.03 | 10.9 |
|  |  |  |  |  |  |  |  |  |  |  |  |  |  |  |  | 13 |  |  |
|  |  |  |  |  |  |  |  |  |  |  |  |  |  |  |  |  |  | 3913 |
| **Good Start Essentials Soy with iron, liquid concentrate, Nestle (infant formula)** - *1 fl oz* | 31 | 40 | 23.4 | 4.4 | 3.5 |  | 0 |  | 14 | 41 | 4 | 0.35 |  | 31 | 5 | 0.02 | 0.5 | 0.12 |
|  |  | 1.0 | 2.0 | 0.9 | 0.6 | 0.4 | 0 |  | 45 | 25 | 0.71 | 0.047 | 0.8 | 118 | 0.6 | 0.04 | 0.02 | 10.8 |
|  |  |  |  |  |  |  |  |  |  |  |  |  |  |  |  | 26 |  |  |
|  |  |  |  |  |  |  |  |  |  |  |  |  |  |  |  |  |  | 3926 |
| **Good Start Essentials Soy with iron, powder, Nestle (infant formula)** - *1 scoop* | 4.3 | 22 | 0.1 | 2.4 | 1.9 |  | 0 |  | 8 | 23 | 2 | 0.19 |  | 20 | 3 | 0.01 | 0.3 | 0.06 |
|  |  | 0.5 | 1.1 | 0.5 | 0.3 | 0.3 | 0 |  | 25 | 14 | 0.39 | 0.026 | 0.4 | 65 | 0.3 | 0.02 | 0.01 | 5.8 |
|  |  |  |  |  |  |  |  |  |  |  |  |  |  |  |  | 13 |  |  |
|  |  |  |  |  |  |  |  |  |  |  |  |  |  |  |  |  |  | 3928 |
| **Good Start Essentials Soy with iron, ready-to-feed Nestle (infant formula)** - *1 fl oz* | 31 | 20 | 27.1 | 2.2 | 1.8 |  | 0 |  | 7 | 21 | 2 | 0.19 |  | 16 | 2 | 0.01 | 0.3 | 0.06 |
|  |  | 0.5 | 1.0 | 0.4 | 0.3 | 0.2 | 0 |  | 23 | 13 | 0.39 | 0.024 | 0.5 | 60 | 0.3 | 0.02 | 0.01 | 5.3 |
|  |  |  |  |  |  |  |  |  |  |  |  |  |  |  |  | 13 |  |  |
|  |  |  |  |  |  |  |  |  |  |  |  |  |  |  |  |  |  | 3925 |
| **Good Start with iron, Carnation (infant formula)** - *1 fl oz* | 31 | 20 | 27.1 | 2.3 | 1.6 |  | 0 |  | 6 | 13 | 2 | 0.16 |  | 19 | 2 | 0.02 | 0.2 | 0.07 |
|  |  | 0.4 | 1.0 | 0.5 | 0.3 | 0.2 | 1 |  | 22 | 7 | 0.31 | 0.016 | 0.4 | 62 | 0.3 | 0.03 | 0.02 | 5.3 |
|  |  |  |  |  |  |  |  |  |  |  |  |  |  |  |  | 13 |  |  |
|  |  |  |  |  |  |  |  |  |  |  |  |  |  |  |  |  |  | 3800 |
| **Good Start with iron, liquid concentrate, Carnation (infant formula)** - *1 fl oz* | 31 | 39 | 23.5 | 4.4 | 3.0 |  | 0 |  | 11 | 25 | 3 | 0.32 |  | 35 | 3 | 0.04 | 0.4 | 0.13 |
|  |  | 0.9 | 2.0 | 0.9 | 0.6 | 0.4 | 1 |  | 42 | 14 | 0.59 | 0.031 | 0.5 | 118 | 0.6 | 0.06 | 0.03 | 9.9 |
|  |  |  |  |  |  |  |  |  |  |  |  |  |  |  |  | 24 |  |  |
|  |  |  |  |  |  |  |  |  |  |  |  |  |  |  |  |  |  | 3801 |
| **Good Start with iron, powder, Carnation (infant formula)** *1 scoop* | 9 | 46 | 0.2 | 5.2 | 3.5 |  | 0 |  | 12 | 31 | 3 | 0.37 |  | 41 | 4 | 0.05 | 0.5 | 0.10 |
|  |  | 1.0 | 2.3 | 1.0 | 0.8 | 0.5 | 3 |  | 50 | 17 | 0.69 | 0.037 | 0.9 | 138 | 0.7 | 0.06 | 0.03 | 11.8 |
|  |  |  |  |  |  |  |  |  |  |  |  |  |  |  |  | 27 |  |  |
|  |  |  |  |  |  |  |  |  |  |  |  |  |  |  |  |  |  | 3802 |
| **Isomil with iron, liquid concentrate, Abbott (infant formula)** *1 fl oz* | 31 | 40 | 23.5 | 4.1 | 4.1 |  | 0 |  | 17 | 42 | 3 | 0.30 | 0.010 | 35 | 4 | 0.02 | 0.5 | 0.18 |
|  |  | 1.0 | 2.2 | 0.7 | 0.8 | 0.5 | 0 |  | 43 | 30 | 0.71 | 0.030 | 0.8 | 118 | 0.4 | 0.04 | 0.02 | 10.2 |
|  |  |  |  |  |  |  |  |  |  |  |  |  |  | 0.3 |  | 24 |  |  |
|  |  |  |  |  |  |  |  |  |  |  |  |  |  |  |  |  |  | 3842 |
| **Isomil with iron, powder, Abbott (infant formula)** - *1 scoop* | 9 | 47 | 0.2 | 4.8 | 4.8 |  | 0 |  | 20 | 49 | 4 | 0.35 | 0.012 | 42 | 4 | 0.03 | 0.6 | 0.21 |
|  |  | 1.1 | 2.5 | 0.8 | 1.0 | 0.6 | 0 |  | 50 | 35 | 0.83 | 0.035 | 1.0 | 139 | 0.5 | 0.04 | 0.03 | 11.8 |
|  |  |  |  |  |  |  |  |  |  |  |  |  |  | 0.3 |  | 27 |  |  |
|  |  |  |  |  |  |  |  |  |  |  |  |  |  |  |  |  |  | 3843 |
| **Isomil with iron, ready-to-feed, Abbott (infant formula)** *1 fl oz* | 31 | 20 | 27.1 | 2.1 | 2.1 |  | 0 |  | 9 | 21 | 2 | 0.15 | 0.005 | 18 | 2 | 0.01 | 0.3 | 0.09 |
|  |  | 0.5 | 1.1 | 0.4 | 0.4 | 0.3 | 0 |  | 22 | 15 | 0.37 | 0.015 | 0.4 | 61 | 0.4 | 0.02 | 0.01 | 5.3 |
|  |  |  |  |  |  |  |  |  |  |  |  |  |  | 0.2 |  | 12 |  |  |
|  |  |  |  |  |  |  |  |  |  |  |  |  |  |  |  |  |  | 3841 |
| **Lophlex powder (phe-free), Nutricia (child/adult formula)** *1 packet* | 14 | 41 |  | 0.1 |  |  |  |  | 2 | 296 | 76 | 2.30 | 0.440 | 167 | 16 | 0.23 | 1.4 | 0.79 |
|  |  | 10.0 | 0 |  |  |  |  |  | 3 | 285 | 3.70 | 0.204 | 14.4 | 557 | 3.1 | 0.24 | 0.40 | 209.1 |
|  |  | 470 | 730 | 1240 | 840 | 200 | 310 | 20 | 0 | 33 | 9 | 6.6 |  | 1.2 | 1 | 83 | 20.40 |  |
|  |  | 0 | 1120 | 610 | 240 | 800 | 830 | 10 |  |  |  |  |  | 6 | 103 | 20 |  | NTRI7 |
| **Milupa PKU 2 (L-amino acid, phe-free), powder, Nutricia (child formula)** - *¼ cup* | 35 | 103 |  | 2.2 |  |  |  |  | 224 | 458 | 55 | 2.80 | 0.245 | 547 | 28 | 0.49 | 8.4 | 1.05 |
|  |  | 23.4 | 0 |  |  |  |  |  | 465 | 354 | 5.25 | 0.700 |  | 1820 | 4.2 | 0.70 | 0.52 | 238.0 |
|  |  | 630 | 1575 | 2660 | 1890 | 630 | 630 |  | 346 | 42 | 11 |  |  | 3.8 | 6 | 458 | 58.45 |  |
|  |  | 0 | 1575 | 1260 | 490 | 1890 | 945 |  |  |  |  |  |  | 105 | 91 | 105 |  | NTRI11 |

| | WT (g) | Macronutrients and Amino Acids | | | | | | | Minerals | | | | | Vitamins | | | | |
|---|---|---|---|---|---|---|---|---|---|---|---|---|---|---|---|---|---|---|
| | | KCAL | $H_2O$ (g) | CHO (g) | TSUG (g) | ASUG (g) | DFIB (g) | | Na (mg) | Ca (mg) | Mg (mg) | Zn (mg) | Mn (mg) | A (mcg RAE) | C (mg) | B-1 (mg) | NIA (mg) | B-12 (mcg) |
| | | PRO (g) | FAT (g) | SFA (g) | MUFA (g) | PUFA (g) | CHOL (mg) | | K (mg) | P (mg) | Fe (mg) | Cu (mg) | Se (mcg) | A (IU) | E (mg ATE) | B-2 (mg) | B-6 (mg) | FOL (mcg DFE) |
| | | HIS (mg) | ISO (mg) | LEU (mg) | LYS (mg) | MET (mg) | CYS (mg) | TAU (mg) | Cl (mg) | I (mcg) | Mo (mcg) | Cr (mcg) | | PANT (mg) | E (IU) | D (IU) | K (mcg) | |
| | | PHE (mg) | TYR (mg) | THR (mg) | TRY (mg) | VAL (mg) | ARG (mg) | CAR (mg) | | | | | | BIO (mcg) | CHLN (mg) | INOS (mg) | | REF |
| **MSUD Analog** (iso-, leu-, & val-free), powder, Nutricia (infant formula) - *¼ cup* | 30 | 142 | | 17.7 | | | | | 36 | 180 | 12 | 2.40 | 0.180 | 158 | 12 | 0.15 | 1.4 | 0.38 |
| | | 3.9 | 6.3 | 2.0 | 2.8 | 1.1 | | | 126 | 150 | 3.00 | 0.135 | 4.5 | 528 | 1.0 | 0.18 | 0.16 | 19.4 |
| | | 228 | 0 | 0 | 414 | 96 | 147 | 6 | 87 | 14 | 4 | 4.5 | | 0.8 | 1 | 102 | 6.30 | |
| | | 270 | 270 | 300 | 120 | 0 | 402 | 3 | | | | | | 8 | 15 | 30 | | NTRI37 |
| **MSUD Maxamaid** (iso-, leu-, & val-free), powder, Nutricia (child formula) - *¼ cup* | 35 | 113 | | 19.6 | | | | | 203 | 284 | 45 | 3.85 | 0.665 | 175 | 22 | 0.28 | 1.8 | 0.70 |
| | | 8.8 | 0 | | | | | | 294 | 284 | 4.90 | 0.350 | 14.0 | 583 | 3.4 | 0.28 | 0.28 | 142.8 |
| | | 522 | 0 | 0 | 941 | 220 | 336 | 49 | 158 | 50 | 12 | 7.5 | | 1.1 | 5 | 168 | 16.80 | |
| | | 612 | 612 | 679 | 269 | 0 | 910 | 7 | | | | | | 6 | 88 | 20 | | NTRI17 |
| **MSUD Maxamum** (iso-, leu-, & val- free), powder, Nutricia (child/adult formula) *¼ cup* | 35 | 107 | | 11.9 | | | | | 196 | 414 | 107 | 3.15 | 0.630 | 234 | 22 | 0.32 | 2.0 | 1.08 |
| | | 14.0 | 0.2 | | | | | | 245 | 398 | 5.14 | 0.287 | 20.3 | 780 | 4.3 | 0.34 | 0.56 | 292.1 |
| | | 805 | 0 | 0 | 1470 | 346 | 560 | 49 | 196 | 46 | 13 | 9.1 | | 1.7 | 6 | 116 | 28.70 | |
| | | 980 | 980 | 1085 | 455 | 0 | 1435 | 14 | | | | | | 9 | 150 | 28 | | NTRI18 |
| **Neocate Infant** (amino acid-based), powder, Nutricia (infant formula) - *⅓ cup* | 35 | 147 | | 17.3 | | | | | 55 | 183 | 18 | 2.45 | 0.133 | 181 | 14 | 0.14 | 2.3 | 0.38 |
| | | 4.6 | 6.7 | | | | | | 229 | 137 | 2.73 | 0.182 | 5.5 | 602 | 1.1 | 0.20 | 0.18 | 25.6 |
| | | | | | | | | | 114 | 23 | 7 | 5.2 | | 0.9 | 2 | 88 | 12.95 | |
| | | | | | | | | | | | | | | 5 | 19 | 34 | | NTRI19 |
| **Neocate Infant w/DHA & ARA** (amino acid-based), powder, Nutricia (infant formula) *⅓ cup* | 35 | 147 | | 17.3 | | | | | 55 | 183 | 18 | 2.45 | 0.133 | 181 | 14 | 0.14 | 2.3 | 0.38 |
| | | 4.6 | 6.7 | | | | | | 229 | 137 | 2.73 | 0.182 | 5.5 | 602 | 1.1 | 0.20 | 0.18 | 25.6 |
| | | | | | | | | | 114 | 23 | 7 | 5.2 | | 0.9 | 2 | 88 | 12.95 | |
| | | | | | | | | | | | | | | 5 | 19 | 34 | | NTRI20 |
| **Neocate Jr** (amino acid-based), powder, Nutricia (child formula) - *⅓ cup* | 34 | 163 | | 16.8 | | | | | 67 | 184 | 26 | 1.60 | 0.211 | 122 | 15 | 0.16 | 1.5 | 0.31 |
| | | 5.4 | 8.2 | | | | | | 222 | 113 | 2.52 | 0.180 | 4.9 | 406 | 1.8 | 0.16 | 0.16 | 82.7 |
| | | | | | | | | | 102 | 29 | 7 | 6.1 | | 0.6 | 3 | 71 | 6.53 | |
| | | | | | | | | | | | | | | 3 | 49 | 36 | | NTRI21 |
| **Neocate One+** (amino acid-based), powder Nutricia (child formula) - *⅓ cup* | 31 | 124 | | 18.1 | | | | | 25 | 77 | 11 | 0.96 | 0.124 | 43 | 4 | 0.07 | 1.1 | 0.09 |
| | | 3.1 | 4.3 | | | | | | 115 | 77 | 0.96 | 0.124 | 1.9 | 144 | 0.7 | 0.08 | 0.10 | 12.6 |
| | | | | | | | | | 43 | 7 | 4 | 3.7 | | 0.3 | 1 | 38 | 1.86 | |
| | | | | | | | | | | | | | | 2 | 23 | 2 | | NTRI22 |
| **Next Step Prosobee**, powder, Mead Johnson - *1 scoop* | 9 | 43 | 0.3 | 5.1 | 5.0 | | 0 | | 15 | 83 | 5 | 0.51 | 0.022 | 39 | 5 | 0.03 | 0.4 | 0.13 |
| | | 1.4 | 1.9 | 0.8 | 0.7 | 0.4 | 0 | | 51 | 56 | 0.86 | 0.032 | 1.2 | 128 | 0.4 | 0.04 | 0.03 | 11.6 |
| | | | | | | | | | | | | | | | | 25 | | |
| | | | | | | | | | | | | | | | | | | 3929 |
| **Nursoy with iron**, dry powder, Wyeth-Ayerst (infant formula) - *1 scoop* | 9 | 46 | 0.2 | 4.7 | 4.7 | | 0 | | 14 | 41 | 5 | 0.34 | | 43 | 4 | 0.04 | 0.3 | 0.14 |
| | | 1.2 | 2.4 | 1.1 | 1.0 | 0.3 | 0 | | 48 | 29 | 0.82 | 0.032 | 1.0 | 142 | 0.3 | 0.07 | 0.03 | 5.8 |
| | | | | | | | | | | | | | | | | 26 | | |
| | | | | | | | | | | | | | | | | | | 3893 |
| **Nursoy with iron**, liquid concentrate, Wyeth-Ayerst (infant formula) - *½ fl oz* | 15 | 19 | 11.4 | 1.8 | 1.8 | | 0 | | 5 | 18 | 2 | 0.16 | | 18 | 2 | 0.02 | 0.1 | 0.06 |
| | | 0.5 | 1.0 | 0.5 | 0.4 | 0.2 | 0 | | 21 | 12 | 0.35 | 0.014 | 0.5 | 59 | 0.1 | 0.03 | 0.01 | 2.6 |
| | | | | | | | | | | | | | | | | 13 | | |
| | | | | | | | | | | | | | | | | | | 3891 |
| **Nursoy with iron**, ready-to-feed, Wyeth-Ayerst (infant formula) - *1 fl oz* | 31 | 20 | 27.3 | 1.9 | 1.9 | | 0 | | 6 | 18 | 2 | 0.16 | | 18 | 2 | 0.02 | 0.2 | 0.06 |
| | | 0.6 | 1.1 | 0.5 | 0.4 | 0.2 | 0 | | 21 | 13 | 0.37 | 0.014 | 0.4 | 77 | 0.1 | 0.03 | 0.01 | 2.8 |
| | | | | | | | | | | | | | | | | 13 | | |
| | | | | | | | | | | | | | | | | | | 3890 |
| **Nutramigen LIPIL**, 20 cal/fl oz, Mead Johnson - *1 fl oz* | 31 | 21 | | 2.2 | | | | | 10 | 20 | 2 | 0.21 | 0.005 | | 3 | 0.02 | 0.2 | 0.06 |
| | | 0.6 | 1.1 | | | | | | 23 | 11 | 0.38 | 0.016 | 0.6 | 62 | | 0.02 | 0.01 | 5.7 |
| | | | | | | | | 1 | 18 | 3 | | | | 0.1 | 0 | 11 | 1.67 | |
| | | | | | | | | 0 | | | | | | 1 | 5 | 4 | | MDJN56 |
| **Pedialyte**, Abbott (medical formula) *1 fl oz* | 31 | 3 | | | | | | | 30 | | | | | | | | | |
| | | | | | | | | | 23 | | | | | | | | | |
| | | | | | | | | | 37 | | | | | | | | | |
| | | | | | | | | | | | | | | | | | | RSSM45 |
| **PediaSure**, Abbott (medical formula) - *1 fl oz* | 31 | 237 | 200.0 | 31.0 | | | | | 90 | 230 | 47 | 1.40 | 0.360 | | 24 | 0.64 | 2.4 | 1.40 |
| | | 7.0 | 9.0 | | | | | | 310 | 200 | 3.30 | 0.240 | 7.6 | 380 | | 0.50 | 0.62 | 120.7 |
| | | | | | | | | 17 | 240 | 23 | 8 | 7.1 | | 2.4 | 5 | 120 | 14.00 | |
| | | | | | | | | 4 | | | | | | 45 | 71 | 19 | | RSSM46 |
| **PediaSure Enteral Formula**, Abbott (medical formula) *8 fl oz (240 ml)* | 245 | 237 | 202.0 | 31.4 | | | | | 90 | 230 | 47 | 1.40 | 0.360 | | 24 | 0.64 | 2.4 | 1.40 |
| | | 7.1 | 9.4 | | | | | | 310 | 200 | 3.30 | 0.240 | 7.6 | 380 | | 0.50 | 0.62 | 120.7 |
| | | | | | | | | 17 | 240 | 23 | 8 | 7.1 | | 2.4 | 5 | 120 | 14.00 | |
| | | | | | | | | 4 | | | | | | 45 | 71 | 19 | | RSSM31 |

| | WT | Macronutrients and Amino Acids | | | | | | | Minerals | | | | | Vitamins | | | | |
|---|---|---|---|---|---|---|---|---|---|---|---|---|---|---|---|---|---|---|
| | (g) | KCAL | $H_2O$ (g) | CHO (g) | TSUG (g) | ASUG (g) | DFIB (g) | | Na (mg) | Ca (mg) | Mg (mg) | Zn (mg) | Mn (mg) | A (mcg RAE) | C (mg) | B-1 (mg) | NIA (mg) | B-12 (mcg) |
| | | PRO (g) | FAT (g) | SFA (g) | MUFA (g) | PUFA (g) | CHOL (mg) | | K (mg) | P (mg) | Fe (mg) | Cu (mg) | Se (mcg) | A (IU) | E (mg ATE) | B-2 (mg) | B-6 (mg) | FOL (mcg DFE) |
| | | HIS (mg) | ISO (mg) | LEU (mg) | LYS (mg) | MET (mg) | CYS (mg) | TAU (mg) | Cl (mg) | I (mcg) | Mo (mcg) | Cr (mcg) | | PANT (mg) | E (IU) | D (IU) | K (mcg) | |
| | | PHE (mg) | TYR (mg) | THR (mg) | TRY (mg) | VAL (mg) | ARG (mg) | CAR (mg) | | | | | | BIO (mcg) | CHLN (mg) | INOS (mg) | | REF |
| **PediaSure w/fiber**, Abbott (medical formula) - *8 fl oz (240 ml)* | 246 | 237 | 199.0 | 32.0 | | | 1.2 | | 90 | 230 | 47 | 1.40 | 0.360 | | 24 | 0.64 | 2.4 | 1.40 |
| | | 7.0 | 9.0 | | | | | | 310 | 200 | 3.30 | 0.240 | 7.6 | 380 | | 0.50 | 0.62 | 120.7 |
| | | | | | | | | 17 | 240 | 23 | 8 | 7.1 | | 2.4 | 5 | 120 | 14.00 | |
| | | | | | | | | 4 | | | | | | 45 | 71 | 19 | | RSSM32 |
| **Pepdite Junior** (free amino acids, non-dairy hydrolysates), powder, Nutricia (child formula) - *1 packet* | 51 | 240 | | 25.5 | | | | | 98 | 271 | 43 | 3.30 | 0.480 | 175 | 22 | 0.24 | 2.9 | 0.48 |
| | | 7.4 | 12.0 | | | | | | 327 | 225 | 3.30 | 0.265 | 7.1 | 582 | 2.6 | 0.24 | 0.24 | 122.4 |
| | | | | | | | | | 151 | 23 | 11 | 9.0 | | 1.0 | 4 | 78 | 6.50 | |
| | | | | | | | | | | | | | | 5 | 90 | 53 | | NTRI23 |
| **Periflex Advance** (phe-free), powder, Nutricia (child/adult formula) - *¼ cup* | 32 | 123 | | 10.6 | | | | | 157 | 331 | 86 | 2.53 | 0.512 | 188 | 17 | 0.26 | 1.6 | 0.86 |
| | | 11.2 | 4.0 | 0.4 | 2.5 | 0.9 | | | 196 | 318 | 4.13 | 0.230 | 16.3 | 624 | 3.5 | 0.27 | 0.45 | 233.9 |
| | | 480 | 768 | 1280 | 992 | 205 | 307 | 38 | 157 | 37 | 10 | 7.3 | | 1.4 | 5 | 93 | 22.98 | |
| | | | | | | | | | | | | | | | | | | NTRI24 |
| **Periflex Jr** (phe-free), powder, Nutricia(child formula) *¼ cup* | 30 | 118 | | 12.6 | | | | | 174 | 243 | 38 | 3.30 | 0.570 | 150 | 19 | 0.24 | 1.5 | 0.60 |
| | | 7.5 | 4.2 | 0.5 | 2.7 | 0.9 | | | 252 | 243 | 4.20 | 0.300 | 12.0 | 500 | 2.9 | 0.24 | 0.24 | 122.4 |
| | | 168 | 540 | 600 | 600 | 153 | 225 | 195 | 135 | 43 | 10 | 6.4 | | 1.0 | 4 | 144 | 14.40 | |
| | | 0 | 690 | 300 | 102 | 540 | 243 | 9 | | | | | | 5 | 75 | 17 | | NTRI25 |
| **Pregestimil**, 20 cal/fl oz, Mead Johnson - *1 fl oz* | 31 | 21 | | 2.1 | | | | | 10 | 24 | 3 | 0.23 | 0.006 | | 3 | 0.02 | 0.2 | 0.06 |
| | | 0.6 | 1.2 | | | | | | 23 | 16 | 0.39 | 0.023 | 0.6 | 81 | | 0.02 | 0.01 | 5.7 |
| | | | | | | | | 1 | 18 | 2 | | | | 0.1 | 1 | 11 | 3.94 | |
| | | | | | | | | 0 | | | | | | 1 | 3 | 4 | | MDJN57 |
| **Pregestimil**, 24 cal/fl oz, Mead Johnson - *1 fl oz* | 31 | 25 | | 2.6 | | | | | 12 | 29 | 3 | 0.28 | 0.007 | | 3 | 0.02 | 0.3 | 0.07 |
| | | 0.7 | 1.4 | | | | | | 28 | 19 | 0.47 | 0.028 | 0.7 | 96 | | 0.02 | 0.02 | 6.9 |
| | | | | | | | | 2 | 22 | 3 | | | | 0.1 | 1 | 13 | 4.74 | |
| | | | | | | | | 1 | | | | | | 1 | 3 | 4 | | MDJN50 |
| **Similac**, low iron, liquid concentrate, Abbott (infant formula) - *1 fl oz* | 31 | 39 | 23.6 | 4.3 | 4.3 | | 0 | | 10 | 31 | 2 | 0.30 | 0.002 | 35 | 4 | 0.04 | 0.4 | 0.10 |
| | | 0.8 | 2.1 | 0.7 | 0.8 | 0.5 | 1 | | 42 | 17 | 0.28 | 0.036 | 0.9 | 118 | 0.4 | 0.06 | 0.02 | 10.2 |
| | | | | | | | | | | | | | | 0.2 | | 24 | | |
| | | | | | | | | | | | | | | | | | | 3856 |
| **Similac low iron**, powder, Abbott (infant formula) - *1 scoop* | 9 | 47 | 0.2 | 4.9 | 4.9 | | 0 | | 11 | 37 | 3 | 0.35 | 0.002 | 43 | 4 | 0.05 | 0.5 | 0.12 |
| | | 1.0 | 2.6 | 0.9 | 0.9 | 0.6 | 1 | | 50 | 20 | 0.33 | 0.043 | 1.0 | 142 | 0.5 | 0.07 | 0.03 | 12.1 |
| | | | | | | | | | | | | | | 0.2 | | 27 | | |
| | | | | | | | | | | | | | | | | | | 3858 |
| **Similac Natural Care**, low Fe, Abbott (infant formula) *1 fl oz* | 31 | 24 | 26.4 | 2.6 | 2.5 | | 0 | | 11 | 51 | 3 | 0.36 | 0.003 | 91 | 9 | 0.06 | 1.2 | 0.13 |
| | | 0.7 | 1.3 | 0.8 | 0.1 | 0.3 | 1 | | 31 | 28 | 0.09 | 0.060 | 0.4 | 302 | 0.6 | 0.15 | 0.06 | 15.2 |
| | | | | | | | | | | | | | | 0.5 | | 36 | | |
| | | | | | | | | | | | | | | | | | | 3839 |
| **Similac PM 60/40**, low Fe, powder, Abbott (infant formula) *1 scoop* | 9 | 47 | 0.2 | 4.9 | 4.7 | | 0 | | 11 | 26 | 3 | 0.35 | 0.002 | 42 | 4 | 0.05 | 0.5 | 0.12 |
| | | 1.0 | 2.6 | 1.1 | 0.5 | 1.0 | 2 | | 37 | 13 | 0.10 | 0.042 | 0.9 | 139 | 0.8 | 0.07 | 0.03 | 11.8 |
| | | | | | | | | | | | | | | 0.2 | | 27 | | |
| | | | | | | | | | | | | | | | | | | 3837 |
| **Similac Special Care Advance 24** w/Fe, ARA, & DHA, ready-to-feed, Abbott (infant formula) - *1 fl oz* | 31 | 22 | 26.5 | 2.6 | 2.6 | | 0 | | 11 | 44 | 3 | 0.37 | 0.003 | 91 | 9 | 0.06 | 1.2 | 0.13 |
| | | 0.6 | 1.0 | 0.7 | 0.1 | 0.2 | 1 | | 31 | 24 | 0.44 | 0.061 | 0.4 | 304 | 0.7 | 0.15 | 0.06 | 15.2 |
| | | | | | | | | | | | | | | 0.5 | | 33 | | |
| | | | | | | | | | | | | | | | | | | 3840 |
| **Similac with iron**, Abbott (infant formula) - *1 fl oz* | 30 | 20 | 26.3 | 2.1 | 2.1 | | 0 | | 5 | 15 | 1 | 0.15 | 0.001 | 18 | 2 | 0.02 | 0.2 | 0.05 |
| | | 0.4 | 1.1 | 0.4 | 0.4 | 0.2 | 1 | | 21 | 8 | 0.35 | 0.018 | 0.4 | 59 | 0.4 | 0.03 | 0.01 | 5.1 |
| | | | | | | | | | | | | | | 0.1 | | 12 | | |
| | | | | | | | | | | | | | | | | | | 3850 |
| **Similac with iron**, liquid concentrate, Abbott (infant formula) *1 fl oz* | 31 | 39 | 23.6 | 4.3 | 4.3 | | 0 | | 10 | 31 | 2 | 0.30 | 0.002 | 35 | 4 | 0.04 | 0.4 | 0.10 |
| | | 0.8 | 2.1 | 0.7 | 0.8 | 0.5 | 1 | | 42 | 17 | 0.71 | 0.036 | 0.9 | 118 | 0.4 | 0.06 | 0.02 | 10.2 |
| | | | | | | | | | | | | | | 0.2 | | 24 | | |
| | | | | | | | | | | | | | | | | | | 3851 |
| **Similac with iron**, powder, Abbott (infant formula) - *1 scoop* | 9 | 47 | 0.2 | 4.9 | 4.9 | | 0 | | 11 | 37 | 3 | 0.35 | 0.002 | 43 | 4 | 0.05 | 0.5 | 0.12 |
| | | 1.0 | 2.6 | 0.9 | 0.9 | 0.6 | 1 | | 50 | 20 | 0.85 | 0.043 | 1.0 | 142 | 0.5 | 0.07 | 0.03 | 12.1 |
| | | | | | | | | | | | | | | 0.2 | | 27 | | |
| | | | | | | | | | | | | | | | | | | 3853 |
| **Vital Jr.**, Abbott (medical formula) *8 fl oz (240 ml)* | 249 | 237 | 200.0 | 31.7 | | | 0.7 | | 170 | 250 | 47 | 1.40 | 0.360 | | 24 | 0.64 | 2.4 | 1.40 |
| | | 7.1 | 9.6 | | | | | | 320 | 200 | 3.30 | 0.240 | 7.6 | 380 | | 0.50 | 0.62 | 120.7 |
| | | | | | | | | 17 | 240 | 23 | 8 | 7.1 | | 2.4 | 5 | 120 | 14.00 | |
| | | | | | | | | 4 | | | | | | 45 | 71 | | | RSSM48 |

| | WT | Macronutrients and Amino Acids | | | | | | | Minerals | | | | | Vitamins | | | | |
|---|---|---|---|---|---|---|---|---|---|---|---|---|---|---|---|---|---|---|
| | (g) | KCAL | $H_2O$ (g) | CHO (g) | TSUG (g) | ASUG (g) | DFIB (g) | | Na (mg) | Ca (mg) | Mg (mg) | Zn (mg) | Mn (mg) | A (mcg RAE) | C (mg) | B-1 (mg) | NIA (mg) | B-12 (mcg) |
| | | PRO (g) | FAT (g) | SFA (g) | MUFA (g) | PUFA (g) | CHOL (mg) | | K (mg) | P (mg) | Fe (mg) | Cu (mg) | Se (mcg) | A (IU) | E (mg ATE) | B-2 (mg) | B-6 (mg) | FOL (mcg DFE) |
| | | HIS (mg) | ISO (mg) | LEU (mg) | LYS (mg) | MET (mg) | CYS (mg) | TAU (mg) | Cl (mg) | I (mcg) | Mo (mcg) | Cr (mcg) | | PANT (mg) | E (IU) | D (IU) | K (mcg) | |
| | | PHE (mg) | TYR (mg) | THR (mg) | TRY (mg) | VAL (mg) | ARG (mg) | CAR (mg) | | | | | | BIO (mcg) | CHLN (mg) | INOS (mg) | | REF |
| **Wyeth-Ayerst infant formula** with iron liquid concentrate *1 fl oz* | 31 | 40 | 23.6 | 4.3 | 4.3 | | 0 | | 9 | 26 | 3 | 0.33 | | 37 | 3 | 0.04 | 0.3 | 0.08 |
| | | 0.9 | 2.2 | 1.0 | 0.9 | 0.3 | 2 | | 34 | 17 | 0.73 | 0.029 | 0.8 | 122 | 0.3 | 0.06 | 0.02 | 5.3 |
| | | | | | | | | | | | | | | | | | | |
| | | | | | | | | | | | | | | | | | | 3881 |
| **Wyeth-Ayerst infant formula with** iron, powder - *1 scoop* | 8 | 42 | 0.2 | 4.5 | 4.5 | | 0 | | 9 | 26 | 3 | 0.31 | | 38 | 3 | 0.04 | 0.3 | 0.08 |
| | | 1.0 | 2.2 | 1.0 | 0.9 | 0.3 | 3 | | 35 | 18 | 0.76 | 0.030 | 0.9 | 126 | 0.3 | 0.06 | 0.03 | 5.3 |
| | | | | | | | | | | | | | | | | | | |
| | | | | | | | | | | | | | | | | | | 3883 |
| **XLeu Analog** (leu-free), powder, Nutricia (infant formula) *¼ cup* | 30 | 142 | | 17.7 | | | | | 36 | 180 | 12 | 2.40 | 0.180 | 158 | 12 | 0.15 | 1.4 | 0.38 |
| | | 3.9 | 6.3 | 2.0 | 2.8 | 1.1 | | | 126 | 150 | 3.00 | 0.135 | 4.5 | 528 | 1.0 | 0.18 | 0.16 | 19.4 |
| | | 198 | 147 | 0 | 354 | 84 | 126 | 6 | 87 | 14 | 4 | 4.5 | | 0.8 | 1 | 102 | 6.30 | |
| | | 231 | 231 | 258 | 102 | 165 | 300 | 3 | | | | | | 8 | 15 | 30 | | NTRI29 |
| **XLeu Maxamaid** (leu-free), powder, Nutricia (child formula) *¼ cup* | 35 | 113 | | 19.6 | | | | | 203 | 284 | 45 | 3.85 | 0.665 | 175 | 22 | 0.28 | 1.8 | 0.70 |
| | | 8.8 | 0 | | | | | | 294 | 284 | 4.90 | 0.350 | 14.0 | 583 | 3.4 | 0.28 | 0.28 | 142.8 |
| | | 448 | 273 | 0 | 682 | 189 | 287 | 49 | 158 | 50 | 12 | 7.5 | | 1.1 | 5 | 168 | 16.80 | |
| | | 525 | 507 | 462 | 175 | 304 | 777 | 7 | | | | | | 6 | 88 | 20 | | NTRI30 |
| **XLeu Maxamum (leu-free),** powder, Nutricia (child/ adult formula) - *¼ cup* | 35 | 107 | | 11.9 | | | | | 196 | 414 | 107 | 3.15 | 0.630 | 234 | 22 | 0.32 | 2.0 | 1.08 |
| | | 14.0 | 0.2 | | | | | | 245 | 398 | 5.14 | 0.287 | 20.3 | 780 | 4.3 | 0.34 | 0.56 | 292.1 |
| | | 735 | 420 | 0 | 1050 | 301 | 455 | 49 | 196 | 46 | 13 | 9.1 | | 1.7 | 6 | 116 | 28.70 | |
| | | 805 | 805 | 735 | 276 | 490 | 1260 | 14 | | | | | | 9 | 150 | 28 | | NTRI31 |
| **XLys, XTry Analog** (lye- and try-free), powder, Nutricia (infant formula) - *¼ cup* | 30 | 142 | | 17.7 | | | | | 36 | 180 | 12 | 2.40 | 0.180 | 158 | 12 | 0.15 | 1.4 | 0.38 |
| | | 3.9 | 6.3 | 2.0 | 2.8 | 1.1 | | | 126 | 150 | 3.00 | 0.135 | 4.5 | 528 | 1.0 | 0.18 | 0.16 | 19.4 |
| | | 195 | 309 | 525 | 0 | 81 | 129 | 6 | 87 | 14 | 4 | 4.5 | | 0.8 | 1 | 102 | 6.30 | |
| | | 231 | 231 | 258 | 0 | 336 | 330 | 3 | | | | | | 8 | 15 | 30 | | NTRI32 |
| **XLys, XTry Maxamaid** (lys- and try-free), powder, Nutricia (child formula) - *¼ cup* | 35 | 113 | | 19.6 | | | | | 203 | 284 | 45 | 3.85 | 0.665 | 175 | 22 | 0.28 | 5.1 | 0.70 |
| | | 8.8 | 0 | | | | | | 294 | 284 | 4.90 | 0.350 | 14.0 | 583 | 3.4 | 0.28 | 0.28 | 142.8 |
| | | 444 | 700 | 1197 | 0 | 186 | 290 | 49 | 158 | 50 | 12 | 7.5 | | 1.1 | 5 | 168 | 16.80 | |
| | | 528 | 528 | 588 | 0 | 763 | 780 | 7 | | | | | | 6 | 88 | 20 | | NTRI33 |
| **XLys, XTry Maxamum** (lys- and try-free), powder, Nutricia (child/adult formula) *¼ cup* | 35 | 107 | | 11.9 | | | | | 196 | 414 | 107 | 3.15 | 0.630 | 234 | 22 | 0.32 | 4.2 | 1.08 |
| | | 14.0 | 0.2 | | | | | | 245 | 398 | 5.14 | 0.287 | 20.3 | 780 | 4.3 | 0.34 | 0.56 | 292.1 |
| | | 700 | 1085 | 1855 | 0 | 287 | 455 | 49 | 196 | 46 | 13 | 9.1 | | 1.7 | 6 | 116 | 28.70 | |
| | | 805 | 805 | 910 | 0 | 1190 | 1225 | 14 | | | | | | 9 | 150 | 28 | | NTRI34 |
| **XMet Analog** (met-free), powder, Nutricia (infant formula) *¼ cup* | 30 | 142 | | 17.7 | | | | | 36 | 180 | 12 | 2.40 | 0.180 | 158 | 12 | 0.15 | 1.4 | 0.38 |
| | | 3.9 | 6.3 | 2.0 | 2.8 | 1.1 | | | 126 | 150 | 3.00 | 0.135 | 4.5 | 528 | 1.0 | 0.18 | 0.16 | 19.4 |
| | | 180 | 279 | 477 | 324 | 0 | 117 | 6 | 87 | 14 | 4 | 4.5 | | 0.8 | 1 | 102 | 6.30 | |
| | | 210 | 240 | 234 | 93 | 303 | 300 | 3 | | | | | | 8 | 15 | 30 | | NTRI35 |
| **XMet Maxamaid** (met-free), powder, Nutricia (child formula) - *¼ cup* | 35 | 113 | | 19.6 | | | | | 203 | 284 | 45 | 3.85 | 0.665 | 175 | 22 | 0.28 | 1.8 | 0.70 |
| | | 8.8 | 0 | | | | | | 294 | 284 | 4.90 | 0.350 | 14.0 | 583 | 3.4 | 0.28 | 0.28 | 142.8 |
| | | 406 | 634 | 1085 | 735 | 0 | 262 | 49 | 158 | 50 | 12 | 7.5 | | 1.1 | 5 | 168 | 16.80 | |
| | | 480 | 480 | 532 | 214 | 690 | 714 | 7 | | | | | | 6 | 88 | 20 | | NTRI36 |
| **XMTVI Analogue** (met-, thr-, and val- free; iso-low), powder, Nutricia (infant formula) *¼ cup* | 30 | 142 | | 17.7 | | | | | 36 | 180 | 12 | 2.40 | 0.180 | 158 | 12 | 0.15 | 1.4 | 0.38 |
| | | 3.9 | 6.3 | 2.0 | 2.8 | 1.1 | | | 126 | 150 | 3.00 | 0.135 | 4.5 | 528 | 1.0 | 0.18 | 0.16 | 19.4 |
| | | 270 | 0 | 600 | 408 | 0 | 147 | 6 | 87 | 14 | 4 | 4.5 | | 0.8 | 1 | 102 | 6.30 | |
| | | 264 | 264 | 0 | 117 | 0 | 399 | 3 | | | | | | 8 | 15 | 30 | | NTRI38 |
| **XMTVI Maxamaid** (met-, thr-, and val- free; iso-low), powder, Nutricia (child formula) *¼ cup* | 35 | 113 | | 19.6 | | | | | 203 | 284 | 45 | 3.85 | 0.665 | 175 | 22 | 0.28 | 1.8 | 0.70 |
| | | 8.8 | 0 | | | | | | 294 | 284 | 4.90 | 0.350 | 14.0 | 583 | 3.4 | 0.28 | 0.28 | 142.8 |
| | | 612 | 12 | 1365 | 927 | 0 | 332 | 49 | 158 | 50 | 12 | 7.5 | | 1.1 | 5 | 168 | 16.80 | |
| | | 602 | 602 | 0 | 266 | 0 | 906 | 7 | | | | | | 6 | 88 | 20 | | NTRI39 |
| **XMTVI Maxamum** (met-, thr-, and val- free; iso-low), powder, Nutricia (child/adult formula) - *¼ cup* | 35 | 107 | | 11.9 | | | | | 196 | 414 | 107 | 3.15 | 0.630 | 234 | 22 | 0.32 | 2.0 | 1.08 |
| | | 14.0 | 0 | | | | | | 245 | 398 | 5.14 | 0.287 | 20.3 | 780 | 4.3 | 0.34 | 0.56 | 292.1 |
| | | 980 | 12 | 2170 | 1470 | 0 | 525 | 49 | 196 | 46 | 13 | 9.1 | | 1.7 | 6 | 116 | 28.70 | |
| | | 945 | 945 | 0 | 420 | 0 | 1435 | 14 | | | | | | 9 | 150 | 28 | | NTRI40 |
| **XPhe Analog** (phe-free), powder, Nutricia (infant formula) *¼ cup* | 30 | 142 | | 17.7 | | | | | 36 | 180 | 12 | 2.40 | 0.180 | 158 | 12 | 0.15 | 1.4 | 0.38 |
| | | 3.9 | 6.3 | 2.0 | 2.8 | 1.1 | | | 126 | 150 | 3.00 | 0.135 | 4.5 | 528 | 1.0 | 0.18 | 0.16 | 19.4 |
| | | 177 | 270 | 465 | 318 | 75 | 114 | 6 | 87 | 14 | 4 | 4.5 | | 0.8 | 1 | 102 | 6.30 | |
| | | 0 | 411 | 228 | 90 | 297 | 309 | 3 | | | | | | 8 | 15 | 30 | | NTRI41 |
| **XPhe Maxamaid** (phe-free), powder, Nutricia (child formula) - *¼ cup* | 35 | 113 | | 19.6 | | | | | 203 | 284 | 45 | 3.85 | 0.665 | 175 | 22 | 0.28 | 1.8 | 0.70 |
| | | 8.8 | 0 | | | | | | 294 | 284 | 4.90 | 0.350 | 14.0 | 583 | 3.4 | 0.28 | 0.28 | 142.8 |
| | | 444 | 595 | 1018 | 777 | 168 | 248 | 49 | 158 | 50 | 12 | 7.5 | | 1.1 | 5 | 168 | 16.80 | |
| | | 0 | 896 | 497 | 200 | 648 | 774 | 7 | | | | | | 6 | 88 | 20 | | NTRI42 |

| | WT (g) | KCAL / PRO(g) / HIS(mg) / PHE(mg) | H2O(g) / FAT(g) / ISO(mg) / TYR(mg) | CHO(g) / SFA(g) / LEU(mg) / THR(mg) | TSUG(g) / MUFA(g) / LYS(mg) / TRY(mg) | ASUG(g) / PUFA(g) / MET(mg) / VAL(mg) | DFIB(g) / CHOL(mg) / CYS(mg) / ARG(mg) | TAU(mg) / CAR(mg) | Na(mg) / K(mg) / Cl(mg) | Ca(mg) / P(mg) / I(mcg) | Mg(mg) / Fe(mg) / Mo(mcg) | Zn(mg) / Cu(mg) / Cr(mcg) | Mn(mg) / Se(mcg) | A(mcg RAE) / A(IU) / PANT(mg) / BIO(mcg) | C(mg) / E(mg ATE) / E(IU) / CHLN(mg) | B-1(mg) / B-2(mg) / D(IU) / INOS(mg) | NIA(mg) / B-6(mg) / K(mcg) | B-12(mcg) / FOL(mcg DFE) / REF |
|---|---|---|---|---|---|---|---|---|---|---|---|---|---|---|---|---|---|---|
| **XPhe Maxamum Drink (phe-free),** | 259 | 160 | | 13.8 | | | | | 210 | 400 | 114 | 3.50 | 0.700 | 250 | 23 | 0.35 | 2.1 | 1.20 |
| Nutricia (child/adult | | 15.0 | 5.0 | 0.8 | 3.0 | 1.0 | | | 263 | 288 | 5.50 | 0.310 | 21.8 | 833 | 4.8 | 0.38 | 0.60 | 312.8 |
| formula) - 250 ml drink box | | 730 | 1130 | 1950 | 1500 | 330 | 480 | 80 | 210 | 49 | 14 | 9.8 | | 1.9 | 7 | 130 | 30.80 | |
| (8.5 fl oz) | | 0 | 1730 | 950 | 380 | 1250 | 1280 | 10 | | | | | | 9 | 161 | 30 | | NTRI43 |
| **XPhe Maxamum powder (phe-free),** | 35 | 107 | | 11.9 | | | | | 196 | 414 | 107 | 3.15 | 0.630 | 234 | 22 | 0.32 | 2.0 | 1.08 |
| Nutricia (child/adult | | 14.0 | 0.4 | | | | | | 245 | 398 | 5.14 | 0.287 | 20.3 | 780 | 4.3 | 0.34 | 0.56 | 292.1 |
| formula) - ¼ cup | | 595 | 945 | 1610 | 1225 | 256 | 385 | 49 | 196 | 46 | 13 | 9.1 | | 1.7 | 6 | 116 | 28.70 | |
| | | 0 | 1400 | 770 | 312 | 1015 | 1050 | 14 | | | | | | 9 | 150 | 28 | | NTRI44 |
| **XPhe, XTry Analog, powder,** | 30 | 142 | | 17.7 | | | | | 36 | 180 | 12 | 2.40 | 0.180 | 158 | 12 | 0.15 | 1.4 | 0.38 |
| Nutricia (infant formula) | | 3.9 | 6.3 | 2.0 | 2.8 | 1.1 | | | 126 | 150 | 3.00 | 0.135 | 4.5 | 528 | 1.0 | 0.18 | 0.16 | 19.4 |
| ¼ cup | | 195 | 300 | 516 | 351 | 81 | 126 | 6 | 87 | 14 | 4 | 4.5 | | 0.8 | 1 | 102 | 6.30 | |
| | | 0 | 0 | 252 | 102 | 330 | 339 | 3 | | | | | | 8 | 15 | 30 | | NTRI45 |
| **XPhe, XTyr Maxamaid (phe- and** | 35 | 113 | | 19.6 | | | | | 203 | 284 | 45 | 3.85 | 0.665 | 175 | 22 | 0.28 | 1.8 | 0.70 |
| tyr-free), powder, Nutricia | | 8.8 | 0 | | | | | | 294 | 284 | 4.90 | 0.350 | 14.0 | 583 | 3.4 | 0.28 | 0.28 | 142.8 |
| (child formula) - ¼ cup | | 441 | 686 | 1176 | 798 | 189 | 287 | 49 | 158 | 50 | 12 | 7.5 | | 1.1 | 5 | 168 | 16.80 | |
| | | 0 | 0 | 574 | 231 | 749 | 774 | 7 | | | | | | 6 | 88 | 20 | | NTRI46 |
| **XPhen, Try Maxamaid (phe- and** | 35 | 108 | | 17.8 | | | | | 203 | 284 | 70 | 4.55 | 0.560 | 184 | 47 | 0.38 | 4.2 | 1.36 |
| tyr-free), powder, Nutricia | | 8.8 | 0 | | | | | | 294 | 284 | 4.20 | 0.630 | 14.0 | 612 | 1.5 | 0.42 | 0.49 | 142.8 |
| (child formula) - ¼ cup | | 462 | 721 | 1236 | 840 | 196 | 301 | 35 | 158 | 35 | 35 | 14.0 | | 1.3 | 2 | 168 | 10.50 | |
| | | 0 | 0 | 605 | 242 | 788 | 808 | 7 | | | | | | 42 | 38 | 19 | | NTRI47 |
| **XPhen, Try Maxamum (phe- and** | 35 | 104 | | 11.9 | | | | | 196 | 234 | 100 | 4.76 | 0.735 | 248 | 31 | 0.49 | 4.8 | 1.26 |
| tyr-free), powder, Nutricia | | 13.6 | 0 | | | | | | 245 | 234 | 8.22 | 0.490 | 17.5 | 827 | 1.8 | 0.49 | 0.74 | 297.5 |
| (child/adult formula) | | 700 | 1085 | 1855 | 1400 | 298 | 455 | 52 | 196 | 37 | 37 | 17.5 | | 1.8 | 3 | 109 | 24.50 | |
| ¼ cup | | 0 | 0 | 910 | 350 | 1190 | 1225 | 7 | | | | | | 49 | 112 | 30 | | NTRI48 |
| **XPTM Analog (phe-, try-, and met-** | 30 | 142 | | 17.7 | | | | | 36 | 180 | 12 | 2.40 | 0.180 | 158 | 12 | 0.15 | 1.4 | 0.38 |
| free), powder, Nutricia | | 3.9 | 6.3 | 2.0 | 2.8 | 1.1 | | | 126 | 150 | 3.00 | 0.135 | 4.5 | 528 | 1.0 | 0.18 | 0.16 | 19.4 |
| (infant formula) - ¼ cup | | 198 | 306 | 525 | 357 | 0 | 129 | 6 | 87 | 14 | 4 | 4.5 | | 0.8 | 1 | 102 | 6.30 | |
| | | 0 | 0 | 258 | 102 | 336 | 345 | 3 | | | | | | 8 | 15 | 30 | | NTRI49 |

## 32.2 MEDICAL FOODS FOR ADULTS

| | WT (g) | C1 | C2 | C3 | C4 | C5 | C6 | C7 | M1 | M2 | M3 | M4 | M5 | V1 | V2 | V3 | V4 | V5 |
|---|---|---|---|---|---|---|---|---|---|---|---|---|---|---|---|---|---|---|
| **Complete Amino Acid Mix** | 10 | 33 | | 0 | | | | | | | | | | | | | | |
| (essential and non-essential), | | 8.2 | 0 | | | | | | | | | | | | | | | |
| powder, Nutricia - 1 T | | 438 | 595 | 1022 | 755 | 165 | 240 | | | | | | | | | | | |
| | | 450 | 430 | 500 | 200 | 650 | 766 | | | | | | | | | | | NTRI2 |
| **Enlive!, Abbott (medical formula)** | 266 | 300 | 192.0 | 65.0 | 15.0 | | 0 | | 60 | 60 | 8 | 3.80 | 0.900 | | 24 | 0.38 | 2.0 | 1.20 |
| 8.1 fl oz (243 ml) | | 10.0 | 0 | 0 | | | 2 | | 40 | 20 | 2.70 | 0.300 | 14.0 | 1250 | | 0.34 | 0.40 | 102.0 |
| | | | | | | | | | 310 | 45 | 32 | 18.0 | | 0.8 | 9 | 60 | 20.00 | |
| | | | | | | | | | | | | | | 30 | | | | RSSM3 |
| **Ensure, Abbott (medical formula)** | 255 | 250 | 200.0 | 40.0 | 23.0 | | 0 | | 200 | 300 | 100 | 3.80 | 1.200 | | 30 | 0.38 | 5.0 | 1.50 |
| 8 fl oz (240 ml) | | 9.0 | 6.0 | 1.0 | 2.0 | 3.0 | 5 | | 370 | 250 | 4.50 | 0.500 | 18.0 | 1250 | | 0.43 | 0.50 | 170.0 |
| | | | | | | | | | 210 | 38 | 38 | 30.0 | | 2.5 | 8 | 100 | 20.00 | |
| | | | | | | | | | | | | | | 75 | 83 | | | RSSM14 |
| **Ensure Fiber with scFOS, Abbott** | 252 | 250 | 195.0 | 42.0 | 14.0 | | 2.8 | | 200 | 350 | 100 | 3.80 | 1.200 | | 30 | 0.38 | 5.0 | 1.50 |
| (medical formula) - 8 fl oz | | 8.8 | 6.1 | 1.0 | 2.0 | 3.0 | 2 | | 370 | 300 | 4.50 | 0.500 | 18.0 | 1250 | | 0.43 | 0.50 | 170.0 |
| (240 ml) | | | | | | | | | 320 | 38 | 38 | 30.0 | | 2.5 | 8 | 100 | 20.00 | |
| | | | | | | | | | | | | | | 75 | 100 | | | RSSM4 |
| **Ensure High Pro, Abbott (medical** | 252 | 230 | 203.0 | 31.0 | 19.0 | | 0 | | 290 | 300 | 100 | 5.70 | 1.200 | | 30 | 0.38 | 5.0 | 1.50 |
| formula) - 8 fl oz (240 ml) | | 12.0 | 6.0 | 1.0 | 2.0 | 3.0 | 2 | | 500 | 250 | 4.50 | 0.500 | 18.0 | 1250 | | 0.43 | 0.50 | 170.0 |
| | | | | | | | | | 375 | 38 | 38 | 30.0 | | 2.5 | 12 | 100 | 20.00 | |
| | | | | | | | | | | | | | | 75 | 100 | | | RSSM6 |
| **Ensure Plus, Abbott (medical** | 255 | 350 | 180.0 | 50.0 | 20.0 | | | | 240 | 300 | 100 | 4.50 | 1.200 | | 36 | 0.38 | 5.0 | 1.50 |
| formula) - 8 fl oz (240 ml) | | 13.0 | 11.0 | 1.0 | 5.0 | 4.5 | 10 | | 420 | 300 | 4.50 | 0.500 | 21.0 | 1250 | | 0.43 | 0.50 | 170.0 |
| | | | | | | | | | 270 | 38 | 45 | 30.0 | | 2.5 | 9 | 100 | 20.00 | |
| | | | | | | | | | | | | | | 75 | 83 | | | RSSM11 |
| **Ensure powder, Abbott (medical** | 252 | 250 | 178.0 | 34.0 | 13.0 | | | | 200 | 150 | 60 | 3.00 | 0.600 | | 36 | 0.38 | 5.0 | 1.50 |
| formula) - ½ cup w/ | | 9.0 | 9.0 | 1.5 | | | 2 | | 370 | 150 | 2.70 | 0.300 | 10.5 | 750 | | 0.43 | 0.50 | 170.0 |
| ¾ cup water (8 fl oz) | | | | | | | | | 340 | 22 | 19 | 18.0 | | 2.5 | 6 | 60 | 12.00 | |
| | | | | | | | | | | | | | | 75 | 75 | | | RSSM12 |

| | WT (g) | Macronutrients and Amino Acids | | | | | | | Minerals | | | | | Vitamins | | | | |
|---|---|---|---|---|---|---|---|---|---|---|---|---|---|---|---|---|---|---|
| | | KCAL | $H_2O$ (g) | CHO (g) | TSUG (g) | ASUG (g) | DFIB (g) | | Na (mg) | Ca (mg) | Mg (mg) | Zn (mg) | Mn (mg) | A (mcg RAE) | C (mg) | B-1 (mg) | NIA (mg) | B-12 (mcg) |
| | | PRO (g) | FAT (g) | SFA (g) | MUFA (g) | PUFA (g) | CHOL (mg) | | K (mg) | P (mg) | Fe (mg) | Cu (mg) | Se (mcg) | A (IU) | E (mg ATE) | B-2 (mg) | B-6 (mg) | FOL (mcg DFE) |
| | | HIS (mg) | ISO (mg) | LEU (mg) | LYS (mg) | MET (mg) | CYS (mg) | TAU (mg) | Cl (mg) | I (mcg) | Mo (mcg) | Cr (mcg) | | PANT (mg) | E (IU) | D (IU) | K (mcg) | |
| | | PHE (mg) | TYR (mg) | THR (mg) | TRY (mg) | VAL (mg) | ARG (mg) | CAR (mg) | | | | | | BIO (mcg) | CHLN (mg) | INOS (mg) | | REF |
| **Ensure pudding**, Abbott (medical food) - *4 fl oz (120 ml)* | 113 | 170 | 76.0 | 27.0 | 20.0 | | 1.0 | | 170 | 100 | 40 | 3.00 | 0.600 | | 9 | 0.23 | 3.0 | 1.20 |
| | | 4.0 | 5.0 | 1.0 | | | 2 | | 180 | 150 | 2.70 | 0.200 | 10.5 | 500 | | 0.26 | 0.30 | 102.0 |
| | | | | | | | | | 68 | 45 | 30 | 12.0 | | 2.0 | 6 | 40 | 12.00 | |
| | | | | | | | | | | | | | | 60 | | | | RSSM13 |
| **Essential Amino Acid Mix**, powder, Nutricia - *1 T* | 9 | 28 | | 0 | | | | | | | | | | | | | | |
| | | 7.1 | 0 | | | | | | | | | | | | | | | |
| | | 340 | 936 | 1455 | 1192 | 340 | 340 | | | | | | | | | | | |
| | | 510 | 851 | 1021 | 212 | 1310 | | | | | | | | | | | | NTRI4 |
| **Glucerna**, Abbott (medical formula) - *8 fl oz (240 ml)* | 248 | 237 | 202.0 | 22.8 | | | 3.4 | | 220 | 170 | 67 | 3.80 | 0.840 | | 50 | 0.38 | 5.0 | 1.50 |
| | | 9.9 | 12.9 | | | | | | 370 | 170 | 3.00 | 0.340 | 12.0 | 1500 | | 0.43 | 0.50 | 170.0 |
| | | | | | | | | 25 | 340 | 25 | 25 | 20.0 | | 2.5 | 8 | 67 | 14.00 | |
| | | | | | | | | 34 | | | | | | 75 | 100 | 200 | | RSSM20 |
| **Glucerna Select**, Abbott (medical formula) - *8 fl oz (240 ml)* | 256 | 237 | 199.0 | 22.8 | | | 5.0 | | 220 | 170 | 67 | 3.80 | 0.840 | | 50 | 0.38 | 5.0 | 1.50 |
| | | 11.9 | 12.9 | | | | | | 430 | 170 | 3.00 | 0.340 | 12.0 | 1495 | | 0.43 | 0.50 | 170.0 |
| | | | | | | | | 25 | 320 | 25 | 25 | 20.0 | | 2.5 | 8 | 67 | 24.00 | |
| | | | | | | | | 34 | | | | | | 76 | 100 | 200 | | RSSM42 |
| **Glucerna Shake**, Abbott (medical food) - *8 fl oz (240 ml)* | 248 | 220 | 200.0 | 29.3 | 7.0 | | 2.8 | | 210 | 250 | 100 | 3.80 | 1.000 | | 60 | 0.38 | 5.0 | 3.00 |
| | | 9.9 | 8.6 | 1.0 | | | 2 | | 370 | 250 | 4.50 | 0.500 | 18.0 | 1750 | | 0.43 | 1.00 | 340.0 |
| | | | | | | | | | 355 | 38 | 38 | 120.0 | | 2.5 | 30 | 100 | 20.00 | |
| | | | | | | | | | | | | | | 75 | 100 | | | RSSM18 |
| **Glucerna Snack Bar**, Abbott (medical food) - *1 bar* | 40 | 150 | | 25.0 | 3.0 | | 1.0 | | 150 | 20 | | | | | 15 | | | |
| | | 6.0 | 4.0 | 3.0 | | | 0 | | 80 | | 1.10 | | | 1000 | | | | |
| | | | | | | | | | | | | 30.0 | | | 30 | | | |
| | | | | | | | | | | | | | | | | | | RSSM19 |
| **Hi-Cal**, Abbott (medical formula) *8 fl oz (240 ml)* | 259 | 475 | 166.0 | 51.3 | | | 21.2 | | 345 | 200 | 80 | 4.50 | 1.000 | | 12 | 0.30 | 4.0 | 1.20 |
| | | 19.8 | 21.2 | | | | | | 580 | 200 | 3.60 | 0.400 | 14.0 | 1000 | | 0.34 | 0.40 | 136.0 |
| | | | | | | | | | 340 | 30 | 30 | 24.0 | | 2.0 | 9 | 80 | 16.00 | |
| | | | | | | | | | | | | | | 60 | 75 | | | RSSM43 |
| **Jevity 1 Cal**, Abbott (medical formula) - *8 fl oz (240 ml)* | 253 | 250 | 197.0 | 36.5 | | | 3.4 | | 220 | 215 | 72 | 4.30 | 0.900 | | 55 | 0.41 | 5.5 | 1.70 |
| | | 10.4 | 8.2 | | | | | | 375 | 180 | 3.30 | 0.370 | 13.0 | 895 | | 0.48 | 0.55 | 187.0 |
| | | | | | | | | 28 | 310 | 28 | 28 | 22.0 | | 2.9 | 8 | 72 | 15.00 | |
| | | | | | | | | 28 | | | | | | 82 | 110 | | | RSSM23 |
| **Jevity 1.2 Cal**, Abbott (medical formula) - *8 fl oz (240 ml)* | 257 | 285 | 191.0 | 40.2 | | | 4.3 | | 325 | 285 | 96 | 5.50 | 1.200 | | 72 | 0.55 | 7.2 | 2.20 |
| | | 13.2 | 9.3 | | | | | | 440 | 285 | 4.30 | 0.480 | 17.0 | 1190 | | 0.62 | 0.72 | 246.5 |
| | | | | | | | | 36 | 360 | 36 | 36 | 29.0 | | 3.6 | 11 | 96 | 20.00 | |
| | | | | | | | | 36 | | | | | | 110 | 145 | | | RSSM22 |
| **Jevity 1.5 Cal**, Abbott (medical formula) - *8 fl oz (240 ml)* | 260 | 355 | 180.0 | 51.1 | | | 5.3 | | 330 | 285 | 95 | 5.40 | 1.200 | | 72 | 0.54 | 7.2 | 2.20 |
| | | 15.1 | 11.8 | | | | | | 510 | 285 | 4.30 | 0.480 | 17.0 | 1185 | | 0.61 | 0.72 | 246.5 |
| | | | | | | | | 36 | 320 | 36 | 36 | 29.0 | | 3.6 | 11 | 95 | 19.00 | |
| | | | | | | | | 36 | | | | | | 110 | 145 | | | RSSM44 |
| **KetoCal** (for intractable epilepsy), powder, Nutricia (child/adult formula) - *amt to make 100 ml* | 20 | 144 | | 0.6 | | | | | 60 | 160 | 22 | 1.16 | 0.320 | 76 | 12 | 0.13 | 1.5 | 0.26 |
| | | 3.0 | 14.4 | | | | | | 216 | 130 | 2.20 | 0.120 | 6.8 | 253 | 1.5 | 0.13 | 0.13 | 64.6 |
| | | | | | | | | | 100 | 16 | 5 | 3.8 | | 0.5 | 2 | 42 | 8.00 | |
| | | | | | | | | | | | | | | 2 | 96 | 27 | | NTRI5 |
| **Lanaflex**, powder (phe-free), Nutricia (adult formula) *1 packet* | 16 | 40 | | 4.4 | | | | | 5 | 474 | 122 | 3.70 | 0.730 | 268 | 25 | 0.36 | 2.2 | 1.30 |
| | | 5.2 | 0.2 | | | | | | 4 | 456 | 5.90 | 0.332 | 23.1 | 892 | 5.0 | 0.38 | 0.65 | 334.9 |
| | | 920 | 460 | 460 | 460 | 920 | | | 0 | 52 | 15 | 10.6 | | 1.9 | 7 | 135 | 32.70 | |
| | | | 920 | 460 | 920 | 460 | | | | | | | | 10 | 165 | 32 | | NTRI6 |
| **Milupa HOM 2** (L-amino acids, met-free), powder, Nutricia (child/adult formula) *¼ cup* | 37 | 107 | | 1.4 | | | | | 237 | 485 | 58 | 2.96 | 0.259 | 578 | 30 | 0.52 | 8.9 | 1.11 |
| | | 25.5 | 0 | | | | | | 492 | 374 | 5.55 | 0.740 | | 1924 | 4.4 | 0.74 | 0.55 | 251.6 |
| | | 666 | 1665 | 2812 | 1998 | 0 | 1258 | | 366 | 44 | 12 | | | 4.1 | 7 | 485 | 61.79 | |
| | | 1184 | 1443 | 1332 | 518 | 1998 | 999 | | | | | | | 111 | 96 | 111 | | NTRI8 |
| **Milupa MSUD 2** (L-amino acids; iso-, leu-, and val-free), powder, Nutricia (child/adult formula) - *¼ cup* | 40 | 120 | | 8.4 | | | | | 256 | 524 | 62 | 3.12 | 0.280 | 625 | 32 | 0.56 | 9.6 | 1.20 |
| | | 21.6 | 0 | | | | | | 532 | 404 | 6.00 | 0.800 | | 2080 | 4.8 | 0.80 | 0.60 | 272.0 |
| | | 720 | 0 | 0 | 2160 | 720 | 720 | | 396 | 48 | 13 | | | 4.4 | 7 | 524 | 66.80 | |
| | | 1280 | 1560 | 1440 | 560 | 0 | 1080 | | | | | | | 120 | 104 | 120 | | NTRI9 |
| **Milupa OS 2** (L-amino acids; iso-, leu-, and val-free), powder, Nutricia (child/adult formula) - *¼ cup* | 40 | 120 | | 7.6 | | | | | 256 | 524 | 62 | 3.12 | 0.280 | 625 | 32 | 0.56 | 9.6 | 1.20 |
| | | 22.5 | 0 | | | | | | 532 | 404 | 6.00 | 0.800 | | 2080 | 4.8 | 0.80 | 0.60 | 272.0 |
| | | 720 | 0 | 3040 | 2160 | 0 | 720 | | 396 | 48 | 13 | | | 4.4 | 7 | 524 | 66.80 | |
| | | 1280 | 1560 | 0 | 560 | 0 | 1080 | | | | | | | 120 | 104 | 120 | | NTRI10 |

| | WT (g) | KCAL | H₂O (g) | CHO (g) | TSUG (g) | ASUG (g) | DFIB (g) | Na (mg) | Ca (mg) | Mg (mg) | Zn (mg) | Mn (mg) | A (mcg RAE) | C (mg) | B-1 (mg) | NIA (mg) | B-12 (mcg) |
|---|---|---|---|---|---|---|---|---|---|---|---|---|---|---|---|---|---|
| | | PRO (g) | FAT (g) | SFA (g) | MUFA (g) | PUFA (g) | CHOL (mg) | K (mg) | P (mg) | Fe (mg) | Cu (mg) | Se (mcg) | A (IU) | E (mg ATE) | B-2 (mg) | B-6 (mg) | FOL (mcg DFE) |
| | | HIS (mg) | ISO (mg) | LEU (mg) | LYS (mg) | MET (mg) | CYS (mg) | TAU (mg) Cl (mg) | I (mcg) | Mo (mcg) | Cr (mcg) | | PANT (mg) | E (IU) | D (IU) | K (mcg) | |
| | | PHE (mg) | TYR (mg) | THR (mg) | TRY (mg) | VAL (mg) | ARG (mg) | CAR (mg) | | | | | BIO (mcg) | CHLN (mg) | INOS (mg) | | REF |
| **Milupa PKU 2 Tom** (low phe), powder, Nutricia (child/adult formula) - *1 packet* | 45 | 185 | | 25.8 | | | | 753 | 252 | 54 | 2.90 | 0.400 | 162 | 16 | 0.27 | 2.0 | 0.50 |
| | | 10.0 | 4.5 | 1.8 | 1.7 | 0.8 | | 211 | 148 | 3.00 | 0.207 | 9.0 | 540 | 2.2 | 0.31 | 0.36 | 75.0 |
| | | 270 | 720 | 1170 | 860 | 270 | 270 | 0 / 1025 | 35 | 13 | 6.0 | | 1.2 | 3 | 64 | 7.60 | |
| | | 9 | 720 | 590 | 230 | 860 | 410 | 20 | | | | | 10 | 94 | 47 | | NTRI12 |
| **Milupa PKU 3** (L-amino acids, phe-free), powder, Nutricia (child/adult formula) - *¼ cup* | 35 | 98 | | 0.6 | | | | 224 | 458 | 189 | 8.40 | 1.680 | 420 | 35 | 0.63 | 6.3 | 1.75 |
| | | 23.8 | 0 | | | | | 465 | 354 | 7.35 | 1.260 | | 1400 | 2.8 | 0.63 | 1.12 | 565.2 |
| | | 630 | 1575 | 2660 | 1890 | 630 | 630 | 350 | 50 | 168 | 224.0 | | 2.9 | 4 | 168 | 58.45 | |
| | | 0 | 2100 | 1260 | 490 | 1890 | 945 | | | | | | 63 | 91 | 105 | | NTRI13 |
| **Milupa TYR 2** (L-amino acids, tyr-, and phe-free), powder, Nutricia (child/adult formula) - *¼ cup* | 37 | 109 | | 4.0 | | | | 237 | 485 | 58 | 2.96 | 0.259 | 578 | 30 | 0.52 | 8.9 | 1.11 |
| | | 23.3 | 0 | | | | | 492 | 374 | 5.55 | 0.740 | | 1924 | 4.4 | 0.74 | 0.55 | 251.6 |
| | | 666 | 1665 | 2812 | 1998 | 666 | 666 | 366 | 44 | 12 | | | 4.1 | 7 | 485 | 61.79 | |
| | | 0 | 0 | 1332 | 518 | 1998 | 999 | | | | | | 111 | 96 | 111 | | NTRI14 |
| **Milupa UCD 2** (L-amino acids for ureacycle disorders), powder, Nutricia (child/adult formula - *¼ cup* | 34 | 99 | 0.7 | 1.5 | | | | 218 | 445 | 0 | 2.65 | 0.238 | 530 | 27 | 0.48 | 8.2 | 1.02 |
| | | 22.8 | 0 | | | | | 452 | 343 | 5.10 | 0.680 | | 1768 | 4.1 | 0.68 | 0.51 | 231.2 |
| | | 1224 | 3026 | 5100 | 3638 | 2414 | 0 | 337 | 41 | 11 | | | 3.7 | 6 | 445 | 56.78 | |
| | | 4794 | 0 | 2414 | 952 | 3638 | 0 | | | | | | 102 | 88 | 102 | | NTRI15 |
| **Monogen** (low-fat, high medium chain triglycerides), powder, Nutricia (child/adult formula) - *amt to make 100 ml* | 18 | 76 | | 12.2 | | | | 36 | 46 | 6 | 0.59 | 0.059 | 58 | 6 | 0.06 | 0.7 | 0.15 |
| | | 2.1 | 2.1 | | | | | 65 | 36 | 0.76 | 0.061 | 1.9 | 195 | 0.5 | 0.09 | 0.07 | 14.4 |
| | | | | | | | | 39 | 7 | 4 | 1.8 | | 0.3 | 1 | 48 | 3.78 | |
| | | | | | | | | | | | | | 4 | 10 | 15 | | NTRI16 |
| **Nepro**, Abbott (medical formula) *8 fl oz (240 ml)* | 259 | 425 | 170.0 | 39.4 | 5.9 | | 3.7 | 250 | 250 | 50 | 6.40 | 0.500 | | 25 | 0.56 | 7.5 | 2.30 |
| | | 19.1 | 22.7 | | | | | 250 | 165 | 4.50 | 0.500 | 18.0 | 750 | | 0.64 | 2.00 | 425.0 |
| | | | | | | | | 38 / 200 | 38 | 19 | 30.0 | | 3.8 | 23 | 20 | 20.00 | |
| | | | | | | | | 63 | | | | | 115 | 150 | | | RSSM24 |
| **Optimental**, Abbott (medical formula) - *8 fl oz (240 ml)* | 250 | 237 | 197.0 | 32.9 | | | 1.2 | 250 | 250 | 100 | 3.80 | 0.840 | | 50 | 0.50 | 6.7 | 2.00 |
| | | 12.2 | 6.7 | | | | | 415 | 250 | 3.00 | 0.340 | | 1950 | | 0.57 | 0.67 | 229.5 |
| | | | | | | | | 25 / 320 | 38 | 25 | 20.0 | | 3.4 | 50 | 67 | 20.00 | |
| | | | | | | | | 25 | | | | | 100 | 100 | | | RSSM26 |
| **Osmolite 1 Cal**, Abbott (medical formula) - *8 fl oz (240 ml)* | 252 | 250 | 199.0 | 33.9 | | | | 220 | 180 | 72 | 4.10 | 0.900 | | 54 | 0.41 | 5.4 | 1.70 |
| | | 10.5 | 8.2 | | | | | 370 | 180 | 3.30 | 0.360 | 13.0 | 895 | | 0.46 | 0.54 | 187.0 |
| | | | | | | | | 27 / 340 | 27 | 27 | 22.0 | | 2.7 | 8 | 72 | 15.00 | |
| | | | | | | | | 27 | | | | | 81 | 110 | | | RSSM28 |
| **Osmolite**, Abbott (medical formula) *8 fl oz (240 ml)* | 252 | 250 | 199.0 | 35.6 | | | | 150 | 125 | 50 | 2.90 | 0.620 | | 38 | 0.38 | 5.0 | 1.50 |
| | | 8.8 | 8.2 | | | | | 240 | 125 | 2.30 | 0.250 | 9.0 | 625 | | 0.43 | 0.50 | 170.0 |
| | | | | | | | | 19 / 200 | 19 | 19 | 15.0 | | 2.5 | 6 | 50 | 10.00 | |
| | | | | | | | | 19 | | | | | 75 | 75 | | | RSSM29 |
| **Oxepa**, Abbott (medical formula) *8 fl oz (240 ml)* | 248 | 355 | 186.0 | 25.0 | | | | 310 | 250 | 100 | 5.70 | 1.300 | | 205 | 0.75 | 10.0 | 3.00 |
| | | 14.8 | 22.2 | | | | | 465 | 250 | 4.50 | 0.500 | 18.0 | 2840 | | 0.85 | 1.00 | 340.0 |
| | | | | | | | | 75 / 400 | 38 | 38 | 30.0 | | 5.0 | 75 | 100 | 20.00 | |
| | | | | | | | | 43 | | | | | 150 | 150 | | | RSSM30 |
| **Perative**, Abbott (medical formula) *8 fl oz (240 ml)* | 254 | 237 | 200.0 | 31.7 | | | 0.7 | 170 | 250 | 47 | 1.40 | 0.360 | | 24 | 0.64 | 2.4 | 1.40 |
| | | 7.1 | 9.6 | | | | | 320 | 200 | 3.30 | 0.240 | 7.6 | 380 | | 0.50 | 0.62 | 120.7 |
| | | | | | | | | 17 / 240 | 23 | 8 | 7.1 | | 2.4 | 5 | 120 | 14.00 | |
| | | | | | | | | 4 | | | | | 45 | 71 | 19 | | RSSM33 |
| **Pivot 1.5 Cal**, Abbott (medical formula) - *8 fl oz (240 ml)* | 255 | 355 | 180.0 | 40.9 | | | 1.8 | 330 | 240 | 95 | 6.00 | 1.200 | | 72 | 0.54 | 7.1 | 2.20 |
| | | 22.2 | 12.0 | | | | | 475 | 240 | 4.30 | 0.480 | 17.0 | 2370 | | 0.61 | 0.71 | 246.5 |
| | | | | | | | | 36 / 380 | 36 | 36 | 29.0 | | 3.6 | 60 | 95 | 19.00 | |
| | | | | | | | | 36 | | | | | 110 | 145 | | | RSSM47 |
| **Polycal** (carbohydrate supplement w/maltodextrins), powder, Nutricia - *¼ cup* | 32 | 123 | | 30.7 | | | | 1 | | | | | | | | | |
| | | | | | | | | | | | | | | | | | |
| | | | | | | | | | | | | | | | | | |
| | | | | | | | | | | | | | | | | | NTRI26 |
| **Polycose**, Abbott (medical formula) *3.3 fl oz (100 ml)* | 120 | 380 | 6.0 | 94.0 | | | | 130 | 30 | | | | | | | | |
| | | | | | | | | 10 | 15 | | | | | | | | |
| | | | | | | | | 223 | | | | | | | | | |
| | | | | | | | | | | | | | | | | | RSSM34 |
| **Promote**, Abbott (medical formula) *8 fl oz (240 ml)* | 250 | 237 | 198.0 | 30.8 | | | | 240 | 285 | 95 | 5.70 | 1.200 | | 82 | 0.54 | 7.2 | 2.20 |
| | | 14.8 | 6.2 | | | | | 470 | 285 | 4.30 | 0.480 | 17.0 | 1720 | | 0.61 | 0.72 | 246.5 |
| | | | | | | | | 36 / 300 | 36 | 36 | 29.0 | | 3.6 | 11 | 95 | 19.00 | |
| | | | | | | | | 36 | | | | | 110 | 145 | | | RSSM37 |

| Food | WT (g) | KCAL<br>PRO (g)<br>HIS (mg)<br>PHE (mg) | $H_2O$ (g)<br>FAT (g)<br>ISO (mg)<br>TYR (mg) | CHO (g)<br>SFA (g)<br>LEU (mg)<br>THR (mg) | TSUG (g)<br>MUFA (g)<br>LYS (mg)<br>TRY (mg) | ASUG (g)<br>PUFA (g)<br>MET (mg)<br>VAL (mg) | DFIB (g)<br>CHOL (mg)<br>CYS (mg)<br>ARG (mg) | <br><br>TAU (mg)<br>CAR (mg) | Na (mg)<br>K (mg)<br>Cl (mg) | Ca (mg)<br>P (mg)<br>I (mcg) | Mg (mg)<br>Fe (mg)<br>Mo (mcg) | Zn (mg)<br>Cu (mg)<br>Cr (mcg) | Mn (mg)<br>Se (mcg) | A (mcg RAE)<br>A (IU)<br>PANT (mg)<br>BIO (mcg) | C (mg)<br>E (mg ATE)<br>E (IU)<br>CHLN (mg) | B-1 (mg)<br>B-2 (mg)<br>D (IU)<br>INOS (mg) | NIA (mg)<br>B-6 (mg)<br>K (mcg) | B-12 (mcg)<br>FOL (mcg DFE)<br><br>REF |
|---|---|---|---|---|---|---|---|---|---|---|---|---|---|---|---|---|---|---|
| Protifar, powder, Nutricia — ¼ cup | 16 | 60 | | 0.1 | | | | | 5 | 216 | 3 | | | | | | | |
| | | 14.2 | 0.3 | | | | | | 8 | 112 | | | | | | | | |
| | | | | | | | | | 16 | | | | | | | | | |
| | | | | | | | | | | | | | | | | | | NTRI27 |
| Pulmocare, Abbott (medical formula) - 8 fl oz (240 ml) | 248 | 355 | 186.0 | 25.0 | | | | | 310 | 250 | 100 | 5.70 | 1.300 | | 75 | 0.75 | 10.0 | 3.00 |
| | | 14.8 | 22.1 | | | | | | 465 | 250 | 4.50 | 0.500 | 18.0 | 2840 | | 0.85 | 1.00 | 340.0 |
| | | | | | | | 36 | | 400 | 38 | 38 | 30.0 | | 5.0 | 20 | 100 | 20.00 | |
| | | | | | | | 36 | | | | | | | 150 | 150 | | | RSSM38 |
| Super Soluble Duocal (calorie supplement), powder, Nutricia - ¼ cup | 30 | 148 | | 21.8 | | | | | 3 | 1 | | | | | | | | |
| | | | 6.7 | 4.1 | 0.8 | 1.4 | | | 1 | 1 | | | | | | | | |
| | | | | | | | | | 3 | | | | | | | | | |
| | | | | | | | | | | | | | | | | | | |
| Suplena, Abbott (medical formula) 8 fl oz (240 ml) | 260 | 425 | 174.0 | 47.8 | 7.2 | | 3.7 | | 185 | 250 | 50 | 6.40 | 0.500 | | 25 | 0.60 | 7.5 | 2.30 |
| | | 10.6 | 22.7 | | | | | | 265 | 165 | 4.50 | 0.500 | 18.0 | 750 | | 0.60 | 2.00 | 425.0 |
| | | | | | | | 38 | | 220 | 38 | 19 | 30.0 | | 3.8 | 23 | 20 | 20.00 | |
| | | | | | | | 63 | | | | | | | 115 | 150 | | | RSSM39 |
| TwoCal HN, Abbott (medical formula) - 8 fl oz (240 ml) | 260 | 475 | 166.0 | 51.8 | | | 1.2 | | 345 | 250 | 100 | 5.70 | 1.300 | | 75 | 0.60 | 8.0 | 2.40 |
| | | | | | | | | | | | | | | | | | | |
| | | | | | | | 38 | 430 | 38 | 38 | 30.0 | 4.0 | | 12 | 100 | 20.00 | | |
| | | | | | | | 38 | | | | | | | 120 | 150 | | | RSSM40 |
| Vital High N, dry packet in water, Abbott (medical formula) 1 pkt in 8.6 fl oz wtr (300 ml) | 332 | 300 | 260.0 | 55.4 | | | | | 170 | 200 | 80 | 4.50 | 1.000 | | 60 | 0.60 | 8.0 | 2.40 |
| | | 12.5 | 3.3 | | | | | | 420 | 200 | 3.60 | 0.400 | 14.0 | 1000 | | 0.68 | 0.80 | 272.0 |
| | | | | | | | | | 310 | 30 | 30 | 24.0 | | 4.0 | 9 | 80 | 16.00 | |
| | | | | | | | | | | | | | | 120 | 120 | | | RSSM41 |

## 32.3 SPORT, ENERGY, AND WEIGHT REDUCTION FOODS

| Food | WT (g) | KCAL<br>PRO<br>HIS<br>PHE | $H_2O$<br>FAT<br>ISO<br>TYR | CHO<br>SFA<br>LEU<br>THR | TSUG<br>MUFA<br>LYS<br>TRY | ASUG<br>PUFA<br>MET<br>VAL | DFIB<br>CHOL<br>CYS<br>ARG | <br><br>TAU<br>CAR | Na<br>K<br>Cl | Ca<br>P<br>I | Mg<br>Fe<br>Mo | Zn<br>Cu<br>Cr | Mn<br>Se | A<br>A(IU)<br>PANT<br>BIO | C<br>E(ATE)<br>E(IU)<br>CHLN | B-1<br>B-2<br>D<br>INOS | NIA<br>B-6<br>K | B-12<br>FOL<br><br>REF |
|---|---|---|---|---|---|---|---|---|---|---|---|---|---|---|---|---|---|---|
| cereal bar, high protein, chocolate, South Beach Diet 1.2 oz bar | 35 | 140 | | 15.0 | 7.0 | | 3.0 | | 150 | 150 | | | | | 0 | | | |
| | | 10.0 | 5.0 | 4.0 | | | 0 | | | | 1.80 | | | 750 | | | | |
| | | | | | | | | | | | | | | | | | | |
| | | | | | | | | | | | | | | | | | | NBSC177 |
| cereal bar, high protein, cinnamon raisin, South Beach Diet 1.2 oz bar | 35 | 140 | | 15.0 | 7.0 | | 3.0 | | 150 | 150 | | | | | 0 | | | |
| | | 10.0 | 5.0 | 3.0 | | | 0 | | | | 1.80 | | | 750 | | | | |
| | | | | | | | | | | | | | | | | | | |
| | | | | | | | | | | | | | | | | | | NBSC180 |
| cereal bar, high protein, cranberry, South Beach Diet 1.2 oz bar | 35 | 140 | | 15.0 | 7.0 | | 3.0 | | 135 | 150 | | | | | 0 | | | |
| | | 10.0 | 5.0 | 2.0 | | | 0 | | | | 1.80 | | | 750 | | | | |
| | | | | | | | | | | | | | | | | | | |
| | | | | | | | | | | | | | | | | | | NBSC181 |
| cereal bar, high protein, maple nut, South Beach Diet - 1.2 oz bar | 35 | 140 | | 15.0 | 7.0 | | 3.0 | | 160 | 150 | | | | | 0 | | | |
| | | 10.0 | 5.0 | 2.5 | | | 5 | | | | 1.80 | | | 750 | | | | |
| | | | | | | | | | | | | | | | | | | |
| | | | | | | | | | | | | | | | | | | NBSC178 |
| cereal bar, high protein, peanut butter, South Beach Diet 1.2 oz bar | 35 | 140 | | 15.0 | 6.0 | | 3.0 | | 160 | 150 | | | | | 0 | | | |
| | | 10.0 | 5.0 | 2.0 | | | 0 | | | | 1.80 | | | 750 | | | | |
| | | | | | | | | | | | | | | | | | | |
| | | | | | | | | | | | | | | | | | | NBSC179 |
| CocoaVia Snack Bar, chocolate 0.78 oz bar | 22 | 72 | | 12.7 | 7.3 | | 1.0 | | 57 | 266 | | | | | 9 | | | 0.90 |
| | | 1.4 | 2.0 | 0.9 | | | 0 | | | | 0.41 | | | 7 | | | 0.30 | 102.1 |
| | | | | | | | | | | | | | | | | | | |
| | | | | | | | | | | | | | | | | | | |
| Luna Nutrition Bar, cherry-covered chocolate - 1.7 oz bar | 48 | 180 | | | | | | | | 350 | | | | | 60 | | | |
| | | | 4.0 | 3.0 | | | | | | | 6.30 | | | | | | | |
| | | | | | | | | | | | | | | | | | | |
| | | | | | | | | | | | | | | | | | | CLIF4 |
| Luna Nutrition Bar, chocolate pecan pie - 1.7 oz bar | 48 | 180 | | 24.0 | 12.0 | | 2.0 | | 125 | 350 | | | | | 60 | | | |
| | | 10.0 | 4.5 | 3.0 | 1.0 | | 0 | | | | 6.30 | | | 1250 | | | | |
| | | | | | | | | | | | | | | | | | | |
| | | | | | | | | | | | | | | | | | | 25018 |

| | WT | Macronutrients and Amino Acids | | | | | | | Minerals | | | | | Vitamins | | | | |
|---|---|---|---|---|---|---|---|---|---|---|---|---|---|---|---|---|---|---|
| | (g) | KCAL | $H_2O$ (g) | CHO (g) | TSUG (g) | ASUG (g) | DFIB (g) | | Na (mg) | Ca (mg) | Mg (mg) | Zn (mg) | Mn (mg) | A (mcg RAE) | C (mg) | B-1 (mg) | NIA (mg) | B-12 (mcg) |
| | | PRO (g) | FAT (g) | SFA (g) | MUFA (g) | PUFA (g) | CHOL (mg) | | K (mg) | P (mg) | Fe (mg) | Cu (mg) | Se (mcg) | A (IU) | E (mg ATE) | B-2 (mg) | B-6 (mg) | FOL (mcg DFE) |
| | | HIS (mg) | ISO (mg) | LEU (mg) | LYS (mg) | MET (mg) | CYS (mg) | TAU (mg) | Cl (mg) | I (mcg) | Mo (mcg) | Cr (mcg) | | PANT (mg) | E (IU) | D (IU) | K (mcg) | |
| | | PHE (mg) | TYR (mg) | THR (mg) | TRY (mg) | VAL (mg) | ARG (mg) | CAR (mg) | | | | | | BIO (mcg) | CHLN (mg) | INOS (mg) | | REF |
| **Luna Nutrition Bar**, nutz over | 48 | 180 | | 24.0 | 12.0 | | 2.0 | | 100 | 350 | | | | | 60 | | | |
| chocolate - *1.7 oz bar* | | 10.0 | 4.5 | 2.5 | 0 | | 0 | | | | 6.30 | | | 1250 | | | | |
| | | | | | | | | | | | | | | | | | | |
| | | | | | | | | | | | | | | | | | | CLIF5 |
| **Luna Nutrition Bar**, s'mores | 48 | 180 | | 26.0 | 12.0 | | 2.0 | | 125 | 350 | | | | | 60 | | | |
| *1.7 oz bar* | | 10.0 | 4.5 | 3.0 | 0 | | 0 | | | | 6.30 | | | 1250 | | | | |
| | | | | | | | | | | | | | | | | | | |
| | | | | | | | | | | | | | | | | | | CLIF6 |
| **PowerBar**, chocolate | 68 | 247 | 6.7 | 47.3 | 20.4 | | 3.9 | | 99 | 343 | 169 | 6.77 | 1.095 | 0 | 63 | 5.48 | 22.2 | 3.81 |
| *2.4 oz bar* | | 9.6 | 2.1 | 0.9 | 0.7 | 0.4 | 0 | | 246 | 418 | 7.96 | 0.972 | 5.3 | 0 | 5.6 | 1.31 | 1.50 | 711.3 |
| | | 245 | 449 | 904 | 666 | 197 | 150 | | | | | | | 10.8 | | | | |
| | | 503 | 184 | 367 | 129 | 564 | 415 | | | | | | | | | | | 25017 |
| **Snickers Marathon Energy Bar** | 55 | 212 | 7.7 | 27.7 | 15.8 | | 3.7 | | 211 | 415 | 174 | 6.53 | 0.582 | 34 | 269 | 1.62 | 24.9 | 6.73 |
| all flavors - *1.9 oz bar* | | 12.1 | 5.9 | 2.6 | 2.2 | 1.1 | 2 | | 193 | 250 | 8.97 | 0.249 | 2.5 | 115 | 15.1 | 1.84 | 2.49 | 606.1 |
| | | 267 | 458 | 773 | 535 | 146 | 130 | | | | | | | 12.4 | | | | |
| | | 537 | 405 | 375 | 122 | 494 | 918 | | | | | | | | | | | 25016 |
| **Snickers Marathon Energy Bar** | 80 | 322 | 7.2 | 42.4 | 23.0 | | 8.0 | | 180 | 500 | 140 | 5.25 | 1.058 | 10 | 60 | 1.50 | 20.0 | 6.00 |
| caramel nut rush - *2.8 oz bar* | | 20.0 | 8.0 | 3.5 | 2.1 | 2.3 | 5 | | 240 | 300 | 8.10 | 0.782 | 3.1 | 34 | 100.0 | 1.70 | 2.00 | 616.8 |
| | | 537 | 925 | 1550 | 1131 | 276 | 266 | | | | | | | 10.0 | | | | |
| | | 1070 | 798 | 765 | 251 | 966 | 1806 | | | | | | | | | | | 25015 |
| **Snickers Marathon Energy Bar** | 55 | 218 | 7.1 | 26.0 | 18.1 | | 1.4 | | 254 | 531 | 140 | 5.25 | | | 79 | 1.50 | 20.0 | 6.00 |
| chewy chocolate peanut | | 13.4 | 7.2 | 2.6 | | | 2 | | | 250 | | | | 2000 | 13.5 | 1.70 | 2.00 | 679.8 |
| *1.9 oz bar* | | | | | | | | | | | | | | 10.0 | | | | |
| | | | | | | | | | | | | | | | | | | 25004 |
| **Snickers Marathon Energy Bar** | 44 | 151 | 6.2 | 23.1 | 10.0 | | 4.6 | | 147 | 658 | 139 | 5.97 | | | 78 | | 19.9 | 5.97 |
| double chocolate nut | | 9.8 | 4.0 | 2.1 | | | 2 | | | 249 | 7.90 | | | 1956 | 13.4 | | 1.99 | 676.7 |
| *1.6 oz bar* | | | | | | | | | | | | | | 10.0 | | | | |
| | | | | | | | | | | | | | | | | | | 25006 |
| **Snickers Marathon Energy Bar** | 44 | 166 | 4.2 | 23.9 | 11.6 | | 4.8 | | 140 | | 139 | 5.23 | | | 78 | 1.49 | 19.9 | 5.97 |
| honey nut oat - *1.6 oz bar* | | 9.9 | 3.5 | 2.0 | | | | | | | 7.99 | 0.199 | | 1958 | 13.4 | 1.69 | 1.99 | 676.3 |
| | | | | | | | | | | | | | | 10.0 | | | | |
| | | | | | | | | | | | | | | | | | | 25008 |
| **Snickers Marathon Energy Bar** | 55 | 223 | 4.4 | 30.3 | 18.2 | | 1.5 | | 230 | 524 | 140 | 5.25 | | | 79 | 1.50 | 20.0 | 6.00 |
| multi-grain crunch | | 10.2 | 7.2 | 2.6 | | | 2 | | | 250 | 8.07 | | | 1750 | 13.5 | 1.70 | 2.00 | 679.8 |
| *1.9 oz bar* | | | | | | | | | | | | | | 10.0 | | | | |
| | | | | | | | | | | | | | | | | | | 25005 |

# SUPPLEMENTARY DATABASES FOR THE COMPOSITION OF FOODS

# Alcohol, Ethyl (Ethanol)

| | SERVING SIZE (g) | ALCOHOL (g/serving) | SR21 CODE/ SOURCE[1] |
|---|---|---|---|
| **COCKTAILS** | | | |
| bloody Mary (tomato juice, vodka, and lemon juice) | 5 fl oz (148 g) | 13.9 | USDA Handbook 8–14 |
| bourbon and soda | 4 fl oz (116 g) | 15.1 | USDA Handbook 8–14 |
| daiquiri (rum, lime juice, and sugar) | 2 fl oz cocktail (60 g) | 13.9 | 14010 |
| daiquiri (rum, lime juice, and sugar), canned | 6.8 fl oz can (207 g) | 19.9 | 14009 |
| gin and tonic (tonic water, gin, and lime juice) | 7.5 fl oz (225 g) | 16.0 | USDA Handbook 8–14 |
| Manhattan (whiskey and vermouth) | 2 fl oz (57 g) | 17.4 | USDA Handbook 8–14 |
| martini (Gin and vermouth) | 2.5 fl oz (70 g) | 22.4 | USDA Handbook 8–14 |
| pina colada (pineapple juice, rum, sugar, and coconut cream) | 4.5 fl oz cocktail (141 g) | 14.0 | 14017 |
| pina colada (pineapple juice, rum, sugar, and coconut cream), canned | 6.8 fl oz can (222 g) | 20.0 | 14015 |
| screwdriver (orange juice and vodka) | 7 fl oz (213 g) | 14.1 | USDA Handbook 8–14 |
| tequila sunrise (orange juice, tequila, lime juice, and grenadine), canned | 6.8 fl oz can (211 g) | 19.8 | 14019 |
| whiskey sour (lemon juice, whiskey, and sugar), canned | 6.8 fl oz can (209 g) | 19.9 | 14027 |
| whiskey sour (lemon juice, whiskey, and sugar), from dry mix | 17 g packet 1.5 fl oz water, and 1.5 fl oz whiskey (103 g) | 15.0 | 14025 |
| whiskey sour (lemon juice, whiskey, and sugar), from liquid mix | 2 fl oz mix and 1.5 fl oz whiskey (106 g) | 15.4 | 14029 |
| **DISTILLED SPIRITS** | | | |
| distilled spirits, all types, 100 proof | 1.5 fl oz jigger (42 g) | 17.9 | 14533 |
| distilled spirits, all types, 80 proof | 1.5 fl oz jigger (42 g) | 14.0 | 14037 |
| distilled spirits, all types, 86 proof | 1.5 fl oz jigger(42 g) | 15.1 | 14550 |
| distilled spirits, all types, 90 proof | 1.5 fl oz jigger (42 g) | 15.9 | 14551 |
| distilled spirits, all types, 94 proof | 1.5 fl oz jigger (42 g) | 16.7 | 14532 |
| gin, 90 proof | 1.5 fl oz jigger (42 g) | 15.9 | 14049 |
| rum, 80 proof | 1.5 fl oz jigger (42 g) | 14.0 | 14050 |
| vodka, 80 proof | 1.5 fl oz jigger (42 g) | 14.0 | 14051 |
| whiskey, 86 proof | 1.5 fl oz jigger (42 g) | 15.1 | 14052 |
| **LIQUEURS** | | | |
| liqueur, coffee with cream, 34 proof | 1.5 fl oz (47 g) | 6.5 | 14415 |
| liqueur, coffee, 53 proof | 1.5 fl oz (52 g) | 11.3 | 14414 |
| liqueur, coffee, 63 proof | 1.5 fl oz (52 g) | 13.5 | 14534 |
| liqueur, crème de menthe, 72 proof | 1.5 fl oz (50 g) | 14.9 | 14034 |
| **MALT BEVERAGES** | | | |
| beer | 12 fl oz (356 g) | 13.9 | 14003 |
| beer, Bud Light, Anheuser-Busch | 12 fl oz (354 g) | 11.7 | 14007 |
| beer, Budweiser Select, light, Anheuser-Busch | 12 fl oz (354 g) | 12.0 | 14005 |
| beer, Budweiser, Anheuser-Busch | 12 fl oz (356 g) | 13.9 | 14004 |
| beer, light | 12 fl oz (354 g) | 11.0 | 14006 |
| beer, Michelob Ultra, light, Anheuser-Busch | 12 fl oz (354 g) | 11.7 | 14013 |
| malt beverage, no alcohol | 12 fl oz (356 g) | 1.1 | 14305 |
| **WINE** | | | |
| sake (Japanese alcoholic beverage made from rice) | 3.5 fl oz (103 g) | 16.6 | 43479 |
| wine, cooking | 3.5 fl oz (103 g) | 3.4 | 43154 |
| wine, dessert, dry | 3.5 fl oz (103 g) | 15.8 | 14536 |
| wine, dessert, sweet | 3.5 fl oz (103 g) | 15.8 | 14057 |
| wine, red | 3.5 fl oz (103 g) | 10.9 | 14096 |
| wine, red, Burgundy | 3.5 fl oz (103 g) | 10.6 | 14152 |
| wine, red, Cabernet Sauvignon | 3.5 fl oz (103 g) | 10.8 | 14097 |
| wine, red, Claret | 3.5 fl oz (103 g) | 10.5 | 14105 |
| wine, red, Merlot | 3.5 fl oz (103 g) | 10.9 | 14602 |
| wine, red, Zinfandel | 3.5 fl oz (103 g) | 11.4 | 14102 |
| wine, table, all types | 3.5 fl oz (103 g) | 10.7 | 14084 |
| wine, white | 3.5 fl oz (103 g) | 10.6 | 14106 |
| wine, white, Pinot Blanc | 3.5 fl oz (103 g) | 10.9 | 14138 |

| | SERVING SIZE (g) | ALCOHOL (g/serving) | SR21 CODE/ SOURCE[1] |
|---|---|---|---|
| wine, white, Pinot Gris/Grigio | 3.5 fl oz (103 g) | 11.0 | 14113 |
| wine, white, Riesling | 3.5 fl oz (103 g) | 9.8 | 14132 |
| wine, white, Sauvignon Blanc | 3.5 fl oz (103 g) | 10.8 | 14134 |
| **OTHER FOODS** | | | |
| cheese fondue (table wine, Swiss cheese, and white flour) | ½ cup (108 g) | 0.3 | 01163 |
| vanilla extract | 1 T (13 g) | 4.5 | 02050 |
| vanilla extract, imitation with alcohol | 1 T (13 g) | 4.3 | 02051 |

[1]Code numbers for foods in the USDA National Nutrient Database for Standard Reference, Release 21, 2008.

Sources:
USDA Agriculture Handbook No. 8–14, Revised. *Composition of Foods, Raw, Processed, Prepared. Beverages.* US Department of Agriculture: Washington, DC, May, 1986.
USDA National Nutrient Database for Standard Reference, Release 21, 2008. Available at: http://www.nal.usda.gov/fnic/foodcomp/search/.

# Amines—Histamine

| | HISTAMINE[1] (mg/100 g) | SOURCE | | HISTAMINE[1] (mg/100 g) | SOURCE |
|---|---|---|---|---|---|
| **BEVERAGES** | | | **CREAM** | | |
| beer, light | 0.6 | Souci et al, 2000 | sour cream | 0.0 | Souci et al, 2000 |
| beer, no alcohol | 0.0 | Souci et al, 2000 | whipping cream | 0.2 | Souci et al, 2000 |
| beer, pale | 0.5 | Souci et al, 2000 | | | |
| beer, pilsener lager | 0.0 | Souci et al, 2000 | **FRUITS** | | |
| grape juice | tr | Souci et al, 2000 | caperberries, raw | 3.8 | Garcia-Garcia et al, 2001 |
| wine, Hungarian | 0.1 | Kovacs et al, 1999 | | | |
| wine, white, German | 0.7 | Souci et al, 2000 | **MEAT AND FISH** | | |
| | | | mackerel, raw | 0.0 | Souci et al, 2000 |
| **CHEESE** | | | sausage, raw | 63.8 | Kovacs et al, 1999 |
| appenzeller cheese, 11% fat | 15.0 | Souci et al, 2000 | | | |
| appenzeller cheese, 32% fat | 17.0 | Souci et al, 2000 | **MILK AND YOGURT** | | |
| blue cheese | 86.4 | Chin et al, 1989 | buttermilk | 0.0 | Souci et al, 2000 |
| blue/Roquefort cheese | 50.0 | Voigt et al, 1974 | milk, whole | 0.1 | Souci et al, 2000 |
| Camembert cheese | 7.0 | Voigt et al, 1974 | yogurt, whole fat | 0.0 | Souci et al, 2000 |
| cheddar cheese, extra sharp | 21.0 | Voigt et al, 1974 | | | |
| cheddar cheese, medium | 14.0 | Voigt et al, 1974 | **SAUCES** | | |
| cheddar cheese, mild | 19.0 | Voigt et al, 1974 | soy sauce | 22.0 | Chin et al, 1989 |
| cheddar cheese, sharp | 11.0 | Voigt et al, 1974 | tamari sauce | 239.2 | Chin et al, 1989 |
| colby cheese | 7.0 | Voigt et al, 1974 | | | |
| Emmental cheese | 2.3 | Souci et al, 2000 | **VEGETABLES** | | |
| Gouda cheese | 7.5 | Voigt et al, 1974 | chives, raw | 0.0 | Kovacs et al, 1999 |
| Gruyere cheese | 6.6 | Souci et al, 2000 | eggplant, baked | 2.6 | Feldman, 1983 |
| Parmesan cheese | 10.7 | Chin et al, 1989 | sauerkraut | 7.0 | Souci et al, 2000 |
| Parmesan cheese | 18.5 | Feldman, 1983 | spinach, raw | 6.0 | Feldman, 1983 |
| Roguefort cheese | 6.5 | Souci et al, 2000 | spinach, raw | 1.0–7.0 | Lavizzari et al, 2007 |
| quark (fresh cheese) | 0.0 | Souci et al, 2000 | | | |
| Sap-Sago (schabziger) cheese | 260.0 | Voigt et al, 1974 | | | |
| tilsit cheese | 27.0 | Souci et al, 2000 | | | |

[1]Histamine, which occurs in foods primarily from the conversion of the amino acid histidine to histamine, may result from fermentation as in the production of cheeses, fermented soy products, sauerkraut, alcoholic beverages, and vinegars, and may result from microbial action when foods begin to spoil as in fish. The histamine content of foods is variable, and the data presented here should be considered as estimates. Different values for some foods are presented from different sources.

Sources:
Chin KW, MM Garriga, DD Metcalfe. The histamine content of Oriental foods. *Food Chem Toxicol* 27:283-287, 1989.
Feldman JM. Histaminuria from histamine-rich foods. *Arch Intern Med* 143:2099-2102, 1983.
Garcia-Garcia P, M Brenes-Balbuena, C Romero-Barranco, A Garrido-Fernandez. Biogenic amines in packed table olives and pickles. *J Food Prot* 64:374-378, 2001.
Kovacs A, L Simon-Sarkadi, K Ganzler. Determination of biogenic amines by capillary electrophoresis. *J Chromatography A* 836:305-313, 1999.
Lavizzari T, MT Veciana-Nougues, O Weingart, S Bover-Cid, A Marine-Font, MC Vidal-Carou. Occurrence of biogenic amines and polyamines in spinach and changes during storage under refrigeration. *J Agric Food Chem* 55:9514-9519, 2007.
Souci SW, W Fachmann, H Kraut. *Food Composition and Nutrition Tables.* Medpharm GmbH-Scientific Publishers, Stuttgart, Germany and CRC Press, Washington, DC, 2000.
Voigt MN, RR Eitenmiller, PE Koehler, MK Hamdy. Tyramine, histamine, and tryptamine content of cheese. *J Milk Food Technol* 37:377-381, 1974.
Additional reference for histamine:
Bodmer X, C Imark, M Kneubuhl. Biogenic amines in foods: Histamine and food processing. *Inflamm Res* 48:296-300, 1999.
Fremont S, DA Moneret-Vautrin, N Zitouni, G Kanny, JP Nicolas. Histamine content of peanuts. *Allergy* 54:528-2-529, 1999.
Ganowiak Z, R Gajewska, A Lebiedzinska. Histamine content in fishers and fish products. *Rocz Panstw Zakl Hig* 32:217-221, 1981.
Kan K, H Ushiyama, T Shindo, K Saito. Survey of histamine content in seafood on the market. *Shokuhin Eiseigaku Zasshi* 46:127-132, 2005.
Kanny G, V Gerbaux, A Olszewski, S Fremont, F Empereur, F Nabet, JC Cabanis, DA Moneret-Vautrin. No correlation between wine intolerance and histamine content of wine. *J Allergy Clin Immunol* 107:375-578, 2001.
Samaha IA, MM Elgassar, AI El-Atabany. Histamine content in sardine and its products. *J Egypt Public Health Assoc* 72:471-478, 1997.

# Amines—Serotonin

| FRUITS[2] | SEROTONIN[1] (mg/100 g) | | SEROTONIN[1] (mg/100 g) |
|---|---|---|---|
| | | filberts, raw | 0.21 |
| | | pecans, raw | 2.90 |
| banana, raw | 1.50 | pignuts, sweet | 2.50 |
| cantaloupe, raw | 0.09 | walnuts, black, raw | 30.40 |
| date, dried | 0.13 | walnuts, English | 8.70 |
| fig, raw | 0.02 | | |
| grapefruit, raw | 0.09 | **VEGETABLES[2]** | |
| honeydew melon, raw | 0.06 | avocado, California Haas, raw | 0.16 |
| kiwifruit, raw | 0.58 | avocado, California Fuerte, raw | 0.15 |
| pineapple, raw | 1.70 | avocado, Florida Booth, raw | 0.02 |
| plum, blue-red, raw | 3.60 | broccoli, raw | 0.02 |
| plum, blue, raw | 4.30 | cauliflower, raw | 0.01 |
| plum, red, raw | 5.70 | eggplant, raw | 0.02 |
| | | plantain, raw | 3.00 |
| **NUTS[2]** | | spinach, raw | 0.01 |
| almonds, beech nuts, cashews, coconut, macadamia nuts, raw | 0.02–0.06 | tomato, raw | 0.32 |
| | | **OTHER FOODS[2]** | |
| Brazil nuts, raw | 0.13 | olives, black | 0.02 |
| butternuts, raw | 39.80 | | |

[1]Serotonin (5-hydroxytryptamine) is synthesized from the amino acid tryptophan in a metabolic pathway using tryptophan hydroxylase and amino acid decarboxylase.

[2]The following contained <0.01 mg serotonin/100 g food: Fruits (apple; blueberries; cherries; crabapple; cranberries; grapes, Tokay; kumquat; lemon; lime; mango; orange; papaya; peach; pear; persimmon; pomegranate; raspberries; strawberries; tangerine); Nuts and Seeds (acorns; chestnuts, American; horse chestnuts; peanuts; pine nuts; pistachio nuts; sunflower seeds); Vegetables (asparagus; carrot; corn; cucumber; green snap beans; lettuce, iceberg; lima beans; peas, green; pepper, sweet, red; potato; radish; soybeans); Other Foods (beef steak, broiled; beer; chicken, baked; coffee; fish, broiled; ham, baked; milk; nutmeg; parmesan cheese; rice; tea; wheat germ; wine, Chianti).

Source:
Feldman JM, EM Lee. Serotonin content of foods: Effect on urinary excretion of 5-hydroxyindoleacetic acid. *Am J Clin Nutr* 42:639-643, 1985.

# Amines—Tryptamine

| | TRYPTAMINE (mg/100 g) | SOURCE | | TRYPTAMINE (mg/100 g) | SOURCE |
|---|---|---|---|---|---|
| **BEVERAGES** | | | orange, raw | 0.10 | Souci et al, 2000 |
| wine, Hungarian | 0.01 | Kovacs et al, 1999 | pineapple, raw | 0.62 | Badria, 2002 |
| | | | pomegranate, raw | 0.47 | Badria, 2002 |
| **CHEESE** | | | strawberries, raw | 0.47 | Badria, 2002 |
| blue/Roquefort cheese | 20.0 | Voigt et al, 1974 | | | |
| camembert cheese | 2.00 | Voigt et al, 1974 | **GRAINS** | | |
| cheddar cheese | 0.10 | Voigt et al, 1974 | barley, raw | 2.54 | Badria, 2002 |
| cheddar cheese, extra sharp | 2.00 | Voigt et al, 1974 | rice, raw | 4.01 | Badria, 2002 |
| cheddar cheese, medium | 2.00 | Voigt et al, 1974 | | | |
| cheddar cheese, mild | 3.00 | Voigt et al, 1974 | **MEAT AND FISH** | | |
| cheddar cheese, sharp | 4.00 | Voigt et al, 1974 | sausage, raw | 36.00 | Kovacs et al, 1999 |
| colby cheese | 13.00 | Voigt et al, 1974 | tuna, canned in oil | 0.10 | Souci et al, 2000 |
| Edam cheese | 8.00 | Voigt et al, 1974 | | | |
| Gouda cheese | 7.00 | Voigt et al, 1974 | **SPICES** | | |
| limburger cheese | 16.00 | Voigt et al, 1974 | garlic, dried | 1.39 | Badria, 2002 |
| mozzarella cheese | 10.00 | Voigt et al, 1974 | ginger, ground | 3.71 | Badria, 2002 |
| muenster cheese | 6.00 | Voigt et al, 1974 | | | |
| port-salut cheese | 12.00–28.00 | Voigt et al, 1974 | **VEGETABLES** | | |
| Sap-Sago cheese | 15.00 | Voigt et al, 1974 | cabbage, raw | 0.77 | Badria, 2002 |
| Swiss cheese | 19.00 | Voigt et al, 1974 | carrot, raw | 1.58 | Badria, 2002 |
| | | | cauliflower, raw | 1.98 | Badria, 2002 |
| **FRUITS** | | | chives, raw | 0.00 | Kovacs et al, 1999 |
| apple, raw | 0.53 | Badria, 2002 | corn, raw | 6.17 | Badria, 2002 |
| banana, raw | 1.13 | Badria, 2002 | cucumber, raw | 1.28 | Badria, 2002 |

| | TRYPTAMINE (mg/100 g) | SOURCE | | TRYPTAMINE (mg/100 g) | SOURCE |
|---|---|---|---|---|---|
| onion, raw | 0.92 | Badria, 2002 | tomato, raw | 0.40 | Souci et al, 2000 |
| potato, raw | 0.00 | Badria, 2002 | tomato, raw | 0.93 | Badria, 2002 |
| radish, raw | 1.47 | Badria, 2002 | turnip, raw | 2.12 | Badria, 2002 |

[1]Tryptamine occurs in foods from the conversion of the amino acid tryptophan to tryptamine. Tryptamine may result from fermentation as in the production of cheeses and may result from microbial action when foods begin to spoil. The tryptamine content of foods is variable, and the data presented here should be considered as estimates.

Sources:
Badria FA. Melatonin, serotonin, and tryptamine in some Egyptian food and medicinal plants. *J Medicinal Food* 5:153-157, 2002.
Kovacs A, L Simon-Sarkadi, K Ganzler. Determination of biogenic amines by capillary electrophoresis. *J Chromatography A* 836:305-313, 1999.
Souci SW, W Fachmann, H Kraut. *Food Composition and Nutrition Tables.* Medpharm GmbH Scientific Publishers, Stuttgart, Germany and CRC Press, Washington, DC, 2000.
Voigt MN, RR Eitenmiller, PE Koehler, MK Hamdy. Tyramine, histamine, and tryptamine content of cheese. *J Milk Food Technol* 37:377-381, 1974.

# Amines—Tyramine

| | TYRAMINE (mg/100 g) | SOURCE | | TYRAMINE (mg/100 g)S | SOURCE |
|---|---|---|---|---|---|
| **BEVERAGES** | | | muenster cheese | 14 | Voigt et al, 1974 |
| | | | parmesan cheese | 28 | Voigt et al, 1974 |
| beer, no alcohol | 0.12 | Souci et al, 2000 | Port-salut cheese | 12–18 | Voigt et al, 1974 |
| beer, pilsener, German | 0.14 | Souci et al, 2000 | quark cheese | 0 | Souci et al, 2000 |
| wine, Hungarian | 0.06 | Kovacs et al, 1999 | Romano cheese | 14 | Voigt et al, 1974 |
| | | | Sap-Sago cheese | 52 | Voigt et al, 1974 |
| **CANDY** | | | stilton cheese | 46 | Voigt et al, 1974 |
| dark chocolate | 0.07 | Jalon et al, 1983 | Swiss cheese | 41 | Voigt et al, 1974 |
| milk chocolate | 0.03 | Jalon et al, 1983 | tilsit cheese | 3 | Souci et al, 2000 |
| | | | | | |
| **CHEESE** | | | **CREAMS** | | |
| appenzeller cheese, 12% fat | 5 | Souci et al, 2000 | sour cream | 0.14 | Souci et al, 2000 |
| appenzeller cheese, 32% fat | 6 | Souci et al, 2000 | whipping cream | 0.17 | Souci et al, 2000 |
| blue/Roquefort cheese | 36 | Voigt et al, 1974 | | | |
| brick cheese | 52 | McCabe, 1986 | **FRUITS** | | |
| brie cheese | 4–26 | Voigt et al, 1974 | avocado, raw | 2 | Sullivan and Shulman, 1984 |
| Camembert cheese | 12 | Voigt et al, 1974 | | | |
| cheddar cheese, extra sharp | 27 | Voigt et al, 1974 | banana, raw | 1 | Souci et al, 2000 |
| cheddar cheese, medium | 24 | Voigt et al, 1974 | orange, raw | 1 | Souci et al, 2000 |
| cheddar cheese, milk | 9 | Voigt et al, 1974 | raspberries, raw | 5 | Souci et al, 2000 |
| cheddar cheese, processed | 11 | Voigt et al, 1974 | | | |
| cheddar cheese, sharp | 21 | Voigt et al, 1974 | **MEAT AND FISH** | | |
| cheddar cheese, smoked | 12 | Voigt et al, 1974 | chicken liver | 10 | Souci et al, 2000 |
| colby cheese | 21 | Voigt et al, 1974 | ox liver | 27 | Souci et al, 2000 |
| cottage cheese | 0 | Voigt et al, 1974 | sausage | 12 | Kovacs et al, 1999 |
| cream cheese | 0 | McCabe, 1986 | sausage, air-dried | 25 | Walker et al, 1996 |
| Edam cheese | 31 | Voigt et al, 1974 | tuna, canned in oil | 0 | Souci et al, 2000 |
| Emmental cheese | 4 | Souci et al, 2000 | | | |
| fontinella cheese | 10 | Voigt et al, 1974 | **MILK AND YOGURT** | | |
| gjetost cheese | 12 | Voigt et al, 1974 | buttermilk | 0.22 | Souci et al, 2000 |
| Gouda cheese | 29 | Voigt et al, 1974 | yogurt, whole milk | 0.13 | Souci et al, 2000 |
| Gruyere cheese | 52 | McCabe, 1986 | | | |
| jack cheese | 13 | Voigt et al, 1974 | **VEGETABLES** | | |
| limburger cheese | 12 | Voigt et al, 1974 | olives, raw | 1 | Kovacs et al, 1999 |
| mozzarella cheese | 16 | Voigt et al, 1974 | sauerkraut | 2 | Souci et al, 2000 |

| | TYRAMINE (mg/100 g) | SOURCE |
|---|---|---|
| sauerkraut | 3 | Walker et al, 1996 |
| tomato, raw | 0.40 | Souci et al, 2000 |

| | | TYRAMINE (mg/100 g) | SOURCE |
|---|---|---|---|
| **OTHER FOODS** | | | |
| cocoa powder, sweetened | | 0.06 | Jalon et al, 1983 |
| soy sauce | | 0.18 | Sullivan and Shulman, 1984 |

[1]Tyramine occurs in foods primarily from the conversion of the amino acid tyrosine to tyramine. Tyramine is generally produced during fermentation, aging, or spoiling of food products. Foods that may contain tyramine include tap beer and ale; Chianti; vermouth; aged cheeses; avocados; overripe and dried fruit; sauerkraut; meats that are aged, processed, cured, or pickled; and fermented soy products. A class of antidepressants called monoamine oxidase inhibitors (MAOIs) can increase the sensitivity to tyramine and may result in hypertensive crises causing stroke or cardiac arrhythmia. Tyramine may trigger migraines in sensitive individuals. The tyramine content of foods is variable, and the data presented here should just be considered as estimates. Different values for some foods are presented from different sources. Professional guidance from a registered dietitian is encouraged for those seeking to avoid tyramine in their diets.

Sources:
Jalon M, C Santos-Buelga, JC Rivas-Gonzalo, A Marine-Font. Tyramine in cocoa and derivatives. *J Food Sci* 48:545-547, 1983.
Kovacs A, L Simon Sarkadi, K Ganzler. Determination of biogenic amines by capillary electrophoresis. *J Chromatography A* 836:305-313, 1999.
McCabe BJ. Dietary tyramine and other pressor amines in MAOI regimes: A review. *J Am Diet Assoc* 86:1059-1064, 1986.
Souci SW, W Fachmann, H Kraut. *Food Composition and Nutrition Tables.* Medpharm GmbH Scientific Publishers, Stuttgart, Germany and CRC Press, Washington, DC, 2000.
Sullivan EA, KI Shulman. Diet and monoamine oxidase inhibitors: A re-examination. *Can J Psychiatry* 29:707-711, 1984.
Voigt MN, RER Eitenmiller, PE Koehler, MK Hamdy. Tyramine, histamine, and tryptamine content of cheese. *J Milk Food Technol* 37:377-381, 1974.
Walker SE, KI Shulman, SA Tailor, D Gardner. Tyramine content of previously restricted foods in monoamine oxidase inhibitor diets. *J Clin Psychopharmacol* 16:383-388, 1996.
Additional reference for tyramine:
Kayaalp SO, N Renda, S Kaymakcalan, A Ozer. Tyramine content of some cheeses. *Toxicol Appl Pharmacol* 16:459-460, 1970.
Vidaud ZE, J Chaviano, E Gonzales, MOG Roche. Tyramine content of some Cuban cheeses. *Nahrung* 31:221-224, 1987.
Additional references for amines:
Center for Food Safety and Applied Nutrition, US Food and Drug Administration. Processing parameters needed to control pathogens in cold smoked fish. Chapter IV. Potential hazards in cold-smoked fish: Biogenic amines. Available at: http://vm.cfsan.fda.gov/~comm/ift2amin.html.
Chang SF, JW Ayres, WE Sandine. Analysis of cheese for histamine, tyramine, tryptamine, histidine, tyrosine, and tryptophan. *J Dairy Sci* 68:2840-2846, 1985.
Edwards RA, RH Dainty, Cm Hibbard, SV Ramantanis. Amines in fresh beef of normal pH and the role of bacteria in changes in concentration observed during storage in vacuum packs at chill temperatures. *J Appl Bacteriol* 63:427-434, 1987.
El-Zayat AI. Tryptamine, tyramine and histamine content of Domiati, Ras and Roquefort cheese. *Z Gesamte Hyg* 32:410-411, 1986.
Ferreira IM, O Pinho. Biogenic amines in Portuguese traditional foods and wines. *J Food Prot* 69:2293-2303, 2006.
Garai G, MT Duenas, A Irastorza, MPJ Martin-Alvarez, MV Moreno-Arribas. Biogenic amines in natural ciders. *J Food Prot* 69:3006-3012, 2006.
Garcia-Garcia P, M Brenes-Balbuena, D Hornero-Mendez, A Garcia-Borrego, A Garrido-Fernandez. Content of biogenic amines in table olives. *J Food Prot* 63:111-116, 2000.
Gloria MBA, BT Watson, L Simon-Sarkadi, MA Daeschel. A survey of biogenic amines in Oregon Pinot noir and Cabernet Sauvignon wines. *Am J Enol Vitic* 49(3):279-282, 1998.
Lorenzo JM, S Martinez, I Franco, J Carballo. Biogenic amine content in relation to physicochemical parameters and microbial counts in two kinds of Spanish traditional sausages. *Archiv fur Lebensmittelhygiene* 59:70-75, 2008.
Mafra I, P Herbert, L Santos, P Barros, A Alves. Evaluation of biogenic amines in some Portuguese quality wines by HPLC Fluorescence detection of OPA derivatives. *Am J Enol Vitic* 50(1):128-132, 1999.
Novella-Rodriguez S, MT Veciana-Nogues, AX Roig-Sagues, AJ Trujillo-Mesa, MC Vidal-Carou. Influence of starter and nonstarter on the formation of biogenic amine in goat cheese during ripening. *J Dairy Sci* 85:2471-2478, 2002.
Pechanek U, W Pfannhauser, H Woidich. Content of biogenic amines in four food groups of the Austrian marketplace. *Z Lebensm Unters Forsch* 176:335-340, 1983.
Ruiz-Capillas C, A Moral. Free amino acids and biogenic amines in red and white muscle of tuna stored in controlled atmospheres. *Amino Acids* 26:125-132, 2004.
Sander JE, T Cai, N Dale, LW Bennett. Development of biogenic amines during fermentation of poultry carcasses. *J Appl Poultry Res* 5:161-166, 1996.
Suzzi G, F Gardini. Biogenic amines in dry fermented sausages: A review. Int *J Food Microbiol* 88:41-54, 2003.

# *Amino Acids*

| | WT (g) | TRY | THR | ISO | LEU | LYS | MET | CYS | PHE | TYR | VAL | ARG | HIS | REF |
|---|---|---|---|---|---|---|---|---|---|---|---|---|---|---|
| | | | | | | | (mg/serving) | | | | | | | |
| **1. BEVERAGES** | | | | | | | | | | | | | | |
| **COFFEE AND COFFEE BEVERAGES** | | | | | | | | | | | | | | |
| **cereal coffee** | | | | | | | | | | | | | | |
| powder—*1 round t* | 1.8 | 0 | 2 | 2 | 6 | 1 | 0 | 3 | 3 | 2 | 4 | 1 | 2 | 14222 |
| prep—*1 t powder in 6 fl oz milk* | 185 | 85 | 278 | 368 | 598 | 481 | 154 | 57 | 296 | 294 | 409 | 224 | 165 | 14421 |
| **coffee** | | | | | | | | | | | | | | |
| brewed—*8 fl oz* | 237 | 0 | 2 | 5 | 12 | 2 | 0 | 5 | 7 | 5 | 7 | 2 | 5 | 14209 |
| decaffeinated, brewed—*8 fl oz* | 237 | 0 | 2 | 5 | 12 | 2 | 0 | 5 | 7 | 5 | 7 | 2 | 5 | 14201 |
| powder—*1 round t* | 1.5 | 0 | 2 | 3 | 7 | 1 | 0 | 3 | 4 | 2 | 4 | 1 | 2 | 14214 |
| powder, decaf—*1 round t* | 1.8 | 1 | 2 | 3 | 8 | 2 | 0 | 3 | 4 | 3 | 5 | 1 | 3 | 14218 |
| **LIQUEURS** | | | | | | | | | | | | | | |
| **liqueur**, coffee with cream, 34 proof—*1.5 fl oz* | 47 | 19 | 60 | 80 | 129 | 105 | 33 | 12 | 64 | 64 | 88 | 48 | 36 | 14415 |
| **2. CANDY** | | | | | | | | | | | | | | |
| **caramels** | 71 | 43 | 136 | 183 | 296 | 240 | 76 | 28 | 146 | 146 | 202 | 110 | 82 | 19074 |
| **dark chocolate** | | | | | | | | | | | | | | |
| bar, sweet—*1.45 oz* | 41 | 24 | 63 | 62 | 97 | 80 | 16 | 20 | 77 | 60 | 96 | 91 | 27 | 19081 |
| chips, semi-sweet—*¼ cup* | 42 | 26 | 71 | 69 | 108 | 89 | 18 | 22 | 86 | 67 | 107 | 101 | 31 | 19080 |
| **Kit Kat, Hershey's**—*2.8 oz bar* | 78 | 70 | 148 | 218 | 406 | 218 | 125 | 94 | 211 | 117 | 281 | 156 | 86 | 19109 |

| | WT (g) | TRY | THR | ISO | LEU | LYS | MET | CYS | PHE | TYR | VAL | ARG | HIS | REF |
|---|---|---|---|---|---|---|---|---|---|---|---|---|---|---|
| | | | | | | | (mg/serving) | | | | | | | |
| **marshmallow** | | | | | | | | | | | | | | |
| miniature—*10 pieces* | 7 | 0 | 2 | 2 | 5 | 5 | 1 | 0 | 3 | 1 | 4 | 10 | 1 | 19116 |
| regular—*1 piece* | 7 | 0 | 2 | 2 | 5 | 5 | 1 | 0 | 3 | 1 | 4 | 10 | 1 | 19116 |
| **peanut bar**—*1.6 oz bar* | 45 | 67 | 234 | 240 | 444 | 245 | 83 | 87 | 354 | 278 | 287 | 818 | 173 | 19147 |
| **Tootsie Roll**—*6 pieces* | 40 | 76 | 16 | 24 | 44 | 36 | 4 | 0 | 20 | 8 | 32 | 24 | 12 | 19064 |

### 3. CEREALS AND GRAINS, COOKED

| | WT (g) | TRY | THR | ISO | LEU | LYS | MET | CYS | PHE | TYR | VAL | ARG | HIS | REF |
|---|---|---|---|---|---|---|---|---|---|---|---|---|---|---|
| **amaranth**, whole grain, dry—*1 cup* | 195 | 353 | 1088 | 1135 | 1714 | 1457 | 441 | 372 | 1057 | 642 | 1324 | 2067 | 759 | 20001 |
| **barley** | | | | | | | | | | | | | | |
| pearled, cooked—*1 cup* | 157 | 60 | 121 | 130 | 242 | 132 | 68 | 78 | 199 | 102 | 174 | 177 | 80 | 20006 |
| whole grain, dry—*1 cup* | 184 | 383 | 780 | 839 | 1560 | 856 | 442 | 508 | 1288 | 659 | 1126 | 1150 | 517 | 20004 |
| **buckwheat groats** | | | | | | | | | | | | | | |
| dry—*1 cup* | 170 | 326 | 860 | 847 | 1414 | 1142 | 292 | 389 | 884 | 410 | 1153 | 1669 | 525 | 20008 |
| roasted, cooked—*1 cup* | 168 | 82 | 217 | 213 | 356 | 289 | 74 | 97 | 223 | 104 | 291 | 420 | 133 | 20010 |
| roasted, dry—*1 cup* | 164 | 279 | 735 | 723 | 1207 | 976 | 251 | 331 | 756 | 349 | 984 | 1425 | 448 | 20009 |
| **bulgur**, cooked—*1 cup* | 182 | 87 | 162 | 207 | 379 | 155 | 87 | 129 | 264 | 164 | 253 | 262 | 129 | 20013 |
| **corn grits, white** | | | | | | | | | | | | | | |
| quick/reg, cooked—*1 cup* | 242 | 24 | 128 | 123 | 421 | 97 | 73 | 63 | 169 | 140 | 174 | 172 | 104 | 8091 |
| **corn grits, yellow** | | | | | | | | | | | | | | |
| quick/reg, cooked—*1 cup* | 242 | 24 | 128 | 123 | 421 | 97 | 73 | 63 | 169 | 140 | 174 | 172 | 104 | 8164 |
| **corn, whole grain**, dry—*3.5 oz* | 100 | 67 | 354 | 337 | 1155 | 265 | 197 | 170 | 463 | 383 | 477 | 470 | 287 | 20014 |
| **couscous**, cooked—*1 cup* | 157 | 77 | 157 | 231 | 407 | 115 | 93 | 168 | 289 | 157 | 254 | 220 | 121 | 20029 |
| **Cream of Rice cereal**, cooked *1 cup* | 244 | 32 | 107 | 37 | 178 | 90 | 63 | 37 | 90 | 120 | 139 | 176 | 63 | 8101 |
| **millet**, cooked—*1 cup* | 174 | 66 | 197 | 258 | 776 | 117 | 122 | 117 | 322 | 188 | 320 | 212 | 130 | 20032 |
| **millet**, dry—*1 cup* | 200 | 238 | 706 | 930 | 2800 | 424 | 442 | 424 | 1160 | 680 | 1156 | 764 | 472 | 20031 |
| **oat bran**, cooked—*1 cup* | 219 | 125 | 188 | 250 | 515 | 285 | 125 | 217 | 339 | 250 | 361 | 480 | 153 | 20034 |
| **oatmeal** | | | | | | | | | | | | | | |
| instant, dry—*1 oz packet* | 28 | 50 | 102 | 139 | 269 | 189 | 60 | 122 | 185 | 106 | 197 | 235 | 80 | 8122 |
| instant, prepared—*1 cup* | 234 | 94 | 194 | 246 | 468 | 316 | 94 | 201 | 304 | 199 | 353 | 414 | 133 | 8123 |
| quick/reg, cooked—*1 cup* | 234 | 94 | 225 | 271 | 505 | 316 | 108 | 227 | 332 | 236 | 374 | 391 | 126 | 8121 |
| quick/reg, dry—*⅓ cup 0.95 oz* | 27 | 49 | 103 | 136 | 265 | 172 | 56 | 123 | 180 | 107 | 186 | 230 | 74 | 8120 |
| **oats, whole grain**, dry—*1 cup* | 156 | 365 | 897 | 1083 | 2003 | 1094 | 487 | 636 | 1396 | 894 | 1462 | 1860 | 632 | 20038 |
| **quinoa**, dry—*1 cup* | 170 | 284 | 716 | 857 | 1428 | 1302 | 525 | 345 | 1008 | 454 | 1010 | 1855 | 692 | 20035 |
| **rice, brown** | | | | | | | | | | | | | | |
| long grain, boiled—*1 cup* | 195 | 64 | 185 | 213 | 417 | 193 | 113 | 60 | 259 | 189 | 294 | 382 | 129 | 20037 |
| medium grain, boiled—*1 cup* | 195 | 58 | 166 | 191 | 372 | 172 | 101 | 55 | 232 | 170 | 265 | 341 | 115 | 20041 |
| **rice, white** | | | | | | | | | | | | | | |
| dry—*½ up* | 98 | 81 | 250 | 302 | 577 | 253 | 165 | 143 | 373 | 233 | 426 | 582 | 165 | 20044 |
| glutinous, boiled—*1 cup* | 174 | 40 | 125 | 151 | 291 | 127 | 82 | 71 | 188 | 117 | 214 | 292 | 82 | 20055 |
| long grain, boiled—*1 cup* | 186 | 58 | 179 | 216 | 413 | 180 | 117 | 102 | 268 | 167 | 305 | 417 | 117 | 20045 |
| long grain, instant, boiled—*1 cup* | 165 | 50 | 132 | 165 | 317 | 101 | 86 | 74 | 190 | 107 | 228 | 315 | 87 | 20049 |
| long grain, parboiled, boiled—*1 cup* | 175 | 68 | 187 | 233 | 450 | 144 | 123 | 105 | 268 | 150 | 324 | 448 | 123 | 20047 |
| medium grain, boiled—*1 cup* | 186 | 52 | 158 | 192 | 366 | 160 | 104 | 91 | 236 | 149 | 270 | 368 | 104 | 20051 |
| short grain, boiled—*1 cup* | 186 | 50 | 156 | 190 | 363 | 158 | 104 | 89 | 234 | 147 | 268 | 366 | 104 | 20053 |
| **rye, whole grain**, dry—*1 cup* | 169 | 260 | 899 | 928 | 1656 | 1022 | 419 | 556 | 1139 | 573 | 1262 | 1374 | 620 | 20062 |
| **sorghum grain**, dry—*1 cup* | 192 | 238 | 664 | 831 | 2863 | 440 | 324 | 244 | 1048 | 616 | 1077 | 682 | 472 | 20067 |
| **wheat cereal, Cream of Wheat** | | | | | | | | | | | | | | |
| inst, ap, ban, mpl—*1 pkt prep* | 150 | 34 | 78 | 106 | 186 | 64 | 46 | 56 | 132 | 78 | 118 | 110 | 57 | 8111 |
| inst, prep—*1 cup* | 240 | 60 | 139 | 192 | 334 | 113 | 82 | 98 | 238 | 139 | 214 | 190 | 101 | 8107 |
| Mix and Eat, prep—*1 pkt prep* | 142 | 38 | 87 | 121 | 209 | 72 | 51 | 62 | 149 | 88 | 135 | 122 | 62 | 8109 |
| quick, cooked—*1 cup* | 239 | 50 | 115 | 160 | 275 | 93 | 67 | 81 | 196 | 115 | 177 | 158 | 84 | 8105 |
| regular, cooked—*1 cup* | 242 | 51 | 114 | 160 | 276 | 94 | 68 | 82 | 198 | 116 | 177 | 157 | 85 | 8103 |
| **wild rice**, boiled—*1 cup* | 164 | 80 | 208 | 274 | 453 | 279 | 195 | 77 | 320 | 277 | 380 | 505 | 171 | 20089 |

### 4. CEREALS, READY-TO-EAT

| | WT (g) | TRY | THR | ISO | LEU | LYS | MET | CYS | PHE | TYR | VAL | ARG | HIS | REF |
|---|---|---|---|---|---|---|---|---|---|---|---|---|---|---|
| **All-Bran,** Kellogg's—*½ cup (1.1 oz)* | 31 | 68 | 118 | 108 | 217 | 108 | 53 | 74 | 149 | 46 | 161 | 189 | 87 | 8001 |
| **Apple Jacks,** Kellogg's—*1 cup (1.1 oz)* | 30 | 15 | 45 | 48 | 116 | 33 | 21 | 24 | 62 | 33 | 65 | 51 | 36 | 8003 |
| **Bran flakes,** Ralston—*¾ cup (1 oz)* | 29 | 40 | 107 | 99 | 196 | 44 | 37 | 58 | 133 | 57 | 135 | 114 | 69 | 8504 |
| **Cheerios,** General Mills—*1 cup (1.1 oz)* | 30 | 47 | 118 | 121 | 256 | 103 | 50 | 59 | 176 | 103 | 165 | 229 | 74 | 8013 |
| **Cinnamon Toast Crunch,** Mills—*¾ cup (1.1 oz)* | 30 | 22 | 52 | 56 | 108 | 25 | 25 | 28 | 71 | 40 | 74 | 86 | 37 | 8272 |
| **Cocoa Krispies,** Kellogg's—*¾ cup (1.1 oz)* | 31 | 25 | 50 | 50 | 105 | 40 | 28 | 28 | 71 | 19 | 74 | 87 | 28 | 8014 |
| **Corn Biscuits,** Ralston—*1 cup (1.1 oz)* | 31 | 9 | 75 | 78 | 321 | 16 | 32 | 27 | 125 | 59 | 92 | 49 | 51 | 8505 |
| **Corn Flakes,** Kellogg's—*1 cup (1.1 oz)* | 30 | 12 | 60 | 66 | 276 | 21 | 36 | 36 | 99 | 21 | 81 | 30 | 45 | 8020 |
| **Corn Flakes,** Ralston—*1 cup (1.1 oz)* | 31 | 11 | 72 | 77 | 314 | 13 | 34 | 34 | 121 | 52 | 94 | 41 | 53 | 8506 |
| **Crispix,** Kellogg's—*1 cup (1 oz)* | 29 | 21 | 71 | 80 | 226 | 25 | 39 | 38 | 110 | 50 | 110 | 98 | 50 | 8259 |
| **Crispy Hexagons,** Ralston—*1 cup (1 oz)* | 28 | 19 | 70 | 74 | 224 | 38 | 38 | 32 | 105 | 52 | 95 | 84 | 46 | 8507 |
| **Crispy Rice,** Ralston—*1 cup (1 oz)* | 28 | 27 | 80 | 84 | 166 | 48 | 39 | 37 | 113 | 67 | 122 | 151 | 46 | 8025 |

| | WT | TRY | THR | ISO | LEU | LYS | MET | CYS | PHE | TYR | VAL | ARG | HIS | REF |
|---|---|---|---|---|---|---|---|---|---|---|---|---|---|---|
| | (g) | | | | | | (mg/serving) | | | | | | | |
| Froot Loops, Kellogg's—*1 cup (1.1 oz)* | 30 | 26 | 48 | 45 | 124 | 29 | 22 | 26 | 70 | 41 | 57 | 51 | 29 | 8030 |
| Frosted Flakes, Kellogg's—*¾ cup (1.1 oz)* | 31 | 7 | 34 | 38 | 164 | 7 | 17 | 17 | 58 | 24 | 51 | 22 | 29 | 8069 |
| Golden Puffs, Malt-O-Meal—*1 cup (1.3 oz)* | 37 | 46 | 64 | 75 | 159 | 19 | 34 | 19 | 117 | 53 | 91 | 46 | 53 | 8478 |
| granola, homemade—*½ cup (2.2 oz)* | 61 | 120 | 329 | 357 | 640 | 392 | 156 | 176 | 450 | 266 | 459 | 834 | 238 | 8037 |
| Kix, General Mills—*1⅓ cups (1.1 oz)* | 30 | 16 | 73 | 67 | 253 | 46 | 35 | 35 | 108 | 70 | 86 | 64 | 48 | 8048 |
| Lucky Charms, General Mills—*1 cup (1.1 oz)* | 30 | 30 | 68 | 68 | 149 | 63 | 33 | 39 | 104 | 57 | 95 | 140 | 42 | 8050 |
| puffed rice—*1 cup (0.49 oz)* | 14 | 13 | 45 | 47 | 74 | 38 | 26 | 15 | 38 | 50 | 58 | 73 | 27 | 8156 |
| puffed wheat—*1 cup (0.42 oz)* | 12 | 27 | 54 | 75 | 128 | 49 | 31 | 35 | 91 | 53 | 84 | 85 | 46 | 8157 |
| Raisin Bran, Kellogg's—*1 cup (2.1 oz)* | 59 | 73 | 150 | 167 | 329 | 73 | 55 | 78 | 212 | 100 | 228 | 189 | 123 | 8060 |
| Raisin Bran, Post—*1 cup (2.1 oz)* | 59 | 83 | 148 | 148 | 295 | 112 | 59 | 106 | 218 | 59 | 206 | 248 | 106 | 8061 |
| Rice Krispies, Kellogg's—*1¼ cups (1.2 oz)* | 33 | 30 | 83 | 89 | 175 | 50 | 45 | 44 | 115 | 54 | 128 | 147 | 49 | 8065 |
| Shredded Wheat, Post | | | | | | | | | | | | | | |
| *1 rectangular biscuit (0.85 oz)* | 24 | 34 | 74 | 82 | 163 | 77 | 41 | 58 | 110 | 31 | 108 | 108 | 55 | 8147 |
| Tasteeos, Ralston—*1 cup (1 oz)* | 28 | 46 | 128 | 137 | 263 | 114 | 46 | 79 | 202 | 82 | 186 | 212 | 73 | 8074 |
| Total, General Mills—*¾ cup (1.1 oz)* | 30 | 39 | 69 | 78 | 156 | | 43 | 45 | 105 | 24 | 102 | 75 | 48 | 8077 |
| wheat and malted barley nuggets—*¼ cup* | 28 | 53 | 109 | 115 | 238 | 50 | 42 | 56 | 168 | 84 | 148 | 115 | 81 | 8038 |

## 5. CHEESE, CHEESE PRODUCTS, AND CHEESE SUBSTITUTES

### CHEESE

| | WT | TRY | THR | ISO | LEU | LYS | MET | CYS | PHE | TYR | VAL | ARG | HIS | REF |
|---|---|---|---|---|---|---|---|---|---|---|---|---|---|---|
| American processed cheese—*1 oz* | 28 | 90 | 201 | 287 | 548 | 615 | 160 | 40 | 315 | 339 | 371 | 260 | 253 | 1042 |
| blue cheese—*1 oz* | 28 | 87 | 220 | 315 | 537 | 519 | 164 | 30 | 304 | 363 | 436 | 199 | 212 | 1004 |
| brick cheese—*1 oz* | 28 | 91 | 247 | 318 | 628 | 595 | 158 | 37 | 345 | 312 | 412 | 245 | 230 | 1005 |
| brie cheese—*1 oz* | 28 | 90 | 210 | 284 | 540 | 518 | 166 | 32 | 324 | 336 | 375 | 206 | 200 | 1006 |
| camembert cheese—*1 oz* | 28 | 86 | 201 | 271 | 515 | 494 | 158 | 31 | 309 | 321 | 358 | 196 | 191 | 1007 |
| caraway cheese—*1 oz* | 28 | 91 | 251 | 438 | 675 | 587 | 185 | 35 | 371 | 340 | 471 | 267 | 248 | 1008 |
| cheddar cheese—*1 oz* | 28 | 90 | 248 | 433 | 668 | 580 | 183 | 35 | 367 | 337 | 466 | 263 | 245 | 1009 |
| cheddar cheese/colby cheese | | | | | | | | | | | | | | |
| low sodium—*1 oz* | 28 | 80 | 223 | 389 | 601 | 522 | 165 | 31 | 330 | 302 | 419 | 237 | 220 | 1169 |
| lowfat—*1 oz* | 28 | 80 | 223 | 389 | 601 | 522 | 165 | 31 | 330 | 302 | 419 | 237 | 220 | 1168 |
| cheshire cheese—*1 oz* | 28 | 84 | 233 | 406 | 627 | 545 | 171 | 33 | 345 | 316 | 437 | 247 | 230 | 1010 |
| colby cheese—*1 oz* | 28 | 85 | 237 | 413 | 637 | 554 | 174 | 33 | 350 | 321 | 444 | 251 | 234 | 1011 |
| cottage cheese | | | | | | | | | | | | | | |
| <.5% fat—*1 cup* | 226 | 310 | 1051 | 1241 | 2344 | 1962 | 565 | 138 | 1211 | 1268 | 1571 | 1044 | 685 | 1014 |
| 1% fat—*1 cup* | 226 | 312 | 1243 | 1645 | 2879 | 2265 | 843 | 260 | 1510 | 1492 | 1733 | 1277 | 931 | 1016 |
| 2% fat—*1 cup* | 226 | 353 | 1202 | 1422 | 2685 | 2246 | 646 | 158 | 1388 | 1453 | 1799 | 1196 | 782 | 1015 |
| 4% fat, creamed—*1 cup* | 226 | 267 | 1064 | 1410 | 2466 | 1941 | 723 | 224 | 1293 | 1279 | 1485 | 1096 | 798 | 1013 |
| creamed, large curd—*1 cup* | 225 | 331 | 1125 | 1330 | 2511 | 2102 | 605 | 148 | 1298 | 1359 | 1683 | 1118 | 734 | 1012 |
| creamed, small curd—*1 cup* | 225 | 331 | 1125 | 1330 | 2511 | 2102 | 605 | 148 | 1298 | 1359 | 1683 | 1118 | 734 | 1012 |
| cream cheese—*1 T* | 15 | 10 | 35 | 49 | 99 | 85 | 29 | 6 | 44 | 45 | 59 | 35 | 26 | 1017 |
| fat-free—*1 oz* | 28 | 51 | 172 | 240 | 486 | 420 | 141 | 31 | 215 | 225 | 293 | 174 | 130 | 1186 |
| lowfat—*1 oz* | 28 | 25 | 86 | 120 | 243 | 210 | 71 | 15 | 108 | 112 | 146 | 87 | 65 | 43274 |
| edam cheese—*1 oz* | 28 | 99 | 261 | 366 | 720 | 745 | 202 | 71 | 402 | 408 | 507 | 270 | 290 | 1018 |
| feta cheese—*1 oz* | 28 | 56 | 178 | 225 | 391 | 341 | 103 | 23 | 189 | 187 | 298 | 132 | 111 | 1019 |
| fontina cheese—*1 oz* | 28 | 101 | 262 | 388 | 746 | 652 | 198 | 73 | 419 | 427 | 539 | 234 | 269 | 1020 |
| gjetost cheese—*1 oz* | 28 | 38 | 110 | 145 | 278 | 228 | 89 | 16 | 151 | 151 | 214 | 92 | 82 | 1021 |
| goat milk cheese | | | | | | | | | | | | | | |
| hard—*1 oz* | 28 | 90 | 319 | 354 | 737 | 613 | 228 | 39 | 340 | 333 | 588 | 253 | 233 | 1156 |
| semi-soft—*1 oz* | 28 | 64 | 225 | 250 | 521 | 434 | 161 | 27 | 241 | 236 | 416 | 179 | 165 | 1157 |
| soft—*1 oz* | 28 | 55 | 193 | 214 | 447 | 372 | 138 | 24 | 206 | 202 | 357 | 154 | 141 | 1159 |
| gouda cheese—*1 oz* | 28 | 99 | 260 | 366 | 718 | 743 | 201 | 71 | 401 | 407 | 506 | 269 | 289 | 1022 |
| gruyere cheese—*1 oz* | 28 | 118 | 305 | 451 | 869 | 759 | 230 | 85 | 488 | 497 | 628 | 272 | 313 | 1023 |
| Limburger cheese—*1 oz* | 28 | 81 | 207 | 341 | 586 | 469 | 173 | 31 | 312 | 335 | 403 | 195 | 162 | 1024 |
| Mexican cheese | | | | | | | | | | | | | | |
| quesa asadero—*1 oz* | 28 | 75 | 206 | 343 | 594 | 433 | 166 | 29 | 333 | 297 | 399 | 213 | 194 | 1166 |
| quesa anejo—*1 oz* | 28 | 60 | 205 | 295 | 565 | 407 | 151 | 24 | 313 | 333 | 375 | 196 | 190 | 1165 |
| quesa chihuahua—*1 oz* | 28 | 55 | 229 | 301 | 565 | 430 | 170 | 40 | 290 | 285 | 354 | 218 | 167 | 1167 |
| monterey jack cheese—*1 oz* | 28 | 88 | 244 | 425 | 656 | 570 | 179 | 34 | 361 | 331 | 458 | 259 | 241 | 1025 |
| mozzarella cheese | | | | | | | | | | | | | | |
| part skim—*1 oz* | 28 | 95 | 259 | 326 | 662 | 690 | 190 | 40 | 354 | 393 | 425 | 292 | 256 | 1028 |
| part skim, low moisture—*1 oz* | 28 | 169 | 322 | 372 | 599 | 316 | 169 | 38 | 332 | 342 | 433 | 169 | 169 | 1029 |
| whole milk—*1 oz* | 28 | 144 | 275 | 318 | 511 | 270 | 144 | 32 | 283 | 292 | 370 | 144 | 144 | 1026 |
| whole milk, low moisture—*1 oz* | 28 | 85 | 230 | 290 | 590 | 614 | 169 | 36 | 316 | 350 | 378 | 260 | 228 | 1027 |
| muenster cheese—*1 oz* | 28 | 92 | 249 | 321 | 633 | 599 | 159 | 37 | 347 | 314 | 415 | 247 | 232 | 1030 |
| Neufchatel cheese—*1 oz* | 28 | 30 | 101 | 140 | 284 | 245 | 82 | 18 | 125 | 131 | 171 | 102 | 76 | 1031 |
| parmesan cheese | | | | | | | | | | | | | | |
| grated—*1 T* | 5 | 26 | 73 | 98 | 186 | 149 | 51 | 6 | 104 | 116 | 126 | 78 | 55 | 1032 |
| hard—*1 oz* | 28 | 135 | 369 | 530 | 967 | 926 | 268 | 66 | 538 | 559 | 687 | 369 | 388 | 1033 |
| pimiento cheese, processed—*1 oz* | 28 | 90 | 201 | 286 | 548 | 615 | 160 | 40 | 315 | 339 | 371 | 259 | 253 | 1043 |

| | WT | TRY | THR | ISO | LEU | LYS | MET | CYS | PHE | TYR | VAL | ARG | HIS | REF |
|---|---|---|---|---|---|---|---|---|---|---|---|---|---|---|
| | (g) | (mg/serving) | | | | | | | | | | | | |
| **port de salut cheese**—*1 oz* | 28 | 96 | 245 | 405 | 695 | 556 | 206 | 38 | 370 | 398 | 478 | 232 | 192 | 1034 |
| **provolone cheese**—*1 oz* | 43 | 148 | 422 | 469 | 988 | 1138 | 295 | 50 | 553 | 654 | 705 | 439 | 479 | 1035 |
| **ricotta cheese** | | | | | | | | | | | | | | |
| part nonfat—*½ cup* | 124 | 157 | 649 | 739 | 1531 | 1678 | 352 | 124 | 697 | 739 | 868 | 792 | 575 | 1037 |
| whole milk—*½ cup* | 124 | 155 | 641 | 730 | 1514 | 1659 | 348 | 123 | 689 | 730 | 858 | 784 | 569 | 1036 |
| **romano cheese**—*1 oz* | 28 | 120 | 328 | 472 | 860 | 823 | 239 | 59 | 479 | 497 | 611 | 328 | 345 | 1038 |
| **roquefort cheese** (from sheepmilk)—*1 oz* | 28 | 85 | 270 | 341 | 592 | 517 | 156 | 35 | 286 | 283 | 452 | 200 | 169 | 1039 |
| **Swiss cheese**—*1 oz* | 28 | 112 | 291 | 430 | 829 | 724 | 220 | 81 | 465 | 474 | 599 | 260 | 298 | 1040 |
| processed—*1 oz* | 28 | 101 | 225 | 320 | 612 | 687 | 179 | 45 | 352 | 379 | 415 | 290 | 282 | 1044 |
| **tilsit cheese**, whole milk—*1 oz* | 28 | 99 | 252 | 416 | 713 | 571 | 211 | 39 | 380 | 408 | 491 | 238 | 197 | 1041 |
| **CHEESE PRODUCTS AND CHEESE SUBSTITUTES** | | | | | | | | | | | | | | |
| **American cheese food**, cold pack—*1 oz* | 28 | 80 | 179 | 255 | 487 | 546 | 143 | 35 | 280 | 301 | 330 | 230 | 224 | 1045 |
| **American processed cheese food** | | | | | | | | | | | | | | |
| *1 oz* | 28 | 74 | 220 | 262 | 487 | 398 | 116 | 53 | 253 | 255 | 309 | 188 | 137 | 1046 |
| **cheese fondue** (table wine, Swiss | | | | | | | | | | | | | | |
| cheese, flour)—*½ cup* | 108 | 193 | 503 | 744 | 1434 | 1253 | 380 | 139 | 806 | 820 | 1038 | 449 | 515 | 1163 |
| **cheese sauce**, homemade—*2 T* | 30 | 37 | 106 | 173 | 271 | 232 | 73 | 17 | 145 | 136 | 188 | 105 | 93 | 1164 |
| **cheese spread**, American—*1 oz* | 28 | 67 | 176 | 233 | 498 | 422 | 151 | 29 | 261 | 249 | 382 | 153 | 143 | 1048 |
| **mozzarella cheese substitute**—*1 oz* | 28 | 42 | 111 | 160 | 259 | 222 | 79 | 14 | 147 | 160 | 190 | 109 | 80 | 1161 |
| **Swiss cheese food**—*1 oz* | 28 | 89 | 199 | 284 | 543 | 609 | 159 | 39 | 312 | 336 | 368 | 257 | 250 | 1047 |
| **6. CREAMS AND CREAMERS (CREAM SUBSTITUTES)** | | | | | | | | | | | | | | |
| **cream** | | | | | | | | | | | | | | |
| **half & half**—*1 T (½ fl oz container)* | 15 | 6 | 20 | 27 | 44 | 35 | 11 | 4 | 21 | 21 | 30 | 16 | 12 | 1049 |
| **light** (coffee/table)—*1 T* | 15 | 6 | 18 | 24 | 40 | 32 | 10 | 4 | 20 | 20 | 27 | 15 | 11 | 1050 |
| **creamer** | | | | | | | | | | | | | | |
| liq/frozen, hydrg veg oils—*1 T (½ fl oz)* | 15 | 2 | 6 | 8 | 13 | 10 | 2 | 3 | 8 | 6 | 8 | 12 | 4 | 1067 |
| liq/frozen, lauric acid—*1 T (½ fl oz)* | 15 | 2 | 6 | 9 | 15 | 12 | 4 | 1 | 8 | 9 | 11 | 6 | 4 | 1068 |
| powdered—*1 T* | 6 | 4 | 12 | 18 | 28 | 23 | 9 | 1 | 15 | 16 | 21 | 11 | 9 | 1069 |
| **sour cream**, cultured—*2 T* | 24 | 8 | 29 | 33 | 66 | 56 | 16 | 6 | 32 | 31 | 40 | 24 | 19 | 1056 |
| imitation—*1 oz* | 28 | 9 | 28 | 41 | 66 | 54 | 20 | 3 | 36 | 38 | 48 | 27 | 20 | 1074 |
| reduced-fat—*1 T* | 15 | 6 | 20 | 27 | 43 | 35 | 11 | 4 | 21 | 21 | 30 | 16 | 12 | 1055 |
| **whipped topping** | | | | | | | | | | | | | | |
| from mix, prepared w/whole | | | | | | | | | | | | | | |
| milk—*1 T* | 4 | 2 | 6 | 9 | 14 | 11 | 4 | 1 | 7 | 7 | 10 | 5 | 4 | 1071 |
| frozen—*1 T* | 4 | 1 | 2 | 3 | 5 | 4 | 2 | 0 | 3 | 3 | 4 | 2 | 1 | 1073 |
| pressurized—*1 T* | 4 | 1 | 2 | 2 | 4 | 3 | 1 | 0 | 2 | 2 | 3 | 2 | 1 | 1072 |
| heavy fluid—*1 T* | 15 | 4 | 14 | 19 | 30 | 24 | 8 | 3 | 15 | 15 | 21 | 11 | 8 | 1053 |
| light fluid—*1 T* | 15 | 5 | 15 | 20 | 32 | 26 | 8 | 3 | 16 | 16 | 22 | 12 | 9 | 1052 |
| **whipping cream**, pressurized—1 T | 3 | 1 | 4 | 6 | 9 | 8 | 2 | 1 | 5 | 5 | 6 | 3 | 3 | 1054 |
| **7. DESSERTS** | | | | | | | | | | | | | | |
| Brownies and Bars | | | | | | | | | | | | | | |
| **brownie**—*1 brownie (2¾″ × ⅞″)* | 56 | 37 | 111 | 137 | 211 | 152 | 66 | 61 | 141 | 97 | 154 | 150 | 60 | 18151 |
| homemade—*1 brownie (2¾″ × ⅞″)* | 56 | 44 | 128 | 148 | 250 | 158 | 74 | 70 | 167 | 120 | 181 | 242 | 76 | 18154 |
| Little Debbie—*1 twin wrapped pkg* | 61 | 37 | 111 | 137 | 211 | 152 | 66 | 61 | 141 | 97 | 154 | 150 | 60 | 18151 |
| **CAKES AND SNACK CAKES** | | | | | | | | | | | | | | |
| **angel food cake**—*1⁄12 cake (1 oz)* | 28 | 21 | 69 | 87 | 135 | 102 | 51 | 42 | 94 | 61 | 99 | 85 | 37 | 18086 |
| from mix—*1⁄12 cake of 10″ cake* | 50 | 38 | 130 | 162 | 248 | 190 | 96 | 77 | 172 | 113 | 184 | 158 | 67 | 18088 |
| **Boston cream pie/cake**, frozen | | | | | | | | | | | | | | |
| *⅙ of 19.5 oz cake* | 92 | 31 | 86 | 106 | 175 | 125 | 50 | 42 | 109 | 82 | 121 | 104 | 50 | 18090 |
| **cheesecake**—*⅙ of 17 oz cake* from | 80 | 51 | 178 | 225 | 371 | 298 | 109 | 57 | 206 | 178 | 251 | 201 | 106 | 18147 |
| mix, no-bake type—*⅛ of 9″ cake* | 99 | 65 | 207 | 266 | 463 | 359 | 115 | 68 | 261 | 218 | 299 | 200 | 146 | 18148 |
| **cherry fudge cake** with chocolate | | | | | | | | | | | | | | |
| icing—*⅛ of 20 oz cake* | 71 | 21 | 74 | 77 | 128 | 105 | 33 | 28 | 70 | 53 | 88 | 79 | 33 | 18095 |
| **chocolate cake** | | | | | | | | | | | | | | |
| homemade—*1⁄12 of 9″ cake* | 95 | 65 | 192 | 228 | 387 | 255 | 110 | 93 | 252 | 187 | 269 | 240 | 114 | 18101 |
| with chocolate icing—*⅛ of 18 oz cake* | 64 | 36 | 106 | 123 | 198 | 151 | 54 | 47 | 130 | 99 | 151 | 133 | 56 | 18096 |
| **chocolate creme-filled snack cake** | | | | | | | | | | | | | | |
| with icing—*1.8 oz snack cake* | 50 | 28 | 78 | 79 | 130 | 98 | 26 | 31 | 78 | 58 | 97 | 78 | 34 | 18127 |
| **chocolate cupcake** with icing, | | | | | | | | | | | | | | |
| lowfat—*1.5 oz cupcake* | 43 | 26 | 71 | 89 | 143 | 100 | 45 | 41 | 98 | 66 | 104 | 89 | 40 | 18452 |
| **coffeecake** | | | | | | | | | | | | | | |
| cinn w/crumb topping | | | | | | | | | | | | | | |
| *⅑ of 20 oz cake* | 63 | 52 | 143 | 181 | 315 | 164 | 77 | 80 | 204 | 137 | 200 | 195 | 97 | 18104 |
| from mix—*⅛ of 8″ × 5¾″ cake* | 56 | 37 | 106 | 137 | 236 | 128 | 67 | 62 | 152 | 104 | 154 | 125 | 69 | 18108 |

| | WT (g) | TRY | THR | ISO | LEU | LYS | MET | CYS | PHE | TYR | VAL | ARG | HIS | REF |
|---|---|---|---|---|---|---|---|---|---|---|---|---|---|---|
| | | (mg/serving) | | | | | | | | | | | | |
| cream/neufchatel cheese | | | | | | | | | | | | | | |
| *1/6 of 16 oz cake* | 76 | 58 | 198 | 248 | 432 | 305 | 109 | 84 | 268 | 200 | 274 | 227 | 141 | 18103 |
| crème-filled with choc icing | | | | | | | | | | | | | | |
| *1/6 of 19 oz cake* | 90 | 52 | 145 | 183 | 326 | 151 | 83 | 92 | 218 | 139 | 206 | 186 | 101 | 18105 |
| with fruit—*1/8 of 14 oz cake* | 50 | 29 | 82 | 104 | 182 | 94 | 47 | 49 | 124 | 76 | 119 | 126 | 56 | 18106 |
| **fruitcake**—*0.5 oz piece* | 43 | 18 | 44 | 52 | 89 | 52 | 25 | 27 | 60 | 41 | 62 | 113 | 31 | 18110 |
| **gingerbread**, homemade | | | | | | | | | | | | | | |
| *1/9 of 8″ square cake* | 74 | 35 | 92 | 112 | 206 | 97 | 59 | 61 | 144 | 92 | 128 | 128 | 64 | 18116 |
| **pineapple upside-down cake** | | | | | | | | | | | | | | |
| homemade—*1/9 of 8″ square cake* | 115 | 49 | 135 | 169 | 304 | 164 | 85 | 76 | 199 | 139 | 192 | 170 | 93 | 18119 |
| **pound cake** | | | | | | | | | | | | | | |
| fat-free | 28 | 20 | 60 | 77 | 122 | 89 | 42 | 34 | 81 | 55 | 87 | 72 | 34 | 18451 |
| made w/butter—*1/10 of 10.6 oz cake* | 30 | 22 | 63 | 78 | 129 | 92 | 40 | 34 | 82 | 59 | 89 | 78 | 37 | 18120 |
| made w/veg shortening | | | | | | | | | | | | | | |
| *1/10 of 10.6 oz cake* | 30 | 21 | 59 | 73 | 121 | 85 | 38 | 33 | 78 | 55 | 83 | 74 | 34 | 18121 |
| **pound snack cake**—*1.1 oz snack cake* | 30 | 21 | 59 | 73 | 121 | 85 | 38 | 33 | 78 | 55 | 83 | 74 | 34 | 18121 |
| **shortcake**, biscuit-type, homemade | | | | | | | | | | | | | | |
| *1 oz shortcake* | 28 | 21 | 52 | 67 | 126 | 55 | 32 | 32 | 85 | 57 | 76 | 67 | 39 | 18126 |
| **sponge cake**—*1/12 of 16 oz cake* | 38 | 27 | 81 | 95 | 159 | 113 | 48 | 45 | 100 | 71 | 107 | 100 | 45 | 18133 |
| homemade—*1/12 of 16 oz cake* | 38 | 34 | 117 | 133 | 224 | 159 | 73 | 61 | 142 | 105 | 150 | 154 | 65 | 18134 |
| **sponge snack cake**, crème-filled | | | | | | | | | | | | | | |
| *1.5 oz snack cake* | 43 | 16 | 52 | 60 | 103 | 71 | 28 | 30 | 59 | 34 | 71 | 61 | 28 | 18128 |
| **white cake** | | | | | | | | | | | | | | |
| homemade—*1/12 of 9″ cake* | 74 | 50 | 141 | 180 | 310 | 178 | 95 | 82 | 208 | 141 | 204 | 174 | 92 | 18139 |
| with coconut icing, homemade | | | | | | | | | | | | | | |
| *1/12 of 9″ cake* | 112 | 60 | 176 | 223 | 379 | 228 | 120 | 102 | 255 | 172 | 256 | 239 | 111 | 18102 |
| **yellow cake** | | | | | | | | | | | | | | |
| homemade—*1/12 of 8″ cake* | 68 | 45 | 130 | 160 | 282 | 167 | 82 | 70 | 181 | 130 | 182 | 162 | 84 | 18146 |
| mix—*2 oz* | 56 | 34 | 77 | 105 | 182 | 110 | 45 | 44 | 114 | 81 | 119 | 91 | 53 | 18144 |
| w/chocolate icing—*1/8 of 18 oz cake* | 64 | 32 | 93 | 111 | 182 | 134 | 52 | 47 | 118 | 88 | 132 | 118 | 52 | 18140 |
| w/vanilla icing—*1/8 of 18 oz cake* | 64 | 29 | 91 | 113 | 186 | 138 | 56 | 43 | 111 | 87 | 127 | 104 | 52 | 18141 |
| COOKIES | | | | | | | | | | | | | | |
| **animal crackers**—*2 oz box (23 pcs)* | 57 | 56 | 110 | 150 | 268 | 138 | 66 | 85 | 185 | 112 | 173 | 150 | 80 | 18150 |
| **anisette sponge**—*1 piece* | 11 | 15 | 51 | 57 | 95 | 75 | 29 | 25 | 56 | 45 | 64 | 67 | 27 | 18423 |
| **arrowroot cookie**—*2 oz box (23 pcs)* | 57 | 56 | 110 | 150 | 268 | 138 | 66 | 85 | 185 | 112 | 173 | 150 | 80 | 18150 |
| **Breakfast Treat**—*1 piece* | 11 | 15 | 51 | 57 | 95 | 75 | 29 | 25 | 56 | 45 | 64 | 67 | 27 | 18423 |
| **butter cookie**—*5 cookies (1 oz)* | 28 | 24 | 60 | 78 | 132 | 86 | 37 | 34 | 84 | 59 | 88 | 73 | 38 | 18155 |
| **chocolate chip cookie** | | | | | | | | | | | | | | |
| from refrig dough—*1 cookie* | 12 | 8 | 20 | 25 | 44 | 27 | 12 | 12 | 29 | 19 | 29 | 24 | 12 | 18164 |
| higher fat—*1 cookie (2¼″ dia)* | 12 | 9 | 16 | 18 | 35 | 8 | 3 | 12 | 26 | 9 | 24 | 19 | 9 | 18159 |
| homemade w/butter | | | | | | | | | | | | | | |
| *1 cookie (2¼″ dia)* | 16 | 12 | 31 | 36 | 63 | 34 | 17 | 18 | 43 | 30 | 45 | 60 | 20 | 18378 |
| homemade w/margarine | | | | | | | | | | | | | | |
| *1 cookie (2¼″ dia)* | 16 | 12 | 31 | 36 | 63 | 34 | 17 | 18 | 43 | 30 | 45 | 60 | 20 | 18165 |
| lower fat—*1 cookie (2¼″ dia)* | 10 | 8 | 17 | 23 | 42 | 22 | 10 | 11 | 28 | 18 | 27 | 22 | 12 | 18158 |
| soft type—*1 cookie* | 15 | 8 | 18 | 23 | 40 | 23 | 10 | 10 | 27 | 18 | 27 | 21 | 11 | 18160 |
| **chocolate sandwich cookie** | | | | | | | | | | | | | | |
| w/crème filling—*1 cookie* | 17 | 10 | 25 | 26 | 44 | 31 | 9 | 11 | 30 | 22 | 35 | 31 | 12 | 18167 |
| w/crème filling, | | | | | | | | | | | | | | |
| choc-covered—*1 cookie* | 10 | 9 | 15 | 17 | 32 | 5 | 8 | 9 | 23 | 10 | 23 | 14 | 9 | 18166 |
| w/extra crème filling—*1 cookie* | 13 | 7 | 15 | 18 | 32 | 18 | 7 | 9 | 22 | 14 | 22 | 20 | 9 | 18168 |
| **chocolate wafer**—*5 wafers (1 oz)* | 28 | 27 | 62 | 73 | 125 | 79 | 29 | 36 | 86 | 57 | 90 | 80 | 36 | 18157 |
| **fig bar**—*2 square bars* | 31 | 14 | 35 | 41 | 69 | 43 | 16 | 23 | 45 | 38 | 48 | 38 | 21 | 18170 |
| **fortune cookie**—*1 cookie* | 8 | 5 | 10 | 13 | 24 | 13 | 6 | 7 | 16 | 10 | 15 | 13 | 7 | 18171 |
| **fudge cookie**, cake type—*1 cookie* | 21 | 12 | 31 | 37 | 64 | 47 | 15 | 14 | 43 | 28 | 47 | 56 | 18 | 18156 |
| **gingersnap**—*1 sm cookie* | 7 | 6 | 11 | 15 | 27 | 14 | 7 | 8 | 18 | 11 | 17 | 15 | 8 | 18172 |
| **graham cracker**—*2 crackers (2½″ sq)* | 14 | 13 | 27 | 34 | 66 | 23 | 17 | 21 | 48 | 29 | 40 | 41 | 22 | 18173 |
| chocolate-covered—*2½″ sq* | 14 | 10 | 28 | 35 | 64 | 32 | 15 | 12 | 42 | 30 | 42 | 30 | 16 | 18174 |
| **ice cream cone** | | | | | | | | | | | | | | |
| cake/wafer (cone only)—1 cone | 4 | 4 | 9 | 12 | 22 | 6 | 6 | 7 | 16 | 9 | 14 | 11 | 7 | 18271 |
| sugar, rolled (cone only)—1 cone | 10 | 9 | 21 | 29 | 55 | 15 | 14 | 18 | 39 | 22 | 33 | 28 | 17 | 18272 |
| waffle (cone only)—1 cone | 4 | 4 | 9 | 12 | 22 | 6 | 6 | 7 | 16 | 9 | 14 | 11 | 7 | 18271 |
| **ladyfinger**—*1 ladyfinger* | 11 | 15 | 51 | 57 | 95 | 75 | 29 | 25 | 56 | 45 | 64 | 67 | 27 | 18423 |
| with lemon juice and rind | | | | | | | | | | | | | | |
| *1 ladyfinger* | 11 | 15 | 51 | 57 | 95 | 75 | 29 | 25 | 56 | 45 | 64 | 67 | 27 | 18175 |
| **macaroon**, homemade | | | | | | | | | | | | | | |
| *1 cookie (2″ dia)* | 24 | 10 | 34 | 41 | 66 | 49 | 24 | 19 | 45 | 29 | 51 | 73 | 18 | 18169 |

| | WT | TRY | THR | ISO | LEU | LYS | MET | CYS | PHE | TYR | VAL | ARG | HIS | REF |
|---|---|---|---|---|---|---|---|---|---|---|---|---|---|---|
| | (g) | | | | | | (mg/serving) | | | | | | | |
| **marshmallow pie** | | | | | | | | | | | | | | |
| 1 small cookie (1¾″ × ¾″) | 13 | 5 | 17 | 17 | 29 | 26 | 6 | 6 | 18 | 11 | 22 | 31 | 8 | 18176 |
| **molasses cookie**—1 cookie | 20 | 16 | 31 | 42 | 75 | 39 | 19 | 24 | 53 | 32 | 49 | 42 | 23 | 18177 |
| Little Debbie—1 cookie | 20 | 16 | 31 | 42 | 75 | 39 | 19 | 24 | 53 | 32 | 49 | 42 | 23 | 18177 |
| **oatmeal cookie** | 18 | 18 | 31 | 40 | 78 | 43 | 22 | 30 | 53 | 36 | 54 | 66 | 26 | 18178 |
| fat-free—2 cookies (1 oz) | 28 | 22 | 49 | 61 | 111 | 60 | 30 | 37 | 78 | 49 | 77 | 84 | 37 | 18456 |
| from refrig dough—1 cookie | 12 | 12 | 24 | 30 | 55 | 34 | 16 | 20 | 37 | 26 | 39 | 45 | 17 | 18183 |
| homemade—1 cookie (2⅝″ dia) | 15 | 13 | 35 | 42 | 76 | 41 | 21 | 23 | 53 | 34 | 52 | 59 | 24 | 18377 |
| soft type—1 cookie | 15 | 14 | 29 | 36 | 68 | 41 | 20 | 25 | 45 | 32 | 47 | 56 | 21 | 18179 |
| **oatmeal raisin cookie**, homemade | | | | | | | | | | | | | | |
| 1 cookie (2⅝″ diameter) | 15 | 12 | 33 | 38 | 70 | 38 | 20 | 21 | 48 | 32 | 48 | 57 | 23 | 18184 |
| **peanut butter cookie** | 15 | 16 | 48 | 54 | 98 | 57 | 22 | 24 | 73 | 53 | 64 | 128 | 34 | 18185 |
| from refrig dough—1 cookie | 12 | 13 | 37 | 43 | 75 | 45 | 17 | 19 | 54 | 39 | 50 | 83 | 25 | 18188 |
| homemade—1 cookie (3″ dia) | 20 | 20 | 60 | 68 | 125 | 64 | 30 | 30 | 92 | 66 | 79 | 147 | 43 | 18189 |
| soft type—1 cookie | 15 | 9 | 26 | 30 | 54 | 30 | 10 | 13 | 40 | 29 | 35 | 69 | 19 | 18186 |
| **peanut butter sandwich cookie** | | | | | | | | | | | | | | |
| 1 cookie | 14 | 15 | 42 | 48 | 86 | 49 | 18 | 23 | 62 | 45 | 56 | 100 | 29 | 18190 |
| **pecan shortbread cookie** | | | | | | | | | | | | | | |
| 1 cookie (2″ diameter) | 14 | 11 | 20 | 27 | 47 | 25 | 13 | 16 | 33 | 21 | 31 | 39 | 15 | 18193 |
| **raisin cookie**, soft type—1 cookie | 15 | 8 | 21 | 25 | 43 | 27 | 13 | 13 | 28 | 19 | 29 | 28 | 14 | 18191 |
| **shortbread cookie** | | | | | | | | | | | | | | |
| 1 cookie (1⅝″ square) | 8 | 7 | 16 | 20 | 36 | 20 | 10 | 11 | 24 | 15 | 23 | 21 | 10 | 18192 |
| **sugar cookie** | 15 | 11 | 27 | 34 | 58 | 38 | 16 | 16 | 38 | 26 | 39 | 33 | 17 | 18204 |
| from refrig dough—1 cookie | 15 | 10 | 23 | 30 | 51 | 31 | 14 | 16 | 34 | 22 | 34 | 31 | 15 | 18206 |
| homemade w/margarine | | | | | | | | | | | | | | |
| 1 cookie (3″ diameter) | 14 | 10 | 26 | 32 | 60 | 27 | 17 | 17 | 42 | 27 | 37 | 35 | 19 | 18208 |
| **sugar wafer** with crème filling | | | | | | | | | | | | | | |
| 8 small wafers (1 oz) | 28 | 17 | 32 | 44 | 79 | 40 | 20 | 25 | 54 | 33 | 51 | 44 | 23 | 18209 |
| **vanilla sandwich** with crème filling | | | | | | | | | | | | | | |
| 1 round cookie (1¾″ diameter) | 10 | 6 | 12 | 17 | 31 | 16 | 8 | 10 | 21 | 13 | 20 | 17 | 9 | 18210 |
| **vanilla wafer** | | | | | | | | | | | | | | |
| 12%–17% fat—7 wafers (1 oz) | 28 | 19 | 47 | 60 | 102 | 64 | 29 | 31 | 68 | 45 | 68 | 62 | 30 | 18212 |
| 18%–21% fat—5 wafers (1 oz) | 28 | 17 | 37 | 47 | 85 | 46 | 20 | 26 | 56 | 34 | 54 | 46 | 24 | 18213 |
| **DOUGHNUTS** | | | | | | | | | | | | | | |
| **cruller**, glazed—3″ dia | 41 | 18 | 43 | 54 | 95 | 60 | 23 | 25 | 60 | 41 | 61 | 56 | 28 | 18253 |
| **doughnut**—3¼″ dia | 47 | 31 | 81 | 95 | 174 | 97 | 40 | 56 | 107 | 49 | 110 | 113 | 54 | 18248 |
| choc, glazed/sugared—3″ dia | 42 | 24 | 71 | 86 | 142 | 98 | 40 | 38 | 94 | 66 | 98 | 95 | 42 | 18251 |
| choc coating/icing—3″ dia | 43 | 26 | 73 | 89 | 157 | 99 | 34 | 42 | 96 | 56 | 103 | 100 | 48 | 18249 |
| yeast-raised, glazed—3¾″ dia | 60 | 36 | 102 | 125 | 226 | 130 | 50 | 70 | 136 | 67 | 142 | 136 | 68 | 18255 |
| yeast-raised w/crème filling | | | | | | | | | | | | | | |
| 1 oval doughnut (3½″ × 2½″) | 85 | 66 | 182 | 230 | 407 | 205 | 100 | 108 | 264 | 173 | 256 | 230 | 125 | 18254 |
| yeast-raised w/jelly filling | | | | | | | | | | | | | | |
| 1 oval doughnut (3½″ × 2½″) | 85 | 60 | 165 | 207 | 366 | 178 | 89 | 100 | 241 | 156 | 229 | 212 | 112 | 18256 |
| yeast-raised, wheat, | | | | | | | | | | | | | | |
| glazed/sugared—3″ dia | 45 | 40 | 98 | 123 | 215 | 128 | 51 | 54 | 133 | 96 | 140 | 132 | 67 | 18252 |
| yeast-raised, glazed/sugared—3″ dia | 45 | 31 | 85 | 104 | 182 | 115 | 47 | 45 | 110 | 82 | 117 | 107 | 54 | 18250 |
| **FROZEN DESSERTS** | | | | | | | | | | | | | | |
| **frozen yogurt** | | | | | | | | | | | | | | |
| soft serve, choc—½ cup | 72 | 40 | 123 | 154 | 248 | 201 | 60 | 29 | 136 | 128 | 184 | 118 | 69 | 19393 |
| soft serve, vanilla—½ cup | 72 | 38 | 122 | 164 | 265 | 215 | 68 | 25 | 130 | 130 | 181 | 98 | 73 | 19293 |
| **ice cream** | | | | | | | | | | | | | | |
| French vanilla, soft serve—½ cup | 86 | 41 | 145 | 185 | 304 | 255 | 78 | 31 | 151 | 146 | 207 | 148 | 85 | 19090 |
| vanilla, low/reduced cal (½ the | | | | | | | | | | | | | | |
| fat), soft serve—½ cup | 88 | 52 | 173 | 229 | 373 | 309 | 96 | 34 | 186 | 180 | 257 | 163 | 103 | 19096 |
| vanilla, regular (10% fat)—½ cup | 66 | 30 | 96 | 129 | 209 | 170 | 53 | 19 | 104 | 102 | 143 | 82 | 58 | 19095 |
| vanilla, rich (16% fat)—½ cup | 107 | 44 | 148 | 195 | 319 | 265 | 81 | 29 | 159 | 152 | 219 | 144 | 89 | 19089 |
| **GELATIN DESSERTS** | | | | | | | | | | | | | | |
| **gelatin dessert** | | | | | | | | | | | | | | |
| from mix with sugar, all flavors | | | | | | | | | | | | | | |
| ½ cup | 135 | 0 | 32 | 26 | 53 | 76 | 14 | 0 | 38 | 7 | 45 | 143 | 15 | 19173 |
| mix with aspartame—0.35 oz pkt | 10 | 0 | 107 | 84 | 177 | 250 | 44 | 0 | 126 | 22 | 150 | 478 | 48 | 19704 |
| mix with sugar, all flavors—3 oz pkt | 85 | 0 | 128 | 100 | 213 | 301 | 53 | 0 | 150 | 26 | 181 | 575 | 58 | 19172 |
| **PASTRIES, SWEET ROLLS, COBBLERS, STRUDELS, AND TURNOVERS** | | | | | | | | | | | | | | |
| **apple strudel**—2.5 oz piece | 71 | 28 | 84 | 104 | 182 | 109 | 48 | 41 | 107 | 82 | 116 | 96 | 54 | 18354 |

| | WT | TRY | THR | ISO | LEU | LYS | MET | CYS | PHE | TYR | VAL | ARG | HIS | REF |
|---|---|---|---|---|---|---|---|---|---|---|---|---|---|---|
| | (g) | (mg/serving) | | | | | | | | | | | | |
| **cream puff** | | | | | | | | | | | | | | |
| shell, homemade—*1 shell* | 66 | 73 | 242 | 284 | 474 | 328 | 157 | 131 | 308 | 221 | 320 | 312 | 138 | 18237 |
| w/custard fill, homemade—*1 puff* | 130 | 108 | 368 | 441 | 725 | 534 | 233 | 173 | 445 | 343 | 495 | 439 | 208 | 18238 |
| **croissant**—*1 med* | 57 | 56 | 162 | 208 | 355 | 188 | 100 | 98 | 237 | 154 | 234 | 193 | 107 | 18239 |
| apple—*1 med* | 57 | 49 | 146 | 185 | 317 | 181 | 86 | 80 | 205 | 139 | 210 | 176 | 95 | 18240 |
| cheese—*1 med* | 57 | 62 | 173 | 232 | 394 | 211 | 107 | 100 | 259 | 172 | 258 | 207 | 121 | 18241 |
| **Danish pastry** | | | | | | | | | | | | | | |
| cinnamon—*4¼″ dia* | 65 | 55 | 159 | 202 | 346 | 192 | 90 | 90 | 226 | 151 | 224 | 203 | 104 | 18244 |
| cream/neufchatel chs—*4¼″ dia* | 71 | 63 | 208 | 263 | 457 | 305 | 124 | 97 | 285 | 208 | 293 | 230 | 146 | 18245 |
| fruit—*4¼″ dia* | 71 | 45 | 121 | 159 | 283 | 126 | 78 | 84 | 190 | 118 | 179 | 148 | 84 | 18246 |
| lemon—*4¼″ dia* | 71 | 45 | 121 | 159 | 283 | 126 | 78 | 84 | 190 | 118 | 179 | 148 | 84 | 18433 |
| nut—*4¼″ dia* | 65 | 57 | 155 | 198 | 344 | 176 | 90 | 90 | 219 | 153 | 226 | 280 | 108 | 18247 |
| raspberry—*4¼″ dia* | 71 | 45 | 121 | 159 | 283 | 126 | 78 | 84 | 190 | 118 | 179 | 148 | 84 | 18435 |
| **éclair** w/custard filling, choc glaze, homemade—*1 éclair (5″ long)* | 100 | 80 | 271 | 324 | 532 | 392 | 169 | 127 | 328 | 253 | 365 | 325 | 152 | 18257 |
| **puff pastry**, frozen—*1 pastry* | 40 | 34 | 79 | 110 | 206 | 58 | 52 | 67 | 147 | 82 | 125 | 104 | 63 | 18211 |
| **sweet roll** | | | | | | | | | | | | | | |
| cheese (cream/neufchatel)—*1 roll* | 66 | 51 | 173 | 211 | 366 | 256 | 94 | 74 | 226 | 169 | 234 | 207 | 121 | 18355 |
| cinn raisin—*1 roll* | 60 | 44 | 127 | 155 | 275 | 146 | 70 | 72 | 180 | 120 | 175 | 170 | 87 | 18356 |
| cinn w/icing, from refrig dough—*1 roll* | 30 | 20 | 48 | 58 | 115 | 42 | 29 | 34 | 80 | 50 | 67 | 65 | 36 | 18358 |
| **toaster pastry** | | | | | | | | | | | | | | |
| apple/blueberry/cherry/strawberry *1 pastry* | 52 | 22 | 54 | 72 | 137 | 56 | 30 | 54 | 88 | 27 | 86 | 74 | 42 | 18362 |
| brown sugar cinn—*1 pastry* | 50 | 28 | 73 | 84 | 162 | 68 | 40 | 47 | 107 | 67 | 94 | 87 | 49 | 18361 |
| PIES, PIE CRUSTS, AND PIE FILLINGS | | | | | | | | | | | | | | |
| **apple pie**—*⅛ of 9″ pie* | 125 | 32 | 68 | 91 | 161 | 88 | 40 | 50 | 110 | 68 | 105 | 92 | 48 | 18301 |
| Dutch—*4.8 oz slice* | 137 | 37 | 86 | 111 | 216 | 59 | 70 | 78 | 142 | 71 | 138 | 115 | 74 | 18944 |
| homemade—*⅛ of 9″ pie* | 155 | 45 | 102 | 129 | 254 | 87 | 65 | 78 | 183 | 112 | 150 | 149 | 82 | 18302 |
| **banana cream pie** | | | | | | | | | | | | | | |
| from mix—*⅛ of 9″ pie* | 92 | 42 | 126 | 155 | 262 | 186 | 61 | 46 | 148 | 121 | 167 | 144 | 77 | 18303 |
| homemade—*⅛ of 9″ pie* | 144 | 79 | 238 | 292 | 516 | 334 | 132 | 98 | 297 | 242 | 330 | 268 | 167 | 18304 |
| **blueberry pie**—*⅛ of 9″ pie* | 125 | 31 | 64 | 86 | 156 | 78 | 39 | 49 | 107 | 64 | 100 | 90 | 46 | 18305 |
| homemade—*⅛ of 9″ pie* | 147 | 43 | 107 | 132 | 263 | 84 | 68 | 75 | 187 | 106 | 159 | 166 | 82 | 18306 |
| **cherry pie** | 125 | 35 | 98 | 129 | 216 | 150 | 54 | 39 | 124 | 100 | 149 | 127 | 62 | 18308 |
| filling, canned—*⅛ can* | 74 | 1 | 7 | 7 | 10 | 12 | 1 | 1 | 6 | 4 | 9 | 5 | 4 | 19314 |
| homemade—*⅛ of 9″ pie* | 180 | 56 | 130 | 158 | 306 | 121 | 77 | 90 | 223 | 135 | 187 | 180 | 103 | 18309 |
| **cherry snack pie**, fried *1 snack pie (5″ × 3¾″)* | 128 | 54 | 114 | 154 | 270 | 155 | 67 | 76 | 177 | 115 | 177 | 143 | 79 | 18444 |
| **chocolate creme pie**—*⅙ of 8″ pie* | 113 | 38 | 99 | 107 | 186 | 128 | 40 | 47 | 128 | 81 | 141 | 155 | 54 | 18310 |
| **chocolate mousse pie**, from mix *⅛ of 9″ pie* | 95 | 46 | 132 | 157 | 264 | 191 | 59 | 48 | 158 | 126 | 180 | 159 | 78 | 18312 |
| **coconut cream pie**—*⅙ of 7″ pie* | 64 | 19 | 50 | 66 | 111 | 76 | 28 | 19 | 63 | 52 | 77 | 69 | 33 | 18313 |
| from mix—*⅛ of 9″ pie* | 94 | 35 | 103 | 129 | 222 | 149 | 55 | 39 | 122 | 102 | 145 | 112 | 63 | 18314 |
| **coconut custard pie**—*⅙ of 8″ pie* | 104 | 82 | 225 | 297 | 501 | 348 | 126 | 88 | 285 | 233 | 343 | 295 | 146 | 18316 |
| **egg custard pie**—*⅙ of 8″ pie* | 105 | 75 | 236 | 295 | 478 | 365 | 145 | 104 | 282 | 225 | 331 | 264 | 133 | 18317 |
| **fruit snack pie**, fried *1 snack pie (5″ × 3¾″)* | 128 | 54 | 114 | 154 | 270 | 155 | 67 | 76 | 177 | 115 | 177 | 143 | 79 | 18319 |
| **lemon meringue pie**—*⅙ of 8″ pie* | 133 | 25 | 80 | 88 | 154 | 112 | 40 | 39 | 88 | 72 | 98 | 108 | 45 | 18320 |
| homemade—*⅛ of 9″ pie* | 127 | 58 | 182 | 215 | 371 | 230 | 117 | 105 | 246 | 171 | 244 | 243 | 110 | 18321 |
| **lemon snack pie**, fried *1 snack pie (5″ × 3¾″)* | 128 | 54 | 114 | 154 | 270 | 155 | 67 | 76 | 177 | 115 | 177 | 143 | 79 | 18445 |
| **mince pie**, homemade—*⅛ of 9″ pie* | 165 | 45 | 116 | 122 | 246 | 96 | 87 | 84 | 185 | 116 | 158 | 201 | 106 | 18322 |
| **peach pie**—*⅙ of 8″ pie* | 117 | 26 | 67 | 78 | 143 | 75 | 41 | 41 | 95 | 61 | 101 | 77 | 43 | 18323 |
| **pecan pie**—*⅙ of 8″ pie* | 113 | 56 | 165 | 192 | 350 | 141 | 90 | 90 | 232 | 102 | 243 | 328 | 119 | 18324 |
| homemade—*⅛ of 9″ pie* | 122 | 84 | 231 | 272 | 454 | 303 | 152 | 135 | 305 | 217 | 311 | 396 | 142 | 18325 |
| **pie crust** | | | | | | | | | | | | | | |
| chocolate cookie, Ready Crust *6.4 oz crust* | 182 | 146 | 373 | 410 | 695 | 446 | 133 | 197 | 504 | 298 | 575 | 528 | 204 | 18943 |
| chocolate wafer, homemade *⅛ of 9″ crust* | 28 | 21 | 49 | 58 | 99 | 64 | 24 | 27 | 67 | 46 | 72 | 62 | 28 | 18398 |
| from mix—*⅛ of 9″ crust* | 20 | 15 | 36 | 49 | 92 | 26 | 23 | 30 | 66 | 36 | 56 | 46 | 28 | 18333 |
| frozen—*⅛ of 9″ crust* | 16 | 10 | 21 | 37 | 74 | 23 | 17 | 21 | 47 | 23 | 46 | 38 | 18 | 18335 |
| graham cracker, Ready Crust *6.5 oz crust* | 183 | 102 | 243 | 324 | 619 | 253 | 135 | 240 | 395 | 121 | 384 | 333 | 187 | 18942 |
| graham, homemade *⅛ of 9″ crust* | 30 | 16 | 36 | 46 | 88 | 33 | 22 | 26 | 62 | 39 | 53 | 52 | 28 | 18330 |
| homemade—*⅛ of 9″ crust* | 23 | 18 | 40 | 51 | 102 | 33 | 26 | 31 | 75 | 45 | 59 | 60 | 33 | 18336 |

| | WT | TRY | THR | ISO | LEU | LYS | MET | CYS | PHE | TYR | VAL | ARG | HIS | REF |
|---|---|---|---|---|---|---|---|---|---|---|---|---|---|---|
| | (g) | (mg/serving) | | | | | | | | | | | | |
| refrigerated, baked | | | | | | | | | | | | | | |
| *7 oz crust* | 198 | 69 | 131 | 238 | 436 | 139 | 99 | 131 | 287 | 139 | 287 | 218 | 119 | 18946 |
| vanilla wafer, homemade | | | | | | | | | | | | | | |
| *1/8 of 9″ crust* | 22 | 11 | 28 | 35 | 60 | 39 | 17 | 17 | 39 | 27 | 40 | 35 | 17 | 18401 |
| **pumpkin pie**—*1/6 of 8″ pie* | 109 | 52 | 168 | 172 | 324 | 209 | 271 | 68 | 191 | 129 | 230 | 168 | 96 | 18326 |
| homemade—*1/8 of 9″ pie* | 155 | 91 | 279 | 350 | 583 | 428 | 163 | 104 | 339 | 290 | 392 | 308 | 169 | 18327 |
| mix, canned—*1 cup* | 270 | 35 | 84 | 92 | 135 | 159 | 32 | 8 | 95 | 122 | 103 | 157 | 46 | 11426 |
| **vanilla cream pie**, homemade | | | | | | | | | | | | | | |
| *1/8 of 9″ pie* | 126 | 76 | 232 | 287 | 500 | 335 | 130 | 89 | 282 | 238 | 321 | 256 | 147 | 18328 |
| **PUDDINGS AND CUSTARDS** | | | | | | | | | | | | | | |
| **banana pudding** from instant mix | | | | | | | | | | | | | | |
| with 2% milk—*1/2 cup* | 140 | 55 | 175 | 234 | 379 | 307 | 98 | 36 | 188 | 188 | 259 | 140 | 105 | 19121 |
| with whole milk—*1/2 cup* | 147 | 56 | 182 | 243 | 392 | 319 | 101 | 37 | 194 | 194 | 269 | 146 | 109 | 19319 |
| **banana pudding** from regular mix | | | | | | | | | | | | | | |
| with 2% milk—*1/2 cup* | 140 | 57 | 183 | 245 | 398 | 322 | 102 | 38 | 196 | 196 | 272 | 148 | 109 | 19122 |
| with whole milk—*1/2 cup* | 140 | 56 | 182 | 242 | 393 | 318 | 101 | 36 | 195 | 193 | 269 | 146 | 109 | 19321 |
| **chocolate pudding** from instant mix | | | | | | | | | | | | | | |
| with lowfat milk—*1/2 cup* | 147 | 65 | 204 | 268 | 434 | 351 | 109 | 44 | 222 | 218 | 306 | 178 | 121 | 19123 |
| with whole milk—*1/2 cup* | 147 | 62 | 194 | 254 | 410 | 332 | 101 | 43 | 210 | 206 | 290 | 169 | 115 | 19185 |
| **chocolate pudding** from regular mix | | | | | | | | | | | | | | |
| with 2% milk—*1/2 cup* | 142 | 65 | 206 | 267 | 432 | 349 | 108 | 45 | 224 | 217 | 307 | 182 | 119 | 19190 |
| **chocolate rennin dessert**, from mix | | | | | | | | | | | | | | |
| with 2% milk—*1/2 cup* | 136 | 61 | 196 | 257 | 418 | 340 | 106 | 41 | 212 | 208 | 291 | 169 | 116 | 19213 |
| with whole milk—*1/2 cup* | 136 | 60 | 194 | 256 | 412 | 336 | 105 | 41 | 209 | 205 | 287 | 166 | 114 | 19221 |
| **coconut cream pudding** from instant | | | | | | | | | | | | | | |
| mix with 2% milk—*1/2 cup* | 147 | 56 | 182 | 243 | 395 | 318 | 101 | 40 | 197 | 194 | 272 | 169 | 110 | 19191 |
| with whole milk—*1/2 cup* | 147 | 56 | 181 | 241 | 391 | 313 | 100 | 40 | 196 | 191 | 269 | 168 | 109 | 19323 |
| **coconut cream pudding**, from reg mix | | | | | | | | | | | | | | |
| with 2% milk—*1/2 cup* | 140 | 57 | 183 | 244 | 396 | 318 | 101 | 39 | 197 | 193 | 273 | 172 | 111 | 19219 |
| with whole milk—*1/2 cup* | 140 | 56 | 181 | 241 | 392 | 314 | 101 | 39 | 196 | 192 | 270 | 171 | 109 | 19325 |
| **egg custard**, from mix | | | | | | | | | | | | | | |
| with 2% milk—*1/2 cup* | 133 | 76 | 263 | 318 | 520 | 432 | 133 | 64 | 247 | 246 | 347 | 221 | 141 | 19205 |
| with whole milk—*1/2 cup* | 133 | 74 | 262 | 315 | 515 | 428 | 132 | 63 | 245 | 243 | 343 | 218 | 140 | 19170 |
| **flan**, from mix | | | | | | | | | | | | | | |
| with 2% milk—*1/2 cup* | 133 | 56 | 180 | 239 | 390 | 315 | 100 | 37 | 193 | 193 | 266 | 145 | 108 | 19231 |
| with whole milk—*1/2 cup* | 133 | 55 | 178 | 237 | 384 | 311 | 98 | 36 | 190 | 190 | 262 | 142 | 106 | 19232 |
| **lemon pudding**, from instant mix | | | | | | | | | | | | | | |
| with 2% milk—*1/2 cup* | 147 | 57 | 184 | 245 | 398 | 322 | 103 | 38 | 197 | 197 | 272 | 147 | 110 | 19204 |
| with whole milk—*1/2 cup* | 147 | 53 | 172 | 232 | 375 | 304 | 96 | 35 | 185 | 185 | 256 | 138 | 104 | 19331 |
| **rice pudding**, from regular mix | | | | | | | | | | | | | | |
| with 2% milk—*1/2 cup* | 144 | 56 | 181 | 243 | 393 | 318 | 101 | 37 | 194 | 194 | 269 | 145 | 108 | 19208 |
| with whole milk—*1/2 cup* | 144 | 56 | 180 | 240 | 389 | 315 | 101 | 36 | 192 | 192 | 265 | 144 | 108 | 19195 |
| **tapioca pudding**, from regular mix | | | | | | | | | | | | | | |
| with 2% milk—*1/2 cup* | 141 | 58 | 183 | 244 | 398 | 321 | 103 | 38 | 196 | 196 | 271 | 149 | 110 | 19209 |
| with whole milk—*1/2 cup* | 141 | 56 | 182 | 243 | 392 | 317 | 102 | 37 | 193 | 193 | 268 | 147 | 109 | 19199 |
| **vanilla pudding**, from instant mix | | | | | | | | | | | | | | |
| with whole milk—*1/2 cup* | 142 | 51 | 166 | 224 | 362 | 294 | 92 | 34 | 179 | 179 | 247 | 133 | 101 | 19203 |
| **vanilla pudding**, from regular mix | | | | | | | | | | | | | | |
| with 2% milk—*1/2 cup* | 140 | 57 | 185 | 246 | 405 | 323 | 104 | 39 | 199 | 199 | 274 | 150 | 112 | 19212 |
| **vanilla rennin dessert**, from mix | | | | | | | | | | | | | | |
| with 2% milk—*1/2 cup* | 133 | 57 | 184 | 246 | 399 | 323 | 102 | 39 | 197 | 197 | 273 | 148 | 110 | 19214 |
| with whole milk—*1/2 cup* | 133 | 56 | 182 | 243 | 394 | 319 | 101 | 37 | 194 | 194 | 269 | 145 | 109 | 19223 |
| **SAUCES, SYRUPS, AND TOPPINGS FOR DESSERTS** | | | | | | | | | | | | | | |
| **butterscotch/caramel dessert** | | | | | | | | | | | | | | |
| topping—*2 T* | 41 | 8 | 27 | 36 | 59 | 48 | 15 | 5 | 29 | 29 | 40 | 22 | 16 | 19364 |
| **icing/frosting**, choc | | | | | | | | | | | | | | |
| ready-to-spread—*2 T* | 41 | 7 | 18 | 17 | 27 | 22 | 5 | 5 | 21 | 17 | 27 | 25 | 8 | 19226 |
| from mix, made w/butter | | | | | | | | | | | | | | |
| *1/12 pkg prep* | 42 | 7 | 19 | 19 | 30 | 25 | 5 | 5 | 23 | 18 | 29 | 26 | 8 | 19241 |
| from mix, made w/margarine | | | | | | | | | | | | | | |
| *1/12 pkg prep* | 42 | 7 | 19 | 19 | 30 | 25 | 5 | 5 | 23 | 18 | 29 | 26 | 8 | 19372 |
| **icing/frosting**, vanilla, from mix | | | | | | | | | | | | | | |
| made w/margarine—*1/12 pkg prep* | 43 | 1 | 5 | 6 | 16 | 5 | 3 | 3 | 6 | 5 | 7 | 6 | 4 | 19371 |
| **icing/frosting**, white fluffy, from mix | | | | | | | | | | | | | | |
| made with water—*1/12 pkg prep* | 26 | 4 | 17 | 21 | 31 | 26 | 12 | 9 | 22 | 14 | 24 | 24 | 8 | 19247 |
| **nuts in syrup dessert topping**—*2 T* | 41 | 24 | 57 | 72 | 127 | 50 | 36 | 44 | 80 | 56 | 92 | 269 | 46 | 19367 |

| | WT (g) | TRY | THR | ISO | LEU | LYS | MET | CYS | PHE | TYR | VAL | ARG | HIS | REF |
|---|---|---|---|---|---|---|---|---|---|---|---|---|---|---|
| | | | | | | | (mg/serving) | | | | | | | |

**8. EGGS, EGG DISHES, AND EGG SUBSTITUTES**

**chicken egg**

| | WT (g) | TRY | THR | ISO | LEU | LYS | MET | CYS | PHE | TYR | VAL | ARG | HIS | REF |
|---|---|---|---|---|---|---|---|---|---|---|---|---|---|---|
| boiled, hard—*1 large egg* | 50 | 76 | 302 | 343 | 538 | 452 | 196 | 146 | 334 | 256 | 384 | 378 | 149 | 1129 |
| dried—*1 T* | 5 | 39 | 118 | 151 | 212 | 163 | 78 | 57 | 136 | 100 | 173 | 154 | 58 | 1134 |
| fried—*1 large egg* | 46 | 83 | 276 | 334 | 540 | 454 | 189 | 135 | 338 | 248 | 427 | 408 | 154 | 1128 |
| omelet, plain—*1 large egg* | 61 | 85 | 285 | 345 | 558 | 468 | 195 | 140 | 349 | 256 | 441 | 422 | 159 | 1130 |
| poached—*1 large egg* | 50 | 83 | 277 | 335 | 542 | 455 | 190 | 136 | 339 | 249 | 428 | 409 | 154 | 1131 |
| raw—*1 large egg* | 50 | 84 | 278 | 336 | 544 | 457 | 190 | 136 | 340 | 250 | 430 | 410 | 154 | 1123 |
| scrambled w/milk—*1 large egg* | 61 | 83 | 322 | 371 | 582 | 488 | 207 | 149 | 356 | 279 | 414 | 393 | 161 | 1132 |
| **chicken egg white**, raw—*1 large egg* | 33 | 41 | 148 | 218 | 335 | 266 | 132 | 95 | 226 | 151 | 267 | 214 | 96 | 1124 |
| **chicken egg yolk**, raw—*1 large egg* | 17 | 30 | 117 | 147 | 238 | 207 | 64 | 45 | 116 | 115 | 161 | 187 | 71 | 1125 |
| **duck egg**, raw—*1 egg* | 70 | 182 | 515 | 419 | 768 | 666 | 403 | 199 | 588 | 429 | 620 | 536 | 224 | 1138 |
| **egg substitute** | | | | | | | | | | | | | | |
| frozen—*¼ cup* | 60 | 98 | 290 | 396 | 583 | 428 | 232 | 137 | 387 | 274 | 475 | 346 | 154 | 1142 |
| liquid—*1.5 fl oz* | 47 | 90 | 260 | 352 | 509 | 370 | 200 | 137 | 360 | 233 | 417 | 368 | 139 | 1143 |
| **goose egg**, raw—*1 egg* | 144 | 406 | 1148 | 932 | 1711 | 1483 | 899 | 445 | 1310 | 956 | 1380 | 1192 | 498 | 1139 |
| **quail egg**, raw—*1 egg* | 9 | 19 | 58 | 73 | 103 | 79 | 38 | 28 | 66 | 49 | 85 | 75 | 28 | 1140 |
| **turkey egg**, raw—*1 egg* | 79 | 173 | 531 | 675 | 949 | 730 | 349 | 258 | 611 | 450 | 778 | 692 | 261 | 1141 |

**9. ENTREES AND MEALS**

**CANNED ENTREES**

| | WT (g) | TRY | THR | ISO | LEU | LYS | MET | CYS | PHE | TYR | VAL | ARG | HIS | REF |
|---|---|---|---|---|---|---|---|---|---|---|---|---|---|---|
| **baked beans** with beef—*1 cup (9.1 oz)* | 259 | 199 | 694 | 723 | 1321 | 1171 | 269 | 176 | 852 | 471 | 855 | 1039 | 471 | 16007 |
| **baked beans** with frankurters *1 cup (9.1 oz)* | 259 | 199 | 723 | 769 | 1383 | 1222 | 272 | 192 | 904 | 492 | 894 | 1106 | 492 | 16008 |
| **beef stew**—*8.2 oz* | 232 | 118 | 462 | 476 | 875 | 812 | 255 | 128 | 443 | 369 | 541 | 675 | 346 | 22905 |
| **chili con carne** (no beans)—*7.8 oz* | 222 | | 686 | 662 | 1241 | 872 | 229 | | 630 | 417 | 839 | 901 | 373 | 22911 |
| **chili with beans** (no meat)—*1 cup (9 oz)* | 256 | 177 | 614 | 640 | 1167 | 1047 | 243 | 156 | 748 | 420 | 753 | 922 | 420 | 16059 |
| **corned beef hash**—*1 cup (8.3 oz)* | 236 | 111 | 526 | 597 | 1015 | 1071 | 323 | 172 | 540 | 439 | 680 | 819 | 401 | 22908 |
| **macaroni and cheese**—*8.9 oz* | 252 | 116 | 302 | 413 | 716 | 403 | 149 | 116 | 441 | 262 | 459 | 315 | 237 | 22247 |
| **pasta with franks** in tomato sauce *1 cup (8.9 oz)* | 252 | 96 | 310 | 328 | 577 | 481 | 149 | 106 | 330 | 219 | 368 | 408 | 229 | 22522 |
| **pasta with meatballs** in tomato sce *1 cup (8.9 oz)* | 252 | 121 | 363 | 413 | 723 | 570 | 171 | 131 | 426 | 290 | 449 | 549 | 265 | 22907 |

**FROZEN ENTREES, SANDWICHES, AND MEALS**

| | WT (g) | TRY | THR | ISO | LEU | LYS | MET | CYS | PHE | TYR | VAL | ARG | HIS | REF |
|---|---|---|---|---|---|---|---|---|---|---|---|---|---|---|
| **beef pot pie**—*7 oz pot pie* | 198 | 152 | 529 | 537 | 1024 | 830 | 263 | 210 | 592 | 396 | 626 | 796 | 370 | 22529 |
| **burrito** | | | | | | | | | | | | | | |
| bean and cheese—*5 oz burrito* | 143 | 114 | 276 | 369 | 685 | 327 | 174 | 167 | 473 | 305 | 423 | 383 | 227 | 22918 |
| beef and bean—*4.9 oz burrito* | 139 | 111 | 299 | 373 | 713 | 345 | 185 | 190 | 493 | 303 | 431 | 456 | 239 | 22917 |
| **chicken pot pie**—*7.7 oz pot pie* | 217 | 154 | 458 | 482 | 907 | 679 | 208 | 193 | 529 | 369 | 542 | 671 | 360 | 22906 |
| **chicken wings, glazed, bbq** | | | | | | | | | | | | | | |
| microwaved—*3.4 oz* | 96 | 223 | 920 | 922 | 1580 | 1672 | 512 | 228 | 898 | 610 | 1001 | 1469 | 571 | 5313 |
| oven-heated—*2.6 oz* | 74 | 151 | 622 | 623 | 1069 | 1131 | 346 | 154 | 607 | 413 | 677 | 994 | 386 | 5320 |
| **lasagna**, cheese, heated—*10.5 oz* | 297 | 193 | 609 | 594 | 1574 | 1069 | 431 | 312 | 846 | 698 | 757 | 653 | 431 | 22910 |
| **rice bowl** with chicken—*12 oz* | 340 | 224 | 853 | 908 | 1567 | 1442 | 456 | 279 | 867 | 537 | 1044 | 1316 | 636 | 22958 |
| **spaghetti Bolognese**, Hlthy Chc—*10 oz* | 283 | 224 | 594 | 679 | 1245 | 577 | 207 | 286 | 826 | 376 | 750 | 756 | 399 | 22401 |
| **turkey and gravy**—*5 oz* | 142 | 95 | 372 | 435 | 666 | 787 | 241 | 87 | 331 | 329 | 443 | 582 | 260 | 5286 |
| **turkey**, stuffing, mshd pot, grvy, mxd veg, microwaved—*14.9 oz meal* | 422 | 304 | 1101 | 1291 | 1988 | 2152 | 663 | 316 | 1047 | 971 | 1334 | 1777 | 747 | 22957 |

**FROZEN PIZZA**

| | WT (g) | TRY | THR | ISO | LEU | LYS | MET | CYS | PHE | TYR | VAL | ARG | HIS | REF |
|---|---|---|---|---|---|---|---|---|---|---|---|---|---|---|
| **cheese**, regular crust, heated *3.6 oz slice* | 103 | 175 | 390 | 483 | 897 | 607 | 190 | 109 | 545 | 330 | 614 | 410 | 287 | 21224 |
| **cheese**, rising crust, heated *4.9 oz slice* | 139 | 261 | 627 | 801 | 1497 | 902 | 288 | 182 | 919 | 531 | 991 | 659 | 459 | 21225 |

**HOMEMADE AND UNSPECIFIED ENTREES**

| | WT (g) | TRY | THR | ISO | LEU | LYS | MET | CYS | PHE | TYR | VAL | ARG | HIS | REF |
|---|---|---|---|---|---|---|---|---|---|---|---|---|---|---|
| **acorn stew**, Apache—*3.5 oz* | 100 | 40 | 360 | 350 | 620 | 580 | 160 | 90 | 330 | 250 | 390 | 470 | 230 | 35182 |
| **hominy and mutton stew**, Navajo *3½ oz* | | | | | | | | | | | | | | |
| **mutton, corn, and squash stew**, Navajo—*3.5 oz* | 100 | 57 | 306 | 336 | 678 | 560 | 211 | 90 | 330 | 233 | 385 | 470 | 217 | 35146 |
| **tamale**, Navajo, homemade—*3.5 oz* | 100 | 52 | 239 | 271 | 568 | 427 | 150 | 83 | 275 | 204 | 318 | 391 | 196 | 35147 |

**10. FAST FOODS AND RESTAURANT FOODS**

**GENERIC FAST FOODS**

| | WT (g) | TRY | THR | ISO | LEU | LYS | MET | CYS | PHE | TYR | VAL | ARG | HIS | REF |
|---|---|---|---|---|---|---|---|---|---|---|---|---|---|---|
| **animal crackers**—*1 box* | 67 | 54 | 135 | 175 | 318 | 153 | 85 | 80 | 211 | 145 | 200 | 174 | 99 | 21029 |

| | WT (g) | TRY | THR | ISO | LEU | LYS | MET | CYS | PHE | TYR | VAL | ARG | HIS | REF |
|---|---|---|---|---|---|---|---|---|---|---|---|---|---|---|
| | | | | | | | (mg/serving) | | | | | | | |
| **biscuit** | | | | | | | | | | | | | | |
| w/egg—*4.8 oz* | 136 | 143 | 479 | 566 | 938 | 662 | 307 | 248 | 598 | 439 | 636 | 601 | 271 | 21002 |
| w/egg, bacon—*5.3 oz* | 150 | 216 | 680 | 822 | 1312 | 1024 | 422 | 294 | 810 | 594 | 952 | 936 | 430 | 21003 |
| w/egg, cheese—*5.2 oz* | 146 | 218 | 588 | 781 | 1244 | 927 | 383 | 266 | 803 | 585 | 937 | 775 | 410 | 21104 |
| w/egg, cheese, bacon—*5.1 oz* | 144 | 235 | 720 | 742 | 1341 | 1001 | 425 | 300 | 808 | 566 | 916 | 850 | 436 | 21007 |
| w/egg, ham—*6.8 oz* | 192 | 273 | 876 | 1000 | 1657 | 1386 | 540 | 376 | 996 | 735 | 1083 | 1190 | 597 | 21004 |
| w/egg, sausage—*6.3 oz* | 180 | 243 | 803 | 783 | 1397 | 1094 | 396 | 347 | 828 | 572 | 959 | 1004 | 482 | 21005 |
| w/egg, steak—*5.2 oz* | 148 | 229 | 747 | 872 | 1428 | 1183 | 460 | 296 | 829 | 641 | 980 | 1014 | 502 | 21006 |
| w/ham—*4 oz* | 113 | 166 | 544 | 580 | 1059 | 924 | 327 | 221 | 618 | 452 | 602 | 768 | 432 | 21008 |
| w/sausage—*4.4 oz serving* | 124 | 130 | 438 | 444 | 820 | 646 | 201 | 190 | | 305 | 516 | | 310 | 21009 |
| **brownie**—*1 brownie (2" square)* | 60 | 34 | 95 | 119 | 203 | 134 | 49 | 36 | 124 | 100 | 142 | 106 | 60 | 21027 |
| **burrito** | | | | | | | | | | | | | | |
| apple/cherry—*1 small burrito* | 74 | 30 | 67 | 87 | 169 | 58 | 44 | 53 | 124 | 74 | 100 | 100 | 56 | 21069 |
| bean—*2 burritos* | 217 | 171 | 529 | 586 | 1094 | 744 | 232 | 213 | 762 | 417 | 692 | 779 | 373 | 21060 |
| bean and cheese—*2 burritos* | 186 | 177 | 506 | 711 | 1179 | 915 | 290 | 151 | 733 | 538 | 787 | 660 | 426 | 21061 |
| bean and chili pepper—*2 burritos* | 204 | 192 | 557 | 620 | 1134 | 738 | 247 | 247 | 798 | 453 | 716 | 830 | 402 | 21062 |
| bean and meat—*2 burritos* | 231 | 270 | 827 | 896 | 1679 | 1372 | 439 | 293 | 982 | 665 | 1028 | 1289 | 621 | 21063 |
| bean, cheese, and beef—*2 burritos* | 203 | 175 | 530 | 658 | 1145 | 932 | 292 | 164 | 678 | 489 | 737 | 751 | 414 | 21064 |
| bean, cheese, and chili pepper *2 burritos* | 336 | 396 | 1109 | 1482 | 2574 | 1804 | 625 | 407 | 1663 | 1126 | 1673 | 1488 | 900 | 21065 |
| beef—*2 burritos* | 220 | 323 | 988 | 1060 | 2000 | 1720 | 563 | 341 | 1087 | 807 | 1206 | 1566 | 763 | 21066 |
| beef and chili pepper—*2 burritos* | 201 | 261 | 822 | 868 | 1628 | 1473 | 462 | 261 | 858 | 653 | 985 | 1306 | 629 | 21067 |
| beef, cheese, and chili pepper *2 burritos* | 304 | 492 | 1505 | 1745 | 3137 | 2797 | 879 | 447 | 1684 | 1325 | 1952 | 2298 | 1207 | 21068 |
| **cheese and deli meats sub**—*8 oz* | 228 | 249 | 743 | 903 | 1589 | 1288 | 438 | 287 | 987 | 750 | 1097 | 1015 | 620 | 21124 |
| **cheeseburger, large** | | | | | | | | | | | | | | |
| double meat, lettuce, tom *1 sandwich* | 258 | 472 | 1465 | 1618 | 2990 | 2905 | 846 | 392 | 1551 | 1244 | 1886 | 2273 | 1182 | 21100 |
| ham, lettuce, tom—*1 sandwich* | 254 | 498 | 1516 | 1702 | 3129 | 3040 | 899 | 434 | 1681 | 1351 | 1963 | 2289 | 1267 | 21099 |
| large, triple meat—*1 sandwich* | 304 | 696 | 2225 | 2405 | 4466 | 4420 | 1274 | 568 | 2262 | 1827 | 2785 | 3490 | 1763 | 21101 |
| **cheeseburger, regular** | | | | | | | | | | | | | | |
| double meat—*1 sandwich* | 155 | 352 | 1048 | 1192 | 2213 | 2159 | 629 | 276 | 1169 | 972 | 1410 | 1593 | 888 | 21092 |
| double meat, 3-pc bun—*1 sandwich* | 160 | 278 | 813 | 942 | 1738 | 1613 | 485 | 235 | 946 | 749 | 1117 | 1230 | 682 | 21094 |
| double meat, 3-pc bun, lettuce, tom—*1 sandwich* | 228 | 374 | 1099 | 1272 | 2332 | 2164 | 652 | 317 | 1272 | 1003 | 1507 | 1660 | 917 | 21095 |
| double meat, lettuce, tom *1 sandwich* | 166 | 267 | 802 | 911 | 1682 | 1642 | 476 | 212 | 895 | 737 | 1076 | 1213 | 676 | 21093 |
| lettuce, tom—*1 sandwich* | 154 | 225 | 645 | 759 | 1388 | 1223 | 379 | 202 | 779 | 590 | 906 | 964 | 537 | 21091 |
| **chicken, breaded, fried** | | | | | | | | | | | | | | |
| dark meat—*drumstick and thigh* | 148 | 337 | 1212 | 1462 | 2170 | 2324 | 780 | 419 | 1184 | 962 | 1443 | 1843 | 861 | 21035 |
| light meat—*side breast and wing* | 163 | 399 | 1439 | 1738 | 2577 | 2760 | 926 | 497 | 1405 | 1143 | 1715 | 2189 | 1024 | 21036 |
| **chicken fillet sandwich**—*1 sandwich* | 182 | 282 | 952 | 1212 | 1780 | 1744 | 608 | 333 | 1008 | 761 | 1199 | 1352 | 697 | 21102 |
| w/cheese—*1 sandwich* | 228 | 347 | 1081 | 1370 | 2177 | 2107 | 702 | 383 | 1261 | 1005 | 1475 | 1585 | 857 | 21103 |
| **chili con carne**—*8.9 oz (1 cup)* | 253 | 293 | 992 | 1020 | 1860 | 1839 | 481 | 253 | 1012 | 716 | 1161 | 1543 | 719 | 21042 |
| **chimichanga, beef**—*1 chimichanga* | 174 | 238 | 759 | 809 | 1514 | 1345 | 430 | 245 | 807 | 607 | 917 | 1197 | 578 | 21070 |
| w/cheese—*1 chimichanga* | 183 | 242 | 727 | 880 | 1570 | 1321 | 437 | 232 | 867 | 670 | 985 | 1076 | 586 | 21071 |
| w/cheese, red chilies—*1 chimichanga* | 180 | 175 | 518 | 598 | 1089 | 900 | 299 | 180 | 616 | 457 | 673 | 788 | 410 | 21073 |
| w/red chilies—*1 chimichanga* | 190 | 224 | 692 | 737 | 1383 | 1210 | 386 | 230 | 752 | 555 | 836 | 1094 | 530 | 21072 |
| **chocolate chip cookies**—*1 box* | 55 | 35 | 80 | 96 | 183 | 75 | 45 | 53 | 135 | 86 | 120 | 118 | 59 | 21030 |
| **cinnamon roll**, mini—*2 rolls* | 50 | 27 | 109 | 138 | 255 | 90 | 55 | 79 | 167 | 106 | 167 | 130 | 81 | 21388 |
| **clams**, breaded, fried—*¾ cup* | 115 | 151 | 457 | 536 | 891 | 620 | 261 | 215 | 558 | 381 | 596 | 699 | 261 | 21043 |
| **coleslaw**—*¾ cup* | 99 | 18 | 52 | 68 | 81 | 71 | 20 | 19 | 50 | 32 | 64 | 87 | 30 | 21127 |
| **corn**, yellow, on cob, boiled, buttered—*1 ear* | 146 | 32 | 180 | 180 | 483 | 191 | 93 | 36 | 209 | 171 | 258 | 181 | 124 | 21128 |
| **corndog**—*1 corndog* | 175 | 150 | 635 | 751 | 1414 | 1150 | 364 | 236 | 660 | 555 | 802 | 1115 | 507 | 21120 |
| **crabcake**—*2.1 oz cake* | 60 | 155 | 450 | 547 | 886 | 914 | 308 | 139 | 488 | 371 | 545 | 923 | 230 | 21046 |
| **croissant** | | | | | | | | | | | | | | |
| w/egg, cheese—*1 sandwich* | 127 | 184 | 476 | 634 | 1074 | 932 | 333 | 188 | 663 | 577 | 763 | 611 | 395 | 21011 |
| w/egg, cheese, bacon—*1 sandwich* | 129 | 224 | 606 | 787 | 1336 | 1186 | 415 | 231 | 815 | 702 | 948 | 800 | 498 | 21012 |
| w/egg, cheese, ham—*1 sandwich* | 154 | 259 | 778 | 915 | 1560 | 1392 | 500 | 311 | 933 | 741 | 1024 | 1055 | 594 | 21013 |
| w/egg, cheese, sausage—*1 sandwich* | 160 | 261 | 789 | 947 | 1602 | 1410 | 512 | 301 | 947 | 779 | 1106 | 1077 | 581 | 21014 |
| **Danish pastry** | | | | | | | | | | | | | | |
| cheese—*3.2 oz pastry* | 91 | 73 | 207 | 265 | 456 | 277 | 128 | 96 | 288 | 217 | 298 | 281 | 144 | 21015 |
| cinnamon—*3.1 oz pastry* | 88 | 63 | 167 | 214 | 365 | 197 | 106 | 97 | 244 | 167 | 245 | 220 | 112 | 21016 |
| fruit—*3.3 oz pastry* | 94 | 63 | 165 | 212 | 361 | 195 | 104 | 95 | 242 | 165 | 242 | 217 | 111 | 21017 |
| **egg drop soup**, Chinese Restaurant *8 fl oz* | 241 | 60 | 89 | 67 | 113 | 125 | 46 | 63 | 67 | 46 | 89 | 89 | 31 | 27000 |
| **eggs, scrambled**—*2 eggs* | 94 | 199 | 618 | 786 | 1114 | 858 | 401 | 289 | 705 | 528 | 902 | 786 | 306 | 21018 |

| | WT (g) | TRY | THR | ISO | LEU | LYS | MET | CYS | PHE | TYR | VAL | ARG | HIS | REF |
|---|---|---|---|---|---|---|---|---|---|---|---|---|---|---|
| | | | | | | | (mg/serving) | | | | | | | |
| **enchilada** | | | | | | | | | | | | | | |
| w/cheese, beef—*1 enchilada* | 192 | 132 | 459 | 528 | 1081 | 785 | 261 | 132 | 516 | 434 | 612 | 670 | 372 | 21075 |
| w/cheese, sour cream—*1 enchilada* | 163 | 99 | 324 | 461 | 879 | 570 | 205 | 83 | 440 | 390 | 526 | 380 | 287 | 21074 |
| **enchirito w**/cheese, beef, beans | | | | | | | | | | | | | | |
| *1 enchirito* | 193 | 197 | 674 | 786 | 1550 | 1183 | 376 | 181 | 774 | 627 | 905 | 977 | 540 | 21076 |
| **English muffin, toasted** | | | | | | | | | | | | | | |
| buttered—*1 muffin* | 63 | 60 | 153 | 187 | 344 | 161 | 88 | 95 | 242 | 157 | 215 | 209 | 112 | 21019 |
| w/cheese, sausage—*1 sandwich* | 115 | 167 | 549 | 572 | 1070 | 791 | 270 | 213 | 627 | 417 | 681 | 673 | 389 | 21020 |
| w/egg, cheese, Canadian bacon | | | | | | | | | | | | | | |
| *1 sandwich* | 137 | 240 | 715 | 756 | 1366 | 982 | 418 | 297 | 832 | 551 | 918 | 829 | 448 | 21021 |
| w/egg, cheese, sausage—*1 sandwich* | 165 | 269 | 863 | 891 | 1614 | 1238 | 474 | 327 | 970 | 668 | 1077 | 1077 | 544 | 21022 |
| **fish fillet,** battered/breaded, fried | | | | | | | | | | | | | | |
| *3.2 oz fillet* | 91 | 153 | 570 | 615 | 1083 | 1135 | 379 | 159 | 548 | 450 | 692 | 775 | 387 | 21047 |
| **fish sandwich,** tartar sauce | | | | | | | | | | | | | | |
| *5.6 oz sandwich* | 158 | 196 | 673 | 758 | 1322 | 1217 | 433 | 221 | 724 | 525 | 874 | 921 | 458 | 21105 |
| w/cheese—*6.5 oz sandwich* | 183 | 245 | 796 | 924 | 1634 | 1554 | 525 | 245 | 900 | 701 | 1082 | 1082 | 593 | 21106 |
| **frankfurter in bun**—*4 oz sandwich* | 114 | 112 | 410 | 516 | 877 | 731 | 227 | 168 | 475 | 321 | 551 | 759 | 336 | 21118 |
| with chili—*4 oz sandwich* | 114 | 129 | 465 | 567 | 972 | 831 | 253 | 179 | 528 | 359 | 609 | 836 | 372 | 21119 |
| **French fries**—*20 to 25 fries (regular size)* | 134 | 51 | 161 | 161 | 252 | 302 | 78 | 44 | 276 | 117 | 239 | 240 | 88 | 21138 |
| **French toast with butter**—*2 slices* | 135 | 143 | 405 | 532 | 817 | 506 | 246 | 200 | 536 | 346 | 625 | 518 | 235 | 21023 |
| **frijoles with cheese**—*1 cup* | 167 | 130 | 431 | 513 | 873 | 760 | 185 | 102 | 563 | 351 | 586 | 600 | 316 | 21077 |
| **ham and cheese sandwich**—*1 sandwich* | 146 | 270 | 739 | 911 | 1667 | 1572 | 486 | 250 | 993 | 821 | 1073 | 1016 | 705 | 21116 |
| **ham, egg, and cheese sandwich** | | | | | | | | | | | | | | |
| *1 sandwich* | 143 | 265 | 752 | 935 | 1572 | 1404 | 493 | 290 | 958 | 764 | 1091 | 1014 | 599 | 21117 |
| **hamburger** | | | | | | | | | | | | | | |
| ¼ lb—*6.1 oz sandwich* | 176 | 248 | 801 | 864 | 1577 | 1433 | 436 | 236 | 831 | 598 | 996 | 1248 | 598 | 21113 |
| large, double meat, lettuce, | | | | | | | | | | | | | | |
| tomato—*8 oz sandwich* | 226 | 414 | 1354 | 1442 | 2649 | 2504 | 746 | 371 | 1354 | 1012 | 1648 | 2133 | 1017 | 21114 |
| large, triple meat—*9.1 oz sandwich* | 259 | 614 | 2015 | 2129 | 3942 | 3838 | 1121 | 523 | 1958 | 1515 | 2427 | 3217 | 1523 | 21115 |
| reg, double meat—*6.2 oz sandwich* | 176 | 363 | 1172 | 1260 | 2321 | 2158 | 651 | 327 | 1192 | 884 | 1448 | 1853 | 889 | 21110 |
| reg, lettuce, tom—*3.9 oz sandwich* | 110 | 156 | 482 | 544 | 981 | 799 | 264 | 163 | 549 | 366 | 634 | 739 | 358 | 21109 |
| **hot and sour soup,** Chinese | | | | | | | | | | | | | | |
| restaurant—*8 fl oz* | 233 | 44 | 259 | 186 | 352 | 356 | 91 | 91 | 198 | 142 | 214 | 310 | 135 | 27001 |
| **hush puppies**—*5 pieces* | 78 | 52 | 201 | 227 | 520 | 226 | 119 | 90 | 245 | 201 | 283 | 257 | 135 | 21129 |
| **ice milk,** soft serve in cone—*1 cone* | 103 | 52 | 160 | 213 | 350 | 268 | 90 | 40 | 181 | 171 | 237 | 137 | 100 | 21028 |
| **nachos** | | | | | | | | | | | | | | |
| w/cheese—*6 to 8 nachos* | 113 | 77 | 329 | 376 | 1019 | 375 | 197 | 129 | 442 | 376 | 485 | 420 | 279 | 21078 |
| w/cheese and jalapenos—*6 to 8 nachos* | 204 | 151 | 594 | 745 | 1795 | 812 | 369 | 208 | 812 | 702 | 918 | 728 | 522 | 21079 |
| w/cheese, beans, ground beef, | | | | | | | | | | | | | | |
| peppers—*6 to 8 nachos* | 255 | 196 | 711 | 885 | 1912 | 1117 | 423 | 219 | 918 | 768 | 1056 | 913 | 599 | 21080 |
| w/cinnamon and sugar—*6 to 8 nachos* | 109 | 51 | 270 | 257 | 882 | 203 | 150 | 130 | 353 | 293 | 365 | 359 | 220 | 21081 |
| **onion rings,** breaded, fried—*8 to 9 rings* | 83 | 49 | 105 | 148 | 242 | 105 | 56 | 75 | 168 | 109 | 150 | 225 | 76 | 21130 |
| **oysters,** battered/breaded, fried | | | | | | | | | | | | | | |
| *6 oysters* | 139 | 149 | 470 | 528 | 880 | 681 | 267 | 206 | 531 | 388 | 573 | 739 | 256 | 21048 |
| **pancakes** w/butter and syrup—*2 pancakes* | 232 | 102 | 304 | 385 | 712 | 420 | 174 | 128 | 401 | 318 | 452 | 350 | 206 | 21025 |
| **pizza** | | | | | | | | | | | | | | |
| cheese, reg crust—*3.6 oz slice* | 103 | 132 | 422 | 581 | 1173 | 793 | 272 | 168 | 684 | 538 | 742 | 501 | 366 | 21299 |
| cheese, thick crust—*3.7 oz slice* | 106 | 139 | 423 | 588 | 1149 | 855 | 304 | 276 | 719 | 517 | 745 | 672 | 348 | 21300 |
| cheese, thin crust—*2.2 oz slice* | 63 | 92 | 324 | 414 | 841 | 606 | 202 | 126 | 489 | 381 | 532 | 349 | 227 | 21301 |
| meat and veg, reg crust—*4.8 oz slice* | 136 | 148 | 543 | 656 | 1255 | 836 | 295 | 242 | 752 | 524 | 787 | 691 | 454 | 21304 |
| pepperoni, reg crust—*3.8 oz slice* | 108 | 129 | 436 | 562 | 1116 | 798 | 284 | 184 | 652 | 504 | 700 | 563 | 377 | 21302 |
| pepperoni, thick crust—*3.7 oz slice* | 106 | 120 | 389 | 517 | 1048 | 741 | 270 | 287 | 642 | 440 | 646 | 523 | 340 | 21303 |
| **potato,** baked w/cheese sce—*1 potato* | 296 | 189 | 494 | 758 | 1157 | 1045 | 314 | 104 | 690 | 616 | 873 | 559 | 423 | 21131 |
| w/bacon—*1 potato* | 299 | 233 | 646 | 939 | 1453 | 1346 | 404 | 141 | 855 | 750 | 1085 | 777 | 541 | 21132 |
| w/broc—*1 potato* | 339 | 173 | 461 | 688 | 1034 | 946 | 281 | 98 | 620 | 546 | 797 | 542 | 380 | 21133 |
| w/chili—*1 potato* | 395 | 292 | 810 | 1153 | 1821 | 1671 | 490 | 178 | 1063 | 912 | 1327 | 995 | 672 | 21134 |
| **potato,** baked w/sour cream, | | | | | | | | | | | | | | |
| chives—*1 potato* | 302 | 100 | 257 | 305 | 468 | 435 | 121 | 79 | 299 | 263 | 390 | 290 | 154 | 21135 |
| **potato, hashed brown**—*½ cup serving* | 72 | 22 | 78 | 66 | 117 | 114 | 24 | 27 | 82 | 60 | 91 | 89 | 32 | 21026 |
| **potato, mashed**—*1 cup* | 240 | 84 | 211 | 250 | 382 | 358 | 101 | 65 | 250 | 218 | 324 | 240 | 127 | 21139 |
| **potato salad**—*⅓ cup* | 95 | 16 | 69 | 78 | 130 | 96 | 34 | 22 | 99 | 66 | 86 | 82 | 35 | 21140 |
| **roast beef sandwich**—*1 sandwich* | 139 | 245 | 874 | 944 | 1655 | 1544 | 509 | 265 | 881 | 680 | 1049 | 1262 | 680 | 21121 |
| w/cheese—*1 sandwich* | 176 | 373 | 1281 | 1417 | 2506 | 2392 | 762 | 378 | 1345 | 1084 | 1598 | 1827 | 1044 | 21122 |
| **roast beef sub**—*8 oz sub* | 216 | 324 | 1147 | 1248 | 2177 | 1979 | 659 | 363 | 1179 | 888 | 1393 | 1639 | 881 | 21125 |
| **salad, veg** | | | | | | | | | | | | | | |
| no dressing—*1½ cups* | 207 | 21 | 104 | 137 | 141 | 143 | 29 | 29 | 95 | 56 | 122 | 135 | 46 | 21052 |
| w/cheese, egg, no dressing—*1½ cups* | 217 | 102 | 341 | 499 | 690 | 599 | 200 | 102 | 414 | 330 | 527 | 401 | 226 | 21053 |
| w/chicken, no dressing—*1½ cups* | 218 | 198 | 735 | 924 | 1284 | 1445 | 460 | 222 | 689 | 576 | 863 | 1036 | 521 | 21054 |

| | WT | TRY | THR | ISO | LEU | LYS | MET | CYS | PHE | TYR | VAL | ARG | HIS | REF |
|---|---|---|---|---|---|---|---|---|---|---|---|---|---|---|
| | (g) | | | | | | (mg/serving) | | | | | | | |
| w/pasta, seafood, no dressing | | | | | | | | | | | | | | |
| 1½ cups | 417 | 192 | 613 | 746 | 1197 | 1059 | 367 | 254 | 688 | 492 | 780 | 934 | 384 | 21055 |
| w/shrimp, no dressing—1½ cups | 236 | 198 | 604 | 734 | 1123 | 1149 | 392 | 198 | 637 | 486 | 741 | 1130 | 297 | 21056 |
| w/turkey, ham, cheese, | | | | | | | | | | | | | | |
| no dressing—1½ cups | 326 | 303 | 1073 | 1343 | 2090 | 2142 | 675 | 287 | 1134 | 988 | 1389 | 1487 | 808 | 21057 |
| **scallops**, breaded, fried—6 scallops | 144 | 186 | 609 | 674 | 1109 | 916 | 343 | 251 | 652 | 494 | 723 | 966 | 317 | 21058 |
| **shake** | | | | | | | | | | | | | | |
| chocolate—12 fl oz | 250 | 120 | 385 | 515 | 835 | 675 | 213 | 78 | 410 | 410 | 570 | 308 | 232 | 14346 |
| strawberry—12 fl oz | 282 | 133 | 429 | 575 | 928 | 750 | 237 | 87 | 457 | 457 | 634 | 341 | 259 | 14428 |
| vanilla—12 fl oz | 250 | 145 | 380 | 395 | 885 | 670 | 238 | 95 | 422 | 308 | 485 | 262 | 225 | 14347 |
| **shrimp**, breaded, fried—6 to 8 shrimp | 164 | 253 | 707 | 868 | 1433 | 1269 | 477 | 274 | 846 | 607 | 902 | 1348 | 392 | 21059 |
| **steak sandwich,** lettuce, tomato, | | | | | | | | | | | | | | |
| mayo—1 sandwich | 204 | 369 | 1204 | 1287 | 2360 | 2217 | 663 | 335 | 1210 | 904 | 1475 | 1893 | 904 | 21123 |
| **sundae** | | | | | | | | | | | | | | |
| caramel—1 sundae | 155 | 98 | 313 | 422 | 680 | 550 | 174 | 64 | 336 | 336 | 467 | 251 | 191 | 21032 |
| hot fudge—1 sundae | 158 | 71 | 216 | 272 | 436 | 354 | 104 | 51 | 240 | 226 | 324 | 209 | 122 | 21033 |
| strawberry—1 sundae | 153 | 83 | 266 | 352 | 571 | 462 | 144 | 55 | 283 | 285 | 390 | 217 | 161 | 21034 |
| **taco** | | | | | | | | | | | | | | |
| 6 oz taco (small) | 263 | 352 | 1176 | 1486 | 2733 | 2249 | 707 | 279 | 1360 | 1168 | 1667 | 1625 | 981 | 21082 |
| 9.3 oz taco (large) | 263 | 352 | 1176 | 1486 | 2733 | 2249 | 707 | 279 | 1360 | 1168 | 1667 | 1625 | 981 | 21082 |
| **taco salad**—1½ cups | 198 | 148 | 503 | 616 | 1087 | 962 | 287 | 119 | 548 | 459 | 679 | 707 | 398 | 21083 |
| w/chili con carne—1½ cups | 261 | 193 | 647 | 817 | 1449 | 1216 | 363 | 159 | 770 | 613 | 911 | 882 | 519 | 21084 |
| **tostada** | | | | | | | | | | | | | | |
| w/beans, beef, cheese—1 tostada | 225 | 173 | 598 | 720 | 1370 | 1048 | 322 | 160 | 722 | 556 | 826 | 830 | 475 | 21086 |
| w/beans, cheese—1 tostada | 144 | 101 | 353 | 433 | 827 | 580 | 176 | 96 | 465 | 333 | 503 | 465 | 275 | 21085 |
| w/beef, cheese—1 tostada | 163 | 218 | 738 | 833 | 1581 | 1402 | 424 | 183 | 763 | 639 | 945 | 1105 | 588 | 21087 |
| w/guacamole—2 tostadas | 261 | 123 | 415 | 556 | 1073 | 676 | 251 | 120 | 540 | 457 | 645 | 483 | 337 | 21088 |
| **tuna salad sub**—9 oz sub | 256 | 343 | 1183 | 1334 | 2322 | 2156 | 755 | 384 | 1267 | 919 | 1526 | 1620 | 804 | 21126 |
| **wonton soup,** Chinese Restaurant—8 fl oz | 223 | 29 | 181 | 134 | 268 | 138 | 67 | 98 | 156 | 109 | 158 | 194 | 87 | 27002 |
| **BURGER KING** | | | | | | | | | | | | | | |
| **cheeseburger**—4.7 oz sandwich | 133 | 106 | 665 | 745 | 1450 | 1250 | 399 | 266 | 878 | 572 | 864 | 1024 | 492 | 21251 |
| Double Whopper—15 oz sandwich | 426 | 426 | 1704 | 2513 | 4516 | 4303 | 1235 | 469 | 2599 | 1619 | 2939 | 3238 | 1576 | 21255 |
| Whopper—13.9 oz sandwich | 395 | 356 | 1738 | 2014 | 3792 | 3318 | 1027 | 434 | 2212 | 1501 | 2370 | 2726 | 1264 | 21253 |
| **chicken sandwich**—7.2 oz sandwich | 204 | 306 | 775 | 1163 | 1979 | 1714 | 571 | 449 | 1183 | 694 | 1285 | 1448 | 775 | 21259 |
| **chicken tenders** | | | | | | | | | | | | | | |
| 2.7 oz (5 pieces) | 77 | 150 | 650 | 1039 | 1385 | 1406 | 452 | 176 | 767 | 492 | 883 | 1065 | 650 | 21256 |
| 4.3 oz (8 pieces) | 123 | 150 | 650 | 1039 | 1385 | 1406 | 452 | 176 | 767 | 492 | 883 | 1065 | 650 | 21256 |
| **Chicken Whopper sandwich** | | | | | | | | | | | | | | |
| 9.6 oz sandwich | 272 | 272 | 1115 | 1360 | 2475 | 2339 | 680 | 354 | 1387 | 789 | 1469 | 1659 | 1006 | 21257 |
| **croissant** | | | | | | | | | | | | | | |
| w/egg and cheese—4 oz Croissan'wich | 112 | 112 | 403 | 544 | 969 | 614 | 259 | 221 | 591 | 441 | 679 | 542 | 295 | 21385 |
| w/sausage and cheese | | | | | | | | | | | | | | |
| 3.8 oz Croissan'wich | 107 | 119 | 514 | 618 | 1120 | 876 | 279 | 190 | 628 | 495 | 735 | 727 | 440 | 21384 |
| w/sausage, egg, cheese | | | | | | | | | | | | | | |
| 5.5 oz Croissan'wich | 157 | 168 | 688 | 867 | 1553 | 1234 | 416 | 295 | 889 | 685 | 1064 | 1039 | 565 | 21383 |
| **French fries** | | | | | | | | | | | | | | |
| 2.6 oz serving (small) | 74 | 41 | 164 | 229 | 252 | 392 | 89 | 16 | 215 | 143 | 243 | 268 | 95 | 21249 |
| 4.1 oz serving (medium) | 117 | 41 | 164 | 229 | 252 | 392 | 89 | 16 | 215 | 143 | 243 | 268 | 95 | 21249 |
| 5.6 oz serving (large) | 160 | 41 | 164 | 229 | 252 | 392 | 89 | 16 | 215 | 143 | 243 | 268 | 95 | 21249 |
| 6.8 oz serving (king) | 194 | 41 | 164 | 229 | 252 | 392 | 89 | 16 | 215 | 143 | 243 | 268 | 95 | 21249 |
| **French toast sticks**—4 oz (5 sticks) | 113 | 54 | 201 | 264 | 497 | 174 | 97 | 153 | 334 | 209 | 314 | 292 | 165 | 21386 |
| **hamburger**—4.3 oz sandwich | 121 | 82 | 543 | 649 | 1235 | 960 | 330 | 57 | 755 | 407 | 751 | 908 | 431 | 21250 |
| Double Whopper—14 oz sandwich | 401 | 401 | 1644 | 2206 | 3930 | 3810 | 1083 | 481 | 2246 | 1363 | 2526 | 3088 | 1444 | 21254 |
| Whopper—10.7 oz sandwich | 304 | 213 | 1137 | 1049 | 2316 | 1803 | 632 | | 1401 | 815 | 1265 | 1745 | 769 | 21252 |
| **Hash Brown Rounds** | | | | | | | | | | | | | | |
| 2.6 oz | 75 | 36 | 124 | 131 | 185 | 180 | 38 | 43 | 129 | 94 | 144 | 139 | 51 | 21387 |
| 4.5 oz | 128 | 36 | 124 | 131 | 185 | 180 | 38 | 43 | 129 | 94 | 144 | 139 | 51 | 21387 |
| **DOMINO'S** | | | | | | | | | | | | | | |
| **pizza** | | | | | | | | | | | | | | |
| cheese, Deep Dish Crust—3.7 oz slice | 106 | 121 | 404 | 545 | 991 | 673 | 298 | 175 | 690 | 504 | 686 | 868 | 382 | 21278 |
| cheese, Thin Crust—1.4 oz slice | 39 | 41 | 164 | 228 | 469 | 343 | 129 | 60 | 271 | 197 | 293 | 197 | 143 | 21279 |
| Extravaganzza, Hand-Tossed | | | | | | | | | | | | | | |
| Crust—5.3 oz slice | 151 | 125 | 482 | 657 | 1293 | 802 | 343 | 207 | 791 | 509 | 799 | 698 | 581 | 21282 |
| Hand-Tossed Crust—4.2 oz slice | 120 | 97 | 367 | 503 | 990 | 674 | 254 | 198 | 635 | 361 | 610 | 523 | 322 | 21280 |
| pepperoni, Deep Dish Crust | | | | | | | | | | | | | | |
| 4.5 oz slice | 127 | 144 | 456 | 591 | 1217 | 834 | 312 | 236 | 761 | 464 | 744 | 607 | 382 | 21281 |

| | WT (g) | TRY | THR | ISO | LEU | LYS | MET | CYS | PHE | TYR | VAL | ARG | HIS | REF |
|---|---|---|---|---|---|---|---|---|---|---|---|---|---|---|
| | | | | | | | (mg/serving) | | | | | | | |
| **LITTLE CAESAR'S PIZZA** | | | | | | | | | | | | | | |
| **pizza** | | | | | | | | | | | | | | |
| cheese, deep dish crust—*3.6 oz slice* | 102 | 159 | 444 | 645 | 1306 | 1134 | 319 | 482 | 781 | 516 | 822 | 630 | 297 | 21290 |
| cheese, regular crust—*3.1 oz slice* | 89 | 134 | 350 | 487 | 1012 | 465 | 267 | 298 | 638 | 448 | 623 | 457 | 320 | 21287 |
| cheese, thin crust—*1.7 oz slice* | 48 | 65 | 267 | 383 | 794 | 637 | 221 | 209 | 462 | 393 | 504 | 336 | 123 | 21292 |
| meat and veg, reg crust—*4.1 oz slice* | 115 | 130 | 452 | 637 | 1178 | 662 | 322 | 397 | 695 | 514 | 744 | 664 | 402 | 21289 |
| pepperoni, deep dish crust—*3.7 oz slice* | 104 | 114 | 384 | 536 | 1109 | 827 | 286 | 482 | 687 | 474 | 666 | 541 | 356 | 21291 |
| pepperoni, regular crust—*3.2 oz slice* | 90 | 117 | 387 | 561 | 1098 | 834 | 291 | 318 | 678 | 447 | 699 | 543 | 354 | 21288 |
| **McDONALD'S** | | | | | | | | | | | | | | |
| **shake** | | | | | | | | | | | | | | |
| chocolate—*12 fl oz* | 250 | 120 | 385 | 515 | 835 | 675 | 213 | 78 | 410 | 410 | 570 | 308 | 232 | 14346 |
| vanilla—*12 fl oz* | 250 | 145 | 380 | 395 | 885 | 670 | 238 | 95 | 422 | 308 | 485 | 262 | 225 | 14347 |
| **PAPA JOHN'S** | | | | | | | | | | | | | | |
| **pizza** | | | | | | | | | | | | | | |
| cheese, thin crust—*3.1 oz slice* | 87 | 124 | 416 | 476 | 961 | 644 | 196 | 113 | 577 | 422 | 607 | 396 | 287 | 21286 |
| pepperoni, regular crust—*4.3 oz slice* | 123 | 156 | 590 | 648 | 1316 | 857 | 261 | 191 | 806 | 556 | 806 | 621 | 412 | 21284 |
| The Works, regular crust—*5.4 oz slice* | 153 | 161 | 604 | 635 | 1270 | 834 | 256 | 214 | 796 | 517 | 765 | 673 | 421 | 21285 |
| **PIZZA HUT** | | | | | | | | | | | | | | |
| **pizza, cheese** | | | | | | | | | | | | | | |
| regular crust—*3.7 oz slice* | 106 | 136 | 436 | 599 | 1208 | 817 | 280 | 173 | 705 | 553 | 764 | 516 | 376 | 21271 |
| regular crust, 14″ dia—*3.5 oz slice* | 100 | 148 | 477 | 518 | 1037 | 660 | 207 | 132 | 610 | 407 | 652 | 432 | 312 | 21293 |
| thick crust, 14″ dia—*3.4 oz slice* | 95 | 136 | 472 | 513 | 1036 | 672 | 201 | 130 | 603 | 401 | 648 | 423 | 315 | 21294 |
| Thin n' Crispy—*2.8 oz slice* | 85 | 134 | 427 | 592 | 1180 | 844 | 276 | 144 | 676 | 583 | 766 | 495 | 363 | 21273 |
| Thin n' Crispy, 14″ dia—*2.7 oz slice* | 76 | 144 | 464 | 507 | 1018 | 683 | 205 | 106 | 585 | 420 | 636 | 407 | 306 | 21295 |
| **pizza, pepperoni** | | | | | | | | | | | | | | |
| regular crust, 14″ dia—*3.6 oz slice* | 101 | 157 | 525 | 535 | 1063 | 785 | 207 | 144 | 618 | 424 | 656 | 525 | 343 | 21296 |
| regular crust—*4.1 oz slice* | 116 | 143 | 485 | 624 | 1239 | 886 | 316 | 204 | 725 | 560 | 777 | 624 | 419 | 21274 |
| thick crust, 14″ dia—*3.5 oz slice* | 85 | 129 | 425 | 446 | 869 | 597 | 178 | 116 | 503 | 329 | 533 | 425 | 285 | 21297 |
| **pizza, Super Supreme** | | | | | | | | | | | | | | |
| regular crust—*4.9 oz slice* | 139 | 146 | 534 | 674 | 1294 | 987 | 296 | 213 | 758 | 591 | 833 | 739 | 449 | 21276 |
| regular crust, 14″ dia—*4.5 oz slice* | 127 | 175 | 640 | 669 | 1240 | 903 | 254 | 169 | 724 | 484 | 792 | 678 | 420 | 21298 |
| **TACO BELL** | | | | | | | | | | | | | | |
| **burrito** | | | | | | | | | | | | | | |
| bean—*7 oz burrito* | 198 | 178 | 590 | 618 | 1192 | 927 | 228 | 184 | 772 | 485 | 742 | 723 | 416 | 21264 |
| Supreme, beef—*8.7 oz burrito* | 247 | 193 | 741 | 746 | 1425 | 1193 | 324 | 237 | 889 | 585 | 897 | 961 | 516 | 21265 |
| Supreme, chicken—*8.7 oz burrito* | 247 | 272 | 921 | 946 | 1719 | 1549 | 440 | 272 | 1037 | 699 | 1084 | 1168 | 699 | 21266 |
| Supreme, steak—*8.7 oz burrito* | 247 | 267 | 921 | 921 | 1714 | 1522 | 408 | 272 | 1028 | 674 | 1057 | 1144 | 613 | 21267 |
| **nachos**—*3.2 oz* | 90 | 47 | 171 | 166 | 498 | 225 | 87 | 69 | 237 | 166 | 214 | 183 | 124 | 21268 |
| Supreme—*6.8 oz* | 194 | 146 | 568 | 545 | 1187 | 879 | 239 | 155 | 706 | 423 | 630 | 743 | 378 | 21269 |
| **taco** | | | | | | | | | | | | | | |
| beef—*2.75 oz taco* | 78 | 76 | 353 | 332 | 701 | 593 | 168 | 86 | 367 | 263 | 404 | 463 | 239 | 21260 |
| salad—*16.8 oz salad* | 475 | 408 | 1264 | 1273 | 2465 | 2095 | 570 | 370 | 1615 | 1036 | 1477 | 1643 | 855 | 21270 |
| soft, beef—*3.5 oz taco* | 99 | 104 | 365 | 373 | 714 | 618 | 193 | 119 | 415 | 297 | 449 | 484 | 257 | 21261 |
| soft, chicken—*3.5 oz taco* | 99 | 151 | 562 | 590 | 1062 | 987 | 312 | 156 | 583 | 438 | 675 | 713 | 446 | 21262 |
| soft, steak—*4.5 oz taco* | 127 | 184 | 638 | 635 | 1177 | 1035 | 320 | 187 | 692 | 493 | 714 | 785 | 413 | 21263 |
| **Wendy's** | | | | | | | | | | | | | | |
| **cheeseburger** | | | | | | | | | | | | | | |
| Classic Double—*10.9 oz sandwich* | 310 | 496 | 1767 | 1829 | 3286 | 3131 | 1054 | 558 | 1767 | 1085 | 2108 | 2511 | 1178 | 21243 |
| Classic Single—*8.3 oz sandwich* | 236 | 283 | 1062 | 1109 | 2006 | 1841 | 590 | 330 | 1109 | 637 | 1251 | 1487 | 732 | 21240 |
| Junior—*4.6 oz sandwich* | 129 | 168 | 568 | 619 | 1122 | 903 | 322 | 206 | 645 | 335 | 710 | 748 | 387 | 21242 |
| **chicken fillet sandwich** | | | | | | | | | | | | | | |
| *8.1 oz sandwich* | 230 | 345 | 1150 | 1242 | 2139 | 1909 | 667 | 414 | 1173 | 621 | 1357 | 1495 | 874 | 21244 |
| **chicken grill sandwich** | | | | | | | | | | | | | | |
| *6.6 oz sandwich* | 188 | 320 | 1072 | 1166 | 1955 | 1861 | 602 | 357 | 1053 | 602 | 1241 | 1429 | 790 | 21245 |
| **Chicken Nuggets** | | | | | | | | | | | | | | |
| *2.1 oz kid's meal (4 pieces)* | 60 | 111 | 406 | 476 | 745 | 736 | 241 | 119 | 392 | 240 | 466 | 567 | 317 | 21246 |
| *2.6 oz (5 pieces)* | 75 | 111 | 406 | 476 | 745 | 736 | 241 | 119 | 392 | 240 | 466 | 567 | 317 | 21246 |
| **French fries** | | | | | | | | | | | | | | |
| *3.2 oz serving (kid's meal size)* | 91 | 65 | 185 | 238 | 288 | 258 | 80 | 65 | 223 | 112 | 262 | 255 | 90 | 21247 |
| *5 oz serving (medium)* | 142 | 65 | 185 | 238 | 288 | 258 | 80 | 65 | 223 | 112 | 262 | 255 | 90 | 21247 |
| *5.6 oz serving (Biggie)* | 159 | 65 | 185 | 238 | 288 | 258 | 80 | 65 | 223 | 112 | 262 | 255 | 90 | 21247 |
| *6.7 oz serving (Great Biggie)* | 190 | 65 | 185 | 238 | 288 | 258 | 80 | 65 | 223 | 112 | 262 | 255 | 90 | 21247 |

| | WT | TRY | THR | ISO | LEU | LYS | MET | CYS | PHE | TYR | VAL | ARG | HIS | REF |
|---|---|---|---|---|---|---|---|---|---|---|---|---|---|---|
| | (g) | | | | | | (mg/serving) | | | | | | | |
| **frosty dairy dessert** | | | | | | | | | | | | | | |
| 6 fl oz (junior) | 113 | 85 | 319 | 447 | 617 | 532 | 149 | 85 | 298 | 255 | 383 | 234 | 170 | 21248 |
| 12 fl oz (small) | 227 | 85 | 319 | 447 | 617 | 532 | 149 | 85 | 298 | 255 | 383 | 234 | 170 | 21248 |
| 16 fl oz (medium) | 298 | 85 | 319 | 447 | 617 | 532 | 149 | 85 | 298 | 255 | 383 | 234 | 170 | 21248 |
| **hamburger** | | | | | | | | | | | | | | |
| Classic Single—7.7 oz sandwich | 218 | 290 | 1001 | 1001 | 1803 | 1676 | 523 | 334 | 1005 | 547 | 1142 | 1452 | 656 | 21239 |
| Junior—4.2 oz sandwich | 117 | 137 | 480 | 497 | 914 | 723 | 260 | 187 | 536 | 246 | 565 | 661 | 331 | 21241 |

## 11. FATS, OILS, SHORTENINGS, AND SPREADS

### ANIMAL FATS

| | WT | TRY | THR | ISO | LEU | LYS | MET | CYS | PHE | TYR | VAL | ARG | HIS | REF |
|---|---|---|---|---|---|---|---|---|---|---|---|---|---|---|
| **beef** | | | | | | | | | | | | | | |
| **fat**, cooked—1 oz | 28 | 20 | 119 | 136 | 237 | 252 | 78 | 38 | 118 | 95 | 148 | 193 | 95 | 13020 |
| **suet**, raw—1 oz | 28 | 3 | 17 | 19 | 33 | 36 | 11 | 5 | 17 | 13 | 21 | 27 | 13 | 13335 |
| **lamb fat**, cooked—1 oz | 28 | 40 | 146 | 164 | 265 | 300 | 87 | 41 | 139 | 115 | 184 | 202 | 108 | 17006 |
| **pork** | | | | | | | | | | | | | | |
| **backfat**, raw—1 oz | 28 | 10 | 37 | 38 | 66 | 74 | 22 | 10 | 33 | 29 | 44 | 51 | 33 | 10004 |
| **fat**, cooked—1 oz | 28 | 26 | 111 | 122 | 211 | 230 | 68 | 29 | 104 | 94 | 130 | 165 | 107 | 10007 |
| **fat**, raw—1 oz | 28 | 17 | 73 | 80 | 139 | 151 | 45 | 19 | 69 | 62 | 85 | 108 | 70 | 10006 |
| **salt pork**, raw—1 oz | 28 | 5 | 46 | 37 | 99 | 117 | 21 | 12 | 53 | 23 | 68 | 146 | 16 | 10165 |
| Spreads | | | | | | | | | | | | | | |
| **butter**—1 T | 14 | 2 | 5 | 7 | 12 | 9 | 3 | 1 | 6 | 6 | 8 | 4 | 3 | 1001 |
| sweet (unsalted)—1 T | 14 | 2 | 5 | 7 | 12 | 9 | 3 | 1 | 6 | 6 | 8 | 4 | 3 | 1145 |
| whipped—1 T | 9 | 1 | 3 | 5 | 7 | 6 | 2 | 1 | 4 | 4 | 5 | 3 | 2 | 1002 |
| **margarine** | | | | | | | | | | | | | | |
| liquid—1 T | 14 | 4 | 12 | 16 | 26 | 21 | 7 | 3 | 13 | 13 | 18 | 10 | 7 | 4105 |
| unspecified oils—1 T | 14 | 2 | 5 | 7 | 12 | 10 | 3 | 1 | 6 | 6 | 8 | 4 | 3 | 4132 |
| **mayonnaise** | | | | | | | | | | | | | | |
| diet, no cholesterol—1 T | 15 | 2 | 7 | 8 | 12 | 9 | 3 | 2 | 6 | 6 | 8 | 9 | 3 | 43599 |
| safflower and soy—1 T | 14 | 2 | 8 | 9 | 13 | 10 | 5 | 3 | 8 | 6 | 10 | 10 | 4 | 4026 |
| soy—1 T | 14 | 2 | 8 | 9 | 13 | 10 | 5 | 3 | 8 | 6 | 10 | 10 | 4 | 4025 |
| **sandwich spread** (mayo-based)—1 T | 15 | 2 | 7 | 8 | 12 | 9 | 3 | 2 | 6 | 6 | 8 | 9 | 3 | 4030 |

## 12. FISH AND SEAFOOD

### CRUSTACEA

| | WT | TRY | THR | ISO | LEU | LYS | MET | CYS | PHE | TYR | VAL | ARG | HIS | REF |
|---|---|---|---|---|---|---|---|---|---|---|---|---|---|---|
| **crab, Alaska king** | | | | | | | | | | | | | | |
| cooked by moist heat—3 oz | 85 | 229 | 666 | 797 | 1306 | 1431 | 463 | 184 | 694 | 547 | 774 | 1436 | 334 | 15137 |
| imitation, made from surimi—3 oz | 85 | 64 | 242 | 196 | 516 | 601 | 222 | 68 | 221 | 186 | 243 | 415 | 133 | 15138 |
| raw—3 oz | 85 | 217 | 630 | 754 | 1234 | 1353 | 438 | 174 | 657 | 518 | 732 | 1358 | 316 | 15136 |
| **crab, blue** | | | | | | | | | | | | | | |
| canned—3 oz | 85 | 243 | 706 | 846 | 1384 | 1518 | 491 | 196 | 737 | 581 | 820 | 1524 | 354 | 15141 |
| cooked by moist heat—3 oz | 85 | 239 | 695 | 832 | 1363 | 1494 | 484 | 192 | 725 | 571 | 808 | 1500 | 348 | 15140 |
| raw—3 oz | 85 | 213 | 621 | 744 | 1218 | 1336 | 432 | 172 | 649 | 511 | 722 | 1340 | 312 | 15139 |
| **crab, dungeness** | | | | | | | | | | | | | | |
| ckd by moist heat—3 oz | 85 | 264 | 765 | 917 | 1503 | 1648 | 535 | 212 | 798 | 632 | 889 | 1654 | 386 | 15226 |
| raw—3 oz | 85 | 206 | 599 | 717 | 1174 | 1288 | 416 | 166 | 625 | 492 | 696 | 1293 | 301 | 15143 |
| **crab, queen** | | | | | | | | | | | | | | |
| cooked by moist heat—3 oz | 85 | 280 | 813 | 974 | 1596 | 1752 | 568 | 226 | 848 | 671 | 945 | 1758 | 410 | 15227 |
| raw—3 oz | 85 | 219 | 637 | 762 | 1248 | 1368 | 443 | 176 | 664 | 524 | 740 | 1374 | 320 | 15144 |
| **crabcake**—2.1 oz cake | 60 | 169 | 497 | 598 | 970 | 1040 | 341 | 143 | 522 | 409 | 588 | 1038 | 248 | 15142 |
| **crayfish, farmed** | | | | | | | | | | | | | | |
| ckd by moist heat—3 oz | 85 | 207 | 601 | 720 | 1180 | 1295 | 420 | 167 | 626 | 496 | 699 | 1299 | 303 | 15243 |
| raw—3 oz | 85 | 176 | 509 | 610 | 1000 | 1096 | 355 | 141 | 531 | 420 | 592 | 1101 | 257 | 15242 |
| **crayfish, wild** | | | | | | | | | | | | | | |
| ckd by moist heat—3 oz | 85 | 199 | 575 | 689 | 1130 | 1238 | 401 | 160 | 600 | 474 | 668 | 1244 | 290 | 15146 |
| raw—3 oz | 85 | 189 | 547 | 656 | 1075 | 1180 | 382 | 152 | 571 | 452 | 637 | 1184 | 276 | 15145 |
| **lobster, northern** | | | | | | | | | | | | | | |
| ckd by moist heat—3 oz | 85 | 242 | 706 | 845 | 1383 | 1516 | 490 | 196 | 736 | 580 | 819 | 1522 | 354 | 15148 |
| raw—3 oz | 85 | 223 | 647 | 774 | 1268 | 1391 | 450 | 179 | 675 | 532 | 751 | 1396 | 325 | 15147 |
| **shrimp** | | | | | | | | | | | | | | |
| breaded and fried—3 oz (11 large) | 85 | 254 | 731 | 886 | 1443 | 1499 | 502 | 219 | 789 | 611 | 871 | 1516 | 371 | 15150 |
| canned—3 oz | 85 | 158 | 700 | 828 | 1429 | 1541 | 473 | 206 | 804 | 688 | 795 | 1386 | 412 | 15152 |
| ckd by moist heat—3 oz | 85 | 247 | 719 | 862 | 1410 | 1547 | 501 | 199 | 751 | 592 | 836 | 1552 | 361 | 15151 |
| imitation, made from surimi—3 oz | 85 | 64 | 509 | 492 | 834 | 962 | 357 | 113 | 413 | 424 | 534 | 700 | 242 | 15153 |
| raw—3 oz | 85 | 241 | 699 | 837 | 1370 | 1503 | 486 | 194 | 729 | 575 | 813 | 1509 | 351 | 15149 |
| **spiny lobster** | | | | | | | | | | | | | | |
| ckd by dry heat—3 oz | 85 | 313 | 905 | 1085 | 1778 | 1951 | 632 | 252 | 944 | 747 | 1052 | 1958 | 456 | 15228 |
| raw—3 oz | 85 | 244 | 709 | 848 | 1389 | 1523 | 493 | 196 | 740 | 582 | 824 | 1529 | 355 | 15154 |

| | WT (g) | TRY | THR | ISO | LEU | LYS | MET | CYS | PHE | TYR | VAL | ARG | HIS | REF |
|---|---|---|---|---|---|---|---|---|---|---|---|---|---|---|
| | | | | | | | (mg/serving) | | | | | | | |
| **FINFISH** | | | | | | | | | | | | | | |
| **anchovies**, canned in olive oil | | | | | | | | | | | | | | |
| canned in olive oil—*5 anchovies* | 20 | 65 | 253 | 266 | 470 | 531 | 171 | 62 | 226 | 195 | 298 | 346 | 170 | 15002 |
| raw—*3 oz* | 85 | 194 | 758 | 797 | 1406 | 1589 | 512 | 185 | 675 | 584 | 891 | 1034 | 509 | 15001 |
| **bass, freshwater** | | | | | | | | | | | | | | |
| ckd by dry heat—*3 oz* | 85 | 230 | 901 | 947 | 1670 | 1888 | 609 | 220 | 802 | 694 | 1059 | 1230 | 605 | 15187 |
| raw—*3 oz* | 85 | 179 | 703 | 739 | 1303 | 1472 | 474 | 172 | 626 | 541 | 825 | 959 | 472 | 15003 |
| **bass, striped** | | | | | | | | | | | | | | |
| ckd by dry heat—*3 oz* | 85 | 217 | 847 | 890 | 1571 | 1775 | 572 | 207 | 754 | 652 | 995 | 1156 | 569 | 15188 |
| raw—*3 oz* | 85 | 169 | 660 | 694 | 1225 | 1384 | 446 | 162 | 588 | 509 | 777 | 902 | 444 | 15004 |
| **bluefish** | | | | | | | | | | | | | | |
| ckd by dry heat—*3 oz* | 85 | 245 | 957 | 1006 | 1775 | 2006 | 646 | 234 | 853 | 737 | 1125 | 1306 | 643 | 15189 |
| raw—*3 oz* | 85 | 190 | 746 | 785 | 1385 | 1564 | 504 | 183 | 665 | 575 | 877 | 1019 | 502 | 15005 |
| **burbot** | | | | | | | | | | | | | | |
| ckd by dry heat—*3 oz* | 85 | 235 | 922 | 970 | 1710 | 1933 | 623 | 225 | 821 | 711 | 1084 | 1259 | 620 | 15190 |
| raw—*3 oz* | 85 | 184 | 720 | 756 | 1334 | 1508 | 486 | 176 | 641 | 554 | 846 | 983 | 484 | 15006 |
| **butterfish** | | | | | | | | | | | | | | |
| ckd by dry heat—*3 oz* | 85 | 211 | 825 | 868 | 1531 | 1730 | 558 | 201 | 735 | 636 | 970 | 1127 | 554 | 15191 |
| raw—*3 oz* | 85 | 165 | 644 | 677 | 1194 | 1349 | 435 | 157 | 574 | 496 | 756 | 879 | 433 | 15007 |
| **carp** | | | | | | | | | | | | | | |
| ckd by dry heat—*3 oz* | 85 | 218 | 852 | 896 | 1579 | 1785 | 575 | 208 | 759 | 656 | 1001 | 1163 | 572 | 15009 |
| raw—*3 oz* | 85 | 170 | 665 | 699 | 1232 | 1392 | 449 | 162 | 592 | 512 | 781 | 907 | 446 | 15008 |
| **catfish, channel** | | | | | | | | | | | | | | |
| breaded and fried—*3 oz* | 85 | 170 | 672 | 711 | 1282 | 1357 | 448 | 174 | 617 | 529 | 802 | 915 | 450 | 15011 |
| farmed, cooked by dry heat—*3 oz* | 85 | 178 | 698 | 733 | 1293 | 1461 | 471 | 171 | 621 | 537 | 819 | 952 | 468 | 15235 |
| farmed, raw—*3 oz* | 85 | 148 | 580 | 609 | 1074 | 1215 | 391 | 142 | 516 | 446 | 681 | 791 | 389 | 15234 |
| wild, ckd by dry heat—*3 oz* | 85 | 176 | 688 | 723 | 1277 | 1442 | 465 | 168 | 613 | 530 | 809 | 940 | 462 | 15233 |
| wild, raw—*3 oz* | 85 | 156 | 610 | 642 | 1131 | 1278 | 412 | 150 | 543 | 470 | 717 | 833 | 410 | 15010 |
| **cisco** | | | | | | | | | | | | | | |
| raw—*3 oz* | 85 | 181 | 707 | 744 | 1312 | 1482 | 478 | 173 | 630 | 545 | 831 | 966 | 475 | 15013 |
| smoked—*3 oz* | 85 | 156 | 609 | 641 | 1130 | 1278 | 411 | 149 | 543 | 469 | 717 | 832 | 410 | 15014 |
| **cod, Atlantic** | | | | | | | | | | | | | | |
| cnd, solids and liquids—*3 oz* | 85 | 217 | 848 | 892 | 1572 | 1777 | 573 | 207 | 756 | 653 | 997 | 1158 | 570 | 15017 |
| ckd by dry heat—*3 oz* | 85 | 218 | 851 | 894 | 1578 | 1782 | 575 | 208 | 757 | 655 | 1000 | 1161 | 571 | 15016 |
| dried and salted—*3 oz* | 85 | 598 | 2341 | 2461 | 4340 | 4904 | 1580 | 572 | 2084 | 1803 | 2751 | 3195 | 1572 | 15018 |
| raw—*3 oz* | 85 | 169 | 664 | 698 | 1230 | 1390 | 448 | 162 | 591 | 511 | 779 | 906 | 445 | 15015 |
| **cod, Pacific** | | | | | | | | | | | | | | |
| ckd by dry heat—*3 oz* | 85 | 218 | 855 | 898 | 1585 | 1792 | 577 | 209 | 762 | 659 | 1005 | 1167 | 575 | 15192 |
| raw—*3 oz* | 85 | 170 | 667 | 701 | 1237 | 1397 | 450 | 163 | 594 | 513 | 784 | 910 | 448 | 15019 |
| **croaker, Atlantic** | | | | | | | | | | | | | | |
| breaded and fried—*3 oz* | 85 | 177 | 670 | 720 | 1258 | 1335 | 446 | 184 | 631 | 528 | 805 | 902 | 446 | 15021 |
| raw—*3 oz* | 85 | 169 | 663 | 696 | 1228 | 1388 | 447 | 162 | 590 | 510 | 779 | 904 | 445 | 15020 |
| **cusk** | | | | | | | | | | | | | | |
| ckd by dry heat—*3 oz* | 85 | 232 | 907 | 954 | 1682 | 1901 | 613 | 222 | 808 | 699 | 1066 | 1238 | 609 | 15193 |
| raw—*3 oz* | 85 | 181 | 708 | 744 | 1312 | 1482 | 478 | 173 | 631 | 545 | 832 | 966 | 475 | 15022 |
| **dolphinfish** | | | | | | | | | | | | | | |
| ckd by dry heat—*3 oz* | 85 | 226 | 884 | 929 | 1639 | 1851 | 597 | 216 | 787 | 681 | 1039 | 1206 | 593 | 15194 |
| raw—*3 oz* | 85 | 176 | 689 | 724 | 1278 | 1444 | 466 | 168 | 614 | 531 | 810 | 941 | 463 | 15023 |
| **drum, freshwater** | | | | | | | | | | | | | | |
| ckd by dry heat—*3 oz* | 85 | 214 | 838 | 881 | 1554 | 1755 | 566 | 205 | 746 | 645 | 985 | 1144 | 563 | 15195 |
| raw—*3 oz* | 85 | 167 | 654 | 687 | 1211 | 1369 | 441 | 160 | 582 | 503 | 768 | 892 | 439 | 15024 |
| **eel** | | | | | | | | | | | | | | |
| ckd by dry heat—*3 oz* | 85 | 225 | 881 | 927 | 1634 | 1845 | 595 | 215 | 785 | 678 | 1035 | 1203 | 592 | 15026 |
| raw—*3 oz* | 85 | 176 | 688 | 722 | 1274 | 1440 | 464 | 168 | 612 | 530 | 808 | 938 | 462 | 15025 |
| **fish sticks/pieces**, frozen, reheated | | | | | | | | | | | | | | |
| *1 stick (4″ × 1″ × ½″)* | 28 | 47 | 164 | 181 | 320 | 300 | 106 | 55 | 171 | 134 | 202 | 220 | 111 | 15027 |
| **flounder/sole** (flatfish) | | | | | | | | | | | | | | |
| ckd by dry heat—*3 oz* | 85 | 230 | 900 | 946 | 1669 | 1886 | 608 | 220 | 802 | 694 | 1058 | 1229 | 604 | 15029 |
| raw—*3 oz* | 85 | 179 | 702 | 738 | 1302 | 1471 | 474 | 172 | 626 | 541 | 825 | 959 | 472 | 15028 |
| **gefiltefish** with broth, sweet | 42 | 36 | 205 | 204 | 340 | 354 | 107 | 47 | 207 | 160 | 230 | 250 | 110 | 15030 |
| **grouper** | | | | | | | | | | | | | | |
| ckd by dry heat—*3 oz* | 85 | 236 | 926 | 973 | 1716 | 1940 | 625 | 226 | 824 | 713 | 1088 | 1264 | 621 | 15032 |
| raw—*3 oz* | 85 | 184 | 722 | 759 | 1339 | 1512 | 488 | 177 | 643 | 556 | 848 | 985 | 484 | 15031 |
| **haddock** | | | | | | | | | | | | | | |
| ckd by dry heat—*3 oz* | 85 | 231 | 904 | 949 | 1675 | 1893 | 610 | 221 | 804 | 695 | 1062 | 1233 | 607 | 15034 |
| raw—*3 oz* | 85 | 180 | 705 | 740 | 1306 | 1476 | 476 | 173 | 627 | 542 | 828 | 961 | 473 | 15033 |
| smoked—*3 oz* | 85 | 241 | 940 | 988 | 1742 | 1969 | 635 | 230 | 837 | 724 | 1105 | 1283 | 632 | 15035 |

| | WT | TRY | THR | ISO | LEU | LYS | MET | CYS | PHE | TYR | VAL | ARG | HIS | REF |
|---|---|---|---|---|---|---|---|---|---|---|---|---|---|---|
| | (g) | | | | | | (mg/serving) | | | | | | | |
| **halibut, Alaskan**, cooked with | | | | | | | | | | | | | | |
| skin—*3 oz* | 85 | 285 | 875 | 864 | 1465 | 1668 | 732 | 326 | 752 | 641 | 946 | 1108 | 457 | 35188 |
| **halibut, Atlantic and Pacific** | | | | | | | | | | | | | | |
| ckd by dry heat—*3 oz* | 85 | 254 | 994 | 1046 | 1844 | 2083 | 672 | 243 | 886 | 766 | 1169 | 1357 | 668 | 15037 |
| raw—*3 oz* | 85 | 198 | 775 | 815 | 1438 | 1624 | 524 | 190 | 691 | 598 | 911 | 1058 | 521 | 15036 |
| **halibut, Greenland** | | | | | | | | | | | | | | |
| ckd by dry heat—*3 oz* | 85 | 175 | 687 | 722 | 1272 | 1438 | 463 | 167 | 611 | 529 | 807 | 937 | 461 | 15196 |
| raw—*3 oz* | 85 | 137 | 536 | 563 | 993 | 1122 | 361 | 131 | 477 | 412 | 629 | 731 | 360 | 15038 |
| **herring, Atlantic** | | | | | | | | | | | | | | |
| ckd by dry heat—*3 oz* | 85 | 219 | 858 | 902 | 1591 | 1798 | 580 | 210 | 764 | 661 | 1009 | 1171 | 576 | 15040 |
| kippered—*3 oz* | 40 | 110 | 431 | 453 | 799 | 903 | 291 | 106 | 384 | 332 | 506 | 588 | 290 | 15042 |
| pickled—*3 oz* | 15 | 24 | 93 | 98 | 173 | 195 | 63 | 23 | 83 | 72 | 110 | 127 | 63 | 15041 |
| raw—*3 oz* | 85 | 171 | 669 | 704 | 1241 | 1402 | 452 | 164 | 596 | 515 | 786 | 914 | 450 | 15039 |
| **herring, Pacific** | | | | | | | | | | | | | | |
| ckd by dry heat—*3 oz* | 85 | 200 | 783 | 823 | 1452 | 1640 | 529 | 191 | 697 | 603 | 921 | 1068 | 526 | 15197 |
| raw—*3 oz* | 85 | 156 | 611 | 642 | 1132 | 1280 | 412 | 150 | 544 | 470 | 718 | 834 | 411 | 15043 |
| **ling** | | | | | | | | | | | | | | |
| ckd by dry heat—*3 oz* | 85 | 232 | 907 | 954 | 1682 | 1901 | 613 | 222 | 808 | 699 | 1066 | 1238 | 609 | 15198 |
| raw—*3 oz* | 85 | 181 | 707 | 744 | 1312 | 1482 | 478 | 173 | 630 | 545 | 831 | 966 | 475 | 15044 |
| **lingcod** | | | | | | | | | | | | | | |
| ckd by dry heat—*3 oz* | 85 | 216 | 844 | 887 | 1564 | 1767 | 570 | 207 | 751 | 649 | 991 | 1152 | 567 | 15199 |
| raw—*3 oz* | 85 | 168 | 658 | 692 | 1220 | 1379 | 445 | 161 | 586 | 507 | 774 | 898 | 442 | 15045 |
| **mackerel, Atlantic** | | | | | | | | | | | | | | |
| ckd by dry heat—*3 oz* | 85 | 227 | 888 | 934 | 1647 | 1862 | 600 | 218 | 791 | 684 | 1044 | 1213 | 597 | 15047 |
| raw—*3 oz* | 85 | 177 | 693 | 728 | 1285 | 1452 | 468 | 169 | 617 | 534 | 814 | 946 | 466 | 15046 |
| **mackerel, jack**, canned, drained—*1 cup* | 190 | 494 | 1932 | 2031 | 3582 | 4047 | 1303 | 473 | 1720 | 1488 | 2270 | 2637 | 1298 | 15048 |
| **mackerel, king** | | | | | | | | | | | | | | |
| ckd by dry heat—*3 oz* | 85 | 247 | 969 | 1018 | 1796 | 2030 | 654 | 237 | 863 | 746 | 1139 | 1323 | 650 | 15200 |
| raw—*3 oz* | 85 | 193 | 756 | 795 | 1401 | 1584 | 510 | 184 | 673 | 582 | 888 | 1032 | 507 | 15049 |
| **mackerel, Pacific/jack** | | | | | | | | | | | | | | |
| ckd by dry heat—*3 oz* | 85 | 245 | 959 | 1008 | 1777 | 2009 | 648 | 235 | 854 | 739 | 1127 | 1309 | 644 | 15201 |
| raw—*3 oz* | 85 | 191 | 748 | 786 | 1386 | 1567 | 505 | 183 | 666 | 576 | 879 | 1021 | 502 | 15050 |
| **mackerel, Spanish** | | | | | | | | | | | | | | |
| ckd by dry heat—*3 oz* | 85 | 224 | 879 | 924 | 1629 | 1841 | 593 | 215 | 783 | 677 | 1033 | 1199 | 590 | 15052 |
| raw—*3 oz* | 85 | 184 | 719 | 756 | 1333 | 1505 | 485 | 176 | 640 | 553 | 845 | 981 | 483 | 15051 |
| **milkfish** | | | | | | | | | | | | | | |
| ckd by dry heat—*3 oz* | 85 | 251 | 981 | 1031 | 1818 | 2054 | 662 | 240 | 874 | 756 | 1153 | 1339 | 659 | 15202 |
| raw—*3 oz* | 85 | 196 | 765 | 804 | 1419 | 1603 | 517 | 187 | 682 | 589 | 899 | 1045 | 513 | 15053 |
| **monkfish** | | | | | | | | | | | | | | |
| ckd by dry heat—*3 oz* | 85 | 177 | 692 | 727 | 1283 | 1449 | 467 | 169 | 616 | 533 | 813 | 944 | 465 | 15203 |
| raw—*3 oz* | 85 | 138 | 540 | 567 | 1000 | 1130 | 365 | 132 | 480 | 416 | 634 | 737 | 362 | 15054 |
| **mullet, striped** | | | | | | | | | | | | | | |
| ckd by dry heat—*3 oz* | 85 | 236 | 925 | 972 | 1714 | 1936 | 624 | 226 | 823 | 711 | 1086 | 1261 | 620 | 15056 |
| raw—*3 oz* | 85 | 184 | 721 | 758 | 1337 | 1510 | 487 | 176 | 642 | 555 | 847 | 984 | 484 | 15055 |
| **ocean perch, Atlantic** | | | | | | | | | | | | | | |
| ckd by dry heat—*3 oz* | 85 | 227 | 890 | 935 | 1650 | 1864 | 601 | 218 | 792 | 685 | 1046 | 1215 | 598 | 15058 |
| raw—*3 oz* | 85 | 178 | 694 | 729 | 1287 | 1454 | 468 | 170 | 618 | 535 | 816 | 948 | 466 | 15057 |
| **orange roughy** | | | | | | | | | | | | | | |
| ckd by dry heat—*3 oz* | 85 | 196 | 876 | 899 | 1527 | 1778 | 619 | 204 | 739 | 679 | 921 | 1231 | 403 | 15232 |
| raw—*3 oz* | 85 | 156 | 629 | 652 | 1099 | 1266 | 447 | 148 | 532 | 484 | 671 | 883 | 287 | 15073 |
| **perch** | | | | | | | | | | | | | | |
| ckd by dry heat—*3 oz* | 85 | 236 | 927 | 973 | 1717 | 1941 | 626 | 226 | 824 | 713 | 1089 | 1264 | 622 | 15061 |
| raw—*3 oz* | 85 | 184 | 722 | 759 | 1340 | 1514 | 488 | 177 | 643 | 557 | 849 | 986 | 485 | 15060 |
| **pike, northern** | | | | | | | | | | | | | | |
| ckd by dry heat—*3 oz* | 85 | 235 | 920 | 967 | 1706 | 1927 | 621 | 225 | 819 | 708 | 1081 | 1255 | 618 | 15063 |
| raw—*3 oz* | 85 | 184 | 717 | 754 | 1330 | 1503 | 484 | 175 | 639 | 552 | 843 | 979 | 482 | 15062 |
| **pike, walleye** | | | | | | | | | | | | | | |
| ckd by dry heat—*3 oz* | 85 | 234 | 915 | 961 | 1695 | 1916 | 617 | 224 | 814 | 704 | 1074 | 1248 | 614 | 15204 |
| raw—*3 oz* | 85 | 182 | 713 | 750 | 1322 | 1494 | 481 | 174 | 635 | 549 | 838 | 973 | 479 | 15064 |
| **pollock, Atlantic** | | | | | | | | | | | | | | |
| ckd by dry heat—*3 oz* | 85 | 237 | 929 | 976 | 1722 | 1946 | 627 | 227 | 827 | 715 | 1091 | 1267 | 624 | 15205 |
| raw—*3 oz* | 85 | 185 | 724 | 762 | 1343 | 1518 | 490 | 177 | 645 | 558 | 852 | 989 | 486 | 15065 |
| **pollock, walleye** | | | | | | | | | | | | | | |
| ckd by dry heat—*3 oz* | 85 | 224 | 876 | 921 | 1624 | 1835 | 592 | 214 | 780 | 675 | 1029 | 1196 | 588 | 15067 |
| raw—*3 oz* | 85 | 163 | 640 | 673 | 1187 | 1341 | 433 | 156 | 570 | 493 | 752 | 874 | 430 | 15066 |
| **pompano, Florida** | | | | | | | | | | | | | | |
| ckd by dry heat—*3 oz* | 85 | 225 | 882 | 928 | 1636 | 1849 | 596 | 216 | 786 | 680 | 1037 | 1204 | 592 | 15069 |
| raw—*3 oz* | 85 | 176 | 688 | 723 | 1277 | 1442 | 465 | 168 | 613 | 530 | 809 | 940 | 462 | 15068 |

| | WT (g) | TRY | THR | ISO | LEU | LYS | MET | CYS | PHE | TYR | VAL | ARG | HIS | REF |
|---|---|---|---|---|---|---|---|---|---|---|---|---|---|---|
| | | | | | | | (mg/serving) | | | | | | | |
| **pout, ocean** | | | | | | | | | | | | | | |
| ckd by dry heat—*3 oz* | 85 | 203 | 795 | 836 | 1474 | 1665 | 536 | 195 | 708 | 612 | 934 | 1085 | 534 | 15206 |
| raw—*3 oz* | 85 | 158 | 620 | 652 | 1149 | 1299 | 418 | 151 | 552 | 478 | 728 | 847 | 416 | 15059 |
| **rockfish, Pacific** | | | | | | | | | | | | | | |
| ckd by dry heat—*3 oz* | 85 | 229 | 896 | 942 | 1661 | 1877 | 605 | 219 | 797 | 690 | 1052 | 1222 | 602 | 15071 |
| raw—*3 oz* | 85 | 178 | 699 | 734 | 1295 | 1464 | 472 | 171 | 622 | 538 | 821 | 954 | 469 | 15070 |
| **sablefish** | | | | | | | | | | | | | | |
| ckd by dry heat—*3 oz* | 85 | 164 | 641 | 673 | 1187 | 1342 | 433 | 156 | 570 | 493 | 753 | 875 | 430 | 15208 |
| raw—*3 oz* | 85 | 128 | 500 | 525 | 927 | 1047 | 337 | 122 | 445 | 385 | 587 | 683 | 336 | 15074 |
| smoked—*3 oz* | 85 | 168 | 658 | 692 | 1220 | 1379 | 445 | 161 | 586 | 507 | 774 | 898 | 442 | 15075 |
| **salmon, Atlantic** | | | | | | | | | | | | | | |
| farmed, ckd by dry heat—*3 oz* | 85 | 211 | 824 | 865 | 1527 | 1725 | 556 | 201 | 734 | 634 | 968 | 1124 | 553 | 15237 |
| farmed, raw—*3 oz* | 85 | 178 | 731 | 823 | 1373 | 1590 | 532 | 186 | 718 | 645 | 941 | 1038 | 467 | 15236 |
| wild, cooked by dry heat—*3 oz* | 85 | 242 | 948 | 996 | 1757 | 1986 | 640 | 232 | 844 | 730 | 1114 | 1294 | 637 | 15209 |
| wild, raw—*3 oz* | 85 | 189 | 740 | 777 | 1371 | 1549 | 499 | 181 | 659 | 570 | 869 | 1009 | 496 | 15076 |
| **salmon, chinook** | | | | | | | | | | | | | | |
| ckd by dry heat—*3 oz* | 85 | 245 | 958 | 1007 | 1776 | 2008 | 647 | 235 | 853 | 738 | 1126 | 1308 | 643 | 15210 |
| raw—*3 oz* | 85 | 191 | 747 | 785 | 1386 | 1566 | 505 | 183 | 666 | 575 | 878 | 1020 | 502 | 15078 |
| smoked (lox)—*3 oz* | 85 | 174 | 681 | 716 | 1263 | 1427 | 460 | 167 | 607 | 524 | 801 | 930 | 457 | 15077 |
| **salmon, chum** | | | | | | | | | | | | | | |
| cnd w/bone, drained—*3 oz* | 85 | 204 | 799 | 840 | 1481 | 1673 | 539 | 196 | 711 | 615 | 938 | 1090 | 536 | 15080 |
| ckd by dry heat—*3 oz* | 85 | 246 | 962 | 1012 | 1784 | 2015 | 649 | 235 | 857 | 741 | 1130 | 1313 | 646 | 15211 |
| raw—*3 oz* | 85 | 192 | 751 | 789 | 1391 | 1572 | 507 | 184 | 668 | 578 | 881 | 1024 | 504 | 15079 |
| **salmon, coho** | | | | | | | | | | | | | | |
| farmed, ckd by dry heat—*3 oz* | 85 | 231 | 905 | 952 | 1679 | 1897 | 611 | 221 | 807 | 697 | 1064 | 1236 | 608 | 15239 |
| farmed, raw—*3 oz* | 85 | 202 | 792 | 833 | 1470 | 1660 | 535 | 194 | 706 | 610 | 932 | 1082 | 532 | 15238 |
| wild, cooked by dry heat—*3 oz* | 85 | 224 | 874 | 919 | 1620 | 1831 | 590 | 213 | 778 | 673 | 1027 | 1193 | 586 | 15247 |
| wild, cooked by moist heat—*3 oz* | 85 | 260 | 1020 | 1072 | 1890 | 2136 | 688 | 249 | 908 | 785 | 1198 | 1391 | 685 | 15082 |
| wild, raw—*3 oz* | 85 | 206 | 806 | 847 | 1493 | 1687 | 544 | 197 | 717 | 620 | 947 | 1100 | 541 | 15081 |
| **salmon, pink** | | | | | | | | | | | | | | |
| canned with bone—*3 oz* | 85 | 189 | 737 | 775 | 1367 | 1544 | 498 | 180 | 656 | 568 | 866 | 1006 | 495 | 15084 |
| ckd by dry heat—*3 oz* | 85 | 243 | 953 | 1001 | 1766 | 1996 | 643 | 233 | 848 | 734 | 1119 | 1300 | 640 | 15212 |
| raw—*3 oz* | 85 | 190 | 743 | 781 | 1378 | 1556 | 502 | 182 | 661 | 572 | 873 | 1014 | 499 | 15083 |
| **salmon, sockeye** | | | | | | | | | | | | | | |
| cnd w/bone, drained—*3 oz* | 85 | 238 | 1065 | 948 | 1538 | 1728 | 584 | 151 | 842 | 727 | 1096 | 1244 | 537 | 15087 |
| ckd by dry heat—*3 oz* | 85 | 260 | 1017 | 1069 | 1886 | 2132 | 687 | 249 | 906 | 784 | 1196 | 1389 | 683 | 15086 |
| raw—*3 oz* | 85 | 203 | 794 | 835 | 1471 | 1663 | 536 | 194 | 707 | 611 | 932 | 1084 | 533 | 15085 |
| **sardines, Atlantic**, cnd in soy oil—*2 sardines* | 24 | 66 | 259 | 272 | 480 | 542 | 175 | 63 | 231 | 199 | 304 | 354 | 174 | 15088 |
| **sardines, Pacific**, cnd in tom sce—*1 sardine* | 38 | 60 | 302 | 302 | 516 | 532 | 181 | 53 | 301 | 238 | 352 | 399 | 258 | 15089 |
| **scup** | | | | | | | | | | | | | | |
| ckd by dry heat—*3 oz* | 85 | 230 | 902 | 948 | 1672 | 1890 | 609 | 220 | 803 | 694 | 1060 | 1231 | 606 | 15213 |
| raw—*3 oz* | 85 | 179 | 703 | 740 | 1304 | 1473 | 475 | 172 | 626 | 541 | 826 | 960 | 473 | 15090 |
| **sea bass** | | | | | | | | | | | | | | |
| ckd by dry heat—*3 oz* | 85 | 225 | 881 | 926 | 1633 | 1844 | 594 | 215 | 785 | 678 | 1034 | 1202 | 592 | 15092 |
| raw—*3 oz* | 85 | 175 | 687 | 722 | 1273 | 1439 | 464 | 168 | 612 | 529 | 808 | 938 | 462 | 15091 |
| **seatrout** | | | | | | | | | | | | | | |
| ckd by dry heat—*3 oz* | 85 | 204 | 800 | 841 | 1482 | 1675 | 540 | 196 | 712 | 616 | 940 | 1091 | 537 | 15214 |
| raw—*3 oz* | 85 | 160 | 624 | 656 | 1157 | 1307 | 422 | 152 | 556 | 480 | 734 | 852 | 419 | 15093 |
| **shad, American** | | | | | | | | | | | | | | |
| ckd by dry heat—*3 oz* | 85 | 207 | 809 | 850 | 1499 | 1694 | 546 | 198 | 720 | 623 | 950 | 1104 | 543 | 15215 |
| raw—*3 oz* | 85 | 162 | 631 | 663 | 1170 | 1322 | 426 | 155 | 562 | 486 | 741 | 861 | 423 | 15094 |
| **shark** | | | | | | | | | | | | | | |
| batter-dipped and fried—*3 oz* | 85 | 180 | 717 | 737 | 1288 | 1389 | 460 | 180 | 638 | 538 | 820 | 930 | 457 | 15096 |
| raw—*3 oz* | 85 | 200 | 782 | 822 | 1449 | 1637 | 528 | 191 | 696 | 602 | 919 | 1067 | 525 | 15095 |
| **sheefish**, dried | 28 | 59 | 263 | 241 | 426 | 510 | 176 | 56 | 238 | 190 | 280 | 367 | 146 | 35169 |
| **sheepshead** | | | | | | | | | | | | | | |
| ckd by dry heat—*3 oz* | 85 | 247 | 970 | 1019 | 1798 | 2032 | 654 | 237 | 864 | 746 | 1139 | 1323 | 651 | 15098 |
| raw—*3 oz* | 85 | 192 | 753 | 791 | 1397 | 1578 | 508 | 184 | 671 | 580 | 885 | 1028 | 506 | 15097 |
| **smelt**, dried—*3 oz* | 28 | 143 | 669 | 602 | 1070 | 1033 | 347 | 129 | 563 | 440 | 745 | 868 | 283 | 35184 |
| **smelt, rainbow** | | | | | | | | | | | | | | |
| ckd by dry heat—*3 oz* | 85 | 215 | 842 | 885 | 1561 | 1765 | 569 | 206 | 750 | 649 | 989 | 1149 | 565 | 15100 |
| raw—*3 oz* | 85 | 167 | 657 | 690 | 1218 | 1376 | 444 | 161 | 585 | 506 | 772 | 897 | 441 | 15099 |
| **snapper** | | | | | | | | | | | | | | |
| ckd by dry heat—*3 oz* | 85 | 250 | 980 | 1030 | 1816 | 2053 | 661 | 240 | 873 | 755 | 1152 | 1337 | 658 | 15102 |
| raw—*3 oz* | 85 | 196 | 764 | 803 | 1417 | 1601 | 516 | 187 | 681 | 588 | 898 | 1043 | 513 | 15101 |
| **spot** | | | | | | | | | | | | | | |
| ckd by dry heat—*3 oz* | 85 | 226 | 884 | 930 | 1640 | 1852 | 597 | 216 | 787 | 681 | 1040 | 1207 | 594 | 15216 |
| raw—*3 oz* | 85 | 176 | 690 | 725 | 1279 | 1445 | 466 | 168 | 615 | 531 | 811 | 942 | 463 | 15103 |

| | WT (g) | TRY | THR | ISO | LEU | LYS | MET | CYS | PHE | TYR | VAL | ARG | HIS | REF |
|---|---|---|---|---|---|---|---|---|---|---|---|---|---|---|
| | | | | | | | (mg/serving) | | | | | | | |
| **sturgeon** | | | | | | | | | | | | | | |
| ckd by dry heat—*3 oz* | 85 | 197 | 771 | 811 | 1430 | 1616 | 521 | 189 | 687 | 594 | 906 | 1052 | 518 | 15105 |
| raw—*3 oz* | 85 | 154 | 602 | 632 | 1115 | 1261 | 406 | 147 | 536 | 463 | 707 | 821 | 404 | 15104 |
| smoked—*3 oz* | 85 | 297 | 1163 | 1222 | 2156 | 2435 | 785 | 284 | 1035 | 895 | 1366 | 1587 | 781 | 15106 |
| **sucker, white** | | | | | | | | | | | | | | |
| ckd by dry heat—*3 oz* | 85 | 205 | 801 | 842 | 1484 | 1677 | 541 | 196 | 713 | 616 | 941 | 1093 | 538 | 15217 |
| raw—*3 oz* | 85 | 160 | 625 | 656 | 1158 | 1308 | 422 | 153 | 556 | 481 | 734 | 853 | 419 | 15107 |
| **sunfish, pumpkinseed** | | | | | | | | | | | | | | |
| ckd by dry heat—*3 oz* | 85 | 237 | 927 | 974 | 1719 | 1941 | 626 | 227 | 825 | 714 | 1089 | 1265 | 622 | 15218 |
| raw—*3 oz* | 85 | 184 | 722 | 760 | 1340 | 1515 | 488 | 177 | 643 | 557 | 849 | 987 | 485 | 15108 |
| **surimi**, cooked—*3 oz* | 85 | 78 | 624 | 603 | 1022 | 1179 | 438 | 139 | 506 | 520 | 654 | 857 | 298 | 15109 |
| **swordfish** | | | | | | | | | | | | | | |
| ckd by dry heat—*3 oz* | 85 | 241 | 946 | 994 | 1754 | 1982 | 638 | 231 | 842 | 728 | 1112 | 1291 | 635 | 15111 |
| raw—*3 oz* | 85 | 189 | 738 | 775 | 1368 | 1545 | 498 | 180 | 657 | 568 | 867 | 1007 | 496 | 15110 |
| **tilapia**, cooked by dry heat—*3 oz* | 85 | 225 | 983 | 1037 | 1734 | 1968 | 651 | 225 | 892 | 740 | 1088 | 1352 | 497 | 15262 |
| **tilefish** | | | | | | | | | | | | | | |
| ckd by dry heat—*3 oz* | 85 | 233 | 913 | 959 | 1692 | 1912 | 616 | 224 | 813 | 703 | 1073 | 1245 | 613 | 15113 |
| raw—*3 oz* | 85 | 167 | 652 | 685 | 1209 | 1366 | 440 | 160 | 581 | 502 | 767 | 890 | 438 | 15112 |
| **trout** | | | | | | | | | | | | | | |
| ckd by dry heat—*3 oz* | 85 | 253 | 992 | 1043 | 1839 | 2079 | 670 | 242 | 884 | 764 | 1166 | 1354 | 666 | 15219 |
| raw—*3 oz* | 85 | 198 | 774 | 813 | 1435 | 1621 | 523 | 190 | 689 | 596 | 910 | 1057 | 519 | 15114 |
| **trout, rainbow** | | | | | | | | | | | | | | |
| farmed, ckd by dry heat—*3 oz* | 85 | 231 | 904 | 950 | 1676 | 1895 | 610 | 221 | 805 | 696 | 1062 | 1234 | 607 | 15241 |
| farmed, raw—*3 oz* | 85 | 199 | 778 | 818 | 1442 | 1629 | 525 | 190 | 693 | 598 | 914 | 1062 | 522 | 15240 |
| wild, cooked by dry heat—*3 oz* | 85 | 218 | 854 | 898 | 1584 | 1789 | 577 | 209 | 761 | 658 | 1004 | 1166 | 574 | 15116 |
| wild, raw—*3 oz* | 85 | 195 | 763 | 802 | 1414 | 1599 | 515 | 187 | 679 | 587 | 897 | 1041 | 513 | 15115 |
| **tuna, bluefin** | | | | | | | | | | | | | | |
| ckd by dry heat—*3 oz* | 85 | 285 | 1114 | 1171 | 2066 | 2335 | 752 | 273 | 993 | 858 | 1310 | 1522 | 748 | 15118 |
| raw—*3 oz* | 85 | 222 | 870 | 914 | 1612 | 1821 | 586 | 212 | 774 | 669 | 1022 | 1187 | 584 | 15117 |
| **tuna, light** | | | | | | | | | | | | | | |
| canned in oil—*3 oz* | 85 | 277 | 1085 | 1141 | 2013 | 2274 | 733 | 265 | 966 | 836 | 1276 | 1482 | 729 | 15119 |
| canned in water—*3 oz* | 85 | 243 | 950 | 999 | 1762 | 1992 | 642 | 232 | 847 | 732 | 1117 | 1298 | 638 | 15121 |
| **tuna salad**, homemade | 85 | 153 | 596 | 628 | 1099 | 1238 | 400 | 146 | 532 | 458 | 700 | 822 | 397 | 15128 |
| **tuna, skipjack** | | | | | | | | | | | | | | |
| ckd by dry heat—*3 oz* | 85 | 269 | 1051 | 1105 | 1949 | 2202 | 710 | 257 | 936 | 809 | 1235 | 1435 | 706 | 15220 |
| raw—*3 oz* | 85 | 209 | 819 | 862 | 1520 | 1717 | 553 | 201 | 730 | 632 | 963 | 1119 | 551 | 15123 |
| **tuna, white** | | | | | | | | | | | | | | |
| canned in oil—*3 oz* | 85 | 252 | 989 | 1040 | 1833 | 2071 | 667 | 241 | 881 | 762 | 1162 | 1350 | 664 | 15124 |
| canned in water—*3 oz* | 85 | 225 | 880 | 925 | 1632 | 1844 | 594 | 215 | 784 | 677 | 1034 | 1201 | 591 | 15126 |
| **tuna, yellowfin** | | | | | | | | | | | | | | |
| ckd by dry heat—*3 oz* | 85 | 286 | 1117 | 1174 | 2071 | 2340 | 754 | 273 | 994 | 860 | 1312 | 1525 | 750 | 15221 |
| raw—*3 oz* | 85 | 223 | 871 | 915 | 1615 | 1825 | 588 | 213 | 776 | 671 | 1023 | 1189 | 585 | 15127 |
| **turbot, European** | | | | | | | | | | | | | | |
| ckd by dry heat—*3 oz* | 85 | 196 | 767 | 806 | 1421 | 1606 | 518 | 188 | 683 | 591 | 901 | 1046 | 515 | 15222 |
| raw—*3 oz* | 85 | 153 | 598 | 629 | 1109 | 1253 | 404 | 146 | 533 | 461 | 703 | 816 | 402 | 15129 |
| **whitefish** | | | | | | | | | | | | | | |
| ckd by dry heat—*3 oz* | 85 | 233 | 912 | 959 | 1691 | 1911 | 615 | 223 | 812 | 702 | 1072 | 1245 | 613 | 15223 |
| dried—*1 oz* | 28 | 162 | 692 | 633 | 1151 | 1336 | 487 | 140 | 655 | 487 | 731 | 1011 | 364 | 35165 |
| raw—*3 oz* | 85 | 182 | 711 | 748 | 1318 | 1490 | 480 | 174 | 633 | 547 | 836 | 971 | 478 | 15130 |
| smoked—*3 oz* | 85 | 223 | 872 | 916 | 1617 | 1827 | 589 | 213 | 777 | 672 | 1025 | 1190 | 586 | 15131 |
| **whiting** | | | | | | | | | | | | | | |
| ckd by dry heat—*3 oz* | 85 | 224 | 875 | 920 | 1622 | 1833 | 591 | 214 | 779 | 674 | 1028 | 1194 | 587 | 15133 |
| raw—*3 oz* | 85 | 174 | 683 | 717 | 1265 | 1430 | 461 | 167 | 608 | 525 | 802 | 932 | 458 | 15132 |
| **wolffish** | | | | | | | | | | | | | | |
| ckd by dry heat—*3 oz* | 85 | 213 | 836 | 879 | 1550 | 1752 | 564 | 205 | 745 | 643 | 983 | 1142 | 562 | 15224 |
| raw—*3 oz* | 85 | 167 | 652 | 685 | 1209 | 1366 | 440 | 160 | 581 | 502 | 767 | 890 | 438 | 15134 |
| **yellowtail** | | | | | | | | | | | | | | |
| ckd by dry heat—*3 oz* | 85 | 282 | 1106 | 1162 | 2049 | 2316 | 746 | 270 | 984 | 852 | 1299 | 1509 | 742 | 15225 |
| raw—*3 oz* | 85 | 220 | 863 | 906 | 1599 | 1807 | 582 | 211 | 768 | 664 | 1013 | 1177 | 579 | 15135 |
| **FISH EGGS** | | | | | | | | | | | | | | |
| **caviar, black and red**, granular—*1 T* | 16 | 52 | 202 | 166 | 341 | 293 | 103 | 72 | 171 | 155 | 202 | 254 | 104 | 15012 |
| **roe, mixed species** | | | | | | | | | | | | | | |
| ckd by dry heat—*1 oz* | 28 | 105 | 365 | 410 | 703 | 610 | 199 | 140 | 392 | 403 | 469 | 459 | 218 | 15207 |
| raw—*1 oz* | 28 | 82 | 285 | 320 | 548 | 476 | 155 | 109 | 306 | 314 | 366 | 358 | 170 | 15072 |
| **whitefish roe/eggs**—*1 oz* | 28 | 78 | 283 | 300 | 459 | 448 | 157 | 64 | 252 | 213 | 358 | 297 | 148 | 35158 |

| | WT (g) | TRY | THR | ISO | LEU | LYS | MET | CYS | PHE | TYR | VAL | ARG | HIS | REF |
|---|---|---|---|---|---|---|---|---|---|---|---|---|---|---|
| | | | | | | | (mg/serving) | | | | | | | |
| **MOLLUSKS AND JELLYFISH** | | | | | | | | | | | | | | |
| **abalone** | | | | | | | | | | | | | | |
| fried—*3 oz* | 85 | 190 | 712 | 726 | 1178 | 1218 | 375 | 222 | 608 | 533 | 731 | 1199 | 321 | 15156 |
| mixed species, raw—*3 oz* | 85 | 163 | 626 | 632 | 1023 | 1086 | 328 | 190 | 521 | 465 | 635 | 1061 | 279 | 15155 |
| **clams** | | | | | | | | | | | | | | |
| breaded and fried—*3 oz (9 small)* | 85 | 143 | 512 | 541 | 870 | 843 | 275 | 173 | 467 | 394 | 552 | 837 | 238 | 15158 |
| canned, drained—*3 oz* | 85 | 243 | 934 | 945 | 1528 | 1623 | 490 | 285 | 778 | 694 | 949 | 1584 | 416 | 15160 |
| cooked by moist heat—*3 oz (19 small)* | 85 | 243 | 934 | 945 | 1528 | 1623 | 490 | 285 | 778 | 694 | 949 | 1584 | 416 | 15159 |
| raw—*3 oz (4 large or 9 small)* | 85 | 122 | 468 | 473 | 764 | 811 | 245 | 143 | 389 | 348 | 474 | 792 | 208 | 15157 |
| **cuttlefish** | | | | | | | | | | | | | | |
| ckd by moist heat—*3 oz* | 85 | 309 | 1188 | 1202 | 1944 | 2063 | 623 | 362 | 989 | 883 | 1206 | 2014 | 530 | 15229 |
| raw—*3 oz* | 85 | 155 | 594 | 601 | 972 | 1031 | 311 | 181 | 495 | 442 | 603 | 1007 | 265 | 15163 |
| **mussels, blue** | | | | | | | | | | | | | | |
| ckd by moist heat—*3 oz* | 85 | 227 | 871 | 881 | 1425 | 1512 | 456 | 265 | 725 | 648 | 884 | 1476 | 388 | 15165 |
| raw—*3 oz* | 85 | 113 | 435 | 440 | 712 | 756 | 228 | 133 | 362 | 324 | 442 | 738 | 194 | 15164 |
| **octopus** | | | | | | | | | | | | | | |
| ckd by moist heat—*3 oz* | 85 | 284 | 1091 | 1103 | 1784 | 1894 | 572 | 332 | 909 | 811 | 1108 | 1850 | 487 | 15230 |
| raw—*3 oz* | 85 | 142 | 546 | 552 | 892 | 947 | 286 | 167 | 454 | 405 | 553 | 925 | 243 | 15166 |
| **oysters, eastern** | | | | | | | | | | | | | | |
| breaded and fried—*3 oz (6 med)* | 88 | 92 | 321 | 348 | 561 | 512 | 175 | 115 | 310 | 255 | 360 | 515 | 154 | 15168 |
| canned—*3 oz (~11 oysters)* | 85 | 67 | 258 | 261 | 422 | 449 | 135 | 79 | 215 | 192 | 262 | 438 | 116 | 15170 |
| farmed, ckd by dry heat—*6 med* | 59 | 46 | 178 | 180 | 291 | 309 | 93 | 54 | 148 | 132 | 181 | 301 | 79 | 15246 |
| farmed, raw—*6 med* | 84 | 50 | 189 | 191 | 309 | 328 | 99 | 58 | 157 | 140 | 192 | 320 | 84 | 15245 |
| wild, ckd by dry heat—*6 med* | 59 | 54 | 209 | 212 | 343 | 363 | 110 | 64 | 175 | 156 | 212 | 355 | 93 | 15244 |
| wild, ckd by moist—*6 med* | 42 | 66 | 255 | 258 | 417 | 442 | 134 | 78 | 212 | 189 | 259 | 432 | 114 | 15169 |
| wild, raw—*6 med* | 84 | 66 | 255 | 258 | 417 | 443 | 134 | 77 | 213 | 190 | 259 | 432 | 113 | 15167 |
| **oysters, Pacific** | | | | | | | | | | | | | | |
| ckd by moist heat—*3 oz* | 85 | 180 | 691 | 700 | 1131 | 1200 | 362 | 211 | 575 | 514 | 702 | 1172 | 309 | 15231 |
| raw—*3 oz* | 85 | 90 | 346 | 349 | 565 | 600 | 181 | 105 | 288 | 257 | 351 | 586 | 154 | 15171 |
| **scallops** | | | | | | | | | | | | | | |
| breaded and fried—*2 large* | 31 | 65 | 238 | 248 | 401 | 397 | 126 | 78 | 213 | 182 | 254 | 392 | 110 | 15173 |
| imitation, made from surimi—*3 oz* | 85 | 66 | 524 | 507 | 859 | 992 | 368 | 116 | 426 | 438 | 551 | 721 | 250 | 15174 |
| raw—*3 oz* | 85 | 160 | 614 | 620 | 1004 | 1066 | 322 | 187 | 511 | 456 | 623 | 1040 | 274 | 15172 |
| **squid** | | | | | | | | | | | | | | |
| fried—*3 oz* | 85 | 172 | 649 | 663 | 1077 | 1114 | 343 | 206 | 558 | 490 | 668 | 1096 | 296 | 15176 |
| raw—*3 oz* | 85 | 148 | 570 | 576 | 932 | 989 | 298 | 173 | 474 | 423 | 578 | 966 | 254 | 15175 |
| **whelks** | | | | | | | | | | | | | | |
| ckd by moist heat—*3 oz* | 85 | 525 | 1816 | 1407 | 3236 | 2490 | 1024 | 318 | 1401 | 1290 | 1764 | 4196 | 830 | 15178 |
| raw—*3 oz* | 85 | 263 | 908 | 704 | 1618 | 1245 | 513 | 159 | 700 | 645 | 881 | 2098 | 415 | 15177 |
| **13. FLOUR, MEALS, AND GRAIN FRACTIONS** | | | | | | | | | | | | | | |
| **arrowroot flour**—*1 cup* | 128 | 5 | 15 | 13 | 24 | 17 | 8 | 8 | 15 | 12 | 18 | 15 | 5 | 20003 |
| **barley** | | | | | | | | | | | | | | |
| flour/meal—*1 cup* | 148 | 259 | 527 | 567 | 1055 | 579 | 299 | 343 | 872 | 445 | 762 | 778 | 349 | 20130 |
| malt flour—*1 cup* | 162 | 214 | 659 | 585 | 1209 | 867 | 476 | 254 | 364 | 552 | 815 | 1354 | 446 | 20131 |
| **buckwheat flour**, whole groat—*1 cup* | 120 | 220 | 578 | 569 | 950 | 768 | 197 | 262 | 594 | 276 | 775 | 1122 | 353 | 20011 |
| **corn flour, yellow** | | | | | | | | | | | | | | |
| masa harina, enr—*1 cup* | 114 | 75 | 400 | 381 | 1306 | 300 | 223 | 192 | 523 | 433 | 539 | 531 | 325 | 20017 |
| whole grain—*1 cup* | 117 | 57 | 305 | 290 | 994 | 228 | 170 | 146 | 398 | 330 | 411 | 404 | 247 | 20016 |
| **cornmeal, white** | | | | | | | | | | | | | | |
| bolted, enr, self-rising—*1 cup* | 122 | 71 | 379 | 361 | 1238 | 284 | 212 | 182 | 497 | 411 | 511 | 504 | 309 | 20323 |
| bolted, enr, self-rising w/wht flour—*1 cup* | 170 | 110 | 518 | 510 | 1654 | 391 | 294 | 264 | 704 | 564 | 706 | 697 | 423 | 20324 |
| whole grain—*1 cup* | 122 | 70 | 372 | 355 | 1215 | 278 | 207 | 178 | 487 | 403 | 501 | 494 | 303 | 20320 |
| **cornmeal, yellow** | | | | | | | | | | | | | | |
| bolted, enr, self-rising—*1 cup* | 122 | 71 | 379 | 361 | 1238 | 284 | 212 | 182 | 497 | 411 | 511 | 504 | 309 | 20023 |
| bolted, enr, self-rising w/wht flour—*1 cup* | 170 | 110 | 518 | 510 | 1654 | 391 | 294 | 264 | 704 | 564 | 706 | 697 | 423 | 20024 |
| degermed, enr—*1 cup* | 138 | 54 | 243 | 341 | 1416 | 148 | 229 | 224 | 516 | 264 | 475 | 337 | 243 | 20022 |
| whole grain—*1 cup* | 122 | 70 | 372 | 355 | 1215 | 278 | 207 | 178 | 487 | 403 | 501 | 494 | 303 | 20020 |
| **cottonseed** | | | | | | | | | | | | | | |
| flour, lowfat—*1 cup* | 94 | 707 | 1732 | 1688 | 3200 | 2377 | 760 | 1229 | 2917 | 1688 | 2404 | 6328 | 1476 | 12008 |
| flour, partially defatted—*1 cup* | 80 | 494 | 1212 | 1181 | 2238 | 1663 | 532 | 859 | 2040 | 1181 | 1682 | 4426 | 1033 | 12007 |
| meal, partially defatted—*3 oz* | 85 | 630 | 1544 | 1504 | 2851 | 2118 | 677 | 1095 | 2598 | 1504 | 2142 | 5638 | 1315 | 12011 |
| **oat bran**—*1 cup* | 94 | 315 | 472 | 628 | 1292 | 714 | 315 | 541 | 854 | 628 | 906 | 1202 | 385 | 20033 |
| **peanut flour**, defatted—*1 cup* | 60 | 304 | 1073 | 1102 | 2030 | 1124 | 385 | 401 | 1623 | 1273 | 1313 | 3746 | 791 | 16099 |
| **potato flour**—*1 cup* | 160 | 184 | 448 | 478 | 680 | 661 | 171 | 112 | 506 | 358 | 570 | 598 | 266 | 11413 |
| **rice bran**—*1 cup* | 118 | 127 | 655 | 670 | 1206 | 767 | 361 | 374 | 749 | 485 | 1040 | 1248 | 419 | 20060 |

| | WT | TRY | THR | ISO | LEU | LYS | MET | CYS | PHE | TYR | VAL | ARG | HIS | REF |
|---|---|---|---|---|---|---|---|---|---|---|---|---|---|---|
| | (g) | | | | | | (mg/serving) | | | | | | | |
| **rice flour** | | | | | | | | | | | | | | |
| brown—*1 cup* | 158 | 145 | 419 | 483 | 945 | 436 | 258 | 139 | 589 | 428 | 670 | 866 | 291 | 20090 |
| white—*1 cup* | 158 | 114 | 332 | 386 | 771 | 327 | 228 | 169 | 501 | 496 | 550 | 815 | 235 | 20061 |
| **rye flour** | | | | | | | | | | | | | | |
| dark—*1 cup* | 128 | 204 | 622 | 692 | 1242 | 622 | 268 | 355 | 909 | 355 | 900 | 813 | 401 | 20063 |
| light—*1 cup* | 102 | 97 | 297 | 330 | 592 | 297 | 128 | 168 | 432 | 168 | 428 | 388 | 191 | 20065 |
| medium—*1 cup* | 102 | 108 | 332 | 369 | 662 | 332 | 143 | 189 | 484 | 189 | 479 | 434 | 213 | 20064 |
| **sesame** | | | | | | | | | | | | | | |
| flour, high fat—*3 oz* | 85 | 573 | 1086 | 1125 | 2004 | 839 | 864 | 528 | 1387 | 1096 | 1461 | 3880 | 770 | 12170 |
| flour, lowfat—*3 oz* | 85 | 932 | 1769 | 1833 | 3265 | 1367 | 1408 | 860 | 2259 | 1785 | 2380 | 6321 | 1255 | 12033 |
| flour, partially defatted—*3 oz* | 85 | 750 | 1423 | 1474 | 2625 | 1099 | 1131 | 692 | 1817 | 1436 | 1914 | 5082 | 1009 | 12032 |
| meal, partially defatted—*3 oz* | 85 | 315 | 598 | 620 | 1104 | 462 | 476 | 291 | 764 | 604 | 805 | 2138 | 424 | 12034 |
| **soy** | | | | | | | | | | | | | | |
| flour, defatted—*1 cup* | 100 | 683 | 2042 | 2281 | 3828 | 3129 | 634 | 757 | 2453 | 1778 | 2346 | 3647 | 1268 | 16117 |
| flour, full-fat—*1 cup* | 84 | 422 | 1260 | 1407 | 2362 | 1930 | 391 | 467 | 1514 | 1097 | 1448 | 2250 | 782 | 16115 |
| flour, full-fat, roasted—*1 cup* | 85 | 430 | 1284 | 1435 | 2409 | 1969 | 399 | 477 | 1544 | 1119 | 1476 | 2295 | 797 | 16116 |
| meal, defatted—*1 cup* | 122 | 797 | 2381 | 2660 | 4465 | 3649 | 739 | 883 | 2862 | 2074 | 2736 | 4254 | 1479 | 16119 |
| **sunflower flour**, partially defatted—*1 cup* | 64 | 470 | 1254 | 1538 | 2240 | 1265 | 668 | 609 | 1578 | 900 | 1776 | 3244 | 853 | 12041 |
| **triticale flour**, whole grain—*1 cup* | 130 | 205 | 532 | 629 | 1196 | 480 | 268 | 361 | 837 | 503 | 800 | 881 | 408 | 20070 |
| **wheat bran**, crude—*1 cup* | 58 | 164 | 290 | 282 | 538 | 348 | 136 | 215 | 345 | 253 | 421 | 630 | 249 | 20077 |
| **wheat flour** | | | | | | | | | | | | | | |
| white, enr, all-purpose—*1 cup* | 125 | 159 | 351 | 446 | 888 | 285 | 229 | 274 | 650 | 390 | 519 | 521 | 288 | 20081 |
| white, enr, bread—*1 cup* | 137 | 190 | 438 | 608 | 1134 | 316 | 288 | 369 | 810 | 449 | 688 | 570 | 348 | 20083 |
| white, enr, cake—*1 cup* | 137 | 162 | 311 | 426 | 764 | 390 | 189 | 244 | 532 | 321 | 493 | 430 | 229 | 20084 |
| white, enr, self-rising—*1 cup* | 125 | 151 | 336 | 428 | 850 | 274 | 219 | 262 | 622 | 372 | 496 | 499 | 275 | 20082 |
| white, enr, tortilla mix—*1 cup* | 111 | 132 | 292 | 371 | 737 | 236 | 190 | 228 | 539 | 323 | 431 | 433 | 239 | 20086 |
| whole wheat—*1 cup* | 120 | 254 | 474 | 610 | 1111 | 454 | 254 | 380 | 775 | 480 | 742 | 770 | 380 | 20080 |
| **wheat germ** | | | | | | | | | | | | | | |
| crude—*½ cup* | 57 | 181 | 552 | 483 | 895 | 837 | 260 | 261 | 529 | 401 | 683 | 1064 | 367 | 20078 |
| toasted—*½ cup* | 56 | 223 | 682 | 597 | 1107 | 1034 | 321 | 323 | 654 | 496 | 844 | 1315 | 454 | 8084 |
| **wheat semolina**, enriched—*1 cup* | 167 | 271 | 559 | 818 | 1448 | 406 | 331 | 598 | 1029 | 556 | 902 | 780 | 429 | 20066 |

## 14. FRUIT AND VEGETABLE JUICES AND JUICE DRINKS

| | WT | TRY | THR | ISO | LEU | LYS | MET | CYS | PHE | TYR | VAL | ARG | HIS | REF |
|---|---|---|---|---|---|---|---|---|---|---|---|---|---|---|
| **beef broth and tomato juice**, canned | | | | | | | | | | | | | | |
| 5.5 fl oz | 168 | 2 | 18 | 15 | 30 | 37 | 7 | 2 | 22 | 5 | 25 | 69 | 10 | 14114 |
| **clam and tomato juice**, canned—*5.5 fl oz* | 166 | 7 | 17 | 18 | 25 | 22 | 7 | 5 | 17 | 10 | 18 | 38 | 12 | 14187 |
| **grape jce** | | | | | | | | | | | | | | |
| cnd/btld—*8 fl oz* | 253 | | 40 | 18 | 30 | 25 | 3 | | 30 | 8 | 25 | 119 | 18 | 9135 |
| swtnd, from frzn conc—*8 fl oz* | 250 | | 12 | 5 | 10 | 8 | | | 10 | 2 | 8 | 40 | 5 | 9137 |
| **lime juice**, raw | | | | | | | | | | | | | | |
| yield from 1 lime (1.2 fl oz) | 38 | 1 | 1 | 1 | 6 | 6 | 1 | 1 | 4 | 1 | 4 | 6 | 1 | 9160 |
| **orange juice** | | | | | | | | | | | | | | |
| canned/bottled—*8 fl oz* | 249 | 5 | 20 | 17 | 32 | 22 | 7 | 12 | 20 | 7 | 25 | 115 | 7 | 9207 |
| from frzn conc—*8 fl oz* | 249 | 5 | 20 | 17 | 32 | 22 | 7 | 12 | 20 | 10 | 27 | 112 | 7 | 9215 |
| raw—*8 fl oz* | 248 | 5 | 20 | 20 | 32 | 22 | 7 | 12 | 22 | 10 | 27 | 117 | 7 | 9206 |
| refrigerated—*8 fl oz* | 248 | 2 | 12 | 12 | 22 | 15 | 5 | 7 | 15 | 7 | 17 | 77 | 5 | 9209 |
| **tangerine juice** | | | | | | | | | | | | | | |
| raw—*8 fl oz* | 247 | 2 | 15 | 12 | 25 | 17 | 5 | 10 | 15 | 7 | 20 | 84 | 5 | 9221 |
| swtnd, canned/bottled—*8 fl oz* | 249 | 2 | 15 | 12 | 25 | 17 | 5 | 10 | 15 | 7 | 20 | 85 | 5 | 9223 |
| swtnd, from frzn conc—*8 fl oz* | 241 | 2 | 12 | 12 | 19 | 14 | 5 | 7 | 12 | 5 | 17 | 70 | 5 | 9225 |
| swtnd, frzn conc—*8 fl oz* | 241 | 10 | 41 | 39 | 70 | 48 | 17 | 27 | 43 | 19 | 58 | 243 | 14 | 9224 |
| **tomato juice**, canned/bottled—*8 fl oz* | 243 | 12 | 41 | 36 | 51 | 53 | 10 | 10 | 39 | 24 | 36 | 36 | 29 | 11886 |

## 15. FRUITS

| | WT | TRY | THR | ISO | LEU | LYS | MET | CYS | PHE | TYR | VAL | ARG | HIS | REF |
|---|---|---|---|---|---|---|---|---|---|---|---|---|---|---|
| **apple** | | | | | | | | | | | | | | |
| dried—*1 ring* | 6 | 1 | 2 | 2 | 3 | 3 | 1 | 1 | 2 | 1 | 3 | 2 | 1 | 9011 |
| dried, cooked—*1 cup sliced* | 171 | 3 | 14 | 14 | 22 | 22 | 3 | 5 | 10 | 7 | 17 | 12 | 5 | 9012 |
| frozen, unsweetened—*1 cup sliced* | 171 | 5 | 17 | 19 | 29 | 29 | 5 | 7 | 14 | 9 | 22 | 15 | 7 | 9014 |
| peeled, microwaved—*1 cup sliced* | 170 | 5 | 17 | 19 | 29 | 31 | 5 | 7 | 14 | 8 | 22 | 15 | 7 | 9006 |
| peeled, raw—*1 medium (2¾″ dia)* | 128 | 1 | 8 | 8 | 18 | 17 | 1 | 1 | 9 | 1 | 15 | 8 | 6 | 9004 |
| raw—*1 medium (2¾″ dia)* | 138 | 1 | 8 | 8 | 18 | 17 | 1 | 1 | 8 | 1 | 17 | 8 | 7 | 9003 |
| sliced, swtnd, cnd, drained—*1 cup* | 204 | 4 | 12 | 14 | 22 | 22 | 4 | 4 | 10 | 6 | 16 | 12 | 6 | 9007 |
| **applesauce** | | | | | | | | | | | | | | |
| sweetened, cnd/btld—*1 cup* | 255 | 5 | 18 | 18 | 28 | 28 | 5 | 5 | 13 | 8 | 20 | 15 | 8 | 9020 |
| unsweetened, cnd/btld—*1 cup* | 244 | 5 | 15 | 15 | 24 | 24 | 5 | 5 | 12 | 7 | 20 | 12 | 7 | 9019 |
| **apricot** | | | | | | | | | | | | | | |
| canned in juice—*1 cup halves* | 244 | 27 | 56 | 46 | 90 | 107 | 7 | 5 | 63 | 37 | 56 | 59 | 24 | 9024 |
| canned in light syrup—*1 cup halves* | 253 | 23 | 48 | 40 | 78 | 94 | 8 | 5 | 56 | 30 | 48 | 53 | 23 | 9026 |

| | WT | TRY | THR | ISO | LEU | LYS | MET | CYS | PHE | TYR | VAL | ARG | HIS | REF |
|---|---|---|---|---|---|---|---|---|---|---|---|---|---|---|
| | (g) | | | | | | (mg/serving) | | | | | | | |
| canned in water—*1 cup halves* | 227 | 30 | 59 | 50 | 95 | 111 | 9 | 5 | 68 | 39 | 59 | 64 | 27 | 9022 |
| dried—*½ cup halves* | 65 | 10 | 47 | 41 | 68 | 54 | 10 | 12 | 40 | 25 | 51 | 43 | 31 | 9032 |
| peeled, canned in water | | | | | | | | | | | | | | |
| *1 cup whole* | 227 | 27 | 57 | 48 | 91 | 109 | 7 | 5 | 64 | 36 | 57 | 61 | 25 | 9023 |
| peeled, cnd in heavy syrup | | | | | | | | | | | | | | |
| *1 cup whole* | 258 | 23 | 46 | 41 | 77 | 93 | 8 | 5 | 54 | 31 | 49 | 52 | 21 | 9028 |
| raw—*3 apricots* | 105 | 16 | 49 | 43 | 81 | 102 | 6 | 3 | 55 | 30 | 49 | 47 | 28 | 9021 |
| sweetened, frozen—*1 cup* | 242 | 19 | 58 | 48 | 94 | 119 | 7 | 5 | 63 | 36 | 58 | 53 | 31 | 9035 |
| **avocado** | | | | | | | | | | | | | | |
| California, raw—*1 med (6.1 oz)* | 173 | 43 | 125 | 144 | 244 | 223 | 64 | 47 | 394 | 83 | 182 | 151 | 83 | 9038 |
| Florida, raw—*1 med (10.7 oz)* | 304 | 85 | 249 | 286 | 486 | 447 | 128 | 94 | 790 | 164 | 365 | 301 | 167 | 9039 |
| raw—*1 cup sliced* | 146 | 36 | 107 | 123 | 209 | 193 | 55 | 39 | 339 | 72 | 156 | 128 | 72 | 9037 |
| **banana chips**—*1 oz* | 28 | 8 | 21 | 21 | 44 | 30 | 7 | 11 | 24 | 15 | 29 | 29 | 50 | 19400 |
| **banana**, raw—*1 medium (7" to 8" long)* | 118 | 11 | 33 | 33 | 80 | 59 | 9 | 11 | 58 | 11 | 55 | 58 | 91 | 9040 |
| **blueberries** | | | | | | | | | | | | | | |
| canned in heavy syrup—*1 cup* | 256 | 8 | 46 | 51 | 100 | 31 | 26 | 18 | 59 | 20 | 69 | 84 | 26 | 9052 |
| frozen—*1 cup* | 155 | 3 | 19 | 20 | 39 | 12 | 11 | 6 | 23 | 8 | 28 | 34 | 9 | 9054 |
| frozen, sweetened—*1 cup* | 230 | 5 | 25 | 28 | 53 | 16 | 14 | 9 | 32 | 12 | 39 | 46 | 14 | 9055 |
| raw—*1 cup* | 145 | 4 | 29 | 33 | 64 | 19 | 17 | 12 | 38 | 13 | 45 | 54 | 16 | 9050 |
| **cantaloupe**, raw—*1 cup pieces* | 177 | 4 | 30 | 37 | 51 | 53 | 21 | 4 | 41 | 25 | 58 | 51 | 27 | 9181 |
| **carambola** (star fruit), raw | | | | | | | | | | | | | | |
| *1 medium (3⅝" diameter)* | 91 | 7 | 40 | 40 | 70 | 70 | 19 | | 34 | 40 | 46 | 19 | 7 | 9060 |
| **cherries, sweet**, raw—*1 cup* | 117 | 11 | 26 | 23 | 35 | 37 | 12 | 12 | 28 | 16 | 28 | 21 | 18 | 9070 |
| **crabapples**, raw—*1 cup sliced* | 110 | 4 | 15 | 18 | 28 | 28 | 4 | 6 | 12 | 9 | 21 | 14 | 7 | 9077 |
| **cranberries**, raw—*1 cup whole* | 95 | 3 | 27 | 31 | 50 | 37 | 3 | 3 | 34 | 30 | 43 | 53 | 17 | 9078 |
| **date** | | | | | | | | | | | | | | |
| dried—*4 dates* | 32 | 4 | 14 | 16 | 27 | 21 | 7 | 21 | 16 | 5 | 23 | 44 | 10 | 9087 |
| medjool, dried—*1 date* | 24 | 2 | 10 | 11 | 20 | 13 | 4 | 11 | 12 | 4 | 16 | 14 | 7 | 9421 |
| **elderberries**, raw—*1 cup* | 145 | 19 | 39 | 39 | 87 | 38 | 20 | 22 | 58 | 74 | 48 | 68 | 22 | 9088 |
| **fig** | | | | | | | | | | | | | | |
| canned in heavy syrup | | | | | | | | | | | | | | |
| *1 fig with liquid* | 28 | 1 | 3 | 3 | 5 | 4 | 1 | 2 | 3 | 4 | 4 | 3 | 1 | 9092 |
| dried—*1 fig* | 19 | 4 | 16 | 17 | 24 | 17 | 6 | 7 | 14 | 8 | 23 | 15 | 7 | 9094 |
| raw—*1 medium (2¼" dia)* | 50 | 3 | 12 | 12 | 16 | 15 | 3 | 6 | 9 | 16 | 14 | 8 | 6 | 9089 |
| **grapefruit** | | | | | | | | | | | | | | |
| canned in juice—*1 cup* | 249 | 17 | 30 | 17 | 32 | 42 | 17 | 17 | 105 | 17 | 35 | 197 | 17 | 9120 |
| canned in light syrup—*1 cup* | 254 | 15 | 25 | 15 | 28 | 36 | 13 | 15 | 86 | 15 | 28 | 160 | 15 | 9121 |
| pink and red, raw | | | | | | | | | | | | | | |
| *½ medium (3¾" diameter)* | 123 | 10 | 16 | 10 | 18 | 23 | 9 | 10 | 57 | 10 | 18 | 107 | 10 | 9112 |
| raw—*½ medium (3¾" diameter)* | 118 | 7 | 13 | 8 | 14 | 19 | 7 | 7 | 45 | 7 | 14 | 83 | 7 | 9111 |
| white, raw—*½ medium (3¾" diameter)* | 118 | 8 | 14 | 8 | 15 | 20 | 8 | 8 | 48 | 8 | 17 | 92 | 8 | 9116 |
| **grapes, American** (slip skin), all | | | | | | | | | | | | | | |
| colors, raw—*1 cup* | 92 | 3 | 16 | 5 | 12 | 13 | 19 | 9 | 12 | 10 | 16 | 42 | 21 | 9131 |
| **grapes, green** | | | | | | | | | | | | | | |
| canned in water—*1 cup* | 245 | 5 | 34 | 10 | 24 | 27 | 42 | 20 | 24 | 22 | 34 | 91 | 44 | 9133 |
| Thompson seedless, | | | | | | | | | | | | | | |
| cnd in heavy syrup—*1 cup* | 256 | 5 | 33 | 10 | 26 | 28 | 41 | 20 | 26 | 20 | 33 | 90 | 46 | 9134 |
| **grapes, red/green**, European, | | | | | | | | | | | | | | |
| seedless, raw—*1 cup* | 160 | 18 | 35 | 18 | 35 | 43 | 14 | 16 | 30 | 16 | 35 | 208 | 35 | 9132 |
| **guava**, raw—*1 medium (3.2 oz)* | 90 | 20 | 86 | 84 | 154 | 65 | 14 | | 5 | 28 | 78 | 58 | 20 | 9139 |
| **honeydew melon**, raw—*1 cup pieces* | 177 | 9 | 23 | 23 | 28 | 32 | 9 | 9 | 27 | 18 | 32 | 25 | 9 | 9184 |
| **kiwifruit**, raw—*1 medium (2.7 oz)* | 76 | 11 | 36 | 39 | 50 | 46 | 18 | 24 | 33 | 26 | 43 | 62 | 21 | 9148 |
| **longan**, dried—*1 oz* | 28 | | 36 | 27 | 57 | 48 | 14 | | 31 | 26 | 61 | 37 | 13 | 9173 |
| **loquat**, raw—*1 medium* | 16 | 1 | 2 | 2 | 4 | 4 | 1 | 1 | 2 | 2 | 3 | 2 | 1 | 9174 |
| **mandarin oranges** | | | | | | | | | | | | | | |
| cnd in juice—*1 cup* | 249 | 15 | 25 | 42 | 37 | 77 | 32 | 15 | 50 | 25 | 65 | 107 | 27 | 9219 |
| cnd in light syrup—*1 cup* | 252 | 10 | 18 | 30 | 28 | 58 | 25 | 13 | 38 | 20 | 48 | 78 | 20 | 9220 |
| **mango**, raw—*1 medium (7.3 oz)* | 207 | 17 | 39 | 37 | 64 | 85 | 10 | | 35 | 21 | 54 | 39 | 25 | 9176 |
| **nectarine**, raw—*1 medium (2½" dia)* | 136 | 7 | 12 | 12 | 19 | 22 | 8 | 7 | 15 | 10 | 18 | 12 | 11 | 9191 |
| **orange** | | | | | | | | | | | | | | |
| all varieties, raw—*1 med (2⅝" dia)* | 131 | 12 | 20 | 33 | 30 | 62 | 26 | 13 | 41 | 21 | 52 | 85 | 24 | 9200 |
| California navel, raw | | | | | | | | | | | | | | |
| *1 med (2⅞" dia)* | 140 | 13 | 25 | 24 | 41 | 53 | 13 | 14 | 74 | 18 | 36 | 161 | 18 | 9202 |
| California Valencia, raw | | | | | | | | | | | | | | |
| *1 med (2⅝" dia)* | 121 | 12 | 21 | 34 | 31 | 64 | 27 | 13 | 41 | 22 | 53 | 88 | 24 | 9201 |
| Florida, raw—*1 med (2⅝" dia)* | 141 | 10 | 16 | 27 | 24 | 49 | 21 | 10 | 32 | 17 | 42 | 69 | 18 | 9203 |
| **papaya**, raw | | | | | | | | | | | | | | |
| *1 medium (5⅛" long × 3" diameter)* | 304 | 24 | 33 | 24 | 49 | 76 | 6 | | 27 | 15 | 30 | 30 | 15 | 9226 |

| | WT (g) | TRY | THR | ISO | LEU | LYS | MET | CYS | PHE | TYR | VAL | ARG | HIS | REF |
|---|---|---|---|---|---|---|---|---|---|---|---|---|---|---|
| | | | | | | | (mg/serving) | | | | | | | |
| **peach** | | | | | | | | | | | | | | |
| canned in heavy syrup, solids and liquid—*1 cup* | 262 | 3 | 47 | 34 | 68 | 39 | 29 | 10 | 37 | 31 | 66 | 31 | 21 | 9241 |
| canned in juice—*1 cup* | 250 | 5 | 62 | 45 | 90 | 50 | 38 | 12 | 50 | 40 | 85 | 40 | 30 | 9238 |
| canned in light syrup—*1 cup* | 251 | 3 | 45 | 33 | 63 | 35 | 28 | 10 | 35 | 30 | 63 | 28 | 20 | 9240 |
| canned in water—*1 cup* | 244 | 2 | 41 | 32 | 61 | 34 | 27 | 10 | 34 | 27 | 59 | 27 | 20 | 9237 |
| dried—*1 cup halves* | 160 | 16 | 226 | 166 | 326 | 186 | 139 | 46 | 182 | 150 | 315 | 147 | 107 | 9246 |
| raw—*1 med (2½″ dia)* | 98 | 10 | 16 | 17 | 26 | 29 | 10 | 12 | 19 | 14 | 22 | 18 | 13 | 9236 |
| spiced, cnd in heavy syrup—*1 cup* | 242 | 2 | 39 | 29 | 56 | 31 | 24 | 7 | 31 | 27 | 56 | 24 | 19 | 9243 |
| sweetened, frozen—*1 cup* | 250 | 5 | 60 | 45 | 88 | 50 | 38 | 12 | 50 | 40 | 85 | 40 | 30 | 9250 |
| **pear, Asian**, raw | | | | | | | | | | | | | | |
| *1 pear (2½″ long, 2½″ dia)* | 122 | 6 | 16 | 17 | 30 | 21 | 7 | 6 | 16 | 5 | 22 | 11 | 6 | 9340 |
| **pear** | | | | | | | | | | | | | | |
| canned in light syrup—*1 cup halves* | 251 | | 13 | 15 | 25 | 18 | 5 | 5 | 13 | 5 | 18 | 8 | 5 | 9256 |
| cnd in heavy syrup, solids and liquid—*1 cup halves* | 266 | | 13 | 16 | 27 | 19 | 5 | 5 | 13 | 5 | 19 | 8 | 5 | 9257 |
| cnd in juice—*1 cup halves* | 248 | | 22 | 25 | 42 | 30 | 10 | 7 | 22 | 7 | 30 | 15 | 10 | 9254 |
| cnd in water—*1 cup halves* | 244 | | 12 | 12 | 22 | 17 | 5 | 5 | 12 | 5 | 17 | 7 | 5 | 9253 |
| dried—*10 halves* | 175 | | 86 | 94 | 164 | 116 | 38 | 31 | 86 | 28 | 116 | 56 | 35 | 9259 |
| raw—*1 med (2½″ dia)* | 166 | 3 | 18 | 18 | 32 | 28 | 3 | 3 | 18 | 3 | 28 | 17 | 3 | 9252 |
| **persimmon, Japanese** | | | | | | | | | | | | | | |
| dried—*1 medium* | 34 | 8 | 24 | 20 | 34 | 27 | 4 | 10 | 21 | 13 | 24 | 20 | 9 | 9264 |
| raw—*1 medium (2½″ dia)* | 168 | 17 | 50 | 42 | 71 | 55 | 8 | 22 | 44 | 27 | 50 | 42 | 20 | 9263 |
| **persimmon**, raw—*1 medium* | 25 | 4 | 10 | 9 | 14 | 11 | 2 | 4 | 9 | 6 | 10 | 8 | 4 | 9265 |
| **pineapple** | | | | | | | | | | | | | | |
| cnd in heavy syrup *1 cup pieces* | 254 | 13 | 23 | 23 | 33 | 41 | 23 | 3 | 23 | 20 | 28 | 30 | 20 | 9270 |
| cnd in juice, solids and liquid—*1 cup pieces* | 249 | 12 | 25 | 25 | 40 | 47 | 27 | 2 | 25 | 25 | 32 | 35 | 22 | 9268 |
| raw—*1 cup pieces* | 155 | 8 | 29 | 29 | 37 | 40 | 19 | 22 | 33 | 29 | 37 | 29 | 16 | 9266 |
| **plum** | | | | | | | | | | | | | | |
| canned in heavy syrup, solids and liquid—*1 plum with liquid* | 46 | | 4 | 3 | 5 | 4 | 1 | 1 | 4 | 1 | 4 | 3 | 3 | 9284 |
| canned in juice *1 plum with liquid* | 46 | | 5 | 5 | 6 | 5 | 2 | 1 | 5 | 2 | 6 | 4 | 4 | 9282 |
| raw—*1 medium (2⅛″ dia)* | 66 | 6 | 7 | 9 | 10 | 11 | 5 | 1 | 9 | 5 | 11 | 6 | 6 | 9279 |
| **prune**, dried—*2 prunes* | 16 | 4 | 8 | 7 | 11 | 8 | 3 | 2 | 17 | 3 | 9 | 6 | 4 | 9291 |
| **raisins**, seedless | | | | | | | | | | | | | | |
| *1.5 oz box (snack size)* | 43 | 22 | 33 | 25 | 41 | 36 | 9 | 8 | 60 | 5 | 36 | 178 | 31 | 9298 |
| **sapodilla**, raw—*1 medium* | 170 | 8 | 20 | 26 | 41 | 66 | 5 | | 22 | 24 | 27 | 29 | 27 | 9313 |
| **sapote**, raw—*1 medium* | 225 | 52 | 130 | 104 | 189 | 216 | 36 | | 119 | 124 | 173 | 124 | 94 | 9314 |
| **strawberries** | | | | | | | | | | | | | | |
| raw—*1 cup whole* | 144 | 12 | 29 | 23 | 49 | 37 | 3 | 9 | 27 | 32 | 27 | 40 | 17 | 9316 |
| swtnd, frzn, thawed—*1 cup* | 255 | 15 | 41 | 31 | 66 | 54 | 3 | 10 | 38 | 43 | 38 | 56 | 26 | 9319 |
| unswtnd, frzn, thawed—*1 cup* | 221 | 11 | 29 | 22 | 49 | 38 | 2 | 9 | 27 | 31 | 27 | 40 | 18 | 9318 |
| **strawberry guava**, raw—*1 cup* | 244 | 12 | 54 | 51 | 95 | 39 | 10 | | 2 | 17 | 49 | 37 | 12 | 9140 |
| **tangerine**, raw—*1 medium (2⅜″ dia)* | 84 | 2 | 13 | 14 | 24 | 27 | 2 | 2 | 15 | 13 | 18 | 57 | 9 | 9218 |
| **watermelon**, raw—*1 cup pieces* | 152 | 11 | 41 | 29 | 27 | 94 | 9 | 3 | 23 | 18 | 24 | 90 | 9 | 9326 |
| **16. GRAIN- AND VEGETABLE-BASED SNACK FOODS** | | | | | | | | | | | | | | |
| **cheese puffs/twists**—*1 oz* | 28 | 18 | 64 | 74 | 182 | 87 | 36 | 24 | 78 | 66 | 90 | 71 | 49 | 19008 |
| **corn-based cones**—*1 oz* | 28 | 11 | 61 | 59 | 200 | 46 | 34 | 29 | 80 | 66 | 83 | 81 | 50 | 19005 |
| nacho—*1 oz* | 28 | 16 | 71 | 74 | 212 | 73 | 39 | 29 | 89 | 77 | 98 | 85 | 56 | 19006 |
| **corn-based onion flavor snack food** | | | | | | | | | | | | | | |
| *1 oz* | 28 | 17 | 81 | 80 | 254 | 67 | 43 | 38 | 106 | 87 | 108 | 113 | 65 | 19007 |
| **corn chips** | 28 | 13 | 69 | 66 | 225 | 52 | 38 | 33 | 90 | 74 | 93 | 91 | 56 | 19003 |
| barbecue—*1 oz* | 28 | 18 | 78 | 78 | 209 | 80 | 38 | 33 | 93 | 76 | 100 | 104 | 56 | 19004 |
| **crisped rice bar w/choc chips**—*1 oz* | 28 | 21 | 46 | 56 | 109 | 56 | 29 | 34 | 73 | 55 | 80 | 109 | 32 | 19010 |
| **granola bar** | | | | | | | | | | | | | | |
| almond, hard—*0.85 oz bar* | 24 | 34 | 53 | 69 | 140 | 75 | 32 | 55 | 94 | 68 | 97 | 143 | 43 | 19016 |
| chocolate chip, hard—*0.85 oz bar* | 24 | 32 | 51 | 66 | 132 | 75 | 32 | 53 | 88 | 66 | 95 | 124 | 39 | 19017 |
| chocolate chip, soft—*1 oz bar* | 28 | 16 | 53 | 62 | 122 | 60 | 29 | 40 | 82 | 53 | 85 | 108 | 39 | 19404 |
| chocolate chip, soft, chocolate-covered—*1 oz bar* | 28 | 20 | 63 | 76 | 133 | 81 | 32 | 18 | 81 | 68 | 97 | 67 | 29 | 19024 |
| chocolate, graham, and marshmallow, soft—*1 oz bar* | 28 | 24 | 58 | 69 | 128 | 69 | 33 | 39 | 89 | 59 | 94 | 127 | 41 | 19405 |
| hard—*1 oz bar* | 28 | 50 | 74 | 99 | 203 | 112 | 50 | 85 | 134 | 99 | 142 | 189 | 60 | 19015 |

| | WT (g) | TRY | THR | ISO | LEU | LYS | MET | CYS | PHE | TYR | VAL | ARG | HIS | REF |
|---|---|---|---|---|---|---|---|---|---|---|---|---|---|---|
| | | | | | | | (mg/serving) | | | | | | | |
| nut and raisin, soft—*1 oz bar* | 28 | 28 | 73 | 84 | 152 | 84 | 38 | 45 | 108 | 73 | 111 | 178 | 52 | 19406 |
| peanut butter and choc | | | | | | | | | | | | | | |
|   chip, soft—*1 oz bar* | 28 | 28 | 92 | 97 | 179 | 100 | 37 | 38 | 139 | 109 | 121 | 293 | 66 | 19027 |
| peanut butter, hard—*0.85 oz bar* | 24 | 31 | 74 | 84 | 163 | 90 | 35 | 48 | 120 | 92 | 109 | 234 | 57 | 19420 |
| peanut butter, soft—*1 oz bar* | 28 | 31 | 98 | 105 | 195 | 105 | 41 | 43 | 149 | 117 | 130 | 310 | 72 | 19021 |
| peanut butter, soft, choc | | | | | | | | | | | | | | |
|   covered—*1.3 oz bar* | 37 | 46 | 143 | 169 | 297 | 192 | 64 | 45 | 189 | 159 | 205 | 255 | 84 | 19026 |
| peanut, hard—*1 oz bar* | 28 | 48 | 93 | 113 | 224 | 124 | 51 | 78 | 158 | 118 | 154 | 272 | 73 | 19019 |
| raisin, soft—*1 oz bar* | 28 | 30 | 72 | 85 | 158 | 84 | 39 | 48 | 110 | 71 | 115 | 164 | 51 | 19022 |
| soft—*1 oz bar* | 28 | 28 | 67 | 82 | 150 | 82 | 36 | 46 | 107 | 70 | 111 | 137 | 46 | 19020 |
| **Oriental snack mix**, rice-based—*1 oz* | 28 | 54 | 179 | 189 | 347 | 191 | 69 | 71 | 272 | 208 | 223 | 589 | 132 | 19031 |
| **popcorn,** | | | | | | | | | | | | | | |
|   94% fat-free, microwaved—*1 oz* | 28 | 22 | 104 | 109 | 414 | 98 | 56 | 52 | 148 | 113 | 146 | 86 | 67 | 25000 |
|   air-popped—*1 oz (~3.5 cups)* | 28 | 24 | 127 | 121 | 412 | 95 | 71 | 61 | 165 | 137 | 170 | 167 | 103 | 19034 |
|   cake—*0.35 oz cake* | 10 | 9 | 36 | 37 | 105 | 31 | 21 | 16 | 49 | 39 | 52 | 58 | 28 | 19036 |
|   caramel-coated—*1 oz* | 28 | 13 | 42 | 44 | 80 | 79 | 20 | 11 | 43 | 31 | 50 | 66 | 31 | 19039 |
|   caramel-coated w/peanuts | | | | | | | | | | | | | | |
|     *1 oz (~⅔ cup)* | 28 | 15 | 65 | 64 | 179 | 56 | 31 | 29 | 90 | 73 | 85 | 137 | 51 | 19038 |
|   cheese—*1 oz (~2.6 cups)* | 28 | 26 | 117 | 113 | 287 | 124 | 53 | 45 | 113 | 98 | 137 | 109 | 71 | 19040 |
|   oil-popped—*1 oz (~2.6 cups)* | 28 | 18 | 95 | 90 | 309 | 71 | 53 | 46 | 124 | 102 | 127 | 125 | 77 | 19035 |
|   oil-popped, microwaved | | | | | | | | | | | | | | |
|     *1 oz (~2.6 cups)* | 28 | 18 | 95 | 90 | 309 | 71 | 53 | 46 | 124 | 102 | 127 | 125 | 77 | 19035 |
| **potato chips** | | | | | | | | | | | | | | |
|   *1 oz* | 28 | 30 | 71 | 79 | 117 | 119 | 31 | 25 | 87 | 73 | 110 | 90 | 43 | 19411 |
|   barbeque—*1 oz* | 28 | 30 | 90 | 96 | 142 | 140 | 36 | 30 | 94 | 77 | 119 | 106 | 49 | 19042 |
|   cheese—*1 oz* | 28 | 20 | 102 | 110 | 166 | 155 | 32 | 29 | 109 | 92 | 140 | 112 | 54 | 19421 |
|   cheese, from dried | | | | | | | | | | | | | | |
|     potatoes—*1 oz* | 28 | 18 | 81 | 92 | 143 | 133 | 31 | 23 | 90 | 79 | 115 | 90 | 48 | 19412 |
|   from dried potatoes—*1 oz* | 28 | 13 | 72 | 73 | 109 | 104 | 19 | 21 | 76 | 65 | 97 | 80 | 37 | 19410 |
|   light—*1 oz* | 28 | 31 | 73 | 81 | 120 | 122 | 32 | 26 | 89 | 74 | 113 | 92 | 44 | 19422 |
|   reduced fat, from dried | | | | | | | | | | | | | | |
|     potatoes—*1 oz* | 28 | 12 | 69 | 69 | 103 | 99 | 18 | 20 | 72 | 62 | 92 | 76 | 35 | 19045 |
|   sour cream n' onion—*1 oz* | 28 | 33 | 119 | 113 | 183 | 161 | 39 | 36 | 76 | 67 | 118 | 72 | 42 | 19043 |
|   sour creamn' onion, from | | | | | | | | | | | | | | |
|     dried potatoes—*1 oz* | 28 | 20 | 80 | 88 | 136 | 122 | 29 | 21 | 81 | 71 | 106 | 86 | 41 | 19046 |
| **pretzel** | | | | | | | | | | | | | | |
|   chocolate-covered—*0.39 oz* | 11 | 11 | 28 | 32 | 58 | 28 | 14 | 16 | 39 | 26 | 37 | 34 | 18 | 19048 |
|   hard—*10 twists (2.1 oz)* | 60 | 58 | 150 | 244 | 454 | 154 | 106 | 102 | 312 | 194 | 288 | 218 | 132 | 19047 |
|   whole wheat—*2 oz* | 57 | 98 | 185 | 235 | 428 | 175 | 101 | 144 | 298 | 187 | 287 | 321 | 147 | 19050 |
| **rice cake, brown rice** | | | | | | | | | | | | | | |
|   *0.32 oz cake* | 9 | 9 | 27 | 31 | 61 | 28 | 17 | 9 | 38 | 28 | 43 | 56 | 19 | 19051 |
|   and buckwheat—*0.32 oz cake* | 9 | 11 | 31 | 32 | 57 | 37 | 14 | 12 | 36 | 21 | 44 | 61 | 20 | 19052 |
|   and corn—*0.32 oz cake* | 9 | 8 | 28 | 30 | 70 | 26 | 16 | 10 | 38 | 29 | 42 | 51 | 20 | 19413 |
|   and multigrain—*0.32 oz cake* | 9 | 10 | 27 | 32 | 61 | 28 | 16 | 10 | 38 | 27 | 43 | 56 | 19 | 19414 |
|   and rye—*0.32 oz cake* | 9 | 9 | 26 | 30 | 56 | 28 | 15 | 11 | 36 | 23 | 41 | 50 | 18 | 19416 |
|   and sesame—*0.32 oz cake* | 9 | 9 | 25 | 29 | 56 | 26 | 16 | 8 | 35 | 26 | 40 | 54 | 17 | 19053 |
| **sesame sticks**, wheat-based—*1 oz* | 28 | 40 | 92 | 118 | 215 | 101 | 54 | 56 | 153 | 99 | 131 | 182 | 73 | 19418 |
| **Sunchips**, Frito Lay—*1 oz* | 28 | 20 | 64 | 50 | 246 | 56 | 42 | 34 | 95 | 48 | 78 | 95 | 45 | 25013 |
| **sweet potato chips**—*1 oz* | 28 | 17 | 68 | 69 | 101 | 67 | 34 | 11 | 82 | 57 | 90 | 64 | 26 | 25012 |
| **taro chips**—*10 chips (0.8 oz)* | 23 | 8 | 24 | 19 | 40 | 24 | 7 | 11 | 29 | 20 | 29 | 37 | 12 | 19524 |
| **tortilla chips** | | | | | | | | | | | | | | |
|   nacho—*1 oz* | 28 | 18 | 79 | 83 | 247 | 81 | 46 | 35 | 105 | 89 | 113 | 108 | 67 | 19057 |
|   nacho, reduced-fat—*1 oz* | 28 | 19 | 88 | 93 | 277 | 88 | 51 | 39 | 117 | 99 | 125 | 120 | 73 | 19424 |
|   ranch—*1 oz* | 28 | 16 | 80 | 78 | 244 | 69 | 43 | 37 | 100 | 83 | 106 | 108 | 62 | 19058 |
|   taco flavor—*1 oz* | 28 | 19 | 82 | 88 | 249 | 84 | 46 | 36 | 108 | 89 | 115 | 112 | 67 | 19063 |
|   white corn—*1 oz* | 28 | 16 | 104 | 125 | 352 | 69 | 46 | 16 | 140 | 142 | 114 | 157 | 67 | 19056 |

## 17. GRAIN PRODUCTS

### BAGELS

**bagel**

| | WT (g) | TRY | THR | ISO | LEU | LYS | MET | CYS | PHE | TYR | VAL | ARG | HIS | REF |
|---|---|---|---|---|---|---|---|---|---|---|---|---|---|---|
| cinnamon raisin | | | | | | | | | | | | | | |
|   *3.7 oz bagel (3½" diameter)* | 105 | 120 | 299 | 385 | 705 | 250 | 188 | 220 | 498 | 286 | 445 | 397 | 228 | 18005 |
| egg (egg in bagel dough) | | | | | | | | | | | | | | |
|   *3.7 oz bagel (4" diameter)* | 105 | 131 | 321 | 432 | 785 | 274 | 200 | 243 | 549 | 323 | 484 | 414 | 243 | 18003 |
| oat bran | | | | | | | | | | | | | | |
|   *3.7 oz bagel (4" diameter)* | 105 | 145 | 316 | 426 | 795 | 302 | 197 | 266 | 552 | 337 | 506 | 483 | 245 | 18007 |
| plain/onion/poppyseed/sesame | | | | | | | | | | | | | | |
|   seed—*3.7 oz bagel (4" diameter)* | 105 | 130 | 316 | 424 | 772 | 264 | 197 | 236 | 545 | 316 | 479 | 403 | 238 | 18001 |

| | WT | TRY | THR | ISO | LEU | LYS | MET | CYS | PHE | TYR | VAL | ARG | HIS | REF |
|---|---|---|---|---|---|---|---|---|---|---|---|---|---|---|
| | (g) | | | | | | (mg/serving) | | | | | | | |
| **BISCUITS** | | | | | | | | | | | | | | |
| **biscuit dough**, mixed grain, refrig | | | | | | | | | | | | | | |
| *1.6 oz biscuit (2½″ diameter)* | 44 | 33 | 74 | 94 | 187 | 63 | 47 | 58 | 134 | 80 | 110 | 113 | 61 | 18017 |
| **biscuit mix**, buttermilk—*1 biscuit* | 35 | 34 | 82 | 101 | 197 | 75 | 50 | 57 | 137 | 85 | 117 | 110 | 62 | 18010 |
| **biscuit**, plain buttermilk | | | | | | | | | | | | | | |
| *1.8 oz biscuit* | 51 | 39 | 90 | 115 | 222 | 85 | 57 | 63 | 157 | 98 | 134 | 125 | 71 | 18009 |
| from mix—*1 oz biscuit* | 28 | 25 | 66 | 83 | 154 | 75 | 39 | 37 | 99 | 69 | 95 | 79 | 47 | 18011 |
| from refrig dough (12% to | | | | | | | | | | | | | | |
| 28% fat)—*1 oz biscuit* | 27 | 19 | 50 | 63 | 115 | 60 | 28 | 36 | 70 | 30 | 75 | 62 | 35 | 18015 |
| from refrig dough (2% to 12% fat) | | | | | | | | | | | | | | |
| *0.7 oz biscuit* | 21 | 20 | 44 | 56 | 113 | 36 | 29 | 35 | 82 | 49 | 66 | 66 | 36 | 18013 |
| homemade—*2.1 oz biscuit (2½″ dia)* | 60 | 52 | 127 | 164 | 308 | 136 | 79 | 79 | 208 | 139 | 188 | 165 | 97 | 18016 |
| **BREADS, QUICK** | | | | | | | | | | | | | | |
| **banana bread**, homemade w/marg | | | | | | | | | | | | | | |
| *2.1 oz slice* | 60 | 32 | 90 | 109 | 196 | 108 | 56 | 54 | 131 | 89 | 125 | 119 | 68 | 18019 |
| **Boston brown bread**, canned | | | | | | | | | | | | | | |
| *1.6 oz slice* | 45 | 33 | 73 | 84 | 158 | 70 | 41 | 52 | 105 | 67 | 105 | 115 | 58 | 18021 |
| **cornbread** | | | | | | | | | | | | | | |
| from mix—*2.1 oz piece* | 60 | 47 | 160 | 186 | 388 | 190 | 98 | 82 | 215 | 161 | 223 | 200 | 109 | 18023 |
| homemade w/2% milk—*2.3 oz piece* | 65 | 44 | 168 | 188 | 441 | 192 | 99 | 76 | 214 | 174 | 232 | 203 | 118 | 18024 |
| **hush puppies**, homemade—*0.8 oz* | 22 | 18 | 61 | 71 | 156 | 68 | 37 | 32 | 84 | 64 | 85 | 77 | 43 | 18270 |
| **Irish soda bread**, homemade—*1 oz slice* | 28 | 20 | 56 | 66 | 122 | 61 | 39 | 34 | 84 | 56 | 79 | 81 | 45 | 18032 |
| **BREADS, YEAST** | | | | | | | | | | | | | | |
| **breadcrumbs**, dry, grated—*1 cup* | 108 | 175 | 461 | 588 | 1040 | 464 | 251 | 300 | 707 | 430 | 648 | 596 | 320 | 18079 |
| seasoned—*1 cup* | 120 | 205 | 509 | 703 | 1208 | 535 | 280 | 282 | 844 | 432 | 868 | 724 | 382 | 18376 |
| **cracked wheat bread**—*0.9 oz slice* | 25 | 28 | 65 | 84 | 152 | 61 | 37 | 48 | 105 | 63 | 97 | 87 | 48 | 18025 |
| **croutons**—*1 cup* | 30 | 42 | 101 | 137 | 250 | 83 | 63 | 78 | 176 | 101 | 154 | 129 | 76 | 18242 |
| seasoned—*1 cup* | 40 | 50 | 130 | 171 | 310 | 138 | 78 | 87 | 210 | 132 | 195 | 161 | 98 | 18243 |
| **egg bread**—*1.4 oz slice (5″ × 3″ × ½″)* | 40 | 45 | 122 | 158 | 277 | 124 | 76 | 83 | 190 | 117 | 177 | 154 | 84 | 18027 |
| **French bread**—*small slice (2″ × 2½″ × 1 ¾″)* | 32 | 39 | 91 | 120 | 220 | 94 | 49 | 75 | 156 | 60 | 137 | 117 | 68 | 18029 |
| **French toast** | | | | | | | | | | | | | | |
| frozen—*2.1 oz piece* | 59 | 55 | 166 | 200 | 345 | 218 | 99 | 84 | 216 | 158 | 224 | 198 | 101 | 18268 |
| homemade w/2% milk—*2.3 oz piece* | 65 | 61 | 198 | 244 | 404 | 268 | 122 | 101 | 253 | 183 | 272 | 237 | 116 | 18269 |
| **Italian bread**—*1.1 oz slice (4½″ × 3¼″ × ¾″)* | 30 | 31 | 74 | 100 | 184 | 59 | 47 | 58 | 130 | 74 | 113 | 95 | 56 | 18033 |
| **mixed-/whole-/7-grain bread** | | | | | | | | | | | | | | |
| *0.92 oz slice* | 26 | 32 | 70 | 84 | 145 | 75 | 36 | 46 | 101 | 61 | 103 | 126 | 51 | 18035 |
| **oat bran bread**—*1.1 oz slice* | 30 | 39 | 90 | 120 | 220 | 89 | 54 | 70 | 155 | 97 | 138 | 134 | 68 | 18037 |
| red cal—*0.81 oz slice* | 23 | 24 | 59 | 74 | 130 | 67 | 32 | 31 | 38 | 89 | 84 | 88 | 42 | 18049 |
| **oatmeal bread**—*0.95 oz slice* | 27 | 31 | 67 | 88 | 164 | 73 | 41 | 56 | 112 | 71 | 106 | 107 | 50 | 18039 |
| red cal—*0.81 oz slice* | 23 | 22 | 54 | 72 | 129 | 60 | 32 | 37 | 88 | 58 | 83 | 75 | 39 | 18051 |
| **protein/gluten bread**—*0.67 oz slice* | 19 | 28 | 70 | 89 | 163 | 71 | 38 | 47 | 113 | 69 | 98 | 104 | 51 | 18043 |
| **pumpernickel bread**—*0.92 oz slice* | 26 | 25 | 69 | 87 | 157 | 64 | 40 | 49 | 110 | 62 | 103 | 93 | 51 | 18044 |
| **raisin bread**—*0.92 oz slice* | 26 | 22 | 58 | 75 | 134 | 52 | 33 | 40 | 94 | 53 | 86 | 94 | 43 | 18047 |
| **rice bran bread**—*0.95 oz slice* | 27 | 29 | 72 | 94 | 168 | 70 | 42 | 51 | 119 | 73 | 109 | 102 | 53 | 18059 |
| **rye bread**—*1.1 oz slice* | 32 | 31 | 82 | 102 | 185 | 75 | 44 | 55 | 132 | 68 | 121 | 104 | 58 | 18060 |
| red cal—*0.81 oz slice* | 23 | 25 | 65 | 82 | 147 | 74 | 36 | 41 | 105 | 66 | 95 | 109 | 48 | 18053 |
| **wheat bran bread**—*1.3 oz slice* | 36 | 40 | 92 | 120 | 217 | 85 | 55 | 69 | 151 | 91 | 139 | 129 | 71 | 18066 |
| **wheat germ bread**—*1 oz slice* | 28 | 32 | 85 | 108 | 192 | 91 | 48 | 53 | 128 | 82 | 123 | 111 | 60 | 18068 |
| **wheat/wheat berry bread**—*0.88 oz slice* | 25 | 20 | 43 | 54 | 97 | 45 | 22 | 32 | 66 | 34 | 65 | 65 | 32 | 18064 |
| red cal—*0.81 oz slice* | 23 | 25 | 63 | 82 | 147 | 60 | 37 | 43 | 102 | 63 | 92 | 78 | 45 | 18055 |
| **white bread**—*0.88 oz slice* | 25 | 22 | 56 | 74 | 133 | 51 | 34 | 40 | 93 | 55 | 84 | 70 | 41 | 18069 |
| homemade w/2% milk | | | | | | | | | | | | | | |
| *1.5 oz thick slice* | 42 | 41 | 102 | 131 | 242 | 113 | 62 | 62 | 163 | 110 | 149 | 133 | 76 | 18073 |
| homemade w/nonfat milk | | | | | | | | | | | | | | |
| *1.6 oz thick slice* | 44 | 42 | 98 | 125 | 239 | 94 | 62 | 68 | 169 | 107 | 144 | 136 | 77 | 18071 |
| red cal—*0.81 oz slice* | 23 | 24 | 66 | 88 | 151 | 82 | 37 | 35 | 96 | 68 | 96 | 78 | 46 | 18057 |
| toasted—*0.78 oz slice* | 22 | 23 | 59 | 78 | 140 | 54 | 35 | 42 | 98 | 57 | 87 | 76 | 43 | 18070 |
| **whole wheat bread**—*1 oz slice* | 28 | 23 | 43 | 55 | 100 | 41 | 23 | 34 | 70 | 43 | 67 | 70 | 34 | 18075 |
| homemade—*1.6 oz thick slice* | 46 | 56 | 114 | 144 | 264 | 112 | 63 | 86 | 185 | 116 | 172 | 176 | 89 | 18077 |
| **BREADSTICKS AND CRACKERS** | | | | | | | | | | | | | | |
| **breadstick** | | | | | | | | | | | | | | |
| *0.35 oz breadstick (7 ⅝″ × ⅜″)* | 10 | 14 | 34 | 46 | 84 | 28 | 21 | 26 | 59 | 34 | 52 | 43 | 26 | 18080 |
| **cheese cracker**—*0.5 oz* | 14 | 18 | 41 | 59 | 104 | 59 | 27 | 24 | 69 | 48 | 67 | 54 | 34 | 18214 |
| w/cheese filling—*6 crackers* | 39 | 43 | 129 | 139 | 249 | 151 | 59 | 60 | 136 | 97 | 149 | 114 | 68 | 18927 |
| w/peanut butter filling—*2 crackers* | 7 | 9 | 29 | 32 | 59 | 29 | 13 | 14 | 45 | 33 | 37 | 81 | 21 | 18215 |

| | WT | TRY | THR | ISO | LEU | LYS | MET | CYS | PHE | TYR | VAL | ARG | HIS | REF |
|---|---|---|---|---|---|---|---|---|---|---|---|---|---|---|
| | (g) | | | | | | (mg/serving) | | | | | | | |
| **cracker meal**—*1 cup* | 115 | 123 | 284 | 393 | 735 | 206 | 186 | 239 | 524 | 291 | 446 | 369 | 225 | 18236 |
| **cracker, round** | | | | | | | | | | | | | | |
| *0.5 oz (~5 crackers)* | 14 | 12 | 27 | 34 | 66 | 14 | 16 | 24 | 46 | 22 | 41 | 35 | 20 | 18229 |
| w/cheese filling—*2 crackers* | 7 | 8 | 19 | 24 | 45 | 21 | 12 | 13 | 31 | 20 | 28 | 25 | 14 | 18230 |
| w/peanut butter filling—*2 crackers* | 7 | 9 | 25 | 28 | 53 | 24 | 12 | 13 | 41 | 29 | 33 | 65 | 19 | 18231 |
| **crispbread, rye**—*1 crispbread* | 10 | 9 | 28 | 32 | 56 | 30 | 12 | 16 | 40 | 17 | 40 | 37 | 18 | 18216 |
| **melba toast**—*1 toast (3 ¾″ × 1 ¾″ × ⅛″)* | 5 | 7 | 17 | 23 | 42 | 14 | 11 | 13 | 30 | 17 | 26 | 22 | 13 | 18220 |
| rye/pumpernickel—*1 toast* | 5 | 7 | 18 | 22 | 40 | 17 | 10 | 12 | 28 | 14 | 26 | 23 | 13 | 18221 |
| wheat—*1 toast* | 5 | 9 | 19 | 24 | 44 | 17 | 11 | 14 | 31 | 19 | 29 | 27 | 14 | 18222 |
| **milk cracker**—*1 cracker* | 11 | 11 | 24 | 32 | 60 | 27 | 15 | 17 | 41 | 26 | 37 | 34 | 18 | 18223 |
| **rusk**—*1 rusk* | 10 | 17 | 51 | 61 | 101 | 68 | 29 | 27 | 67 | 47 | 68 | 65 | 31 | 18224 |
| **rye cracker** w/cheese filling | | | | | | | | | | | | | | |
| *2 crackers* | 7 | 8 | 20 | 25 | 45 | 23 | 11 | 13 | 31 | 19 | 29 | 28 | 15 | 18225 |
| **saltine**—*5 crackers (0.49 oz)* | 14 | 16 | 38 | 47 | 91 | 24 | 21 | 32 | 63 | 25 | 56 | 49 | 28 | 18228 |
| fat-free, low sodium—*6 crackers* | 30 | 41 | 86 | 113 | 215 | 87 | 54 | 67 | 154 | 93 | 132 | 124 | 67 | 18457 |
| unsalted top—*5 crackers* | 15 | 18 | 38 | 50 | 95 | 39 | 24 | 30 | 68 | 41 | 58 | 55 | 30 | 18426 |
| **soda crackers**—*5 crackers (0.5 oz)* | 14 | 17 | 38 | 48 | 95 | 32 | 25 | 29 | 69 | 42 | 56 | 57 | 31 | 18425 |
| **wheat crackers**—*0.5 oz (~7 thin* | | | | | | | | | | | | | | |
| *squares)* | 14 | 17 | 34 | 44 | 81 | 33 | 19 | 27 | 58 | 35 | 52 | 52 | 27 | 18232 |
| w/cheese filling—*2 crackers* | 7 | 9 | 21 | 27 | 49 | 24 | 12 | 14 | 33 | 21 | 31 | 29 | 15 | 18233 |
| w/peanut butter filling—*2 crackers* | 7 | 11 | 29 | 34 | 64 | 31 | 14 | 17 | 47 | 32 | 40 | 72 | 22 | 18234 |
| **whole wheat crackers**—*0.5 oz* | | | | | | | | | | | | | | |
| *(~3.5 crackers)* | 14 | 19 | 36 | 46 | 84 | 34 | 19 | 29 | 59 | 36 | 56 | 58 | 29 | 18235 |
| **ENGLISH MUFFINS** | | | | | | | | | | | | | | |
| **English muffin**—*2 oz* | 57 | 62 | 189 | 230 | 372 | 256 | 87 | 104 | 238 | 147 | 259 | 233 | 115 | 18258 |
| mixed grain/granola—*2.3 oz muffin* | 66 | 78 | 184 | 238 | 428 | 192 | 104 | 131 | 296 | 185 | 279 | 291 | 133 | 18260 |
| raisin cinn/apple cinn—*2 oz muffin* | 57 | 51 | 153 | 181 | 295 | 197 | 69 | 83 | 196 | 109 | 207 | 208 | 94 | 18262 |
| wheat—*2 oz muffin* | 57 | 64 | 152 | 194 | 340 | 154 | 83 | 103 | 235 | 145 | 223 | 205 | 110 | 18264 |
| whole wheat—*2.3 oz muffin* | 66 | 85 | 187 | 232 | 403 | 204 | 93 | 125 | 275 | 180 | 273 | 275 | 135 | 18266 |
| **ETHNIC GRAIN PRODUCTS** | | | | | | | | | | | | | | |
| **chow mein noodles**—*1 cup* | 45 | 48 | 99 | 145 | 256 | 72 | 58 | 106 | 182 | 99 | 160 | 138 | 76 | 20113 |
| **eggroll wrapper**—*7″ square wrapper* | 32 | 36 | 86 | 118 | 219 | 65 | 56 | 71 | 156 | 87 | 133 | 111 | 67 | 18368 |
| **matzo**—*1 oz* | 28 | 32 | 75 | 104 | 194 | 54 | 49 | 63 | 138 | 77 | 118 | 97 | 60 | 18217 |
| egg (egg in matzo dough)—*1 oz* | 28 | 42 | 108 | 132 | 248 | 109 | 69 | 75 | 175 | 111 | 152 | 152 | 78 | 18218 |
| egg, onion (egg, onion in matzo | | | | | | | | | | | | | | |
| dough)—*1 oz* | 28 | 34 | 83 | 104 | 197 | 79 | 53 | 60 | 140 | 88 | 119 | 122 | 62 | 18400 |
| whole wheat—*1 oz* | 28 | 58 | 107 | 137 | 249 | 104 | 57 | 86 | 174 | 108 | 167 | 177 | 87 | 18219 |
| **phyllo dough**—*1 sheet* | 19 | 17 | 37 | 47 | 93 | 30 | 24 | 29 | 68 | 41 | 54 | 55 | 30 | 18338 |
| **pita bread** | | | | | | | | | | | | | | |
| white—*1 large (6½″ dia)* | 60 | 63 | 154 | 209 | 380 | 131 | 96 | 118 | 268 | 154 | 236 | 197 | 117 | 18041 |
| whole wheat—*1 large (6½″ dia)* | 64 | 95 | 180 | 235 | 429 | 170 | 98 | 146 | 301 | 187 | 282 | 291 | 145 | 18042 |
| **rice noodles** | | | | | | | | | | | | | | |
| cellophane, Chinese, dry—*1 cup* | 140 | 3 | 7 | 10 | 18 | 15 | 3 | 1 | 14 | 7 | 11 | 15 | 7 | 16082 |
| cooked—*1 cup* | 176 | 19 | 58 | 69 | 132 | 58 | 37 | 33 | 86 | 53 | 99 | 134 | 37 | 20134 |
| **soba** (Japanese noodles), ckd—*1 cup* | 114 | 82 | 202 | 222 | 376 | 244 | 82 | 107 | 247 | 120 | 284 | 361 | 136 | 20115 |
| **somen** (Japanese noodles), ckd—*1 cup* | 176 | 90 | 187 | 273 | 482 | 136 | 109 | 199 | 341 | 185 | 301 | 260 | 143 | 20117 |
| **taco shell**, from corn tortilla | | | | | | | | | | | | | | |
| *1 medium (5″ dia)* | 13 | 5 | 30 | 29 | 109 | 26 | 23 | 18 | 38 | 29 | 37 | 37 | 22 | 18360 |
| **tortilla** | | | | | | | | | | | | | | |
| corn—*1 medium (6″ dia)* | 24 | 10 | 52 | 50 | 171 | 39 | 29 | 25 | 68 | 57 | 71 | 69 | 42 | 18363 |
| flour—*1 medium (7″ to 8″ dia)* | 46 | 49 | 113 | 141 | 276 | 98 | 71 | 83 | 200 | 122 | 164 | 164 | 90 | 18364 |
| **wonton wrapper**—*7″ square wrapper* | 32 | 36 | 86 | 118 | 219 | 65 | 56 | 71 | 156 | 87 | 133 | 111 | 67 | 18368 |
| **MUFFINS** | | | | | | | | | | | | | | |
| **blueberry muffin**, homemade | | | | | | | | | | | | | | |
| w/2% milk—*2 oz muffin* | 57 | 46 | 125 | 157 | 284 | 150 | 78 | 71 | 185 | 129 | 179 | 158 | 86 | 18278 |
| **corn muffin**—*4.9 oz muffin* | 139 | 95 | 314 | 357 | 717 | 388 | 163 | 153 | 413 | 303 | 409 | 443 | 210 | 18279 |
| from mix—*1 oz muffin* | 28 | 23 | 76 | 89 | 185 | 90 | 46 | 39 | 103 | 77 | 106 | 95 | 52 | 18280 |
| homemade with 2% milk | | | | | | | | | | | | | | |
| *2 oz muffin (2 ¾″ × 2″)* | 57 | 44 | 149 | 173 | 373 | 173 | 89 | 72 | 200 | 154 | 207 | 182 | 104 | 18282 |
| **muffin**, homemade with 2% milk | | | | | | | | | | | | | | |
| *2 oz muffin* | 57 | 49 | 132 | 165 | 298 | 159 | 82 | 74 | 195 | 137 | 188 | 165 | 91 | 18273 |
| **oat bran muffin**—*4.9 oz muffin* | 139 | 146 | 292 | 364 | 703 | 385 | 171 | 253 | 481 | 325 | 506 | 656 | 217 | 18283 |
| **raisin bran muffin**, toasted—*1 muffin* | 34 | 25 | 67 | 74 | 134 | 85 | 32 | 36 | 89 | 61 | 85 | 110 | 46 | 18388 |
| **toaster muffin**, blueberry, toasted | | | | | | | | | | | | | | |
| *1 muffin* | 31 | 20 | 60 | 68 | 116 | 86 | 22 | 25 | 75 | 53 | 72 | 100 | 38 | 18386 |

| | WT (g) | TRY | THR | ISO | LEU | LYS | MET | CYS | PHE | TYR | VAL | ARG | HIS | REF |
|---|---|---|---|---|---|---|---|---|---|---|---|---|---|---|
| | | | | | | | (mg/serving) | | | | | | | |
| **PANCAKES** | | | | | | | | | | | | | | |
| **pancake** | | | | | | | | | | | | | | |
| blueberry, homemade | | | | | | | | | | | | | | |
| *4" diameter pancake* | 38 | 29 | 86 | 107 | 185 | 115 | 53 | 42 | 115 | 86 | 121 | 102 | 55 | 18294 |
| buttermilk, homemade | | | | | | | | | | | | | | |
| *4" diameter pancake* | 38 | 31 | 97 | 120 | 207 | 133 | 59 | 46 | 129 | 94 | 138 | 112 | 62 | 18390 |
| from complete mix | | | | | | | | | | | | | | |
| *4" diameter pancake* | 38 | 22 | 71 | 82 | 169 | 80 | 40 | 36 | 97 | 69 | 98 | 84 | 48 | 18290 |
| from incomplete mix | | | | | | | | | | | | | | |
| *4" diameter pancake* | 38 | 36 | 113 | 142 | 250 | 154 | 68 | 54 | 146 | 111 | 163 | 130 | 71 | 18292 |
| frozen | | | | | | | | | | | | | | |
| *4" diameter pancake* | 41 | 21 | 62 | 82 | 146 | 82 | 33 | 42 | 88 | 40 | 97 | 71 | 43 | 18288 |
| homemade | | | | | | | | | | | | | | |
| *4" diameter pancake* | 38 | 30 | 90 | 113 | 195 | 122 | 56 | 44 | 121 | 91 | 127 | 106 | 58 | 18293 |
| whole wheat, from incomplete | | | | | | | | | | | | | | |
| mix—*4" diameter pancake* | 44 | 52 | 139 | 174 | 297 | 193 | 80 | 73 | 184 | 137 | 206 | 190 | 90 | 18300 |
| **PASTA** | | | | | | | | | | | | | | |
| **macaroni** | | | | | | | | | | | | | | |
| enr, boiled—*1 cup elbow-shaped* | 140 | 116 | 288 | 319 | 616 | 186 | 91 | 158 | 416 | 151 | 367 | 295 | 185 | 20100 |
| prot-fortified, enr, boiled | | | | | | | | | | | | | | |
| *1 cup elbow-shaped* | 140 | 144 | 319 | 447 | 780 | 267 | 181 | 308 | 547 | 308 | 496 | 441 | 237 | 20102 |
| vegetable, enr, boiled | | | | | | | | | | | | | | |
| *1 cup spiral-shaped* | 134 | 78 | 163 | 234 | 414 | 125 | 94 | 168 | 292 | 161 | 260 | 225 | 123 | 20106 |
| whole wheat, boiled | | | | | | | | | | | | | | |
| *1 cup elbow shaped* | 140 | 97 | 200 | 290 | 510 | 165 | 120 | 155 | 371 | 195 | 323 | 263 | 175 | 20108 |
| **noodles, egg** | | | | | | | | | | | | | | |
| enr, boiled (egg in dough)—*1 cup* | 160 | 69 | 221 | 304 | 584 | 219 | 138 | 154 | 384 | 150 | 352 | 307 | 194 | 20110 |
| enr, dry (egg in dough)—*1 cup* | 57 | 76 | 245 | 338 | 649 | 245 | 153 | 170 | 426 | 167 | 391 | 342 | 215 | 20109 |
| homemade, ckd (egg in dough) | | | | | | | | | | | | | | |
| *4 oz* | 112 | 75 | 186 | 250 | 428 | 185 | 113 | 160 | 293 | 175 | 277 | 250 | 124 | 20097 |
| spinach, enr, boiled (egg and | | | | | | | | | | | | | | |
| spinach in dough)—*1 cup* | 160 | 107 | 251 | 349 | 582 | 242 | 149 | 213 | 402 | 238 | 390 | 344 | 170 | 20112 |
| **pasta** | | | | | | | | | | | | | | |
| fresh, refrig—*4.5 oz* | 128 | 183 | 378 | 552 | 977 | 274 | 223 | 403 | 694 | 375 | 609 | 526 | 289 | 20093 |
| homemade, ckd—*4 oz* | 112 | 73 | 150 | 221 | 390 | 109 | 88 | 160 | 277 | 150 | 243 | 209 | 115 | 20094 |
| homemade wo/egg, ckd—*4 oz* | 112 | 63 | 130 | 189 | 335 | 94 | 76 | 138 | 237 | 129 | 208 | 180 | 100 | 20098 |
| made from corn, bld—*1 cup* | 140 | 27 | 139 | 132 | 451 | 104 | 77 | 66 | 181 | 150 | 186 | 183 | 112 | 20092 |
| spinach, fresh, refrig—*4.5 oz* | 128 | 192 | 451 | 625 | 1041 | 430 | 266 | 380 | 717 | 425 | 696 | 614 | 303 | 20095 |
| spinach, refrig, ckd—*4 oz* | 112 | 75 | 177 | 245 | 409 | 169 | 104 | 150 | 282 | 167 | 274 | 242 | 120 | 20096 |
| **spaghetti** | | | | | | | | | | | | | | |
| enr, boiled—*1 cup* | 140 | 113 | 284 | 314 | 608 | 183 | 90 | 157 | 410 | 150 | 361 | 291 | 183 | 20121 |
| enr, dry—*2 oz* | 57 | 105 | 263 | 291 | 563 | 170 | 84 | 145 | 381 | 139 | 335 | 270 | 170 | 20120 |
| pro-fort, enr, boiled—*1 cup* | 140 | 144 | 319 | 447 | 780 | 267 | 181 | 308 | 547 | 308 | 496 | 441 | 237 | 20123 |
| spinach, boiled—*1 cup* | 140 | 81 | 172 | 248 | 437 | 132 | 99 | 176 | 308 | 171 | 274 | 238 | 130 | 20127 |
| whole wheat, boiled—*1 cup* | 140 | 97 | 200 | 290 | 510 | 165 | 120 | 155 | 371 | 195 | 323 | 263 | 175 | 20125 |
| **ROLLS** | | | | | | | | | | | | | | |
| **dinner roll** | | | | | | | | | | | | | | |
| *1 oz roll (2" square, 2" high)* | 28 | 23 | 80 | 94 | 204 | 65 | 41 | 64 | 142 | 81 | 112 | 106 | 62 | 18342 |
| homemade with 2% milk | | | | | | | | | | | | | | |
| *1.2 oz roll (2½" diameter)* | 35 | 37 | 99 | 124 | 224 | 116 | 61 | 57 | 149 | 103 | 141 | 127 | 69 | 18396 |
| made with egg | | | | | | | | | | | | | | |
| *1.2 oz roll (2½" diameter)* | 35 | 39 | 108 | 138 | 240 | 115 | 65 | 70 | 163 | 102 | 155 | 134 | 73 | 18344 |
| wheat—*1 oz roll* | 28 | 33 | 67 | 90 | 166 | 57 | 41 | 56 | 117 | 69 | 106 | 99 | 54 | 18347 |
| whole wheat | | | | | | | | | | | | | | |
| *1.3 oz roll (2½" diameter)* | 36 | 48 | 94 | 120 | 216 | 96 | 50 | 71 | 148 | 94 | 145 | 147 | 73 | 18348 |
| **frankfurter roll**—*1.5 oz roll* | 43 | 44 | 113 | 149 | 265 | 104 | 67 | 80 | 185 | 110 | 167 | 141 | 82 | 18350 |
| **French roll**—*1.3 oz roll* | 38 | 38 | 97 | 128 | 231 | 88 | 58 | 69 | 160 | 95 | 144 | 122 | 71 | 18349 |
| **hamburger roll**—*1.5 oz roll* | 43 | 44 | 113 | 149 | 265 | 104 | 67 | 80 | 185 | 110 | 167 | 141 | 82 | 18350 |
| mixed grain—*1.5 oz roll* | 43 | 52 | 121 | 154 | 282 | 109 | 69 | 92 | 197 | 114 | 183 | 174 | 91 | 18351 |
| **hard/kaiser roll** | | | | | | | | | | | | | | |
| *2 oz roll (3½"diameter)* | 57 | 67 | 162 | 218 | 395 | 138 | 100 | 123 | 279 | 162 | 246 | 205 | 122 | 18353 |
| **oat bran roll**—*1.2 oz roll* | 33 | 40 | 90 | 121 | 222 | 89 | 54 | 71 | 157 | 98 | 140 | 135 | 68 | 18345 |
| **pumpernickel roll**—*1.3 oz roll* | 36 | 38 | 98 | 125 | 229 | 84 | 55 | 71 | 164 | 82 | 148 | 127 | 71 | 43441 |
| **rye roll**—*1.3 oz roll* | 36 | 43 | 113 | 143 | 256 | 102 | 62 | 77 | 184 | 94 | 168 | 145 | 81 | 18346 |

| | WT (g) | TRY | THR | ISO | LEU | LYS | MET | CYS | PHE | TYR | VAL | ARG | HIS | REF |
|---|---|---|---|---|---|---|---|---|---|---|---|---|---|---|
| | | | | | | | (mg/serving) | | | | | | | |
| **STUFFINGS AND COATINGS** | | | | | | | | | | | | | | |
| **bread stuffing**, from mix—½ *cup* | 100 | 41 | 97 | 120 | 228 | 96 | 57 | 64 | 161 | 101 | 137 | 136 | 74 | 18082 |
| **cornbread stuffing** dry—*1 oz* | 28 | 29 | 90 | 102 | 244 | 78 | 52 | 55 | 139 | 96 | 125 | 123 | 70 | 18084 |
| from mix—½ *cup* | 100 | 31 | 95 | 108 | 256 | 85 | 55 | 57 | 145 | 101 | 132 | 128 | 73 | 18085 |
| **WAFFLES** | | | | | | | | | | | | | | |
| **waffle** | | | | | | | | | | | | | | |
| buttermilk, frozen, toasted | | | | | | | | | | | | | | |
| *1 waffle (4" square)* | | 33 | 27 | 82 | 103 | 180 | 109 | 49 | 57 | 111 | 57 | 119 | 104 | 52 | 18933 |
| frozen, toasted | | | | | | | | | | | | | | |
| *1 waffle (4" square)* | 33 | 28 | 83 | 98 | 174 | 103 | 44 | 57 | 102 | 49 | 111 | 95 | 49 | 18403 |
| homemade | | | | | | | | | | | | | | |
| *1 round waffle (7" diameter)* | 75 | 74 | 217 | 272 | 472 | 288 | 134 | 109 | 296 | 220 | 307 | 259 | 140 | 18367 |
| **18. INFANT, JUNIOR, AND TODDLER FOODS** | | | | | | | | | | | | | | |
| **INFANT, JUNIOR, AND TODDLER BAKED PRODUCTS** | | | | | | | | | | | | | | |
| **teething biscuit**—*0.4 oz biscuit* | 11 | 13 | 42 | 49 | 90 | 56 | 21 | 16 | 46 | 38 | 55 | 38 | 24 | 3216 |
| **INFANT, JUNIOR, AND TODDLER CEREALS** | | | | | | | | | | | | | | |
| **barley infant cereal** | | | | | | | | | | | | | | |
| dry—*1 T* | 2.4 | 3 | 9 | 10 | 19 | 9 | 5 | 6 | 16 | 10 | 14 | 14 | 6 | 3181 |
| prep w/whole milk—*1 oz* | 28 | 17 | 52 | 66 | 113 | 78 | 29 | 19 | 67 | 56 | 79 | 54 | 32 | 3681 |
| **cereal and egg yolks** | | | | | | | | | | | | | | |
| junior—*6 oz jar* | 170 | 46 | 139 | 170 | 292 | 216 | 87 | 48 | 156 | 143 | 207 | 177 | 76 | 3198 |
| strained—*4 oz jar* | 113 | 31 | 93 | 113 | 194 | 144 | 58 | 32 | 104 | 95 | 138 | 118 | 51 | 3197 |
| **high pro infant cereal**, prep w/ | | | | | | | | | | | | | | |
| whole milk—*1 oz* | 28 | 36 | 102 | 127 | 211 | 170 | 47 | 40 | 124 | 102 | 137 | 156 | 67 | 3682 |
| **mixed cereal** | | | | | | | | | | | | | | |
| dry, infant—*1 T* | 2.5 | 4 | 10 | 12 | 26 | 10 | 6 | 9 | 17 | 12 | 16 | 18 | 7 | 3185 |
| prep w/whole milk, infant—*1 oz* | 28 | 18 | 53 | 68 | 123 | 80 | 30 | 23 | 68 | 60 | 81 | 60 | 34 | 3685 |
| w/applesauce and | | | | | | | | | | | | | | |
| bananas, junior—*6 oz jar* | 170 | 22 | 58 | 73 | 146 | 60 | 41 | 44 | 105 | 73 | 99 | 110 | 46 | 3188 |
| w/applesauce and | | | | | | | | | | | | | | |
| bananas, strained—*4 oz jar* | 113 | 15 | 40 | 50 | 99 | 41 | 28 | 31 | 71 | 50 | 67 | 76 | 32 | 3187 |
| w/bananas, dry, infant—*1 T* | 2.5 | 3 | 9 | 11 | 24 | 12 | 5 | 5 | 14 | 11 | 15 | 13 | 8 | 3186 |
| w/bananas, prep w/ | | | | | | | | | | | | | | |
| whole milk, infant—*1 oz* | 28 | 17 | 52 | 66 | 119 | 82 | 29 | 16 | 62 | 57 | 79 | 51 | 35 | 3686 |
| **oatmeal** | | | | | | | | | | | | | | |
| prep w/whole milk, infant | | | | | | | | | | | | | | |
| cereal—*1 oz* | 28 | 19 | 56 | 72 | 125 | 87 | 31 | 29 | 62 | 62 | 87 | 75 | 32 | 3689 |
| w/applesauce and bananas, | | | | | | | | | | | | | | |
| junior—*6 oz jar* | 170 | 29 | 78 | 83 | 170 | 92 | 53 | 51 | 114 | 88 | 117 | 160 | 58 | 3192 |
| w/applesauce and bananas, | | | | | | | | | | | | | | |
| strained—*4 oz jar* | 113 | 19 | 52 | 55 | 112 | 60 | 34 | 33 | 75 | 59 | 77 | 105 | 38 | 3191 |
| w/bananas, dry, infant | | | | | | | | | | | | | | |
| cereal—*1 T* | 2 | 3 | 8 | 10 | 20 | 11 | 5 | 5 | 12 | 10 | 14 | 14 | 7 | 3190 |
| w/bananas, prep w/whole | | | | | | | | | | | | | | |
| milk, infant cereal—*1 oz* | 28 | 18 | 54 | 69 | 120 | 87 | 32 | 19 | 66 | 60 | 83 | 60 | 37 | 3690 |
| **rice cereal** | | | | | | | | | | | | | | |
| dry, infant—*1 T* | 2 | 2 | 6 | 6 | 11 | 6 | 4 | 3 | 7 | 6 | 9 | 13 | 4 | 3194 |
| prep w/whole milk, infant—*1 oz* | 28 | 15 | 49 | 60 | 101 | 75 | 28 | 15 | 54 | 52 | 72 | 57 | 30 | 3694 |
| w/applesce and bananas, | | | | | | | | | | | | | | |
| Gerber 2nd Foods—*4.25 oz jar* | 120 | 14 | 48 | 58 | 139 | 82 | 24 | 17 | 70 | 67 | 82 | 48 | 38 | 3195 |
| w/applesce and bananas, | | | | | | | | | | | | | | |
| Heinz Strained-2—*4.25 oz jar* | 120 | 14 | 48 | 58 | 139 | 82 | 24 | 17 | 70 | 67 | 82 | 48 | 38 | 3195 |
| w/bananas, dry, infant—*1 T* | 2 | 3 | 9 | 9 | 16 | 9 | 5 | 4 | 8 | 7 | 11 | 12 | 5 | 3212 |
| w/bananas, prep w/whole | | | | | | | | | | | | | | |
| milk, infant—*1 oz* | 28 | 18 | 55 | 68 | 113 | 82 | 30 | 15 | 55 | 54 | 76 | 55 | 33 | 3712 |
| w/mixed fruit, Gerber 3rd | | | | | | | | | | | | | | |
| Foods—*6 oz jar* | 170 | 24 | 70 | 80 | 160 | 71 | 46 | 36 | 102 | 100 | 114 | 165 | 48 | 3210 |
| **INFANT, JUNIOR, AND TODDLER DESSERTS** | | | | | | | | | | | | | | |
| **Dutch apple dessert**, junior—*6 oz jar* | 170 | 3 | 12 | 14 | 20 | 22 | 3 | 5 | 10 | 7 | 15 | 10 | 5 | 3221 |
| **orange pudding**, strained—*4 oz jar* | 113 | | 51 | 64 | 128 | 102 | 17 | | 47 | 51 | 79 | 96 | 35 | 3226 |
| **van custard pudding**, Bch-Nut Stg 2/ | | | | | | | | | | | | | | |
| Gerber 2nd Fds/Heinz Str-2 | | | | | | | | | | | | | | |
| *4 oz jar* | 113 | | 67 | 85 | 67 | 129 | 52 | | 82 | 67 | 99 | 70 | 46 | 3245 |

| | WT | TRY | THR | ISO | LEU | LYS | MET | CYS | PHE | TYR | VAL | ARG | HIS | REF |
|---|---|---|---|---|---|---|---|---|---|---|---|---|---|---|
| | (g) | | | | | | (mg/serving) | | | | | | | |

**INFANT, JUNIOR, AND TODDLER DINNERS**

| | WT | TRY | THR | ISO | LEU | LYS | MET | CYS | PHE | TYR | VAL | ARG | HIS | REF |
|---|---|---|---|---|---|---|---|---|---|---|---|---|---|---|
| **beef lasagna**, toddler—*6 oz jar* | 170 | 80 | 277 | 350 | 551 | 505 | 139 | 82 | 309 | 224 | 393 | 430 | 173 | 3043 |
| **beef noodle**, Beech-Nut Stage 3/ | | | | | | | | | | | | | | |
| Gerber 3rd Fds/Heinz Jr-3—*6 oz jar* | 170 | 46 | 168 | 235 | 354 | 314 | 90 | 49 | 199 | 158 | 224 | 267 | 126 | 3287 |
| **beef, rice**, toddler—*6 oz jar* | 170 | 78 | 340 | 416 | 666 | 639 | 209 | 92 | 335 | 274 | 468 | 575 | 218 | 3049 |
| **beef stew**, Beech-Nut Table Time | | | | | | | | | | | | | | |
| *6 oz jar* | 170 | 90 | 357 | 418 | 660 | 670 | 241 | 90 | 342 | 270 | 462 | 600 | 218 | 3052 |
| **chicken stew**, toddler—*6 oz jar* | 170 | 97 | 376 | 437 | 688 | 697 | 190 | 88 | 362 | 292 | 496 | 563 | 218 | 3072 |
| **macaroni and cheese**, junior | | | | | | | | | | | | | | |
| *6 oz jar* | 170 | 54 | 133 | 221 | 398 | 252 | 153 | 54 | 224 | 209 | 250 | 173 | 105 | 3090 |
| **macaroni, tomato, beef**, Bch-Nut | | | | | | | | | | | | | | |
| Stg 3/Gerber 3rd Fds—*6 oz jar* | 170 | 48 | 153 | 201 | 337 | 253 | 66 | 58 | 190 | 139 | 216 | 226 | 109 | 3045 |
| **spaghetti, tomato, meat**, toddler | | | | | | | | | | | | | | |
| *6 oz jar* | 170 | 110 | 335 | 456 | 702 | 532 | 177 | 112 | 410 | 313 | 486 | 483 | 240 | 3051 |
| **vegetables, beef** | | | | | | | | | | | | | | |
| Bch-Nut Stg 2/Gerber | | | | | | | | | | | | | | |
| 2nd Fds/Heinz Str-2—*4 oz jar* | 113 | 23 | 110 | 125 | 218 | 208 | 69 | 37 | 116 | 97 | 144 | 185 | 84 | 3053 |
| Bch-Nut Stg 3/Gerber 3rd | | | | | | | | | | | | | | |
| Fds/Heinz Jr-3—*6 oz jar* | 170 | 34 | 151 | 168 | 289 | 279 | 88 | 51 | 165 | 133 | 196 | 245 | 112 | 3054 |
| Earth's Best—*4 oz jar* | 113 | 23 | 110 | 125 | 218 | 208 | 69 | 37 | 116 | 97 | 144 | 185 | 84 | 3053 |
| **vegetables, lamb**, junior—*6 oz jar* | 170 | 41 | 131 | 162 | 264 | 262 | 53 | 31 | 141 | 112 | 173 | 240 | 82 | 3067 |
| **vegetables, turkey**, toddler—*6 oz jar* | 170 | 102 | 316 | 423 | 661 | 563 | 150 | 88 | 340 | 296 | 473 | 502 | 194 | 3086 |

**INFANT, JUNIOR, AND TODDLER MEATS**

| | WT | TRY | THR | ISO | LEU | LYS | MET | CYS | PHE | TYR | VAL | ARG | HIS | REF |
|---|---|---|---|---|---|---|---|---|---|---|---|---|---|---|
| **chicken** | | | | | | | | | | | | | | |
| Bch-Nut Stg 1/Gerber 2nd Fds/ | | | | | | | | | | | | | | |
| Heinz Str-2—*2.5 oz jar* | 71 | 111 | 437 | 458 | 751 | 812 | 261 | 128 | 396 | 312 | 489 | 679 | 295 | 3012 |
| Gerber 3rd Fds/Heinz Jr-3 | | | | | | | | | | | | | | |
| *2.5 oz jar* | 71 | 119 | 469 | 492 | 807 | 872 | 280 | 137 | 425 | 334 | 525 | 730 | 316 | 3013 |
| **chicken sticks**, Gerber Graduates | | | | | | | | | | | | | | |
| *2.5 oz jar* | 71 | 83 | 406 | 518 | 811 | 824 | 229 | 90 | 478 | 353 | 542 | 712 | 328 | 3014 |
| **ham** | | | | | | | | | | | | | | |
| Gerber 2nd Foods—*2.5 oz jar* | 71 | 98 | 428 | 469 | 789 | 838 | 252 | 121 | 376 | 331 | 508 | 667 | 335 | 3008 |
| junior—*2.5 oz jar* | 71 | 106 | 466 | 510 | 858 | 911 | 274 | 132 | 409 | 359 | 553 | 726 | 365 | 3009 |
| **lamb**, junior—*2.5 oz jar* | 71 | 107 | 492 | 507 | 852 | 958 | 338 | 148 | 425 | 378 | 547 | 707 | 273 | 3011 |
| **meat sticks**, Gerber Graduates | | | | | | | | | | | | | | |
| *2.5 oz jar* | 71 | 65 | 413 | 474 | 740 | 734 | 219 | 52 | 431 | 370 | 491 | 618 | 327 | 3021 |
| **pork**, strained—*2.5 oz jar* | 71 | 97 | 438 | 483 | 800 | 822 | 283 | 109 | 405 | 362 | 498 | 673 | 317 | 3007 |
| **turkey**, Bch-Nut Stg 1/Gerber 2nd | | | | | | | | | | | | | | |
| Fds/Heinz Str-2—*2.5 oz jar* | 71 | 106 | 449 | 509 | 808 | 841 | 315 | 124 | 419 | 357 | 516 | 645 | 260 | 3015 |
| **turkey sticks**, Gerber Graduates | | | | | | | | | | | | | | |
| *2.5 oz jar* | 71 | 72 | 388 | 447 | 760 | 835 | 216 | 87 | 433 | 343 | 462 | 627 | 261 | 3017 |

**INFANT, JUNIOR, AND TODDLER VEGETABLES**

| | WT | TRY | THR | ISO | LEU | LYS | MET | CYS | PHE | TYR | VAL | ARG | HIS | REF |
|---|---|---|---|---|---|---|---|---|---|---|---|---|---|---|
| **beets**, Gerber 2nd Fds/Heinz Str-2 | | | | | | | | | | | | | | |
| *4 oz jar* | 113 | 14 | 36 | 43 | 52 | 38 | 11 | 8 | 20 | 40 | 51 | 34 | 24 | 3098 |
| **carrots** | | | | | | | | | | | | | | |
| Bch-Nut Baby's 1st/Gerber 1st | | | | | | | | | | | | | | |
| Fds/Heinz Beginner-1 | | | | | | | | | | | | | | |
| *2.5 oz jar* | 71 | 8 | 16 | 17 | 23 | 14 | 6 | 4 | 17 | 13 | 21 | 36 | 9 | 3099 |
| Bch-Nut Stg 1/Gerber 2nd Fds/ | | | | | | | | | | | | | | |
| Heinz Str-2—*2.5 oz jar* | 71 | 8 | 16 | 17 | 23 | 14 | 6 | 4 | 17 | 13 | 21 | 36 | 9 | 3099 |
| Bch-Nut Stg 3/Gerber 3rd Fds/ | | | | | | | | | | | | | | |
| Heinz Jr-3—*6 oz jar* | 170 | 19 | 39 | 41 | 56 | 36 | 15 | 10 | 42 | 34 | 53 | 88 | 22 | 3100 |
| Earth's Best—*2.5 oz jar* | 71 | 8 | 16 | 17 | 23 | 14 | 6 | 4 | 17 | 13 | 21 | 36 | 9 | 3099 |
| **corn and sweet potatoes**, strained | | | | | | | | | | | | | | |
| *4.5 oz jar* | 128 | 22 | 67 | 76 | 146 | 84 | 42 | 22 | 68 | 72 | 95 | 73 | 49 | 3934 |
| **corn, yellow, creamed** | | | | | | | | | | | | | | |
| Bch-Nut Stg 2/Gerber 2nd Fds/ | | | | | | | | | | | | | | |
| Heinz Str-2—*4 oz jar* | 113 | 17 | 59 | 73 | 158 | 92 | 45 | 20 | 55 | 76 | 87 | 68 | 52 | 3119 |
| Heinz Jr-3—*6 oz jar* | 170 | 26 | 88 | 110 | 240 | 139 | 68 | 31 | 83 | 116 | 133 | 102 | 78 | 3120 |
| **garden vegetables**, strained—*4 oz jar* | 113 | 31 | 82 | 97 | 162 | 131 | 49 | 23 | 99 | 107 | 112 | 221 | 51 | 3283 |
| **green beans** | | | | | | | | | | | | | | |
| Bch-Nut Stg 1/Gerber 2nd | | | | | | | | | | | | | | |
| Fds/Heinz Str-2—*2.5 oz jar* | 71 | 11 | 39 | 41 | 60 | 46 | 13 | 8 | 38 | 33 | 50 | 51 | 26 | 3091 |
| Beech-Nut Stage 3—*6 oz jar* | 170 | 24 | 87 | 92 | 133 | 100 | 31 | 17 | 83 | 71 | 110 | 112 | 56 | 3092 |
| Gerber 1st Fds/Heinz | | | | | | | | | | | | | | |
| Beginner-1—*2.5 oz jar* | 71 | 11 | 39 | 41 | 60 | 46 | 13 | 8 | 38 | 33 | 50 | 51 | 26 | 3091 |

| | WT (g) | TRY | THR | ISO | LEU | LYS | MET | CYS | PHE | TYR | VAL | ARG | HIS | REF |
|---|---|---|---|---|---|---|---|---|---|---|---|---|---|---|
| | | | | | | | (mg/serving) | | | | | | | |
| **mixed vegetables** | | | | | | | | | | | | | | |
| junior—*6 oz jar* | 170 | 26 | 76 | 95 | 155 | 80 | 36 | 48 | 94 | 88 | 117 | 158 | 53 | 3282 |
| strained—*4 oz jar* | 113 | 15 | 43 | 53 | 87 | 45 | 20 | 27 | 53 | 50 | 66 | 89 | 29 | 3286 |
| **spinach, creamed,** Gerber 2nd Fds—*4 oz jar* | 113 | 41 | 114 | 127 | 250 | 167 | 62 | 35 | 108 | 130 | 171 | 172 | 72 | 3127 |
| **sweet potatoes** | | | | | | | | | | | | | | |
| Bch-Nut Baby's 1st/Gerber 1st Fds/Hnz Bgnr-1—*2.5 oz jar* | 71 | 16 | 38 | 36 | 55 | 31 | 17 | 11 | 44 | 29 | 52 | 38 | 18 | 3108 |
| Bch-Nut Stg 1/Gerber 2nd Fds/Heinz Str-2—*2.5 oz jar* | 71 | 16 | 38 | 36 | 55 | 31 | 17 | 11 | 44 | 29 | 52 | 38 | 18 | 3108 |
| Bch-Nut Stg 3/Gerber 3rd Fds/Heinz Jr-3—*6 oz jar* | 170 | 36 | 90 | 85 | 129 | 73 | 39 | 26 | 104 | 68 | 121 | 90 | 42 | 3109 |
| Earth's Best—*2.5 oz jar* | 71 | 16 | 38 | 36 | 55 | 31 | 17 | 11 | 44 | 29 | 52 | 38 | 18 | 3108 |
| **19. MEATS** | | | | | | | | | | | | | | |
| **BEEF** | | | | | | | | | | | | | | |
| **beef bottom sirloin tri-tip roast** | | | | | | | | | | | | | | |
| 0″ trim, lean, roasted—*3 oz* | 85 | 150 | 909 | 1034 | 1809 | 1922 | 592 | 293 | 898 | 724 | 1128 | 1470 | 726 | 13985 |
| 0″ trim, lean and fat, brld—*3 oz* | 85 | 275 | 1176 | 1313 | 2249 | 2388 | 722 | 274 | 1103 | 932 | 1376 | 1715 | 822 | 23545 |
| 0″ trim, lean, broiled—*3 oz* | 85 | 281 | 1205 | 1346 | 2305 | 2447 | 740 | 280 | 1130 | 955 | 1410 | 1757 | 841 | 13987 |
| **beef brisket, flat half, 0″ trim** | | | | | | | | | | | | | | |
| lean and fat, braised—*3 oz* | 85 | 184 | 1117 | 1272 | 2224 | 2363 | 728 | 361 | 1105 | 891 | 1387 | 1808 | 892 | 13369 |
| lean, braised—*3 oz* | 85 | 186 | 1130 | 1286 | 2249 | 2389 | 736 | 365 | 1117 | 901 | 1402 | 1828 | 902 | 13370 |
| **beef brisket, flat half, choice,** ⅛″ trim | | | | | | | | | | | | | | |
| lean and fat, braised—*3 oz* | 85 | 154 | 936 | 1065 | 1863 | 1979 | 609 | 303 | 925 | 746 | 1162 | 1514 | 747 | 13806 |
| lean, braised—*3 oz* | 85 | 122 | 736 | 839 | 1466 | 1558 | 480 | 238 | 728 | 587 | 915 | 1193 | 588 | 23613 |
| **beef brisket, flat half, select,** ⅛″ trim | | | | | | | | | | | | | | |
| lean and fat, braised—*3 oz* | 85 | 99 | 604 | 687 | 1201 | 1277 | 394 | 195 | 597 | 481 | 749 | 977 | 482 | 23659 |
| lean, braised—*3 oz* | 85 | 120 | 728 | 830 | 1450 | 1541 | 475 | 235 | 720 | 581 | 904 | 1179 | 582 | 23632 |
| **beef brisket, point half, 0″ trim** | | | | | | | | | | | | | | |
| lean and fat, braised—*3 oz* | 85 | 224 | 874 | 899 | 1580 | 1663 | 512 | 224 | 780 | 672 | 972 | 1264 | 685 | 13371 |
| lean, braised—*3 oz* | 85 | 267 | 1041 | 1072 | 1884 | 1984 | 610 | 267 | 931 | 801 | 1159 | 1507 | 816 | 13372 |
| **beef brisket, whole** (flat and point halves) 0″ trim, lean and fat, braised—*3 oz* | 85 | 150 | 910 | 1036 | 1811 | 1924 | 593 | 294 | 899 | 726 | 1130 | 1472 | 727 | 13367 |
| 0″ trim, lean, braised—*3 oz* | 85 | 167 | 1010 | 1151 | 2012 | 2137 | 659 | 326 | 999 | 806 | 1255 | 1635 | 807 | 13368 |
| **beef chuck arm pot roast, choice** | | | | | | | | | | | | | | |
| 0″ trim, lean, braised—*3 oz* | 85 | 186 | 1133 | 1290 | 2256 | 2397 | 739 | 366 | 1120 | 904 | 1407 | 1833 | 905 | 13377 |
| ⅛″ trim, lean and fat, braised—*3 oz* | 85 | 105 | 633 | 721 | 1261 | 1340 | 413 | 205 | 626 | 505 | 786 | 1025 | 506 | 13811 |
| ⅛″ trim, lean, braised—*3 oz* | 85 | 122 | 745 | 849 | 1484 | 1577 | 486 | 241 | 737 | 595 | 926 | 1207 | 596 | 23612 |
| **beef chuck arm pot roast, select** | | | | | | | | | | | | | | |
| 0″ trim, lean and fat, braised—*3 oz* | 85 | 163 | 993 | 1130 | 1976 | 2100 | 647 | 320 | 982 | 792 | 1232 | 1606 | 793 | 13375 |
| 0″ trim, lean, braised—*3 oz* | 85 | 186 | 1133 | 1290 | 2256 | 2397 | 739 | 366 | 1120 | 904 | 1407 | 1834 | 905 | 13378 |
| ⅛″ trim, lean and fat, braised—*3 oz* | 85 | 108 | 656 | 747 | 1306 | 1388 | 428 | 212 | 649 | 524 | 815 | 1062 | 524 | 13813 |
| ⅛″ trim, lean, braised—*3 oz* | 85 | 124 | 756 | 861 | 1504 | 1599 | 493 | 244 | 747 | 603 | 938 | 1223 | 604 | 23631 |
| **beef chuck blade roast, choice** | | | | | | | | | | | | | | |
| 0″ trim, lean and fat, braised—*3 oz* | 85 | 257 | 1001 | 1031 | 1812 | 1908 | 587 | 257 | 895 | 771 | 1115 | 1449 | 785 | 13380 |
| 0″ trim, lean, braised—*3 oz* | 85 | 296 | 1153 | 1187 | 2087 | 2196 | 676 | 296 | 1031 | 887 | 1284 | 1669 | 904 | 13383 |
| ⅛″ trim, lean and fat, braised—*3 oz* | 85 | 162 | 631 | 649 | 1141 | 1201 | 370 | 162 | 564 | 485 | 702 | 912 | 494 | 13817 |
| **beef chuck blade roast, select** | | | | | | | | | | | | | | |
| 0″ trim, lean and fat, braised—*3 oz* | 85 | 296 | 1153 | 1187 | 2087 | 2196 | 676 | 296 | 1031 | 887 | 1284 | 1669 | 904 | 13384 |
| 0″ trim, lean and fat, braised—*3 oz* | 85 | 263 | 1024 | 1055 | 1854 | 1952 | 600 | 263 | 915 | 788 | 1141 | 1482 | 803 | 13381 |
| ⅛″ trim, lean and fat, braised—*3 oz* | 85 | 165 | 645 | 664 | 1167 | 1228 | 378 | 165 | 576 | 496 | 718 | 933 | 506 | 13819 |
| **beef chuck clod roast, choice** | | | | | | | | | | | | | | |
| 0″ trim, lean and fat, roasted—*3 oz* | 85 | 226 | 965 | 1075 | 1842 | 1955 | 592 | 225 | 904 | 764 | 1127 | 1406 | 676 | 23528 |
| 0″ trim, lean, roasted—*3 oz* | 85 | 238 | 1019 | 1139 | 1950 | 2070 | 626 | 237 | 956 | 808 | 1193 | 1486 | 711 | 13937 |
| **beef chuck clod roast, select** | | | | | | | | | | | | | | |
| 0″ trim, lean and fat, roasted—*3 oz* | 85 | 251 | 1071 | 1195 | 2048 | 2173 | 657 | 249 | 1005 | 849 | 1252 | 1561 | 749 | 23531 |
| 0″ trim, lean, roasted—*3 oz* | 85 | 258 | 1103 | 1233 | 2111 | 2241 | 677 | 257 | 1035 | 876 | 1291 | 1609 | 770 | 13940 |
| **beef chuck clod steak, choice** | | | | | | | | | | | | | | |
| 0″ trim, lean and fat, braised—*3 oz* | 85 | 258 | 1101 | 1227 | 2102 | 2231 | 675 | 257 | 1031 | 872 | 1286 | 1604 | 770 | 23533 |
| 0″ trim, lean, braised—*3 oz* | 85 | 271 | 1159 | 1295 | 2218 | 2354 | 711 | 269 | 1088 | 920 | 1357 | 1691 | 809 | 13943 |
| **beef chuck clod steak, select** | | | | | | | | | | | | | | |
| 0″ trim, lean and fat, braised—*3 oz* | 85 | 274 | 1171 | 1308 | 2240 | 2377 | 719 | 273 | 1099 | 929 | 1370 | 1708 | 818 | 23536 |
| 0″ trim, lean, braised—*3 oz* | 85 | 279 | 1193 | 1333 | 2282 | 2422 | 732 | 277 | 1119 | 946 | 1396 | 1739 | 832 | 13946 |
| **beef chuck shldr medallion, choice** | | | | | | | | | | | | | | |
| 0″ trim, lean, grilled—*3 oz* | 85 | 117 | 711 | 809 | 1415 | 1504 | 463 | 230 | 703 | 567 | 882 | 1150 | 568 | 23036 |
| **beef chuck shldr medallion, select** | | | | | | | | | | | | | | |
| 0″ trim, lean, grilled—*3 oz* | 85 | 146 | 890 | 1014 | 1773 | 1884 | 581 | 287 | 881 | 710 | 1106 | 1441 | 711 | 23054 |

| | WT | TRY | THR | ISO | LEU | LYS | MET | CYS | PHE | TYR | VAL | ARG | HIS | REF |
|---|---|---|---|---|---|---|---|---|---|---|---|---|---|---|
| | (g) | | | | | | (mg/serving) | | | | | | | |
| **beef chuck shldr top blade steak,** | | | | | | | | | | | | | | |
| **choice** 0″ trim, lean and fat, grld—*3 oz* | 85 | 108 | 658 | 750 | 1311 | 1392 | 429 | 212 | 651 | 525 | 818 | 1065 | 526 | 23043 |
| **beef chuck shldr top blade steak,** | | | | | | | | | | | | | | |
| **select** 0″ trim, lean and fat, grld—*3 oz* | 85 | 106 | 645 | 734 | 1284 | 1364 | 421 | 208 | 638 | 514 | 801 | 1044 | 515 | 23059 |
| **beef chuck shldr top/center steak,** | | | | | | | | | | | | | | |
| **select** 0″ trim, lean and fat, grld—*3 oz* | 85 | 145 | 885 | 1008 | 1763 | 1873 | 577 | 286 | 876 | 706 | 1099 | 1433 | 707 | 23038 |
| **beef chuck shldr top/center steak,** | | | | | | | | | | | | | | |
| **select** 0″ trim, lean, grld—*3 oz* | 85 | 147 | 893 | 1017 | 1778 | 1889 | 582 | 288 | 883 | 712 | 1109 | 1445 | 713 | 23058 |
| **beef chuck, tender steak, choice** | | | | | | | | | | | | | | |
| 0″ trim, lean and fat, broiled—*3 oz* | 85 | 236 | 1011 | 1130 | 1934 | 2053 | 620 | 235 | 949 | 802 | 1183 | 1474 | 706 | 23519 |
| 0″ trim, lean, broiled—*3 oz* | 85 | 236 | 1012 | 1130 | 1935 | 2054 | 620 | 235 | 949 | 802 | 1183 | 1474 | 706 | 13961 |
| **beef chuck, tender steak, select** | | | | | | | | | | | | | | |
| 0″ trim, lean and fat, broiled—*3 oz* | 85 | 239 | 1024 | 1144 | 1959 | 2080 | 629 | 238 | 961 | 813 | 1198 | 1493 | 715 | 23521 |
| 0″ trim, lean, broiled—*3 oz* | 85 | 240 | 1027 | 1147 | 1964 | 2084 | 630 | 239 | 963 | 814 | 1201 | 1497 | 716 | 13963 |
| **beef chuck, top blade, choice** | | | | | | | | | | | | | | |
| 0″ trim, lean and fat, brld—*3 oz* | 85 | 236 | 1012 | 1130 | 1935 | 2054 | 620 | 235 | 949 | 802 | 1183 | 1476 | 706 | 23523 |
| 0″ trim, lean, broiled—*3 oz* | 85 | 240 | 1026 | 1146 | 1962 | 2082 | 630 | 238 | 962 | 813 | 1200 | 1495 | 716 | 13965 |
| **beef chuck, top blade, select** | | | | | | | | | | | | | | |
| 0″ trim, lean and fat, broiled—*3 oz* | 85 | 235 | 1007 | 1125 | 1926 | 2044 | 618 | 235 | 944 | 799 | 1178 | 1469 | 704 | 23525 |
| 0″ trim, lean, broiled—*3 oz* | 85 | 240 | 1028 | 1148 | 1966 | 2087 | 631 | 239 | 964 | 815 | 1203 | 1499 | 717 | 13967 |
| **beef flank, choice,** 0″ trim | | | | | | | | | | | | | | |
| lean and fat, broiled—*3 oz* | 85 | 154 | 935 | 1065 | 1862 | 1979 | 609 | 302 | 925 | 746 | 1162 | 1514 | 747 | 13067 |
| lean, braised—*3 oz* | 85 | 156 | 951 | 1084 | 1895 | 2013 | 620 | 308 | 941 | 759 | 1182 | 1540 | 760 | 13069 |
| lean, broiled—*3 oz* | 85 | 156 | 944 | 1076 | 1881 | 1998 | 615 | 305 | 934 | 753 | 1173 | 1529 | 755 | 13070 |
| **beef flank, select,** 0″ trim | | | | | | | | | | | | | | |
| lean and fat, broiled—*3 oz* | 85 | 156 | 944 | 1074 | 1878 | 1996 | 615 | 305 | 932 | 752 | 1171 | 1527 | 754 | 13949 |
| lean, broiled—*3 oz* | 85 | 156 | 949 | 1081 | 1890 | 2009 | 619 | 307 | 938 | 757 | 1179 | 1537 | 758 | 23655 |
| **beef, ground, 10% fat** | | | | | | | | | | | | | | |
| crumbles, pan-browned—*3 oz* | 85 | 134 | 946 | 1063 | 1884 | 2009 | 631 | 252 | 934 | 753 | 1186 | 1548 | 796 | 23565 |
| loaf, baked—*3 oz piece* | 85 | 126 | 885 | 995 | 1763 | 1879 | 590 | 236 | 874 | 705 | 1109 | 1448 | 745 | 23566 |
| patty, broiled—*3 oz patty* | 85 | 123 | 868 | 976 | 1729 | 1844 | 579 | 232 | 858 | 691 | 1088 | 1420 | 731 | 23563 |
| patty, pan-broiled—*3 oz patty* | 85 | 119 | 838 | 943 | 1669 | 1780 | 558 | 224 | 828 | 667 | 1051 | 1371 | 706 | 23564 |
| **beef, ground, 15% fat** | | | | | | | | | | | | | | |
| crumbles, pan-browned—*3 oz* | 85 | 122 | 913 | 1040 | 1837 | 1952 | 607 | 243 | 917 | 726 | 1157 | 1529 | 767 | 23570 |
| loaf, baked—*3 oz piece* | 85 | 113 | 854 | 973 | 1718 | 1826 | 568 | 227 | 858 | 679 | 1082 | 1431 | 717 | 23571 |
| patty, broiled—*3 oz patty* | 85 | 113 | 853 | 973 | 1718 | 1825 | 568 | 227 | 858 | 679 | 1082 | 1431 | 717 | 23568 |
| patty, pan-broiled—*3 oz patty* | 85 | 108 | 811 | 924 | 1631 | 1733 | 539 | 216 | 815 | 644 | 1028 | 1358 | 681 | 23569 |
| **beef, ground, 20% fat** | | | | | | | | | | | | | | |
| crumbles, pan-browned—*3 oz* | 85 | 107 | 879 | 1018 | 1789 | 1895 | 583 | 233 | 902 | 698 | 1129 | 1514 | 736 | 23575 |
| loaf, baked—*3 oz piece* | 85 | 100 | 822 | 952 | 1673 | 1771 | 545 | 218 | 843 | 653 | 1056 | 1415 | 688 | 23576 |
| patty, broiled—*3 oz patty* | 85 | 102 | 838 | 972 | 1706 | 1806 | 556 | 222 | 859 | 666 | 1076 | 1443 | 701 | 23573 |
| patty, pan-broiled—*3 oz patty* | 85 | 95 | 783 | 907 | 1592 | 1686 | 518 | 207 | 802 | 621 | 1005 | 1347 | 655 | 23574 |
| **beef, ground, 25% fat** | | | | | | | | | | | | | | |
| crumbles, pan-browned—*3 oz* | 85 | 92 | 844 | 997 | 1742 | 1837 | 558 | 223 | 887 | 669 | 1101 | 1500 | 704 | 23580 |
| loaf, baked—*3 oz piece* | 85 | 86 | 789 | 932 | 1628 | 1716 | 521 | 208 | 829 | 626 | 1028 | 1402 | 658 | 23581 |
| patty, broiled—*3 oz patty* | 85 | 89 | 821 | 970 | 1694 | 1787 | 542 | 217 | 863 | 651 | 1071 | 1459 | 684 | 23578 |
| patty, pan-broiled—*3 oz patty* | 85 | 82 | 753 | 890 | 1554 | 1639 | 497 | 199 | 791 | 597 | 983 | 1339 | 628 | 23579 |
| **beef, ground, 30% fat** | | | | | | | | | | | | | | |
| broiled—*3 oz* | 85 | 74 | 802 | 969 | 1682 | 1765 | 527 | 210 | 867 | 634 | 1066 | 1482 | 665 | 13497 |
| crumbles, pan-browned—*3 oz* | 85 | 74 | 808 | 976 | 1694 | 1777 | 530 | 211 | 873 | 638 | 1073 | 1492 | 670 | 13494 |
| patty, baked—*3 oz patty* | 85 | 70 | 754 | 911 | 1582 | 1661 | 496 | 197 | 815 | 597 | 1002 | 1393 | 626 | 13495 |
| patty, pan-broiled—*3 oz patty* | 85 | 66 | 722 | 873 | 1516 | 1590 | 475 | 189 | 781 | 571 | 960 | 1334 | 599 | 13496 |
| **beef, ground, 5% fat** | | | | | | | | | | | | | | |
| crumbles, pan-browned—*3 oz* | 85 | 147 | 978 | 1086 | 1932 | 2065 | 654 | 263 | 951 | 779 | 1214 | 1568 | 826 | 23560 |
| loaf, baked—*3 oz piece* | 85 | 138 | 916 | 1017 | 1809 | 1933 | 611 | 246 | 891 | 729 | 1136 | 1468 | 774 | 23561 |
| patty, broiled—*3 oz patty* | 85 | 132 | 881 | 979 | 1741 | 1861 | 589 | 236 | 858 | 702 | 1094 | 1413 | 745 | 23558 |
| patty, pan-broiled—*3 oz patty* | 85 | 130 | 865 | 960 | 1708 | 1826 | 578 | 232 | 842 | 688 | 1074 | 1386 | 730 | 23559 |
| **beef ribeye, small end (ribs 10 to 12)** | | | | | | | | | | | | | | |
| choice, 0″ trim, lean and fat, brld—*3 oz* | 85 | 167 | 650 | 669 | 1176 | 1238 | 381 | 167 | 581 | 500 | 724 | 941 | 510 | 13095 |
| choice, 0″ trim, lean, brld—*3 oz* | 85 | 191 | 747 | 769 | 1352 | 1424 | 438 | 191 | 668 | 575 | 832 | 1081 | 586 | 13097 |
| select, 0″ trim, lean and fat, brld—*3 oz* | 85 | 152 | 926 | 1055 | 1844 | 1958 | 604 | 299 | 915 | 739 | 1150 | 1499 | 740 | 13952 |
| select, 0″ trim, lean, brld—*3 oz* | 85 | 167 | 1017 | 1158 | 2024 | 2150 | 662 | 328 | 1005 | 811 | 1262 | 1646 | 812 | 13490 |
| **beef ribs, large end (ribs 6 to 9)** | | | | | | | | | | | | | | |
| choice, 0″ trim, lean and fat, rstd—*3 oz* | 85 | 217 | 847 | 871 | 1532 | 1612 | 496 | 217 | 756 | 651 | 943 | 1225 | 664 | 13386 |
| choice, 0″ trim, lean, rstd—*3 oz* | 85 | 262 | 1023 | 1052 | 1850 | 1947 | 599 | 262 | 914 | 786 | 1138 | 1479 | 802 | 13389 |
| **beef ribs, shortribs** | | | | | | | | | | | | | | |
| lean and fat, braised—*3 oz* | 85 | 121 | 733 | 834 | 1459 | 1550 | 478 | 236 | 724 | 584 | 910 | 1186 | 585 | 13148 |
| lean, braised—*3 oz* | 85 | 172 | 1045 | 1189 | 2080 | 2210 | 681 | 337 | 1033 | 833 | 1297 | 1691 | 835 | 13150 |

| | WT (g) | TRY | THR | ISO | LEU | LYS | MET | CYS | PHE | TYR | VAL | ARG | HIS | REF |
|---|---|---|---|---|---|---|---|---|---|---|---|---|---|---|
| | | | | | | | (mg/serving) | | | | | | | |
| **beef ribs, small end (ribs 10 to 12)** | | | | | | | | | | | | | | |
| choice, 0" trim, lean and fat, brld—3 oz | 85 | 235 | 918 | 945 | 1662 | 1749 | 538 | 235 | 821 | 706 | 1023 | 1329 | 720 | 13392 |
| choice, 0" trim, lean, brld—3 oz | 85 | 267 | 1041 | 1072 | 1884 | 1983 | 610 | 267 | 931 | 801 | 1159 | 1506 | 816 | 13395 |
| choice, ⅛" trim, lean and fat, brld—3 oz | 85 | 106 | 649 | 739 | 1291 | 1371 | 422 | 209 | 641 | 517 | 805 | 1049 | 518 | 13853 |
| choice, ⅛" trim, lean, brld—3 oz | 85 | 165 | 1005 | 1144 | 2000 | 2125 | 654 | 325 | 993 | 802 | 1247 | 1626 | 802 | 23638 |
| select, 0" trim, lean and fat, brld—3 oz | 85 | 237 | 925 | 952 | 1674 | 1761 | 542 | 237 | 826 | 711 | 1030 | 1338 | 725 | 13393 |
| select, 0" trim, lean, broiled—3 oz | 85 | 267 | 1041 | 1072 | 1884 | 1983 | 610 | 267 | 931 | 801 | 1159 | 1506 | 816 | 13396 |
| select, ⅛" trim, lean and fat, rstd—3 oz | 85 | 159 | 621 | 640 | 1125 | 1184 | 365 | 159 | 555 | 478 | 692 | 899 | 487 | 13859 |
| select, ⅛" trim, lean and fat, rstd—3 oz | 85 | 230 | 896 | 922 | 1621 | 1706 | 525 | 230 | 801 | 689 | 997 | 1296 | 702 | 13860 |
| select, ⅛" trim, lean, broiled—3 oz | 85 | 123 | 751 | 855 | 1496 | 1590 | 490 | 242 | 743 | 599 | 933 | 1216 | 600 | 23623 |
| **beef ribs, small end (ribs 20 to 12)** | | | | | | | | | | | | | | |
| choice, ⅛" trim, lean and fat, rstd—3 oz | 85 | 137 | 833 | 949 | 1658 | 1762 | 543 | 269 | 824 | 665 | 1034 | 1348 | 666 | 13854 |
| **beef round, bottom, choice, 0" trim** | | | | | | | | | | | | | | |
| lean and fat, braised—3 oz | 85 | 183 | 1112 | 1266 | 2213 | 2351 | 724 | 359 | 1099 | 887 | 1380 | 1799 | 888 | 13401 |
| lean and fat, roasted—3 oz | 85 | 150 | 909 | 1035 | 1810 | 1923 | 592 | 293 | 898 | 725 | 1129 | 1471 | 726 | 13402 |
| lean, braised—3 oz | 85 | 184 | 1123 | 1279 | 2236 | 2377 | 732 | 363 | 1111 | 896 | 1395 | 1818 | 898 | 13410 |
| lean, roasted—3 oz | 85 | 152 | 925 | 1053 | 1841 | 1956 | 603 | 298 | 915 | 738 | 1148 | 1497 | 739 | 13411 |
| **beef round, bottom, choice, ⅛" trim** | | | | | | | | | | | | | | |
| lean and fat, braised—3 oz | 85 | 116 | 703 | 801 | 1401 | 1488 | 458 | 227 | 695 | 561 | 874 | 1138 | 562 | 13871 |
| lean and fat, roasted—3 oz | 85 | 184 | 1115 | 1271 | 2221 | 2360 | 727 | 360 | 1103 | 890 | 1386 | 1805 | 891 | 13872 |
| lean, braised—3 oz | 85 | 126 | 767 | 873 | 1526 | 1621 | 500 | 247 | 757 | 611 | 952 | 1240 | 612 | 23594 |
| lean, roasted—3 oz | 85 | 124 | 754 | 859 | 1502 | 1595 | 492 | 244 | 745 | 602 | 937 | 1221 | 603 | 23618 |
| **beef round, bottom, select, 0" trim** | | | | | | | | | | | | | | |
| lean and fat, braised—3 oz | 85 | 192 | 1168 | 1330 | 2326 | 2470 | 762 | 377 | 1154 | 932 | 1450 | 1890 | 933 | 13404 |
| lean and fat, roasted—3 oz | 85 | 157 | 954 | 1086 | 1899 | 2017 | 621 | 308 | 943 | 761 | 1184 | 1544 | 762 | 13405 |
| lean, braised—3 oz | 85 | 196 | 1186 | 1351 | 2362 | 2509 | 774 | 383 | 1173 | 946 | 1473 | 1920 | 948 | 13413 |
| lean, roasted—3 oz | 85 | 158 | 960 | 1094 | 1912 | 2032 | 626 | 310 | 949 | 766 | 1193 | 1555 | 768 | 13414 |
| **beef round, bottom, select, ⅛" trim** | | | | | | | | | | | | | | |
| lean and fat, braised—3 oz | 85 | 116 | 702 | 800 | 1398 | 1486 | 458 | 227 | 694 | 560 | 872 | 1136 | 561 | 13874 |
| lean and fat, roasted—3 oz | 85 | 165 | 1001 | 1141 | 1994 | 2118 | 653 | 324 | 990 | 799 | 1244 | 1621 | 800 | 13875 |
| lean, braised—3 oz | 85 | 191 | 1162 | 1323 | 2314 | 2458 | 757 | 376 | 1149 | 927 | 1443 | 1881 | 928 | 23622 |
| lean, roasted—3 oz | 85 | 159 | 966 | 1100 | 1924 | 2043 | 630 | 312 | 955 | 770 | 1199 | 1564 | 772 | 23590 |
| **beef round, eye of, choice, 0" trim** | | | | | | | | | | | | | | |
| lean and fat, roasted—3 oz | 85 | 160 | 971 | 1105 | 1932 | 2053 | 632 | 314 | 960 | 774 | 1205 | 1571 | 775 | 13416 |
| lean, roasted—3 oz | 85 | 161 | 976 | 1111 | 1943 | 2065 | 636 | 315 | 965 | 779 | 1212 | 1579 | 779 | 13419 |
| **beef round, eye of, choice, ⅛" trim** | | | | | | | | | | | | | | |
| lean and fat, roasted—3 oz | 85 | 122 | 736 | 839 | 1466 | 1558 | 480 | 238 | 728 | 587 | 915 | 1192 | 588 | 13879 |
| lean, roasted—3 oz | 85 | 167 | 1014 | 1155 | 2020 | 2146 | 661 | 328 | 1003 | 809 | 1260 | 1642 | 810 | 23620 |
| **beef round, eye of, select, 0" trim** | | | | | | | | | | | | | | |
| lean and fat, roasted—3 oz | 85 | 166 | 1007 | 1148 | 2006 | 2132 | 657 | 326 | 996 | 804 | 1251 | 1631 | 805 | 13417 |
| lean, roasted—3 oz | 85 | 167 | 1016 | 1157 | 2023 | 2149 | 662 | 328 | 1005 | 810 | 1261 | 1645 | 812 | 13420 |
| **beef round, eye of, select, ⅛" trim** | | | | | | | | | | | | | | |
| lean and fat, roasted—3 oz | 85 | 119 | 723 | 824 | 1440 | 1530 | 472 | 234 | 715 | 577 | 898 | 1170 | 578 | 13881 |
| lean, roasted—3 oz | 85 | 165 | 1005 | 1144 | 2001 | 2126 | 655 | 325 | 994 | 802 | 1248 | 1627 | 802 | 23591 |
| **beef round, full cut, choice, ⅛" trim** | | | | | | | | | | | | | | |
| lean and fat, broiled—3 oz | 85 | 196 | 763 | 785 | 1381 | 1454 | 447 | 196 | 683 | 587 | 850 | 1104 | 598 | 13864 |
| lean and fat, broiled—3 oz | 85 | 196 | 763 | 785 | 1381 | 1454 | 447 | 196 | 682 | 587 | 850 | 1104 | 598 | 13866 |
| **beef round, knuckle tip cntr steak** | | | | | | | | | | | | | | |
| choice, 0" trim, lean and fat, grilled—3 oz | 85 | 117 | 712 | 811 | 1419 | 1507 | 464 | 230 | 705 | 568 | 885 | 1153 | 569 | 23047 |
| select, 0" trim, lean and fat, grilled—3 oz | 85 | 117 | 711 | 809 | 1415 | 1504 | 463 | 230 | 703 | 567 | 883 | 1151 | 568 | 23061 |
| **beef round, knuckle tip side steak** | | | | | | | | | | | | | | |
| choice, 0" trim, lean and fat, grilled—3 oz | 85 | 163 | 993 | 1130 | 1977 | 2100 | 647 | 320 | 982 | 792 | 1233 | 1607 | 793 | 23033 |
| select, 0" trim, lean and fat, grilled—3 oz | 85 | 162 | 988 | 1125 | 1966 | 2089 | 643 | 319 | 977 | 788 | 1227 | 1598 | 789 | 23056 |
| **beef round, outside bottom steak** | | | | | | | | | | | | | | |
| choice, 0" trim, lean and fat, grld—3 oz | 85 | 124 | 752 | 857 | 1498 | 1591 | 490 | 243 | 744 | 600 | 934 | 1217 | 601 | 23051 |
| select, 0" trim, lean and fat, grilled—3 oz | 85 | 121 | 733 | 835 | 1459 | 1550 | 478 | 237 | 725 | 585 | 910 | 1187 | 586 | 23063 |
| **beef round, tip, choice, 0" trim** | | | | | | | | | | | | | | |
| lean and fat, roasted—3 oz | 85 | 151 | 917 | 1045 | 1827 | 1941 | 598 | 297 | 907 | 732 | 1139 | 1485 | 733 | 13422 |
| lean, roasted—3 oz | 85 | 155 | 940 | 1070 | 1872 | 1988 | 613 | 303 | 929 | 750 | 1167 | 1522 | 751 | 13425 |
| **beef round, tip, choice, ⅛" trim** | | | | | | | | | | | | | | |
| lean and fat, roasted—3 oz | 85 | 185 | 723 | 745 | 1308 | 1377 | 424 | 185 | 646 | 556 | 805 | 1046 | 567 | 13885 |
| **beef round, tip, select, 0" trim** | | | | | | | | | | | | | | |
| lean and fat, roasted—3 oz | 85 | 149 | 902 | 1028 | 1796 | 1908 | 588 | 292 | 892 | 720 | 1120 | 1460 | 721 | 13423 |
| lean, roasted—3 oz | 85 | 153 | 929 | 1058 | 1850 | 1966 | 606 | 300 | 919 | 741 | 1154 | 1504 | 742 | 13426 |
| **beef round, tip, select, ⅛" trim** | | | | | | | | | | | | | | |
| lean and fat, roasted—3 oz | 85 | 188 | 733 | 755 | 1326 | 1397 | 429 | 188 | 655 | 564 | 816 | 1061 | 575 | 13887 |
| **beef round, top, choice, 0" trim** | | | | | | | | | | | | | | |
| lean and fat, braised—3 oz | 85 | 339 | 1323 | 1361 | 2393 | 2519 | 775 | 339 | 1182 | 1017 | 1472 | 1913 | 1036 | 13430 |
| lean and fat, broiled—3 oz | 85 | 177 | 1074 | 1224 | 2139 | 2273 | 700 | 347 | 1062 | 857 | 1334 | 1739 | 858 | 13968 |

| | WT | TRY | THR | ISO | LEU | LYS | MET | CYS | PHE | TYR | VAL | ARG | HIS | REF |
|---|---|---|---|---|---|---|---|---|---|---|---|---|---|---|
| | (g) | | | | | | (mg/serving) | | | | | | | |
| lean, braised—3 *oz* | 85 | 344 | 1341 | 1380 | 2427 | 2555 | 786 | 344 | 1198 | 1032 | 1493 | 1941 | 1051 | 13436 |
| lean, broiled—3 *oz* | 85 | 177 | 1076 | 1226 | 2143 | 2277 | 701 | 348 | 1064 | 858 | 1336 | 1742 | 860 | 13492 |
| **beef round, top, choice, ⅛" trim** | | | | | | | | | | | | | | |
| lean and fat, braised—3 *oz* | 85 | 122 | 745 | 848 | 1483 | 1576 | 485 | 241 | 737 | 594 | 925 | 1206 | 595 | 13894 |
| lean and fat, broiled—3 *oz* | 85 | 325 | 1266 | 1303 | 2290 | 2411 | 742 | 325 | 1131 | 973 | 1409 | 1831 | 992 | 13895 |
| lean and fat, panfried—3 *oz* | 85 | 171 | 1037 | 1181 | 2065 | 2193 | 676 | 335 | 1025 | 827 | 1288 | 1678 | 828 | 13896 |
| lean, broiled—3 *oz* | 85 | 128 | 778 | 886 | 1549 | 1646 | 507 | 252 | 769 | 620 | 966 | 1259 | 621 | 23609 |
| **beef round, top, select, 0" trim** | | | | | | | | | | | | | | |
| lean and fat, braised—3 *oz* | 85 | 339 | 1323 | 1361 | 2393 | 2519 | 775 | 339 | 1182 | 1017 | 1472 | 1913 | 1036 | 13432 |
| lean and fat, broiled—3 *oz* | 85 | 177 | 1074 | 1224 | 2139 | 2273 | 700 | 347 | 1062 | 857 | 1334 | 1739 | 858 | 13969 |
| lean, braised—3 *oz* | 85 | 344 | 1341 | 1380 | 2427 | 2555 | 786 | 344 | 1198 | 1032 | 1493 | 1941 | 1051 | 13438 |
| lean, broiled—3 *oz* | 85 | 177 | 1076 | 1226 | 2143 | 2277 | 701 | 348 | 1064 | 858 | 1336 | 1742 | 860 | 13493 |
| **beef round, top, select, ⅛" trim** | | | | | | | | | | | | | | |
| lean and fat, braised—3 *oz* | 85 | 171 | 1037 | 1182 | 2066 | 2195 | 677 | 335 | 1026 | 827 | 1289 | 1679 | 829 | 13900 |
| lean and fat, broiled—3 *oz* | 85 | 212 | 825 | 850 | 1494 | 1572 | 484 | 212 | 738 | 635 | 920 | 1194 | 647 | 13901 |
| lean, broiled—3 *oz* | 85 | 179 | 1088 | 1239 | 2167 | 2302 | 709 | 351 | 1076 | 868 | 1351 | 1761 | 869 | 23621 |
| **beef sandwich steaks, flaked, chpd** | | | | | | | | | | | | | | |
| formed, thinly sliced—2 *oz steak* | 56 | 115 | 393 | 402 | 752 | 783 | 219 | 90 | 356 | 293 | 455 | 633 | 298 | 13342 |
| **beef short loin porterhouse steak** | | | | | | | | | | | | | | |
| choice, ⅛" trim, lean and fat—3 *oz* | 85 | 179 | 698 | 718 | 1263 | 1329 | 409 | 179 | 624 | 537 | 777 | 1010 | 547 | 23001 |
| select, 0" trim, lean, broiled—3 *oz* | 85 | 239 | 1024 | 1144 | 1959 | 2080 | 629 | 238 | 960 | 813 | 1198 | 1493 | 714 | 13466 |
| select, ⅛" trim, lean and fat, brld—3 *oz* | 85 | 197 | 769 | 791 | 1391 | 1465 | 450 | 197 | 688 | 592 | 857 | 1113 | 603 | 23003 |
| **beef short loin, select, ⅛" trim** | | | | | | | | | | | | | | |
| lean, broiled—3 *oz* | 85 | 164 | 1000 | 1138 | 1991 | 2115 | 652 | 323 | 989 | 797 | 1241 | 1618 | 798 | 23589 |
| **beef short loin T-bone steak** | | | | | | | | | | | | | | |
| choice, 0" trim, lean, broiled—3 *oz* | 85 | 247 | 1021 | 1141 | 1952 | 2072 | 626 | 237 | 958 | 742 | 1194 | 1396 | 712 | 13481 |
| choice, ⅛" trim, lean and fat, brld—3 *oz* | 85 | 183 | 712 | 734 | 1289 | 1357 | 417 | 183 | 637 | 548 | 794 | 1031 | 558 | 23005 |
| select, 0" trim, lean, broiled—3 *oz* | 85 | 247 | 1022 | 1142 | 1954 | 2074 | 627 | 237 | 958 | 743 | 1195 | 1397 | 712 | 13484 |
| select, ⅛" trim, lean and fat, brld—3 *oz* | 85 | 190 | 739 | 760 | 1336 | 1406 | 433 | 190 | 660 | 568 | 822 | 1068 | 579 | 23007 |
| **beef short loin, top, choice, 0" trim** | | | | | | | | | | | | | | |
| lean and fat, broiled—3 *oz* | 85 | 159 | 966 | 1100 | 1924 | 2043 | 630 | 312 | 955 | 771 | 1199 | 1564 | 772 | 13446 |
| lean, broiled—3 *oz* | 85 | 162 | 982 | 1118 | 1955 | 2077 | 640 | 317 | 971 | 783 | 1219 | 1590 | 785 | 13449 |
| **beef short loin, top, choice, ⅛" trim** | | | | | | | | | | | | | | |
| lean and fat, broiled—3 *oz* | 85 | 116 | 700 | 797 | 1395 | 1482 | 456 | 226 | 693 | 558 | 870 | 1134 | 559 | 13911 |
| lean, broiled—3 *oz* | 85 | 128 | 774 | 881 | 1540 | 1636 | 504 | 250 | 765 | 617 | 960 | 1252 | 618 | 23627 |
| **beef short loin, top, select, 0" trim** | | | | | | | | | | | | | | |
| lean and fat, broiled—3 *oz* | 85 | 164 | 994 | 1133 | 1980 | 2105 | 649 | 321 | 983 | 793 | 1235 | 1610 | 795 | 13447 |
| lean, broiled—3 *oz* | 85 | 165 | 1005 | 1144 | 2001 | 2126 | 655 | 325 | 994 | 802 | 1248 | 1626 | 802 | 13450 |
| **beef short loin, top, select, ⅛" trim** | | | | | | | | | | | | | | |
| lean and fat, broiled—3 *oz* | 85 | 181 | 706 | 726 | 1277 | 1344 | 413 | 181 | 631 | 542 | 785 | 1021 | 552 | 13915 |
| **beef skirt steak, inside, 0" trim** | | | | | | | | | | | | | | |
| lean and fat, broiled—3 *oz* | 85 | 240 | 1026 | 1145 | 1961 | 2082 | 629 | 239 | 962 | 813 | 1199 | 1495 | 717 | 23540 |
| lean, broiled—3 *oz* | 85 | 245 | 1047 | 1170 | 2003 | 2127 | 643 | 243 | 983 | 830 | 1226 | 1527 | 730 | 13977 |
| **beef skirt steak, outside, 0" trim** | | | | | | | | | | | | | | |
| lean and fat, broiled—3 *oz* | 85 | 216 | 922 | 1029 | 1763 | 1871 | 566 | 215 | 864 | 731 | 1079 | 1345 | 645 | 23541 |
| lean, broiled—3 *oz* | 85 | 222 | 950 | 1062 | 1817 | 1929 | 583 | 221 | 891 | 753 | 1112 | 1385 | 662 | 13979 |
| **beef tenderloin, choice, 0" trim** | | | | | | | | | | | | | | |
| lean and fat, broiled—3 *oz* | 85 | 156 | 949 | 1082 | 1891 | 2009 | 619 | 307 | 939 | 757 | 1180 | 1538 | 759 | 13440 |
| lean, broiled—3 *oz* | 85 | 162 | 983 | 1119 | 1958 | 2079 | 641 | 318 | 972 | 784 | 1221 | 1591 | 785 | 13443 |
| **beef tenderloin, choice, ⅛" trim** | | | | | | | | | | | | | | |
| lean and fat, broiled—3 *oz* | 85 | 110 | 673 | 767 | 1340 | 1424 | 439 | 218 | 666 | 537 | 836 | 1090 | 538 | 13920 |
| lean and fat, roasted—3 *oz* | 85 | 148 | 898 | 1023 | 1788 | 1899 | 585 | 290 | 887 | 716 | 1114 | 1453 | 717 | 13921 |
| lean, broiled—3 *oz* | 85 | 123 | 751 | 855 | 1496 | 1590 | 490 | 242 | 743 | 599 | 933 | 1216 | 600 | 23624 |
| **beef tenderloin, select, 0" trim** | | | | | | | | | | | | | | |
| lean and fat, broiled—3 *oz* | 85 | 152 | 923 | 1051 | 1838 | 1952 | 602 | 298 | 913 | 736 | 1146 | 1494 | 737 | 13441 |
| lean, broiled—3 *oz* | 85 | 157 | 954 | 1085 | 1898 | 2017 | 621 | 308 | 943 | 761 | 1184 | 1543 | 762 | 13444 |
| **beef tenderloin, select, ⅛" trim** | | | | | | | | | | | | | | |
| lean and fat, broiled—3 *oz* | 85 | 108 | 658 | 749 | 1310 | 1391 | 428 | 212 | 650 | 524 | 817 | 1065 | 525 | 13923 |
| lean and fat, roasted—3 *oz* | 85 | 144 | 876 | 997 | 1744 | 1853 | 571 | 283 | 866 | 699 | 1087 | 1418 | 700 | 13924 |
| lean, broiled—3 *oz* | 85 | 123 | 749 | 853 | 1491 | 1584 | 488 | 242 | 740 | 598 | 930 | 1212 | 598 | 23583 |
| **beef top sirloin, choice, 0" trim** | | | | | | | | | | | | | | |
| lean and fat, broiled—3 *oz* | 85 | 162 | 985 | 1122 | 1962 | 2085 | 643 | 319 | 974 | 786 | 1224 | 1595 | 787 | 13452 |
| lean, broiled—3 *oz* | 85 | 169 | 1028 | 1171 | 2048 | 2176 | 671 | 332 | 1017 | 820 | 1278 | 1665 | 822 | 13455 |
| **beef top sirloin, choice, ⅛" trim** | | | | | | | | | | | | | | |
| lean and fat, broiled—3 *oz* | 85 | 108 | 658 | 749 | 1310 | 1391 | 428 | 212 | 650 | 524 | 817 | 1065 | 525 | 13931 |
| lean and fat, pan-fried—3 *oz* | 85 | 156 | 951 | 1083 | 1893 | 2011 | 620 | 307 | 940 | 758 | 1181 | 1539 | 760 | 13932 |
| lean, broiled—3 *oz* | 85 | 122 | 744 | 847 | 1482 | 1574 | 485 | 241 | 735 | 593 | 924 | 1204 | 594 | 23625 |
| **beef top sirloin, select, 0" trim** | | | | | | | | | | | | | | |
| lean and fat, broiled—3 *oz* | 85 | 166 | 1006 | 1147 | 2004 | 2129 | 656 | 326 | 995 | 803 | 1250 | 1629 | 804 | 13453 |
| lean, broiled—3 *oz* | 85 | 172 | 1046 | 1191 | 2082 | 2213 | 682 | 337 | 1034 | 834 | 1299 | 1693 | 836 | 13456 |

| | WT | TRY | THR | ISO | LEU | LYS | MET | CYS | PHE | TYR | VAL | ARG | HIS | REF |
|---|---|---|---|---|---|---|---|---|---|---|---|---|---|---|
| | **(g)** | | | | | | (mg/serving) | | | | | | | |
| **beef top sirloin, select,** ⅛″ trim | | | | | | | | | | | | | | |
| lean and fat, broiled—*3 oz* | 85 | 116 | 702 | 800 | 1398 | 1486 | 457 | 227 | 694 | 560 | 872 | 1136 | 561 | 13934 |
| lean, broiled—*3 oz* | 85 | 124 | 756 | 861 | 1505 | 1600 | 493 | 244 | 747 | 604 | 939 | 1224 | 604 | 23584 |
| **breakfast strips, beef,** cooked | | | | | | | | | | | | | | |
| *3 slices (1.2 oz)* | 34 | 97 | 402 | 460 | 782 | 816 | 247 | 136 | 383 | 347 | 468 | 657 | 339 | 13345 |
| **corned beef** (cured beef brisket) | | | | | | | | | | | | | | |
| cooked—*3 oz* | 85 | 101 | 617 | 703 | 1228 | 1306 | 402 | 199 | 610 | 492 | 766 | 999 | 493 | 13347 |
| **beef sausage** (fresh), pan-fried—*3 oz* | 85 | 100 | 684 | 734 | 1268 | 1366 | 347 | 177 | 639 | 492 | 841 | 1028 | 555 | 7956 |
| | | | | | | | | | | | | | | |
| **GAME AND AMPHIBIANS** | | | | | | | | | | | | | | |
| **antelope,** roasted—*3 oz* | 85 | | 1158 | 957 | 2116 | 2093 | 712 | 223 | 991 | 869 | 1114 | 1647 | 1191 | 17145 |
| **beaver,** roasted—*3 oz* | 85 | | 1128 | 1266 | 2337 | 2754 | 673 | | 1204 | 924 | 1209 | 1820 | 1166 | 17151 |
| **bison** | | | | | | | | | | | | | | |
| chuck shoulder clod, lean | | | | | | | | | | | | | | |
| braised—*3 oz* | 85 | 217 | 1303 | 1386 | 2463 | 2664 | 777 | 343 | 1219 | 977 | 1545 | 1955 | 1052 | 17333 |
| ground, grass-fed, pan-fried | | | | | | | | | | | | | | |
| *3 oz* | 85 | 163 | 982 | 1045 | 1856 | 2008 | 585 | 258 | 919 | 736 | 1164 | 1473 | 793 | 17148 |
| ground, pan-broiled | | | | | | | | | | | | | | |
| *3 oz* | 85 | 153 | 916 | 975 | 1733 | 1874 | 547 | 241 | 858 | 688 | 1087 | 1375 | 740 | 17331 |
| ribeye steak, lean, broiled | | | | | | | | | | | | | | |
| *3 oz* | 85 | 190 | 1136 | 1209 | 2148 | 2322 | 677 | 298 | 1062 | 852 | 1346 | 1704 | 917 | 17335 |
| top round steak, lean, broiled | | | | | | | | | | | | | | |
| *3 oz* | 85 | 194 | 1164 | 1238 | 2201 | 2380 | 694 | 306 | 1089 | 873 | 1380 | 1746 | 940 | 17336 |
| top sirloin steak, lean, broiled | | | | | | | | | | | | | | |
| *3 oz* | 85 | 180 | 1082 | 1151 | 2045 | 2213 | 645 | 284 | 1012 | 811 | 1283 | 1623 | 874 | 17332 |
| **boar, wild,** roasted—*3 oz* | 85 | 323 | 1131 | 1162 | 1955 | 2371 | 592 | 312 | 962 | 858 | 1289 | 1670 | 1220 | 17159 |
| **buffalo top round steak,** broiled—*3 oz* | 85 | 290 | 1094 | 1196 | 2204 | 1926 | 769 | 295 | 1063 | 929 | 1236 | 1640 | 908 | 35176 |
| **caribou,** roasted—*3 oz* | 85 | 389 | 1082 | 1145 | 2088 | 2292 | 565 | 182 | 1125 | 830 | 1189 | 1505 | 1002 | 17163 |
| **deer** | | | | | | | | | | | | | | |
| all cuts, roasted—*3 oz* | 85 | | 1208 | 1015 | 2181 | 2243 | 633 | 287 | 1048 | 909 | 1200 | 1849 | 1270 | 17165 |
| ground, pan-broiled—*3 oz* | 85 | 199 | 848 | 963 | 1707 | 1822 | 524 | 209 | 848 | 701 | 1089 | 1340 | 670 | 17344 |
| loin steak, lean, broiled—*3 oz* | 85 | 229 | 976 | 1108 | 1964 | 2097 | 603 | 241 | 976 | 808 | 1254 | 1543 | 771 | 17345 |
| shoulder clod, lean, braised—*3 oz* | 85 | 270 | 1153 | 1310 | 2320 | 2477 | 711 | 285 | 1153 | 954 | 1480 | 1822 | 911 | 17346 |
| tenderloin, lean, broiled—*3 oz* | 85 | 226 | 963 | 1094 | 1938 | 2069 | 595 | 238 | 963 | 796 | 1237 | 1522 | 761 | 17347 |
| top round steak, lean, broiled—*3 oz* | 85 | 240 | 1023 | 1163 | 2060 | 2199 | 632 | 252 | 1023 | 847 | 1314 | 1618 | 808 | 17348 |
| **elk** | | | | | | | | | | | | | | |
| eye of round, cooked—*3 oz* | 85 | 300 | 981 | 1255 | 2315 | 2032 | 848 | 332 | 1124 | 988 | 2013 | 1735 | 947 | 35178 |
| ground, pan-broiled—*3 oz* | 85 | 202 | 910 | 950 | 1688 | 1850 | 556 | 223 | 829 | 708 | 1051 | 1355 | 698 | 17339 |
| ground patty, cooked—*3 oz* | 85 | 230 | 1025 | 1173 | 2250 | 1945 | 774 | 310 | 1092 | 934 | 1269 | 1692 | 849 | 35172 |
| loin, lean, broiled—*3 oz* | 85 | 235 | 1059 | 1106 | 1964 | 2153 | 647 | 258 | 965 | 824 | 1223 | 1576 | 812 | 17340 |
| roasted—*3 oz* | 85 | 463 | 1118 | 827 | 2164 | 2383 | 616 | | 1018 | 919 | 906 | 1762 | 819 | 17167 |
| round, lean, broiled—*3 oz* | 85 | 235 | 1057 | 1103 | 1961 | 2148 | 646 | 258 | 963 | 822 | 1221 | 1573 | 810 | 17341 |
| tenderloin, lean, broiled—*3 oz* | 85 | 234 | 1051 | 1097 | 1949 | 2136 | 642 | 257 | 957 | 817 | 1214 | 1564 | 806 | 17342 |
| **emu** | | | | | | | | | | | | | | |
| fan fillet, broiled—*3 oz* | 85 | 176 | 762 | 864 | 1467 | 1564 | 504 | 192 | 758 | 567 | 885 | 1196 | 582 | 5624 |
| flat fillet, raw—*3 oz* | 85 | 125 | 542 | 615 | 1044 | 1113 | 359 | 137 | 540 | 404 | 630 | 851 | 414 | 5625 |
| full rump, broiled—*3 oz* | 85 | 189 | 820 | 930 | 1580 | 1684 | 542 | 207 | 817 | 610 | 953 | 1289 | 626 | 5627 |
| ground, pan-broiled—*3 oz* patty | 85 | 160 | 693 | 785 | 1334 | 1422 | 458 | 174 | 689 | 516 | 805 | 1088 | 530 | 5622 |
| inside drum, broiled—*3 oz* | 85 | 182 | 789 | 894 | 1520 | 1619 | 522 | 199 | 785 | 587 | 916 | 1238 | 603 | 5629 |
| outside drum, raw—*3 oz* | 85 | 130 | 563 | 638 | 1083 | 1154 | 372 | 142 | 560 | 418 | 654 | 883 | 429 | 5630 |
| oyster, raw—*3 oz* | 85 | 128 | 556 | 630 | 1070 | 1141 | 368 | 140 | 553 | 414 | 646 | 873 | 424 | 5631 |
| top loin, broiled—*3 oz* | 85 | 163 | 708 | 803 | 1364 | 1454 | 468 | 178 | 705 | 527 | 823 | 1112 | 541 | 5632 |
| **goat,** roasted—*3 oz* | 85 | 343 | 1096 | 1165 | 1919 | 1714 | 617 | 275 | 800 | 708 | 1234 | 1691 | 480 | 17169 |
| **horse,** roasted—*3 oz* | 85 | 297 | 1073 | 1134 | 1897 | 2038 | 530 | 334 | 983 | 750 | 1239 | 1567 | 919 | 17171 |
| **moose,** roasted—*3 oz* | 85 | | 1142 | 1194 | 2190 | 2257 | 637 | | 1074 | 915 | 1353 | 1608 | 836 | 17173 |
| **muskrat,** roasted—*3 oz* | 85 | | 1051 | 974 | 2017 | 2005 | 426 | | 1056 | 700 | 1137 | 1227 | 761 | 17175 |
| **ostrich** | | | | | | | | | | | | | | |
| ground, pan-broiled—*3 oz* | 85 | 198 | 975 | 1056 | 1806 | 1963 | 621 | 229 | 917 | 722 | 1097 | 1520 | 558 | 5642 |
| inside leg, cooked—*3 oz* | 85 | 220 | 1081 | 1171 | 2003 | 2178 | 689 | 253 | 1017 | 802 | 1218 | 1686 | 620 | 5645 |
| inside strip, cooked—*3 oz* | 85 | 223 | 1095 | 1186 | 2028 | 2204 | 698 | 257 | 1030 | 812 | 1232 | 1708 | 627 | 5647 |
| outside strip, cooked—*3 oz* | 85 | 217 | 1064 | 1153 | 1972 | 2143 | 678 | 249 | 1001 | 789 | 1198 | 1659 | 609 | 5650 |
| oyster, cooked—*3 oz* | 85 | 218 | 1074 | 1164 | 1990 | 2162 | 684 | 252 | 1011 | 796 | 1210 | 1674 | 615 | 5652 |
| tip, trimmed, cooked—*3 oz* | 85 | 216 | 1062 | 1151 | 1968 | 2139 | 677 | 249 | 1000 | 788 | 1196 | 1656 | 609 | 5656 |
| top loin, cooked—*3 oz* | 85 | 213 | 1048 | 1136 | 1942 | 2111 | 668 | 246 | 987 | 777 | 1181 | 1635 | 600 | 5658 |
| **rabbit, domesticated** | | | | | | | | | | | | | | |
| raw—*3 oz* | 85 | 225 | 762 | 808 | 1328 | 1493 | 427 | 214 | 700 | 607 | 866 | 1053 | 478 | 17177 |
| roasted—*3 oz* | 85 | 326 | 1105 | 1172 | 1924 | 2162 | 618 | 310 | 1014 | 880 | 1255 | 1526 | 693 | 17178 |
| stewed—*3 oz* | 85 | 341 | 1155 | 1225 | 2012 | 2261 | 646 | 325 | 1060 | 920 | 1312 | 1595 | 724 | 17179 |

| | WT | TRY | THR | ISO | LEU | LYS | MET | CYS | PHE | TYR | VAL | ARG | HIS | REF |
|---|---|---|---|---|---|---|---|---|---|---|---|---|---|---|
| | (g) | | | | | | (mg/serving) | | | | | | | |
| rabbit, wild hare raw—3 oz | 85 | 245 | 829 | 879 | 1443 | 1622 | 463 | 233 | 761 | 660 | 942 | 1144 | 519 | 17180 |
| stewed—3 oz | 85 | 371 | 1255 | 1332 | 2187 | 2457 | 702 | 353 | 1152 | 1000 | 1426 | 1734 | 787 | 17181 |
| seal, bearded | | | | | | | | | | | | | | |
| dried—1 oz | 28 | 223 | 904 | 878 | 1788 | 1873 | 472 | 124 | 917 | 603 | 904 | 1303 | 825 | 35055 |
| dried in oil—1 oz | 28 | 95 | 386 | 375 | 764 | 801 | 202 | 53 | 392 | 258 | 386 | 557 | 353 | 35164 |
| squirrel, roasted—3 oz | 85 | | 996 | 996 | 1879 | 1891 | 574 | | 1012 | 783 | 1034 | 1364 | 683 | 17184 |
| water buffalo, roasted—3 oz | 85 | 278 | 1091 | 1144 | 1963 | 1800 | 571 | 365 | 914 | 915 | 1213 | 1429 | 755 | 17161 |

### LAMB, DOMESTIC US

| | WT | TRY | THR | ISO | LEU | LYS | MET | CYS | PHE | TYR | VAL | ARG | HIS | REF |
|---|---|---|---|---|---|---|---|---|---|---|---|---|---|---|
| **lamb foreshank, choice,** ¼″ trim | | | | | | | | | | | | | | |
| lean and fat, braised—3 oz | 85 | 282 | 1032 | 1164 | 1876 | 2129 | 619 | 288 | 982 | 811 | 1301 | 1433 | 764 | 17008 |
| lean, braised—3 oz | 85 | 308 | 1128 | 1272 | 2050 | 2328 | 677 | 314 | 1073 | 886 | 1422 | 1566 | 835 | 17010 |
| **lamb, ground,** broiled—3 oz | 85 | 246 | 900 | 1015 | 1636 | 1858 | 540 | 251 | 857 | 707 | 1135 | 1250 | 666 | 17225 |
| **lamb leg and shoulder,** cubed, lean, | | | | | | | | | | | | | | |
| braised—3 oz | 85 | 335 | 1226 | 1381 | 2227 | 2529 | 735 | 342 | 1166 | 962 | 1545 | 1702 | 907 | 17060 |
| broiled—3 oz | 85 | 279 | 1022 | 1152 | 1856 | 2107 | 612 | 285 | 972 | 802 | 1288 | 1418 | 756 | 17061 |
| **lamb leg, shank half, choice,** ¼″ trim | | | | | | | | | | | | | | |
| lean and fat, roasted—3 oz | 85 | 263 | 960 | 1083 | 1746 | 1982 | 576 | 268 | 914 | 755 | 1211 | 1334 | 711 | 17016 |
| lean, roasted—3 oz | 85 | 280 | 1025 | 1155 | 1862 | 2115 | 615 | 286 | 975 | 805 | 1292 | 1423 | 758 | 17018 |
| **lamb leg, sirloin half, choice,** ¼″ trim | | | | | | | | | | | | | | |
| lean and fat, roasted—3 oz | 85 | 245 | 896 | 1010 | 1629 | 1849 | 537 | 250 | 853 | 704 | 1130 | 1244 | 663 | 17020 |
| lean, roasted—3 oz | 85 | 281 | 1032 | 1163 | 1874 | 2128 | 619 | 287 | 981 | 810 | 1300 | 1431 | 763 | 17022 |
| **lamb leg, whole, choice,** ¼″ trim | | | | | | | | | | | | | | |
| lean and fat, roasted—3 oz | 85 | 254 | 930 | 1048 | 1689 | 1918 | 558 | 259 | 884 | 730 | 1172 | 1290 | 688 | 17012 |
| lean, roasted—3 oz | 85 | 281 | 1029 | 1160 | 1871 | 2124 | 617 | 287 | 979 | 808 | 1298 | 1429 | 762 | 17014 |
| **lamb loin, choice,** ¼″ trim | | | | | | | | | | | | | | |
| lean and fat, broiled—3 oz | 85 | 250 | 915 | 1032 | 1664 | 1890 | 549 | 255 | 871 | 719 | 1154 | 1272 | 677 | 17024 |
| lean and fat, roasted—3 oz | 85 | 224 | 820 | 925 | 1491 | 1692 | 492 | 229 | 780 | 644 | 1034 | 1139 | 607 | 17025 |
| lean, broiled—3 oz | 85 | 298 | 1091 | 1230 | 1982 | 2251 | 654 | 304 | 1038 | 857 | 1375 | 1515 | 808 | 17027 |
| lean, roasted—3 oz | 85 | 264 | 967 | 1091 | 1758 | 1996 | 580 | 269 | 921 | 760 | 1220 | 1343 | 716 | 17028 |
| **lamb rib, choice,** ¼″ trim | | | | | | | | | | | | | | |
| lean and fat, broiled—3 oz | 85 | 210 | 768 | 866 | 1396 | 1585 | 461 | 214 | 731 | 604 | 968 | 1066 | 569 | 17031 |
| lean and fat, roasted—3 oz | 85 | 144 | 528 | 595 | 960 | 1090 | 317 | 147 | 502 | 415 | 666 | 733 | 391 | 17029 |
| lean, broiled—3 oz | 85 | 230 | 839 | 946 | 1525 | 1731 | 503 | 234 | 798 | 659 | 1057 | 1164 | 621 | 17240 |
| lean, roasted—3 oz | 85 | 217 | 794 | 895 | 1442 | 1638 | 476 | 221 | 755 | 623 | 1000 | 1102 | 587 | 17241 |
| **lamb shoulder, arm, choice,** ¼″ trim | | | | | | | | | | | | | | |
| lean and fat, braised—3 oz | 85 | 302 | 1106 | 1246 | 2009 | 2281 | 663 | 309 | 1051 | 869 | 1394 | 1535 | 819 | 17044 |
| lean and fat, broiled—3 oz | 85 | 243 | 889 | 1002 | 1616 | 1834 | 533 | 248 | 846 | 698 | 1121 | 1234 | 658 | 17045 |
| lean and fat, roasted—3 oz | 85 | 224 | 819 | 924 | 1490 | 1692 | 491 | 229 | 779 | 643 | 1034 | 1138 | 607 | 17046 |
| lean, braised—3 oz | 85 | 353 | 1293 | 1458 | 2349 | 2667 | 775 | 360 | 1230 | 1015 | 1630 | 1794 | 957 | 17048 |
| lean, broiled—3 oz | 85 | 275 | 1008 | 1136 | 1832 | 2080 | 604 | 281 | 959 | 791 | 1271 | 1399 | 746 | 17049 |
| lean, roasted—3 oz | 85 | 253 | 927 | 1044 | 1683 | 1911 | 555 | 258 | 881 | 728 | 1168 | 1286 | 686 | 17050 |
| **lamb shoulder, blade, choice,** ¼″ trim | | | | | | | | | | | | | | |
| lean and fat, braised—3 oz | 85 | 283 | 1037 | 1170 | 1885 | 2140 | 622 | 289 | 987 | 814 | 1308 | 1440 | 768 | 17052 |
| lean and fat, broiled—3 oz | 85 | 230 | 840 | 946 | 1526 | 1732 | 503 | 234 | 799 | 660 | 1058 | 1165 | 621 | 17053 |
| lean and fat, roasted—3 oz | 85 | 221 | 809 | 912 | 1470 | 1669 | 485 | 226 | 770 | 636 | 1020 | 1124 | 599 | 17054 |
| lean, braised—3 oz | 85 | 321 | 1177 | 1327 | 2139 | 2428 | 706 | 328 | 1119 | 924 | 1484 | 1634 | 871 | 17056 |
| lean, broiled—3 oz | 85 | 253 | 927 | 1045 | 1685 | 1912 | 556 | 258 | 881 | 728 | 1169 | 1287 | 686 | 17057 |
| lean, roasted—3 oz | 85 | 245 | 895 | 1009 | 1627 | 1848 | 537 | 250 | 852 | 703 | 1129 | 1243 | 663 | 17058 |
| **lamb shoulder, whole, choice,** ¼″ trim | | | | | | | | | | | | | | |
| lean and fat, braised—3 oz | 85 | 285 | 1043 | 1176 | 1896 | 2152 | 626 | 291 | 992 | 819 | 1315 | 1448 | 772 | 17036 |
| lean and fat, broiled—3 oz | 85 | 242 | 888 | 1001 | 1615 | 1833 | 533 | 248 | 845 | 698 | 1120 | 1233 | 658 | 17037 |
| lean and fat, roasted—3 oz | 85 | 224 | 819 | 923 | 1488 | 1690 | 491 | 229 | 779 | 643 | 1033 | 1136 | 606 | 17038 |
| lean, braised—3 oz | 85 | 326 | 1193 | 1346 | 2169 | 2462 | 716 | 333 | 1136 | 938 | 1504 | 1657 | 883 | 17040 |
| lean, broiled—3 oz | 85 | 269 | 987 | 1112 | 1793 | 2036 | 592 | 275 | 938 | 774 | 1244 | 1369 | 730 | 17041 |
| lean, roasted—3 oz | 85 | 247 | 907 | 1023 | 1649 | 1872 | 544 | 253 | 863 | 712 | 1144 | 1260 | 672 | 17042 |
| **mutton,** roasted—3 oz | 85 | 218 | 1193 | 1350 | 2349 | 2549 | 780 | 296 | 1189 | 988 | 1426 | 1851 | 829 | 35141 |

### LAMB, IMPORTED FROM AUSTRALIA

| | WT | TRY | THR | ISO | LEU | LYS | MET | CYS | PHE | TYR | VAL | ARG | HIS | REF |
|---|---|---|---|---|---|---|---|---|---|---|---|---|---|---|
| **lamb foreshank,** ⅛″ trim | | | | | | | | | | | | | | |
| lean and fat, braised—3 oz | 85 | 246 | 899 | 1017 | 1638 | 1860 | 539 | 252 | 856 | 707 | 1136 | 1250 | 667 | 17287 |
| lean, braised—3 oz | 85 | 273 | 999 | 1130 | 1817 | 2065 | 598 | 280 | 950 | 785 | 1261 | 1387 | 740 | 17289 |
| **lamb leg, whole,** ⅛″ trim | | | | | | | | | | | | | | |
| lean and fat, roasted—3 oz | 85 | 250 | 914 | 1034 | 1663 | 1889 | 547 | 257 | 869 | 718 | 1153 | 1269 | 677 | 17291 |
| lean, roasted—3 oz | 85 | 271 | 992 | 1122 | 1805 | 2050 | 594 | 279 | 944 | 780 | 1252 | 1378 | 735 | 17293 |
| **lamb loin,** ⅛″ trim | | | | | | | | | | | | | | |
| lean and fat, broiled—3 oz | 85 | 253 | 926 | 1047 | 1685 | 1914 | 555 | 260 | 881 | 728 | 1169 | 1286 | 687 | 17311 |
| lean, broiled—3 oz | 85 | 264 | 964 | 1090 | 1754 | 1992 | 577 | 270 | 916 | 758 | 1216 | 1339 | 715 | 17313 |

| | WT (g) | TRY | THR | ISO | LEU | LYS | MET | CYS | PHE | TYR | VAL | ARG | HIS | REF |
|---|---|---|---|---|---|---|---|---|---|---|---|---|---|---|
| | | | | | | | (mg/serving) | | | | | | | |
| **lamb retail cuts,** ⅛" trim | | | | | | | | | | | | | | |
| lean and fat, cooked—*3 oz* | 85 | 243 | 891 | 1007 | 1621 | 1841 | 534 | 250 | 847 | 700 | 1124 | 1238 | 660 | 17281 |
| lean, cooked—*3 oz* | 85 | 265 | 970 | 1097 | 1765 | 2005 | 581 | 273 | 923 | 763 | 1224 | 1348 | 719 | 17283 |
| **lamb rib,** ⅛" trim | | | | | | | | | | | | | | |
| lean and fat, roasted—*3 oz* | 85 | 221 | 808 | 914 | 1470 | 1669 | 484 | 227 | 768 | 635 | 1019 | 1122 | 599 | 17315 |
| lean, roasted—*3 oz* | 85 | 245 | 894 | 1012 | 1628 | 1850 | 536 | 252 | 851 | 704 | 1129 | 1243 | 663 | 17317 |
| **lamb shoulder, whole** | | | | | | | | | | | | | | |
| lean and fat, braised—*3 oz* | 85 | 234 | 856 | 969 | 1559 | 1771 | 513 | 241 | 814 | 673 | 1081 | 1190 | 635 | 17319 |
| lean, braised—*3 oz* | 85 | 192 | 703 | 795 | 1279 | 1454 | 422 | 197 | 669 | 552 | 887 | 977 | 521 | 17320 |
| **LAMB, IMPORTED FROM NEW ZEALAND** | | | | | | | | | | | | | | |
| **lamb foreshank** | | | | | | | | | | | | | | |
| lean and fat, braised—*3 oz* | 85 | 268 | 981 | 1106 | 1783 | 2025 | 588 | 274 | 933 | 770 | 1237 | 1362 | 726 | 17069 |
| lean, braised—*3 oz* | 85 | 305 | 1119 | 1261 | 2033 | 2309 | 671 | 312 | 1064 | 879 | 1411 | 1553 | 828 | 17071 |
| **lamb leg, whole** | | | | | | | | | | | | | | |
| lean and fat, roasted—*3 oz* | 85 | 246 | 903 | 1017 | 1640 | 1862 | 541 | 252 | 858 | 709 | 1137 | 1253 | 668 | 17073 |
| lean, roasted—*3 oz* | 85 | 275 | 1007 | 1135 | 1830 | 2077 | 604 | 280 | 958 | 790 | 1270 | 1397 | 745 | 17075 |
| **lamb loin** | | | | | | | | | | | | | | |
| lean and fat, broiled—*3 oz* | 85 | 233 | 853 | 960 | 1549 | 1759 | 511 | 238 | 811 | 669 | 1074 | 1183 | 631 | 17077 |
| lean, broiled—*3 oz* | 85 | 292 | 1066 | 1202 | 1938 | 2200 | 639 | 298 | 1014 | 837 | 1344 | 1480 | 789 | 17079 |
| **lamb retail cuts** | | | | | | | | | | | | | | |
| lean and fat, cooked—*3 oz* | 85 | 242 | 888 | 1001 | 1615 | 1833 | 533 | 248 | 845 | 698 | 1120 | 1233 | 658 | 17063 |
| lean, cooked—*3 oz* | 85 | 294 | 1077 | 1214 | 1957 | 2221 | 645 | 300 | 1024 | 846 | 1357 | 1494 | 796 | 17065 |
| **lamb rib** | | | | | | | | | | | | | | |
| lean and fat, roasted—*3 oz* | 85 | 189 | 690 | 779 | 1255 | 1425 | 414 | 193 | 657 | 542 | 870 | 958 | 511 | 17081 |
| lean, roasted—*3 oz* | 85 | 242 | 888 | 1001 | 1615 | 1833 | 533 | 248 | 845 | 698 | 1120 | 1233 | 658 | 17083 |
| **lamb shoulder, whole** | | | | | | | | | | | | | | |
| lean and fat, braised—*3 oz* | 85 | 280 | 1026 | 1157 | 1865 | 2117 | 615 | 286 | 976 | 806 | 1294 | 1425 | 760 | 17085 |
| lean, braised—*3 oz* | 85 | 338 | 1239 | 1397 | 2252 | 2556 | 743 | 345 | 1178 | 973 | 1562 | 1720 | 917 | 17087 |
| **PORK** | | | | | | | | | | | | | | |
| **Canadian bacon** (cured pork) | | | | | | | | | | | | | | |
| grilled—*2 slices* | 47 | 113 | 457 | 430 | 802 | 897 | 310 | 142 | 370 | 345 | 454 | 621 | 414 | 10131 |
| unheated—*2 slices* | 57 | 117 | 473 | 444 | 828 | 926 | 320 | 147 | 382 | 356 | 469 | 642 | 428 | 10130 |
| **pork bacon** | | | | | | | | | | | | | | |
| cured, broiled/pan-fried | | | | | | | | | | | | | | |
| *3 medium slices* | 19 | 61 | 285 | 342 | 567 | 604 | 162 | 81 | 289 | 228 | 388 | 472 | 274 | 10124 |
| cured, raw—*3 medium slices* | 68 | 66 | 309 | 370 | 614 | 654 | 175 | 88 | 313 | 247 | 420 | 511 | 296 | 10123 |
| **ham, cured** (purchased fully ckd) | | | | | | | | | | | | | | |
| lean (4% fat), canned—*3 oz* | 85 | 178 | 702 | 677 | 1222 | 1351 | 410 | 186 | 606 | 516 | 705 | 973 | 621 | 10137 |
| lean (4% fat), canned, roasted—*3 oz* | 85 | 204 | 802 | 774 | 1398 | 1545 | 469 | 212 | 694 | 590 | 806 | 1114 | 711 | 10138 |
| lean (5% fat), roasted—*3 oz* | 85 | 213 | 791 | 780 | 1412 | 1509 | 470 | 268 | 768 | 584 | 772 | 1156 | 638 | 10134 |
| reg (11% fat), roasted—*3 oz* | 85 | 202 | 750 | 740 | 1338 | 1430 | 445 | 253 | 728 | 553 | 731 | 1096 | 604 | 10136 |
| reg (13% fat), canned—*3 oz* | 85 | 164 | 644 | 621 | 1122 | 1239 | 377 | 171 | 557 | 473 | 646 | 893 | 570 | 10139 |
| reg (13% fat), canned, roasted—*3 oz* | 85 | 198 | 779 | 751 | 1357 | 1499 | 455 | 207 | 672 | 572 | 782 | 1080 | 689 | 10140 |
| cntr slice, lean and fat, unheated—*3 oz* | 85 | 206 | 762 | 751 | 1361 | 1454 | 452 | 258 | 740 | 563 | 744 | 1114 | 615 | 10142 |
| whole, lean and fat, roasted—*3 oz* | 85 | 208 | 800 | 780 | 1442 | 1551 | 468 | 268 | 784 | 580 | 800 | 1240 | 625 | 10151 |
| whole, lean and fat, unheated—*3 oz* | 85 | 178 | 685 | 669 | 1237 | 1330 | 402 | 230 | 672 | 496 | 686 | 1062 | 536 | 10150 |
| whole, lean, roasted—*3 oz* | 85 | 255 | 947 | 933 | 1690 | 1805 | 562 | 320 | 920 | 699 | 923 | 1383 | 763 | 10153 |
| whole, lean, unheated—*3 oz* | 85 | 228 | 843 | 831 | 1505 | 1608 | 501 | 286 | 819 | 622 | 822 | 1232 | 680 | 10152 |
| **ham patties, cured** | | | | | | | | | | | | | | |
| grilled—*2 oz patty* | 60 | 93 | 355 | 349 | 631 | 678 | 211 | 107 | 338 | 262 | 347 | 515 | 291 | 10147 |
| unheated—*2.3 oz patty* | 65 | 97 | 370 | 363 | 656 | 706 | 219 | 112 | 352 | 272 | 361 | 536 | 303 | 10146 |
| **ham steak,** extra lean, cured, | | | | | | | | | | | | | | |
| unheated—*3 oz* | 85 | 200 | 740 | 729 | 1319 | 1409 | 439 | 251 | 718 | 545 | 721 | 1080 | 596 | 10149 |
| **pork arm, picnic, cured** | | | | | | | | | | | | | | |
| lean and fat, roasted—*3 oz* | 85 | 193 | 752 | 732 | 1362 | 1469 | 439 | 250 | 740 | 541 | 760 | 1193 | 581 | 10168 |
| lean, roasted—*3 oz* | 85 | 254 | 943 | 930 | 1683 | 1798 | 560 | 319 | 916 | 695 | 920 | 1377 | 760 | 10169 |
| **pork arm, picnic** | | | | | | | | | | | | | | |
| lean and fat, braised—*3 oz* | 85 | 281 | 1054 | 1068 | 1873 | 2112 | 602 | 293 | 939 | 790 | 1268 | 1538 | 891 | 10075 |
| lean and fat, roasted—*3 oz* | 85 | 232 | 877 | 886 | 1562 | 1765 | 499 | 243 | 785 | 654 | 1059 | 1301 | 734 | 10076 |
| lean, braised—*3 oz* | 85 | 348 | 1252 | 1284 | 2200 | 2466 | 726 | 349 | 1095 | 955 | 1488 | 1704 | 1096 | 10078 |
| lean, roasted—*3 oz* | 85 | 288 | 1035 | 1062 | 1820 | 2039 | 600 | 289 | 905 | 790 | 1230 | 1410 | 906 | 10079 |
| **pork backribs,** lean and fat, roasted—*3 oz* | 85 | 262 | 942 | 966 | 1655 | 1855 | 546 | 263 | 823 | 718 | 1119 | 1282 | 824 | 10193 |
| **pork blade roll, cured,** lean and fat | | | | | | | | | | | | | | |
| roasted—*3 oz* | 85 | 176 | 653 | 643 | 1165 | 1245 | 388 | 221 | 634 | 482 | 637 | 954 | 526 | 10171 |
| **pork Boston blade** | | | | | | | | | | | | | | |
| lean and fat, braised—*3 oz* | 85 | 224 | 957 | 1049 | 1816 | 1976 | 587 | 246 | 896 | 811 | 1114 | 1418 | 921 | 10081 |

| | WT | TRY | THR | ISO | LEU | LYS | MET | CYS | PHE | TYR | VAL | ARG | HIS | REF |
|---|---|---|---|---|---|---|---|---|---|---|---|---|---|---|
| | (g) | | | | | | (mg/serving) | | | | | | | |
| lean and fat, broiled—*3 oz* | 85 | 276 | 993 | 1018 | 1744 | 1955 | 575 | 277 | 868 | 757 | 1180 | 1352 | 869 | 10082 |
| lean and fat, roasted—*3 oz* | 85 | 241 | 883 | 900 | 1561 | 1754 | 508 | 246 | 779 | 667 | 1056 | 1247 | 759 | 10083 |
| lean, braised—*3 oz* | 85 | 238 | 1014 | 1112 | 1924 | 2095 | 622 | 261 | 949 | 859 | 1181 | 1503 | 976 | 10085 |
| lean, broiled—*3 oz* | 85 | 289 | 1038 | 1064 | 1823 | 2044 | 602 | 290 | 907 | 792 | 1233 | 1413 | 908 | 10086 |
| lean, roasted—*3 oz* | 85 | 262 | 940 | 964 | 1652 | 1851 | 545 | 263 | 822 | 717 | 1117 | 1279 | 822 | 10087 |
| **pork breakfast strips**, cured | | | | | | | | | | | | | | |
| cooked—*3 slices (1.2 oz)* | 34 | 95 | 378 | 400 | 685 | 731 | 217 | 101 | 379 | 287 | 474 | 601 | 284 | 10129 |
| raw—*3 slices (2.4 oz)* | 68 | 77 | 307 | 324 | 556 | 592 | 176 | 82 | 308 | 233 | 384 | 488 | 230 | 10128 |
| **pork breast**, lean and fat, broiled—*3 oz* | 85 | 288 | 1064 | 1146 | 1992 | 2152 | 663 | 273 | 1006 | 959 | 1224 | 1559 | 984 | 10959 |
| **pork center loin (chops)** w/bone | | | | | | | | | | | | | | |
| lean and fat, braised—*3 oz* | 85 | 292 | 1068 | 1090 | 1887 | 2122 | 615 | 298 | 943 | 808 | 1278 | 1505 | 919 | 10037 |
| lean and fat, broiled—*3 oz* | 85 | 230 | 977 | 1071 | 1855 | 2019 | 599 | 252 | 915 | 829 | 1137 | 1448 | 940 | 10038 |
| lean and fat, pan-fried—*3 oz* | 85 | 312 | 1143 | 1165 | 2020 | 2271 | 658 | 319 | 1009 | 865 | 1367 | 1612 | 983 | 10179 |
| lean, braised—*3 oz* | 85 | 321 | 1156 | 1186 | 2032 | 2276 | 671 | 323 | 1011 | 882 | 1374 | 1573 | 1012 | 10041 |
| lean, broiled—*3 oz* | 85 | 240 | 1021 | 1119 | 1937 | 2110 | 626 | 263 | 956 | 865 | 1188 | 1513 | 983 | 10042 |
| lean, pan-fried—*3 oz* | 85 | 348 | 1250 | 1281 | 2195 | 2460 | 724 | 349 | 1092 | 953 | 1484 | 1701 | 1093 | 10176 |
| **pork center loin (roasts)** | | | | | | | | | | | | | | |
| lean and fat, roasted—*3 oz* | 85 | 276 | 1009 | 1029 | 1780 | 2001 | 581 | 281 | 888 | 764 | 1204 | 1413 | 870 | 10039 |
| lean, roasted—*3 oz* | 85 | 298 | 1069 | 1096 | 1878 | 2105 | 620 | 298 | 935 | 816 | 1271 | 1456 | 936 | 10043 |
| **pork center rib (chops)** w/bone | | | | | | | | | | | | | | |
| lean and fat, braised—*3 oz* | 85 | 278 | 1019 | 1039 | 1801 | 2026 | 586 | 284 | 900 | 771 | 1219 | 1438 | 876 | 10045 |
| lean and fat, broiled—*3 oz* | 85 | 218 | 932 | 1022 | 1768 | 1925 | 572 | 240 | 872 | 790 | 1085 | 1381 | 897 | 10046 |
| lean, braised—*3 oz* | 85 | 306 | 1100 | 1128 | 1934 | 2167 | 638 | 308 | 962 | 840 | 1307 | 1498 | 962 | 10049 |
| lean, broiled—*3 oz* | 85 | 230 | 984 | 1079 | 1867 | 2033 | 604 | 253 | 921 | 834 | 1146 | 1459 | 947 | 10050 |
| lean, pan-fried—*3 oz* | 85 | 267 | 984 | 1002 | 1741 | 1958 | 565 | 274 | 870 | 743 | 1178 | 1397 | 843 | 10197 |
| **pork center rib (roasts)** | | | | | | | | | | | | | | |
| lean and fat, roasted—*3 oz* | 85 | 288 | 1053 | 1075 | 1857 | 2087 | 607 | 293 | 927 | 798 | 1256 | 1470 | 910 | 10047 |
| lean, roasted—*3 oz* | 85 | 310 | 1114 | 1143 | 1958 | 2195 | 646 | 311 | 974 | 851 | 1324 | 1517 | 975 | 10051 |
| **pork, ground**, cooked—*3 oz* | 85 | 277 | 997 | 1023 | 1752 | 1964 | 578 | 279 | 871 | 761 | 1185 | 1357 | 872 | 10220 |
| **pork leg (rump and shank half)** | | | | | | | | | | | | | | |
| lean and fat, roasted—*3 oz* | 85 | 275 | 1018 | 1035 | 1804 | 2032 | 584 | 283 | 903 | 768 | 1221 | 1459 | 869 | 10009 |
| lean, roasted—*3 oz* | 85 | 318 | 1142 | 1170 | 2006 | 2248 | 662 | 319 | 998 | 871 | 1356 | 1554 | 999 | 10011 |
| **pork loin blade (chops)** w/bone | | | | | | | | | | | | | | |
| lean and fat, braised—*3 oz* | 85 | 212 | 813 | 819 | 1453 | 1644 | 462 | 225 | 732 | 604 | 985 | 1225 | 676 | 10029 |
| lean and fat, broiled—*3 oz* | 85 | 221 | 839 | 847 | 1495 | 1691 | 478 | 233 | 752 | 626 | 1013 | 1249 | 702 | 10030 |
| lean and fat, panfried—*3 oz* | 85 | 207 | 795 | 799 | 1421 | 1610 | 450 | 220 | 717 | 589 | 964 | 1208 | 657 | 10178 |
| lean, braised—*3 oz* | 85 | 270 | 972 | 996 | 1707 | 1912 | 564 | 271 | 849 | 741 | 1154 | 1323 | 850 | 10033 |
| lean, broiled—*3 oz* | 85 | 274 | 984 | 1009 | 1729 | 1938 | 570 | 275 | 860 | 751 | 1170 | 1340 | 861 | 10034 |
| lean, panfried—*3 oz* | 85 | 267 | 960 | 984 | 1687 | 1891 | 557 | 269 | 840 | 733 | 1141 | 1307 | 840 | 10120 |
| **pork loin blade (roasts)** | | | | | | | | | | | | | | |
| lean and fat, roasted—*3 oz* | 85 | 236 | 891 | 901 | 1584 | 1788 | 507 | 247 | 796 | 666 | 1073 | 1309 | 750 | 10031 |
| lean, roasted—*3 oz* | 85 | 287 | 1033 | 1059 | 1815 | 2033 | 598 | 288 | 903 | 788 | 1227 | 1406 | 904 | 10035 |
| **pork loin, whole** | | | | | | | | | | | | | | |
| lean and fat, braised—*3 oz* | 85 | 286 | 1045 | 1066 | 1843 | 2071 | 602 | 292 | 920 | 791 | 1247 | 1461 | 902 | 10021 |
| lean and fat, broiled—*3 oz* | 85 | 287 | 1049 | 1071 | 1850 | 2079 | 605 | 292 | 923 | 796 | 1252 | 1465 | 907 | 10022 |
| lean and fat, panfried—*3 oz* | 85 | 290 | 1047 | 1072 | 1843 | 2067 | 606 | 292 | 918 | 797 | 1246 | 1439 | 912 | 10023 |
| lean, braised—*3 oz* | 85 | 309 | 1109 | 1137 | 1948 | 2184 | 643 | 309 | 969 | 846 | 1318 | 1510 | 970 | 10025 |
| lean, broiled—*3 oz* | 85 | 309 | 1109 | 1137 | 1948 | 2184 | 643 | 309 | 969 | 846 | 1318 | 1510 | 970 | 10026 |
| lean, panfried—*3 oz* | 85 | 309 | 1111 | 1139 | 1952 | 2188 | 644 | 310 | 972 | 847 | 1320 | 1512 | 972 | 10027 |
| **pork petite tender**, lean and fat, | | | | | | | | | | | | | | |
| broiled—*3 oz* | 85 | 278 | 1027 | 1106 | 1922 | 2077 | 640 | 264 | 970 | 925 | 1182 | 1504 | 949 | 10960 |
| **pork, raw**—*3 oz* | 85 | 190 | 697 | 710 | 1232 | 1386 | 400 | 194 | 615 | 526 | 834 | 986 | 598 | 10003 |
| **pork rump** | | | | | | | | | | | | | | |
| lean and fat, roasted—*3 oz* | 85 | 301 | 1104 | 1125 | 1951 | 2194 | 636 | 308 | 975 | 836 | 1320 | 1556 | 949 | 10013 |
| lean, roasted—*3 oz* | 85 | 334 | 1201 | 1232 | 2110 | 2365 | 696 | 336 | 1050 | 916 | 1426 | 1635 | 1051 | 10015 |
| **pork sausage (fresh)** | | | | | | | | | | | | | | |
| pan-fried—*1.1 oz patty (3 ⅞" dia)* | 27 | 42 | 207 | 191 | 352 | 399 | 128 | 53 | 175 | 151 | 211 | 310 | 151 | 7064 |
| raw—*3 oz* | 85 | 89 | 506 | 535 | 915 | 1013 | 267 | 133 | 461 | 348 | 592 | 752 | 467 | 7063 |
| **pork shank** | | | | | | | | | | | | | | |
| lean and fat, roasted—*3 oz* | 85 | 256 | 956 | 970 | 1697 | 1915 | 547 | 266 | 851 | 718 | 1150 | 1389 | 811 | 10017 |
| lean, roasted—*3 oz* | 85 | 304 | 1095 | 1123 | 1924 | 2156 | 635 | 306 | 957 | 836 | 1300 | 1491 | 958 | 10019 |
| **pork shoulder, whole** | | | | | | | | | | | | | | |
| lean and fat, roasted—*3 oz* | 85 | 236 | 881 | 893 | 1561 | 1760 | 504 | 245 | 783 | 661 | 1057 | 1273 | 747 | 10071 |
| lean, roasted—*3 oz* | 85 | 274 | 983 | 1008 | 1727 | 1936 | 570 | 275 | 859 | 751 | 1168 | 1339 | 860 | 10073 |
| **pork sirloin (chops)** with bone | | | | | | | | | | | | | | |
| lean and fat, braised—*3 oz* | 85 | 263 | 967 | 985 | 1710 | 1924 | 556 | 269 | 855 | 731 | 1158 | 1371 | 830 | 10053 |
| lean and fat, broiled—*3 oz* | 85 | 277 | 1017 | 1037 | 1799 | 2023 | 586 | 284 | 899 | 769 | 1217 | 1439 | 874 | 10054 |
| braised—*3 oz* | 85 | 292 | 1048 | 1074 | 1841 | 2064 | 608 | 292 | 916 | 800 | 1245 | 1426 | 917 | 10057 |
| broiled—*3 oz* | 85 | 308 | 1105 | 1133 | 1941 | 2175 | 641 | 309 | 966 | 843 | 1312 | 1504 | 966 | 10058 |

| | WT (g) | TRY | THR | ISO | LEU | LYS | MET | CYS | PHE | TYR | VAL | ARG | HIS | REF |
|---|---|---|---|---|---|---|---|---|---|---|---|---|---|---|
| | | | | | | | (mg/serving) | | | | | | | |
| **pork sirloin (roasts)** | | | | | | | | | | | | | | |
| lean and fat, roasted—*3 oz* | 85 | 238 | 1017 | 1114 | 1929 | 2100 | 624 | 261 | 952 | 862 | 1183 | 1506 | 978 | 10055 |
| lean, roasted—*3 oz* | 85 | 248 | 1060 | 1162 | 2012 | 2190 | 650 | 273 | 993 | 898 | 1234 | 1572 | 1020 | 10059 |
| **pork sirloin tip roast**, lean and fat | | | | | | | | | | | | | | |
| braised—*3 oz* | 85 | 314 | 1163 | 1252 | 2176 | 2352 | 725 | 298 | 1098 | 1047 | 1337 | 1703 | 1075 | 10962 |
| **pork spareribs**, lean and fat, braised—*3 oz* | 85 | 314 | 1128 | 1157 | 1982 | 2221 | 654 | 315 | 986 | 861 | 1340 | 1535 | 987 | 10089 |
| **pork tenderloin** | | | | | | | | | | | | | | |
| lean and fat, broiled—*3 oz* | 85 | 320 | 1154 | 1182 | 2031 | 2278 | 668 | 322 | 1012 | 879 | 1374 | 1586 | 1005 | 10221 |
| lean and fat, roasted—*3 oz* | 85 | 233 | 994 | 1089 | 1886 | 2053 | 609 | 255 | 931 | 842 | 1157 | 1473 | 956 | 10222 |
| lean, broiled—*3 oz* | 85 | 328 | 1181 | 1210 | 2075 | 2326 | 684 | 330 | 1032 | 901 | 1402 | 1607 | 1033 | 10223 |
| lean, roasted—*3 oz* | 85 | 234 | 999 | 1095 | 1895 | 2063 | 613 | 257 | 935 | 847 | 1162 | 1480 | 960 | 10061 |
| **pork top loin (chops)** | | | | | | | | | | | | | | |
| lean and fat, braised—*3 oz* | 85 | 293 | 1068 | 1091 | 1884 | 2117 | 616 | 298 | 940 | 810 | 1275 | 1490 | 924 | 10063 |
| lean and fat, braised—*3 oz* | 85 | 238 | 1015 | 1113 | 1926 | 2097 | 622 | 261 | 950 | 860 | 1182 | 1504 | 977 | 10064 |
| lean and fat, pan-fried—*3 oz* | 85 | 305 | 1114 | 1136 | 1964 | 2207 | 642 | 310 | 980 | 844 | 1329 | 1555 | 962 | 10186 |
| lean, braised—*3 oz* | 85 | 314 | 1128 | 1157 | 1982 | 2222 | 654 | 315 | 986 | 861 | 1340 | 1536 | 987 | 10067 |
| lean, broiled—*3 oz* | 85 | 246 | 1052 | 1153 | 1997 | 2174 | 645 | 270 | 985 | 892 | 1225 | 1560 | 1012 | 10068 |
| lean, pan-fried—*3 oz* | 85 | 329 | 1183 | 1213 | 2078 | 2330 | 686 | 331 | 1034 | 903 | 1405 | 1611 | 1035 | 10181 |
| **pork top loin (roasts)** | | | | | | | | | | | | | | |
| lean and fat, roasted—*3 oz* | 85 | 236 | 1010 | 1107 | 1915 | 2085 | 619 | 259 | 945 | 856 | 1175 | 1496 | 971 | 10065 |
| lean, roasted—*3 oz* | 85 | 244 | 1040 | 1139 | 1972 | 2146 | 638 | 267 | 973 | 881 | 1210 | 1540 | 1000 | 10069 |
| **pork w/beef sausage** (fresh) | | | | | | | | | | | | | | |
| pan-fried—*1 oz patty* | 27 | 36 | 150 | 143 | 263 | 294 | 89 | 38 | 129 | 109 | 160 | 230 | 111 | 7065 |
| **VEAL** | | | | | | | | | | | | | | |
| **veal breast, plate half**, bone out | | | | | | | | | | | | | | |
| lean and fat, braised—*3 oz* | 85 | 223 | 962 | 1085 | 1753 | 1816 | 515 | 250 | 888 | 701 | 1216 | 1297 | 800 | 17273 |
| **veal breast, point half**, bone out | | | | | | | | | | | | | | |
| lean and fat, braised—*3 oz* | 85 | 242 | 1048 | 1182 | 1908 | 1977 | 560 | 272 | 967 | 763 | 1325 | 1413 | 871 | 17274 |
| **veal breast, whole**, bone out, | | | | | | | | | | | | | | |
| lean and fat, braised—*3 oz* | 85 | 231 | 1001 | 1130 | 1823 | 1889 | 536 | 260 | 924 | 729 | 1266 | 1350 | 832 | 17272 |
| **veal breast, whole**, bone out | | | | | | | | | | | | | | |
| lean, braised—*3 oz* | 85 | 260 | 1125 | 1270 | 2049 | 2123 | 602 | 292 | 1039 | 820 | 1423 | 1517 | 936 | 17275 |
| **veal, ground**, broiled—*3 oz* | 85 | 210 | 905 | 1021 | 1649 | 1708 | 484 | 234 | 836 | 660 | 1145 | 1219 | 752 | 17143 |
| **veal leg (top round)** | | | | | | | | | | | | | | |
| lean and fat, braised—*3 oz* | 85 | 311 | 1343 | 1514 | 2446 | 2533 | 717 | 347 | 1240 | 980 | 1699 | 1808 | 1116 | 17095 |
| lean and fat, breaded, pan-fried—*3 oz* | 85 | 241 | 996 | 1138 | 1837 | 1822 | 536 | 279 | 960 | 734 | 1285 | 1341 | 813 | 17096 |
| lean and fat, pan-fried—*3 oz* | 85 | 273 | 1179 | 1329 | 2148 | 2224 | 630 | 304 | 1089 | 860 | 1492 | 1587 | 979 | 17097 |
| lean and fat, roasted—*3 oz* | 85 | 238 | 1028 | 1159 | 1874 | 1940 | 549 | 266 | 950 | 751 | 1301 | 1385 | 854 | 17098 |
| lean, braised—*3 oz* | 85 | 316 | 1363 | 1537 | 2484 | 2571 | 728 | 352 | 1259 | 994 | 1725 | 1835 | 1132 | 17100 |
| lean, breaded, pan-fried—*3 oz* | 85 | 251 | 1038 | 1185 | 1912 | 1900 | 558 | 289 | 998 | 764 | 1337 | 1397 | 847 | 17101 |
| lean, pan-fried—*3 oz* | 85 | 286 | 1232 | 1389 | 2244 | 2324 | 658 | 318 | 1138 | 899 | 1559 | 1658 | 1023 | 17102 |
| lean, roasted—*3 oz* | 85 | 241 | 1042 | 1175 | 1899 | 1966 | 557 | 269 | 963 | 761 | 1319 | 1403 | 866 | 17103 |
| **veal leg and shoulder**, cubed for | | | | | | | | | | | | | | |
| stew lean, braised—*3 oz* | 85 | 301 | 1298 | 1463 | 2364 | 2447 | 693 | 335 | 1198 | 947 | 1641 | 1747 | 1078 | 17141 |
| **veal loin** | | | | | | | | | | | | | | |
| lean and fat, braised—*3 oz* | 85 | 260 | 1121 | 1264 | 2043 | 2114 | 598 | 290 | 1035 | 818 | 1418 | 1509 | 932 | 17105 |
| lean and fat, roasted—*3 oz* | 85 | 213 | 921 | 1038 | 1678 | 1737 | 492 | 238 | 851 | 672 | 1165 | 1240 | 765 | 17106 |
| lean, braised—*3 oz* | 85 | 289 | 1246 | 1405 | 2271 | 2351 | 666 | 322 | 1152 | 910 | 1577 | 1678 | 1035 | 17108 |
| lean, roasted—*3 oz* | 85 | 226 | 977 | 1102 | 1781 | 1844 | 522 | 252 | 903 | 713 | 1237 | 1316 | 812 | 17109 |
| **veal ribs** | | | | | | | | | | | | | | |
| lean and fat, braised—*3 oz* | 85 | 279 | 1204 | 1357 | 2194 | 2272 | 643 | 311 | 1113 | 879 | 1524 | 1622 | 1000 | 17111 |
| lean and fat, roasted—*3 oz* | 85 | 207 | 890 | 1003 | 1621 | 1678 | 475 | 230 | 822 | 649 | 1125 | 1198 | 740 | 17112 |
| lean, braised—*3 oz* | 85 | 297 | 1278 | 1442 | 2330 | 2412 | 683 | 331 | 1182 | 933 | 1618 | 1721 | 1062 | 17114 |
| lean, roasted—*3 oz* | 85 | 222 | 956 | 1078 | 1742 | 1804 | 511 | 247 | 884 | 698 | 1210 | 1288 | 795 | 17115 |
| **veal shank (fore and hind)** | | | | | | | | | | | | | | |
| lean and fat, braised—*3 oz* | 85 | 270 | 1170 | 1321 | 2132 | 2209 | 626 | 219 | 1080 | 853 | 1479 | 1578 | 973 | 17277 |
| lean, braised—*3 oz* | 85 | 276 | 1196 | 1350 | 2178 | 2257 | 640 | 311 | 1104 | 872 | 1511 | 1612 | 994 | 17279 |
| **veal shoulder, arm** | | | | | | | | | | | | | | |
| lean and fat, braised—*3 oz* | 85 | 289 | 1249 | 1408 | 2275 | 2355 | 667 | 323 | 1153 | 911 | 1579 | 1681 | 1038 | 17123 |
| lean and fat, roasted—*3 oz* | 85 | 219 | 945 | 1066 | 1723 | 1783 | 505 | 244 | 874 | 690 | 1196 | 1273 | 785 | 17124 |
| lean, braised—*3 oz* | 85 | 308 | 1327 | 1496 | 2417 | 2502 | 709 | 343 | 1226 | 968 | 1679 | 1786 | 1102 | 17126 |
| lean, roasted—*3 oz* | 85 | 225 | 971 | 1094 | 1768 | 1830 | 518 | 251 | 897 | 708 | 1227 | 1306 | 807 | 17127 |
| **veal shoulder, blade** | | | | | | | | | | | | | | |
| lean and fat, braised—*3 oz* | 85 | 269 | 1161 | 1309 | 2115 | 2190 | 620 | 300 | 1073 | 847 | 1469 | 1563 | 965 | 17129 |
| lean and fat, roasted—*3 oz* | 85 | 217 | 934 | 1052 | 1702 | 1761 | 499 | 241 | 863 | 682 | 1182 | 1257 | 776 | 17130 |
| lean, braised—*3 oz* | 85 | 281 | 1213 | 1367 | 2209 | 2287 | 648 | 314 | 1120 | 885 | 1534 | 1633 | 1007 | 17132 |
| lean, roasted—*3 oz* | 85 | 220 | 952 | 1073 | 1734 | 1795 | 508 | 246 | 880 | 694 | 1204 | 1282 | 791 | 17133 |

| | WT | TRY | THR | ISO | LEU | LYS | MET | CYS | PHE | TYR | VAL | ARG | HIS | REF |
|---|---|---|---|---|---|---|---|---|---|---|---|---|---|---|
| | (g) | | | | | | (mg/serving) | | | | | | | |
| **veal shoulder, whole** | | | | | | | | | | | | | | |
| lean and fat, braised—3 oz | 85 | 276 | 1191 | 1342 | 2169 | 2246 | 636 | 308 | 1100 | 869 | 1506 | 1603 | 989 | 17117 |
| lean and fat, roasted—3 oz | 85 | 218 | 940 | 1060 | 1713 | 1774 | 502 | 243 | 869 | 686 | 1190 | 1266 | 781 | 17118 |
| lean, braised—3 oz | 85 | 290 | 1250 | 1409 | 2278 | 2359 | 668 | 323 | 1155 | 913 | 1582 | 1684 | 1039 | 17120 |
| lean, roasted—3 oz | 85 | 222 | 959 | 1080 | 1747 | 1808 | 512 | 247 | 886 | 700 | 1213 | 1290 | 796 | 17121 |
| **veal sirloin** | | | | | | | | | | | | | | |
| lean and fat, braised—3 oz | 85 | 269 | 1161 | 1308 | 2115 | 2190 | 620 | 300 | 1073 | 847 | 1469 | 1562 | 965 | 17135 |
| lean and fat, roasted—3 oz | 85 | 216 | 933 | 1052 | 1701 | 1761 | 499 | 241 | 863 | 682 | 1182 | 1257 | 776 | 17136 |
| lean, braised—3 oz | 85 | 292 | 1261 | 1421 | 2298 | 2378 | 673 | 326 | 1165 | 921 | 1595 | 1697 | 1048 | 17138 |
| lean, roasted—3 oz | 85 | 226 | 977 | 1102 | 1781 | 1844 | 522 | 252 | 903 | 713 | 1237 | 1316 | 813 | 17139 |
| **INTERNAL ORGANS AND OTHER PARTS** | | | | | | | | | | | | | | |
| **beef brain**, pan-fried—3 oz | 85 | 88 | 507 | 414 | 802 | 639 | 222 | 190 | 540 | 379 | 524 | 583 | 272 | 13319 |
| **beef liver**, braised—3 oz | 85 | 313 | 1033 | 1149 | 2270 | 1910 | 645 | 447 | 1288 | 959 | 1497 | 1475 | 747 | 13326 |
| **beef liver**, pan-fried—3 oz | 85 | 285 | 942 | 1048 | 2070 | 1741 | 588 | 407 | 1175 | 875 | 1365 | 1345 | 682 | 13327 |
| **beef liver**, raw—3 oz | 85 | 224 | 739 | 822 | 1624 | 1366 | 462 | 320 | 921 | 686 | 1071 | 1055 | 535 | 13325 |
| **beef lungs**, braised—3 oz | 85 | 158 | 647 | 827 | 1273 | 1229 | 347 | 266 | 705 | 391 | 854 | 1049 | 527 | 13329 |
| **beef pancreas** (sweetbread) braised | | | | | | | | | | | | | | |
| 3 oz | 85 | 298 | 1068 | 1164 | 1799 | 1699 | 416 | 295 | 958 | 1006 | 1235 | 1316 | 453 | 13332 |
| **beef spleen**, braised—3 oz | 85 | 222 | 840 | 823 | 1884 | 1543 | 393 | 618 | 857 | 608 | 1284 | 1236 | 765 | 13334 |
| **beef thymus** (sweetbread) braised—3 oz | 85 | 143 | 672 | 633 | 1239 | 1545 | 258 | 238 | 532 | 386 | 805 | 1224 | 327 | 13338 |
| **calf brain**, raw—3 oz | 85 | 88 | 434 | 357 | 677 | 544 | 193 | 92 | 462 | 340 | 417 | 481 | 219 | 17188 |
| **calf heart**, raw—3 oz | 85 | 156 | 646 | 700 | 1147 | 1257 | 333 | 157 | 633 | 479 | 763 | 907 | 393 | 17193 |
| **calf kidney**, raw—3 oz | 85 | 172 | 611 | 570 | 1085 | 891 | 280 | 149 | 636 | 513 | 708 | 825 | 324 | 17197 |
| **calf liver**, raw—3 oz | 85 | 233 | 742 | 823 | 1619 | 1383 | 478 | 316 | 930 | 674 | 1078 | 1187 | 536 | 17202 |
| **calf lung**, raw—3 oz | 85 | 110 | 515 | 575 | 791 | 1027 | 220 | 118 | 492 | 292 | 590 | | | 17207 |
| **calf spleen**, raw—3 oz | 85 | 153 | 630 | 715 | 988 | 1151 | 339 | 184 | 552 | 424 | 722 | | | 17216 |
| **calf tongue**, raw—3 oz | 85 | 157 | 587 | 626 | 1052 | 1074 | 301 | 145 | 575 | 438 | 670 | 854 | 333 | 17222 |
| **lamb brain**, braised—3 oz | 85 | 110 | 478 | 424 | 833 | 684 | 212 | 111 | 514 | 390 | 508 | 719 | 283 | 17186 |
| **lamb brain**, pan-fried—3 oz | 85 | 149 | 646 | 574 | 1127 | 925 | 287 | 150 | 695 | 528 | 687 | 972 | 382 | 17187 |
| **lamb heart**, braised—3 oz | 85 | 230 | 1001 | 920 | 1805 | 1599 | 465 | 178 | 918 | 661 | 1057 | 1388 | 485 | 17192 |
| **lamb heart**, raw—3 oz | 85 | 151 | 660 | 607 | 1191 | 1054 | 307 | 117 | 605 | 436 | 696 | 915 | 320 | 17191 |
| **lamb kidney**, braised—3 oz | 85 | 271 | 946 | 800 | 1509 | 1303 | 408 | 230 | 931 | 708 | 1179 | 1160 | 506 | 17196 |
| **lamb liver**, braised—3 oz | 85 | 302 | 1124 | 1119 | 2122 | 1405 | 564 | 272 | 1160 | 927 | 1431 | 1457 | 610 | 17200 |
| **lamb liver**, pan-fried—3 oz | 85 | 252 | 938 | 935 | 1773 | 1174 | 471 | 228 | 969 | 774 | 1194 | 1217 | 510 | 17201 |
| **lamb liver**, raw—3 oz | 85 | 201 | 750 | 746 | 1415 | 937 | 376 | 182 | 774 | 618 | 954 | 972 | 407 | 17199 |
| **lamb lung**, braised—3 oz | 85 | 173 | 621 | 534 | 1352 | 1093 | 305 | 265 | 696 | 476 | 931 | 1017 | 425 | 17206 |
| **lamb pancreas** (sweetbread) | | | | | | | | | | | | | | |
| braised—3 oz | 85 | 248 | 714 | 683 | 1242 | 1676 | 280 | 248 | 652 | 466 | 838 | 1148 | 558 | 17211 |
| **lamb spleen**, braised—3 oz | 85 | 248 | 918 | 1425 | 2001 | 1742 | 428 | 288 | 1022 | 655 | 1468 | 1421 | 749 | 17215 |
| **lamb tongue**, braised—3 oz | 85 | 185 | 829 | 717 | 1305 | 1298 | 388 | 201 | 684 | 543 | 878 | 1208 | 405 | 17221 |
| **pork brain**, braised—3 oz | 85 | 132 | 482 | 477 | 899 | 811 | 205 | 182 | 525 | 433 | 587 | 540 | 277 | 10097 |
| **pork brain**, raw—3 oz | 85 | 112 | 408 | 404 | 762 | 687 | 173 | | 445 | 366 | 498 | 457 | 235 | 10096 |
| **pork ears**, simmered—3 oz | 111 | 34 | 529 | 405 | 971 | 813 | 142 | 158 | 566 | 354 | 708 | 1416 | 212 | 10101 |
| **pork heart**, braised—3 oz | 129 | 351 | 1335 | 1467 | 2748 | 2518 | 779 | 546 | 1344 | 1042 | 1612 | 2046 | 774 | 10104 |
| **pork heart**, raw—3 oz | 85 | 169 | 643 | 706 | 1324 | 1214 | 376 | 263 | 648 | 502 | 777 | 986 | 373 | 10103 |
| **pork jowl**, raw—3 oz | 85 | 18 | 178 | 143 | 379 | 449 | 81 | 48 | 203 | 88 | 259 | 560 | 61 | 10105 |
| **pork kidney**, braised—3 oz | 85 | 280 | 895 | 1153 | 1938 | 1555 | 463 | 473 | 1019 | 777 | 1244 | 1327 | 518 | 10107 |
| **pork kidney**, raw—3 oz | 85 | 181 | 580 | 747 | 1255 | 1007 | 300 | 307 | 660 | 503 | 806 | 859 | 336 | 10106 |
| **pork liver**, braised—3 oz | 85 | 311 | 941 | 1122 | 1971 | 1706 | 548 | 417 | 1083 | 754 | 1366 | 1363 | 602 | 10111 |
| **pork liver**, raw—3 oz | 85 | 256 | 774 | 922 | 1620 | 1402 | 450 | 343 | 890 | 620 | 1123 | 1119 | 495 | 10110 |
| **pork lung**, braised—3 oz | 85 | 124 | 496 | 564 | 1095 | 1029 | 228 | 222 | 587 | 400 | 840 | 734 | 357 | 10113 |
| **pork lung**, raw—3 oz | 85 | 105 | 422 | 479 | 929 | 873 | 194 | 188 | 498 | 338 | 712 | 622 | 303 | 10112 |
| **pork pancreas** (sweetbread) | | | | | | | | | | | | | | |
| braised—3 oz | 85 | 531 | 1089 | 1272 | 1810 | 1670 | 400 | 310 | 1039 | 1016 | 1306 | 1396 | 469 | 10116 |
| **pork (pig) feet**, cured, pickled—3 oz | 85 | 20 | 267 | 168 | 435 | 425 | 109 | 87 | 286 | 158 | 247 | 741 | 109 | 10132 |
| **pork spleen**, braised—3 oz | 85 | 246 | 959 | 1070 | 1960 | 1791 | 445 | 307 | 1024 | 672 | 1304 | 1308 | 571 | 10118 |
| **pork spleen**, raw—3 oz | 85 | 156 | 607 | 677 | 1241 | 1134 | 281 | 195 | 649 | 425 | 825 | 828 | 362 | 10117 |
| **pork tail**, simmered—3 oz | 85 | 87 | 506 | 332 | 809 | 867 | 260 | 187 | 434 | 289 | 434 | 997 | 260 | 10175 |
| **pork tongue**, braised—3 oz | 85 | 236 | 865 | 934 | 1642 | 1674 | 459 | | 849 | | 1065 | 1265 | 514 | 10122 |
| **pork tongue**, raw—3 oz | 85 | 160 | 586 | 632 | 1111 | 1133 | 310 | 200 | 574 | 422 | 721 | 856 | 348 | 10121 |
| **sheep spleen**, raw—3 oz | 85 | 162 | 597 | 927 | 1300 | 1132 | 278 | 187 | 665 | 426 | 955 | 924 | 486 | 17214 |
| **veal brain**, braised—3 oz | 85 | 98 | 483 | 397 | 753 | 604 | 214 | 102 | 513 | 378 | 464 | 535 | 244 | 17189 |
| **veal brain**, pan-fried—3 oz | 85 | 123 | 609 | 501 | 950 | 762 | 270 | 128 | 648 | 477 | 586 | 675 | 309 | 17190 |
| **veal heart**, braised—3 oz | 85 | 264 | 1095 | 1186 | 1944 | 2131 | 564 | 266 | 1074 | 812 | 1295 | 1537 | 666 | 17194 |
| **veal kidney**, braised—3 oz | 85 | 287 | 1020 | 951 | 1811 | 1488 | 469 | 248 | 1061 | 858 | 1183 | 1379 | 541 | 17198 |
| **veal liver**, braised—3 oz | 85 | 307 | 977 | 1083 | 2131 | 1820 | 629 | 416 | 1224 | 887 | 1419 | 1562 | 705 | 17203 |
| **veal liver**, pan-fried—3 oz | 85 | 295 | 940 | 1043 | 2052 | 1753 | 605 | 400 | 1179 | 854 | 1366 | 1505 | 678 | 17204 |

| | WT (g) | TRY | THR | ISO | LEU | LYS | MET | CYS | PHE | TYR | VAL | ARG | HIS | REF |
|---|---|---|---|---|---|---|---|---|---|---|---|---|---|---|
| | | | | | | | (mg/serving) | | | | | | | |
| **veal lung**, braised—*3 oz* | 85 | 127 | 592 | 660 | 910 | 1180 | 252 | 136 | 565 | 337 | 677 | | | 17208 |
| **veal spleen**, braised—*3 oz* | 85 | 201 | 829 | 940 | 1300 | 1515 | 446 | 241 | 727 | 558 | 950 | | | 17217 |
| **veal tongue**, braised—*3 oz* | 85 | 237 | 884 | 942 | 1584 | 1616 | 453 | 218 | 865 | 658 | 1008 | 1285 | 501 | 17223 |

## 20. MEATS, LUNCHEON AND SNACK

### FRANKFURTERS AND OTHER LUNCHEON-TYPE SAUSAGES

| | WT (g) | TRY | THR | ISO | LEU | LYS | MET | CYS | PHE | TYR | VAL | ARG | HIS | REF |
|---|---|---|---|---|---|---|---|---|---|---|---|---|---|---|
| **beef sausage**, smoked, pan-fried | | | | | | | | | | | | | | |
|   *1.5 oz sausage* | 43 | 55 | 229 | 262 | 445 | 465 | 141 | 78 | 218 | 198 | 267 | 375 | 193 | 13357 |
| **blood sausage** (blood/black | | | | | | | | | | | | | | |
|   pudding, blutwurst)—*0.9 slice* | 25 | 45 | 142 | 80 | 348 | 262 | 50 | 45 | 205 | 85 | 255 | 170 | 178 | 7005 |
| **bockwurst** (pork, veal, milk, eggs), | | | | | | | | | | | | | | |
|   raw *3.2 oz sausage* | 91 | 139 | 558 | 616 | 1007 | 1061 | 303 | 147 | 506 | 411 | 698 | 746 | 467 | 7006 |
| **bratwurst** | | | | | | | | | | | | | | |
|   beef and pork, smoked—*2.3 oz* | 66 | 71 | 307 | 320 | 535 | 596 | 240 | 69 | 267 | 255 | 306 | 505 | 261 | 7922 |
|   pork, beef, and turkey, | | | | | | | | | | | | | | |
|     lite, smoked—*2.3 oz* | 66 | 96 | 373 | 405 | 689 | 721 | 220 | 102 | 343 | 296 | 436 | 564 | 281 | 7924 |
|   veal, cooked—*3 oz* | 85 | 121 | 519 | 586 | 946 | 980 | 278 | 134 | 479 | 379 | 657 | 700 | 432 | 7910 |
| **brotwurst**, pork and beef w/nonfat | | | | | | | | | | | | | | |
|   dry milk—*2.5 oz link (7/lb)* | 70 | 91 | 420 | 427 | 756 | 798 | 259 | 112 | 378 | 308 | 476 | 665 | 308 | 7015 |
| **chicken, beef, and pork sausage** | | | | | | | | | | | | | | |
|   skinless—*1 link* | 84 | 122 | 475 | 515 | 877 | 917 | 281 | 130 | 436 | 376 | 555 | 718 | 358 | 7928 |
| **chorizo**, pork and beef | | | | | | | | | | | | | | |
|   *2.1 oz link (4" long)* | 60 | 167 | 884 | 1324 | 1025 | 1448 | 282 | 166 | 689 | 449 | 548 | 1016 | 433 | 7019 |
| **frankfurter**—*1.8 oz* | 52 | 58 | 246 | 276 | 472 | 501 | 151 | 57 | 231 | 196 | 289 | 359 | 172 | 7950 |
|   beef—*1.5 oz* | 43 | 52 | 223 | 249 | 427 | 454 | 137 | 52 | 209 | 177 | 261 | 326 | 156 | 7022 |
|   beef and pork—*1.6 oz* | 45 | 53 | 209 | 213 | 380 | 409 | 121 | 55 | 189 | 158 | 240 | 318 | 163 | 7023 |
|   beef, heated—*1.8 oz* | 52 | 65 | 277 | 310 | 530 | 563 | 170 | 64 | 260 | 220 | 324 | 404 | 193 | 7945 |
|   chicken—*1.6 oz* | 45 | 46 | 260 | 206 | 461 | 493 | 154 | 58 | 231 | 176 | 241 | 401 | 163 | 7024 |
|   heated—*1.8 oz* | 52 | 55 | 235 | 263 | 449 | 477 | 144 | 55 | 220 | 186 | 275 | 343 | 164 | 7949 |
|   pork—*2.7 oz* | 76 | 114 | 426 | 434 | 761 | 853 | 243 | 118 | 382 | 321 | 515 | 619 | 357 | 7939 |
|   pork, beef, Am cheese | | | | | | | | | | | | | | |
|     (cheesefurter)—*1.5 oz* | 43 | 64 | 232 | 267 | 473 | 499 | 155 | 64 | 241 | 224 | 297 | 361 | 202 | 7016 |
|   turkey—*1.6 oz* | 45 | 51 | 307 | 243 | 523 | 557 | 181 | 47 | 266 | 228 | 263 | 419 | 244 | 7025 |
| **Italian sausage** | | | | | | | | | | | | | | |
|   pork, cooked—*2.4 oz link* | 67 | 108 | 531 | 490 | 900 | 1020 | 326 | 135 | 449 | 387 | 539 | 792 | 387 | 7089 |
|   sweet, cooked—*3 oz link* | 84 | 93 | 350 | 368 | 638 | 674 | 203 | 92 | 317 | 276 | 411 | 484 | 280 | 7914 |
|   turkey, smoked—*2 oz link* | 56 | 117 | 458 | 529 | 822 | 948 | 293 | 114 | 413 | 402 | 551 | 724 | 314 | 7927 |
| **kielbasa** (pork, beef w/nonfat | | | | | | | | | | | | | | |
|   dry milk) cooked—*0.9 oz slice* | 26 | 36 | 112 | 166 | 227 | 263 | 72 | 58 | 130 | 127 | 166 | 245 | 82 | 7037 |
| **knockwurst/knackwurst**, pork, | | | | | | | | | | | | | | |
|   beef *2.5 oz sausage* | 72 | 99 | 311 | 460 | 629 | 727 | 199 | 162 | 361 | 353 | 460 | 678 | 226 | 7038 |
| **Polish sausage** | | | | | | | | | | | | | | |
|   beef w/chicken, hot, cooked | | | | | | | | | | | | | | |
|     *5 pcs* | 55 | 76 | 325 | 336 | 592 | 610 | 208 | 86 | 296 | 244 | 373 | 509 | 244 | 7915 |
|   pork and beef, smoked—*2.7 oz* | 76 | 81 | 353 | 369 | 616 | 686 | 277 | 80 | 308 | 293 | 353 | 581 | 300 | 7916 |
|   pork, cooked | | | | | | | | | | | | | | |
|     *8 oz sausage (10" long, 1¼" dia)* | 227 | 313 | 1342 | 1387 | 2443 | 2520 | 860 | 356 | 1224 | 1008 | 1541 | 2100 | 1008 | 7059 |
| **pork and beef sausage** w/cheddar | | | | | | | | | | | | | | |
|   cheese, smoked—*2.7 oz* | 77 | 116 | 416 | 477 | 847 | 893 | 277 | 116 | 431 | 400 | 531 | 647 | 362 | 7917 |
| **Smokie** (smoked sausage) | | | | | | | | | | | | | | |
|   pork, beef w/flour and nfdm | | | | | | | | | | | | | | |
|     *2.4 oz link (4" long)* | 68 | 95 | 389 | 422 | 732 | 734 | 244 | 110 | 367 | 312 | 460 | 591 | 295 | 7076 |
|   pork, beef w/nfdm | | | | | | | | | | | | | | |
|     *2.4 oz link (4" long)* | 68 | 92 | 375 | 411 | 710 | 709 | 234 | 103 | 354 | 307 | 449 | 553 | 282 | 7077 |
| **turkey sausage**, hot, smoked—*2 oz* | 56 | 96 | 375 | 438 | 671 | 794 | 244 | 88 | 334 | 333 | 448 | 588 | 263 | 7929 |
| **Vienna sausage**, beef and pork, cnd | | | | | | | | | | | | | | |
|   *0.6 oz sausage (2" long, ⅞" dia)* | 16 | 17 | 57 | 89 | 128 | 127 | 42 | 28 | 68 | 55 | 92 | 113 | 44 | 7083 |

### LUNCH MEATS AND SPREADS

| | WT (g) | TRY | THR | ISO | LEU | LYS | MET | CYS | PHE | TYR | VAL | ARG | HIS | REF |
|---|---|---|---|---|---|---|---|---|---|---|---|---|---|---|
| **barbeque loaf lunch meat**—*0.8 oz slice* | 23 | 39 | 157 | 168 | 295 | 303 | 91 | 45 | 147 | 124 | 183 | 224 | 119 | 7001 |
| **beef** | | | | | | | | | | | | | | |
|   chopped, smoked—*1 oz slice* | 28 | 46 | 237 | 232 | 422 | 461 | 137 | 67 | 212 | 171 | 260 | 382 | 164 | 13358 |
|   loaf lunch meat—*1 oz slice* | 28 | 29 | 157 | 151 | 278 | 309 | 89 | 42 | 142 | 108 | 174 | 279 | 106 | 7042 |
|   lunch meat, jellied—*1 oz slice* | 28 | 38 | 208 | 200 | 368 | 409 | 118 | 55 | 188 | 143 | 231 | 368 | 140 | 13353 |
| **beerwurst**, pork and beef—*1 oz slice* | 28 | 49 | 187 | 191 | 337 | 364 | 108 | 50 | 167 | 142 | 215 | 274 | 150 | 7931 |
| **berliner**, pork and beef—*0.8 oz slice* | 23 | 25 | 107 | 112 | 186 | 208 | 84 | 24 | 93 | 89 | 107 | 176 | 91 | 7004 |

| | WT | TRY | THR | ISO | LEU | LYS | MET | CYS | PHE | TYR | VAL | ARG | HIS | REF |
|---|---|---|---|---|---|---|---|---|---|---|---|---|---|---|
| | (g) | | | | | | (mg/serving) | | | | | | | |
| **bologna** | | | | | | | | | | | | | | |
| beef and pork—*1 oz slice* | 28 | 60 | 216 | 227 | 388 | 420 | 125 | 59 | 193 | 170 | 260 | 288 | 181 | 7008 |
| pork—*1 oz slice* | 28 | 42 | 179 | 186 | 327 | 337 | 115 | 48 | 164 | 135 | 206 | 281 | 135 | 7010 |
| pork and turkey, light—*1 oz slice* | 28 | 28 | 100 | 117 | 200 | 186 | 61 | 42 | 113 | 85 | 132 | 176 | 66 | 7936 |
| pork, turkey, beef—*1 oz slice* | 28 | 35 | 143 | 151 | 262 | 287 | 83 | 38 | 133 | 109 | 172 | 254 | 101 | 7937 |
| turkey—*1 oz slice* | 28 | 36 | 139 | 159 | 249 | 285 | 89 | 38 | 128 | 121 | 167 | 234 | 95 | 7011 |
| **braunschweiger** (pork liver sausage) | | | | | | | | | | | | | | |
| *0.6 oz slice (2½″ dia, ¼″ thick)* | 18 | 26 | 96 | 87 | 186 | 164 | 56 | 45 | 100 | 77 | 111 | 138 | 58 | 7014 |
| **chicken breast** | | | | | | | | | | | | | | |
| fat-free, mesquite flavor—*2 slices* | 42 | 77 | 288 | 341 | 504 | 561 | 184 | 96 | 271 | 221 | 339 | 452 | 201 | 7932 |
| fat-free, oven-roasted—*2 slices* | 42 | 77 | 288 | 341 | 504 | 561 | 184 | 96 | 271 | 221 | 339 | 452 | 201 | 7933 |
| **chicken breast roll**, oven-roasted—*2 oz* | 56 | 90 | 334 | 398 | 587 | 654 | 214 | 111 | 315 | 258 | 393 | 520 | 235 | 7935 |
| **chicken roll**, light meat | | | | | | | | | | | | | | |
| *2 slices (2 oz)* | 57 | 121 | 454 | 537 | 794 | 883 | 289 | 152 | 426 | 348 | 533 | 711 | 316 | 7017 |
| **chicken spread**, canned—*1 oz* | 28 | 55 | 204 | 246 | 360 | 403 | 131 | 66 | 192 | 159 | 241 | 313 | 145 | 7018 |
| **chicken/turkey salad spread** | | | | | | | | | | | | | | |
| *1 oz (~2T)* | 28 | 36 | 139 | 164 | 246 | 283 | 90 | 39 | 127 | 115 | 165 | 218 | 97 | 7067 |
| **corned beef** | | | | | | | | | | | | | | |
| canned—*0.7 oz slice* | 21 | 52 | 215 | 246 | 418 | 436 | 132 | 73 | 205 | 186 | 250 | 351 | 181 | 13348 |
| jellied loaf—*1 oz slice* | 28 | 46 | 250 | 241 | 444 | 493 | 142 | 67 | 227 | 172 | 278 | 444 | 168 | 7020 |
| **ham** | | | | | | | | | | | | | | |
| chopped, canned—*0.7 oz slice* | 21 | 38 | 151 | 145 | 262 | 290 | 88 | 40 | 131 | 111 | 151 | 209 | 134 | 7026 |
| minced—*0.7 oz slice* | 21 | 33 | 154 | 147 | 264 | 286 | 96 | 40 | 135 | 113 | 157 | 215 | 127 | 7030 |
| salad spread—*1 oz (about 2 T)* | 28 | 25 | 115 | 113 | 203 | 216 | 64 | 14 | 99 | 78 | 125 | 166 | 98 | 7031 |
| sliced, lean (5% fat)—*1 oz slice* | 28 | 65 | 241 | 237 | 430 | 459 | 143 | 81 | 234 | 178 | 235 | 352 | 194 | 7028 |
| sliced, reg (11% fat)—*1 oz slice* | 28 | 43 | 156 | 160 | 276 | 311 | 89 | 45 | 139 | 118 | 188 | 234 | 134 | 7029 |
| **ham and cheese loaf**—*1 oz slice* | 28 | 58 | 201 | 211 | 379 | 422 | 123 | 66 | 193 | 157 | 225 | 313 | 190 | 7032 |
| Oscar Mayer—*1 oz slice* | 28 | 63 | 188 | 219 | 397 | 446 | 123 | 47 | 212 | 205 | 269 | 257 | 188 | 7211 |
| **ham and cheese spread** | | | | | | | | | | | | | | |
| *1 oz (about 2 T)* | 28 | 104 | 191 | 217 | 421 | 413 | 133 | 71 | 216 | 186 | 284 | 250 | 167 | 7033 |
| **honey loaf**, pork and beef | | | | | | | | | | | | | | |
| *1 oz slice* | 28 | 32 | 129 | 132 | 228 | 250 | 73 | 35 | 114 | 96 | 151 | 179 | 118 | 7035 |
| **honey roll sausage**, beef | | | | | | | | | | | | | | |
| *0.8 oz slice* | 23 | 35 | 179 | 175 | 319 | 349 | 103 | 51 | 160 | 129 | 196 | 289 | 124 | 7088 |
| **liver cheese**, pork—*1.3 oz slice* | 38 | 78 | 247 | 240 | 506 | 448 | 130 | 125 | 272 | 177 | 306 | 315 | 149 | 7040 |
| **liver pate** | | | | | | | | | | | | | | |
| canned—*1 oz (~2 T)* | 28 | 44 | 159 | 155 | 294 | 235 | 80 | 48 | 163 | 127 | 215 | 251 | 83 | 7055 |
| chicken, canned—*1 oz (2 T)* | 28 | 55 | 168 | 206 | 335 | 267 | 95 | 61 | 194 | 137 | 242 | 228 | 97 | 7053 |
| goose, smoked, canned—*1 oz (~2 T)* | 28 | 45 | 142 | 170 | 288 | 242 | 76 | 43 | 159 | 112 | 201 | 196 | 85 | 7054 |
| truffle flavor—*2 oz* | 56 | 88 | 318 | 310 | 588 | 469 | 159 | 95 | 326 | 254 | 430 | 501 | 167 | 7942 |
| **liverwurst** | | | | | | | | | | | | | | |
| pork—*1 oz* | 28 | 42 | 188 | 183 | 319 | 323 | 80 | 42 | 173 | 101 | 240 | 227 | 125 | 7041 |
| spread—*4 T* | 55 | 83 | 369 | 359 | 626 | 635 | 157 | 82 | 339 | 199 | 471 | 447 | 246 | 7911 |
| **luxury loaf**, pork—*1 oz slice* | 28 | 60 | 246 | 228 | 425 | 463 | 131 | 43 | 201 | 180 | 250 | 328 | 184 | 7060 |
| **macaroni and cheese loaf** | | | | | | | | | | | | | | |
| chicken, pork, and beef—*1 slice* | 38 | 55 | 169 | 206 | 344 | 274 | 101 | 68 | 189 | 144 | 225 | 242 | 123 | 7940 |
| **mortadella**, beef and pork | | | | | | | | | | | | | | |
| *0.5 oz slice* | 15 | 23 | 95 | 106 | 182 | 189 | 59 | 31 | 90 | 80 | 110 | 154 | 78 | 7050 |
| **mother's loaf**, pork—*0.7 oz slice* | 21 | 36 | 127 | 134 | 236 | 247 | 75 | 43 | 120 | 94 | 140 | 191 | 112 | 7061 |
| **olive loaf**, pork—*1 oz slice* | 28 | 29 | 132 | 118 | 244 | 227 | 84 | 40 | 117 | 107 | 142 | 163 | 82 | 7051 |
| **pastrami** | | | | | | | | | | | | | | |
| beef—*1 oz slice* | 28 | 39 | 240 | 273 | 478 | 507 | 156 | 78 | 237 | 191 | 298 | 389 | 192 | 13355 |
| beef, 98% fat-free—*6 slices* | 57 | 89 | 371 | 425 | 722 | 754 | 228 | 126 | 354 | 321 | 433 | 607 | 313 | 7925 |
| turkey—*2 slices* | 57 | 116 | 455 | 523 | 810 | 947 | 292 | 117 | 408 | 396 | 543 | 735 | 313 | 7052 |
| **pepperoni**, pork and beef | | | | | | | | | | | | | | |
| *0.2 oz slice (1 ⅜″ dia, ⅛″ thick)* | 6 | 14 | 52 | 54 | 94 | 99 | 31 | 14 | 47 | 40 | 59 | 78 | 41 | 7057 |
| **pickle and pimento loaf**, pork | | | | | | | | | | | | | | |
| *1 oz slice* | 28 | 31 | 116 | 125 | 209 | 223 | 72 | 38 | 110 | 92 | 134 | 240 | 87 | 7058 |
| **picnic loaf**, pork and beef | | | | | | | | | | | | | | |
| *1 oz slice* | 28 | 40 | 184 | 163 | 321 | 334 | 106 | 45 | 150 | 128 | 180 | 249 | 122 | 7062 |
| **pork and beef loaf**, Dutch Brand | | | | | | | | | | | | | | |
| *1.3 slice* | 38 | 65 | 289 | 324 | 538 | 586 | 180 | 90 | 273 | 226 | 349 | 446 | 229 | 7021 |
| **pork and beef** lunch meat—*2 oz slice* | 57 | 76 | 310 | 367 | 597 | 675 | 164 | 131 | 291 | 286 | 406 | 527 | 231 | 7047 |
| **pork and beef luncheon sausage** | | | | | | | | | | | | | | |
| *0.8 oz slice (4″ dia, ⅛″ thick)* | 23 | 37 | 153 | 181 | 294 | 333 | 81 | 65 | 143 | 141 | 200 | 260 | 114 | 7090 |
| **pork and beef sausage**, New England | | | | | | | | | | | | | | |
| Brand—*0.8 oz slice (4″ dia, ⅛″ thick)* | 23 | 44 | 174 | 175 | 313 | 348 | 103 | 57 | 157 | 123 | 185 | 276 | 150 | 7091 |
| **pork** lunch meat, canned—*.7 oz slice* | 21 | 26 | 102 | 120 | 200 | 196 | 70 | 45 | 103 | 80 | 137 | 182 | 75 | 7045 |

| | WT (g) | TRY | THR | ISO | LEU | LYS | MET | CYS | PHE | TYR | VAL | ARG | HIS | REF |
|---|---|---|---|---|---|---|---|---|---|---|---|---|---|---|
| | | | | | | (mg/serving) | | | | | | | | |
| **salami** | | | | | | | | | | | | | | |
| beef—*2 slices (1.6 oz)* | 46 | 63 | 261 | 299 | 508 | 530 | 161 | 88 | 249 | 226 | 305 | 427 | 220 | 7068 |
| beef and pork—*2 slices (1.6 oz)* | 46 | 52 | 240 | 310 | 427 | 509 | 138 | 90 | 221 | 254 | 307 | 393 | 165 | 7069 |
| beef and pork, less sodium—*1 oz* | 28 | 32 | 146 | 189 | 260 | 310 | 84 | 55 | 135 | 155 | 187 | 239 | 101 | 7913 |
| beerwurst, pork—*2 slices (1.6 oz)* | 46 | 52 | 260 | 223 | 434 | 475 | 163 | 49 | 207 | 185 | 235 | 372 | 193 | 7003 |
| dry/hard, Italian, pork, beef, 50% less sodium—*3 slices (1 oz)* | 28 | 59 | 269 | 272 | 485 | 511 | 166 | 73 | 243 | 199 | 303 | 424 | 196 | 7941 |
| dry/hard, pork—*3 slices (1 oz)* | 27 | 68 | 273 | 293 | 439 | 507 | 127 | 78 | 254 | 185 | 302 | 371 | 166 | 7071 |
| Italian, pork—*1 oz* | 28 | 71 | 283 | 304 | 455 | 526 | 132 | 81 | 263 | 192 | 314 | 384 | 172 | 7926 |
| turkey—*2 slices (2 oz)* | 57 | 99 | 388 | 454 | 695 | 822 | 253 | 91 | 346 | 345 | 463 | 608 | 272 | 7070 |
| **sandwich spread**, pork and beef—*1 oz (~2T)* | 28 | 23 | 94 | 94 | 168 | 186 | 55 | 30 | 84 | 66 | 100 | 148 | 78 | 7073 |
| **Swisswurst**, pork, beef, Swiss cheese, smoked—*2.7 oz* | 77 | 116 | 416 | 477 | 847 | 893 | 277 | 116 | 431 | 400 | 531 | 647 | 362 | 7920 |
| **turkey breast** lunch meat *0.7 oz slice (3½″ square)* | 21 | 41 | 159 | 186 | 286 | 338 | 104 | 37 | 142 | 142 | 190 | 250 | 112 | 7079 |
| **turkey ham** (cured thigh meat) lunch meat—*2 slices* | 57 | 109 | 432 | 497 | 770 | 902 | 279 | 109 | 388 | 376 | 516 | 698 | 298 | 7080 |
| **turkey roll** light and dark meat—*2 slices* | 57 | 114 | 451 | 518 | 803 | 940 | 291 | 114 | 405 | 392 | 538 | 729 | 311 | 7082 |
| light meat—*2 slices* | 57 | 117 | 465 | 534 | 827 | 968 | 299 | 117 | 417 | 404 | 555 | 752 | 320 | 7081 |
| **MEAT-BASED SNACKS** | | | | | | | | | | | | | | |
| **bacon and beef sticks**—*1 oz* | 28 | 59 | 269 | 272 | 485 | 511 | 166 | 73 | 243 | 199 | 303 | 424 | 196 | 7921 |
| **beef, dried**—*5 slices (0.7 oz)* | 21 | 40 | 241 | 275 | 480 | 510 | 157 | 78 | 238 | 192 | 299 | 390 | 193 | 13350 |
| **beef sticks**, smoked—*0.7 oz stick* | 20 | 37 | 166 | 164 | 295 | 304 | 91 | 58 | 160 | 119 | 190 | 304 | 106 | 19407 |
| **pork skins**—*1 oz* | 28 | 33 | 510 | 387 | 930 | 779 | 134 | 148 | 543 | 337 | 678 | 1355 | 203 | 19041 |
| barbecue—*1 oz* | 28 | 37 | 494 | 384 | 902 | 755 | 133 | 144 | 526 | 332 | 654 | 1273 | 201 | 19408 |
| **summer sausage sticks**, pork, beef cheddar cheese—*1 oz* | 28 | 42 | 151 | 174 | 308 | 325 | 101 | 42 | 157 | 146 | 193 | 235 | 132 | 7918 |
| **21. MEAT SUBSTITUTES, TOFU, AND RELATED SOY PRODUCTS** | | | | | | | | | | | | | | |
| **MEAT SUBSTITUTES** | | | | | | | | | | | | | | |
| **bacon**, simulated meat product *3 strips (0.6 oz)* | 16 | 26 | 72 | 89 | 146 | 116 | 23 | 28 | 98 | 64 | 95 | 140 | 48 | 16104 |
| **meat extender**, simulated meat product *1 oz* | 28 | 161 | 452 | 559 | 914 | 727 | 146 | 176 | 611 | 400 | 592 | 874 | 299 | 16106 |
| **sausage meat substitute**, pan-fried *0.9 oz link* | 25 | 70 | 196 | 242 | 397 | 316 | 63 | 76 | 265 | 174 | 257 | 380 | 130 | 16107 |
| **TOFU AND RELATED SOY PRODUCTS** | | | | | | | | | | | | | | |
| **fuyu** (salted, fermented tofu) prep w/calcium sulfate—*0.4 oz block* | 11 | 14 | 37 | 44 | 68 | 59 | 11 | 12 | 44 | 30 | 45 | 60 | 26 | 16432 |
| **miso** (soybean paste)—*1 oz* | 28 | 43 | 134 | 142 | 230 | 134 | 36 | 0 | 136 | 99 | 153 | 220 | 68 | 16112 |
| **natto** (boiled, fermented soybeans) *1 cup (6.2 oz)* | 175 | 390 | 1423 | 1629 | 2641 | 2004 | 364 | 385 | 1647 | 973 | 1782 | 1591 | 896 | 16113 |
| **okara** (soybean pulp)—*1 cup (4.3 oz)* | 122 | 61 | 160 | 194 | 298 | 259 | 50 | 54 | 192 | 132 | 198 | 261 | 113 | 16130 |
| **tempeh**, uncooked—*1 cup (5.9 oz)* | 166 | 322 | 1321 | 1461 | 2374 | 1507 | 290 | 320 | 1482 | 1102 | 1527 | 2078 | 774 | 16114 |
| **tofu, extra firm** prep w/nigari (MgCl)—*3 oz* | 85 | 131 | 343 | 416 | 638 | 553 | 107 | 116 | 409 | 281 | 424 | 558 | 245 | 16159 |
| silken, lite, Mori-Nu—*3 oz* | 85 | 82 | 202 | 275 | 462 | 364 | 75 | 79 | 309 | 213 | 273 | 448 | 149 | 16165 |
| silken, Mori-Nu—*3 oz* | 85 | 105 | 263 | 326 | 543 | 421 | 80 | 108 | 366 | 267 | 339 | 452 | 155 | 16163 |
| **tofu, firm** prep w/calcium sulfate—*3 oz* | 85 | 209 | 547 | 665 | 1019 | 883 | 172 | 185 | 653 | 449 | 677 | 892 | 390 | 16426 |
| prep w/calcium sulfate and nigari (MgCl)—*3 oz* | 85 | 105 | 349 | 377 | 619 | 393 | 94 | 26 | 371 | 312 | 387 | 609 | 191 | 16126 |
| prep w/nigari (MgCl)—*3 oz* | 85 | 168 | 439 | 534 | 819 | 710 | 138 | 149 | 524 | 360 | 544 | 717 | 314 | 16160 |
| silken, lite, Mori-Nu—*3 oz* | 85 | 81 | 187 | 252 | 426 | 326 | 65 | 67 | 274 | 195 | 243 | 400 | 133 | 16164 |
| silken, Mori-Nu—*3 oz* | 85 | 72 | 243 | 297 | 498 | 390 | 90 | 85 | 335 | 254 | 327 | 439 | 144 | 16162 |
| **tofu**, fried—*0.5 oz piece* | 13 | 35 | 91 | 111 | 170 | 147 | 29 | 31 | 109 | 75 | 113 | 149 | 65 | 16129 |
| **tofu**, frozen, dried (koyadofu, kori tofu, tung tou-fu)—*1 piece* | 17 | 127 | 333 | 404 | 619 | 537 | 104 | 113 | 397 | 273 | 411 | 542 | 237 | 16128 |
| prep w/calcium sulfate—*0.6 oz piece* | 17 | 127 | 333 | 404 | 619 | 537 | 104 | 113 | 397 | 273 | 411 | 542 | 237 | 16428 |
| **tofu**, prep w/calcium sulfate, fried *0.5 oz piece* | 13 | 35 | 91 | 111 | 170 | 147 | 29 | 31 | 109 | 75 | 113 | 149 | 65 | 16429 |
| **tofu**, regular, prep w/calcium sulfate—*3 oz* | 85 | 107 | 280 | 340 | 522 | 452 | 88 | 95 | 334 | 230 | 347 | 457 | 200 | 16427 |
| **tofu, soft** prep w/calcium sulfate and nigari (MgCl)—*3 oz* | 85 | 87 | 228 | 275 | 423 | 366 | 71 | 77 | 271 | 186 | 281 | 371 | 162 | 16127 |
| soft, silken, Mori-Nu—*3 oz* | 85 | 58 | 183 | 198 | 237 | 290 | 63 | 61 | 258 | 164 | 251 | 326 | 99 | 16161 |
| **yufu** (salted, fermented tofu)—*0.4 oz block* | 11 | 14 | 37 | 44 | 68 | 59 | 11 | 12 | 44 | 30 | 45 | 60 | 26 | 16132 |

| | WT | TRY | THR | ISO | LEU | LYS | MET | CYS | PHE | TYR | VAL | ARG | HIS | REF |
|---|---|---|---|---|---|---|---|---|---|---|---|---|---|---|
| | (g) | | | | | | (mg/serving) | | | | | | | |

**22. MILKS, MILK BEVERAGES, AND YOGURT**

**COW MILK**

**buttermilk**
| | WT | TRY | THR | ISO | LEU | LYS | MET | CYS | PHE | TYR | VAL | ARG | HIS | REF |
|---|---|---|---|---|---|---|---|---|---|---|---|---|---|---|
| cultured—*8 fl oz* | 245 | 88 | 387 | 500 | 806 | 679 | 198 | 76 | 426 | 341 | 595 | 309 | 233 | 1088 |
| dry—*1 T* | 7 | 34 | 108 | 145 | 235 | 190 | 60 | 22 | 116 | 116 | 161 | 87 | 65 | 1094 |

**condensed milk,** sweetened,
| | WT | TRY | THR | ISO | LEU | LYS | MET | CYS | PHE | TYR | VAL | ARG | HIS | REF |
|---|---|---|---|---|---|---|---|---|---|---|---|---|---|---|
| canned—*1 fl oz* | 38 | 43 | 136 | 182 | 294 | 238 | 75 | 28 | 145 | 145 | 201 | 109 | 81 | 1095 |

**evaporated milk,** canned
| | WT | TRY | THR | ISO | LEU | LYS | MET | CYS | PHE | TYR | VAL | ARG | HIS | REF |
|---|---|---|---|---|---|---|---|---|---|---|---|---|---|---|
| nonfat—*1 fl oz* | 32 | 34 | 109 | 146 | 237 | 192 | 60 | 22 | 116 | 116 | 162 | 87 | 66 | 1097 |
| whole—*1 fl oz* | 32 | 31 | 98 | 132 | 213 | 173 | 55 | 20 | 105 | 105 | 146 | 79 | 59 | 1096 |
| **milk, lowfat,** 1% fat—*8 fl oz* | 244 | 98 | 217 | 456 | 915 | 700 | 203 | 283 | 407 | 346 | 529 | 234 | 205 | 1082 |
| pro-fortified—*8 fl oz* | 246 | 135 | 435 | 585 | 947 | 768 | 244 | 89 | 467 | 467 | 647 | 349 | 263 | 1084 |
| w/ndms—*8 fl oz* | 245 | 120 | 385 | 517 | 835 | 676 | 213 | 78 | 412 | 412 | 571 | 309 | 230 | 1083 |
| **milk, nonfat**—*8 fl oz* | 245 | 98 | 201 | 368 | 801 | 617 | 152 | 301 | 355 | 363 | 441 | 176 | 184 | 1085 |
| pro-fortified—*8 fl oz* | 246 | 138 | 440 | 590 | 954 | 772 | 244 | 91 | 470 | 470 | 652 | 352 | 263 | 1087 |
| w/ndms—*8 fl oz* | 245 | 122 | 394 | 529 | 858 | 693 | 220 | 81 | 421 | 421 | 586 | 316 | 238 | 1086 |

**milk powder,** nonfat
| | WT | TRY | THR | ISO | LEU | LYS | MET | CYS | PHE | TYR | VAL | ARG | HIS | REF |
|---|---|---|---|---|---|---|---|---|---|---|---|---|---|---|
| calcium-reduced—*1 oz* | 28 | 140 | 449 | 601 | 974 | 788 | 249 | 92 | 480 | 480 | 665 | 360 | 270 | 1093 |
| instant w/vit A—*1 ⅓ cups (3.2 oz pkt)* | 91 | 450 | 1441 | 1933 | 3129 | 2533 | 801 | 296 | 1542 | 1542 | 2138 | 1157 | 866 | 1092 |
| regular w/o vit A—*¼ cup* | 30 | 153 | 490 | 656 | 1063 | 860 | 272 | 100 | 524 | 524 | 726 | 393 | 294 | 1091 |
| **milk powder,** whole—*¼ cup* | 32 | 119 | 380 | 509 | 825 | 668 | 211 | 78 | 407 | 407 | 564 | 305 | 228 | 1090 |
| **milk, reduced fat,** 2% fat | 244 | 98 | 251 | 447 | 808 | 569 | 203 | 261 | 395 | 373 | 532 | 261 | 178 | 1079 |
| pro-fortified—*8 fl oz* | 246 | 138 | 438 | 588 | 952 | 770 | 244 | 91 | 470 | 470 | 649 | 352 | 263 | 1081 |
| w/ndms—*8 fl oz* | 245 | 120 | 385 | 517 | 835 | 676 | 213 | 78 | 412 | 412 | 571 | 309 | 230 | 1080 |
| **milk, whole,** 3.25% fat—*8 fl oz* | 244 | 183 | 349 | 403 | 647 | 342 | 183 | 41 | 359 | 371 | 468 | 183 | 183 | 1077 |
| **milk, whole,** 3.7% fat—*8 fl oz* | 244 | 112 | 361 | 483 | 783 | 634 | 200 | 73 | 386 | 386 | 537 | 290 | 217 | 1078 |
| **milk, whole,** low sodium—*8 fl oz* | 244 | 107 | 342 | 459 | 742 | 600 | 190 | 71 | 366 | 366 | 505 | 273 | 205 | 1089 |

**COW MILK BEVERAGES**

**carob-flavored milk,** from carob mix
| | WT | TRY | THR | ISO | LEU | LYS | MET | CYS | PHE | TYR | VAL | ARG | HIS | REF |
|---|---|---|---|---|---|---|---|---|---|---|---|---|---|---|
| in whole milk—*8 fl oz* | 256 | 182 | 348 | 402 | 648 | 343 | 182 | 41 | 358 | 371 | 468 | 182 | 182 | 14169 |

**chocolate malted milk,** whole milk
| | WT | TRY | THR | ISO | LEU | LYS | MET | CYS | PHE | TYR | VAL | ARG | HIS | REF |
|---|---|---|---|---|---|---|---|---|---|---|---|---|---|---|
| *8 fl oz* | 265 | 196 | 379 | 437 | 710 | 376 | 196 | 61 | 398 | 403 | 511 | 225 | 204 | 14318 |
| with added nutrients—*8 fl oz* | 265 | 183 | 347 | 403 | 647 | 342 | 183 | 40 | 358 | 368 | 469 | 183 | 183 | 14316 |

**chocolate milk**
| | WT | TRY | THR | ISO | LEU | LYS | MET | CYS | PHE | TYR | VAL | ARG | HIS | REF |
|---|---|---|---|---|---|---|---|---|---|---|---|---|---|---|
| 1% milk—*8 fl oz* | 250 | 115 | 365 | 490 | 792 | 642 | 202 | 75 | 390 | 390 | 542 | 292 | 220 | 1104 |
| reduced fat—*8 fl oz* | 250 | 112 | 350 | 350 | 688 | 575 | 175 | 75 | 350 | 300 | 450 | 262 | 200 | 1103 |
| whole milk—*8 fl oz* | 250 | 112 | 357 | 480 | 778 | 628 | 198 | 72 | 382 | 382 | 530 | 288 | 215 | 1102 |
| w/chocolate syrup—*8 fl oz* | 282 | 192 | 372 | 426 | 685 | 372 | 189 | 48 | 389 | 395 | 505 | 217 | 192 | 14182 |
| w/instant mix—*8 fl oz* | 266 | 192 | 372 | 426 | 684 | 372 | 189 | 48 | 388 | 394 | 505 | 218 | 194 | 14177 |

**eggnog**
| | WT | TRY | THR | ISO | LEU | LYS | MET | CYS | PHE | TYR | VAL | ARG | HIS | REF |
|---|---|---|---|---|---|---|---|---|---|---|---|---|---|---|
| from mix w/whole milk | | | | | | | | | | | | | | |
| nonalcoholic—*8 fl oz* | 272 | 182 | 351 | 405 | 653 | 348 | 185 | 41 | 362 | 373 | 473 | 188 | 185 | 14245 |
| nonalcoholic—*8 fl oz* | 254 | 137 | 444 | 584 | 937 | 757 | 221 | 97 | 462 | 462 | 643 | 378 | 241 | 1057 |

**hot chocolate,** homemade w/2%
| | WT | TRY | THR | ISO | LEU | LYS | MET | CYS | PHE | TYR | VAL | ARG | HIS | REF |
|---|---|---|---|---|---|---|---|---|---|---|---|---|---|---|
| milk—*8 fl oz* | 250 | 92 | 238 | 422 | 762 | 538 | 190 | 248 | 375 | 352 | 503 | 248 | 168 | 1105 |
| **malted milk,** whole milk—*8 fl oz* | 265 | 209 | 411 | 477 | 790 | 408 | 217 | 90 | 443 | 437 | 554 | 273 | 231 | 14312 |

**strawberry flavored mix** in whole
| | WT | TRY | THR | ISO | LEU | LYS | MET | CYS | PHE | TYR | VAL | ARG | HIS | REF |
|---|---|---|---|---|---|---|---|---|---|---|---|---|---|---|
| milk—*8 fl oz* | 266 | 112 | 364 | 487 | 787 | 638 | 202 | 74 | 388 | 388 | 537 | 290 | 218 | 14351 |

**COW MILK YOGURT**

**yogurt,** lowfat
| | WT | TRY | THR | ISO | LEU | LYS | MET | CYS | PHE | TYR | VAL | ARG | HIS | REF |
|---|---|---|---|---|---|---|---|---|---|---|---|---|---|---|
| fruit—*8 oz container* | 227 | 57 | 406 | 540 | 999 | 890 | 293 | 91 | 540 | 502 | 822 | 300 | 245 | 1121 |
| fruit w/low-cal | | | | | | | | | | | | | | |
| sweetener—*8 oz container* | 227 | 61 | 454 | 602 | 1112 | 990 | 325 | 100 | 602 | 556 | 913 | 331 | 272 | 1203 |
| plain—*8 oz container* | 227 | 68 | 490 | 649 | 1201 | 1069 | 352 | 109 | 649 | 602 | 985 | 359 | 295 | 1117 |
| strawberry—*8 oz container* | 227 | 50 | 370 | 493 | 910 | 810 | 266 | 82 | 493 | 456 | 747 | 272 | 225 | 1120 |
| vanilla—*8 oz container* | 227 | 64 | 459 | 611 | 1128 | 1003 | 329 | 102 | 611 | 565 | 926 | 336 | 277 | 1119 |
| **yogurt,** nonfat | | | | | | | | | | | | | | |
| fruit—*8 oz container* | 227 | 64 | 459 | 611 | 1126 | 997 | 329 | 102 | 613 | 561 | 924 | 343 | 277 | 43261 |
| plain—*8 oz container* | 227 | 73 | 533 | 711 | 1310 | 1167 | 384 | 118 | 711 | 656 | 1076 | 390 | 322 | 1118 |
| **yogurt,** whole, plain—*8 oz container* | 227 | 45 | 322 | 429 | 794 | 706 | 232 | 73 | 429 | 397 | 651 | 236 | 195 | 1116 |

**OTHER MAMMAL MILKS**

| | WT | TRY | THR | ISO | LEU | LYS | MET | CYS | PHE | TYR | VAL | ARG | HIS | REF |
|---|---|---|---|---|---|---|---|---|---|---|---|---|---|---|
| **ewe (sheep) milk**—*8 fl oz* | 245 | 206 | 657 | 828 | 1438 | 1257 | 380 | 86 | 696 | 688 | 1098 | 485 | 409 | 1109 |
| **goat milk**—*8 fl oz* | 244 | 107 | 398 | 505 | 766 | 708 | 195 | 112 | 378 | 437 | 586 | 290 | 217 | 1106 |
| **human milk**—*1 fl oz* | 31 | 5 | 14 | 17 | 29 | 21 | 7 | 6 | 14 | 16 | 20 | 13 | 7 | 1107 |
| **Indian buffalo milk**—*8 fl oz* | 244 | 129 | 444 | 495 | 893 | 683 | 237 | 117 | 395 | 447 | 534 | 278 | 190 | 1108 |

| | WT (g) | TRY | THR | ISO | LEU | LYS | MET | CYS | PHE | TYR | VAL | ARG | HIS | REF |
|---|---|---|---|---|---|---|---|---|---|---|---|---|---|---|
| | | | | | | (mg/serving) | | | | | | | | |
| **NON-DAIRY MILK-LIKE BEVERAGES AND YOGURTS** | | | | | | | | | | | | | | |
| **soymilk**—*8 fl oz* | 245 | 93 | 265 | 279 | 456 | 321 | 66 | 0 | 277 | 218 | 287 | 458 | 149 | 16120 |
| chocolate, unfortified—*8 fl oz* | 243 | 92 | 262 | 277 | 452 | 318 | 66 | 0 | 275 | 216 | 284 | 454 | 148 | 16166 |
| **23. NUTS AND SEEDS** | | | | | | | | | | | | | | |
| **NUTS, NUT PRODUCTS, AND NUT-LIKE PRODUCTS** | | | | | | | | | | | | | | |
| **acorn flour**, full-fat—*3.5 oz* | 100 | 90 | 288 | 348 | 596 | 468 | 126 | 133 | 328 | 227 | 421 | 577 | 208 | 12060 |
| **acorns** | | | | | | | | | | | | | | |
| dried—*1 oz* | 28 | 27 | 87 | 105 | 180 | 141 | 38 | 40 | 99 | 69 | 127 | 174 | 63 | 12059 |
| raw—*1 oz* | 28 | 21 | 66 | 80 | 137 | 108 | 29 | 31 | 75 | 52 | 97 | 132 | 48 | 12058 |
| **almond butter**—*1 T* | 16 | 43 | 89 | 105 | 188 | 81 | 28 | 43 | 135 | 85 | 124 | 302 | 68 | 12195 |
| **almonds** | | | | | | | | | | | | | | |
| dry-roasted—*1 oz (~22 nuts)* | 28 | 56 | 197 | 201 | 428 | 175 | 55 | 82 | 334 | 154 | 233 | 717 | 172 | 12063 |
| honey-roasted—*1 oz (~22 nuts)* | 28 | 79 | 161 | 190 | 339 | 145 | 50 | 79 | 244 | 154 | 225 | 545 | 122 | 12206 |
| oil-roasted—*1 oz (22 nuts)* | 28 | 54 | 190 | 193 | 411 | 168 | 53 | 79 | 321 | 148 | 223 | 690 | 166 | 12065 |
| raw—*1 oz* | 28 | 60 | 167 | 197 | 417 | 162 | 42 | 53 | 314 | 127 | 229 | 685 | 156 | 12061 |
| **beechnuts**, dried—*1 oz* | 28 | 19 | 62 | 69 | 103 | 103 | 41 | 55 | 73 | 48 | 97 | 124 | 48 | 12077 |
| **brazilnuts**, raw—*1 oz (6–8 nuts)* | 28 | 39 | 101 | 144 | 323 | 138 | 282 | 103 | 176 | 118 | 212 | 601 | 108 | 12078 |
| **butternuts**, dried—*1 oz (about 9 nuts)* | 28 | 102 | 263 | 330 | 616 | 216 | 171 | 136 | 404 | 274 | 431 | 1361 | 226 | 12084 |
| **cashew butter**—*1 T* | 16 | 44 | 109 | 134 | 236 | 150 | 50 | 52 | 145 | 90 | 191 | 320 | 73 | 12088 |
| **cashews** | | | | | | | | | | | | | | |
| dry-roasted—*1 oz* | 28 | 66 | 166 | 205 | 360 | 229 | 77 | 79 | 221 | 137 | 291 | 487 | 112 | 12085 |
| oil-roasted—*1 oz (18 nuts)* | 28 | 74 | 178 | 204 | 381 | 240 | 94 | 102 | 246 | 131 | 283 | 550 | 118 | 12086 |
| raw—*1 oz* | 28 | 80 | 193 | 221 | 412 | 260 | 101 | 110 | 266 | 142 | 306 | 594 | 128 | 12087 |
| **chestnuts, Chinese** | | | | | | | | | | | | | | |
| boiled, steamed—*1 oz* | 28 | 10 | 32 | 30 | 50 | 44 | 20 | 21 | 36 | 24 | 42 | 83 | 23 | 12095 |
| dried—*1 oz* | 28 | 22 | 76 | 71 | 118 | 104 | 46 | 50 | 87 | 57 | 100 | 196 | 55 | 12094 |
| raw—*1 oz* | 28 | 14 | 47 | 44 | 73 | 64 | 28 | 31 | 53 | 35 | 62 | 120 | 34 | 12093 |
| roasted—*1 oz* | 28 | 15 | 50 | 47 | 77 | 68 | 30 | 33 | 57 | 38 | 66 | 129 | 36 | 12096 |
| **chestnuts, European** | | | | | | | | | | | | | | |
| boiled, steamed—*1 oz* | 28 | 6 | 20 | 22 | 33 | 33 | 13 | 18 | 24 | 15 | 31 | 40 | 15 | 12101 |
| dried—*1 oz* | 28 | 20 | 64 | 71 | 106 | 106 | 42 | 57 | 76 | 50 | 100 | 128 | 50 | 12099 |
| raw—*1 oz* | 28 | 8 | 24 | 27 | 40 | 40 | 16 | 22 | 29 | 19 | 38 | 48 | 19 | 12097 |
| roasted—*1 oz (3 nuts)* | 28 | 10 | 32 | 35 | 53 | 53 | 21 | 28 | 38 | 25 | 50 | 64 | 25 | 12167 |
| **chestnuts, Japanese** | | | | | | | | | | | | | | |
| boiled, steamed—*1 oz* | 28 | 3 | 9 | 11 | 14 | 15 | 6 | 7 | 9 | 6 | 14 | 15 | 6 | 12203 |
| dried—*1 oz* | 28 | 21 | 59 | 72 | 91 | 96 | 35 | 43 | 57 | 42 | 87 | 97 | 37 | 12175 |
| raw—*1 oz* | 28 | 9 | 25 | 31 | 39 | 41 | 15 | 18 | 25 | 18 | 38 | 41 | 16 | 12202 |
| roasted—*1 oz* | 28 | 12 | 33 | 41 | 52 | 54 | 20 | 24 | 32 | 24 | 49 | 55 | 21 | 12204 |
| **coconut cream** | | | | | | | | | | | | | | |
| raw—*8 fl oz* | 240 | 101 | 317 | 341 | 646 | 384 | 163 | 173 | 442 | 269 | 528 | 1428 | 199 | 12115 |
| sweetened, canned—*8 fl oz* | 296 | 38 | 127 | 136 | 258 | 154 | 65 | 68 | 178 | 107 | 210 | 568 | 80 | 12116 |
| **coconut, dried**—*1 oz* | 28 | 23 | 70 | 76 | 143 | 85 | 36 | 38 | 98 | 60 | 117 | 316 | 44 | 12108 |
| creamed—*1 oz* | 28 | 17 | 54 | 58 | 110 | 66 | 28 | 29 | 75 | 46 | 90 | 244 | 34 | 12177 |
| sweetened, flaked, canned—*1 oz* | 28 | 11 | 34 | 37 | 70 | 41 | 18 | 18 | 48 | 29 | 57 | 154 | 22 | 12110 |
| sweetened, flaked, pkgd—*1 oz* | 28 | 6 | 24 | 19 | 53 | 41 | 17 | 8 | 37 | 16 | 34 | 150 | 21 | 12109 |
| sweetened, shredded—*1 oz* | 28 | 10 | 29 | 32 | 60 | 36 | 15 | 16 | 41 | 25 | 49 | 132 | 18 | 12179 |
| toasted—*1 oz* | 28 | 17 | 54 | 58 | 110 | 66 | 28 | 29 | 75 | 46 | 90 | 244 | 34 | 12114 |
| **coconut milk** | | | | | | | | | | | | | | |
| canned—*8 fl oz* | 226 | 54 | 167 | 179 | 339 | 201 | 86 | 90 | 231 | 140 | 276 | 748 | 104 | 12118 |
| frozen—*8 fl oz* | 240 | 46 | 142 | 151 | 286 | 170 | 72 | 77 | 197 | 120 | 235 | 634 | 89 | 12176 |
| raw—*8 fl oz* | 240 | 65 | 199 | 216 | 408 | 242 | 103 | 108 | 278 | 170 | 334 | 902 | 127 | 12117 |
| **coconut**, raw—*1.6 oz piece (2″ × 2″ × ½″)* | 45 | 18 | 54 | 59 | 111 | 66 | 28 | 30 | 76 | 46 | 91 | 246 | 35 | 12104 |
| **coconut water**—*8 fl oz* | 240 | 19 | 62 | 67 | 127 | 77 | 31 | 34 | 89 | 53 | 106 | 283 | 41 | 12119 |
| **filberts (hazelnuts)** | | | | | | | | | | | | | | |
| dried—*1 oz (20 nuts)* | 28 | 54 | 139 | 153 | 298 | 118 | 62 | 78 | 186 | 101 | 196 | 619 | 121 | 12120 |
| dry-roasted—*1 oz* | 28 | 54 | 140 | 153 | 299 | 118 | 62 | 78 | 187 | 102 | 197 | 622 | 122 | 12122 |
| **ginkgo nuts** | | | | | | | | | | | | | | |
| canned—*1 oz (14 nuts)* | 28 | 11 | 40 | 31 | 47 | 31 | 8 | 3 | 25 | 9 | 42 | 62 | 15 | 12129 |
| dried—*1 oz* | 28 | 48 | 179 | 140 | 211 | 138 | 37 | 15 | 114 | 41 | 190 | 281 | 68 | 12128 |
| raw—*1 oz* | 28 | 20 | 75 | 59 | 88 | 58 | 15 | 6 | 48 | 17 | 79 | 118 | 29 | 12127 |
| **hickorynuts**, dried—*1 oz (~9 to 10 nuts)* | 28 | 39 | 118 | 161 | 288 | 139 | 84 | 76 | 200 | 127 | 204 | 584 | 109 | 12130 |
| **macadamia nuts** | | | | | | | | | | | | | | |
| dry-roasted—*1 oz (10 to 12 nuts)* | 28 | 18 | 102 | 87 | 166 | 5 | 6 | 1 | 183 | 141 | 100 | 386 | 54 | 12132 |
| raw—*1 oz (10 to 12 nuts)* | 28 | 19 | 104 | 88 | 169 | 5 | 6 | 2 | 186 | 143 | 102 | 393 | 55 | 12131 |
| **mixed nuts** | | | | | | | | | | | | | | |
| dry-roasted—*1 oz* | 28 | 74 | 167 | 208 | 384 | 199 | 64 | 80 | 267 | 189 | 262 | 628 | 134 | 12135 |

| | WT | TRY | THR | ISO | LEU | LYS | MET | CYS | PHE | TYR | VAL | ARG | HIS | REF |
|---|---|---|---|---|---|---|---|---|---|---|---|---|---|---|
| | (g) | | | | | | (mg/serving) | | | | | | | |
| oil-roasted—*1 oz* | 28 | 69 | 159 | 203 | 376 | 184 | 95 | 82 | 258 | 183 | 262 | 567 | 132 | 12137 |
| w/o peanuts, oil-roasted—*1 oz* | 28 | 71 | 159 | 197 | 354 | 191 | 97 | 85 | 230 | 143 | 267 | 557 | 116 | 12138 |
| **peanut butter** | | | | | | | | | | | | | | |
| chunk style/crunchy—*2 T* | 32 | 73 | 166 | 195 | 488 | 215 | 84 | 72 | 379 | 262 | 247 | 874 | 176 | 16097 |
| smooth—*2 T* | 32 | 73 | 165 | 194 | 486 | 214 | 84 | 72 | 378 | 260 | 246 | 870 | 175 | 16098 |
| **peanut flour**, lowfat—*1 cup* | 60 | 197 | 695 | 713 | 1315 | 728 | 249 | 260 | 1051 | 824 | 851 | 2425 | 512 | 16100 |
| **peanuts**, all types | | | | | | | | | | | | | | |
| boiled—*½ cup (33 nuts)* | 28 | 37 | 129 | 133 | 245 | 136 | 46 | 48 | 196 | 154 | 158 | 452 | 95 | 16088 |
| dry-roasted—*1 oz (28 nuts)* | 28 | 64 | 227 | 233 | 430 | 238 | 81 | 85 | 344 | 270 | 278 | 793 | 168 | 16090 |
| oil-roasted—*1 oz* | 28 | 65 | 171 | 274 | 507 | 265 | 81 | 105 | 400 | 282 | 321 | 909 | 183 | 16089 |
| raw—*1 oz* | 28 | 70 | 247 | 254 | 468 | 259 | 89 | 93 | 374 | 294 | 303 | 864 | 183 | 16087 |
| **peanuts, Spanish** | | | | | | | | | | | | | | |
| oil-roasted—*1 oz* | 28 | 76 | 269 | 276 | 508 | 281 | 96 | 101 | 407 | 319 | 329 | 938 | 198 | 16092 |
| raw—*1 oz* | 28 | 71 | 251 | 258 | 475 | 263 | 90 | 94 | 380 | 298 | 307 | 876 | 185 | 16091 |
| **peanuts, Valencia** | | | | | | | | | | | | | | |
| oil-roasted—*1 oz* | 28 | 74 | 259 | 266 | 491 | 272 | 93 | 97 | 393 | 308 | 318 | 906 | 192 | 16094 |
| raw—*1 oz* | 28 | 68 | 241 | 247 | 456 | 252 | 86 | 90 | 364 | 286 | 295 | 840 | 178 | 16093 |
| **peanuts, Virginia** | | | | | | | | | | | | | | |
| oil-roasted—*1 oz* | 28 | 70 | 248 | 255 | 470 | 260 | 89 | 93 | 375 | 295 | 304 | 866 | 183 | 16096 |
| raw—*1 oz* | 28 | 69 | 242 | 248 | 457 | 253 | 87 | 90 | 366 | 287 | 296 | 844 | 178 | 16095 |
| **pecans** | | | | | | | | | | | | | | |
| dried—*1 oz (20 halves)* | 28 | 26 | 86 | 94 | 167 | 80 | 51 | 43 | 119 | 60 | 115 | 330 | 73 | 12142 |
| dry-roasted—*1 oz (20 halves)* | 28 | 27 | 89 | 97 | 173 | 83 | 53 | 44 | 123 | 62 | 119 | 342 | 76 | 12143 |
| oil-roasted—*1 oz (15 halves)* | 28 | 26 | 86 | 94 | 168 | 81 | 51 | 43 | 120 | 60 | 116 | 331 | 73 | 12144 |
| **pilinuts**, dried—*1 oz (15 nuts)* | 28 | 53 | 114 | 135 | 249 | 103 | 111 | 53 | 139 | 107 | 196 | 424 | 71 | 12145 |
| **pine nuts** | | | | | | | | | | | | | | |
| pignolia, dried—*1 oz (15 to 16 nuts)* | 28 | 30 | 104 | 152 | 277 | 151 | 73 | 81 | 147 | 143 | 192 | 676 | 95 | 12147 |
| pinyon, dried—*1 oz* | 28 | 41 | 103 | 126 | 234 | 122 | 58 | 59 | 124 | 119 | 167 | 630 | 78 | 12149 |
| **pistachios** | | | | | | | | | | | | | | |
| dried—*1 oz (47 nuts)* | 28 | 76 | 188 | 252 | 435 | 322 | 95 | 100 | 297 | 116 | 347 | 568 | 142 | 12151 |
| dry-roasted—*1 oz (47 nuts)* | 28 | 80 | 196 | 262 | 452 | 335 | 98 | 104 | 309 | 121 | 361 | 590 | 148 | 12152 |
| **soy nuts** | | | | | | | | | | | | | | |
| dry-roasted—*1 oz* | 28 | 161 | 481 | 538 | 902 | 738 | 150 | 179 | 578 | 419 | 553 | 860 | 299 | 16111 |
| roasted—*1 cup* | 172 | 881 | 2632 | 2939 | 4933 | 4032 | 817 | 975 | 3161 | 2291 | 3024 | 4699 | 1634 | 16110 |
| **trail mix**—*1 oz* | | 46 | 135 | 144 | 249 | 144 | 57 | 61 | 184 | 128 | 184 | 426 | 100 | 19059 |
| tropical—*1 oz* | 28 | 21 | 62 | 62 | 101 | 63 | 41 | 32 | 73 | 45 | 83 | 164 | 59 | 19061 |
| unsalted—*1 oz* | 28 | 46 | 135 | 144 | 249 | 144 | 57 | 61 | 184 | 128 | 184 | 426 | 100 | 19821 |
| with chocolate chips—*1 oz* | 28 | 46 | 140 | 155 | 267 | 164 | 61 | 53 | 192 | 142 | 197 | 419 | 100 | 19062 |
| **walnuts, black**, dried—*1 oz* | 28 | 89 | 202 | 270 | 472 | 200 | 131 | 129 | 306 | 207 | 356 | 1013 | 188 | 12154 |
| **walnuts, English/Persian**, dried | | | | | | | | | | | | | | |
| *1 oz (14 halves)* | 28 | 48 | 167 | 175 | 328 | 119 | 66 | 58 | 199 | 114 | 211 | 638 | 109 | 12155 |
| **wheat-base formulated nuts** | | | | | | | | | | | | | | |
| flavored—*1 oz* | 28 | 48 | 155 | 155 | 272 | 248 | 77 | 63 | 164 | 136 | 199 | 275 | 106 | 12200 |
| macadamia-flavored—*1 oz* | 28 | 39 | 133 | 136 | 239 | 214 | 67 | 52 | 143 | 120 | 174 | 228 | 91 | 12199 |
| unflavored—*1 oz* | 28 | 46 | 162 | 155 | 277 | 255 | 78 | 71 | 169 | 136 | 204 | 298 | 110 | 12140 |
| **SEEDS AND SEED PRODUCTS** | | | | | | | | | | | | | | |
| **breadfruit seeds** | | | | | | | | | | | | | | |
| boiled—*1 oz* | 28 | 25 | 77 | 89 | 113 | 114 | 19 | 23 | 160 | 109 | 107 | 99 | 41 | 12003 |
| raw—*1 oz* | 28 | 34 | 108 | 124 | 158 | 160 | 27 | 32 | 223 | 152 | 150 | 138 | 58 | 12001 |
| roasted—*1 oz* | 28 | 29 | 90 | 104 | 132 | 134 | 23 | 27 | 187 | 128 | 125 | 116 | 48 | 12158 |
| **cottonseed kernels**, roasted—*1 T* | 10 | 49 | 120 | 117 | 223 | 165 | 53 | 86 | 203 | 117 | 167 | 440 | 103 | 12160 |
| **flaxseeds**—*1 T* | 12 | 36 | 92 | 108 | 148 | 103 | 44 | 41 | 115 | 59 | 129 | 231 | 57 | 12220 |
| **lotus seeds** | | | | | | | | | | | | | | |
| dried—*1 oz (42 seeds)* | 28 | 62 | 209 | 214 | 340 | 276 | 75 | 56 | 215 | 105 | 277 | 353 | 120 | 12013 |
| raw—*1 oz* | 28 | 17 | 56 | 57 | 91 | 74 | 20 | 15 | 58 | 28 | 74 | 95 | 32 | 12205 |
| **pumpkin and squash seed kernels** | | | | | | | | | | | | | | |
| dried—*1 oz (142 seeds)* | 28 | 121 | 253 | 354 | 582 | 513 | 154 | 84 | 342 | 285 | 552 | 1129 | 191 | 12014 |
| roasted—*1 oz* | 28 | 162 | 340 | 475 | 782 | 690 | 207 | 113 | 460 | 383 | 742 | 1517 | 256 | 12016 |
| **safflower seed** | | | | | | | | | | | | | | |
| kernels, dried—*1 oz* | 28 | 51 | 164 | 201 | 323 | 150 | 80 | 87 | 226 | 149 | 287 | 490 | 127 | 12021 |
| meal, partially defatted—*1 oz* | 28 | 113 | 361 | 442 | 711 | 329 | 175 | 192 | 497 | 327 | 632 | 1078 | 279 | 12022 |
| **sesame butter (tahini)** | | | | | | | | | | | | | | |
| from roasted, toasted kernels—*1 T* | 15 | 56 | 106 | 110 | 195 | 82 | 84 | 51 | 135 | 107 | 142 | 378 | 75 | 12166 |
| from unroasted kernels—*1 T* | 14 | 55 | 104 | 108 | 192 | 81 | 83 | 51 | 133 | 105 | 140 | 373 | 74 | 12171 |
| paste—*1 T* | 16 | 63 | 120 | 124 | 222 | 93 | 96 | 58 | 153 | 121 | 162 | 429 | 85 | 12169 |
| **sesame seed kernels** | | | | | | | | | | | | | | |
| dried—*1 T* | 8 | 26 | 58 | 60 | 120 | 52 | 70 | 35 | 75 | 63 | 78 | 260 | 44 | 12201 |
| toasted—*1 oz* | 28 | 104 | 197 | 204 | 364 | 152 | 157 | 96 | 252 | 199 | 265 | 704 | 140 | 12029 |

| | WT (g) | TRY | THR | ISO | LEU | LYS | MET | CYS | PHE | TYR | VAL | ARG | HIS | REF |
|---|---|---|---|---|---|---|---|---|---|---|---|---|---|---|
| | | | | | | | (mg/serving) | | | | | | | |
| **sesame seeds, whole** | | | | | | | | | | | | | | |
| dried—*1 T* | 9 | 35 | 66 | 69 | 122 | 51 | 53 | 32 | 85 | 67 | 89 | 237 | 47 | 12023 |
| roasted, toasted—*1 oz* | 28 | 104 | 197 | 204 | 364 | 152 | 157 | 96 | 252 | 199 | 265 | 704 | 140 | 12024 |
| **sunflower seed butter**—*1 T* | 16 | 48 | 128 | 157 | 229 | 129 | 68 | 62 | 161 | 92 | 182 | 332 | 87 | 12040 |
| **sunflower seed kernels** | | | | | | | | | | | | | | |
| dried—*1 cup without hulls* | 144 | 501 | 1336 | 1640 | 2389 | 1349 | 711 | 649 | 1683 | 959 | 1894 | 3460 | 910 | 12036 |
| dry-roasted—*1 oz* | 28 | 83 | 221 | 271 | 394 | 223 | 118 | 107 | 278 | 158 | 312 | 571 | 150 | 12037 |
| oil-roasted—*1 oz* | 28 | 86 | 229 | 281 | 409 | 231 | 122 | 111 | 288 | 164 | 324 | 592 | 156 | 12038 |
| toasted—*1 oz* | 28 | 74 | 197 | 241 | 351 | 198 | 105 | 95 | 247 | 141 | 278 | 508 | 134 | 12039 |
| **watermelon seeds**, dried | | | | | | | | | | | | | | |
| *1 oz (95 large seeds)* | 28 | 109 | 311 | 376 | 602 | 248 | 234 | 123 | 569 | 284 | 436 | 1371 | 217 | 12174 |

## 24. POULTRY

### CHICKEN, BROILER/FRYER PARTS

| | WT (g) | TRY | THR | ISO | LEU | LYS | MET | CYS | PHE | TYR | VAL | ARG | HIS | REF |
|---|---|---|---|---|---|---|---|---|---|---|---|---|---|---|
| **chicken (broiler/fryer) back** w/skin | | | | | | | | | | | | | | |
| flour-coated, fried—*½ back (2.5 oz)* | 72 | 226 | 822 | 1001 | 1463 | 1599 | 529 | 272 | 790 | 647 | 973 | 1235 | 587 | 5050 |
| stewed—*¼ cup (1.4 oz)* | 40 | 96 | 362 | 429 | 634 | 705 | 231 | 121 | 341 | 278 | 426 | 567 | 253 | 5052 |
| **chicken (broiler/fryer) breast** w/skin | | | | | | | | | | | | | | |
| rotisseried—*3 oz* | 85 | 270 | 632 | 1108 | 2131 | 2519 | 774 | 277 | 1025 | 854 | 1163 | 1649 | 952 | 5348 |
| battered, fried—*½ breast (4.9 oz)* | 140 | 399 | 1431 | 1753 | 2562 | 2758 | 920 | 475 | 1387 | 1137 | 1702 | 2121 | 1022 | 5058 |
| flour-coated, fried—*½ breast (3.5 oz)* | 98 | 357 | 1300 | 1599 | 2306 | 2581 | 845 | 410 | 1228 | 1028 | 1531 | 1915 | 940 | 5059 |
| roasted—*½ breast (3.5 oz)* | 98 | 333 | 1219 | 1494 | 2154 | 2424 | 791 | 382 | 1146 | 960 | 1432 | 1800 | 879 | 5060 |
| stewed—*½ breast (3.9 oz)* | 110 | 343 | 1257 | 1541 | 2221 | 2499 | 815 | 395 | 1181 | 990 | 1476 | 1858 | 906 | 5061 |
| **chicken (broiler/fryer) breast** w/o skin | | | | | | | | | | | | | | |
| flour-coated, fried—*½ breast (3 oz)* | 86 | 335 | 1214 | 1518 | 2158 | 2439 | 796 | 368 | 1142 | 970 | 1427 | 1733 | 892 | 5063 |
| roasted—*½ breast (3 oz)* | 86 | 311 | 1127 | 1409 | 2002 | 2266 | 739 | 341 | 1059 | 900 | 1324 | 1609 | 828 | 5064 |
| stewed—*½ breast (3.4 oz)* | 95 | 322 | 1163 | 1454 | 2066 | 2339 | 762 | 352 | 1092 | 929 | 1365 | 1661 | 855 | 5065 |
| **chicken (broiler/fryer) drumstick** | | | | | | | | | | | | | | |
| w/skin battered, fried—*2.5 oz drumstick* | 72 | 181 | 650 | 798 | 1165 | 1253 | 418 | 216 | 631 | 518 | 774 | 962 | 465 | 5067 |
| flour-coated, fried—*1.7 oz drmstk* | 49 | 150 | 549 | 672 | 972 | 1085 | 355 | 174 | 518 | 432 | 646 | 815 | 395 | 5068 |
| roasted—*1.8 oz drumstick* | 52 | 158 | 583 | 708 | 1028 | 1152 | 376 | 186 | 548 | 456 | 684 | 876 | 417 | 5069 |
| rotisseried—*1.8 oz drumstick* | 52 | 126 | 443 | 579 | 1077 | 1228 | 395 | 141 | 490 | 418 | 643 | 892 | 399 | 5349 |
| stewed—*2 oz drumstick* | 57 | 163 | 599 | 730 | 1057 | 1187 | 388 | 191 | 563 | 470 | 704 | 897 | 429 | 5070 |
| **chicken (broiler/fryer) drumstick** | | | | | | | | | | | | | | |
| w/o skin roasted—*1.6 oz drumstick* | 44 | 145 | 526 | 657 | 934 | 1057 | 345 | 159 | 494 | 420 | 617 | 751 | 386 | 5073 |
| **chicken (broiler/fryer) leg** w/skin | | | | | | | | | | | | | | |
| flour-coated, fried—*4 oz leg* | 112 | 340 | 1245 | 1520 | 2205 | 2452 | 804 | 400 | 1180 | 980 | 1467 | 1858 | 893 | 5077 |
| roasted—*4 oz leg* | 114 | 332 | 1226 | 1487 | 2160 | 2421 | 791 | 393 | 1153 | 959 | 1440 | 1847 | 876 | 5078 |
| stewed—*4.4 oz leg* | 125 | 339 | 1252 | 1520 | 2208 | 2474 | 808 | 401 | 1178 | 980 | 1471 | 1884 | 894 | 5079 |
| **chicken (broiler/fryer) leg** w/o skin | | | | | | | | | | | | | | |
| stewed—*3.6 oz leg* | 101 | 310 | 1120 | 1401 | 1991 | 2253 | 734 | 339 | 1052 | 896 | 1316 | 1600 | 823 | 5083 |
| **chicken (broiler/fryer) neck** w/skin | | | | | | | | | | | | | | |
| battered, fried—*1.5 oz neck* | 43 | 92 | 340 | 398 | 603 | 632 | 213 | 123 | 332 | 262 | 406 | 543 | 232 | 5085 |
| flour-coated, fried—*1.3 oz neck* | 36 | 92 | 346 | 403 | 608 | 658 | 218 | 122 | 331 | 264 | 410 | 559 | 237 | 5086 |
| simmered—*1.3 oz neck* | 38 | 76 | 295 | 331 | 510 | 557 | 183 | 107 | 278 | 218 | 347 | 500 | 196 | 5087 |
| simmered—*0.63 neck* | 18 | 52 | 187 | 233 | 332 | 375 | 122 | 57 | 175 | 149 | 219 | 267 | 137 | 5090 |
| **chicken (broiler/fryer) thigh** w/skin | | | | | | | | | | | | | | |
| flour-coated, fried—*2.2 oz thigh* | 62 | 187 | 685 | 835 | 1214 | 1345 | 442 | 222 | 652 | 539 | 808 | 1027 | 490 | 5093 |
| roasted—*2.2 oz thigh* | 62 | 174 | 643 | 779 | 1133 | 1269 | 415 | 206 | 604 | 502 | 755 | 971 | 458 | 5094 |
| rotisseried—*3 oz* | 85 | 172 | 652 | 846 | 1539 | 1737 | 568 | 197 | 683 | 575 | 929 | 1278 | 600 | 5351 |
| stewed—*2.4 oz thigh* | 68 | 177 | 654 | 792 | 1153 | 1291 | 422 | 211 | 615 | 511 | 768 | 990 | 466 | 5095 |
| **chicken (broiler/fryer) thigh** | | | | | | | | | | | | | | |
| w/o skin roasted—*1.8 oz thigh* | 52 | 158 | 570 | 712 | 1012 | 1146 | 373 | 173 | 535 | 456 | 669 | 814 | 419 | 5098 |
| **chicken (broiler/fryer) wing** w/skin | | | | | | | | | | | | | | |
| battered, fried—*1.7 oz wing* | 49 | 107 | 390 | 461 | 696 | 722 | 245 | 141 | 385 | 304 | 467 | 611 | 268 | 5101 |
| flour-coated, fried—*1.1 oz wing* | 32 | 90 | 338 | 396 | 592 | 650 | 214 | 116 | 321 | 258 | 398 | 538 | 233 | 5102 |
| roasted—*1.2 oz wing* | 34 | 98 | 370 | 432 | 645 | 714 | 234 | 126 | 348 | 281 | 435 | 592 | 255 | 5103 |
| rotisseried—*3 oz* | 85 | 201 | 559 | 903 | 1573 | 1635 | 636 | 216 | 740 | 592 | 1028 | 1301 | 632 | 5352 |
| stewed—*1.4 oz wing* | 40 | 98 | 370 | 434 | 646 | 716 | 235 | 125 | 348 | 282 | 435 | 588 | 256 | 5104 |

### CHICKEN, BROILER/FRYERS

| | WT (g) | TRY | THR | ISO | LEU | LYS | MET | CYS | PHE | TYR | VAL | ARG | HIS | REF |
|---|---|---|---|---|---|---|---|---|---|---|---|---|---|---|
| **chicken (broiler/fryer) dark meat** | | | | | | | | | | | | | | |
| w/skin, roasted—*3 oz* | 85 | 246 | 910 | 1095 | 1601 | 1789 | 585 | 296 | 856 | 707 | 1069 | 1389 | 645 | 5037 |
| w/skin, stewed—*3 oz* | 85 | 222 | 824 | 992 | 1449 | 1620 | 530 | 267 | 774 | 641 | 968 | 1255 | 584 | 5038 |
| w/o skin, fried—*3 oz* | 85 | 289 | 1038 | 1299 | 1850 | 2075 | 679 | 319 | 983 | 831 | 1222 | 1481 | 762 | 5044 |
| w/o skin, roasted—*3 oz* | 85 | 272 | 983 | 1228 | 1745 | 1976 | 643 | 298 | 923 | 785 | 1153 | 1403 | 722 | 5045 |
| w/o skin, stewed—*3 oz* | 85 | 258 | 932 | 1165 | 1657 | 1875 | 611 | 282 | 876 | 745 | 1095 | 1331 | 685 | 5046 |
| **chicken (broiler/fryer) light and dark meat** w/skin, battered, fried—*3 oz* | 85 | 218 | 784 | 956 | 1405 | 1500 | 502 | 264 | 764 | 622 | 935 | 1171 | 557 | 5007 |

| | WT | TRY | THR | ISO | LEU | LYS | MET | CYS | PHE | TYR | VAL | ARG | HIS | REF |
|---|---|---|---|---|---|---|---|---|---|---|---|---|---|---|
| | (g) | | | | | | (mg/serving) | | | | | | | |
| w/skin, flour-coated, fried—3 oz | 85 | 275 | 1004 | 1223 | 1778 | 1972 | 648 | 325 | 953 | 789 | 1183 | 1501 | 718 | 5008 |
| w/skin, roasted—3 oz | 85 | 259 | 959 | 1158 | 1688 | 1890 | 617 | 309 | 902 | 747 | 1126 | 1454 | 682 | 5009 |
| w/skin, stewed—3 oz | 85 | 235 | 867 | 1048 | 1527 | 1709 | 558 | 280 | 815 | 677 | 1019 | 1313 | 617 | 5010 |
| w/o skin, flour-coated, fried—3 oz | 85 | 304 | 1096 | 1370 | 1950 | 2196 | 717 | 334 | 1034 | 876 | 1289 | 1563 | 805 | 5012 |
| w/o skin, roasted—3 oz | 85 | 287 | 1039 | 1299 | 1845 | 2089 | 681 | 314 | 976 | 830 | 1220 | 1483 | 763 | 5013 |
| w/o skin, stewed—3 oz | 85 | 271 | 980 | 1225 | 1741 | 1970 | 642 | 297 | 921 | 783 | 1150 | 1399 | 720 | 5014 |
| **chicken (broiler/fryer) light meat** | | | | | | | | | | | | | | |
| w/skin, flour-coated, fried—3 oz | 85 | 292 | 1073 | 1306 | 1896 | 2114 | 693 | 344 | 1013 | 842 | 1262 | 1605 | 768 | 5031 |
| w/skin, roasted—3 oz | 85 | 277 | 1022 | 1239 | 1801 | 2018 | 660 | 327 | 960 | 799 | 1200 | 1539 | 729 | 5032 |
| w/skin, stewed—3 oz | 85 | 250 | 921 | 1119 | 1624 | 1821 | 594 | 295 | 866 | 721 | 1082 | 1385 | 658 | 5033 |
| w/o skin, fried—3 oz | 85 | 326 | 1178 | 1472 | 2094 | 2366 | 772 | 357 | 1108 | 942 | 1384 | 1681 | 865 | 5040 |
| w/o skin, roasted—3 oz | 85 | 307 | 1109 | 1387 | 1971 | 2232 | 727 | 337 | 1042 | 887 | 1303 | 1584 | 815 | 5041 |
| w/o skin, stewed—3 oz | 85 | 286 | 1037 | 1296 | 1842 | 2086 | 679 | 314 | 974 | 829 | 1218 | 1481 | 762 | 5042 |
| **CHICKEN, ROASTERS** | | | | | | | | | | | | | | |
| **chicken (roaster) dark meat** | | | | | | | | | | | | | | |
| w/o skin, roasted—3 oz | 85 | 231 | 835 | 1044 | 1483 | 1679 | 547 | 253 | 785 | 667 | 980 | 1192 | 614 | 5120 |
| **chicken (roaster) light and dark meat** | | | | | | | | | | | | | | |
| w/skin, roasted—3 oz | 85 | 226 | 841 | 1012 | 1478 | 1653 | 541 | 272 | 790 | 654 | 988 | 1280 | 596 | 5112 |
| w/o skin, roasted—3 oz | 85 | 248 | 898 | 1123 | 1595 | 1806 | 589 | 272 | 844 | 717 | 1054 | 1283 | 660 | 5114 |
| **chicken (roaster) light** meat w/o skin | | | | | | | | | | | | | | |
| roasted—3 oz | 85 | 269 | 974 | 1218 | 1731 | 1959 | 638 | 295 | 915 | 779 | 1144 | 1391 | 716 | 5118 |
| **CHICKEN, STEWERS** | | | | | | | | | | | | | | |
| **chicken (stewer) dark meat** w/o skin | | | | | | | | | | | | | | |
| stewed—3 oz | 85 | 280 | 1011 | 1263 | 1795 | 2032 | 662 | 306 | 949 | 808 | 1187 | 1443 | 743 | 5132 |
| **chicken (stewer) light and dark meat** | | | | | | | | | | | | | | |
| w/skin, stewed—3 oz | 85 | 256 | 946 | 1146 | 1667 | 1867 | 609 | 303 | 889 | 739 | 1111 | 1428 | 674 | 5124 |
| w/o skin, stewed—3 oz | 85 | 303 | 1092 | 1365 | 1941 | 2197 | 716 | 331 | 1026 | 873 | 1283 | 1560 | 802 | 5126 |
| **chicken (stewer) light** meat w/o skin | | | | | | | | | | | | | | |
| stewed—3 oz | 85 | 328 | 1187 | 1482 | 2107 | 2386 | 777 | 360 | 1114 | 948 | 1393 | 1694 | 871 | 5130 |
| **CHICKEN, UNSPECIFIED TYPES** | | | | | | | | | | | | | | |
| chicken, canned with broth—5 oz can | 142 | 345 | 1271 | 1541 | 2241 | 2505 | 815 | 422 | 1196 | 993 | 1494 | 1924 | 903 | 5277 |
| chicken, raw—3 oz | 85 | 212 | 768 | 960 | 1364 | 1545 | 503 | 233 | 722 | 614 | 902 | 1096 | 564 | 5011 |
| **TURKEY, ROASTERS** | | | | | | | | | | | | | | |
| **turkey (roaster) back** | | | | | | | | | | | | | | |
| w/skin, roasted—3 oz | 85 | 237 | 949 | 1065 | 1675 | 1936 | 603 | 260 | 855 | 802 | 1130 | 1584 | 638 | 5214 |
| w/o skin, roasted—½ back (3.5 oz) | 99 | 315 | 1234 | 1442 | 2210 | 2614 | 803 | 288 | 1101 | 1096 | 1473 | 1934 | 865 | 5216 |
| **turkey (roaster) breast** | | | | | | | | | | | | | | |
| w/skin, roasted—3 oz | 85 | 274 | 1082 | 1246 | 1928 | 2261 | 698 | 269 | 969 | 944 | 1291 | 1737 | 747 | 5218 |
| w/o skin, roasted—3 oz | 85 | 291 | 1136 | 1329 | 2036 | 2408 | 740 | 266 | 1014 | 1010 | 1357 | 1782 | 797 | 5220 |
| **turkey (roaster) dark meat** | | | | | | | | | | | | | | |
| w/skin, roasted—3 oz | 85 | 258 | 1024 | 1173 | 1822 | 2129 | 659 | 261 | 919 | 887 | 1221 | 1661 | 704 | 5208 |
| w/o skin, roasted—3 oz | 85 | 279 | 1091 | 1275 | 1953 | 2310 | 710 | 255 | 973 | 969 | 1302 | 1710 | 765 | 5212 |
| **turkey (roaster) leg** | | | | | | | | | | | | | | |
| w/skin, roasted—8.6 oz leg | 245 | 779 | 3067 | 3545 | 5473 | 6431 | 1982 | 752 | 2744 | 2688 | 3660 | 4902 | 2127 | 5222 |
| w/o skin, roasted—7.9 oz leg | 224 | 744 | 2908 | 3400 | 5210 | 6162 | 1893 | 681 | 2594 | 2583 | 3472 | 4561 | 2041 | 5224 |
| **turkey (roaster) light meat** | | | | | | | | | | | | | | |
| w/skin, roasted—3 oz | 85 | 269 | 1063 | 1217 | 1890 | 2209 | 683 | 271 | 954 | 921 | 1268 | 1725 | 730 | 5206 |
| w/o skin, roasted—3 oz | 85 | 292 | 1142 | 1334 | 2044 | 2418 | 743 | 267 | 1018 | 1014 | 1363 | 1790 | 801 | 5210 |
| **turkey (roaster) skin, roasted** | | | | | | | | | | | | | | |
| 1.2 oz (yield from 1 lb of turkey) | 34 | 57 | 254 | 229 | 418 | 425 | 142 | 118 | 240 | 162 | 300 | 549 | 137 | 5204 |
| **turkey (roaster) wing** | | | | | | | | | | | | | | |
| w/skin, roasted—3.2 oz wing | 90 | 262 | 1053 | 1173 | 1855 | 2134 | 666 | 297 | 951 | 881 | 1255 | 1781 | 703 | 5226 |
| w/o skin, roasted—2.1 oz wing | 60 | 210 | 823 | 962 | 1475 | 1744 | 536 | 193 | 734 | 731 | 983 | 1291 | 578 | 5228 |
| **TURKEY, YOUNG HEN** | | | | | | | | | | | | | | |
| **turkey (young hen) back** w/skin | | | | | | | | | | | | | | |
| roasted—3 oz | 85 | 243 | 968 | 1098 | 1716 | 1996 | 619 | 256 | 870 | 829 | 1154 | 1592 | 659 | 5246 |
| **turkey (young hen) breast** w/skin | | | | | | | | | | | | | | |
| roasted—3 oz | 85 | 273 | 1074 | 1240 | 1916 | 2250 | 694 | 265 | 961 | 939 | 1282 | 1720 | 745 | 5248 |
| **turkey (young hen) dark meat** | | | | | | | | | | | | | | |
| w/skin, roasted—3 oz | 85 | 258 | 1017 | 1169 | 1810 | 2121 | 655 | 255 | 911 | 885 | 1213 | 1638 | 701 | 5240 |
| w/o skin, roasted—3 oz | 85 | 275 | 1074 | 1256 | 1925 | 2277 | 700 | 252 | 959 | 955 | 1284 | 1686 | 754 | 5244 |
| **turkey (young hen) leg** w/skin | | | | | | | | | | | | | | |
| roasted—3 oz | 85 | 264 | 1038 | 1202 | 1853 | 2180 | 672 | 253 | 928 | 911 | 1238 | 1653 | 721 | 5250 |

|  | WT | TRY | THR | ISO | LEU | LYS | MET | CYS | PHE | TYR | VAL | ARG | HIS | REF |
|---|---|---|---|---|---|---|---|---|---|---|---|---|---|---|
|  | (g) |  |  |  |  |  | (mg/serving) |  |  |  |  |  |  |  |
| **turkey (young hen) light and dark meat** |  |  |  |  |  |  |  |  |  |  |  |  |  |  |
| w/skin, roasted—*3 oz* | 85 | 264 | 1044 | 1200 | 1859 | 2178 | 672 | 261 | 935 | 909 | 1245 | 1680 | 720 | 5232 |
| w/o skin, roasted—*3 oz* | 85 | 282 | 1106 | 1293 | 1981 | 2343 | 720 | 258 | 987 | 983 | 1321 | 1734 | 776 | 5234 |
| **turkey (young hen) light meat** |  |  |  |  |  |  |  |  |  |  |  |  |  |  |
| w/skin, roasted—*3 oz* | 85 | 269 | 1064 | 1225 | 1896 | 2222 | 686 | 266 | 954 | 927 | 1270 | 1714 | 734 | 5238 |
| w/o skin, roasted—*3 oz* | 85 | 289 | 1130 | 1321 | 2025 | 2394 | 736 | 264 | 1008 | 1004 | 1350 | 1772 | 793 | 5242 |
| **turkey (young hen) wing** w/skin |  |  |  |  |  |  |  |  |  |  |  |  |  |  |
| roasted—*3 oz* | 85 | 251 | 999 | 1130 | 1768 | 2054 | 638 | 265 | 898 | 852 | 1190 | 1647 | 677 | 5252 |
| **TURKEY, YOUNG TOM** |  |  |  |  |  |  |  |  |  |  |  |  |  |  |
| **turkey (young tom) back** w/skin |  |  |  |  |  |  |  |  |  |  |  |  |  |  |
| roasted—*3 oz* | 85 | 246 | 980 | 1109 | 1736 | 2016 | 626 | 260 | 881 | 836 | 1169 | 1617 | 666 | 5270 |
| **turkey (young tom) breast** w/skin |  |  |  |  |  |  |  |  |  |  |  |  |  |  |
| roasted—*3 oz* | 85 | 269 | 1062 | 1221 | 1891 | 2215 | 684 | 267 | 952 | 924 | 1267 | 1714 | 732 | 5272 |
| **turkey (young tom) dark meat** |  |  |  |  |  |  |  |  |  |  |  |  |  |  |
| w/skin, roasted—*3 oz* | 85 | 277 | 1085 | 1267 | 1942 | 2298 | 706 | 253 | 967 | 963 | 1295 | 1701 | 761 | 5268 |
| w/o skin, roasted—*3 oz* | 85 | 259 | 1023 | 1176 | 1822 | 2134 | 660 | 258 | 917 | 890 | 1221 | 1652 | 706 | 5264 |
| **turkey (young tom) leg** w/skin |  |  |  |  |  |  |  |  |  |  |  |  |  |  |
| roasted—*3 oz* | 85 | 265 | 1043 | 1204 | 1860 | 2186 | 675 | 256 | 933 | 913 | 1245 | 1668 | 723 | 5274 |
| **turkey (young tom) light and dark meat** |  |  |  |  |  |  |  |  |  |  |  |  |  |  |
| w/skin, roasted—*3 oz* | 85 | 264 | 1042 | 1196 | 1854 | 2170 | 671 | 263 | 934 | 904 | 1243 | 1683 | 717 | 5256 |
| w/o skin, roasted—*3 oz* | 85 | 283 | 1110 | 1298 | 1988 | 2352 | 722 | 259 | 990 | 986 | 1325 | 1741 | 779 | 5258 |
| **turkey (young tom) light meat** |  |  |  |  |  |  |  |  |  |  |  |  |  |  |
| w/skin, roasted—*3 oz* | 85 | 267 | 1056 | 1210 | 1878 | 2197 | 679 | 267 | 946 | 915 | 1259 | 1707 | 726 | 5262 |
| w/o skin, roasted—*3 oz* | 85 | 288 | 1130 | 1321 | 2024 | 2394 | 735 | 264 | 1008 | 1004 | 1349 | 1772 | 792 | 5266 |
| **turkey (young tom) wing** w/skin |  |  |  |  |  |  |  |  |  |  |  |  |  |  |
| roasted—*3 oz* | 85 | 251 | 1000 | 1129 | 1769 | 2051 | 638 | 269 | 901 | 850 | 1192 | 1659 | 677 | 5276 |
| **TURKEY, UNSPECIFIED TYPES** |  |  |  |  |  |  |  |  |  |  |  |  |  |  |
| **turkey breast**, raw—*3 oz* | 85 | 206 | 813 | 934 | 1448 | 1697 | 524 | 204 | 728 | 707 | 970 | 1310 | 561 | 5191 |
| **turkey breast** w/skin, prebasted |  |  |  |  |  |  |  |  |  |  |  |  |  |  |
| roasted—*3 oz* | 85 | 209 | 822 | 949 | 1466 | 1719 | 530 | 208 | 737 | 718 | 982 | 1321 | 568 | 5293 |
| **turkey**, canned with broth—*5 oz can* | 142 | 371 | 1461 | 1680 | 2603 | 3043 | 939 | 378 | 1309 | 1271 | 1744 | 2361 | 1005 | 5284 |
| **turkey**, diced, seasoned—*1 oz* | 28 | 58 | 228 | 262 | 405 | 474 | 146 | 59 | 204 | 198 | 272 | 368 | 157 | 5285 |
| **turkey**, ground, cooked—*2.9 oz patty* | 82 | 251 | 987 | 1152 | 1766 | 2089 | 643 | 230 | 880 | 876 | 1178 | 1547 | 693 | 5306 |
| **turkey patty**, breaded/battered, |  |  |  |  |  |  |  |  |  |  |  |  |  |  |
| fried—*3.3 oz patty* | 94 | 157 | 562 | 673 | 1049 | 1091 | 359 | 164 | 556 | 509 | 696 | 858 | 391 | 5292 |
| **turkey**, raw—*3 oz* | 85 | 210 | 823 | 962 | 1475 | 1743 | 536 | 192 | 734 | 731 | 983 | 1290 | 577 | 5167 |
| **turkey roast**, boneless, frozen |  |  |  |  |  |  |  |  |  |  |  |  |  |  |
| seasoned, roasted—*3 oz* | 85 | 206 | 806 | 943 | 1443 | 1708 | 524 | 189 | 719 | 717 | 962 | 1264 | 565 | 5296 |
| **turkey sausage** (fresh) |  |  |  |  |  |  |  |  |  |  |  |  |  |  |
| breakfast, mild—*2 links (2 oz)* | 56 | 98 | 384 | 449 | 688 | 814 | 250 | 90 | 343 | 341 | 459 | 603 | 269 | 7919 |
| pan-fried—*2 oz* | 56 | 104 | 500 | 556 | 939 | 1055 | 298 | 129 | 485 | 417 | 581 | 809 | 323 | 7958 |
| reduced fat brown and serve, |  |  |  |  |  |  |  |  |  |  |  |  |  |  |
| cooked—*2 oz* | 56 | 108 | 408 | 464 | 736 | 805 | 239 | 116 | 395 | 352 | 489 | 691 | 273 | 7066 |
| **turkey skin**—*1 oz* | 28 | 29 | 127 | 115 | 209 | 212 | 71 | 59 | 120 | 81 | 150 | 274 | 68 | 5169 |
| **turkey sticks**, breaded/battered, |  |  |  |  |  |  |  |  |  |  |  |  |  |  |
| fried—*2.25 oz stick* | 64 | 109 | 388 | 465 | 726 | 748 | 248 | 114 | 387 | 351 | 481 | 591 | 269 | 5300 |
| **turkey thigh** w/skin, prebasted, |  |  |  |  |  |  |  |  |  |  |  |  |  |  |
| roasted—*3 oz* | 85 | 178 | 700 | 811 | 1250 | 1468 | 452 | 174 | 626 | 614 | 836 | 1119 | 485 | 5294 |
| **OTHER POULTRY** |  |  |  |  |  |  |  |  |  |  |  |  |  |  |
| **Cornish game hen** |  |  |  |  |  |  |  |  |  |  |  |  |  |  |
| w/skin, roasted—*3 oz* | 85 | 210 | 779 | 935 | 1368 | 1529 | 500 | 253 | 732 | 604 | 914 | 1190 | 551 | 5308 |
| w/o skin, roasted—*3 oz* | 85 | 231 | 836 | 1046 | 1486 | 1683 | 548 | 253 | 786 | 669 | 983 | 1194 | 615 | 5310 |
| **duck** |  |  |  |  |  |  |  |  |  |  |  |  |  |  |
| w/skin, roasted—*3 oz* | 85 | 197 | 657 | 741 | 1245 | 1263 | 404 | 254 | 639 | 544 | 797 | 1091 | 393 | 5140 |
| w/o skin, roasted—*3 oz* | 85 | 278 | 853 | 1025 | 1686 | 1708 | 540 | 307 | 836 | 760 | 1044 | 1274 | 527 | 5142 |
| **duckling, white pekin breast,** |  |  |  |  |  |  |  |  |  |  |  |  |  |  |
| boneless w/skin, roasted—*3 oz* | 85 | 286 | 883 | 1060 | 1742 | 1766 | 557 | 316 | 866 | 786 | 1080 | 1316 | 547 | 5315 |
| w/o skin, roasted—*3 oz* | 85 | 323 | 994 | 1193 | 1964 | 1989 | 626 | 357 | 976 | 886 | 1216 | 1482 | 615 | 5316 |
| **duckling, white pekin leg,** bone in | 85 | 313 | 964 | 1157 | 1902 | 1928 | 608 | 346 | 946 | 858 | 1179 | 1437 | 597 | 5317 |
| w/skin, roasted—*3 oz* | 85 | 313 | 964 | 1157 | 1902 | 1928 | 608 | 346 | 946 | 858 | 1179 | 1437 | 597 | 5317 |
| w/o skin, roasted—*3 oz* | 85 | 340 | 1049 | 1259 | 2070 | 2098 | 661 | 376 | 1029 | 934 | 1283 | 1563 | 649 | 5318 |
| **goose** |  |  |  |  |  |  |  |  |  |  |  |  |  |  |
| w/skin, roasted—*3 oz* | 85 | 282 | 955 | 1006 | 1793 | 1690 | 517 | 332 | 897 | 684 | 1047 | 1331 | 595 | 5147 |
| w/o skin, roasted—*3 oz* | 85 | 343 | 1052 | 1265 | 2080 | 2108 | 666 | 378 | 1032 | 938 | 1289 | 1572 | 650 | 5149 |
| **Guinea hen** w/o skin, raw—*3 oz* | 85 | 205 | 741 | 927 | 1317 | 1491 | 485 | 224 | 696 | 592 | 870 | 1058 | 545 | 5152 |

| | WT (g) | TRY | THR | ISO | LEU | LYS | MET | CYS | PHE | TYR | VAL | ARG | HIS | REF |
|---|---|---|---|---|---|---|---|---|---|---|---|---|---|---|
| | | | | | | | (mg/serving) | | | | | | | |
| **pheasant** | | | | | | | | | | | | | | |
| w/skin, raw—*3 oz* | 85 | 258 | 942 | 1044 | 1590 | 1713 | 547 | 259 | 745 | 615 | 1046 | 1200 | 734 | 5153 |
| w/o skin, raw—*3 oz* | 85 | 279 | 1003 | 1125 | 1696 | 1833 | 583 | 263 | 782 | 657 | 1109 | 1218 | 798 | 5154 |
| **squab** (pigeon), w/o skin, raw—*3 oz* | 85 | 233 | 745 | 812 | 1276 | 1302 | 471 | 259 | 645 | 690 | 807 | 943 | 564 | 5161 |
| **POULTRY INTERNAL ORGANS AND OTHER PARTS** | | | | | | | | | | | | | | |
| **chicken giblets** fried—*3 oz* | 85 | 317 | 1247 | 1386 | 2211 | 1996 | 688 | 371 | 1258 | 907 | 1476 | 1835 | 645 | 5021 |
| simmered—*3 oz* | 85 | 93 | 382 | 428 | 796 | 701 | 228 | 143 | 434 | 343 | 525 | 575 | 267 | 5022 |
| **chicken heart**, simmered—*3 oz* | 85 | 287 | 1017 | 1203 | 1958 | 1882 | 542 | 305 | 1006 | 804 | 1272 | 1440 | 589 | 5026 |
| **chicken liver** | | | | | | | | | | | | | | |
| raw—*3 oz* | 85 | 150 | 616 | 691 | 1285 | 1132 | 367 | 231 | 700 | 555 | 848 | 929 | 431 | 5027 |
| simmered—*3 oz* | 85 | 211 | 868 | 972 | 1809 | 1594 | 517 | 326 | 986 | 781 | 1194 | 1308 | 607 | 5028 |
| **duck liver**, raw—*3 oz* | 85 | 224 | 708 | 846 | 1437 | 1205 | 377 | 214 | 792 | 561 | 1004 | 976 | 423 | 5143 |
| **goose liver** | | | | | | | | | | | | | | |
| pate (pate de foie gras) | | | | | | | | | | | | | | |
| smoked, canned—*2 T* | 26 | 42 | 132 | 158 | 268 | 224 | 70 | 40 | 147 | 104 | 187 | 182 | 79 | 5282 |
| raw—*3 oz* | 85 | 196 | 619 | 740 | 1255 | 1053 | 330 | 187 | 693 | 490 | 877 | 853 | 370 | 5150 |
| **25. SALAD DRESSINGS** | | | | | | | | | | | | | | |
| **LOW AND REDUCED CALORIE SALAD DRESSINGS** | | | | | | | | | | | | | | |
| **French salad dressing** | | | | | | | | | | | | | | |
| low/reduced calorie—*1 T* | 16 | 0 | 2 | 2 | 2 | 3 | 0 | 0 | 3 | 1 | 2 | 2 | 1 | 4020 |
| **Italian salad dressing** | | | | | | | | | | | | | | |
| low/reduced calorie—*1 T* | 15 | 1 | 2 | 2 | 4 | 3 | 1 | 1 | 2 | 1 | 3 | 8 | 1 | 4021 |
| **Russian salad dressing** | | | | | | | | | | | | | | |
| low/reduced calorie—*2 T* | 32 | 2 | 9 | 9 | 14 | 11 | 4 | 3 | 7 | 7 | 10 | 11 | 4 | 4022 |
| **REGULAR SALAD DRESSINGS** | | | | | | | | | | | | | | |
| **French salad dressing**—*1 T* | 16 | 1 | 3 | 4 | 5 | 3 | 2 | 1 | 3 | 1 | 4 | 9 | 2 | 4120 |
| **mayonnaise type salad dressing**—*2 T* | 15 | 2 | 7 | 8 | 12 | 9 | 3 | 2 | 6 | 6 | 8 | 9 | 3 | 4018 |
| **homemade salad dressing**, ckd—*1 T* | 16 | 10 | 29 | 41 | 72 | 53 | 21 | 21 | 41 | 33 | 51 | 39 | 19 | 4134 |
| **sesame seed salad dressing**—*1 T* | 15 | 7 | 7 | 7 | 12 | 21 | 4 | 0 | 13 | 15 | 10 | 60 | 5 | 4016 |
| **26. SAUCES, GRAVIES, AND CONDIMENTS** | | | | | | | | | | | | | | |
| **CONDIMENT SAUCES** | | | | | | | | | | | | | | |
| **catsup** (ketchup)—*1 T* | 15 | 3 | 10 | 8 | 11 | 12 | 2 | 2 | 9 | 5 | 8 | 8 | 7 | 11935 |
| low sodium—*1 T* | 15 | 3 | 10 | 8 | 11 | 12 | 2 | 2 | 9 | 5 | 8 | 8 | 7 | 11949 |
| **hot pepper sauce**—*1 t* | 4.7 | 0 | 1 | 1 | 1 | 1 | 0 | 0 | 1 | 1 | 1 | 1 | 0 | 6168 |
| **mustard**—*1 t* | 5 | 0 | 9 | 8 | 15 | 14 | 4 | 4 | 8 | 7 | 10 | 13 | 6 | 2046 |
| **soy sauce** | | | | | | | | | | | | | | |
| soy and wheat (shoyu)—*1 T* | 16 | 14 | 41 | 48 | 80 | 57 | 15 | 18 | 53 | 36 | 50 | 69 | 26 | 16123 |
| soy (tamari)—*1 T* | 18 | 33 | 73 | 88 | 132 | 132 | 30 | 19 | 96 | 62 | 94 | 73 | 39 | 16124 |
| **tabasco sauce**, McIlhenny—*1 t* | 4.7 | 1 | 2 | 2 | 3 | 3 | 1 | 1 | 2 | 1 | 3 | 3 | 1 | 6169 |
| **ENTRÉE SAUCES AND GRAVIES** | | | | | | | | | | | | | | |
| **guava sauce**—*1 cup* | 238 | 7 | 29 | 29 | 50 | 21 | 5 | | 2 | 10 | 26 | 19 | 7 | 9143 |
| **tomato sauce**, bottled—*½ cup* | 122 | 12 | 50 | 33 | 46 | 50 | 10 | 17 | 122 | 24 | 33 | 38 | 27 | 11549 |
| Spanish style—*½ cup* | 122 | 12 | 40 | 34 | 49 | 50 | 9 | 11 | 37 | 23 | 35 | 35 | 28 | 11649 |
| w/herbs and cheese—*½ cup* | 122 | 26 | 72 | 85 | 138 | 135 | 34 | 20 | 85 | 73 | 100 | 109 | 61 | 11555 |
| w/mushrooms—*½ cup* | 122 | 21 | 52 | 45 | 67 | 90 | 17 | 9 | 48 | 28 | 50 | 51 | 34 | 11551 |
| w/onions—*½ cup* | 122 | 20 | 45 | 51 | 60 | 72 | 12 | 22 | 44 | 35 | 41 | 139 | 30 | 11553 |
| w/onions, grn pepper, celery—*½ cup* | 125 | 10 | 28 | 26 | 35 | 38 | 6 | 9 | 26 | 18 | 25 | 46 | 19 | 11557 |
| w/tomato pieces—*½ cup* | 122 | 11 | 37 | 32 | 45 | 46 | 9 | 10 | 34 | 22 | 33 | 33 | 26 | 11559 |
| **white sauce** | | | | | | | | | | | | | | |
| medium, homemade—*½ cup* | 125 | 54 | 173 | 232 | 375 | 304 | 96 | 35 | 185 | 185 | 256 | 139 | 104 | 6166 |
| thick, homemade—*½ cup* | 125 | 50 | 161 | 216 | 350 | 284 | 89 | 32 | 173 | 173 | 239 | 129 | 98 | 6167 |
| thin, homemade—*½ cup* | 125 | 58 | 184 | 248 | 400 | 324 | 102 | 38 | 196 | 196 | 274 | 148 | 111 | 6165 |
| **beef gravy**, Heinz Home Style—*½ cup* | 114 | 8 | 33 | 35 | 68 | 55 | 14 | 8 | 39 | 22 | 43 | 63 | 25 | 6985 |
| **OLIVES AND PICKLES** | | | | | | | | | | | | | | |
| **olives, black**, cnd/bottled—*1 jumbo* | 8.3 | | 3 | 3 | 5 | 3 | 1 | | 3 | 2 | 4 | 6 | 2 | 9194 |
| **dill pickle**—*1 spear* | 30 | 2 | 5 | 6 | 8 | 8 | 2 | 1 | 5 | 3 | 6 | 12 | 3 | 11937 |
| **pickle relish** | | | | | | | | | | | | | | |
| hamburger—*½ cup* | 122 | 9 | 23 | 26 | 37 | 34 | 9 | 9 | 23 | 15 | 27 | 51 | 15 | 11958 |
| hot dog—*½ cup* | 122 | 23 | 57 | 61 | 92 | 84 | 22 | 23 | 56 | 39 | 68 | 118 | 37 | 11944 |
| sweet—*1 T* | 15 | 1 | 2 | 2 | 3 | 2 | 1 | 0 | 2 | 1 | 2 | 3 | 1 | 11945 |
| **sour pickle**—*1 medium (3 ¾" long)* | 65 | 2 | 6 | 6 | 9 | 9 | 2 | 1 | 6 | 4 | 7 | 14 | 3 | 11941 |
| **sweet gherkin pickle**—*1 small (2½" long)* | 15 | 2 | 3 | 3 | 4 | 5 | 2 | 2 | 3 | 2 | 3 | 5 | 1 | 11940 |

| | WT (g) | TRY | THR | ISO | LEU | LYS | MET | CYS | PHE | TYR | VAL | ARG | HIS | REF |
|---|---|---|---|---|---|---|---|---|---|---|---|---|---|---|
| | | | | | | | (mg/serving) | | | | | | | |

**27. SOUPS**

**CONDENSED SOUPS**

| | WT (g) | TRY | THR | ISO | LEU | LYS | MET | CYS | PHE | TYR | VAL | ARG | HIS | REF |
|---|---|---|---|---|---|---|---|---|---|---|---|---|---|---|
| **celery soup, cream of**, cond, cnd | | | | | | | | | | | | | | |
| *10.8 oz can* | 305 | 46 | 143 | 189 | 302 | 180 | 73 | 46 | 189 | 131 | 217 | 143 | 95 | 6010 |
| **cheese soup**, cond, cnd—*11 oz can* | 312 | 175 | 462 | 783 | 1245 | 924 | 284 | 109 | 677 | 605 | 924 | 393 | 356 | 6011 |
| **chicken soup, cream of**, cond, cnd | | | | | | | | | | | | | | |
| *10.8 oz can* | 305 | 104 | 317 | 415 | 640 | 522 | 195 | 122 | 372 | 287 | 421 | 406 | 223 | 6016 |
| **minestrone soup**, cond, cnd—*½ cup* | 123 | 31 | 105 | 130 | 236 | 183 | 44 | 33 | 154 | 85 | 180 | 198 | 74 | 6040 |
| **mushroom soup, cream of**, cond, | | | | | | | | | | | | | | |
| cnd—*10.8 oz can* | 305 | 70 | 189 | 235 | 384 | 265 | 95 | 61 | 226 | 183 | 262 | 204 | 113 | 6043 |
| **tomato soup**, cond, cnd—*10.8 oz can* | 305 | 49 | 125 | 143 | 241 | 122 | 55 | 67 | 171 | 104 | 162 | 146 | 88 | 6159 |
| **vegetable beef soup**, cond, cnd | | | | | | | | | | | | | | |
| *½ cup (4 fl oz)* | 125 | 48 | 174 | 210 | 356 | 342 | 94 | 39 | 204 | 145 | 246 | 260 | 122 | 6071 |
| **vegetarian vegetable soup**, cond | | | | | | | | | | | | | | |
| cnd—*½ cup (4 fl oz)* | 123 | 15 | 75 | 100 | 149 | 100 | 25 | 25 | 100 | 49 | 100 | 100 | 49 | 6068 |

**CONDENSED SOUPS, PREPARED WITH MILK**

| | WT (g) | TRY | THR | ISO | LEU | LYS | MET | CYS | PHE | TYR | VAL | ARG | HIS | REF |
|---|---|---|---|---|---|---|---|---|---|---|---|---|---|---|
| **asparagus soup, cream of**, cond, cnd | | | | | | | | | | | | | | |
| prep w/milk—*1 cup (8 fl oz)* | 248 | 84 | 260 | 340 | 558 | 432 | 144 | 67 | 290 | 270 | 384 | 231 | 159 | 6201 |
| **celery soup, cream of**, cond, cnd | | | | | | | | | | | | | | |
| prep w/milk—*1 cup (8 fl oz)* | 248 | 74 | 241 | 322 | 518 | 394 | 131 | 55 | 273 | 248 | 360 | 206 | 149 | 6210 |
| **cheese soup**, cond, cnd, prep w/ | | | | | | | | | | | | | | |
| milk—*1 cup (8 fl oz)* | 251 | 128 | 371 | 567 | 906 | 700 | 218 | 83 | 474 | 444 | 650 | 309 | 256 | 6211 |
| **chicken soup, cream of**, cond, cnd | | | | | | | | | | | | | | |
| prep w/milk—*1 cup (8 fl oz)* | 248 | 99 | 312 | 414 | 657 | 533 | 181 | 87 | 347 | 312 | 444 | 312 | 201 | 6216 |
| **green pea soup**, cond, cnd, prep w/ | | | | | | | | | | | | | | |
| milk—*1 cup (8 fl oz)* | 254 | 130 | 485 | 541 | 1016 | 831 | 206 | 117 | 572 | 447 | 711 | 853 | 279 | 6249 |
| **potato soup, cream of**, cond, cnd | | | | | | | | | | | | | | |
| prep w/milk—*1 cup (8 fl oz)* | 248 | 82 | 243 | 320 | 513 | 402 | 131 | 64 | 278 | 255 | 362 | 221 | 149 | 6253 |
| **tomato bisque**, cond, cnd, prep w/ | | | | | | | | | | | | | | |
| milk—*1 cup (8 fl oz)* | 251 | 80 | 248 | 321 | 520 | 409 | 131 | 60 | 271 | 254 | 356 | 211 | 153 | 6358 |

**CONDENSED SOUPS, PREPARED WITH WATER**

| | WT (g) | TRY | THR | ISO | LEU | LYS | MET | CYS | PHE | TYR | VAL | ARG | HIS | REF |
|---|---|---|---|---|---|---|---|---|---|---|---|---|---|---|
| **asparagus soup, cream of**, cond, cnd | | | | | | | | | | | | | | |
| prep w/water—*1 cup (8 fl oz)* | 244 | 29 | 78 | 98 | 163 | 112 | 41 | 29 | 95 | 76 | 115 | 85 | 49 | 6401 |
| **bean with frankurters soup**, cond, | | | | | | | | | | | | | | |
| cnd prep w/water—*1 cup (8 fl oz)* | 250 | 105 | 412 | 488 | 822 | 680 | 125 | 110 | 558 | 298 | 550 | 525 | 260 | 6406 |
| **cheese soup**, cond, cnd, prep w/ | | | | | | | | | | | | | | |
| water—*1 cup (8 fl oz)* | 247 | 72 | 190 | 321 | 511 | 380 | 116 | 44 | 279 | 249 | 380 | 163 | 146 | 6411 |
| **chicken and dumplings soup**, cond | | | | | | | | | | | | | | |
| cnd, prep w/water—*1 cup (8 fl oz)* | 241 | 53 | 193 | 243 | 407 | 378 | 108 | 72 | 224 | 142 | 277 | 292 | 137 | 6412 |
| **chicken gumbo**, cond, cnd, prep w/ | | | | | | | | | | | | | | |
| water—*1 cup (8 fl oz)* | 244 | 22 | 83 | 100 | 168 | 161 | 46 | 17 | 98 | 68 | 117 | 122 | 59 | 6417 |
| **chicken soup, cream of**, cond, cnd | | | | | | | | | | | | | | |
| prep w/water—*1 cup (8 fl oz)* | 244 | 41 | 129 | 171 | 264 | 215 | 81 | 51 | 154 | 117 | 173 | 166 | 93 | 6416 |
| **chicken vegetable soup**, cond, cnd | | | | | | | | | | | | | | |
| prep w/water—*1 cup (8 fl oz)* | 241 | 31 | 113 | 135 | 231 | 222 | 60 | 24 | 133 | 94 | 159 | 169 | 80 | 6425 |
| **minestrone soup**, cond, cnd, prep | | | | | | | | | | | | | | |
| w/water—*1 cup (8 fl oz)* | 241 | 31 | 104 | 130 | 236 | 183 | 43 | 34 | 154 | 84 | 178 | 198 | 72 | 6440 |
| **potato soup, cream of**, cond, cnd | | | | | | | | | | | | | | |
| prep w/water—*1 cup (8 fl oz)* | 244 | 24 | 61 | 76 | 117 | 83 | 29 | 27 | 83 | 61 | 93 | 76 | 39 | 6453 |
| **split pea with ham soup**, cond, cnd | | | | | | | | | | | | | | |
| prep w/water—*1 cup (8 fl oz)* | 253 | 101 | 364 | 435 | 711 | 696 | 139 | 134 | 455 | 319 | 491 | 703 | 215 | 6451 |
| **stockpot soup**, cond, cnd, prep | | | | | | | | | | | | | | |
| w/water—*1 cup (8 fl oz)* | 247 | 42 | 151 | 183 | 311 | 299 | 82 | 35 | 178 | 126 | 215 | 227 | 109 | 6460 |
| **tomato bisque**, cond, cnd, prep | | | | | | | | | | | | | | |
| w/water—*1 cup (8 fl oz)* | 247 | 22 | 67 | 77 | 126 | 89 | 30 | 25 | 77 | 59 | 86 | 67 | 44 | 6558 |
| **turkey noodle soup**, cond, cnd, prep | | | | | | | | | | | | | | |
| w/water—*1 cup (8 fl oz)* | 244 | 37 | 124 | 151 | 254 | 212 | 73 | 46 | 156 | 102 | 168 | 159 | 90 | 6465 |
| **turkey vegetable soup**, cond, cnd | | | | | | | | | | | | | | |
| prep w/water—*1 cup (8 fl oz)* | 241 | 27 | 96 | 116 | 198 | 190 | 53 | 22 | 113 | 82 | 135 | 145 | 67 | 6466 |

**DEHYDRATED SOUPS**

| | WT (g) | TRY | THR | ISO | LEU | LYS | MET | CYS | PHE | TYR | VAL | ARG | HIS | REF |
|---|---|---|---|---|---|---|---|---|---|---|---|---|---|---|
| **chicken noodle soup**, dehydrated | 11 | 16 | 67 | 76 | 127 | 89 | 29 | 18 | 80 | 52 | 84 | 97 | 44 | 6128 |
| **ramen noodle soup**, beef flavor | | | | | | | | | | | | | | |
| dehydrated—*amt for 1 serving* | 43 | 21 | 129 | 158 | 288 | 92 | 46 | 61 | 197 | 122 | 181 | 159 | 85 | 6982 |
| **ramen noodle soup**, chicken flavor | | | | | | | | | | | | | | |
| dehydrated—*amt for 1 serving* | 43 | 13 | 127 | 149 | 277 | 90 | 45 | 60 | 193 | 115 | 173 | 150 | 82 | 6983 |

| | WT (g) | TRY | THR | ISO | LEU | LYS | MET | CYS | PHE | TYR | VAL | ARG | HIS | REF |
|---|---|---|---|---|---|---|---|---|---|---|---|---|---|---|
| | | | | | | | (mg/serving) | | | | | | | |
| **DEHYDRATED SOUPS, RECONSTITUTED** | | | | | | | | | | | | | | |
| **oxtail soup**, dehydrated, reconstituted | | | | | | | | | | | | | | |
| 1 cup (8 fl oz) | 253 | 33 | 89 | 121 | 197 | 144 | 35 | 38 | 134 | 94 | 119 | 197 | 66 | 6495 |
| **READY-TO-SERVE SOUPS** | | | | | | | | | | | | | | |
| **beef, chunky soup**, cnd, rts—1 cup (8 fl oz) | 240 | 113 | 466 | 593 | 898 | 929 | 247 | 122 | 482 | 353 | 636 | 610 | 276 | 6070 |
| **chicken broth**, 99% fat-free, cnd / | | | | | | | | | | | | | | |
| carton Swanson—1 cup (8 fl oz) | 227 | 16 | 16 | 16 | 32 | 43 | 16 | 16 | 16 | 16 | 16 | 36 | 23 | 6984 |
| **chicken soup**, chunky, cnd, rts | | | | | | | | | | | | | | |
| 1 cup (8 fl oz) | 240 | 118 | 418 | 528 | 883 | 816 | 233 | 156 | 482 | 312 | 600 | 631 | 298 | 6015 |
| **split pea with ham soup**, chunky, | | | | | | | | | | | | | | |
| cnd rts—1 cup (8 fl oz) | 240 | 110 | 391 | 468 | 766 | 749 | 149 | 144 | 490 | 343 | 526 | 758 | 233 | 6050 |
| **turkey soup**, chunky, cnd, rts | | | | | | | | | | | | | | |
| 1 cup (8 fl oz) | 236 | 99 | 404 | 514 | 781 | 809 | 215 | 106 | 418 | 307 | 552 | 531 | 238 | 6064 |
| **vegetable soup**, chunky, cnd, rts | | | | | | | | | | | | | | |
| 1 cup (8 fl oz) | 240 | 26 | 108 | 161 | 271 | 190 | 26 | 26 | 161 | 82 | 190 | 190 | 82 | 6067 |
| **28. SPICES, HERBS, AND FLAVORINGS** | | | | | | | | | | | | | | |
| **basil** | | | | | | | | | | | | | | |
| dried—1 T | 4.5 | 10 | 26 | 26 | 49 | 28 | 9 | 7 | 33 | 19 | 32 | 30 | 13 | 2003 |
| raw—1 T | 5 | 2 | 5 | 5 | 10 | 6 | 2 | 1 | 6 | 4 | 6 | 6 | 3 | 2044 |
| **caraway seeds**—1 T | 7 | 17 | 53 | 58 | 85 | 72 | 25 | 23 | 61 | 45 | 73 | 88 | 38 | 2005 |
| **chives** | | | | | | | | | | | | | | |
| freeze-dried—¼ cup | 0.8 | 2 | 7 | 7 | 10 | 8 | 2 | | 5 | 5 | 7 | 12 | 3 | 11615 |
| raw—1 T chopped | 3 | 1 | 4 | 4 | 6 | 5 | 1 | | 3 | 3 | 4 | 7 | 2 | 11156 |
| **cinnamon**, ground—1 T | 7 | 3 | 10 | 10 | 18 | 17 | 5 | 4 | 10 | 10 | 16 | 12 | 8 | 2010 |
| **dill seeds**—1 T | 7 | | 40 | 54 | 65 | 73 | 10 | | 47 | | 78 | 88 | 22 | 2016 |
| **dill weed**, raw—1 cup sprigs | 9 | 1 | 6 | 18 | 14 | 22 | 1 | 2 | 6 | 9 | 14 | 13 | 6 | 2045 |
| **fennel seeds**—1 T | 6 | 15 | 36 | 42 | 60 | 45 | 18 | 13 | 39 | 25 | 55 | 41 | 20 | 2018 |
| **fenugreek seeds**—1 T | 11 | 43 | 99 | 137 | 193 | 185 | 37 | 41 | 120 | 84 | 121 | 271 | 73 | 2019 |
| **garlic powder**—1 T | 8 | 17 | 37 | 52 | 82 | 46 | 27 | 14 | 39 | 17 | 57 | 134 | 25 | 2020 |
| **ginger**, ground—1 T | 5 | 3 | 9 | 13 | 19 | 15 | 3 | 2 | 12 | 5 | 19 | 11 | 8 | 2021 |
| **ginger root**, raw—1 T | 5 | 1 | 2 | 3 | 4 | 3 | 1 | 0 | 2 | 1 | 4 | 2 | 2 | 11216 |
| **mustard seeds**, yellow—1 T | 11 | 58 | 120 | 119 | 196 | 167 | 53 | 64 | 117 | 82 | 146 | 192 | 84 | 2024 |
| **onion flakes**, dehydrated—¼ cup | 14 | 18 | 30 | 44 | 44 | 60 | 10 | 22 | 32 | 31 | 29 | 168 | 20 | 11284 |
| **onion powder**—1 T | 7 | 8 | 14 | 21 | 23 | 33 | 6 | 13 | 17 | 16 | 17 | 94 | 10 | 2026 |
| **peppermint**, raw—2 T | 3.2 | 2 | 5 | 5 | 9 | 5 | 2 | 1 | 6 | 4 | 6 | 6 | 2 | 2064 |
| **poppy seeds**—2 T | 9 | 17 | 62 | 74 | 119 | 86 | 45 | 27 | 68 | 65 | 99 | 175 | 42 | 2033 |
| **rosemary**, raw—1 T | 1.7 | 1 | 2 | 2 | 4 | 2 | 1 | 1 | 3 | 2 | 3 | 3 | 1 | 2063 |
| **shallots**, freeze-dried—¼ cup | 3.6 | 5 | 17 | 19 | 26 | 22 | 5 | | 14 | 13 | 20 | 32 | 8 | 11640 |
| **spearmint** | | | | | | | | | | | | | | |
| dried—1 T | 1.6 | 5 | 13 | 13 | 24 | 14 | 4 | 4 | 16 | 10 | 16 | 15 | 6 | 2066 |
| raw—1 T | 11 | 6 | 15 | 15 | 27 | 16 | 5 | 4 | 18 | 11 | 18 | 17 | 7 | 2065 |
| **29. SUGARS, SYRUPS, AND OTHER SWEETENERS** | | | | | | | | | | | | | | |
| **honey**—1 T | 21 | 1 | 1 | 2 | 2 | 2 | 0 | 1 | 2 | 2 | 2 | 1 | 0 | 19296 |
| **jam/preserves**—1 T | 20 | 2 | 5 | 3 | 7 | 6 | 0 | 1 | 4 | 5 | 4 | 6 | 3 | 19297 |
| **malt syrup**—1 T | 24 | 18 | 50 | 50 | 91 | 64 | 26 | 16 | 62 | 41 | 73 | 68 | 32 | 19352 |
| **marmalade**, orange—1 T | 20 | 1 | 1 | 2 | 1 | 3 | 1 | 1 | 2 | 1 | 3 | 4 | 1 | 19303 |
| **sugar substitute**, Equal, Nutrasweet—1 pkt | 1 | 0 | 0 | 0 | 0 | 0 | 0 | 0 | 12 | 0 | 0 | 0 | 0 | 19337 |
| **30. VEGETABLES AND VEGETABLE DISHES** | | | | | | | | | | | | | | |
| **FLOWER, STEM, AND STALK VEGETABLES** | | | | | | | | | | | | | | |
| **asparagus** boiled, drained—1 cup (12 pieces) | 180 | 52 | 166 | 148 | 252 | 203 | 61 | 61 | 148 | 103 | 225 | 178 | 95 | 11012 |
| canned, drained—1 cup | 242 | 51 | 145 | 191 | 225 | 244 | 51 | 60 | 123 | 82 | 198 | 242 | 80 | 11015 |
| frozen—1 cup | 180 | 56 | 162 | 214 | 252 | 275 | 56 | 68 | 137 | 92 | 223 | 272 | 90 | 11018 |
| frozen, boiled, drained—1 cup | 180 | 52 | 148 | 196 | 230 | 252 | 50 | 63 | 126 | 85 | 205 | 248 | 83 | 11019 |
| raw—1 cup | 134 | 36 | 113 | 100 | 172 | 139 | 42 | 42 | 100 | 70 | 154 | 122 | 66 | 11011 |
| **broccoflower** | | | | | | | | | | | | | | |
| boiled, drained—⅕ head | 90 | 36 | 99 | 104 | 160 | 147 | 39 | 32 | 97 | 59 | 138 | 131 | 55 | 11967 |
| raw—1 cup pieces | 64 | 25 | 68 | 72 | 110 | 101 | 27 | 22 | 67 | 41 | 95 | 91 | 38 | 11965 |
| **broccoli** boiled, drained—1 med stalk | 180 | 61 | 173 | 166 | 265 | 279 | 77 | 56 | 209 | 108 | 248 | 360 | 113 | 11091 |
| chopped, frozen—1 cup | 156 | 45 | 142 | 170 | 204 | 220 | 53 | 31 | 133 | 98 | 200 | 228 | 78 | 11092 |
| chopped, raw—1 cup | 91 | 30 | 80 | 72 | 117 | 123 | 35 | 25 | 106 | 46 | 114 | 174 | 54 | 11090 |
| chopped, frozen, boiled drained—1 cup | 184 | 59 | 186 | 223 | 267 | 287 | 68 | 40 | 173 | 129 | 261 | 296 | 101 | 11093 |
| florets, raw—1 cup | 71 | 21 | 65 | 77 | 93 | 100 | 24 | 14 | 60 | 45 | 91 | 103 | 36 | 11740 |
| spears, frozen, boiled, drained—1 cup | 184 | 59 | 186 | 223 | 267 | 287 | 68 | 40 | 173 | 129 | 261 | 296 | 101 | 11095 |

| | WT (g) | TRY | THR | ISO | LEU | LYS | MET | CYS | PHE | TYR | VAL | ARG | HIS | REF |
|---|---|---|---|---|---|---|---|---|---|---|---|---|---|---|
| | | | | | | | (mg/serving) | | | | | | | |
| **cauliflower** | | | | | | | | | | | | | | |
| boiled, drained—*1 cup pieces* | 124 | 30 | 83 | 87 | 133 | 123 | 32 | 26 | 82 | 50 | 114 | 110 | 46 | 11136 |
| frozen—*1 cup pieces* | 180 | 47 | 131 | 139 | 212 | 194 | 50 | 41 | 130 | 79 | 182 | 175 | 74 | 11137 |
| frozen, boiled, drained—*1 cup pcs* | 180 | 38 | 106 | 110 | 169 | 155 | 41 | 34 | 104 | 63 | 146 | 140 | 59 | 11138 |
| raw—*1 cup pieces* | 100 | 26 | 72 | 75 | 116 | 106 | 28 | 23 | 71 | 43 | 99 | 95 | 40 | 11135 |
| **celery** | | | | | | | | | | | | | | |
| boiled, drained—*1 cup diced* | 150 | 16 | 36 | 38 | 58 | 48 | 10 | 8 | 36 | 16 | 50 | 36 | 21 | 11144 |
| raw—*1 medium stalk (7.5" long)* | 40 | 4 | 8 | 8 | 13 | 11 | 2 | 2 | 8 | 4 | 11 | 8 | 5 | 11143 |
| **hearts of palm** (heart palm), cnd—*1 cup* | 146 | 34 | 142 | 147 | 247 | 133 | 61 | 28 | 143 | 72 | 166 | 260 | 80 | 11961 |
| **kohlrabi** | | | | | | | | | | | | | | |
| boiled, drained—*1 cup slices* | 165 | 18 | 86 | 137 | 117 | 97 | 23 | 12 | 68 | | 87 | 183 | 33 | 11242 |
| raw—*1 cup slices* | 135 | 14 | 66 | 105 | 90 | 76 | 18 | 9 | 53 | | 68 | 142 | 26 | 11241 |
| **leek** | | | | | | | | | | | | | | |
| boiled, drained—*1 leek* | 124 | 7 | 42 | 35 | 64 | 52 | 12 | 17 | 37 | 27 | 38 | 52 | 17 | 11247 |
| raw—*1 leek (~1 cup)* | 89 | 11 | 56 | 46 | 85 | 69 | 16 | 22 | 49 | 36 | 50 | 69 | 22 | 11246 |
| **scallions** (green/spring onions), raw | | | | | | | | | | | | | | |
| *1 cup chopped* | 100 | 20 | 72 | 77 | 109 | 91 | 20 | | 59 | 53 | 81 | 132 | 32 | 11291 |
| **sesbania flower**, steamed—*1 cup* | 104 | 18 | 53 | 63 | 99 | 59 | 15 | 11 | 64 | | 72 | 64 | 24 | 11448 |
| | | | | | | | | | | | | | | |
| **FRUIT (SEED-CONTAINING) VEGETABLES** | | | | | | | | | | | | | | |
| **acorn winter squash** | | | | | | | | | | | | | | |
| baked—*1 cup cubed* | 205 | 33 | 68 | 90 | 131 | 84 | 29 | 20 | 90 | 78 | 98 | 127 | 43 | 11483 |
| boiled—*1 cup mashed* | 245 | 24 | 49 | 64 | 93 | 61 | 20 | 15 | 64 | 56 | 71 | 91 | 32 | 11484 |
| raw—*1 cup cubed* | 140 | 15 | 34 | 43 | 63 | 41 | 14 | 10 | 43 | 38 | 48 | 62 | 21 | 11482 |
| **ancho pepper**, dried—*1 pepper* | 17 | 26 | 72 | 63 | 103 | 88 | 24 | 37 | 61 | 42 | 83 | 94 | 39 | 11978 |
| **breadfruit**, raw—*¼ small* | 96 | | 50 | 61 | 62 | 36 | 10 | 9 | 25 | 18 | 45 | | | 9059 |
| **butternut winter squash** | | | | | | | | | | | | | | |
| baked—*1 cup cubed* | 205 | 27 | 55 | 72 | 105 | 68 | 23 | 16 | 72 | 62 | 80 | 102 | 35 | 11486 |
| cooked—*1 cup cubed* | 140 | 18 | 38 | 49 | 71 | 46 | 15 | 11 | 49 | 42 | 55 | 70 | 24 | 11866 |
| frozen, boiled—*1 cup mashed* | 240 | 41 | 89 | 115 | 168 | 108 | 36 | 26 | 115 | 98 | 127 | 163 | 55 | 11488 |
| raw—*1 cup cubed* | 140 | 20 | 42 | 55 | 80 | 52 | 17 | 13 | 55 | 48 | 60 | 78 | 27 | 11485 |
| **calabash gourd**, white-flowered | | | | | | | | | | | | | | |
| boiled, drained—*1 cup cubed* | 146 | 4 | 25 | 47 | 51 | 29 | 6 | | 20 | | 38 | 20 | 6 | 11219 |
| **chayote** | | | | | | | | | | | | | | |
| boiled, drained—*1 cup pieces* | 160 | 13 | 50 | 53 | 93 | 48 | 2 | | 58 | 38 | 75 | 42 | 18 | 11150 |
| raw—*1 cup pieces* | 132 | 15 | 53 | 58 | 102 | 51 | 1 | | 62 | 42 | 83 | 46 | 20 | 11149 |
| **chili pepper, green** | | | | | | | | | | | | | | |
| canned—*1 cup* | 139 | 14 | 36 | 32 | 53 | 44 | 13 | 19 | 31 | 21 | 42 | 47 | 19 | 11980 |
| hot, cnd, solids and liq—*1 pepper* | 73 | 9 | 24 | 21 | 34 | 29 | 8 | 12 | 20 | 14 | 28 | 31 | 13 | 11329 |
| hot, raw—*1 pepper* | 45 | 12 | 33 | 29 | 47 | 40 | 11 | 17 | 28 | 19 | 38 | 43 | 18 | 11670 |
| **chili pepper, red** | | | | | | | | | | | | | | |
| hot, cnd, solids and liq—*1 pepper* | 73 | 9 | 24 | 21 | 34 | 29 | 8 | 12 | 20 | 14 | 28 | 31 | 13 | 11820 |
| hot, raw—*1 pepper* | 45 | 12 | 33 | 29 | 47 | 40 | 11 | 17 | 28 | 19 | 38 | 43 | 18 | 11819 |
| hot, sun-dried—*1 pepper* | 0.5 | 1 | 2 | 2 | 3 | 2 | 1 | 1 | 2 | 1 | 2 | 3 | 1 | 11962 |
| **crook/straightneck summer squash** | | | | | | | | | | | | | | |
| boiled, drained—*1 cup sliced* | 180 | 14 | 40 | 59 | 95 | 90 | 23 | 18 | 58 | 43 | 74 | 68 | 36 | 11468 |
| canned, drained—*1 cup sliced* | 216 | 11 | 32 | 48 | 78 | 73 | 19 | 13 | 48 | 35 | 60 | 56 | 28 | 11471 |
| frzn, boiled, drained—*1 cup sliced* | 192 | 21 | 60 | 88 | 144 | 136 | 35 | 27 | 86 | 65 | 111 | 104 | 54 | 11474 |
| raw—*1 cup sliced* | 130 | 10 | 30 | 44 | 72 | 68 | 18 | 13 | 43 | 32 | 55 | 52 | 26 | 11467 |
| **cucumber**, raw—*1 large (8¼" long)* | 301 | 15 | 57 | 63 | 87 | 87 | 18 | 12 | 57 | 33 | 66 | 132 | 30 | 11205 |
| peeled—*1 medium* | 201 | 14 | 24 | 24 | 50 | 50 | 24 | 14 | 62 | 4 | 24 | 62 | 4 | 11206 |
| **eggplant (aubergine)** | | | | | | | | | | | | | | |
| boiled, drained—*1 cup* | 99 | 8 | 30 | 36 | 51 | 39 | 9 | 4 | 35 | 22 | 43 | 46 | 19 | 11210 |
| raw—*1 cup* | 82 | 7 | 30 | 37 | 52 | 39 | 9 | 5 | 35 | 22 | 43 | 47 | 19 | 11209 |
| **green snap beans** | | | | | | | | | | | | | | |
| boiled, drained—*1 cup* | 125 | 25 | 102 | 86 | 145 | 114 | 29 | 22 | 86 | 55 | 116 | 95 | 44 | 11053 |
| canned, drained—*1 cup* | 135 | 16 | 68 | 57 | 96 | 74 | 19 | 15 | 57 | 36 | 77 | 62 | 30 | 11056 |
| frozen—*1 cup* | 124 | 24 | 98 | 82 | 138 | 108 | 27 | 22 | 82 | 52 | 110 | 91 | 42 | 11060 |
| frzn, boiled, drained—*1 cup* | 135 | 22 | 88 | 73 | 123 | 97 | 24 | 19 | 73 | 46 | 99 | 81 | 38 | 11061 |
| frzn, microwaved—*1 cup* | 111 | 21 | 88 | 73 | 123 | 97 | 24 | 20 | 73 | 47 | 99 | 81 | 38 | 11062 |
| raw—*1 cup* | 110 | 21 | 87 | 73 | 123 | 97 | 24 | 20 | 74 | 46 | 99 | 80 | 37 | 11052 |
| **hubbard winter squash** | | | | | | | | | | | | | | |
| baked—*1 cup cubed* | 205 | 43 | 90 | 119 | 172 | 113 | 37 | 27 | 119 | 102 | 131 | 168 | 57 | 11490 |
| boiled—*1 cup mashed* | 236 | 50 | 104 | 137 | 198 | 130 | 42 | 31 | 137 | 118 | 151 | 194 | 66 | 11491 |
| raw—*1 cup cubed* | 116 | 32 | 70 | 90 | 132 | 86 | 29 | 20 | 90 | 78 | 100 | 129 | 43 | 11489 |
| **Hungarian pepper**, raw—*1 pepper* | 27 | 3 | 8 | 7 | 11 | 10 | 3 | 4 | 7 | 5 | 9 | 11 | 4 | 11981 |
| **jalapeno pepper** | | | | | | | | | | | | | | |
| cnd, solids and liq—*1 pepper* | 22 | 3 | 7 | 7 | 11 | 9 | 3 | 4 | 6 | 4 | 9 | 10 | 4 | 11632 |
| raw—*1 pepper* | 14 | 2 | 7 | 6 | 10 | 9 | 2 | 4 | 6 | 4 | 8 | 9 | 4 | 11979 |

| | WT | TRY | THR | ISO | LEU | LYS | MET | CYS | PHE | TYR | VAL | ARG | HIS | REF |
|---|---|---|---|---|---|---|---|---|---|---|---|---|---|---|
| | (g) | | | | | | (mg/serving) | | | | | | | |
| **okra** bld, drained—*8 pods (3" long)* | 85 | 14 | 52 | 55 | 83 | 64 | 17 | 15 | 52 | 69 | 72 | 66 | 25 | 11279 |
| frzn, cooked, drained—*1 cup* | 184 | 31 | 125 | 132 | 201 | 155 | 40 | 37 | 125 | 167 | 175 | 160 | 61 | 11281 |
| raw—*1 cup sliced* | 100 | 17 | 65 | 69 | 105 | 81 | 21 | 19 | 65 | 87 | 91 | 84 | 31 | 11278 |
| **pimiento pepper**, canned—*1 T* | 12 | 2 | 5 | 4 | 7 | 6 | 2 | 3 | 4 | 3 | 6 | 6 | 3 | 11943 |
| **plantain**, cooked—*1 cup sliced* | 154 | 14 | 32 | 34 | 55 | 57 | 15 | 18 | 42 | 31 | 43 | 102 | 60 | 9278 |
| **pumpkin winter squash** | | | | | | | | | | | | | | |
| boiled, drained—*1 cup mashed* | 245 | 22 | 51 | 56 | 83 | 96 | 20 | 5 | 56 | 74 | 61 | 96 | 27 | 11423 |
| canned—*1 cup mashed* | 245 | 32 | 78 | 83 | 125 | 147 | 29 | 7 | 86 | 113 | 93 | 145 | 42 | 11424 |
| raw—*1 cup cubed* | 116 | 14 | 34 | 36 | 53 | 63 | 13 | 3 | 37 | 49 | 41 | 63 | 19 | 11422 |
| **scallop summer squash** | | | | | | | | | | | | | | |
| boiled, drained—*1 cup sliced* | 180 | 16 | 45 | 67 | 110 | 103 | 27 | 20 | 65 | 50 | 85 | 79 | 40 | 11476 |
| raw—*1 cup sliced* | 130 | 14 | 38 | 56 | 91 | 87 | 22 | 17 | 55 | 42 | 70 | 66 | 34 | 11475 |
| **snow peas** boiled, drained—*1 cup* | 160 | 51 | 184 | 301 | 427 | 376 | 21 | 59 | 168 | 184 | 510 | 251 | 32 | 11301 |
| frzn, boiled, drained—*1 cup* | 160 | 54 | 197 | 323 | 458 | 403 | 22 | 64 | 179 | 197 | 547 | 269 | 35 | 11303 |
| raw—*1 cup whole* | 63 | 17 | 62 | 101 | 144 | 127 | 7 | 20 | 57 | 62 | 172 | 84 | 11 | 11300 |
| **spaghetti winter squash** | | | | | | | | | | | | | | |
| boiled/baked—*1 cup* | 155 | 14 | 28 | 37 | 53 | 34 | 11 | 8 | 37 | 31 | 40 | 51 | 17 | 11493 |
| **summer squash**, all varieties | | | | | | | | | | | | | | |
| boiled, drained—*1 cup sliced* | 180 | 14 | 40 | 59 | 95 | 90 | 23 | 18 | 58 | 43 | 74 | 68 | 36 | 11642 |
| raw—*1 cup sliced* | 113 | 12 | 32 | 47 | 78 | 73 | 19 | 14 | 46 | 35 | 60 | 56 | 28 | 11641 |
| **sweet pepper**, green | | | | | | | | | | | | | | |
| boiled, drained—*1 cup* | 135 | 16 | 46 | 40 | 65 | 55 | 15 | 24 | 39 | 26 | 53 | 59 | 26 | 11334 |
| cnd, solids and liq—*1 cup halves* | 140 | 14 | 41 | 36 | 59 | 50 | 14 | 21 | 35 | 24 | 48 | 53 | 22 | 11335 |
| frozen—*3.5 oz* | 100 | 14 | 40 | 35 | 56 | 48 | 13 | 21 | 33 | 22 | 45 | 52 | 22 | 11337 |
| frzn, boiled, drained—*1 cup chopped* | 135 | 16 | 47 | 42 | 66 | 57 | 15 | 24 | 39 | 27 | 54 | 61 | 26 | 11338 |
| raw—*1 med (2 ¾" long)* | 119 | 14 | 43 | 29 | 43 | 46 | 8 | 14 | 109 | 14 | 43 | 32 | 12 | 11333 |
| **sweet pepper**, red | | | | | | | | | | | | | | |
| boiled, drained—*1 cup* | 135 | 16 | 46 | 40 | 65 | 55 | 15 | 24 | 39 | 26 | 53 | 59 | 26 | 11823 |
| frzn, boiled, drained—*1 cup chopped* | 135 | 15 | 53 | 27 | 46 | 46 | 7 | 24 | 65 | 12 | 39 | 46 | 22 | 11918 |
| raw—*1 med (2 ¾" long)* | 119 | 14 | 48 | 25 | 43 | 43 | 7 | 23 | 60 | 11 | 37 | 43 | 20 | 11821 |
| **sweet pepper**, yellow, raw | | | | | | | | | | | | | | |
| *1 large (3 ¾" long)* | 186 | 24 | 69 | 60 | 97 | 82 | 22 | 35 | 58 | 39 | 78 | 89 | 37 | 11951 |
| **tomato**, green, raw | | | | | | | | | | | | | | |
| *1 medium (2 ⅜" diameter)* | 123 | 11 | 37 | 36 | 54 | 54 | 12 | 20 | 38 | 26 | 38 | 36 | 22 | 11527 |
| **tomato**, orange, raw—*1 tomato* | 111 | 9 | 32 | 30 | 47 | 47 | 11 | 17 | 33 | 22 | 33 | 32 | 20 | 11695 |
| **tomato paste**, canned—*6 oz* | 170 | 53 | 226 | 151 | 211 | 228 | 46 | 78 | 558 | 112 | 150 | 173 | 121 | 11546 |
| **tomato puree**, canned—*½ cup* | 125 | 14 | 46 | 39 | 58 | 60 | 11 | 12 | 42 | 26 | 41 | 40 | 31 | 11547 |
| **tomato**, red | | | | | | | | | | | | | | |
| boiled—*1 cup* | 240 | 19 | 65 | 62 | 94 | 94 | 22 | 34 | 67 | 43 | 65 | 62 | 38 | 11530 |
| canned—*1 cup* | 240 | 19 | 106 | 55 | 70 | 70 | 19 | 19 | 70 | 46 | 41 | 58 | 38 | 11531 |
| cherry, raw—*1 tomato* | 62 | 4 | 17 | 11 | 16 | 17 | 4 | 6 | 42 | 9 | 11 | 13 | 9 | 11529 |
| Italian, raw—*1 tomato* | 62 | 4 | 17 | 11 | 16 | 17 | 4 | 6 | 42 | 9 | 11 | 13 | 9 | 11529 |
| plum, raw—*1 tomato* | 62 | 4 | 17 | 11 | 16 | 17 | 4 | 6 | 42 | 9 | 11 | 13 | 9 | 11529 |
| raw—*1 tomato* | 62 | 4 | 17 | 11 | 16 | 17 | 4 | 6 | 42 | 9 | 11 | 13 | 9 | 11529 |
| stewed—*1 cup* | 255 | 48 | 138 | 163 | 270 | 158 | 61 | 74 | 191 | 105 | 191 | 171 | 92 | 11660 |
| stewed, canned—*1 cup* | 255 | 18 | 59 | 56 | 89 | 89 | 20 | 31 | 64 | 41 | 64 | 56 | 36 | 11533 |
| sun-dried—*1 cup* | 54 | 56 | 193 | 183 | 279 | 280 | 66 | 99 | 198 | 131 | 195 | 185 | 116 | 11955 |
| sun-dried, cnd in oil, drained *1 cup* | 110 | 41 | 141 | 133 | 204 | 205 | 48 | 73 | 144 | 96 | 143 | 135 | 85 | 11956 |
| **tomato**, yellow, raw—*1 tomato* | 212 | 15 | 51 | 49 | 76 | 76 | 17 | 28 | 53 | 36 | 53 | 51 | 32 | 11696 |
| **winter squash**, all varieties | | | | | | | | | | | | | | |
| baked—*1 cup cubed* | 205 | 27 | 55 | 72 | 102 | 68 | 23 | 16 | 72 | 62 | 78 | 100 | 35 | 11644 |
| raw—*1 cup cubed* | 116 | 24 | 50 | 66 | 95 | 61 | 21 | 15 | 66 | 57 | 72 | 94 | 31 | 11643 |
| **yellow snap beans** | | | | | | | | | | | | | | |
| boiled, drained—*1 cup* | 125 | 25 | 102 | 86 | 145 | 114 | 29 | 22 | 86 | 55 | 116 | 95 | 44 | 11724 |
| canned, drained—*1 cup* | 135 | 16 | 68 | 57 | 96 | 74 | 19 | 15 | 57 | 36 | 77 | 62 | 30 | 11932 |
| frozen, drained—*1 cup* | 135 | 22 | 88 | 73 | 123 | 97 | 24 | 19 | 73 | 46 | 99 | 81 | 38 | 11732 |
| **zucchini summer squash** | | | | | | | | | | | | | | |
| baby, raw—*1 medium* | 11 | 3 | 7 | 11 | 17 | 17 | 4 | 3 | 11 | 8 | 14 | 13 | 6 | 11953 |
| boiled, drained—*1 cup slices* | 180 | 11 | 27 | 41 | 67 | 63 | 16 | 13 | 40 | 31 | 52 | 49 | 25 | 11478 |
| frozen, bld, drained—*1 cup slices* | 223 | 22 | 62 | 91 | 149 | 143 | 36 | 27 | 89 | 69 | 116 | 107 | 56 | 11480 |
| Italian style, canned—*1 cup* | 227 | 20 | 57 | 84 | 136 | 129 | 34 | 25 | 82 | 61 | 104 | 98 | 50 | 11481 |
| raw—*1 cup slices* | 113 | 11 | 33 | 50 | 80 | 76 | 20 | 14 | 49 | 36 | 61 | 58 | 29 | 11477 |
| **LEAFY VEGETABLES** | | | | | | | | | | | | | | |
| **agave**, raw—*3.5 oz* | 100 | 8 | 14 | 14 | 25 | 28 | 9 | 8 | 19 | 9 | 22 | 106 | 8 | 35192 |
| **amaranth leaves** | | | | | | | | | | | | | | |
| boiled, drained—*1 cup* | 132 | 36 | 112 | 135 | 220 | 144 | 41 | 33 | 150 | 90 | 156 | 137 | 58 | 11004 |
| raw—*1 cup* | 28 | 9 | 28 | 33 | 55 | 36 | 10 | 8 | 37 | 22 | 38 | 34 | 15 | 11003 |

| | WT (g) | TRY | THR | ISO | LEU | LYS | MET | CYS | PHE | TYR | VAL | ARG | HIS | REF |
|---|---|---|---|---|---|---|---|---|---|---|---|---|---|---|
| | | | | | | | (mg/serving) | | | | | | | |
| **beet greens** | | | | | | | | | | | | | | |
| boiled, drained—*1 cup* | 144 | 58 | 109 | 76 | 166 | 108 | 30 | 35 | 98 | 88 | 109 | 105 | 56 | 11087 |
| raw—*1 cup* | 38 | 13 | 25 | 17 | 37 | 24 | 7 | 8 | 22 | 20 | 25 | 24 | 13 | 11086 |
| **broccoli raab** (rapini) | | | | | | | | | | | | | | |
| boiled—*3.5 oz* | 100 | 52 | 128 | 125 | 206 | 239 | 58 | 47 | 154 | 90 | 184 | 207 | 80 | 11097 |
| raw—*1 cup chopped* | 40 | 17 | 42 | 42 | 68 | 79 | 19 | 16 | 51 | 30 | 61 | 69 | 26 | 11096 |
| **Brussels sprouts** | | | | | | | | | | | | | | |
| boiled, drained—*1 cup* | 156 | 44 | 142 | 156 | 178 | 181 | 37 | 25 | 115 | | 183 | 239 | 89 | 11099 |
| frozen—*1 cup* | 155 | 65 | 209 | 229 | 264 | 267 | 56 | 37 | 170 | | 268 | 352 | 132 | 11100 |
| frozen, bld, drained—*1 cup* | 155 | 62 | 202 | 222 | 254 | 257 | 54 | 36 | 164 | | 259 | 338 | 127 | 11101 |
| raw—*1 cup* | 88 | 33 | 106 | 116 | 134 | 136 | 28 | 19 | 86 | | 136 | 179 | 67 | 11098 |
| **cabbage**, green/white | | | | | | | | | | | | | | |
| boiled, drained—*1 cup shredded* | 150 | 16 | 53 | 45 | 62 | 64 | 18 | 16 | 48 | 28 | 63 | 111 | 33 | 11110 |
| raw—*1 cup shredded* | 70 | 8 | 25 | 21 | 29 | 31 | 8 | 8 | 22 | 13 | 29 | 52 | 15 | 11109 |
| **cabbage**, red/purple | | | | | | | | | | | | | | |
| boiled, drained—*1 cup shredded* | 150 | 20 | 62 | 54 | 74 | 76 | 21 | 20 | 57 | 34 | 75 | 132 | 39 | 11113 |
| raw—*1 cup shredded* | 70 | 8 | 27 | 24 | 32 | 34 | 10 | 8 | 25 | 15 | 34 | 58 | 17 | 11112 |
| **cabbage**, savoy | | | | | | | | | | | | | | |
| boiled, drained—*1 cup shredded* | 145 | 26 | 90 | 132 | 135 | 123 | 26 | 22 | 84 | 45 | 112 | 148 | 54 | 11115 |
| raw—*1 cup shredded* | 70 | 14 | 48 | 71 | 72 | 66 | 14 | 12 | 45 | 24 | 60 | 80 | 29 | 11114 |
| **cabbage**, swamp (skunk cabbage) | | | | | | | | | | | | | | |
| boiled, drained—*1 cup* | 98 | | 110 | 81 | 114 | 85 | 34 | 23 | 100 | 63 | 106 | 116 | 36 | 11504 |
| raw—*1 cup* | 56 | | 78 | 58 | 82 | 61 | 25 | 16 | 71 | 45 | 76 | 83 | 26 | 11503 |
| **celtuce leaves**, raw—*12 leaves* | 100 | 6 | 39 | 55 | 52 | 55 | 10 | 10 | 36 | 21 | 46 | 46 | 15 | 11145 |
| **chicory greens**, raw—*1 cup chopped* | 180 | 56 | 85 | 182 | 133 | 121 | 18 | | 74 | | 139 | 223 | 52 | 11152 |
| **Chinese cabbage**, pak choi | | | | | | | | | | | | | | |
| boiled, drained—*1 cup shredded* | 170 | 26 | 87 | 151 | 155 | 158 | 15 | 29 | 78 | 51 | 117 | 148 | 46 | 11117 |
| raw—*1 cup shredded* | 70 | 10 | 34 | 60 | 62 | 62 | 6 | 12 | 31 | 20 | 46 | 59 | 18 | 11116 |
| **Chinese cabbage**, pe-tsai | | | | | | | | | | | | | | |
| boiled, drained—*1 cup shredded* | 119 | 18 | 58 | 101 | 105 | 106 | 11 | 20 | 52 | 35 | 79 | 100 | 31 | 11120 |
| raw—*1 cup shredded* | 76 | 9 | 30 | 52 | 53 | 54 | 5 | 10 | 27 | 17 | 40 | 51 | 16 | 11119 |
| **coleslaw**, homemade—*½ cup* | 60 | 10 | 29 | 37 | 49 | 43 | 11 | 9 | 28 | 20 | 37 | 42 | 17 | 11159 |
| **collards** | | | | | | | | | | | | | | |
| boiled, drained—*1 cup chopped* | 190 | 51 | 141 | 163 | 247 | 192 | 53 | 42 | 142 | 106 | 198 | 205 | 76 | 11162 |
| frozen—*1 cup chopped* | 170 | 60 | 162 | 185 | 284 | 218 | 63 | 46 | 163 | 124 | 223 | 235 | 87 | 11163 |
| frozen, bld, drained—*1 cup chopped* | 170 | 65 | 178 | 206 | 313 | 240 | 68 | 51 | 178 | 136 | 246 | 258 | 97 | 11164 |
| raw—*1 cup chopped* | 36 | 11 | 31 | 36 | 54 | 42 | 12 | 9 | 31 | 24 | 43 | 45 | 17 | 11161 |
| **cornsalad** (lamb's lettuce), raw—*1 cup* | 56 | 15 | 42 | 55 | 74 | 57 | 14 | 11 | 51 | 20 | 55 | 51 | 20 | 11190 |
| **endive**, raw—*1 cup chopped* | 50 | 2 | 25 | 36 | 49 | 32 | 7 | 5 | 26 | 20 | 32 | 31 | 12 | 11213 |
| **horseradish tree leafy tips** | | | | | | | | | | | | | | |
| chopped, boiled, drained—*1 cup* | 42 | 34 | 97 | 106 | 186 | 126 | 29 | 33 | 115 | 82 | 144 | 125 | 46 | 11223 |
| **jute** (potherb) | | | | | | | | | | | | | | |
| boiled, drained—*1 cup* | 87 | 21 | 113 | 152 | 266 | 151 | 44 | 28 | 146 | 101 | 171 | 171 | 76 | 11232 |
| raw—*1 cup* | 28 | 8 | 46 | 62 | 109 | 61 | 18 | 11 | 59 | 41 | 69 | 69 | 31 | 11231 |
| **kale** | | | | | | | | | | | | | | |
| boiled, drained—*1 cup chopped* | 130 | 30 | 111 | 148 | 173 | 148 | 23 | 32 | 126 | 87 | 135 | 138 | 52 | 11234 |
| frozen, bld, drained—*1 cup chopped* | 130 | 46 | 165 | 221 | 259 | 221 | 35 | 49 | 190 | 131 | 203 | 205 | 78 | 11236 |
| raw—*1 cup chopped* | 67 | 27 | 98 | 132 | 155 | 132 | 21 | 29 | 113 | 78 | 121 | 123 | 46 | 11233 |
| **kale, Scotch** (curly leaves), boiled, drained—*1 cup chopped* | 130 | 30 | 111 | 147 | 172 | 147 | 23 | 32 | 126 | 87 | 135 | 136 | 52 | 11623 |
| **lambsquarters**, boiled drained—*1 cup* | 180 | 52 | 223 | 347 | 481 | 486 | 67 | 122 | 227 | 241 | 310 | 347 | 158 | 11245 |
| **lettuce**, butterhead, raw—*1 cup* | 55 | 7 | 23 | 21 | 39 | 31 | 8 | 5 | 29 | 10 | 30 | 28 | 9 | 11250 |
| **lettuce**, iceberg, raw—*1 cup* | 55 | 5 | 14 | 10 | 14 | 13 | 3 | 3 | 13 | 4 | 13 | 8 | 5 | 11252 |
| **lettuce**, looseleaf (leaf), raw—*1 cup* | 56 | 5 | 33 | 47 | 44 | 47 | 9 | 9 | 31 | 18 | 39 | 40 | 12 | 11253 |
| **mustard greens** | | | | | | | | | | | | | | |
| boiled, drained—*1 cup chopped* | 140 | 35 | 84 | 115 | 97 | 144 | 29 | 48 | 84 | 167 | 123 | 231 | 56 | 11271 |
| frozen—*1 cup chopped* | 146 | 39 | 96 | 133 | 111 | 165 | 34 | 54 | 96 | 193 | 142 | 264 | 66 | 11272 |
| frozen, bld, drained—*1 cup chopped* | 150 | 38 | 90 | 124 | 105 | 154 | 32 | 51 | 90 | 180 | 132 | 249 | 62 | 11273 |
| raw—*1 cup chopped* | 56 | 17 | 40 | 55 | 46 | 69 | 14 | 22 | 40 | 80 | 59 | 110 | 27 | 11270 |
| **parsley**, raw—*10 sprigs* | 10 | 4 | 12 | 12 | 20 | 18 | 4 | 1 | 14 | 8 | 17 | 12 | 6 | 11297 |
| **pumpkin leaves**, boiled, drained—*1 cup* | 71 | 25 | 96 | 96 | 195 | 123 | 33 | 19 | 105 | 96 | 111 | 133 | 31 | 11419 |
| **purslane** | | | | | | | | | | | | | | |
| boiled, drained—*1 cup* | 115 | 18 | 58 | 61 | 105 | 75 | 16 | 12 | 67 | 28 | 83 | 66 | 26 | 11428 |
| raw—*1 cup* | 43 | 6 | 19 | 20 | 34 | 25 | 5 | 4 | 22 | 9 | 27 | 22 | 9 | 11427 |
| **romaine** (cos lettuce), raw—*1 cup* | 56 | 6 | 24 | 25 | 43 | 36 | 8 | 3 | 36 | 14 | 31 | 30 | 12 | 11251 |
| **sauerkraut**, canned, solids and liquid *1 cup* | 142 | 11 | 36 | 30 | 41 | 44 | 13 | 11 | 33 | 20 | 43 | 75 | 23 | 11439 |

| | WT | TRY | THR | ISO | LEU | LYS | MET | CYS | PHE | TYR | VAL | ARG | HIS | REF |
|---|---|---|---|---|---|---|---|---|---|---|---|---|---|---|
| | (g) | | | | | | (mg/serving) | | | | | | | |
| **sorrel** (dock) | | | | | | | | | | | | | | |
| boiled, drained—*1 cup chopped* | 133 | | 114 | 124 | 202 | 140 | 43 | | 138 | 100 | 161 | 130 | 65 | 11617 |
| raw—*1 cup chopped* | 133 | | 125 | 136 | 222 | 153 | 47 | | 152 | 110 | 177 | 144 | 72 | 11616 |
| **spinach** boiled, drained—*1 cup* | 180 | 72 | 229 | 274 | 416 | 328 | 99 | 63 | 241 | 203 | 302 | 302 | 119 | 11458 |
| canned, drained—*1 cup* | 214 | 81 | 257 | 308 | 469 | 368 | 111 | 73 | 272 | 227 | 338 | 340 | 133 | 11461 |
| frozen—*1 cup* | 156 | 156 | 339 | 197 | 315 | 392 | 81 | 45 | 323 | 335 | 278 | 750 | 76 | 11463 |
| frozen, bld, drained—*1 cup* | 190 | 192 | 418 | 243 | 390 | 486 | 101 | 55 | 401 | 416 | 344 | 929 | 93 | 11464 |
| raw—*1 cup* | 30 | 12 | 37 | 44 | 67 | 52 | 16 | 11 | 39 | 32 | 48 | 49 | 19 | 11457 |
| souffle, homemade—*1 cup* | 136 | 147 | 420 | 613 | 964 | 760 | 282 | 129 | 554 | 477 | 688 | 498 | 313 | 11658 |
| **Swiss chard**, raw—*1 cup* | 36 | 6 | 30 | 53 | 47 | 36 | 7 | | 40 | | 40 | 42 | 13 | 11147 |
| **taro leaves**, steamed—*1 cup* | 145 | 38 | 132 | 206 | 310 | 194 | 62 | 51 | 155 | 141 | 203 | 174 | 90 | 11521 |
| **turnip greens and root**, frozen, boiled | | | | | | | | | | | | | | |
| drained—*1 cup* | 163 | 80 | 254 | 246 | 419 | 305 | 106 | 52 | 279 | 178 | 315 | 287 | 114 | 11577 |
| **turnip greens** | | | | | | | | | | | | | | |
| boiled, drained—*1 cup* | 144 | 29 | 91 | 85 | 151 | 107 | 37 | 19 | 101 | 63 | 112 | 104 | 40 | 11569 |
| canned, solids and liq—*1 cup* | 234 | 54 | 173 | 164 | 290 | 206 | 73 | 35 | 194 | 124 | 215 | 199 | 77 | 11570 |
| frozen—*1 cup* | 164 | 71 | 221 | 210 | 371 | 264 | 92 | 46 | 249 | 157 | 276 | 253 | 98 | 11574 |
| frozen, bld, drained—*1 cup chopped* | 164 | 95 | 302 | 284 | 503 | 358 | 125 | 62 | 338 | 213 | 374 | 344 | 133 | 11575 |
| raw—*1 cup* | 55 | 14 | 45 | 43 | 75 | 54 | 19 | 9 | 51 | 32 | 56 | 52 | 20 | 11568 |
| **vinespinach**, raw—*3.5 oz* | 100 | 28 | 55 | 53 | 101 | 86 | 19 | 27 | 85 | 48 | 65 | 70 | 39 | 11587 |
| **watercress**, raw—*1 cup* | 34 | 10 | 45 | 32 | 56 | 46 | 7 | 2 | 39 | 21 | 47 | 51 | 14 | 11591 |
| **winged bean leaves**, raw—*3.5 oz* | 100 | 116 | 182 | 204 | 359 | 228 | 64 | 75 | 188 | 126 | 245 | 178 | 82 | 11597 |
| **LEGUMES (BEANS AND PEAS)** | | | | | | | | | | | | | | |
| **adzuki beans**, mature | | | | | | | | | | | | | | |
| boiled—*1 cup* | 230 | 166 | 586 | 690 | 1454 | 1304 | 182 | 161 | 915 | 515 | 890 | 1118 | 455 | 16002 |
| dry—*½ cup* | 99 | 189 | 667 | 783 | 1651 | 1482 | 208 | 182 | 1041 | 585 | 1013 | 1271 | 519 | 16001 |
| sweetened (yokan)—*1 slice* | 14 | 4 | 16 | 18 | 39 | 35 | 5 | 4 | 24 | 14 | 24 | 30 | 12 | 16004 |
| canned—*1 slice* | 296 | 107 | 382 | 447 | 944 | 847 | 118 | 104 | 595 | 334 | 580 | 728 | 296 | 16003 |
| **baked beans** | | | | | | | | | | | | | | |
| homemade—*1 cup* | 253 | 170 | 577 | 612 | 1083 | 959 | 218 | 157 | 726 | 392 | 713 | 901 | 387 | 16005 |
| vegetarian, canned—*1 cup* | 254 | 130 | 378 | 574 | 1029 | 757 | 119 | 94 | 678 | 307 | 660 | 582 | 335 | 16006 |
| w/pork, cnd—*1 cup* | 253 | 157 | 559 | 587 | 1063 | 913 | 202 | 144 | 721 | 374 | 696 | 825 | 372 | 16009 |
| w/pork in sweet sauce, cnd—*1 cup* | 253 | 159 | 564 | 592 | 1073 | 921 | 205 | 147 | 726 | 377 | 703 | 832 | 374 | 16010 |
| w/pork in tomato sauce, cnd—*1 cup* | 253 | 190 | 354 | 564 | 969 | 827 | 101 | 106 | 602 | 299 | 640 | 582 | 299 | 16011 |
| **black beans**, mature | | | | | | | | | | | | | | |
| boiled—*1 cup* | 172 | 181 | 642 | 673 | 1218 | 1046 | 229 | 165 | 824 | 430 | 798 | 944 | 425 | 16015 |
| dry—*½ cup* | 97 | 248 | 882 | 925 | 1673 | 1439 | 315 | 228 | 1133 | 590 | 1096 | 1297 | 583 | 16014 |
| **black turtle beans**, mature | | | | | | | | | | | | | | |
| boiled—*1 cup* | 185 | 179 | 636 | 668 | 1208 | 1040 | 228 | 165 | 818 | 426 | 792 | 938 | 422 | 16017 |
| canned—*1 cup* | 240 | 170 | 610 | 638 | 1154 | 994 | 218 | 158 | 782 | 408 | 756 | 895 | 403 | 16018 |
| **broadbeans** (fava beans), immature | | | | | | | | | | | | | | |
| boiled, drained—*1 cup* | 170 | 82 | 303 | 366 | 629 | 532 | 63 | 112 | 332 | 286 | 400 | 675 | 196 | 11089 |
| raw—*1 cup* | 109 | 61 | 227 | 274 | 471 | 399 | 47 | 84 | 249 | 214 | 299 | 505 | 146 | 11088 |
| **broadbeans** (fava beans), mature | | | | | | | | | | | | | | |
| boiled—*1 cup* | 170 | 122 | 459 | 520 | 972 | 826 | 105 | 165 | 546 | 410 | 575 | 1193 | 328 | 16053 |
| canned—*1 cup* | 256 | 133 | 497 | 566 | 1052 | 896 | 115 | 179 | 591 | 443 | 622 | 1293 | 356 | 16054 |
| dry—*½ cup* | 75 | 185 | 696 | 790 | 1473 | 1253 | 160 | 251 | 827 | 620 | 871 | 1808 | 498 | 16052 |
| **chickpeas** (garbanzo beans), mature | | | | | | | | | | | | | | |
| boiled—*1 cup* | 164 | 139 | 540 | 623 | 1035 | 973 | 190 | 195 | 779 | 361 | 610 | 1369 | 400 | 16057 |
| canned—*1 cup* | 240 | 115 | 442 | 509 | 845 | 794 | 156 | 161 | 636 | 295 | 499 | 1118 | 326 | 16058 |
| dry—*½ cup* | 100 | 185 | 716 | 828 | 1374 | 1291 | 253 | 259 | 1034 | 479 | 809 | 1819 | 531 | 16056 |
| **cowpeas** (blackeyed peas), immature | | | | | | | | | | | | | | |
| boiled, drained—*1 cup* | 165 | 61 | 195 | 280 | 373 | 345 | 74 | 78 | 287 | 214 | 304 | 366 | 170 | 11192 |
| frozen—*1 cup* | 160 | 165 | 536 | 770 | 1024 | 944 | 205 | 214 | 789 | 589 | 832 | 1006 | 464 | 11195 |
| frzn, boiled, drained—*1 cup* | 170 | 167 | 537 | 774 | 1030 | 949 | 206 | 214 | 792 | 592 | 836 | 1012 | 466 | 11196 |
| raw—*1 cup* | 168 | 57 | 185 | 265 | 354 | 326 | 71 | 74 | 272 | 203 | 287 | 348 | 160 | 11191 |
| **cowpeas** (blackeyed peas), mature | | | | | | | | | | | | | | |
| boiled—*1 cup* | 172 | 163 | 506 | 540 | 1018 | 900 | 189 | 146 | 776 | 430 | 633 | 920 | 413 | 16063 |
| canned—*1 cup* | 240 | 139 | 432 | 463 | 871 | 770 | 161 | 125 | 665 | 367 | 542 | 787 | 353 | 16064 |
| dry—*½ cup* | 84 | 244 | 752 | 803 | 1514 | 1336 | 281 | 218 | 1153 | 638 | 942 | 1368 | 613 | 16062 |
| w/pork, canned—*1 cup* | 240 | 82 | 250 | 269 | 504 | 446 | 94 | 72 | 384 | 214 | 314 | 456 | 204 | 16065 |
| **cowpeas, catjang**, mature, boiled—*1 cup* | 171 | 171 | 528 | 564 | 1065 | 941 | 198 | 154 | 812 | 450 | 662 | 963 | 431 | 16061 |
| **cranberry beans** (Roman beans), mature | | | | | | | | | | | | | | |
| boiled—*1 cup* | 177 | 196 | 696 | 729 | 1320 | 1135 | 248 | 181 | 894 | 466 | 866 | 1023 | 460 | 16020 |
| canned—*1 cup* | 260 | 172 | 606 | 637 | 1152 | 991 | 216 | 156 | 780 | 406 | 754 | 892 | 400 | 16021 |
| **falafel**, from mature broadbeans | | | | | | | | | | | | | | |
| homemade—*0.6 oz patty (2¼″ dia)* | 17 | 23 | 84 | 96 | 160 | 146 | 32 | 31 | 120 | 58 | 96 | 218 | 62 | 16138 |

| | WT | TRY | THR | ISO | LEU | LYS | MET | CYS | PHE | TYR | VAL | ARG | HIS | REF |
|---|---|---|---|---|---|---|---|---|---|---|---|---|---|---|
| | (g) | | | | | | (mg/serving) | | | | | | | |
| **French beans**, mature, boiled—*1 cup* | 177 | 147 | 526 | 550 | 997 | 857 | 188 | 136 | 674 | 352 | 653 | 773 | 347 | 16023 |
| **great northern beans**, mature | | | | | | | | | | | | | | |
| boiled—*1 cup* | 177 | 175 | 621 | 651 | 1177 | 1012 | 221 | 161 | 798 | 416 | 772 | 913 | 411 | 16025 |
| canned—*1 cup* | 262 | 231 | 710 | 914 | 1640 | 1352 | 252 | 181 | 1140 | 456 | 1114 | 1058 | 529 | 16026 |
| dry—½ *cup* | 92 | 238 | 846 | 888 | 1605 | 1380 | 303 | 219 | 1087 | 566 | 1052 | 1245 | 559 | 16024 |
| **green peas** | | | | | | | | | | | | | | |
| boiled, drained—*1 cup* | 160 | 59 | 322 | 309 | 512 | 502 | 130 | 51 | 317 | 179 | 371 | 677 | 168 | 11305 |
| canned, drained—*1 cup* | 170 | 51 | 280 | 270 | 449 | 440 | 114 | 44 | 277 | 158 | 326 | 593 | 148 | 11308 |
| frozen—*1 cup* | 144 | 52 | 281 | 269 | 448 | 439 | 114 | 45 | 276 | 157 | 325 | 593 | 147 | 11312 |
| frzn, boiled, drained—*1 cup* | 160 | 56 | 309 | 296 | 491 | 483 | 125 | 48 | 304 | 173 | 357 | 651 | 162 | 11313 |
| raw—*1 cup* | 145 | 54 | 294 | 283 | 468 | 460 | 119 | 46 | 290 | 165 | 341 | 621 | 155 | 11304 |
| w/onions, red peppers garlic, cnd, solids and liq—*1 cup* | 228 | 48 | 264 | 253 | 420 | 413 | 107 | 41 | 260 | 148 | 306 | 556 | 139 | 11310 |
| **hummus** from chickpeas, homemade | | | | | | | | | | | | | | |
| *1 T* | 15 | 9 | 27 | 31 | 52 | 44 | 12 | 11 | 38 | 20 | 32 | 75 | 20 | 16137 |
| **hyacinth beans**, immature | | | | | | | | | | | | | | |
| boiled, drained—*1 cup* | 87 | | 108 | 175 | 267 | 177 | 23 | 17 | 57 | 46 | 190 | 175 | 108 | 11225 |
| **hyacinth beans**, mature, boiled—*1 cup* | 194 | 132 | 611 | 757 | 1341 | 1079 | 126 | 184 | 795 | 565 | 819 | 1160 | 452 | 16068 |
| **kidney beans**, all types, mature, | | | | | | | | | | | | | | |
| boiled—*1 cup* | 176 | 183 | 561 | 722 | 1295 | 1068 | 199 | 143 | 899 | 361 | 880 | 836 | 419 | 16028 |
| canned—*1 cup* | 256 | 161 | 494 | 635 | 1139 | 940 | 174 | 125 | 791 | 317 | 773 | 735 | 369 | 16029 |
| dry—½ *cup* | 92 | 257 | 913 | 958 | 1731 | 1489 | 327 | 236 | 1173 | 611 | 1134 | 1343 | 604 | 16027 |
| **kidney beans**, California red, mature | | | | | | | | | | | | | | |
| boiled—*1 cup* | 256 | 276 | 983 | 1032 | 1866 | 1605 | 351 | 253 | 1265 | 658 | 1224 | 1446 | 650 | 16031 |
| **kidney beans**, red, mature | | | | | | | | | | | | | | |
| boiled—*1 cup* | 177 | 182 | 646 | 678 | 1227 | 1053 | 230 | 166 | 830 | 432 | 804 | 950 | 428 | 16033 |
| dry—½ *cup* | 92 | 246 | 872 | 915 | 1655 | 1423 | 312 | 225 | 1121 | 583 | 1085 | 1283 | 577 | 16032 |
| **kidney beans**, royal red, mature, | | | | | | | | | | | | | | |
| boiled—*1 cup* | 177 | 198 | 706 | 742 | 1340 | 1152 | 253 | 182 | 908 | 473 | 878 | 1039 | 467 | 16036 |
| **lentils**, mature, boiled—*1 cup* | 198 | 160 | 640 | 772 | 1295 | 1247 | 152 | 234 | 881 | 477 | 887 | 1380 | 503 | 16070 |
| **lentils**, pink, mature, dry—½ *cup* | 96 | 214 | 859 | 1035 | 1737 | 1670 | 204 | 314 | 1181 | 640 | 1188 | 1851 | 674 | 16144 |
| **lima beans**, immature | | | | | | | | | | | | | | |
| baby, frzn, boiled, drained—*1 cup* | 180 | 157 | 508 | 770 | 940 | 790 | 119 | 146 | 590 | 385 | 747 | 801 | 407 | 11040 |
| baby, frozen—*1 cup* | 164 | 164 | 528 | 800 | 979 | 823 | 123 | 151 | 613 | 400 | 777 | 833 | 423 | 11039 |
| boiled, drained—*1 cup* | 170 | 151 | 491 | 745 | 910 | 765 | 116 | 141 | 571 | 372 | 722 | 775 | 393 | 11032 |
| green, cnd, solids & liq—*1 cup* | 248 | 134 | 429 | 647 | 791 | 665 | 99 | 122 | 496 | 325 | 630 | 675 | 342 | 11715 |
| green Fordhook, frozen, boiled, drained—*1 cup* | 170 | 136 | 437 | 663 | 811 | 682 | 102 | 126 | 508 | 332 | 644 | 690 | 350 | 11038 |
| **lima beans**, mature | | | | | | | | | | | | | | |
| baby, boiled—*1 cup* | 182 | 173 | 632 | 770 | 1263 | 981 | 186 | 162 | 843 | 517 | 881 | 897 | 448 | 16075 |
| dry—½ *cup* | 101 | 246 | 900 | 1096 | 1796 | 1396 | 264 | 230 | 1200 | 736 | 1252 | 1277 | 636 | 16074 |
| large, boiled—*1 cup* | 184 | 169 | 620 | 756 | 1238 | 962 | 182 | 158 | 826 | 508 | 863 | 880 | 438 | 16072 |
| large, canned—*1 cup* | 241 | 140 | 513 | 624 | 1024 | 795 | 149 | 130 | 684 | 419 | 713 | 728 | 364 | 16073 |
| large, dry—½ *cup* | 89 | 226 | 825 | 1005 | 1646 | 1280 | 241 | 211 | 1100 | 676 | 1149 | 1170 | 584 | 16071 |
| **lupins**, mature | | | | | | | | | | | | | | |
| boiled—*1 cup* | 166 | 208 | 951 | 1154 | 1960 | 1381 | 183 | 319 | 1026 | 971 | 1079 | 2771 | 735 | 16077 |
| dry—½ *cup* | 83 | 240 | 1105 | 1340 | 2277 | 1604 | 212 | 370 | 1191 | 1129 | 1253 | 3218 | 855 | 16076 |
| **mung beans**, mature | | | | | | | | | | | | | | |
| boiled—*1 cup* | 202 | 154 | 465 | 600 | 1099 | 990 | 170 | 125 | 858 | 424 | 735 | 994 | 414 | 16081 |
| dry—½ *cup* | 103 | 268 | 805 | 1038 | 1902 | 1714 | 295 | 216 | 1486 | 735 | 1274 | 1722 | 716 | 16080 |
| **mungo beans**, mature | | | | | | | | | | | | | | |
| boiled—*1 cup* | 180 | 140 | 472 | 693 | 1125 | 900 | 198 | 126 | 792 | 421 | 761 | 884 | 380 | 16084 |
| dry—½ *cup* | 103 | 271 | 901 | 1326 | 2152 | 1724 | 378 | 241 | 1517 | 806 | 1458 | 1691 | 727 | 16083 |
| **navy beans**, mature | | | | | | | | | | | | | | |
| boiled—*1 cup* | 182 | 182 | 526 | 704 | 1274 | 946 | 202 | 138 | 857 | 359 | 917 | 755 | 375 | 16038 |
| canned—*1 cup* | 262 | 236 | 726 | 933 | 1674 | 1381 | 257 | 186 | 1163 | 466 | 1137 | 1082 | 542 | 16039 |
| dry—½ *cup* | 104 | 257 | 739 | 990 | 1792 | 1331 | 284 | 194 | 1204 | 503 | 1291 | 1061 | 527 | 16037 |
| **peas, split**, mature, boiled—*1 cup* | 196 | 182 | 580 | 674 | 1172 | 1180 | 167 | 249 | 753 | 474 | 772 | 1458 | 398 | 16086 |
| **peas, split**, yellow and green, mature | | | | | | | | | | | | | | |
| dry—½ *cup* | 98 | 270 | 855 | 994 | 1725 | 1737 | 246 | 366 | 1109 | 697 | 1136 | 2144 | 585 | 16085 |
| **pigeon peas** | | | | | | | | | | | | | | |
| boiled—*1 cup* | 168 | 111 | 402 | 412 | 811 | 796 | 128 | 131 | 973 | 282 | 491 | 680 | 405 | 16102 |
| dry—½ *cup* | 103 | 218 | 790 | 809 | 1595 | 1567 | 250 | 258 | 1914 | 554 | 965 | 1338 | 797 | 16101 |
| **pink beans**, mature | | | | | | | | | | | | | | |
| boiled—*1 cup* | 169 | 181 | 644 | 676 | 1222 | 1051 | 230 | 167 | 828 | 431 | 801 | 948 | 426 | 16041 |
| dry—½ *cup* | 105 | 260 | 926 | 971 | 1757 | 1510 | 331 | 239 | 1190 | 620 | 1151 | 1363 | 612 | 16040 |
| **pinto beans**, mature | | | | | | | | | | | | | | |
| boiled—*1 cup* | 171 | 185 | 566 | 728 | 1308 | 1077 | 200 | 144 | 908 | 364 | 887 | 845 | 422 | 16043 |

| | WT | TRY | THR | ISO | LEU | LYS | MET | CYS | PHE | TYR | VAL | ARG | HIS | REF |
|---|---|---|---|---|---|---|---|---|---|---|---|---|---|---|
| | (g) | | | | | | (mg/serving) | | | | | | | |
| canned—*1 cup* | 240 | 139 | 492 | 514 | 931 | 802 | 178 | 127 | 631 | 326 | 612 | 725 | 324 | 16044 |
| dry—*½ cup* | 96 | 228 | 778 | 836 | 1496 | 1302 | 249 | 180 | 1051 | 410 | 958 | 1052 | 534 | 16042 |
| **refried beans**, canned—*1 cup* | 252 | 164 | 582 | 610 | 1104 | 950 | 209 | 151 | 748 | 391 | 723 | 857 | 386 | 16103 |
| **soybeans,** green/immature (edamame) | | | | | | | | | | | | | | |
| boiled, drained—*1 cup* | 180 | 270 | 886 | 977 | 1589 | 1330 | 270 | 203 | 1006 | 797 | 988 | 1789 | 598 | 11451 |
| frozen, heated—*1 cup* | 155 | 195 | 513 | 465 | 1155 | 1155 | 219 | 192 | 756 | 521 | 502 | 1122 | 414 | 11212 |
| raw—*1 cup* | 256 | 402 | 1321 | 1459 | 2371 | 1984 | 402 | 302 | 1500 | 1188 | 1475 | 2668 | 891 | 11450 |
| **soybeans,** mature, boiled—*1 cup* | 172 | 416 | 1244 | 1388 | 2331 | 1906 | 385 | 461 | 1495 | 1084 | 1429 | 2221 | 772 | 16109 |
| dry—*½ cup* | 93 | 550 | 1642 | 1833 | 3077 | 2517 | 509 | 609 | 1973 | 1431 | 1887 | 2932 | 1020 | 16108 |
| **white beans**, mature, boiled—*1 cup* | 179 | 206 | 732 | 768 | 1389 | 1196 | 261 | 190 | 942 | 490 | 911 | 1078 | 485 | 16050 |
| canned—*1 cup* | 262 | 225 | 799 | 838 | 1517 | 1305 | 286 | 207 | 1027 | 534 | 996 | 1176 | 529 | 16051 |
| dry—*½ cup* | 101 | 280 | 993 | 1041 | 1884 | 1619 | 355 | 257 | 1276 | 665 | 1234 | 1460 | 656 | 16049 |
| **white beans**, small, mature | | | | | | | | | | | | | | |
| boiled—*1 cup* | 179 | 190 | 675 | 709 | 1282 | 1103 | 242 | 175 | 868 | 453 | 840 | 993 | 448 | 16046 |
| dry—*½ cup* | 107 | 268 | 950 | 997 | 1803 | 1550 | 339 | 246 | 1221 | 636 | 1181 | 1398 | 629 | 16045 |
| **winged beans**, mature | | | | | | | | | | | | | | |
| boiled—*1 cup* | 172 | 401 | 619 | 771 | 1311 | 1121 | 187 | 286 | 750 | 765 | 803 | 991 | 415 | 16136 |
| dry—*½ cup* | 90 | 686 | 1061 | 1321 | 2247 | 1922 | 320 | 491 | 1286 | 1311 | 1377 | 1697 | 711 | 16135 |
| **yardlong bean**, immature, boiled, | | | | | | | | | | | | | | |
| drained—*1 cup sliced* | 104 | 30 | 98 | 140 | 187 | 173 | 37 | 40 | 145 | 107 | 152 | 184 | 85 | 11200 |
| **yardlong bean**, mature, boiled | | | | | | | | | | | | | | |
| *1 cup sliced* | 171 | 174 | 540 | 576 | 1086 | 959 | 202 | 156 | 828 | 458 | 675 | 982 | 439 | 16134 |
| **yellow beans**, mature, boiled—*1 cup* | 177 | 191 | 683 | 717 | 1296 | 1113 | 244 | 177 | 878 | 457 | 848 | 1004 | 451 | 16048 |
| **yellow snap beans**, raw—*1 cup* | 110 | 21 | 87 | 73 | 123 | 97 | 24 | 20 | 74 | 46 | 99 | 80 | 37 | 11722 |

## SPROUT AND SHOOT VEGETABLES

| | WT | TRY | THR | ISO | LEU | LYS | MET | CYS | PHE | TYR | VAL | ARG | HIS | REF |
|---|---|---|---|---|---|---|---|---|---|---|---|---|---|---|
| **bamboo shoots** | | | | | | | | | | | | | | |
| boiled, drained—*1 cup* | 120 | 19 | 60 | 61 | 98 | 95 | 20 | 16 | 64 | | 74 | 68 | 30 | 11027 |
| canned, drained—*1 cup* | 131 | 24 | 75 | 76 | 122 | 117 | 26 | 18 | 79 | | 93 | 84 | 37 | 11028 |
| raw—*1 cup* | 151 | 41 | 130 | 133 | 211 | 202 | 45 | 33 | 136 | | 160 | 146 | 63 | 11026 |
| **kidney bean sprouts**, bld, drained | | | | | | | | | | | | | | |
| *1 cup* | 125 | 62 | 254 | 268 | 434 | 344 | 62 | 69 | 304 | 208 | 310 | 329 | 169 | 11030 |
| **lentil sprouts**, stir-fried—*1 cup* | 125 | | 402 | 400 | 771 | 872 | 129 | 410 | 542 | 310 | 489 | 750 | 315 | 11249 |
| **mung bean sprouts** | | | | | | | | | | | | | | |
| boiled, drained—*1 cup* | 124 | 35 | 72 | 122 | 161 | 153 | 31 | 15 | 107 | 47 | 120 | 181 | 64 | 11044 |
| canned, drained—*1 cup* | 125 | 24 | 50 | 84 | 111 | 106 | 21 | 11 | 75 | 32 | 84 | 126 | 45 | 11626 |
| raw—*1 cup* | 104 | 38 | 81 | 137 | 182 | 173 | 35 | 18 | 122 | 54 | 135 | 205 | 73 | 11043 |
| stir-fried—*1 cup* | 124 | 72 | 151 | 257 | 341 | 324 | 66 | 32 | 227 | 100 | 253 | 383 | 135 | 11045 |
| **navy bean sprouts**, bld, drained—*1 cup* | 125 | 92 | 371 | 392 | 635 | 504 | 92 | 100 | 446 | 304 | 454 | 481 | 248 | 11047 |
| **pea sprouts**, bld, drained—*1 cup* | 125 | | 300 | 276 | 591 | 621 | 111 | 250 | 406 | 205 | 356 | 784 | 271 | 11317 |
| **soybean sprouts** | | | | | | | | | | | | | | |
| raw—*1 cup* | 70 | 111 | 352 | 406 | 657 | 526 | 97 | 110 | 449 | 334 | 434 | 634 | 244 | 11452 |
| steamed—*1 cup* | 94 | 97 | 306 | 352 | 571 | 457 | 84 | 96 | 390 | 290 | 377 | 550 | 212 | 11453 |
| stir-fried—*1 cup* | 125 | 199 | 629 | 726 | 1174 | 940 | 173 | 196 | 801 | 598 | 775 | 1131 | 435 | 11454 |

## TUBER AND ROOT VEGETABLES

| | WT | TRY | THR | ISO | LEU | LYS | MET | CYS | PHE | TYR | VAL | ARG | HIS | REF |
|---|---|---|---|---|---|---|---|---|---|---|---|---|---|---|
| **beet** | | | | | | | | | | | | | | |
| boiled, drained—*½ cup sliced* | 85 | 17 | 42 | 42 | 60 | 51 | 16 | 17 | 41 | 34 | 50 | 37 | 19 | 11081 |
| canned, drained—*1 cup* | 170 | 19 | 46 | 46 | 66 | 56 | 17 | 19 | 44 | 37 | 54 | 41 | 20 | 11084 |
| Harvard, cnd, solids and liq—*1 cup* | 246 | 25 | 62 | 62 | 86 | 74 | 25 | 25 | 59 | 49 | 71 | 54 | 27 | 11605 |
| pickled, cnd, solids and liq—*1 cup* | 227 | 20 | 54 | 54 | 77 | 66 | 20 | 23 | 52 | 43 | 64 | 48 | 25 | 11609 |
| raw—*½ cup sliced* | 68 | 13 | 32 | 33 | 46 | 39 | 12 | 13 | 31 | 26 | 38 | 29 | 14 | 11080 |
| **burdock root**, bld, drained—*1 cup slices* | 125 | 10 | 44 | 51 | 55 | 115 | 15 | 10 | 56 | 30 | 58 | 180 | 52 | 11105 |
| **carrot** | | | | | | | | | | | | | | |
| baby, raw—*1 medium* | 10 | 1 | 3 | 3 | 4 | 3 | 1 | 1 | 3 | 2 | 4 | 4 | 1 | 11960 |
| boiled, drained—*½ cup sliced* | 78 | 8 | 122 | 49 | 66 | 65 | 13 | 53 | 39 | 27 | 44 | 58 | 26 | 11125 |
| canned, drained—*1 cup sliced* | 146 | 12 | 193 | 77 | 102 | 102 | 20 | 83 | 61 | 42 | 70 | 92 | 39 | 11128 |
| frozen, bld, drained—*½ cup sliced* | 146 | 10 | 174 | 70 | 92 | 92 | 19 | 74 | 55 | 38 | 63 | 83 | 36 | 11131 |
| raw—*1 carrot (7½" long)* | 72 | 9 | 138 | 55 | 73 | 73 | 14 | 60 | 44 | 31 | 50 | 66 | 29 | 11124 |
| **cassava**, raw—*1 cup* | 206 | 39 | 58 | 56 | 80 | 91 | 23 | 58 | 54 | 35 | 72 | 282 | 41 | 11134 |
| **potato, French fries** | | | | | | | | | | | | | | |
| extruded, frzn, heated—*10 pieces* | 50 | 24 | 80 | 76 | 107 | 94 | 20 | 12 | 76 | 44 | 90 | 84 | 30 | 11409 |
| frzn—*10 pieces* | 50 | 10 | 39 | 39 | 66 | 66 | 18 | 18 | 48 | 38 | 62 | 64 | 23 | 11402 |
| frzn, baked—*10 pieces* | 50 | 12 | 46 | 46 | 78 | 78 | 21 | 21 | 56 | 46 | 74 | 76 | 27 | 11403 |
| **garlic**, raw—*3 cloves* | 9 | 6 | 14 | 20 | 28 | 25 | 7 | 6 | 16 | 7 | 26 | 57 | 10 | 11215 |
| **jicama (yambean)** | | | | | | | | | | | | | | |
| boiled, drained—*3.5 oz* | 100 | | 18 | 16 | 25 | 26 | 7 | 6 | 17 | 12 | 22 | 37 | 19 | 11604 |
| raw—*½ cup sliced* | 120 | | 22 | 19 | 30 | 31 | 8 | 7 | 20 | 14 | 26 | 44 | 23 | 11603 |

| | WT | TRY | THR | ISO | LEU | LYS | MET | CYS | PHE | TYR | VAL | ARG | HIS | REF |
|---|---|---|---|---|---|---|---|---|---|---|---|---|---|---|
| | (g) | (mg/serving) | | | | | | | | | | | | |
| **lotus root** | | | | | | | | | | | | | | |
| boiled, drained—*10 slices (2½″ dia)* | 89 | 11 | 28 | 29 | 37 | 51 | 12 | 12 | 25 | 15 | 30 | 47 | 20 | 11255 |
| raw—*10 slices (2½″ dia)* | 81 | 16 | 41 | 44 | 56 | 76 | 18 | 18 | 38 | 23 | 45 | 71 | 31 | 11254 |
| **mountain yam**, Hawaiian, steamed | | | | | | | | | | | | | | |
| *1 cup cubed* | 145 | 20 | 88 | 86 | 158 | 97 | 33 | 30 | 116 | 67 | 102 | 209 | 55 | 11259 |
| **onion rings**, breaded, parfried, frzn | | | | | | | | | | | | | | |
| heated—*10 med rings (2″ to 3″ dia)* | 60 | 42 | 90 | 128 | 210 | 91 | 49 | 65 | 146 | 94 | 130 | 195 | 65 | 11296 |
| **onion**, white | | | | | | | | | | | | | | |
| boiled, drained—*1 cup chopped* | 210 | 42 | 69 | 101 | 101 | 136 | 23 | 50 | 74 | 71 | 65 | 384 | 46 | 11283 |
| canned, sol and liq—*1 cup chopped* | 224 | 27 | 45 | 65 | 63 | 87 | 16 | 34 | 47 | 45 | 43 | 244 | 29 | 11285 |
| frozen, bld, drained—*1 cup chopped* | 210 | 23 | 38 | 57 | 57 | 76 | 13 | 29 | 42 | 40 | 38 | 214 | 25 | 11288 |
| raw—*1 cup chopped* | 160 | 22 | 34 | 22 | 40 | 62 | 3 | 6 | 40 | 22 | 34 | 166 | 22 | 11282 |
| **onion, Welsh**, raw—*1 cup chopped* | 160 | 34 | 118 | 130 | 181 | 152 | 34 | | 98 | 88 | 134 | 219 | 53 | 11293 |
| **potato**, baked—1 med (2¼″ dia) | 173 | 67 | 157 | 175 | 260 | 263 | 67 | 54 | 192 | 159 | 244 | 199 | 93 | 11674 |
| peeled—*1 potato (2⅓″ × 4¾″)* | 156 | 47 | 111 | 125 | 184 | 186 | 48 | 39 | 136 | 114 | 172 | 140 | 67 | 11363 |
| **potato**, cottage fries, frzn, heated | | | | | | | | | | | | | | |
| *10 pieces* | 50 | 23 | 78 | 74 | 104 | 92 | 20 | 10 | 74 | 43 | 88 | 82 | 29 | 11407 |
| **potato**, hashed brown | | | | | | | | | | | | | | |
| frozen, prep—*1 cup* | 156 | 66 | 223 | 212 | 296 | 262 | 55 | 31 | 211 | 123 | 251 | 232 | 83 | 11391 |
| homemade—*1 cup* | 156 | 73 | 170 | 192 | 282 | 284 | 73 | 61 | 207 | 175 | 262 | 217 | 105 | 11370 |
| **potato**, mashed | 240 | 82 | 178 | 202 | 305 | 262 | 82 | 50 | 206 | 185 | 264 | 187 | 103 | 11657 |
| from flakes w/o milk—*1 cup* | 210 | 57 | 141 | 153 | 246 | 191 | 71 | 36 | 200 | 134 | 208 | 149 | 78 | 11379 |
| from granules w/milk—*1 cup* | 210 | 65 | 204 | 235 | 370 | 284 | 88 | 44 | 214 | 204 | 281 | 172 | 109 | 11383 |
| homemade w/whole milk | | | | | | | | | | | | | | |
| and butter—*1 cup* | 210 | 71 | 162 | 183 | 277 | 242 | 76 | 46 | 189 | 166 | 239 | 170 | 94 | 11371 |
| **potato**, microwaved | | | | | | | | | | | | | | |
| *1 potato (2½″ diameter)* | 202 | 77 | 180 | 200 | 297 | 301 | 79 | 63 | 220 | 184 | 279 | 228 | 109 | 11675 |
| **potato pancake**, homemade—*1 pancake* | 76 | 38 | 87 | 100 | 151 | 141 | 40 | 35 | 112 | 90 | 135 | 125 | 55 | 11672 |
| **potato**, peeled | | | | | | | | | | | | | | |
| boiled—*1 med (2¼″ to 3¼″ dia)* | 167 | 45 | 104 | 117 | 172 | 174 | 45 | 37 | 127 | 107 | 160 | 132 | 63 | 11367 |
| canned, drained—*1 cup* | 180 | 40 | 92 | 103 | 153 | 155 | 40 | 32 | 113 | 94 | 144 | 117 | 56 | 11376 |
| microwaved—*1 potato (2⅓″ × 4¾″)* | 156 | 51 | 119 | 133 | 197 | 200 | 51 | 42 | 145 | 122 | 184 | 151 | 72 | 11368 |
| **potato puffs**, frzn, htd—*1 cup (18 puffs)* | 128 | 26 | 106 | 111 | 196 | 173 | 41 | 47 | 127 | 96 | 159 | 166 | 59 | 11399 |
| **potato**, raw—*1 med (2¼″ to 3¼″ dia)* | 213 | 68 | 160 | 179 | 264 | 268 | 70 | 55 | 196 | 164 | 249 | 202 | 96 | 11352 |
| **potato**, red-skinned | | | | | | | | | | | | | | |
| baked—*1 small (1¾″ to 2½″ dia)* | 138 | 33 | 112 | 106 | 160 | 167 | 51 | 40 | 222 | 86 | 161 | 163 | 55 | 11358 |
| raw—*1 medium (2¼″ to 3¼″ dia)* | 213 | 36 | 128 | 119 | 192 | 192 | 55 | 38 | 343 | 72 | 190 | 187 | 62 | 11355 |
| **potato**, russet | | | | | | | | | | | | | | |
| baked—*1 small (1¾″ to 2½″ dia)* | 138 | 34 | 102 | 106 | 150 | 175 | 47 | 37 | 241 | 97 | 171 | 155 | 57 | 11356 |
| raw—*1 medium (2¼″ to 3¼″ dia)* | 213 | 38 | 117 | 124 | 183 | 215 | 66 | 45 | 383 | 75 | 207 | 192 | 75 | 11353 |
| **potato salad**, homemade—*1 cup* | 250 | 105 | 290 | 352 | 505 | 428 | 165 | 127 | 338 | 260 | 430 | 380 | 155 | 11414 |
| **potato**, scalloped, homemade—*1 cup* | 245 | 103 | 282 | 353 | 551 | 470 | 142 | 83 | 331 | 296 | 426 | 289 | 172 | 11372 |
| **potato**, white-skinned | | | | | | | | | | | | | | |
| baked—*1 small (1¾″ to 2½″ dia)* | 138 | 33 | 94 | 92 | 132 | 148 | 43 | 32 | 203 | 69 | 139 | 139 | 47 | 11357 |
| raw—*1 medium (2¼″ to 3¼″ dia)* | 213 | 34 | 117 | 113 | 166 | 181 | 58 | 45 | 320 | 62 | 179 | 177 | 60 | 11354 |
| **potatoes** au gratin, homemade—*1 cup* | 245 | 172 | 470 | 696 | 1085 | 933 | 287 | 108 | 622 | 564 | 796 | 497 | 370 | 11373 |
| **potatoes O'Brien** | | | | | | | | | | | | | | |
| frozen, prepared—*⅔ cup* | 85 | 29 | 68 | 76 | 111 | 112 | 29 | 26 | 81 | 67 | 102 | 94 | 41 | 11397 |
| homemade—*1 cup* | 194 | 68 | 173 | 213 | 328 | 279 | 83 | 58 | 206 | 178 | 258 | 211 | 105 | 11671 |
| **radish**, Oriental | | | | | | | | | | | | | | |
| boiled, drained—*1 cup sliced* | 147 | 6 | 41 | 43 | 51 | 49 | 9 | 7 | 32 | 19 | 46 | 57 | 19 | 11431 |
| dried—*1 cup* | 116 | 50 | 378 | 399 | 479 | 456 | 87 | 72 | 304 | 174 | 423 | 529 | 173 | 11432 |
| raw—*1 radish (7″ long)* | 338 | 10 | 84 | 88 | 105 | 101 | 20 | 17 | 68 | 37 | 95 | 118 | 37 | 11430 |
| **radish**, red, raw—*½ cup sliced* | 58 | 5 | 13 | 12 | 18 | 19 | 6 | 6 | 21 | 5 | 20 | 22 | 8 | 11429 |
| **radish**, white icicle, raw—*½ cup sliced* | 50 | 3 | 22 | 24 | 29 | 28 | 5 | 4 | 18 | 10 | 26 | 32 | 10 | 11637 |
| **rutabaga (swede)** | | | | | | | | | | | | | | |
| boiled, drained—*1 cup cubed* | 170 | 24 | 85 | 90 | 70 | 71 | 17 | 20 | 58 | 42 | 87 | 270 | 54 | 11436 |
| raw—*1 cup cubed* | 140 | 18 | 64 | 70 | 53 | 55 | 14 | 15 | 43 | 32 | 67 | 207 | 42 | 11435 |
| **shallots**, raw—*4 T chopped* | 40 | 11 | 39 | 42 | 60 | 50 | 11 | | 32 | 29 | 44 | 72 | 17 | 11677 |
| **sweet potato** | | | | | | | | | | | | | | |
| baked—*1 med (2″ dia, 5″ long)* | 114 | 46 | 122 | 80 | 135 | 96 | 42 | 32 | 130 | 50 | 125 | 80 | 44 | 11508 |
| candied, homemade | | | | | | | | | | | | | | |
| *1 piece (2″ dia, 2½″ long)* | 105 | 12 | 45 | 46 | 68 | 46 | 22 | 7 | 55 | 38 | 60 | 42 | 18 | 11659 |
| cnd in light syrup, drained—*1 cup* | 196 | 31 | 125 | 125 | 184 | 123 | 63 | 20 | 151 | 104 | 165 | 118 | 47 | 11647 |
| canned, mashed—*1 cup* | 255 | 61 | 250 | 252 | 370 | 247 | 125 | 41 | 303 | 207 | 329 | 235 | 94 | 11514 |
| canned, vacuum pack—*1 cup pieces* | 200 | 66 | 176 | 114 | 194 | 138 | 60 | 46 | 188 | 72 | 180 | 116 | 64 | 11512 |
| frozen—*1 cup cubed* | 176 | 37 | 150 | 150 | 220 | 148 | 74 | 25 | 180 | 123 | 197 | 139 | 56 | 11516 |
| frozen, baked—*1 cup cubed* | 176 | 37 | 150 | 151 | 222 | 148 | 74 | 25 | 181 | 123 | 197 | 141 | 56 | 11517 |

| | WT | TRY | THR | ISO | LEU | LYS | MET | CYS | PHE | TYR | VAL | ARG | HIS | REF |
|---|---|---|---|---|---|---|---|---|---|---|---|---|---|---|
| | (g) | | | | | | (mg/serving) | | | | | | | |
| peeled, boiled—*1 cup mashed* | 328 | 92 | 239 | 157 | 266 | 190 | 82 | 62 | 256 | 98 | 246 | 157 | 89 | 11510 |
| raw—*1 medium (5" long)* | 130 | 40 | 108 | 72 | 120 | 86 | 38 | 29 | 116 | 44 | 112 | 72 | 40 | 11507 |
| **taro** | | | | | | | | | | | | | | |
| cooked—*1 cup sliced* | 132 | 11 | 32 | 25 | 50 | 30 | 9 | 15 | 37 | 25 | 37 | 48 | 16 | 11519 |
| raw—*1 cup* | 104 | 24 | 72 | 56 | 115 | 70 | 21 | 33 | 85 | 57 | 85 | 107 | 35 | 11518 |
| **turnip** | | | | | | | | | | | | | | |
| boiled, drained—*1 cup cubed* | 156 | 11 | 31 | 45 | 41 | 44 | 14 | 6 | 22 | 17 | 36 | 30 | 17 | 11565 |
| frozen, boiled, drained—*1 cup* | 156 | 23 | 66 | 97 | 89 | 95 | 30 | 14 | 47 | 36 | 80 | 64 | 37 | 11567 |
| raw—*1 cup cubed* | 130 | 12 | 32 | 47 | 43 | 47 | 14 | 6 | 22 | 17 | 39 | 31 | 18 | 11564 |
| **yam**, baked/bld, drained—*1 cup cubed* | 136 | 16 | 71 | 68 | 128 | 79 | 27 | 24 | 94 | 53 | 82 | 169 | 45 | 11602 |

## VEGETABLE COMBINATIONS

| | WT | TRY | THR | ISO | LEU | LYS | MET | CYS | PHE | TYR | VAL | ARG | HIS | REF |
|---|---|---|---|---|---|---|---|---|---|---|---|---|---|---|
| **corn, yellow** w/red and green peppers | | | | | | | | | | | | | | |
| cnd, solids and liquid—*1 cup* | 227 | 39 | 211 | 211 | 558 | 225 | 109 | 45 | 243 | 197 | 300 | 216 | 143 | 11184 |
| **green peas and carrots** | | | | | | | | | | | | | | |
| canned, solids and liq—*1 cup* | 255 | 41 | 207 | 201 | 319 | 314 | 79 | 33 | 201 | 115 | 240 | 418 | 107 | 11318 |
| frozen, drained—*½ cup* | 80 | 17 | 125 | 93 | 148 | 146 | 36 | 33 | 91 | 54 | 106 | 186 | 50 | 11323 |
| **green peas and onions** | | | | | | | | | | | | | | |
| canned, solids and liq—*1 cup* | 120 | 29 | 144 | 142 | 229 | 228 | 58 | 26 | 143 | 84 | 166 | 324 | 77 | 11324 |
| frozen, bld, drained—*1 cup* | 180 | 34 | 167 | 164 | 266 | 265 | 67 | 31 | 166 | 97 | 193 | 376 | 88 | 11327 |
| **mixed vegetables** | | | | | | | | | | | | | | |
| canned, drained—*1 cup* | 163 | 42 | 170 | 205 | 280 | 251 | 51 | 39 | 176 | 109 | 220 | 284 | 108 | 11581 |
| frozen—*1 cup* | 182 | 62 | 242 | 295 | 402 | 360 | 73 | 55 | 253 | 157 | 317 | 410 | 155 | 11583 |
| frozen, boiled, drained—*1 cup* | 182 | 53 | 209 | 253 | 346 | 309 | 62 | 47 | 218 | 135 | 271 | 351 | 133 | 11584 |
| frozen, drained—*1 cup* | 182 | 53 | 209 | 253 | 346 | 309 | 62 | 47 | 218 | 135 | 271 | 351 | 133 | 11584 |
| **succotash** (corn and lima beans) | | | | | | | | | | | | | | |
| boiled, drained—*1 cup* | 192 | 109 | 405 | 549 | 856 | 570 | 131 | 106 | 470 | 332 | 591 | 568 | 309 | 11496 |
| canned, solids and liq—*1 cup* | 255 | 74 | 275 | 375 | 584 | 388 | 89 | 71 | 321 | 227 | 403 | 388 | 212 | 11499 |
| frozen, bld, drained—*1 cup* | 170 | 82 | 304 | 413 | 644 | 428 | 99 | 80 | 354 | 250 | 445 | 427 | 233 | 11502 |
| w/cream style corn, cnd—*1 cup* | 266 | 80 | 293 | 396 | 617 | 410 | 93 | 77 | 338 | 239 | 426 | 410 | 223 | 11497 |

## OTHER VEGETABLES

| | WT | TRY | THR | ISO | LEU | LYS | MET | CYS | PHE | TYR | VAL | ARG | HIS | REF |
|---|---|---|---|---|---|---|---|---|---|---|---|---|---|---|
| **corn pudding**, homemade—*1 cup* | 250 | 130 | 480 | 522 | 1020 | 598 | 278 | 150 | 535 | 445 | 642 | 495 | 272 | 11656 |
| **corn, white**, steamed—*1 cup* | 164 | 92 | 500 | 581 | 1712 | 495 | 379 | 233 | 704 | 330 | | | | 35135 |
| **corn, yellow** | | | | | | | | | | | | | | |
| boiled, drained—*1 baby ear* | 8 | 2 | 11 | 11 | 29 | 11 | 6 | 2 | 12 | 10 | 15 | 11 | 7 | 11168 |
| canned, drained—*1 cup* | 164 | 41 | 133 | 139 | 549 | 415 | 102 | 67 | 205 | 171 | 208 | 184 | 120 | 11172 |
| canned, vacuum pack—*1 cup* | 210 | 36 | 204 | 204 | 546 | 214 | 105 | 42 | 235 | 193 | 290 | 206 | 139 | 11176 |
| creamed, canned—*1 cup* | 256 | 31 | 179 | 179 | 481 | 189 | 92 | 36 | 207 | 169 | 256 | 182 | 123 | 11174 |
| frozen—*1 cup* | 164 | 44 | 144 | 151 | 595 | 449 | 110 | 74 | 221 | 185 | 225 | 200 | 130 | 11178 |
| frozen, boiled, drained—*1 cup* | 164 | 51 | 189 | 225 | 412 | 251 | 112 | 62 | 215 | 174 | 274 | 207 | 110 | 11179 |
| frozen, microwaved—*1 cup* | 141 | 47 | 154 | 162 | 637 | 481 | 118 | 79 | 237 | 197 | 241 | 213 | 138 | 11182 |
| raw—*1 cup* | 154 | 35 | 199 | 199 | 536 | 211 | 103 | 40 | 231 | 189 | 285 | 202 | 137 | 11167 |
| **hominy, canned** | | | | | | | | | | | | | | |
| white—*1 cup* | 165 | 13 | 82 | 96 | 333 | 54 | 51 | 54 | 125 | 92 | 127 | 112 | 74 | 20030 |
| yellow—*1 cup* | 160 | 13 | 80 | 93 | 323 | 53 | 50 | 53 | 122 | 90 | 123 | 109 | 72 | 20330 |
| **kelp** (kombu/tangle), raw (seaweed)—*2 T* | 10 | 5 | 6 | 8 | 8 | 8 | 2 | 10 | 4 | 3 | 7 | 6 | 2 | 11445 |
| **laver** (nori), raw (seaweed)—*2 T (~4 sheets)* | 10 | 4 | 23 | 26 | 50 | 22 | 14 | 10 | 27 | 25 | 40 | 28 | 14 | 11446 |
| **mushrooms, common white** | | | | | | | | | | | | | | |
| boiled, drained—*1 cup pieces* | 156 | 37 | 117 | 83 | 131 | 117 | 34 | 14 | 94 | 48 | 254 | 86 | 62 | 11261 |
| canned, drained—*1 cup pieces* | 156 | 33 | 101 | 72 | 112 | 101 | 30 | 11 | 81 | 41 | 218 | 73 | 53 | 11264 |
| raw—*1 cup pieces* | 70 | 25 | 75 | 53 | 84 | 75 | 22 | 8 | 60 | 31 | 162 | 55 | 40 | 11260 |
| **mushrooms, crimini, italian**, brown, | | | | | | | | | | | | | | |
| raw—*1 piece* | 14 | 8 | 16 | 14 | 21 | 35 | 7 | 1 | 14 | 8 | 16 | 17 | 9 | 11266 |
| **mushrooms, enoki**, raw—*1 large* | 5 | 2 | 6 | 4 | 6 | 6 | 2 | 1 | 8 | 7 | 12 | 6 | 4 | 11950 |
| **mushrooms, oyster**, raw—*1 large* | 148 | 62 | 207 | 166 | 249 | 186 | 62 | 41 | 166 | 124 | 292 | 269 | 104 | 11987 |
| **mushrooms, portabella**, raw | | | | | | | | | | | | | | |
| *1 medium (3.9 oz)* | 110 | 34 | 75 | 54 | 88 | 68 | 20 | 13 | 60 | 47 | 169 | 75 | 47 | 11265 |
| **mushrooms, shitake** | | | | | | | | | | | | | | |
| cooked—*4 mushrooms* | 72 | 3 | 49 | 40 | 67 | 34 | 18 | 19 | 48 | 32 | 48 | 64 | 16 | 11269 |
| dried—*4 mushrooms* | 15 | 5 | 75 | 61 | 102 | 51 | 27 | 29 | 73 | 48 | 73 | 97 | 24 | 11268 |
| **nopales** (prickly pear) | | | | | | | | | | | | | | |
| cooked—*1 cup sliced* | 149 | 21 | 63 | 77 | 122 | 94 | 24 | 12 | 77 | 45 | 92 | 82 | 39 | 11964 |
| raw—*1 cup sliced* | 86 | 12 | 34 | 42 | 66 | 51 | 13 | 7 | 42 | 25 | 51 | 45 | 22 | 11963 |
| **spirulina** (seaweed) | | | | | | | | | | | | | | |
| dried—*1 cup* | 15 | 139 | 446 | 481 | 742 | 454 | 172 | 99 | 417 | 388 | 527 | 622 | 163 | 11667 |
| raw—*1 oz* | 28 | 27 | 86 | 93 | 143 | 87 | 33 | 19 | 80 | 74 | 101 | 120 | 31 | 11666 |
| **wakame** (seaweed), raw—*2 T* | 10 | 4 | 16 | 9 | 26 | 11 | 6 | 3 | 11 | 5 | 21 | 9 | 2 | 11669 |

| | WT (g) | TRY | THR | ISO | LEU | LYS | MET | CYS | PHE | TYR | VAL | ARG | HIS | REF |
|---|---|---|---|---|---|---|---|---|---|---|---|---|---|---|
| | | | | | | | (mg/serving) | | | | | | | |

### 31. MISCELLANEOUS FOOD INGREDIENTS

| | WT (g) | TRY | THR | ISO | LEU | LYS | MET | CYS | PHE | TYR | VAL | ARG | HIS | REF |
|---|---|---|---|---|---|---|---|---|---|---|---|---|---|---|
| **baking chocolate** (unsweetened)—*1 oz* | 28 | 36 | 104 | 115 | 195 | 132 | 39 | 63 | 147 | 119 | 183 | 228 | 60 | 19078 |
| liquid—*1 oz packet* | 28 | 51 | 135 | 132 | 206 | 171 | 35 | 41 | 164 | 128 | 204 | 193 | 59 | 19077 |
| **carob powder**—*1 cup* | 103 | 49 | 279 | 215 | 455 | 202 | 83 | 30 | 156 | 124 | 459 | 134 | 126 | 16055 |
| **cocoa powder**, unsweetened—*1 T* | 5.4 | 16 | 42 | 41 | 64 | 53 | 11 | 13 | 51 | 40 | 64 | 60 | 18 | 19165 |
| processed w/alkali (dutched)—*1 T* | 5.4 | 15 | 39 | 38 | 59 | 49 | 10 | 12 | 47 | 37 | 59 | 55 | 17 | 19166 |
| **cornstarch**—*¼ cup* | 32 | 0 | 3 | 3 | 12 | 2 | 2 | 2 | 4 | 3 | 4 | 4 | 3 | 20027 |
| **gelatin**, dry, unsweetened | | | | | | | | | | | | | | |
| 1 oz packet (4 T) | 28 | 0 | 413 | 324 | 687 | 969 | 170 | 0 | 486 | 85 | 583 | 1852 | 185 | 19177 |
| **soy pro concentrate** | | | | | | | | | | | | | | |
| acid wash—*1 oz* | 28 | 234 | 693 | 824 | 1377 | 1100 | 228 | 248 | 918 | 644 | 858 | 1300 | 442 | 16420 |
| alcohol extraction—*1 oz* | 28 | 234 | 693 | 824 | 1377 | 1100 | 228 | 248 | 918 | 644 | 858 | 1300 | 442 | 16121 |
| **soy protein isolate**—*1 oz* | 28 | 312 | 878 | 1191 | 1899 | 1492 | 316 | 293 | 1286 | 902 | 1147 | 1868 | 645 | 16122 |
| potassium type | 28 | 312 | 878 | 1191 | 1899 | 1492 | 316 | 293 | 1286 | 902 | 1147 | 1868 | 645 | 16422 |
| ProPlus, Protein Tech Intl—*1 oz* | 28 | 308 | 924 | 1176 | 1988 | 1512 | 308 | 308 | 1260 | 924 | 1232 | 1820 | 616 | 16176 |
| Supro, Protein Tech Intl—*1 oz* | 28 | 308 | 924 | 1204 | 2016 | 1540 | 322 | 322 | 1288 | 924 | 1260 | 1876 | 644 | 16175 |
| **tapioca**, pearl, dry—*1 cup* | 152 | 5 | 6 | 6 | 9 | 9 | 3 | 6 | 6 | 3 | 8 | 29 | 5 | 20068 |
| **whey, acid** | | | | | | | | | | | | | | |
| dry—*1 cup* | 57 | 137 | 336 | 331 | 636 | 575 | 126 | 120 | 220 | 171 | 330 | 186 | 131 | 1113 |
| fluid—*1 cup* | 246 | 39 | 93 | 93 | 177 | 160 | 34 | 34 | 62 | 47 | 93 | 52 | 37 | 1112 |
| **whey, sweet** | | | | | | | | | | | | | | |
| dry—*1 cup* | 145 | 297 | 1185 | 1043 | 1720 | 1494 | 349 | 367 | 590 | 526 | 1011 | 544 | 344 | 1115 |
| fluid—*1 cup* | 246 | 32 | 133 | 116 | 192 | 167 | 39 | 42 | 66 | 59 | 113 | 62 | 39 | 1114 |
| **yeast, baker's** | | | | | | | | | | | | | | |
| active dry—*0.25 oz package* | 7 | 34 | 139 | 152 | 214 | 221 | 53 | 36 | 130 | 111 | 164 | 148 | 70 | 18375 |
| compressed—*0.6 oz cake* | 17 | 18 | 74 | 81 | 114 | 117 | 28 | 19 | 69 | 59 | 87 | 79 | 37 | 18374 |

# Caffeine and Theobromine

| | CAFFEINE (mg/100 g) | THEOBROMINE (mg/100 g) | SERVING SIZE (g) | CAFFEINE (mg/serving) | THEOBROMINE (mg/serving) | SOURCE (SR21 CODE NUMBER) |
|---|---|---|---|---|---|---|
| **BEVERAGES** | | | | | | |
| **CARBONATED, LOW CALORIE BEVERAGES** | | | | | | |
| Cherry Coke Zero | 10 | | 12 fl oz (355 g) | 36 | | COLA |
| Coca-Cola Zero | 10 | | 12 fl oz (355 g) | 36 | | COLA |
| Diet Cherry Coke | 10 | | 12 fl oz (355 g) | 36 | | COLA |
| diet chocolate soda | 12 | 0 | 12 fl oz (355 g) | 43 | 0 | FNDDS |
| Diet Coke | 13 | | 12 fl oz (355 g) | 46 | | COLA |
| Diet Coke with lime | 13 | | 12 fl oz (355 g) | 46 | | COLA |
| Diet Coke with Splenda | 10 | | 12 fl oz (355 g) | 36 | | COLA |
| diet cola with aspartame | 12 | 0 | 12 fl oz (355 g) | 43 | 0 | SR21 (14416) |
| diet cola with sodium saccharin | 11 | 0 | 12 fl oz (355 g) | 39 | 0 | SR21 (14166) |
| diet fruit-flavored soda with caffeine | 15 | 0 | 12 fl oz (355 g) | 53 | 0 | FNDDS |
| Diet Inca Cola | 11 | | 12 fl oz (355 g) | 39 | | COLA |
| Diet Mello Yello | 9 | 0 | 12 fl oz (355 g) | 32 | 0 | COLA |
| Diet Mr. Pibb | 8 | 0 | 12 fl oz (355 g) | 28 | 0 | COLA |
| diet pepper-type soda | 12 | 0 | 12 fl oz (355 g) | 43 | 0 | FNDDS |
| Diet RC | 9 | 0 | 12 fl oz (355 g) | 33 | 0 | Bunker and McWilliams, 1979 |
| Diet-Rite | 9 | 0 | 12 fl oz (355 g) | 32 | 0 | Bunker and McWilliams, 1979 |
| Pibb Zero | 11 | | 12 fl oz (355 g) | 39 | | COLA |
| Tab | 13 | | 12 fl oz (355 g) | 46 | | COLA |
| Vanilla Coke Zero | 10 | | 12 fl oz (355 g) | 36 | | COLA |
| **CARBONATED, SUGAR-SWEETENED BEVERAGES** | | | | | | |
| Cherry Coke | 9 | | 12 fl oz (370 g) | 33 | | COLA |
| cherry cola, Shasta | 12 | 0 | 12 fl oz (370 g) | 44 | 0 | SHST |
| chocolate-flavored soda | 2 | 63 | 12 fl oz (369 g) | 7 | 232 | SR21 (14552) |
| Coca-Cola Blak | 19 | | 12 fl oz (370 g) | 70 | | COLA |
| Coca-Cola Classic | 9 | | 12 fl oz (370 g) | 33 | | COLA |
| Coca-Cola with lime | 9 | | 12 fl oz (370 g) | 33 | | COLA |
| cola with fruit/vanilla flavor | 8 | 0 | 12 fl oz (370 g) | 30 | 0 | FNDDS |
| cola with higher caffeine (e.g., Jolt Cola) | 27 | 0 | 12 fl oz (370 g) | 100 | 0 | SR21 (14148) |

| | CAFFEINE (mg/100 g) | THEOBROMINE (mg/100 g) | SERVING SIZE (g) | CAFFEINE (mg/serving) | THEOBROMINE (mg/serving) | SOURCE (SR21 CODE NUMBER) |
|---|---|---|---|---|---|---|
| Cola | 8 | 0 | 12 fl oz (370 g) | 30 | 0 | SR21 (14400) |
| Dr. Pepper | 16 | 0 | 12 fl oz (370 g) | 61 | 0 | Bunker and McWilliams, 1979 |
| Floatz, Barq's | 6 | | 12 fl oz (370 g) | 22 | | COLA |
| fruit-flavored soda with caffeine | 15 | 0 | 12 fl oz (370 g) | 56 | 0 | FNDDS |
| Inca Cola | 10 | | 12 fl oz (370 g) | 37 | | COLA |
| lemon-lime soda with caffeine | 15 | 0 | 12 fl oz (368 g) | 55 | 0 | SR21 (14144) |
| Mello Yello | 14 | | 12 fl oz (370 g) | 52 | | COLA |
| Mello Yello cherry | 14 | | 12 fl oz (370 g) | 52 | | COLA |
| Mello Yello melon | 14 | | 12 fl oz (370 g) | 52 | | COLA |
| Moon Mist | 14 | 0 | 12 fl oz (370 g) | 52 | 0 | SHST |
| Mountain Dew | 15 | 0 | 12 fl oz (370 g) | 55 | 0 | Bunker and McWilliams, 1979 |
| Mr. Pibb | 7 | 0 | 12 fl oz (370 g) | 26 | 0 | COLA |
| pepper-type soda | 10 | 0 | 12 fl oz (368 g) | 37 | 0 | SR21 (14153) |
| Pepsi-Cola | 12 | 0 | 12 fl oz (370 g) | 43 | 0 | Bunker and McWilliams, 1979 |
| Pibb Xtra | 11 | | 12 fl oz (370 g) | 41 | | COLA |
| RC Cola | 9 | 0 | 12 fl oz (370 g) | 34 | 0 | Bunker and McWilliams, 1979 |
| Red Flash | 11 | | 12 fl oz (370 g) | 41 | | COLA |
| root beer, Barq's | 6 | | 12 fl oz (370 g) | 22 | | COLA |
| Surge | 9 | 0 | 12 fl oz (370 g) | 33 | 0 | COLA |
| Vanilla Coke | 9 | | 12 fl oz (370 g) | 33 | | COLA |

**COFFEE BEVERAGES**

| | CAFFEINE (mg/100 g) | THEOBROMINE (mg/100 g) | SERVING SIZE (g) | CAFFEINE (mg/serving) | THEOBROMINE (mg/serving) | SOURCE (SR21 CODE NUMBER) |
|---|---|---|---|---|---|---|
| Caffe Americano, Starbucks | 47 | | grande; 16 fl oz (475 g) | 223 | | STAR |
| Caffe Latte with 2% milk, Starbucks | 31 | | grande; 16 fl oz (480 g) | 149 | | STAR |
| Caffe Mocha with 2% milk and whipped cream, Starbucks | 36 | 0 | grande; 16 fl oz (480 g) | 173 | 0 | STAR |
| café con leche with sugar | 18 | 0 | 8 fl oz (245 g) | 44 | 0 | FNDDS |
| cappuccino | 20 | 0 | 4 fl oz (120 g) | 24 | 0 | FNDDS |
| cappuccino with 2% milk, Starbucks | 31 | | grande; 16 fl oz (480 g) | 149 | | STAR |
| Caramel Macchiato with 2% milk, Starbucks | 31 | | grande; 16 fl oz (480 g) | 149 | | STAR |
| Caramocha, Planet Java | 23 | 0 | 9.5 fl oz (285 g) | 66 | 0 | COLA |
| coffee and chicory instant powder | 2063 | 0 | 1 round t (1.8 g) | 37 | 0 | SR21 (14222) |
| coffee and chicory, brewed | 3142 | 0 | 8 fl oz (237 g) | 7447 | 0 | SR21 (14222) |
| coffee and cocoa instant powder with whitener and low-calorie sweetener | 476 | 390 | 1 t (6 g) | 29 | 23 | SR21 (43343) |
| coffee and cocoa instant powder, decaffeinated, with whitener and low-calorie sweetener | 25 | 324 | 1 t (6 g) | 2 | 19 | SR21 (14204) |
| coffee instant powder | 3142 | 0 | 1 round t (1.5 g) | 47 | 0 | SR21 (14214) |
| coffee instant powder, cappuccino flavor with sugar | 302 | 0 | 2 round t (14 g) | 42 | 0 | SR21 (14228) |
| coffee instant powder, decaffeinated | 122 | 0 | 1 round t (1.8 g) | 2 | 0 | SR21 (14218) |
| coffee instant powder, French flavor with sugar | 246 | 0 | 2 round t (12 g) | 30 | 0 | SR21 (14229) |
| coffee instant powder, mocha flavor with sugar | 360 | 294 | 2 round t (12 g) | 43 | 35 | SR21 (14224) |
| coffee, acid neutralized, from instant powder | 29 | 0 | 8 fl oz (237 g) | 69 | 0 | FNDDS |
| coffee, brewed | 40 | 0 | 8 fl oz (237 g) | 95 | 0 | SR21 (14209) |
| coffee, decaffeinated, brewed | 1 | 0 | 8 fl oz (237 g) | 2 | 0 | SR21 (14201) |
| coffee, decaffeinated, from instant powder | 1 | 0 | 8 fl oz (237 g) | 2 | 0 | SR21 (14219) |
| coffee, dripolated | 104 | 0 | 8 fl oz (237 g) | 245 | 0 | Bunker and McWilliams, 1979 |
| coffee, from instant powder | 26 | 0 | 8 fl oz (237 g) | 62 | 0 | SR21 (14215) |
| coffee, from liquid concentrate | 19 | 0 | 8 fl oz (237 g) | 45 | 0 | FNDDS |
| coffee, percolated | 78 | 0 | 8 fl oz (237 g) | 185 | 0 | Bunker and McWilliams, 1979 |
| espresso, decaffeinated | 1 | 0 | 6 fl oz (178 g) | 2 | 0 | SR21 (14202) |
| espresso, from restaurant | 212 | 0 | 6 fl oz (178 g) | 377 | 0 | SR21 (14210) |
| espresso, Starbucks | 250 | | solo; 5 fl oz (150 g) | 375 | | STAR |
| Frappuccino, caramel with whipped cream, Starbucks | 23 | | grande; 16 fl oz (480 g) | 110 | | STAR |

| | CAFFEINE (mg/100 g) | THEOBROMINE (mg/100 g) | SERVING SIZE (g) | CAFFEINE (mg/serving) | THEOBROMINE (mg/serving) | SOURCE (SR21 CODE NUMBER) |
|---|---|---|---|---|---|---|
| Frappuccino, caramel, light, Starbucks | 20 | | grande; 16 fl oz (480 g) | 96 | | STAR |
| Frappuccino, cinnamon dolce with whipped cream, Starbucks | 23 | | grande; 16 fl oz (480 g) | 110 | | STAR |
| Frappuccino, mocha with whipped cream, Starbucks | 24 | | grande; 16 fl oz (480 g) | 115 | | STAR |
| Frappuccino, mocha, light, Starbucks | 20 | | grande; 16 fl oz (480 g) | 96 | | STAR |
| Frappuccino, vanilla with whipped cream, Starbucks | 24 | | grande; 16 fl oz (480 g) | 115 | | STAR |
| Frappuccino, vanilla, light, Starbucks | 21 | | grande; 16 fl oz (480 g) | 101 | | STAR |
| Iced Caffe Latte with 2% milk, Starbucks | 31 | | grande; 16 fl oz (480 g) | 149 | | STAR |
| Iced Caffe Mocha with 2% milk and whipped cream, Starbucks | 36 | | grande; 16 fl oz (480 g) | 173 | | STAR |
| latte | 76 | 0 | 8 fl oz (240 g) | 182 | 0 | FNDDS |
| latte, cinnamon dolce, with 2% milk and whipped cream, Starbucks | 31 | | grande; 16 fl oz (480 g) | 149 | | STAR |
| latte, vanilla, skinny (with sugar-free syrup and nonfat milk), Starbucks | 31 | | grande; 16 fl oz (480 g) | 149 | | STAR |
| latte, vanilla, with 2% milk, Starbucks | 31 | | grande; 16 fl oz (480 g) | 149 | | STAR |
| white chocolate mocha with 2% milk and whipped cream, Starbucks | 31 | | grande; 16 fl oz (480 g) | 149 | | STAR |
| **LIQUEURS** | | | | | | |
| liqueur, coffee with cream, 34 proof | 8 | 0 | 1.5 fl oz (47 g) | 4 | 0 | SR21 (14415) |
| liqueur, coffee, 53 proof | 26 | 0 | 1.5 fl oz (52 g) | 14 | 0 | SR21 (14414) |
| liqueur, coffee, 63 proof | 26 | 0 | 1.5 fl oz (52 g) | 14 | 0 | SR21 (14535) |
| **SPORT AND ENERGY BEVERAGES** | | | | | | |
| KMX, blue | 15 | 0 | 8.4 fl oz (252 g) | 38 | 0 | COLA |
| KMX, orange | 15 | 0 | 8.4 fl oz (252 g) | 38 | 0 | COLA |
| Red Bull, added caffeine and vitamins | 30 | 0 | 8 fl oz (240 g) | 72 | 0 | SR21 (14154) |
| Red Bull, sugar free, added caffeine and vitamins | 30 | 0 | 8 fl oz (240 g) | 72 | 0 | SR21 (14156) |
| **TEA** | | | | | | |
| iced tea instant powder, decaffeinated | 169 | 11 | 1 t (11 g) | 19 | 1 | SR21 (14353) |
| iced tea instant powder, lemon flavor | 2066 | 40 | 2 round T (11 g) | 227 | 4 | SR21 (14368) |
| iced tea instant powder, lemon flavor with sodium saccharin | 2240 | 24 | 4 T (14 g) | 314 | 3 | SR21 (14375) |
| iced tea instant powder, lemon flavor with sugar | 35 | 1 | 3 heaping t (23 g) | 8 | 0 | SR21 (14370) |
| iced tea with lemon, canned/bottled, Nestea | 3 | 0 | 8 fl oz (240 g) | 7 | 0 | SR21 (14137) |
| iced tea, canned/bottled, Cool from Nestea | 5 | 0 | 8 fl oz (237 g) | 12 | 0 | COLA |
| iced tea, diet lemon, canned/bottled, Nestea | 5 | 0 | 8 fl oz (238 g) | 12 | 0 | COLA |
| iced tea, diet, canned/bottled, Cool from Nestea | 3 | 0 | 8 fl oz (240 g) | 7 | 0 | COLA |
| iced tea, Earl Grey, canned/bottled, Nestea | 14 | 0 | 8 fl oz (240 g) | 34 | 0 | COLA |
| iced tea, from instant | 11 | 0 | 8 fl oz (237 g) | 26 | 0 | SR21 (14367) |
| iced tea, lemon flavor with sodium saccharin, from instant | 11 | 0 | 8 fl oz (237 g) | 26 | 0 | SR21 (14376) |
| iced tea, lemon flavor with sugar, from instant | 3 | 0 | 8 fl oz (259 g) | 8 | 0 | SR21 (14371) |

| | CAFFEINE (mg/100 g) | THEOBROMINE (mg/100 g) | SERVING SIZE (g) | CAFFEINE (mg/serving) | THEOBROMINE (mg/serving) | SOURCE (SR21 CODE NUMBER) |
|---|---|---|---|---|---|---|
| iced tea, lemon flavor with sugar, from instant, Lipton | 42 | 0 | 8 fl oz (259 g) | 109 | 0 | Groisser, 1978 |
| iced tea, lemon flavor with sugar, from instant, Nestea | 37 | 0 | 8 fl oz (259 g) | 96 | 0 | Groisser, 1978 |
| iced tea, lemon flavor, from instant | 11 | 0 | 8 fl oz (238 g) | 26 | 0 | SR18 (14369) |
| iced tea, lemon flavor, sugar-sweetened, canned/bottled, Arizona | 5 | 0 | 8 fl oz (227 g) | 11 | 0 | SR21 (14475) |
| iced tea, lemon flavor, sugar-sweetened, canned/bottled, Lipton Brisk | 2 | 0 | 8 fl oz (245 g) | 5 | 0 | SR21 (14476) |
| iced tea, lemon green, canned/bottled, Mad River | 10 | 0 | 8 fl oz (240 g) | 24 | 0 | COLA |
| iced tea, lemon/peach/raspberry, canned/bottled, Nestea | 5 | 0 | 8 fl oz (240 g) | 12 | 0 | COLA |
| iced tea, no ice, Wendy's | 8 | 1 | 12 fl oz (356 g) | 28 | 4 | SR21 (14601) |
| iced tea, oolong with honey, canned/bottled, Mad River | 13 | 0 | 8 fl oz (240 g) | 31 | 0 | COLA |
| iced tea, red, canned/bottled, Mad River | 10 | 0 | 8 fl oz (240 g) | 24 | 0 | COLA |
| iced tea, unsweetened, canned/bottled, Nestea | 7 | 0 | 8 fl oz (240 g) | 17 | 0 | COLA |
| lemonade with Tazo Zen green tea, Starbucks | 5 | | grande; 16 fl oz (475 g) | 24 | | STAR |
| tea, black, brewed 1 minute from bag | 20 | 0 | 8 fl oz (237 g) | 47 | 0 | Bunker and McWilliams, 1979 |
| tea, black, brewed 3 minutes | 20 | 2 | 8 fl oz (237 g) | 47 | 5 | SR21 (14355) |
| tea, black, brewed 4 minutes from bag, Lipton | 21 | 0 | 8 fl oz (237 g) | 50 | 0 | Groisser, 1978 |
| tea, black, brewed 4 minutes from bag, Red Rose | 25 | 0 | 8 fl oz (237 g) | 60 | 0 | Groisser, 1978 |
| tea, black, brewed 4 minutes from bag, Salada | 22 | 0 | 8 fl oz (237 g) | 52 | 0 | Groisser, 1978 |
| tea, black, brewed 4 minutes from bag, Tetley | 14 | 0 | 8 fl oz (237 g) | 33 | 0 | Groisser, 1978 |
| tea, black, brewed 4 minutes from bag, Twinings Darjeeling | 36 | 0 | 8 fl oz (237 g) | 85 | 0 | Groisser, 1978 |
| tea, black, brewed 4 minutes from bag, Twinings English Breakfast | 29 | 0 | 8 fl oz (239 g) | 68 | 0 | Groisser, 1978 |
| tea, black, brewed 4 minutes from loose tea, Twining | 43 | 0 | 8 fl oz (237 g) | 101 | 0 | Groisser, 1978 |
| tea, black, brewed 5 minutes from bag | 33 | 0 | 8 fl oz (237 g) | 77 | 0 | Bunker and McWilliams, 1979 |
| tea, black, brewed 5 minutes from loose tea | 28 | 0 | 8 fl oz (237 g) | 67 | 0 | Bunker and McWilliams, 1979 |
| tea, black, brewed, with low calorie sweetener | 20 | 2 | 8 fl oz (237 g) | 47 | 5 | FNDDS |
| tea, black, brewed, with sugar | 19 | 2 | 8 fl oz (237 g) | 46 | 5 | FNDDS |
| tea, black, decaffeinated, brewed | 1 | 0 | 8 fl oz (237 g) | 2 | 0 | FNDDS |
| tea, black, decaffeinated, brewed 3 minutes | 1 | 0 | 8 fl oz (237 g) | 2 | 0 | SR21 (14352) |
| tea, black, from frozen concentrate | 20 | 2 | 8 fl oz (237 g) | 47 | 5 | FNDDS |
| tea, black, from instant powder | 11 | 0 | 8 fl oz (237 g) | 26 | 0 | Ahuja and Perloff, 2001 |
| tea, black, from instant powder, Lipton | 34 | 0 | 8 fl oz (237 g) | 81 | 0 | Groisser, 1978 |
| tea, black, from instant powder, Nestea | 27 | 0 | 8 fl oz (237 g) | 63 | 0 | Groisser, 1978 |
| tea, black oolong, brewed 4 minutes from loose tea, Jackson Formosa | 23 | 0 | 8 fl oz (237 g) | 55 | 0 | Groisser, 1978 |
| tea, green, brewed 5 minutes from loose tea | 25 | 0 | 8 fl oz (237 g) | 59 | 0 | Bunker and McWilliams, 1979 |
| tea, green, Chinese, brewed 4 minutes from bag | 20 | 0 | 8 fl oz (237 g) | 47 | 0 | Groisser, 1978 |

| | CAFFEINE (mg/100 g) | THEOBROMINE (mg/100 g) | SERVING SIZE (g) | CAFFEINE (mg/serving) | THEOBROMINE (mg/serving) | SOURCE (SR21 CODE NUMBER) |
|---|---|---|---|---|---|---|
| tea, green, Japanese, brewed 5 minutes | 14 | 0 | 8 fl oz (237 g) | 34 | 0 | Bunker and McWilliams, 1979 |
| **OTHER BEVERAGES** | | | | | | |
| Mountain berry, Mad River | 2 | 0 | 8 fl oz (250 g) | 5 | 0 | COLA |
| orange carrot medley, Mad River | 2 | 0 | 8 fl oz (250 g) | 5 | 0 | COLA |
| **CANDY** | | | | | | |
| After Eight Mints, Nestle | 20 | 142 | 5 mints (41 g) | 8 | 58 | SR18 (19153) |
| almonds, chocolate-covered | 6 | 62 | 1 oz (28 g) | 2 | 17 | FNDDS |
| Baby Ruth, Nestle | 4 | 119 | 0.7 oz bar (21 g) | 1 | 25 | SR21 (19111) |
| Bar None | 11 | 0 | 2 oz (57 g) | 6 | 0 | CSFII |
| Butterfinger, Nestle | 1 | 36 | 0.7 oz bar (21 g) | 0 | 8 | SR21 (19069) |
| caramel and chocolate-flavored roll | 7 | 75 | 2.25 oz bar (64 g) | 4 | 48 | SR21 (19076) |
| caramels with nuts, chocolate-covered | 19 | 113 | 1 oz (28 g) | 5 | 32 | SR21 (43031) |
| caramels, chocolate-covered | 5 | 47 | 1 oz (28 g) | 1 | 13 | FNDDS |
| chocolate discs, sugar-coated | 14 | 143 | 1 oz (28 g) | 4 | 40 | FNDDS |
| chocolate, Mexican | 14 | 231 | 1 oz (28 g) | 4 | 65 | SR21 (19124) |
| chocolate-covered nougat | 6 | 57 | 1 oz (28 g) | 2 | 16 | FNDDS |
| chocolate-covered nougat and caramel | 6 | 64 | 1 oz (28 g) | 2 | 18 | FNDDS |
| Chunky, Nestle | 29 | 157 | 1.4 oz piece (40 g) | 12 | 63 | SR18 (19119) |
| coconut candy, chocolate-covered | 17 | 130 | 1 oz (28 g) | 5 | 36 | FNDDS |
| Crunch, Nestle | 30 | 168 | 4 fun size bars (40 g) | 12 | 67 | SR21 (19145) |
| dark chocolate chips, semi-sweet | 62 | 486 | ¼ cup (42 g) | 26 | 204 | SR21 (19080) |
| dark chocolate, 45%–59% cacao | 43 | 493 | 1 oz (28 g) | 12 | 138 | SR21 (19902) |
| dark chocolate, 60%–69% cacao | 86 | 632 | 1 oz (28 g) | 24 | 177 | SR21 (19903) |
| dark chocolate, 70%–85% cacao | 80 | 802 | 1 oz (28 g) | 22 | 225 | SR21 (19904) |
| dark chocolate, Hershey Special Dark | 76 | 476 | 2.6 oz bar (73 g) | 55 | 347 | HRSH |
| dark chocolate, sweet | 66 | 426 | 1.45 oz bar (41 g) | 27 | 175 | SR21 (19081) |
| dark chocolate-coated coffee beans | 839 | 368 | 28 pieces (40 g) | 336 | 147 | SR21 (19268) |
| Demet's Turtles, Nestle | 4 | 48 | 6 oz package (170 g) | 7 | 82 | SR18 (19158) |
| Fifth Avenue, Hershey | 5 | 79 | 2 oz bar (56 g) | 3 | 44 | SR21 (19098) |
| fondant, chocolate-covered | 10 | 185 | 1 large patty (43 g) | 4 | 80 | SR21 (19083) |
| fruit, chocolate-covered | 1 | 22 | 1 oz (28 g) | 0 | 6 | FNDDS |
| fudge, caramel with nuts, chocolate-coated | 4 | 44 | 1 oz (28 g) | 1 | 12 | FNDDS |
| fudge, chocolate marshmallow with nuts, homemade | 16 | 129 | 0.78 oz piece (22 g) | 4 | 28 | SR21 (19301) |
| fudge, chocolate marshmallow, homemade | 18 | 139 | 0.7 oz piece (20 g) | 4 | 28 | SR21 (19379) |
| fudge, chocolate with nuts, homemade | 7 | 112 | 0.67 oz piece (19 g) | 1 | 21 | SR21 (19101) |
| fudge, chocolate, chocolate-covered | 12 | 152 | 1 oz (28 g) | 3 | 43 | FNDDS |
| fudge, chocolate, homemade | 8 | 130 | 0.6 oz piece (17 g) | 1 | 22 | SR21 (19100) |
| gumdrops, chocolate-covered | 6 | 57 | 1 oz (28 g) | 2 | 16 | FNDDS |
| honeycombed peanut butter, chocolate-covered | 5 | 79 | 1 oz (28 g) | 1 | 22 | FNDDS |
| Hundred Grand, Nestle (candy) | 8 | 55 | 1.5 oz bar (43 g) | 3 | 24 | SR21 (19144) |
| Kisses, Hershey | 26 | 212 | 9 pieces; (43 g) | 11 | 91 | HRSH |
| Kit Kat, Hershey | 14 | 116 | 2.8 oz bar (78 g) | 11 | 90 | SR21 (19109) |
| Krackel, Hershey | 17 | 151 | 2 oz bar (56 g) | 10 | 85 | HRSH |
| M&M's almond chocolate candies | 7 | 73 | 1.31 oz bag (37 g) | 3 | 27 | SR21 (42227) |
| M&M's peanut butter chocolate candies | 6 | 63 | 1.63 oz bag (46 g) | 3 | 29 | SR21 (42148) |
| M&M's Peanut | 10 | 108 | 25 pieces (49 g) | 5 | 53 | SR21 (19140) |
| M&M's Plain | 14 | 143 | 1.69 oz package; 69 pieces (48 g) | 7 | 69 | SR21 (19141) |
| Mars Almond, M&M's/Mars | 4 | 29 | 1.76 oz bar (50 g) | 2 | 15 | SR21 (19115) |
| marshmallow, chocolate covered | 20 | 128 | 1 oz (28 g) | 6 | 36 | FNDDS |
| milk chocolate chips | 20 | 205 | ¼ cup (42 g) | 8 | 86 | SR21 (19120) |
| milk chocolate with almonds | 18 | 183 | 1.55 oz bar (44 g) | 8 | 81 | SR21 (19132) |
| milk chocolate with crisped rice | 20 | 203 | 1.55 oz bar (44 g) | 9 | 89 | SR21 (19134) |

| | CAFFEINE (mg/100 g) | THEOBROMINE (mg/100 g) | SERVING SIZE (g) | CAFFEINE (mg/serving) | THEOBROMINE (mg/serving) | SOURCE (SR21 CODE NUMBER) |
|---|---|---|---|---|---|---|
| milk chocolate with peanuts | 20 | 0 | 1 oz (28 g) | 6 | 0 | CSFII |
| milk chocolate, Hershey | 23 | 200 | 1.55 oz bar (43 g) | 10 | 86 | HRSH |
| milk chocolate-coated coffee beans | 800 | 178 | 28 pieces (40 g) | 320 | 71 | SR21 (19279) |
| Milky Way, dark | 30 | 238 | 1.76 oz bar (50 g) | 15 | 119 | SR21 (42196) |
| Milky Way | 8 | 92 | 0.6 oz bar (18 g) | 1 | 17 | SR18 (19135) |
| Milky Way, Midnight Bar | 30 | 238 | 1.1 oz bar (60 g) | 18 | 143 | FNDDS |
| Mounds, Hershey | 17 | 130 | 1.9 oz bar (53 g) | 9 | 69 | SR21 (19142) |
| Mr. Goodbar, Hershey | 18 | 198 | 1.75 oz bar (49 g) | 9 | 97 | SR21 (19143) |
| Oh Henry!, Nestle | 4 | 44 | 2 oz bar (57 g) | 2 | 25 | SR21 (19118) |
| peanuts, chocolate-covered | 14 | 145 | 10 pieces (40 g) | 6 | 58 | SR21 (19126) |
| peanuts, chocolate-covered, Goobers | 22 | 109 | 1.38 oz package (39 g) | 9 | 43 | SR18 (19105) |
| Pot of Gold almond chocolate bar, Hershey | 21 | 137 | 2.8 oz bar (78 g) | 16 | 107 | HRSH |
| Pot of Gold Solitaires, Hershey | 15 | 144 | 2.8 oz bar (78 g) | 12 | 112 | HRSH |
| raisins, chocolate-covered | 10 | 122 | ¼ cup (45 g) | 5 | 55 | SR21 (19127) |
| Reese's Fast Break, Hershey | 6 | 60 | 2 oz bar (56 g) | 3 | 34 | SR21 (19896) |
| Reese's Peanut Butter Cups, Hershey | 7 | 72 | 2 pieces; (45 g) | 3 | 32 | SR21 (19150) |
| Reesesticks, Hershey | 0 | 48 | 1.5 oz piece (42 g) | 0 | 20 | SR21 (19249) |
| Rolo caramels with milk chocolate, Hershey | 6 | 52 | 1.9 oz package (54 g) | 3 | 28 | SR21 (19152) |
| Sixlets, Hershey | 14 | 143 | 1 packet (6.3 g) | 1 | 9 | FNDDS |
| Skor Toffee Bar, Hershey | 8 | 59 | 1.4 oz bar (39 g) | 3 | 23 | HRSH |
| Snickers | 8 | 85 | 2 oz bar (57 g) | 5 | 48 | SR21 (19155) |
| Sweet Escapes, caramel and peanut butter, Hershey | 7 | 0 | 0.7 oz bar (20 g) | 1 | 0 | HRSH |
| Sweet Escapes, chocolate toffee, Hershey | 21 | 0 | 1.4 oz bar (39 g) | 8 | 0 | HRSH |
| Sweet Escapes, triple chocolate wafer, Hershey | 18 | 0 | 1.4 oz bar (39 g) | 7 | 0 | HRSH |
| Three Musketeers | 7 | 106 | 2.13 oz bar (60 g) | 4 | 64 | SR21 (19159) |
| Toblerone (milk chocolate with honey and almond nougat) | 17 | 174 | 2 oz (56 g) | 10 | 97 | FNDDS |
| toffee with nuts, chocolate-covered | 5 | 56 | 1 oz (28 g) | 1 | 16 | FNDDS |
| toffee, chocolate-covered (Heath Bar) | 5 | 55 | 1 oz (28 g) | 1 | 15 | FNDDS |
| Tootsie Roll | 7 | 75 | 6 pieces (40 g) | 3 | 30 | SR21 (19064) |
| truffles | 14 | 148 | 1 oz (28 g) | 4 | 41 | FNDDS |
| truffles, homemade | 15 | 152 | 0.42 oz piece (12 g) | 2 | 18 | SR21 (19138) |
| Twix Cookie Bar, caramel | 7 | 70 | 2 bars (58 g) | 4 | 41 | SR21 (19160) |
| Twix Cookie Bar, chocolate fudge | 10 | 212 | 2 bars (58 g) | 6 | 123 | FNDDS |
| Twix Cookie Bar, peanut butter | 7 | 70 | 2 bars (58 g) | 4 | 41 | SR21 (19161) |
| Whatchamacallit, Hershey | 10 | 100 | 1.7 oz bar (48 g) | 5 | 48 | SR21 (19162) |

**CEREALS, READY-TO-EAT**

| | CAFFEINE (mg/100 g) | THEOBROMINE (mg/100 g) | SERVING SIZE (g) | CAFFEINE (mg/serving) | THEOBROMINE (mg/serving) | SOURCE (SR21 CODE NUMBER) |
|---|---|---|---|---|---|---|
| Cocoa Blasts, Quaker | 21 | 188 | 1 cup (33 g) | 7 | 62 | SR21 (08294) |
| Cocoa Crispy Rice, Kountry Fresh | 4 | 45 | 1 oz (28 g) | 1 | 13 | Caudle and Bell, 2000 |
| Cocoa Crunchies, Kountry Fresh | 6 | 67 | 1 oz (28 g) | 2 | 19 | Caudle and Bell, 2000 |
| Cocoa Frosted Flakes, Kellogg | 1 | 11 | 1 oz (28 g) | 0 | 3 | Caudle and Bell, 2000 |
| Cocoa Krispies, Kellogg's | 3 | 66 | ¾ cup (31 g) | 1 | 20 | SR21 (08014) |
| Cocoa Pebbles, Post | 4 | 57 | ¾ cup (29 g) | 1 | 17 | Caudle and Bell, 2000 |
| Cocoa Puffs, General Mills | 2 | 22 | 1 cup (30 g) | 1 | 7 | SR21 (08271) |
| Coco-Roos, Malt-O-Meal | 4 | 136 | ¾ cup (30 g) | 1 | 41 | SR21 (08206) |
| Cookie Crisp, chocolate chip/vanilla, General Mills | 2 | 22 | 1 cup (30 g) | 1 | 7 | SR21 (08017) |
| Count Chocula, General Mills | 3 | 95 | 1 cup (30 g) | 1 | 29 | SR21 (08270) |
| Dyno-Bites, cocoa, Malt-O-Meal | 1 | 35 | ¾ cup (29 g) | 0 | 10 | SR21 (08495) |
| Oreo O's, Post | 11 | 130 | ¾ cup (27 g) | 3 | 35 | Caudle and Bell, 2000 |
| Smorz, Kellogg's | 4 | 41 | 1 cup (30 g) | 1 | 12 | SR21 (08530) |

**DESSERTS**

| | CAFFEINE (mg/100 g) | THEOBROMINE (mg/100 g) | SERVING SIZE (g) | CAFFEINE (mg/serving) | THEOBROMINE (mg/serving) | SOURCE (SR21 CODE NUMBER) |
|---|---|---|---|---|---|---|
| brownie, fast food | 2 | 79 | 2″ square brownie (60 g) | 1 | 47 | SR21 (21027) |
| brownie, from mix | 13 | 85 | brownie 2¾″ × ⅞″ (56 g) | 7 | 48 | Shively and Tarka, 1984 |

| | CAFFEINE (mg/100 g) | THEOBROMINE (mg/100 g) | SERVING SIZE (g) | CAFFEINE (mg/serving) | THEOBROMINE (mg/serving) | SOURCE (SR21 CODE NUMBER) |
|---|---|---|---|---|---|---|
| brownie, Little Debbie | 2 | 78 | 1 twin wrapped package (61 g) | 1 | 48 | SR21 (18151) |
| cake batter, chocolate | 7 | 156 | 1 oz (28 g) | 2 | 44 | FNDDS |
| cake, cherry fudge with chocolate icing | 0 | 5 | 1/8 of 20 oz cake (71 g) | 0 | 4 | SR21 (18095) |
| cake, chocolate, from mix | 7 | 86 | 1/8 of 18 oz cake (64 g) | 4 | 55 | Shively and Tarka, 1984 |
| cake, pound, chocolate | 6 | 95 | 1/10 of 10.6 oz cake (30 g) | 2 | 29 | FNDDS |
| cake, pound, chocolate, fat-free, cholesterol-free | 3 | 105 | 1 oz (28 g) | 1 | 29 | FNDDS |
| cake, sponge, chocolate with icing | 10 | 108 | 1/12 of 12 oz cake (38 g) | 4 | 41 | FNDDS |
| cake, sponge, chocolate without icing | 8 | 75 | 1/12 of 12 oz cake (38 g) | 3 | 29 | FNDDS |
| Caramel Delights cookie, Snackwell's | 8 | 101 | 1 cookie (18 g) | 1 | 18 | SR18 (18650) |
| cheesecake, chocolate | 5 | 87 | 1/6 of 17 oz cake (80 g) | 4 | 70 | FNDDS |
| chocolate syrup | 6 | 190 | 2 T (39 g) | 2 | 74 | SR21 (14181) |
| cookie, chocolate chip, 12%–17% fat | 7 | 55 | 2¼″ diameter cookie (10 g) | 1 | 6 | SR21 (18158) |
| cookie, chocolate chip, fast food | 11 | 83 | 1 box (55 g) | 6 | 46 | SR21 (21030) |
| cookie, chocolate chip, homemade with margarine | 16 | 127 | 2¼″ diameter cookie (16 g) | 3 | 20 | SR21 (18165) |
| cookie, chocolate chunk pecan, Pepperidge Farm | 11 | 83 | 2¼″ diameter cookie (12 g) | 1 | 10 | SR21 (18159) |
| cookie, chocolate devil's food, fat-free, Snackwell's | 8 | 95 | 1 cookie (16 g) | 1 | 15 | SR21 (18651) |
| cookie, chocolate sandwich with chocolate filling | 4 | 0 | 1 cookie (17 g) | 1 | 0 | CSFII |
| cookie, chocolate sandwich with crème filling | 1 | 26 | 1 cookie (17 g) | 0 | 4 | SR21 (18167) |
| cookie, chocolate sandwich with crème filling, chocolate-covered | 13 | 430 | 1 cookie (10 g) | 1 | 43 | SR21 (18166) |
| cookie, chocolate wafer | 7 | 223 | 5 wafers (28 g) | 2 | 62 | SR21 (18157) |
| cookie bar with chocolate, nuts, and graham crackers | 9 | 69 | 2 bars (58 g) | 5 | 40 | FNDDS |
| cookie with peanut butter filling, chocolate-covered | 4 | 135 | 1 oz cookie (28 g) | 1 | 38 | FNDDS |
| cookie, vanilla with caramel, coconut, and chocolate coating | 2 | 78 | 1 oz cookie (28 g) | 1 | 22 | FNDDS |
| cupcake, chocolate with fruit/cream filling, lowfat | 5 | 157 | 1.5 oz cupcake (43 g) | 2 | 68 | FNDDS |
| cupcake, chocolate with icing, lowfat | 2 | 83 | 1.5 oz cupcake (43 g) | 1 | 36 | SR21 (18452) |
| cupcake, chocolate with icing/filling | 6 | 215 | 1.5 oz cupcake (43 g) | 3 | 92 | FNDDS |
| cookie, marshmallow pie | 5 | 159 | small cookie 1¾″ × ¾″ (13 g) | 1 | 21 | SR21 (18176) |
| cookie, oatmeal chocolate chip | 11 | 88 | 1 oz cookie (28 g) | 3 | 25 | FNDDS |
| cookie, shortbread with chocolate filling | 12 | 97 | 1 cookie (25 g) | 3 | 24 | FNDDS |
| cookie, sugar with chocolate | 1 | 10 | 1 oz cookie (28 g) | 0 | 3 | FNDDS |
| dessert topping, chocolate fudge | 7 | 247 | 2 T (38 g) | 3 | 94 | SR21 (19348) |
| doughnut, chocolate with chocolate icing | 7 | 183 | 1 oval doughnut (85 g) | 6 | 156 | FNDDS |
| doughnut, chocolate, glazed/sugared | 1 | 21 | 3″ diameter doughnut (42 g) | 0 | 9 | SR21 (18251) |
| doughnut with chocolate coating/icing | 2 | 53 | 3″ diameter doughnut (43 g) | 1 | 23 | SR21 (18249) |
| doughnut, yeast-raised with chocolate coating | 9 | 0 | 1 oval doughnut (85 g) | 8 | 0 | CSFII |
| doughnut, yeast-raised, chocolate | 10 | 0 | 1 oval doughnut (85 g) | 9 | 0 | CSFII |
| doughnut, yeast-raised, chocolate with chocolate icing | 19 | 0 | 1 oval doughnut (85 g) | 16 | 0 | CSFII |

| | CAFFEINE (mg/100 g) | THEOBROMINE (mg/100 g) | SERVING SIZE (g) | CAFFEINE (mg/serving) | THEOBROMINE (mg/serving) | SOURCE (SR21 CODE NUMBER) |
|---|---|---|---|---|---|---|
| éclair with custard filling and chocolate glaze, homemade | 2 | 14 | 5″ long éclair (100 g) | 2 | 14 | SR21 (18257) |
| frozen dessert, chocolate | 2 | 0 | ½ cup (72 g) | 1 | 0 | CSFII |
| frozen tofu, chocolate (e.g., Tofutti) | 7 | 0 | ½ cup (72 g) | 5 | 0 | CSFII |
| frozen yogurt, nonfat with low calorie sweetener, chocolate | 3 | 106 | ½ cup (72 g) | 2 | 76 | SR21 (42185) |
| frozen yogurt, soft serve, chocolate | 3 | 106 | ½ cup (72 g) | 2 | 76 | SR21 (19393) |
| frozen yogurt, whole fat, chocolate | 3 | 106 | ½ cup (72 g) | 2 | 76 | SR21 (42186) |
| Fudgesicle Pop, no added sugar, Good Humor (frozen dessert) | 0 | 5 | 1 pop (84 g) | 0 | 4 | SR21 (19871) |
| graham cracker, chocolate-covered | 46 | 363 | 2½″ square (14 g) | 6 | 51 | SR21 (18174) |
| ice cream bar, chocolate covered | 0 | 34 | 1 bar (50 g) | 0 | 17 | Shively and Tarka, 1984 |
| ice cream, chocolate | 3 | 62 | ½ cup (66 g) | 2 | 41 | SR21 (19270) |
| ice cream, chocolate, light | 2 | 69 | ½ cup (67 g) | 1 | 46 | SR21 (19114) |
| ice cream, chocolate, light, soft serve | 2 | 56 | ½ cup (71 g) | 1 | 40 | FNDDS |
| ice cream, chocolate, rich | 4 | 120 | 1 cup (148 g) | 6 | 178 | SR21 (43541) |
| icing/frosting, chocolate, from mix made with butter | 5 | 145 | 1/12 package prepared (42 g) | 2 | 61 | SR21 (19241) |
| icing/frosting, chocolate, from mix made with margarine | 5 | 145 | 1/12 package prepared (42 g) | 2 | 61 | SR21 (19372) |
| icing/frosting, chocolate, ready-to-serve | 2 | 79 | 2 T (41 g) | 1 | 32 | SR21 (19226) |
| mousse, chocolate | 7 | 45 | ½ cup (202 g) | 14 | 91 | SR21 (19182) |
| pie/cake, Boston cream, frozen | 0 | 6 | ⅙ of 19.5 oz cake (92 g) | 0 | 6 | SR21 (18090) |
| pie, chocolate creme | 0 | 13 | ⅙ of 8″ pie (113 g) | 0 | 15 | SR21 (18310) |
| pie, chocolate mousse, from mix | 1 | 8 | ⅛ of 9″ pie (95 g) | 1 | 8 | SR21 (18312) |
| pie crust, chocolate cookie, Ready Crust | 15 | 100 | 6.4 oz crust (182 g) | 27 | 182 | SR21 (18943) |
| pie crust, chocolate wafer, homemade | 5 | 166 | ⅛ of 9″ crust (28 g) | 1 | 46 | SR21 (18398) |
| pudding, chocolate, from instant mix with lowfat milk | 1 | 39 | ½ cup (147 g) | 1 | 57 | SR21 (19123) |
| pudding, chocolate, from instant mix with whole milk | 2 | 62 | ½ cup (147 g) | 3 | 91 | SR21 (19185) |
| pudding, chocolate, from regular mix with 2% milk | 2 | 63 | ½ cup (142 g) | 3 | 89 | SR21 (19190) |
| pudding, chocolate, from regular mix with whole milk | 2 | 63 | ½ cup (142 g) | 3 | 89 | SR21 (19189) |
| pudding, chocolate, ready-to-eat | 2 | 70 | 5 oz serving (142 g) | 3 | 99 | SR21 (19183) |
| pudding, tapioca, chocolate | 7 | 62 | 5 oz (142 g) | 10 | 88 | FNDDS |
| rennin dessert, chocolate, from mix with 2% milk | 1 | 42 | ½ cup (136 g) | 1 | 57 | SR21 (19213) |
| rennin dessert, chocolate, from mix with whole milk | 1 | 42 | ½ cup (136 g) | 1 | 57 | SR21 (19221) |
| shake, chocolate, McDonald's | 1 | 45 | 12 fl oz (250 g) | 3 | 113 | SR21 (14346) |
| snack cake, chocolate crème-filled with icing | 6 | 215 | 1.8 oz snack cake (50 g) | 3 | 108 | SR21 (18127) |
| sundae, hot fudge, fast food | 1 | 49 | 1 sundae (158 g) | 2 | 77 | SR21 (21033) |
| **GRAIN PRODUCTS** | | | | | | |
| granola bar, coconut, chocolate-covered | 3 | 41 | 1 oz bar (28 g) | 1 | 11 | SR21 (42272) |
| granola bar, peanut butter, soft, chocolate-covered | 6 | 42 | 1.3 oz bar (37 g) | 2 | 16 | SR21 (19026) |
| muffin, chocolate | 8 | 132 | 2 oz muffin (57 g) | 5 | 75 | FNDDS |
| muffin, chocolate chip | 6 | 49 | 2 oz muffin (57 g) | 3 | 28 | FNDDS |
| pretzel, hard, chocolate-covered | 6 | 57 | 0.39 oz (11 g) | 1 | 6 | FNDDS |
| **MILK BEVERAGES AND YOGURT** | | | | | | |
| chocolate malted milk, whole milk | 3 | 28 | 8 fl oz (265 g) | 8 | 74 | SR21 (14318) |
| chocolate malted milk, whole milk with added nutrients | 2 | 28 | 8 fl oz (265 g) | 5 | 74 | SR21 (14316) |
| chocolate milk, 1% milk | 2 | 23 | 8 fl oz (250 g) | 5 | 58 | SR21 (01104) |

| | CAFFEINE (mg/100 g) | THEOBROMINE (mg/100 g) | SERVING SIZE (g) | CAFFEINE (mg/serving) | THEOBROMINE (mg/serving) | SOURCE (SR21 CODE NUMBER) |
|---|---|---|---|---|---|---|
| chocolate milk, from cocoa and sugar mix | 3 | 100 | 8 fl oz (250 g) | 7 | 250 | Ahuja and Perloff, 2001 |
| chocolate milk, from instant mix | 2 | | 8 fl oz (250 g) | 5 | | Shively and Tarka, 1984 |
| chocolate milk, from instant mix with aspartame | 2 | 73 | 6 fl oz (204 g) | 4 | 149 | SR21 (14423) |
| chocolate milk, reduced fat | 1 | 22 | 8 fl oz (250 g) | 3 | 55 | SR21 (01103) |
| chocolate milk, whole milk | 2 | 23 | 8 fl oz (250 g) | 5 | 58 | SR21 (01102) |
| chocolate milk, whole milk with chocolate syrup | 2 | 64 | 8 fl oz (282 g) | 6 | 180 | SR21 (14182) |
| chocolate milk, whole milk with instant mix | 3 | 104 | 8 fl oz (266 g) | 8 | 277 | SR21 (14177) |
| cocoa (hot chocolate), from mix with aspartame, prepared with water | 2 | 51 | 1 packet in 6 fl oz water (192 g) | 4 | 98 | SR21 (14390) |
| cocoa (hot chocolate), from mix, prepared with water | 2 | 44 | 1 oz packet in 6 fl oz water (206 g) | 4 | 91 | SR21 (14194) |
| cocoa (hot chocolate), homemade with 2% milk | 2 | 68 | 8 fl oz (250 g) | 5 | 170 | SR21 (01105) |
| cocoa (hot chocolate) with 2% milk and whipped cream, Starbucks | 5 | | grande; 16 fl oz (480 g) | 24 | | STAR |
| chocolate malted mix for milk | 37 | 345 | 3 heaping t (21 g) | 8 | 72 | SR21 (14317) |
| chocolate mix for milk | 36 | 424 | 2 T (21 g) | 8 | 89 | SR21 (14175) |
| chocolate mix with aspartame for milk | 25 | 833 | 0.75 oz packet (21 g) | 5 | 175 | SR21 (14422) |
| cocoa mix for milk | 18 | 323 | 3–4 heaping t (28 g) | 5 | 90 | SR21 (14192) |
| Instant Breakfast mix with low calorie sweetener, chocolate | 52 | 608 | 1 packet (20 g) | 10 | 122 | SR21 (43260) |
| Instant Breakfast mix, chocolate | 25 | 290 | 1 packet (37 g) | 9 | 107 | SR21 (43205) |
| malted milk mix, chocolate | 37 | 345 | 3 heaping t (21 g) | 8 | 72 | FNDDS |
| malted milk mix, chocolate with added nutrients | 28 | 345 | 4–5 heaping t (21 g) | 6 | 72 | FNDDS |
| soymilk, chocolate, unfortified | 2 | 23 | 8 fl oz (243 g) | 5 | 56 | SR21 (16166) |
| yogurt, nonfat, chocolate | 2 | 23 | 8 oz container (227 g) | 5 | 52 | SR21 (01187) |
| **OTHER FOODS** | | | | | | |
| baking chocolate (unsweetened) | 80 | 1297 | 1 oz (28 g) | 22 | 363 | SR21 (19078) |
| baking chocolate (unsweetened), liquid | 47 | 1597 | 1 oz packet (28 g) | 13 | 447 | SR21 (19077) |
| chocolate liquor | 214 | 1220 | 1 fl oz (30 g) | 64 | 366 | Shively and Tarka, 1984 |
| cocoa powder, unsweetened | 230 | 2057 | 1 T (5.4 g) | 12 | 111 | SR21 (19165) |
| cocoa powder, unsweetened, processed with alkali (dutched) | 78 | 2634 | 1 T (5.4 g) | 4 | 142 | SR21 (19166) |
| filbert (hazelnut) spread, chocolate-flavored | 7 | 230 | 2 T (37 g) | 3 | 85 | SR21 (19125) |
| gravy, redeye | 41 | 0 | ¼ cup (60 g) | 25 | 0 | FNDDS |
| mole poblano sauce | 2 | 29 | ¼ cup (60 g) | 1 | 17 | FNDDS |
| Snickers Marathon Energy Bar, all flavors | 6 | 57 | 1.9 oz bar (55 g) | 3 | 31 | SR21 (25016) |
| Snickers Marathon Energy Bar, caramel nut rush | 3 | 28 | 2.8 oz bar (80 g) | 2 | 22 | SR21 (25015) |
| wheat cereal with chocolate flavor, cooked with milk | 1 | 40 | 1 cup (243 g ) | 2 | 97 | FNDDS |

Sources:
COLA = The CocaCola Company
HRSH = Hershey Foods Corporation
SHST = Shasta Sales, Incorporated
STAR = Starbucks
Bunker ML, M Mc Williams. Caffeine content of common beverages. *J Am Diet Assoc* 74:28-32, 1979.
Caudle AG, LN Bell. Caffeine and the theobromine contents of ready-to-eat chocolate cereals. *J Am Diet Assoc* 100:690-692, 2000.
Groisser DS. A study of caffeine in tea. I. A new spectrophotometric micro-method> II. Concentration of caffeine in various strength, brands, blends, and types of teas. *Am J Clin Nutr* 31:1727-1731, 1978.
Shively CA, SM Tarka. Methylxanthine composition and consumption patterns of cocoa and chocolate products. *The Methylxanthine Beverages and Foods: Chemistry, Consumption, and Health Effects.* Alan R. Liss, Inc, New York , NY, 1984.
USDA. Continuing Survey of the Food Intake of Individuals (CSFII) 1994-1996 Survey Nutrient Database, 1998.
USDA. Food and Nutrient Database for Dietary Studies 3.0, 2008. Available at: http://www.ars.usda.gov/Services/docs.htm?docid=12089.
USDA National Nutrient Database for Standard Reference, Release 18 (SR18), 2005.
USDA National Nutrient Database for Standard Reference, Release 21 (SR21), 2008. Available at: http://www.nal.usda.gov/fnic/foddcomp/serch/.

# Carotenoids—Alpha-Carotene, Beta-Carotene, Beta-Cryptoxanthin, Lutein + Zeaxanthin, and Lycopene

| | ALPHA-CAROTENE (mcg/100 g) | BETA-CAROTENE (mcg/100 g) | BETA-CRYPTOXANTHIN (mcg/100 g) | LUTEIN + ZEAXANTHIN (mcg/100 g) | LYCOPENE (mcg/100 g) | SR21 CODE NUMBER[1] |
|---|---|---|---|---|---|---|
| **CANDY** | | | | | | |
| dark chocolate, 45%–59% cacao | 7 | 26 | 1 | 31 | 0 | 19902 |
| Reesesticks, Hershey | 0 | 4 | 0 | 45 | 0 | 19249 |
| toffee, homemade | 0 | 64 | 0 | 0 | 0 | 19383 |
| **CEREALS AND GRAINS, COOKED** | | | | | | |
| barley, pearled, cooked | 0 | 5 | 0 | 56 | 0 | 20006 |
| buckwheat groats, roasted, cooked | 0 | 0 | 0 | 60 | 0 | 20010 |
| bulgur, cooked | 0 | 1 | 0 | 54 | 0 | 20013 |
| corn grits, butter flavor, instant, enriched, prepared, Quaker | | 124 | | | | 08238 |
| corn grits, yellow, regular/quick, enriched, cooked | 9 | 14 | 0 | 197 | 0 | 08164 |
| millet, cooked | 0 | 2 | 0 | 70 | 0 | 20032 |
| Nestum cereal (wheat with honey), prepared, Nestle | 3 | 5 | 0 | 73 | 0 | 43306 |
| oatmeal, quick/regular, cooked | 0 | 0 | 0 | 180 | 0 | 08121 |
| Whole Wheat Hot Natural Cereal, cooked | 0 | 0 | 0 | 41 | 0 | 08145 |
| wild rice, boiled | 0 | 2 | 0 | 64 | 0 | 20089 |
| **CEREALS, READY-TO-EAT** | | | | | | |
| All-Bran, Kellogg's | 0 | 4 | 0 | 180 | 0 | 08001 |
| Apple Jacks, Kellogg's | 20 | 31 | 0 | 448 | 0 | 08003 |
| Basic 4, General Mills | 16 | 34 | 2 | 357 | 0 | 08262 |
| Boo Berry, General Mills | 18 | 27 | 0 | 375 | 0 | 08273 |
| Cap'n Crunch, Quaker | 43 | 66 | 0 | 986 | 0 | 08010 |
| Cheerios, General Mills | 0 | 0 | 0 | 176 | 0 | 08013 |
| Cinnamon Oatmeal Squares, Quaker | 0 | 0 | 1 | 137 | 0 | 08215 |
| Cinnamon Toast Crunch, General Mills | 0 | 1 | 0 | 55 | 0 | 08272 |
| Cocoa Blasts, Quaker | 30 | 46 | 0 | 644 | 0 | 08294 |
| Cocoa Puffs, General Mills | 8 | 13 | 0 | 184 | 0 | 08271 |
| Coco-Roos, Malt-O-Meal | 28 | 43 | 0 | 609 | 0 | 08206 |
| Cookie Crisp, chocolate chip/vanilla, General Mills | 15 | 23 | 0 | 347 | 0 | 08017 |
| Corn Biscuits, Ralston | 0 | 73 | 66 | | 0 | 08505 |
| Corn Bursts, Malt-O-Meal | 39 | 60 | 0 | 842 | 0 | 08083 |
| Corn Chex, General Mills | 54 | 82 | 0 | 1154 | 0 | 08019 |
| Corn Flakes, Country, General Mills | 54 | 82 | 0 | 1154 | 0 | 08269 |
| Corn Flakes, Kellogg's | 19 | 162 | 50 | 339 | 0 | 08020 |
| Corn Pops, Kellogg's | 26 | 40 | 0 | 556 | 0 | 08068 |
| Count Chocula, General Mills | 15 | 22 | 0 | 336 | 0 | 08270 |
| Cracklin' Oat Bran, Kellogg's | 0 | 0 | 0 | 49 | 0 | 08023 |
| Crispix, Kellogg's | 0 | 39 | 34 | 196 | 0 | 08259 |
| Crunchy Bran, Quaker | 46 | 70 | 0 | 943 | 0 | 08018 |
| Fiber One, General Mills | 10 | 19 | 0 | 782 | 0 | 08244 |
| Frankenberry, General Mills | 17 | 27 | 0 | 372 | 0 | 08268 |
| French Toast Crunch, General Mills | 27 | 42 | 0 | 583 | 0 | 08086 |
| Froot Loops, Kellogg's | 20 | 30 | 0 | 425 | 0 | 08030 |
| Frosted Flakes, Kellogg's | 34 | 52 | 0 | 731 | 0 | 08069 |
| Golden Grahams, General Mills | 12 | 20 | 0 | 324 | 0 | 08035 |
| Golden Puffs, Malt-O-Meal | 0 | 2 | 0 | 94 | 0 | 08478 |
| GoLean, Kashi | 21 | 47 | 0 | 413 | 0 | 08393 |
| granola with raisins, lowfat, 100% natural, Quaker | 5 | 8 | 0 | 183 | 0 | 08220 |
| Honey Crunch Corn Flakes, Kellogg's | 37 | 56 | 0 | 784 | 0 | 08309 |

| | ALPHA-CAROTENE (mcg/100 g) | BETA-CAROTENE (mcg/100 g) | BETA-CRYPTOXANTHIN (mcg/100 g) | LUTEIN + ZEAXANTHIN (mcg/100 g) | LYCOPENE (mcg/100 g) | SR21 CODE NUMBER[1] |
|---|---|---|---|---|---|---|
| Honey Nut Chex, General Mills | 20 | 30 | 0 | 419 | 0 | 08057 |
| Honey Puffs Kashi | 0 | 0 | 0 | 135 | 0 | 08389 |
| King Vitaman, Quaker | 52 | 80 | 0 | 1124 | 0 | 08047 |
| Kix, General Mills | 33 | 51 | 0 | 794 | 0 | 08048 |
| Life, oat, Quaker | 12 | 19 | 0 | 120 | 0 | 08049 |
| Lucky Charms, General Mills | 0 | 0 | 0 | 81 | 0 | 08050 |
| Multi-Bran Chex, General Mills | 30 | 46 | 0 | 724 | 0 | 08345 |
| Natural Cereal, 100% with oats and honey, Quaker | 0 | 2 | 0 | 112 | 0 | 08054 |
| Oat Bran Flakes, Health Valley | 2 | 4 | 0 | 163 | 0 | 43495 |
| Oatmeal Crisp, almond, General Mills | 0 | 2 | 3 | 108 | 0 | 08202 |
| Product 19, Kellogg's | 43 | 66 | 0 | 942 | 0 | 08058 |
| Puffs, Kashi | 0 | 3 | 0 | 134 | 0 | 08388 |
| Raisin Bran, Kellogg's | 0 | 3 | 0 | 120 | 0 | 08060 |
| Raisin Nut Bran, General Mills | 1 | 4 | 0 | 150 | 0 | 08261 |
| Reese's Peanut Butter Puffs, General Mills | 21 | 33 | 0 | 458 | 0 | 08194 |
| Special K, fruit and yogurt, Kellogg's | 0 | 8 | 5 | 52 | 0 | 08531 |
| Sweet Crunch/Quisp, Quaker | 26 | 39 | 0 | 572 | 0 | 08059 |
| Toasted Oatmeal, honey nut, Quaker | 0 | 1 | 0 | 134 | 0 | 08219 |
| Tootie Fruities, Malt-O-Meal | 30 | 46 | 0 | 651 | 0 | 08349 |
| Total, corn, General Mills | 46 | 70 | 0 | 977 | 0 | 08246 |
| Total, General Mills | 0 | 4 | 0 | 172 | 0 | 08077 |
| Total, raisin bran, General Mills | 2 | 4 | 0 | 158 | 0 | 08247 |
| Trix, General Mills | 15 | 22 | 0 | 315 | 0 | 08078 |
| Weetabix | 0 | 0 | 0 | 238 | 0 | 42237 |
| Wheat Bran Flakes, Kellogg's Complete | 0 | 0 | 0 | 171 | 0 | 08028 |
| Wheat Chex, General Mills | 0 | 5 | 0 | 207 | 0 | 08082 |
| Wheaties, General Mills | 0 | 4 | 0 | 173 | 0 | 08089 |

**CHEESE, CHEESE PRODUCTS, AND CHEESE SUBSTITUTES**

| | | | | | | |
|---|---|---|---|---|---|---|
| American cheese spread | 0 | 55 | 0 | 0 | 0 | 01048 |
| American processed cheese | 0 | 82 | 0 | 0 | 0 | 01042 |
| American processed cheese food | 0 | 65 | 0 | 0 | 0 | 01046 |
| blue cheese | 0 | 74 | 0 | 0 | 0 | 01004 |
| brick cheese | 0 | 76 | 0 | 0 | 0 | 01005 |
| cheddar cheese | 0 | 85 | 0 | 0 | 0 | 01009 |
| colby cheese | 0 | 82 | 0 | 0 | 0 | 01011 |
| cream cheese | 0 | 41 | 0 | 0 | 0 | 01017 |
| fontina cheese | 0 | 32 | 0 | 0 | 0 | 01020 |
| goat milk cheese, semi-soft | 0 | 77 | 0 | 0 | 0 | 01157 |
| gruyere cheese | 0 | 33 | 0 | 0 | 0 | 01023 |
| monterey jack cheese | 0 | 78 | 0 | 0 | 0 | 01025 |
| mozzarella cheese, part skim, low moisture | 0 | 44 | 0 | 0 | 0 | 01029 |
| mozzarella cheese, whole milk, low moisture | 0 | 63 | 0 | 0 | 0 | 01027 |
| Neufchatel cheese | 0 | 27 | 0 | | 0 | 01031 |
| parmesan cheese, grated | 0 | 31 | 0 | 0 | 0 | 01032 |
| parmesan cheese, hard | 0 | 28 | 0 | 0 | 0 | 01033 |
| pimiento cheese, processed | 12 | 151 | 0 | 20 | 0 | 01043 |
| port de salut cheese | 0 | 29 | 0 | 0 | 0 | 01034 |
| provolone cheese | 0 | 68 | 0 | 0 | 0 | 01035 |
| ricotta cheese, part nonfat | 0 | 20 | 0 | 0 | 0 | 01037 |
| ricotta cheese, whole milk | 0 | 33 | 0 | 0 | 0 | 01036 |
| Romano cheese | 0 | 69 | 0 | 0 | 0 | 01038 |
| soy cheese | 0 | 25 | 0 | 0 | 0 | 43299 |
| Swiss cheese | 0 | 70 | 0 | 0 | 0 | 01040 |
| Swiss processed cheese | 0 | 63 | 0 | 0 | 0 | 01044 |

**CREAMS AND CREAMERS**

| | | | | | | |
|---|---|---|---|---|---|---|
| cream, half and half | 0 | 22 | 0 | 0 | 0 | 01049 |
| cream, light (coffee/table) | 0 | 37 | 0 | 0 | 0 | 01050 |

| | ALPHA-CAROTENE (mcg/100 g) | BETA-CAROTENE (mcg/100 g) | BETA-CRYPTOXANTHIN (mcg/100 g) | LUTEIN + ZEAXANTHIN (mcg/100 g) | LYCOPENE (mcg/100 g) | SR21 CODE NUMBER[1] |
|---|---|---|---|---|---|---|
| creamer, powdered | 0 | 20 | 0 | 0 | 0 | 01069 |
| sour cream, cultured | 0 | 26 | 0 | 0 | 0 | 01056 |
| sour cream, cultured, reduced-fat | 0 | 23 | 0 | 0 | 0 | 01055 |
| sour cream, light | 0 | 21 | 0 | 0 | 0 | 01179 |
| sour cream, reduced fat | 0 | 27 | 0 | 0 | 0 | 01178 |
| whipped topping, from mix, prepared with whole milk | 0 | 32 | 0 | 0 | 0 | 01071 |
| whipped topping, frozen | 0 | 86 | 0 | 0 | 0 | 01073 |
| whipped topping, pressurized | 0 | 47 | 0 | 0 | 0 | 01072 |
| whipping cream, heavy fluid | 0 | 72 | 0 | 0 | 0 | 01053 |
| whipping cream, light fluid | 0 | 60 | 0 | 0 | 0 | 01052 |
| whipping cream, pressurized | 0 | 43 | 0 | 0 | 0 | 01054 |

**DESSERTS**

| | ALPHA-CAROTENE | BETA-CAROTENE | BETA-CRYPTOXANTHIN | LUTEIN + ZEAXANTHIN | LYCOPENE | SR21 CODE NUMBER[1] |
|---|---|---|---|---|---|---|
| apple crisp, homemade | 0 | 30 | 8 | 19 | 0 | 19186 |
| apple strudel | 1 | 5 | 3 | 42 | 0 | 18354 |
| cake, cherry fudge with chocolate icing | 0 | 131 | 0 | 33 | 0 | 18095 |
| cake, sponge | 1 | 4 | 2 | 85 | 0 | 18133 |
| chocolate mousse, homemade | 3 | 27 | 3 | 94 | 0 | 19182 |
| coffeecake, cinnamon with crumb topping, from mix | 0 | 2 | 2 | 44 | 0 | 18108 |
| cookie, butter | 0 | 35 | 1 | 22 | 0 | 18155 |
| cookie, chocolate chip, homemade with margarine | | 150 | | | | 18165 |
| cookie, oatmeal | 0 | 0 | 0 | 31 | 0 | 18178 |
| cookie, raisin, soft type | 0 | 1 | 1 | 37 | 0 | 18191 |
| cookie, shortbread | 8 | 13 | 1 | 203 | 0 | 18192 |
| cookie, sugar | 0 | 1 | 1 | 38 | 0 | 18204 |
| cookie, vanilla wafer, 12%–17% fat | 0 | 1 | 1 | 41 | 0 | 18212 |
| cream puff shell, homemade | 0 | 164 | 4 | 157 | 0 | 18237 |
| cream puff with custard filling, homemade | 0 | 84 | 2 | 80 | 0 | 18238 |
| croissant | 0 | 38 | 1 | 74 | 0 | 18239 |
| croissant, cheese | 0 | 89 | 0 | 43 | 0 | 18241 |
| custard, egg, homemade | 0 | 6 | 2 | 59 | 0 | 19168 |
| Danish pastry, cinnamon | 0 | 2 | 1 | 52 | 0 | 18244 |
| doughnut, yeast-raised, glazed | 1 | 3 | 1 | 36 | 0 | 18255 |
| doughnut, yeast-raised with crème filling | 0 | 2 | 1 | 33 | 0 | 18254 |
| doughnut, yeast-raised with jelly filling | 3 | 8 | 3 | 108 | 0 | 18256 |
| éclair with custard filling and chocolate glaze, homemade | 0 | 117 | 3 | 112 | 0 | 18257 |
| flan (crème caramel, caramel custard), homemade | 0 | 5 | 2 | 65 | 0 | 19094 |
| fruit juice bar, frozen | 0 | 11 | 0 | 34 | 0 | 19263 |
| fruitcake | 1 | 3 | 1 | 21 | 0 | 18110 |
| graham cracker | 0 | 1 | 0 | 61 | 0 | 18173 |
| ice cream, chocolate | 0 | 19 | 0 | 0 | 0 | 19270 |
| ice cream, chocolate, rich | 0 | 31 | 0 | 2 | 0 | 43541 |
| ice cream, French vanilla, soft serve | 5 | 30 | 5 | 151 | 0 | 19090 |
| ice cream, vanilla, rich (16% fat) | 1 | 32 | 1 | 34 | 0 | 19089 |
| icing/frosting, chocolate, from mix made with butter | | 55 | | | | 19241 |
| icing/frosting, vanilla, from mix made with margarine | | 91 | | | | 19371 |
| ladyfinger with lemon juice and rind | 9 | 22 | 8 | 266 | 0 | 18175 |
| orange juice bar (frozen dessert) | 0 | 12 | 0 | 39 | 0 | 43346 |
| pie, banana cream, homemade | 5 | 21 | 1 | 46 | 0 | 18304 |
| pie, blueberry | 0 | 39 | 0 | 15 | 0 | 18305 |
| pie, cherry | 0 | 69 | 0 | 20 | 0 | 18308 |
| pie crust, chocolate wafer, homemade | 0 | 156 | 0 | 8 | 0 | 18398 |
| pie crust, graham, homemade | 0 | 131 | 0 | 29 | 0 | 18330 |

| | ALPHA-CAROTENE (mcg/100 g) | BETA-CAROTENE (mcg/100 g) | BETA-CRYPTOXANTHIN (mcg/100 g) | LUTEIN + ZEAXANTHIN (mcg/100 g) | LYCOPENE (mcg/100 g) | SR21 CODE NUMBER[1] |
|---|---|---|---|---|---|---|
| pie crust, vanilla wafer, homemade | 0 | 197 | 1 | 27 | 0 | 18401 |
| pie, custard, egg | 0 | 9 | 1 | 50 | 0 | 18317 |
| pie, Dutch apple | 0 | 10 | 11 | 42 | 1 | 18944 |
| pie filling, cherry, low-calorie, canned | 0 | 125 | 0 | 70 | 0 | 43098 |
| pie, peach | 0 | 64 | 25 | 15 | 0 | 18323 |
| pie, pumpkin | 686 | 1023 | 3 | 20 | 0 | 18326 |
| pie, vanilla cream, homemade | 2 | 22 | 1 | 52 | 0 | 18328 |
| pudding, lemon, from regular mix with sugar, egg yolk, and water | 2 | 4 | 1 | 44 | 0 | 19333 |
| sweet roll, cinnamon raisin | 1 | 5 | 2 | 70 | 0 | 18356 |

### EGGS, EGG DISHES, AND EGG SUBSTITUTES

| | | | | | | |
|---|---|---|---|---|---|---|
| duck egg, whole | 0 | 14 | 12 | 459 | 0 | 01138 |
| chicken egg yolk, raw | 38 | 88 | 33 | 1094 | 0 | 01125 |
| chicken egg, boiled, hard | 0 | 11 | 10 | 353 | 0 | 01129 |
| chicken egg, fried | 0 | 46 | 10 | 358 | 0 | 01128 |
| chicken egg, omelet, plain | 0 | 36 | 8 | 279 | 0 | 01130 |
| chicken egg, poached | 0 | 10 | 9 | 330 | 0 | 01131 |
| chicken egg, raw | 0 | 10 | 9 | 331 | 0 | 01123 |
| chicken egg, scrambled with milk | 0 | 33 | 7 | 245 | 0 | 01132 |
| egg substitute, frozen | 0 | 135 | 0 | 0 | 0 | 01142 |
| egg substitute, liquid | 0 | 216 | 0 | 0 | 0 | 01143 |
| goose egg, raw | 0 | 13 | 12 | 442 | 0 | 01139 |
| quail egg, raw | 0 | 11 | 10 | 369 | 0 | 01140 |

### ENTREES

| | | | | | | |
|---|---|---|---|---|---|---|
| baked beans with frankfurters, canned | 0 | 52 | 0 | 13 | 409 | 16008 |
| beef macaroni, frozen entrée, Healthy Choice | 1 | 98 | 0 | 39 | 5535 | 22402 |
| beef, sliced, gravy, mashed potatoes, and carrots, frozen meal, Freezer Queen | 1120 | 1930 | | | | 22710 |
| beef stew, canned | 356 | 811 | 19 | 215 | 3 | 22905 |
| burrito, beef and bean, frozen | 1 | 126 | 1 | 22 | 8444 | 22917 |
| chili with beans (no meat), canned | 0 | 180 | 43 | 107 | 1069 | 16059 |
| pasta with franks in tomato sauce, canned | 0 | 70 | 1 | 5 | 7506 | 22522 |
| pasta with meatballs in tomato sauce, canned | 0 | 109 | 0 | 1 | 7669 | 22907 |
| pizza, cheese, regular crust, frozen, heated | 0 | 88 | 0 | 34 | 1829 | 21224 |
| pizza, cheese, rising crust, frozen, heated | 0 | 93 | 0 | 24 | 1925 | 21225 |
| spaghetti Bolognese, frozen entrée, Healthy Choice | 0 | 104 | 0 | 7 | 3200 | 22401 |
| turkey pot pie, frozen | | 1060 | | | | 22528 |

### FAST FOODS AND RESTAURANT FOODS

| | | | | | | |
|---|---|---|---|---|---|---|
| bagel with egg, sausage patty, and cheese | 0 | 0 | 0 | 119 | 0 | 21410 |
| bagel with ham, egg, and cheese | 0 | 18 | 4 | 141 | 0 | 21409 |
| biscuit with egg and bacon | 0 | 14 | 3 | 107 | 0 | 21003 |
| biscuit with egg and ham | 0 | 14 | 3 | 108 | 0 | 21004 |
| biscuit with egg and sausage | 0 | 39 | 3 | 102 | 0 | 21005 |
| burrito, bean, Taco Bell | 0 | 40 | 0 | | | 21264 |
| Burrito Supreme, beef, Taco Bell | 0 | 49 | 0 | | | 21265 |
| Burrito Supreme, steak, Taco Bell | 0 | 43 | 0 | | | 21267 |
| cheeseburger sandwich, regular, single meat | 2 | 64 | 4 | 19 | 0 | 21090 |
| egg, scrambled | 0 | 62 | 6 | 233 | 0 | 21018 |
| English muffin (toasted) with cheese and sausage | 1 | 24 | 1 | 60 | 1 | 21020 |
| griddle cake sandwich with egg, cheese, and bacon | 0 | 16 | 2 | 94 | 0 | 21307 |

| | ALPHA-CAROTENE (mcg/100 g) | BETA-CAROTENE (mcg/100 g) | BETA-CRYPTOXANTHIN (mcg/100 g) | LUTEIN + ZEAXANTHIN (mcg/100 g) | LYCOPENE (mcg/100 g) | SR21 CODE NUMBER[1] |
|---|---|---|---|---|---|---|
| griddle cake sandwich with egg, cheese, and sausage | 0 | 15 | 2 | 81 | 0 | 21305 |
| Nachos Supreme, Taco Bell | 0 | 42 | 0 | | | 21269 |
| pizza, cheese, regular crust | 0 | 92 | 0 | 58 | 1915 | 21299 |
| pizza, meat and vegetable, regular crust | 0 | 81 | 0 | 26 | 1689 | 21304 |
| pizza, pepperoni, regular crust | 0 | 94 | 0 | 24 | 1957 | 21302 |
| sauce, spicy buffalo, McDonald's | | 617 | | | | 21314 |
| taco salad, Taco Bell | 0 | 37 | 0 | | | 21270 |
| taco, soft, beef, Taco Bell | 0 | 48 | 0 | | | 21261 |
| **FATS, OILS, SHORTENINGS, AND SPREADS** | | | | | | |
| butter | 0 | 158 | 0 | 0 | 0 | 01001 |
| butter, whipped | 0 | 158 | 0 | 0 | 0 | 01002 |
| margarine, liquid | 0 | 610 | 0 | 0 | 0 | 04105 |
| margarine, stick/tub composite, 60% fat | 0 | 610 | 0 | 0 | 0 | 04614 |
| margarine-butter blend (60% corn oil, 40% butter) | 0 | 610 | 0 | 0 | 0 | 04585 |
| mayonnaise, diet, no cholesterol | 1 | 94 | 27 | 87 | 0 | 43599 |
| mayonnaise, soy | 0 | 6 | 5 | 190 | 0 | 04025 |
| sandwich spread (mayonnaise-based) | 1 | 94 | 27 | 87 | 0 | 04030 |
| **FISH AND SEAFOODS** | | | | | | |
| caviar, black and red, granular | 0 | 0 | 0 | 648 | 0 | 15012 |
| fish sticks/pieces, frozen, reheated | 0 | 2 | 1 | 43 | 0 | 15027 |
| roe (fish eggs), mixed species, raw | 0 | 0 | 0 | 214 | 0 | 15072 |
| sardines, Pacific, canned in tomato sauce, drained | 0 | 21 | 0 | 0 | 1515 | 15089 |
| **FLOUR, MEALS, AND GRAIN FRACTIONS** | | | | | | |
| barley flour/meal | 0 | 0 | 0 | 160 | 0 | 20130 |
| buckwheat flour, whole groats | 0 | 0 | 0 | 220 | 0 | 20011 |
| corn bran | 21 | 32 | 0 | 1355 | 0 | 20015 |
| corn flour, yellow, whole grain | 63 | 97 | 0 | 1355 | 0 | 20016 |
| oat bran | 0 | 0 | 0 | 180 | 0 | 20033 |
| oat flour | 0 | 0 | 0 | 180 | 0 | 20132 |
| rice bran | 0 | 0 | 0 | 220 | 0 | 20060 |
| rye flour, medium | 0 | 0 | 0 | 210 | 0 | 20064 |
| soy flour, full-fat | 0 | 72 | 0 | 0 | 0 | 16115 |
| wheat bran, crude | 0 | 6 | 0 | 240 | 0 | 20077 |
| wheat flour, white, enriched, bread | 0 | 1 | 0 | 79 | 0 | 20083 |
| wheat flour, whole wheat | 0 | 5 | 0 | 220 | 0 | 20080 |
| wheat germ, toasted | 0 | 62 | 0 | 790 | 0 | 08084 |
| **FRUIT AND VEGETABLE JUICES AND JUICE DRINKS** | | | | | | |
| acerola juice, raw | 0 | 305 | 0 | 17 | 0 | 09002 |
| apricot nectar, canned/bottled | 0 | 786 | 7 | 14 | 0 | 09036 |
| blackberry juice, canned | 0 | 74 | 0 | 68 | 0 | 09043 |
| carrot juice, canned | 4342 | 9303 | 0 | 333 | 2 | 11655 |
| clam and tomato juice, canned | 0 | 89 | 0 | 20 | 2982 | 14187 |
| cranberry juice, unsweetened | 0 | 27 | 0 | 68 | 0 | 43382 |
| grape juice, canned/bottled | 0 | 5 | 0 | 35 | 0 | 09135 |
| mango nectar, canned | 0 | 402 | 26 | 0 | 0 | 09436 |
| mixed vegetable and fruit juice drink | 144 | 1178 | 0 | 12 | 0 | 14119 |
| orange apricot juice drink, canned | 2 | 79 | 60 | 47 | 0 | 14327 |
| orange grapefruit juice, canned/bottled | 4 | 20 | 98 | 73 | 0 | 09217 |
| orange juice drink, canned/bottled | 1 | 7 | 37 | 29 | 0 | 42270 |
| orange juice, canned/bottled | 5 | 29 | 148 | 115 | 0 | 09207 |
| orange juice, from frozen concentrate | 3 | 17 | 91 | 115 | 0 | 09215 |
| orange juice, raw | 6 | 33 | 169 | 115 | 0 | 09206 |
| orange strawberry banana juice | 3 | 17 | 68 | 58 | 0 | 42149 |
| papaya nectar, canned | 0 | 91 | 251 | 25 | 0 | 09229 |

| | ALPHA-CAROTENE (mcg/100 g) | BETA-CAROTENE (mcg/100 g) | BETA-CRYPTOXANTHIN (mcg/100 g) | LUTEIN + ZEAXANTHIN (mcg/100 g) | LYCOPENE (mcg/100 g) | SR21 CODE NUMBER[1] |
|---|---|---|---|---|---|---|
| passion fruit juice, purple, raw | 0 | 419 | 23 | 0 | 0 | 09232 |
| passion fruit juice, yellow, raw | 35 | 525 | 47 | 0 | 0 | 09233 |
| peach nectar, canned/bottled | 0 | 128 | 53 | 37 | 0 | 09251 |
| prune juice, canned/bottled | 0 | 2 | 0 | 40 | 0 | 09294 |
| tangerine juice, sweetened, canned/bottled | 14 | 38 | 214 | 166 | 0 | 09223 |
| tangerine juice, sweetened, frozen concentrate | | 277 | 2767 | | | 09224 |
| tomato juice, canned/bottled | 0 | 270 | 0 | 60 | 9037 | 11540 |
| vegetable juice, canned/bottled | 210 | 830 | 0 | 80 | 9660 | 11578 |

**FRUITS**

| | ALPHA-CAROTENE (mcg/100 g) | BETA-CAROTENE (mcg/100 g) | BETA-CRYPTOXANTHIN (mcg/100 g) | LUTEIN + ZEAXANTHIN (mcg/100 g) | LYCOPENE (mcg/100 g) | SR21 CODE NUMBER[1] |
|---|---|---|---|---|---|---|
| abiyuch, raw | 0 | 60 | | | | 09427 |
| apricot, canned in light syrup, solids and liquid | 0 | 789 | 7 | 26 | 0 | 09026 |
| apricot, dried | 0 | 2163 | 0 | 0 | 0 | 09032 |
| apricot, raw | 19 | 1094 | 104 | 89 | 0 | 09021 |
| avocado, California, raw | 24 | 63 | 27 | 271 | 0 | 09038 |
| avocado, Florida, raw | 27 | 53 | 36 | | | 09039 |
| banana, raw | 25 | 26 | 0 | 22 | 0 | 09040 |
| blackberries, canned in heavy syrup, solids and liquid | 0 | 131 | 0 | 79 | 0 | 09046 |
| blackberries, frozen, unsweetened | 0 | 68 | 0 | 118 | 0 | 09048 |
| blackberries, raw | 0 | 128 | 0 | 118 | 0 | 09042 |
| blueberries, canned in heavy syrup, solids and liquid | 0 | 22 | 0 | 53 | 0 | 09052 |
| blueberries, frozen | 0 | 28 | 0 | 68 | 0 | 09054 |
| blueberries, raw | 0 | 32 | 0 | 80 | 0 | 09050 |
| boysenberries, frozen, unsweetened | 0 | 40 | 0 | 118 | 0 | 09057 |
| cantaloupe, raw | 16 | 2020 | 1 | 26 | 0 | 09181 |
| carambola (star fruit), raw | 24 | 25 | 0 | 66 | 0 | 09060 |
| cherries, maraschino, canned, drained | 0 | 27 | 0 | 59 | 0 | 09328 |
| cherries, sour, canned in water, solids and liquid | 0 | 452 | 0 | 57 | 0 | 09064 |
| cherries, sour, frozen | 0 | 522 | 0 | 61 | 0 | 09068 |
| cherries, sour, raw | 0 | 770 | 0 | 85 | 0 | 09063 |
| cherries, sweet, canned in juice, solids and liquid | 0 | 75 | 0 | 57 | 0 | 09072 |
| cherries, sweet, raw | 0 | 38 | 0 | 85 | 0 | 09070 |
| cherries, sweet, sweetened, frozen | 0 | 113 | 0 | 85 | 0 | 09076 |
| cranberries, dried, sweetened | 0 | 0 | 0 | 33 | 0 | 09079 |
| cranberries, raw | 0 | 36 | 0 | 91 | 0 | 09078 |
| cranberry sauce, jellied, canned | 0 | 25 | 0 | 63 | 0 | 09081 |
| currants, red/white, raw | 0 | 25 | 0 | 47 | 0 | 09084 |
| currants, zante, dried | 1 | 43 | 1 | 0 | 0 | 09085 |
| date, dried | 0 | 6 | 0 | 75 | 0 | 09087 |
| date, medjool, dried | 0 | 89 | 0 | 23 | 0 | 09421 |
| fig, raw | 0 | 85 | 0 | 9 | 0 | 09089 |
| fruit cocktail, canned in juice, solids and liquid | 0 | 154 | 58 | 75 | 0 | 09097 |
| fruit roll (dried fruit) | 1 | 34 | 0 | 41 | 0 | 19014 |
| fruit salad, canned in heavy syrup, solids and liquid | 0 | 254 | 96 | 75 | 0 | 09105 |
| grapefruit, pink and red, raw | 3 | 686 | 6 | 5 | 1419 | 09112 |
| grapefruit, white, raw | 8 | 14 | 3 | 10 | 0 | 09116 |
| grapes, American (slip skin), all colors, raw | 1 | 59 | 0 | 72 | 0 | 09131 |
| grapes, green, Thompson seedless, canned in heavy syrup, solids and liquid | 1 | 38 | 0 | 48 | 0 | 09134 |
| grapes, red/green, European, seedless, raw | 1 | 39 | 0 | 72 | 0 | 09132 |
| guava, raw | 0 | 374 | 0 | 0 | 5204 | 09139 |
| honeydew melon, raw | 0 | 30 | 0 | 27 | 0 | 09184 |
| kiwifruit, raw | 0 | 52 | 0 | 122 | 0 | 09148 |

| | ALPHA-CAROTENE (mcg/100 g) | BETA-CAROTENE (mcg/100 g) | BETA-CRYPTOXANTHIN (mcg/100 g) | LUTEIN + ZEAXANTHIN (mcg/100 g) | LYCOPENE (mcg/100 g) | SR21 CODE NUMBER[1] |
|---|---|---|---|---|---|---|
| kumquat, raw | 155 | 0 | 193 | 129 | 0 | 09149 |
| lemon peel, raw | 1 | 7 | 45 | 18 | 0 | 09156 |
| lemon, raw | 1 | 3 | 20 | 11 | 0 | 09150 |
| lime, raw | 0 | 30 | 0 | 0 | 0 | 09159 |
| loganberries, frozen | 0 | 21 | 0 | 118 | 0 | 09167 |
| mandarin oranges, canned, juice pack | 133 | 193 | 503 | 163 | 0 | 09219 |
| mango, raw | 17 | 445 | 11 | 0 | 0 | 09176 |
| mulberries, raw | 12 | 9 | 0 | 136 | 0 | 09190 |
| nectarine, raw | 0 | 150 | 98 | 130 | 0 | 09191 |
| orange, California navel, raw | 7 | 87 | 116 | 129 | 0 | 09202 |
| orange, Florida, raw | 11 | 71 | 116 | 129 | 0 | 09203 |
| papaya, raw | 0 | 276 | 761 | 75 | 0 | 09226 |
| passion fruit (granadilla), purple, raw | 0 | 743 | 41 | 0 | 0 | 09231 |
| peach, canned in juice, solids and liquid | 1 | 189 | 78 | 61 | 0 | 09238 |
| peach, raw | 0 | 162 | 67 | 91 | 0 | 09236 |
| pear, Asian, raw | 0 | 0 | 0 | 50 | 0 | 09340 |
| pear, canned in juice, solids and liquid | 0 | 3 | 0 | 34 | 0 | 09254 |
| pear, raw | 0 | 13 | 2 | 45 | 0 | 09252 |
| persimmon, Japanese, raw | 0 | 253 | 1447 | 834 | 159 | 09263 |
| pineapple, raw | 0 | 35 | 0 | 0 | 0 | 09266 |
| plum, canned in juice, solids and liquid | 0 | 554 | 102 | 49 | 0 | 09282 |
| plum, raw | 0 | 190 | 35 | 73 | 0 | 09279 |
| prune, dried | 57 | 394 | 93 | 148 | 0 | 09291 |
| raspberries, raw | 16 | 12 | 0 | 136 | 0 | 09302 |
| raspberries, sweetened, frozen | 29 | 21 | 0 | 113 | 0 | 09306 |
| rowal, raw (fruit) | 0 | 230 | | | | 09428 |
| salmonberries, raw | 41 | 277 | 0 | | 0 | 35154 |
| tangerine, raw | 101 | 155 | 407 | 138 | 0 | 09218 |
| watermelon, raw | 0 | 303 | 78 | 8 | 4532 | 09326 |
| **GRAIN- AND VEGETABLE-BASED SNACK FOODS** | | | | | | |
| cheese puffs/twists | 0 | 0 | 0 | 643 | 0 | 19008 |
| corn chips | 0 | 0 | 0 | 212 | 0 | 19003 |
| corn-based onion flavor snack food | 33 | 51 | 0 | 879 | 0 | 19007 |
| granola bar, coconut, chocolate-covered | 0 | 0 | 0 | 48 | 0 | 42272 |
| granola bar, fruit-filled, nonfat | 0 | 173 | 242 | 103 | 1 | 19435 |
| granola bar, oat, fruits, and nut | 0 | 1 | 0 | 59 | 0 | 19023 |
| popcorn cake | 21 | 33 | 0 | 537 | 0 | 19036 |
| popcorn, 94% fat-free, microwaved | 7 | 75 | 160 | 1259 | 0 | 25000 |
| popcorn, air-popped | 58 | 89 | 0 | 1450 | 0 | 19034 |
| popcorn, oil-popped | 46 | 70 | 0 | 829 | 0 | 19035 |
| sweet potato chips | 0 | 14,204 | 0 | 0 | 0 | 25012 |
| tortilla chips, from white corn, unsalted | 24 | 37 | 0 | 507 | 0 | 43364 |
| **GRAIN PRODUCTS** | | | | | | |
| bagel, plain/onion/poppyseed/ sesame seed | 0 | 0 | 0 | 52 | 0 | 18001 |
| bread, banana, homemade with margarine | | 102 | | | | 18019 |
| bread, Boston brown, canned | 1 | 2 | 0 | 71 | 0 | 18021 |
| bread, Italian | 0 | 0 | 0 | 48 | 0 | 18033 |
| bread, mixed grain/whole grain/ 7-grain | 0 | 0 | 0 | 94 | 0 | 18035 |
| bread, oat bran | 0 | 0 | 0 | 46 | 0 | 18037 |
| bread, oatmeal | 0 | 0 | 0 | 72 | 0 | 18039 |
| bread, pumpernickel | 0 | 0 | 0 | 46 | 0 | 18044 |
| bread, raisin | 0 | 0 | 0 | 44 | 0 | 18047 |
| bread, rice bran | 0 | 0 | 0 | 49 | 0 | 18059 |

| | ALPHA-CAROTENE (mcg/100 g) | BETA-CAROTENE (mcg/100 g) | BETA-CRYPTOXANTHIN (mcg/100 g) | LUTEIN + ZEAXANTHIN (mcg/100 g) | LYCOPENE (mcg/100 g) | SR21 CODE NUMBER[1] |
|---|---|---|---|---|---|---|
| bread, rye | 0 | 4 | 1 | 54 | 0 | 18060 |
| bread, wheat bran | 0 | 0 | 0 | 54 | 0 | 18066 |
| bread, wheat germ | 0 | 2 | 0 | 55 | 0 | 18068 |
| bread, wheat/wheat berry | 0 | 0 | 0 | 44 | 0 | 18064 |
| bread, whole wheat | 0 | 2 | 0 | 76 | 0 | 18075 |
| breadcrumbs, dry, grated, seasoned | 0 | 116 | 0 | | 0 | 18376 |
| breadstick | 0 | 1 | 0 | 65 | 0 | 18080 |
| cracker meal | 0 | 0 | 0 | 76 | 0 | 18236 |
| crackers, rye | 1 | 2 | 0 | 245 | 0 | 18226 |
| crackers, wheat | 0 | 0 | 0 | 81 | 0 | 18232 |
| crackers, whole wheat | 0 | 0 | 0 | 179 | 0 | 18235 |
| crispbread, rye | 0 | 0 | 0 | 194 | 0 | 18216 |
| croutons, seasoned | 0 | 6 | 0 | 45 | 0 | 18243 |
| English muffin | 0 | 0 | 0 | 42 | 0 | 18258 |
| French toast, homemade with 2% milk | | 66 | | | | 18269 |
| hush puppies, homemade | 17 | 27 | 1 | 401 | 0 | 18270 |
| macaroni, vegetable, enriched, boiled | 0 | 55 | 0 | 13 | 245 | 20106 |
| macaroni, whole wheat, boiled | 0 | 2 | 0 | 81 | 0 | 20108 |
| melba toast | 0 | 0 | 0 | 74 | 0 | 18220 |
| muffin, corn | 12 | 20 | 0 | 263 | 0 | 18279 |
| noodles, chow mein | 0 | 1 | 0 | 56 | 0 | 20113 |
| noodles, egg and spinach, enriched, boiled (egg and spinach in the noodle dough) | 0 | 51 | 0 | 2232 | 0 | 20112 |
| noodles, egg, enriched, boiled (egg in the noodle dough) | 0 | 1 | 0 | 38 | 0 | 20110 |
| noodles, egg, enriched, dry (egg in pasta dough) | 0 | 2 | 1 | 110 | 0 | 20109 |
| pancake, frozen | 0 | 1 | 0 | 20 | 0 | 18288 |
| pita bread, white | 0 | 0 | 0 | 53 | 0 | 18041 |
| pita bread, whole wheat | 0 | 0 | 0 | 53 | 0 | 18042 |
| roll, dinner, wheat (white) | 0 | 0 | 0 | 65 | 0 | 18347 |
| roll, dinner, whole wheat | 0 | 0 | 0 | 115 | 0 | 18348 |
| roll, frankfurter | 0 | 0 | 0 | 45 | 0 | 18350 |
| roll, French | 0 | 0 | 0 | 50 | 0 | 18349 |
| roll, hamburger | 0 | 0 | 0 | 45 | 0 | 18350 |
| roll, hard/kaiser | 0 | 0 | 0 | 58 | 0 | 18353 |
| roll, oat bran | 0 | 0 | 0 | 44 | 0 | 18345 |
| roll, pumpernickel | 0 | 0 | 0 | 46 | 0 | 43441 |
| roll, rye | 0 | 4 | 1 | 54 | 0 | 18346 |
| spaghetti, whole wheat, boiled | 0 | 2 | 0 | 81 | 0 | 20125 |
| stuffing, bread, from mix | 0 | 88 | 0 | 18 | 0 | 18082 |
| stuffing, cornbread, from mix | 0 | 58 | 0 | 0 | 0 | 18085 |
| taco shell, from corn tortilla | 3 | 3 | 13 | 106 | 3 | 18360 |
| waffle, buttermilk, frozen, toasted | 0 | 2 | 2 | 66 | 0 | 18933 |
| waffle, frozen, toasted | 0 | 1 | 1 | 51 | 0 | 18403 |

### INFANT, JUNIOR, AND TODDLER FOODS
### BAKED PRODUCTS

| | | | | | | |
|---|---|---|---|---|---|---|
| baby/infant pretzel | 1 | 4 | 1 | 72 | 0 | 03215 |
| crackers, vegetable, infant food | 636 | 1825 | 1 | 359 | 1883 | 03209 |
| fruit cookie, infant food | 810 | 1002 | 2 | 175 | 0 | 03206 |
| teething biscuit | 6 | 13 | 0 | 169 | 0 | 03216 |

### CEREALS

| | | | | | | |
|---|---|---|---|---|---|---|
| barley infant cereal, dry | 0 | 0 | 0 | 170 | 0 | 03181 |
| mixed cereal with bananas, dry, infant food | 49 | 51 | 0 | 96 | 0 | 03186 |
| mixed cereal, dry, infant food | 6 | 9 | 0 | 148 | 0 | 03185 |
| oatmeal with applesauce and bananas, strained infant cereal | 2 | 13 | 8 | 90 | 0 | 03191 |
| oatmeal with bananas, dry infant cereal | 27 | 28 | 0 | 157 | 0 | 03190 |
| oatmeal, dry, infant cereal | 0 | 0 | 0 | 185 | 0 | 03189 |

| | ALPHA-CAROTENE (mcg/100 g) | BETA-CAROTENE (mcg/100 g) | BETA-CRYPTOXANTHIN (mcg/100 g) | LUTEIN + ZEAXANTHIN (mcg/100 g) | LYCOPENE (mcg/100 g) | SR21 CODE NUMBER[1] |
|---|---|---|---|---|---|---|
| rice cereal with bananas, dry, infant food | 11 | 12 | 0 | 39 | 0 | 03212 |
| whole wheat cereal with apples, dry, infant cereal | 0 | 10 | 4 | 203 | 0 | 03184 |
| **DESSERTS** | | | | | | |
| blueberry yogurt dessert, strained infant food | 0 | 23 | 0 | 64 | 0 | 43537 |
| cherry vanilla pudding, strained infant food | 0 | 145 | 0 | 9 | 0 | 03224 |
| fruit dessert, Gerber 2nd Foods | 2 | 64 | 27 | 43 | 0 | 03235 |
| peach cobbler, Gerber 3rd Foods | 0 | 68 | 28 | 39 | 0 | 03228 |
| tutti fruit, strained infant food | 1 | 35 | 89 | 21 | 0 | 43006 |
| vanilla custard pudding, Beech-Nut Stage 2/Gerber 2nd Foods/Heinz Strained-2 | 1 | 2 | 1 | 39 | 0 | 03245 |
| **DINNERS** | | | | | | |
| apples and sweet potatoes dinner, Gerber 2nd Foods | 0 | 1225 | 9 | 13 | 0 | 03154 |
| beef and vegetables dinner, infant food | 993 | 2165 | 0 | 58 | 0 | 03055 |
| beef noodle dinner, Beech-Nut Stage 2/Gerber 2nd Foods/ Heinz Strained-2 | 159 | 350 | 0 | 23 | 476 | 03047 |
| beef stew dinner, Beech-Nut Table Time | 346 | 816 | 0 | 26 | 2575 | 03052 |
| broccoli and chicken dinner, Gerber 2nd Foods/Heinz Strained-2 | 9 | 278 | 0 | 511 | 0 | 03298 |
| carrots and beef dinner, Gerber 2nd Food | 3716 | 6813 | 0 | 139 | 1 | 03290 |
| chicken and rice, infant food | 260 | 571 | 0 | 105 | 0 | 43008 |
| chicken noodle dinner, Beech-Nut Stage 2/Gerber 2nd Foods/ Heinz Strained-2 | 495 | 1060 | 0 | 40 | 0 | 03068 |
| macaroni, tomato, and beef, Beech-Nut Stage 2/Gerber 2nd Foods/Heinz Strained-2 | 213 | 420 | 0 | 0 | 42 | 03044 |
| pasta with vegetables, Gerber | 39 | 282 | 0 | 341 | 290 | 03077 |
| ravioli, cheese and tomato sauce, infant food | 2 | 230 | 3 | 69 | 1632 | 03046 |
| spaghetti, tomato, and beef, Beech-Nut Stage 3/Gerber 3nd Foods/Heinz Junior-3 | 304 | 601 | 0 | 0 | 0 | 03050 |
| sweet potatoes and chicken, Beech-Nut Stage 2 | 0 | 2590 | 0 | 0 | 0 | 03303 |
| turkey and rice, Beech-Nut Stage 2/Gerber 2nd Foods/ Heinz Strained-2 | 368 | 789 | 0 | 38 | 0 | 03082 |
| vegetables and bacon, Gerber 2nd Foods/Heinz Strained-2 | 515 | 1112 | 0 | 225 | 1 | 03059 |
| vegetables and beef, Beech-Nut Stage 3/Gerber 3rd Foods/ Heinz Junior-3 | 810 | 2545 | 11 | 51 | 627 | 03054 |
| vegetables and chicken dinner, Beech-Nut Stage 3/Gerber 3rd Foods | 592 | 1270 | 0 | 36 | 0 | 03274 |
| vegetables and ham dinner, Beech-Nut Stage 2/Gerber 2nd Foods/Heinz Strained-2 | 645 | 1401 | 0 | 49 | 685 | 03061 |
| vegetables and lamb dinner, Beech-Nut Stage 2/Heinz Strained-2 | 443 | 976 | 0 | 34 | 947 | 03066 |
| vegetables and turkey dinner, Gerber 2nd Foods | 998 | 2139 | 0 | 76 | 0 | 03084 |

| | ALPHA-CAROTENE (mcg/100 g) | BETA-CAROTENE (mcg/100 g) | BETA-CRYPTOXANTHIN (mcg/100 g) | LUTEIN + ZEAXANTHIN (mcg/100 g) | LYCOPENE (mcg/100 g) | SR21 CODE NUMBER[1] |
|---|---|---|---|---|---|---|
| **FRUIT JUICES** | | | | | | |
| apple cranberry juice, infant food | 0 | 17 | 0 | 49 | 0 | 03169 |
| apple peach juice, infant food | 0 | 31 | 13 | 29 | 0 | 03168 |
| apple plum juice, infant food | 0 | 24 | 5 | 21 | 0 | 03170 |
| apple sweet potato juice, infant food | 0 | 1849 | 0 | 6 | 0 | 42266 |
| orange apple banana juice, Heinz Strained | 1 | 5 | 22 | 59 | 0 | 03174 |
| orange carrot juice, infant food | 395 | 863 | 135 | 135 | 0 | 42267 |
| orange juice, Beech-Nut Stage 3/ Gerber 2nd Foods/Heinz Strained | 2 | 9 | 47 | 113 | 0 | 03172 |
| **FRUITS** | | | | | | |
| applesauce and apricots, Beech-Nut Stage 2/Gerber 2nd Foods/Heinz Strained-2 | 3 | 189 | 26 | 28 | 0 | 03142 |
| applesauce and cherries, strained infant food | 0 | 25 | 4 | 56 | 0 | 03144 |
| apricots with tapioca, Gerber 2nd Foods | 7 | 412 | 39 | 11 | 0 | 03118 |
| mango with tapioca, Gerber | 10 | 262 | 6 | 0 | 0 | 03140 |
| peaches, Beech-Nut Baby's First/ Gerber 1st Foods/Heinz Beginner-1 | 0 | 378 | 68 | 163 | 0 | 03130 |
| plums with tapioca, Gerber 2nd Foods/Heinz Strained-2 | 0 | 78 | 14 | 30 | 0 | 03134 |
| plums, bananas, and rice, strained infant food | 0 | 73 | 13 | 65 | 0 | 03293 |
| prunes with tapioca, Gerber 2nd Foods | 33 | 228 | 54 | 39 | 0 | 03136 |
| **VEGETABLES** | | | | | | |
| butternut squash and corn, Gerber 2nd Foods | 362 | 1476 | 38 | 970 | 0 | 03114 |
| carrots, Beech-Nut Baby's First/ Gerber 1st Foods/Heinz Beginner-1 | 2602 | 5575 | 0 | 0 | 0 | 03099 |
| corn and sweet potatoes, strained infant food | 12 | 1488 | 3 | 215 | 0 | 03934 |
| corn, yellow, creamed, Heinz Junior-3 | 10 | 13 | 3 | 423 | 0 | 03120 |
| garden vegetables, strained infant food | 740 | 3270 | 0 | 1374 | 0 | 03283 |
| green beans, Beech-Nut Stage 3 | 0 | 292 | 0 | 493 | 0 | 03092 |
| green peas, Beech-Nut Baby's First/Gerber 1st Foods | 11 | 124 | 0 | 1465 | 0 | 03121 |
| mixed vegetables, strained infant food | 699 | 1550 | 0 | 381 | 0 | 03286 |
| peas and brown rice, infant food | 11 | 227 | 0 | 1256 | 0 | 42279 |
| spinach, creamed, Gerber 2nd Foods | 0 | 2456 | 0 | 4505 | 0 | 03127 |
| squash, yellow, Beech-Nut Baby's First/Gerber 1st Foods/Heinz Beginner-1 | 242 | 896 | 9 | 3527 | 0 | 03104 |
| sweet potatoes, Beech-Nut Stage 1/Gerber 2nd Foods/ Heinz Strained-2 | 0 | 3863 | 0 | 0 | 0 | 03108 |
| **MEAT AND POULTRY ORGANS** | | | | | | |
| beef brain, simmered | 0 | 70 | 0 | 0 | 0 | 13320 |
| beef liver, pan-fried | 11 | 182 | 21 | 0 | 0 | 13327 |
| chicken liver, simmered | 11 | 30 | 11 | 83 | 21 | 05028 |
| **MEATS, LUNCHEON AND SNACK** | | | | | | |
| beef sticks, smoked | | 150 | | | | 19407 |

| | ALPHA-CAROTENE (mcg/100 g) | BETA-CAROTENE (mcg/100 g) | BETA-CRYPTOXANTHIN (mcg/100 g) | LUTEIN + ZEAXANTHIN (mcg/100 g) | LYCOPENE (mcg/100 g) | SR21 CODE NUMBER[1] |
|---|---|---|---|---|---|---|
| bockwurst (pork, veal, milk, eggs), raw | 0 | 148 | 2 | 108 | 0 | 07006 |
| pickle and pimento loaf, pork | 4 | 147 | 46 | 87 | 0 | 07058 |
| **NUTS AND SEEDS** | | | | | | |
| pecans, dry-roasted | 0 | 84 | | | | 12143 |
| pistachios, dry-roasted | 0 | 157 | 0 | 1205 | 0 | 12152 |
| soy nuts, roasted | 0 | 120 | 0 | 0 | 0 | 16110 |
| flaxseeds | 0 | 0 | 0 | 651 | 0 | 12220 |
| pumpkin and squash seed kernels, roasted | 0 | 228 | 0 | 0 | 0 | 12016 |
| sesame butter (tahini), from roasted and toasted kernels | 0 | 40 | 0 | 0 | 0 | 12166 |
| sesame seed kernels, dried | 0 | 40 | 0 | 0 | 0 | 12201 |
| sunflower seed kernels, dried | 0 | 30 | 0 | 0 | 0 | 12036 |
| **SALAD DRESSINGS** | | | | | | |
| bacon and tomato salad dressing | 0 | 92 | 52 | 29 | 2597 | 43331 |
| buttermilk salad dressing, lite | 2 | 4 | 2 | 49 | 0 | 43215 |
| coleslaw salad dressing | 2 | 4 | 1 | 48 | 0 | 43016 |
| French salad dressing | 0 | 232 | 92 | 0 | 373 | 04120 |
| French salad dressing, reduced calorie | 4 | 120 | 0 | 0 | 3843 | 42171 |
| homemade salad dressing, cooked | 0 | 3 | 1 | 50 | 0 | 04134 |
| mayonnaise-type salad dressing | 1 | 94 | 27 | 87 | 0 | 04018 |
| mayonnaise-type salad dressing, low calorie | 1 | 94 | 27 | 87 | 0 | 43329 |
| Russian salad dressing | 2 | 320 | 49 | 173 | 3576 | 04015 |
| thousand island salad dressing | 0 | 92 | 52 | 29 | 2597 | 04017 |
| thousand island salad dressing, low/reduced calorie | 0 | 154 | 65 | 100 | 3097 | 04023 |
| **SAUCES, GRAVIES, AND CONDIMENTS** | | | | | | |
| barbeque sauce | 4 | 139 | 0 | 0 | 4431 | 06150 |
| catsup (ketchup) | 0 | 560 | 0 | 0 | 16,709 | 11935 |
| hot pepper sauce, ready-to-serve | 6 | 91 | 7 | 121 | 0 | 06168 |
| olives, black, canned/bottled | 0 | 204 | 8 | 510 | 0 | 09194 |
| olives, green, canned/bottled | 0 | 231 | 9 | 510 | 0 | 09195 |
| pickle (cucumber), dill | 19 | 78 | 45 | 41 | 0 | 11937 |
| pickle (cucumber), sour | 20 | 81 | 47 | 43 | 0 | 11941 |
| pickle (cucumber), sweet gherkin | 81 | 325 | 186 | 170 | 0 | 11940 |
| salsa | 0 | 175 | 0 | 0 | 10,515 | 06164 |
| sweet and sour sauce, homemade | 2 | 65 | 0 | 1 | 2032 | 06285 |
| tabasco sauce, McIlhenny | 62 | 919 | 68 | 10 | 0 | 06169 |
| tomato sauce, bottled | 0 | 259 | 3 | 23 | 13,979 | 11549 |
| **SOUPS, CANNED, READY-TO-SERVE** | | | | | | |
| beef stroganoff soup, chunky | 49 | 365 | 1 | 386 | 14 | 06980 |
| beef, chunky soup | 234 | 536 | 0 | 36 | 1325 | 06070 |
| chicken noodle soup, chunky | 266 | 593 | 14 | 58 | 0 | 06018 |
| chicken rice soup, chunky | 529 | 1183 | 1 | 96 | 13 | 06022 |
| chicken vegetable soup with potato and cheese, chunky | 77 | 186 | 0 | 33 | 54 | 06208 |
| clam chowder, Manhattan, chunky | 270 | 662 | 0 | 33 | 5112 | 06027 |
| gazpacho | 1 | 69 | 8 | 26 | 915 | 06036 |
| minestrone soup, chunky | 370 | 885 | 0 | 45 | 5963 | 06039 |
| split pea soup, Progresso Healthy Classics | 35 | 313 | 1 | 1286 | 7 | 06192 |
| split pea with ham soup, chunky | 445 | 995 | 0 | 78 | 0 | 06050 |
| vegetable soup, chunky | 512 | 1198 | 3 | 124 | 2953 | 06067 |
| **SPICES, HERBS, AND FLAVORINGS** | | | | | | |
| basil, dried | 0 | 5584 | 81 | 1150 | 393 | 02003 |
| basil, raw | 0 | 3142 | 46 | 5650 | 0 | 02044 |
| black pepper | 0 | 156 | 48 | 205 | 6 | 02030 |
| capers, canned | 0 | 83 | 0 | 0 | 0 | 02054 |

| | ALPHA-CAROTENE (mcg/100 g) | BETA-CAROTENE (mcg/100 g) | BETA-CRYPTOXANTHIN (mcg/100 g) | LUTEIN + ZEAXANTHIN (mcg/100 g) | LYCOPENE (mcg/100 g) | SR21 CODE NUMBER[1] |
|---|---|---|---|---|---|---|
| caraway seeds | 0 | 189 | 58 | 205 | 6 | 02005 |
| chili powder | 2090 | 15,000 | 3490 | 310 | 21 | 02009 |
| chives, raw | 0 | 2612 | 0 | 323 | 0 | 11156 |
| cilantro leaves, dried | 31 | 3407 | 175 | 5530 | 0 | 02012 |
| cinnamon, ground | 1 | 112 | 129 | 222 | 15 | 02010 |
| cloves, ground | 0 | 84 | 468 | 0 | 0 | 02011 |
| cumin | 0 | 762 | 0 | 448 | 0 | 02014 |
| curry powder | 0 | 592 | 0 | 0 | 0 | 02015 |
| ginger, ground | 0 | 88 | 0 | 0 | 0 | 02021 |
| marjoram, dried | 0 | 4806 | 70 | 862 | 0 | 02023 |
| mustard seeds, yellow | 0 | 37 | 0 | 448 | 0 | 02024 |
| nutmeg, ground | 0 | 16 | 90 | 0 | 0 | 02025 |
| oregano, dried, ground | 0 | 4112 | 60 | 862 | 0 | 02027 |
| paprika | 0 | 27,679 | 7923 | 13,157 | 0 | 02028 |
| parsley, dried | 1430 | 5380 | 30 | 5530 | 397 | 02029 |
| poultry seasoning | 0 | 1568 | 23 | 503 | 2 | 02034 |
| pumpkin pie spice | 0 | 36 | 241 | 189 | 13 | 02035 |
| red/cayenne pepper | 0 | 21,840 | 6252 | 13,157 | 0 | 02031 |
| sage, ground | 0 | 3485 | 109 | 862 | 0 | 02038 |
| thyme, ground | 0 | 2264 | 33 | 862 | 0 | 02042 |

**VEGETABLES AND VEGETABLE DISHES**

**FRUIT, STEM, AND STALK VEGETABLES**

| | | | | | | |
|---|---|---|---|---|---|---|
| artichoke, boiled | 0 | 8 | 0 | 464 | 0 | 11008 |
| asparagus, boiled | 0 | 604 | 0 | 771 | 30 | 11012 |
| asparagus, canned | 0 | 493 | 0 | 630 | 24 | 11015 |
| broccoflower, raw | 0 | 93 | 0 | 42 | 0 | 11965 |
| broccoli, boiled | 0 | 929 | 0 | 1080 | 0 | 11091 |
| broccoli, raw | 25 | 361 | 1 | 1403 | 0 | 11090 |
| broccoli, spears, frozen, boiled | 19 | 597 | 1 | 1095 | 0 | 11095 |
| celery, boiled | 0 | 313 | 0 | 329 | 0 | 11144 |
| celery, raw | 0 | 270 | 0 | 283 | 0 | 11143 |
| Chinese broccoli (Chinese kale), boiled | 0 | 983 | 0 | 912 | 0 | 11969 |
| leek, boiled | 0 | 487 | 0 | 925 | 0 | 11247 |
| rhubarb, cooked, sweetened, frozen | 0 | 44 | 0 | 123 | 0 | 09310 |
| scallions (green/spring onions), raw | 0 | 598 | 0 | 1137 | 0 | 11291 |

**FRUIT (SEED-CONTAINING) VEGETABLES**

| | | | | | | |
|---|---|---|---|---|---|---|
| acorn winter squash, boiled | 0 | 490 | 0 | 66 | 0 | 11484 |
| balsam pear (bitter melon/bitter gourd) pods, boiled | 0 | 68 | 0 | 1323 | 0 | 11025 |
| banana pepper, raw | 39 | 184 | 0 | 0 | 0 | 11976 |
| butternut winter squash, baked | 1130 | 4570 | 3116 | 0 | 0 | 11486 |
| chili pepper, green, hot, canned, solids and liquid | 14 | 410 | 30 | 444 | 0 | 11329 |
| chili pepper, green, hot, raw | 23 | 671 | 50 | 725 | 0 | 11670 |
| chili pepper, red, hot, canned, solids and liquid | 446 | 6664 | 495 | 444 | 0 | 11820 |
| chili pepper, red, hot, raw | 36 | 534 | 40 | 709 | 0 | 11819 |
| chili pepper, red, hot, sun-dried | 994 | 14,844 | 1103 | 5494 | 0 | 11962 |
| crookneck/straightneck summer squash, boiled | 0 | 98 | 0 | 315 | 0 | 11468 |
| crookneck/straightneck summer squash, canned | 0 | 61 | 0 | 198 | 0 | 11471 |
| cucumber, raw | 11 | 45 | 26 | 23 | 0 | 11205 |
| eggplant (aubergine), boiled | 0 | 22 | 0 | 0 | 0 | 11210 |
| green snap beans, boiled | 0 | 420 | 0 | 709 | 0 | 11053 |
| green snap beans, canned | 156 | 122 | 24 | 441 | 0 | 11056 |
| hubbard winter squash, boiled | 529 | 2139 | 0 | 0 | 0 | 11491 |
| jalapeno pepper, canned, solids and liquid | 32 | 968 | 72 | 657 | 0 | 11632 |
| jalapeno pepper, raw | 15 | 455 | 34 | 492 | 0 | 11979 |
| okra, boiled, drained | 0 | 170 | 0 | 390 | 0 | 11279 |
| pimiento pepper, canned | 238 | 1474 | 0 | 366 | 0 | 11943 |

| | ALPHA-CAROTENE (mcg/100 g) | BETA-CAROTENE (mcg/100 g) | BETA-CRYPTOXANTHIN (mcg/100 g) | LUTEIN + ZEAXANTHIN (mcg/100 g) | LYCOPENE (mcg/100 g) | SR21 CODE NUMBER[1] |
|---|---|---|---|---|---|---|
| plantain, cooked | 353 | 369 | 0 | 28 | 0 | 09278 |
| pumpkin winter squash, boiled | 348 | 2096 | 1450 | 1014 | 0 | 11423 |
| pumpkin winter squash, canned | 4795 | 6940 | 0 | 0 | 0 | 11424 |
| scallop summer squash, boiled | 0 | 51 | 0 | 250 | 0 | 11476 |
| serrano pepper, raw | 18 | 534 | 40 | 544 | 0 | 11977 |
| snow peas, boiled | 42 | 597 | 0 | 702 | 0 | 11301 |
| snow peas, raw | 44 | 630 | 0 | 740 | 0 | 11300 |
| spaghetti winter squash, boiled/baked | 15 | 59 | 0 | 0 | 0 | 11493 |
| summer squash, all varieties, boiled | 0 | 127 | 0 | 2249 | 0 | 11642 |
| sweet pepper, green, boiled | 26 | 264 | 8 | 431 | 0 | 11334 |
| sweet pepper, green, raw | 21 | 208 | 7 | 341 | 0 | 11333 |
| sweet pepper, red, boiled | 18 | 1525 | 460 | 47 | 0 | 11823 |
| sweet pepper, red, raw | 20 | 1624 | 490 | 51 | 0 | 11821 |
| sweet pepper, yellow, raw | | 120 | | | | 11951 |
| tomatillo, raw | 10 | 63 | 0 | 467 | 0 | 11954 |
| tomato paste, canned | 29 | 901 | 0 | 0 | 28,764 | 11546 |
| tomato puree, canned | 0 | 306 | 0 | 0 | 21,754 | 11547 |
| tomato, green, raw | 78 | 346 | 0 | 0 | 0 | 11527 |
| tomato, red, boiled | 0 | 293 | 0 | 94 | 3041 | 11530 |
| tomato, red, canned | 0 | 70 | 0 | 86 | 2767 | 11531 |
| tomato, red, raw | 101 | 449 | 0 | 123 | 2573 | 11529 |
| tomato, red, sun-dried | 0 | 524 | 0 | 1419 | 45,902 | 11955 |
| waxgourd (Chinese preserving melon), boiled | 0 | 0 | 0 | 197 | 0 | 11594 |
| winter squash, all varieties, baked | 682 | 2793 | 0 | 1415 | 0 | 11644 |
| yellow snap beans, boiled | 0 | 49 | 0 | 709 | 0 | 11724 |
| yellow snap beans, canned | 0 | 63 | 0 | 441 | 0 | 11932 |
| zucchini summer squash, boiled | 0 | 670 | 0 | 1150 | 0 | 11478 |

**LEAFY VEGETABLES**

| | | | | | | |
|---|---|---|---|---|---|---|
| arugula, raw | 0 | 1424 | 0 | 3555 | 0 | 11959 |
| balsam pear (bitter melon/bitter gourd) leafy tips, boiled | 0 | 1450 | 0 | 2638 | 0 | 11023 |
| beet greens, boiled | 4 | 4590 | 0 | 1819 | 0 | 11087 |
| broccoli raab (rapini) | 0 | 2720 | 0 | 1683 | 0 | 11097 |
| Brussels sprouts, boiled | 0 | 465 | 0 | 1290 | 0 | 11099 |
| cabbage, green/white, boiled | 0 | 48 | 0 | 27 | 0 | 11110 |
| cabbage, green/white, raw | 33 | 42 | 0 | 30 | 0 | 11109 |
| cabbage, napa, boiled | 49 | 133 | 0 | | 0 | 11970 |
| cabbage, red/purple, raw | 0 | 670 | 0 | 329 | 20 | 11112 |
| cabbage, savoy, raw | 0 | 600 | 0 | 77 | 0 | 11114 |
| chicory greens, raw | 0 | 3430 | 0 | 10,300 | 0 | 11152 |
| Chinese cabbage, pak choi, boiled | 1 | 2549 | 0 | 38 | 0 | 11117 |
| Chinese cabbage, pak choi, raw | 1 | 2681 | 0 | 40 | 0 | 11116 |
| Chinese cabbage, pe-tsai, raw | 1 | 190 | 0 | 48 | 0 | 11119 |
| cilantro, raw | 36 | 3930 | 202 | 865 | 0 | 11165 |
| coleslaw, homemade | | 138 | | | | 11159 |
| collards, boiled | 90 | 4814 | 20 | 7694 | 0 | 11162 |
| dandelion greens, boiled | 244 | 3940 | 82 | 9158 | 0 | 11208 |
| endive, raw | 0 | 1300 | 0 | 0 | 0 | 11213 |
| fiddlehead ferns, raw | 261 | 2040 | | | | 11995 |
| garden cress, boiled | 0 | 2790 | 0 | 8402 | 0 | 11204 |
| garden cress, raw | 0 | 4150 | 0 | 12,500 | 0 | 11203 |
| garland chrysanthemum, boiled | 0 | 1543 | 0 | 3467 | 0 | 11158 |
| garland chrysanthemum, raw | 0 | 1380 | 24 | 3834 | | 11157 |
| grape leaves, canned | 629 | 2838 | 0 | | | 11975 |
| grape leaves, raw | 629 | 16,194 | 9 | 1747 | 0 | 11974 |
| horseradish tree leafy tips, chopped, boiled | 0 | 4208 | 0 | 1747 | 0 | 11223 |
| jute (potherb), boiled | 0 | 3111 | 0 | 1747 | 0 | 11232 |
| kale, boiled | 0 | 8173 | 0 | 18246 | 0 | 11234 |
| lambsquarters, boiled | 4 | 4688 | 0 | 1857 | 0 | 11245 |
| lettuce, butterhead, raw | 0 | 1987 | 0 | 1223 | 0 | 11250 |
| lettuce, iceberg, raw | 4 | 299 | 0 | 277 | 0 | 11252 |
| lettuce, looseleaf (leaf), raw | 0 | 4443 | 0 | 1730 | 0 | 11253 |

| | ALPHA-CAROTENE (mcg/100 g) | BETA-CAROTENE (mcg/100 g) | BETA-CRYPTOXANTHIN (mcg/100 g) | LUTEIN + ZEAXANTHIN (mcg/100 g) | LYCOPENE (mcg/100 g) | SR21 CODE NUMBER[1] |
|---|---|---|---|---|---|---|
| mustard greens, boiled | 0 | 3794 | 0 | 5962 | 0 | 11271 |
| parsley, raw | 0 | 5054 | 0 | 5561 | 0 | 11297 |
| pumpkin leaves, boiled | 0 | 960 | 0 | 1747 | 0 | 11419 |
| radicchio, raw | 0 | 16 | 0 | 8832 | 0 | 11952 |
| romaine (cos lettuce), raw | 0 | 5226 | 0 | 2312 | 0 | 11251 |
| sauerkraut, canned, solids and liquid | 5 | 8 | 0 | 295 | 0 | 11439 |
| spinach au gratin, frozen, Budget Gourmet | | 2620 | | | | 22603 |
| spinach soufflé, homemade | 3 | 1493 | 2 | 3249 | 0 | 11658 |
| spinach, boiled | 0 | 6288 | 0 | 11,308 | 0 | 11458 |
| spinach, canned | 0 | 5881 | 0 | 10,575 | 0 | 11461 |
| spinach, raw | 0 | 5626 | 0 | 12,198 | 0 | 11457 |
| sweet potato leaves, steamed | 0 | 550 | 0 | 2633 | 0 | 11506 |
| Swiss chard, boiled | 45 | 3652 | 0 | 11,015 | 0 | 11148 |
| turnip greens and root, frozen, boiled | 0 | 5167 | 0 | 9532 | 0 | 11577 |
| turnip greens, boiled | 0 | 4575 | 0 | 8440 | 0 | 11569 |
| turnip greens, frozen, boiled | 0 | 6459 | 0 | 11,915 | 0 | 11575 |
| watercress, raw | 0 | 1914 | 0 | 5767 | 0 | 11591 |
| **LEGUMES (BEANS AND PEAS)** | | | | | | |
| baked beans with pork in tomato sauce, canned | 0 | 50 | 0 | 14 | 322 | 16011 |
| broadbeans (fava beans) in pod, immature, raw | 0 | 196 | 9 | | | 11973 |
| chili beans, barbecue ranch style | 0 | 7 | 0 | 13 | 297 | 43112 |
| green peas, canned | 9 | 514 | 0 | 1350 | 0 | 11308 |
| green peas, frozen, boiled | 20 | 1250 | 0 | 2400 | 0 | 11313 |
| lima beans, immature, baby, frozen, boiled | 0 | 100 | 0 | 0 | 0 | 11040 |
| lima beans, immature, boiled | 0 | 182 | 0 | 0 | 0 | 11032 |
| lima beans, immature, green Fordhook, frozen, boiled | 0 | 114 | 0 | 0 | 0 | 11038 |
| mungo beans, mature, boiled | 0 | 19 | 0 | 0 | 0 | 16084 |
| peas, split, yellow and green, mature, dry | 0 | 89 | 0 | 0 | 0 | 16085 |
| pigeon peas, immature, boiled | 0 | 30 | 0 | 141 | 0 | 11345 |
| shellie (shell) beans, canned, solids and liquid | 0 | 137 | 0 | 331 | 0 | 11050 |
| **SPROUT AND SHOOT VEGETABLES** | | | | | | |
| alfalfa sprouts, raw | 6 | 87 | 6 | 0 | 0 | 11001 |
| pokeberry shoots (poke), boiled | 0 | 5220 | 0 | 1747 | 0 | 11351 |
| **TUBER AND ROOT VEGETABLES** | | | | | | |
| carrot, baby, raw | 3767 | 6391 | 0 | 358 | 0 | 11960 |
| carrot, boiled | 3776 | 8332 | 0 | 687 | 0 | 11125 |
| carrot, canned | 2743 | 5331 | 0 | 0 | 0 | 11128 |
| carrot, frozen, boiled | 3716 | 8199 | 199 | 676 | 0 | 11131 |
| carrot, raw | 3477 | 8285 | 0 | 256 | 1 | 11124 |
| potato, hashed brown, homemade | 0 | 3 | 0 | 16 | 0 | 11370 |
| potato, mashed, from granules with milk | 0 | 33 | 0 | 7 | 0 | 11383 |
| potato, mashed, homemade with whole milk and butter | 0 | 30 | 0 | 7 | 0 | 11371 |
| potato pancake, homemade | 0 | 4 | 2 | 87 | 0 | 11672 |
| potato puffs, frozen, heated | 0 | 3 | 0 | 16 | 0 | 11399 |
| potato, red-skinned, baked | 0 | 6 | 0 | 31 | 0 | 11358 |
| potato, russet, baked | 0 | 6 | 0 | 20 | 0 | 11356 |
| potato salad, homemade | | 36 | | | | 11414 |
| sweet potato, baked | 43 | 11,509 | 0 | 0 | 0 | 11508 |
| sweet potato, canned in light syrup, drained | 0 | 5501 | 0 | 0 | 0 | 11647 |
| sweet potato, canned, mashed | 0 | 5219 | 0 | 0 | 0 | 11514 |
| sweet potato, canned, vacuum pack | 0 | 4790 | 0 | 0 | 0 | 11512 |

| | ALPHA-CAROTENE (mcg/100 g) | BETA-CAROTENE (mcg/100 g) | BETA-CRYPTOXANTHIN (mcg/100 g) | LUTEIN + ZEAXANTHIN (mcg/100 g) | LYCOPENE (mcg/100 g) | SR21 CODE NUMBER[1] |
|---|---|---|---|---|---|---|
| sweet potato, frozen, baked | 47 | 12,498 | 0 | 0 | 0 | 11517 |
| taro, cooked | 0 | 39 | 22 | 0 | 0 | 11519 |
| **VEGETABLE COMBINATIONS** | | | | | | |
| green peas and carrots, frozen | 1868 | 4725 | 99 | 1538 | 0 | 11323 |
| green peas and onions, frozen, boiled | 10 | 626 | 0 | 1202 | 0 | 11327 |
| mixed vegetables, canned | 2636 | 5670 | 5 | 493 | 0 | 11581 |
| mixed vegetables, frozen, boiled | 968 | 2082 | 0 | 637 | 0 | 11584 |
| succotash (corn and lima beans), frozen, boiled | 9 | 82 | 61 | 342 | 0 | 11502 |
| **VEGETABLES, OTHER** | | | | | | |
| corn pudding, homemade | 11 | 37 | 76 | 458 | 0 | 11656 |
| corn, yellow, boiled | 23 | 66 | 161 | 906 | 0 | 11168 |
| corn, yellow, canned, vacuum pack | 26 | 33 | 6 | 1045 | 0 | 11176 |
| corn, yellow, creamed, canned | 23 | 30 | 6 | 949 | 0 | 11174 |
| nopales (prickly pear), cooked | 47 | 242 | 0 | 0 | 0 | 11964 |
| seaweed, Irish moss, raw | 0 | 71 | 0 | 0 | 0 | 11444 |
| seaweed, kelp (kombu/tangle), raw | 0 | 70 | 0 | 0 | 0 | 11445 |
| seaweed, laver (nori), raw | 0 | 3121 | 0 | 0 | 0 | 11446 |
| seaweed, spirulina, dried | 0 | 342 | 0 | 0 | 0 | 11667 |
| seaweed, wakame, raw | 0 | 216 | 0 | 0 | 0 | 11669 |
| **OTHER FOODS** | | | | | | |
| baking chocolate (unsweetened) | 0 | 0 | 0 | 38 | 0 | 19078 |
| cocoa powder, unsweetened | 0 | 0 | 0 | 38 | 0 | 19165 |
| jam/preserves, apricot | 2 | 116 | 11 | 9 | 0 | 19719 |
| marmalade, orange | 5 | 15 | 38 | 58 | 0 | 19303 |

[1]Code numbers for foods in the USDA National Nutrient Database for Standard References, Release 21, 2008.

Source:
USDA National Nutrient Database for Standard Reference, Release 21, 2008. Available at: http://www.nal.usda.gov/fnic/foodcomp.search/.

# Carotenoids—Zeaxanthin

| | ZEAXANTHIN (mcg/100 g) | SR21 CODE NUMBER[1] | | ZEAXANTHIN (mcg/100 g) | SR21 CODE NUMBER[1] |
|---|---|---|---|---|---|
| **FRUITS AND FRUIT JUICES** | | | corn, sweet, yellow, canned | 528 | 11172 |
| orange, all varieties, raw | 74 | 09200 | green snap beans, canned | 44 | 11056 |
| orange juice, from frozen concentrate | 80 | 09215 | kale, boiled | 173 | 11234 |
| | | | lettuce, romaine (cos), raw | 187 | 11251 |
| peach, canned in heavy syrup | 19 | 09370 | lettuce, iceberg, raw | 70 | 11252 |
| peach, raw | 6 | 09236 | peas, green, canned | 58 | 11308 |
| persimmon, Japanese, raw | 488 | 09263 | spinach, boiled | 179 | 11458 |
| tangerine, raw | 112 | 09218 | spinach, raw | 331 | 11457 |
| | | | turnip greens, boiled | 267 | 11569 |
| **VEGETABLES** | | | | | |
| broccoli, boiled | 23 | 11091 | **OTHER FOODS** | | |
| carrot, baby, raw | 23 | 11960 | egg, whole, raw | 23 | 01123 |
| celery, boiled | 8 | 11144 | cornmeal, degermed, yellow, enriched | 457 | 20022 |
| celery, raw | 3 | 11143 | | | |
| collards, boiled | 266 | 11162 | | | |

[1]Code numbers for foods in the USDA National Nutrient Database for Standard Reference, Release 21, 2008.

Source:
USDA National Nutrient Database for Standard Reference, Release 21, 2008. Available at: http://www.nal.usda.gov/fnic/foodcomp/search/.

# Coenzyme Q (Ubiquinone)

| | COENZYME Q $(\mu g/100\ g)^1$ | SOURCE | | COENZYME Q $(\mu g/100\ g)^1$ | SOURCE |
|---|---|---|---|---|---|
| **CHEESE** | | | sardines, raw | 1190 | Kubo et al, 2008 |
| cheese, edam | 120 | Mattila and Kumpulainen, 2001 | sardines, raw | 6430 | Kamei et al, 1986 |
| cheese, emmental | 130 | Mattila and Kumpulainen, 2001 | scallops, minced, raw | 495 | Kubo et al, 2008 |
| cheese, full fat | 141 | Kubo et al, 2008 | shrimp, raw | 166 | Kubo et al, 2008 |
| cheese, full fat | 210 | Kamei et al, 1986 | tuna, canned | 1490 | Kubo et al, 2008 |
| | | | tuna, canned | 1620 | Mattila and Kumpulainen, 2001 |
| **EGGS, CHICKEN** | | | tuna, raw | 487 | Kubo et al, 2008 |
| egg, raw | 73 | Kubo et al, 2008 | yellowtail, five-ray, skin removed, raw | 1280 | Kubo et al, 2008 |
| egg, raw | 120 | Mattila and Kumpulainen, 2001 | | | |
| egg, raw | 370 | Kamei et al, 1986 | yellowtail, raw | 2100 | Kamei et al, 1986 |
| | | | yellowtail, young, raw | 3340 | Kubo et al, 2008 |
| **FATS AND OILS** | | | | | |
| butter | 710 | Kamei et al, 1986 | **FRUITS** | | |
| canola (rapeseed) oil | 6350 | Mattila and Kumpulainen, 2001 | apple, peeled, raw | 121 | Kubo et al, 2008 |
| canola (rapeseed) oil | 7550 | Kamei et al, 1986 | apple, raw | 150 | Mattila and Kumpulainen, 2001 |
| coconut oil | 0 | Kamei et al, 1986 | blackcurrants, raw | 420 | Mattila and Kumpulainen, 2001 |
| corn oil | 19,920 | Kamei et al, 1986 | banana, raw | 82 | Kubo et al, 2008 |
| cottonseed oil | 7640 | Kamei et al, 1986 | clementine, raw | 90 | Mattila and Kumpulainen, 2001 |
| lard | 1000 | Kamei et al, 1986 | grapefruit, raw | 130 | Kubo et al, 2008 |
| olive oil | 1060 | Kamei et al, 1986 | lingonberries, raw | 380 | Mattila and Kumpulainen, 2001 |
| rice bran oil | 400 | Kamei et al, 1986 | orange, raw | 102 | Kubo et al, 2008 |
| safflower oil | 2920 | Kamei et al, 1986 | orange, raw | 140 | Mattila and Kumpulainen, 2001 |
| sesame oil | 3200 | Kamei et al, 1986 | persimmon, raw | 77 | Kubo et al, 2008 |
| soy oil | 5380 | Kubo et al, 2008 | strawberries, raw | 51 | Kubo et al, 2008 |
| soy oil | 10,030 | Kamei et al, 1986 | strawberries, raw | 150 | Mattila and Kumpulainen, 2001 |
| | | | | | |
| **FISH AND SEAFOOD** | | | **FRUIT JUICES** | | |
| cattlefish, raw | 2440 | Kamei et al, 1986 | lingonberry juice, fresh | 8 | Mattila and Kumpulainen, 2001 |
| cod, raw | 370 | Kubo et al, 2008 | orange juice, fresh | 30 | Mattila and Kumpulainen, 2001 |
| crab, raw | 400 | Farbu and Lambertsen, 1979 | | | |
| cuttlefish, raw | 467 | Kubo et al, 2008 | **GRAINS AND GRAIN PRODUCTS** | | |
| eel, raw | 1110 | Kamei et al, 1986 | barley, whole grain, raw | 1050 | Kamei et al, 1986 |
| fish sausage, raw | 125 | Kubo et al, 2008 | buckwheat, whole grain, raw | 1920 | Kamei et al, 1986 |
| flatfish, raw | 180 | Kubo et al, 2008 | corn grain, raw | 2250 | Kamei et al, 1986 |
| flatfish, raw | 550 | Kamei et al, 1986 | Job's tears, raw (Asian grain) | 1210 | Kamei et al, 1986 |
| halibut, red muscle, raw | 4490 | Farbu and Lambertsen, 1979 | millet, whole grain, raw | 1560 | Kamei et al, 1986 |
| halibut, white muscle, raw | 202 | Farbu and Lambertsen, 1979 | oats, whole grain, raw | 1230 | Kamei et al, 1986 |
| | | | rice bran | 3380 | Kamei et al, 1986 |
| herring, Baltic, raw | 1120 | Mattila et al, 2000 | rice, brown, raw | 420 | Kamei et al, 1986 |
| | | | rice, white, raw | 230 | Kamei et al, 1986 |
| herring, Baltic, raw | 1590 | Mattila and Kumpulainen, 2001 | rye bread | 470 | Mattila and Kumpulainen, 2001 |
| | | | rye crispbread | 470 | Mattila and Kumpulainen, 2001 |
| herring, raw | 1940 | Souchet and Laplante, 2007 | rye flour | 320 | Mattila et al, 2000 |
| horse mackerel | 13,000 | Kubo et al, 2008 | wheat bread | 210 | Mattila and Kumpulainen, 2001 |
| horse mackerel | 2070 | Kamei et al, 1986 | wheat flour | 130 | Kamei et al, 1986 |
| mackerel, raw | 1060 | Kubo et al, 2008 | wheat germ | 10,260 | Kamei et al, 1986 |
| mackerel, raw | 4330 | Kamei et al, 1986 | wheat grain, raw | 590 | Kamei et al, 1986 |
| mackerel, red muscle, raw | 6760 | Souchet and Laplante, 2007 | | | |
| mackerel, red muscle, raw | 2420 | Farbu and Lambertsen, 1979 | **MEATS** | | |
| mackerel, white muscle, raw | 1390 | Souchet and Laplante, 2007 | beef heart, raw | 11,330 | Mattila and Kumpulainen, 2001 |
| mackerel, white muscle, raw | 360 | Farbu and lambertsen, 1979 | beef liver, raw | 5050 | Kubo et al, 2008 |
| mussel, blue, raw | 401 | Farbu and Lambertsen, 1979 | beef liver, raw | 4060 | Mattila and Kumpulainen, 2001 |
| mussel, horse, raw | 154 | Farbu and Lambertsen, 1979 | beef, raw | 1700 | Mattila et al, 2000 |
| octopus leg, minced, raw | 342 | Kubo et al, 2008 | beef, raw | 3690 | Mattila and Kumpulainen, 2001 |
| oysters, raw | 342 | Kubo et al, 2008 | beef, raw | 3100 | Kamei et al, 1986 |
| pollack, frozen, raw | 1600 | Mattila and Kumpulainen, 2001 | beef shoulder, raw | 4010 | Kubo et al, 2008 |
| rainbow trout, raw | 880 | Mattila and Kumpulainen, 2001 | beef thigh, raw | 3030 | Kubo et al, 2008 |
| saithe (pollack species), red muscle, raw | 8250 | Farbu and Lambertsen, 1979 | pork, ham, raw | 2090 | Mattila and Kumpulainen, 2001 |
| | | | pork heart, raw | 6300 | Mattila et al, 2000 |
| saithe (pollack species), white muscle, raw | 184 | Farbu and Lambertsen, 1979 | pork heart, raw | 12,990 | Mattila and Kumpulainen, 2001 |
| | | | pork liver, raw | 2390 | Mattila and Kumpulainen, 2001 |
| salmon, raw | 573 | Kubo et al, 2008 | pork shoulder, raw | 4500 | Kubo et al, 2008 |
| | | | pork thigh, raw | 1380 | Kubo et al, 2008 |
| | | | reindeer meat, raw | 16,640 | Mattila and Kumpulainen, 2001 |

| | COENZYME Q (μg/100 g)[1] | SOURCE |
|---|---|---|
| **MILK AND YOGURT (COW)** | | |
| milk, lowfat (1.5% fat) | 10 | Mattila and Kumpulainen, 2001 |
| milk, whole | 31 | Kubo et al, 2008 |
| milk, whole | 60 | Kamei et al, 1986 |
| yogurt, whole milk | 26 | Kubo et al, 2008 |
| yogurt, whole milk | 240 | Mattila and Kumpulainen, 2001 |
| **NUTS AND SEEDS** | | |
| almonds, raw | 499 | Kubo et al, 2008 |
| almonds, roasted | 1990 | Kamei et al, 1986 |
| chestnuts, raw | 660 | Kamei et al, 1986 |
| hazelnuts, roasted | 1670 | Kamei et al, 1986 |
| peanuts, roasted | 2670 | Kamei et al, 1986 |
| pistachio nuts, roasted | 2010 | Kamei et al, 1986 |
| sesame seeds, roasted | 1760 | Kubo et al, 2008 |
| sesame seeds, roasted | 2300 | Kamei et al, 1986 |
| walnuts, raw | 1900 | Kamei et al, 1986 |
| **POULTRY** | | |
| chicken breast, raw | 1710 | Kubo et al, 2008 |
| chicken heart, raw | 19,200 | Kubo et al, 2008 |
| chicken, raw | 1440 | Mattila and Kumpulainen, 2001 |
| chicken, raw | 2100 | Kamei et al, 1986 |
| chicken thigh, without skin, raw | 2500 | Kubo et al, 2008 |
| **SOY PRODUCTS** | | |
| kinako (roasted and ground soybeans) | 5010 | Kamei et al, 1986 |
| miso | 245 | Kubo et al, 2008 |
| natto | 557 | Kubo et al, 2008 |
| natto | 1000 | Kamei et al, 1986 |
| soymilk | 250 | Kubo et al, 2008 |
| tofu | 286 | Kubo et al, 2008 |
| **VEGETABLES** | | |
| adzuki beans, dry | 1810 | Kamei et al, 1986 |
| adzuki beans, raw | 231 | Kubo et al, 2008 |
| asparagus, raw | 216 | Kubo et al, 2008 |
| avocado, raw | 948 | Kubo et al, 2008 |
| basella leaves, raw | 450 | Kamei et al, 1986 |
| broccoli, raw | 701 | Kubo et al, 2008 |
| broccoli, raw | 890 | Kamei et al, 1986 |
| burdock root, raw | 360 | Kamei et al, 1986 |
| cabbage, raw | 307 | Kubo et al, 2008 |
| cabbage, raw | 160 | Kamei et al, 1986 |
| carrot, raw | 170 | Mattila and Kumpulainen, 2001 |
| carrot, raw | 220 | Kamei et al, 1986 |

| | COENZYME Q (μg/100 g)[1] | SOURCE |
|---|---|---|
| cauliflower, raw | 663 | Kubo et al, 2008 |
| cauliflower, raw | 274 | Mattila and Kumpulainen, 2001 |
| cauliflower, raw | 140 | Kamei et al, 1986 |
| Chinese cabbage, raw | 448 | Kubo et al, 2008 |
| Chinese cabbage, raw | 210 | Kamei et al, 1986 |
| common beans, raw | 186 | Mattila and Kumpulainen, 2001 |
| corn, sweet, raw | 760 | Kamei et al, 1986 |
| cucumber, raw | 8 | Kubo et al, 2008 |
| cucumber, raw | 130 | Kamei et al, 1986 |
| eggplant, raw | 101 | Kubo et al, 2008 |
| eggplant, raw | 210 | Kamei et al, 1986 |
| garland chrysanthemum, raw | 170 | Kamei et al, 1986 |
| garlic, raw | 345 | Kubo et al, 2008 |
| garlic, raw | 280 | Kamei et al, 1986 |
| lettuce, raw | 140 | Kamei et al, 1986 |
| lotus root, raw | 96 | Kubo et al, 2008 |
| mushrooms, raw | 0 | Kubo et al, 2008 |
| mustard spinach, raw | 203 | Kubo et al, 2008 |
| okra, raw | 0 | Kubo et al, 2008 |
| onion, raw | 67 | Kubo et al, 2008 |
| onion, raw | 100 | Kamei et al, 1986 |
| onion, Welsh, raw | 107 | Kubo et al, 2008 |
| parsley, raw | 747 | Kubo et al, 2008 |
| peas, raw | 234 | Kubo et al, 2008 |
| peas, raw | 280 | Mattila and Kumpulainen, 2001 |
| pepper, sweet, raw | 350 | Kamei et al, 1986 |
| perilla (Asian herb), raw | 207 | Kubo et al, 2008 |
| perilla (Asian herb), raw | 1020 | Kamei et al, 1986 |
| potato, white, peeled, raw | 105 | Kubo et al, 2008 |
| potato, white, raw | 50 | Mattila and Kumpulainen, 2001 |
| potato, white, raw | 100 | Kamei et al, 1986 |
| pumpkin, raw | 0 | Kubo et al, 2008 |
| pumpkin, raw | 220 | Kamei et al, 1986 |
| radish, Japanese, raw | 71 | Kubo et al, 2008 |
| radish, Japanese, raw | 100 | Kamei et al, 1986 |
| radish leaves, Japanese, raw | 330 | Kamei et al, 1986 |
| soybean sprouts, raw | 106 | Kubo et al, 2008 |
| soybeans, boiled | 1210 | Kamei et al, 1986 |
| soybeans, dry | 1900 | Kamei et al, 1986 |
| soybeans, green, raw | 1870 | Kamei et al, 1986 |
| soybeans, raw | 682 | Kubo et al, 2008 |
| spinach, raw | 44 | Kubo et al, 2008 |
| spinach, raw | 1020 | Kamei et al, 1986 |
| sweet potato, peeled, raw | 301 | Kubo et al, 2008 |
| sweet potato, raw | 360 | Kamei et al, 1986 |
| taro, Japanese, peeled, raw | 80 | Kubo et al, 2008 |
| tomato, raw | 0 | Kubo et al, 2008 |
| tomato, raw | 90 | Mattila and Kumpulainen, 2001 |

[1]The values reflect somewhat different measures of coenzyme Q (CoQ) because one reference provided total CoQ, two provided only CoQ10, and three provided CoQ9 and CoQ10 separately (see notes with references). CoQ9 and CoQ10 were summed for the three references that provided both. Other sources of variation may be the differences in the species of foods from various countries (country of data origin noted with references) and differences in analytical methods and sample preparations.

Sources:
Farbu T, G Lambertsen. Ubiquinone analyses in fish tissues and in some marine invertebrates. Comp Biochem Physiol 63B:395-397, 1979. [Norway; total CoQ]
Kamei M, T Fujita, T Kanbe, K Sasaki, K Oshiba, S Otani, I Matsui-Yuasa, S Morishita. The distribution and content of ubiquinone in foods. *Internat J Vit Nutr Res* 56:57-63, 1986. [Japan; CoQ9 and CoQ10 separately]
Kubo H, K Fujii, T Kawabe, S Matsumoto, H Kishida, K Hosoe. Food content of ubiquinol-10 and ubiquinone-10 in the Japanese diet. *J Food Comp Anal* 21:199-210, 2008. [Japan; only CoQ10]
Mattila P, J Kumpulainen. Coenzyme Q9 and Q10: Contents in foods and dietary intake. J Food Comp Anal 14:409-417, 2001. [Finland; CoQ9 and CoQ10 separately]
Mattila P, M Lehtonen, J Kumpulainen. Comparison of in-line connected diode array and electrochemical detectors in the high-performance liquid chromatographic analysis of coenzymes Q9 and Q10 in food materials. J Agric Food Chem 48:1229-1233, 2000. [Finland; CoQ9 and CoQ10 separately; authors report results by in-line connected electrochemical (EC) and diode array (DAD) detection; the DAD results are used here.]
Souchet N, S Laplante. Seasonal variation of co-enzyme Q10 content in pelagic fish tissues from Eastern Quebec. J Food Comp Anal 20:403-410, 2007. [Canada; CoQ10 only]

# *Dietary Fiber Components—Lignin And Pectin*

| | LIGNIN (g/100 g) | PECTIN[1] (g/100 g) | SOURCE | | LIGNIN (g/100 g) | PECTIN[1] (g/100 g) | SOURCE |
|---|---|---|---|---|---|---|---|
| **CEREALS, READY-TO-EAT** | | | | date, dried | 8.0 | 2.0 | Marlett and Cheung, 1997 |
| All Bran | 4.3 | 1.0 | Marlett, 1992 | fig, dried | 2.2 | 2.3 | Marlett and Cheung, 1997 |
| bran flakes, 40% | 1.5 | 0.7 | Marlett, 1992 | fruit cocktail, canned | 0.2 | 0.1 | Marlett and Cheung, 1997 |
| Corn Chex | 1.4 | Tr | Marlett and Cheung, 1997 | gooseberries, raw | 0.2 | | Souci et al, 2000 |
| corn flakes | 0.7 | 0.1 | Marlett, 1992 | grapefruit, pink, Florida | Tr | 0.7 | Marlett, 1992 |
| corn flakes, sugar-frosted | 0.4 | Tr | Marlett and Cheung, 1997 | grapefruit, white, Florida | Tr | 0.3 | Marlett, 1992 |
| Frosted Miniwheats | 1.0 | 0.2 | Marlett, 1992 | grapes, black/red, raw | 0.4 | 0.2 | Marlett and Cheung, 1997 |
| Golden Grahams | 0.4 | Tr | Marlett and Cheung, 1997 | grapes, green, Thompson, raw | 0.2 | 0.3 | Marlett, 1992 |
| granola | 0.4 | 0.4 | Marlett and Cheung, 1997 | honeydew melon, raw | Tr | 0.2 | Marlett and Cheung, 1997 |
| Grape-Nuts | 0.7 | Tr | Marlett and Cheung, 1997 | kiwifruit, raw | 0.8 | 0.4 | Marlett and Cheung, 1997 |
| Grape-Nuts Flakes | 0.7 | Tr | Marlett and Cheung, 1997 | lemon, peeled, raw | Tr | 0.7 | Marlett and Cheung, 1997 |
| Life | 1.8 | Tr | Marlett and Cheung, 1997 | nectarine, raw | 0.1 | 0.3 | Marlett, 1992 |
| Product 19 | 1.5 | 0.2 | Marlett, 1992 | orange, navel, raw | Tr | 0.7 | Marlett, 1992 |
| puffed rice | 0.7 | Tr | Marlett and Cheung, 1997 | orange, Florida, raw | Tr | 0.9 | Marlett, 1992 |
| puffed wheat | 0.7 | Tr | Marlett and Cheung, 1997 | papaya, raw | Tr | 0.7 | Marlett and Cheung, 1997 |
| Rice Krispies | 0.6 | 0.1 | Marlett, 1992 | peach, raw | 0.1 | 0.5 | Marlett and Cheung, 1997 |
| shredded wheat | 0.9 | 0.3 | Marlett, 1992 | pear, Bartlett, raw | 0.4 | 0.7 | Marlett, 1992 |
| Special K | 0.9 | 0.1 | Marlett, 1992 | pear canned in light syrup | 0.2 | 0.3 | Marlett, 1992 |
| Wheat Chex | 0.4 | 0.4 | Marlett and Cheung, 1997 | plum, canned | 0.2 | 0.6 | Marlett and Cheung, 1997 |
| Wheaties | 1.4 | 0.6 | Marlett, 1992 | plum, prune, raw | 0.4 | 0.7 | Marlett and Cheung, 1997 |
| Total | 1.6 | 0.1 | Marlett, 1992 | plum, raw | 0.2 | 0.5 | Marlett, 1992 |
| | | | | prune, dried | 1.2 | 2.4 | Marlett and Cheung, 1997 |
| **DESSERTS** | | | | raisins, dried | 1.8 | 0.9 | Marlett, 1992 |
| brownie | 1.0 | Tr | Marlett and Cheung, 1997 | raspberries, raw | 2.3 | 0.5 | Marlett and Cheung, 1997 |
| brownie with nuts | 1.5 | Tr | Marlett and Cheung, 1997 | strawberries, raw | 0.5 | 0.5 | Marlett, 1992 |
| cake, devil's food | 1.0 | 0.3 | Marlett and Cheung, 1997 | tangerine, raw | 0.1 | 0.8 | Marlett, 1992 |
| cake, gingerbread | 0.3 | Tr | Marlett and Cheung, 1997 | | | | |
| cake, pound/sponge | 0.3 | Tr | Marlett and Cheung, 1997 | **GRAINS AND GRAIN PRODUCTS** | | | |
| cinnamon roll | 0.4 | 0.1 | Marlett, 1992 | bread, Italian | 0.7 | 0.1 | Marlett, 1992 |
| coffeecake | 0.2 | Tr | Marlett and Cheung, 1997 | bread, raisin | 0.8 | Tr | Marlett and Cheung, 1997 |
| cookie, date | 1.7 | 0.3 | Marlett and Cheung, 1997 | bread, rye | 0.4 | Tr | Marlett and Cheung, 1997 |
| cookie, fig | 1.0 | 1.7 | Marlett and Cheung, 1997 | bread, white | 0.5 | 0.1 | Marlett, 1992 |
| cookie, gingersnap | 0.4 | Tr | Marlett, 1992 | bread, whole wheat | 1.4 | Tr | Marlett and Cheung, 1997 |
| cookie, graham cracker | 0.4 | 0.1 | Marlett, 1992 | cornbread | 0.4 | 0.1 | Marlett, 1992 |
| cookie, oatmeal | 0.7 | Tr | Marlett and Cheung, 1997 | crackers, cheese with peanut butter | 0.7 | Tr | Marlett and Cheung, 1997 |
| cookie, peanut | Tr | 0.4 | Marlett and Cheung, 1997 | crackers, saltines | 0.5 | Tr | Marlett, 1992 |
| doughnut, glazed | 0.5 | Tr | Marlett and Cheung, 1997 | crackers, Triscuits | 0.7 | Tr | Marlett and Cheung, 1997 |
| éclair, frozen | 0.5 | Tr | Marlett and Cheung, 1997 | English muffin | 0.7 | 0.1 | Marlett, 1992 |
| ice cream cone (cone only) | 0.5 | Tr | Marlett, 1992 | hush puppy, homemade | 0.4 | 0.2 | Marlett and Cheung, 1997 |
| pie crust | 0.6 | Tr | Marlett, 1992 | macaroni, boiled | 0.7 | Tr | Marlett, 1992 |
| pie filling, apple, canned | Tr | 0.3 | Marlett and Cheung, 1997 | muffin | 0.4 | Tr | Marlett, 1992 |
| pie, pecan | 0.2 | 0.1 | Marlett and Cheung, 1997 | muffin, blueberry | 0.8 | Tr | Marlett and Cheung, 1997 |
| pie, rhubarb | 0.1 | 0.3 | Marlett and Cheung, 1997 | muffin, wheat bran | 0.5 | Tr | Marlett and Cheung, 1997 |
| sweet roll with nuts | 0.3 | 0.1 | Marlett and Cheung, 1997 | muffin, wheat bran, homemade | 0.8 | Tr | Marlett and Cheung, 1997 |
| sweet roll with raisins | 0.6 | Tr | Marlett and Cheung, 1997 | noodles, egg, boiled | 0.4 | Tr | Marlett, 1992 |
| | | | | oat bran | 3.5 | 0.3 | Marlett and Cheung, 1997 |
| **FRUITS** | | | | oatmeal, regular, cooked | 0.5 | 0.1 | Marlett, 1992 |
| apple, Granny Smith, raw | 0.1 | 0.8 | Marlett, 1992 | pancake | 0.2 | Tr | Marlett and Cheung, 1997 |
| apple, peeled, raw | 0.1 | 0.5 | Marlett and Cheung, 1997 | pancake, buckwheat | 1.7 | Tr | Marlett and Cheung, 1997 |
| apple, Red Delicious, peeled, raw | 0.1 | 0.5 | Marlett, 1992 | pancake mix | 0.6 | 0.1 | Marlett, 1992 |
| apple, Red Delicious, raw | 0.2 | 0.7 | Marlett, 1992 | popcorn, popped | 1.7 | Tr | Marlett and Cheung, 1997 |
| applesauce, canned | 0.1 | 0.3 | Marlett and Cheung, 1997 | roll, dinner | 0.4 | Tr | Marlett and Cheung, 1997 |
| apricot, canned in syrup | 0.1 | 0.6 | Marlett, 1992 | roll, hamburger | 0.2 | Tr | Marlett, 1992 |
| apricot, dried | 0.7 | 1.4 | Marlett and Cheung, 1997 | roll, hard | 1.2 | Tr | Marlett and Cheung, 1997 |
| banana, raw | 0.6 | 0.4 | Marlett, 1992 | roll, submarine | 0.9 | Tr | Marlett and Cheung, 1997 |
| blackberries, frozen | 3.0 | 0.9 | Marlett and Cheung, 1997 | taco shell | 0.9 | 0.3 | Marlett, 1992 |
| blueberries, raw | 0.9 | 0.6 | Marlett, 1992 | tortilla, flour | 0.3 | Tr | Marlett, 1992 |
| cantaloupe, raw | Tr | 0.3 | Marlett, 1992 | waffle | 0.4 | Tr | Marlett and Cheung, 1997 |
| cherries, tart, canned | 0.2 | 0.3 | Marlett, 1992 | wheat germ | 1.2 | 0.8 | Marlett, 1992 |
| cranberry sauce, canned | 0.3 | 0.1 | Marlett and Cheung, 1997 | wheat flour, white | 0.2 | 0.1 | Marlett, 1992 |
| currants, black, raw | 1.5 | | Souci et al, 2000 | | | | |
| currants, red, raw | 0.7 | | Souci et al, 2000 | | | | |

| | LIGNIN (g/100 g) | PECTIN[1] (g/100 g) | SOURCE | | LIGNIN (g/100 g) | PECTIN[1] (g/100 g) | SOURCE |
|---|---|---|---|---|---|---|---|
| **NUTS AND SEEDS** | | | | okra, boiled | 0.7 | 0.5 | Marlett and Cheung, 1997 |
| | | | | onion, green, raw | 0.2 | 0.8 | Marlett, 1992 |
| almonds, raw | 1.9 | 1.6 | Marlett, 1992 | onion rings, frozen, heated | 0.1 | 0.4 | Marlett and Cheung, 1997 |
| cashews, roasted | 1.1 | 0.7 | Marlett and Cheung, 1997 | | | | |
| coconut, shredded | 0.0 | 0.3 | Marlett, 1992 | onion, yellow, raw | Tr | 0.5 | Marlett, 1992 |
| peanut butter | 0.8 | 1.0 | Marlett, 1992 | parsnip, boiled | 1.3 | 1.2 | Marlett and Cheung, 1997 |
| peanuts | 0.7 | 1.2 | Marlett, 1992 | pepper, sweet green, raw | 0.3 | 0.4 | Marlett, 1992 |
| pumpkin seeds | 8.0 | Tr | Marlett and Cheung, 1997 | | | | |
| pecans | 1.4 | 1.1 | Marlett and Cheung, 1997 | potato, baked | 0.3 | 0.3 | Marlett, 1992 |
| walnuts, English | 0.9 | 0.7 | Marlett, 1992 | potato, French fried | 0.1 | 0.4 | Marlett, 1992 |
| | | | | potato, peeled, boiled | Tr | 0.2 | Marlett, 1992 |
| **SOUPS AND ENTREES** | | | | potato, red-skinned, boiled | 0.1 | 0.3 | Marlett and Cheung, 1997 |
| corn beef hash, canned | 0.0 | 0.1 | Marlett and Cheung, 1997 | | | | |
| lasagna with meat sauce, frozen | 0.3 | 0.2 | Marlett and Cheung, 1997 | potato, red-skinned, peeled, boiled | Tr | 0.2 | Marlett and Cheung, 1997 |
| | | | | | | | |
| soup, pea, canned, prepared | 0.2 | 0.1 | Marlett and Cheung, 1997 | potato salad | Tr | 0.2 | Marlett and Cheung, 1997 |
| | | | | potato, scalloped, frozen, heated | Tr | 0.2 | Marlett and Cheung, 1997 |
| soup, vegetable beef, canned, prepared | 0.1 | 0.1 | Marlett and Cheung, 1997 | | | | |
| | | | | pumpkin, canned | 0.2 | 0.8 | Marlett, 1992 |
| soup, vegetarian vegetable, canned, prepared | 0.1 | 0.3 | Marlett, 1992 | radish, red, raw | Tr | 0.4 | Marlett, 1992 |
| | | | | rhubarb, cooked with sugar | 0.1 | 0.2 | Marlett and Cheung, 1997 |
| | | | | | | | |
| **VEGETABLES** | | | | rutabaga, boiled | 0.1 | 0.8 | Marlett and Cheung, 1997 |
| artichoke, boiled | 0.1 | 1.0 | Marlett and Cheung, 1997 | sauerkraut, canned | Tr | 0.8 | Marlett and Cheung, 1997 |
| asparagus, boiled | 0.1 | 0.6 | Marlett, 1992 | spinach, boiled/canned | 0.3 | 0.5 | Marlett and Cheung, 1997 |
| asparagus spears, canned | 0.2 | 0.2 | Marlett, 1992 | summer squash, zucchini, raw | Tr | 0.2 | Marlett, 1992 |
| avocado, raw | 0.1 | 1.0 | Marlett, 1992 | | | | |
| bean sprouts, canned | 0.1 | 0.2 | Marlett, 1992 | Swiss chard, boiled | 0.2 | 0.6 | Marlett and Cheung, 1997 |
| beet, canned | Tr | 0.5 | Marlett, 1992 | sweet potato, canned in light syrup | 0.1 | 0.3 | Marlett, 1992 |
| beet greens, boiled | 0.1 | 0.6 | Marlett and Cheung, 1997 | | | | |
| broccoli, boiled | 0.3 | 0.9 | Marlett, 1992 | tomato, canned | 0.1 | 0.3 | Marlett, 1992 |
| broccoli, raw | 0.3 | 0.7 | Marlett, 1992 | tomato sauce, canned | 0.6 | 0.6 | Marlett and Cheung, 1997 |
| Brussels sprouts, boiled | 0.1 | 1.0 | Marlett, 1992 | turnip greens, frozen | 0.1 | 0.9 | Marlett, 1992 |
| cabbage, green, boiled | 0.1 | 0.7 | Marlett and Cheung, 1997 | winter squash, acorn/ butternut, baked | Tr | 0.6 | Marlett and Cheung, 1997 |
| cabbage, green, raw | Tr | 0.6 | Marlett, 1992 | | | | |
| carrot, raw | 0.1 | 0.8 | Marlett, 1992 | | | | |
| cauliflower, boiled | Tr | 0.6 | Marlett, 1992 | **VEGETABLES—LEGUMES** | | | |
| cauliflower, raw | 0.1 | 0.6 | Marlett, 1992 | baked beans with pork, canned | 0.2 | 0.6 | Marlett and Cheung, 1997 |
| celery, boiled | Tr | 0.6 | Marlett, 1992 | | | | |
| celery, raw | Tr | 0.6 | Marlett, 1992 | black beans, boiled | 0.5 | 0.2 | Marlett and Cheung, 1997 |
| Chinese cabbage, raw | Tr | 0.3 | Marlett and Cheung, 1997 | blackeye peas, canned | 0.5 | 0.3 | Marlett, 1992 |
| collards, boiled | 0.2 | 1.1 | Marlett and Cheung, 1997 | crowder peas, canned | 0.4 | 0.4 | Marlett and Cheung, 1997 |
| corn, creamed, canned | 0.2 | Tr | Marlett and Cheung, 1997 | great northern beans, boiled | 0.1 | 0.8 | Marlett and Cheung, 1997 |
| corn, whole kernel, canned | 0.5 | 0.1 | Marlett, 1992 | | | | |
| | | | | kidney beans, canned | 0.3 | 0.6 | Marlett and Cheung, 1997 |
| corn, whole kernel, frozen | 0.3 | 0.1 | Marlett, 1992 | lentils, boiled | 0.2 | 0.2 | Marlett and Cheung, 1997 |
| | | | | lima beans, green, canned | 0.1 | 0.4 | Marlett, 1992 |
| cucumber, raw | 0.1 | 0.2 | Marlett, 1992 | | | | |
| endive, raw | 0.4 | 1.2 | Marlett and Cheung, 1997 | navy beans, boiled | 0.1 | 0.4 | Marlett and Cheung, 1997 |
| escarole, raw | 0.4 | 0.4 | Marlett and Cheung, 1997 | peas, green, canned | 0.1 | 0.5 | Marlett, 1992 |
| green snap beans, canned | 0.2 | 0.4 | Marlett, 1992 | peas, green, frozen | Tr | 0.7 | Marlett, 1992 |
| | | | | pigeon peas, canned | 1.0 | 0.4 | Marlett and Cheung, 1997 |
| kale, boiled | 0.3 | 1.4 | Marlett and Cheung, 1997 | white beans, dry | 1.4 | | Souci et al, 2000 |
| kohlrabi, boiled | Tr | 0.5 | Marlett and Cheung, 1997 | | | | |
| lettuce, leaf/romaine, iceberg, raw | 0.2 | 0.4 | Marlett and Cheung, 1997 | **OTHER FOODS** | | | |
| | | | | catsup | 0.2 | 0.3 | Marlett, 1992 |
| mushrooms, canned | Tr | 0.3 | Marlett and Cheung, 1997 | olives, black | 0.6 | 0.3 | Marlett, 1992 |
| mushrooms, raw | 0.3 | Tr | Marlett and Cheung, 1997 | olives, green with pimento | 0.4 | 0.3 | Marlett, 1992 |
| mustard greens, boiled | 0.1 | 1.1 | Marlett and Cheung, 1997 | pickle, dill | 0.1 | 0.3 | Marlett, 1992 |
| | | | | potato chips | 0.0 | 0.7 | Marlett and Cheung, 1997 |

[1]Pectin is the sum of soluble and insoluble pectin for Marlett, 1992, and Marlett and Cheung, 1997.

Sources:
Marlett JA. Content and composition of dietary fiber in 117 frequently consumed foods. *J Am Diet Assoc* 92:175-186, 1992.
Marlett JA, T-F Cheung. Database and quick methods of assessing typical dietary fiber intakes using data for 228 commonly consumed foods. *J Am Diet Assoc* 97:1139-1148, 1997.
Souci SW, W Fachmann, H Kraut. *Food Composition and Nutrition Tables.* Medpharm GmbH Scientific Publishers, Stuttgart, Germany and CRC Press, Washington, DC, 2000.

# *Fatty Acids—Omega-3 Fatty Acids*

| | | OMEGA-3 FATTY ACIDS (g/serving) | OMEGA-3 FATTY ACIDS (g/100 g) | SR21 CODE NUMBER[1] |
|---|---|---|---|---|
| **DESSERTS** | | | | |
| brownie, homemade | brownie 2¾" × ⅞" (56 g) | 0.526 | 0.939 | 18154 |
| nuts in syrup dessert topping | 2 T (41 g) | 0.992 | 2.420 | 19367 |
| pie, cherry snack, fried | 1 snack pie (128 g) | 0.727 | 0.568 | 18444 |
| pie, fruit snack, fried | 1 snack pie (128 g) | 0.727 | 0.568 | 18319 |
| pie, lemon snack, fried | 1 snack pie (128 g) | 0.727 | 0.568 | 18445 |
| puff pastry, frozen | 1 pastry (40 g) | 1.035 | 2.588 | 18211 |
| **FAST FOODS** | | | | |
| Big Breakfast (scrambled eggs, sausage patty, hash brown piece, and biscuit), McDonald's | 9.3 oz breakfast (266 g) | 0.513 | 0.193 | 21341 |
| biscuit with egg and bacon, fast food | 5.3 oz serving (150 g) | 0.534 | 0.356 | 21003 |
| biscuit with egg and ham, fast food | 6.8 oz serving (192 g) | 0.501 | 0.261 | 21004 |
| cheeseburger sandwich, Double Whopper, Burger King | 15 oz sandwich (426 g) | 1.670 | 0.392 | 21255 |
| cheeseburger sandwich, regular, double meat, double-decker bun with lettuce and tomato, fast food | 1 sandwich (228 g) | 0.650 | 0.285 | 21095 |
| cheeseburger sandwich, regular, single meat with lettuce and tomato, fast food | 1 sandwich (154 g) | 0.551 | 0.358 | 21091 |
| cheeseburger sandwich, Whopper, Burger King | 13.9 oz sandwich (395 g) | 1.853 | 0.469 | 21253 |
| Chicken (crispy) Classic Sandwich, McDonald's | 8.2 oz sandwich (232 g) | 0.701 | 0.302 | 21403 |
| chicken fillet sandwich, fast food | 1 sandwich (182 g) | 0.959 | 0.527 | 21102 |
| chicken fillet sandwich, Wendy's | 8.1 oz sandwich (230 g) | 0.536 | 0.233 | 21244 |
| chicken sandwich, Burger King | 7.2 oz sandwich (204 g) | 1.281 | 0.628 | 21259 |
| Chicken Selects (breast strips), McDonald's | 5 pieces (221 g) | 0.807 | 0.365 | 21308 |
| Chicken Whopper sandwich, Burger King | 9.6 oz sandwich (272 g) | 1.423 | 0.523 | 21257 |
| coleslaw, fast food | ¾ cup (99 g) | 0.773 | 0.781 | 21127 |
| corn dog, fast food (frankfurter with cornmeal coating) | 1 corn dog (175 g) | 0.730 | 0.417 | 21120 |
| fish sandwich with tartar sauce and cheese, fast food | 6.5 oz sandwich (183 g) | 0.959 | 0.524 | 21106 |
| fish sandwich with tartar sauce, fast food | 5.6 oz sandwich (158 g) | 0.630 | 0.399 | 21105 |
| hamburger sandwich, Double Whopper, Burger King | 14 oz sandwich (401 g) | 1.263 | 0.315 | 21254 |
| hamburger, Whopper, Burger King | 10.7 oz sandwich (304 g) | 0.836 | 0.275 | 21252 |
| sauce, creamy ranch, McDonald's | 1.5 oz (221 g) | 1.391 | 3.235 | 21311 |
| **FATS, OILS, AND SPREADS** | | | | |
| seal (bearded) oil | 1 T (14 g) | 3.998 | 28.555 | 35057 |
| seal (spotted) oil | 1 T (14 g) | 2.055 | 14.680 | 35156 |
| whale (beluga) oil | 1 T (14 g) | 1.232 | 8.800 | 35014 |
| cod liver oil | 1 T (14 g) | 2.763 | 19.736 | 04589 |
| herring oil | 1 T (14 g) | 1.661 | 11.861 | 04590 |
| menhaden oil | 1 T (14 g) | 3.939 | 28.135 | 04591 |
| salmon oil | 1 T (14 g) | 4.943 | 35.307 | 04593 |
| sardine oil | 1 T (14 g) | 3.373 | 24.093 | 04594 |
| mayonnaise, soy | 1 T (14 g) | 0.658 | 4.702 | 04025 |
| canola oil | 1 T (14 g) | 1.279 | 9.137 | 04582 |
| corn and canola oil | 1 T (14 g) | 0.812 | 5.798 | 42289 |
| mustard oil | 1 T (14 g) | 0.826 | 5.899 | 04583 |
| soy (hydrogenated) and cottonseed oil (for bread) | 1 T (14 g) | 0.560 | 4.000 | 04546 |
| soy lecithin | 1 T (14 g) | 0.719 | 5.136 | 04531 |
| soy oil, salad/cooking | 1 T (14 g) | 0.950 | 6.789 | 04044 |

| | | OMEGA-3 FATTY ACIDS (g/serving) | OMEGA-3 FATTY ACIDS (g/100 g) | SR21 CODE NUMBER[1] |
|---|---|---|---|---|
| walnut oil | 1 T (14 g) | 1.456 | 10.400 | 04528 |
| wheat germ oil | 1 T (14 g) | 0.966 | 6.900 | 04038 |
| **FISH AND SHELLFISH** | | | | |
| anchovies, raw | 3 oz (85 g) | 1.256 | 1.478 | 15001 |
| bass, freshwater, cooked by dry heat | 3 oz (85 g) | 0.861 | 1.013 | 15187 |
| bass, freshwater, raw | 3 oz (85 g) | 0.672 | 0.790 | 15003 |
| bass, striped, cooked by dry heat | 3 oz (85 g) | 0.838 | 0.986 | 15188 |
| bass, striped, raw | 3 oz (85 g) | 0.654 | 0.769 | 15004 |
| bluefish, cooked by dry heat | 3 oz (85 g) | 0.907 | 1.067 | 15189 |
| bluefish, raw | 3 oz (85 g) | 0.708 | 0.833 | 15005 |
| carp, cooked by dry heat | 3 oz (85 g) | 0.767 | 0.902 | 15009 |
| carp, raw | 3 oz (85 g) | 0.598 | 0.704 | 15008 |
| caviar, black and red, granular | 1 T (16 g) | 1.086 | 6.787 | 15012 |
| cisco, smoked (finfish) | 3 oz (85 g) | 1.291 | 1.519 | 15014 |
| drum, freshwater, cooked by dry heat | 3 oz (85 g) | 0.845 | 0.994 | 15195 |
| drum, freshwater, raw | 3 oz (85 g) | 0.659 | 0.775 | 15024 |
| eel, cooked by dry heat | 3 oz (85 g) | 0.712 | 0.838 | 15026 |
| eel, raw | 3 oz (85 g) | 0.555 | 0.653 | 15025 |
| halibut, Alaskan, cooked with skin | 3 oz (85 g) | 0.567 | 0.667 | 35188 |
| halibut, Atlantic and Pacific, cooked by dry heat | 3 oz (85 g) | 0.569 | 0.669 | 15037 |
| halibut, Greenland, cooked by dry heat | 3 oz (85 g) | 1.145 | 1.347 | 15196 |
| halibut, Greenland, raw | 3 oz (85 g) | 0.893 | 1.051 | 15038 |
| herring, Atlantic, cooked by dry heat | 3 oz (85 g) | 1.884 | 2.217 | 15040 |
| herring, Atlantic, kippered | piece 5″ × 1¾″ × ¼″ (40 g) | 0.946 | 2.365 | 15042 |
| herring, Atlantic, raw | 3 oz (85 g) | 1.470 | 1.729 | 15039 |
| herring, Pacific, cooked by dry heat | 3 oz (85 g) | 2.055 | 2.418 | 15197 |
| herring, Pacific, raw | 3 oz (85 g) | 1.604 | 1.887 | 15043 |
| mackerel, Atlantic, cooked by dry heat | 3 oz (85 g) | 1.209 | 1.422 | 15047 |
| mackerel, Atlantic, raw | 3 oz (85 g) | 2.270 | 2.670 | 15046 |
| mackerel, jack, canned, drained | 1 cup (190 g) | 2.616 | 1.377 | 15048 |
| mackerel, Pacific/jack, cooked by dry heat | 3 oz (85 g) | 1.760 | 2.070 | 15201 |
| mackerel, Pacific/jack, raw | 3 oz (85 g) | 1.372 | 1.614 | 15050 |
| mackerel, salted | 1 oz (28 g) | 1.438 | 5.134 | 83110 |
| mackerel, Spanish, cooked by dry heat | 3 oz (85 g) | 1.238 | 1.457 | 15052 |
| mackerel, Spanish, raw | 3 oz (85 g) | 1.255 | 1.476 | 15051 |
| mussels, blue, cooked by moist heat | 3 oz (85 g) | 0.736 | 0.866 | 15165 |
| oysters, eastern, breaded and fried | 6 medium (88 g) | 0.549 | 0.624 | 15168 |
| oysters, eastern, wild, cooked by moist heat | 6 medium (42 g) | 0.565 | 1.345 | 15169 |
| oysters, eastern, wild, raw | 6 medium (84 g) | 0.564 | 0.672 | 15167 |
| oysters, Pacific, cooked by moist heat | 3 oz (85 g) | 1.258 | 1.480 | 15231 |
| oysters, Pacific, raw | 3 oz (85 g) | 0.629 | 0.740 | 15171 |
| pompano, Florida, cooked by dry heat | 3 oz (85 g) | 0.839 | 0.987 | 15069 |
| pompano, Florida, raw | 3 oz (85 g) | 0.655 | 0.770 | 15068 |
| roe (fish eggs), mixed species, cooked by dry heat | 1 oz (28 g) | 0.874 | 3.120 | 15207 |
| roe (fish eggs), mixed species, raw | 1 oz (28 g) | 0.682 | 2.434 | 15072 |
| sablefish, cooked by dry heat | 3 oz (85 g) | 1.806 | 2.125 | 15208 |
| sablefish, raw | 3 oz (85 g) | 1.410 | 1.659 | 15074 |
| sablefish, smoked | 3 oz (85 g) | 1.856 | 2.183 | 15075 |
| salmon, Atlantic, farmed, cooked by dry heat | 3 oz (85 g) | 1.921 | 2.260 | 15237 |
| salmon, Atlantic, farmed, raw | 3 oz (85 g) | 2.147 | 2.526 | 15236 |
| salmon, Atlantic, wild, cooked by dry heat | 3 oz (85 g) | 2.198 | 2.586 | 15209 |
| salmon, Atlantic, wild, raw | 3 oz (85 g) | 1.715 | 2.018 | 15076 |
| salmon, chinook, cooked by dry heat | 3 oz (85 g) | 1.822 | 2.143 | 15210 |
| salmon, chinook, raw | 3 oz (85 g) | 1.991 | 2.342 | 15078 |
| salmon, chum, canned with bone, drained | 3 oz (85 g) | 1.117 | 1.314 | 15080 |
| salmon, chum, cooked by dry heat | 3 oz (85 g) | 0.807 | 0.949 | 15211 |

| | | OMEGA-3 FATTY ACIDS (g/serving) | OMEGA-3 FATTY ACIDS (g/100 g) | SR21 CODE NUMBER[1] |
|---|---|---|---|---|
| salmon, chum, raw | 3 oz (85 g) | 0.629 | 0.740 | 15079 |
| salmon, coho, farmed, cooked by dry heat | 3 oz (85 g) | 1.152 | 1.355 | 15239 |
| salmon, coho, farmed, raw | 3 oz (85 g) | 1.089 | 1.281 | 15238 |
| salmon, coho, wild, cooked by dry heat | 3 oz (85 g) | 0.947 | 1.114 | 15247 |
| salmon, coho, wild, cooked by moist heat | 3 oz (85 g) | 1.587 | 1.867 | 15082 |
| salmon, coho, wild, raw | 3 oz (85 g) | 1.253 | 1.474 | 15081 |
| salmon, pink, canned with bone | 3 oz (85 g) | 1.493 | 1.757 | 15084 |
| salmon, pink, cooked by dry heat | 3 oz (85 g) | 1.237 | 1.455 | 15212 |
| salmon, pink, raw | 3 oz (85 g) | 0.965 | 1.135 | 15083 |
| salmon, sockeye, canned with bone, drained | 3 oz (85 g) | 1.425 | 1.676 | 15087 |
| salmon, sockeye, cooked by dry heat | 3 oz (85 g) | 1.210 | 1.424 | 15086 |
| salmon, sockeye, raw | 3 oz (85 g) | 1.108 | 1.303 | 15085 |
| sardines, Pacific, canned in tomato sauce, drained | 1 sardine (38 g) | 0.643 | 1.693 | 15089 |
| sea bass, cooked by dry heat | 3 oz (85 g) | 0.730 | 0.859 | 15092 |
| sea bass, raw | 3 oz (85 g) | 0.570 | 0.671 | 15091 |
| shad, American, raw | 3 oz (85 g) | 2.252 | 2.649 | 15094 |
| shark, batter-dipped and fried | 3 oz (85 g) | 0.823 | 0.968 | 15096 |
| shark, raw | 3 oz (85 g) | 0.833 | 0.980 | 15095 |
| shrimp, canned | 3 oz (85 g) | 0.514 | 0.605 | 15152 |
| smelt, dried | 1 oz (28 g) | 0.664 | 2.370 | 35184 |
| smelt, rainbow, cooked by dry heat | 3 oz (85 g) | 0.829 | 0.975 | 15100 |
| smelt, rainbow, raw | 3 oz (85 g) | 0.646 | 0.760 | 15099 |
| spot, cooked by dry heat | 3 oz (85 g) | 0.840 | 0.988 | 15216 |
| spot, raw | 3 oz (85 g) | 0.655 | 0.770 | 15103 |
| squid, fried | 3 oz (85 g) | 0.549 | 0.646 | 15176 |
| sucker, white, cooked by dry heat | 3 oz (85 g) | 0.660 | 0.776 | 15217 |
| sucker, white, raw | 3 oz (85 g) | 0.513 | 0.604 | 15107 |
| swordfish, cooked by dry heat | 3 oz (85 g) | 0.898 | 1.057 | 15111 |
| swordfish, raw | 3 oz (85 g) | 0.701 | 0.825 | 15110 |
| tilefish, cooked by dry heat | 3 oz (85 g) | 0.891 | 1.048 | 15113 |
| trout, cooked by dry heat | 3 oz (85 g) | 1.165 | 1.370 | 15219 |
| trout, rainbow, farmed, cooked by dry heat | 3 oz (85 g) | 1.051 | 1.236 | 15241 |
| trout, rainbow, farmed, raw | 3 oz (85 g) | 0.838 | 0.986 | 15240 |
| trout, rainbow, wild, cooked by dry heat | 3 oz (85 g) | 0.999 | 1.175 | 15116 |
| trout, rainbow, wild, raw | 3 oz (85 g) | 0.690 | 0.812 | 15115 |
| trout, raw | 3 oz (85 g) | 0.908 | 1.068 | 15114 |
| trout, steelhead, boiled, canned | 3 oz (85 g) | 0.932 | 1.097 | 35181 |
| tuna, bluefin, cooked by dry heat | 3 oz (85 g) | 1.414 | 1.664 | 15118 |
| tuna, bluefin, raw | 3 oz (85 g) | 1.103 | 1.298 | 15117 |
| tuna, white, canned in water, drained | 3 oz (85 g) | 0.808 | 0.951 | 15126 |
| whitefish, cooked by dry heat | 3 oz (85 g) | 1.748 | 2.056 | 15223 |
| whitefish, raw | 3 oz (85 g) | 1.363 | 1.604 | 15130 |
| wolffish, Atlantic, cooked by dry heat | 3 oz (85 g) | 0.735 | 0.865 | 15224 |
| wolffish, Atlantic, raw | 3 oz (85 g) | 0.574 | 0.675 | 15134 |

### GRAINS AND GRAIN PRODUCTS

| | | | | |
|---|---|---|---|---|
| chow mein noodles | 1 cup (45 g) | 0.889 | 1.976 | 20113 |
| noodles, crunchy, Chinese restaurant | 1 cup (45 g) | 0.910 | 2.022 | 20118 |
| oat bran muffin | 4.9 oz muffin (139 g) | 0.637 | 0.458 | 18283 |
| Optimum, Nature's Path (RTE cereal) | 1 cup (55 g) | 1.029 | 1.870 | 08502 |
| quinoa, dry | 1 cup (170 g) | 0.522 | 0.307 | 20035 |
| soy flour, full-fat | 1 cup (84 g) | 1.158 | 1.378 | 16115 |
| soy flour, full-fat, roasted | 1 cup (85 g) | 1.239 | 1.458 | 16116 |
| Uncle Sam Cereal (RTE cereal) | 1 cup (55 g) | 3.300 | 6.000 | 08435 |
| waffle, homemade | 7″ diameter round waffle (74 g) | 0.592 | 0.789 | 18367 |

### MEATS AND POULTRY

| | | | | |
|---|---|---|---|---|
| beef brain, pan-fried | 3 oz (85 g) | 0.859 | 1.010 | 13319 |
| beef brain, raw | 3 oz (85 g) | 1.041 | 1.225 | 13318 |
| beef brain, simmered | 3 oz (85 g) | 1.052 | 1.238 | 13320 |
| lamb brain, braised | 3 oz (85 g) | 0.629 | 0.740 | 17186 |
| lamb brain, pan-fried | 3 oz (85 g) | 1.369 | 1.610 | 17187 |

| | | OMEGA-3 FATTY ACIDS (g/serving) | OMEGA-3 FATTY ACIDS (g/100 g) | SR21 CODE NUMBER[1] |
|---|---|---|---|---|
| lamb, rib, choice, ¼″ trim, lean and fat, roasted | 3 oz (85 g) | 0.527 | 0.620 | 17029 |
| lamb tongue, braised | 3 oz (85 g) | 0.519 | 0.610 | 17221 |
| pork brain, braised | 3 oz (85 g) | 0.680 | 0.800 | 10097 |
| pork brain, raw | 3 oz (85 g) | 0.672 | 0.790 | 10096 |
| pork breakfast strips, cured, raw | 3 slices (68 g) | 0.612 | 0.900 | 10128 |
| Polish sausage, pork, cooked | sausage 10″ long, 1¼″ diameter (227 g) | 0.658 | 0.290 | 07059 |
| turkey nuggets/sticks, breaded, Louis Rich | 3 pieces (85 g) | 0.544 | 0.640 | 07265 |
| **NUTS AND SEEDS** | | | | |
| butternuts, dried | ~9 nuts (28 g) | 2.441 | 8.718 | 12084 |
| flaxseeds | 1 T (12 g) | 2.738 | 22.813 | 12220 |
| soy nuts, roasted | 1 cup (172 g) | 2.914 | 1.694 | 16110 |
| walnuts, black, dried | 1 oz (28 g) | 0.562 | 2.006 | 12154 |
| walnuts, English/Persian, dried | 14 halves (28 g) | 2.542 | 9.080 | 12155 |
| **SALAD DRESSINGS** | | | | |
| Caesar salad dressing | 1 T (15 g) | 0.582 | 3.877 | 43015 |
| peppercorn salad dressing | 1 T (13 g) | 0.503 | 3.872 | 42137 |
| ranch salad dressing | 2 T (30 g) | 0.919 | 3.063 | 04639 |
| Russian salad dressing | 2 T (30 g) | 0.522 | 1.741 | 04015 |
| **VEGETABLES AND VEGETABLE DISHES** | | | | |
| baked beans with frankfurters, canned | 1 cup (259 g) | 0.539 | 0.208 | 16008 |
| chili beans, barbecue ranch style | 1 cup (253 g) | 0.858 | 0.339 | 43112 |
| French beans, mature, boiled | 1 cup (177 g) | 0.508 | 0.287 | 16023 |
| mungo beans, mature, boiled | 1 cup (180 g) | 0.603 | 0.335 | 16084 |
| mungo beans, mature, dry | ½ cup (103 g) | 1.029 | 0.999 | 16083 |
| natto (boiled, fermented soybeans) | 1 cup (175 g) | 1.285 | 0.734 | 16113 |
| navy beans, mature, dry | ½ cup (104 g ) | 0.560 | 0.538 | 16037 |
| potato pancake, homemade | 1 pancake (76 g) | 0.661 | 0.870 | 11672 |
| potato salad, homemade | 1 cup (250 g) | 0.925 | 0.370 | 11414 |
| potato, hashed brown, homemade | 1 cup (156 g) | 0.527 | 0.338 | 11370 |
| soybeans, green/immature (edamame), boiled, drained | 1 cup (180 g) | 0.637 | 0.354 | 11451 |
| soybeans, green/immature (edamame), frozen, heated | 1 cup (155 g) | 0.560 | 0.361 | 11212 |
| soybeans, green/immature (edamame), raw | 1 cup (256 g) | 0.963 | 0.376 | 11450 |
| soybeans, mature, boiled | 1 cup (172 g) | 1.029 | 0.598 | 16109 |
| soybeans, mature, dry | ½ cup (93 g) | 1.237 | 1.330 | 16108 |
| soybean sprouts, stir-fried | 1 cup (125 g) | 0.590 | 0.472 | 11454 |
| spinach, frozen, boiled, drained | 1 cup (190 g) | 0.705 | 0.371 | 11464 |
| **OTHER FOODS** | | | | |
| agutuk with fish and shortening, Alaskan | 3½ oz (100 g) | 16.100 | 16.100 | 35002 |
| agutuk with fish, berry, and seal oil, Alaskan | 3½ oz (100 g) | 0.530 | 0.530 | 35001 |
| fruit and nut squares, soft (candy) | 4 pieces (56 g) | 0.736 | 1.315 | 19866 |
| goose egg, raw | 1 egg (144 g) | 0.798 | 0.554 | 01139 |
| shark fin soup, from restaurant | 1 cup (216 g) | 0.570 | 0.264 | 06180 |
| tofu, firm, prepared with nigari | 3 oz (85 g) | 0.567 | 0.667 | 16160 |

[1]Code numbers for foods in the USDA National Nutrient Database for Standard Reference, Release 21, 2008.

Sources:
USDA National Nutrient Database for Standard Reference, Release 21, 2008. Available at: http://www.nal.usda.gov/fnic/foodcomp/search/.

# *Fatty Acids—Trans Fatty Acids*

| | TRANS FATTY ACIDS (g/100 g) | SERVING SIZE (g) | *TRANS* FATTY ACIDS (g/serving) | SOURCE (SR21 CODE NUMBER)[1] |
|---|---|---|---|---|
| **CANDY** | | | | |
| caramel and chocolate-flavored roll | 0.726 | 2.25 oz bar (64 g) | 0.465 | SR21 (19076) |
| dark chocolate, 45%–59% cacao | 0.112 | 1 oz (28 g) | 0.031 | SR21 (19902) |
| dark chocolate, 60%–69% cacao | 0.078 | 1 oz (28 g) | 0.022 | SR21 (19903) |
| dark chocolate, 70%–85% cacao | 0.030 | 1 oz (28 g) | 0.008 | SR21 (19904) |
| fudge, chocolate marshmallow with nuts, homemade | 0.270 | 0.78 oz piece (22g) | 0.059 | SR21 (19301) |
| fudge, chocolate marshmallow, homemade | 0.291 | 0.7 oz piece (20 g) | 0.058 | SR21 (19379) |
| Kit Kat, Hershey | 0.099 | 2.8 oz bar (78 g) | 0.077 | SR21 (19109) |
| taffy, homemade | 0.119 | 0.53 oz piece (15 g) | 0.018 | SR21 (19382) |
| toffee, homemade | 0.613 | 0.42 oz piece (12 g) | 0.074 | SR21 (19383) |
| Tootsie Roll | 0.719 | 6 pieces (40 g) | 0.288 | SR21 (19064) |
| **CEREALS, READY-TO-EAT** | | | | |
| Apple Jacks, Kellogg's | 0.011 | 1 cup (30 g) | 0.003 | SR21 (08003) |
| Cheerios, General Mills | 0.007 | 1 cup (30 g) | 0.002 | SR21 (08013) |
| Cinnamon Toast Crunch, General Mills | 0.112 | ¾ cup (30 g) | 0.034 | SR21 (08272) |
| Golden Puffs, Malt-O-Meal | 0.028 | 1 cup (37 g) | 0.010 | SR21 (0478) |
| Kix, General Mills | 0.025 | 1⅓ cups (30 g) | 0.008 | SR21 (08048) |
| Lucky Charms, General Mills | 0.005 | 1 cup (30 g) | 0.002 | SR21 (08050) |
| Raisin Bran, Kellogg's | 0.035 | 1 cup (59 g) | 0.021 | SR21 (08060) |
| Rice Krispies, Kellogg's | 0.002 | 1¼ cups (33 g) | 0.001 | SR21 (08065) |
| wheat and malted barley nuggets | 0.007 | ¼ cup (28 g) | 0.002 | SR21 (08038) |
| **CHEESE** | | | | |
| cheese 'n salsa dip, mild/medium Old El Paso | 3.448 | 2 T (29 g) | 1.000 | GENM |
| **DESSERTS** | | | | |
| cake, butter pecan, from mix, SuperMoist | 1.299 | 1/12 cake (77 g) | 1.000 | GENM |
| cake, carrot, from mix, SuperMoist | 1.205 | 1/10 cake (83 g) | 1.000 | GENM |
| cake, cherry chip, from mix, SuperMoist | 1.807 | 1/10 cake (83 g) | 1.500 | GENM |
| cake, chocolate, butter recipe, from mix, SuperMoist | 1.316 | 1/12 cake (76 g) | 1.000 | GENM |
| cake, chocolate devil's food, from mix, SuperMoist | 1.250 | 1/12 cake (80 g) | 1.000 | GENM |
| cake, chocolate fudge, from mix, SuperMoist | 1.250 | 1/12 cake (80 g) | 1.000 | GENM |
| cake, French vanilla, from mix, SuperMoist | 1.299 | 1/12 cake (77g) | 1.000 | GENM |
| cake, German chocolate, from mix, SuperMoist | 1.250 | 1/12 cake (80 g) | 1.000 | GENM |
| cake, golden vanilla, from mix, SuperMoist | 1.299 | 1/12 cake (77 g) | 1.000 | GENM |
| cake, lemon, from mix, SuperMoist | 1.333 | 1/12 cake (75 g) | 1.000 | GENM |
| cake, milk chocolate, from mix, SuperMoist | 1.299 | 1/12 cake (77 g) | 1.000 | GENM |
| cake, pineapple, from mix, Betty Crocker Classic | 2.756 | ⅙ cake (127 g) | 3.500 | GENM |
| cake, pound, from mix, Betty Crocker Classic | 2.439 | ⅛ cake (82 g) | 2.000 | GENM |
| cake, rainbow chip, from mix, SuperMoist | 1.807 | 1/10 cake (83 g) | 1.500 | GENM |
| cake, spice, from mix, SuperMoist | 1.299 | 1/12 cake (77 g) | 1.000 | GENM |
| cake, strawberry, from mix, SuperMoist | 1.299 | 1/12 cake (77 g) | 1.000 | GENM |
| cake, white, from mix, SuperMoist | 1.389 | 1/12 cake (72 g) | 1.000 | GENM |
| cake, yellow, butter recipe, from mix, SuperMoist | 1.299 | 1/12 cake (77 g) | 1.000 | GENM |
| cookie, chocolate chip, higher fat | 0.090 | 2¼″ diameter cookie (12 g) | 0.011 | SR21 (18159) |
| cookie, chocolate chip, soft type | 0.090 | 1 cookie (15 g) | 0.014 | SR21 (18160) |
| cookie, chocolate sandwich with crème filling, chocolate-covered | 0.034 | 1 cookie (10 g) | 0.003 | SR21 (18166) |
| cookie, holiday shapes, from refrigerated dough, Pillsbury | 9.615 | .9 oz cookie (26 g) | 2.500 | GENM |
| cookie, peanut butter, from refrigerated dough, Pillsbury | 3.448 | 1 oz cookie (29 g) | 1.000 | GENM |
| cookie, sugar, from mix, Betty Crocker | 3.030 | 2 cookies (33 g) | 1.000 | GENM |
| cookie, sugar, from refrigerated dough, Pillsbury | 5.172 | 2 cookies (29 g) | 1.500 | GENM |
| gingerbread, from mix, Betty Crocker Classic | 1.829 | ⅛ cake (82 g) | 1.500 | GENM |
| icing/frosting, chocolate, ready-to-spread, Betty Crocker Creamy Deluxe | 6.061 | 2 T (33 g) | 2.000 | GENM |
| icing/frosting, vanilla, whipped, ready-to-spread, Betty Crocker | 6.250 | 2 T (24 g) | 1.500 | GENM |
| lemon bar from mix, Betty Crocker Sunkist | 2.500 | 1 bar (40 g) | 1.000 | GENM |
| sweet roll, caramel, from refrigerated dough, Pillsbury | 5.102 | 1.7 oz roll (49 g) | 2.500 | GENM |

| | TRANS FATTY ACIDS (g/100 g) | SERVING SIZE (g) | *TRANS* FATTY ACIDS (g/serving) | SOURCE (SR21 CODE NUMBER)[1] |
|---|---|---|---|---|
| sweet roll, cinnamon with cream cheese icing, from refrigerated dough, Pillsbury | 4.545 | 1.6 oz roll (44 g) | 2.000 | GENM |
| toaster pastry, apple/blueberry/cherry/strawberry | 2.668 | 1 pastry (52 g) | 1.387 | SR21 (18362) |
| Toaster Strudel Pastries (average for 11 flavors), frozen, Pillsbury | 1.929 | 1.9 oz strudel (54 g) | 1.042 | GENM |
| turnover, apple, from refrigerated dough, Pillsbury | 5.263 | 2 oz turnover (57 g) | 3.000 | GENM |
| turnover, cherry, from refrigerated dough, Pillsbury | 5.263 | 2 oz turnover (57 g) | 3.000 | GENM |

**ENTREES**

| | | | | |
|---|---|---|---|---|
| Chicken Helper, cheddar and broccoli, prepared | 0.866 | 1 cup (231 g) | 2.000 | GENM |
| Chicken Helper, chicken and stuffing, prepared | 0.469 | 1 cup (213 g) | 1.000 | GENM |
| Chicken Helper, fettuccini alfredo, prepared | 0.617 | 1 cup (243 g) | 1.500 | GENM |
| clam chowder, New England, condensed, canned, prepared with milk | 0.040 | 1 cup (248 g) | 0.099 | SR21 (06230) |
| fajitas, prepared, Old El Paso Dinner Kit | 1.721 | 2 fajitas (208 g) | 1.500 | GENM |
| gordita with ranch sauce, prepared, Old El Paso Dinner Kit | 1.056 | 1 gordita (142 g) | 1.500 | GENM |
| Hamburger Helper, cheeseburger macaroni, prepared | 0.218 | 1 cup (229 g) | 0.500 | GENM |
| Hamburger Helper, chili macaroni, prepared | 0.209 | 1 cup (239 g) | 0.500 | GENM |
| Hamburger Helper, four cheese lasagna, prepared | 0.227 | 1 cup (220 g) | 0.500 | GENM |
| Hamburger Helper, rice oriental, prepared | 0.213 | 1 cup (235 g) | 0.500 | GENM |
| Hamburger Helper, stroganoff, prepared | 0.238 | 1 cup (210 g) | 0.500 | GENM |
| herb chicken vegetable rice, dry packaged entree, Bowl Appetit, Betty Crocker | 1.471 | 2.4 oz bowl (68 g) | 1.000 | GENM |
| Nachos, Stuffed, cheese, frozen, Totino's | 1.190 | 6 nachos (84 g) | 1.000 | GENM |
| pierogies, broccoli and cheddar, Mrs. Ts | 0.833 | 3 pierogies (120 g) | 1.000 | ATCO |
| pierogies, sour cream and chive, Mrs. Ts | 0.417 | 3 pierogies (120 g) | 0.500 | ATCO |
| pizza rolls, sausage, frozen, Totino's | 1.765 | 6 rolls (85 g) | 1.500 | GENM |
| pizza, cheese, frozen, Jeno's Crisp 'N Tasty | 2.308 | 6.9 oz pizza (195 g) | 4.500 | GENM |
| pizza, combination, frozen, Jeno's Crisp 'N Tasty | 2.273 | 7 oz pizza (198g) | 4.500 | GENM |
| pizza, sausage, frozen, Jeno's Crisp 'N Tasty | 2.273 | 7 oz pizza (198 g) | 4.500 | GENM |
| pizza, Supreme, frozen, Jeno's Crisp 'N Tasty | 2.206 | 7.2 oz pizza (204 g) | 4.500 | GENM |
| potato, broccoli, and cheese chowder, canned, ready-to-serve, Progresso | 0.198 | 1 cup; 8 fl oz (252 g) | 0.500 | GENM |
| tacos, soft with ground beef, prepared, Old El Paso Dinner Kit | 1.136 | 1 tacos (176 g) | 2.000 | GENM |
| Toaster Scrambles Pastries, cheese, egg, and bacon, frozen, Pillsbury | 2.128 | 1.66 oz entrée (47 g) | 1.000 | GENM |
| Toaster Scrambles Pastries, cheese, egg, and ham, frozen, General Mills | 2.128 | 1.66 oz entrée (47 g) | 1.000 | GENM |
| Toaster Scrambles Pastries, cheese, egg, and sausage, frozen, Pillsbury | 3.191 | 1.66 oz entrée (47 g) | 1.5000 | GENM |
| Tuna Helper, creamy pasta, prepared | 0.813 | 1 cup (246 g) | 2.000 | GENM |
| Tuna Helper, tetrazzini, prepared | 0.837 | 1 cup (239 g) | 2.000 | GENM |
| Tuna Helper, tuna melt, prepared | 0.630 | 1 cup (238 g) | 1.500 | GENM |

**FAST FOODS**

| | | | | |
|---|---|---|---|---|
| apple dumpling pie, Bob Evans | 2.089 | 9 oz slice (383 g) | 8.000 | BOBE |
| apple pie, Boston Market | 2.941 | 6 oz slice (170 g) | 5.000 | BOST |
| apple turnover, Arby's | 4.688 | 4.5 oz turnover (128 g) | 6.000 | ARBY |
| Arby's Melt on bun, Arby's | 0.685 | 5.2 oz sandwich (146 g) | 1.000 | ARBY |
| Bacon Beef'n Cheddar on bun, Arby's | 0.943 | 7.5 oz sandwich (212 g) | 2.000 | ARBY |
| BBQ Bacon'n Jack 2for, Arby's | 0.592 | 6 oz sandwich (169 g) | 1.000 | ARBY |
| beef sirloin sandwich, Boston Market | 1.872 | 13.2 oz sandwich (374 g) | 7.000 | BOST |
| beef sirloin, roasted, Boston Market | 0.704 | 5 oz (142 g) | 1.000 | BOST |
| Beef'n Cheddar on bun, Arby's | 0.513 | 6.9 oz sandwich (195 g) | 1.000 | ARBY |
| biscuit with chicken fingers, Arby's | 0.758 | 4.7 oz sandwich (132 g) | 1.000 | ARBY |
| blackberry cobbler, Bob Evans | 3.524 | 8 oz piece (227 g) | 8.000 | BOBE |
| BLT sandwich, Arby's | 0.340 | 10.4 oz sandwich (294 g) | 1.000 | ARBY |
| brownie, cheesecake, Au Bon Pain | 2.655 | 4 oz brownie (113 g) | 3.000 | AUBN |
| brownie, chocolate chip, Au Bon Pain | 2.655 | 4 oz brownie (113 g) | 3.000 | AUBN |
| brownie, hazelnut mocha, Au Bon Pain | 3.097 | 4 oz brownie (113 g) | 3.500 | AUBN |
| brownie, rocky road, Au Bon Pain | 2.655 | 4 oz brownie (113 g) | 3.000 | AUBN |
| burrito, border scramble, Bob Evans | 0.217 | 16.2 oz (460 g) | 1.000 | BOBE |
| butter crumb cake, Au Bon Pain | 1.176 | 6 oz slice (170 g) | 2.000 | AUBN |
| calzone, breakfast, Au Bon Pain | 0.524 | 6.8 oz calzone (191 g) | 1.000 | AUBN |
| cheddar cheese potato soup, Bob Evans | 0.990 | 14.3 fl oz bowl (404 g) | 4.000 | BOBE |
| Cheddar Fries, Arby's | 2.941 | 6 oz medium (170 g)) | 5.000 | ARBY |

| | TRANS FATTY ACIDS (g/100 g) | SERVING SIZE (g) | *TRANS* FATTY ACIDS (g/serving) | SOURCE (SR21 CODE NUMBER)[1] |
|---|---|---|---|---|
| Cheese Curds, A&W | 0.704 | 5 oz (142 g) | 1.000 | AANW |
| Cheese Fries, A&W | 2.353 | 6 oz (170 g) | 4.000 | AANW |
| cheeseburger with bacon, Bob Evans | 0.851 | 8.3 oz sandwich (235 g) | 2.000 | BOBE |
| cheeseburger, bacon double, A&W | 1.320 | 10.7 oz sandwich (303 g) | 4.000 | AANW |
| cheeseburger, bacon, A&W | 1.570 | 7.9 oz sandwich (223 g) | 3.500 | AANW |
| cheeseburger, Bob Evans | 0.909 | 7.8 oz sandwich (220 g) | 2.000 | BOBE |
| cheeseburger, double, A&W | 1.389 | 10.2 oz sandwich (288 g) | 4.000 | AANW |
| cheeseburger, kids, A&W | 2.000 | 6.2 oz sandwich (175 g) | 3.500 | AANW |
| cheesecake, New York, Au Bon Pain | 0.752 | 4.7 oz slice (133 g) | 1.000 | AUBN |
| cherry turnover, Arby's | 4.688 | 4.5 oz turnover (128 g) | 6.000 | ARBY |
| chicken (crispy) sandwich, A&W | 2.055 | 7.7 oz sandwich (219 g) | 4.500 | AANW |
| chicken (fried) club sandwich, Bob Evans | 0.379 | 9.3 oz sandwich (264 g) | 1.000 | BOBE |
| chicken (grilled) club sandwich, Bob Evans | 0.412 | 8.6 oz sandwich (243 g) | 1.000 | BOBE |
| chicken (grilled) sandwich, A&W | 1.408 | 7.5 oz sandwich (213 g) | 3.000 | AANW |
| chicken cordon bleu sandwich, crispy, Arby's | 0.412 | 8.6 oz sandwich (243 g) | 1.000 | ARBY |
| chicken fillet sandwich, crispy, Arby's | 0.420 | 8.4 oz sandwich (238 g) | 1.000 | ARBY |
| chicken sandwich, SW Chipotle, crispy, Arby's | 0.372 | 9.5 oz sandwich (269 g) | 1.000 | ARBY |
| Chicken Strips | 1.258 | 3 pieces;(159 g)) | 2.000 | AANW |
| Chicken Tenders, Arby's | 0.917 | 5 pieces (218 g) | 2.000 | ARBY |
| Chicken Tenders, Arby's | 1.000 | 2 kids meal pieces (100 g) | 1.000 | ARBY |
| chicken, bacon, Swiss, crispy on bun, Arby's | 0.467 | 7.6 oz sandwich (214 g) | 1.000 | ARBY |
| Chili Cheese Fries, A&W | 2.020 | 7 oz (198 g) | 4.000 | AANW |
| Chili Fries, A&W | 2.353 | 6 oz (170g) | 4.000 | AANW |
| chocolate cake, Boston Market | 3.103 | 5.1 of slice (145 g) | 4.500 | BOST |
| chocolate chip cookie, Arby's | 4.444 | 1.6 oz cookie (45 g) | 2.000 | ARBY |
| Cinnamon Twist, TJ Cinnamons | 5.634 | 2.5 oz piece (71 g) | 4.000 | ARBY |
| cornbread, Boston Market | 2.222 | 1.6 oz piece (45 g) | 1.000 | BOST |
| Corned Beef Reuben sandwich, Arby's | 0.324 | 10.9 oz sandwich (309 g) | 1.000 | ARBY |
| croissant, raspberry cheese, Au Bon Pain | 0.485 | 3.6 oz croissant (103 g) | 0.500 | AUBN |
| croissant, sweet cheese, Au Bon Pain | 0.971 | 3.6 oz croissant (103 g) | 1.000 | AUBN |
| Curly Fries, Arby's | 2.830 | 3.7 oz; small (106 g) | 3.000 | ARBY |
| Curly Fries, Arby's | 3.030 | 7 oz; large (198 g) | 6.000 | ARBY |
| Curly Fries, Arby's | 3.125 | 4.5 oz; medium (128 g) | 4.000 | ARBY |
| Danish pastry, cherry, Au Bon Pain | 0.935 | 3.8 oz pastry (107 g) | 1.000 | AUBN |
| Danish pastry, lemon, Au Bon Pain | 0.926 | 3.8 oz pastry (108 g) | 1.000 | AUBN |
| Danish pastry, sweet cheese, Au Bon Pain | 0.935 | 3.8 oz pastry (107 g) | 1.000 | AUBN |
| diet root beer float, A&W | 0.063 | large (794 g) | 0.500 | AANW |
| fish sandwich, Bob Evans | 0.606 | 11.6 oz sandwich (330 g) | 2.000 | BOBE |
| frankfurter in bun (hot dog), A&W | 1.111 | 3.2 oz sandwich (90 g) | 1.000 | AANW |
| frankfurter in bun with cheese (Cheese Dog), A&W | 0.794 | 4.4 oz sandwich (126 g) | 1.000 | AANW |
| frankfurter in bun with chili (Coney Dog), A&W | 0.794 | 4.4 oz sandwich (126 g) | 1.000 | AANW |
| frankfurter in bun with chili and cheese (Coney Cheese Dog), A&W | 0.649 | 5.4 oz sandwich (154 g) | 1.000 | AANW |
| French dip and Swiss on French roll, Arby's | 0.446 | 7.9 oz sandwich (224 g) | 1.000 | ARBY |
| French dip on French roll, Arby's | 0.505 | 7 oz sandwich (198 g) | 1.000 | ARBY |
| French dip sub with au jus, Arby's | 0.356 | 9.9 oz sub (281 g) | 1.000 | ARBY |
| French fries, A&W | 3.526 | large (156 g) | 5.500 | AANW |
| French fries, A&W | 3.540 | kids size (133 g) | 4.000 | AANW |
| fries, homestyle, Arby's | 2.347 | large (213 g) | 5.000 | ARBY |
| fries, homestyle, Arby's | 2.655 | small (113 g) | 3.000 | ARBY |
| fries, homestyle, Arby's | 2.817 | medium (142 g) | 4.000 | ARBY |
| ham and Swiss cheese sandwich, Arby's | 0.279 | 12.7 oz sandwich (359 g) | 1.000 | ARBY |
| hamburger, Bob Evans | 1.042 | 6.8 oz sandwich (192 g) | 2.000 | BOBE |
| hamburger, kids, A&W | 2.174 | 5.7 oz sandwich (161 g) | 3.500 | AANW |
| hamburger, Papa Burger, A&W | 1.389 | 10.2 oz sandwich (288 g) | 4.000 | AANW |
| hot chocolate with 2% milk and whipped cream, Starbucks | 0.104 | grande; 16 fl oz (480 g) | 0.500 | STAR |
| Iced Caffe Mocha with 2% milk and whipped cream, Starbucks | 0.104 | grande; 16 fl oz (480 g) | 0.500 | STAR |
| Italian sub, Arby's | 0.361 | 9.8 oz sub (277 g) | 1.000 | ARBY |
| Jalapeno Bites, Arby's | 0.790 | large (22 g) | 0.170 | ARBY |
| key lime crumb cake, Au Bon Pain | 1.869 | 3.8 oz square (107 g) | 2.000 | AUBN |
| Latte, cinnamon dolce, with 2% milk and whipped cream, Starbucks | 0.104 | grande; 16 fl oz (480 g) | 0.500 | STAR |
| macaroni and cheese, Boston Market (fast food) | 0.226 | 7.8 oz (221 g) | 0.500 | BOST |
| meat loaf sandwich, Bob Evans | 0.213 | 16.6 oz sandwich (470 g) | 1.000 | BOBE |
| Mozzarella Sticks, Arby's | 1.825 | large (274 g) | 5.000 | ARBY |
| omelet, bacon and cheese, Bob Evans | 0.341 | 10.3 oz (293 g) | 1.000 | BOBE |
| omelet, Border Scramble, Bob Evans | 0.228 | 15.5 oz (438 g) | 1.000 | BOBE |

| | TRANS FATTY ACIDS (g/100 g) | SERVING SIZE (g) | *TRANS* FATTY ACIDS (g/serving) | SOURCE (SR21 CODE NUMBER)[1] |
|---|---|---|---|---|
| omelet, Farmer's Market, Bob Evans | 0.460 | 15.3 oz (435 g) | 2.000 | BOBE |
| omelet, Garden harvest, Bob Evans | 0.444 | 15.9 oz (450 g) | 2.000 | BOBE |
| omelet, ham and cheese, Bob Evans | 0.307 | 11.5 oz (326 g) | 1.000 | BOBE |
| omelet, sausage and cheese, Bob Evans | 0.310 | 11.4 oz (323 g) | 1.000 | BOBE |
| omelet, three cheese, Bob Evans | 0.373 | 9.4 oz (268 g) | 1.000 | BOBE |
| omelet, turkey Florentine, Bob Evans | 0.246 | 14.4 oz (407 g) | 1.000 | BOBE |
| omelet, western, Bob Evans | 0.254 | 13.9 oz (394 g) | 1.000 | BOBE |
| Onion Petals, Arby's | 0.707 | large (293 g) | 2.000 | ARBY |
| onion rings, A&W | 3.982 | 4 oz (113 g ) | 4.500 | AANW |
| pastry, almond Artisan, Au Bon pan | 1.709 | 4.1 oz pastry (117 g) | 2.000 | AUBN |
| pastry, blueberry sweet cheese Artisan, Au Bon Pain | 1.154 | 4.6 oz pastry (130 g) | 1.500 | AUBN |
| pastry, Danish apple nun, Au Bon Pain | 3.158 | 3.4 oz pastry (95 g) | 3.000 | AUBN |
| pastry, Danish pretzel, Au Bon Pain | 0.629 | 6 oz pastry (159 g) | 1.000 | AUBN |
| pastry, hurricane, Au Bon Pain | 4.348 | 6.5 oz pastry (184 g) | 8.000 | AUBN |
| pastry, strawberry puff, Au Bon Pain | 1.685 | 3.1 oz pastry (89 g) | 1.500 | AUBN |
| Philly Beef and Swiss cheese sub, Arby's | 0.326 | 10.8 oz sub (307 g) | 1.000 | ARBY |
| Polar Swirl, M&M, A&W | 0.147 | medium (340 g) | 0.500 | AANW |
| Polar Swirl, Oreo, A&W | 0.294 | medium (340 g) | 1.000 | AANW |
| Polar Swirl, Reese's A&W | 0.147 | medium (340 g) | 0.500 | AANW |
| pork loin sandwich, Bob Evans | 0.219 | 16.1 oz sandwich (457 g) | 1.000 | BOBE |
| Potato Bites, loaded, Arby's | 6.818 | large (44 g) | 3.000 | ARBY |
| Potato Cakes, Arby's | 3.333 | 3 cakes (150 g) | 5.000 | ARBY |
| potato, baked with broccoli and cheddar cheese, Arby's | 0.503 | 14 oz (398 g) | 2.000 | ARBY |
| potato, baked with sour cream, butter, cheddar cheese, and bacon bits, Arby's | 0.277 | 12.7 oz (361 g) | 1.000 | ARBY |
| pumpkin pie, Bob Evans | 1.382 | 7.7 oz slice (217 g) | 3.000 | BOBE |
| raspberry cookie, Au Bon Pain | 0.794 | 2.2 oz cookie (63 g) | 0.500 | AUBN |
| roast beef and Swiss cheese sandwich, Arby's | 0.758 | 9.3 oz sandwich (264 g) | 2.000 | ARBY |
| roast beef sandwich on bun, large, Arby's | 0.712 | 9.9 oz sandwich (281 g) | 2.000 | ARBY |
| roast beef sandwich on bun, medium, Arby's | 0.476 | 7.4 oz sandwich (210 g) | 1.000 | ARBY |
| roast beef sandwich on bun, regular, Arby's | 0.649 | 5.4 oz sandwich (154 g) | 1.000 | ARBY |
| roast beef sandwich on bun, super, Arby's | 0.505 | 7 oz sandwich (198 g) | 1.000 | ARBY |
| roast beef sub, Arby's | 0.667 | 10.6 oz sub (300 g) | 2.000 | ARBY |
| root beer float, A&W | 0.063 | large (794 g) | 0.500 | AANW |
| Root Beer Freeze, A&W | 0.098 | medium (510 g) | 0.500 | AANW |
| salad dressing, Caesar, Boston Market | 0.704 | 2.5 oz (71 g) | 0.500 | BOST |
| salad, Chicken Club, Arby's | 0.489 | 14.4 oz salad (409 g) | 2.000 | ARBY |
| salad, chopped with dressing, Boston Market | 0.178 | 19.9 oz salad (563 g) | 1.000 | BOST |
| salad, Santa Fe with chicken fingers, Arby's | 0.538 | 13.1 oz salad (372 g) | 2.000 | ARBY |
| shake, chocolate, A&W | 0.211 | medium (475 g) | 1.000 | AANW |
| shake, chocolate, Arby's | 0.196 | large 510 g) | 1.000 | ARBY |
| shake, jamocha, Arby's | 0.196 | regular (510 g) | 1.000 | ARBY |
| shake, strawberry, A&W) | 0.211 | medium (475 g) | 1.000 | AANW |
| shake, strawberry, Arby's | 0.196 | large (510 g) | 1.000 | ARBY |
| shake, vanilla, A&W | 0.211 | medium (475 g) | 1.000 | AANW |
| shake, vanilla, Arby's | 0.214 | large (468 g) | 1.000 | ARBY |
| steak burger, Bob Evans | 0.559 | 12.6 oz sandwich (358 g) | 2.000 | BOBE |
| strudel, apple, Au Bon Pain | 3.731 | 4.8 oz piece (134 g) | 5.000 | AUBN |
| strudel, cherry, Au Bon Pain | 4.425 | 4 oz piece (113 g) | 5.000 | AUBN |
| sweet roll, pecan, Au Bon Pain | 1.504 | 4.7 oz roll (133 g) | 2.000 | AUBN |
| Swiss Melt with roast beef on bun, Arby's | 0.685 | 5.2 oz sandwich (146 g) | 1.000 | ARBY |
| Tangy Southwest sauce, Arby's | 1.754 | 2 oz (57 g) | 1.000 | ARBY |
| turkey and Swiss cheese sandwich, Arby's | 0.279 | 12.7 oz sandwich (359 g) | 1.000 | ARBY |
| Turkey Ranch and Bacon sandwich, Arby's | 0.262 | 13.5 oz sandwich (382 g) | 1.000 | ARBY |
| Turkey Reuben sandwich on rye bread, Arby's | 0.324 | 10.9 oz sandwich (309 g) | 1.000 | ARBY |
| turkey sandwich, Bob Evans | 0.243 | 14.5 oz sandwich (411 g) | 1.000 | BOBE |
| turkey sub, Arby's | 0.351 | 10.1 oz sub (285 g) | 1.000 | ARBY |
| white chocolate mocha with 2% milk and whipped cream, Starbucks | 0.104 | grande; 16 fl oz (480 g) | 0.555 | STAR |
| white hot chocolate with 2% milk and whipped cream, Starbucks | 0.104 | grande; 16 fl oz (480 g) | 0.555 | STAR |
| wrap (flour tortilla) with bacon, egg, potato, and American cheese, Arby's | 1.064 | 6.6 oz wrap (188 g) | 2.000 | ARBY |
| wrap (flour tortilla) with bacon, lettuce, tomato, and mayonnaise, Arby's | 0.402 | 8.8 oz wrap (249 g) | 1.000 | ARBY |
| wrap (flour tortilla) with chicken, jack and cheddar cheeses, lettuce, onion, and ranch sauce, Arby's | 0.398 | 8.9 oz wrap (251 g) | 1.000 | ARBY |

| | TRANS FATTY ACIDS (g/100 g) | SERVING SIZE (g) | *TRANS* FATTY ACIDS (g/serving) | SOURCE (SR21 CODE NUMBER)[1] |
|---|---|---|---|---|
| wrap (flour tortilla) with ham, egg, potato, and American cheese, Arby's | 0.877 | 8 oz wrap (228 g) | 2.000 | ARBY |
| wrap (flour tortilla) with sausage, egg, potato, and American cheese, Arby's | 0.889 | 7.9 oz wrap (225 g) | 2.000 | ARBY |
| wrap (flour tortilla) with turkey, cheddar cheese, bacon, onion, tomato, lettuce, and ranch spread, Arby's | 0.315 | 11.2 oz wrap (317 g) | 1.000 | ARBY |
| wrap (flour tortilla), corned beef Reuben, Arby's | 0.357 | 9.9 oz wrap (280 g) | 1.000 | ARBY |
| wrap (flour tortilla), roast turkey Reuben, Arby's | 0.357 | 9.9 oz wrap (280 g) | 1.000 | ARBY |
| wrap, Thai chicken, Au Bon Pain | 0.243 | 14.5 oz wrap (411 g) | 1.000 | AUBN |
| cheeseburger sandwich, regular, single meat, fast food | 0.547 | 1 sandwich (113 g) | 0.618 | SR21 (21090) |
| egg drop soup, Chinese Restaurant | 0.001 | 8 fl oz (241 g) | 0.002 | SR21 (27000) |
| French fries, fast food | 3.764 | regular (134 g) | 5.044 | SR21 (21138) |
| hamburger sandwich, regular, single meat with condiments, fast food | 0.456 | 3.2 oz sandwich (90 g) | 0.410 | SR21 (21108) |
| noodles, crunchy, Chinese restaurant | 0.136 | 1 cup (45 g) | 0.061 | SR21 (20118) |
| wonton soup, Chinese Restaurant | 0.001 | 8 fl oz (223 g) | 0.002 | SR21 (27002) |
| cheeseburger, Burger King | 0.672 | 4.7 oz sandwich (133 g) | 0.894 | SR21 (21251) |
| cheeseburger, Double Whopper, Burger King | 0.620 | 15 oz sandwich (426 g) | 2.641 | SR21 (21255) |
| cheeseburger, Whopper, Burger King | 0.425 | 13.9 oz sandwich (395 g) | 1.679 | SR21 (21253) |
| chicken sandwich, Burger King | 0.775 | 7.2 oz sandwich (204 g) | 1.581 | SR21 (21259) |
| chicken tenders, Burger King | 2.934 | 5 pieces (77 g) | 2.259 | SR21 (21256) |
| chicken tenders, Burger King | 2.934 | 8 pieces (123 g) | 3.609 | SR21 (21256) |
| Chicken Whopper sandwich, Burger King | 0.161 | 9.6 oz sandwich (272 g) | 0.438 | SR21 (21257) |
| French fries, Burger King | 4.659 | 2.6 oz small (74 g) | 3.448 | SR21 (21249) |
| French fries, Burger King | 4.659 | 4.1 oz medium (117 g) | 5.451 | SR21 (21249) |
| French fries, Burger King | 4.659 | 5.6 oz large (160 g) | 7.454 | SR21 (21240) |
| French fries, Burger King | 4.659 | 6.8 oz king (194) | 9.038 | SR21 (21240) |
| hamburger sandwich, Burger King | 0.542 | 4.3 oz sandwich (121 g) | 0.656 | SR21 (21250) |
| hamburger sandwich, Double Whopper, Burger King | 0.346 | 14 oz sandwich (401 g) | 1.387 | SR21 (21254) |
| hamburger, Whopper, Burger King | 0.436 | 10.7 oz sandwich (304 g) | 1.325 | SR21 (21252) |
| shake, vanilla, Burger King | 0.296 | medium (397 g) | 1.175 | SR21 (21141) |
| apple pie, baked, McDonald's | 6.126 | 2.7 oz pie (77 g) | 4.717 | SR21 (21324) |
| biscuit, McDonald's | 0.125 | 2.4 oz biscuit (69 g) | 0.086 | SR21 (21317) |
| Chicken McNugget sauce, barbeque, McDonald's | 0.005 | 1 oz packet (28 g) | 0.001 | SR21 (21310) |
| Chicken McNugget sauce, honey mustard, McDonald's | 0.014 | 0.5 oz packet (14 g) | 0.002 | SR21 (21316) |
| Chicken McNugget sauce, hot mustard, McDonald's | 0.042 | 1 oz packet (28 g) | 0.012 | SR21 (21313) |
| Chicken McNugget sauce, sweet'n sour, McDonald's | 0.011 | 1 oz packet (28 g) | 0.003 | SR21 (21315) |
| chocolate chip cookie, McDonald's | 0.885 | 2 oz bag (57 g) | 0.504 | SR21 (21325) |
| cinnamon roll, McDonald's | 4.233 | 3.4 oz roll (99 g) | 4.191 | SR21 (21322) |
| French fries, McDonald's | 0.131 | 2.4 oz small (68 g) | 0.089 | SR21 (21238) |
| McDonaldland cookies, McDonald's | 4.329 | 2 oz bag (57 g) | 2.468 | SR21 (21326) |
| potato, hashed brown, McDonald's | 0.106 | 1.9 oz (53 g) | 0.056 | SR21 (21319) |
| sausage patty, McDonald's | 0.396 | 1.5 oz (43 g) | 0.170 | SR21 (21323) |
| caramel sauce, lowfat, McDonald's | 0.038 | 0.8 oz (21 g) | 0.000 | SR21 (21343) |
| Chicken McNuggets, McDonald's | 0.164 | 6 pieces (108 g) | 0.177 | SR21 (21309) |
| Chicken Selects (breast strips), McDonald's | 0.116 | 5 pieces (221 g) | 0.256 | SR21 (21308) |
| sauce, creamy ranch, McDonald's | 0.191 | 1.5 oz (43 g) | 0.082 | SR21 (21311) |
| sauce, spicy buffalo, McDonald's | 0.056 | 1.5 oz (43 g) | 0.024 | SR21 (21314) |
| cheeseburger sandwich, Junior, Wendy's | 0.421 | 4.6 oz sandwich (129 g) | 0.543 | SR21 (21242) |
| hamburger sandwich, Junior, Wendy's | 0.232 | 4.2 oz hamburger (117 g) | 0.271 | SR21 (21241) |
| biscuit, McDonald's | 0.125 | 3.2 oz biscuit; large (90 g) | 0.113 | SR21 (21460) |
| cheeseburger, Classic Single, Wendy's | 0.343 | 8.3 oz sandwich (236 g) | 0.809 | SR21 (21240) |
| chicken fillet sandwich, Wendy's | 0.394 | 8.1 oz sandwich (230 g) | 0.906 | SR21 (21244) |
| **FATS, OILS, AND SPREADS** | | | | |
| butter | 2.982 | 1 T (14 g) | 0.417 | SR21 (01001) |
| butter, sweet (unsalted) | 2.982 | 1 T (14 g) | 0.417 | SR21 (1145) |
| canola oil | 0.395 | 1 T (14 g) | 0.055 | SR21 (04582) |
| canola oil, Natreon | 0.240 | 1 T (14 g) | 0.034 | SR21 (04678) |
| corn and canola oil | 0.334 | 1 T (14 g) | 0.047 | SR21 (42289) |
| margarine, corn and soy, 80% fat, stick | 14.890 | 1 T (14 g) | 2.085 | SR21 (04628) |
| margarine, fat-free, tub | 0.168 | 1 T (15 g) | 0.025 | SR21 (04631) |
| margarine, soy, 70% fat | 14.785 | 1 T (14 g) | 2.070 | SR21 (04629) |
| margarine, stick/tub composite, 60% fat | 6.885 | 1 T (14 g) | 0.964 | SR21 (04614) |
| margarine, unspecified oils | 14.890 | 1 T (14 g) | 2.085 | SR21 (04132) |
| margarine-butter blend (60% corn oil, 40% butter) | 14.279 | 1 T (14 g) | 1.999 | SR21 (04585) |
| pork fat, cooked | 0.719 | 1 oz (28 g) | 0.201 | SR21 (10007) |
| pork fat, raw | 0.786 | 1 oz (28 g) | 0.220 | SR21 (10006) |

| | TRANS FATTY ACIDS (g/100 g) | SERVING SIZE (g) | *TRANS* FATTY ACIDS (g/serving) | SOURCE (SR21 CODE NUMBER)[1] |
|---|---|---|---|---|
| Smart Balance Light Buttery Spread | 0.281 | 1 T (14 g) | 0.039 | SR21 (04674) |
| soy oil, salad/cooking | 0.533 | 1 T (14 g) | 0.075 | SR21 (04044) |
| **FISH AND SHELLFISH** | | | | |
| crab, Alaska king, imitation, made from surimi | 0.007 | 3 oz (85 g) | 0.006 | SR21 (15138) |
| fish sticks/pieces, frozen, reheated | 0.855 | stick 4″ × 1″ × ½″ (28 g) | 0.239 | SR21 (15027) |
| **GRAIN- AND VEGETABLE-BASED SNACKS** | | | | |
| cheese puffs/twists | 0.812 | 1 oz (28 g) | 0.227 | SR21 (19008) |
| Chex Mix | 0.444 | ⅔ cup (28 g) | 0.124 | SR21 (19033) |
| corn chips | 0.442 | 1 oz (28 g) | 0.124 | SR21 (19003) |
| Gardetto's Snack Mix | 4.082 | 1.7 oz pouch (49 g) | 2.000 | GENM |
| plantain chips | 0.251 | 1 oz (28 g) | 0.070 | SR21 (25027) |
| popcorn, 94% fat-free, microwaved | 0.885 | 1 oz (28 g) | 0.248 | SR21 (25000) |
| popcorn, butter, popped, PopSecret | 16.667 | 1 cup (6g) | 1.000 | GENM |
| popcorn, extra butter, popped, PopSecret | 14.286 | 1 cup (7 g) | 1.000 | GENM |
| potato chips, from dried potatoes | 0.199 | 1 oz (28 g) | 0.056 | SR21 (19410) |
| potato chips, reduced fat, from dried potatoes | 0.139 | 1 oz (28 g) | 0.039 | SR21 (19045) |
| Sunchips, Frito Lay | 0.088 | 1 oz (28 g) | 0.025 | SR21 (25013) |
| tortilla chips | 0.069 | 1 oz (28 g) | 0.019 | SR21 (25028) |
| tortilla chips, nacho | 0.216 | 1 oz (28 g) | 0.060 | SR21 (19057) |
| tortilla chips, ranch | 0.345 | 1 oz (28 g) | 0.097 | SR21 (19058) |
| Veggie Crisps, sundried tomato and pesto, Snyder | 1.786 | 1 oz (28 g) | 0.500 | SNYD |
| **GRAINS AND GRAIN PRODUCTS** | | | | |
| biscuit, Butter Tastin, from refrigerated dough, Grands! | 5.172 | 2 oz biscuit (58 g) | 3.000 | GENM |
| biscuit, buttermilk, from refrigerated dough, Grands! | 5.172 | 2 oz biscuit (58 g) | 3.000 | GENM |
| biscuit, extra rich, from refrigerated dough, Grands! | 5.738 | 2.15 oz biscuit (61 g) | 3.500 | GENM |
| biscuit, flaky layer buttermilk, from refrigerated dough, Pillsbury | 2.344 | 2.3 oz biscuit (64 g) | 1.500 | GENM |
| biscuit, flaky, from refrigerated dough, Grands! | 5.172 | 2.15 oz biscuit (58 g) | 3.000 | GENM |
| biscuit, southern style, from refrigerated dough, Grands! | 5.172 | 2 oz biscuit (58 g) | 3.000 | GENM |
| biscuit, wheat, reduced fat, from refrigerated dough, Grands! | 4.098 | 2.15 oz biscuit (61 g) | 2.500 | GENM |
| breadstick, Italian garlic and herb, from refrigerated dough, Pillsbury | 2.500 | 2 pieces; 2.1 oz (60 g) | 1.500 | GENM |
| cornbread breadstick twists, from refrigerated dough, Pillsbury | 4.878 | 1.45 oz piece (41 g) | 2.000 | GENM |
| crackers, Ritz, Nabisco | 1.050 | 1 cracker (16 g) | 0.168 | SR21 (18621) |
| crackers, round | 0.862 | ~5 crackers (14 g) | 0.121 | SR21 (18229) |
| oatmeal, instant, dry | 0.004 | 1 oz packet (28 g) | 0.001 | SR21 (08122) |
| oatmeal, instant, prepared | 0.001 | 1 cup (234 g) | 0.002 | SR21 (08123) |
| saltines | 0.442 | 5 crackers (14 g) | 0.062 | SR21 (18228) |
| soda crackers | 0.442 | 5 crackers (14 g) | 0.062 | SR21 (18425) |
| taco shell, from corn tortilla | 4.783 | 5″ diameter shell (13 g) | 0.622 | SR21 (18360) |
| tortilla, flour, Old El Paso | 2.439 | 8″ diameter tortilla (41 g) | 1.000 | GENM |
| **MEATS** | | | | |
| beef chuck shoulder medallion, choice, 0″ trim, lean, grilled | 0.214 | 3 oz (85 g) | 0.182 | SR21 (23036) |
| beef chuck shoulder medallion, select, 0″ trim, lean, grilled | 0.273 | 3 oz (85 g) | 0.232 | SR21 (23054) |
| beef chuck shoulder top blade steak, choice, 0″ trim, lean and fat, grilled | 0.335 | 3 oz (85 g) | 0.285 | SR21 (23043) |
| beef chuck shoulder top blade steak, select, 0″ trim, lean and fat, grilled | 0.371 | 3 oz (85 ) | 0.315 | SR21 (23059) |
| beef chuck shoulder top/center steak, select, 0″ trim, lean and fat, grilled | 0.290 | 3 oz (85 g) | 0.247 | SR21 (23038) |
| beef chuck shoulder top/center steak, select, 0″ trim, lean, grilled | 0.275 | 3 oz (85 g) | 0.234 | SR21 (230058) |
| beef round, knuckle tip center steak, choice, 0″ trim, lean and fat, grilled | 0.206 | 3 oz (85 g) | 0.175 | SR21 (23047) |
| beef round, knuckle tip center steak, select, 0″ trim, lean and fat, grilled | 0.209 | 3 oz (85 g) | 0.178 | SR21 (23061) |
| beef round, knuckle tip side steak, choice, 0″ trim, lean and fat, grilled | 0.114 | 3 oz (85 g) | 0.097 | SR21 (23033) |
| beef round, knuckle tip side steak, select, 0″ trim, lean and fat, grilled | 0.169 | 3 oz (85 g) | 0.144 | SR21 (23056) |
| beef round, outside bottom steak, choice, 0″ trim, lean and fat, grilled | 0.136 | 3 oz (85 g) | 0.116 | SR21 (23051) |

| | TRANS FATTY ACIDS (g/100 g) | SERVING SIZE (g) | *TRANS* FATTY ACIDS (g/serving) | SOURCE (SR21 CODE NUMBER)[1] |
|---|---|---|---|---|
| beef round, outside bottom steak, select, 0" trim, lean and fat, grilled | 0.169 | 3 oz (85 g) | 0.144 | SR21 (23063) |
| beef, ground, 15% fat, patty, broiled | 0.947 | 3 oz patty (85 g) | 0.805 | SR21 (23568) |
| beef, ground, 30% fat, broiled | 0.891 | 3 oz (85 g) | 0.757 | SR21 (13497) |
| buffalo top round steak, broiled | 0.088 | 3 oz (85 g) | 0.075 | SR21 (35176) |
| elk, eye of round, cooked | 0.040 | 3 oz (85 g) | 0.034 | SR21 (35178) |
| elk, ground patty, cooked | 0.065 | 3 oz (85 g) | 0.055 | SR21 (35172) |
| pork Boston blade (steaks and roasts), lean and fat, braised | 0.154 | 3 oz (85 g) | 0.131 | SR21 (10081) |
| pork Boston blade (steaks and roasts), lean, braised | 0.102 | 3 oz (85 g) | 0.087 | SR21 (10085) |
| pork breast, lean and fat, broiled | 0.020 | 3 oz (85 g) | 0.017 | SR21 (10959) |
| pork center loin (chops) with bone, lean and fat, broiled | 0.107 | 3 oz (85 g) | 0.091 | SR21 (10038) |
| pork center loin (chops) with bone, lean, broiled | 0.064 | 3 oz (85 g) | 0.054 | SR21 (10042) |
| pork center rib (chops) with bone, lean and fat, broiled | 0.120 | 3 oz (85 g) | 0.102 | SR21 (10046) |
| pork center rib (chops) with bone, lean, broiled | 0.067 | 3 oz (85 g) | 0.057 | SR21 (10050) |
| pork petite tender, lean and fat, broiled | 0.022 | 3 oz (85 g) | 0.019 | SR21 (10960) |
| pork sirloin (roasts), lean and fat, roasted | 0.102 | 3 oz (85 g) | 0.087 | SR21 (10055) |
| pork sirloin (roasts), lean, roasted | 0.063 | 3 oz (85 g) | 0.054 | SR21 (10059) |
| pork sirloin tip roast, lean and fat braised | 0.012 | 3 oz (85 g) | 0.010 | SR21 (10962) |
| pork tenderloin, lean and fat, roasted | 0.038 | 3 oz (85 g) | 0.032 | SR21 (10222) |
| pork tenderloin, lean, roasted | 0.033 | 3 oz (85 g) | 0.028 | SR21 (10061) |
| pork top loin (chops), lean and fat, broiled | 0.087 | 3 oz (85 g) | 0.074 | SR21 (10064) |
| pork top loin (chops), lean, broiled | 0.052 | 3 oz (85 g) | 0.044 | SR21 (0068) |
| pork top loin (roasts), lean and fat, roasted | 0.079 | 3 oz (85 g) | 0.067 | SR21 (10065) |
| pork top loin (roasts), lean, roasted | 0.051 | 3 oz (85 g) | 0.043 | SR21 (10069) |
| pork feet, cured, pickled | 0.065 | 3 oz (85 g) | 0.055 | SR21 (10132) |

**MEATS, LUNCHEON**

| | | | | |
|---|---|---|---|---|
| beef, thin sliced lunch meat | 0.127 | 5 slices (21 g) | 0.027 | SR21 (07043) |
| chicken roll, light meat (lunch meat) | 0.038 | 2 slices (57 g) | 0.022 | SR21 (07017) |
| frankfurter, chicken | 0.148 | 1.6 oz frankfurter (45 g) | 0.067 | SR21 (07024) |
| frankfurter, turkey | 0.789 | 1.6 oz frankfurter (45 g) | 0.355 | SR21 (07025) |
| ham, sliced, lean (5% fat) (lunch meat) | 0.016 | 1 oz slice (28 g) | 0.004 | SR21 (07028) |
| kielbasa (pork and beef with nonfat dry milk solids), cooked | 0.358 | 0.9 oz slice (26 g) | 0.093 | SR21 (07037) |
| pepperoni, pork and beef | 1.634 | slice 1⅜" diameter, ⅛" thick (6 g) | 0.098 | SR21 (07057) |
| salami, beef and pork | 0.586 | 2 slices (46 g) | 0.270 | SR21 (07069) |
| Smokie (smoked sausage), pork | 0.231 | link 4" long (68 g) | 0.157 | SR21 (07074) |
| turkey roll, light meat (lunch meat) | 0.053 | 2 slices (57 g) | 0.030 | SR21 (07081) |

**MILKS AND MILK BEVERAGES**

| | | | | |
|---|---|---|---|---|
| cocoa (hot chocolate), homemade with 2% milk | 0.072 | 8 fl oz (250 g) | 0.180 | SR21 (01105) |
| milk, lowfat, 1% fat | 0.037 | 8 fl oz (244 g) | 0.090 | SOURCE (01082) |
| milk, reduced fat, 2% fat | 0.078 | 8 fl oz (244 g) | 0.190 | SR21 (01079) |

**NUTS AND SEEDS**

| | | | | |
|---|---|---|---|---|
| almonds, raw | 0.017 | 1 oz (28 g) | 0.005 | SR21 (12061) |
| coconut, dried, sweetened, flaked, packaged | 0.002 | 1 oz (28 g) | 0.001 | SR21 (12109) |
| sunflower seed kernels, oil-roasted without salt | 0.158 | 1 oz (28 g) | 0.044 | SR21 (12038) |

**VEGETABLES**

| | | | | |
|---|---|---|---|---|
| potato, cheesy scalloped, from mix, Betty Crocker Specialty Potatoes | 0.350 | ½ cup prepared (143 g) | 0.500 | GENM |
| potato, mashed, four cheese, from mix, Betty Crocker | 0.476 | 1 cup prepared (210 g) | 1.000 | GENM |
| potato, mashed, roasted garlic, from mix, Betty Crocker | 0.952 | ½ cup prepared (105 g) | 1.000 | GENM |
| potato, mashed, sour cream and chives, from mix, Betty Crocker | 0.952 | ½ cup prepared (105 g) | 1.000 | GENM |
| potato, sour cream 'n chive, from mix, Betty Crocker Specialty Potatoes | 0.360 | ½ cup prepared (139 g) | 0.500 | GENM |
| potatoes au gratin, from mix, Betty Crocker Specialty Potatoes | 0.709 | ½ cup prepared (141 g) | 1.000 | GENM |
| refried beans, vegetarian, canned | 0.003 | 1 cup (242 g) | 0.007 | SR21 (16171) |
| refried beans, canned | 0.025 | 1 cup (252 g) | 0.063 | SR21 (16103) |
| soybeans, green/immature (edamame), frozen, heated | 0.009 | 1 cup (155 g) | 0.014 | SR21 (11212) |
| sweet potato, candied, frozen, Green Giant | 1.095 | ¾ cup (137 g) | 1.500 | GENM |

| | TRANS FATTY ACIDS (g/100 g) | SERVING SIZE (g) | *TRANS* FATTY ACIDS (g/serving) | SOURCE (SR21 CODE NUMBER)[1] |
|---|---|---|---|---|
| **OTHER FOODS** | | | | |
| Ensure pudding, Abbott (medical food) | 1.770 | 4 fl oz (113 g) | 2.000 | RSSM |
| Fruit Gushers, all flavors, Betty Crocker | 2.000 | 0.9 oz pouch (25 g) | 0.500 | GENM |
| mustard (prepared condiment sauce) | 0.013 | 1 t (5 g) | 0.001 | SR21 (02046) |
| PowerBar, chocolate (energy food) | 0.010 | 2.4 oz bar (68 g) | 0.007 | SR21 (25017) |
| white sauce, thin, homemade with butter | 0.089 | ½ cup (125 g) | 0.111 | SR21 (06264) |

Sources:
AANW = A&W
ARBY = Arby's
ATCO = Ateeco, Incorporated
AUBN = Au Bon Pain
BOBE = Bob Evans
BOST = Boston Market
GENM = General Mills, Incorporated
RSSM = Ross Products Division, Abbott Labs, Medical Foods
SARG = Sargento
STAR = Starbucks
USDA National Nutrient Database for Standard Reference, Release 21 (SR21), 2008. Available at: http://www.nal.usda.gov/fnic/foodcomp/serarch/.

# *Flavonoids—Anthocyanins*

| | CYANIDIN (mg/100 g) | DELPHINIDIN (mg/100 g) | MALVIDIN (mg/100 g) | PELARGONIDIN (mg/100 g) | PEONIDIN (mg/100 g) | PETUNIDIN (mg/100 g) | SR21 CODE NUMBER[1] |
|---|---|---|---|---|---|---|---|
| **BEVERAGES** | | | | | | | |
| wine, red | 0.40 | 1.04 | 7.00 | | 0.84 | 0.93 | 14096 |
| wine, white | 0.00 | | 0.06 | | | | 14106 |
| **FRUITS AND FRUIT JUICES** | | | | | | | |
| apple, peeled, raw | 1.81 | 0.01 | 0.00 | 0.01 | 0.00 | 0.00 | 09004 |
| apple, raw | 2.44 | 0.00 | 0.00 | 0.00 | 0.01 | 0.00 | 09003 |
| banana, raw | 0.00 | 7.39 | 0.00 | 0.00 | 0.00 | 0.00 | 09040 |
| blackberries, raw | 90.31 | 0.00 | 0.00 | 0.15 | 0.00 | 0.00 | 09042 |
| blueberries, frozen | 4.36 | 21.59 | 49.65 | 0.02 | 0.47 | 18.16 | 09054 |
| blueberries, raw | 16.97 | 47.40 | 61.35 | 0.00 | 11.38 | 26.42 | 09050 |
| cherries, sour, raw | 6.64 | | | | | | 09063 |
| cherries, sweet, raw | 75.18 | 0.00 | 0.00 | 0.54 | 4.47 | 0.00 | 09070 |
| cranberries, dried, sweetened | 0.60 | 0.10 | | 0.02 | | | 09079 |
| cranberries, raw | 41.81 | 7.66 | 0.31 | 0.00 | 42.10 | 0.00 | 09078 |
| cranberry juice cocktail, canned/bottled | 0.38 | 0.03 | | 0.03 | | | 14242 |
| cranberry sauce, jelled, canned | 0.10 | 0.02 | | 0.02 | | | 09081 |
| currants, black, raw | 85.63 | 181.11 | | 1.17 | 0.66 | 3.87 | 09083 |
| date, dried | 1.70 | 0.00 | 0.00 | 0.00 | 0.00 | 0.00 | 09087 |
| elderberries, raw | 758.48 | | | 1.13 | | | 09088 |
| gooseberries, raw | 3.61 | | | | 0.13 | | 09107 |
| grape juice, canned/bottled | 0.56 | 0.47 | | 0.02 | | | 09135 |
| grapes, red, raw | 1.46 | 3.67 | 34.71 | 0.02 | 2.89 | 2.11 | 97074 |
| honeydew melon, raw | 0.00 | 0.00 | 0.00 | 0.00 | 0.00 | 0.00 | 09184 |
| mango, raw | 0.10 | 0.02 | | 0.02 | | | 09176 |
| nectarine, raw | 1.81 | 0.00 | 0.00 | 0.00 | 0.00 | 0.00 | 09191 |
| peach, raw | 1.61 | 0.00 | 0.00 | 0.00 | 0.00 | 0.00 | 09236 |
| pear, raw | 12.18 | 0.00 | 0.00 | 0.00 | 0.00 | 0.00 | 09252 |
| plum, raw | 12.02 | 0.00 | 0.00 | 0.00 | 0.00 | 0.00 | 09279 |
| prune, dried | 0.71 | 0.04 | 0.00 | 0.00 | 0.00 | 0.00 | 09291 |
| raisins, seedless | 0.03 | 0.01 | 0.00 | 0.01 | 0.00 | 0.00 | 09298 |
| raspberries, raw | 35.84 | 0.29 | 0.70 | 1.85 | 0.00 | 0.00 | 09302 |
| strawberries, raw | 1.96 | 0.32 | 0.00 | 31.27 | 0.00 | 0.08 | 09316 |
| strawberries, unsweetened, frozen, thawed | 1.27 | 0.02 | | 19.32 | | | 09318 |
| **NUTS** | | | | | | | |
| almonds, raw | 2.46 | 0.00 | 0.00 | 0.00 | 0.00 | 0.00 | 12061 |
| filberts (hazelnuts), dried | 6.71 | 0.00 | 0.00 | 0.00 | 0.00 | 0.00 | 12120 |
| pecans, dried | 10.74 | 7.28 | 0.00 | 0.00 | 0.00 | 0.00 | 12142 |
| pistachios, dried | 6.06 | 0.00 | 0.00 | 0.00 | 0.00 | 0.00 | 12151 |
| walnuts, English/Persian, dried | 2.71 | 0.00 | 0.00 | 0.00 | 0.00 | 0.00 | 12155 |
| **VEGETABLES** | | | | | | | |
| avocado, raw | 0.33 | 0.00 | 0.00 | 0.00 | 0.00 | 0.00 | 09037 |
| black beans, mature, dry | | 11.98 | 6.45 | | | 9.57 | 16014 |
| cabbage, red/purple, raw | 72.86 | 0.10 | | 0.02 | | | 11112 |
| Chinese cabbage, pak choi, boiled, drained | 0.02 | 0.02 | | 0.02 | | | 11117 |
| cowpeas (blackeye peas), mature, dry | 94.72 | 94.60 | 34.28 | | 11.07 | 27.82 | 16062 |
| eggplant (aubergine), raw | 0.02 | 13.76 | | 0.02 | | | 11209 |
| green peas, frozen, boiled, drained | 0.03 | 0.03 | | 0.02 | | | 11313 |
| green snap beans, boiled, drained | 0.02 | 0.02 | | 0.02 | | | 11053 |
| kidney beans, red, mature, dry | 1.19 | | | 2.42 | | | 16032 |
| lettuce, looseleaf (leaf), raw | 0.29 | 0.00 | 0.00 | 0.00 | 0.00 | 0.00 | 11253 |
| lettuce, red leaf, raw | 2.77 | 0.00 | 0.00 | 0.00 | 0.00 | 0.00 | 11257 |
| radish, red, raw | 0.00 | 0.00 | 0.00 | 25.66 | 0.00 | 0.00 | 11429 |
| yardlong bean, immature, boiled, drained | 1.10 | 0.02 | | 0.02 | | | 11200 |
| **OTHER FOODS** | | | | | | | |
| vinegar, red wine | 0.00 | 0.08 | 0.43 | | 0.07 | 0.08 | 99109 |

[1]Code numbers for foods in the USDA National Nutrient Database for Standard Reference, Release 21, 2008.

Source:
USDA Database for the Flavonoid Content of Selected Foods, Release 2.1, 2007. Available at: http://www.ars.usda.gov/Services/docs.htm?docid=6231.

# Flavonoids—Flavan-3-ols—Catechins

| | (−)-EPICATECHIN (mg/100 g) | (−)-EPICATECHIN 3-GALLATE (mg/100 g) | (−)-EPIGALLO-CATECHIN (mg/100 g) | (−)-EPIGALLOCATECHIN 3-GALLATE (mg/100 g) | (+)-CATECHIN (mg/100 g) | (+)-CATECHIN 3-GALLATE (mg/100 g) | (+)-GALLOCATE-CHIN (mg/100 g) | SR21 CODE NUMBER[1] |
|---|---|---|---|---|---|---|---|---|
| **BEVERAGES** | | | | | | | | |
| beer | 0.33 | 0.00 | 0.00 | 0.00 | 2.07 | | 0.08 | 14003 |
| coffee, brewed | 0.04 | 0.00 | 0.04 | 0.00 | 0.00 | | 0.00 | 14209 |
| tea, black, brewed 3 minutes | 2.13 | 5.87 | 7.93 | 9.26 | 1.47 | | 1.20 | 14355 |
| tea, black, decaffeinated, brewed 3 minutes | 0.49 | 0.64 | 0.55 | 1.01 | | | | 14352 |
| tea, iced, from instant | 0.31 | 0.24 | 0.61 | 0.86 | | | | 14367 |
| tea leaves, black, dry | 255.19 | 688.27 | 956.81 | 1121.92 | 137.82 | 50.83 | 91.73 | 99060 |
| tea leaves, black dry, decaffeinated | 77.53 | 81.99 | 51.45 | 136.86 | 0.00 | | | 99345 |
| tea leaves, green dry | 811.72 | 1491.29 | 2057.98 | 7115.98 | 57.12 | 7.07 | 258.11 | 99061 |
| tea leaves, green, dry, decaffeinated | 423.02 | 522.01 | 1153.49 | 1843.64 | | | | 99346 |
| tea leaves, oolong, dry | 248.42 | 627.25 | 750.80 | 3412.62 | 30.63 | 19.89 | 305.69 | 99062 |
| wine, red | 3.28 | 0.01 | 0.06 | 0.00 | 7.02 | | 0.10 | 14096 |
| wine, sherry | 1.25 | | | | 1.60 | | | 99075 |
| wine, white | 0.55 | 0.00 | 0.00 | 0.00 | 0.77 | | 0.00 | 14106 |
| **FRUITS AND FRUIT JUICES** | | | | | | | | |
| apple juice, canned/bottled | 4.71 | 0.00 | 0.00 | 0.00 | 1.25 | | 0.00 | 09016 |
| apple, peeled, raw | 6.15 | 0.00 | 0.25 | 0.05 | 1.32 | | 0.00 | 09004 |
| apple, raw | 6.07 | 0.01 | 0.36 | 0.26 | 0.89 | | 0.00 | 09003 |
| applesauce, unsweetened, canned/bottled | 5.41 | 0.00 | 0.00 | 0.00 | 0.69 | | 0.00 | 09019 |
| apricot, raw | 5.47 | 0.00 | 0.00 | 0.00 | 4.79 | | 0.00 | 09021 |
| banana, raw | 0.02 | 0.00 | 0.00 | 0.00 | 6.10 | | 0.00 | 09040 |
| blackberries, raw | 4.66 | 0.00 | 0.10 | 0.68 | 37.06 | | 0.00 | 09042 |
| blueberries, raw | 13.69 | 0.00 | 0.66 | 0.00 | 37.24 | | 0.12 | 09050 |
| cherries, sour, raw | 3.83 | | | | 0.30 | | | 09063 |
| cherries, sweet, raw | 6.97 | 0.05 | 0.34 | 0.00 | 1.31 | | 0.00 | 09070 |
| cranberries, raw | 4.37 | 0.00 | 0.74 | 0.97 | 0.39 | | 0.00 | 09078 |
| cranberry juice cocktail, canned/bottled | | | | | 0.19 | | | 14242 |
| currants, black, raw | 0.47 | 0.00 | 0.00 | 0.00 | 0.70 | | 0.00 | 09083 |
| custard apple (bullock's heart), raw | 5.63 | 0.04 | 0.00 | 0.00 | 0.58 | | 0.00 | 09086 |
| fig, raw | 0.02 | 0.00 | 0.00 | 0.00 | 0.15 | | 0.00 | 09089 |
| gooseberries, raw | 0.00 | 0.00 | 0.00 | 0.00 | 1.67 | | 0.44 | 09107 |
| grape juice, canned/bottled | 0.00 | 0.00 | 0.00 | 0.00 | 0.19 | | 0.00 | 09135 |
| grapes, red, raw | 1.20 | 0.17 | 0.08 | 0.00 | 0.82 | | 0.00 | 97074 |
| grapes, white or green, raw | 1.70 | 0.25 | 0.02 | 0.00 | 3.73 | | 0.01 | 99047 |
| honeydew melon, raw | 0.01 | 0.00 | 0.04 | 0.00 | 0.00 | | 0.00 | 09184 |
| kiwifruit, raw | 0.27 | 0.01 | 0.00 | 0.09 | 0.00 | | 0.00 | 09148 |
| mango, raw | 0.00 | 0.00 | 0.00 | 0.00 | 1.72 | | 0.00 | 09176 |
| nectarine, raw | 2.54 | 0.00 | 0.00 | 0.00 | 2.98 | | 0.00 | 09191 |
| peach, canned in heavy syrup, drained | 0.00 | 0.00 | 0.00 | 0.00 | 1.87 | | 0.00 | 09370 |
| peach, raw | 2.34 | 0.00 | 1.04 | 0.30 | 4.92 | | 0.00 | 09236 |

| | (−)-EPICATE-CHIN (mg/100 g) | (−)-EPICATECHIN 3-GALLATE (mg/100 g) | (−)-EPIGALLO-CATECHIN (mg/100 g) | (−)-EPIGALLOCATECHIN 3-GALLATE (mg/100 g) | (+)-CATECHIN (mg/100 g) | (+)-CATECHIN 3-GALLATE (mg/100 g) | (+)-GALLOCATE-CHIN (mg/100 g) | SR21 CODE NUMBER[1] |
|---|---|---|---|---|---|---|---|---|
| pear, raw | 3.76 | 0.02 | 0.59 | 0.17 | 0.27 | | 0.00 | 09252 |
| persimmon, raw | 0.00 | 0.00 | 0.00 | 0.00 | 0.63 | | 0.17 | 97088 |
| plum, raw | 3.2 | 0.76 | 0.24 | 0.40 | 2.89 | | 0.09 | 09279 |
| pomegranate, raw | 0.08 | 0.00 | 0.16 | 0.00 | 0.40 | | 0.17 | 09286 |
| quince, raw | 0.67 | 0.00 | 0.00 | 0.00 | 0.75 | | 0.00 | 09296 |
| raisins, seedless | 0.10 | 0.00 | 0.00 | 0.00 | 0.42 | | 0.00 | 09298 |
| raspberries, raw | 4.07 | 0.00 | 0.46 | 0.54 | 1.56 | | 0.00 | 09302 |
| strawberries, raw | 0.12 | 0.15 | 0.78 | 0.11 | 3.32 | | 0.03 | 09316 |
| **MILK AND MILK BEVERAGES** | | | | | | | | |
| chocolate milk, reduced fat | 0.26 | 0.00 | 0.00 | 0.00 | 0.82 | | 0.00 | 01103 |
| cocoa (hot chocolate), from mix, prepared with water | 0.59 | 0.00 | 0.00 | 0.00 | 0.74 | | 0.00 | 14194 |
| **NUTS** | | | | | | | | |
| almonds, raw | 0.60 | 0.00 | 2.59 | 0.00 | 1.28 | | 0.00 | 12061 |
| cashews, oil-roasted | 0.93 | 0.15 | 0.00 | 0.00 | 0.90 | | 0.00 | 12086 |
| chestnut, European, raw, peeled | 0.00 | 0.00 | 0.00 | 0.00 | 0.01 | | 0.01 | 12098 |
| filberts (hazelnuts), dried | 0.22 | 0.00 | 2.78 | 1.06 | 1.19 | | 0.00 | 12120 |
| peanuts, all types, oil-roasted | 0.00 | 0.00 | 0.66 | 0.00 | 0.00 | | 0.00 | 16089 |
| pecans, dried | 0.82 | 0.00 | 5.63 | 2.30 | 7.24 | | 0.00 | 12142 |
| pine nuts, pinyon, dried | 0.00 | 0.00 | 0.49 | 0.00 | 0.00 | | 0.00 | 12149 |
| pistachios, dried | 0.83 | 0.00 | 2.05 | 0.40 | 3.57 | | 0.00 | 12151 |
| **VEGETABLES** | | | | | | | | |
| avocado, raw | 0.37 | 0.00 | 0.00 | 0.15 | 0.00 | | 0.00 | 09037 |
| broadbeans (fava beans), immature, boiled, drained | 7.82 | 0.00 | 4.65 | 0.00 | 8.16 | | 0.00 | 11089 |
| broadbeans (fava beans), immature, raw | 28.96 | 0.00 | 15.47 | 0.00 | 14.29 | | 4.15 | 11088 |
| green peas, raw | 0.01 | 0.00 | 0.00 | 0.00 | 0.01 | | 0.00 | 11304 |
| kidney beans, all types, mature, canned | 0.35 | 0.00 | 0.00 | 0.00 | 1.66 | | 0.00 | 16029 |
| lentils, mature, dry | 0.00 | 0.00 | 0.00 | 0.00 | 0.35 | | 0.14 | 16069 |
| pinto beans, mature, dry | 0.14 | 0.00 | 0.05 | 0.00 | 5.07 | | 0.00 | 16042 |
| rhubarb, raw | 0.51 | 0.60 | 0.00 | 0.00 | 2.17 | | 0.00 | 09307 |
| soybeans, mature, dry | 37.41 | | | | | | | 16108 |
| Swiss chard, raw | | | | | 2.15 | | | 11147 |
| white beans, mature, dry | 0.09 | 0.00 | 0.00 | 0.00 | 0.01 | | 0.00 | 16049 |
| **OTHER FOODS** | | | | | | | | |
| buckwheat flour, whole groats | 3.53 | | | | | | | 20011 |
| carob powder | | 30.06 | | 109.46 | 50.75 | | | 16055 |
| jam/preserves, apricot | 0.50 | 0.00 | 0.00 | 0.00 | 0.47 | | 0.00 | 19719 |
| jam/preserves, cherry | 0.90 | 0.00 | 0.00 | 0.00 | 0.16 | | 0.00 | 99114 |
| jam/preserves, strawberry | 0.00 | 0.00 | 0.00 | 0.00 | 0.90 | | 0.00 | 99064 |
| milk chocolate chips | 6.31 | 0.00 | 0.00 | 0.00 | 2.07 | | 0.00 | 19120 |
| vinegar, red wine | 2.20 | | | | | | | 99109 |
| vinegar, white wine | 0.60 | | | | 3.60 | | | 99108 |

[1]Code numbers for foods in the USDA National Nutrient Database for Standard Reference, Release 21, 2008.

Source:
USDA Database for the Flavonoid Content of Selected Foods, Release 2.1, 2007. Available at http://www.ars.usda.gov/Services/docs.htm?docid=6231.

# Flavonoids—Flavan-3-ols—Theaflavins and Thearubigins

| | THEAFLAVIN-3, 3'-DIGALLATE (mg/100 g) | THEAFLAVIN-3'-GALLATE (mg/100 g) | THEAFLAVIN-3-GALLATE (mg/100 g) | THEARUBIGINS (mg/100 g) | SR21 CODE NUMBER[1] |
|---|---|---|---|---|---|
| **BEVERAGES** | | | | | |
| iced tea, from instant | 0.01 | 0.00 | 0.01 | 23.65 | 14367 |
| tea, black, brewed 3 minutes | 1.75 | 1.51 | 1.25 | 81.30 | 14355 |
| tea, black, decaffeinated, brewed 3 minutes | 0.43 | 0.18 | 0.41 | 49.03 | 14352 |

[1]Code numbers for foods in the USDA National Nutrient Database for Standard Reference, Release 21, 2008.

Source:
USDA Database for the Flavonoid Content of Selected Foods, Release 2.1, 2007. Available at http://www.ars.usda.gov/Services/docs.htm?docid=6231.

# Flavonoids—Flavones

| | APIGENIN (mg/100 g) | LUTEOLIN (mg/100 g) | SR21 CODE NUMBER[1] | | APIGENIN (mg/100 g) | LUTEOLIN (mg/100 g) | SR21 CODE NUMBER[1] |
|---|---|---|---|---|---|---|---|
| **FRUITS** | | | | cabbage, green/white, raw | 0.08 | 0.10 | 11109 |
| apple, peeled, raw | 0.00 | 0.01 | 09004 | cabbage, red/purple, raw | 0.01 | 0.10 | 11112 |
| apple, raw | 0.00 | 0.17 | 09003 | carrot, raw | 0.00 | 0.13 | 11124 |
| blueberries, frozen | 0.01 | 1.80 | 09054 | cauliflower, raw | 0.03 | 0.07 | 11135 |
| blueberries, raw | 0.00 | 0.20 | 09050 | celeriac (celery root), raw | 2.41 | 0.00 | 11141 |
| cantaloupe, raw | 0.00 | 0.64 | 09181 | celery, raw | 2.34 | 0.63 | 11143 |
| cranberries, dried, sweetened | 0.01 | 0.02 | 09079 | chicory greens, raw | 0.77 | 1.30 | 11152 |
| cranberry juice cocktail, canned/bottled | 0.01 | 0.03 | 14242 | chili pepper, green, hot, raw | 1.40 | 3.87 | 11670 |
| cranberry sauce, jelled, canned | 0.01 | 0.02 | 09081 | Chinese cabbage, pak choi, boiled, drained | 0.01 | 0.02 | 11117 |
| grape juice, canned/bottled | 0.01 | 0.01 | 09135 | Chinese cabbage, pak choi, raw | 0.65 | 0.20 | 11116 |
| grapefruit, pink and red, raw | 0.00 | 0.60 | 09112 | Chinese cabbage, pe-tsai, raw | 0.01 | 0.02 | 11119 |
| grapes, red, raw | 0.00 | 1.30 | 97074 | chives, raw | 0.00 | 0.15 | 11156 |
| kiwifruit, raw | 0.00 | 1.12 | 09148 | eggplant (aubergine), raw | 0.01 | 0.02 | 11209 |
| kumquat, raw | 21.87 | | 09149 | green peas, frozen, boiled, drained | 0.01 | 0.40 | 11313 |
| lemon juice, canned/bottled | | 1.83 | 09153 | jalapeno pepper, raw | | 1.34 | 11979 |
| lemon, raw | 0.00 | 1.90 | 09150 | kohlrabi, raw | 0.00 | 1.30 | 11241 |
| mango, raw | 0.01 | 0.02 | 09176 | lettuce, iceberg, raw | 0.13 | 0.03 | 11252 |
| orange, all varieties, raw | 0.01 | 1.13 | 09200 | lettuce, looseleaf (leaf), raw | 0.16 | 0.50 | 11253 |
| orange, California navel, raw | 0.00 | 0.70 | 09202 | lettuce, red leaf, raw | 0.00 | 1.58 | 11257 |
| papaya, raw | 0.01 | 0.02 | 09226 | pumpkin winter squash, raw | 0.00 | 1.63 | 11422 |
| strawberries, unsweetened, frozen, thawed | 0.01 | 0.02 | 09318 | romaine (cos lettuce), raw | 0.00 | 0.06 | 11251 |
| watermelon, raw | 0.00 | 0.61 | 09326 | rutabaga (Swede), raw | 3.85 | 0.00 | 11435 |
| | | | | serrano pepper, raw | | 4.14 | 11977 |
| **SPICES AND HERBS** | | | | spinach, raw | 0.00 | 0.74 | 11457 |
| marjoram, dried | 3.50 | 0.00 | 02023 | sweet pepper, green, raw | 0.00 | 4.98 | 11333 |
| parsley, dried | 13506.22 | 19.75 | 02029 | sweet pepper, red, raw | 0.00 | 0.61 | 11821 |
| parsley, raw | 225.93 | 1.24 | 11297 | sweet pepper, yellow, raw | 0.00 | 1.02 | 11951 |
| peppermint, raw (herb) | 8.71 | 11.33 | 02064 | sweet potato leaves, raw | 0.06 | 0.11 | 11505 |
| rosemary, raw | 0.55 | 2.00 | 02063 | sweet potato, raw | 0.01 | 0.02 | 11507 |
| thyme, raw | 2.00 | 45.25 | 02049 | tomato, red, canned | 0.01 | 0.02 | 11531 |
| | | | | vinespinach, raw | 62.2 | | 11587 |
| **VEGETABLES** | | | | watercress, raw | 0.01 | 0.02 | 11591 |
| artichoke, raw | 4.70 | 2.27 | 11007 | yardlong bean, immature, boiled, drained | 0.01 | 0.02 | 11200 |
| beet, raw | 0.00 | 0.37 | 11080 | | | | |
| broccoli, raw | 0.00 | 0.86 | 11090 | **OTHER FOODS** | | | |
| Brussels sprouts, raw | 0.00 | 0.34 | 11098 | buckwheat groats, roasted, dry | 0.28 | | 20009 |
| cabbage, green/white, boiled, drained | 0.01 | 0.02 | 11110 | wine, red | 1.33 | 0.00 | 14096 |

[1]Code numbers for foods in the USDA National Nutrient Database for Standard Reference, Release 21, 2008.

Source:
USDA Database for the Flavonoid Content Tof Selected Foods, Release 2.1, 2007. Available at http://www.ars.usda.gov/Services/docs.htm?docid=6231.

# Flavonoids—Flavonols

| | ISORHAMNETIN (mg/100 g) | KAEMPFEROL (mg/100 g) | MYRICETIN (mg/100 g) | QUERCETIN (mg/100 g) | SR21 CODE NUMBER[1] |
|---|---|---|---|---|---|
| **BEVERAGES** | | | | | |
| beer | | 0.81 | 0.03 | 0.02 | 14003 |
| coffee, brewed | | 0.00 | 0.05 | 0.05 | 14209 |
| tea, black, brewed 3 minutes | | 1.31 | 0.45 | 1.99 | 14355 |
| tea, black, decaffeinated, brewed 3 minutes | | 0.88 | 0.89 | 2.74 | 14352 |
| tea, iced, from instant | | 0.32 | 0.21 | 0.87 | 14367 |
| wine, red | 0.07 | 0.24 | 0.94 | 2.16 | 14096 |
| wine, white | 0.00 | 0.01 | 0.03 | 0.09 | 14106 |
| **FRUITS AND FRUIT JUICES** | | | | | |
| apple juice, canned/bottled | | 0.00 | 0.01 | 0.62 | 09016 |
| apple, peeled, raw | | 0.01 | 0.01 | 0.96 | 09004 |
| apple, raw | | 0.02 | 0.00 | 4.27 | 09003 |
| applesauce, unsweetened, canned/bottled | | 0.00 | 0.00 | 2.00 | 09019 |
| apricot, raw | | 0.00 | 0.00 | 2.08 | 09021 |
| blackberries, raw | | 0.06 | 0.67 | 1.76 | 09042 |
| blueberries, frozen | | 1.1 | 1.76 | 4.64 | 09054 |
| blueberries, raw | | 1.81 | 2.66 | 5.05 | 09050 |
| cherries, sour, raw | | 0.00 | 0.00 | 2.92 | 09063 |
| cherries, sweet, raw | | 0.00 | 0.00 | 2.64 | 09070 |
| cranberries, dried, sweetened | | 0.01 | 2.40 | 4.50 | 09079 |
| cranberries, raw | | 0.09 | 6.78 | 15.09 | 09078 |
| cranberry juice cocktail, canned/bottled | | 0.01 | 0.51 | 1.27 | 14242 |
| cranberry sauce, jelled, canned | | 0.01 | 2.70 | 2.40 | 09081 |
| currants, black, raw | | 0.50 | 6.64 | 5.55 | 09083 |
| date, dried | | | 0.00 | 0.93 | 09087 |
| elderberries, raw | | | | 42.00 | 09088 |
| fig, raw | | | 0.00 | 0.93 | 09089 |
| gooseberries, raw | | 0.88 | 0.00 | 1.23 | 09107 |
| grape juice, canned/bottled | | 0.01 | 0.21 | 0.64 | 09135 |
| grapefruit juice, canned/bottled | | | | 0.90 | 09123 |
| grapefruit juice, raw | | 0.00 | 0.05 | 0.05 | 09128 |
| grapefruit, pink and red, raw | | 0.01 | 0.01 | 0.33 | 09112 |
| grapes, red, raw | | 0.00 | 0.01 | 1.38 | 97074 |
| grapes, white or green, raw | | 0.00 | 0.30 | 1.62 | 99047 |
| lemon juice, raw | | 0.00 | 0.03 | 0.37 | 09152 |
| lemon, raw | | 0.00 | 0.00 | 1.52 | 09150 |
| lime juice, raw | | | | 0.51 | 09160 |
| lime, raw | | | | 0.40 | 09159 |
| mango, raw | | 0.01 | 0.03 | 0.00 | 09176 |
| mulberries, raw | | 0.00 | | 2.47 | 09190 |
| nectarine, raw | | | 0.00 | 0.69 | 09191 |
| orange juice, raw | | 0.00 | 0.05 | 0.27 | 09206 |
| orange juice, refrigerated | | | | 0.61 | 09209 |
| orange, all varieties, raw | | 0.01 | 0.02 | 0.58 | 09200 |
| orange, California navel, raw | | 0.01 | 0.01 | 0.20 | 09202 |
| papaya, raw | | 0.01 | 0.03 | 0.00 | 09226 |
| peach, raw | | 0.00 | 0.00 | 0.68 | 09236 |
| pear, raw | 0.30 | 0.00 | 0.00 | 4.51 | 09252 |
| pineapple, raw | | 0.01 | 0.01 | 0.00 | 09266 |
| plum, raw | | 0.00 | 0.00 | 3.45 | 09279 |
| prickly pear, raw | 0.65 | 0.18 | | 4.86 | 09287 |
| prune, dried | | 0.01 | 0.01 | 1.80 | 09291 |
| raisins, seedless | | 0.01 | 0.01 | 0.25 | 09298 |
| raspberries, raw | | 0.09 | 0.00 | 1.23 | 09302 |
| strawberries, raw | | 0.46 | 0.00 | 1.14 | 09316 |
| strawberries, unsweetened, frozen, thawed | | 0.49 | 0.35 | 0.46 | 09318 |
| tangerine juice, raw | | 0.00 | | 0.29 | 09221 |
| **GRAIN FRACTIONS** | | | | | |
| buckwheat flour, whole groats | | | | 3.15 | 20011 |
| buckwheat groats, dry | | | | 23.09 | 20008 |
| buckwheat groats, roasted, dry | | | | 7.16 | 20009 |

| | ISORHAMNETIN (mg/100 g) | KAEMPFEROL (mg/100 g) | MYRICETIN (mg/100 g) | QUERCETIN (mg/100 g) | SR21 CODE NUMBER[1] |
|---|---|---|---|---|---|
| **NUTS** | | | | | |
| almonds, raw | 7.05 | 0.52 | 0.00 | 0.36 | 12061 |
| pistachios, dried | | | 0.00 | 1.46 | 12151 |
| **SPICES, HERBS, AND FLAVORINGS** | | | | | |
| bay leaves, dried | | 4.82 | 0.00 | 3.19 | 02004 |
| capers, canned | | 131.34 | | 172.55 | 02054 |
| chives, raw | 6.75 | 10.00 | 0.00 | 4.77 | 11156 |
| cilantro, raw | 0.00 | 0.00 | | 52.90 | 11165 |
| dill weed, raw | 43.5 | 13.33 | 0.70 | 55.15 | 02045 |
| parsley, dried | 331.24 | 0.00 | | | 02029 |
| parsley, raw | 0.00 | 1.49 | 8.08 | 0.33 | 11297 |
| **VEGETABLES** | | | | | |
| alfalfa sprouts, raw | | 0.00 | 0.00 | 1.70 | 11001 |
| arugula, raw | | 72.45 | | 6.95 | 11959 |
| asparagus, boiled, drained | | | | 7.61 | 11012 |
| asparagus, raw | | | | 12.40 | 11011 |
| beet, raw | | 0.00 | 0.00 | 0.13 | 11080 |
| broadbeans (fava beans), immature, raw | | 0.00 | 2.6 | 2.00 | 11088 |
| broadbeans (fava beans), mature, canned | | 0.35 | 0.00 | 0.55 | 16054 |
| broccoli raab (rapini), boiled | | | 0.00 | 1.05 | 11097 |
| broccoli raab (rapini), raw | | | 0.00 | 2.25 | 11096 |
| broccoli, boiled, drained | | 1.38 | 0.00 | 0.21 | 11091 |
| broccoli, frozen | | 2.49 | | 2.40 | 11092 |
| broccoli, raw | | 4.01 | 0.01 | 2.51 | 11090 |
| Brussels sprouts, raw | | 0.95 | 0.00 | 0.30 | 11098 |
| cabbage, green/white, boiled, drained | | 0.01 | 0.03 | 0.01 | 11110 |
| cabbage, green/white, raw | | 0.15 | 0.00 | 0.30 | 11109 |
| cabbage, red/purple, raw | | 0.00 | 0.20 | 0.38 | 11112 |
| carrot, raw | | 0.01 | 0.07 | 0.31 | 11124 |
| cauliflower, frozen | | 0.25 | | 0.83 | 11137 |
| cauliflower, raw | | 0.38 | 0.00 | 0.66 | 11135 |
| celeriac (celery root), raw | | 0.00 | 0.00 | 0.18 | 11141 |
| celery, raw | | | 0.00 | 0.39 | 11143 |
| chicory greens, raw | | 2.45 | 0.00 | 4.82 | 11152 |
| chili pepper, green, hot, raw | | 0.00 | 1.20 | 14.70 | 11670 |
| Chinese cabbage, pak choi, boiled, drained | | 2.40 | 0.03 | 0.30 | 11117 |
| Chinese cabbage, pak choi, raw | | 8.32 | 0.03 | 5.58 | 11116 |
| Chinese cabbage, pe-tsai, raw | | 0.10 | 0.03 | 0.01 | 11119 |
| cowpeas (blackeye peas), mature, dry | | 1.92 | 2.60 | 17.22 | 16062 |
| cucumber, raw | | 0.06 | 0.00 | 0.04 | 11205 |
| dishcloth (towel) gourd, raw (vegetable) | | 0.00 | 0.13 | 0.03 | 11220 |
| eggplant (aubergine), raw | | 0.01 | 0.03 | 0.00 | 11209 |
| endive, raw | | 10.10 | 0.00 | 0.00 | 11213 |
| garden cress, raw | 1.00 | 13.00 | | 0.00 | 11203 |
| green peas, canned, drained | | 0.00 | 0.00 | 0.11 | 11308 |
| green peas, frozen | | 0.00 | | 0.15 | 11312 |
| green peas, frozen, boiled, drained | | 0.07 | 0.03 | 0.12 | 11313 |
| green peas, raw | | 0.00 | 0.00 | 14.27 | 11304 |
| green snap beans, boiled, drained | | | | 3.09 | 11053 |
| green snap beans, canned, drained | | 0.02 | 0.00 | 1.49 | 11056 |
| green snap beans, frozen | | 0.24 | | 1.30 | 11060 |
| green snap beans, frozen, boiled, drained | | 0.26 | | 1.25 | 11061 |
| green snap beans, raw | | 0.40 | 0.00 | 2.88 | 11052 |
| jalapeno pepper, raw | | | | 5.07 | 11979 |
| kale, raw | | 26.74 | 0.00 | 7.71 | 11233 |
| kohlrabi, raw | | 2.43 | 0.00 | 0.40 | 11241 |
| leek, raw | | 2.95 | 0.00 | 0.10 | 11246 |

| | ISORHAMNETIN (mg/100 g) | KAEMPFEROL (mg/100 g) | MYRICETIN (mg/100 g) | QUERCETIN (mg/100 g) | SR21 CODE NUMBER[1] |
|---|---|---|---|---|---|
| lettuce, butterhead, raw | | 0.02 | 0.00 | 2.73 | 11250 |
| lettuce, iceberg, raw | | 0.15 | 0.06 | 1.42 | 11252 |
| lettuce, looseleaf (leaf), raw | | 0.02 | 0.09 | 5.63 | 11253 |
| lettuce, red leaf, raw | | 0.00 | 0.00 | 11.99 | 11257 |
| okra, raw | | | | 24.26 | 11278 |
| onion, white, boiled, drained | | 0.34 | | 24.36 | 11283 |
| onion, white, raw | 5.01 | 0.62 | 0.02 | 21.42 | 11282 |
| onions, Welsh, raw | | 24.95 | | | 11293 |
| parsnip, raw | | 0.00 | 0.00 | 0.99 | 11298 |
| pepper, serrano, raw | | | | 15.98 | 11977 |
| pepper, sweet green, raw | | 0.00 | 0.00 | 2.40 | 11333 |
| pepper, sweet red, raw | | 0.00 | 0.00 | 0.25 | 11821 |
| pepper, sweet yellow, raw | | 0.00 | | 1.35 | 11951 |
| potato, raw | | 0.03 | 0.00 | 0.84 | 11352 |
| potato, red-skinned, baked | | | 0.00 | 1.43 | 11358 |
| potato, red-skinned, raw | | | 0.00 | 0.65 | 11355 |
| potato, russet, baked | | | 0.00 | 0.73 | 11356 |
| potato, russet, raw | | | 0.00 | 1.65 | 11353 |
| potato, white-skinned, baked | | | 0.00 | 1.19 | 11357 |
| potato, white-skinned, raw | | | 0.00 | 0.49 | 11354 |
| radish seed sprouts, raw | | 21.85 | | | 11676 |
| radish, red, raw | | 0.86 | 0.00 | 0.00 | 11429 |
| romaine (cos lettuce), raw | | | 0.00 | 4.49 | 11251 |
| rutabaga (Swede), raw | | 0.57 | 2.13 | 0.08 | 11435 |
| scallions (green/spring onions), raw | | 1.16 | 0.00 | 18.33 | 11291 |
| sorrel (dock), raw (vegetable) | 0.00 | 10.30 | 5.70 | 86.20 | 11616 |
| spinach, raw | | 7.64 | 0.01 | 4.11 | 11457 |
| sweet potato leaves, raw | | 0.25 | 4.89 | 11.57 | 11505 |
| sweet potato, raw | | 0.01 | 0.03 | 0.01 | 11507 |
| Swiss chard, raw | | 4.30 | 1.35 | 2.63 | 11147 |
| taro, raw | | | | 2.87 | 11518 |
| tomato juice, canned/bottled | | 0.06 | 0.05 | 1.46 | 11886 |
| tomato puree, canned | | 0.08 | | 4.12 | 11547 |
| tomato sauce, marinara, bottled | | 0.01 | | 0.91 | 06931 |
| tomato, red, boiled | | 0.01 | 0.01 | 0.70 | 11530 |
| tomato, red, canned | | 0.01 | 0.03 | 0.50 | 11531 |
| tomato, red, raw | | 0.08 | 0.15 | 0.59 | 11529 |
| tomato, yellow, raw | | 0.04 | | 0.21 | 11696 |
| turnip greens, raw | | 11.87 | 0.00 | 0.73 | 11568 |
| watercress, raw | 0.00 | 1.40 | 0.20 | 7.44 | 11591 |
| white beans, mature, dry | | 3.40 | | | 16049 |
| yardlong bean, immature, boiled, drained | | 0.50 | 0.03 | 5.30 | 11200 |
| yellow snap beans, raw | | 0.42 | | 3.03 | 11722 |
| zucchini summer squash, boiled, drained | | | | 0.47 | 11478 |
| zucchini summer squash, raw | | | | 0.66 | 11477 |

**OTHER FOODS**

| | ISORHAMNETIN (mg/100 g) | KAEMPFEROL (mg/100 g) | MYRICETIN (mg/100 g) | QUERCETIN (mg/100 g) | SR21 CODE NUMBER[1] |
|---|---|---|---|---|---|
| carob powder | | 0.44 | 6.73 | 38.78 | 16055 |
| catsup (ketchup) | | 0.01 | | 0.86 | 11935 |
| chocolate milk, reduced fat | | 0.00 | 0.05 | 0.12 | 01103 |
| cocoa powder, unsweetened | | | | 20.13 | 19165 |
| jam/preserves, apricot | | 0.11 | | 0.71 | 19719 |
| jam/preserves, strawberry | | 0.64 | | 0.45 | 99064 |
| tomato soup, canned, condensed | | 0.00 | | 0.14 | 06159 |

[1]Code numbers for foods in the USDA National Nutrient Database for Standard Reference, Release 21, 2008.

Source:
USDA Database for the Flavonoid Content of Selected Foods, Release 2.1, 2007. Available at http://www.ars.usda.gov/Services/docs.htm?docid=6231.

# Flavonoids—Flavanones

| | ERIODICTYOL (mg/100 g) | HESPERETIN (mg/100 g) | NARINGENIN (mg/100 g) | SR21 CODE NUMBER[1] |
|---|---|---|---|---|
| **BEVERAGES** | | | | |
| wine, red | | 0.63 | 1.77 | 14096 |
| wine, white | | 0.40 | 0.38 | 14106 |
| **FRUITS AND FRUIT JUICES** | | | | |
| grapefruit juice, canned/bottled | | 1.15 | 18.07 | 09123 |
| grapefruit juice, from frozen concentrate | | | 31.18 | 09126 |
| grapefruit juice, pink, raw | 0.00 | 0.78 | 17.19 | 09404 |
| grapefruit juice, raw | 0.65 | 3.42 | 20.06 | 09128 |
| grapefruit, pink and red, raw | | 0.35 | 32.64 | 09112 |
| grapefruit, white, raw | | 0.64 | 21.34 | 09116 |
| kumquat, raw | | | 57.39 | 09149 |
| lemon juice, canned/bottled | 10.56 | 13.43 | 0.00 | 09153 |
| lemon juice, raw | 4.88 | 14.47 | 1.38 | 09152 |
| lemon, raw | 21.36 | 27.9 | 0.55 | 09150 |
| lime juice, raw | 2.19 | 8.97 | 0.38 | 09160 |
| lime, raw | | 43.00 | 3.40 | 09159 |
| orange juice, from frozen concentrate | | 26.21 | 3.27 | 09215 |
| orange juice, raw | 0.17 | 11.26 | 2.19 | 09206 |
| orange juice, refrigerated | | 5.52 | 1.55 | 09209 |
| orange, all varieties, raw | | 27.25 | 15.32 | 09200 |
| orange, California navel, raw | | 21.87 | 7.10 | 09202 |
| pummelo, raw | | 8.40 | 24.72 | 09295 |
| strawberries, raw | | 0.00 | 0.26 | 09316 |
| tangerine juice, raw | 0.02 | 9.56 | 1.20 | 09221 |
| tangerine juice, sweetened, from frozen concentrate | | 22.01 | 3.61 | 09225 |
| tangerine, raw | | 7.94 | 10.02 | 09218 |
| yuzu, raw | | 28.73 | 24.82 | 99361 |
| **NUTS** | | | | |
| almonds, raw | 0.25 | 0.00 | 0.13 | 12061 |
| **SPICES AND HERBS** | | | | |
| peppermint, raw | 30.92 | 9.52 | | 02064 |
| rosemary, raw | | 0.00 | 24.86 | 02063 |
| **VEGETABLES** | | | | |
| artichoke, raw | | | 12.51 | 11007 |
| tomato, red, raw | | 0.00 | 0.68 | 11529 |

[1]Code numbers for foods in the USDA National Nutrient Database for Standard Reference, Release 21, 2008.

Source:
USDA Database for the Flavonoid Content of Selected Foods, Release 2.1, 2007. Available at http://www.ars.usda.gov/Services/docs.htm?docid=6231.

# Flavonoids—Proanthocyanidins

| | MONOMERS (mg/100 g) | DIMMERS (mg/100 g) | TRIMERS (mg/100 g) | 4–6MERS (mg/100 g) | 10MERS (mg/100 g) | POLYMERS (>10 MERS) (mg/100 g) | SR21 CODE NUMBER[1] |
|---|---|---|---|---|---|---|---|
| **BEVERAGES** | | | | | | | |
| coffee, brewed | 0.11 | 0.00 | 0.00 | | | | 14209 |
| beer | 0.63 | 0.85 | 0.15 | 0.40 | 0.00 | 0.00 | 14003 |
| tea, black, brewed 3 minutes | 9.30 | 3.74 | 0.38 | | | | 14355 |
| wine, red | 16.64 | 20.49 | 1.80 | 6.70 | 5.00 | 11.00 | 14096 |
| wine, rose | 1.33 | 0.86 | 0.01 | | | | 14104 |
| wine, sherry, white | 3.62 | 4.56 | | | | | 97002 |
| wine, white | 0.59 | 0.21 | 0.01 | | | | 14106 |

| | MONOMERS (mg/100 g) | DIMMERS (mg/100 g) | TRIMERS (mg/100 g) | 4–6MERS (mg/100 g) | 10MERS (mg/100 g) | POLYMERS (>10 MERS) (mg/100 g) | SR21 CODE NUMBER[1] |
|---|---|---|---|---|---|---|---|
| **CANDY** | | | | | | | |
| dark chocolate | 79.79 | 59.05 | 32.25 | 48.10 | 14.38 | | 99321 |
| milk chocolate chips | 23.47 | 23.10 | 14.65 | 40.72 | 17.63 | 32.82 | 19120 |
| **CEREALS AND GRAINS** | | | | | | | |
| barley, whole grain, dry | 3.13 | 46.11 | 50.00 | | | | 20004 |
| sorghum grain, dry | 9.09 | 22.10 | 28.43 | 157.37 | 223.4 | 1461.99 | 20067 |
| **FLOUR AND MEALS** | | | | | | | |
| buckwheat flour, whole groats | 3.79 | 46.51 | | | | | 20011 |
| **FRUIT JUICES** | | | | | | | |
| apple juice, canned/bottled | 4.96 | 4.04 | 2.74 | 0.38 | 0.10 | 0.00 | 09016 |
| cranberry juice cocktail, canned/bottled | 0.56 | 2.71 | 1.59 | 4.58 | 3.84 | 8.33 | 14242 |
| grape juice, canned/bottled | 1.69 | 3.18 | 1.78 | 7.49 | 6.46 | 28.37 | 09135 |
| grape juice, white, canned | 0.16 | 0.24 | 0.00 | | | | 97082 |
| **FRUITS** | | | | | | | |
| apple, Fuji, raw | 6.46 | 9.92 | 6.09 | 19.09 | 13.81 | 14.22 | 97066 |
| apple, Gala, raw | 5.94 | 9.55 | 6.24 | 21.28 | 18.73 | 30.68 | 97067 |
| apple, Golden Delicious, raw | 3.71 | 7.59 | 4.73 | 21.77 | 18.75 | 26.46 | 97069 |
| apple, Granny Smith, raw | 5.68 | 12.76 | 8.24 | 32.90 | 30.12 | 46.31 | 97070 |
| apple, peeled, raw | 7.50 | 9.50 | | | | | 09004 |
| apple, Red Delicious, raw | 6.46 | 11.76 | 7.86 | 19.06 | 16.75 | 27.03 | 97072 |
| apricot, raw | 1.32 | 1.33 | 0.77 | 4.90 | 2.20 | 0.80 | 09021 |
| avocado, California, raw | 0.96 | 1.46 | 1.36 | 3.17 | 0.44 | 0.00 | 09038 |
| banana, raw | 0.13 | 0.43 | 0.49 | 2.32 | 0.00 | 0.00 | 09040 |
| blackberries, raw | 3.73 | 4.45 | 2.11 | 7.27 | 4.24 | 1.51 | 09042 |
| blueberries, raw | 3.46 | 5.71 | 4.15 | 19.57 | 14.55 | 129.05 | 09050 |
| blueberries, wild, raw | 3.23 | 8.45 | 6.56 | 25.99 | 29.31 | 255.09 | 97085 |
| cherries, sweet, raw | 5.11 | 3.25 | 2.39 | 6.51 | 1.87 | 0.00 | 09070 |
| chokeberries, raw | 5.20 | 12.50 | 10.30 | 40.30 | 52.90 | 542.60 | 97012 |
| cranberries, raw | 7.26 | 25.93 | 18.93 | 70.27 | 62.90 | 233.48 | 09078 |
| currants, black, raw | 0.90 | 2.90 | 3.00 | 10.60 | 9.90 | 122.40 | 09083 |
| currants, red, raw | 3.23 | 1.90 | 0.00 | | | | 99044 |
| custard apple (bullock's heart), raw | 6.25 | 14.20 | 4.49 | | | | 09086 |
| date, dried | 0.00 | 1.84 | 3.02 | 5.88 | 0.00 | 0.00 | 09087 |
| fig, raw | 0.03 | 0.01 | 0.00 | 0.00 | 0.00 | 0.00 | 09089 |
| grapes, green, raw | 0.96 | 2.33 | 1.88 | 8.35 | 9.15 | 58.87 | 97073 |
| grapes, red, raw | 1.36 | 2.38 | 1.01 | 6.07 | 6.23 | 44.56 | 97074 |
| kiwifruit, gold, raw | 1.10 | 1.61 | 1.16 | 5.00 | 5.03 | 0.00 | 97079 |
| kiwifruit, raw | 0.51 | 0.61 | 0.52 | 1.32 | 0.20 | 0.00 | 09148 |
| mango, raw | 2.30 | 1.80 | 1.40 | 7.20 | 0.00 | 0.00 | 09176 |
| marionberries (northwest blackberries), raw | 0.90 | 3.40 | 2.40 | 2.20 | 0.00 | 0.00 | 97011 |
| nectarine, raw | 5.57 | 5.00 | 1.75 | 5.98 | 3.57 | 7.31 | 09191 |
| peach, canned in heavy syrup, drained | 0.62 | 1.82 | 0.00 | 0.00 | 0.00 | 0.00 | 09370 |
| peach, raw | 4.48 | 12.24 | 4.41 | 17.66 | 10.94 | 22.02 | 09236 |
| pear, red anjou, raw | 2.67 | 2.81 | 2.29 | 6.47 | 4.57 | 13.11 | 97076 |
| persimmon, raw | 0.80 | 0.44 | 0.04 | | | | 97088 |
| plum, raw | 10.88 | 38.54 | 22.25 | 58.04 | 33.79 | 57.28 | 09279 |
| pomegranate, raw | 0.81 | 0.29 | 0.00 | | | | 09286 |
| quince, raw | 1.42 | 2.61 | 1.22 | | | | 09296 |
| raspberries, raw | 3.91 | 8.64 | 3.92 | 7.70 | 0.90 | 0.00 | 09302 |
| strawberries, raw | 3.71 | 5.26 | 4.90 | 28.14 | 23.88 | 75.78 | 09316 |
| **INFANT, JUNIOR, AND TODDLER** | | | | | | | |
| apple blueberry, junior food | 2.90 | 5.10 | 2.80 | 7.80 | 5.20 | 2.20 | 03165 |
| apple juice, Earth's Best | 0.09 | 0.19 | 0.19 | 0.47 | 0.09 | 0.00 | 03166 |
| apples, organic, strained infant food | 3.80 | 8.90 | 5.10 | 17.80 | 12.30 | 14.80 | 97018 |

| | MONOMERS (mg/100 g) | DIMMERS (mg/100 g) | TRIMERS (mg/100 g) | 4–6MERS (mg/100 g) | 10MERS (mg/100 g) | POLYMERS (>10 MERS) (mg/100 g) | SR21 CODE NUMBER[1] |
|---|---|---|---|---|---|---|---|
| apples, strawberries, and bananas, strained infant food | 3.00 | 7.30 | 4.30 | 14.90 | 10.60 | 14.00 | 97020 |
| applesauce, Earth's Best | 3.40 | 6.40 | 3.60 | 9.80 | 6.10 | 0.00 | 03116 |
| apricots with pears and apples, strained infant food | 1.70 | 3.40 | 2.30 | 7.60 | 4.60 | 0.00 | 97021 |
| bananas and strawberries, strained infant food | 0.40 | 1.00 | 0.90 | 3.80 | 3.30 | 2.80 | 97024 |
| bananas, plums, and grapes, strained infant food | 1.10 | 2.50 | 1.90 | 8.10 | 7.10 | 4.40 | 97022 |
| barley infant cereal, dry | 4.80 | 9.30 | 4.50 | 4.10 | 0.00 | 0.00 | 03181 |
| blueberry buckle dessert, strained infant food | 0.70 | 1.80 | 1.30 | 5.30 | 4.40 | 4.40 | 97025 |
| cherry vanilla pudding, junior food | 1.60 | 2.70 | 1.70 | 5.20 | 2.90 | 0.00 | 03225 |
| peaches, strained infant food | 1.85 | 3.80 | 2.80 | 8.75 | 5.75 | 0.00 | 97019 |
| pear juice, infant food | 0.03 | 0.09 | 0.09 | 0.00 | 0.00 | 0.00 | 43408 |
| pears, Earth's Best | 1.55 | 2.65 | 1.80 | 5.70 | 3.65 | 0.00 | 03132 |
| plums with apples, strained infant food | 1.40 | 4.00 | 2.70 | 10.30 | 7.40 | 7.30 | 97023 |
| white grape juice, infant food | 0.09 | 0.19 | 0.19 | 0.37 | 0.00 | 0.00 | 97064 |
| **MILK BEVERAGES** | | | | | | | |
| chocolate milk, whole milk | 0.40 | 2.18 | 0.00 | 0.00 | 0.00 | 0.00 | 01102 |
| chocolate malted mix for milk | 35.90 | 20.60 | 8.77 | 12.10 | 0.77 | | 14317 |
| **NUTS** | | | | | | | |
| almonds, raw | 7.77 | 9.52 | 8.82 | 39.97 | 37.68 | 80.26 | 12061 |
| cashews, raw | 6.66 | 2.02 | 0.00 | 0.00 | 0.00 | 0.00 | 12087 |
| filberts (hazelnuts), dried | 9.83 | 12.51 | 13.56 | 67.72 | 74.6 | 322.44 | 12120 |
| peanut butter, smooth | 2.03 | 3.00 | 8.14 | 0.00 | 0.00 | 0.00 | 16098 |
| peanuts, all types, oil-roasted | 5.11 | 4.07 | 3.67 | 2.77 | 0.00 | 0.00 | 16089 |
| pecans, dried | 17.22 | 42.13 | 26.03 | 101.43 | 84.23 | 223.01 | 12142 |
| pistachios, dried | 10.94 | 13.26 | 10.51 | 42.24 | 37.93 | 122.46 | 12151 |
| walnuts, English/Persian, dried | 6.93 | 5.65 | 7.19 | 22.05 | 5.41 | 20.02 | 12155 |
| **SPICES AND HERBS** | | | | | | | |
| cinnamon, ground | 23.92 | 256.29 | 1252.20 | 2608.63 | 1458.32 | 2508.78 | 02010 |
| curry powder | 0.00 | 9.50 | 22.88 | 41.78 | 0.00 | 0.00 | 02015 |
| **VEGETABLES—LEGUMES** | | | | | | | |
| black beans, mature, dry | 2.90 | 5.20 | 0.00 | 0.00 | 0.00 | 0.00 | 16014 |
| broadbeans (fava beans), mature, dry | 80.84 | 73.48 | 0.13 | | | | 16052 |
| cowpeas (blackeye peas), mature, dry | 14.00 | 6.00 | 6.10 | 7.30 | 0.00 | 0.00 | 16062 |
| kidney beans, red, mature, dry | 16.25 | 22.90 | 23.60 | 98.85 | 90.50 | 258.15 | 16032 |
| lentils, mature, dry | 0.53 | 1.20 | 0.11 | | | | 16069 |
| pinto beans, mature, boiled | 1.75 | 4.40 | 3.91 | 10.52 | 4.32 | 1.41 | 16043 |
| pinto beans, mature, dry | 10.72 | 19.22 | 16.18 | 125.90 | 135.62 | 459.63 | 16042 |
| **OTHER FOODS** | | | | | | | |
| baking chocolate (unsweetened) | 198.54 | 206.51 | 130.88 | 332.62 | 216.39 | 551 | 19078 |
| cocoa powder, unsweetened | 316.83 | 183.49 | 159.54 | 524.53 | 188.93 | | 19165 |

[1]Code number for food in the USDA National Nutrient Database for Standard Reference (SR), Release 21.

Source:
USDA Database for the Proanthocyanidin Content of Selected Foods. Prepared by Nutrient Data Laboratory, Beltsville Human Nutrition Research Center, Agricultural Research Service, US Department of Agriculture in collaboration with Arkansas Children's Nutrition Center, ARS, USDA, Little Rock, AR; Mars, Inc., Hackettstown, NY; and Ocean Spray Cranberries, Inc., Lakeville, MA. August 2004. Available at: http://www.nal.usda.goav/fnic/foodcomp.

# *Flavonoids-Isoflavones (Daidzein, Genistein, and Glycitein)*

| | DAIDZEIN (mg/100g) | GENISTEIN (mg/100 g) | GLYCITEIN (mg/100 g) | TOTAL ISOFLAVONES (mg/100 g) | SR21 CODE NUMBER[1] |
|---|---|---|---|---|---|
| **CEREALS, GRAINS, AND GRAIN PRODUCTS** | | | | | |
| bread, mixed grain/whole grain/7-grain | 0.20 | 0.15 | 0.00 | 0.38 | 18035 |
| bread, wheat germ | 0.25 | 0.23 | | 0.49 | 18068 |
| bread, white | 0.06 | 0.13 | 0.00 | 0.19 | 18069 |
| breadcrumbs, dry, grated | 0.40 | 0.30 | 0.00 | 0.70 | 18079 |
| GoLean, Kashi (RTE cereal) | 8.40 | 7.70 | 1.40 | 17.40 | 08393 |
| granola bar, hard | 0.05 | 0.08 | | 0.13 | 19015 |
| Smart Start, soy protein, Kellogg's (RTE cereal) | 41.90 | 41.90 | 10.20 | 93.90 | 08385 |
| soy flour, defatted | 64.55 | 87.31 | 15.08 | 150.94 | 16117 |
| soy flour, full-fat | 72.92 | 98.77 | 16.12 | 178.10 | 16115 |
| soy flour, full-fat, roasted | 89.46 | 85.12 | 16.40 | 165.04 | 16116 |
| soy meal, defatted | 80.77 | 114.71 | 16.12 | 209.58 | 16119 |
| **DESSERTS** | | | | | |
| cake, chocolate creme-filled snack with icing | 0.13 | 0.15 | 0.00 | 0.28 | 18127 |
| cake, sponge | 0.10 | 0.10 | 0.00 | 0.20 | 18133 |
| doughnut | 2.58 | 2.44 | 0.29 | 5.31 | 18248 |
| doughnut with chocolate coating/icing | 1.90 | 1.65 | 0.20 | 3.70 | 18249 |
| doughnut, yeast-raised, glazed | 0.30 | 0.20 | 0.00 | 0.60 | 18255 |
| doughnut, yeast-raised, glazed/sugared | 0.50 | 0.50 | 0.10 | 1.10 | 18250 |
| sweet roll, cinnamon, McDonald's | 4.40 | 0.90 | 0.70 | 6.00 | 21322 |
| sweet roll, cinnamon raisin | 0.70 | 0.65 | 0.10 | 1.50 | 18356 |
| **ENTREES** | | | | | |
| chili con carne (no beans), canned | 1.00 | 1.10 | 0.17 | 2.20 | 22911 |
| chili con carne with beans, canned | 1.25 | 1.03 | 0.15 | 2.43 | 22904 |
| chili with beans, vegetarian, canned, Hormel | 1.90 | 1.20 | 0.20 | 3.30 | 22720 |
| ramen noodle soup, beef flavor, dehydrated | 0.73 | 0.43 | 0.07 | 1.23 | 06982 |
| ramen noodle soup, chicken flavor, dehydrated | 0.00 | 0.30 | 0.00 | 0.40 | 06983 |
| Spaghetti O's, canned, Campbell's | 0.20 | 0.30 | 0.00 | 0.60 | 22932 |
| taco, beef monster, Jack In The Box | 2.60 | 13.10 | 0.20 | 15.90 | 99555 |
| **FRUITS** | | | | | |
| currants, black, raw | 0.02 | 0.06 | 0.00 | 0.07 | 09083 |
| grapefruit, white, raw | 0.04 | 0.03 | | 0.06 | 09116 |
| raisins, seedless | 0.03 | 0.05 | 0.00 | 0.08 | 09298 |
| **MEATS, FISH, AND EGGS** | | | | | |
| beef patty with vegetable protein, frozen, cooked | 0.67 | 1.09 | 0.10 | 1.86 | 23501 |
| beef patty with vegetable protein, frozen, raw | 0.35 | 0.77 | 0.02 | 1.14 | 23506 |
| crab, Alaska king, imitation, made from surimi | 0.05 | 0.05 | 0.00 | 0.10 | 15138 |
| egg, raw | 0.03 | 0.02 | | 0.05 | 01123 |
| frankfurter, beef | 1.00 | 0.80 | 0.10 | 1.90 | 07022 |
| frankfurter, beef and pork | 0.05 | 0.05 | 0.00 | 0.15 | 07023 |
| Smokie (smoked sausage), pork and beef | 0.25 | 0.40 | 0.00 | 0.70 | 07075 |
| tuna, light, canned in water | 0.04 | 0.05 | 0.00 | 0.09 | 15184 |
| tuna, white, canned in oil | 0.12 | 0.15 | 0.02 | 0.28 | 15185 |
| **MEAT SUBSTITUTES, TOFU, AND OTHER SOY PRODUCTS** | | | | | |
| bacon, simulated meat product | 2.20 | 5.66 | 1.50 | 9.36 | 16104 |
| Big Franks, canned, Loma Linda/Worthington Foods | 1.00 | 2.05 | 0.30 | 3.35 | 22126 |
| Breakfast Patty, frozen, Morningstar Farms | 2.00 | 2.30 | 0.30 | 4.60 | 22122 |
| Chik Patty, frozen, Morningstar Farms | 1.80 | 2.20 | 0.40 | 4.40 | 16557 |
| frankfurter, simulated meat product | 5.78 | 6.43 | 0.06 | 12.27 | 43130 |
| FriChik, canned, Worthington Foods | 3.45 | 7.90 | 0.85 | 12.20 | 16513 |
| sausage meat substitute, pan-fried | 4.46 | 9.23 | 2.30 | 14.34 | 16107 |
| miso (soybean paste) | 16.43 | 23.24 | 3.00 | 41.45 | 16112 |
| natto (boiled, fermented soybeans) | 33.22 | 37.66 | 10.55 | 82.29 | 16113 |
| okara (soybean pulp) | 3.62 | 4.47 | 1.30 | 9.39 | 16130 |
| soy beverage powder | 40.07 | 62.18 | 10.90 | 109.51 | 99018 |
| soy protein concentrate, alcohol extraction | 5.78 | 5.26 | 1.57 | 11.49 | 16121 |
| soy protein isolate | 30.81 | 57.28 | 8.54 | 91.05 | 16122 |

| | DAIDZEIN (mg/100g) | GENISTEIN (mg/100 g) | GLYCITEIN (mg/100 g) | TOTAL ISOFLAVONES (mg/100 g) | SR21 CODE NUMBER[1] |
|---|---|---|---|---|---|
| soy yogurt | 5.70 | 9.40 | 1.20 | 16.30 | 43476 |
| tempeh, cooked (soy product) | 13.12 | 21.14 | 1.39 | 35.64 | 16174 |
| tempeh, uncooked (soy product) | 22.66 | 36.15 | 3.82 | 60.61 | 16114 |
| tofu, extra firm, prepared with nigari | 8.23 | 12.45 | 1.95 | 22.63 | 16159 |
| tofu, firm, prepared with calcium sulfate and nigari | 12.31 | 16.10 | 2.75 | 30.41 | 16126 |
| tofu, firm, silken, Mori-Nu | 12.42 | 16.95 | 2.40 | 29.97 | 16162 |
| tofu, fried | 13.80 | 18.43 | 2.93 | 34.78 | 16129 |
| tofu, frozen, dried (koyadofu, kori tofu, tung tou-fu) | 29.59 | 51.04 | 3.44 | 83.20 | 16128 |
| tofu, regular, prepared with calcium sulfate | 8.56 | 12.99 | 1.98 | 22.73 | 16427 |
| tofu, salted and fermented (fuyu) | 20.72 | 23.83 | 4.95 | 48.51 | 16132 |
| tofu, soft, prepared with calcium sulfate and nigari | 9.49 | 11.91 | 1.68 | 22.61 | 16127 |
| Veggie Sausage Links, frozen, Morningstar Farms | 1.18 | 2.45 | 0.30 | 3.93 | 16546 |
| **NUTS AND SEEDS** | | | | | |
| flaxseeds | 0.02 | 0.04 | 0.06 | 0.07 | 12220 |
| peanuts, raw | 0.02 | 0.24 | | 0.26 | 16087 |
| pistachios, dried | 1.875 | 1.75 | 0.00 | 3.63 | 12151 |
| soy nuts, dry-roasted | 62.14 | 75.78 | 13.33 | 148.50 | 16111 |
| **SAUCES, GRAVIES, AND CONDIMENTS** | | | | | |
| hoisin sauce | 6.10 | 3.25 | 0.55 | 9.90 | 06175 |
| soy sauce made with hydrolyzed vegetable protein | 0.10 | 0.00 | 0.00 | 0.10 | 16125 |
| soy sauce made with soy and wheat (shoyu) | 0.78 | 0.39 | 0.14 | 1.18 | 16123 |
| Worcestershire sauce | 0.10 | 0.00 | 0.00 | 0.20 | 06971 |
| gravy, turkey, canned | 0.15 | 0.15 | 0.05 | 0.35 | 06125 |
| **VEGETABLES—LEGUMES** | | | | | |
| adzuki beans, mature, dry | 0.36 | 0.23 | 0.00 | 0.59 | 16001 |
| broadbeans (fava beans), mature, dry | 0.33 | 0.15 | 0.28 | 0.63 | 16052 |
| chickpeas (garbanzo beans), mature, dry | 0.23 | 0.06 | 0.22 | 0.38 | 16056 |
| lentils, mature, dry | 0.01 | 0.05 | 0.00 | 0.06 | 16069 |
| lima beans, mature, large, boiled | 0.01 | 0.03 | | 0.01 | 16072 |
| lupins, mature, dry | 0.10 | 0.15 | 0.00 | 0.25 | 16076 |
| mung bean sprouts, raw | 0.06 | 0.08 | 0.00 | 0.10 | 11043 |
| mung beans, mature, dry | 0.00 | 0.09 | 0.00 | 0.09 | 16080 |
| navy beans, mature, dry | 0.01 | 0.20 | | 0.21 | 16037 |
| peas, split, yellow and green, mature, dry | 0.33 | 0.11 | 0.00 | 0.44 | 16085 |
| pigeon peas, mature, dry | 0.02 | 0.54 | | 0.56 | 16101 |
| pinto beans, mature, dry | 0.01 | 0.17 | | 0.18 | 16042 |
| soybean sprouts, raw | 12.87 | 18.77 | 2.88 | 34.39 | 11452 |
| soybean sprouts, steamed | 5.00 | 6.70 | 0.80 | 12.50 | 11453 |
| soybeans, green/immature (edamame), boiled, drained | 7.41 | 7.06 | 4.60 | 17.92 | 11451 |
| soybeans, green/immature (edamame), raw | 20.34 | 22.57 | 7.57 | 48.95 | 11450 |
| soybeans, mature, boiled | 30.76 | 31.26 | 3.75 | 65.11 | 16109 |
| soybeans, mature, dry | 62.90 | 81.35 | 15.29 | 155.76 | 16108 |
| white beans, small, mature, dry | 0.00 | 0.37 | | 0.37 | 16045 |
| **SPECIAL DIETARY FOODS** | | | | | |
| Clif Bar, crunchy peanut butter | 13.3 | 13.00 | 0.60 | 26.90 | 99538 |
| Ensure | 1.40 | 2.58 | 0.28 | 4.33 | 99485 |
| Ensure Plus | 0.20 | 0.35 | 0.00 | 0.60 | 43528 |
| infant formula, Isomil with iron, powder, Abbott | 6.03 | 12.23 | 2.73 | 25.82 | 03843 |
| infant formula, Isomil with iron, ready-to-feed, Abbott | 0.73 | 1.37 | 0.12 | 2.21 | 03841 |
| infant formula, Nursoy with iron, dry powder, Wyeth-Ayerst | 5.70 | 13.55 | 2.05 | 28.01 | 03893 |
| infant formula, Nursoy with iron, liquid concentrate, Wyeth-Ayerst | 0.98 | 2.69 | 0.35 | 3.81 | 03891 |
| infant formula, Nursoy with iron, ready-to-feed, Wyeth-Ayerst | 0.75 | 1.60 | 0.28 | 2.63 | 03890 |
| Luna Bar, nuts over chocolate | 8.10 | 8.40 | 1.20 | 17.70 | 99539 |
| PowerBar, chocolate | 1.80 | 3.27 | | 5.07 | 25017 |
| **OTHER FOODS** | | | | | |
| licorice, black, soft | 0.16 | 0.31 | 0.00 | 0.47 | 99474 |
| olive oil, extra-virgin | 0.01 | 0.03 | 0.00 | 0.04 | 99423 |

[1]Code numbers for foods in the USDA National Nutrient Database for Standard References, Release 21, 2008.

Source:
USDA Database for the Isoflavone Content of Selected Foods, Release 2.0, 2008. Available at http://www.ars.usda.gov/Srvices/docs.htm?docid=6382.

# *Flavonoids—Biochanin, Coumestrol, and Formononetin*

| | BIOCHANIN A (mg/100 g) | COUMESTROL (mg/100 g) | FORMONONETIN (mg/100 g) | SR21 CODE NUMBER[1] |
|---|---|---|---|---|
| **FRUITS AND FRUIT JUICES** | | | | |
| apricot, dried | 0.05 | 0.00 | 0.01 | 09032 |
| grapefruit, white, raw | 0.05 | 0.05 | 0.05 | 09116 |
| orange juice, refrigerated | 0.05 | 0.03 | 0.03 | 09209 |
| **NUTS AND SEEDS** | | | | |
| almonds, raw | | 0.02 | 0.00 | 12061 |
| fenugreek seeds | 0.01 | 0.00 | 0.01 | 02019 |
| flaxseeds | 0.00 | 0.02 | 0.02 | 12220 |
| peanuts, raw | 0.01 | 0.00 | 0.00 | 16087 |
| pistachios, dried | | 0.01 | 0.00 | 12151 |
| sunflower seed kernels, dried | 0.01 | 0.01 | 0.03 | 12036 |
| **SOY PRODUCTS** | | | | |
| soy flour, full-fat | 0.02 | 0.00 | 0.01 | 16115 |
| soy nuts, dry-roasted | 0.00 | 0.02 | 0.03 | 16111 |
| soy sauce made with soy and wheat (shoyu) | 0.00 | 0.02 | 0.00 | 16123 |
| soymilk | | 0.81 | 0.00 | 16120 |
| tofu, firm, prepared with calcium sulfate and nigari | 0.00 | 0.11 | 0.00 | 16126 |
| **VEGETABLES** | | | | |
| alfalfa sprouts, raw | 0.03 | 1.60 | 1.43 | 11001 |
| asparagus, raw | 0.00 | 0.05 | 0.00 | 11011 |
| broadbeans (fava beans), mature, dry | 0.12 | 0.00 | 0.01 | 16052 |
| chickpeas (garbanzo beans), mature, dry | 1.54 | 0.01 | 0.12 | 16056 |
| cowpeas (blackeye peas), mature, dry | 0.58 | 0.01 | 0.00 | 16062 |
| garlic, raw | 0.05 | 0.00 | 0.00 | 11215 |
| green snap beans, boiled, drained | 0.04 | 0.00 | 0.01 | 11053 |
| green snap beans, raw | 0.04 | 0.00 | 0.15 | 11052 |
| great northern beans, mature, dry | 0.60 | 0.00 | 0.00 | 16024 |
| kidney beans, all types, mature, boiled | 0.41 | 0.00 | 0.00 | 16028 |
| kidney beans, all types, mature, dry | 0.04 | 0.00 | 0.00 | 16027 |
| kidney beans, red, mature, dry | 0.01 | 0.00 | 0.00 | 16032 |
| lima beans, mature, baby, dry | 0.37 | 0.00 | 0.55 | 16074 |
| lima beans, mature, large, dry | 0.27 | 0.14 | 0.32 | 16071 |
| mung bean sprouts, raw | 0.01 | 0.93 | 0.01 | 11043 |
| mungo beans, mature, dry | 0.02 | 0.00 | 0.00 | 16083 |
| navy beans, mature, dry | 0.02 | 0.00 | 0.00 | 16037 |
| peas, split, yellow and green, mature, dry | 0.09 | 0.81 | 0.00 | 16085 |
| pigeon peas, mature, dry | 0.10 | 0.01 | 0.02 | 16101 |
| pinto beans, mature, dry | 0.28 | 1.81 | 0.01 | 16042 |
| soybean sprouts, raw | 0.00 | 0.34 | 0.03 | 11452 |
| soybeans, mature, dry | 0.00 | 0.02 | 8.46 | 16108 |
| **OTHER FOODS** | | | | |
| coffee, brewed | 0.00 | 0.03 | 0.00 | 14209 |
| egg, raw | 0.05 | 0.00 | 0.05 | 01123 |
| PowerBar, chocolate | 0.00 | 0.09 | 0.00 | 25017 |

[1]Code numbers for foods in the USDA National Nutrient Database for Standard References, Release 21, 2008.

Source:
USDA Database for the Isoflavone Content of Selected Foods, Release 2.0, 2008. Available at http://www.ars.usda.gov/Srvices/docs.htm?docid=6382.

# Glutathione

| | GLUTATHIONE (mg/100 g) | SOURCE | | GLUTATHIONE (mg/100 g) | SOURCE |
|---|---|---|---|---|---|
| **FRUITS AND FRUIT JUICES** | | | mustard greens, raw | 4.92 | Mills et al, 1997 |
| apple, raw | 0.61 | Souci et al, 2000 | okra, raw | 7.99 | Mills et al, 1997 |
| banana, raw | 0.71 | Souci et al, 2000 | onion, yellow, raw | 2.27 | Mills et al, 1997 |
| orange, raw | 4.00 | Souci et al, 2000 | parsley, raw | 12.00 | Souci et al, 2000 |
| orange juice | 0.89 | Souci et al, 2000 | pepper, sweet green, raw | 4.30 | Mills et al, 1997 |
| pear | 1.20 | Souci et al, 2000 | potato, raw | 10.76 | Mills et al, 1997 |
| | | | purslane, chamber-grown, raw | 14.81 | Simopoulos et al, 1992 |
| **VEGETABLES** | | | purslane, wild, raw | 11.90 | Simopoulos et al, 1992 |
| asparagus spears, raw | 18.75 | Mills et al, 1997 | radish, raw | 4.61 | Mills et al, 1997 |
| asparagus tips, raw | 28.58 | Mills et al, 1997 | spinach, raw | 13.52 | Mills et al, 1997 |
| beet, raw | 3.07 | Mills et al, 1997 | spinach, raw | 9.65 | Simopoulos et al, 1992 |
| broccoli flower, raw | 25.82 | Mills et al, 1997 | squash, summer, zucchini, raw | 6.76 | Mills et al, 1997 |
| broccoli stalk, raw | 9.20 | Mills et al, 1997 | squash, winter, acorn, raw | 5.53 | Mills et al, 1997 |
| Brussels sprouts, raw | 34.42 | Mills et al, 1997 | squash, yellow, raw | 8.61 | Mills et al, 1997 |
| cabbage core, raw | 19.05 | Mills et al, 1997 | sweet potato, raw | 6.15 | Mills et al, 1997 |
| cabbage leaves, raw | 2.61 | Mills et al, 1997 | tomato, raw | 3.69 | Mills et al, 1997 |
| carrot, raw | 1.91 | Mills et al, 1997 | turnip raw | 2.46 | Mills et al, 1997 |
| cauliflower, raw | 9.20 | Mills et al, 1997 | turnip greens, raw | 5.53 | Mills et al, 1997 |
| celery, raw | 0.65 | Mills et al, 1997 | | | |
| collard greens, raw | 2.83 | Mills et al, 1997 | **OTHER FOODS** | | |
| cucumber, raw | 1.63 | Mills et al, 1997 | beef muscle, raw | 20.00 | Souci et al, 2000 |
| corn, raw | 14.14 | Mills et al, 1997 | bread, rye | 0.65 | Souci et al, 2000 |
| eggplant, raw | 1.63 | Mills et al, 1997 | chicken breast with skin, raw | 9.50 | Souci et al, 2000 |
| green snap beans, raw | 4.30 | Mills et al, 1997 | corn flour | 3.90 | Souci et al, 2000 |
| kale, raw | 3.38 | Mills et al, 1997 | milk, whole | 0.33 | Souci et al, 2000 |
| lettuce, iceberg | 0.00 | Mills et al, 1997 | peanuts, raw | 2.10 | Souci et al, 2000 |
| mushrooms, common white (*Agaricus bisporus*) | 0.98 | Souci et al, 2000 | | | |

Sources:
Mills BJ, CT Stinson, MC Liu, CA Lang. Glutathione and cyst(e)ine profiles of vegetables using high performance liquid chromatography with dual electrochemical detection. *J Food Comp Anal* 10:90-101, 1997. (Values were converted from micromoles per 100 grams to milligrams per 100 gram by multiplying by 307.77, the molecular weight of glutathione, and dividing by 100.)
Souci SW, W Fachmann, H Kraut. *Food Composition and Nutrition Tables.* Medpharm GmbH Scientific Publishers, Stuttgart, Germany and CRC Press, Washington, DC, 2000.
Simopoulos AP, HA Normal, JE Gillaspy, JA Duke. Common purslane: A source of omega-3 fatty acids and antioxidants. *J Am Coll Nutr* 11:374-382, 1992.

# Gluten

**GLUTEN-CONTAINING FOODS AND INGREDIENTS[1]**

barley, barley flour, malt barley, pearl barley
bran (wheat bran)
breaded/creamed foods (e.g., fish, meat, vegetables)
breads/baked goods prepared from wheat, barley, or rye flour
bulgur
cereals made from wheat, rye, or barley
chapatti flour (ingredient of Indian flatbread)
couscous (endosperm of durum wheat)
cracked wheat
farina (hot wheat cereal also called semolina or Cream of Wheat)
gluten, gluten flour
graham flour, graham crackers
gravies prepared with wheat, rye, or barley flour
kamut (type of wheat)
malt, malt extract, malt flavoring, malt syrup, malt vinegar, malted barley
matzoh meal, matzoh balls
orzo (rice-shaped pasta made from hard wheat semolina)
pasta prepared from wheat, rye, barley, or semolina flour
rye, rye flour

salad dressings containing wheat, rye, or barley flour
sauces prepared with wheat, rye, or barley flour
semolina (endosperm of hard or soft wheat)
soups containing wheat or rye flour or barley
spelt (type of wheat)
triticale (wheat-rye hybrid)
wheat, wheat bran, wheat flour, wheat germ

**GLUTEN-FREE FOODS**

amaranth
animal-based foods (eggs; fish, meat, poultry; milk, cheese, yogurt)
arrowroot
beans, peas, bean flours
bread/baked goods prepared from corn, potato, rice, soy flours or gluten-free flour
buckwheat, buckwheat flour, buckwheat noodles (soba)[2]
cereals prepared from corn, cornmeal, hominy, rice, quinoa, or soy
corn, cornmeal, cornstarch
fruits
gluten-free products

hominy
kasha (buckwheat groats, buckwheat porridge)
lima bean flour
millet
nuts, nut flour, nut meal, peanut butter
oats, oatmeal (uncontaminated)[3]
pasta prepared from rice or gluten-free ingredients
potato, potato flour, potato starch
quinoa

rice, rice bran, rice flour, rice noodles
sago (palm starch)
sorghum, sorghum flour
soybeans, soy flour, soy products
tapioca (manioc, cassava, yucca)
teff (cereal grass cultivated in Eritrea, Ethiopia, India, and Australia)
vegetables
wild rice

---

[1]Celiac disease (also called sprue, nontropical sprue, and celiac sprue) is a genetic disorder of the small intestine caused by intolerance of the protein gluten, which is present in wheat, rye, and barley. Gluten consumption by persons with celiac disease results in immune reactions that damage the lining of the small intestine. Symptoms may include abdominal bloating and pain, diarrhea, fatigue, anemia, bone or joint pain, osteoporosis, behavior changes, numbness in the legs, muscle cramps, seizures, mouth ulcers, and itchy rash (dermatitis herpetiformia). A gluten-free diet stops the symptoms and allows for healing of the intestinal damage.

[2]Buckwheat (despite its name) is not a type of wheat.

[3]Oats may be contaminated with gluten due to crop rotation and milling with wheat.

Sources:

Biagi F, J Campanella, S Martucci, et al. A milligram of gluten a day keeps the mucosal recovery away. *Nutr Rev* 62:360-363, 2004.
Collin P, L Thorell, K Kaukinen, M Maki. The safe threshold for gluten contamination in gluten-free products. Can trace amounts be accepted in the treatment of celiac disease? *Aliment Pharmacol Ther* 19:1277-1283, 2004.
Collin P, M Maki, K Kaukinen. It is the compliance, not milligrams of gluten, that is essential in the treatment of celiac disease (Letter to the Editor). *Nutr Rev* 62:490-491, 2004.
Fasano A, C Catassi. Current approaches to diagnosis and treatment of celiac disease: An evolving spectrum. *Gastroenterology* 120:636-651, 2001.
Gluten-Free drugs for celiac disease patients. *The Medical Letter* 50:19-20, 2008.
National Digestive Diseases Information Clearinghouse. Celiac Disease. http://digestive.niddk.nih.gov/ddiseases/pubs/celiac/index.htm.
National Institutes of Health. NIH Consensus Development Conference on Celiac Disease. http://consensus.nih.gov/2004/2004CeliacDisease118html.htm. 2004.
Niewinski MM. Advances in celiac disease and gluten-free diet. *J Am Diet Assoc* 108:661-672, 2008.
Pietzak MM. Recognizing and managing celiac disease. *Nutrition & the MD* 29:1-4, 2003.
Storsrud S, YI Malmheden, RA Lenner. Gluten contamination in oat products and products naturally free from gluten. *Eur Food Res Technol* 217:481-485, 2003.
Thompson T. Case problem: Questions regarding the acceptability of buckwheat, amaranth, quinoa, and oats from a patient with celiac disease. *J Am Diet Assoc* 101:586-587, 2001.
Thompson T. Oats and the gluten-free diet. *J Am Diet Assoc* 103:376-379, 2003.
Thompson T. Questionable foods and the gluten-free diet: Survey of current recommendations. *J Am Diet Assoc* 100:463-465, 2000.
Thompson T. Wheat starch, gliadin, and the gluten-free diet. *J Am Diet Assoc* 101:1456-1459, 2001.

# *Minerals—Fluoride*

| | FLUORIDE (µg/100 g) | SR21 CODE NUMBER[1] | | FLUORIDE (µg/100 g) | SR21 CODE NUMBER[1] |
|---|---|---|---|---|---|
| **BEVERAGES** | | | pepper-type soda, canned/bottled | 36 | 14153 |
| **CARBONATED BEVERAGES** | | | Pepsi One, all regions | 40 | 97531 |
| carbonated water, fruit-flavored | 105 | 97541 | Pepsi One, mid-west | 47 | 97532 |
| Coca-Cola, all regions | 49 | 97516 | Pepsi One, northeast | 31 | 97533 |
| Coca-Cola, mid-west | 46 | 97517 | Pepsi One, south | 56 | 97534 |
| Coca-Cola, northeast | 53 | 97518 | Pepsi One, west | 18 | 97535 |
| Coca-Cola, south | 57 | 97519 | Pepsi, all regions | 32 | 97511 |
| Coca-Cola, west | 36 | 97520 | Pepsi, mid-west | 36 | 97512 |
| cola without ice, fast-food type | 74 | 97510 | Pepsi, northeast | 27 | 97513 |
| cola, cherry flavor | 41 | 97624 | Pepsi, south | 45 | 97514 |
| cream soda | 35 | 14130 | Pepsi, west | 13 | 97515 |
| Diet Coke, all regions | 60 | 97526 | root beer | 71 | 14157 |
| Diet Coke, mid-west | 69 | 97527 | Sprite, mid-west | 47 | 97537 |
| Diet Coke, northeast | 58 | 97528 | Sprite, northeast | 48 | 97538 |
| Diet Coke, south | 72 | 97529 | Sprite, south | 59 | 97539 |
| Diet Coke, west | 33 | 97530 | Sprite, west | 29 | 97540 |
| diet cola without ice, fast-food type | 78 | 97509 | tonic water | 83 | 14155 |
| diet lemon-lime soda | 15 | 97625 | | | |
| Diet Pepsi, all regions | 48 | 97521 | **COFFEE AND COFFEE BEVERAGES** | | |
| Diet Pepsi, mid-west | 46 | 97522 | cereal coffee (grain beverage), instant, with water | 125 | 14237 |
| Diet Pepsi, northeast | 46 | 97523 | coffee, brewed | 91 | 14209 |
| Diet Pepsi, south | 66 | 97524 | coffee, decaffeinated, brewed | 52 | 14201 |
| Diet Pepsi, west | 25 | 97525 | | | |
| ginger ale, canned/bottled | 69 | 14136 | **DISTILLED SPIRITS** | | |
| grape soda, canned/bottled | 86 | 14142 | distilled spirits, all types, 80 proof | 9 | 14037 |
| lemon-lime soda with caffeine, canned/bottled | 42 | 14144 | | | |
| lemon-lime soda without ice, fast-food type | 64 | 97536 | **MALT BEVERAGES** | | |
| lemon-lime soda, canned/bottled | 48 | 14145 | beer | 44 | 14003 |
| orange soda, canned/bottled | 81 | 14150 | beer, light | 45 | 14006 |

| | FLUORIDE (µg/100 g) | SR21 CODE NUMBER[1] |
|---|---|---|
| **TEA** | | |
| iced tea instant powder, lemon flavor with sugar | 584 | 14370 |
| iced tea with lemon, canned/bottled, Nestea | 90 | 14137 |
| iced tea, from instant | 335 | 14367 |
| iced tea, lemon flavor with sugar, from instant | 116 | 14371 |
| iced tea, lemon flavor, sugar-sweetened, canned/bottled, Arizona | 123 | 14475 |
| iced tea, lemon flavor, sugar-sweetened, canned/bottled, Lipton Brisk | 72 | 14476 |
| tea, black, brewed 3 minutes | 373 | 14355 |
| tea, black, brewed, mid-west | 393 | 97558 |
| tea, black, brewed, northeast | 357 | 97559 |
| tea, black, brewed, south | 380 | 97560 |
| tea, black, brewed, west | 355 | 97561 |
| tea, black, decaffeinated, brewed 3 minutes | 269 | 14352 |
| tea, black, decaffeinated, brewed, mid-west | 293 | 97554 |
| tea, black, decaffeinated, brewed, northeast | 279 | 97555 |
| tea, black, decaffeinated, brewed, south | 264 | 97556 |
| tea, black, decaffeinated, brewed, west | 247 | 97557 |
| tea, black, microwaved, all regions | 322 | 97549 |
| tea, black, microwaved, mid-west | 319 | 97550 |
| tea, black, microwaved, northeast | 309 | 97551 |
| tea, black, microwaved, south | 338 | 97552 |
| tea, black, microwaved, west | 310 | 97553 |
| tea, chamomile, brewed | 13 | 14545 |
| tea, green decaffeinated, brewed | 272 | 97630 |
| tea, green, brewed | 115 | 97629 |
| tea, peppermint, brewed | 9 | 97631 |
| **WATER** | | |
| Very Fine Fruit 20 Water | 6 | 97573 |
| water, bottled, Aquafina | 5 | 14433 |
| water, bottled, Calistoga | 7 | 14437 |
| water, bottled, Crystal Geyser | 24 | 14438 |
| water, bottled, Dannon | 11 | 14432 |
| water, bottled, Dannon Fluoride To Go | 78 | 14440 |
| water, bottled, Dasani | 7 | 14434 |
| water, bottled, Evian | 10 | 14559 |
| water, bottled, Naya | 14 | 14439 |
| water, bottled, Perrier | 31 | 14384 |
| water, bottled, Poland Spring | 10 | 14385 |
| water, bottled, Saratoga | 20 | 97572 |
| water, bottled, Volvic | 34 | 97574 |
| water, municipal/well tap, all regions | 71 | 97577 |
| water, municipal/well tap, mid-west | 88 | 97579 |
| water, municipal/well tap, northeast | 69 | 97582 |
| water, municipal/well tap, south | 76 | 97585 |
| water, municipal/well tap, west | 47 | 97588 |
| water, municipal tap, all regions | 81 | 14429 |
| water, municipal tap, mid-west | 99 | 97580 |
| water, municipal tap, northeast | 74 | 97583 |
| water, municipal tap, south | 93 | 97586 |
| water, municipal tap, west | 51 | 97589 |
| water, well tap, mid-west | 53 | 97581 |
| water, well tap, northeast | 9 | 97584 |
| water, well tap, south | 10 | 97587 |
| water, well tap, west | 24 | 97590 |
| water, well, all regions | 26 | 97578 |

| | FLUORIDE (µg/100 g) | SR21 CODE NUMBER[1] |
|---|---|---|
| **WINE** | | |
| wine, red | 105 | 14096 |
| wine, white | 202 | 14106 |
| **CANDY** | | |
| caramels | 27 | 19074 |
| M&M's Plain | 17 | 19141 |
| milk chocolate chips | 5 | 19120 |
| Reese's Peanut Butter Cups, Hershey | 89 | 19150 |
| Snickers | 36 | 19155 |
| **CEREALS AND GRAINS, COOKED** | | |
| corn grits, white, quick, enriched, cooked | 56 | 08161 |
| corn grits, white, regular/quick, enriched, cooked | 56 | 08091 |
| oatmeal, quick/regular, cooked | 72 | 08121 |
| rice, white, long grain, enriched, boiled | 41 | 20045 |
| wheat cereal (farina), enriched, cooked | 51 | 08113 |
| **CEREALS, READY-TO-EAT** | | |
| Cheerios, General Mills | 68 | 08013 |
| Corn Flakes, Country, General Mills | 17 | 08269 |
| Corn Flakes, Kellogg's | 17 | 08020 |
| Crispix, Kellogg's | 31 | 08259 |
| Crispy Rice, Malt-O-Meal | 19 | 08348 |
| Crispy Rice, Ralston | 19 | 08025 |
| granola cereal with raisins, lowfat, Kellogg's | 33 | 08284 |
| granola with raisins, lowfat, 100% natural, Quaker | 33 | 08220 |
| puffed rice | 19 | 08156 |
| Puffed Rice, Quaker | 19 | 08066 |
| puffed wheat | 27 | 08157 |
| Puffed Wheat, Kellogg's | 27 | 08379 |
| Raisin Bran, Kellogg's | 65 | 08060 |
| Raisin Bran, Post | 65 | 08061 |
| Rice Krispies, Kellogg's | 19 | 08065 |
| Shredded Wheat Miniatures, Kellogg's | 27 | 08384 |
| Shredded Wheat, Post | 27 | 08147 |
| Total, corn, General Mills | 17 | 08246 |
| Wheaties Raisin Bran, General Mills | 65 | 08026 |
| Wheaties, General Mills | 27 | 08089 |
| **CHEESE AND CHEESE PRODUCTS** | | |
| American processed cheese | 35 | 01042 |
| American processed cheese food | 35 | 01046 |
| cheddar cheese | 35 | 01009 |
| cheddar cheese/colby cheese, low sodium | 35 | 01169 |
| cheddar cheese/colby cheese, lowfat | 35 | 01168 |
| cheese sauce, ready-to-serve | 29 | 06930 |
| cheese spread, American | 35 | 01048 |
| cottage cheese, 2% fat | 32 | 01015 |
| cottage cheese, 4% fat, creamed with fruit | 32 | 01013 |
| cottage cheese, creamed, small curd | 32 | 01012 |
| **DESSERTS** | | |
| cookie, oatmeal raisin, homemade | 69 | 18184 |
| éclair with custard filling and chocolate glaze, homemade | 13 | 18257 |
| frozen yogurt, flavors other than chocolate | 26 | 42187 |
| frozen yogurt, whole fat, chocolate | 40 | 42186 |
| gelatin dessert, from mix with sugar, all flavors | 69 | 19173 |

| | FLUORIDE (μg/100 g) | SR21 CODE NUMBER[1] | | FLUORIDE (μg/100 g) | SR21 CODE NUMBER[1] |
|---|---|---|---|---|---|
| ice cream sandwich with chocolate ice cream, Klondike Slim-A-Bear | 27 | 19888 | cranberry apple juice drink, low-calorie, bottled | 70 | 43404 |
| ice cream sandwich with mint ice cream, Klondike Slim-A-Bear | 27 | 19889 | cranberry grape juice drink, bottled | 65 | 14241 |
| ice cream sandwich with vanilla ice cream, Klondike Slim-A-Bear | 27 | 19887 | cranberry juice cocktail, canned/bottled | 67 | 14242 |
| | | | cranberry juice cocktail, from frozen concentrate | 67 | 14431 |
| ice cream, chocolate | 23 | 19270 | cranberry juice cocktail, low calorie, with added calcium, bottled | 70 | 1423 |
| ice cream, vanilla, regular (10% fat) | 15 | 19095 | | | |
| ice pop (frozen dessert) | 74 | 19283 | fruit drink, ready-to-drink, Capri-Sun | 71 | 14272 |
| ice pop with low-calorie sweetener (frozen dessert) | 89 | 43514 | fruit drink, ready-to-drink, Hawaiian Punch | 44 | 97543 |
| orange juice bar (frozen dessert) | 77 | 43346 | fruit drink, ready-to-drink, Hi-C | 22 | 97544 |
| pie, apple | 13 | 18301 | grape juice drink, canned/bottled | 32 | 14282 |
| pie, pumpkin | 32 | 18326 | grape juice, canned/bottled | 72 | 09135 |
| pudding, banana, from instant mix with whole milk | 22 | 19319 | grapefruit juice, canned/bottled | 45 | 09123 |
| pudding, chocolate, from instant mix with whole milk | 22 | 19185 | mixed vegetable and fruit juice drink, canned/bottled | 12 | 14119 |
| pudding, lemon, from instant mix with whole milk | 22 | 19331 | orange juice drink, canned/bottled | 55 | 42270 |
| | | | orange juice, canned/bottled | 52 | 09207 |
| pudding, vanilla, from instant mix with whole milk | | | orange juice, canned/bottled | 31 | 09207 |
| | | | orange juice, from frozen concentrate | 58 | 09215 |
| | | | prune juice, canned/bottled | 60 | 09294 |
| | | | tomato juice, canned/bottled | 7 | 11540 |
| **EGGS** | | | **FRUITS** | | |
| egg, boiled, hard/fried/omelet/poached/ scrambled with milk | 5 | 01129/01128/ 01130/01131/ 01132 | applesauce, sweetened, canned/bottled | 5 | 09020 |
| | | | fruit cocktail, canned in heavy syrup, solids and liquid | 9 | 09100 |
| egg, raw | 1 | 01123 | grapes, red/green, European, seedless, raw | 8 | 09132 |
| **ENTREES** | | | peach, canned in heavy syrup, solids and liquid | 7 | 09241 |
| beef ravioli in tomato and meat sauce, canned, Chef Boyardee | 13 | 22515 | peach, raw | 4 | 09236 |
| beef stew, canned | 57 | 22905 | pear, canned in heavy syrup, drained | 8 | 09374 |
| chicken pot pie, frozen | 58 | 22906 | pear, canned in heavy syrup, solids and liquid | 8 | 09257 |
| chili con carne with beans, canned | 45 | 22904 | prune, dried | 4 | 09291 |
| pizza, cheese, regular crust, frozen, heated | 31 | 21224 | raisins, seedless | 233 | 09298 |
| spaghetti Bolognese, frozen entrée, Healthy Choice | 38 | 22401 | strawberries, raw | 4 | 09316 |
| **FAST FOODS AND RESTAURANT FOODS** | | | **GRAIN- AND VEGETABLE-BASED SNACKS** | | |
| French fries, McDonald's | 115 | 21238 | popcorn, oil-popped, microwaved | 6 | 19035 |
| hamburger sandwich, large, single meat, fast food | 28 | 21202 | potato chips | 61 | 19411 |
| shake, vanilla, McDonald's | 14 | 14347 | potato chips, baked | 106 | 42283 |
| steak sandwich with lettuce, tomato, and mayonnaise, fast food | 37 | 21123 | tortilla chips | 52 | 19056 |
| **FISH AND SEAFOOD** | | | **GRAIN PRODUCTS** | | |
| crab, blue, canned | 210 | 15141 | biscuit, plain/buttermilk, from refrigerated dough (12%–28% fat) | 26 | 18015 |
| fish sticks/pieces, frozen, reheated | 134 | 15027 | biscuit, plain/buttermilk, from refrigerated dough (2%–12% fat) | 26 | 18013 |
| shrimp, breaded and fried | 166 | 15150 | bread, rye | 51 | 18060 |
| shrimp, canned | 201 | 15152 | bread stuffing, from mix | 51 | 18082 |
| tuna, light, canned in oil, drained | 31 | 15119 | bread, white | 49 | 18069 |
| tuna, light, canned in water, drained | 19 | 15121 | bread, whole wheat | 49 | 18075 |
| tuna, white, canned in oil, drained | 31 | 15124 | cornbread, from mix | 11 | 18023 |
| | | | macaroni, enriched, boiled | 7 | 20100 |
| **FRUIT AND VEGETABLE JUICES AND JUICE DRINKS** | | | macaroni, enriched, dry | 18 | 20099 |
| | | | noodles, egg, enriched, boiled (egg in the noodle dough) | 6 | 20110 |
| carrot juice | 7 | 97634 | pancake, frozen | 20 | 18288 |
| cranberry apple juice drink, bottled | 83 | 14238 | | | |

| | FLUORIDE (µg/100 g) | SR21 CODE NUMBER[1] |
|---|---|---|
| roll, hamburger | 25 | 18350 |
| spaghetti, enriched, boiled | 7 | 20121 |
| spaghetti, enriched, dry | 18 | 20120 |
| tortilla, flour | 33 | 18364 |

**INFANT, JUNIOR, AND TODDLER FOODS**

| | FLUORIDE (µg/100 g) | SR21 CODE NUMBER[1] |
|---|---|---|
| apple cranberry juice, infant food | 10 | 03169 |
| apple grape juice, Earth's Best | 45 | 03265 |
| apple juice, Earth's Best | 12 | 03166 |
| apple peach juice, infant food | 19 | 03168 |
| apple prune juice, infant food | 13 | 03171 |
| bananas with pineapple and tapioca, Gerber 3rd Foods/Heinz Junior-3 | 16 | 03156 |
| bananas with tapioca, Gerber 3rd Foods/ Heinz Junior-3 | 36 | 03280 |
| carrots, Beech-Nut Stage 3/Gerber 3rd Foods/Heinz Junior-3 | 12 | 03100 |
| chicken noodle dinner, Beech-Nut Stage 3/ Gerber 3rd Foods/Heinz Junior-3 | 29 | 03069 |
| fruit dessert, Gerber 3rd Foods/Heinz Junior-3 | 18 | 03236 |
| green beans, Beech-Nut Stage 3 | 12 | 03092 |
| green beans, Gerber 1st Foods/Heinz Beginner-1 | 16 | 03091 |
| green peas, Beech-Nut Stage 1/Gerber 2nd Foods | 25 | 03121 |
| lamb, junior food | 10 | 03011 |
| macaroni and cheese, junior food | 6 | 03090 |
| mango with tapioca, Gerber | 12 | 03140 |
| oatmeal with applesauce and bananas, junior cereal | 8 | 03192 |
| peach cobbler, Gerber 3rd Foods | 8 | 03228 |
| pears, Beech-Nut Stage 3/Gerber 3rd Foods/ Heinz Junior-3 | 9 | 03133 |
| plums with tapioca, Gerber 3rd Foods | 34 | 03135 |
| rice cereal with applesauce and bananas, Heinz Strained-2 | 16 | 03195 |
| squash, yellow, Gerber 3rd Foods | 5 | 03105 |
| sweet potatoes, Beech-Nut Stage 3/Gerber 3rd Foods/Heinz Junior-3 | 10 | 03109 |
| turkey and rice, Beech-Nut Stage 3/Gerber 3rd Foods/Heinz Junior-3 | 20 | 03083 |
| turkey, Gerber 3rd Foods | 44 | 03016 |
| vanilla custard pudding, Beech-Nut Stage 3/ Gerber 3rd Foods/Heinz Junior-3 | 4 | 03246 |
| vegetables and beef, Beech-Nut Stage 3/ Gerber 3rd Foods/Heinz Junior-3 | 21 | 03054 |
| vegetables and ham dinner, Gerber 3rd Foods/ Heinz Junior-3 | 14 | 03062 |
| vegetables and turkey dinner, Gerber 3rd Foods | 8 | 03085 |

**MEATS**

| | FLUORIDE (µg/100 g) | SR21 CODE NUMBER[1] |
|---|---|---|
| bacon, pork, cured, broiled/pan-fried | 34 | 10124 |
| beef liver, pan-fried | 5 | 13327 |
| ham, cured (fully cooked as purchased), whole, lean and fat, roasted | 20 | 10151 |
| sausage (fresh), pork, pan-fried | 16 | 07064 |
| veal leg (top round), lean and fat, breaded, pan-fried | 21 | 17096 |
| veal liver, pan-fried | 5 | 17204 |

**MEATS, LUNCHEON**

| | FLUORIDE (µg/100 g) | SR21 CODE NUMBER[1] |
|---|---|---|
| bologna, beef | 36 | 07007 |
| bologna, beef and pork | 36 | 07008 |
| bologna, pork | 36 | 07010 |
| bologna, pork, turkey, beef | 36 | 07937 |
| bologna, turkey | 36 | 07011 |
| frankfurter, beef | 48 | 07022 |
| ham and cheese loaf (lunch meat) | 36 | 07032 |

**MILKS, MILK BEVERAGES, AND YOGURT**

| | FLUORIDE (µg/100 g) | SR21 CODE NUMBER[1] |
|---|---|---|
| buttermilk, cultured | 4 | 01088 |
| chocolate milk, reduced fat/whole milk | 5 | 01103/01102 |
| cocoa (hot chocolate), from mix, prepared with water | 48 | 14194 |
| evaporated milk, nonfat/whole, canned | 8 | 01097/01096 |
| milk, lowfat, 1% fat | 3 | 01082 |
| milk, nonfat/reduced fat/lowfat | 3 | 01085/01079/ 01121 |
| yogurt, lowfat, plain | 12 | 01117 |
| yogurt, lowfat, strawberry | 9 | 01120 |
| yogurt, lowfat, vanilla | 12 | 01119 |
| yogurt, nonfat, chocolate | 12 | 01187 |
| yogurt, nonfat/whole, plain | 12 | 01118/01116 |

**NUTS AND SEEDS**

| | FLUORIDE (µg/100 g) | SR21 CODE NUMBER[1] |
|---|---|---|
| peanuts, all types, dry-roasted, salted | 16 | 16090 |
| pecans, dried | 10 | 12142 |

**POULTRY**

| | FLUORIDE (µg/100 g) | SR21 CODE NUMBER[1] |
|---|---|---|
| turkey (young hen) light and dark meat with skin, roasted | 21 | 05232 |
| turkey (young tom) light and dark meat with skin, roasted | 21 | 05256 |

**SAUCES, GRAVIES, AND CONDIMENTS**

| | FLUORIDE (µg/100 g) | SR21 CODE NUMBER[1] |
|---|---|---|
| catsup (ketchup) | 15 | 11935 |
| gravy, beef, canned | 99 | 06116 |
| pickle (cucumber), dill | 30 | 11937 |
| tomato sauce, bottled | 35 | 11549 |
| tomato sauce, marinara, bottled | 22 | 06931 |

**SOUPS**

| | FLUORIDE (µg/100 g) | SR21 CODE NUMBER[1] |
|---|---|---|
| chicken broth, condensed, canned, prepared with water | 61 | 06413 |
| chicken corn chowder, canned, ready-to-serve | 132 | 06725 |
| chicken noodle soup, condensed, canned, prepared with water | 35 | 06419 |
| tomato soup, canned, condensed, prepared with milk | 7 | 06359 |

**SUGARS, SYRUPS, AND OTHER SWEETENERS**

| | FLUORIDE (µg/100 g) | SR21 CODE NUMBER[1] |
|---|---|---|
| honey | 7 | 19296 |
| jam/preserves | 19 | 19297 |
| jelly | 73 | 19300 |
| pancake/waffle syrup | 44 | 19129 |

**VEGETABLES**

| | FLUORIDE (µg/100 g) | SR21 CODE NUMBER[1] |
|---|---|---|
| asparagus, boiled, drained | 22 | 11012 |
| avocado, raw | 7 | 09037 |
| beet, canned, drained | 26 | 11084 |
| baked beans with pork, canned | 54 | 16009 |
| carrot, boiled, drained | 47 | 11125 |
| coleslaw, homemade | 11 | 11159 |

| | FLUORIDE (μg/100 g) | SR21 CODE NUMBER[1] | | FLUORIDE (μg/100 g) | SR21 CODE NUMBER[1] |
|---|---|---|---|---|---|
| corn, yellow, creamed, canned | 28 | 11174 | potato, scalloped, homemade | 31 | 11372 |
| corn, yellow, creamed, Heinz Junior-3 | 32 | 03120 | radish, red, raw | 6 | 11429 |
| corn, yellow, frozen | 15 | 11178 | sauerkraut, canned, solids and liquid | 7 | 11439 |
| French fries, frozen, baked | 26 | 11403 | sweet potato, candied, homemade | 8 | 11659 |
| green snap beans, raw | 19 | 11052 | spinach, boiled, drained | 38 | 11458 |
| lima beans, immature, green Fordhook, frozen, boiled, drained | 7 | 11038 | tomato, red, canned | 5 | 11531 |
| mixed vegetables, canned, drained | 37 | 11581 | **SPECIAL DIETARY FOODS** | | |
| mushrooms, common white, canned, drained | 10 | 11264 | Gatorade, fruit flavor, Quaker Oats | 34 | 14460 |
| onion rings, breaded, parfried, frozen, heated | 55 | 11296 | Powerade, lemon-lime flavor, Coca-Cola | 62 | 14461 |
| potato puffs, frozen, heated | 6 | 11399 | | | |
| potato, cottage fries, frozen, heated | 26 | 11407 | **OTHER FOODS** | | |
| potato, mashed, homemade with whole milk and butter | 39 | 11371 | creamer, powdered | 112 | 01069 |
| | | | mayonnaise, safflower and soy/soy | 9 | 04026/04025 |
| potato, russet, baked | 45 | 11356 | | | |

[1]Code numbers for foods in the USDA National Nutrient Database for Standard Reference, Release 21, 2008.

Source:
USDA National Fluoride Database of Selected Beverages and Foods, Release 2. Prepared by Nutrient Data laboratory, USDA in collaboration with University of Minnesota, Nutrition Coordinating Center; University of Iowa, College of Dentistry; Virginia Polytechnic Institute and State University, Food Analysis Laboratory Control Center; national Agricultural Statistics Services, USDA; and Food Composition laboratory, USDA, December 2005. Available at: http://www.ars.usda.gov/Services/Services.htm?modecode=12-35-45-00.

# Minerals—Iodine

| | IODINE[1] (μg/100 g) | SOURCE | | IODINE[1] (μg/100 g) | SOURCE |
|---|---|---|---|---|---|
| **BEVERAGES** | | | **CHEESE** | | |
| beer | 0.4 | FDA, 2007 | American cheese | 53.1 | FDA, 2007 |
| coffee, brewed | 0.0 | FDA, 2007 | cheddar cheese, sharp/mild | 56.6 | FDA, 2007 |
| cola | 0.0 | FDA, 2007 | cottage cheese, 2% fat | 40.0 | FDA, 2007 |
| cola, low-calorie | 0.4 | FDA, 2007 | cottage cheese, 4% fat | 27.0 | Pennington et al, 1995 |
| fruit drink, canned | 0.9 | FDA, 2007 | cream cheese | 45.6 | FDA, 2007 |
| fruit drink, from powder | 0.0 | FDA, 2007 | Swiss cheese | 115.0 | FDA, 2007 |
| fruit flavored soda | 0.0 | FDA, 2007 | | | |
| lemonade, from frozen concentrate | 0.0 | FDA, 2007 | **CREAM** | | |
| tea, brewed from bag | 0.0 | FDA, 2007 | half and half | 41.1 | FDA, 2007 |
| wine, table, dry | 0.0 | FDA, 2007 | cream substitute, frozen | 0.7 | FDA, 2007 |
| | | | cream substitute, powdered | 7.0 | Pennington et al, 1995 |
| **CANDY** | | | sour cream | 43.9 | FDA, 2007 |
| caramels | 35.0 | Pennington et al, 1995 | sour cream dip | 40.8 | FDA, 2007 |
| chocolate, nougat, and nut bar | 22.8 | FDA, 2007 | | | |
| milk chocolate candy | 71.5 | FDA, 2007 | **DESSERTS** | | |
| sucker | 42.4 | FDA, 2007 | brownie, ready-to-eat | 21.6 | FDA, 2007 |
| | | | cake, chocolate with chocolate icing, ready-to-eat/frozen | 44.8 | FDA, 2007 |
| **CEREALS, COOKED** | | | cake, yellow with white icing, from mix | 87.8 | FDA, 2007 |
| corn grits, enriched cooked | 0.5 | FDA, 2007 | chocolate syrup | 0.0 | FDA, 2007 |
| farina, enriched, cooked | 0.0 | FDA, 2007 | coffeecake, ready-to-eat/frozen | 29.0 | Pennington et al, 1995 |
| oatmeal, cooked | 1.4 | FDA, 2007 | cookie, chocolate chip | 2.3 | FDA, 2007 |
| rice, white, enriched, cooked | 0.0 | FDA, 2007 | cookie, chocolate with crème filling | 76.0 | Pennington et al, 1995 |
| | | | cookie, sandwich with crème filling | 0.0 | FDA, 2007 |
| **CEREALS, READY-TO-EAT** | | | cookie, sugar | 4.2 | FDA, 2007 |
| corn flakes | 93.0 | Pennington et al, 1995 | Danish/sweet roll, ready-to-eat/frozen | 59.9 | FDA, 2007 |
| crisped rice | 2.0 | FDA, 2007 | doughnut with icing, from doughnut store | 31.8 | FDA, 2007 |
| fruit-flavored, sweetened | 0.9 | FDA, 2007 | | | |
| granola with raisins | 12.3 | FDA, 2007 | doughnut, cake type, ready-to-eat/frozen | 25.0 | Pennington et al, 1995 |
| oat ring | 8.5 | FDA, 2007 | | | |
| raisin bran | 7.7 | FDA, 2007 | gelatin dessert, strawberry, from instant mix | 0.0 | FDA, 2007 |
| shredded wheat | 6.8 | FDA, 2007 | | | |

| | IODINE[1] (µg/100 g) | SOURCE | | IODINE[1] (µg/100 g) | SOURCE |
|---|---|---|---|---|---|
| ice cream, chocolate | 45.0 | Pennington et al, 1995 | pizza, cheese and pepperoni, regular crust, fast food | 21.7 | FDA, 2007 |
| ice cream sandwich | 59.0 | Pennington et al, 1995 | shake, chocolate, fast food | 51.4 | FDA, 2007 |
| ice cream, vanilla | 57.7 | FDA, 2007 | taco/tostada, from Mexican carry-out | 8.6 | FDA, 2007 |
| ice cream, vanilla, light | 72.3 | FDA, 2007 | | | |
| pie, apple, frozen, heated | 0.0 | FDA, 2007 | **FATS, OILS, AND SPREADS** | | |
| pie, pumpkin, frozen, heated | 19.0 | FDA, 2007 | butter | 7.3 | FDA, 2007 |
| popsicle | 45.7 | FDA, 2007 | corn oil | 1.0 | Pennington et al, 1995 |
| pudding, chocolate, from instant made with whole milk | 37.0 | Pennington et al, 1995 | margarine, stick type | 1.0 | FDA, 2007 |
| pudding, flavor other than chocolate, ready-to-eat | 17.0 | FDA, 2007 | mayonnaise | 2.0 | FDA, 2007 |
| sherbet, fruit flavor | 147.0 | FDA, 2007 | **FISH AND SHELLFISH** | | |
| | | | catfish, pan-fried | 0.7 | FDA, 2007 |
| **EGGS** | | | cod/haddock fillet, baked | 116.0 | Pennington et al, 1995 |
| egg, fried | 52.0 | Pennington et al, 1995 | fish sticks, frozen, heated | 60.5 | FDA, 2007 |
| egg, scrambled with milk | 52.6 | FDA, 2007 | salmon steak/filet, fresh/frozen, baked | 21.5 | FDA, 2007 |
| egg, soft-boiled | 39.9 | FDA, 2007 | shrimp, boiled | 14.2 | FDA, 2007 |
| | | | shrimp, breaded and fried, homemade | 41.0 | Pennington et al, 1995 |
| **ENTREES** | | | tuna, canned in oil | 20.0 | Pennington et al, 1995 |
| beef and vegetable stew, canned | 0.3 | FDA, 2007 | tuna, canned in water | 5.2 | FDA, 2007 |
| beef and vegetable stew, homemade | 18.0 | Pennington et al, 1995 | | | |
| beef stroganoff, homemade | 11.3 | FDA, 2007 | **FRUIT AND VEGETABLE JUICES** | | |
| chicken, fried, with mashed potatoes, cornbread, and vegetable, frozen dinner | 24.0 | Pennington et al, 1995 | apple juice, bottled | 2.7 | FDA, 2007 |
| chicken noodle casserole, homemade | 25.0 | Pennington et al, 1995 | cranberry juice cocktail, canned/bottled | 0.0 | FDA, 2007 |
| chicken pot pie, frozen, heated | 3.7 | FDA, 2007 | grape juice, from frozen concentrate | 0.0 | FDA, 2007 |
| chili con carne with beans, canned | 1.3 | FDA, 2007 | grapefruit juice, from frozen concentrate | 0.0 | FDA, 2007 |
| hamburger, ¼ lb with garnish, fast food | 2.3 | FDA, 2007 | orange juice, bottled/carton | 9.4 | FDA, 2007 |
| lasagna with meat, frozen, heated | 12.7 | FDA, 2007 | fruit juice blend, 100% juice, canned/bottled | 0.7 | FDA, 2007 |
| lasagna with meat, homemade | 33.0 | Pennington et al, 1995 | orange juice, from frozen concentrate | 1.7 | FDA, 2007 |
| macaroni and cheese, from box mix | 16.2 | FDA, 2007 | pineapple juice, from frozen concentrate | 3.1 | FDA, 2007 |
| meatloaf, homemade | 23.1 | FDA, 2007 | prune juice, bottled | 3.9 | FDA, 2007 |
| pizza, cheese, frozen, heated | 95.0 | Pennington et al, 1995 | tomato juice, bottled | 2.9 | FDA, 2007 |
| pork chow mein, homemade | 9.0 | Pennington et al, 1995 | | | |
| spaghetti in tomato sauce, canned | 23.0 | Pennington et al, 1995 | **FRUITS** | | |
| spaghetti with meat sauce, homemade | 1.2 | FDA, 2007 | applesauce, canned | 0.0 | FDA, 2007 |
| tuna noodle casserole, homemade | 14.6 | FDA, 2007 | apple, raw | 0.0 | FDA, 2007 |
| | | | apricot, canned in heavy/light syrup | 1.6 | FDA, 2007 |
| **FAST FOODS AND RESTAURANT FOODS** | | | banana, raw | 0.0 | FDA, 2007 |
| | | | cantaloupe, raw | 0.0 | FDA, 2007 |
| beef with vegetables in sauce, from Chinese carry-out | 0.3 | FDA, 2007 | fruit cocktail, canned in heavy syrup | 10.8 | FDA, 2007 |
| burrito, beef, beans, and cheese, from Mexican carry-out | 6.1 | FDA, 2007 | grapefruit, raw | 0.0 | FDA, 2007 |
| cheeseburger, ¼ lb, fast food | 8.6 | FDA, 2007 | grapes, red/green, raw | 0.0 | FDA, 2007 |
| chicken breast, fried, fast food | 2.3 | FDA, 2007 | orange, raw | 0.4 | FDA, 2007 |
| chicken filet (broiled) sandwich, fast food | 26.8 | FDA, 2007 | peach, canned in light/medium syrup | 0.7 | FDA, 2007 |
| chicken leg, fried, fast food | 0.3 | FDA, 2007 | peach, raw | 0.0 | FDA, 2007 |
| chicken nuggets, fast food | 0.0 | FDA, 2007 | pear, canned in light syrup | 0.5 | FDA, 2007 |
| chicken with vegetables in sauce, from Chinese carry-out | 1.1 | FDA, 2007 | pear, raw | 0.0 | FDA, 2007 |
| egg, cheese, and ham on English muffin, fast food | 25.4 | FDA, 2007 | pineapple, canned in syrup | 3.2 | FDA, 2007 |
| | | | prune, dried | 30.0 | Pennington et al, 1995 |
| fish sandwich, fast food | 29.9 | FDA, 2007 | raisins, dried | 0.0 | FDA, 2007 |
| French fries, fast food | 0.0 | FDA, 2007 | strawberries, raw | 0.0 | FDA, 2007 |
| fried rice, from Chinese carry-out | 3.6 | FDA, 2007 | watermelon, raw | 0.0 | FDA, 2007 |

| | IODINE[1] (μg/100 g) | SOURCE |
|---|---|---|
| **GRAIN PRODUCTS** | | |
| bagel | 46.2 | FDA, 2007 |
| biscuit, from refrigerated dough | 7.0 | FDA, 2007 |
| bread, cracked wheat | 51.2 | FDA, 2007 |
| bread, rye | 2.6 | FDA, 2007 |
| bread, white | 83.1 | FDA, 2007 |
| bread, whole wheat | 16.3 | FDA, 2007 |
| breakfast tart/toaster pastry | 52.3 | FDA, 2007 |
| cornbread, homemade | 28.3 | FDA, 2007 |
| corn chips | 1.5 | FDA, 2007 |
| crackers, butter type | 3.6 | FDA, 2007 |
| crackers, saltines | 0.0 | FDA, 2007 |
| English muffin, toasted | 1.2 | FDA, 2007 |
| graham crackers | 2.3 | FDA, 2007 |
| granola bar with raisins | 6.0 | FDA, 2007 |
| macaroni, enriched, boiled | 19.0 | Pennington et al, 1995 |
| macaroni salad, from grocery/deli | 3.6 | FDA, 2007 |
| muffin, blueberry/plain | 12.3 | FDA, 2007 |
| noodles, egg, enriched, boiled | 2.4 | FDA, 2007 |
| pancake, frozen, heated | 17.1 | FDA, 2007 |
| popcorn, butter flavor, microwave popped | 1.1 | FDA, 2007 |
| popcorn, popped in oil | 27.0 | Pennington et al, 1995 |
| pretzel, hard | 0.4 | FDA, 2007 |
| roll, white, enriched | 81.0 | Pennington et al, 1995 |
| spaghetti, enriched, boiled | 1.2 | FDA, 2007 |
| tortilla, flour | 1.3 | FDA, 2007 |
| **INFANT, JUNIOR, AND TODDLER FOODS** | | |
| cereal, mixed, prepared with whole milk | 17.0 | Pennington et al, 1995 |
| cereal, oatmeal, prepared with water | 0.0 | FDA, 2007 |
| cereal, rice, prepared with water | 0.0 | FDA, 2007 |
| cereal, rice with apples, prepared with water | 6.4 | FDA, 2007 |
| dessert, fruit dessert/pudding | 1.8 | FDA, 2007 |
| dessert, pudding/custard | 18.2 | FDA, 2007 |
| dinner, vegetables and beef | 0.0 | FDA, 2007 |
| dinner, chicken noodle | 0.0 | FDA, 2007 |
| dinner, macaroni, tomatoes, and beef | 1.2 | FDA, 2007 |
| dinner, vegetables and chicken | 0.0 | FDA, 2007 |
| dinner, vegetables and ham | 0.4 | FDA, 2007 |
| dinner, turkey and rice | 0.5 | FDA, 2007 |
| fruit juice, apple juice | 1.9 | FDA, 2007 |
| fruit, bananas with tapioca | 0.0 | FDA, 2007 |
| fruit juice, orange juice | 0.0 | FDA, 2007 |
| fruit, applesauce | 1.5 | FDA, 2007 |
| fruit, peaches | 0.0 | FDA, 2007 |
| fruit, pears | 0.0 | FDA, 2007 |
| infant formula, milk-based, high iron, ready-to-feed | 13.7 | FDA, 2007 |
| infant formula, milk-based, low iron, ready-to-feed | 14.9 | FDA, 2007 |
| infant formula, soy-based, ready-to-feed | 11.3 | FDA, 2007 |
| meat, beef | 0.0 | FDA, 2007 |
| meat, chicken | 4.7 | FDA, 2007 |
| meat, lamb and broth/gravy | 1.1 | FDA, 2007 |
| meat, pork | 7.0 | Pennington et al, 1995 |
| meat, turkey and broth/gravy | 0.0 | FDA, 2007 |
| meat, veal and broth/gravy | 0.7 | FDA, 2007 |
| teething biscuits | 48.5 | FDA, 2007 |
| vegetables, carrots | 0.0 | FDA, 2007 |

| | IODINE[1] (μg/100 g) | SOURCE |
|---|---|---|
| vegetables, creamed corn | 4.0 | Pennington et al, 1995 |
| vegetables, creamed spinach | 10.0 | Pennington et al, 1995 |
| vegetables, green beans | 0.0 | FDA, 2007 |
| vegetables, mixed vegetables | 0.0 | FDA, 2007 |
| vegetables, peas, green | 0.3 | FDA, 2007 |
| vegetable, squash | 0.8 | FDA, 2007 |
| vegetables, sweet potatoes | 0.7 | FDA, 2007 |
| yogurt, lowfat, fruit-flavored | 39.6 | FDA, 2007 |
| **MEATS** | | |
| beef/calf liver, pan-fried | 8.8 | FDA, 2007 |
| beef chuck roast, baked | 1.2 | FDA, 2007 |
| beef, ground, patty, pan-fried | 2.0 | FDA, 2007 |
| beef loin/sirloin steak, pan-fried | 15.0 | Pennington et al, 1995 |
| beef round steak, stewed | 18.0 | Pennington et al, 1995 |
| beef steak, loin/sirloin, broiled | 0.7 | FDA, 2007 |
| lamb chop, pan-fried | 0.0 | FDA, 2007 |
| meatloaf, baked, homemade | 38.0 | Pennington et al, 1995 |
| pork bacon, pan-fried | 0.0 | FDA, 2007 |
| pork chop, pan-fried | 0.0 | FDA, 2007 |
| pork, ham, cured, baked | 0.0 | FDA, 2007 |
| pork roast loin, baked | 0.0 | FDA, 2007 |
| pork sausage, pan-fried | 0.5 | FDA, 2007 |
| veal cutlet, breaded, pan-fried | 19.0 | Pennington et al, 1995 |
| **MEATS, LUNCHEON** | | |
| bologna | 24.3 | FDA, 2007 |
| chicken/turkey lunch meat | 1.9 | FDA, 2007 |
| frankfurter, boiled | 7.3 | FDA, 2007 |
| ham lunch meat, sliced | 0.0 | FDA, 2007 |
| salami | 22.1 | FDA, 2007 |
| **MILKS AND YOGURT** | | |
| buttermilk | 24.0 | Pennington et al, 1995 |
| chocolate milk | 45.3 | FDA, 2007 |
| evaporated milk | 38.0 | Pennington et al, 1995 |
| milk, nonfat | 42.6 | FDA, 2007 |
| milk, 2% fat | 45.2 | FDA, 2007 |
| milk, whole | 45.2 | FDA, 2007 |
| yogurt, 2% fat, plain | 33.0 | Pennington et al, 1995 |
| yogurt, 2% fat, strawberry | 20.0 | Pennington et al, 1995 |
| **NUTS AND SEEDS** | | |
| peanut butter, creamy | 3.6 | FDA, 2007 |
| peanuts, dry-roasted | 4.4 | FDA, 2007 |
| pecans, packaged | 8.0 | Pennington et al, 1995 |
| sunflower seeds, roasted | 5.1 | FDA, 2007 |
| **POULTRY** | | |
| chicken breast, roasted | 0.5 | FDA, 2007 |
| chicken drumstick and breast, breaded, fried, homemade | 17.0 | Pennington et al, 1995 |
| chicken thigh, oven-roasted, skin removed | 0.0 | FDA, 2007 |
| turkey breast, baked | 0.4 | FDA, 2007 |
| **SAUCES, GRAVY, AND SALAD DRESSINGS** | | |
| gravy, brown, from mix | 3.0 | Pennington et al, 1995 |
| gravy, brown, canned/bottled | 1.3 | FDA, 2007 |
| salad dressing, creamy/buttermilk | 7.7 | FDA, 2007 |
| salad dressing, Italian | 1.0 | Pennington et al, 1995 |
| white sauce, medium, homemade | 19.0 | Pennington et al, 1995 |

| | IODINE[1] (µg/100 g) | SOURCE |
|---|---|---|
| **SOUPS** | | |
| bean with bacon/pork soup, condensed, prepared with water | 0.4 | FDA, 2007 |
| beef bouillon, condensed, prepared with water | 2.0 | Pennington et al, 1995 |
| chicken noodle soup, condensed, prepared with water | 0.8 | FDA, 2007 |
| clam chowder, New England, ready-to-eat | 30.5 | FDA, 2007 |
| Oriental/ramen noodles, prepared with water | 0.5 | FDA, 2007 |
| tomato soup, condensed, prepared with whole milk | 1.2 | FDA, 2007 |
| vegetable beef soup, condensed, prepared with water | 0.0 | FDA, 2007 |
| **SUGARS, SYRUPS, AND SWEETENERS** | | |
| honey | 1.4 | FDA, 2007 |
| jelly | 2.9 | FDA, 2007 |
| sugar, white, granulated | 0.0 | FDA, 2007 |
| syrup, pancake | 0.0 | FDA, 2007 |
| **VEGETABLES** | | |
| asparagus, fresh/frozen, boiled | 0.3 | FDA, 2007 |
| avocado, raw | 0.0 | FDA, 2007 |
| beans, refried, canned | 1.0 | FDA, 2007 |
| beans with pork, canned | 0.0 | FDA, 2007 |
| beet, canned | 1.7 | FDA, 2007 |
| broccoli, fresh/frozen, boiled | 0.0 | FDA, 2007 |
| Brussels sprouts, boiled | 0.0 | FDA, 2007 |
| cabbage, fresh, boiled | 0.0 | FDA, 2007 |
| carrot, baby, raw | 0.0 | FDA, 2007 |
| carrot, boiled | 0.5 | FDA, 2007 |
| cauliflower, fresh/frozen, boiled | 0.0 | FDA, 2007 |
| celery, raw | 0.3 | FDA, 2007 |
| coleslaw with dressing, from grocery/deli | 0.9 | FDA, 2007 |
| coleslaw with dressing, homemade | 4.0 | Pennington et al, 1995 |
| collards, fresh/frozen, boiled | 0.7 | FDA, 2007 |
| corn, raw, frozen, boiled | 0.4 | FDA, 2007 |
| corn, canned | 0.3 | FDA, 2007 |
| corn, creamed, canned | 11.0 | Pennington et al, 1995 |
| cowpeas, boiled | 26.0 | Pennington et al, 1995 |
| cucumber, raw | 0.0 | FDA, 2007 |
| eggplant, boiled | 0.0 | FDA, 2007 |
| green snap beans, canned | 0.7 | FDA, 2007 |
| green snap beans, raw/frozen, boiled | 0.0 | FDA, 2007 |

| | IODINE[1] (µg/100 g) | SOURCE |
|---|---|---|
| lettuce, iceberg raw | 0.0 | FDA, 2007 |
| lettuce, leaf, raw | 0.4 | FDA, 2007 |
| lima beans, immature, frozen, boiled | 0.4 | FDA, 2007 |
| lima beans, mature, boiled | 9.0 | Pennington et al, 1995 |
| navy beans, boiled | 39.0 | Pennington et al, 1995 |
| mushrooms, raw | 0.3 | FDA, 2007 |
| mixed vegetables, frozen, boiled | 0.6 | FDA, 2007 |
| okra, boiled | 0.5 | FDA, 2007 |
| onion, mature, raw | 0.0 | FDA, 2007 |
| onion rings, breaded and fried, frozen, heated | 30.0 | Pennington et al, 1995 |
| peas, green, canned | 4.0 | Pennington et al, 1995 |
| peas, green, frozen, boiled | 4.0 | Pennington et al, 1995 |
| pepper, green, raw | 0.4 | FDA, 2007 |
| pinto beans, boiled | 0.0 | FDA, 2007 |
| potato, French fried, frozen, heated | 0.4 | FDA, 2007 |
| potato, mashed, from instant | 51.0 | Pennington et al, 1995 |
| potato, mashed, homemade | 10.8 | FDA, 2007 |
| potato, scalloped, homemade | 31.0 | Pennington et al, 1995 |
| potato salad, from grocery/deli | 2.0 | FDA, 2007 |
| potato, peeled, boiled | 0.0 | FDA, 2007 |
| potato with peel, baked | 0.8 | FDA, 2007 |
| red beans, boiled | 21.0 | Pennington et al, 1995 |
| spinach, canned | 5.0 | Pennington et al, 1995 |
| spinach, fresh/frozen, boiled | 3.0 | FDA, 2007 |
| summer squash, boiled | 0.0 | FDA, 2007 |
| sweet potato, candied, homemade | 15.0 | Pennington et al, 1995 |
| sweet potato, canned | 0.8 | FDA, 2007 |
| tomato, raw | 0.0 | FDA, 2007 |
| tomato salsa, canned | 3.7 | FDA, 2007 |
| tomato sauce, canned | 0.4 | FDA, 2007 |
| turnip, boiled | 0.4 | FDA, 2007 |
| white beans, boiled | 0.0 | FDA, 2007 |
| winter squash, baked, mashed | 0.6 | FDA, 2007 |
| **OTHER FOODS** | | |
| catsup (ketchup) | 0.6 | FDA, 2007 |
| chocolate powder for milk | 10.0 | Pennington et al, 1995 |
| meal replacement liquid, ready-to-drink | 152.0 | FDA, 2007 |
| mustard, yellow | 0.5 | FDA, 2007 |
| olives, black | 0.0 | FDA, 2007 |
| pickle, dill | 0.0 | FDA, 2007 |
| potato chips | 1.0 | FDA, 2007 |
| salt, Lite, iodized, Morton | 6500.0 | MORT |
| salt, iodized, Morton | 6500.0 | MORT |
| sweet and sour sauce | 0.5 | FDA, 2007 |

[1]Foods higher in iodine may contain erythrosine (a red food dye that is high in iodine), iodine-containing dough conditioners, or iodine from iodophor cleaning solutions that are commonly used in the dairy industry.

Sources:
MORT = Morton Salt Company (values for Morton salt and Lite Morton salt)
Food and Drug Administration (FDA). Total Diet Study Statistics on Element Results. 2007. Available at: http://www.cfsan.fda.gov/~comm/tds-res.html.
Pennington JAT, SA Schoen, GD Salmon, B Young, RD Johnson, RW Marts. Composition of core foods of the US food supply, 1982-1991. III. Copper, manganese, selenium, and iodine. *J Food Comp Anal* 8:171-217, 1995.

# Minerals—Molybdenum

| | MOLYBDENUM (μg/100 g) | SOURCE | | MOLYBDENUM (μg/100 g) | SOURCE |
|---|---|---|---|---|---|
| **BEVERAGES** | | | **GRAINS AND GRAIN PRODUCTS** | | |
| tea, instant powder, dry | 990 | Varo et al, 1980d | macaroni, dry | 20 | Varo et al, 1980c |
| wine apple | 1 | Varo et al, 1980d | pancake, oven-baked | 10 | Varo et al, 1980c |
| wine, red, Hungarian | 1 | Varo et al, 1980d | rice, parboiled | 40 | Varo et al, 1980c |
| wine, red, Spanish | 2 | Varo et al, 1980d | rice, whole grain/polished, dry | 20 | Varo et al, 1980c |
| wine, white, Bordeaux | 2 | Varo et al, 1980d | rye-crisp crackers | 20 | Varo et al, 1980c |
| | | | wheat bran | 20 | Varo et al, 1980c |
| **CEREALS, READY-TO-EAT** | | | wheat flour, whole grain | 20 | Varo et al, 1980c |
| oats, puffed | 20 | Varo et al, 1980c | wheat germ | 30 | Varo et al, 1980c |
| rice, puffed | 20 | Varo et al, 1980c | | | |
| | | | **MEATS** | | |
| **CHEESE** | | | beef liver, raw | 170 | Nuurtamo et al, 1980b |
| blue cheese | 6 | Varo et al, 1980a | beef kidney, raw | 60 | Nuurtamo et al, 1980b |
| cottage cheese | 5 | Varo et al, 1980a | beef liver, raw | 160 | Nuurtamo et al, 1980b |
| Edam cheese, 20%/40% fat | 5/6 | Varo et al, 1980a | liver paste | 50 | Nuurtamo et al, 1980b |
| Emmenthal cheese | 10 | Varo et al, 1980a | pork kidney, raw | 70 | Nuurtamo et al, 1980b |
| Gouda cheese | 6 | Varo et al, 1980a | pork liver, raw | 200 | Nuurtamo et al, 1980b |
| Gruyere cheese | 10 | Varo et al, 1980a | pork, short plate, raw | 10 | Nuurtamo et al, 1980b |
| processed cheese | 6 | Varo et al, 1980a | rabbit meat, raw | 10 | Nuurtamo et al, 1980b |
| quark cheese | 7 | Varo et al, 1980a | salami, dry | 10 | Nuurtamo et al, 1980b |
| | | | sheep liver, raw | 70 | Nuurtamo et al, 1980b |
| **CREAM** | | | | | |
| coffee cream | 5 | Varo et al, 1980a | **MILKS** | | |
| half and half | 5 | Varo et al, 1980a | infant formula, milk-based | 10 | Varo et al, 1980a |
| whipping cream | 20 | Varo et al, 1980a | milk, human | 1 | Varo et al, 1980a |
| | | | milk, whole | 5 | Varo et al, 1980a |
| **ENTREES** | | | milk, whole, dry | 40 | Varo et al, 1980a |
| green pea soup | 20 | Varo et al, 1980e | | | |
| hamburger sandwich | 20 | Varo et al, 1980e | **VEGETABLES** | | |
| meat balls with gravy | 10 | Varo et al, 1980e | cabbage, red, pickled | 10 | Varo et al, 1980b |
| meat and cabbage casserole | 10 | Varo et al, 1980e | green snap beans, raw | 20 | Varo et al, 1980b |
| | | | green snap beans, frozen | 20 | Varo et al, 1980b |
| **FISH AND SHELLFISH** | | | leek, raw | 10 | Varo et al, 1980b |
| herring, salted | 10 | Nuurtamo et al, 1980a | mushrooms, raw | 20 | Varo et al, 1980b |
| mussels, canned in water | 30 | Nuurtamo et al, 1980a | onion, red, raw | 30 | Varo et al, 1980b |
| salmon, canned in oil | 10 | Nuurtamo et al, 1980a | parsley, raw | 10 | Varo et al, 1980b |
| | | | parsnip, raw | 10 | Varo et al, 1980b |
| **FRUITS** | | | peas, green, dried | 70 | Varo et al, 1980b |
| cloudberries, raw | 10 | Varo et al, 1980b | peas, green, frozen | 20 | Varo et al, 1980b |
| cranberries, raw | 10 | Varo et al, 1980b | peas, green, raw | 20 | Varo et al, 1980b |
| currants, black/red, raw | 10 | Varo et al, 1980b | pepper, sweet red, raw | 70 | Varo et al, 1980b |
| | | | sauerkraut | 10 | Varo et al, 1980b |
| | | | turnip, raw | 10 | Varo et al, 1980b |

Sources:

Nuurtamo M, P Varo, E Saari, P Koivistoinen. Mineral element composition of Finnish foods. VI. Fish and fish products. *Acta Agric Scanda*, Suppl 22:77-87, 1980a.

Nuurtamo M, P Vaor, E Saari, P Koivistoinen. Mineral element composition of Finnish foods. V. Meat and meat products. *Acta Agric Scand*, Suppl 22:57-76, 1980b.

Varo P, M Nuurtamo, E Saari, P Koivistoinen. Mineral element composition of Finnish foods. VII. Dairy products, eggs, and margarine. *Acta Agric Scand*, Suppl 22:115-126, 1980a.

Varo P, O Lahelma, M Nuurtamo, E Saari, P Koivistoinen. Mineral element composition of Finnish foods. VII. Potato, vegetables, fruits, berries, nuts and mushrooms. *Acta Agric Scand*, Suppl 22:89-113, 1980b.

Varo P, M Nuurtamo, E Saari, P Koivistoinen. Mineral element composition of Finish foods. IV. Flours and bakery products. *Acta Agric Scand*, Suppl 22:37-55, 1980c.

Varo P, M Nuurtamo, E Saari, P Koivistoinen. Mineral element composition of Finnish foods. IX. Beverages, confectionaires, sugar and condiments. *Acta Agric Scand*, Suppl 22:127-139, 1980d.

Varo P, M Nuurtamo, E Saari, P Koisivtoinen. Mineral element composition of Finnish foods. X. Industrial convenience foods, quantity service foods and baby foods. *Acta Agric Scand*, Suppl 22:141-160, 1980c.

# Plant Acids—Oxalic Acid

| | OXALIC ACID (mg/100g) | SOURCE | | OXALIC ACID (mg/100g) | SOURCE |
|---|---|---|---|---|---|
| **FLOURS AND MEALS** | | | cabbage, green, raw | 100 | USDA, 2005 |
| barley flour | 56 | Chai and Liebman, 2005 | chicory, raw | 210 | USDA, 2005 |
| buckheat flour | 269 | Chai and Liebman, 2005 | Chinese cabbage, raw | 6 | Judprasong et al, 2006 |
| corn meal | 54 | Chai and Liebman, 2005 | Chinese kale, raw | 23 | Judprasong et al, 2006 |
| rice flour, brown | 37 | Chai and Liebman, 2005 | chives, raw | 1480 | USDA, 2005 |
| rye flour, dark | 51 | Chai and Liebman, 2005 | collards, raw | 450 | USDA, 2005 |
| semolina flour | 48 | Chai and Liebman, 2005 | coriander, raw | 10 | USDA, 2005 |
| soy flour | 183 | Chai and Liebman, 2005 | endive, raw | 110 | USDA, 2005 |
| wheat flour, white, unbleached | 40 | Chai and Liebman, 2005 | kale, raw | 20 | USDA, 2005 |
| wheat flour, whole | 67 | Chai and Liebman, 2005 | lettuce, raw | 330 | USDA, 2005 |
| | | | parsley, raw | 1700 | USDA, 2005 |
| **FRUITS** | | | purslane, raw | 1310 | USDA, 2005 |
| bitter melon, raw | 71 | Judprasong et al, 2006 | spinach, raw | 970 | USDA, 2005 |
| papaya, raw | 5 | Judprasong et al, 2006 | turnip greens, raw | 50 | USDA, 2005 |
| | | | watercress, raw | 310 | USDA, 2005 |
| **NUTS** | | | | | |
| almonds, roasted | 469 | Chai and Liebman, 2005 | **LEGUMES (BEANS AND PEAS)** | | |
| cashews, roasted | 262 | Chai and Liebman, 2005 | anasazi beans, boiled | 80 | Chai and Liebman, 2005 |
| hazelnuts, raw | 222 | Chai and Liebman, 2005 | azuki beans, boiled | 25 | Chai and Liebman, 2005 |
| macadamia nuts, raw | 42 | Chai and Liebman, 2005 | black beans, boiled | 72 | Chai and Liebman, 2005 |
| peanuts, raw | 142 | Judprasong et al, 2006 | cowpeas (blackeye peas), boiled | 4 | Chai and Liebman, 2005 |
| pecans, raw | 64 | Chai and Liebman, 2005 | garbanzo beans, boiled | 9 | Chai and Liebman, 2005 |
| pine nuts, raw | 198 | Chai and Liebman, 2005 | great northern beans, boiled | 75 | Chai and Liebman, 2005 |
| pine nuts, roasted | 140 | Chai and Liebman, 2005 | kidney beans, red, boiled | 16 | Chai and Liebman, 2005 |
| pistachio nuts, roasted | 49 | Chai and Liebman, 2005 | lentils, boiled | 8 | Chai and Liebman, 2005 |
| walnuts, raw | 74 | Chai and Liebman, 2005 | lima beans, large, boiled | 8 | Chai and Liebman, 2005 |
| | | | mung beans, boiled | 8 | Chai and Liebman, 2005 |
| **VEGETABLES** | | | navy beans, boiled | 57 | Chai and Liebman, 2005 |
| **FLOUR, STEM, AND STALK VEGETABLES** | | | peas, green, split, boiled | 6 | Chai and Liebman, 2005 |
| asparagus, raw | 130 | USDA, 2005 | peas, raw | 50 | USDA, 2005 |
| broccoli, raw | 190 | USDA, 2005 | peas, yellow, split, boiled | 5 | Chai and Liebman, 2005 |
| cauliflower, raw | 150 | USDA, 2005 | pink beans, boiled | 75 | Chai and Liebman, 2005 |
| celery, raw | 190 | USDA, 2005 | pinto beans, boiled | 27 | Chai and Liebman, 2005 |
| | | | red beans, boiled | 35 | Chai and Liebman, 2005 |
| **FRUIT (SEED-CONTAINING) VEGETABLES** | | | soybeans, boiled | 56 | Chai and Liebman, 2005 |
| cucumber, raw | 20 | USDA, 2005 | white beans, small, boiled | 78 | Chai and Liebman, 2005 |
| eggplant, raw | 190 | USDA, 2005 | | | |
| eggplant, green, long, raw | 55 | Judprasong et al, 2006 | **TUBER AND ROOT VEGETABLES** | | |
| okra, raw | 50 | USDA, 2005 | carrot, raw | 500 | USDA, 2005 |
| pepper, raw | 40 | USDA, 2005 | cassava root, raw | 1260 | USDA, 2005 |
| snap beans, raw | 360 | USDA, 2005 | parsnip, raw | 40 | USDA, 2005 |
| squash, raw | 20 | USDA, 2005 | potato, raw | 50 | USDA, 2005 |
| tomato, raw | 50 | USDA, 2005 | radish, raw | 480 | USDA, 2005 |
| yard long beans, green, raw | 38 | Judprasong et al, 2006 | rutabaga, raw | 30 | USDA, 2005 |
| | | | sweet potato, raw | 240 | USDA, 2005 |
| **LEAFY VEGETABLES** | | | turnip, raw | 210 | USDA, 2005 |
| amaranth leaves, raw | 1090 | USDA, 2005 | **OTHER VEGETABLES** | | |
| beet leaves, raw | 610 | USDA, 2005 | corn, sweet, raw | 10 | USDA, 2005 |
| Brussels sprouts, raw | 360 | USDA, 2005 | garlic, raw | 360 | USDA, 2005 |
| | | | onion, raw | 50 | USDA, 2005 |

Sources:
Chai W, M Liebman. Oxlate content of legumes, nuts, and grain-based flours. *J Food Comp Anal* 18:723-729, 2007.
Judprasong K, S Charoenkiatkul, P Sungpuag, K Vasanachitt, Y Nakjamanong. Total and soluble oxalate contents in Thai vegetables, cereal grains and legume seeds and their changes after cooking. *J Food Comp Anal* 19:340-347, 2006. (Thailand)
United States Department of Agriculture (USDA). Oxalic acid content of selected vegetables. http://www.ars.usda.gov/Services/docs.htm?docid=9444. Last modified September 26, 2005.

# *Plant Acids—Phytic Acid*

| | PHYTIC ACID (mg/100 g) | SOURCE | | PHYTIC ACID (mg/100 g) | SOURCE |
|---|---|---|---|---|---|
| **BEVERAGES** | | | **VEGETABLES** | | |
| coffee, brewed | 5 | Harland and Oberleas, 1985 | carrot, raw | 9 | Oberleas and Harland, 1981 |
| coffee, from instant powder | 0 | Harland and Oberleas, 1985 | corn, sweet, yellow, canned | 31 | Oberleas and Harland, 1981 |
| coffee, ground roast | 370 | Harland and Oberleas, 1985 | green snap beans, canned | 91 | Oberleas and Harland, 1981 |
| coffee, instant powder | 200 | Harland and Oberleas, 1985 | potato, boiled, peeled | 81 | Oberleas and Harland, 1981 |
| tea, brewed | 1 | Harland and Oberleas, 1985 | tomato, canned | 6 | Oberleas and Harland, 1981 |
| tea, from instant powder | 1 | Harland and Oberleas, 1985 | | | |
| tea, instant powder | 260 | Harland and Oberleas, 1985 | **VEGETABLES—LEGUMES** | | |
| | | | blackeye peas, boiled | 995/986 | Reddy et al, 1982/Davies and Warrington, 1986 |
| **CEREALS** | | | | | |
| corn flakes | 48 | Oberleas and Harland, 1981 | blackeye peas, canned | 98 | Reddy et al, 1982 |
| farina, regular, cooked | 4 | Oberleas and Harland, 1981 | blackeye peas, dry | 1148/1205 | Reddy et al, 1982/Davies and Warrington, 1986 |
| granola | 625 | Oberleas and Harland, 1981 | | | |
| oatmeal, cooked | 111 | Oberleas and Harland, 1981 | black gram, ground, cooked | 888 | Davies and Warrington, 1986 |
| rice flakes | 232 | Oberleas and Harland, 1981 | black gram, ground, dry | 934 | Davies and Warrington, 1986 |
| wheat flakes | 1467 | Oberleas and Harland, 1981 | black gram, whole, boiled | 688 | Davies and Warrington, 1986 |
| wheat, shredded | 1481 | Oberleas and Harland, 1981 | black gram, whole, dry | 794 | Davies and Warrington, 1986 |
| | | | chickpea flour | 788 | Davies and Warrington, 1986 |
| **FRUITS** | | | chickpeas, green | 280 | Souci et al, 2000 |
| apple, raw | 63 | Oberleas and Harland, 1981 | chickpeas, split, boiled | 769 | Davies and Warrington, 1986 |
| avocado, raw | 17 | Souci et al, 2000 | chickpeas, split, dry | 1053 | Davies and Warrington, 1986 |
| banana, raw | 20 | Souci et al, 2000 | chickpeas, whole, boiled | 580 | Davies and Warrington, 1986 |
| | | | chickpeas, whole, dry | 560 | Davies and Warrington, 1986 |
| **GRAINS AND GRAIN FRACTIONS** | | | common Mexican beans, boiled | 756 | Hernandez-Unzon and Ortega-Delgado, 1989 |
| barley, whole grain, raw | 1070 | Souci et al, 2000 | | | |
| corn, whole grain, raw | 940 | Souci et al, 2000 | green gram, ground, cooked | 663 | Davies and Warrington, 1986 |
| cornmeal, blue | 1870 | Kuhnlein et al, 1979 | green gram, ground, dry | 863 | Davies and Warrington, 1986 |
| cornmeal, pink, | 1250 | Kuhnlein et al, 1979 | green gram, whole, boiled | 695 | Davies and Warrington, 1986 |
| cornmeal, white | 1740 | Kuhnlein et al, 1979 | green gram, whole, dry | 809 | Davies and Warrington, 1986 |
| oats, whole grain, raw | 400 | Souci et al, 2000 | kidney beans, boiled | 778 | Davies and Warrington, 1986 |
| quinoa (pigweed), raw | 541 | Souci et al, 2000 | kidney beans, dry | 893 | Davies and Warrington, 1986 |
| rice, polished, raw | 2539 | Oberleas and Harland, 1981 | kidney beans, red, boiled | 1080 | Reddy et al, 1982 |
| wheat bran, crude | 3011 | Oberleas and Harland, 1981 | kidney beans, red, canned | 260 | Reddy et al, 1982 |
| wheat germ | 4071 | Oberleas and Harland, 1981 | kidney beans, red, dry | 1170 | Reddy et al, 1982 |
| wheat flour, white all-purpose | 282 | Oberleas and Harland, 1981 | lentils, pappadum | 673 | Davies and Warrington, 1986 |
| wheat flour, whole | 845 | Oberleas and Harland, 1981 | lentils, split, boiled | 235 | Davies and Warrington, 1986 |
| | | | lentils, split, dry | 526 | Davies and Warrington, 1986 |
| **GRAIN PRODUCTS** | | | lentils, whole, boiled | 252 | Davies and Warrington, 1986 |
| bread, rye | 942 | Oberleas and Harland, 1981 | lentils, whole, dry | 495 | Davies and Warrington, 1986 |
| bread, white | 69 | Oberleas and Harland, 1981 | lima beans, dry | 1011 | Oberleas and Harland, 1981 |
| bread, whole wheat | 390 | Oberleas and Harland, 1981 | mung beans, boiled | 130 | Reddy et al, 1982 |
| chapatti, dark flour | 341 | Davies and Warrington, 1986 | mung beans, canned | 66 | Reddy et al, 1982 |
| chapatti, light flour | 254 | Davies and Warrington, 1986 | mung beans, dry | 204 | Reddy et al, 1982 |
| chapatti, whole wheat | 513 | Davies and Warrington, 1986 | navy beans, boiled | 346 | Oberleas and Harland, 1981 |
| chapatti flour, dark | 695 | Davies and Warrington, 1986 | navy beans, dry | 615 | Oberleas and Harland, 1981 |
| chapatti flour, light | 578 | Davies and Warrington, 1986 | peas, green, canned | 28 | Oberleas and Harland, 1981 |
| chapatti flour, whole wheat | 669 | Davies and Warrington, 1986 | pink beans, boiled | 370 | Reddy et al, 1982 |
| crackers, saltines | 172 | Oberleas and Harland, 1981 | pink beans, canned | 126 | Reddy et al, 1982 |
| corn chips | 635 | Oberleas and Harland, 1981 | pink beans, dry | 503 | Reddy et al, 1982 |
| macaroni, boiled | 81 | Oberleas and Harland, 1981 | red gram, ground, cooked | 650 | Davies and Warrington, 1986 |
| popcorn, popped, plain | 614 | Oberleas and Harland, 1981 | red gram, ground, dry | 1107 | Davies and Warrington, 1986 |
| | | | soybean meal | 3441 | Mohamed et al, 1991 |
| **NUTS** | | | white beans, dry | 800 | Souci et al, 2000 |
| peanut butter | 1252 | Oberleas and Harland, 1981 | | | |
| peanuts, roasted | 175 | Oberleas and Harland, 1981 | **OTHER FOODS** | | |
| | | | cocoa mix | 270 | Harland and Oberleas, 1985 |
| | | | cocoa powder | 1880 | Oberleas and Harland, 1981 |

Sources:
Davies NT, S Warrington. The phytic acid, mineral, trace element, protein, and moisture content of UK Asian immigrant foods. *Hum Nutr Appl Nutr* 40A:49-59, 1986
Harland BF, D Oberleas. Phytate and zinc conents of coffees, cocoas, and teas. *J Food Sci* 50:832-833, 1985.
Harnandez-Unzon HY, ML Ortega-Delgado. Phytic acid in stored common bean seeds (*Phaseolus vulgaris* L.). *Plant Foods Hum Nutr* 39:209-221, 1989.
Mohamed AI, T Mebrahtu, M Rangappa. Nutrient composition and anti-nutritional factors in selected vegetable soybean (*Glycine Max L. Merr.*). *Plant Foods Hum Nutr* 41:89-100, 1991.
Oberleas D, BF Harland. Phytate content of foods: Effect on dietary zinc bioavailability. *J Am Diet Assoc* 79:433-436, 1981.
Reddy NR, SK Sathe, DK Salunkhe. Phytates in legumes and cereals. *Advances Food Res* 28:1-92, 1982.
Souci SW, W Fachmann, H Kraut. *Food Composition and NutritionTables.* Medpharm GmbH Scientific Publishers, Stuttgart, Germany and CRC Press, Washington, DC, 2000.

# *Plant Acids—Salicylic Acid*

| | SALICYLIC ACID (mg/100 g) | | SALICYLIC ACID (mg/100 g) |
|---|---|---|---|
| **BEVERAGES** | | currants, black, frozen | 3.06 |
| | | currants, dried | 5.80 |
| ale, stout | 0.30 | currants, red, frozen | 5.06 |
| brandy | 0.40 | custard apple, raw | 0.21 |
| Coca-Cola | 0.25 | date, dried | 4.50 |
| coffee instant powder | 0.29 | fig, canned | 0.25 |
| gin | 0.40 | fig, dried | 0.64 |
| hard cider | 0.17 | fig, raw | 0.18 |
| liqueur | 3.05 | grapefruit, raw | 0.68 |
| port | 2.80 | grapes, canned | 0.16 |
| rum | 1.02 | grapes, red, raw | 0.94 |
| sherry | 0.50 | grapes, green, raw | 1.88 |
| tea bag, black, Tetley | 5.57 | guava, canned | 2.02 |
| tea bag/leaves, black, Twinings | 3.70 | kiwifruit, raw | 0.32 |
| tea bag, herbal | 0.48 | lemon, raw | 0.18 |
| wine, Cabernet Sauvignon | 0.86 | loganberries, canned | 4.40 |
| wine, champagne | 1.02 | loquat, raw | 0.26 |
| wine, claret | 0.63 | lychee, canned | 0.36 |
| Wine, Riesling | 0.84 | mango, raw | 0.11 |
| wine, rose | 0.37 | mulberries, raw | 0.76 |
| wine, vermouth, dry | 0.46 | nectarine, raw | 0.49 |
| wine, white, dry | 0.10 | orange, raw | 2.39 |
| | | papaya (pawpaw), raw | 0.08 |
| **CANDY** | | passion fruit (granadilla), raw | 0.14 |
| caramels | 0.12 | peach, raw | 0.58 |
| licorice | 8.87 | peach, canned | 0.68 |
| peppermints, Lifesavers | 0.86 | pear, raw | 0.27 |
| | | persimmon, raw | 0.18 |
| **CHEESE** | | pineapple, canned | 136 |
| blue vein cheese | 0.05 | pineapple, raw | 2.10 |
| Camembert cheese | 0.01 | plum, green, raw | 0.10 |
| mozzarella cheese | 0.02 | plum, red, canned | 1.16 |
| | | plum, red prune, canned | 6.87 |
| **FISH AND SHELLFISH** | | plum, red, raw | 0.21 |
| prawn, raw | 0.04 | pomegranate, raw | 0.07 |
| scallops, raw | 0.02 | raspberries, frozen | 3.88 |
| | | raspberries, raw | 5.14 |
| **FRUIT JUICES** | | raisins, dried | 6.62 |
| apple juice | 0.19 | raisins, sultana, dried | 7.80 |
| apricot nectar | 0.14 | strawberries, raw | 1.36 |
| grapefruit juice | 0.42 | tamarillo, raw | 0.10 |
| grape juice, dark | 0.88 | tangelo, raw | 0.72 |
| grape juice, light | 0.18 | tangerine, raw | 0.56 |
| orange juice | 0.18 | watermelon, raw | 0.48 |
| peach nectar | 0.10 | youngberries, canned | 3.06 |
| pineapple juice | 0.16 | | |
| | | **NUTS AND SEEDS** | |
| **FRUITS** | | almonds, raw | 3.00 |
| apple, canned | 0.55 | Brazil nuts, raw | 0.46 |
| apple, raw, Granny Smith | 0.59 | cashews, raw | 0.07 |
| apple, raw, red varieties | 0.46 | coconut, dried | 0.26 |
| apricot, canned | 1.42 | hazelnuts, raw | 0.14 |
| apricot, raw | 2.58 | macadamia nuts, raw | 0.52 |
| avocado, raw | 0.60 | peanut butter | 0.23 |
| blackberries, canned | 1.86 | peanuts, raw | 1.12 |
| blueberries, canned | 2.76 | pecans, raw | 0.12 |
| boysenberries, canned | 2.04 | pine nuts, raw | 0.51 |
| cantaloupe, raw | 1.50 | pistachios, raw | 0.55 |
| cherries, sweet, canned | 2.78 | sesame seeds, dry | 0.23 |
| cherries, sweet, raw | 0.85 | sunflower seeds, dry | 0.12 |
| cherries, sour, canned | 0.30 | walnuts, raw | 0.30 |
| cranberries, canned | 1.64 | | |
| cranberry sauce, canned | 1.44 | | |

|  | SALICYLIC ACID (mg/100 g) |
|---|---|
| **SAUCES AND CONDIMENTS** | |
| horseradish, canned | 0.18 |
| olives, black, canned | 0.34 |
| olives, green, canned | 1.29 |
| pickle, gherkin | 6.14 |
| tabasco sauce, McIlhenny | 0.45 |
| Worcestershire sauce | 64.3 |
| **SPICES AND HERBS** | |
| allspice | 5.20 |
| aniseed | 22.80 |
| bay leaves | 2.52 |
| basil, ground | 3.40 |
| canella | 42.60 |
| cardamom | 7.70 |
| caraway seeds, ground | 2.82 |
| cayenne powder | 17.60 |
| celery seed powder | 10.10 |
| chili flakes | 1.38 |
| chili powder | 1.30 |
| cinnamon, ground | 15.20 |
| cloves | 5.74 |
| coriander leaves, raw | 0.20 |
| cumin powder | 45.00 |
| curry powder | 218.00 |
| dill seed, raw | 6.90 |
| dill seed, ground | 94.40 |
| fennel, ground | 0.80 |
| fenugreek seeds, ground | 12.20 |
| gram masala powder | 66.80 |
| ginger root, raw | 4.50 |
| mace powder | 32.20 |
| mint, raw | 9.40 |
| mustard powder | 26.00 |
| nutmeg | 2.40 |
| oregano | 66.00 |
| paprika, hot | 203.00 |
| paprika, sweet | 5.70 |
| parsley, raw | 0.08 |
| pepper, black | 6.20 |
| pepper, white | 1.10 |
| pimiento powder | 4.90 |
| rosemary, ground | 68.00 |
| sage leaves, dried | 21.70 |
| tarragon, ground | 34.80 |
| turmeric, ground | 76.40 |
| thyme, dry | 183.00 |
| vanilla flavoring, liquid | 1.44 |
| **SWEETENERS** | |
| honey | 6.30 |
| molasses | 0.22 |
| pancake syrup | 0.10 |
| **VEGETABLES** | |
| alfalfa sprouts, raw | 0.70 |
| asparagus, canned | 0.32 |

|  | SALICYLIC ACID (mg/100 g) |
|---|---|
| beet, canned | 0.32 |
| broadbeans, raw | 0.73 |
| broccoli, raw | 0.65 |
| Brussels sprouts, raw | 0.07 |
| cabbage, red, raw | 0.08 |
| carrot, raw | 0.23 |
| cauliflower, raw | 0.16 |
| chayote, raw | 0.01 |
| chicory, raw | 1.02 |
| chives, raw | 0.03 |
| corn, sweet, canned | 0.26 |
| corn, sweet, creamed, canned | 0.39 |
| cucumber, peeled, raw | 0.78 |
| eggplant, raw | 0.88 |
| endive, raw | 1.90 |
| garlic, raw | 0.10 |
| green beans, French, raw | 0.11 |
| leek, raw | 0.08 |
| mung bean sprouts, raw | 0.06 |
| mushrooms, champignon, raw | 1.26 |
| mushrooms, common white, raw | 0.24 |
| okra, canned | 0.59 |
| onion, raw | 0.16 |
| parsnip, raw | 0.45 |
| peas, green, raw | 0.04 |
| peas, yellow, split, dry | 0.02 |
| pepper, green chili, raw | 0.64 |
| pepper, green sweet, raw | 1.20 |
| pepper, red chili, raw | 1.20 |
| pepper, yellow-green chili, raw | 0.62 |
| pimiento, red, canned | 0.15 |
| potato, raw | 0.12 |
| pumpkin, raw | 0.12 |
| radish, red, raw | 1.24 |
| rhubarb, raw | 0.13 |
| shallot, raw | 0.03 |
| spinach, frozen | 0.16 |
| spinach, raw | 0.58 |
| squash, marrow, raw | 0.17 |
| squash, winter, raw | 0.63 |
| squash, zucchini, raw | 1.04 |
| sweet potato, yellow, raw | 0.48 |
| tomato, canned | 0.53 |
| tomato juice, canned | 0.13 |
| tomato paste, canned | 0.81 |
| tomato, raw | 0.13 |
| tomato sauce, canned | 1.52 |
| turnip, raw | 0.16 |
| water chestnuts, canned | 2.92 |
| **OTHER FOODS** | |
| cornmeal | 0.43 |
| liver, unspecified, raw | 0.05 |
| tomato soup | 0.47 |
| vinegar, white | 1.33 |

Source:
Swain AR, Dutton SP, Truswell AS. Salicylates in foods. *J Am Diet Assoc* 85:950–960, 1985.
See also: Perry CA, J Dwyer, JA Gelfand, RR Couris, WW McCloskey. Health effects of salicylates in foods and drugs. *Nutr Rev* S2:225–240, 1996 for information on the salicylate content of various medication.

# *Plant Sterols—Phytosterol*

| | PHYTOSTEROL (mg/100 g) | SR21 CODE NUMBER[1] | | PHYTOSTEROL (mg/100 g) | SR21 CODE NUMBER[1] |
|---|---|---|---|---|---|
| **CREAMS AND CREAMERS** | | | sesame oil | 865 | 04058 |
| creamer, liquid/frozen with hydrogenated vegetable oils | 13 | 01067 | sheanut oil (sheanut butter) | 357 | 04536 |
| creamer, liquid/frozen with lauric acid oils | 9 | 01068 | soy (hydrogenated) and cottonseed oil | 152 | 04543 |
| creamer, powdered | 32 | 01069 | soy (hydrogenated) and cottonseed oil (for bread) | 200 | 04546 |
| sour cream, cultured, imitation | 18 | 01074 | soy oil (hydrogenated) | 132 | 04034 |
| whipped topping, frozen | 23 | 01073 | sunflower oil, <60% linoleic acid | 100 | 04060 |
| whipped topping, pressurized | 20 | 01072 | sunflower oil, >60% linoleic acid | 100 | 04506 |
| | | | walnut oil | 176 | 04528 |
| **EGGS AND EGG SUBSTITUTES** | | | wheat germ oil | 553 | 04038 |
| egg, fried | 8 | 01128 | | | |
| egg substitute, frozen | 95 | 01142 | **FRUITS** | | |
| egg substitute, liquid | 4 | 01143 | apple, raw | 12 | 09003 |
| | | | apricot, raw | 18 | 09021 |
| **FATS—SHORTENINGS** | | | banana, raw | 16 | 09040 |
| shortening, beef tallow and cottonseed (for frying) | 32 | 04550 | cantaloupe, raw | 10 | 09181 |
| shortening, hydrogenated coconut oil and palm kernel oil (for confectionery) | 86 | 04551 | cherries, sweet, raw | 12 | 09070 |
| | | | fig, raw | 31 | 09089 |
| | | | grapefruit, white, raw | 17 | 09116 |
| shortening, lard and vegetable oil | 13 | 04544 | grapes, red/green, European, seedless, raw | 4 | 09132 |
| shortening, palm (for confectionery) | 49 | 04570 | lemon peel, raw | 35 | 09156 |
| | | | loquat, raw | 2 | 09174 |
| shortening, soy (hydrogenated) and cottonseed | 200 | 04547 | orange peel, raw | 34 | 09216 |
| | | | orange, California navel, raw | 24 | 09202 |
| shortening, soy (hydrogenated) and cottonseed (household) | 200 | 04031 | peach, raw | 10 | 09236 |
| | | | pear, raw | 8 | 09252 |
| shortening, soy (hydrogenated) and palm (household) | 148 | 04559 | persimmon, Japanese, raw | 4 | 09263 |
| | | | pineapple, raw | 6 | 09266 |
| shortening, soy (hydrogenated), 30% linoleic acid | 132 | 04552 | plum, raw | 7 | 09279 |
| | | | strawberries, raw | 12 | 09316 |
| shortening, sunflower oil, hydrogenated | 10 | 04545 | watermelon, raw | 2 | 09326 |
| | | | | | |
| | | | **GRAIN- AND VEGETABLE-BASED SNACK FOODS** | | |
| **FATS—SPREADS** | | | cheese puffs/twists (snack food) | 313 | 19008 |
| margarine, liquid | 174 | 04105 | Oriental snack mix, rice-based | 25 | 19031 |
| mayonnaise, diet, no cholesterol | 97 | 43599 | potato chips, from dried potatoes | 34 | 19410 |
| mayonnaise, imitation, soy | 62 | 04027 | sweet potato chips | 12 | 25012 |
| mayonnaise, safflower and soy | 347 | 04026 | | | |
| sandwich spread (mayonnaise-based) | 75 | 04030 | **GRAINS AND GRAIN PRODUCTS** | | |
| Smart Balance Omega Plus Spread with plant sterols and fish oil | 3 | 04677 | amaranth, whole grain, dry | 24 | 20001 |
| | | | biscuit, plain/buttermilk, homemade | 30 | 18016 |
| | | | bread, banana, homemade with margarine | 34 | 18019 |
| **FATS—VEGETABLE OILS** | | | bread, Irish soda, homemade | 13 | 18032 |
| almond oil | 266 | 04529 | bread, egg | 7 | 18027 |
| apricot kernel oil | 266 | 04530 | breadcrumbs, dry, grated | 8 | 18079 |
| babassu oil | 95 | 04534 | cornbread, homemade with 2% milk | 12 | 18024 |
| cocoa oil (cocoa butter) | 201 | 04501 | | | |
| coconut oil | 86 | 04047 | crackers, cheese with cheese filling | 44 | 18927 |
| corn oil | 968 | 04518 | | | |
| cottonseed oil | 324 | 04502 | crackers, round with peanut butter filling | 49 | 18231 |
| grapeseed oil | 180 | 04517 | | | |
| hazelnut oil | 120 | 04532 | English muffin, raisin cinnamon/apple cinnamon | 2 | 18262 |
| olive oil | 221 | 04053 | | | |
| palm kernel oil | 95 | 04513 | noodles, egg, homemade, cooked (egg in pasta dough) | 1 | 20097 |
| peanut oil | 207 | 04042 | | | |
| poppyseed oil | 276 | 04514 | pasta, homemade without egg, cooked | 2 | 20098 |
| rice bran oil | 1190 | 04037 | roll, pumpernickel | 3 | 43441 |
| safflower oil, >70% linoleic acid | 444 | 04510 | toaster pastry, apple/blueberry/ cherry/strawberry | 13 | 18362 |
| safflower oil, >70% oleic acid | 444 | 04511 | | | |

| | PHYTOSTEROL (mg/100 g) | SR21 CODE NUMBER[1] |
|---|---|---|
| **MEATS AND FISH** | | |
| fish sticks/pieces, frozen, reheated | 3 | 15027 |
| pork center loin (chops) with bone, lean and fat, pan-fried | 2 | 10179 |
| pork center loin (chops) with bone, lean, pan-fried | 3 | 10176 |
| pork center rib (chops) with bone, lean, pan-fried | 3 | 10197 |
| pork loin blade (chops) with bone, lean and fat, pan-fried | 3 | 10178 |
| pork loin blade (chops) with bone, lean, pan-fried | 4 | 10120 |
| pork top loin (chops), lean and fat, pan-fried | 2 | 10186 |
| pork top loin (chops), lean, pan-fried | 3 | 10181 |
| veal leg (top round), lean and fat, breaded, pan-fried | 3 | 17096 |
| veal leg (top round), lean, breaded, pan-fried | 3 | 17101 |
| **MEATS, LUNCHEON AND SNACK** | | |
| frankfurter, pork | 1 | 07939 |
| frankfurter, pork and beef with American cheese (cheesefurter) | 3 | 07016 |
| beerwurst, pork and beef | 3 | 07931 |
| bologna, turkey | 2 | 07011 |
| ham, sliced, regular (11% fat) | 5 | 07029 |
| pepperoni, pork and beef | 5 | 07057 |
| pickle and pimento loaf, pork | 21 | 07058 |
| pork and beef loaf, Dutch Brand | 3 | 07021 |
| **NUTS AND SEEDS** | | |
| almonds, dry-roasted | 118 | 12063 |
| almonds, oil-roasted | 130 | 12065 |
| cashews, dry-roasted | 158 | 12085 |
| chestnuts, European, raw | 22 | 12097 |
| coconut milk, raw | 1 | 12117 |
| coconut, raw | 47 | 12104 |
| filberts (hazelnuts), dried | 96 | 12120 |
| filberts (hazelnuts), dry-roasted | 110 | 12122 |
| macadamia nuts, dry-roasted | 114 | 12132 |
| macadamia nuts, raw | 116 | 12131 |
| peanut butter, chunk style/crunchy | 102 | 16097 |
| peanut butter, smooth | 102 | 16098 |
| peanuts, raw | 220 | 16087 |
| pecans, dried | 102 | 12142 |
| pecans, dry-roasted without salt | 85 | 12143 |
| pecans, oil-roasted | 108 | 12144 |
| pine nuts, pignolia, dried | 141 | 12147 |
| pistachios, dried | 214 | 12151 |
| pistachios, dry-roasted | 214 | 12152 |
| sesame seeds, whole, dried | 714 | 12023 |
| sunflower seed kernels, dried | 534 | 12036 |
| trail mix, tropical | 80 | 19061 |
| walnuts, black, dried | 108 | 12154 |
| walnuts, English/Persian, dried | 72 | 12155 |

| | PHYTOSTEROL (mg/100 g) | SR21 CODE NUMBER[1] |
|---|---|---|
| **SALAD DRESSINGS** | | |
| French salad dressing, homemade | 176 | 04133 |
| mayonnaise-type salad dressing | 97 | 04018 |
| Russian salad dressing, low/reduced calorie | 10 | 04022 |
| salad dressing, homemade, cooked | 24 | 04134 |
| vinegar and oil salad dressing, homemade | 66 | 04135 |
| **SAUCES, GRAVIES, AND CONDIMENTS** | | |
| catsup (ketchup) | 7 | 11935 |
| horseradish | 9 | 02055 |
| white sauce, medium, homemade | 29 | 06166 |
| white sauce, thick, homemade | 40 | 06167 |
| white sauce, thin, homemade | 16 | 06165 |
| pickle (cucumber), dill | 14 | 11937 |
| pickle (cucumber), sour | 14 | 11941 |
| pickle (cucumber), sweet gherkin | 14 | 11940 |
| **SPICES, HERBS, AND FLAVORINGS** | | |
| allspice, ground | 61 | 02001 |
| basil, dried | 106 | 02003 |
| black pepper | 92 | 02030 |
| capers, canned | 48 | 02054 |
| caraway seeds | 76 | 02005 |
| cardamon (cardamom) | 46 | 02006 |
| celery seeds | 60 | 02007 |
| chili powder | 83 | 02009 |
| chives, raw | 9 | 11156 |
| cinnamon, ground | 26 | 02010 |
| cloves, ground | 256 | 02011 |
| coriander seeds | 46 | 02013 |
| cumin (spice) | 68 | 02014 |
| curry powder | 72 | 02015 |
| dill seeds | 124 | 02016 |
| fennel seeds | 66 | 02018 |
| fenugreek seeds | 140 | 02019 |
| garlic powder | 8 | 02020 |
| ginger root, raw | 15 | 11216 |
| ginger, ground | 83 | 02021 |
| lemon grass (citronella), raw | 6 | 11972 |
| mace, ground | 73 | 02022 |
| marjoram, dried | 60 | 02023 |
| mustard seeds, yellow | 118 | 02024 |
| nutmeg, ground | 62 | 02025 |
| onion powder | 87 | 02026 |
| oregano, dried, ground | 203 | 02027 |
| paprika | 175 | 02028 |
| peppermint, raw | 13 | 02064 |
| poppy seeds | 89 | 02033 |
| poultry seasoning | 96 | 02034 |
| pumpkin pie spice | 71 | 02035 |
| red/cayenne pepper | 83 | 02031 |
| rosemary, raw | 44 | 02063 |
| sage, ground | 244 | 02038 |
| savory, ground | 31 | 02039 |
| spearmint, dried | 82 | 02066 |
| spearmint, raw | 10 | 02065 |
| tarragon, ground | 81 | 02041 |
| thyme, ground | 163 | 02042 |
| turmeric, ground | 82 | 02043 |
| white pepper | 55 | 02032 |

| | PHYTOSTEROL (mg/100 g) | SR21 CODE NUMBER[1] |
|---|---|---|
| **VEGETABLES** | | |
| **FLOWER, STEM, AND STALK VEGETABLES** | | |
| asparagus, raw | 24 | 11011 |
| cauliflower, raw | 18 | 11135 |
| celery, boiled, drained | 7 | 11144 |
| celery, raw | 6 | 11143 |
| **FRUIT (SEED-CONTAINING) VEGETABLES** | | |
| banana pepper, raw | 3 | 11976 |
| cucumber, raw | 14 | 11205 |
| eggplant (aubergine), raw | 7 | 11209 |
| okra, raw | 24 | 11278 |
| pimiento pepper, canned | 9 | 11943 |
| pumpkin winter squash, raw | 12 | 11422 |
| serrano pepper, raw | 6 | 11977 |
| sweet pepper, green, boiled, drained | 9 | 11334 |
| sweet pepper, green, raw | 9 | 11333 |
| sweet pepper, red, boiled, drained | 9 | 11823 |
| tomato, orange, raw | 4 | 11695 |
| tomato, red, boiled | 9 | 11530 |
| tomato, red, cherry, raw | 7 | 11529 |
| tomato, red, Italian, raw | 7 | 11529 |
| tomato, red, plum, raw | 7 | 11529 |
| tomato, red, raw | 7 | 11529 |
| tomato, red, stewed | 14 | 11660 |
| tomato, yellow, raw | 6 | 11696 |
| **LEAFY VEGETABLES** | | |
| beet greens, raw | 21 | 11086 |
| Brussels sprouts, raw | 24 | 11098 |
| cabbage, green/white, boiled, drained | 10 | 11110 |
| cabbage, green/white, raw | 11 | 11109 |
| celtuce leaves, raw | 11 | 11145 |
| cilantro (coriander), raw | 5 | 11165 |
| grape leaves, raw | 21 | 11974 |
| lettuce, iceberg, raw | 10 | 11252 |
| lettuce, looseleaf (leaf), raw | 38 | 11253 |
| parsley, raw | 5 | 11297 |
| spinach soufflé, homemade | 2 | 11658 |
| spinach, raw | 9 | 11457 |
| turnip greens, raw | 12 | 11568 |
| **LEGUMES (BEANS AND PEAS)** | | |
| adzuki beans, mature, dry | 76 | 16001 |
| broadbeans (fava beans) in pod, immature, raw | 22 | 11973 |
| broadbeans (fava beans), mature, dry | 124 | 16052 |
| chickpeas (garbanzo beans), mature, dry | 35 | 16056 |

| | PHYTOSTEROL (mg/100 g) | SR21 CODE NUMBER[1] |
|---|---|---|
| hummus from chickpeas (garbanzo beans), homemade | 11 | 16137 |
| kidney beans, all types, mature, dry | 127 | 16027 |
| lentils, pink, mature, dry | 57 | 16144 |
| mung beans, mature, dry | 23 | 16080 |
| peas, split, yellow and green, mature, dry | 135 | 16085 |
| soybeans, green/immature (edamame), boiled, drained | 50 | 11451 |
| soybeans, green/immature (edamame), raw | 50 | 11450 |
| soybeans, mature, dry | 161 | 16108 |
| **SPROUT AND SHOOT VEGETABLES** | | |
| bamboo shoots, raw | 19 | 11026 |
| mung bean sprouts, raw | 15 | 11043 |
| **TUBER AND ROOT VEGETABLES** | | |
| beet, raw | 25 | 11080 |
| onion, white, boiled, drained | 18 | 11283 |
| onion, white, raw | 15 | 11282 |
| potato pancake, homemade | 9 | 11672 |
| potato, mashed, from granules with milk | 13 | 11383 |
| potato, mashed, homemade with whole milk and butter | 19 | 11371 |
| potato, raw | 5 | 11352 |
| potato, russet, raw | 5 | 11353 |
| potato, white-skinned, raw | 4 | 11354 |
| radish, red, raw | 7 | 11429 |
| shallots, raw | 5 | 11677 |
| sweet potato, raw | 12 | 11507 |
| taro, raw | 19 | 11518 |
| turnip, raw | 7 | 11564 |
| **MISCELLANEOUS FOODS** | | |
| biscuit with egg, fast food | 13 | 21002 |
| cheese sauce, homemade | 11 | 01164 |
| icing/frosting, chocolate, from mix made with margarine | 29 | 19372 |
| icing/frosting, chocolate, ready-to-serve | 34 | 19226 |
| jam/preserves | 12 | 19297 |
| oxtail soup, dehydrated, reconstituted | 2 | 06495 |
| Snickers Marathon Energy Bar, caramel nut rush (sport food) | 7 | 25015 |
| zwieback toast, Gerber | 31 | 03217 |

[1]Code numbers for foods in the USDA National Nutrient Database for Standard Reference, Release 21, 2008.

Source:
USDA National Nutrient Database for Standard Reference, Release 21, 2008. Available at: http://www.nal.usda.gov/fnic/foodcomp.search/.

# Plant Sterols—Beta-Sitosterol, Campesterol, and Stigmasterol

| | BETA-SITOSTEROL (mg/100 g) | CAMPESTEROL (mg/100 g) | STIGMASTEROL (mg/100 g) | SOURCE/SR21 CODE NUMBER[1] |
|---|---|---|---|---|
| **CANDY** | | | | |
| milk chocolate | 37 | 6 | 16 | 19120 |
| milk chocolate chips | 37 | 6 | 16 | 19120 |
| **CEREALS, GRAINS, AND GRAIN-BASED PRODUCTS** | | | | |
| amaranth, whole grain, dry | | | 2 | Souci et al, 2000 |
| buckwheat flour, whole groats | 16 | 4 | 1 | Souci et al, 2000 |
| buckwheat groats, dry | 164 | 20 | 8 | Souci et al, 2000 |
| cookie, chocolate sandwich with extra crème filling | 34 | 13 | 11 | 18168 |
| corn chips | 148 | 51 | 21 | 19003 |
| corn, whole grain, dry | 120 | 32 | 21 | Souci et al, 2000 |
| crackers, round with peanut butter filling | 0 | 0 | 0 | 18231 |
| tortilla chips | 61 | 24 | 14 | 19056 |
| wheat cereal, whole grain, cooked | 40 | 27 | | Souci et al, 2000 |
| **EGGS AND EGG DISHES** | | | | |
| egg, omelet, plain | 12 | 3 | 2 | 01130 |
| egg, scrambled with milk | 11 | 3 | 1 | 01132 |
| spinach soufflé, homemade | 0 | 0 | 0 | 11658 |
| **FATS, OILS, AND SPREADS** | | | | |
| butter | 4 | 0 | 0 | 01001 |
| butter, sweet (unsalted) | 4 | 0 | 0 | 01145 |
| canola oil | 413 | 241 | 3 | 04582 |
| canola oil, Natreon | 426 | 202 | | 04678 |
| cocoa oil (cocoa butter) | 138 | 22 | 61 | Souci et al, 2000 |
| coconut oil | 48 | 9 | 13 | Souci et al, 2000 |
| corn and canola oil | 419 | 233 | 9 | 42289 |
| corn oil | 595 | 179 | 51 | Souci et al, 2000 |
| cottonseed oil | 303 | 20 | | Souci et al, 2000 |
| grapeseed oil | 255 | 36 | 36 | Souci et al, 2000 |
| linseed oil | 206 | 117 | 30 | Souci et al, 2000 |
| margarine, corn and soy, 80% fat, stick | 275 | 75 | 35 | 04628 |
| margarine, fat-free, tub | 2 | 1 | 1 | 04631 |
| margarine, soy, 70% fat | 81 | 31 | 25 | 04629 |
| margarine, stick/tub composite, 60% fat | 74 | 28 | 25 | 04614 |
| margarine, unspecified oils | 275 | 75 | 35 | 04132 |
| mayonnaise, soy | 102 | 39 | 39 | 04025 |
| olive oil | 119 | 3 | 1 | Souci et al, 2000 |
| Smart Balance Omega Plus Spread with plant sterols and fish oil | 3 | 0 | 0 | 04677 |
| palm kernel oil | 53 | 8 | 10 | Souci et al, 2000 |
| palm oil | 28 | 7 | 4 | Souci et al, 2000 |
| peanut oil | 162 | 29 | 26 | Souci et al, 2000 |
| poppyseed oil | 173 | 58 | 16 | Souci et al, 2000 |
| pumpkinseed oil | 6.7 | 19 | 20 | Souci et al, 2000 |
| safflower oil | 180 | 46 | 30 | Souci et al, 2000 |
| sesame oil | 430 | 164 | 60 | Souci et al, 2000 |
| sheanut oil (sheanut butter) | | | 18 | Souci et al, 2000 |
| soy oil, salad/cooking | 172 | 62 | 59 | 04044 |
| sunflower oil | 210 | 32 | 35 | Souci et al, 2000 |
| walnut oil | 154 | 9 | | Souci et al, 2000 |
| wheat germ oil | 1606 | 611 | 19 | Souci et al, 2000 |
| **FRUITS** | | | | |
| apple, raw | 11 | 1 | | Souci et al, 2000 |
| apricot, raw | 16 | 1 | | Souci et al, 2000 |
| avocado, California, raw | 76 | 5 | 2 | 09038 |
| avocado, raw | 76 | 5 | 2 | 09037 |
| banana, raw | 11 | 2 | 3 | Souci et al, 2000 |
| cantaloupe, raw | 8 | | | Souci et al, 2000 |
| cherries, sweet, raw | 12 | | | Souci et al, 2000 |
| fig, raw | 27 | 1 | 31 | Souci et al, 2000 |
| grapefruit, raw | 13 | 2 | 2 | Souci et al, 2000 |

| | BETA-SITOSTEROL (mg/100 g) | CAMPESTEROL (mg/100 g) | STIGMASTEROL (mg/100 g) | SOURCE/SR21 CODE NUMBER[1] |
|---|---|---|---|---|
| grapes, purple, raw | 3 | | | Souci et al, 2000 |
| lemon, raw | 8 | 2 | 1 | Souci et al, 2000 |
| orange, raw | 17 | 4 | 2 | Souci et al, 2000 |
| peach, raw | 6 | 1 | 3 | Souci et al, 2000 |
| pear, raw | 7 | | | Souci et al, 2000 |
| pineapple, raw | 4 | 1 | | Souci et al, 2000 |
| plum, raw | 6 | | | Souci et al, 2000 |
| pomegranate, raw | 4 | 1 | 0 | 09286 |
| strawberries, raw | 10 | | | Souci et al, 2000 |
| watermelon, raw | 1 | | | Souci et al, 2000 |
| **NUTS AND SEEDS** | | | | |
| almonds, dry-roasted | 110 | 3 | 4 | 12063 |
| almonds, oil-roasted | 118 | 9 | 3 | 12065 |
| almonds, raw | 132 | 5 | 4 | 12061 |
| cashews, raw | 130 | 13 | | Souci et al, 2000 |
| chestnuts, European, raw | 18 | 2 | 2 | Souci et al, 2000 |
| coconut, raw | 27 | 3 | 7 | Souci et al, 2000 |
| filberts (hazelnuts), dried | 89 | 6 | 1 | 12120 |
| filberts (hazelnuts), dry-roasted | 103 | 6 | 1 | 12122 |
| macadamia nuts, dry-roasted | 107 | 7 | 0 | 12132 |
| macadamia nuts, raw | 108 | 8 | 0 | 12131 |
| peanuts, raw | 142 | 24 | 23 | Souci et al, 2000 |
| pecans, dried | 89 | 5 | 3 | 12142 |
| pecans, dry-roasted without salt | 78 | 4 | 2 | 12143 |
| pecans, oil-roasted | 96 | 7 | 5 | 12144 |
| pistachios, dried | 198 | 10 | 5 | 12151 |
| pistachios, dry-roasted | 199 | 10 | 4 | 12152 |
| pistachios, raw | 198 | 10 | 5 | Souci et al, 2000 |
| walnuts, black, dried | 103 | 5 | 0 | 12154 |
| walnuts, English/Persian, dried | 64 | 7 | 1 | 12155 |
| walnuts, English/Persian, raw | 64 | 7 | | Souci et al, 2000 |
| sunflower seed kernels, dried | 95 | 14 | 15 | Souci et al, 2000 |
| **VEGETABLES** | | | | |
| asparagus, raw | 14 | 1 | 4 | Souci et al, 2000 |
| broadbeans (fava beans) in pod, immature, raw | 18 | 3 | 1 | 11973 |
| Brussels sprouts, raw | 17 | 6 | | Souci et al, 2000 |
| carrot, raw | 7 | 1 | 3 | Souci et al, 2000 |
| cauliflower, raw | 12 | 3 | 2 | Souci et al, 2000 |
| cilantro, raw | 2 | 0 | 3 | 11165 |
| cucumber, raw | 14 | | | Souci et al, 2000 |
| eggplant (aubergine), raw | 3 | | 2 | Souci et al, 2000 |
| grape leaves, raw | 20 | | 2 | 11974 |
| green peas, raw | 106 | 10 | 10 | Souci et al, 2000 |
| lemon grass (citronella), raw (herb) | 4 | 1 | 1 | 11972 |
| lentils, pink, mature, dry | 47 | 6 | 4 | 16144 |
| lettuce, looseleaf (leaf), raw | 5 | 1 | 4 | Souci et al, 2000 |
| okra, raw | 15 | 3 | 6 | Souci et al, 2000 |
| onion, white, raw | 12 | 1 | | Souci et al, 2000 |
| pepper, banana, raw | 2 | 1 | 0 | 11976 |
| pepper, serrano, raw | 3 | 2 | 0 | 11977 |
| potato, mashed, homemade with whole milk and butter | 12 | 3 | 2 | 11371 |
| potato, raw | 3 | | 1 | Souci et al, 2000 |
| pumpkin winter squash, raw | 12 | | | Souci et al, 2000 |
| radish, red, raw | 6 | 5 | | Souci et al, 2000 |
| tomato, red, cherry, raw | 3 | 1 | 4 | Souci et al, 2000 |
| tomato, red, Italian, raw | 3 | 1 | 4 | Souci et al, 2000 |
| tomato, red, plum, raw | 3 | 1 | 4 | Souci et al, 2000 |
| tomato, red, raw | 3 | 1 | 4 | Souci et al, 2000 |
| buttermilk salad dressing, lite | 38 | 20 | 9 | 43215 |
| **MISCELLANEOUS FOODS** | | | | |
| baking chocolate (unsweetened) | 85 | 13 | 38 | 19078 |
| Snickers Marathon Energy Bar, caramel nut rush | 5 | 1 | 2 | 25015 |

[1]Code numbers for foods in the USDA National Nutrient Database for Standard Reference, Release 21, 2008.

Sources:
Souci SW, Fachmann W, Kraut H. Food Composition and Nutrition Tables. Medpharm GmbH Scientific Publishers, Stuttgart, Germany, and CRC Press: Washington, DC, 2000.
US Department of Agriculture. Nutrient Database for Standard Reference, Release 21, 2008. Available at: http://www.nal.usda.gov/fnic/foodcomp/search/.

# *Purines*

| | PURINES[1] (mg/100 g) | SOURCE[2] | | PURINES[1] (mg/100 g) | SOURCE[2] |
|---|---|---|---|---|---|
| **BEVERAGES** | | | cherries, sweet, raw | 17 | Souci et al, 2000 |
| beer, light | 14 | Souci et al, 2000 | currants, red, raw | 17 | Souci et al, 2000 |
| beer, no alcohol | 8 | Souci et al, 2000 | date, dried | 35 | Souci et al, 2000 |
| beer, pilsener, German | 13 | Souci et al, 2000 | elderberries, raw | 33 | Souci et al, 2000 |
| | | | fig, dried | 64 | Souci et al, 2000 |
| **CHEESE AND YOGURT** | | | gooseberries, raw | 16 | Souci et al, 2000 |
| brie cheese | 7 | Souci et al, 2000 | grapes, | 27 | Souci et al, 2000 |
| Camembert cheese | 4 | Souci et al, 2000 | kiwifruit, raw | 19 | Souci et al, 2000 |
| cheddar cheese | 7 | Souci et al, 2000 | orange, raw | 19 | Souci et al, 2000 |
| cottage cheese | 8 | Brule et al, 1988 | peach, raw | 21 | Souci et al, 2000 |
| Edam/brie cheese | 6 | Brule et al, 1988 | pear, raw | 12 | Souci et al, 2000 |
| Limburger cheese | 32 | Souci et al, 2000 | pineapple, raw | 19 | Souci et al, 2000 |
| processed cheese | 2 | Brule et al, 1988 | plum, raw | 24 | Souci et al, 2000 |
| yogurt, plain | 7 | Brule et al, 1988 | prune, dried | 64 | Souci et al, 2000 |
| | | | raisins | 107 | Souci et al, 2000 |
| **FISH AND SHELLFISH** | | | raspberries, raw | 18 | Souci et al, 2000 |
| anchovies, canned | 321 | Clifford and Story, 1976 | quince, raw | 30 | Souci et al, 2000 |
| anchovies, raw | 411 | Clifford and Story, 1976 | strawberries, raw | 21 | Souci et al, 2000 |
| carp, raw | 160 | Souci et al, 2000 | | | |
| caviar | 144 | Souci et al, 2000 | **GRAINS AND GRAIN FRACTIONS** | | |
| caviar substitute | 18 | Souci et al, 2000 | barley, whole grain without husk | 94 | Souci et al, 2000 |
| clams, canned | 62 | Clifford and Story, 1976 | millet, shucked grain | 62 | Souci et al, 2000 |
| clams, raw | 136 | Clifford and Story, 1976 | oats, whole grain without husk | 94 | Souci et al, 2000 |
| coalfish (saithe), raw | 163 | Souci et al, 2000 | rice, white, boiled | 6 | Brule et al, 1988 |
| cod, raw | 109 | Souci et al, 2000 | rye, whole grain | 51 | Souci et al, 2000 |
| crayfish, raw | 60 | Souci et al, 2000 | wheat flour | 12 | Brule et al, 1988 |
| eel, raw | 139 | Souci et al, 2000 | wheat, whole grain | 51 | Souci et al, 2000 |
| eel, smoked | 78 | Souci et al, 2000 | | | |
| haddock, boiled | 95 | Brule et al, 1989 | **GRAIN PRODUCTS** | | |
| haddock, broiled | 119/193 | Brule et al, 1989/1992 | bread, crusty | 16 | Brule et al, 1988 |
| haddock, raw | 102 | Brule et al, 1989 | bread, white | 12 | Brule et al, 1988 |
| herring, canned | 378 | Clifford and Story, 1976 | corn cereal | 1 | Brule et al, 1988 |
| herring roe | 190 | Souci et al, 2000 | crispbread | 60 | Souci et al, 2000 |
| lobster, raw | 118 | Souci et al, 2000 | pasta with egg, dry | 40 | Souci et al, 200 |
| mackerel, canned | 246 | Clifford and Story, 1976 | roll | 21 | Souci et al, 2000 |
| mackerel, raw | 194 | Clifford and Story, 1976 | waffle/pancake | 4 | Brule et al, 1988 |
| mussels, raw | 112 | Souci et al, 2000 | | | |
| ocean perch (redfish), raw | 241 | Souci et al, 2000 | **MEATS** | | |
| oysters, canned | 107 | Clifford and Story, 1976 | beef brisket, raw | 90 | Souci et al, 2000 |
| pike, raw | 140 | Souci et al, 2000 | beef chuck, raw | 120 | Souci et al, 2000 |
| pike perch, raw | 110 | Souci et al, 2000 | beef fillet, raw | 110 | Souci et al, 2000 |
| plaice, raw | 93 | Souci et al, 2000 | beef forerib, raw | 120 | Souci et al, 2000 |
| salmon, canned | 88 | Clifford and Story, 1976 | beef, ground, raw | 90 | Brule et al, 1988 |
| salmon, raw | 250 | Clifford and Story, 1976 | beef roast, raw | 125 | Brule et al, 1988 |
| sardines, canned | 399 | Clifford and Story, 1976 | beef roast/stew, raw | 109 | Brule et al, 1988 |
| sardines, raw | 345 | Clifford and Story, 1976 | beef rump, raw | 120 | Souci et al, 2000 |
| scallops, raw | 136 | Souci et al, 2000 | beef roast (sirloin), raw | 110 | Souci et al, 2000 |
| shrimp, canned | 234 | Clifford and Story, 1976 | beef shoulder, raw | 110 | Souci et al, 2000 |
| sole, raw | 131 | Souci et al, 2000 | beef sirloin, raw | 125 | Brule et al, 1988 |
| sprat, smoked | 840 | Souci et al, 2000 | beef steak, boiled | 108/121 | Brule et al, 1988/1989 |
| squid, raw | 135 | Clifford and Story, 1976 | beef steak, raw | 106 | Brule et al, 1989 |
| trout, raw | 297 | Souci et al, 2000 | lamb roast/chop, raw | 128 | Brule et al, 1988 |
| tuna, canned | 142 | Clifford and Story, 1976 | pork, cured | 86 | Brule et al, 1988 |
| whitefish, frozen | 129 | Brule et al, 1988 | pork chop, raw | 145 | Souci et al, 2002 |
| whitefish, raw | 116 | Brule et al, 1988 | pork chuck, raw | 140 | Souci et al, 2000 |
| | | | pork fillet, raw | 150 | Souci et al, 2000 |
| **FRUITS** | | | pork leg, raw | 160 | Souci et al, 2000 |
| apple, raw | 14 | Souci et al, 2000 | pork roast/chop, raw | 120 | Brule et al, 1988 |
| apricot, dried | 73 | Souci et al, 2000 | pork sausage, raw | 101 | Souci et al, 2000 |
| avocado, raw | 19 | Souci et al, 2000 | pork shoulder, raw | 150 | Souci et al, 2000 |
| banana, raw | 57 | Souci et al, 2000 | veal cutlet, raw | 140/143 | Souci et al, 2000/ Brule et al, 1988 |
| bilberries (huckleberries), raw | 22 | Souci et al, 2000 | | | |
| cantaloupe, raw | 33 | Souci et al, 2000 | veal knuckle, raw | 150 | Souci et al, 2000 |
| cherries, morello, raw | 17 | Souci et al, 2000 | veal leg, raw | 150 | Souci et al, 2000 |

| | PURINES[1] (mg/100 g) | SOURCE[2] | | PURINES[1] (mg/100 g) | SOURCE[2] |
|---|---|---|---|---|---|
| veal neck, raw | 150 | Souci et al, 2000 | chicken, broiler, drumstick, raw | 132 | Young, 1980 |
| veal sausage, raw | 91 | Souci et al, 2000 | chicken, broiler, gizzard, raw | 131 | Young, 1980 |
| veal shoulder, raw | 140 | Souci et al, 2000 | chicken, broiler, neck and back, raw | 94 | Young, 1980 |
| | | | chicken, broiler, neck, raw | 123 | Young, 1980 |
| **MEATS, GAME** | | | chicken, broiler, skin, raw | 105 | Young, 1980 |
| hare, raw | 105 | Souci et al, 2000 | chicken, broiler, thigh, raw | 127/152 | Young, 1980/1982 |
| horse, raw | 200 | Souci et al, 2000 | chicken, broiler, thigh, roasted | 149 | Young, 1982 |
| rabbit, raw | 132 | Souci et al, 2000 | chicken heart, raw | 223 | Clifford and Story, 1976 |
| venison, back, raw | 105 | Souci et al, 2000 | chicken liver, raw | 236/243 | Young, 1980/Clifford |
| venison, leg, raw | 138 | Souci et al, 2000 | | | and Story, 1976 |
| | | | chicken, roaster | 115 | Souci et al, 2000 |
| **MEATS, INTERNAL ORGANS** | | | chicken, stewer, breast, raw | 178 | Young, 1983 |
| belly, pork, raw | 100 | Souci et al, 2000 | chicken, stewer, breast, stewed | 184 | Young, 1983 |
| belly, pork, smoked, dried | 127 | Souci et al, 2000 | chicken, stewer, skin, raw | 59 | Young, 1983 |
| brains, beef, raw | 162 | Clifford and Story, 1976 | chicken, stewer, skin, stewed | 94 | Young, 1983 |
| brains, calf, raw | 92 | Souci et al, 2000 | chicken, stewer, thigh, raw | 144 | Young, 1983 |
| brains, ox, raw | 75 | Souci et al, 2000 | chicken, stewer, thigh, stewed | 146 | Young, 1983 |
| brains, pork, raw | 83 | Souci et al, 2000 | duck, raw | 138 | Souci et al, 2000 |
| heart, beef, raw | 171 | Clifford and Story, 1976 | goose, raw | 165 | Souci et al, 2000 |
| heart, lamb, raw | 171 | Clifford and Story, 1976 | turkey with skin, raw | 150 | Souci et al, 2000 |
| heart, ox, raw | 256 | Souci et al, 2000 | | | |
| heart, pork, raw | 530 | Souci et al, 2000 | **VEGETABLES** | | |
| heart, sheep, raw | 241 | Souci et al, 2000 | artichoke, raw | 78 | Souci et al, 2000 |
| kidney, beef, raw | 213 | Clifford and Story, 1976 | asparagus, raw | 23 | Souci et al, 2000 |
| kidney, calf, raw | 218 | Souci et al, 2000 | bamboo shoots, raw | 29 | Souci et al, 2000 |
| kidney, ox, raw | 269 | Souci et al, 2000 | beet, raw | 19 | Souci et al, 2000 |
| kidney, pork, raw | 334 | Souci et al, 2000 | broccoli, raw | 81 | Souci et al, 2000 |
| liver, beef, boiled | 237 | Brule et al, 1989 | Brussels sprouts, raw | 69 | Souci et al, 2000 |
| liver, beef, broiled | 236/184 | Brule et al, 1989/1992 | cabbage, red, raw | 32 | Souci et al, 2000 |
| liver, beef, raw | 202 | Brule et al, 1989 | cabbage, savoy, raw | 37 | Souci et al, 2000 |
| liver, calf, raw | 460 | Souci et al, 2000 | cabbage, white, raw | 22 | Souci et al, 2000 |
| liver, lamb, raw | 147 | Clifford and Story, 1976 | carrot, raw | 17 | Souci et al, 2000 |
| liver, ox, raw | 554 | Souci et al, 2000 | cauliflower, raw | 51 | Souci et al, 2000 |
| liver, pork, raw | 289 | Clifford and Story, 1976 | celeriac, raw | 30 | Souci et al, 2000 |
| lung, calf, raw | 147 | Souci et al, 2000 | chicory, raw | 12 | Souci et al, 2000 |
| lung, ox, raw | 399 | Souci et al, 2000 | Chinese cabbage, raw | 21 | Souci et al, 2000 |
| lung, pork, raw | 434 | Souci et al, 2000 | chives, raw | 67 | Souci et al, 2000 |
| spleen, calf, raw | 343 | Souci et al, 2000 | corn, sweet, raw | 52 | Souci et al, 2000 |
| spleen, ox, raw | 444 | Souci et al, 2000 | cress, raw | 28 | Souci et al, 2000 |
| spleen, pork, raw | 516 | Souci et al, 2000 | cucumber, raw | 7 | Souci et al, 2000 |
| spleen, sheep, raw | 773 | Souci et al, 2000 | eggplant, raw | 21 | Souci et al, 2000 |
| sweetbread (neck), calf, raw | 1260 | Souci et al, 2000 | endive, raw | 17 | Souci et al, 2000 |
| tongue, ox, raw | 160 | Souci et al, 2000 | fennel leaves, raw | 14 | Souci et al, 2000 |
| tongue, pork, raw | 136 | Souci et al, 2000 | kale, raw | 48 | Souci et al, 2000 |
| | | | kohlrabi, raw | 25 | Souci et al, 2000 |
| **MEATS, LUNCHEON** | | | lamb's lettuce, raw | 38 | Souci et al, 2000 |
| black pudding (blutwurst) | 55 | Souci et al, 2000 | leek, raw | 74 | Souci et al, 2000 |
| corned beef | 57 | Souci et al, 2000 | lettuce, raw | 13 | Souci et al, 2000 |
| frankfurter | 89 | Souci et al, 2000 | mushrooms, boletus, dried | 488 | Souci et al, 2000 |
| liverwurst (liver sausage) | 165 | Souci et al, 2000 | mushrooms, boletus, raw | 92 | Souci et al, 2000 |
| ham, cooked | 131 | Souci et al, 2000 | mushrooms, chanterelle, canned | 6 | Souci et al, 2000 |
| mortadella | 96 | Souci et al, 2000 | mushrooms, chanterelle, raw | 17 | Souci et al, 2000 |
| salami | 104 | Souci et al, 2000 | mushrooms, canned | 25 | Brule et al, 1988 |
| Vienna sausage | 78 | Souci et al, 2000 | mushrooms, common white, raw | 58/47 | Souci et al, 2000/ |
| | | | | | Brule et al, 1988 |
| **NUTS AND SEEDS** | | | mushrooms, morel, raw | 30 | Souci et al, 2000 |
| almonds, raw | 37 | Souci et al, 2000 | mushrooms, oyster, raw | 50 | Souci et al, 2000 |
| Brazil nuts, raw | 23 | Souci et al, 2000 | onion, raw | 13 | Souci et al, 2000 |
| hazelnuts, raw | 37 | Souci et al, 2000 | parsley, raw | 57 | Souci et al, 2000 |
| peanuts, raw | 79 | Souci et al, 2000 | pepper, sweet green, raw | 55 | Souci et al, 2000 |
| poppy seeds, dried | 170 | Souci et al, 2000 | potato, raw | 16 | Souci et al, 2000 |
| sesame seeds, dried | 62 | Souci et al, 2000 | potato, baked | 18 | Souci et al, 2000 |
| sunflower seeds, dried | 143 | Souci et al, 2000 | pumpkin, raw | 44 | Souci et al, 2000 |
| walnuts, raw | 25 | Souci et al, 2000 | radish, raw | 13 | Souci et al, 2000 |
| | | | rhubarb, raw | 12 | Souci et al, 2000 |
| **POULTRY** | | | salsify, black (viper's grass), raw | 71 | Souci et al, 2000 |
| chicken, broiler, breast, raw | 131/168 | Young, 1980/1982 | sauerkraut | 16 | Souci et al, 2000 |
| chicken, broiler, breast, roasted | 179 | Young, 1982 | soybean sprouts, raw | 80 | Souci et al, 2000 |

| | PURINES[1] (mg/100 g) | SOURCE[2] | | PURINES[1] (mg/100 g) | SOURCE[2] |
|---|---|---|---|---|---|
| spinach, raw | 57 | Souci et al, 2000 | peas, green, dry | 84 | Souci et al, 2000 |
| squash, zucchini, raw | 24 | Souci et al, 2000 | peas, split, dry | 195 | Clifford and Story, 1976 |
| tomato, raw | 11 | Souci et al, 2000 | pinto beans, dry | 171 | Clifford and Story, 1976 |
| | | | red beans, dry | 162 | Clifford and Story, 1976 |
| **VEGETABLES—LEGUMES** | | | soybeans, boiled | 185 | Brule et al, 1992 |
| chickpeas, dry | 56 | Clifford and Story, 1976 | white beans, small, dry | 202 | Clifford and Story, 1976 |
| cowpeas, dry | 230 | Clifford and Story, 1976 | | | |
| cranberry beans, dry | 75 | Clifford and Story, 1976 | **OTHER FOODS** | | |
| French beans, dry | 45 | Souci et al, 2000 | cocoa powder | 71 | Souci et al, 2000 |
| great northern beans, dry | 213 | Clifford and Story, 1976 | olives, green marinated | 29 | Souci et al, 2000 |
| lentils, dry | 222 | Clifford and Story, 1976 | tofu | 68 | Souci et al, 2000 |
| lima beans, baby, dry | 144 | Clifford and Story, 1976 | yeast, bakers, compressed | 680 | Souci et al, 2000 |
| lima beans, large, dry | 149 | Clifford and Story, 1976 | yeast, brewers, dried | 1810 | Souci et al, 2000 |
| mungo (black gram) beans, dry | 222 | Souci et al, 2000 | | | |

[1]Purine values are the sum of adenine, guanine, xanthine, and hypoxanthine. In gout, uric acid (a metabolite of purines) tends to accumulate and deposit in the toe joint and other joints. Drug treatment is generally prescribed; however, dietary restriction of purine-yielding foods may also be advised. Foods lowest in purines (0–50 mg/100 g) include fruits, fruit juices, and most vegetables (with a few exceptions); nonwhole grain products; nuts; milk and cheeses; eggs; beverages (coffee, tea, sodas); fats; and sweeteners. Foods highest in purines (150–825 mg/100 g) include anchovies, brains, beef kidney, game meats, gravies, herring, calf/beef liver, mackerel, meat extracts, sardines, scallops, and sweetbreads. Other foods that are high in purines (50–150 mg/100 g) include several vegetables (asparagus, cauliflower, mushrooms, green peas, spinach); legumes (beans, lentils, peas); whole grain products; fresh and saltwater fish and shellfish; and meats, meat soups, and poultry.

[2]Values from the sources have been rounded to the nearest whole number. Values from Souci et al, 2000, were expressed as milligrams of uric acid per 100 grams.

Sources:
Brule D, G Sarwar, L Savoie. Changes in serum and urinary uric acid levels in normal human subjects fed purine-rich foods containing different amounts of adenine and hypoxanthine. *J Am Coll Nutr* 11:353-358, 1992.
Brule D, G Sarwar, L Savoie. Effects of methods of cooking on free and total purine bases in meat and fish. *J Inst Can Sci Technol Aliment* 22:248-251, 1989.
Brule D, G Sarwar, L Savoie. Purine content of selected Canadian food products. *J Food Comp Anal* 1:130-138, 1988.
Clifford AJ, Dl Story. Levels of purines in foods and their metabolic effects in rats. *J Nutr* 106:435-442, 1976.
Souci SW, W Fachmann, H Kraut. *Food Composition and Nutrition Tables*. Medpharm GmbH Scientific Publishers, Stuttgart, Germany and CRC Press, Washington, DC, 2000.
Young LL. Effect of stewing on purine content of broiler tissues. *J Fd Sci* 48:315-316, 1983.
Young LL. Evaluation of four purine compounds in poultry products. *J Fd Sci* 45:1064-1067, 1980.
Young LL. Purine content of raw and roasted chicken broiler meat. *J Fd Sci* 47:1374-1375, 1982.

# Resistant Starch

| | RESISTANT STARCH (g/100 g) | | RESISTANT STARCH (g/100 g) |
|---|---|---|---|
| **CEREALS AND GRAINS** | | rice squares | 4.2 |
| barley, pearled, cooked | 2.4 | shredded wheat | 1.2 |
| buckwheat groats, cooked | 1.8 | Smacks, Kellogg's | 1.6 |
| corn polenta (corn porridge), cooked | 0.8 | Special K, Kellogg's | 1.6 |
| corn, sweet, boiled | 0.3 | wheat squares | 1.4 |
| millet, cooked | 1.7 | whole-wheat flakes | 1.0 |
| oats, rolled, uncooked | 11.3 | Weetabix | 0.1 |
| oatmeal, cooked | 0.2 | | |
| rice, brown, boiled | 1.7 | **DESSERTS** | |
| rice porridge (from rice flour) | 0.4 | bread pudding | 0.8 |
| rice, white, boiled | 1.2 | chocolate cookie | 0.8 |
| rice, white, instant parboiled, boiled | 1.3 | fruitcake | 0.1 |
| | | gingersnaps (cookies) | 0.4 |
| **CEREALS, READY-TO-EAT** | | graham cracker (cookie) | 0.3 |
| All Bran, Kellogg's | 0.7 | ice cream cone | 0.3 |
| Alpen, Weetabix | 0.0 | ice cream cone, sugar | 0.5 |
| All-Bran Buds, Kellogg's | 0.6 | oatmeal cookie | 0.2 |
| bran flakes | 0.7 | pastry, choux (light dessert pastry) | 0.5 |
| corn flakes | 3.2 | pie crust, frozen, baked | 0.5 |
| corn puffs | 1.4 | puff pastry shell, frozen, baked | 0.4 |
| corn squares | 1.3 | shortbread cookie | 2.6 |
| granola | 0.1 | sponge cake | 0.2 |
| Grape-Nuts type cereal | 0.8 | sugar cookie | 0.3 |
| muesli | 3.3 | sweet roll with fruit | 0.2 |
| oat bran | 1.0 | vanilla wafers (cookies) | 0.2 |
| oatmeal square | 0.6 | white cake, homemade | 1.8 |
| oats, toasted | 1.2 | | |
| puffed rice | 2.3 | **ENTREES** | |
| puffed wheat | 6.2 | beans in tomato sauce | 1.2 |
| Rice Krispies, Kellogg's | 1.9 | lasagna | 0.1 |

| | RESISTANT STARCH (g/100 g) | | | RESISTANT STARCH (g/100 g) |
|---|---|---|---|---|
| meatloaf made with breadcrumbs | 0.1 | | pizza dough, baked | 2.8 |
| pasta (egg) filled with cheese and tomato, boiled | 0.3 | | pumpernickel bread | 4.5 |
| pasta (egg) filled with cheese, boiled | 0.3 | | rice crackers | 0.4 |
| pasta (egg) filled with green vegetables, herbs, and cheese, boiled | 0.6 | | rice noodles, cooked | 0.9 |
| | | | roll, French | 0.5 |
| pasta (egg) filled with meat, boiled | 0.9 | | roll, white, crusty | 0.3 |
| pasta (egg) filled with mushrooms, boiled | 0.3 | | roll, white, soft | 0.5 |
| | | | roll, whole wheat | 0.4 |
| **FRUITS** | | | rusk toast | 1.8 |
| banana, cooked | 0.8 | | rye bread, whole grain | 3.2 |
| banana, raw | 4.0 | | saltines (crackers) | 0.6 |
| | | | scone, fruit | 0.1 |
| **GRAIN-BASED SNACKS** | | | sourdough bread | 2.1 |
| cereal bar with fruit filling | 2.3 | | spaghetti, boiled | 1.1 |
| cheese puffs (snack food) | 0.2 | | tortilla, corn | 3.0 |
| corn chips, low-fat | 0.7 | | tortilla, flour | 0.0 |
| corn crisps | 0.8 | | waffle, multigrain, frozen, toasted | 0.5 |
| corn puffs (snack food) | 0.0 | | waffle, frozen, toasted | 0.6 |
| granola bar, oats and honey | 0.2 | | wheat crackers, thin | 0.4 |
| popcorn cake | 0.3 | | wheat germ bread | 0.1 |
| potato chips | 3.5 | | white bread | 1.2 |
| pretzel | 1.0 | | white bread, high fiber | 0.9 |
| rice cake, white rice | 0.2 | | whole wheat bread | 1.0 |
| **GRAIN PRODUCTS** | | | **VEGETABLES** | |
| bagel | 0.7 | | black/brown beans, boiled | 1.7 |
| breadstick, hard | 2.3 | | chickpeas (garbanzo beans), boiled | 2.6 |
| brioche (French bread with egg and butter) | 1.7 | | cowpeas, boiled | 0.6 |
| chow mein noodles | 0.4 | | kidney beans, boiled | 2.0 |
| Crispbread, Ryvita (cracker) | 2.8 | | lentils, boiled | 3.4 |
| croissant | 0.4 | | lima beans, boiled | 1.2 |
| croutons | 1.4 | | mung beans, boiled | 1.6 |
| crumpet | 0.3 | | pea soup | 1.9 |
| English muffin | 1.0 | | peas, mature, boiled | 2.6 |
| foccacia (Italian bread made with herbs and cheeses) | 1.2 | | pigeon peas, boiled | 1.0 |
| | | | pinto beans, boiled | 1.9 |
| French bread | 0.5 | | plantain, cooked | 3.5 |
| Italian bread | 1.2 | | potato, baked | 1.0 |
| Italian bread, toasted | 3.8 | | potato, boiled | 1.3 |
| macaroni, boiled | 1.1 | | potato, canned | 1.0 |
| melba rounds (crackers) | 1.5 | | potato croquette (fried, shaped potato snack) | 1.3 |
| muffin, homemade | 1.0 | | potato dumpling | 1.6 |
| multi-grain bread | 0.9 | | potato, fried | 2.8 |
| multi-grain crackers | 0.5 | | potatoes, mashed, from instant | 0.4 |
| naan (Asian round flour flatbread) | 0.3 | | potato pancake (fried shredded potato cake) | 1.1 |
| noodles, egg (egg added as ingredient), boiled | 1.6 | | potato salad | 1.0 |
| | | | potato, slow cooked | 0.3 |
| oatmeal bread | 1.2 | | sweet potato, boiled | 0.7 |
| oyster crackers | 0.5 | | white beans, boiled | 4.2 |
| pasta, whole wheat, boiled | 1.4 | | yam, boiled | 1.5 |
| pita bread, whole wheat | 1.3 | | | |
| pita bread, white | 1.9 | | **MISCELLANEOUS FOODS** | |
| poori (fried Indian flatbread) | 0.6 | | tapioca, boiled | 0.3 |

Source:
Murphy MM, Douglass JS, Birkett A. Resistant starch intakes in the United States. *J Am Diet Assoc* 108:67–78, 2008.

# Sugars—*Fructose, Galactose, Glucose, Lactose, Maltose, and Sucrose*

| | SERVING SIZE (g) | TOTAL SUGARS (g/serving) | FRUCTOSE (g/serving) | GALACTOSE (g/serving) | GLUCOSE (g/serving) | LACTOSE (g/serving) | MALTOSE (g/serving) | SUCROSE (g/serving) | SOURCE (SR21 CODE NUMBER) |
|---|---|---|---|---|---|---|---|---|---|
| **BEVERAGES** | | | | | | | | | |
| beer cooler | 12 fl oz (367 g) | 25.3 | 14.3 | 0.00 | 11.0 | 0.00 | | 0.00 | Matthews et al, 1987 |
| brandy, cherry | 1½ fl oz (42 g) | 13.7 | 6.8 | 0.00 | 6.9 | 0.00 | | 0.00 | Matthews et al, 1987 |
| cappuccino, from instant powder | 8 fl oz (256 g) | 9.5 | | | 0.2 | | 0.00 — | 9.2 | Matthews et al, 1987 |
| cherry drink, canned/ bottled | 8 fl oz (251g) | 26.8 | 10.3 | 0.00 | 13.0 | 0.00 | 1.2 | 2.0 | Matthews et al, 1987 |
| coffee with mocha flavor and sugar, from instant powder | 8 fl oz (251 g) | 6.5 | | | 0.2 | 0.2 | 0.2 | 5.8 | Matthews et al, 1987 |
| cola with higher caffeine (e.g., Jolt Cola) | 12 fl oz (370 g) | 39.1 | 22.6 | | 16.6 | | | 0.00 | SR21 (14148) |
| cola, caffeine-free | 12 fl oz (370 g) | 39.1 | 22.6 | | 16.6 | | | 0.00 | SR21 (14147) |
| cola | 12 fl oz (370 g) | 33.2 | 16.3 | 0.00 | 14.8 | 0.00 | 0.4 | 7.8 | Matthews et al, 1987 |
| Gatorade, fruit flavor, Quaker Oats | 8 fl oz (240 g) | 12.6 | 4.4 | | 5.2 | 0.5 | 0.5 | 2.208 | SR21 (14460) |
| ginger ale | 12 fl oz (366 g) | 31.8 | 13.5 | | 11.3 | | | 6.9 | SR21 (14136) |
| fruit punch drink, canned/bottled | 8 fl oz (248 g) | ~26.8 | 9.2 | 0.00 | 8.4 | 0.00 | 0.00 | 9.2 | Matthews et al, 1987 |
| fruit punch drink, from dry mix | 8 fl oz (262 g) | 30.4 | 11.0 | 0.00 | 10.7 | 0.00 | | 8.9 | Matthews et al, 1987 |
| fruit punch drink, from frozen concentrate | 8 fl oz (247 g) | 25.2 | 5.4 | 0.00 | 7.2 | 0.00 | | 12.6 | Matthews et al, 1987 |
| lemonade, from dry mix | 8 fl oz (264 g) | 26.8 | 0.00 | 0.00 | 0 | 0.00 | | 14.5 | Matthews et al, 1987 |
| lemonade, from frozen concentrate | 8 fl oz (248 g) | 32.6 | 8.7 | 0.00 | 11.4 | 0.00 | | 2.7 | Matthews et al, 1987 |
| lemon-lime soda with caffeine | 12 fl oz (368 g) | 37.5 | 21.6 | | 15.9 | | | 0.00 | SR21 (14144) |
| lemon-lime soda | 12 fl oz (368 g) | 33.0 | 19.1 | | 11.5 | | | 2.4 | SR21 (14145) |
| liqueur, coffee, 53 proof | 1.5 fl oz (52 g) | 24.1 | 2.3 | 0.00 | 2.5 | 0.00 | 0.9 | 14.1 | Matthews et al, 1987 |
| liqueur, coffee with cream, 34 proof | 1.5 fl oz (47 g) | 9.3 | | | | | | 8.1 | Matthews et al, 1987 |
| liqueur, orange | 1.5 fl oz (50 g) | 14.2 | 0.00 | 0.00 | 0.6 | 0.00 | | 13.5 | Matthews et al, 1987 |
| orange drink, canned/ bottled | 8 fl oz (248 g) | 27.3 | 0.00 | 0.00 | 0.00 | 0.00 | 0.00 | 17.8 | Matthews et al, 1987 |
| pepper-type soda | 12 fl oz (368 g) | 36.4 | 16.2 | 0.00 | 19.5 | 0.00 | | 0.7 | Matthews et al, 1987 |
| Powerade, lemon-lime flavor, Coca-Cola | 8 fl oz (240 g) | 14.7 | 7.7 | | 5.3 | 0.5 | 0.5 | 0.48 | SR21 (14461) |
| root beer | 12 fl oz (370 g) | 39.2 | 11.8 | 0.00 | 11.84 | 0.00 | | 20.7 | Matthews et al, 1987 |
| thirst-quencher beverage, bottled | 8 fl oz (241 g) | 13.3 | 5.1 | 0.00 | 5.8 | 0.00 | | 3.374 | Matthews et al, 1987 |
| whiskey sour mix, dry | 0.56 oz packet (17 g) | 16.5 | 0.00 | 0.00 | 0.2 | 0.00 | 0.00 | 12.1 | Matthews et al, 1987 |
| whiskey sour mix, liquid | 2 fl oz (65 g) | 13.9 | 5.3 | 0.00 | 5.1 | 0.00 | 1.5 | 2.5 | Matthews et al, 1987 |
| wine cooler | 12 fl oz (355 g) | 35.5 | 12.8 | 0.00 | 13.1 | 0.00 | | 9.6 | Matthews et al, 1987 |
| wine, dessert, sweet | 3.5 fl oz (103 g) | 8.0 | 5.3 | | 2.7 | | | 0.00 | SR21 (14057) |
| **CANDY** | | | | | | | | | |
| carob candy chips | ¼ cup (42 g) | 15.8 | 3.4 | | 2.0 | 0.00 | 0.00 | 10.4 | Matthews et al, 1987 |
| cashew and honey bar | 1 oz (28 g) | 5.3 | 1.1 | | 1.8 | 0.4 | 1.6 | 0.4 | Matthews et al, 1987 |
| chewing gum, Chiclets | 10 Chiclets (16 g) | 10.6 | | 0.00 | | | 0.00 | 11.9 | Matthews et al, 1987 |
| chocolate-covered mint patty | 1.5 oz patty (43 g) | 27.4 | | | | | | 34.2 | Matthews et al, 1987 |
| chocolate-covered nougat | 1 oz (28 g) | 17.2 | 0.2 | | 2.0 | 1.0 | 2.0 | 10.7 | Matthews et al, 1987 |
| chocolate-covered peanut butter nougat, caramel, and peanuts | 1 oz (28 g) | 12.6 | 0.1 | | 1.8 | 1.2 | 1.7 | 7.7 | Matthews et al, 1987 |
| chocolate-covered peanuts | 1 oz (28 g) | ~9.8 | | | 0.3 | | | 9.5 | Matthews et al, 1987 |
| chocolate-covered wafer cookie bar | 1 oz (28 g) | 12.2 | | | 1.4 | | | 10.9 | Matthews et al, 1987 |

| | SERVING SIZE (g) | TOTAL SUGARS (g/serving) | FRUCTOSE (g/serving) | GALACTOSE (g/serving) | GLUCOSE (g/serving) | LACTOSE (g/serving) | MALTOSE (g/serving) | SUCROSE (g/serving) | SOURCE (SR21 CODE NUMBER) |
|---|---|---|---|---|---|---|---|---|---|
| coconut bar | 1 oz (28 g) | 12.1 | 0.8 | | 3.0 | 0.00 | 0.868 | 7.4 | Matthews et al, 1987 |
| dark chocolate chips, semi-sweet | ¼ cup (42 g) | ~22.7 | | | 1.9 | 0.00 | 0.00 | 20.8 | Matthews et al, 1987 |
| dark chocolate, 45%–59% cacao | 1 oz (28 g) | 13.4 | 0.00 | 0.00 | 0.00 | 0.5 | 0.00 | 12.9 | SR21 (19902) |
| dark chocolate, 60%–69% cacao | 1 oz (28 g) | 10.3 | 0.00 | 0.00 | 0.00 | 0.1 | 0.00 | 10.2 | SR21 (19903) |
| dark chocolate, 70%–85% cacao | 1 oz (28 g) | 6.7 | 0.00 | 0.00 | 0.00 | 0.00 | 0.00 | 6.7 | SR21 (19904) |
| dark chocolate, sweet | 1.45 oz bar (41 g) | 21.1 | 0.00 | | 0.00 | 0.00 | 0.00 | 19.9 | Matthews et al, 1987 |
| fruit and honey bar | 1 oz (28 g) | 7.0 | 2.2 | | 2.8 | 0.00 | 0.672 | 1.3 | Matthews et al, 1987 |
| hard candy | 5 pieces (28 g) | ~18.7 | | 0.00 | | 0.00 | | 18.7 | Matthews et al, 1987 |
| jelly beans | 10 large/ 25 small (28 g) | 19.6 | | 0.00 | | 0.00 | | 16.5 | Matthews et al, 1987 |
| Kit Kat, Hershey (candy bar) | 2.8 oz bar (78 g) | 38.0 | 0.1 | 0.00 | 0.1 | 6.4 | 0.00 | 31.2 | SR21 (19109) |
| milk chocolate | 1 oz (28 g) | 14.4 | 0.00 | 0.00 | 0.00 | 2.1 | 0.00 | 13.1 | Matthews et al, 1987 |
| milk chocolate chips | ¼ cup (42 g) | 21.6 | 0.0 | 0.00 | 0.1 | 3.1 | 0.00 | 19.6 | Matthews et al, 1987 |
| milk chocolate with almonds | 1.55 oz bar (44 g) | ~19.6 | 0.1 | | 0.1 | 2.7 | 0.00 | 16.7 | Matthews et al, 1987 |
| milk chocolate with crisped rice | 1.55 oz bar (44 g) | ~22.1 | 0.1 | | 0.1 | 2.9 | | 19.0 | Matthews et al, 1987 |
| sugar-coated chocolate and peanut discs | 1 oz (28 g) | 13.2 | | | | 1.1 | | 12.1 | Matthews et al, 1987 |
| sugar-coated chocolate discs | 1 oz (28 g) | 16.2 | | | | 1.0 | | 14.4 | Matthews et al, 1987 |
| sunflower and honey bar | 1 oz (28 g) | 5.7 | 1.2 | | 1.7 | 0.4 | 2.0 | 0.4 | Matthews et al, 1987 |
| sunflower candy bar | 1 oz (28 g) | 5.4 | 0.6 | | 0.1 | 0.00 | 0.6 | 4.1 | Matthews et al, 1987 |
| taffy, fruit-flavored | 1 oz (28 g) | 18.5 | 1.0 | | 3.3 | | 2.0 | 10.5 | Matthews et al, 1987 |
| toffee | 1 oz (28 g) | 15.5 | 1.4 | | 1.9 | 0.7 | | 11.4 | Matthews et al, 1987 |
| Tootsie Roll (candy) | 6 pieces (40 g) | 22.5 | 0.2 | 0.00 | 3.1 | 0.9 | 2.6 | 15.7 | SR21 (19064) |
| white chocolate chips | ¼ cup (42 g) | ~26.1 | | | | 4.1 | | 22.1 | Matthews et al, 1987 |
| **CEREALS, READY-TO-EAT** | | | | | | | | | |
| Apple Jacks, Kellogg's | 1 cup (30 g) | 12.5 | 0.2 | 0.00 | 0.2 | 0.00 | 0.00 | 12.0 | SR21 (08003) |
| bran flakes with raisins | ¾ cup (39 g) | 10.4 | 3.2 | 0.00 | 2.8 | 0.00 | 0.00 | 3.9 | Matthews et al, 1987 |
| Bran flakes, Ralston | ¾ cup (29 g) | 5.0 | 0.6 | 0.00 | 0.6 | 0.00 | 0.1 | 3.6 | SR21 (08504) |
| Cap'n Crunch Peanut Butter Crunch, Quaker | ¾ cup (27 g) | 8.9 | | 0.00 | | | | | SR21 (08012) |
| Cinnamon Toast Crunch, General Mills | ¾ cup (30 g) | 9.9 | 2.2 | 0.00 | 0.4 | 0.00 | 0.00 | 7.3 | SR21 (08272) |
| Cocoa Krispies, Kellogg's | ¾ cup (31 g) | 10.5 | 0.1 | 0.00 | 0.6 | 0.00 | 0.00 | 9.8 | SR21 (08014) |
| Froot Loops, Kellogg's | 1 cup (30 g) | 13.5 | 0.00 | 0.00 | 0.00 | 0.00 | 0.1 | 13.3 | SR21 (08030) |
| Frosted Flakes, Kellogg's | ¾ cup (31 g) | 12.0 | 0.4 | 0.00 | 0.4 | 0.00 | 0.1 | 11.0 | SR21 (08069) |
| Frosted Krispies, Kellogg's | ¾ cup (30 g) | ~11.7 | 0.2 | 0.00 | 0.2 | 0.00 | 0.00 | 11.3 | Matthews et al, 1987 |
| Golden Puffs, Malt-O-Meal | 1 cup (37 g) | 19.0 | 1.1 | 0.00 | 3.0 | 0.00 | 1.7 | 13.1 | SR21 (08478) |
| Heartland Natural cereal with raisins, Heartland | ½ cup (56 g) | 15.3 | 2.6 | 0.00 | 2.6 | 0.5 | 0.00 | 9.5 | Matthews et al, 1987 |
| Lucky Charms, General Mills | 1 cup (30 g) | 12.0 | 0.1 | 0.00 | 1.4 | 0.00 | 0.5 | 9.9 | SR21 (08050) |
| puffed wheat, sugar-coated | ⅞ cup (28 g) | 15.1 | 0.4 | 0.00 | 1.0 | 0.00 | 0.5 | 10.6 | Matthews et al, 1987 |
| Raisin Bran, Kellogg's | 1 cup (59 g) | 17.6 | 9.1 | 0.00 | 8.4 | 0.00 | 0.00 | 0.1 | SR21 (08060) |
| raisin bran, Post | 1 cup (59 g) | 16.5 | 7.2 | 0.00 | 8.1 | 0.00 | 0.4 | 0.8 | SR21 (08061) |
| shredded wheat, frosted | 1 rectangular biscuit (24 g) | 5.5 | 0.00 | 0.00 | 0.00 | 0.00 | 0.00 | 5.9 | Matthews et al, 1987 |
| Smacks, Kellogg's | ¾ cup (27 g) | ~15.5 | 0.3 | 0.00 | 3.3 | 0.00 | 0.00 | 11.9 | Matthews et al, 1987 |

| | SERVING SIZE (g) | TOTAL SUGARS (g/serving) | FRUCTOSE (g/serving) | GALACTOSE (g/serving) | GLUCOSE (g/serving) | LACTOSE (g/serving) | MALTOSE (g/serving) | SUCROSE (g/serving) | SOURCE (SR21 CODE NUMBER) |
|---|---|---|---|---|---|---|---|---|---|
| **CHEESE** | | | | | | | | | |
| cottage cheese, 2% fat | 1 cup (226 g) | 8.3 | 0.00 | 0.00 | 1.7 | 6.5 | 0.00 | 0.00 | SR21 (01015) |
| cottage cheese, creamed, large/small curd | 1 cup (225 g) | 6.0 | 0.00 | 0.00 | 0.00 | 6.0 | 0.00 | 0.00 | SR21 (01012) |
| **DESSERTS** | | | | | | | | | |
| animal crackers | 2 oz box (57 g) | 7.9 | 0.6 | 0.00 | 1.0 | 0.00 | 0.2 | 11.2 | Matthews et al, 1987 |
| cake, sponge with jam filling | 1.2 oz piece (32 g) | 15.3 | 1.2 | 0.00 | 2.6 | 0.00 | 0.00 | 11.4 | Matthews et al, 1987 |
| chocolate syrup | 2 T (39 g) | ~13.4 | 3.0 | | 4.9 | 1.9 | 1.7 | 11.9 | Matthews et al, 1987 |
| chocolate wafer | 5 wafers (28 g) | 8.3 | 0.4 | 0.00 | 0.0 | 0.2 | 0.3 | 10.4 | Matthews et al, 1987 |
| cookie, chocolate chip, soft type | 1 cookie (15 g) | 5.7 | 0.8 | 0.00 | 1.1 | 0.00 | 0.1 | 3.6 | SR21 (18160) |
| cookie, chocolate sandwich with extra crème filling | 1 cookie (13 g) | 6.0 | 0 | 0.00 | 0.1 | 0.00 | 0.00 | 5.8 | SR21 (18168) |
| doughnut | 3¼" diameter doughnut (47 g) | 10.6 | | 0.00 | 1.4 | 0.8 | | 5.6 | Matthews et al, 1987 |
| gelatin dessert, from mix with sugar, raspberry | ½ cup (135 g) | 11.7 | | 0.00 | 7.3 | 0.00 | | 4.4 | Matthews et al, 1987 |
| fruitcake | 1.5 oz piece (43 g) | 12.8 | 4.8 | 0.00 | 4.8 | 0.00 | 0.00 | 8.8 | Matthews et al, 1987 |
| ice pop (frozen dessert) | 2 fl oz bar (59 g) | 8.0 | 1.6 | | 2.3 | 0.00 | 0.4 | 3.7 | SR21 (19283) |
| icing/frosting, chocolate | 2 T (41 g) | 23.6 | 0.9 | | 1.5 | 2.2 | 0.6 | 17.6 | Matthews et al, 1987 |
| icing/frosting, flavors other than chocolate, carob, white chocolate | 2 T (41 g) | 29.2 | 0.3 | | 0.6 | 0.00 | 0.5 | 27.8 | Matthews et al, 1987 |
| pie, apple, fried, snack size | 3 oz pie (85 g) | 9.8 | 2.0 | 0.00 | 1.7 | 0.2 | 0.7 | 5.2 | Matthews et al, 1987 |
| pie, cherry, fried, snack size | 1 snack pie (128 g) | 15.1 | 6.6 | 0.00 | 7.4 | 0.00 | 1.0 | | Matthews et al, 1987 |
| pie crust, graham cracker, Ready Crust | 6.5 oz crust (183 g) | 33.2 | 0.00 | | 0.00 | 0.00 | 0.00 | 33.2 | SR21 (18942) |
| pie, Dutch apple | 4.8 oz slice (137 g) | 30.2 | 6.3 | | 6.7 | 0.00 | 2.1 | 15.1 | SR21 (18944) |
| pie, fruit | ⅙ pie (149 g) | 46.0 | 4.2 | 0.00 | 8.5 | 0.00 | 1.3 | 32.0 | Matthews et al, 1987 |
| pie, pecan | ⅛ of 8" pie (113 g) | 28.4 | 0.00 | 0.00 | 6.2 | 0.3 | 5.6 | 16.3 | SR21 (18324) |
| pie, pumpkin | ⅛ of 8" pie (109 g) | 20.6 | 3.1 | 0.00 | 4.1 | 2.2 | 1.0 | 10.1 | SR21 (18326) |
| pudding, chocolate, ready-to-eat | 5 oz serving (142 g) | 24.4 | 0.00 | 0.00 | 0.00 | 2.4 | 0.00 | 22.0 | SR21 (19183) |
| pudding, tapioca, ready-to-eat | 5 oz serving (142 g) | 21.2 | 0.00 | 0.00 | 0.00 | 3.3 | 0.00 | 17.8 | SR21 (19218) |
| pudding, vanilla, ready-to-eat | 4 oz serving (113 g) | 19.2 | 0.00 | 0.00 | 0.00 | 2.0 | 0.00 | 17.1 | SR21 (19201) |
| snack cake, sponge, crème-filled | 1.5 oz snack cake (43 g) | 16.0 | 1.1 | | 2.5 | 0.00 | 0.00 | 12.4 | SR21 (18128) |
| **ENTREES** | | | | | | | | | |
| baked beans with frankfurters, canned | 1 cup (259 g) | 16.9 | 2.3 | | 2.8 | | | 0.00 | Matthews et al, 1987 |
| chicken pot pie, frozen | 7.7 oz pie (217 g) | ~8.2 | 0.2 | | 1.6 | 1.5 | 4.0 | 0.9 | SR21 (22906) |
| lasagna with meat and tomato sauce, low-fat, frozen entrée | 10.9 oz entrée (309 g) | ~6.1 | 2.3 | | 2.3 | | | 1.5 | SR21 (22915) |
| pizza, cheese, rising crust, frozen, heated | 4.9 oz slice (139 g) | 7.1 | 2.1 | | 1.6 | | 3.4 | | SR21 (21225) |
| pizza, meat and vegetable, regular crust, frozen, heated | 4.8 oz slice (136 g) | ~6.6 | 1.8 | 0.2 | 3.4 | | 1.2 | | SR21 (21226) |
| pizza, meat and vegetable, rising crust, frozen, heated | 5.3 oz slice (149 g) | ~10.8 | 2.5 | 0.2 | 4.5 | | 3.6 | | SR21 (21227) |
| pizza, pepperoni, frozen | 5.1 oz serving (146 g) | ~5.7 | 1.5 | | 2.3 | 0.3 | 1.1 | 0.5 | SR21 (22903) |
| rice bowl with chicken, frozen | 12 oz entrée (340 g) | 13.8 | 1.1 | 0.00 | 0.8 | 0.00 | 0.00 | 11.9 | SR21 (22958) |

| | SERVING SIZE (g) | TOTAL SUGARS (g/serving) | FRUCTOSE (g/serving) | GALACTOSE (g/serving) | GLUCOSE (g/serving) | LACTOSE (g/serving) | MALTOSE (g/serving) | SUCROSE (g/serving) | SOURCE (SR21 CODE NUMBER) |
|---|---|---|---|---|---|---|---|---|---|
| turkey, stuffing, mashed potatoes with gravy, mixed vegetables, frozen, microwaved | 14.9 oz meal (422 g) | 20.3 | 4.3 | | 7.1 | 0.00 | 0.00 | 8.9 | SR21 (22957) |

**FAST FOODS**

| | SERVING SIZE (g) | TOTAL SUGARS (g/serving) | FRUCTOSE (g/serving) | GALACTOSE (g/serving) | GLUCOSE (g/serving) | LACTOSE (g/serving) | MALTOSE (g/serving) | SUCROSE (g/serving) | SOURCE (SR21 CODE NUMBER) |
|---|---|---|---|---|---|---|---|---|---|
| apple dippers (slices) with lowfat caramel sauce, McDonald's | 3.1 oz (89 g) | 15.3 | 4.6 | 0.00 | 3.6 | 0.6 | 1.7 | 4.7 | SR21 (21366) |
| apple dippers (slices), McDonald's | 2.4 oz (68 g) | 6.2 | 3.4 | 0.00 | 0.6 | 0.00 | 0.00 | 2.2 | SR21 (21342) |
| bagel with egg, sausage patty, and cheese, fast food | 7.7 oz sandwich (219 g) | 6.3 | 1.7 | 0.00 | 1.8 | 0.8 | 1.9 | 0.00 | SR21 (21410) |
| bagel with ham, egg, and cheese, fast food | 6.7 oz sandwich (191 g) | 7.0 | 1.8 | 0.00 | 2.2 | 0.8 | 1.8 | 0.2 | SR21 (21409) |
| bagel with steak, egg, and cheese, fast food | 7.7 oz sandwich (217 g) | 6.4 | 1.9 | 0.00 | 1.8 | 0.8 | 2.0 | 0.00 | SR21 (21411) |
| Burrito Supreme, beef, Taco Bell | 8.7 oz burrito (247 g) | ~6.7 | 1.6 | | 3.9 | 0.4 | 0.4 | 0.4 | SR21 (21265) |
| caramel sauce, lowfat, McDonald's | 0.8 oz (21 g) | 9.1 | 1.2 | 0.00 | 3.0 | 0.6 | 1.7 | 2.4 | SR21 (21343) |
| cheeseburger, Big Mac, McDonald's | 7.6 oz sandwich (215 g) | 8.5 | 3.6 | 0.00 | 2.2 | 0.7 | 1.0 | 1.0 | SR21 (21237) |
| cheeseburger, Big N' Tasty, McDonald's | 9.3 oz sandwich (247 g) | 9.5 | 4.0 | 0.00 | 3.2 | 0.6 | 1.1 | 0.5 | SR21 (21353) |
| cheeseburger, Burger King | 4.7 oz sandwich (133 g) | 6.0 | 2.5 | 0.2 | 0.00 | 0.1 | 1.0 | 2.2 | SR21 (21251) |
| cheeseburger, Classic Single, Wendy's | 8.3 oz sandwich (236 g) | ~5.7 | 2.6 | | 1.9 | 0.5 | 0.7 | 0.00 | SR21 (21240) |
| cheeseburger, double, McDonald's | 6.1 oz sandwich (173 g) | 8.1 | 3.1 | 0.00 | 2.5 | 1.1 | 1.0 | 0.3 | SR21 (21344) |
| cheeseburger, double quarter pounder, McDonald's | 9.9 oz sandwich (280 g) | 9.8 | 3.8 | 0.00 | 3.3 | 1.1 | 1.3 | 0.4 | SR21 (21345) |
| cheeseburger, Double Whopper, Burger King | 15 oz sandwich (426 g) | 15.4 | 5.4 | 2.2 | 0.00 | 0.3 | 2.3 | 5.1 | SR21 (21255) |
| cheeseburger, Junior, Wendy's | 4.6 oz sandwich (129 g) | ~6.0 | 2.9 | | 2.6 | 0.3 | 0.2 | 0.00 | SR21 (21242) |
| cheeseburger, large, single meat with lettuce and tomato, fast food | 1 sandwich (219 g) | 8.8 | 3.8 | 0.00 | 3.0 | 0.6 | 1.0 | 0.4 | SR21 (21098) |
| cheeseburger, large, triple meat, fast food | 1 sandwich (304 g) | 10.0 | 3.8 | 0.00 | 2.1 | 2.5 | 1.1 | 0.4 | SR21 (21101) |
| cheeseburger, McDonald's | 4.3 oz sandwich (121 g) | 7.5 | 3.1 | 0.00 | 2.4 | 0.6 | 1.0 | 0.3 | SR21 (21233) |
| cheeseburger, regular, double meat and double-decker bun, fast food | 1 sandwich (160 g) | 8.7 | 3.9 | 0.00 | 2.2 | 1.0 | 1.2 | 0.4 | SR21 (21094) |
| cheeseburger, regular, double meat, fast food | 1 sandwich (155 g) | 6.2 | 2.5 | 0.00 | 1.4 | 1.2 | 0.7 | 0.3 | SR21 (21092) |
| cheeseburger, regular, single meat, fast food | 1 sandwich (113 g) | 5.9 | 2.2 | 0.2 | 2.0 | 0.3 | 0.5 | 0.7 | SR21 (21090) |
| cheeseburger, regular, single meat, fast food | 1 sandwich (113 g) | 5.8 | 2.3 | | 2.1 | 0.2 | 1.1 | 0.1 | Matthews et al, 1987 |
| cheeseburger, Quarter Pounder, McDonald's | 7.05 oz sandwich (199 g) | 9.8 | 3.8 | 0.00 | 3.3 | 1.1 | 1.2 | 0.4 | SR21 (21235) |
| cheeseburger, Whopper, Burger King | 13.9 oz sandwich (395 g) | 16.2 | 6.5 | 0.3 | 0.00 | 0.3 | 2.7 | 6.3 | SR21 (21253) |
| Chicken Grill Sandwich, Wendy's | 6.6 oz sandwich (188 g) | ~7.2 | 3.4 | | 3.5 | 0.00 | 0.3 | 0.00 | SR21 (21245) |

| | SERVING SIZE (g) | TOTAL SUGARS (g/serving) | FRUCTOSE (g/serving) | GALACTOSE (g/serving) | GLUCOSE (g/serving) | LACTOSE (g/serving) | MALTOSE (g/serving) | SUCROSE (g/serving) | SOURCE (SR21 CODE NUMBER) |
|---|---|---|---|---|---|---|---|---|---|
| chicken (grilled) Classic Sandwich, McDonald's | 8 oz sandwich (229 g) | 11.5 | 4.8 | 0.00 | 3.9 | 0.00 | 1.8 | 1.0 | SR21 (21402) |
| chicken (grilled) Club Sandwich, McDonald's | 9.4 oz sandwich (269 g) | 12.6 | | | 4.0 | 0.00 | 1.9 | 1.8 | SR21 (21404) |
| chicken (grilled) Ranch BLT Sandwich, McDonald's | 8.5 oz sandwich (242 g) | 12.6 | 4.8 | 0.00 | 3.9 | 0.3 | 1.8 | 1.7 | SR21 (21406) |
| Chicken McNugget sauce, barbeque, McDonald's | 1 oz packet (28 g) | 9.6 | 4.3 | 0.00 | 5.1 | 0.00 | 0.1 | 0.00 | SR21 (21310) |
| Chicken McNugget sauce, honey, McDonald's | 0.5 oz packet (14 g) | 10.4 | 5.3 | 0.00 | 4.5 | 0.00 | 0.4 | 0.1 | SR21 (21312) |
| Chicken McNugget sauce, hot mustard, McDonald's | 1 oz packet (28 g) | 6.1 | 2.7 | 0.00 | 3.1 | 0.00 | 0.1 | 0.2 | SR21 (21313) |
| Chicken McNugget sauce, sweet'n sour, McDonald's | 1 oz packet (28 g) | 10.0 | 4.4 | 0.00 | 5.2 | 0.00 | 0.1 | 0.3 | SR21 (21315) |
| chicken sandwich, Burger King | 7.2 oz sandwich (204 g) | 5.5 | 2.0 | 0.00 | 0.00 | 0.00 | 1.6 | 1.9 | SR21 (21259) |
| Chicken Whopper sandwich, Burger King | 9.6 oz sandwich (272 g) | 9.2 | 3.7 | 0.00 | 0.00 | 0.00 | 2.1 | 3.4 | SR21 (21257) |
| chocolate chip cookie, McDonald's | 2 oz bag (57 g) | 19.3 | 0.1 | 0.00 | 0.5 | 0.4 | 0.00 | 18.3 | SR21 (21325) |
| cinnamon roll, McDonald's | 3.4 oz roll (99 g) | 24.4 | 4.6 | 0.00 | 7.2 | 0.9 | 1.1 | 10.5 | SR21 (21322) |
| cinnamon roll, miniature, fast food | 2 rolls (50 g) | 9.0 | 1.9 | 0.00 | 3.5 | 0.5 | 0.4 | 2.7 | SR21 (21388) |
| cookies, McDonald's | 2 oz bag (57 g) | 13.7 | 0.6 | 0.00 | 0.6 | 0.00 | 0.1 | 12.4 | SR21 (21326) |
| fish sandwich with tartar sauce and cheese, fast food | 6.5 oz sandwich (183 g) | 6.0 | 2.4 | | 1.5 | 0.4 | 1.3 | 0.5 | Matthews et al, 1987 |
| French toast sticks, Burger King | 5 sticks (113 g) | 11.2 | 0.8 | 0.00 | 1.2 | 0.2 | 0.9 | 8.1 | SR21 (21386) |
| French toast sticks, fast food | 5 sticks (141 g) | 13.9 | 1.0 | 0.00 | 1.4 | 0.2 | 1.1 | 10.1 | SR21 (21024) |
| frosty dairy dessert, junior, Wendy's | 6 fl oz (113 g) | ~17.6 | 0.2 | | 0.6 | 6.1 | 1.0 | 9.7 | SR21 (21248) |
| frosty dairy dessert, medium, Wendy's | 16 fl oz (298 g) | ~46.6 | 0.4 | | 1.6 | 16.2 | 2.7 | 25.7 | SR21 (21248) |
| frosty dairy dessert, small, Wendy's | 12 fl oz (227 g) | ~35.6 | 0.3 | | 1.2 | 12.3 | 2.2 | 19.6 | SR21 (21248) |
| fruit and yogurt parfait with granola, McDonald's | 12 oz serving (338 g) | 43.4 | 5.9 | 0.6 | 2.6 | 7.1 | 0.2 | 26.8 | SR21 (21380) |
| fruit and yogurt parfait, McDonald's | 11 oz serving (310 g) | 36.9 | 5.5 | 0.6 | 2.3 | 6.9 | 0.00 | 21.6 | SR21 (21381) |
| griddle cake sandwich with egg, cheese, and bacon, fast food | 5.9 oz sandwich (168 g) | 16.1 | 0.2 | 0.00 | 5.2 | 1.2 | 0.6 | 8.8 | SR21 (21307) |
| griddle cake sandwich with egg, cheese, and sausage, fast food | 7 oz sandwich (199 g) | 15.7 | 0.2 | 0.00 | 5.4 | 1.2 | 0.6 | 8.3 | SR21 (21305) |
| griddle cake sandwich, sausage, fast food | 4.7 oz sandwich (135 g) | 15.1 | 0.2 | 0.00 | 5.3 | 0.7 | 0.6 | 8.3 | SR21 (21306) |
| hamburger, ¼ lb meat, fast food | 6.1 oz sandwich (176 g) | 7.6 | 3.0 | | 3.0 | 0.2 | 1.4 | 0.2 | Matthews et al, 1987 |
| hamburger, Big N' Tasty, McDonald's | 8.85 oz sandwich (232 g) | 8.8 | 3.9 | 0 | 3.1 | 0.1 | 1.1 | 0.5 | SR21 (21351) |
| hamburger, Burger King | 4.3 oz sandwich (121 g) | 5.9 | 2.5 | 0.1 | 0.00 | 0.00 | 0.9 | 2.2 | SR21 (21250) |

| | SERVING SIZE (g) | TOTAL SUGARS (g/serving) | FRUCTOSE (g/serving) | GALACTOSE (g/serving) | GLUCOSE (g/serving) | LACTOSE (g/serving) | MALTOSE (g/serving) | SUCROSE (g/serving) | SOURCE (SR21 CODE NUMBER) |
|---|---|---|---|---|---|---|---|---|---|
| hamburger, Classic Single, Wendy's | 7.7 oz hamburger (218 g) | ~5.9 | 2.9 | | 2.5 | 0.00 | 0.5 | 0.00 | SR21 (21239) |
| hamburger, Double Whopper, Burger King | 14 oz sandwich (401 g) | 14.1 | 5.7 | 0.3 | 0.00 | 0.00 | 2.3 | 5.8 | SR21 (21254) |
| hamburger, Junior, Wendy's | 4.2 oz hamburger (117 g) | ~6.5 | 3.1 | | 2.8 | 0.00 | 0.6 | 0 | SR21 (21241) |
| hamburger, large, single meat, fast food | 6.1 oz sandwich (172 g) | 6.3 | 3.2 | | 2.0 | 0.3 | 0.6 | 0.3 | SR21 (21202) |
| hamburger, McDonald's | 3.8 oz sandwich (105 g) | 6.9 | 3.1 | 0.00 | 2.4 | 0.2 | 1.0 | 0.3 | SR21 (21228) |
| hamburger, Quarter Pounder, McDonald's | 6.1 oz sandwich (171 g) | 8.8 | 3.8 | 0.00 | 3.3 | 0.1 | 1.2 | 0.4 | SR21 (21234) |
| hamburger, regular, double meat, fast food | 6.2 oz sandwich (176 g) | 7.3 | 3.6 | 0.00 | 2.0 | 0.2 | 1.0 | 0.4 | SR21 (21110) |
| hamburger, regular, single meat, fast food | 3.2 oz sandwich (90 g) | 5.2 | 2.5 | 0.00 | 1.5 | 0.2 | 0.7 | 0.3 | SR21 (21107) |
| hamburger, Whopper, Burger King | 10.7 oz sandwich (304 g) | 12.8 | 5.3 | 0.3 | 0.00 | 0.00 | 2.0 | 5.2 | SR21 (21252) |
| ice cream, vanilla (reduced fat) in cone, McDonald's | 3.2 oz cone (90 g) | 17.5 | 0.1 | 0.00 | 0.6 | 5.0 | 0.3 | 11.5 | SR21 (21333) |
| ice milk, soft serve in cake cone, fast food | 1 serving (115 g) | 20.0 | 0.1 | 0.00 | 1.0 | 6.5 | 0.8 | 11.5 | Matthews et al, 1987 |
| ice milk, soft serve in sugar cone, fast food | 1 serving (93 g) | 17.8 | 0.4 | 0.00 | 0.9 | 4.7 | 0.5 | 11.2 | Matthews et al, 1987 |
| McFlurry, M&M's, McDonald's | 12.3 oz serving (348 g) | 84.8 | 0.7 | 0.00 | 2.6 | 21.7 | 1.0 | 58.8 | SR21 (21338) |
| McFlurry, Oreo, McDonald's | 11.9 oz serving (337 g) | 71.4 | 0.6 | 0.00 | 3.0 | 18.9 | 0.9 | 47.8 | SR21 (21339) |
| McGriddles, bacon, egg, and cheese, McDonald's | 5.9 oz entrée (168 g) | 16.1 | 0.2 | 0.00 | 5.2 | 1.2 | 0.6 | 8.8 | SR21 (21327) |
| McGriddles, sausage, egg, and cheese, McDonald's | 7 oz entrée (199 g) | 15.7 | 0.2 | 0.00 | 5.4 | 1.2 | 0.6 | 8.3 | SR21 (21329) |
| McGriddles, sausage, McDonald's | 4.7 oz entrée (135 g) | 15.2 | 0.2 | 0.00 | 5.3 | 0.7 | 0.6 | 8.3 | SR21 (21328) |
| pancakes and sausage, McDonald's | 9.3 oz entrée (264 g) | 45.7 | 0.4 | 0.00 | 11.3 | 5.3 | 11.5 | 17.2 | SR21 (21364) |
| pancakes with margarine and syrup, McDonald's | 8 oz serving (228 g) | 46.9 | 0.4 | 0.00 | 11.5 | 5.4 | 11.8 | 17.7 | SR21 (21365) |
| pie, apple, McDonald's | 2.7 oz pie (77 g) | 13.3 | 3.3 | 0.00 | 3.5 | 0.1 | 0.2 | 6.0 | SR21 (21324) |
| pizza, cheese, regular crust, Papa John's | 4.1 oz slice (117 g) | 6.2 | 2.1 | 0.1 | 1.7 | 0.3 | 1.5 | 0.5 | SR21 (21283) |
| pizza, Extravaganzza Feast, Classic Hand-Tossed Crust | 5.3 oz slice (151 g) | 5.0 | 1.3 | 0.1 | 1.5 | 0.5 | 1.5 | 0.00 | SR21 (21282) |
| pizza, meat and vegetable, regular crust, fast food | 4.8 oz slice (136 g) | 5.1 | 1.5 | 0.1 | 1.4 | 0.2 | 1.6 | 0.1 | SR21 (21304) |
| pizza, pepperoni, regular crust, Papa John's | 4.3 oz slice (123 g) | 5.9 | 2.0 | 0.1 | 1.7 | 0.3 | 1.4 | 0.5 | SR21 (21284) |
| pizza, Super Supreme, regular crust, Pizza Hut | 4.9 oz slice (139 g) | 5.2 | 1.2 | 0.1 | 1.0 | 0.4 | 2.4 | 0.00 | SR21 (21276) |
| pizza, The Works, regular crust, Papa John's | 5.4 oz slice (153 g) | 7.4 | 2.4 | 0.1 | 2.3 | 0.2 | 1.9 | 0.5 | SR21 (21285) |
| salad, bacon ranch with grilled chicken, McDonald's | 11.3 oz salad (321 g) | 5.5 | 2.2 | 0.00 | 1.8 | 0.00 | 0.00 | 1.6 | SR21 (21376) |
| shake, chocolate, triple thick, McDonald's | 16 fl oz (333 g) | 78.7 | 5.5 | 0.00 | 11.5 | 17.7 | 3.8 | 40.1 | SR21 (21331) |

| | SERVING SIZE (g) | TOTAL SUGARS (g/serving) | FRUCTOSE (g/serving) | GALACTOSE (g/serving) | GLUCOSE (g/serving) | LACTOSE (g/serving) | MALTOSE (g/serving) | SUCROSE (g/serving) | SOURCE (SR21 CODE NUMBER) |
|---|---|---|---|---|---|---|---|---|---|
| shake, strawberry, fast food | 12 fl oz (282 g) | 52.4 | 5.1 | | 10.1 | 13.8 | 4.2 | 19.2 | Matthews et al, 1987 |
| shake, strawberry, McDonald's | 16 fl oz (333 g) | 79.1 | 2.3 | 0.00 | 5.1 | 17.6 | 1.8 | 52.2 | SR21 (21332) |
| shake, vanilla, Burger King | 14 fl oz medium (397 g) | 46.3 | 0.00 | 0.5 | 0.00 | 16.9 | 0.00 | 28.9 | SR21 (21141) |
| shake, vanilla, triple thick, McDonald's | 16 fl oz (333 g) | 68.0 | 0.5 | 0.00 | 5.4 | 17.7 | 4.3 | 40.1 | SR21 (21330) |
| sundae, caramel, fast food | 1 sundae (155 g) | 38.7 | 1.2 | | 7.7 | 8.4 | 3.4 | 18.3 | Matthews et al, 1987 |
| sundae, hot caramel, McDonald's | 6.4 oz sundae (182 g) | 42.8 | 1.4 | 0.00 | 5.4 | 9.9 | 3.0 | 23.0 | SR21 (21335) |
| sundae, hot fudge, fast food | 1 sundae (158 g) | 40.1 | 0.8 | | 2.4 | 9.0 | 0.6 | 26.9 | Matthews et al, 1987 |
| sundae, hot fudge, McDonald's | 6.3 oz sundae (179 g) | 48.1 | 0.4 | 0.00 | 1.4 | 10.5 | 0.6 | 35.2 | SR21 (21336) |
| sundae, strawberry, fast food | 1 sundae (153 g) | 41.6 | 5.2 | | 9.5 | 6.9 | | 19.1 | Matthews et al, 1987 |
| sundae, strawberry, McDonald's | 6.3 oz sundae (178 g) | 45.1 | 2.9 | 0.00 | 3.9 | 8.4 | 0.5 | 29.4 | SR21 (21334) |
| taco salad, Taco Bell | 16.8 oz salad (475 g) | ~6.3 | 3.0 | | 1.2 | 0.7 | 0.7 | 0.7 | SR21 (21270) |

**FRUIT JUICES**

| | SERVING SIZE (g) | TOTAL SUGARS (g/serving) | FRUCTOSE (g/serving) | GALACTOSE (g/serving) | GLUCOSE (g/serving) | LACTOSE (g/serving) | MALTOSE (g/serving) | SUCROSE (g/serving) | SOURCE (SR21 CODE NUMBER) |
|---|---|---|---|---|---|---|---|---|---|
| apple juice, canned/bottled | 8 fl oz (248 g) | 23.8 | 14.2 | 0.00 | 6.5 | 0.00 | 0.00 | 3.1 | SR21 (09016) |
| citrus fruit juice drink, from frozen concentrate | 8 fl oz (248 g) | 28.2 | | 0.00 | | 0.00 | | | Matthews et al, 1987 |
| cranberry juice cocktail, canned/bottled | 8 fl oz (253 g) | 30.0 | 12.6 | 0.00 | 17.2 | 0.00 | 0.3 | 0.00 | SR21 (14242) |
| grape juice, canned/bottled | 8 fl oz (253 g) | 35.9 | 18.6 | 0.00 | 17.2 | 0.00 | 0.00 | 0.1 | SR21 (09135) |
| grape juice, sweetened, from frozen concentrate | 8 fl oz (250 g) | 31.6 | 11.0 | | 9.0 | 0.00 | | | Matthews et al, 1987 |
| grapefruit juice, canned/bottled | 8 fl oz (247 g) | 21.9 | | 0.00 | | 0.00 | | | Matthews et al, 1987 |
| grapefruit juice, raw | 8 fl oz (247 g) | 22.5 | 4.4 | 0.00 | 6.7 | 0.00 | | 4.4 | Matthews et al, 1987 |
| guava nectar, canned | 8 fl oz (251 g) | 31.0 | 14.0 | 0.00 | 14.7 | 0.00 | 1.8 | 0.5 | SR21 (09435) |
| mango nectar, canned | 8 fl oz (251 g) | 31.2 | 13.9 | 0.00 | 13.3 | 0.00 | 1.4 | 2.6 | SR21 (09436) |
| orange juice, canned/bottled | 8 fl oz (249 g) | 21.8 | 6.0 | 0.00 | 5.6 | 0.00 | 0.00 | 10.1 | SR21 (09207) |
| orange juice, from frozen concentrate | 8 fl oz (249 g) | 20.9 | 6.4 | 0.00 | 5.8 | 0.00 | 0.00 | 8.7 | SR21 (09215) |
| orange juice, raw | 8 fl oz (248 g) | 20.8 | 7.4 | 0.00 | 6.9 | 0.00 | | 10.2 | Matthews et al, 1987 |
| pear nectar, raw | 8 fl oz (250 g) | 21.7 | 17.7 | 0.00 | 4.0 | 0.00 | | | Matthews et al, 1987 |
| pineapple juice, canned/bottled | 8 fl oz (250 g) | 24.9 | 9.5 | 0.00 | 11.6 | 0.00 | 0.00 | 3.8 | SR21 (09273) |
| pomegranate juice, bottled | 8 fl oz (249 g) | 31.5 | 15.9 | 0.00 | 15.6 | 0.00 | 0.00 | 0.00 | SR21 (09442) |
| prune juice, canned/bottled | 8 fl oz (256 g) | 42.1 | 20.2 | 0.00 | 14.1 | 0.00 | | | Matthews et al, 1987 |
| tamarind nectar, canned | 8 fl oz (251 g) | 31.9 | 15.2 | 0.00 | 14.8 | 0.00 | 1.4 | 0.3 | SR21 (09437) |
| tomato juice, canned/bottled | 8 fl oz (243 g) | 8.6 | 3.7 | | 3.3 | | | 0.6 | SR21 (11886) |
| vegetable juice, canned/bottled | 8 fl oz (242 g) | 8.0 | 4.6 | 0.00 | 3.1 | 0.00 | 0.00 | 0.5 | Matthews et al, 1987 |

**FRUITS**

| | SERVING SIZE (g) | TOTAL SUGARS (g/serving) | FRUCTOSE (g/serving) | GALACTOSE (g/serving) | GLUCOSE (g/serving) | LACTOSE (g/serving) | MALTOSE (g/serving) | SUCROSE (g/serving) | SOURCE (SR21 CODE NUMBER) |
|---|---|---|---|---|---|---|---|---|---|
| abiyuch, raw | ½ cup (114 g) | 9.7 | 4.3 | 0.00 | 5.1 | 0.00 | 0.2 | 0.00 | SR21 (09427) |
| apple, peeled, raw | medium 2¾" diameter (128 g) | 12.9 | 7.7 | 0.00 | 4.2 | 0.00 | 0.00 | 1.0 | SR21 (09004) |
| apple, raw | medium 2¾" diameter (138 g) | 14.3 | 8.1 | 0.00 | 3.3 | 0.00 | 0.00 | 2.8 | SR21 (09003) |
| apple, Red Delicious, raw | medium 2¾" diameter (138 g) | 13.9 | 7.7 | | 2.52 | | | 3.7 | Li et al, 2002 |

| | SERVING SIZE (g) | TOTAL SUGARS (g/serving) | FRUCTOSE (g/serving) | GALACTOSE (g/serving) | GLUCOSE (g/serving) | LACTOSE (g/serving) | MALTOSE (g/serving) | SUCROSE (g/serving) | SOURCE (SR21 CODE NUMBER) |
|---|---|---|---|---|---|---|---|---|---|
| applesauce, sweetened, canned/bottled | 1 cup (255 g) | 37.4 | 18.5 | 0.00 | 14.0 | 0.00 | 2.3 | 2.5 | SR21 (09020) |
| applesauce, unsweetened, canned/bottled | 1 cup (244 g) | 22.9 | 14.3 | 0.00 | 5.6 | 0.00 | 0.2 | 2.7 | SR21 (09019) |
| apricot, dried | ½ cup halves (65 g) | 34.7 | 8.1 | 0.00 | 21.5 | 0.00 | 0.00 | 5.1 | SR21 (09032) |
| apricot, raw | 3 apricots (105 g) | 9.7 | 1.0 | 0.00 | 2.5 | 0.00 | 0.1 | 6.2 | SR21 (09021) |
| avocado, Florida Fuerte, raw | 1 medium (304 g) | 7.3 | 0.8 | | 6.6 | | | | Li et al, 2002 |
| avocado, Florida, raw | 1 medium (304 g) | 7.3 | 0.8 | | 6.6 | 0.00 | 0.00 | 0.00 | SR21 (09039) |
| banana, raw | medium 7–8" long (118 g) | 14.4 | 5.7 | 0.00 | 5.9 | 0.00 | | 2.8 | SR21 (09040) |
| blackberries, raw | 1 cup (144 g) | 7.0 | 3.4 | 0.00 | 3.3 | 0.00 | 0.1 | 0.1 | SR21 (09042) |
| blackberries, wild, raw | 1 cup (144 g) | 5.2 | 2.8 | 0.00 | 2.4 | 0.00 | 0.00 | 0.00 | SR21 (35015) |
| blueberries in light syrup, canned | 1 cup (244 g) | 42.7 | 20.6 | 0.00 | 21.0 | 0.00 | 0.00 | 1.0 | SR21 (09352) |
| blueberries, raw | 1 cup (145 g) | 14.4 | 7.2 | 0.00 | 7.1 | 0.00 | 0.00 | 0.1 | SR21 (09050) |
| blueberries, wild, frozen | 1 cup (140 g) | ~9.9 | 5.2 | | 4.7 | 0.00 | 0.00 | 0.00 | SR21 (09053) |
| blueberries, wild, in heavy syrup, canned | 1 cup (319 g) | 61.5 | 28.8 | 0.00 | 32.3 | 0.00 | 0.4 | 0.00 | SR21 (09053) |
| blueberries, wild, raw | 1 cup (148 g) | 9.6 | 4.9 | 0.00 | 4.6 | 0.00 | 0.00 | 0.00 | SR21 (35155) |
| cantaloupe, raw | 1 cup pieces (177 g) | 13.9 | 3.3 | 0.1 | 2.7 | 0.00 | 0.1 | 7.7 | SR21 (09181) |
| cherries, sour, canned in water, solids and liquid | 1 cup (244 g) | 18.5 | 6.6 | | 9.5 | | | 2.4 | SR21 (09064) |
| cherries, sour, raw | 1cup (103 g) | 8.7 | 3.6 | 0.00 | 4.3 | 0.00 | 0.00 | 0.8 | SR21 (09063) |
| cherries, sweet, raw | 1 cup (117 g) | 15.0 | 6.3 | 0.7 | 7.7 | 0.00 | 0.1 | 0.17 | SR21 (09070) |
| chokecherries, pitted, raw | 3.5 oz (100 g) | 14.2 | 5.4 | 0.00 | 8.8 | 0.00 | 0.00 | 0.00 | SR21 (35179) |
| clementine, raw | 2.6 oz fruit (74 g) | 6.8 | 1.2 | 0.00 | 1.2 | 0.00 | 0.00 | 4.4 | SR21 (09433) |
| currants, black, raw | 1 cup (112 g) | 9.0 | 4.1 | 0.00 | 3.7 | 0.00 | 0.00 | 1.1 | Matthews et al, 1987 |
| currants, red/white, raw | 1 cup (112 g) | 8.2 | 3.9 | | 3.6 | | | 0.7 | SR21 (09084) |
| date, dried | 4 dates (32 g) | 20.3 | 6.2 | 0.00 | 6.3 | 0.00 | 0.00 | 7.6 | SR21 (09087) |
| date, medjool, dried | 1 date (24 g) | 15.9 | 7.7 | 0.00 | 8.1 | 0.00 | 0.00 | 0.1 | SR21 (09421) |
| fig, dried | 1 fig (19 g) | 9.1 | 4.3 | 0.00 | 4.7 | 0.00 | 0.00 | 0.00 | SR21 (09094) |
| fig, raw | 1 medium (50 g) | 8.1 | 1.4 | | 1.8 | 0.00 | | 0.2 | Matthews et al, 1987 |
| fruit cocktail, canned in juice | 1 cup (237 g) | 25.7 | 14.2 | | 14.2 | 0.00 | | 7.8 | Matthews et al, 1987 |
| grapefruit, pink and red, raw | ½ medium (123 g) | 8.5 | 2.2 | 0.00 | 2.0 | 0.00 | 0.00 | 4.3 | SR21 (09112) |
| grapefruit, raw | ½ medium (118 g) | 8.2 | 1.4 | 0.00 | 1.5 | 0.00 | | 4.0 | Matthews et al, 1987 |
| grapefruit, white, raw | ½ medium (118 g) | 8.6 | 1.9 | | 1.9 | | 0.1 | 2.8 | Li et al, 2002 |
| grapes, American (slip skin), all colors, raw | 1 cup (92 g) | 14.9 | 6.3 | | 6.0 | 0.00 | 1.4 | 1.3 | Matthews et al, 1987 |
| grapes, green, Thompson seedless, raw | 1 cup (160 g) | 24.8 | 13.0 | | 11.5 | | 0.00 | 0.2 | Li et al, 2002 |
| grapes, red/green, European, seedless, raw | 1 cup (160 g) | 24.8 | 13.0 | 0.00 | 11.5 | 0.00 | 0.00 | 0.2 | SR21 (09132) |
| guava, raw | 1 medium (90 g) | 8.0 | 1.6 | | 0.7 | | | 1.0 | Li et al, 2002 |
| honeydew melon, raw | 1 cup pieces (177 g) | 14.4 | 5.2 | 0.00 | 4.7 | 0.00 | 0.00 | 4.4 | SR21 (09184) |
| jackfruit, raw | 1 cup sliced (165 g) | 30.4 | 2.3 | 0.00 | 2.3 | 0.00 | | 8.9 | Matthews et al, 1987 |
| kiwifruit, raw | 1 medium (76 g) | 6.8 | 3.3 | 0.1 | 3.1 | 0.00 | 0.1 | 0.1 | SR21 (09148) |
| mango, raw | 1 medium (207 g) | 30.6 | 7.9 | | 1.4 | | | 6.6 | Li et al, 2002 |
| nectarine, raw | 1 medium (136 g) | 10.7 | 1.9 | 0.00 | 2.1 | 0.00 | 0.00 | 6.6 | SR21 (09191) |
| orange, all varieties, raw | 1 medium (131 g) | 12.2 | 3.3 | 0.00 | 2.9 | 0.00 | 0.4 | 5.5 | Matthews et al, 1987 |
| orange, California navel, raw | 1 medium (140 g) | 11.9 | 3.1 | 0.00 | 2.8 | 0.00 | 0.00 | 6.0 | SR21 (09202) |
| papaya, raw | 1 medium (304 g) | 17.9 | 8.2 | 0.00 | 4.2 | 0.00 | 0.00 | 5.5 | Matthews et al, 1987 |
| peach, canned in juice | 1 cup (250 g) | 25.7 | 14.7 | 0.00 | 16.2 | 0.00 | 3.5 | 9.0 | Matthews et al, 1987 |

| | SERVING SIZE (g) | TOTAL SUGARS (g/serving) | FRUCTOSE (g/serving) | GALACTOSE (g/serving) | GLUCOSE (g/serving) | LACTOSE (g/serving) | MALTOSE (g/serving) | SUCROSE (g/serving) | SOURCE (SR21 CODE NUMBER) |
|---|---|---|---|---|---|---|---|---|---|
| peach, dried | 1 cup halves (160 g) | 66.8 | 21.6 | | 20.5 | | | 24.7 | SR21 (09246) |
| peach, peeled, raw | 1 medium (213 g) | 24.1 | 8.3 | | 7.5 | | | 8.3 | Li et al, 2002 |
| peach, raw | 1 medium (98 g) | 8.2 | 1.5 | 0.00 | 1.9 | 0.00 | 0.1 | 4.7 | SR21 (09236) |
| pear, canned in heavy syrup | 1 cup halves (266 g) | ~40.6 | 15.7 | 0.00 | 16.2 | 0.00 | 5.0 | 3.7 | Matthews et al, 1987 |
| pear, canned in heavy syrup, solids and liquid | 1 cup halves (266 g) | 40.4 | 15.7 | | 16.2 | | 5.0 | 3.7 | SR21 (09257) |
| pear, canned in juice | 1 cup halves (248 g) | 24.0 | 14.4 | 0.00 | 8.2 | 0.00 | 0.00 | 1.5 | Matthews et al, 1987 |
| pear, canned in juice, solids and liquid | 1 cup halves (248 g) | 24.0 | 14.4 | | 8.2 | | 0.00 | 1.5 | SR21 (09254) |
| pear, canned in light syrup | 1 cup halves (251 g) | 30.4 | 12.8 | 0.00 | 12.0 | 0.00 | 2.8 | 2.8 | Matthews et al, 1987 |
| pear, canned in light syrup, solids and liquid | 1 cup halves (251 g) | 30.4 | 12.8 | | 12.0 | | 2.8 | 2.8 | SR21 (09256) |
| pear, canned in water | 1 cup halves (244 g) | 14.9 | 9.5 | 0.00 | 4.6 | 0.00 | 0.00 | 0.7 | Matthews et al, 1987 |
| pear, canned in water, solids and liquid | 1 cup halves (244 g) | 14.9 | 9.5 | | 4.6 | | 0.00 | 0.7 | SR21 (09253) |
| pear, raw | 1 medium (166 g) | 16.3 | 10.3 | 0.00 | 4.6 | 0.00 | 0.00 | 1.3 | SR21 (09252) |
| persimmon, Japanese, raw | 1 medium (168 g) | 21.0 | 9.3 | | 9.1 | | | 2.6 | SR21 (09263) |
| pineapple, canned in heavy syrup | 1 cup pieces (254 g) | 42.9 | 18.3 | 0.00 | 19.0 | 0.00 | | 5.6 | Matthews et al, 1987 |
| pineapple, canned in heavy syrup, solids and liquid | 1 cup pieces (254 g) | 42.9 | 18.3 | | 19.0 | | | 5.6 | SR21 (09270) |
| pineapple, canned in juice | 1 cup pieces (249 g) | 36.0 | 16.2 | 0.00 | 19.2 | 0.00 | | 0.6 | Matthews et al, 1987 |
| pineapple, canned in juice, solids and liquid | 1 cup pieces (249 g) | 36.0 | 16.2 | | 19.2 | | | 0.6 | SR21 (09268) |
| pineapple, raw | 1 cup pieces (155 g) | 15.3 | 3.3 | 0.00 | 2.7 | 0.00 | 0.00 | 9.3 | SR21 (09266) |
| plum, prune, raw | 1 cup halves (165 g) | 19.3 | 5.4 | 0.00 | 5.1 | 0.00 | 0.5 | 8.2 | Matthews et al, 1987 |
| plum, raw | 1 medium (66 g) | 6.5 | 2.0 | 0.1 | 3.3 | 0.00 | 0.00 | 1.0 | SR21 (09279) |
| pomegranate, raw | 1 medium (154 g) | 25.5 | 7.2 | 0.00 | 7.7 | 0.00 | 0.00 | 0.6 | Matthews et al, 1987 |
| prune puree | 1 oz (28 g) | 10.9 | 3.9 | | 6.2 | | | | SR21 (09423) |
| prune, dried | 2 prunes (16 g) | 6.1 | 2.0 | 0.00 | 4.1 | 0.00 | 0.00 | 0.00 | SR21 (09291) |
| raisins, seedless | 1.5 oz snack box (43 g) | 25.4 | 12.8 | 0.00 | 11.9 | 0.00 | 0.00 | 0.2 | SR21 (09298) |
| raspberries, raw | 1 cup (123 g) | 5.4 | 2.9 | 0.00 | 2.3 | 0.00 | 0.00 | 0.2 | SR21 (09302) |
| rowal, raw (fruit) | 1 cup (228 g) | 32.1 | 1.1 | 0.00 | 2.5 | 0.00 | 0.00 | 28.5 | SR21 (09428) |
| strawberries, raw | 1 cup whole (144 g) | 7.0 | 3.5 | 0.00 | 2.9 | 0.00 | 0.00 | 0.7 | SR21 (09316) |
| strawberries, unsweetened, frozen, thawed | 1 cup (221 g) | 10.1 | 4.8 | | 4.5 | | | 0.8 | SR21 (09318) |
| tangelo, raw | 4.7 oz (131 g) | 9.7 | | 0.00 | 4.8 | 0.00 | | 4.8 | Matthews et al, 1987 |
| tangerine, raw | 1 medium (84 g) | 8.9 | 2.0 | 0.00 | 1.8 | 0.00 | 0.00 | 5.1 | SR21 (09218) |
| watermelon, raw | 1 cup pieces (152 g) | 9.4 | 5.1 | 0.00 | 2.4 | 0.00 | 0.1 | 1.8 | SR21 (09326) |

**GRAIN PRODUCTS**

| | | | | | | | | | |
|---|---|---|---|---|---|---|---|---|---|
| breadcrumbs, dry, grated | 1 cup (108 g) | 6.7 | 2.6 | 0.00 | 2.0 | 0.00 | 2.1 | 0.00 | SR21 (18079) |
| breadcrumbs, dry, grated, seasoned | 1 cup (120 g) | 6.9 | 2.4 | 0.00 | 2.1 | 0.00 | 2.5 | 0.00 | SR21 (18376) |
| granola bar, chocolate chip, soft | 1 oz bar (28 g) | 8.1 | 0.6 | 0.00 | 1.4 | 0.1 | 1.3 | 4.6 | SR21 (19404) |
| granola bar, hard | 1 oz bar (28 g) | 5.5 | 0.4 | 0.00 | 0.3 | 0.00 | | 4.8 | Matthews et al, 1987 |
| popcorn, caramel-coated | 1 oz (28 g) | 14.9 | 0.2 | | 0.7 | | 0.3 | 9.5 | Matthews et al, 1987 |

| | SERVING SIZE (g) | TOTAL SUGARS (g/serving) | FRUCTOSE (g/serving) | GALACTOSE (g/serving) | GLUCOSE (g/serving) | LACTOSE (g/serving) | MALTOSE (g/serving) | SUCROSE (g/serving) | SOURCE (SR21 CODE NUMBER) |
|---|---|---|---|---|---|---|---|---|---|
| **INFANT, JUNIOR, AND TODDLER FOODS** | | | | | | | | | |
| apple blueberry, junior food | 6 oz jar (170 g) | 15.0 | 8.2 | 0.00 | 6.1 | 0.00 | 0.00 | 0.7 | SR21 (03165) |
| apple raspberry, strained infant food | 4 oz jar (113 g) | 14.6 | | | | | | 0.8 | SR21 (03152) |
| apples and chicken dinner, Beech-Nut Stage 2/Gerber 2nd Foods/ Heinz Strained-2 | 4 oz jar (113 g) | 8.9 | 5.8 | | 2.1 | 0.00 | 0.00 | 1.0 | SR21 (03297) |
| apples and sweet potatoes dinner, Gerber 2nd Foods | 4 oz jar (113 g) | 13.1 | 8.0 | | 3.5 | | 0.9 | 0.7 | SR21 (03154) |
| applesauce and apricots, Beech-Nut Stage 2/ Gerber 2nd Foods/ Heinz Strained-2 | 4 oz jar (113 g) | 10.4 | 5.4 | 0.00 | 3.2 | 0.00 | 0.00 | 1.8 | SR21 (03142) |
| applesauce and apricots, Heinz Junior-3 | 4.5 oz jar (128 g) | 11.2 | 6.7 | 0.00 | 3.6 | 0.00 | 0.00 | 0.9 | SR21 (03143) |
| bananas with pineapple and tapioca, Gerber 2nd Foods/Heinz Strained-2 | 4.25 oz jar (120 g) | 12.9 | 4.1 | 0.00 | 4.0 | 0.00 | 0.00 | 4.7 | SR21 (03157) |
| corn and sweet potatoes, strained infant food | 4.5 oz jar (128 g) | 5.1 | 0.1 | 0.00 | 0.1 | 0.00 | 0.00 | 0.8 | SR21 (03934) |
| Dutch apple dessert, junior food | 6 oz jar (170 g) | 30.4 | 9.0 | | 3.6 | 0.00 | 0.00 | 15.0 | SR21 (03221) |
| mixed cereal with applesauce and bananas, strained infant food | 4 oz jar (113 g) | 8.8 | 3.5 | 0.00 | 3.6 | 0.00 | 0.00 | 1.7 | SR21 (03187) |
| mixed cereal with applesauce and bananas, junior food | 6 oz jar (170 g) | 13.2 | 5.2 | 0.00 | 5.4 | 0.00 | 0.00 | 2.6 | SR21 (03188) |
| peach cobbler, Gerber 2nd Foods/Heinz Strained-2 | 4 oz jar (113 g) | 12.0 | 0.7 | 0.00 | 0.9 | 0.00 | 0.00 | 2.3 | SR21 (03227) |
| peaches, Beech-Nut/ Gerber/Heinz | 4 oz jar (113 g) | 13.0 | 4.5 | 0.00 | 4.6 | 0.00 | 0.00 | 3.8 | SR21 (03130) |
| peaches, Beech-Nut Stage 3/Gerber 3rd Foods/Heinz Junior-3 | 6 oz jar (170 g) | 19.5 | 6.8 | 0.00 | 7.0 | 0.00 | 0.00 | 5.7 | SR21 (03131) |
| pears and pineapple, Gerber 3rd Foods | 6 oz jar (170 g) | 12.5 | 7.2 | 0.00 | 3.4 | 0.00 | 0.00 | 1.9 | SR21 (03159) |
| plums with tapioca, Gerber 2nd Foods/ Heinz Strained-2 | 4 oz jar (113 g) | 15.1 | 4.6 | 0.2 | 7.7 | 0.00 | 0.1 | 2.4 | SR21 (03134) |
| plums, bananas, and rice, strained infant food | 4.5 oz jar (128 g) | 11.9 | 3.7 | 0.1 | 6.0 | 0.00 | 0.1 | 1.9 | SR21 (03293) |
| prunes with tapioca, Gerber 2nd Foods/ Heinz Strained-2 | 4 oz jar (113 g) | 12.4 | 3.7 | 0.00 | 7.7 | 0.00 | 0.00 | 0.00 | SR21 (03136) |
| prunes with tapioca, junior food | 6 oz jar (170 g) | 18.6 | 5.6 | 0.00 | 11.5 | 0.00 | 0.00 | 0.1 | SR21 (03137) |
| squash, yellow, Gerber 3rd Foods | 6 oz jar (170 g) | 5.5 | 1.6 | 0.00 | 1.8 | 0.00 | 0.00 | 2.0 | SR21 (03105) |
| vanilla custard pudding, Beech-Nut Stage 3/ Gerber 3rd Foods/ Heinz Junior-3 | 6 oz jar (170 g) | 20.7 | 0.4 | 0.00 | 0.4 | 2.9 | 0.00 | 15.9 | SR21 (03246) |

| | SERVING SIZE (g) | TOTAL SUGARS (g/serving) | FRUCTOSE (g/serving) | GALACTOSE (g/serving) | GLUCOSE (g/serving) | LACTOSE (g/serving) | MALTOSE (g/serving) | SUCROSE (g/serving) | SOURCE (SR21 CODE NUMBER) |
|---|---|---|---|---|---|---|---|---|---|
| **MILKS, MILK BEVERAGES, AND YOGURT** | | | | | | | | | |
| buttermilk, cultured | 8 fl oz (245 g) | 11.7 | 0.00 | 0.5 | 0.00 | 9.1 | 0.00 | 0.00 | Matthews et al, 1987 |
| chocolate milk made with chocolate malt mix | 8 fl oz (265 g) | 17.7 | 0.8 | | | 10.9 | 5.8 | 0.5 | Matthews et al, 1987 |
| chocolate milk, reduced fat | 8 fl oz (250 g) | 23.9 | 1.0 | | 1.3 | 9.6 | 0.00 | 12.0 | SR21 (01103) |
| cocoa (hot chocolate), homemade with 2% milk | 8 fl oz (250 g) | 24.2 | 0.00 | 0.00 | 0.00 | 11.6 | 0.00 | 0.00 | SR21 (01105) |
| eggnog, nonalcoholic | 8 fl oz (254 g) | 21.4 | 0.00 | 0.00 | 0.1 | 10.6 | 0.00 | 0.00 | SR21 (01057) |
| milk, acidophilus | 8 fl oz (227 g) | 7.5 | 0.00 | 1.6 | 0.00 | 5.9 | 0.00 | 0.00 | Matthews et al, 1987 |
| milk, lowfat, 1% fat | 8 fl oz (244 g) | 12.7 | 0.00 | 0.00 | 0.00 | 12.7 | 0.00 | 0.00 | SR21 (01082) |
| milk, nonfat | 8 fl oz (245 g) | 12.5 | 0.00 | 0.00 | 0.00 | 12.5 | 0.00 | 0.00 | SR21 (01085) |
| milk powder, nonfat, regular without vitamin A | ¼ cup (30 g) | 15.6 | 0.00 | | | 15.1 | | | Matthews et al, 1987 |
| milk, reduced fat, 2% fat | 8 fl oz (244 g) | 12.3 | 0.00 | 0.00 | 0.00 | 12.2 | 0.00 | 0.00 | SR21 (01080) |
| milk, whole, 3.25% fat | 8 fl oz (244 g) | 12.8 | 0.00 | 0.00 | 0.00 | 12.8 | 0.00 | 0.00 | SR21 (01077) |
| yogurt, lowfat, plain | 8 oz container (227 g) | 16.0 | 0.00 | 3.2 | 0.00 | 8.4 | 0.00 | 0.00 | Matthews et al, 1987 |
| yogurt, lowfat, strawberry | 8 oz container (227 g) | 42.3 | 5.9 | 2.3 | 7.7 | 7.5 | 1.6 | 10.0 | Matthews et al, 1987 |
| **NUTS** | | | | | | | | | |
| coconut cream, sweetened, canned | 8 fl oz (296 g) | 152.4 | 0.00 | | 0.00 | 0.00 | 0.00 | 152.4 | SR21 (12116) |
| coconut, dried, sweetened, flaked, canned | 1 oz (28 g) | 9.6 | 0.00 | 0.00 | 0.2 | 0.00 | | | Matthews et al, 1987 |
| coconut, dried, sweetened, flaked, packaged | 1 oz (28 g) | 10.3 | 0.00 | 0.00 | 0.1 | 0.00 | 0.00 | 10.1 | SR21 (12109) |
| coconut, dried, toasted | 1 oz (28 g) | 10.6 | | 0.00 | | 0.00 | | 9.0 | Matthews et al, 1987 |
| **SALAD DRESSINGS** | | | | | | | | | |
| Russian salad dressing, low/reduced calorie | 2 T (32 g) | 6.0 | 3.8 | 0.00 | 5.0 | 0.00 | 0.00 | 0.00 | Matthews et al, 1987 |
| Russian salad dressing | 2 T (30 g) | 6.5 | 0.6 | 0.00 | 5.2 | 0.00 | 1.7 | 1.9 | Matthews et al, 1987 |
| **SUGARS, SYRUPS, AND OTHER SWEETENERS** | | | | | | | | | |
| corn syrup, dark | 2 T (40 g) | 10.7 | 0.5 | | 6.0 | 0.00 | 3.9 | 0.9 | Matthews et al, 1987 |
| corn syrup, high-fructose | 2 T (38 g) | 10.0 | 14.2 | | 13.9 | 0.00 | | 0.3 | Matthews et al, 1987 |
| corn syrup, light (in color) | 2 T (40 g) | 10.7 | | | | | | 0.00 | SR21 (19350) |
| honey | 1 T (21 g) | 17.2 | 8.6 | 0.6 | 7.5 | | 0.3 | 0.2 | SR21 (19296) |
| maple syrup | 2 T (40 g) | 23.8 | 0.3 | | 0.9 | | | 22.5 | SR21 (19353) |
| molasses | 2 T (40 g) | 22.2 | 5.1 | | 4.8 | | | 11.8 | SR21 (19304) |
| molasses, blackstrap | 2 T (40 g) | 17.1 | 3.2 | 0.00 | 3.0 | 0.00 | | 10.8 | Matthews et al, 1987 |
| pancake/waffle syrup | 1 T (20 g) | 6.6 | 1.0 | 0.00 | 3.9 | 0.00 | 2.3 | 2.4 | Matthews et al, 1987 |
| sorghum syrup | 1 T (21 g) | 15.7 | | 0.00 | | 0.00 | | 7.0 | Matthews et al, 1987 |
| sugar, brown | 1T (14 g) | 13.6 | 0.1 | 0.00 | 0.2 | 0.00 | 0.00 | 13.2 | SR21 (19334) |
| sugar, white, caramelized | 1 T (15 g) | 6.8 | | 0.00 | 4.8 | 0.00 | 0.3 | 1.8 | Matthews et al, 1987 |
| sugar, white, powdered | 1 T (8 g) | 7.8 | | 0.00 | | 0.00 | | 7.4 | Matthews et al, 1987 |
| **VEGETABLES** | | | | | | | | | |
| agave, boiled | 3.5 oz (100 g) | 20.9 | 17.6 | 0.00 | 1.6 | 0.00 | 0.00 | 1.7 | SR21 (35193) |
| agave, dried | 1 oz (28 g) | 14.2 | 12.0 | 0.00 | 1.0 | 0.00 | 0.00 | 1.2 | SR21 (35194) |
| baked beans with pork in sweet sauce, canned | 1 cup (253 g) | 21.6 | 3.2 | 0.00 | 3.3 | 0.00 | 0.2 | 13.8 | SR21 (16010) |

| | SERVING SIZE (g) | TOTAL SUGARS (g/serving) | FRUCTOSE (g/serving) | GALACTOSE (g/serving) | GLUCOSE (g/serving) | LACTOSE (g/serving) | MALTOSE (g/serving) | SUCROSE (g/serving) | SOURCE (SR21 CODE NUMBER) |
|---|---|---|---|---|---|---|---|---|---|
| baked beans with pork in tomato sauce, canned | 1 cup (253 g) | 14.3 | 2.6 | 0.00 | 3.0 | 0.00 | 0.2 | 8.5 | SR21 (16011) |
| baked beans, vegetarian, canned | 1 cup (254 g) | 20.2 | 4.0 | 0.00 | 4.0 | 0.00 | 0.00 | 12.2 | SR21 (16006) |
| carrot, frozen, boiled | 1 cup sliced (146 g) | 5.9 | 0.4 | 0.00 | 0.5 | 0.00 | 0.00 | 5.0 | SR21 (11131) |
| carrot, microwaved | 1 cup sliced (146 g) | 10.8 | 0.7 | | 0.7 | | | 9.3 | Li et al, 2002 |
| chickpeas (garbanzo beans), mature, boiled | 1 cup (164 g) | 7.9 | 0.2 | 0.2 | 0.2 | 0.00 | 0.3 | 2.0 | Matthews et al, 1987 |
| corn, white, steamed | 1 cup (164 g) | 10.6 | 1.7 | 0.00 | 1.8 | 0.00 | 0.00 | 7.1 | SR21 (35135) |
| corn, yellow, canned | 1 cup (164 g) | 5.0 | 0.4 | 0.6 | 0.8 | 0.00 | 0.4 | 2.8 | SR21 (11172) |
| corn, yellow, canned, vacuum pack | 1 cup (210 g) | 7.5 | 0.5 | 0.00 | 0.5 | 0.00 | 0.3 | 6.1 | SR21 (11176) |
| corn, yellow, creamed, canned | 1 cup (256 g) | 8.3 | 0.6 | 0.00 | 0.6 | 0.00 | 0.3 | 6.8 | SR21 (11174) |
| corn, yellow, frozen, boiled | 1 cup (164 g) | 5.0 | 0.7 | 0.00 | 0.8 | 0.00 | 0.3 | 3.2 | SR21 (11179) |
| corn, yellow, on cob, from farm, raw | 1 cup kernels (154 g) | 10.2 | 2.4 | | 2.1 | | | 5.6 | Li et al, 2002 |
| cucumber, raw | 1 large (301 g) | 5.0 | 2.6 | 0.00 | 2.3 | 0.00 | 0.00 | 0.1 | SR21 (11205) |
| eggplant (aubergine), fried, not breaded | 1 cup (130 g) | 5.2 | 2.5 | 0.00 | 2.2 | 0.00 | | 0.4 | Matthews et al, 1987 |
| Jerusalem artichoke (sunchoke), raw, freshly harvested | 1 cup chopped (130 g) | 12.5 | 0.3 | 0.00 | 0.00 | 0.00 | 0.00 | 3.0 | Matthews et al, 1987 |
| Jerusalem artichoke (sunchoke), raw, stored | 1 cup chopped (143 g) | 13.7 | 1.1 | 0.00 | 0.8 | 0.00 | 1.0 | 10.7 | Matthews et al, 1987 |
| lima beans, mature, large, boiled | 1 cup (184 g) | 5.3 | 0.4 | | | 0.00 | 0.00 | 0.9 | Matthews et al, 1987 |
| onion, white, boiled, drained | 1 cup chopped (210 g) | 9.9 | 3.0 | 0.00 | 4.6 | 0.00 | 0.00 | 2.3 | SR21 (11283) |
| onion, white, raw | 1 cup chopped (160 g) | 6.8 | 2.1 | 0.00 | 3.1 | 0.00 | 0.00 | 1.6 | SR21 (11282) |
| peas, green, boiled | 1 cup (160 g) | 9.5 | 0.6 | 0.00 | 0.2 | 0.00 | 0.3 | 8.3 | SR21 (11305) |
| peas, green, canned | 1 cup (170 g) | 5.1 | 0.1 | 0.2 | 0.3 | 0.00 | 0.1 | 4.4 | SR21 (11308) |
| peas, green, frozen, boiled | 1 cup (160 g) | 7.4 | 0.2 | 0.00 | 0.2 | 0.00 | 0.2 | 6.9 | SR21 (11313) |
| peas, green, raw | 1 cup (145 g) | 8.2 | 0.6 | 0.00 | 0.2 | 0.00 | 0.2 | 7.2 | SR21 (11304) |
| radish, Oriental, raw | radish 7" long (338g) | 8.4 | | 0.00 | | 0.00 | | | Matthews et al, 1987 |
| rutabaga (Swede), raw | 1 cup cubed (140 g) | 7.84 | 2.0 | 0.00 | 4.5 | 0.00 | | 1.1 | Matthews et al, 1987 |
| soybeans, mature, boiled | 1 cup (172 g) | 5.2 | 0.3 | | 0.2 | 0.00 | 0.00 | 0.9 | Matthews et al, 1987 |
| sweet pepper, red, raw | 1 medium (119 g) | 5.0 | 2.7 | 0.00 | 2.3 | 0.00 | 0.00 | 0.00 | SR21 (11821) |
| sweet potato, baked | 1 medium (114 g) | 7.4 | 0.6 | 0.00 | 0.6 | 0.00 | 3.5 | 2.6 | SR21 (11508) |
| sweet potato, canned, vacuum pack | 1 cup pieces (200 g) | 10.0 | | 0.00 | | 0.00 | | | Matthews et al, 1987 |
| sweet potato, peeled, boiled | 1 cup mashed (328 g) | 18.8 | 1.4 | 0.00 | 1.8 | 0.00 | 10.9 | 4.7 | SR21 (11510) |
| sweet potato, raw | 1 medium (130 g) | 5.4 | 0.9 | 0.00 | 1.2 | 0.00 | 0.00 | 3.3 | SR21 (11507) |
| tomato paste, canned | 6 oz can (170 g) | 20.7 | 9.9 | 0.00 | 9.8 | 0.00 | 0.5 | 0.5 | SR21 (11546) |
| tomato puree, canned | ½ cup (125 g) | 6.0 | 3.0 | 0.00 | 3.1 | 0.00 | 0.00 | 0.00 | SR21 (11547) |
| tomato sauce, bottled | ½ cup (122 g) | 5.2 | 2.0 | 0.00 | 2.8 | 0.00 | 0.00 | 0.3 | SR21 (11549) |
| tomato, red, boiled | 1 cup (240 g) | 6.0 | 3.1 | 0.00 | 2.8 | 0.00 | 0.00 | 0.00 | SR21 (11530) |
| tomato, red, canned | 1 cup (240 g) | 5.7 | 3.0 | 0.00 | 2.6 | 0.00 | 0.00 | 0.00 | SR21 (11531) |
| tomato, red, stewed, canned | 1 cup (255 g) | 9.0 | 4.8 | 0.00 | 4.1 | 0.00 | 0.00 | 0.00 | SR21 (11533) |

| | SERVING SIZE (g) | TOTAL SUGARS (g/serving) | FRUCTOSE (g/serving) | GALACTOSE (g/serving) | GLUCOSE (g/serving) | LACTOSE (g/serving) | MALTOSE (g/serving) | SUCROSE (g/serving) | SOURCE (SR21 CODE NUMBER) |
|---|---|---|---|---|---|---|---|---|---|
| **OTHER FOODS** | | | | | | | | | |
| chocolate malted mix for milk | 3 heaping t (21 g) | 15.0 | 0.9 | | | 1.2 | 5.8 | 0.7 | Matthews et al, 1987 |
| crab, Alaska king, imitation, made from surimi | 3 oz (85 g) | 5.3 | 0.5 | 0.00 | 2.3 | 0.00 | 0.00 | 2.5 | SR21 (15138) |
| mushroom soup, cream of, condensed, canned, prepared with milk | 1 cup (248 g) | 8.2 | 0.00 | 0.00 | 0.00 | 6.6 | 0.00 | 0.00 | SR21 (06243) |
| oatmeal, maple and brown sugar, instant, prepared, Quaker | 1 packet prepared (155 g) | 12.5 | | 0.00 | | 0.00 | | 4.6 | Matthews et al, 1987 |
| PowerBar, chocolate | 2.4 oz bar (68 g) | 20.4 | 10.8 | 0.00 | 8.1 | 0.00 | 1.1 | 0.3 | SR21 (25017) |
| Snickers Marathon Energy Bar, all flavors | 1.9 oz bar (55 g) | 15.8 | 0.3 | 0.00 | 4.7 | 0.00 | 2.9 | 7.8 | SR21 (25016) |
| Snickers Marathon Energy Bar, caramel nut rush | 2.8 oz bar (80 g) | 23.0 | 0.3 | | 7.3 | | 4.5 | 10.8 | SR21 (25015) |
| wheat germ, crude | ½ cup (57 g) | 6.9 | | 0.00 | | 0.00 | 0.00 | 4.2 | Matthews et al, 1987 |
| whey, sweet, fluid | 1 cup (246 g) | 12.6 | 0.00 | 0.00 | 0.00 | 11.1 | | 0.00 | Matthews et al, 1987 |

Sources:
Li BW, Andrews KW, Pehrsson PR. Individual sugars, soluble, and insoluble dietary fiber contents of 70 high consumption foods. *J Food Comp Anal* 15:715–723, 2002.
Matthews RH, Pehrsson PR, Farhat-Sabet M. *Sugars Content of Selected Foods: Individual and Total Sugars.* Home Economics Research Report Number 48, September 1987.
USDA National Nutrient Database for Standard Reference, Release 21 (SR21), 2008. Available at: http://www.nal.usda.gov/fnic/foodcomp.search/.

# Sugars—Raffinose and Stachyose

| | RAFFINOSE (g/100 g) | STACHYOSE (g/100 g) | | RAFFINOSE (g/100 g) | STACHYOSE (g/100 g) |
|---|---|---|---|---|---|
| **GRAINS AND GRAIN FRACTIONS** | | | cauliflower, raw | | 0.1 |
| | | | chicory, raw | 1.2 | 0.3 |
| amaranth grain | 0.3 | | corn, sweet, raw | 0.2 | 0.2 |
| cottonseed flour, defatted | 9.2 | 0.8 | leek, raw | 0.1 | 0.6 |
| millet, proso | 0.1 | | lettuce, romaine (cos), raw | 0.1 | |
| oat bran | 0.3 | 0.2 | onion, raw | 1.4 | 0.7 |
| oat flour | 0.2 | 0.1 | parsley, raw | 0.3 | |
| rice bran | 0.1 | | parsnip, raw | 0.6 | 0.0 |
| sesame flour, defatted | 0.2 | 0.2 | pepper, sweet, green, raw | 0.1 | |
| sorghum grain | 0.1 | | pumpkin, raw | 0.1 | 0.1 |
| sunflower flour, defatted | 3.0 | | salsify, black, raw | 1.6 | 1.1 |
| soy flour, dehulled, defatted | 0.8 | 4.6 | squash, summer, raw | 0.1 | 0.1 |
| wheat bran | 0.1 | | | | |
| wheat flour, white | 0.2 | | **VEGETABLES—LEGUMES** | | |
| wheat flour, whole grain | 0.2 | | adzuki beans, raw | 0.2 | 3.9 |
| | | | blackeye peas (cowpeas), raw | 0.5 | 2.4 |
| **NUTS** | | | broadbeans, boiled | 0.4 | 0.2 |
| peanuts, dried | 0.1 | 0.4 | chickpeas (garbanzo beans), boiled | 0.4 | 0.5 |
| pistachio nuts, dried | 0.6 | 0.1 | common beans, boiled | 0.2 | 0.7 |
| | | | lentils, raw | 0.3 | 1.9 |
| **VEGETABLES** | | | lima beans, raw | 0.4 | 2.5 |
| beet, raw | 0.1 | 0.0 | lupins, raw | 0.7 | 3.7 |
| broccoli, raw | 0.1 | 0.2 | mung beans, boiled | 0.3 | 0.3 |
| Brussels, sprouts, raw | 0.2 | | peas, split, raw | 0.7 | 2.1 |
| cabbage, raw | 0.1 | 0.1 | pigeonpeas, boiled | 0.4 | 0.4 |
| carrot, raw | 0.1 | 0.1 | soybeans, raw | 0.7 | 3.2 |
| | | | winged beans, raw | 1.3 | 2.9 |

Source:
Matthews PH, Pehrsson RP, Farhat-Sabet M. *Sugars Content of Selected Foods: Individual and Total Sugars*, Home Economics Research Report Number 48, September 1987.

# Total Antioxidant Capacity (Oxygen Radical Absorbance Capacity [ORAC])

| | ORAC (μmol TE[1]/100 g) | SR21 CODE NUMBER | | ORAC (μmol TE[1]/100 g) | SR21 CODE NUMBER |
|---|---|---|---|---|---|
| **BEVERAGES** | | | cantaloupe, raw | 315 | 09181 |
| tea, black, brewed | 1128 | 14355 | cranberries, raw | 9584 | 09078 |
| tea, green, brewed | 1253 | 99070 | currants, European black, raw | 7960 | 09083 |
| wine, table, red | 3873 | 14096 | currants, red, raw | 3387 | 99044 |
| wine, table, red, Cabernet Sauvignon | 5034 | 14097 | date, deglet noor | 3895 | 09087 |
| | | | date, medjool | 2387 | 09421 |
| wine, table, rose | 1005 | 99439 | elderberries, raw | 14697 | 09088 |
| wine, table, white | 392 | 14106 | fig, raw | 3383 | 09089 |
| | | | gooseberries, raw | 3277 | 09107 |
| **CANDY** | | | grapefruit, pink and red, raw | 1548 | 09112 |
| dark chocolate | 20823 | 99412 | grapes, red, raw | 1260 | 97074 |
| milk chocolate | 7528 | 19120 | grapes, white/green, raw | 1118 | 99047 |
| semisweet chocolate | 18053 | 19080 | guava, red, raw | 1990 | 99428 |
| | | | guava, white, raw | 2550 | 99429 |
| **CEREALS, READY-TO-EAT** | | | honeydew melon, raw | 241 | 09184 |
| granola, lowfat with raisins | 2294 | 99450 | kiwifruit, raw | 882 | 09148 |
| Life, Quaker | 1517 | 08049 | kiwifruit, gold, raw | 1210 | 97079 |
| oat bran cereal | 2183 | 99452 | lime, raw | 82 | 09159 |
| oat toasted squares | 2143 | 99453 | mango, raw | 1002 | 09176 |
| shredded wheat | 16062 | 08147 | nectarine, raw | 750 | 09191 |
| | | | orange, navel, raw | 1819 | 09202 |
| **FATS AND OILS** | | | peach, canned in heavy syrup | 436 | 09370 |
| peanut oil | 106 | 04042 | peach, dried | 4222 | 99418 |
| olive oil, extra virgin | 1150 | 99423 | peach, raw | 1814 | 09236 |
| | | | pear, dried | 9496 | 99421 |
| **FRUIT JUICES** | | | pear, green, raw | 1911 | 97075 |
| apple juice, canned/bottled | 408 | 09016 | pear, raw | 2941 | 09252 |
| blueberry juice | 2906 | 99430 | pear, red anjou, raw | 1746 | 97076 |
| cranberry juice, red | 865 | 99432 | pineapple, raw | 385 | 09266 |
| cranberry juice, white | 232 | 99433 | pineapple, extra sweet, raw | 884 | 09429 |
| cranberry-concord grape juice | 1480 | 99434 | plum, black, raw | 7581 | 97077 |
| grape juice, concord | 2377 | 99431 | plum, raw | 6259 | 09279 |
| grape juice, red | 1788 | 99436 | prune, dried | 6552 | 09291 |
| grape juice, white | 793 | 99050 | raisins, dried | 3037 | 09298 |
| grapefruit juice | 1238 | 09128 | raspberries, raw | 4882 | 09302 |
| lemon juice | 1225 | 09152 | strawberries, raw | 3577 | 09316 |
| lime juice, raw | 823 | 09160 | tangerine, raw | 1620 | 09218 |
| orange juice, raw | 726 | 09206 | watermelon, raw | 142 | 09326 |
| pear juice | 704 | 97016 | | | |
| pineapple juice, canned | 568 | 09273 | **GRAIN PRODUCTS** | | |
| pomegranate juice | 2341 | 99435 | bread, butternut, whole grain | 2104 | 99449 |
| prune juice, canned | 2036 | 09294 | bread, mixed grain | 1421 | 18035 |
| strawberry juice | 1002 | 99437 | bread, oatnut | 1318 | 99448 |
| | | | bread, pumpernickel | 1963 | 18044 |
| **FRUITS** | | | rice bran | 24287 | 20060 |
| apple, dried | 6681 | 99416 | popcorn, air-popped | 1743 | 19034 |
| apple, Fuji, raw | 2589 | 97066 | tortilla chips, reduced fat | 1704 | 19444 |
| apple, Gala, raw | 2828 | 97067 | | | |
| apple, Golden Delicious, raw | 2670 | 97069 | **INFANT AND JUNIOR FOODS** | | |
| apple, Golden Delicious, raw, peeled | 2210 | 97068 | apple and blueberry, junior | 4822 | 03165 |
| apple, Granny Smith, raw | 3898 | 97070 | applesauce, strained | 4123 | 03116 |
| apple, raw | 3082 | 09003 | bananas, strained | 2658 | 97017 |
| apple, raw, peeled | 2573 | 09004 | peaches, strained | 6257 | 97019 |
| apple, Red Delicious, raw | 4275 | 97072 | peaches, junior | 2551 | 03131 |
| apple, Red Delicious, raw, peeled | 2936 | 97071 | pear juice | 414 | 43408 |
| applesauce, canned | 1965 | 09019 | | | |
| apricot, dried | 3234 | 99417 | **NUTS AND SEEDS** | | |
| apricot, raw | 1115 | 09021 | almonds, raw | 4454 | 12061 |
| banana, raw | 879 | 09040 | Brazil nuts, dried | 1419 | 12078 |
| blackberries, raw | 5347 | 09042 | cashew nuts, raw | 1948 | 12087 |
| blueberries, raw | 6552 | 09050 | hazelnuts (filberts), raw | 9645 | 12120 |

| | ORAC (μmol TE[1]/100 g) | SR21 CODE NUMBER | | ORAC (μmol TE[1]/100 g) | SR21 CODE NUMBER |
|---|---|---|---|---|---|
| macadamia nuts, dry-roasted | 1695 | 12132 | cauliflower, raw | 829 | 11135 |
| peanut butter, smooth | 3432 | 16098 | celery, raw | 497 | 11143 |
| peanuts, raw | 3166 | 16087 | coriander, raw | 5141 | 11165 |
| pecans, raw | 17940 | 12142 | corn, sweet, yellow, canned | 413 | 11170 |
| pine nuts, dried | 616 | 12147 | corn, sweet, yellow, frozen | 522 | 11178 |
| pistachio nuts, raw | 7983 | 12151 | corn, sweet, yellow, raw | 728 | 11167 |
| walnuts, English, raw | 13541 | 12155 | cowpeas, common, mature, raw | 4343 | 16062 |
| | | | cucumber, raw | 214 | 11205 |
| **SPICES AND HERBS** | | | cucumber, raw, peeled | 126 | 11206 |
| basil, raw | 4805 | 02044 | eggplant, boiled | 245 | 11210 |
| basil, dried | 67553 | 02003 | eggplant, raw | 933 | 11209 |
| cardamon | 2764 | 02006 | fennel bulb, raw | 307 | 11957 |
| chili powder | 23636 | 02009 | garden rocket, raw | 1904 | 99414 |
| cinnamon, ground | 267536 | 02010 | green snap beans, canned | 290 | 11054 |
| cloves, ground | 314446 | 02011 | green snap beans, raw | 759 | 11052 |
| cumin seed | 76800 | 02014 | kidney beans, mature, raw | 8459 | 16032 |
| curry powder | 48504 | 02015 | leek, raw | 490 | 11246 |
| dill week, raw | 4392 | 02045 | lentils, raw | 7282 | 16069 |
| garlic powder | 6665 | 02020 | lettuce, butterhead, raw | 1423 | 11250 |
| garlic, raw | 5346 | 11215 | lettuce, green leaf, raw | 1447 | 11253 |
| ginger, ground | 28811 | 02021 | lettuce, iceberg, raw | 438 | 11252 |
| ginger root | 14840 | 11216 | lettuce, red leaf, raw | 2380 | 11257 |
| lemon balm, raw | 5997 | 99112 | lettuce, romaine (cos), raw | 963 | 11251 |
| marjoram, raw | 27297 | 99438 | lima beans, immature, canned | 243 | 11033 |
| mustard seed, yellow | 29257 | 02024 | navy beans, mature, raw | 1520 | 16037 |
| onion powder | 5735 | 02026 | onion, raw | 1034 | 11282 |
| oregano, dried | 200129 | 02027 | onion, red, raw | 1521 | 99055 |
| oregano, raw | 13970 | 99115 | onion, sweet, raw | 614 | 11294 |
| paprika | 17919 | 02028 | onion, white, raw | 863 | 99056 |
| parsley, dried | 74349 | 02029 | onion, yellow, sautéed | 1220 | 11286 |
| parsley, raw | 1301 | 11297 | peas, green, frozen | 600 | 11312 |
| peppermint, raw | 13978 | 02064 | peas, split, mature, raw | 524 | 16085 |
| pepper, black | 27618 | 02030 | peas, yellow, mature, raw | 741 | 99457 |
| poppy seeds | 481 | 02033 | pepper, sweet green, raw | 923 | 11333 |
| sage, raw | 32004 | 99116 | pepper, sweet green sautéed | 615 | 11339 |
| savory, raw | 9465 | 99456 | pepper, sweet orange, raw | 984 | 99451 |
| tarragon, raw | 15542 | 99119 | pepper, sweet red, raw | 791 | 11821 |
| thyme, raw | 27426 | 02049 | pepper, sweet red, sautéed | 847 | 11921 |
| turmeric, ground | 159277 | 02043 | pepper, sweet yellow, grilled | 694 | 99440 |
| | | | pepper, sweet yellow, raw | 965 | 11951 |
| **VEGETABLES** | | | pink beans, mature, raw | 8320 | 16040 |
| agave, cooked | 2938 | 35193 | pinto beans, mature, boiled | 904 | 16043 |
| agave, dried | 7274 | 35194 | pinto beans, mature, raw | 7779 | 16042 |
| agave, raw | 1247 | 35192 | potato, baked | 1058 | 11357 |
| alfalfa seeds, sprouted, raw | 1510 | 11001 | potato, raw | 1058 | 11354 |
| artichoke, raw | 6552 | 11007 | potato, red-skin, baked | 1326 | 11358 |
| artichoke, Ocean Mist, boiled | 9416 | 99362 | potato, red-skin, raw | 1098 | 11355 |
| artichoke, Ocean Mist, microwaved | 9402 | 99363 | potato, Russet, baked | 1680 | 11356 |
| asparagus, boiled | 1644 | 11012 | potato, Russet, raw | 1322 | 11353 |
| avocado, Hass, raw | 1933 | 97080 | pumpkin, raw | 483 | 11422 |
| beet greens, raw | 1946 | 11086 | radish, raw | 1736 | 11429 |
| beet, raw | 1767 | 11080 | radish seeds, sprouted, raw | 2184 | 11676 |
| black beans, mature, raw | 8040 | 16014 | soybeans, mature, raw | 5764 | 16108 |
| black turtle beans, mature, raw | 6416 | 15016 | spinach, chopped/leaf, frozen | 1687 | 11463 |
| broccoli, boiled | 2386 | 11091 | spinach, raw | 1515 | 11457 |
| broccoli, frozen spears | 496 | 11094 | squash, summer, zucchini, raw | 180 | 11477 |
| broccoli, raw | 1362 | 11090 | squash, winter, butternut, raw | 396 | 11485 |
| broccoli raab, boiled | 1552 | 11097 | sweet potato, baked | 2115 | 11508 |
| broccoli raab, raw | 3083 | 11096 | sweet potato, boiled, peeled | 766 | 11510 |
| cabbage, boiled | 856 | 11110 | sweet potato, raw | 902 | 11507 |
| cabbage, raw | 508 | 11109 | tomato, boiled | 406 | 11530 |
| cabbage, red, boiled | 3145 | 11113 | tomato juice, canned | 486 | 11540 |
| cabbage, red, raw | 2252 | 11112 | tomato, plum, raw | 546 | 99051 |
| carrot, baby, raw | 436 | 11960 | tomato, raw | 367 | 11529 |
| carrot, boiled | 317 | 11125 | tomato sauce, canned | 694 | 11549 |
| carrot, raw | 666 | 11124 | vegetable juice cocktail, canned | 548 | 11578 |
| cauliflower, boiled | 620 | 11136 | | | |

| OTHER FOODS | ORAC (μmol TE[1]/100 g) | SR21 CODE NUMBER | | ORAC (μmol TE[1]/100 g) | SR21 CODE NUMBER |
|---|---|---|---|---|---|
| | | | cocoa mix powder | 485 | 14192 |
| baking chocolate, unsweetened | 49926 | 19078 | cocoa powder, unsweetened | 80933 | 19165 |
| catsup | 578 | 11935 | salsa, fresh | 1001 | 06164 |
| chocolate milk, reduced fat | 1263 | 01103 | vinegar, red wine | 410 | 99444 |

[1]TE=Trolox Equivalents

Source:
Oxygen Radical Absorbance Capacity (ORAC) of Selected Foods—2007. Prepared by Nutrient Data laboratory, USDA in collaboration with Arkansas Children's Nutrition Center, USDA. November 2007. Available at: http://www.ars.usda.gov/Services/docs.htm?docid=15866.

# Vitamins/Vitamin-Like Components—Biotin

| | BIOTIN (μg/100 g) | SOURCE | | BIOTIN (μg/100 g) | SOURCE |
|---|---|---|---|---|---|
| **BEVERAGES** | | | **ENTREES** | | |
| beer | 0.1 | Staggs et al, 2004 | beef and vegetable soup, ready-to-serve | 0.1 | Staggs et al, 2004 |
| Coca-Cola | 0.1 | Staggs et al, 2004 | chili, ready-to-serve | 0.5 | Staggs et al, 2004 |
| punch, red fruit | 0.2 | Staggs et al, 2004 | macaroni and cheese, ready-to-serve | 0.1 | Staggs et al, 2004 |
| tea, sweetened | 0.1 | Staggs et al, 2004 | pizza, cheese | 0.1 | Staggs et al, 2004 |
| wine, white | 0.1 | Staggs et al, 2004 | pizza, pepperoni | 0.2 | Staggs et al, 2004 |
| | | | ramen noodles, dry | 0.1 | Staggs et al, 2004 |
| **CANDY** | | | tomato sauce with beef, bottled/canned | 0.1 | Staggs et al, 2004 |
| dark chocolate | 6.0 | Souci et al, 2000 | | | |
| marzipan | 2.0 | Souci et al, 2000 | **FISH AND SHELLFISH** | | |
| milk chocolate | 3.0 | Souci et al, 2000 | catfish, breaded, fried | 0.7 | Staggs et al, 2004 |
| | | | clams, soft, raw | 2.3 | Souci et al, 2000 |
| **CEREALS** | | | cod, raw | 2.2 | Souci et al, 2000 |
| Cheerios | 0.1 | Staggs et al, 2004 | crab, canned | 4.6 | Souci et al, 2000 |
| corn grits, cooked | 0.1 | Staggs et al, 2004 | fish sticks, breaded and fried | 1.0 | Staggs et al, 2004 |
| Frosted Flakes | 0.1 | Staggs et al, 2004 | haddock, raw | 2.5 | Souci et al, 2000 |
| Golden Grahams | 0.1 | Staggs et al, 2004 | halibut, raw | 3.1 | Souci et al, 2000 |
| Kix | 0.1 | Staggs et al, 2004 | lobster, raw | 4.5 | Souci et al, 2000 |
| oatmeal, cooked | 0.2 | Staggs et al, 2004 | mackerel, raw | 4.3 | Souci et al, 2000 |
| | | | oysters, raw | 10.0 | Souci et al, 2000 |
| **CHEESE** | | | salmon, pink, canned in water | 5.9 | Staggs et al, 2004 |
| American cheese | 3.1 | Staggs et al, 2004 | sardines, canned in oil | 9.1 | Souci et al, 2000 |
| cheddar cheese, mild | 1.4 | Staggs et al, 2004 | scallops, raw | 1.1 | Souci et al, 2000 |
| Edam cheese | 1.5 | Souci et al, 2000 | trout, raw | 4.5 | Souci et al, 2000 |
| Emmental cheese | 3.0 | Souci et al, 2000 | tuna, canned in water | 0.7 | Staggs et al, 2004 |
| gorgonzola cheese | 2.0 | Souci et al, 2000 | | | |
| gruyere cheese | 1.3 | Souci et al, 2000 | **FRUIT JUICES** | | |
| Limburger cheese | 8.6 | Souci et al, 2000 | apple juice, canned | 0.1 | Staggs et al, 2004 |
| mozzarella cheese | 2.0 | Souci et al, 2000 | grape juice | 1.2 | Souci et al, 2000 |
| Parmesan cheese | 3.0 | Souci et al, 2000 | elderberry juice | 0.7 | Souci et al, 2000 |
| provolone cheese | 0.1 | Staggs et al, 2004 | lemon juice | 0.3 | Ranganna et al, 1983 |
| | | | orange juice, canned | 0.4 | Staggs et al, 2004 |
| **CREAMS** | | | orange juice, navel | 0.5 | Ranganna et al, 1983 |
| cream, ≥10% fat | 3.4 | Souci et al, 2000 | orange juice, Valencia | 0.8 | Ranganna et al, 1983 |
| sour cream | 3.0 | Souci et al, 2000 | tangerine juice | 0.5 | Ranganna et al, 1983 |
| whipping cream, ≥30% fat | 3.4 | Souci et al, 2000 | | | |
| | | | **FRUITS** | | |
| **DESSERTS** | | | acerola (West Indian cherry), raw | 2.5 | Souci et al, 2000 |
| cake, vanilla with icing | 0.0 | Staggs et al, 2004 | apple, raw | 0.0 | Staggs et al, 2004 |
| cookie, chocolate sandwich | 0.1 | Staggs et al, 2004 | avocado, raw | 1.0 | Staggs et al, 2004 |
| cookie, sugar | 0.3 | Staggs et al, 2004 | banana, raw | 0.1 | Staggs et al, 2004 |
| poptart, blueberry | 0.0 | Staggs et al, 2004 | blueberries, raw | 1.1 | Souci et al, 2000 |
| pudding, banana | 1.0 | Staggs et al, 2004 | cherries, sweet, raw | 0.4 | Souci et al, 2000 |
| | | | currants, black, raw | 2.4 | Souci et al, 2000 |
| **EGGS** | | | currants, red, raw | 2.6 | Souci et al, 2000 |
| chicken egg white, microwaved | 5.8 | Staggs et al, 2004 | gooseberries, raw | 0.5 | Souci et al, 2000 |
| chicken egg, whole, microwaved | 21.4 | Staggs et al, 2004 | grapes, raw | 1.5 | Souci et al, 2000 |
| chicken egg yolk, microwaved | 27.2 | Staggs et al, 2004 | elderberries, black, raw | 1.8 | Souci et al, 2000 |

| | BIOTIN (µg/100 g) | SOURCE | | BIOTIN (µg/100 g) | SOURCE |
|---|---|---|---|---|---|
| lemon, raw | 0.6 | Ranganna et al, 1983 | cow milk, nonfat/whole | 0.1 | Staggs et al, 2004 |
| lemon peel, raw | 2.5 | Ranganna et al, 1983 | ewe (sheep) milk | 0.00 | Souci et al, 2000 |
| orange peel, Valencia | 5.1 | Ranganna et al, 1983 | goat milk | 0.00 | Souci et al, 2000 |
| orange, Valencia, raw | 1.2 | Ranganna et al, 1983 | human milk | 0.8/100 ml | Hartman and Dryden, 1965 |
| peach, canned | 0.2 | Souci et al, 2000 | | | |
| peach, raw | 1.9 | Souci et al, 2000 | yogurt, whole fat | 0.1 | Staggs et al, 2004 |
| pear, raw | 0.1 | Souci et al, 2000 | | | |
| plum, raw | 0.1 | Souci et al, 2000 | **NUTS AND SEEDS** | | |
| raisins, dried | 0.4 | Staggs et al, 2004 | almonds, roasted | 4.4 | Staggs et al, 2004 |
| raspberries, raw | 0.2 | Staggs et al, 2004 | chestnuts, sweet (marone) | 1.5 | Souci et al, 2000 |
| strawberries, raw | 1.5 | Staggs et al, 2004 | peanuts, roasted | 17.5 | Staggs et al, 2004 |
| | | | pecans, raw | 2.0 | Staggs et al, 2004 |
| **GRAIN PRODUCTS** | | | sunflower seeds, roasted | 7.8 | Staggs et al, 2004 |
| bread, white, toasted | 1.2 | Staggs et al, 2004 | walnuts, raw | 2.6 | Staggs et al, 2004 |
| bread, whole wheat | 0.1 | Staggs et al, 2004 | | | |
| crispbread | 7.0 | Souci et al, 2000 | **POULTRY** | | |
| crackers, saltines | 0.3 | Staggs et al, 2004 | chicken liver, microwaved | 187.2 | Staggs et al, 2004 |
| hush puppies | 0.2 | Staggs et al, 2004 | chicken nuggets, breaded, fried fast food | 1.3 | Staggs et al, 2004 |
| noodles, boiled | 0.2 | Staggs et al, 2004 | chicken, roaster, raw | 2.0 | Souci et al, 2000 |
| roll, dinner | 0.0 | Staggs et al, 2004 | chicken strips, breaded, fried, fast food | 0.4 | Staggs et al, 2004 |
| roll, hamburger | 0.3 | Staggs et al, 2004 | frankfurter, chicken and pork, boiled | 3.7 | Staggs et al, 2004 |
| | | | turkey, deli processed, sliced | 0.7 | Staggs et al, 2004 |
| **GRAINS AND GRAIN FRACTIONS** | | | | | |
| corn flour | 6.6 | Souci et al, 2000 | **VEGETABLES** | | |
| oats, rolled | 20.0 | Souci et al, 2000 | asparagus, canned | 1.7 | Souci et al, 2000 |
| rice, brown, raw | 12.0 | Souci et al, 2000 | asparagus, raw | 2.0 | Souci et al, 2000 |
| rice, white, raw | 3.0 | Souci et al, 2000 | broccoli, raw | 0.9 | Staggs et al, 2004 |
| wheat bran | 44.0 | Souci et al, 2000 | Brussels sprouts, raw | 0.4 | Souci et al, 2000 |
| wheat germ | 17.0 | Souci et al, 2000 | cabbage, red, raw | 2.0 | Souci et al, 2000 |
| wheat flour, white | 2.0 | Souci et al, 2000 | cabbage, savoy, raw | 0.1 | Souci et al, 2000 |
| | | | cabbage, white, raw | 3.2 | Souci et al, 2000 |
| **MEATS** | | | carrot, canned | 0.6 | Staggs et al, 2004 |
| beef, corned, raw | 2.0 | Souci et al, 2000 | cauliflower, raw | 0.2 | Staggs et al, 2004 |
| beef filet, raw | 4.6 | Souci et al, 2000 | celery, raw | 0.1 | Souci et al, 2000 |
| beef hamburger patty, pan-fried | 4.5 | Staggs et al, 2004 | chicory, raw | 4.8 | Souci et al, 2000 |
| beef rump, raw | 3.8 | Souci et al, 2000 | corn, whole kernel, canned | 0.0 | Staggs et al, 2004 |
| beef top round, raw | 4.6 | Souci et al, 2000 | cucumber, raw | 0.9 | Souci et al, 2000 |
| mutton brisket, raw | 2.0 | Souci et al, 2000 | fennel leaves, raw | 2.5 | Souci et al, 2000 |
| mutton leg, raw | 6.0 | Souci et al, 2000 | green snap beans, canned | 0.00 | Staggs et al, 2004 |
| pork chop, microwaved | 4.5 | Staggs et al, 2004 | kale, raw | 0.5 | Souci et al, 2000 |
| pork leg, raw | 5.1 | Souci et al, 2000 | kohlrabi, raw | 2.7 | Souci et al, 2000 |
| | | | leek, raw | 1.6 | Souci et al, 2000 |
| **MEAT, INTERNAL ORGANS** | | | lettuce, raw | 1.9 | Souci et al, 2000 |
| brain, calf/ox, raw | 6.1 | Souci et al, 2000 | mungo (black gram) beans, dry | 7.5 | Souci et al, 2000 |
| heart, calf/ox, raw | 7.3 | Souci et al, 2000 | mushrooms, canned | 2.2 | Staggs et al, 2004 |
| heart, pork, raw | 4.0 | Souci et al, 2000 | onion, raw | 3.5 | Souci et al, 2000 |
| kidney, calf, raw | 80.0 | Souci et al, 2000 | parsley, raw | 0.4 | Souci et al, 2000 |
| kidney, ox, raw | 58.0 | Souci et al, 2000 | parsnip, raw | 0.1 | Souci et al, 2000 |
| liver, beef, microwaved | 41.6 | Staggs et al, 2004 | peas, dry | 19.0 | Souci et al, 2000 |
| liver, calf, raw | 75.0 | Souci et al, 2000 | peas, green, canned | 1.5 | Souci et al, 2000 |
| liver, ox, raw | 100.0 | Souci et al, 2000 | peas with pods, green, raw | 5.3 | Souci et al, 2000 |
| liver, pork, raw | 27.0 | Souci et al, 2000 | potato, French fries | 0.3 | Staggs et al, 2004 |
| liver, sheep, raw | 130.0 | Souci et al, 2000 | potato, mashed with gravy | 0.1 | Staggs et al, 2004 |
| lungs, calf/ox, raw | 5.9 | Souci et al, 2000 | potato, tator tots | 0.1 | Staggs et al, 2004 |
| spleen, ox raw | 5.7 | Souci et al, 2000 | pumpkin, raw | 0.4 | Souci et al, 2000 |
| tongue, calf/ox, raw | 3.3 | Souci et al, 2000 | rutabaga (Swede), raw | 0.1 | Souci et al, 2000 |
| | | | salad, mixed garden | 0.3 | Staggs et al, 2004 |
| **MILK AND YOGURT** | | | soybeans, dry | 60.0 | Souci et al, 2000 |
| buffalo milk | 0.00 | Souci et al, 2000 | spinach, frozen | 0.7 | Staggs et al, 2004 |
| cow milk, 2% fat | 0.1 | Staggs et al, 2004 | sweet potato, microwaved | 1.5 | Staggs et al, 2004 |
| cow milk, buttermilk | 0.00 | Souci et al, 2000 | tomato juice | 2.5 | Souci et al, 2000 |
| cow milk, chocolate, lowfat | 0.4 | Staggs et al, 2004 | tomato, raw | 0.7 | Staggs et al, 2004 |
| cow milk, condensed, sweetened, canned | 3.8 | Souci et al, 2000 | turnip, raw | 2.0 | Souci et al, 2000 |

| | BIOTIN (μg/100 g) | SOURCE | | BIOTIN (μg/100 g) | SOURCE |
|---|---|---|---|---|---|
| **OTHER FOODS** | | | salad dressing, ranch | 0.2 | Staggs et al, 2004 |
| | | | whey, dried powder | 43.0 | Souci et al, 2000 |
| cocoa powder | 20.0 | Souci et al, 2000 | whey, sweet | 1.4 | Souci et al, 2000 |
| catsup (ketchup) | 0.1 | Staggs et al, 2004 | yeast | 20.2 | Staggs et al, 2004 |
| mayonnaise | 0.2 | Staggs et al, 2004 | | | |
| potato chips, barbecue, baked | 0.1 | Staggs et al, 2004 | | | |

Sources:

Hartman AM, LP Dryden. *Vitamins in Milk and Milk Products: A Review.* American Dairy Science Association, Champaign IL, 1965.

Ranganna S, Vs Govindarajan, KVR Ramana. *Citrus fruits – Varieties, chemistry, technology, and quality evaluation. Part II. Chemistry, technology, and quality evaluation. A. Chemistry.* Critical Reviews in Food Science and Nutrition. Vol 18, issue 4. CRC Press, Boca Raton, FL, 1983.

Souci SW, W Fachmann, H Kraut. *Food Composition and Nutrition Tables.* Medpharm GmbH Scientific Publishers, Stuttgart, Germany and CRC Press, Washington, DC, 2000.

Staggs, C, WM Sealey, BJ McCabe, AM Teague, DM Mock. Determination of the biotin content of select foods using accurate and sensitive HPLC/avidin binding. *J Fd Comp Anal* 17:767-776, 2004.

# Vitamins/Vitamin-Like Components—Choline and Betaine

| | FREE CHOLINE (mg/100g) | TOTAL CHOLINE (mg/100g) | BETAINE (mg/100g) | SR21 SOURCE CODE[1] |
|---|---|---|---|---|
| **BEVERAGES** | | | | |
| beer | 5.7 | 9.9 | 8.1 | 14003 |
| beer, light | 5.5 | 7.9 | 6.3 | 14006 |
| coffee, brewed | 1.9 | 2.6 | 0.1 | 14209 |
| coffee instant powder, decaffeinated | 94.0 | 100.0 | 0.7 | 14218 |
| cola | 0.00 | 0.4 | 0.1 | 14400 |
| diet cola with aspartame | 0.00 | 0.00 | 0.1 | 14416 |
| lemonade frozen concentrate | 0.4 | 2.0 | 0.4 | 14292 |
| orange soda | 0.00 | 0.6 | 0.1 | 14150 |
| wine, red | 4.5 | 5.7 | 0.3 | 14096 |
| wine, white | 3.4 | 4.7 | 0.2 | 14106 |
| **CANDY** | | | | |
| caramel and chocolate-flavored roll (candy) | 6.2 | 19.0 | 1.4 | 19076 |
| M&M's Plain (candy) | 9.1 | 22.0 | 0.8 | 19141 |
| milk chocolate chips | 9.1 | 46.0 | 2.6 | 19120 |
| **CEREALS AND GRAINS, COOKED** | | | | |
| amaranth, whole grain, dry | 37.0 | 70.0 | 68.0 | 20001 |
| buckwheat groats, roasted, cooked | 11.0 | 20.0 | 0.5 | 20010 |
| buckwheat groats, roasted, dry | 32.0 | 54.0 | 2.6 | 20009 |
| bulgur, cooked | 2.7 | 6.9 | 83 | 20013 |
| corn grits, instant, enriched, dry, Quaker | 4.2 | 14.0 | 1.1 | 08092 |
| corn grits, instant, enriched, prepared, Quaker | 1.0 | 2.6 | 0.2 | 08093 |
| Oat Bran Cereal, dry, Quakers/Mother's | 4.4 | 59.0 | 36.0 | 08231 |
| oatmeal, quick/regular, cooked | 1.3 | 7.4 | 3.1 | 08121 |
| oats, whole grain, dry | 5.0 | 30.0 | 31.0 | 20038 |
| quinoa, dry | 38.0 | 70.0 | 630.0 | 20035 |
| rice, brown, long grain, boiled | 4.7 | 9.2 | 0.5 | 20037 |
| rice, white, long grain, enriched, boiled | 0.7 | 2.1 | 0.3 | 20045 |
| wheat cereal (farina), quick, enriched, cooked, Cream of Wheat | 1.6 | 3.5 | 6.9 | 08105 |
| **CEREALS, READY-TO-EAT** | | | | |
| All-Bran, Kellogg's | 26.0 | 49.0 | 360.0 | 08001 |
| Bran flakes, Ralston | 11.0 | 31.0 | 120.0 | 08504 |
| Cap'n Crunch Peanut Butter Crunch, Quaker | 7.1 | 15.0 | 1.8 | 08012 |
| Cheerios, General Mills | 4.4 | 26.0 | 35.0 | 08013 |
| Cocoa Krispies, Kellogg's | 4.2 | 8.7 | 1.3 | 08014 |
| Corn Biscuits, Ralston | 2.6 | 11.0 | 7.1 | 08505 |
| Corn Flakes, Kellogg's | 1.4 | 3.9 | 0.7 | 08020 |
| Corn flakes, Ralston | 1.6 | 2.2 | 1.2 | 08506 |
| Crispix, Kellogg's | 2.0 | 3.8 | 0.7 | 08259 |
| Froot Loops, Kellogg's | 1.8 | 11.0 | 33.0 | 08030 |
| Honey Puffs Kashi | 8.2 | 30.0 | 68.0 | 08389 |
| Natural Cereal, 100% with oats, honey, and raisins, Quaker | 8.3 | 32.0 | 140.0 | 08218 |
| Oatmeal Crisp, almond, General Mills | 5.0 | 25.0 | 35.0 | 08202 |
| raisin bran, Post | 12.0 | 29.0 | 290.0 | 08061 |

| | FREE CHOLINE (mg/100 g) | TOTAL CHOLINE (mg/100g) | BETAINE (mg/100 g) | SR21 SOURCE CODE[1] |
|---|---|---|---|---|
| Rice Krispies, Kellogg's | 2.0 | 6.0 | 0.5 | 08065 |
| Shredded Wheat, Post | 5.5 | 23.0 | 160.0 | 08147 |
| Special K Red Berries, Kellogg's | 7.5 | 22.0 | 38.0 | 08383 |
| Special K, Kellogg's | 12.0 | 31.0 | 26.0 | 08067 |
| Tasteeos, Ralston | 2.9 | 15.0 | 20.0 | 08074 |
| Total, General Mills | 5.8 | 19.0 | 170.0 | 08077 |
| Uncle Sam Cereal | 12.0 | 50.0 | 250.0 | 08435 |
| wheat bran, toasted, Kretschmer | 54.0 | 81.0 | 320.0 | 08363 |
| Wheaties, General Mills | 11.0 | 33.0 | 200.0 | 08089 |

**CHEESE AND CHEESE PRODUCTS**

| | | | | |
|---|---|---|---|---|
| American processed cheese food | 7.9 | 36.0 | 1.4 | 01046 |
| cheddar cheese | 1.6 | 17.0 | 0.7 | 01009 |
| cottage cheese, <5% fat | 3.7 | 18.0 | 0.9 | 01014 |
| cottage cheese, 2% fat | 2.9 | 16.0 | 0.6 | 01015 |
| cottage cheese, creamed, small curd | 3.6 | 18.0 | 0.7 | 01012 |
| cream cheese | 3.6 | 27.0 | 0.7 | 01017 |
| mozzarella cheese, part skim, low moisture | 2.3.0 | 14.0 | 0.7 | 01029 |
| Swiss cheese | 4.5 | 16.0 | 0.6 | 01040 |

**CREAMS AND CREAMERS**

| | | | | |
|---|---|---|---|---|
| cream, half and half | 3.9 | 19.0 | 0.7 | 01049 |
| creamer, powdered | 0.5 | 2.3 | 0.1 | 01069 |
| sour cream, cultured | 3.9 | 19.0 | 0.6 | 01056 |

**DESSERTS**

| | | | | |
|---|---|---|---|---|
| cake, chocolate, homemade | 5.4 | 130.0 | 48.0 | 18101 |
| cake, yellow with vanilla icing | 4.6 | 36.0 | 19.0 | 18141 |
| cookie, chocolate chunk pecan, Pepperidge Farm | 8.9 | 17.0 | 43.0 | 18159 |
| cupcake, chocolate with icing, lowfat | 5.0 | 21.0 | 22.0 | 18452 |
| Danish pastry, fruit | 8.7 | 22.0 | 14.0 | 18246 |
| doughnut | 4.9 | 37.0 | 38.0 | 18248 |
| doughnut with chocolate coating/icing | 5.4 | 29.0 | 27.0 | 18249 |
| frozen yogurt, flavors other than chocolate | 5.1 | 23.0 | 0.9 | 42187 |
| graham cracker | 13 | 22.0 | 39.0 | 18173 |
| ice cream, chocolate | 5.1 | 23.0 | 0.6 | 19270 |
| ice cream, vanilla, regular (10% fat) | 4.8 | 26.0 | 1.1 | 19095 |
| icing/frosting, chocolate, ready-to-serve | 5.6 | 6.9 | 2.2 | 19226 |
| icing/frosting, vanilla, ready-to-serve | 0.8 | 2.3 | 2.6 | 19230 |
| pie, apple | 4.7 | 7.2 | 16.0 | 18301 |
| pudding, chocolate, ready-to-eat | 4.3 | 9.5 | 0.9 | 19183 |
| toaster pastry, strawberry, frosted, Pop-Tarts | 3.6 | 7.8 | 20.0 | 18489 |
| toaster pastry, strawberry, Pop-Tarts | 4.0 | 8.4 | 21.0 | 18488 |

**EGGS**

| | | | | |
|---|---|---|---|---|
| egg, boiled, hard | 0.7 | 230.0 | 0.6 | 01129 |
| egg, fried | 0.7 | 270.0 | 0.7 | 01128 |
| egg, raw | 0.6 | 250.0 | 0.6 | 01123 |
| egg white, raw | 0.2 | 1.1 | 0.3 | 01124 |
| egg yolk, raw | 1.3 | 680.0 | 0.9 | 01125 |

**ENTREES**

| | | | | |
|---|---|---|---|---|
| acorn stew, Apache | 1.3 | 34.0 | 9.6 | 35182 |
| beef stew, canned | 2.9 | 16.0 | 1.8 | 22905 |
| burrito, bean and cheese, microwaved | 14.0 | 28.0 | 30.0 | 22927 |
| burrito, beef and bean, microwaved | 15.0 | 28.0 | 34.0 | 22928 |
| chicken wings, glazed, barbecue flavored, frozen, microwaved | 5.7 | 74.0 | 17.0 | 05313 |
| chicken wings, glazed, barbecue flavored, frozen, oven heated | 4.0 | 77.0 | 14.0 | 05320 |
| chili con carne with beans, canned | 12.0 | 27.0 | 0.9 | 22904 |
| lasagna with meat sauce, frozen | 5.2 | 17.0 | 6.1 | 22916 |
| macaroni and cheese, boxed, prepared with cheese powder | 4.0 | 14.0 | 12.0 | 98070 |
| macaroni and cheese, boxed, prepared with cheese sauce | 4.3 | 22.0 | 19.0 | 98071 |
| macaroni and cheese, canned | 2.8 | 5.4 | 43.0 | 22247 |
| pizza, meat and vegetable, regular crust, frozen, heated | 11.0 | 25.0 | 25.0 | 21226 |
| pizza, pepperoni, frozen | 11.0 | 26.0 | 20.0 | 22903 |
| pizza, sausage and pepperoni, frozen | 8.1 | 22.0 | 19.0 | 22902 |

| | FREE CHOLINE (mg/100 g) | TOTAL CHOLINE (mg/100g) | BETAINE (mg/100 g) | SR21 SOURCE CODE[1] |
|---|---|---|---|---|
| **FAST FOODS AND RESTAURANT FOODS** | | | | |
| bagel with egg, sausage patty, and cheese | 3.9 | 84.0 | 8.7 | 21410 |
| bagel with ham, egg, and cheese | 3.7 | 98.0 | 11.0 | 21409 |
| bagel with steak, egg, and cheese | 4.0 | 82.0 | 10.0 | 21411 |
| biscuit with egg and sausage | 2.5 | 98.0 | 7.3 | 21005 |
| biscuit with egg, cheese, and bacon | 2.2 | 130.0 | 11.0 | 21007 |
| biscuit with sausage | 3.2 | 27.0 | 9.1 | 21009 |
| burrito, bean, cheese, and beef | 16.0 | 28.0 | 12.0 | 21064 |
| burrito, bean | 16.0 | 27.0 | 15.0 | 21060 |
| cheeseburger sandwich, large, double meat with lettuce and tomato | 5.4 | 39.0 | 30.0 | 21100 |
| cheeseburger sandwich, large, single meat with lettuce and tomato | 3.1 | 29.0 | 12.0 | 21098 |
| chicken fillet sandwich | 5.5 | 35.0 | 29.0 | 21102 |
| cinnamon roll, miniature | 4.5 | 27.0 | 12.0 | 21388 |
| croissant with egg and cheese | 3.2 | 92.0 | 10.0 | 21011 |
| croissant with egg, cheese, and sausage | 3.4 | 84.0 | 8.4 | 21014 |
| egg roll, from restaurant | 3.8 | 18.0 | 22.0 | 98119 |
| English muffin (toasted) with cheese and sausage | 4.5 | 30.0 | 19.0 | 21020 |
| English muffin (toasted) with egg, cheese, and sausage | 2.9 | 100.0 | 10.0 | 21022 |
| fish sandwich with tartar sauce and cheese | 7.4 | 33.0 | 98.0 | 21106 |
| French fries | 11.0 | 21.0 | 0.5 | 21138 |
| French toast sticks | 6.4 | 14.0 | 20.0 | 21024 |
| hamburger sandwich, large, double meat with lettuce and tomato | 9.5 | 41.0 | 46.0 | 21114 |
| hamburger sandwich, large, single meat | 5.0 | 33.0 | 22.0 | 21202 |
| hamburger sandwich, regular, single meat | 5.6 | 34.0 | 41.0 | 21107 |
| nachos with cheese, beans, ground beef, and peppers | 7.5 | 28.0 | 2.0 | 21080 |
| nachos with cheese | 4.8 | 26.0 | 0.7 | 21078 |
| pizza, cheese, regular crust | 5.9 | 16.0 | 28.0 | 21299 |
| pizza, cheese, thick crust | 6.0 | 17.0 | 27.0 | 21300 |
| pizza, cheese, thin crust | 8.8 | 19.0 | 20.0 | 21301 |
| pizza, meat and vegetable, regular crust | 8.3 | 22.0 | 24.0 | 21304 |
| pizza, pepperoni, regular crust | 10.0 | 25.0 | 26.0 | 21302 |
| pizza, pepperoni, thick crust | 9.7 | 25.0 | 28.0 | 21303 |
| potato, hashed brown | 7.2 | 18.0 | 0.3 | 21026 |
| salad, taco salad | 8.8 | 23.0 | 11.0 | 21083 |
| shake, vanilla, McDonald's | 3.9 | 22.0 | 1.2 | 14347 |
| taco, small | 11.0 | 32.0 | 3.3 | 21082 |
| **FATS, OILS, AND SPREADS** | | | | |
| butter | 0.6 | 19.0 | 0.35 | 01001 |
| canola oil | 0.00 | 0.2 | 0.00 | 04582 |
| margarine, canola oil | 0.1 | 11.0 | 0.1 | 98083 |
| margarine, soy, 70% fat | 0.5 | 14.0 | 0.00 | 04629 |
| margarine-butter blend (60% corn oil, 40% butter) | 0.3 | 6.5 | 0.1 | 04585 |
| mayonnaise, imitation, soy | 0.3 | 15.0 | 0.4 | 04027 |
| mayonnaise, soy | 0.00 | 22.0 | 0.00 | 04025 |
| olive oil | 0.00 | 0.3 | 0.1 | 04053 |
| pork fat, cooked | 1.6 | 33.0 | 1.9 | 10007 |
| pork fat, raw | 1.5 | 25.0 | 2.4 | 10006 |
| soy oil, salad/cooking | 0.00 | 0.2 | 0.00 | 04044 |
| **FISH AND SEAFOOD** | | | | |
| cod, Atlantic, cooked by dry heat | 18.0 | 84.0 | 9.7 | 15016 |
| crab, Alaska king, imitation, made from surimi | 0.8 | 13.0 | 1.8 | 15138 |
| crab, blue, canned | 0.1 | 34.0 | 13.0 | 15141 |
| fish sticks/pieces, frozen, reheated | 7.7 | 36.0 | 45.0 | 15027 |
| halibut, Alaskan, cooked with skin | 5.5 | 64.0 | 5.2 | 35188 |
| orange roughy, cooked by dry heat (finfish) | 18.0 | 49.0 | 3.1 | 15232 |
| orange roughy, raw (finfish) | 14.0 | 35.0 | 2.1 | 15073 |
| salmon, Atlantic, farmed, cooked by dry heat | 7.8 | 91.0 | 1.8 | 15237 |
| salmon, Atlantic, farmed, raw | 9.9 | 79.0 | 3.0 | 15236 |
| salmon, sockeye, canned with bone, drained | 4.0 | 83.0 | 3.7 | 15087 |
| salmon, sockeye, cooked by dry heat | 8.6 | 66.0 | 2.1 | 15086 |
| sheefish, raw | 12.0 | 110.0 | 120.0 | 35169 |
| shrimp, canned | 1.5 | 81.0 | 23.0 | 15152 |
| smelt, dried | 170.0 | 300.0 | 15.0 | 35184 |
| tilapia, cooked by dry heat | 21.0 | 83.0 | 25.0 | 15262 |
| trout, steelhead, boiled, canned | 2.6 | 90.0 | 2.5 | 35181 |
| trout, steelhead, dried | 15.0 | 260.0 | 38.0 | 35180 |

| | FREE CHOLINE (mg/100 g) | TOTAL CHOLINE (mg/100g) | BETAINE (mg/100 g) | SR21 SOURCE CODE[1] |
|---|---|---|---|---|
| tuna, light, canned in water, drained | 2.1 | 29.0 | 2.7 | 15121 |
| whitefish, dried | 50.0 | 210.0 | 88.0 | 35165 |
| whitefish roe/eggs | 12.0 | 250.0 | 8.2 | 35158 |
| **FLOUR, MEALS, AND GRAIN FRACTIONS** | | | | |
| barley malt flour | 4.9 | 38.0 | 66.0 | 20131 |
| corn bran | 15.0 | 18.0 | 4.6 | 20015 |
| corn flour (masa), yellow, enriched | 1.9 | 4.3 | 2.0 | 20317 |
| cornmeal, yellow, degermed, enriched | 6.4 | 11.0 | 0.4 | 20022 |
| cornmeal, yellow, whole grain | 11.0 | 22.0 | 12.0 | 20020 |
| oat bran | 4.9 | 32.0 | 20.0 | 20033 |
| rye flour, dark | 8.3 | 30.0 | 150.0 | 20063 |
| soy flour, defatted | 120.0 | 190.0 | 2.8 | 16117 |
| wheat flour, white, enriched, all-purpose | 5.7 | 10.0 | 70.0 | 20081 |
| wheat flour, whole wheat | 13.0 | 31.0 | 73.0 | 20080 |
| wheat germ, toasted | 130.0 | 180.0 | 410.0 | 08084 |
| **FRUIT JUICES** | | | | |
| apple juice, calcium and vitamin C added | 0.7 | 1.8 | 0.1 | 98005 |
| cranberry juice cocktail, canned/bottled | 0.4 | 1.1 | 0.1 | 14242 |
| grape juice, canned/bottled | 3.0 | 3.2 | 0.2 | 09135 |
| guava nectar, canned | 0.5 | 1.1 | 0.1 | 09435 |
| lime juice, raw | 1.1 | 5.1 | 0.2 | 09160 |
| mango nectar, canned | 1.0 | 1.5 | 0.0 | 09436 |
| orange juice, refrigerated | 2.2 | 6.6 | 0.2 | 09209 |
| tamarind nectar, canned | 0.3 | 1.3.0 | 0.1 | 09437 |
| **FRUITS** | | | | |
| apple, raw | 0.3 | 3.4 | 0.1 | 09003 |
| apricot, dried | 7.1 | 14.0 | 0.3 | 09032 |
| avocado, California, raw | 8.6 | 14.0 | 0.7 | 09038 |
| banana, raw | 3.2 | 9.8 | 0.1 | 09040 |
| blackberries, raw | 1.8 | 8.6 | 0.3 | 09042 |
| blackberries, wild, raw | 1.4 | 4.9 | 0.2 | 35015 |
| blueberries, raw | 3.0 | 6.0 | 0.2 | 09050 |
| blueberries, wild, raw | 2.9 | 11.0 | 0.5 | 35155 |
| cantaloupe, raw | 4.1 | 7.6 | 0.1 | 09181 |
| chokecherries, pitted, raw | 6.7 | 11.0 | 0.5 | 35179 |
| clementine, raw | 11.0 | 14.0 | 0.1 | 09433 |
| cranberries, raw | 1.3 | 5.5 | 0.2 | 09078 |
| date, dried | 6.1 | 6.3 | 0.4 | 09087 |
| fig, dried | 13.0 | 16.0 | 0.8 | 09094 |
| grapefruit, pink and red, raw | 3.6 | 7.5 | 0.2 | 09112 |
| grapes, red/green, European, seedless, raw | 4.8 | 5.6 | 0.1 | 09132 |
| kiwifruit, raw | 2.6 | 7.8 | 0.5 | 09148 |
| nectarine, raw | 1.7 | 6.2 | 0.2 | 09191 |
| orange, California navel, raw | 4.7 | 8.4 | 0.1 | 09202 |
| peach, canned in heavy syrup, drained | 0.4 | 3.8 | 0.3 | 09370 |
| peach, raw | 0.8 | 6.1 | 0.3 | 09236 |
| pear, canned in heavy syrup, solids and liquid | 0.6 | 1.9 | 0.3 | 09257 |
| pear, raw | 2.2 | 5.1 | 0.2 | 09252 |
| pineapple, raw | 5.1 | 5.7 | 0.1 | 09429 |
| prune, dried | 6.7 | 10.0 | 0.4 | 09291 |
| raisins, seedless | 9.4 | 11.0 | 0.3 | 09298 |
| raspberries, raw | 3.1 | 12.0 | 0.8 | 09302 |
| strawberries, raw | 0.6 | 5.7 | 0.2 | 09316 |
| tangerine, raw | 5.2 | 10.0 | 0.1 | 09218 |
| watermelon, raw | 3.1 | 4.1 | 0.3 | 09326 |
| **GRAIN- AND VEGETABLE-BASED SNACK FOODS** | | | | |
| cheese puffs/twists | 3.8 | 12.0 | 0.6 | 19008 |
| corn chips | 1.9 | 12.0 | 0.1 | 19003 |
| granola bar, chocolate chip, soft | 7.1 | 17.0 | 22.0 | 19404 |
| granola bar, hard | 4.2 | 22.0 | 6.9 | 19015 |
| popcorn, 94% fat-free, microwaved | 5.4 | 13 | 0.3 | 25000 |
| popcorn, air-popped | 7.2 | 21 | 0.8 | 19034 |
| popcorn, oil-popped, microwaved | 5.6 | 15 | 0.4 | 19035 |
| potato chips | 4.6 | 12 | 0.2 | 19411 |

| | FREE CHOLINE (mg/100 g) | TOTAL CHOLINE (mg/100g) | BETAINE (mg/100 g) | SR21 SOURCE CODE[1] |
|---|---|---|---|---|
| pretzel, hard | 16.0 | 30 | 50 | 19047 |
| Sunchips, Frito Lay | 3.9 | 15 | 39 | 25013 |
| tortilla chips | 4.2 | 19 | 0.4 | 19056 |
| tortilla chips, nacho | 4.5 | 23 | 1.2 | 19057 |
| tortilla chips, nacho cheese, lowfat, made with Olestra | 4.6 | 20 | 0.3 | 19444 |
| tortilla chips, ranch | 4.2 | 18 | 3 | 19058 |
| **GRAIN PRODUCTS** | | | | |
| bagel, plain/onion/poppyseed/sesame seed | 7.7 | 15.0 | 20.0 | 18001 |
| biscuit, plain/buttermilk | 6.9 | 8.9 | 43.0 | 18009 |
| biscuit, plain/buttermilk, from refrigerated dough (2–12% fat) | 17.0 | 20.0 | 45.0 | 18013 |
| bread, French | 6.9 | 15.0 | 55.0 | 18029 |
| bread, wheat/wheat berry | 12.0 | 19.0 | 85.0 | 18064 |
| bread, white | 8.6 | 15.0 | 31.0 | 18069 |
| bread, whole wheat | 18.0 | 27.0 | 38.0 | 18075 |
| crackers, cheese with peanut butter filling | 11.0 | 25.0 | 34.0 | 18215 |
| crackers, cheese with cheese filling | 6.7 | 28.0 | 41.0 | 18927 |
| crackers, round | 8.2 | 14.0 | 52.0 | 18229 |
| crackers, saltines | 13.0 | 20.0 | 55.0 | 18228 |
| crackers, wheat | 19.0 | 27.0 | 58.0 | 18232 |
| English muffin | 5.2 | 14.0 | 33.0 | 18258 |
| English muffin, raisin cinnamon/apple cinnamon | 4.9 | 13.0 | 28.0 | 18262 |
| muffin, homemade with 2% milk | 15.0 | 43.0 | 92.0 | 18273 |
| pancake, from complete mix | 5.5 | 19.0 | 26.0 | 18290 |
| pancake, frozen | 3.5 | 31.0 | 72.0 | 18288 |
| pancake, frozen, microwaved | 4.1 | 28.0 | 69.0 | 18936 |
| noodles, egg, enriched, boiled (egg in noodle dough) | 9.3 | 26.0 | 19.0 | 20110 |
| noodles, egg, enriched, dry (egg in noodle dough) | 50.0 | 79.0 | 130.0 | 20109 |
| spaghetti, enriched, boiled | 3.5 | 6.4 | 68.0 | 20121 |
| spaghetti, enriched, dry | 9.7 | 15.0 | 140.0 | 20120 |
| taco shell, from corn tortilla | 8.1 | 30.0 | 0.6 | 18360 |
| tortilla, corn | 4.1 | 13.0 | 0.4 | 18363 |
| tortilla, flour | 4.6 | 7.9 | 5.3 | 18364 |
| **INFANT, JUNIOR, AND TODDLER FOODS** | | | | |
| beef, Gerber 3rd Foods/Heinz Junior-3 | 1.5 | 38.0 | 3.1 | 03003 |
| broccoli and chicken dinner, Gerber 2nd Foods/Heinz Strained-2 | 6.7 | 31.0 | 2.3 | 03298 |
| chicken, Gerber 3rd Foods/Heinz Junior-3 | 3.3 | 43.0 | 12.0 | 03013 |
| green beans, Gerber 1st Foods/Heinz Beginner-1 | 2.9 | 23.0 | 0.1 | 03091 |
| green peas, Beech-Nut Stage 1/Gerber 2nd Foods | 5.1 | 32.0 | 0.5 | 03121 |
| lamb, junior food | 2.8 | 55.0 | 6.6 | 03011 |
| oatmeal, dry, infant cereal | 5.0 | 32.0 | 21.0 | 03189 |
| peaches, Beech-Nut Stage 1/Gerber 2nd Foods/Heinz Strained-2 | 0.6 | 8.5 | 0.4 | 03130 |
| squash, yellow, Earth's Best | 4.6 | 7.6 | 0.3 | 03104 |
| turkey, Gerber 3rd Foods | 1.7 | 40.0 | 4.7 | 03016 |
| vegetables and beef, Beech-Nut Stage 3/Gerber 3rd Foods/ Heinz Junior-3 | 3.5 | 17.0 | 1.1 | 03054 |
| **MEATS** | | | | |
| beef chuck shoulder medallion, choice, 0" trim, lean, grilled | 0.9 | 85.0 | 12.0 | 23036 |
| beef chuck shoulder top blade steak, choice, 0" trim, lean and fat, grilled | 2.2 | 100.0 | 12.0 | 23043 |
| beef chuck shoulder top/center steak, select, 0" trim, lean and fat, grilled | 0.6 | 94.0 | 16.0 | 23038 |
| beef round, knuckle tip center steak, choice, 0" trim, lean and fat, grilled | 0.6 | 86.0 | 13.0 | 23047 |
| beef round, knuckle tip side steak, choice, 0" trim, lean and fat, grilled | 0.5 | 100.0 | 6.9 | 23033 |
| beef round, outside bottom steak, choice, 0" trim, lean and fat, grilled | 0.9 | 91.0 | 11.0 | 23051 |
| beef, ground, 5% fat, patty, broiled | 2.2 | 85.0 | 6.6 | 23558 |
| beef, ground, 10% fat, patty, broiled | 2.2 | 84.0 | 7.1 | 23563 |
| beef, ground, 15% fat, patty, broiled | 2.2 | 82.0 | 7.5 | 23568 |
| beef, ground, 20% fat, patty, broiled | 2.3 | 81.0 | 8.0 | 23573 |
| beef, ground, 25% fat, patty, broiled | 2.3 | 79.0 | 8.5 | 23578 |
| beef, ground, 30% fat, patty, broiled | 2.3 | 78.0 | 10.0 | 13497 |
| beef liver, braised | 62.0 | 430.0 | 5.6 | 13326 |
| beef liver, pan-fried | 57.0 | 420.0 | 6.3 | 13327 |

| | FREE CHOLINE (mg/100 g) | TOTAL CHOLINE (mg/100 g) | BETAINE (mg/100 g) | SR21 SOURCE CODE[1] |
|---|---|---|---|---|
| beef liver, raw | 56.0 | 330.0 | 4.4 | 13325 |
| beef sausage (fresh), pan-fried | 0.5 | 51.0 | 10.0 | 07956 |
| calf liver, raw | 85.0 | 310.0 | 7.6 | 17202 |
| caribou shoulder meat, dried | 51.0 | 260.0 | 43.0 | 35161 |
| pork bacon, cured, microwaved | 12.0 | 120.0 | 3.0 | 10861 |
| pork bacon, cured, raw | 4.4 | 47.0 | 0.9 | 10123 |
| pork Boston blade (steaks and roasts), lean, braised | 5.5 | 110.0 | 3.5 | 10085 |
| pork tenderloin, lean, roasted | 1.8 | 89.0 | 4.3 | 10061 |
| pork top loin (chops), lean, broiled | 1.1 | 78.0 | 2.8 | 10068 |
| pork, ground, cooked | 3.0 | 87.0 | 4.7 | 10220 |
| pork sausage (fresh), pan-fried | 7.1 | 67.0 | 3.6 | 07064 |
| pork sausage (fresh), raw | 8.0 | 53.0 | 3.4 | 07063 |
| seal (bearded) meat, dried | 17.0 | 120.0 | 16.0 | 35055 |
| seal (bearded) meat, dried in oil | 6.8 | 68.0 | 61.0 | 35164 |
| veal liver, braised | 89.0 | 400.0 | 9.8 | 17203 |
| veal liver, pan-fried | 93.0 | 410.0 | 8.1 | 17204 |

**MEATS, LUNCHEON**

| | | | | |
|---|---|---|---|---|
| bologna, beef | 18.0 | 46.0 | 5.1 | 07007 |
| frankfurter | 6.7 | 44.0 | 3.6 | 07950 |
| frankfurter, beef | 3.9 | 34.0 | 5.0 | 07022 |
| frankfurter, beef, heated | 4.3 | 39.0 | 5.5 | 07945 |
| frankfurter, chicken | 6.2 | 51.0 | 5.1 | 07024 |
| frankfurter, heated | 5.9 | 43.0 | 3.5 | 07949 |
| Smokie (smoked sausage), pork and beef | 23.0 | 51.0 | 2.1 | 07075 |

**MEAT SUBSTITUTES AND TOFU**

| | | | | |
|---|---|---|---|---|
| soy protein burger, frozen | 9.9 | 14.0 | 5.0 | 43133 |
| tofu, firm, prepared with calcium sulfate and nigari (magnesium chloride) | 8.3 | 28.0 | 0.4 | 16126 |
| tofu, soft, prepared with calcium sulfate and nigari (magnesium chloride) | 9.7 | 27.0 | 0.4 | 16127 |

**MILK AND YOGURT**

| | | | | |
|---|---|---|---|---|
| chocolate milk, reduced fat | 5.4 | 17.0 | 0.7 | 01103 |
| milk, lowfat, 1% fat | 4.0 | 18.0 | 0.6 | 01082 |
| milk, nonfat | 2.8 | 16.0 | 1.9 | 01085 |
| milk, reduced fat, 2% fat | 2.8 | 16.0 | 0.9 | 01079 |
| milk, whole, 3.25% fat | 3.7 | 14.0 | 0.6 | 01077 |
| soymilk | 13.0 | 24.0 | 0.8 | 16120 |
| yogurt, lowfat, fruit | 2.1 | 14.0 | 0.8 | 01121 |
| yogurt, lowfat, plain | 2.3 | 15.0 | 0.9 | 01117 |
| yogurt, nonfat, fruit | 3.3 | 16.0 | 0.7 | 43261 |

**NUTS AND SEEDS**

| | | | | |
|---|---|---|---|---|
| almonds, raw | 9.4 | 52.0 | 0.5 | 12061 |
| brazil nuts, raw | 16.0 | 29.0 | 0.4 | 12078 |
| cashew nuts, oil-roasted | 20.0 | 61.0 | 11.0 | 12586 |
| coconut milk, canned | 5.1 | 8.5 | 0.0 | 12118 |
| coconut, dried, sweetened, flaked, packaged | 9.7 | 19.0 | 1.3 | 12109 |
| filberts (hazelnuts), dried | 15.0 | 46.0 | 0.4 | 12120 |
| flaxseeds | 39.0 | 79.0 | 3.1 | 12220 |
| macadamia nuts, dry-roasted | 11.0 | 45.0 | 0.3 | 12632 |
| peanut butter, chunk style/crunchy | 25.0 | 61.0 | 1.0 | 16097 |
| peanut butter, smooth | 26.0 | 66.0 | 0.4 | 16098 |
| peanuts, raw | 18.0 | 53.0 | 0.6 | 16087 |
| pecans, dried | 9.7 | 41.0 | 0.7 | 12142 |
| pine nuts, pignolia, dried | 8.4 | 56.0 | 0.4 | 12147 |
| pistachios, dry-roasted | 11.0 | 71.0 | 0.8 | 12652 |
| sesame seed kernels, dried | 9.6 | 26.0 | 0.7 | 12201 |
| sunflower seed kernels, dried | 18.0 | 55.0 | 35.0 | 12036 |
| walnuts, black, dried | 8.3 | 32.0 | 0.6 | 12154 |
| walnuts, English/Persian, dried | 7.3 | 39.0 | 0.3 | 12155 |

**POULTRY**

| | | | | |
|---|---|---|---|---|
| chicken (broiler/fryer) light and dark meat with skin, roasted | 5.3 | 66.0 | 5.6 | 05009 |

| | FREE CHOLINE (mg/100 g) | TOTAL CHOLINE (mg/100 g) | BETAINE (mg/100 g) | SR21 SOURCE CODE[1] |
|---|---|---|---|---|
| chicken (broiler/fryer) light and dark meat without skin, roasted | 5.7 | 79.0 | 5.7 | 05013 |
| chicken liver, pan-fried | 69.0 | 330.0 | 21.0 | 05661 |
| chicken liver, raw | 49.0 | 190.0 | 17.0 | 05027 |
| chicken liver, simmered | 48.0 | 290.0 | 13.0 | 05028 |
| chicken, raw | 5.8 | 66.0 | 8.5 | 05011 |
| turkey gizzard, simmered | 9.5 | 82.0 | 1.8 | 05174 |
| turkey heart, simmered | 3.9 | 170.0 | 3.1 | 05176 |
| turkey liver, simmered | 9.7 | 220.0 | 2.5 | 05178 |
| turkey sausage (fresh), pan-fried | 2.0 | 63.0 | 8.0 | 07958 |
| **SALAD DRESSINGS** | | | | |
| Italian salad dressing | 1.5 | 2.6 | 0.0 | 04114 |
| **SAUCES AND CONDIMENTS** | | | | |
| catsup (ketchup) | 7.5 | 13.0 | 0.2 | 11935 |
| mustard (prepared condiment sauce) | 12.0 | 22.0 | 0.2 | 02046 |
| pickle (cucumber), dill | 0.9 | 3.4 | 0.0 | 11937 |
| pickle (cucumber), sweet gherkin | 0.9 | 3.1 | 0.3 | 11940 |
| salsa | 7.3 | 12.0 | 0.3 | 06164 |
| soy sauce made with soy and wheat (shoyu) | 18.0 | 18.0 | 30.0 | 16123 |
| tomato sauce, bottled | 6.5 | 9.9 | 0.8 | 11549 |
| tomato sauce, marinara, bottled | 8.5 | 14.0 | 0.6 | 06931 |
| **SOUPS** | | | | |
| chicken noodle soup, condensed, canned | 3.3 | 11.0 | 12.0 | 06019 |
| tomato soup, condensed, canned | 6.1 | 13.0 | 4.2 | 06159 |
| **SPICES AND HERBS** | | | | |
| basil, dried | 50.0 | 55.0 | 16.0 | 02003 |
| basil, raw | 8.0 | 11.0 | 0.4 | 02044 |
| black pepper | 9.4 | 11.0 | 8.9 | 02030 |
| chili powder | 49 | 67.0 | 2.8 | 02009 |
| cinnamon, ground | 7.0 | 11.0 | 3.9 | 02010 |
| cloves, ground | 29.0 | 37.0 | 1.4 | 02011 |
| curry powder | 42.0 | 64.0 | 29.0 | 02015 |
| garlic powder | 42.0 | 68.0 | 6.1 | 02020 |
| ginger, ground | 33.0 | 41.0 | 3.4 | 02021 |
| mustard seeds, yellow | 46.0 | 120.0 | 1.9 | 02024 |
| onion powder | 25.0 | 39.0 | 0.4 | 02026 |
| oregano, dried, ground | 28.0 | 32.0 | 9.8 | 02027 |
| paprika | 34.0 | 52.0 | 7.1 | 02028 |
| parsley, dried | 17.0 | 97.0 | 1.8 | 02029 |
| poppy seeds | 7.2 | 8.8 | 0.9 | 02033 |
| turmeric, ground | 21.0 | 49.0 | 9.7 | 02043 |
| **SWEETENERS** | | | | |
| honey | 1.2 | 2.2 | 1.7 | 19296 |
| jam/preserves | 2.6 | 10.0 | 0.1 | 19297 |
| molasses | 10.0 | 13.0 | 1.0 | 19304 |
| sugar, brown | 2.2 | 2.5 | 0.3 | 19334 |
| **VEGETABLES** | | | | |
| agave, boiled | 5.2 | 8.8 | 0.4 | 35193 |
| alfalfa sprouts, raw | 11.0 | 14.0 | 0.4 | 11001 |
| artichoke, boiled | 4.2 | 34.0 | 0.2 | 11008 |
| artichoke, microwaved | 6.4 | 22.0 | 0.4 | 98010 |
| asparagus, boiled | 6.6 | 26.0 | 0.9 | 11012 |
| asparagus, raw | 12.0 | 16.0 | 0.6 | 11011 |
| baked beans with pork in sweet sauce, canned | 13.0 | 25.0 | 0.1 | 16010 |
| baked beans with pork in tomato sauce, canned | 25.0 | 39.0 | 0.4 | 16011 |
| baked beans, vegetarian, canned | 17.0 | 32.0 | 0.1 | 16006 |
| beet, canned | 0.3 | 7.5 | 260.0 | 11084 |
| beet, raw | 4.1 | 6.0 | 130.0 | 11080 |
| broccoli, boiled | 8.5 | 40.0 | 0.1 | 11091 |
| broccoli, raw | 18.0 | 19.0 | 0.1 | 11090 |

| | FREE CHOLINE (mg/100 g) | TOTAL CHOLINE (mg/100 g) | BETAINE (mg/100 g) | SR21 SOURCE CODE[1] |
|---|---|---|---|---|
| broccoli raab (rapini), boiled | 4.3 | 34.0 | 0.2 | 11097 |
| broccoli raab (rapini), raw | 12.0 | 18.0 | 0.3 | 11096 |
| Brussels sprouts, boiled | 23.0 | 41.0 | 0.2 | 11099 |
| cabbage, green/white, boiled | 7.6 | 20.0 | 0.3 | 11110 |
| cabbage, green/white, raw | 6.1 | 11.0 | 0.4 | 11109 |
| cabbage, red/purple, boiled | 5.0 | 21.0 | 0.1 | 11113 |
| cabbage, red/purple, raw | 9.7 | 17.0 | 0.1 | 11112 |
| carrot, baby, raw | 5.4 | 7.5 | 0.1 | 11960 |
| carrot, boiled | 0.4 | 8.8 | 0.1 | 11125 |
| carrot, raw | 6.8 | 8.8 | 0.4 | 11124 |
| cauliflower, boiled | 25.0 | 39.0 | 0.1 | 11136 |
| celery, raw | 5.3 | 6.1 | 0.1 | 11143 |
| corn, yellow, frozen, boiled | 8.9 | 22.0 | 0.2 | 11179 |
| cucumber, peeled, raw | 3.5 | 5.7 | 0.1 | 11206 |
| cucumber, raw | 4.0 | 6.0 | 0.1 | 11205 |
| green peas, frozen, boiled | 2.2 | 28.0 | 0.2 | 11313 |
| green snap beans, frozen, boiled | 4.0 | 14.0 | 0.1 | 11061 |
| kale, boiled | 0.1 | 0.4 | 0.3 | 11234 |
| kidney beans, red, mature, canned | 17.0 | 33.0 | 0.1 | 16034 |
| lettuce, butterhead, raw | 5.9 | 8.5 | 0.1 | 11250 |
| lettuce, iceberg, raw | 4.8 | 6.7 | 0.1 | 11252 |
| mushrooms, common white, raw | 5.9 | 17.0 | 11 | 11260 |
| navy beans, mature, boiled | 21.0 | 45.0 | 0.1 | 16038 |
| navy beans, mature, canned | 14.0 | 27.0 | 0.1 | 16039 |
| navy beans, mature, dry | 50.0 | 87.0 | 0.1 | 16037 |
| onion, white, raw | 4.4 | 6.1 | 0.1 | 11282 |
| pinto beans, mature, boiled | 11.0 | 35.0 | 0.1 | 16043 |
| pinto beans, mature, dry | 32.0 | 66.0 | 0.4 | 16042 |
| potato, French fries, frozen | 15.0 | 22.0 | 0.7 | 11402 |
| potato, French fries, frozen, baked | 14.0 | 24.0 | 0.7 | 11403 |
| potato, mashed | 8.4 | 14.0 | 0.4 | 11657 |
| potato, red-skinned, baked | 8.5 | 19.0 | 0.2 | 11358 |
| potato, red-skinned, raw | 9.7 | 16.0 | 0.2 | 11355 |
| potato, russet, baked | 8.1 | 15.0 | 0.2 | 11356 |
| potato, russet, raw | 10.0 | 13.0 | 0.2 | 11353 |
| potato, white-skinned, baked | 6.8 | 14.0 | 0.2 | 11357 |
| potato, white-skinned, raw | 7.9 | 11.0 | 0.2 | 11354 |
| radish, red, raw | 4.8 | 6.5 | 0.1 | 11429 |
| romaine (cos lettuce), raw | 7.6 | 9.9 | 0.1 | 11251 |
| sauerkraut, canned, solids and liquid | 8.7 | 10.0 | 0.5 | 11439 |
| soybeans, green/immature (edamame), frozen, heated | 6.9 | 56.0 | 4.5 | 11212 |
| soybeans, mature, dry | 47.0 | 120.0 | 2.1 | 16108 |
| spinach, frozen | 2.3 | 22.0 | 120.0 | 11463 |
| spinach, frozen, boiled, drained | 1.7 | 25.0 | 110.0 | 11464 |
| sweet pepper, green, raw | 3.6 | 5.6 | 0.1 | 11333 |
| sweet pepper, red, raw | 4.0 | 5.6 | 0.1 | 11821 |
| sweet potato, baked | 0.9 | 13.0 | 35.0 | 11508 |
| tomato paste, canned | 26.0 | 39.0 | 0.4 | 11546 |
| tomato, red, raw | 4.4 | 6.7 | 0.1 | 11529 |
| winter squash, all varieties, baked | 2.1 | 11.0 | 0.2 | 11644 |
| zucchini summer squash, boiled | 0.5 | 9.4 | 0.3 | 11478 |
| **SPECIAL DIETARY FOODS** | | | | |
| Luna meal bar | 14.0 | 42.0 | 1.7 | 25021 |
| Optima meal bar, chocolate peanut, Slimfast | 19.0 | 41.0 | 2.2.0 | 25020 |
| PowerBar, chocolate | 7.8 | 18.0 | 4.3 | 25017 |
| **OTHER FOODS** | | | | |
| baking chocolate (unsweetened) | 34.0 | 46.0 | 2.6 | 19078 |
| yeast, baker's, active dry | 6.1 | 32.0 | 3.4 | 18375 |

[1]Code numbers for foods in the USDA National Nutrient Database for Standard Reference, Release 21, 2008.

Source:
USDA Database for the Choline Content of Common Foods, Release Two. Prepared by Patterson KY, Bhagwat SA, Williams JR, et al., in collaboration with Zeisel SH, Dacosta KA, and Mar MH. January 2008. Available at: http://www.nla.usda.gov/fnic/foodcomp/Data/Choline/Choln02.pdf.

# Vitamins/Vitamin-Like Components—Myo-Inositol

| | MYO-INOSITOL (mg/100 g) | SOURCE | | MYO-INOSITOL (mg/100 g) | SOURCE |
|---|---|---|---|---|---|
| **BEVERAGES** | | | pie, chocolate, creme | 52 | Clements and Darnell, 1980 |
| coffee instant powder | 646 | Clements and Darnell, 1980 | pie, lemon | 63 | Clements and Darnell, 1980 |
| coffee, brewed | 5 | Clements and Darnell, 1980 | pie, pecan | 64 | Clements and Darnell, 1980 |
| Diet Pepsi | 1 | Clements and Darnell, 1980 | to pie, sweet potato | 20 | Clements and Darnell, 1980 |
| cola | 0.00 | Clements and Darnell, 1980 | pudding, cranberry | 1 | Clements and Darnell, 1980 |
| fruit punch drink, canned/bottled | 17 | Clements and Darnell, 1980 | sherbet | 7 | Clements and Darnell, 1980 |
| grapefruit soda | 1 | Clements and Darnell, 1980 | **EGGS** | | |
| lemonade | 2 | Clements and Darnell, 1980 | egg, raw | 9 | Clements and Darnell, 1980 |
| orange soda, Shasta | 1 | Clements and Darnell, 1980 | egg, scrambled with milk | 8 | Clements and Darnell, 1980 |
| raspberry soda | 0.00 | Clements and Darnell, 1980 | egg white, raw | 5 | Clements and Darnell, 1980 |
| Seven-Up | 0.00 | Clements and Darnell, 1980 | egg yolk, raw | 34 | Clements and Darnell, 1980 |
| tea, black, brewed | 3 | Clements and Darnell, 1980 | | | |
| **CEREALS AND GRAINS** | | | **FISH AND SHELLFISH** | | |
| barley, pearled, cooked | 3 | Clements and Darnell, 1980 | clams, raw | 3 | Clements and Darnell, 1980 |
| corn grits, enriched, cooked | 10 | Clements and Darnell, 1980 | crab, raw | 5 | Clements and Darnell, 1980 |
| oatmeal, quick, cooked | 34 | Clements and Darnell, 1980 | herring, canned in oil | 0.00 | Clements and Darnell, 1980 |
| oatmeal, regular, cooked | 42 | Clements and Darnell, 1980 | oysters, raw | 25 | Clements and Darnell, 1980 |
| rice, brown, long grain, boiled | 30 | Clements and Darnell, 1980 | salmon, unspecified, canned in oil | 20 | Clements and Darnell, 1980 |
| rice, white, instant, boiled | 2 | Clements and Darnell, 1980 | sardines, unspecified, canned | 12 | Clements and Darnell, 1980 |
| rice, white, medium grain, enriched, boiled | 15 | Clements and Darnell, 1980 | shrimp, broiled | 7 | Clements and Darnell, 1980 |
| wild rice, boiled | 27 | Clements and Darnell, 1980 | trout, broiled | 11 | Clements and Darnell, 1980 |
| | | | tuna salad | 12 | Clements and Darnell, 1980 |
| **CEREALS, READY-TO-EAT** | | | tuna, canned in oil, drained | 11 | Clements and Darnell, 1980 |
| bran flakes, 40% | 274 | Clements and Darnell, 1980 | tuna, canned in water, drained | 15 | Clements and Darnell, 1980 |
| corn flakes | 6 | Clements and Darnell, 1980 | tuna, chunk light, canned in water, drained | 9 | Clements and Darnell, 1980 |
| Cracklin' Bran | 67 | Clements and Darnell, 1980 | whitefish, broiled | 2 | Clements and Darnell, 1980 |
| puffed rice | 5 | Clements and Darnell, 1980 | | | |
| puffed wheat | 8 | Clements and Darnell, 1980 | **FRUIT AND VEGETABLE JUICES AND JUICE DRINKS** | | |
| raisin bran | 107 | Clements and Darnell, 1980 | apple juice, canned/bottled | 21 | Clements and Darnell, 1980 |
| shredded wheat | 35 | Clements and Darnell, 1980 | apple juice, from frozen concentrate | 33 | Clements and Darnell, 1980 |
| Team Flakes | 93 | Clements and Darnell, 1980 | apricot nectar, canned/bottled | 26 | Clements and Darnell, 1980 |
| **CHEESE** | | | carrot juice, canned | 1 | Clements and Darnell, 1980 |
| American processed cheese | 7 | Clements and Darnell, 1980 | cranberry apple juice drink, canned/bottled | 1 | Clements and Darnell, 1980 |
| cheddar cheese | 9 | Clements and Darnell, 1980 | cranberry juice cocktail, canned/bottled | 7 | Clements and Darnell, 1980 |
| cottage cheese, 2% fat | 1 | Clements and Darnell, 1980 | grape juice, from frozen concentrate | 36 | Clements and Darnell, 1980 |
| cottage cheese, creamed, large curd | 2 | Clements and Darnell, 1980 | grapefruit juice, canned/bottled | 41 | Clements and Darnell, 1980 |
| cottage cheese, creamed, small curd | 2 | Clements and Darnell, 1980 | grapefruit juice, from frozen concentrate | 380 | Clements and Darnell, 1980 |
| cream cheese | 7 | Clements and Darnell, 1980 | lemon juice from California lemons, raw | 66 | Ranganna et al, 1983 |
| mozzarella cheese | 5 | Clements and Darnell, 1980 | lemon juice, canned/bottled | 73 | Clements and Darnell, 1980 |
| muenster cheese | 3 | Clements and Darnell, 1980 | lemon juice, raw | 30 | Clements and Darnell, 1980 |
| parmesan cheese | 6 | Clements and Darnell, 1980 | orange juice from navel orange, raw | 156 | Ranganna et al, 1983 |
| Swiss cheese | 5 | Clements and Darnell, 1980 | orange juice from Valencia orange, raw | 159 | Ranganna et al, 1983 |
| **DESSERTS** | | | orange juice, canned/bottled | 200 | Clements and Darnell, 1980 |
| cake, angel food | 2 | Clements and Darnell, 1980 | orange juice, from frozen concentrate | 204 | Clements and Darnell, 1980 |
| cake, chocolate, from mix | 18 | Clements and Darnell, 1980 | orange juice, raw | 35 | Clements and Darnell, 1980 |
| cake, lemon | 19 | Clements and Darnell, 1980 | peach nectar, canned/bottled | 1 | Clements and Darnell, 1980 |
| cake, strawberry shortcake | 69 | Clements and Darnell, 1980 | pineapple juice, canned/bottled | 15 | Clements and Darnell, 1980 |
| cake, yellow with sugar icing | 5 | Clements and Darnell, 1980 | prune juice, canned/bottled | 26 | Clements and Darnell, 1980 |
| cobbler, cherry | 30 | Clements and Darnell, 1980 | tangerine juice, raw | 135 | Ranganna et al, 1983 |
| cookie, sugar | 34 | Clements and Darnell, 1980 | tomato juice, canned/bottled | 48 | Clements and Darnell, 1980 |
| cookie, vanilla wafer, 12%–17% fat | 23 | Clements and Darnell, 1980 | V8 Juice, canned/bottled, Campbell's | 29 | Clements and Darnell, 1980 |
| gelatin dessert, from mix with sugar, all flavors | 7 | Clements and Darnell, 1980 | | | |
| graham cracker | 10 | Clements and Darnell, 1980 | | | |
| ice cream, vanilla | 9 | Clements and Darnell, 1980 | | | |
| pie, apple | 22 | Clements and Darnell, 1980 | | | |

| | MYO-INOSITOL (mg/100 g) | SOURCE |
|---|---|---|
| **FRUITS** | | |
| apple, dried, cooked | 9 | Clements and Darnell, 1980 |
| apple, Red Delicious, raw | 10 | Clements and Darnell, 1980 |
| apple, Rome, raw | 15 | Clements and Darnell, 1980 |
| apple, Yellow Delicious, raw | 24 | Clements and Darnell, 1980 |
| applesauce, unsweetened, canned/bottled | 18 | Clements and Darnell, 1980 |
| apricot, canned in water | 52 | Clements and Darnell, 1980 |
| avocado, raw | 46 | Clements and Darnell, 1980 |
| blackberries, canned in water | 173 | Clements and Darnell, 1980 |
| cantaloupe, raw | 355 | Clements and Darnell, 1980 |
| cherries, sweet, black bing, canned in water | 59 | Clements and Darnell, 1980 |
| cherries, sweet, canned in water | 5 | Clements and Darnell, 1980 |
| cherries, sweet, dark, canned in water | 127 | Clements and Darnell, 1980 |
| cherries, sweet, raw | 14 | Clements and Darnell, 1980 |
| cherries, sweet, Royal Ann, raw | 4 | Clements and Darnell, 1980 |
| cranberries, raw | 15 | Clements and Darnell, 1980 |
| cranberry sauce, canned | 2 | Clements and Darnell, 1980 |
| date, dried | 152 | Clements and Darnell, 1980 |
| fig, calimyrna, dried | 91 | Clements and Darnell, 1980 |
| fruit cocktail, canned in heavy syrup | 19 | Clements and Darnell, 1980 |
| grapefruit, canned in light syrup | 117 | Clements and Darnell, 1980 |
| grapefruit, raw | 199 | Clements and Darnell, 1980 |
| grapes, green, canned in water | 7 | Clements and Darnell, 1980 |
| grapes, green, raw | 16 | Clements and Darnell, 1980 |
| grapes, purple, raw | 15 | Clements and Darnell, 1980 |
| honeydew melon, raw | 46 | Clements and Darnell, 1980 |
| kiwifruit, raw | 136 | Clements and Darnell, 1980 |
| lemon peel from California lemons, raw | 216 | Ranganna et al., 1983 |
| lemon peel, raw | 33 | Clements and Darnell, 1980 |
| lemon, California, raw | 109 | Ranganna et al, 1983 |
| lime, raw | 194 | Clements and Darnell, 1980 |
| mandarin oranges, canned in light syrup | 149 | Clements and Darnell, 1980 |
| mango, raw | 99 | Clements and Darnell, 1980 |
| nectarine, raw | 118 | Clements and Darnell, 1980 |
| orange peel from Valencia orange, raw | 257 | Ranganna et al, 1983 |
| orange, raw | 307 | Clements and Darnell, 1980 |
| orange, Valencia, raw | 204 | Ranganna et al, 1983 |
| papaya, raw | 8 | Clements and Darnell, 1980 |
| peach, cling, canned in water | 34 | Clements and Darnell, 1980 |
| peach, cling, raw | 19 | Clements and Darnell, 1980 |
| peach, dried | 164 | Clements and Darnell, 1980 |
| peach, freestone, raw | 58 | Clements and Darnell, 1980 |
| pear, Bartlett, canned, water pack | 46 | Clements and Darnell, 1980 |
| pear, raw | 73 | Clements and Darnell, 1980 |
| pineapple, canned in water | 16 | Clements and Darnell, 1980 |
| pineapple, raw | 33 | Clements and Darnell, 1980 |
| plum, raw | 11 | Clements and Darnell, 1980 |
| plum, red, raw | 30 | Clements and Darnell, 1980 |
| prune, dried | 470 | Clements and Darnell, 1980 |
| raisins, seedless | 20 | Clements and Darnell, 1980 |
| strawberries, raw | 13 | Clements and Darnell, 1980 |
| watermelon, raw | 31 | Clements and Darnell, 1980 |
| **GRAIN PRODUCTS** | | |
| bread, bran, Orowheat | 81 | Clements and Darnell, 1980 |
| bread, French | 34 | Clements and Darnell, 1980 |
| bread, pumpernickel | 160 | Clements and Darnell, 1980 |
| bread, Roman Meal | 38 | Clements and Darnell, 1980 |
| bread, rye | 47 | Clements and Darnell, 1980 |
| bread, rye cocktail | 39 | Clements and Darnell, 1980 |
| bread, wheat, stone-ground | 115 | Suements and Darnell, 1980 |

| | MYO-INOSITOL (mg/100 g) | SOURCE |
|---|---|---|
| bread, white | 26 | Clements and Darnell, 1980 |
| bread, whole multigrain | 47 | Clements and Darnell, 1980 |
| bread, whole wheat | 142 | Clements and Darnell, 1980 |
| biscuit, plain | 31 | Clements and Darnell, 1980 |
| Cheese Nibs (crackers) | 246 | Clements and Darnell, 1980 |
| cornbread, homemade (quick bread) | 14 | Clements and Darnell, 1980 |
| cornbread stuffing, dry | 8 | Clements and Darnell, 1980 |
| French toast, homemade | 8 | Clements and Darnell, 1980 |
| macaroni, enriched, boiled | 5 | Clements and Darnell, 1980 |
| melba toast | 59 | Clements and Darnell, 1980 |
| muffin | 15 | Clements and Darnell, 1980 |
| noodles, egg, enriched, boiled (egg in the noodle dough) | 18 | Clements and Darnell, 1980 |
| pancake | 23 | Clements and Darnell, 1980 |
| roll, dinner | 23 | Clements and Darnell, 1980 |
| roll, frankfurter | 115 | Clements and Darnell, 1980 |
| roll, hamburger | 478 | Clements and Darnell, 1980 |
| saltines | 47 | Clements and Darnell, 1980 |
| soda crackers, salt-free | 13 | Clements and Darnell, 1980 |
| spaghetti, enriched, boiled | 31 | Clements and Darnell, 1980 |
| waffle | 22 | Clements and Darnell, 1980 |
| Wheat Thins, Nabisco | 89 | Clements and Darnell, 1980 |
| **MEATS** | | |
| beef liver, raw | 64 | Clements and Darnell, 1980 |
| beef roast, choice, raw | 15 | Clements and Darnell, 1980 |
| beef round steak, raw | 15 | Clements and Darnell, 1980 |
| beef round, ground, broiled | 37 | Clements and Darnell, 1980 |
| beef sirloin steak, raw | 30 | Clements and Darnell, 1980 |
| beef tips, braised | 7 | Clements and Darnell, 1980 |
| beef, ground, patty, broiled | 8 | Clements and Darnell, 1980 |
| beef, meatloaf | 30 | Clements and Darnell, 1980 |
| lamb chop, raw | 37 | Clements and Darnell, 1980 |
| pork bacon, cured, broiled/pan-fried | 23 | Clements and Darnell, 1980 |
| pork chop, baked | 6 | Clements and Darnell, 1980 |
| pork chop, barbequed | 42 | Clements and Darnell, 1980 |
| pork chop, broiled | 14 | Clements and Darnell, 1980 |
| pork liver, raw | 17 | Clements and Darnell, 1980 |
| pork roast, raw | 30 | Clements and Darnell, 1980 |
| **MEATS, LUNCHEON** | | |
| bologna | 94 | Clements and Darnell, 1980 |
| corned beef, canned | 19 | Clements and Darnell, 1980 |
| frankfurter | 16 | Clements and Darnell, 1980 |
| ham, deviled, canned | 4 | Clements and Darnell, 1980 |
| ham, spiced | 6 | Clements and Darnell, 1980 |
| liver cheese, pork | 346 | Clements and Darnell, 1980 |
| liver loaf | 22 | Clements and Darnell, 1980 |
| lunch meat, canned | 18 | Clements and Darnell, 1980 |
| luncheon loaf, spiced | 39 | Clements and Darnell, 1980 |
| pastrami, beef | 28 | Clements and Darnell, 1980 |
| salami, beef and pork | 42 | Clements and Darnell, 1980 |
| souse | 54 | Clements and Darnell, 1980 |
| Vienna sausage, beef and pork, canned | 81 | Clements and Darnell, 1980 |
| **MILK AND YOGURT** | | |
| buttermilk, cultured | 1 | Clements and Darnell, 1980 |
| chocolate milk, reduced fat | 19 | Clements and Darnell, 1980 |
| cocoa mix for milk | 31 | Clements and Darnell, 1980 |
| condensed milk, sweetened, canned | 26 | Clements and Darnell, 1980 |
| milk, nonfat | 4 | Clements and Darnell, 1980 |
| milk, whole, 4% fat | 4 | Clements and Darnell, 1980 |
| yogurt, boysenberry | 7 | Clements and Darnell, 1980 |
| yogurt, coffee | 9 | Clements and Darnell, 1980 |

| | MYO-INOSITOL (mg/100 g) | SOURCE |
|---|---|---|
| yogurt, plain | 6 | Clements and Darnell, 1980 |
| yogurt, raspberry | 16 | Clements and Darnell, 1980 |
| yogurt, strawberry | 16 | Clements and Darnell, 1980 |
| yogurt, vanilla | 9 | Clements and Darnell, 1980 |
| **NUTS** | | |
| almonds, raw | 278 | Clements and Darnell, 1980 |
| cashews, raw | 81 | Clements and Darnell, 1980 |
| coconut, dried, sweetened, shredded | 33 | Clements and Darnell, 1980 |
| peanut butter, chunky | 128 | Clements and Darnell, 1980 |
| peanut butter, creamy | 304 | Clements and Darnell, 1980 |
| peanuts, all types, boiled | 134 | Clements and Darnell, 1980 |
| peanuts, raw | 133 | Clements and Darnell, 1980 |
| sunflower seed kernels, dried | 12 | Clements and Darnell, 1980 |
| walnuts, English/Persian, raw | 198 | Clements and Darnell, 1980 |
| **POULTRY** | | |
| chicken, baked | 8 | Clements and Darnell, 1980 |
| chicken breast, raw | 30 | Clements and Darnell, 1980 |
| chicken leg, baked | 39 | Clements and Darnell, 1980 |
| chicken liver, raw | 131 | Clements and Darnell, 1980 |
| turkey breast, raw | 8 | Clements and Darnell, 1980 |
| turkey, roasted | 23 | Clements and Darnell, 1980 |
| **SALAD DRESSINGS** | | |
| blue cheese salad dressing | 8 | Clements and Darnell, 1980 |
| French salad dressing | 7 | Clements and Darnell, 1980 |
| French salad dressing, low/reduced calorie | 8 | Clements and Darnell, 1980 |
| oil and vinegar salad dressing | 4 | Clements and Darnell, 1980 |
| thousand island salad dressing | 50 | Clements and Darnell, 1980 |
| thousand island salad dressing, low/reduced calorie | 8 | Clements and Darnell, 1980 |
| **SAUCES AND CONDIMENTS** | | |
| catsup (ketchup) | 38 | Clements and Darnell, 1980 |
| hot pepper sauce, ready-to-serve | 25 | Clements and Darnell, 1980 |
| tomato sauce, bottled | 81 | Clements and Darnell, 1980 |
| olives, green, canned/bottled | 2 | Clements and Darnell, 1980 |
| **SOUPS** | | |
| beef broth/bouillon cube | 41 | Clements and Darnell, 1980 |
| split pea soup, ready-to-serve | 17 | Clements and Darnell, 1980 |
| tomato soup, canned, ready-to-serve | 7 | Clements and Darnell, 1980 |
| vegetable soup, canned/ homemade | 6 | Clements and Darnell, 1980 |
| **VEGETABLES** | | |
| **FLOWER, STEM, AND STALK VEGETABLES** | | |
| artichoke hearts, canned | 116 | Clements and Darnell, 1980 |
| artichoke, frozen | 80 | Clements and Darnell, 1980 |
| artichoke, raw | 60 | Clements and Darnell, 1980 |
| asparagus, canned | 28 | Clements and Darnell, 1980 |
| asparagus, frozen | 15 | Clements and Darnell, 1980 |
| asparagus, raw | 29 | Clements and Darnell, 1980 |
| asparagus, white, canned | 38 | Clements and Darnell, 1980 |
| broccoli, frozen | 11 | Clements and Darnell, 1980 |
| broccoli, raw | 30 | Clements and Darnell, 1980 |
| cauliflower, frozen | 15 | Clements and Darnell, 1980 |
| cauliflower, raw | 18 | Clements and Darnell, 1980 |
| celery, raw | 5 | Clements and Darnell, 1980 |
| scallions (green/spring onions), raw | 27 | Clements and Darnell, 1980 |

| | MYO-INOSITOL (mg/100 g) | SOURCE |
|---|---|---|
| **FRUIT (SEED-CONTAINING) VEGETABLES** | | |
| acorn winter squash, frozen | 66 | Clements and Darnell, 1980 |
| acorn winter squash, raw | 22 | Clements and Darnell, 1980 |
| banana pepper, raw | 135 | Clements and Darnell, 1980 |
| chili pepper, red, hot, raw | 59 | Clements and Darnell, 1980 |
| cucumber, raw | 15 | Clements and Darnell, 1980 |
| eggplant (aubergine), canned | 84 | Clements and Darnell, 1980 |
| eggplant (aubergine), frozen | 44 | Clements and Darnell, 1980 |
| eggplant (aubergine), raw | 84 | Clements and Darnell, 1980 |
| green beans, canned | 51 | Clements and Darnell, 1980 |
| green beans, French style, canned | 87 | Clements and Darnell, 1980 |
| green beans, French style, frozen | 55 | Clements and Darnell, 1980 |
| green beans, frozen | 55 | Clements and Darnell, 1980 |
| green beans, Italian, canned | 35 | Clements and Darnell, 1980 |
| green beans, pole, frozen | 175 | Clements and Darnell, 1980 |
| green beans, raw | 105 | Clements and Darnell, 1980 |
| hubbard winter squash, raw | 66 | Clements and Darnell, 1980 |
| jalapeno pepper, canned | 30 | Clements and Darnell, 1980 |
| okra, canned | 117 | Clements and Darnell, 1980 |
| okra, fried | 37 | Clements and Darnell, 1980 |
| okra, frozen | 28 | Clements and Darnell, 1980 |
| okra, raw | 33 | Clements and Darnell, 1980 |
| pumpkin winter squash, canned | 62 | Clements and Darnell, 1980 |
| summer squash, green, raw | 17 | Clements and Darnell, 1980 |
| sweet pepper, green, frozen | 29 | Clements and Darnell, 1980 |
| sweet pepper, green, raw | 57 | Clements and Darnell, 1980 |
| tomato paste, canned | 51 | Clements and Darnell, 1980 |
| tomato puree, canned | 77 | Clements and Darnell, 1980 |
| tomato, red, canned | 38 | Clements and Darnell, 1980 |
| tomato, red, cherry, raw | 41 | Clements and Darnell, 1980 |
| tomato, red, raw | 54 | Clements and Darnell, 1980 |
| winter squash, yellow, canned | 6 | Clements and Darnell, 1980 |
| winter squash, yellow, frozen | 25 | Clements and Darnell, 1980 |
| winter squash, yellow, raw | 32 | Clements and Darnell, 1980 |
| yellow snap beans, canned | 144 | Clements and Darnell, 1980 |
| zucchini summer squash, raw | 53 | Clements and Darnell, 1980 |
| **LEAFY VEGETABLES** | | |
| Brussels sprouts, frozen | 81 | Clements and Darnell, 1980 |
| cabbage, green/white, raw | 21 | Clements and Darnell, 1980 |
| cabbage, red/purple, raw | 9 | Clements and Darnell, 1980 |
| cabbage, savoy, raw | 70 | Clements and Darnell, 1980 |
| Chinese cabbage, pak choi, raw | 27 | Clements and Darnell, 1980 |
| collards, canned | 30 | Clements and Darnell, 1980 |
| collards, frozen | 16 | Clements and Darnell, 1980 |
| collards, raw | 64 | Clements and Darnell, 1980 |
| endive, raw | 11 | Clements and Darnell, 1980 |
| lettuce, looseleaf (leaf), raw | 18 | Clements and Darnell, 1980 |
| lettuce, red leaf | 22 | Clements and Darnell, 1980 |
| mustard greens, canned | 9 | Clements and Darnell, 1980 |
| mustard greens, frozen | 17 | Clements and Darnell, 1980 |
| mustard greens, raw | 23 | Clements and Darnell, 1980 |
| parsley, raw | 22 | Clements and Darnell, 1980 |
| poke greens, raw | 43 | Clements and Darnell, 1980 |
| romaine (cos lettuce), raw | 17 | Clements and Darnell, 1980 |
| sauerkraut, canned | 11 | Clements and Darnell, 1980 |
| spinach, canned | 25 | Clements and Darnell, 1980 |
| spinach, frozen | 6 | Clements and Darnell, 1980 |
| spinach, raw | 8 | Clements and Darnell, 1980 |
| turnip greens and root, canned | 8 | Clements and Darnell, 1980 |
| turnip greens, canned | 12 | Clements and Darnell, 1980 |
| turnip greens, frozen | 8 | Clements and Darnell, 1980 |
| turnip greens, raw | 43 | Clements and Darnell, 1980 |

| | MYO-INOSITOL (mg/100 g) | SOURCE | | MYO-INOSITOL (mg/100 g) | SOURCE |
|---|---|---|---|---|---|
| **LEGUMES (BEANS AND PEAS)** | | | **TUBER AND ROOT VEGETABLES** | | |
| baked beans with pork, canned | 86 | Clements and Darnell, 1980 | | | |
| cowpeas (blackeye peas), immature, frozen | 70 | Clements and Darnell, 1980 | beet, canned | 20 | Clements and Darnell, 1980 |
| | | | beet, raw | 12 | Clements and Darnell, 1980 |
| cowpeas (blackeye peas), mature, canned | 117 | Clements and Darnell, 1980 | beet, whole small, canned | 8 | Clements and Darnell, 1980 |
| | | | carrot, canned | 52 | Clements and Darnell, 1980 |
| cowpeas (blackeye peas), mature, dry | 39 | Clements and Darnell, 1980 | carrot, frozen | 10 | Clements and Darnell, 1980 |
| | | | carrot, raw | 12 | Clements and Darnell, 1980 |
| great northern beans, mature, canned | 440 | Clements and Darnell, 1980 | onion, purple, raw | 41 | Clements and Darnell, 1980 |
| | | | onion, white, boiled | 24 | Clements and Darnell, 1980 |
| great northern beans, mature, dry | 327 | Clements and Darnell, 1980 | onion, white, raw | 23 | Clements and Darnell, 1980 |
| green beans, shelled, raw | 193 | Clements and Darnell, 1980 | onion, yellow, cooked | 16 | Clements and Darnell, 1980 |
| green peas, large, canned | 235 | Clements and Darnell, 1980 | onion, yellow, raw | 44 | Clements and Darnell, 1980 |
| green peas, large, frozen | 95 | Clements and Darnell, 1980 | potato, baked | 97 | Clements and Darnell, 1980 |
| green peas, raw | 40 | Clements and Darnell, 1980 | potato, hashed brown, homemade | 57 | Clements and Darnell, 1980 |
| green peas, small, canned | 76 | Clements and Darnell, 1980 | | | |
| green peas, small, frozen | 85 | Clements and Darnell, 1980 | potato, mashed, from instant | 30 | Clements and Darnell, 1980 |
| kidney beans, dark red, mature, canned | 249 | Clements and Darnell, 1980 | potato, mashed, homemade | 19 | Clements and Darnell, 1980 |
| | | | potato, peeled, canned | 47 | Clements and Darnell, 1980 |
| kidney beans, light red, mature, canned | 69 | Clements and Darnell, 1980 | potatoes au gratin, homemade | 24 | Clements and Darnell, 1980 |
| | | | radish, red, raw | 10 | Clements and Darnell, 1980 |
| kidney beans, light red, mature, dry | 60 | Clements and Darnell, 1980 | rutabaga (Swede), canned | 252 | Clements and Darnell, 1980 |
| | | | rutabaga (Swede), raw | 24 | Clements and Darnell, 1980 |
| lentils, mature, dry | 45 | Clements and Darnell, 1980 | sweet potato, baked | 92 | Clements and Darnell, 1980 |
| lima beans, immature, baby green, frozen | 42 | Clements and Darnell, 1980 | | | |
| lima beans, immature, green, canned | 146 | Clements and Darnell, 1980 | **OTHER VEGETABLES** | | |
| | | | corn, white, creamed, canned | 7 | Clements and Darnell, 1980 |
| lima beans, immature, green, frozen | 48 | Clements and Darnell, 1980 | corn, yellow, canned | 24 | Clements and Darnell, 1980 |
| | | | corn, yellow, creamed, canned | 20 | Clements and Darnell, 1980 |
| lima beans, immature, large green, canned | 35 | Clements and Darnell, 1980 | corn, yellow, creamed, frozen | 13 | Clements and Darnell, 1980 |
| | | | corn, yellow, frozen | 11 | Clements and Darnell, 1980 |
| lima beans, immature, small green, canned | 110 | Clements and Darnell, 1980 | green peas and carrots, frozen | 99 | Clements and Darnell, 1980 |
| | | | hominy, white, canned | 43 | Clements and Darnell, 1980 |
| lima beans, mature, baby, dry | 56 | Clements and Darnell, 1980 | hominy, yellow, canned | 17 | Clements and Darnell, 1980 |
| lima beans, mature, large, canned | 23 | Clements and Darnell, 1980 | mixed vegetables, canned | 5 | Clements and Darnell, 1980 |
| lima beans, mature, large, dry | 33 | Clements and Darnell, 1980 | mixed vegetables, frozen | 13 | Clements and Darnell, 1980 |
| lima beans, mature, speckled, dry | 70 | Clements and Darnell, 1980 | mushrooms, common white, canned | 29 | Clements and Darnell, 1980 |
| lima beans, mature, speckled, frozen | 55 | Clements and Darnell, 1980 | mushrooms, common white, raw | 9 | Clements and Darnell, 1980 |
| navy beans, mature, canned | 65 | Clements and Darnell, 1980 | **OTHER FOODS** | | |
| navy beans, mature, dry | 283 | Clements and Darnell, 1980 | honey | 33 | Clements and Darnell, 1980 |
| peas, field, canned | 48 | Clements and Darnell, 1980 | mayonnaise | 4 | Clements and Darnell, 1980 |
| peas, field, frozen | 68 | Clements and Darnell, 1980 | mayonnaise, low calorie | 5 | Clements and Darnell, 1980 |
| peas, purple hull, canned | 98 | Clements and Darnell, 1980 | pancake/waffle syrup | 1 | Clements and Darnell, 1980 |
| peas, purple hull, dry | 38 | Clements and Darnell, 1980 | popcorn, oil-popped | 107 | Clements and Darnell, 1980 |
| peas, split, mature, dry | 128 | Clements and Darnell, 1980 | potato chips | 73 | Clements and Darnell, 1980 |
| pinto beans, mature, canned | 23 | Clements and Darnell, 1980 | potato chips, formed, canned | 58 | Clements and Darnell, 1980 |
| soybeans, mature, dry | 88 | Clements and Darnell, 1980 | sour cream, cultured | 76 | Clements and Darnell, 1980 |

Sources:

Clements RS, Darnell B. Myo-inositol content of common foods: Development of a high-myo-inositol diet. *Am J Clin Nutr* 33:1954–1967, 1980.

Ranganna S, Govindarajan VS, Ramana KVR. Citrus fruits-Varieties, chemistry, technology, and quality evaluation. Part II. Chemistry, technology, and quality evaluation. A. Chemistry. *Crit Rev Food Sci Nut* 18(4):313–386, 1983.

# *Vitamins/Vitamin-Like Components—Vitamin $D_3$*

| | SERVING SIZE (g) | VITAMIN $D_3$ (IU/serving) | VITAMIN $D_3$ (IU/100 g) | SOURCE (SR21 CODE NUMBER) |
|---|---|---|---|---|
| **CEREALS, READY-TO-EAT** | | | | |
| All-Bran Buds, Kellogg's | ⅓ cup (30 g) | 40 | 133 | SR21 (08005) |
| All-Bran with extra fiber, Kellogg's | ½ cup (26 g) | 55 | 210 | SR21 (08253) |
| All-Bran Yogurt Bites, Kellogg's | 1¼ cup (56 g) | 41 | 73 | SR21 (08518) |
| All-Bran, Kellogg's | ½ cup (31 g) | 53 | 170 | SR21 (08001) |
| Alpha-Bits, frosted, Post | 1 cup (32 g) | 40 | 125 | SR21 (08325) |
| Alpha-Bits, marshmallow, Post | 1 cup (29 g) | 40 | 138 | SR21 (08326) |
| Apple Cinnamon O's, organic, Barbara's Bakery | ¾ cup (30 g) | 100 | 333 | BARB |
| Apple Jacks, Kellogg's | 1 cup (30 g) | 38 | 127 | SR21 (08003) |
| Apple Zings, Malt-O-Meal | 1 cup (33 g) | 41 | 123 | SR21 (08493) |
| Banana Nut Crunch, Post | 1 cup (59 g) | 40 | 68 | SR21 (08320) |
| Basic 4, General Mills | 1 cup (55 g) | 40 | 73 | SR21 (08262) |
| Blueberry Morning, Post | 1¼ cups (55 g) | 40 | 73 | SR21 (08321) |
| Blueberry Muffin Tops Cereal, Malt-O-Meal | ¾ cup (30 g) | 48 | 161 | SR21 (08487) |
| Bran Flakes, high fiber, Malt-O-Meal | ¾ cup (29 g) | 72 | 248 | SR21 (08490) |
| Bran Flakes, Post | ¾ cup (30 g) | 40 | 133 | SR21 (08322) |
| Cheerios, apple cinnamon, General Mills | ¾ cup (30 g) | 40 | 133 | SR21 (08263) |
| Cheerios, berry burst, General Mills | 1 cup (30 g) | 60 | 200 | SR21 (08239) |
| Cheerios, Frosted, General Mills | 1 cup (30 g) | 43 | 143 | SR21 (08267) |
| Cheerios, General Mills | 1 cup (30 g) | 40 | 133 | SR21 (08013) |
| Cheerios, honey nut, General Mills | 1 cup (30 g) | 43 | 143 | SR21 (08045) |
| Cheerios, multi-grain, General Mills | 1 cup (30 g) | 41 | 138 | SR21 (08087) |
| Cinnamon Grahams, General Mills | ¾ cup (30 g) | 40 | 133 | SR21 (08139) |
| Cinnamon Mini Swirlz, Kellogg's | 1 cup (30 g) | 40 | 133 | SR21 (08520) |
| Cinnamon Toast Crunch, General Mills | ¾ cup (30 g) | 40 | 133 | SR21 (08272) |
| Cinnamon Toasters, Malt-O-Meal | ¾ cup (30 g) | 44 | 145 | SR21 (08494) |
| Cocoa Krispies, Kellogg's | ¾ cup (31 g) | 40 | 130 | SR21 (08014) |
| Cocoa Pebbles, Post | ¾ cup (29 g) | 40 | 138 | SR21 (08323) |
| Coco-Roos, Malt-O-Meal | ¾ cup (30 g) | 55 | 182 | SR21 (08206) |
| Cookie Crisp, chocolate chip/vanilla, General Mills | 1 cup (30 g) | 40 | 133 | SR21 (08017) |
| Cookie Crisp, peanut butter, General Mills | ¾ cup (30 g) | 40 | 133 | SR21 (08516) |
| Corn Bursts, Malt-O-Meal | 1 cup (31 g) | 44 | 141 | SR21 (08083) |
| Corn Chex, General Mills | 1 cup (30 g) | 40 | 133 | SR21 (08019) |
| Corn Flakes with Bananas, Kellogg's | ¾ cup (26 g) | 46 | 175 | SR21 (08472) |
| Corn Flakes, Country, General Mills | 1 cup (30 g) | 40 | 133 | SR21 (08269) |
| Corn Flakes, honey crisp, Quaker | 1 cup (30 g) | 40 | 133 | SR21 (08396) |
| Corn Flakes, Kellogg's | 1 cup (30 g) | 46 | 152 | SR21 (08020) |
| Corn Flakes, Malt-O-Meal | 1 cup (30 g) | 89 | 296 | SR21 (08497) |
| Corn Flakes, Post Toasties | 1 cup (28 g) | 40 | 143 | SR21 (08338) |
| Corn Pops, Kellogg's | 1 cup (31 g) | 50 | 162 | SR21 (08068) |
| Cracklin' Oat Bran, Kellogg's | ¾ cup (55 g) | 45 | 81 | SR21 (08023) |
| Cranberry Macadamia Nut, Quaker | 1 cup (60 g) | 26 | 43 | SR21 (08400) |
| Cran-Vanilla Crunch, Kellogg's | 1¼ cups (55 g) | 40 | 73 | SR21 (08521) |
| Crispix Cinnamon Crunch, Kellogg's | ¾ cup (30 g) | 40 | 133 | SR21 (08374) |
| Crispix, Kellogg's | 1 cup (29 g) | 40 | 138 | SR21 (08259) |
| Crispy Rice, Malt-O-Meal | 1 cup (33 g) | 44 | 132 | SR21 (09348) |
| Cruncheroos, Kellogg's | 1 cup (30 g) | 49 | 163 | SR21 (08375) |
| Dyno-Bites, cocoa, Malt-O-Meal | ¾ cup (29 g) | 67 | 230 | SR21 (08495) |
| Dyno-Bites, fruity, Malt-O-Meal | ¾ cup (27 g) | 53 | 195 | SR21 (08501) |
| Eggo Crunch, maple flavored, Kellogg's | 1 cup (33 g) | 40 | 121 | SR21 (08524) |
| French Toast Crunch, General Mills | ¾ cup (30 g) | 38 | 125 | SR21 (08086) |
| Froot Loops, ⅓ less sugar, Kellogg's | 1¼ cups (32 g) | 54 | 169 | SR21 (08468) |
| Froot Loops, Kellogg's | 1 cup (30 g) | 38 | 125 | SR21 (08030) |
| Froot Loops, marshmallow blasted, Kellogg's | 1 cup (30 g) | 40 | 133 | SR21 (08376) |
| Froot Loops, marshmallow, rainbow breeze, Kellogg's | 1 cup (30 g) | 40 | 133 | SR21 (08526) |
| Frosted Chex, General Mills | ¾ cup (30 g) | 40 | 133 | SR21 (08514) |
| Frosted Flakes, ⅓ less sugar, Kellogg's | 1 cup (31 g) | 63 | 202 | SR21 (08469) |
| Frosted Flakes, Kellogg's | ¾ cup (31 g) | 40 | 129 | SR21 (08069) |
| Frosted Flakes, Malt-O-Meal | 1 cup (40 g) | 69 | 172 | SR21 (08409) |
| Frosted Krispies, Kellogg's | ¾ cup (30 g) | 40 | 133 | SR21 (08032) |
| Fruit & Fibre (dates, raisins, walnuts), Post | 1 cup (55 g) | 40 | 73 | SR21 (08327) |
| Fruit Harvest, apple cinnamon, Kellogg's | 1 cup (52 g) | 33 | 64 | SR21 (08456) |
| Fruit Harvest, banana berry, Kellogg's | ¾ cup (30 g) | 40 | 133 | SR21 (08470) |

| | SERVING SIZE (g) | VITAMIN $D_3$ (IU/serving) | VITAMIN $D_3$ (IU/100 g) | SOURCE (SR21 CODE NUMBER) |
|---|---|---|---|---|
| Fruit Harvest, peach/strawberry, Kellogg's | ¾ cup (30 g) | 41 | 136 | SR21 (08457) |
| Fruit Harvest, strawberry/blueberry, Kellogg's | ¾ cup (29 g) | 59 | 205 | SR21 (08458) |
| Fruity Brontosaurus Blasts, Quaker | 1 cup (31 g) | 51 | 165 | SR21 (08357) |
| Fruity Pebbles, Post | ¾ cup (27 g) | 40 | 148 | SR21 (08324) |
| Golden Crisp, Post | ¾ cup (27 g) | 40 | 148 | SR21 (08328) |
| Golden Grahams, General Mills | ¾ cup (30 g) | 40 | 133 | SR21 (08035 |
| Golden Puffs, Malt-O-Meal | 1 cup (37 g) | 56 | 151 | SR21 (08478) |
| granola cereal with raisins, lowfat, Kellogg's | ⅗ cup 60 g) | 40 | 67 | SR21 (08284) |
| granola cereal, lowfat, Kellogg's | ½ cup (49 g) | 40 | 82 | SR21 (08189) |
| Grape Nuts Flakes, Post | ¾ cup (29 g) | 40 | 138 | SR21 (08330) |
| Great Grains, crunchy pecan, Post | ⅗ cup (53 g) | 40 | 75 | SR21 (08331) |
| Great Grains, raisin, date, and pecan, Post | ⅗ cup (54 g) | 40 | 74 | SR21 (08332) |
| Harmony, General Mills | 1¼ cups (55 g) | 40 | 73 | SR21 (08398) |
| Healthy Choice, almond crunch with raisins, Kellogg's | 1 cup (55 g) | 76 | 138 | SR21 (08195) |
| Honey Bunches of Oats, almond, Post | ¾ cup (31 g) | 40 | 129 | SR21 (08334) |
| Honey Buzzers, Malt-O-Meal | 1⅓ cups (29 g) | 50 | 171 | SR21 (08476) |
| Honey Crunch 'n Oats, organic, Barbara's Bakery | ⅔ cup (30 g) | 40 | 133 | BARB |
| Honey Crunch Corn Flakes, Kellogg's | ¾ cup (30 g) | 42 | 140 | SR21 (08309) |
| Honey Graham Cereal, Malt-O-Meal | ¾ cup (30 g) | 45 | 149 | SR21 (08481) |
| Honey Nut O's, organic, Barbara's Bakery | ¾ cup (30 g) | 100 | 333 | BARB |
| Honeycomb, Post | 1⅓ cups (29 g) | 40 | 138 | SR21 (08335) |
| Just Right, fruit and nut, Kellogg's | 1 cup (60 g) | 50 | 83 | SR21 (08283) |
| Kaboom, General Mills | 1¼ cups (30 g) | 40 | 133 | SR21 (08278) |
| King Vitaman, Quaker | 1½ cups (31 g) | 41 | 133 | SR21 (08047) |
| Kix, berry berry, General Mills | ¾ cup (30 g) | 40 | 133 | SR21 (08274) |
| Kix, General Mills | 1 ⅓ cups (30 g) | 40 | 133 | SR21 (08048) |
| Lucky Charms, chocolate, General Mills | 1 cup (30 g) | 40 | 133 | SR21 (08513) |
| Lucky Charms, General Mills | 1 cup (30 g) | 44 | 148 | SR21 (08050) |
| Marshmallow Mateys, Malt-O-Meal | 1 cup (30 g) | 53 | 177 | SR21 (08138) |
| Mighty Bites, cinnamon, Kashi | 1 cup (30 g) | 40 | 121 | SR21 (08540) |
| Mighty Bites, honey crunch, Kashi | 1 cup (33 g) | 40 | 121 | SR21 (08541) |
| Mini Swirlz, peanut butter, Kellogg's | 1 cup (30 g) | 40 | 133 | SR21 (08558) |
| MiniSwirlz, fudge ripple, Kellogg's | 1 cup (30 g) | 40 | 133 | SR21 (08536) |
| Mueslix, raisin and almond crunch with dates, Kellogg's | ⅗ cup (55 g) | 16 | 29 | SR21 (08286) |
| Multi-Bran Chex, General Mills | 1 cup (49 g) | 42 | 85 | SR21 (08345) |
| Oat Bran Flakes, Common Sense, Kellogg's | ¾ cup (30 g) | 42 | 140 | SR21 (08258) |
| Oreo O's, Post | ¾ cup; 0.95 oz (27 g) | 40 | 148 | SR21 (08336) |
| Organic Wild Puffs, Barbara's Bakery | 1 cup (27 g) | 100 | 370 | BARB |
| Organic Wild Puffs, caramel, Barbara's Bakery | ¾ cup (30 g) | 100 | 333 | BARB |
| Organic Wild Puffs, cocoa, Barbara's Bakery | 1 cup (30 g) | 100 | 333 | BARB |
| Organic Wild Puffs, fruit punch, Barbara's Bakery | 1 cup (30 g) | 100 | 333 | BARB |
| Peanut Butter Toast Crunch, General Mills | ¾ cup (30 g) | 40 | 133 | SR21 (08517) |
| Product 19, Kellogg's | 1 cup (30 g) | 39 | 131 | SR21 (08058) |
| puffed wheat, sugar-coated | ⅞ cup (28 g) | 41 | 148 | SR21 (08073) |
| Raisin Bran Crunch, Kellogg's | 1 cup (53 g) | 40 | 75 | SR21 (08380) |
| Raisin Bran, Kellogg's | 1 cup (59 g) | 40 | 68 | SR21 (08060) |
| raisin bran, Malt-O-Meal | 1 cup (59 g) | 48 | 82 | SR21 (08484) |
| raisin bran, Para Su Familia, General Mills | 1⅓ cups (55 g) | 40 | 73 | SR21 (08371) |
| raisin bran, Post | 1 cup (59 g) | 40 | 68 | SR21 (08061) |
| Reese's Peanut Butter Puffs, General Mills | ¾ cup (30 g) | 40 | 133 | SR21 (08194) |
| Rice Chex, General Mills | 1¼ cups (31 g) | 46 | 148 | SR21 (08064) |
| Rice Krispies Treats, Kellogg's | ¾ cup (30 g) | 41 | 135 | SR21 (08288) |
| Rice Krispies, berry, Kellogg's | 1 cup (30 g) | 40 | 133 | SR21 (08519) |
| Rice Krispies, Kellogg's | 1¼ cups (33 g) | 41 | 124 | SR21 (08065) |
| Robots, Kellogg's | 1 cup (29 g) | 40 | 138 | SR21 (08527) |
| Scooby-Doo, berry bones, Kellogg's | 1 cup (32 g) | 44 | 138 | SR21 (08466) |
| Smacks, Kellogg's | ¾ cup (27 g) | 40 | 148 | SR21 (08071) |
| Smart Start Healthy Heart, Kellogg's | 1 cup (50 g) | 34 | 67 | SR21 (08528) |
| Smart Start Healthy Heart, maple brown sugar, Kellogg's | 1¼ cups (60 g) | 40 | 67 | SR21 (08529) |
| Smart Start, Kellogg's | 1 cup (50 g) | 40 | 80 | SR21 (08318) |
| Smorz, Kellogg's | 1 cup (30 g) | 40 | 133 | SR21 (08530) |
| Special K, fruit and yogurt, Kellogg's | ¾ cup (32 g) | 13 | 40 | SR21 (08531) |
| SpongeBob SquarePants, Kellogg's | 1 cup (30 g) | 41 | 137 | SR21 (08532) |
| Star Wars, Kellogg's | 1 cup (29 g) | 40 | 138 | SR21 (08533) |
| Tasteeos, Ralston | 1 cup (28 g) | 37 | 133 | SR21 (08074) |
| Team Cheerios, General Mills | ¾ cup (27 g) | 32 | 119 | SR21 (08088) |
| Tiger Power, Kellogg's | 1 cup (30 g) | 36 | 121 | SR21 (08534) |
| Toasted Honey Crunch, Kellogg's | 1¼ cups (58 g) | 40 | 69 | SR21 (08535) |

| | SERVING SIZE (g) | VITAMIN D$_3$ (IU/serving) | VITAMIN D$_3$ (IU/100 g) | SOURCE (SR21 CODE NUMBER) |
|---|---|---|---|---|
| Toasty O's, apple cinnamon, Malt-O-Meal | 1 cup (40 g) | 58 | 145 | SR21 (08408) |
| Toasty O's, honey nut, Malt-O-Meal | 1 cup (30 g) | 54 | 181 | SR21 (08491) |
| Toasty O's, Malt-O-Meal | 1 cup (30 g) | 33 | 111 | SR21 (08350) |
| Tony's Cinnamon Krunchers, Kellogg's | ¾ cup (29 g) | 50 | 172 | SR21 (08460) |
| Tootie Fruities, Malt-O-Meal | 1 cup (32 g) | 47 | 148 | SR21 (08349) |
| Total, corn, General Mills | 1⅓ cups (30 g) | 34 | 114 | SR21 (08246) |
| Total, General Mills | ¾ cup (30 g) | 40 | 133 | SR21 (08077) |
| Total, raisin bran, General Mills | 1 cup (55 g) | 40 | 73 | SR21 (08247) |
| Total, whole grain, General Mills | ¾ cup; 1.1 oz (30 g) | 40 | 133 | GENM |
| Trix, General Mills | 1 cup (30 g) | 38 | 125 | SR21 (08078) |
| wheat and malted barley flakes | ⅞ cup (28 g) | 39 | 138 | SR21 (08039) |
| wheat and malted barley nuggets | ¼ cup (28 g) | 19 | 69 | SR21 (08038) |
| Wheat Bran Flakes, Kellogg's Complete | ⅔ cup (28 g) | 39 | 138 | SR21 (08028) |
| Wheat Chex, General Mills | 1 cup (30 g) | 24 | 80 | SR21 (08082) |
| Wheaties Raisin Bran, General Mills | 1 cup (55 g) | 40 | 73 | SR21 (08026) |
| Wheaties, General Mills | 1 cup (30 g) | 40 | 133 | SR21 (08089) |
| **CHEESE AND CREAMS** | | | | |
| Camembert cheese | 1 oz (28 g) | 3 | 12 | SR21 (01007) |
| cheddar cheese | 1 oz (28 g) | 3 | 12 | SR21 (01009) |
| Edam cheese | 1 oz (28 g) | 10 | 36 | SR21 (01018) |
| parmesan cheese, hard | 1 oz (28 g) | 8 | 28 | SR21 (01033) |
| Swiss cheese | 1 oz (28 g) | 12 | 44 | SR21 (01040) |
| whipped topping, from mix, prepared with whole milk | 1 T (4 g) | 1 | 30 | SR21 (01071) |
| whipping cream, heavy fluid | 1 T (15 g) | 8 | 52 | SR21 (01053) |
| **DESSERTS** | | | | |
| flan (crème caramel/caramel custard), from mix, with 2% milk | ½ cup (133 g) | 48 | 36 | SR21 (19231) |
| flan (crème caramel/caramel custard), from mix, with whole milk | ½ cup (133 g) | 48 | 36 | SR21 (19232) |
| ice cream, chocolate, light | ½ cup (67 g) | 7 | 11 | SR21 (19114) |
| ice cream, vanilla, low/reduced calorie (½ the fat) | ½ cup (66 g) | 17 | 26 | SR21 (19088) |
| ice cream, vanilla, rich (16% fat) | ½ cup (107 g) | 47 | 44 | SR21 (19089) |
| pudding, banana, from instant mix with 2% milk | ½ cup (140 g) | 46 | 33 | SR21 (19121) |
| pudding, banana, from regular mix with 2% milk | ½ cup (140 g) | 49 | 35 | SR21 (19122) |
| pudding, chocolate, from instant mix with lowfat milk | ½ cup (147 g) | 49 | 33 | SR21 (19123) |
| pudding, lemon, from instant mix with 2% milk | ½ cup (147 g) | 49 | 33 | SR21 (19204) |
| pudding, rice, from regular mix with 2% milk | ½ cup (144 g) | 49 | 34 | SR21 (19208) |
| pudding, rice, from regular mix with whole milk | ½ cup (144 g) | 49 | 34 | SR21 (19195) |
| pudding, tapioca, from regular mix with 2% milk | ½ cup (141 g) | 48 | 34 | SR21 (19209) |
| pudding, tapioca, from regular mix with whole milk | ½ cup (141 g) | 48 | 34 | SR21 (19199) |
| pudding, vanilla, from regular mix with 2% milk | ½ cup (140 g) | 49 | 35 | SR21 (19212) |
| rennin dessert, chocolate, from mix with 2% milk | ½ cup (136 g) | 49 | 36 | SR21 (19213) |
| rennin dessert, chocolate, from mix with whole milk | ½ cup (136 g) | 49 | 36 | SR21 (19221) |
| rennin dessert, vanilla, from mix with 2% milk | ½ cup (133 g) | 49 | 37 | SR21 (19214) |
| rennin dessert, vanilla, from mix with whole milk | ½ cup (133 g) | 49 | 37 | SR21 (19223) |
| **EGGS** | | | | |
| egg, fried | 1 large egg (46 g) | 17 | 37 | SR21 (01128) |
| egg, omelet, plain | 1 large egg (61 g) | 18 | 29 | SR21 (01130) |
| egg, poached | 1 large egg (50 g) | 17 | 34 | SR21 (01131) |
| egg, raw | 1 large egg (50 g) | 18 | 35 | SR21 (01123) |
| egg, scrambled with milk | 1 large egg (61 g) | 21 | 34 | SR21 (01132) |
| egg yolk, raw | yolk of 1 large egg (17 g) | 18 | 107 | SR21 (01125) |
| **FAST FOODS** | | | | |
| Burrito Supreme, beef, Taco Bell | 8.7 oz burrito (247 g) | 17 | 7 | SR21 (21265) |
| egg, scrambled, fast food | 2 eggs (94 g) | 64 | 68 | SR21 (21018) |
| English muffin (toasted) with cheese and sausage, fast food | 1 muffin sandwich (115 g) | 6 | 5 | SR21 (21020) |
| English muffin (toasted) with egg, cheese, and Canadian bacon, fast food | 1 muffin sandwich (137 g) | 44 | 32 | SR21 (21021) |
| fish sandwich with tartar sauce and cheese, fast food | 6.5 oz sandwich (183 g) | 37 | 20 | SR21 (21106) |
| hamburger sandwich, regular, double meat, fast food | 6.2 oz sandwich (176 g) | 28 | 16 | SR21 (21110) |
| hamburger sandwich, regular, single meat, fast food | 3.2 oz sandwich (90 g) | 11 | 12 | SR21 (21107) |
| ice milk, soft serve in cone, fast food | 1 cone (103 g) | 8 | 8 | SR21 (21028) |
| shake, chocolate, fast food | 12 fl oz (250 g) | 88 | 35 | SR21 (14346) |
| shake, strawberry, fast food | 12 fl oz (282 g) | 23 | 8 | SR21 (14428) |
| sundae, caramel, fast food | 1 sundae (155 g) | 12 | 8 | SR21 (21032) |
| sundae, hot fudge, fast food | 1 sundae (158 g) | 19 | 12 | SR21 (21033) |

| | SERVING SIZE (g) | VITAMIN D$_3$ (IU/serving) | VITAMIN D$_3$ (IU/100 g) | SOURCE (SR21 CODE NUMBER) |
|---|---|---|---|---|
| sundae, strawberry, fast food | 1 sundae (153 g) | 18 | 12 | SR21 (21034) |
| shake, chocolate, McDonald's | 12 fl oz (250 g) | 88 | 35 | SR21 (14246) |
| **FATS, OILS, AND SPREADS** | | | | |
| butter | 1 T (14 g) | 8 | 56 | SR21 (01001) |
| cod liver oil | 1 T (14 g) | 1400 | 10,000 | SR21 (04589) |
| sardine oil | 1 T (14 g) | 46 | 332 | SR21 (04594) |
| seal (bearded) oil | 1 T (14 g) | 4 | 30 | SR21 (35057) |
| seal (spotted) oil | 1 T (14 g) | 4 | 30 | SR21 (35156) |
| whale (beluga) oil | 1 T (14 g) | 32 | 228 | SR21 (35014) |
| **FISH AND SHELLFISH** | | | | |
| catfish, channel, wild, raw | 3 oz (85 g) | 425 | 500 | SR21 (15010) |
| caviar, black and red, granular | 1 T (16 g) | 37 | 232 | SR21 (15012) |
| clams, raw | 4 large or 9 small (85 g) | 3 | 4 | SR21 (15157) |
| cod, Atlantic, canned, solids and liquid | 3 oz (85 g) | 71 | 84 | SR21 (15017) |
| cod, Atlantic, raw | 3 oz (85 g) | 37 | 44 | SR21 (15015) |
| fish sticks/pieces, frozen, reheated | stick 4″ × 1″ × ½″ (28 g) | 2 | 7 | SR21 (15027) |
| flounder/sole (flatfish), raw | 3 oz (85 g) | 51 | 60 | SR21 (15028) |
| halibut, Greenland, raw | 3 oz (85 g) | 510 | 600 | SR21 (15038) |
| herring, Atlantic, kippered | piece 5″ × 1 ¾″ × ¼″ (40 g) | 48 | 120 | SR21 (15042) |
| herring, Atlantic, pickled | piece 1 ¾″ × ⅞″ × ½″ (15 g) | 102 | 680 | SR21 (15041) |
| herring, Atlantic, raw | 3 oz (85 g) | 1384 | 1,628 | SR21 (15039) |
| mackerel, Atlantic, raw | 3 oz (85 g) | 306 | 360 | SR21 (15046) |
| mackerel, jack, canned, drained | 1 cup (190 g) | 479 | 252 | SR21 (15048) |
| oysters, eastern, wild, raw | 6 medium (84 g) | 269 | 320 | SR21 (15167) |
| salmon, chum, canned with bone, drained | 3 oz (85 g) | 190 | 224 | SR21 (15080) |
| salmon, pink, canned with bone | 3 oz (85 g) | 530 | 624 | SR21 (15084) |
| salmon, sockeye, canned with bone, drained | 3 oz (85 g) | 649 | 763 | SR21 (15087) |
| sardines, Atlantic, canned in soy oil, drained | 2 sardines (24 g) | 65 | 272 | SR21 (15088) |
| sardines, Pacific, canned in tomato sauce, drained | 1 sardine (38 g) | 182 | 480 | SR21 (15089) |
| shrimp, raw | 3 oz (85 g) | 129 | 152 | SR21 (15149) |
| trout, steelhead, boiled, canned | 3 oz (85 g) | 513 | 604 | SR21 (35181) |
| trout, steelhead, dried | 1 oz (28 g) | 176 | 628 | SR21 (35180) |
| tuna, light, canned in oil, drained | 3 oz (85 g) | 201 | 236 | SR21 (15119) |
| **GRAINS, GRAIN-BASED SNACKS, AND OTHER GRAIN PRODUCTS** | | | | |
| breadstick, Italian garlic and herb, from refrigerated dough, Pillsbury | 2 pieces (60 g) | 32 | 53 | GENM |
| cheese puffs/twists (snack food) | 1 oz (28 g) | 0.00 | 1 | SR21 (19008) |
| egg bread (yeast bread) | slice 5″ × 3″ × ½″ (40 g) | 6 | 16 | SR21 (18027) |
| fruit and yogurt bar, apple cinnamon, Barbara's Bakery | 1 bar (42 g) | 40 | 95 | BARB |
| fruit and yogurt bar, blueberry apple, Barbara's Bakery | 1 bar (42 g) | 40 | 95 | BARB |
| fruit and yogurt bar, cherry apple, Barbara's Bakery | 1 bar (42 g) | 40 | 95 | BARB |
| fruit and yogurt bar, strawberry apple, Barbara's Bakery | 1 bar (42 g) | 40 | 95 | BARB |
| Milk 'n Cereal Bar, Cinnamon Toast Crunch, General Mills | 1.6 oz bar (45 g) | 100 | 222 | GENM |
| Milk 'n Cereal Bar, Cocoa Puffs, General Mills | 1.4 oz bar (40 g) | 100 | 250 | GENM |
| Milk 'n Cereal Bar, Honey Nut Cheerios, General Mills | 1.4 oz bar (40 g) | 100 | 250 | GENM |
| Nestum cereal (wheat with honey), prepared, Nestle | 1 cup (240 g) | 101 | 42 | SR21 (43306) |
| **INFANT, JUNIOR, AND TODDLER FOODS** | | | | |
| beef, Beech-Nut Stage 1/Gerber 2nd Foods/Heinz Strained-2 | 2.5 oz jar (71 g) | 11 | 15 | SR21 (03002) |
| beef, Gerber 3rd Foods/Heinz Junior-3 | 2.5 oz jar (71 g) | 11 | 15 | SR21 (03003) |
| broccoli and chicken dinner, Gerber 2nd Foods/Heinz Strained-2 | 4 oz jar (113 g) | 97 | 86 | SR21 (03298) |
| turkey, Beech-Nut Stage 1/Gerber 2nd Foods/Heinz Strained-2 | 2.5 oz jar (71 g) | 24 | 34 | SR21 (03015) |
| turkey, Gerber 3rd Foods | 2.5 oz jar (71 g) | 24 | 34 | SR21 (03016) |
| veal, Beech-Nut Stage 1/Gerber 2nd Foods/Heinz Strained-2 | 2.5 oz jar (71 g) | 18 | 26 | SR21 (03005) |
| vegetables and beef, Beech-Nut Stage 2/Gerber 2nd Foods/Heinz Strained-2 | 4 oz jar (113 g) | 42 | 37 | SR21 (03053) |
| vegetables and beef, Beech-Nut Stage 3/Gerber 3rd Foods/Heinz Junior-3 | 6 oz jar (170 g) | 63 | 37 | SR21 (03054) |
| **MEATS AND LUNCHEON MEATS** | | | | |
| barbeque loaf | 0.8 oz slice (23 g) | 8 | 36 | SR21 (07001) |
| beef kidney, raw | 3 oz (85 g) | 27 | 32 | SR21 (13323) |
| beef liver, raw | 3 oz (85 g) | 14 | 16 | SR21 (13325) |
| bratwurst, pork, cooked | 3 oz (85 g) | 37 | 44 | SR21 (07013) |

| | SERVING SIZE (g) | VITAMIN D₃ (IU/serving) | VITAMIN D₃ (IU/100 g) | SOURCE (SR21 CODE NUMBER) |
|---|---|---|---|---|
| brotwurst, pork and beef with nonfat dry milk | 2.5 oz link (70 g) | 8 | 11 | SR21 (07015) |
| berliner, pork and beef | 0.8 oz slice (23 g) | 3 | 13 | SR21 (07004) |
| bologna, beef and pork | 1 oz slice (28 g) | 9 | 32 | SR21 (07008) |
| bologna, beef, Oscar Mayer | 1 oz slice (28 g) | 9 | 32 | SR21 (07201) |
| bologna, pork | 1 oz slice (28 g) | 16 | 56 | SR21 (07010) |
| bologna, Wisconsin ring, Oscar Mayer | 1 oz slice (28 g) | 11 | 40 | SR21 (07206) |
| braunschweiger (pork liver sausage) | slice 2 ½″ diameter, ¼″ thick (18 g) | 9 | 48 | SR21 (07014) |
| braunschweiger (pork liver sausage), saran tube, Oscar Mayer | 2 oz (56 g) | 18 | 33 | SR21 (07208) |
| braunschweiger (pork liver sausage), sliced, Oscar Mayer | 1 oz (28 g) | 12 | 44 | SR21 (07207) |
| frankfurter, beef | 1.5 oz frankfurter (43 g) | 15 | 36 | SR21 (07022) |
| frankfurter, beef and pork | 1.6 oz frankfurter (45 g) | 16 | 36 | SR21 (07023) |
| frankfurter, beef, Oscar Mayer | 1.6 oz frankfurter (45 g) | 11 | 24 | SR21 (07241) |
| frankfurter, pork and beef with American cheese (cheesefurter) | 1.5 oz frankfurter (43 g) | 5 | 12 | SR21 (07016) |
| frankfurter, turkey, Butcher Boy Meats | 2 oz frankfurter (56 g) | 7 | 12 | SR21 (07269) |
| ham and cheese loaf | 1 oz slice (28 g) | 12 | 44 | SR21 (07032) |
| ham and cheese loaf, Oscar Mayer | 1 oz slice (28 g) | 12 | 42 | SR21 (07211) |
| headcheese, pork, Oscar Mayer | 1 oz slice (28 g) | 13 | 46 | SR21 (07218) |
| honey loaf (pork and beef) | 1 oz slice (28 g) | 11 | 40 | SR21 (07035) |
| honey roll sausage (beef) | 0.8 oz slice (23 g) | 9 | 40 | SR21 (07088) |
| liver cheese, pork, Oscar Mayer | 1.3 oz slice (38 g) | 19 | 49 | SR21 (07220) |
| luxury loaf, pork | 1 oz slice (28 g) | 8 | 28 | SR21 (07060) |
| mother's loaf, pork | 0.7 oz slice (21 g) | 8 | 40 | SR21 (07061) |
| olive loaf, pork | 1 oz slice (28 g) | 12 | 44 | SR21 (07051) |
| peppered loaf, pork and beef | 1 oz slice (28 g) | 9 | 32 | SR21 (07056) |
| pepperoni, pork and beef | slice 1 ⅜″ diameter, ⅛″ thick (6 g) | 1 | 9 | SR21 (07057) |
| pickle and pimento loaf, pork | 1 oz slice (28 g) | 9 | 33 | SR21 (07058) |
| picnic loaf, pork and beef | 1 oz slice (28 g) | 13 | 48 | SR21 (07062) |
| Polish sausage, pork and beef, smoked | 2.7 oz (76 g) | 33 | 44 | SR21 (07916) |
| pork and beef sausage with cheddar cheese, smoked | 2.7 oz (77 g) | 9 | 12 | SR21 (07917) |
| salami, beef | 2 slices (46 g) | 22 | 48 | SR21 (07068) |
| salami, beef and pork, less sodium | 1 oz (28 g) | 9 | 32 | SR21 (07913) |
| salami, beerwurst, pork | 2 slices (46 g) | 17 | 36 | SR21 (07003) |
| salami, beerwurst, pork and beef | 2 slices (46 g) | 17 | 36 | SR21 (07002) |
| salami, dry/hard, beef and pork, Oscar Mayer | 3 slices (27 g) | 17 | 62 | SR21 (07230) |
| salami, turkey | 2 slices (57 g) | 14 | 24 | SR21 (07070) |
| sausage (fresh), pork with beef, pan-fried | patty 3 ⅞″ diameter, ¼″ thick (27 g) | 8 | 28 | SR21 (07065) |
| sausage (fresh), pork, raw | 3 oz (85 g) | 44 | 52 | SR21 (07063) |
| Smokie (smoked sausage), pork and beef | link; 4″ long (68 g) | 30 | 44 | SR21 (07075) |
| summer sausage sticks, pork and beef with cheddar cheese | 1 oz (28 g) | 3 | 12 | SR21 (07918) |
| thuringer (cervelat/summer sausage), beef and pork | 2 slices (46 g) | 20 | 44 | SR21 (07078) |
| thuringer (cervelat/summer sausage), beef, Oscar Mayer | 2 slices (46 g) | 18 | 40 | SR21 (07237) |
| thuringer (cervelat/summer sausage), Oscar Mayer | 2 slices (46 g) | 22 | 47 | SR21 (07238) |

**MILK, MILK BEVERAGES, AND YOGURT**

| | SERVING SIZE (g) | VITAMIN D₃ (IU/serving) | VITAMIN D₃ (IU/100 g) | SOURCE (SR21 CODE NUMBER) |
|---|---|---|---|---|
| chocolate milk, 1% milk | 8 fl oz (250 g) | 100 | 40 | SR21 (01104) |
| chocolate milk, reduced fat | 8 fl oz (250 g) | 100 | 40 | SR21 (01103) |
| chocolate milk, whole milk | 8 fl oz (250 g) | 100 | 40 | SR21 (01102) |
| chocolate mix with aspartame for milk | 0.75 oz packet (21 g) | 39 | 188 | SR21 (14422) |
| cocoa (hot chocolate), homemade with 2% milk | 8 fl oz (250 g) | 100 | 40 | SR21 (01105) |
| evaporated milk, nonfat, canned | 1 fl oz (32 g) | 26 | 80 | SR21 (01097) |
| goat milk | 8 fl oz (244 g) | 29 | 12 | SR21 (01106) |
| human milk | 1 fl oz (31 g) | 1 | 4 | SR21 (01107) |
| milk, lowfat, 1% fat | 8 fl oz (244 g) | 127 | 52 | SR21 (01082) |
| milk, lowfat, 1% fat with nonfat dry milk solids | 8 fl oz (245 g) | 98 | 40 | SR21 (01083) |
| milk, lowfat, 1% fat, protein fortified | 8 fl oz (246 g) | 98 | 40 | SR21 (01084) |
| milk, nonfat | 8 fl oz (245 g) | 100 | 41 | SR21 (01085) |
| milk, nonfat with nonfat dry milk solids | 8 fl oz (245 g) | 98 | 40 | SR21 (01086) |
| milk, nonfat, protein fortified | 8 fl oz (246 g) | 98 | 40 | SR21 (01087) |
| milk powder, nonfat, instant with vitamin A | 1⅓ cups (91 g) | 400 | 440 | SR21 (01092) |
| milk powder, nonfat, regular without vitamin A | ¼ cup (30 g) | 100 | 332 | SR21 (01091) |
| milk powder, whole | ¼ cup (32 g) | 100 | 312 | SR21 (01090) |
| milk, reduced fat, 2% fat | 8 fl oz (244 g) | 105 | 43 | SR21 (01079) |

| | SERVING SIZE (g) | VITAMIN D$_3$ (IU/serving) | VITAMIN D$_3$ (IU/100 g) | SOURCE (SR21 CODE NUMBER) |
|---|---|---|---|---|
| milk, reduced fat, 2% fat with nonfat dry milk solids | 8 fl oz (245 g) | 98 | 40 | SR21 (01080) |
| milk, reduced fat, 2% fat, protein fortified | 8 fl oz (246 g) | 98 | 40 | SR21 (01081) |
| milk, whole, 3.25% fat | 8 fl oz (244 g) | 98 | 40 | SR21 (01077) |
| soymilk, chai, Silk | 8 fl oz (243 g) | 80 | 33 | SR21 (16247) |
| soymilk, chocolate, Silk | 8 fl oz (243 g) | 119 | 49 | SR21 (16237) |
| soymilk, Silk | 8 fl oz (243 g) | 119 | 49 | SR21 (16235) |
| soymilk, vanilla, Silk | 8 fl oz (243 g) | 119 | 49 | SR21 (16236) |
| soy yogurt, Silk | 1 container (227 g) | 120 | 53 | SR21 (16252) |
| yogurt, fruit flavors with Trix, Yoplait | 4 oz container (113 g) | 40 | 35 | GENM |
| yogurt, fruit flavors, Yoplait Go-Gurt | 2.3 oz tube (64 g) | 24 | 38 | GENM |
| yogurt, light, fruit flavors, Yoplait | 6 oz container (170 g) | 80 | 47 | GENM |
| **VEGETABLES AND VEGETABLE DISHES** | | | | |
| corn pudding, homemade | 1 cup (260 g) | 28 | 11 | SR21 (11656) |
| mushrooms, common white, boiled, drained | 1 cup pieces (156 g) | 33 | 21 | SR21 (11261) |
| mushrooms, common white, canned, drained | 1 cup pieces (156 g) | 33 | 21 | SR21 (11264) |
| mushrooms, common white, raw | 1 cup pieces (70 g) | 13 | 18 | SR21 (11260) |
| potato, mashed | 1 cup (240 g) | 14 | 6 | SR21 (11657) |
| potato, mashed, from flakes without milk | 1 cup (210 g) | 25 | 12 | SR21 (11379) |
| potato, mashed, from granules with milk | 1 cup (210 g) | 19 | 9 | SR21 (11383) |
| potato, mashed, homemade with whole milk and butter | 1 cup (210 g) | 13 | 6 | SR21 (11371) |
| spinach soufflé, homemade | 1 cup (136 g) | 34 | 25 | SR21 (11658) |
| **OTHER FOODS** | | | | |
| clam chowder, New England, condensed, canned, prepared with milk | 8 fl oz (248 g) | 55 | 22 | SR21 (06230) |
| orange juice with calcium and vitamin D, refrigerated, Florida's Natural | 8 fl oz (249 g) | 60 | 24 | FLOR |

Sources:
BARB = Barbara's Bakery, Incorporated
FLOR = Florida's Natural
GENM = General Mills, Incorporated
USDA National Nutrient Database for Standard Reference, Release 21, 2008. Available at: http://www.nal.usda.gov/fnic/foodcomp/search/.

# *Vitamins/Vitamin-Like Components—Vitamin K (Phylloquinone)*

| | VITAMIN K (µg/100 g) | SR21 CODE NUMBER[1] | | VITAMIN K (µg/100 g) | SR21 CODE NUMBER[1] |
|---|---|---|---|---|---|
| **DESSERTS** | | | margarine-butter blend (60% corn oil, 40% butter) | 86 | 04585 |
| cookie, chocolate sandwich with crème filling, chocolate-covered | 23 | 18166 | mayonnaise, diet, no cholesterol | 42 | 43599 |
| sugar, homemade with margarine | 26 | 18208 | mayonnaise, fat-free, Kraft | 155 | 04013 |
| cream puff shell, homemade | 24 | 18237 | mayonnaise, imitation, soy | 42 | 04027 |
| pie crust, chocolate wafer, homemade | 25 | 18398 | mayonnaise, light, Kraft Mayo Light | 155 | 04011 |
| pie crust, graham cracker, Ready Crust | 22 | 18942 | mayonnaise, safflower and soy | 25 | 04026 |
| pie crust, graham, homemade | 25 | 18330 | mayonnaise, soy | 42 | 04025 |
| pie crust, vanilla wafer, homemade | 34 | 18401 | Miracle Whip, light, Kraft | 84 | 04012 |
| | | | Miracle Whip, nonfat, Kraft | 84 | 04014 |
| **FAST FOODS** | | | oat oil | 25 | 04588 |
| chicken sandwich, Burger King | 24 | 21259 | olive oil | 60 | 04053 |
| Chicken Whopper sandwich, Burger King | 23 | 21257 | palm kernel oil | 25 | 04513 |
| coleslaw, fast food | 57 | 21127 | rice bran oil | 25 | 04037 |
| pizza, pepperoni, thick crust, 14″ diameter, Pizza Hut | 21 | 21297 | sandwich spread (mayonnaise-based) | 25 | 04030 |
| | | | Smart Balance Buttery Spread | 55 | 04673 |
| taco, soft, steak, Taco Bell | 21 | 21263 | Smart Balance Light Buttery Spread | 47 | 04674 |
| | | | Smart Balance Omega Plus Spread with plant sterols and fish oil | 52 | 04677 |
| **FATS, OILS, AND SPREADS** | | | shortening, hydrogenated coconut oil and palm kernel oil (for confectionery) | 43 | 04551 |
| canola oil | 71 | 04582 | | | |
| cocoa oil (cocoa butter) | 25 | 04501 | shortening, lard and vegetable oil | 21 | 04544 |
| corn and canola oil | 42 | 42289 | shortening, soy (hydrogenated) and cottonseed | 43 | 04547 |
| cottonseed oil | 25 | 04502 | | | |
| margarine, corn and soy, 80% fat, stick | 75 | 04628 | shortening, soy (hydrogenated) and cottonseed (household) | 43 | 04031 |
| margarine, liquid | 106 | 04105 | | | |
| margarine, stick/tub composite, 60% fat | 101 | 04614 | shortening, soy (hydrogenated), 30% linoleic acid | 43 | 04552 |
| margarine, unspecified oils | 93 | 04132 | | | |

| | VITAMIN K (µg/100 g) | SR21 CODE NUMBER[1] |
|---|---|---|
| soy (hydrogenated) and cottonseed oil | 25 | 04543 |
| soy lecithin | 184 | 04531 |
| soy oil (hydrogenated) | 25 | 04034 |
| soy oil, salad/cooking | 184 | 04044 |
| wheat germ oil | 25 | 04038 |
| **FISH AND SHELLFISH** | | |
| abalone, mixed species, raw | 23 | 15155 |
| tuna, light, canned in oil, drained | 44 | 15119 |
| **FRUITS** | | |
| avocado, California, raw | 21 | 09038 |
| avocado, raw | 21 | 09037 |
| blackberries, frozen, unsweetened | 20 | 09048 |
| blackberries, raw | 20 | 09042 |
| blueberries in light syrup, canned | 20 | 09352 |
| chokecherries, pitted, raw | 29 | 35179 |
| kiwifruit, raw | 40 | 09148 |
| pear, dried | 20 | 09259 |
| prune, dried | 59 | 09291 |
| prune, dried, stewed | 26 | 09292 |
| **GRAIN PRODUCTS** | | |
| breadcrumbs, dry, grated, seasoned | 46 | 18376 |
| crackers, cheese with cheese filling | 20 | 18927 |
| crackers, Ritz, Nabisco | 50 | 18621 |
| crackers, round | 42 | 18229 |
| hush puppies, homemade | 24 | 18270 |
| noodles, egg and spinach, enriched, boiled (egg and spinach in the noodle dough) | 101 | 20112 |
| potato chips | 22 | 19411 |
| potato sticks (snack food) | 22 | 19415 |
| sweet potato chips | 24 | 25012 |
| toaster muffin, blueberry, toasted | 21 | 18386 |
| tortilla chips | 21 | 19056 |
| tortilla chips, lowfat, unsalted | 21 | 19833 |
| tortilla chips, nacho cheese, lowfat, made with Olestra | 192 | 19444 |
| soy flour, full-fat | 70 | 16115 |
| soy flour, full-fat, roasted | 71 | 16116 |
| **INFANT AND TODDLER FOODS** | | |
| broccoli and chicken dinner, Gerber 2nd Foods/Heinz Strained-2 | 73 | 03298 |
| crackers, vegetable, infant food | 35 | 03209 |
| garden vegetables, strained infant food | 24 | 03283 |
| green beans, Beech-Nut Stage 1/Gerber 2nd Foods/Heinz Strained-2 | 42 | 03091 |
| green beans, Gerber 1st Foods/Heinz Beginner-1 | 42 | 03091 |
| macaroni, tomato, and beef, Beech-Nut Stage 2/Gerber 2nd Foods/Heinz Strained-2 | 29 | 03044 |
| prunes, strained infant food | 22 | 03139 |
| spinach, creamed, Gerber 2nd Foods | 197 | 03127 |
| **NUTS AND SEEDS** | | |
| cashews, dry-roasted | 35 | 12085 |
| cashews, oil-roasted | 35 | 12086 |
| cashews, raw | 34 | 12087 |
| pine nuts, pignolia, dried | 54 | 12147 |
| pumpkin and squash seed kernels, dried | 51 | 12014 |
| pumpkin and squash seed kernels, roasted | 47 | 12016 |
| soy nuts, dry-roasted | 37 | 16111 |
| soy nuts, roasted | 50 | 16110 |

| | VITAMIN K (µg/100 g) | SR21 CODE NUMBER[1] |
|---|---|---|
| **SALAD DRESSINGS** | | |
| bacon and tomato salad dressing | 69 | 43331 |
| blue cheese salad dressing | 86 | 04539 |
| blue cheese salad dressing, reduced calorie | 91 | 42153 |
| buttermilk salad dressing, lite | 35 | 43215 |
| Caesar salad dressing | 105 | 43015 |
| coleslaw salad dressing | 64 | 43016 |
| coleslaw salad dressing, reduced fat | 39 | 42230 |
| French salad dressing | 121 | 04120 |
| Green Goddess salad dressing | 97 | 43017 |
| Italian salad dressing | 56 | 04114 |
| mayonnaise type salad dressing | 42 | 04018 |
| peppercorn salad dressing | 125 | 42137 |
| ranch salad dressing | 125 | 04639 |
| Russian salad dressing | 54 | 04015 |
| salad dressing, mayonnaise type, fat-free | 25 | 42193 |
| salad dressing, mayonnaise type, low calorie | 25 | 43329 |
| sesame seed salad dressing | 56 | 04016 |
| sweet and sour salad dressing | 40 | 43019 |
| thousand island salad dressing | 69 | 04017 |
| thousand island salad dressing, low/reduced calorie | 28 | 04023 |
| vinegar and oil salad dressing, homemade | 99 | 04135 |
| **SOUPS** | | |
| beef noodle soup, dehydrated | 137 | 06077 |
| beef stroganoff soup, chunky, canned, ready-to-serve | 103 | 06980 |
| split pea soup, canned, Progresso Healthy Classics | 36 | 06192 |
| **HERBS AND SPICES** | | |
| basil, dried | 1714 | 02003 |
| basil, raw | 415 | 02044 |
| black pepper | 164 | 02030 |
| capers, canned | 25 | 02054 |
| chili powder | 106 | 02009 |
| chives, raw | 213 | 11156 |
| cilantro leaves, dried | 1360 | 02012 |
| cinnamon, ground | 31 | 02010 |
| cloves, ground | 142 | 02011 |
| curry powder | 100 | 02015 |
| marjoram, dried | 622 | 02023 |
| oregano, dried, ground | 622 | 02027 |
| paprika | 80 | 02028 |
| parsley, dried | 1359 | 02029 |
| poultry seasoning | 805 | 02034 |
| pumpkin pie spice | 28 | 02035 |
| red/cayenne pepper | 80 | 02031 |
| sage, ground | 1714 | 02038 |
| thyme, ground | 1714 | 02042 |
| **VEGETABLES** | | |
| **FLOWER, STEM, AND STALK VEGETABLES** | | |
| asparagus, boiled | 51 | 11012 |
| asparagus, canned | 41 | 11015 |
| asparagus, frozen, boiled | 80 | 11019 |
| asparagus, raw | 42 | 11011 |
| broccoflower, raw | 20 | 11965 |
| broccoli, boiled | 141 | 11091 |
| broccoli, chopped, frozen, boiled | 88 | 11093 |
| broccoli, frozen | 81 | 11092 |
| broccoli, raw | 102 | 11090 |
| broccoli, spears, frozen, boiled | 88 | 11095 |
| celery, boiled | 38 | 11144 |
| celery, raw | 29 | 11143 |
| Chinese broccoli (Chinese kale), boiled | 85 | 11969 |

| | VITAMIN K (µg/100 g) | SR21 CODE NUMBER[1] | | VITAMIN K (µg/100 g) | SR21 CODE NUMBER[1] |
|---|---|---|---|---|---|
| leek, boiled | 25 | 11247 | mustard greens, raw | 497 | 11270 |
| leek, raw | 47 | 11246 | parsley, raw | 1640 | 11297 |
| rhubarb, cooked, sweetened, frozen | 21 | 09310 | pumpkin leaves, boiled | 108 | 11419 |
| rhubarb, frozen | 29 | 09309 | radicchio, raw | 255 | 11952 |
| rhubarb, raw | 29 | 09307 | romaine (cos lettuce), raw | 102 | 11251 |
| scallions (green/spring onions), raw | 207 | 11291 | spinach soufflé, homemade | 126 | 11658 |
| | | | spinach, boiled | 494 | 11458 |
| **FRUIT (SEED-CONTAINING) VEGETABLES** | | | spinach, canned | 462 | 11461 |
| | | | spinach, frozen | 372 | 11463 |
| chili pepper, red, hot, sun-dried | 108 | 11962 | spinach, frozen, boiled | 541 | 11464 |
| green snap beans, canned | 39 | 11056 | spinach, raw | 483 | 11457 |
| green snap beans, frozen | 45 | 11060 | sweet potato leaves, steamed | 109 | 11506 |
| okra, boiled | 40 | 11279 | Swiss chard, boiled | 327 | 11148 |
| okra, frozen, cooked | 48 | 11281 | Swiss chard, raw | 830 | 11147 |
| okra, raw | 53 | 11278 | turnip greens and root, frozen, boiled | 415 | 11577 |
| snap beans, green, frozen, microwaved | 58 | 11062 | turnip greens, boiled | 368 | 11569 |
| snow peas, boiled | 25 | 11301 | turnip greens, frozen, boiled | 519 | 11575 |
| snow peas, frozen, boiled | 30 | 11303 | turnip greens, raw | 251 | 11568 |
| snow peas, raw | 25 | 11300 | watercress, raw | 250 | 11591 |
| tomato, red, sun-dried | 43 | 11955 | | | |
| | | | **LEGUMES (BEANS AND PEAS)** | | |
| **LEAFY VEGETABLES** | | | cowpeas (blackeye peas), immature, boiled | 27 | 11192 |
| amaranth leaves, raw | 1140 | 11003 | cowpeas (blackeye peas), immature, frozen, boiled | 37 | 11196 |
| arugula, raw | 109 | 11959 | | | |
| balsam pear (bitter melon/bitter gourd) leafy tips, boiled | 163 | 11023 | green peas, boiled | 26 | 11305 |
| | | | green peas, canned | 37 | 11308 |
| beet greens, boiled | 484 | 11087 | green peas, frozen | 28 | 11312 |
| beet greens, raw | 400 | 11086 | green peas, frozen, boiled | 24 | 11313 |
| broccoli raab (rapini), boiled | 256 | 11097 | green peas, raw | 25 | 11304 |
| broccoli raab (rapini), raw | 224 | 11096 | pigeon peas, immature, boiled | 20 | 11345 |
| Brussels sprouts, boiled | 140 | 11099 | soybeans, green/immature (edamame), frozen, heated | 27 | 11212 |
| Brussels sprouts, frozen, boiled | 193 | 11101 | | | |
| Brussels sprouts, raw | 177 | 11098 | soybeans, mature, dry | 47 | 16108 |
| cabbage, green/white, boiled | 109 | 11110 | | | |
| cabbage, green/white, raw | 76 | 11109 | **SPROUT AND SHOOT VEGETABLES** | | |
| cabbage, red/purple, boiled | 48 | 11113 | alfalfa sprouts, raw | 30 | 11001 |
| cabbage, red/purple, raw | 38 | 11112 | mung bean sprouts, boiled | 23 | 11044 |
| cabbage, savoy, raw | 69 | 11114 | mung bean sprouts, raw | 33 | 11043 |
| chicory greens, raw | 298 | 11152 | pokeberry shoots (poke), boiled | 108 | 11351 |
| Chinese cabbage, pak choi, boiled | 34 | 11117 | soybean sprouts, steamed | 71 | 11453 |
| Chinese cabbage, pak choi, raw | 45 | 11116 | | | |
| Chinese cabbage, pe-tsai, raw | 43 | 11119 | **TUBER AND ROOT VEGETABLES** | | |
| cilantro (coriander), raw | 310 | 11165 | celeriac (celery root), raw | 41 | 11141 |
| collards, boiled | 440 | 11162 | parsnip, raw | 22 | 11298 |
| collards, frozen, boiled | 623 | 11164 | | | |
| collards, raw | 511 | 11161 | **OTHER VEGETABLES** | | |
| dandelion greens, boiled | 551 | 11208 | mixed vegetables, frozen, boiled | 23 | 11584 |
| dandelion greens, raw | 778 | 11207 | mixed vegetables, frozen | 23 | 11584 |
| endive, raw | 231 | 11213 | seaweed, agar, dried | 24 | 11663 |
| garden cress, boiled | 383 | 11204 | seaweed, kelp (kombu/tangle), raw | 66 | 11445 |
| garden cress, raw | 542 | 11203 | seaweed, spirulina, dried | 25 | 11667 |
| garland chrysanthemum, boiled | 143 | 11158 | | | |
| garland chrysanthemum, raw | 350 | 11157 | **OTHER FOODS** | | |
| grape leaves, raw | 109 | 11974 | bockwurst (pork, veal, milk, eggs), raw | 70 | 07006 |
| horseradish tree leafy tips, chopped, boiled | 108 | 11223 | Instant Breakfast mix with low calorie sweetener, chocolate | 120 | 43260 |
| jute (potherb), boiled | 108 | 11232 | | | |
| kale, boiled | 817 | 11234 | Instant Breakfast mix, chocolate | 90 | 43205 |
| kale, frozen, boiled | 882 | 11236 | miso (soybean paste) | 29 | 16112 |
| kale, raw | 817 | 11233 | natto (boiled, fermented soybeans) | 23 | 16113 |
| lambsquarters, boiled | 494 | 11245 | pickle (cucumber), dill | 39 | 11937 |
| lettuce, butterhead, raw | 102 | 11250 | pickle (cucumber), sour | 47 | 11941 |
| lettuce, iceberg, raw | 24 | 11252 | pickle (cucumber), sweet gherkin | 47 | 11940 |
| lettuce, looseleaf (leaf), raw | 174 | 11253 | pickle relish, sweet | 84 | 11945 |
| mustard greens, boiled | 299 | 11271 | pickled cabbage, Japanese style | 126 | 43143 |
| mustard greens, frozen, boiled | 335 | 11273 | | | |

[1]Code numbers from the USDA National Nutrient Database for Standard Reference, Release 21, 2008.

Source:
USDA. National Nutrient Database for Standard Reference, Release 21, 2008. Available at: http://www.nal.usda.gov/fnic/foodcomp/search/.

# Scientific Names for Plants and Animals Used as Foods or Food Ingredients[1]

| PLANT FOOD | SCIENTIFIC NAME |
|---|---|
| acerola | *Malpighia punicifolia* |
| acorn squash | *Cucurbita maxima* |
| acorns | *Quercus* spp. |
| adzuki beans | *Phaseolus angularis* |
| agar (seaweed) | *Gelidum corneum; Eucheuma* spp. |
| alfalfa sprouts | *Medicago sativa* |
| allspice | *Pimenta officinalis; P. dioica* |
| almonds | *Prunus amygdalus; P. dulcis* |
| amaranth | *Amaranthus* spp. |
| anise seeds | *Pimpinella anisum* |
| apple | *Malus communis; M. domestica; M. sylvestris; M. pumila* |
| apricot | *Prunus armeniaca* |
| arrowroot | *Maranta arundinacea* |
| artichoke (globe/French artichoke) | *Cynara scolymus* |
| arugula (garden rocket) | *Eruca sativa* |
| asparagus | *Asparagus officinalis* |
| avocado | *Persea Americana* |
| babassu oil | *Orbignya barbosiana* |
| balsam pear (bitter melon/ bitter gourd) | *Momordica charantia* |
| bamboo shoots | *Phyllostachys edulis; P.* spp. |
| banana | *Musa nana; M. sapientum; M. paradisiaca* |
| barley | *Hordeum vulgare; H. distichon* |
| basil | *Ocimum basilicum* |
| bay leaf | *Laurus nobilis* |
| beechnuts | *Fagus* spp. |
| beet (beetroot) | *Beta vulgaris* var *Crassa* |
| blackberries | *Rubus fruticosus; R.* spp. |
| blueberries | *Vaccinium* spp. |
| borage | *Borago officinalis* |
| boysenberries | *Rubus ursinus* var *loganobaccus* |
| Brazil nuts | *Bertholletia excelsa* |
| breadfruit | *Artocarpus altilis; A. incisus; A. communis* |
| broadbeans (fava beans) | *Vicia faba* |
| broccoli | *Brassica oleracea* var *italica* |
| Brussels sprouts | *Brassica oleracea* var *gemmifera* |
| buckwheat | *Fagopyrum esculentum* |
| burdock root | *Arctium lappa* |
| butterbur (fuki) | *Petasites japonicus* |
| butternut squash | *Cucurbita moschata* |
| butternuts | *Juglans cinerea* |
| cabbage, green | *Brassica oleracea* var *capitata* |
| cabbage, red | *Brassica oleracea* var *capitata f. rubra* |
| cabbage, savoy | *Brassica oleracea* var *sabuda* |
| calabash gourd | *Lagenaria siceraria* |
| canola (rapeseed) oil | *Brassica napus; B.* spp. |
| cantaloupe | *Cucumis melo* var *cantalupensis* |
| capers | *Capparis spinosa* |
| carambola (star fruit/starfruit) | *Averrhoa carambola* |
| caraway seeds | *Carum carvi* |
| cardamon (cardamom) | *Elettaria cardamonum* |
| cardoon | *Cynara cardunculus* |
| carissa (natal plum) | *Carissa macrocarpa* |
| carob (locust bean) | *Ceratonia siliqua* |
| carrot | *Daucus carota* |
| casaba melon | *Cucumis melo* |
| cashews | *Anacardium occidentale* |
| cassava (manioc) | *Manihot utilissima; M. esculenta* |
| cauliflower | *Brassica oleraces* var *botrytis* |

| PLANT FOOD | SCIENTIFIC NAME |
|---|---|
| celeriac (celery root) | *Apium graveolens* var *rapaceum* |
| celery | *Apium graveolens* |
| celtuce | *Lactuca sativa* |
| chamomile (camomile) tea leaves | *Matricaria recutita; M. chamomilla* |
| chayote squash (mirliton) | *Sechium edule* |
| cherimoya | *Annona cherimola* |
| cherries, sour | *Prunus cerasus* |
| cherries, sweet | *Prunus avium* |
| chervil | *Anthriscus cerefolium* |
| chestnuts, Chinese | *Castanea mollissima* |
| chestnuts, European | *Castanea sativa* |
| chestnuts, Japanese | *Castanea crenata* |
| chickpeas (garbanzo beans) | *Cicer arietinum* |
| chicory (curly endive; radicchio) | *Cichorium endivia* |
| chicory, whitloof (Belgian endive; whitloof) | *Cichorium intybus* var *foliosum* |
| Chinese cabbage (pak choi, pe-tsai) | *Brassica chinensis; B. rapa* var *chinensis* |
| chili pepper (ancho, banana, pasilla, Hungarian, jalapeno, pimento, Serrano) | *Capsicum frutescens; C. annuum* |
| chili pepper, hot (red, green, yellow) | *Capsicum frutescens* |
| chives | *Allium schoenoprasum* |
| cilantro | *Coriandrum sativum* |
| cinnamon | *Cinnamomum zeylanicum; C. verum; C. aromaticum; C. cassia* |
| cloves | *Eugenia caryophyllata; E. aromatica; Syzygium aromaticum* |
| cocoa (cacao) | *Theobroma cacao* |
| coconut | *Cocos nucifera* |
| coffee | *Coffea Arabica* |
| collards | *Brassica oleracea* var *viridis; B. oleracea* var *acephala* |
| coriander seeds | *Coriandrum sativum* |
| corn, yellow/white | *Zea mays* |
| cornsalad (lamb's lettuce) | *Valerianella olitoria; V. locusta* var *olitoria* |
| cottonseed flour, kernels, meal, oil | *Gossypium* spp. |
| cowpeas (blackeye/ blackeyed peas) | *Vigna unguiculata* |
| cowpeas, catjang | *Vigna unguiculata cylindrical* |
| crabapples | *Malus* spp. |
| cranberries | *Vaccinium oxyoccus; V. macrocarpon* |
| cranberry (Roman) beans | *Phaseolus vulgaris* |
| crookneck/straightneck squash | *Cucurbita maxima* |
| cucumber | *Cucumis sativus* |
| cumin | *Cuminum syminum* |
| currants, black or red | *Ribes nigrum* |
| currants, white | *Ribes rubrum* var *leucocarpum* |
| currants, zante (dried grapes) | *Vitis vinifera* |
| custard apple (bullock's heart) | *Annona reticulate* |
| dandelion greens | *Taraxacum officinale* |
| date | *Phoenix dactylifera* |
| dill seeds/dill weed | *Anethum graveolens* |
| dishcloth (towel) gourd | *Luffa aegyptiaca* |
| durian | *Durio zibethinus* |
| eggplant (aubergine) | *Solanum melongena ovigerum* |
| elderberries | *Sambucus* spp. |

| PLANT FOOD | SCIENTIFIC NAME | PLANT FOOD | SCIENTIFIC NAME |
|---|---|---|---|
| epazote | *Chenopodium ambrosioides* | marjoram | *Orignum majorana;* |
| eppaw | *Perideridia oregana* | | *Majorana hortensis* |
| feijoa | *Feijoa sellowiana* | millet | *Panicum milliaceum* |
| fennel bulb, leaves, seeds | *Foeniculum vulgare* | mothbeans | *Vigna aconitifolia* |
| fenugreek seeds | *Trigonella foenum-graecum* | mountain yam, Hawaiian | *Dioscorea pentaphylla* |
| fiddlehead ferns | *Matteuccia struthiopteris* | mulberries | *Morus nigra* |
| fig | *Ficus carica* | mung beans, mung bean sprouts | *Phaseolus aureau; Vigna radiata* |
| filberts (hazelnuts) | *Corylus avellana; C. maxima* | mungo beans | *Vigna mungo* |
| flaxseeds | *Linum usitatissimum* | mushrooms, common white | *Agaricus bisporus* |
| French (haricot) beans | *Phaseolus vulgaris* | (champignon) | |
| garden cress | *Lepidium sativum* | mushrooms, crimini, Italian, brown | *Agaricus bisporus* |
| garland chrysanthemum | *Chrysanthemum coronarium; C. spatiosum* | mushrooms, enoki | *Flammulina veluptites;* |
| garlic | *Allium sativum* | | *Collybia veluptpes* |
| ginger root | *Zingiber officinale* | mushrooms, oyster | *Pleurotus ostratus* |
| ginko nuts | *Ginko biloba* | mushrooms, portabella | *Agaricus bisporus* |
| gooseberries | *Ribes grossularia; Ribes* spp. | mushrooms, shiitake | *Lentinus edodes* |
| grapefruit | *Citrus paradisi* | mushrooms, straw | *Volvariella volvacea* |
| grapes | *Vitis vinifers; V.* spp. | mustard greens | *Brassica nigra; B. juncea;* |
| great northern beans | *Phaseolus vulgaris* | | *Sinapis alba* |
| green snap beans | *Phaseolus vulgaris* | mustard oil, powder, seeds | *Brassica arvensis* |
| groundcherries | *Physalis* spp. | mustard spinach (tendergreen) | *Brassica rapa* var *perviridis* |
| guava | *Psidium guajava* | navy beans and sprouts | *Phaseolus vulgaris* |
| guava, strawberry | *Psidium cattleianum* | nectarine | *Prunus persica* var *nectarina* |
| hearts of palm (palm heart) | *Sabal palmetto* | New Zealand spinach | *Tetragonia tetragonioides* |
| hickory nuts | *Carya ovata; C.* spp. | nopales (prickly pear) (vegetable) | *Nopalea cochrenillifera* |
| hominy | *Zea mays* | nutmeg | *Myristica fragrans; M. officinalis;* |
| honeydew melon | *Cucumis melo* | | *M. moschata; M. aromatica;* |
| horseradish root | *Armorica rusticana* | | *M. amboinensis* |
| horseradish tree pods | *Moringa oleifera* | oats | *Avena sativa* |
| hubbard squash | *Cucurbita maxima* | oheloberries | *Vaccinium reticulatum* |
| hyacinth beans | *Dolichos purpureus; D. lablab* | okra (lady's finger) | *Hibiscus esculentus* |
| Irish moss (seaweed) | *Gigartina mamillosa; Chondrus crispus* | olives | *Olea europea* |
| jackfruit | *Artocarpur heterophyllus* | onion | *Allium cepa* |
| java plum | *Syzygium cumini* | onion, Welsh | *Allium fistulosum* |
| Jerusalem artichoke (sunchoke) | *Helianthus tuberosus* | orange, navel/Valencia | *Citrus sinensis* |
| jicama (yambean) | *Pachyrhizus* spp. | oregano | *Origanum vulgare* |
| jute | *Corchorus olitorius* | palm oil | *Elacis guineensis* |
| kale, curly | *Brassica oleracea* var *acephala* | papaya (papaw) | *Carica papaya* |
| kale, Scotch | *Brassica napus* var *pabularia* | paprika | *Capsicum anuum; C. tetragonna* |
| kelp (kombu/tangle) (seaweed) | *Laminaria* spp. | parsley | *Petroselinum crispum; P. hortnse;* |
| kidney beans, red | *Phaseolus vulgaris* | | *P. sativum* |
| kiwifruit | *Actinidia chinensis* | parsnip | *Pastinace sativa; Peucadenum sativa* |
| kohlrabi | *Brassica oleracea* var *gongylodes* | passion fruit, purple | *Passiflora edulis* |
| kumquat | *Fortunella* spp. | (purple granadilla) | |
| lambsquarters | *Chenopodium album* | passion fruit, yellow | *Passiflora laurifolis; P. laurifolia* |
| laver (nori) (seaweed) | *Porphyra perforate* | peach | *Prunus persica* |
| leek | *Allium ampeloprasum* var *porrum* | peanuts | *Arachis hypogaea* |
| lemon | *Citrus limon* | pear | *Pyrus communis* |
| lemon grass (citronella) | *Cymbopogon citratus* | pear, Asian | *Pyrus ussuriensis; P. pyrifolia* |
| lentils | *Lens esculenta; L. culinaris* | peas, green/split | *Pisum sativum* |
| lettuce (butterhead, cos, | *Lactuca sativa* | pecans | *Carya pecan; C. illinopensis* |
| crisphead, looseleaf) | | pepeao | *Auricularia polytricha* |
| lichee (lichi/litchee) | *Litchi chinensis* | pepper, black or white (spice) | *Piper nigrum* |
| lima beans | *Phaseolus lunatus* | pepper, red (cayenne/chili) (spice) | *Capicum frutescens* |
| lime | *Citrus aurantifolia* | peppermint | *Mentha piperita* |
| linseeds, linseed oil | *Linum usitatissium* | persimmon | *Diospyros virginiana* |
| loganberries | *Rubus ursinus* var. *loganbaccus* | persimmon, Japanese | *Diopyros kaki* |
| longan | *Dimocarpus longan; Euphoria longan* | pigeon peas | *Cajanus cajan* |
| loquat | *Eriobotrya japonica* | pilinuts (pilinuts-canarytree) | *Canarium ovatum* |
| lotus root | *Nelumbo nucifera* | pine nuts, pignolia | *Pinus pinea* |
| lupins | *Lupinus albus* | pine nuts, pinyon | *Pinus edulis* |
| macadamia nuts | *Macadamia integrifolia;* | pineapple | *Ananas sativus; A. comosus* |
| | *M. tetraphylla* | pink beans | *Phaseolus vulgaris* |
| malabar spinach | *Basella rubra; B. alba* | pinto beans | *Phaseolus vulgaris* |
| mammy apple (mamey) | *Mammea Americana* | pistachio nuts | *Pistacia vera* |
| mandarin orange | *Citrus nobilis deliciosa* | pitanga (Surinam cherry) | *Eugenia unifolora* |
| mango | *Mangifera indica* | plantain | *Musa paradisiaca* |
| mangosteen | *Garcinia mangostana* | plum | *Prunus domestica; P.* spp. |
| maple sugar, maple syrup | *Acer saccharum* | pokeberry sprouts (poke) | *Phytolacca americana* |

| PLANT FOOD | SCIENTIFIC NAME |
|---|---|
| pomegranate | *Punica granatum* |
| popcorn | *Zea mays* var *everta* |
| poppyseeds | *Papaver rhoeas; P. somniferum* |
| potato | *Solanum tuberosum* |
| prickly pear (cactus fig) (fruit) | *Opuntia* spp. |
| prune (dried plum) | *Prunus domestica* |
| pummelo | *Citrus grandis* |
| pumpkin | *Cucurbita pepo; C.* spp. |
| pumpkin seeds | *Cucurbita maxima* |
| purslane | *Portulaca oleracea* |
| quince | *Cydonia oblonga* var *piriformis* |
| quinola | *Chenopodium quinoa* |
| radish, red | *Raphanus sativus* var *radicula* |
| radish, Oriental (daikon) | *Raphanus sativus* var *longipinratus* |
| radish, white icicle | *Raphanus sativus* var *radicula* |
| raisins (dried grapes) | *Vitis vinifera* |
| rambutan | *Nephelium lappaceum* |
| raspberries | *Rubus idaeus; R.* spp. |
| rhubarb | *Rheum rhaponticum; R. rhabarbaum* |
| rice | *Oryza sativa* |
| rose apple | *Syzglum jambos* |
| roselle | *Hibiscus sabdariffa* |
| rosemary | *Rosmarinus officinalis* |
| rowal | *Sorbus aucuparia* |
| rutabaga (Swede) | *Brassica napus* var *napobrassica* |
| rye | *Secale cereale* |
| safflower oil, safflower seeds | *Carthamus tinctorius* |
| saffron | *Crocus sativus* |
| sage | *Salvia officinalis; S. sclarea; S. pratensis* |
| salsify | *Tragopogon porrifolius* |
| sapodilla | *Manikara zapota* |
| sapote | *Pouteria sapota* |
| savory, summer (herb) | *Satureja hortnesis* |
| savory, winter (herb) | *Satureja montana* |
| scallions (green/spring onions) | *Allium cepa* |
| scallop squash | *Cucurbita maxima* |
| semolina | *Triticum vulgare* |
| sesame seeds | *Sesamum indicum; S. orientale* |
| sesbania flower | *Sesbania* spp. |
| shallots | *Allium ascalonicum* |
| sheanut oil | *Butyrospermum paradoxum* |
| snow peas (edible-podded peas) | *Pisum sativum* |
| sorghum | *Sorghum vulgare* var *durra;* |
| | *S. bicolor; S.* spp. |
| sorrel (dock) | *Rumex acetosa* |
| soursop | *Annona muricata* |
| soybeans, soybean sprouts | *Glygine max* |
| sugar (from sugar beets) | *Beta vulgaris* var *Crassa* |
| sugar (from sugar cane) | *Saccharum officinarum* |
| spaghetti squash | *Cucurbita pepo* |
| spearmint | *Mentha spicata* |
| spinach | *Spinacia oleracea* |
| spirulina (seaweed) | *Spirulina* spp. |
| squash, summer | *Cucurbita pepo* |
| squash, winter | *Cucurbita maxima* |
| strawberries | *Fragaria ananassa; F. virginiana* |
| sugar apple | *Annona squamosa* |
| sunflower flour, oil, seeds | *Helianthus annuus* |
| swamp cabbage | *Ipomea aquatic* |
| sweet (bell) pepper (green, red, yellow) | *Capsicum annuum* |
| sweet potato | *Ipomoea batatas* |
| Swiss chard | *Beta vulgaris* var *cicla* |
| tamarind | *Tamarindus indica* |
| tangerine | *Citrus reticulata* |
| taro (dasheen) | *Colocasia antiquorum; C. esculenta* |
| taro, Tahitian | *Alocasia macrorrhiza* |
| tarragon | *Artemisia dracunculus;* |
| | *Tagetes minuta* |

| PLANT FOOD | SCIENTIFIC NAME |
|---|---|
| tea | *Camillia sinensis* |
| thyme | *Thymus vulgaris* |
| tomatillo | *Physalis ixocarpa* |
| tomato | *Lycopersicom esculentun* |
| tree fern | *Cyathea medullaris; C.* spp. |
| triticale flour | *Triticosecale rimpauli* |
| turmeric | *Cucuma domestica; C. longa* |
| turnip | *Brassica rapa* var *rapifera* |
| vanilla | *Vanila fragrans; V. planifolia* |
| vinepinach | *Basella alba* |
| wakame (seaweed) | *Undaria pinnatifida; U.* spp. |
| walnuts | *Juglans regina; J. nigra* |
| wasabi root | *Wasabia japonica* |
| water chestnuts, Chinese (matai) | *Eleocharis tuberose; E. dulcis; Scirpus tuberosa* |
| watercress | *Nasturthium officinale; N. aquaticum* |
| watermelon | *Citrullus lanatus; Cucumis citrullus* |
| waxgourd | *Benincasa hispida* |
| wheat | *Triticum vulgare; T. aestivum* |
| white beans | *Phaseolus vulgaris* |
| wild rice | *Zizania aquatica; Z.* spp. |
| winged beans, winged bean leaves | *Psophocarpus tetragonolobus* |
| yam | *Dioscorea batatas; D. esculenta; A. alata; D.* spp. |
| yardlong bean | *Vigna unguiculata sesquipedalis* |
| yautia | *Xanthosoma* spp. |
| yellow snap beans (wax beans) | *Phaseolus vulgaris* |
| Yuzu (Asian citrus fruit) | *Citrus ichangensis; C. reticulate* var. austera |
| zucchini | *Cucuribita pepo* |

| ANIMAL FOOD | SCIENTIFIC NAME |
|---|---|
| abalone | *Haliotis rufescens* |
| anchovies | *Engraulis encrasicholus; E. mordax; E.* spp. |
| antelope | Subfamily *Hippotraginae* |
| bass, freshwater | *Percichthyidae* spp.; *Centrachidae* spp. |
| bass, striped | *Morone chrysops; M. saxatilis* |
| bear | *Ursus* spp. |
| beaver | *Castor Canadensis* |
| beefalo | Hybrid of *Bison bison* and *Bos taurus* |
| bison | *Bison americanus* |
| bluefish | *Pomatomus saltatrix* |
| boar | *Sus scofa* |
| buffalo, Indian/wild | *Bubalus bubalis* |
| burbot | *Lota lota* |
| butterfish | *Peprilus triacanthus* |
| chicken/eggs | *Gallus domesticus* |
| caribou | *Rangifer caribou* |
| carp | *Cypinus carpio* |
| catfish, channel/farmed/wild | *Ictalurus punctatus* |
| cisco | *Coregonus artedii* |
| clams, mixed species | *Lamellibranchia* spp. |
| cod, Atlantic | *Gadus morhua* |
| cod, Pacific | *Gadux macrocephalus* |
| cow (beef, veal, milk) | *Bos Taurus* |
| crab, Alaska king | *Paralithodes camtschatica* |
| crab, blue | *Callinectes sapidus* |
| crab, Dungeness | *Cancer magister* |
| crab, queen | *Chionoecles opilio* |
| crayfish | *Procambarus clarkii; Astacus* spp.; *Orconectes* spp.; *Procambarus* spp. |
| croaker, Atlantic | *Micropogonias undulates* |
| cusk | *Brosme brosme* |
| cuttlefish | *Sepia* spp. |
| deer | *Odocoileus* spp. |

| ANIMAL FOOD | SCIENTIFIC NAME | ANIMAL FOOD | SCIENTIFIC NAME |
|---|---|---|---|
| drum, freshwater | *Aplodinotus grunniens* | rockfish, Pacific | *Scorpaenidae* family |
| duck, domesticated | *Anas platyhynchos* | sablefish | *Anoplopoma fimbria* |
| eel | *Anguilla* spp.; *A. rostrata* | salmon, Atlantic | *Salmo salar* |
| elk | *Cercus alces* | salmon, chinook | *Oncorhyunchus tshawytscha* |
| emu | *Dromalus novachollandiae* | salmon, chum | *Oncorhyunchus keta* |
| flounder/sole | *Pleuronectes* spp. | salmon, coho | *Oncorhynchus kisutch* |
| goat | *Capra* spp. | salmon, pink | *Oncorhyunchus gorbuscha* |
| goose | *Anser anser* | salmon, sockeye | *Oncorhynchus nerka* |
| grouper, mixed species | *Epinephelus* spp. | sardine, Atlantic | *Clupea harengus harengus* |
| guinea hen | *Numida meleagris* | sardine, Pacific | *Sardinops* spp. |
| haddock | *Melanogrammus aeglefinus* | scallops, bay | *Argopecten irradians* |
| halibut, Atlantic | *Hippoglossus hippoglossus* | scallops, calico | *Argopecten gibbus* |
| halibut, Greenland | *Reinhardtius hippoglossoides* | scallops, mixed species | *Pectinidae* spp. |
| halibut, Pacific | *Hippoglossus stenolepis* | scallops, queen | *Chamys opercularis* |
| herring, Atlantic | *Clupea harengus harengus* | scallops, sea | *Placopecten magellanicus* |
| herring, Pacific | *Clupea harengus pallasi* | scup | *Stenotomus chrysops* |
| horse | *Equus caballus* | sea bass, mixed species | *Centropristes lateolabrax japonicus* |
| lamb/sheep | *Ovis aries* | seatrout | *Cynoscion* spp. |
| ling | *Molva molva* | shad, American | *Alosa sapidissima* |
| lingcod | *Ophiodon elongates* | shark, mako | *Isurus oxyrinchus* |
| lobster, northern | *Homarus americanus* | shark, mixed species | *Squaliformes* |
| mackerel, Atlantic | *Scomber scombrus* | sheefish | *Stednous leucichthys nelma* |
| mackerel, jack | *Trachusus synmetricus* | sheep/lamb | *Ovis aries* |
| mackerel, king | *Scombermorus cavalla* | sheepshead | *Archosargus probatocephalus* |
| mackerel, Pacific | *Scomber japonicus* | shrimp, black tiger | *Penacus monodon* |
| mackerel, Spanish | *Scombermorus maculates* | shrimp, gulf, brown | *Penacus aztecus* |
| menhaden oil | *Brevortia* spp. | shrimp, gulf, pink | *Penacus duoarum* |
| milkfish | *Chanos chanos* | shrimp, gulf, white | *Penaeus setiferus* |
| monkfish | *Lophius americanus; L. piscatorius* | shrimp, mixed species | *Penaeidae; Pandlidae* |
| moose | *Alces Americana* | shrimp, Pacific white | *Penaeus vannamei; P. stylirostris* |
| mullet, striped | *Mugil cerphalus* | shrimp, pink | *Pandalus borealis; P. jordani* |
| muskrat | *Ondatra zibethica* | smelt, rainbow | *Osmerus mordax* |
| mussels, blue | *Mytilus edulis* | snapper, mixed species | *Lutjanidae* |
| ocean perch, Atlantic | *Sebastes marinus* | spiny lobster | *Panulirus* spp.; *Jasus* spp. |
| octopus | *Octopus vulgaris; O.* spp. | spot | *Leiostomus xanthuras* |
| opossum (possum) | *Didilphis virginiana; Trichosurus* spp. | squab (pigeon) | *Columba livia* |
| orange roughy | *Hoplostethus atlanticus* | squid | *Loligoidae pealei; L. opalescens;* |
| ostrich | *Struthio camelus* | | *Illex illecebrosus* |
| oysters, eastern | *Crassostrea virginica* | squirrel | *Sciurus vulgaris* |
| oysters, Pacific | *Crassostrea gigas* | sturgeon, mixed species | *Acipenser* spp. |
| perch, Atlantic | *Sebastes marinus* L | sucker, white | *Catostomus commersoni* |
| perch, mixed species | *Morone americana Gmelin; Perca flavenscens (Mitchill)* | sunfish | *Lepomis gibbosus* |
| | | swordfish | *Xiphias gladius* |
| perch, Pacific | *Sebastes* spp. | tilefish | *Lopholatilus chamaeleonticeps* |
| perch, white | *Mornoe americana* | trout, mixed species | *Salmonidae* spp. |
| pheasant | *Phasianus colchicus* | trout, rainbow | *Salmo gairdneri* |
| pig (pork) | *Sus scrofa* | una, albacore | *Thunnus alalunga* |
| pike, northern | *Esox lucius* | tuna, bluefin | *Thunnus thynnus* |
| pike, walleye | *Stizostedion vitreum* | ttuna, skipjack | *Euthynnus pelamis* |
| pollock (pollack), Atlantic | *Pollachius virens; Gadus virens* | tuna, yellowfin | *Thunnus albacares* |
| pompano | *Trachinotus carolinus* | turbot, European | *Scophthalmus maximus* |
| pout, ocean | *Macrozoarces Gadus virens* | turkey | *Meleagris gallopavo* |
| quail | *Bonsas umbellus; Colinus virginianus* | welks | *Buccinidae* |
| rabbit, domesticated | *Oryctolagus euniculus* | whitefish | *Coregonus clupeaformis* |
| rabbit, wild | *Sylvilagus floridanus* | whiting, mixed species | *Gadidae* |
| raccoon | *Procyon lotor* | yellowtail | *Seriola* spp. |

[1]The terms generally refer to the *Genus species* names for each food. For some foods, the name of the variety (var.) is also provided. The term "spp." is used to indicate that there are various species for the plant or animal. This list is limited to the foods and ingredients included in this nineteenth edition of *Food Values*.

Sources:
Encyclopaedia Britannica, Inc. *Encyclopaedia Britannica*. Chicago, IL: Helen Hemingway Benton, 1974.
Hvass E. *Plants that Feed and Serve Us*. New York: Hippocrene Books, 1975.
Kiple KF, Ornelas KC (eds). *The Cambridge World History of Food*. New York: Cambridge University Press, 2000.
Masefield GB, Wallis M, Harrison SG, et al. *The Oxford Book of Food Plants*. London, England: Oxford Universty Press, 1971.
Nettleton JA. *Seafood Nutrition. Facts, Issues and Marketing of Nutrition in Fish and Shellfish*. Huntington, NY: Osprey Books, 1985.
Rogers J. *What Food Is That? And How Healthy Is It?* Sydney, Australia: Weldon Publishing, 1990.
Tiedjeans VA. *The Vegetable Encyclopedia and Gardner's Guide*. New York: Avehel Books,1943.
United States Department of Agriculture. *National Nutrient Database for Standard Reference, Release 20*. Available at: http://www.nal.usda.gov/fnic/foodcomp/search/.

# Food Name Synonyms and Cross References[1]

| FOR THIS NAME, | SEE THIS INDEXED NAME | FOR THIS NAME, | SEE THIS INDEXED NAME |
|---|---|---|---|
| ahi | tuna, yellowfin | catfish, ocean | wolffish, Atlantic |
| aku | tuna, skipjack | catjang cowpeas | cowpeas, catjang |
| albacore | tuna, white | celery root | celeriac |
| apple, mammy | mammy apple | cervelat | thuringer (cervelat/summer sausage) |
| artichoke, Jerusalem | Jerusalem artichoke | chamomile tea | tea, chamomile |
| ascolano olives | olives, green | champignon mushrooms | mushrooms, common white |
| Asian pear | pear, Asian | chard, Swiss | Swiss chard |
| asparagus bean | yardlong bean | cheesefurter | frankfurter, pork, beef, |
| au gratin potatoes | potatoes au gratin | | and American cheese |
| aubergine | eggplant | chicken frank/frankfurter | frankfurter, chicken |
| awa | milkfish | Chinese chestnuts | chestnuts, Chinese |
| Barbados cherry | acerola | Chinese gooseberry | kiwifruit |
| basella | vinespinach | Chinese kale | Chinese broccoli |
| beans, black | black beans | Chinese parsley | cilantro |
| beans, black turtle | black turtle beans | Chinese pear | pear, Asian |
| beans, cranberry | cranberry beans | Chinese preserving melon | waxgourd |
| beans, French | French beans | Chinese water chestnuts | water chestnuts, Chinese (matai) |
| beans, goa | winged beans | chinook salmon | salmon, Chinook |
| beans, great northern | great northern beans | chocolate, dark | dark chocolate |
| beans, green | green snap beans | chocolate, milk | milk chocolate |
| beans, hyacinth | hyacinth beans | chrysanthemum, garland | garland chrysanthemum |
| beans, kidney | kidney beans | chub | cisco, smoked |
| beans, lima | lima beans | citronella | lemon grass |
| beans, mung | mung beans | cocoa | *See also:* hot chocolate |
| beans, navy | navy beans | cocoa butter | cocoa oil |
| beans, pink | pink beans | Colorado pinyon pines | pinenuts, pinyon |
| beans, pinto | pinto beans | confectioner's sugar | sugar, white, powdered |
| beans, Roman | cranberry beans | corn and lima beans | Succotash |
| beans, white, small | white beans, small | cos lettuce | Romaine |
| beans, winged | winged beans | cottage fries | potato, cottage fries |
| beans, yardlong | yardlong bean | cotto salami | salami, cotto |
| beans, yellow | yellow snap beans | crème caramel | flan (crème caramel/caramel custard) |
| beer salami | salami, beerwurst | crème de menthe | liqueur, crème de menthe |
| beerwurst | salami, beerwurst | cress | garden cress |
| beetroot | beet | crimini mushrooms | mushrooms, crimini |
| Belgian endive | chicory, whitloof | crisphead lettuce | lettuce, crisphead |
| bell pepper | sweet pepper | crowder peas | cowpeas |
| bengal gram | chickpeas | curly endive | chicory greens |
| bitter gourd | balsam pear | curly kale | kale, curly |
| bitter melon | balsam pear | daikon | radish, Oriental |
| black pudding | blood sausage | dasheen | taro |
| blackeye/blackeyed peas | cowpeas | dessert topping | *See:* Sauces, Syrups, and Toppings for |
| blood pudding | blood sausage | | Desserts (Section 7.10) |
| blutwurst | blood sausage | dock | sorrel |
| bologna, Lebanon | Lebanon bologna | dogfish | shark |
| bottled water | water, bottled | edible-podded peas | snow peas |
| bouillon, beef | beef broth/bouillon | egg custard | custard, egg |
| bouillon, chicken | chicken broth/bouillon | endive, Belgian | chicory, witloof |
| breakfast sausage | sausage (fresh), beef; sausage (fresh), | enoki mushrooms | mushrooms, enoki |
| | pork | escalloped potatoes | potatoes, scalloped |
| broth, beef | beef broth/bouillon | European chestnuts | chestnuts, European |
| broth, chicken | chicken broth/bouillon | farina | wheat cereal |
| bullock's heart | custard apple | fava beans | broadbeans |
| butterbeans | lima beans | fish eggs | caviar; roe |
| butterhead lettuce | lettuce, butterhead | flatfish | flounder/sole |
| cabbage, Chinese | Chinese cabbage, pak choi; | fondue | cheese fondue |
| | Chinese cabbage, pe-tsai | Fordhook lima beans | lima beans, immature, green, fordhook |
| cabbage salad | coleslaw | frank | frankfurter |
| cabbage, skunk | swamp cabbage | French artichoke | artichoke |
| cactus fig | pickly pear (fruit) | fries | French fries |
| camomile tea | chamomile tea | frosting | icing/frosting |
| cape gooseberries | groundcherries | fruit leather | fruit roll (dried fruit) |
| caramel custard | flan (crème caramel/caramel custard) | fruit pectin | pectin |
| cardamom | cardamon | fuki | butterbur |

| FOR THIS NAME, | SEE THIS INDEXED NAME | FOR THIS NAME, | SEE THIS INDEXED NAME |
|---|---|---|---|
| garbanzo beans | chickpeas | matai | water chestnuts, Chinese |
| garden rocket | arugula | miriliton | chayote |
| Genoa salami | salami, Genoa | mission olives | olives, black |
| globe artichoke | artichoke | mousse | chocolate mousse |
| goa beans | winged beans | muffins, English | English muffins |
| golden gram | chickpeas | muskmelon | cantaloupe |
| goobers/goober peas | peanuts | natal plum | carissa |
| goosefish | monkfish | navel orange | orange, navel |
| grain beverage | cereal coffee | nori | laver (nori) (seaweed) |
| granadilla, purple | passion fruit, purple | nut pines | pine nuts, pinyon |
| green gram | mung beans | nutmeg butter | nutmeg oil |
| green onions | scallions (green/spring onions) | O'Brien potatoes | potatoes O'Brien |
| green soybeans | edamame | ocean catfish | wolfish |
| Greenland halibut | halibut, Greenland | oranges, mandarin | mandarin oranges |
| grits | corn grits | Oriental radishes | radishes, Oriental |
| groundnuts | peanuts | oyster mushrooms | mushrooms, oyster |
| hake | whiting | oyster plant | salsify |
| ham and cheese roll | ham and cheese loaf | Pacific mackerel | mackerel, Pacific/jack |
| hare | rabbit, wild hare | pak choi | Chinese cabbage, pak choi |
| haricot beans | French beans, mature | palm heart | hearts of palm |
| hash/hashed browns | potato, hashed brown | papaw | papaya |
| Hawaiian mountain yam | mountain yam, Hawaiian | pate | liver pate |
| hazelnuts | filberts | pear pods, balsam | balsam pear pods |
| herbal tea | tea, herbal | pepper, bell | sweet pepper |
| herring, lake | cisco | pepper sauce | hot pepper sauce |
| heart palm | hearts of palm | pepper, sweet | sweet pepper |
| hot chili pepper | chili pepper, green, hot; chili pepper, red, hot | pe-tsai | Chinese cabbage, pe-tsai |
| | | pickerel | pike |
| hot chocolate | *See also:* cocoa | pigeon | squab |
| hot dog | frankfurter | pignolia | pine nuts, pignolia |
| hot sauce | hot pepper sauce | pignon | pine nuts, pinyon |
| ice | *See:* ice pop; Italian ice; lime ice | pinions | pine nuts, pinyon |
| iceberg lettuce | lettuce, iceberg | pinocchios | pine nuts, pinyon |
| infant formula | *See products by brand name in Section 32.1* | pistache nuts | pistachios |
| Italian chestnuts | chestnuts, European | pistachio nuts | pistachios |
| Italian salami | salami, Italian | plum, dried | prune |
| Italian stone pines | pine nuts, pignolia | poha | groundcherries |
| jack | mackerel, jack; mackerel, Pacific/jack | poke | pokeberry sprouts |
| jambolan | java plum | pollack | pollock, Atlantic; pollock, walleye |
| Japanese chestnuts | chestnuts, Japanese | pollock, Alaskan | pollock, walleye |
| Japanese noodles | soba; somen | porgy | scup |
| Japanese pear | pear, Asian | pork fat | *Also see:* lard |
| Japanese persimmon | persimmon, Japanese | pork liver sausage | braunschweiger |
| jerky | beef jerky | portabella mushrooms | mushrooms, portabella |
| Jolt Cola | cola with higher caffeine | possom | opossum |
| Kaiser roll | roll, hard/Kaiser | potatoes, fried | *See:* French fries; potato, cottage fried; potato, hashed brown |
| ketchup | catsup | | |
| kombu | kelp (kombu/tangle) (seaweed) | preserves | jam/preserves |
| knackwurst | knockwurst | prickly pear (vegetable) | nopales |
| kolbassy | kielbasa/kolbassy | purple granadilla | passion fruit, purple |
| lady's finger | okra | purple passion fruit | passion fruit, purple |
| lamb's lettuce | cornsalad | Queensland nuts | macadamia nuts |
| laver | seaweed, laver (nori) | radicchio | chicory greens |
| leaf lettuce | lettuce, looseleaf | raisinets | chocolate-coated raisins, Raisinets |
| litchi | litchee | rapeseed oil | canola oil |
| liver sausage | liverwurst | red kidney beans | kidney beans, red |
| looseleaf lettuce | lettuce, looseleaf | red gram | pigeon peas |
| lox | salmon, Chinook, smoked | redfish | ocean perch, Atlantic |
| lychee | lichee | relish | pickle relish |
| mahimahi | dolphinfish | rice, wild | wild rice |
| mamey | mammy apple | Roman beans | cranberry beans |
| mammee apple | mammy apple | roughy, orange | orange roughy |
| mango squash | chayote | salmon, keta | salmon, chum |
| manioc | cassava | salmon, red | salmon, sockeye |
| manzillo olives | olives, black | sausage, blood | blood sausage |
| marmalade plum | sapote | sausage, liver | liver sausage |
| marrow | squash, summer | scallions | onion, green/spring |
| masa harina | corn flour, yellow, masa harina | scalloped potatoes | potato, scalloped |
| mashed potatoes | potato, mashed | Scotch kale | kale, Scotch |

| FOR THIS NAME, | SEE THIS INDEXED NAME | FOR THIS NAME, | SEE THIS INDEXED NAME |
|---|---|---|---|
| scrod | cod, Atlantic | sweetbread | beef/lamb/pork/veal pancreas; beef/veal thymus |
| sea snails | whelks | | |
| seaweed | *See:* agar, Irish moss, kelp, laver, spirulina, wakame | sweetsop | sugar apple |
| | | tahini | sesame butter |
| semi-sweet chocolate | dark chocolate | Tahitian taro | taro, Tahitian |
| sevailano olives | olives, green | tamari | soy sauce (made with soy, but no wheat) |
| shiitake mushrooms | mushrooms, shiitake | | |
| shoyu | soy sauce with soy and wheat | tangerines, canned | mandarin oranges, canned |
| sim-sim | sesame seeds | tangle | kelp (kombu/tangle) (seaweed) |
| skipjack tuna | tuna, skipjack | tannier | yautia |
| skunk cabbage | swamp cabbage | tap water | water, municipal tap |
| smoked sausage | Smokie | tendergreen | mustard spinach |
| snails, sea | whelks | towel gourd | dishcloth gourd |
| snap beans | green snap beans; yellow snap beans | turbot | halibut, Greenland |
| sodium chloride | salt | turkey frank/frankfurter | frankfurter, turkey |
| sorrel | dock | turkey hot dog | frankfurter, turkey |
| southern peas | cowpeas | turkey pastrami | pastrami, turkey |
| soybean curd | tofu | turtle black beans | black turtle beans |
| soybean paste | miso | Valencia orange | orange, Valencia |
| soybeans, green | edamame | vegetable oyster | salsify |
| spinach, mustard | mustard spinach | vegetable pear | chayote |
| spring onion | scallions (green/spring onions) | vegetables, mixed | mixed vegetables |
| sprouts | *See:* alfalfa sprouts or mung bean sprouts | viper's grass | salsify, black |
| | | wakame | wakame (seaweed) |
| squash seeds | pumpkin and squash seeds | walleye | pollock, walleye |
| St. John's bread | carob | water convulvolus | swamp cabbage |
| star fruit/starfruit | carambola | wax beans | yellow snap beans |
| stone pines | pine nuts, pignolia | Welsh onion | onion, Welsh |
| straightneck squash | crookneck/straightneck squash | West Indian cherry | acerola |
| straw mushrooms | mushrooms, straw | white-flowered gourd | calabash gourd |
| strawberry guava | guava, strawberry | white icicle radish | radish, white icicle |
| string beans | green snap beans | wiener | frankfurter |
| sugar snap peas | snow peas | witloof chicory | chicory, witloof |
| summer sausage | thuringer (cervelat/summer sausage) | yam, mountain, Hawaiian | mountain yam, Hawaiian |
| sunchoke | Jerusalem artichoke | yambean | jicama |
| Surinam cherry | pitanga | yellow passion fruit | passion fruit, yellow |
| Swede | rutabaga | yellowfin tuna | tuna, yellowfin |
| sweet chestnuts | chestnuts, European | yokan | adzuki beans, mature, sweetened |

[1]To assist users in locating foods in the database, this list provides alternative food names in the left-hand column and the term used in this nineteenth edition of *Food Values* in the right-hand column. The names in the right-hand column are listed in the index with the page numbers.

Sources:
Encyclopaedia Britannica, Inc. *Encyclopaedia Britannica.* Chicago, IL: Helen Hemingway Benton, 1974.
Hvass E. *Plants that Feed and Serve Us.* New York: Hippocrene Books, 1975.
Kiple KF, Ornelas KC (eds). *The Cambridge World History of Food.* New York: Cambridge University Press, 2000.
Masefield GV, Wallis M, Harrison SG, et al. *The Oxford Book of Food Plants.* London, England: Oxford University Press, 1971.
Nettleton JA. *Seafood Nutrition. Facts, Issues and Marketing of Nutrition in Fish and Shellfish.* Huntington, NY: Osprey Books, 1985.
Rogers J, *What Food Is That: And How Healthy Is It?* Sydney, Australia: Weldon Publishing, 1990.
Tiedjeans VA. *The Vegetable Encyclopedia and Gardner's Guide.* New York: Avehel Books, 1943.

# *Bibliography For Food Composition Data (July 2003–December 2008)*

Abebe Y, A Bogale, KM Hambidge, BJ Stoecker, K Bailey, RS Gibson. **Phytate, zinc, iron, and calcium** content of selected raw and prepared foods consumed in rural Sidama, Southern Ethiopia and implications for bioavailability. *J Food Comp Anal* 20:161–168, 2007.

Abdul-Hamid A, RRR Sulaiman, A Osman, N Saari. Preliminary study of the chemical composition of **rice milling fractions** stabilized by microwave heating. *J Food Comp Anal* 20:627–637, 2007. [macronutrients, carotenoids, total phenolics, 10 minerals, amino acids]

Abu-Lafi S, JW Dembicki, P Goldshlag, LO Hanus, VM Dembitsky. The use of the 'Cryogenic' GC/MS and on-column injection for study of **organosulfur compounds of the** *Allium Sativum*. *J Food Comp Anal* 17:235–245, 2004.

Agbede JO, VA Aletor. Studies of the chemical composition and protein quality evaluation of differently processed *Canavalia ensiformis* and *Mucuna pruriens* **seed flours**. *J Food Comp Anal* 18:89–103, 2005.

Agbor-Egbe T, IL Mbome, The effects of processing techniques in reducing **cyanogens** levels during the production of some **Cameroonian cassava foods**. *J Food Comp Anal* 19:354–363, 2006.

Aguilera-Morales M, M Casas-Valdez, S Carrillo-Dominguez, B Gonzalez-Acosta, F Perez-Gil. Chemical composition and m icrobiological assays of **marine algae** *Enteromorpha* spp. As a potential food source. *J Food Comp Anal* 18:79–88, 2005.

Ahmed MK, JK Daun, R Przybylski. FI-IR based methodology for quantitation of total **tocopherols, tocotrienols and plastochromanol-8 in vegetable oils**. *J Food Comp Anal* 18:359–364, 2005.

Aimutis WR. **Bioactive properties of milk proteins** with particular focus on anticariogenesis. *J Nutr* 134:989S–995S, 2004.

Alaburda J, AP de Almeida, L Shundo, V Ruvieri, M Sabino. Determination of **folic acid in fortified wheat flours**. *J Food Comp Anal* 21:336–342, 2008.

Alajaji SA, TA El-Adawy. Nutritional composition of **chickpea** (*Cicer arietinum* L.) as affected by microwave cooking and other traditional cooking methods. *J Food Comp Anal* 19:806–812, 2006.

Albers MJ, LJ Harnack, LM Steffern, et al. 2006 Marketplace survey of *trans*-**fatty acid content of margarines and butters, cookies and snack cakes, and savory snacks**. *J Am Diet Assoc* 108:367–370, 2008.

Alfawaz MA. **Chemical composition of hummayd** (*Rumex vesicarius*) grown in Saudi Arabia. *J Food Comp Anal* 19:552–555, 2006.

Almaraz-Abarca N, M da G Campos, JA Avila-Reyes, N Naranjo-Jimenez, JH Corral, LS Gonzalez-Valdez. **Antioxidant activity** of polyphenolic extract of monofloral honeybee-collected **pollen** from mesquite (*Prosopis juliflora*, Leguminosae). *J Food Comp Anal* 20:119–124, 2007.

Almeida-Muradian LB, LC Pamplona, S Coimbra, OM Barth. Chemical composition and botanical evaluation of **dried bee pollen pellets**. *J Food Comp Anal* 18:105–111, 2005.

Al-Saleh, IA, G Billedo, II El-Doush. Levels of **selenium, DL-alpha-tocopherol, DL-gamma-tocopherol, all-trans-retinol, thymoquinone, and thymol** in different brands of *Nigella sativa* **seeds**. *J Food Comp Anal* 19:167–175, 2006.

Altinoz S, S Toptan. Simultaneous determination of **Indigotin and Ponceau-4R** in food samples by using Vierordt's method, ratio spectra first order derivative and derivative UV spectrophotometry. *J Food Comp Anal* 16:517–530, 2003.

Alvarez M, IM Moreno, AM Jos, AM Camean, AG Gonzalez. Study of **mineral profile** of Montilla-Moriles "fino" **wines** using inductively coupled plasma atomic emission spectrometry methods. *J Food Comp Anal* 20:391–395, 2007.

Amir Y, AL Haenni, A Youyou. Physical and biochemical differences in the composition of the seeds of **Algerian leguminous crops**. *J Food Comp Anal* 20:466–471, 2007.

Andreotti G, E Trivellone, A Motta. Characterization of **buffalo milk** by $^{31}$P-nuclear magnetic resonance spectroscopy. *J Food Comp Anal* 19:843–849, 2006.

Anjum FM, I Ahmad, MS Butt, MA Sheikh, I Pasha. **Amino acid** composition of **spring wheats** and losses of **lysine** during **chapati** baking. *J Food Comp Anal* 18:523–532, 2005.

Anli RE, N Vural S Yilmaz, YH Vural. The determination of **biogenic amines in Turkish red wines**. *J Food Comp Anal* 17:53–62, 2004.

Anttonen MJ, Ro Karjalainen. Environmental and genetic variation of **phenolic compounds in red raspberry**. *J Food Comp Anal* 18:759–769, 2005.

Aoun E, J Rima, G Chidiac, K Hanna. High-performance liquid chromatographic and spectrofluorometric determination of **alpha-tocopherol** in a natural plant: Ferula hermonis (**Zalooh root**). *J Food Comp Anal* 18:607–615, 2005.

Applequist WL, B Avula, BT Schaneberg, Y-H Wang, IA Khan. Comparative **fatty acid** content of seeds of four *Cucurbita* species grown in a common (shared) garden. *J Food Comp Anal* 19:606–611, 2006.

Ariefkjohan MW, DA Savaiano, **Chocolate** and cardiovascular health: Is it too good to be true? *Nutr Rev* 63:427–430, 2005.

Askin MA, MF Balta, FE Tekintas, A Kazankaya, F Balta. **Fatty acid** composition affected by kernel weight in **almond** (*Prunus dulcis* (Mill.) Webb.) genetic resources. *J Food Comp Anal* 20:7–12, 2007.

Assuncao RB, AZ Mercadante. **Carotenoids and ascorbic acid** composition from **commercial products of cashew apple (Anacardium occidentale L.)**. *J Food Comp Anal* 16:647–657, 2003.

Athar N, A Hardacre, G Taylor, S Clark, R Harding, J McLaughlin. **Vitamin retention in extruded food products**. *J Food Comp Anal* 19:379–383, 2006. [thiamin, riboflavin, niacin, and pyridoxine in oat maize, and maize+pea cereals]

Atlabachew M, BS Chandravanshi. Levels of major, minor and trace **elements** in commercially available **enset** (*Ensete ventricosum* (Welw.), Cheesman) food products (**kocho** and **bulla**) in Ethiopia. *J Food Comp Anal* 21:545–552, 2008. [K, Na, Ca, Mg, Cu, Zn, Mn, Co, Fe, Cr, Ni, Cd, Pb]

Auerback MH, SAS Craig, JF Howlett, KC Hayes. **Caloric availability of polydextrose**. *Nutr Rev* 65:544–549, 2007.

Avallone S, T-WE Tiemtore, C Mouquet-Rivier, S Treche. Nutritional value of six multi-ingredient **sauces** from Burkina Faso. *J Food Comp Anal* 21:553–558, 2008. [Fe, Zn, beta-carotene, retinol activity, cis-carotene]

Bacigalupo MA, R Longhi, G Meroni. **Alpha-solanine and alpha-chaconine glycoalkaloid** assay in *Solanum tuberosum* extracts by lipsomes and time-resolved fluorescence. *J Food Comp Anal* 17:665–673, 2004.

Badrie N, M Joseph, N Darbasie. Nutritive composition of a **street food 'doubles' channa** (*Cicer arietinum*) **burger** and its components sold in Trinidad, West Indies. *J Food Comp Anal* 18:171–179, 2005.

Balta MF, T Yarilgac, MA Askin M Kucuk, F Balta, K Ozrenk. Determination of **fatty acid** compositions, **oil** contents and some quality traits of **hazelnut** genetic resources grown in eastern Anatolia of Turkey. *J Food Comp Anal* 19:681–686, 2006.

Barikmo I, F Ouattara, A Oshaug. Differences in **micronutrients** content found in **cereals** from various parts of Mali. *J Food Comp Anal* 20:681–687, 2007. [iron, zinc, thiamin, riboflavin, and niacin in millet flour, sorghum flour, rice, wheat flour, and fonio]

Batnett LE, Am Broomfield, Wh Hendriks, MB Hunt, TK McGhie. The in vivo antioxidant action and the reduction of oxidative stress by **boysenberry extract** is dependent on base diet constitutents in rats. *J Med Food* 10:281–289, 2007. [macronutrients, Na, K, phenolics, anthocyanins]

Bastos DHM, EY Ishimoto, MOM Marques, AF Ferri, EAFS Torres. **Essential oil and antioxidant activity of green mate and mate tea** (*Ilex paraguariensis*) infusions. *J Food Comp Anal* 19:538–543, 2006.

Bautista-Ortin AT, JI Fernandez-Fernandez, JM Lopez-Roca, E Gomez-Plaza. The effects of enological practices in **anthocyanins, phenolic compounds** and **wine** colour and their dependence on grape characteristics. *J Food Comp Analal* 20:546–552, 2007.

Baylin A, X Siles, A Donnovan-Palmer, X Fernandez, H Campos. **Fatty acid** composition of **Costa Rican foods** including *trans* **fatty acid** content. *J Food Comp Anal* 20:182–192, 2007.

Beecher GR. Overview of dietary **flavonoids**: Nomenclature, occurrence, and intake. *J Nutr* 133:3248S–3254S, 2003.

Bellomo MG, B Fallico. **Anthocyanins, chlorophylls, and xanthophylls in pistachio nuts** (*Pistacia vera*) of different geographic origin. *J Food Comp Anal* 20:352–359, 2007.

Benatti P, G Peluso, R Nicolai, M Calvani. **Polyunsaturated fatty acids**: Biochemical, nutritional and epigenetic properties. *J Am Col Nutr* 23:281–301, 2004.

Bengtsson A, A Namutebi, ML Alminger, U Svanberg. Effects of various traditional processing methods on the all-*trans*-β-**carotene** content of orange-fleshed **sweet potato**. *J Food Comp Anal* 21:134–143, 2008.

Bernardez MM, JDM Miguelez, JG Queijeiro. HPLC determination of **sugars** in varieties of **chestnut fruits** from Galicia (Spain). *J Food Comp Anal* 17:63–67, 2004.

Bhakta D, IS Silva, C Higgins, L Sevak, T Kassam-Khamis, P Mangtani, H Adlercreutz, A McMichael. A semiquantitative food frequency questionnaire is a valid indicator of the usual intake of **phytoestrogens** by South Asian women in the UK relative to multiple 24-h dietary recalls and multiple plasma samples. *J Nutr* 135:116–123, 2005. [phytoestrogen concentration of some foods commonly consumed by South Asian women in the UK]

Bhandari MR, J Kawabata. Cooking effects on **oxalate, phytate, trypsin, and α-amylase inhibitors of wild yam tubers** of Nepal. *J Food Comp Anal* 19:524–530, 2006.

Bird AR, CF lorry, DA Davies, S Usher, DL Topping. A novel **barley** cultivar (Himalaya 292) with a specific gene mutation in starch synthase IIa raises large bowel starch and short-chain fatty acids in rats. *J Nutr* 134:831–835, 2004.

Blasi F, D Montesano, M De Angelis, a Maurizi, F ventura, L Cossignani, MS Simonetti, P Damiani. Results of stereospecific analysis of **triacylglycerol** fraction from **donkey, cow, ewe, goat and buffalo milk**. *J Food Comp Anal* 21:1–7, 2008.

Blitz C, SP Murphy, DLM Au. Adding **lignan** values to a food composition database. *J Food Comp Anal* 20:99–105, 2007.

Blitz CL, SP Murphy, DYMT Au, KMM Yonemori, JA Foote, LN Kolonel. Creating default codes and assigning nutrient values for non-specific **dietary supplements**. *J Food Comp Anal* 19:453–460, 2006.

Bobrowska-Grzesik W, A Jokobik-Kolon. Leaching of **cadmium** and **lead** from **dried fruits** and **fruit teas** to infusions and decoctions. *J Food Comp Anal* 21:326–331, 2008.

Bohrer D, PC do Nascimento, E Becker, LM de Carvalho, M Dessuy. **Arsenic species** in **solutions for parenteral nutrition**. *J Parenteral Enteral Nutr* 29:1–7, 2005.

Bond B, DR Fernandez, DJ VanderJagt, M Williams, Y-S Huang, L-T Chuang, M Millson, R Andrews, RG Glew. **Fatty acid, amino acid and trace mineral** analysis of three complementary **foods from Jos, Nigeria**. *J Food Comp Anal* 18:675–690, 2005.

Bonfoh B, J Zinsstag, Z Farah, CF Simbe, IO Alfaroukh, R Aebi, R Badertscher, M Collomb, J Meyer, B Rehberger. **Raw milk** composition of Malian Zebu cows (*Bos indicus*) raised under traditional system. *J Food Comp Anal* 18:29–38, 2005.

Bopp M, C Lovelady, C Hunter, T Kinsella. Maternal diet and exercise: Effects on **long-chain polyunsaturated fatty acid** concentrations in breast milk. *J Am Diet Assoc* 105:1098–1102, 2005.

Borges OP, JS Carvalho, PR Correia, AP Silva. **Lipid and fatty acid profiles** of *Castenea sativa* Mill. **chestnuts** of 17 native Portuguese cultivars. *J Food Comp Anal* 20:80–89, 2007.

Bradbury JH. Simple wetting method to reduce **cyanogens** content of cassava flour. *J Food Comp Anal* 19:388–393, 2006.

Brat P, S George, A Bellamy, L Du Chaffaut, A Scalbert, L Mennen, N Arnault, MJ Amiot. Daily **polyphenol** intake in France from **fruit and vegetables**. *J Nutr* 136:2368–2373, 2006. [**total polyphenol content of fruits and vegetables**]

Brooks SPJ, R Mongeau, JR Deeks, BJ Lampi, R Brassard. **Dietary fibre in baby foods of major brands sold in Canada**. *J Food Comp Anal* 19:59–66, 2005.

Brown MJ, MG Ferruzzi, ML Nguyen, DA Cooper, AL Eldridge, SJ Schwartz, WS White. **Carotenoid** bioavailability is higher from **salads** ingested with full-fat than with fat-reduced salad dressing as measured with electrochemical detection. *Am J Clin Nutr* 80:396–403, 2004.

Burrowes JD, NJ Ramer. Removal of **potassium** from **tuberous root vegetables** by leaching. *J Renal Nutr* 16:304–311, 2006.

Busby MG, L Fischer, K-A Da Costa, D Thompson, M-H Mar, SH Zeisel. **Choline-** and **betaine**-defined diets for use in clinical research and for the management of trimethylaminuria. *J Am Diet Assoc* 104:1836–1845, 2004.

Byamukama R, BT Kiremire, OM Andersen, A Steigen. **Anthocyanins** from **fruits of *Rubus pinnatus* and *Rubus rigidus***. *J Food Comp Anal* 18:599–605, 2005.

Cabrera C, R Artacho, R Gimenez. Beneficial effects of **green tea** – A review. *J Am Coll Nutr* 25:79–99, 2006.

Cabrita MJ, AMC Freitas, O Laureano, D Borsa, R Di Stefano. **Aroma compounds** in varietal **wines** from Alentejo, Portugal. *J Food Comp Anal* 20:375–390, 2007.

Cakduribu GAm NE Nabes, **Proximate composition, fatty acids, and cholesterol** content of meat cuts from **tegu lizard** *Tupinambis merianae*. *J Food Comp Anal* 19:711–714, 2006.

Caldwell CR, SJ Britz. Effect of supplemental ultraviolet radiation on the **carotenoid and chlorophyll** composition of green house-grown **leaf lettuce** (*Lactuca sativa* L.) cultivars. *J Food Comp Anal* 19:637–644, 2006.

Campbell JK, K Canene-Adams, BL Lindshield, T W-M Boileau, SK Clinton, JW Erdman. **Tomato phytochemicals** and prostate cancer risk. *J Nutr* 134:3486S–3492S, 2004.

Canales A, J Benedi, M Nus, J Librelotto, JM Sanchez-Montero, FJ Sanchez-Muniz. Effect of **walnut-enriched restructured meat** in the antioxidant status of overweight/obese senior subjects with at least one extra CHD-risk factor. *J Am Col Nutr* 26:225–232, 2007. [**macronutrients, tocopherols, Mg**]

Canas PMI, EG Romero, SG Alonso, MF Gonzalez, MLLP Herreros. **Amino acids and biogenic amines** during spontaneous malolactic fermentation in **Tempranillo red wines**. *J Food Comp Anal* 21:731–735, 2008.

Canas S, V Casanova, AP Belhior. **Antioxidant activity and pheonlic content** of **Portuguese** wine aged **brandies**. *J Food Comp Anal* 21:626–633, 2008.

Canene-Adams K, JK Campbell, S Zariphen, EH Jeffery, JW Erdman. The **tomato** as a functional food. *J Nutr* 135:1226–1230, 2005. [**K, tocopherol, vitamin A, vitamin C, folate, Carotenoids in tomatoes, catsup, tomato juice, tomato sauce, and tomato soup**]

Cano A, A Medina, A Bermejo. **Bioactive compounds** in different **citrus** varieties. Discrimination among cultivars. *J Food Comp Anal* 21:377–381, 2008. [**vitamin C, hesperidin, narirutin**]

Cardoso AP, E Mirione, M Ernesto, F Massaza, J Cliff, MR Haque, JH Bradbury. Processing of **cassava roots** to remove **cyanogens**. *J Food Comp Anal* 18:451–460, 2005.

Cardoso DR, SM Bettin, RV Reche, BS Lima-Neto, DW Franco. HPLC-DAD analysis of **ketones** as their 2,4-dinitrophenylhydrazones in **Brazilian sugar-cane spirits and rum**. *J Food Comp Anal* 16:563–573, 2003.

Cardozo Jr, EL, O Ferrarese-Filho, LC Filho, MLL Ferrarese, CM Donaduzzi, JA Sturion. **Methylxanthines and phenolic compounds in mate** (*Ilex paraguariensis* St. Hil.) progenies grown in Brazil. *J Food Comp Anal* 20:553–558, 2007. [methylxanthines, caffeine, theobromine, phenol chlorogenic acid, caffeic acid]

Case S. The **gluten**-free diet: How to provide effective education and resources. *Gastroenterology* 128:S128–S134, 2005.

Catherwood DJ, GP Savage, SM Mason, JJC Scheffer, JA Douglas. **Oxalate** content of cormels of Japanese **taro** (*Colocasia esculenta* (L.) Shott) and the effect of cooking. *J Food Comp Anal* 20:147–151, 2007.

Ceballos H, T Sanchez, AL Chavez, C Iglesias, D Debouck, G Mafla, J Tohme. Variation in crude **protein** content in **cassava** (*Manihot esculenta* Crantz) roots. *J Food Comp Anal* 19:589–593, 2006.

Cemek M, L Akkaya, YO Birdane, K Seyrek, S Bulut, M Konuk. **Nitrate and nitrite** levels in **fruity and natural mineral waters** marketed in western Turkey. *J Food Comp Anal* 20:236–240, 2007.

Cerklewski FL. **Calcium** fortification of food can add unneeded dietary **phosphorus**. *J Food Comp Anal* 18:595–598, 2005.

Chai W, M Liebman. **Oxalate content of legumes, nuts, and grain-based flour**. *J Food Comp Anal* 18:723–729, 2005.

Chalchat JC, MM Ozcan. Composition of the **essential oil of** *Helichrysum chasmolycicum* growing wilk in Turkey. *J Medicinal Food* 9:287–289, 2006.

Champagne ET. *Rice Chemistry and Technology*, 3rd ed, Am Assoc Cereal Chemists, Inc, St Paul MN, ISBN 1–891127–34–9, 2004.

Chan SSL, EL Ferguson, K Bailey, U Fahmida, TB Harper, RS Gibson. The concentrations of **iron, calcium, zinc and phytate in cereals and legumes** habitually consumed by infants living in East Lombok, Indonesia. *J Food Comp Anal* 20:609–617, 2007.

Chan-Blanco Y, F Vaillant, AM Perez, M Reynes, J-M Brillouet, P Brat. The **noni fruit** (*Morinda citrifolia* L.): A review of agricultural research, nutritional and therapeutic properties. *J Food Comp Anal* 19:645–654, 2006.

Chanlos S, L Joly-Pottuz, M Chatelut, O Vittori, JL Cretier. Determination of **carmoisine, allura red, and ponceau 4R in sweets and soft drinks** by differential pulse polarography. *J Food Comp Anal* 18:503–515, 2005.

Chawla R, R Arora, S Singh, RK Sagar, RK Sharma, R Kumar, A Sharma, ML Gupta, S Singh, J Prasad, HA Khan, A Swaroop, AK Sinha, AK Gupta, RP Tripathi, PS Ahuja. **Radioprotective and antioxidant activity** of fractionated extracts of **berries of** *Hippophae rhamnoids*. *J Med Food* 10:101–109, 2007.

Cheikh-Rouhou S, S Besbes, G Lognay, C Blecker, C Deroanne, H Attia. **Sterol** composition of **black cumin** (*Nigella sativa* L.) and **Aleppo pine** (*Pinus halepensis* Mill.) seed oils. *J Food Comp Anal* 21:162–168, 2008.

Chen M-H, CJ Bergman. A rapid procedure for analysing **rice bran tocopherol, tocotrienol, and gamma-oryzanol** contents. *J Food Comp Anal* 18:139–151, 2005. Republished in *J Food Comp Anal* 18:319–331, 2005.

Chin ST, SAH Nazimah, SY Quek, YBC Man, RA Rahman, DM Hashim. Analysis of **volatile compounds from Malaysian durians** (*Curio zibethinus*) using headspace SPME coupled to fast GC-MS. *J Food Comp Anal* 20:31–44, 2007.

Chinnici F, U Spinabelli, C Riponi, A Amati. Optimization of the determination of **organic acid and sugars in fruit juices** by ion-exclusion liquid chromatography. *J Food Comp Anal* 18:121–130, 2005.

Chirico G, R Marzollo, S Cortinovis, C Fonte, A Gasparoni. **Antiinfective properties of human milk**. *J Nutr* 138:1801S–1806S, 2008.

Cho IK, J Rima, CL Chang, QX Li. Spectrofluorometric and high-performance liquid chromatographic determination of **all-rac-alpha-tocopheryl acetate in virgin olive oil**. *J Food Comp Anal* 20:57–62, 2007.

Cho S, S Kang, J Cho, A Kim, S Park, Y-K Hong, D-H Ahn. **Antioxidant peptide** isolated from **muscle protein of bullfrog**, *Rana catesbeiana* Shaw. *J Med Food* 10:401–407, 2007.

Choi EY, R Graham, J Stangoulis. Semi-quantitative analysis for selecting **Fe-** and **Zn**-dense genotypes of **staple food crops**. *J Food Comp Anal* 20:496–505, 2007.

Choi M-S, KC Rhee. Production and processing of **soybeans** and nutrition and safety of **isoflavone and other soy products** for human health. *J Med Food* 9:1–10, 2006.

Chokeprasert P, AL Chrles, K-H Sue, T-C Huang. **Volatile components of the leaves, fruits, and seeds of wampee** (*Clausena lansium* (Lour.) Skeels). *J Food Comp Anal* 20:52–56, 2007.

Christian KR, MG Nair, JC Jackson. **Antioxidant** and cyclooxygenase inhibitory **activity of sorrel** (Hibiscus sabdariffa). *J Food Comp Anal* 19:778–783, 2006.

Chun J, J Lee, L Y, J Exler, RR Eitenmiller. **Tocopherol and tocotrienol** contents of **raw and processed fruits and vegetables** in the United States diet. *J Food Comp Anal* 19:196–204, 2006.

Chun J, JA Martin, L Chen, J Lee, L Ye, RR Eitenmiller. A differential assay of **folic acid and total folate** in foods containing **enriched cereal-grain products** to calculate mcg dietary folate equivalents (mcg DFE). *J Food Comp Anal* 19:182–187, 2006.

Chung SWC, KP Kwong, JCW Yau, AMC Wong, Y Xiao. **Chloropropanols** levels in foodstuffs marketed in **Hong Kong**. *J Food Comp Anal* 21:569–573, 2008.

Clausen I, L Ovesen. Changes in **fat** content of **pork and beef** after pan-frying under different conditions. *J Food Comp Anal* 18:201–211, 2005.

Clauses I, J Jakobsen, T Leth, L Ovesen. **Vitamin D3 and 25-hydroxyvitamin D3 in raw and cooked pork cuts**. *J Food Comp Anal* 16:575–585, 2003.

Cockell KA, G Bonacci, B Belonje. **Manganese** content of **soy or rice beverages** is high in comparison to **infant formulas**. *J Am Col Nutr* 23:124–130, 2004.

Covas M-I, V Ruiz-Guiterrez, R de la Torre, A Kafatos, RM Lamuela-Raventos, J Osada, RW Owen, F Visioli. Minor components of **olive oil**: Evidence to date of health benefits in humans. Nutr Rev 64:S20–S30, 2006.

Dai J, JD Patel, RJ Mumper. Characterization of **blackberry extract** and its antiproliferative and anti-inflammatory properties. *J Med Food* 10:258–265, 2007. **[anthocyanins, phenolics, total antioxidant capacity]**

Damon M, NZ Zhang, DB Haytowitz, SL Booth. **Phylloguqinone (vitamin K1) content of vegetables**. *J Food Comp Anal* 18:751–758, 2005.

Dancheck B, V Nussenblatt, MO Ricks, N Kumwenda, MC Neville, DT Moncrief, TE Taha, RD Semba. **Breast milk retinol** concentrations are not associated with systemic inflammation among breast-feeding women in Malawi. *J Nutr* 135:223–226, 2005.

Daniel DR, LD Thompson, BJ Shriver, C-K Wu, LC Hoover. Nonhydrogenated **cottonseed oil** can be used as a deep fat frying medium to reduce *trans*-**fatty acid** content in **French fries**. *J Am Diet Assoc* 105:1927–1932, 2005.

Da Silva EGP, V Hatje, WNL dos Santos, LM Costa, ARA Nogueira, SLC Ferreira. Fast method for the determination of **copper, manganese and iron in seafood** samples. *J Food Comp Anal* 21:259–263, 2008.

da Silva LP, M de Lourdes Santorio Ciocca. **Total, insoluble, and soluble dietary fiber** values measured by enzymatic-gravimetric method in **cereal grains**. *J Food Comp Anal* 18:113–120, 2005.

da Silveira, TML, E Tavares, MBA Gloria. Profile and levels of **bioactive amines in instant coffee**. *J Food Comp Anal* 20:451–457, 2007.

Davidson L, KA Jamil, SA Sarker, C Zeder, G Fuchs, R Hurrell. **Human milk** as a source of **ascorbic acid**: No enhancing effect on iron bioavailability from a traditional complementary food consumed by Bangladeshi infants and young children. *Am J Clin Nutr* 79:1073–1077, 2004.

Davis DR, MD Epp, HD Riordan. Changes in USDA food composition data for **43 garden crops**, 1950 to 1999. *J Am Col Nutr* 23:669–682, 1004.

de Azevedo-Meleiro CH, DB Rodriguez-Amaya. **Carotenoids of endive and New Zealand spinach** as affected by maturity, season, and minimal processing. *J Food Comp Anal* 18:845–855, 2005.

de Rosso VV, S Hillebrand, EC Montilla, FO Bobbio, P Winterhalter, AZ Mercadante. Determination of **anthocyanins** from **acerola** (*Malpighia emarginata* DC.) and **acai** (*Euterpe oleracea* Mart.) by HPLC-PDA-MS/MS. *J Food Comp Anal* 21:291–299, 2008.

de Oliveira AN, H de Santana, CTBV Zaia, DAM Zaia. A study of reaction between quinines and thiourea: Determination of **thiourea in orange juice**. *J Food Comp Anal* 17:165–177, 2004.

de Sa MC, DB Rodriguez-Amaya. Optimization of HPLC quantification of **carotenoids in cooked green vegetables** – Comparison of analytical and calculated data. *J Food Comp Anal* 17:37–51, 2004.

de Sousa RA, JCJ Silva, N Baccan, S Cadore. Determination of **metals in bottled coconut water** using an inductively coupled plasma optical emission spectrometer. *J Food Comp Anal* 18:399–408, 2005. (Ca, Mg, Mn, Fe, Zn, Cu)

Deepa N, C Kaur, B Singh, HC Kapoor. **Antioxidant activity** in some **red sweet pepper** cultivars. *J Food Comp Anal* 19:572–578, 2006.

Dinh TTN, JR Blanton Jr, JC Brooks, MF Miller, LD Thompson. A simplified method for **cholesterol** determination in **meat and meat products**. *J Food Comp Anal* 21:306–314, 2008.

Dobrinas S, S Birghila, V Coatu. Assessment of **polycyclic aromatic hydrocarbons in honey and propolis** produced from various flowering trees and plants in Romania. *J Food Comp Anal* 21:71–77, 2008.

Du Q, J Zheng, Y Xu. Composition of **anthocyanins** in **mulberry** and their antioxidant activity. *J Food Comp Anal* 21:390–395, 2008.

Duenas M, JJ Perez-Alonso, C Santos-Buelga, T Escribano-Bailon. **Anthocyanin** composition in **fig** (*Ficus carica* L.). *J Food Comp Anal* 21:107–115, 2008.

Duggan P, KD Cashman, A Flynn, C Bolton-Smith, M Kiely. **Phylloquinone (vitamin K1)** intakes and food sources in 18–64 year old Irish adults. *Brit J Nutr* 91:151–158, 2004.

Duhan A, N Khetarpaul, S Bishnoi. HCl-extractability of **zinc and copper** as affected by soaking, dehulling, cooking and germination of high yielding **pigeon pea cultivars**. *J Food Comp Anal* 17:597–604, 2004.

Dumlu MU, E Gurkan. Elemental and nutritional analysis of *Punica granatum* from Turkey. *J Med Food* 10:392–395, 2007. [**pomegranate: vit C, phytoserol, anthocyanin, K, Na, CA, Mg, Fe, P**]

Dumont JF, J Peterson, D Haytowitz, SL Booth. **Phylloquinone and dihydrophylloquinone contents of mixed dishes, processed meats, soups and cheeses**. *J Food Comp Anal* 16:595–603, 2003.

Dundar MS, H Altundag. **Selenium content of Turkish hazelnut varieties**: Kara Findik, Tombul, and Delisava. *J Food Comp Anal* 17:707–712, 2004.

Duvenage SS, HC Schonfeldt. Impact of South African fortification legislation on product formulation for low-income households. *J Food Comp Anal* 20:688–695, 2007. [**vitamin A, thiamin, riboflavin, niacin, pyridoxine, folic acid, iron, and zinc in maize meal and brown bread**]

Egan MB, A Fragodt, MM Raats, C Hodgkins, M Lumbers. The importance of harmonizing food composition data across Europe (Review). *European J Clin Nutr* 61:813–821, 2007.

Eisele TA, SR Drake. The partial compositional characteristics of **apple juice** from 175 apple varieties. *J Food Comp Anal* 18:213–221, 2005.

Ekholm P, H Reinivuo, P Mattila, H Pakkala, J Koponen, A Happonen, J Hellstrom, M-L Ovaskainen. Changes in the **mineral and trace element** contents of **cereals, fruits and vegetables in Finland**. *J Food Comp Anal* 20:487–495, 2007. [K, Ca, Mg, P, Fe, Cu, Mn, Zn, Co, Ni, Se, Al, Cd, Pb]

Ekvall J, R Stegmark, M Nyman. Optimization of extraction methods for determination of the **raffinose family oligosaccharides in leguminous vine peas** (*Pisum sativum* L.) and effects of blanching. *J Food Comp Anal* 20:13–18, 2007.

El-Arab AE, M Ali, L Hussein. **Vitamin B1** profile of the **Egyptian core foods** and adequacy of intake. *J Food Comp Anal* 17:81–97, 2004.

Ellis PR, CWC Kendall, Y Ren, C Parker, JF Pacy, KW Waldron, DJA Jenkins. Role of cell walls in the bioaccessibility of lipids in **almond seeds**. *Am J Clin Nutr* 80:604–613, 2004. (data for monosaccharides and uronic acids)

Elmastas M, O Isildak, I Turkekul, N Temur. Determination of **antioxidant activity and antioxidant compounds in wild edible mushrooms**. *J Food Comp Anal* 20:337–345, 2007.

Englberger L, W Aalbersberg, J Schierle, GC Marks, MH Fitzgerald, F Muller, A Jekkein, J Alfred, NV Velde. **Carotenoid** content of different edible **pandanus fruit** cultivars of the republic of the Marshall Islands. *J Food Comp Anal* 19:484–494, 2006.

Englberger L, J Schierle, K Kraemer, W Aalbersberg, U Dolodolotawake, J Humphries, R Graham, AP Reid, A Lorens, K Albert, A Levendusky, E Johnson, Y Paul, F Sengebau. **Carotenoid and mineral content** of Micronesian giant swamp **taro** (*Cyrtosperma*) *J Food Comp Anal* 21:93–106, 2008.

Engler MB, MM Engler. The emerging role of **flavonoid-rich cocoa and chocolate** in cardiovascular health and disease. *Nutr Rev* 64:109–118, 2006.

Engler MB, MM Engler, CY Chen, MJ Malloy, A Browne, FY Chiu, H-K Kwak, P Milbury, SM Paul, J Blumberg, ML Mietus-Snyder. **Flavonoid-rich dark chocolate** improves endothelial function and increases plasma epicatechin concentrations in healthy adults. *J Am Col Nutr* 23:197–204, 2004.

Erbas M, MK Uslu, MO Erbas, M Certel. Effects of fermentation and storage on the **organic and fatty acid contents of tarhana**, a Turkish fermented cereal food. *J Food Comp Anal* 19:294–301, 2006.

Esmaillzadeh A, f Tahbaz, I Gaieni, H Alvai-Majd, L Azadbakht. **Concentrated pomegranate juice** improves lipid profiles in diabetic patients with hyperlipidemia. *J Medicinal Food* 7:305–308, 2004.

Espana MSA, EMR Rodriguez, CD Romero. Comparison of **mineral and trace element** concentrations in **two mollusks** from the Strait of Magellan (Chile). *J Food Comp Anal* 20:273–279, 2007.

Fadavi A, M Barzegar, MH Azizi. Determination of **fatty acids and total lipid** content in oilseed of 25 **pomegranates** varieties grown in Iran. *J Food Comp Anal* 19:676–680, 2006.

Falch E, T Rustad, R Jonsdottir, NB Shaw, J Dumay, JP Berge, S Arason, JP Kerry, M Sandbakk, M Aursand. Geographical and seasonal differences in **lipid** composition and relative weight of by-products from **gadiform species**. *J Food Comp Anal* 19:727–736, 2006.

Farfan NB, N Samman. Retention of nutrients in **processed cuts of Creole cattle**. *J Food Comp Anal* 16:459–468, 2003.

Feeney MJ. **Mushrooms** – Intake, composition, and research. *Nutr Today* 41:219–226, 2006.

Feijoo O, A Moreno, E Falque. Content of *trans-* and *cis-*resveratrol in Galician white and red wines. *J Food Comp Anal* 21:608–613, 2008

Felsner ML, CB Cano, RE Bruns, HM Watanabe, LB Almeida-Muradin, JR Matos. Characterization of **monofloral honeys** by **ash** contents through a hierarchical design. *J Food Comp Anal* 17:737–747, 2004.

Fernandes G, A Velangi, TMS Wolever. **Glycemic index of potatoes** commonly consumed in North America. *J Am Diet Assoc* 105:557–562, 2005.

Field CJ. The **immunological components of human milk** and their effects on immune development in infants. *J Nutr* 135:1–4, 2005.

Finley JW. **Bioavailability of selenium** from foods. *Nutr Rev* 64:146–151, 2006.

Finley JW. **Selenium** accumulation in **plant foods**. *Nutr Rev* 63:196–202, 2005.

Finley JW, A Sigrid-Keck, RJ Robbins, KH Hintze. **Selenium** enrichment of **broccoli**: Interactions between selenium and secondary plant compounds. *J Nutr* 135:1236–1238, 2005.

Flood A, AF Subar, SG Hull, TP Zimmerman, DJA Jenkins, A Schatzkin. Methodology for adding **glycemic load values** to the national Cancer Institute Diet History Questionnaire database. *J Am Diet Assoc* 106:393–402, 2006.

Forrester-Anderson IT, J McNitt, R Way, M Way. **Fatty acid** content of pasture-reared fryer **rabbit** meat. *J Food Comp Anal* 19:715–719, 2006.

Fowomola MA, AA Akindahunsi. Nutritional quality of **sandbox tree** (*Hura crepitans* Lin.). *J Med Food* 10:159–164, 2007.

Franco I, MC Escamilla, J Garcia, MCG Fontan, J Carballo. **Fatty acid profile** of the fat from **Celta pig** breed fattened using a traditional feed: Effect of the location in the carcass. *J Food Comp Anal* 19:792–799, 2006.

Franke AA, LJ Custer, C Arakaki, SP Murphy. **Vitamin C and flavonoid levels of fruits and vegetables consumed in Hawaii**. *J Food Comp Anal* 17:1–35, 2004.

Fresco L. Commentary: **Rice** is life. *J Food Comp Anal* 18:249–253, 2005.

Frisen R, SM Innis. *Trans* **fatty acids in human milk in Canada** declined with the introduction of *trans* fat food labeling. *J Nutr* 136:2558–2561, 2006.

Frontela C, FJ Garcia-Alonso, G Ros, C Martinez. **Phytic acid and inositol phosphates** in raw **flours and infant cereals**: The effect of processing. *J Food Comp Anal* 21:343–350, 2008.

Gallaher RN, K Gallaher, AJ Marshall, AC Marshall. **Mineral** analysis of ten types of commercially available **tea**. *J Food Comp Anal* 19:S53–S57, 2006. [**Ca, Cu, Fe, Mg, Mn, P, K, Na, Zn**]

Galvano F, L La Fauci, G Graziani, R Ferracane, R Masella, C Di Giacomo, A Scacco, M D'Archivio, L Vanella, g Galvano. **Phenolic compounds** and **antioxidant activity** of Italian extra virgin **olive oil** Monti Iblei. *J Med Food* 10:650–656, 2007.

Gambelli L, GP Santaroni. **Polyphenols** content in some **Italian red wines of different geographical origins**. *J Food Comp Anal* 17:613–618, 2004.

Garsetti M, S Vinoy, V Lang, S Holt, S Loyer, JC Brand-Miller. The **glycemic and insulinemic index of plain sweet biscuits**: Relationships to in vitro starch digestibility. *J Am Col Nutr* 24:441–447, 2005.

Gezgin S, MM Ozcan, E Atalay. Determination of **minerals** extracted from several **commercial teas** (*Camellia sinensis*) to hot water (infusion). *J Med Food* 9:123–127, 2006. [**Al,As,B,Ba,Ca,Cd,Co,Cr,C,Fe,K,Li,Mg,Mn,Na,Ni,P,Pb,S,Se,Sr,V,Zn**]

Giami SY. Compositional and Nutritional properties of selected newly developed lines of **cowpea** (*Vigna unguiculata* L. Walp). *J Food Comp Anal* 18:665–673, 2005.

Girardi F, RM Cardozo, VLF de Souza, GV de Moraes, CR dos Santos, JV Visentainer, RF Zara, NE de Souza. **Proximate composition and fatty acid profile** of semi confined **young capibara** (*Hydrochoerus hydrochaeris hydrochaeris* L. 1766) meat. *J Food Comp Anal* 18:647–654, 2005.

Glew RH, JH Herbein, I Ma, M Obadofin, WA Wark, DJ VanderJagt. The *trans* **fatty acid and conjugated linoleic acid** content of **Fulani butter oil** in Nigeria. *J Food Comp Anal* 19:704–710, 2006.

Glew RS, DJ VanderJagt, R Bosse, Y-S Huang, L-T Chuang, RH Glew. The nutrient content of **three edible plants of the Republic of Niger**. *J Food Comp Anal* 18:15–27, 2005. [amino acids, fatty acids, minerals in cecego, godilo/gudai, and cabbage leaf]

Glew RS, Dj VanderJaft, Y-S Huang, L-T Chuang, R Bosse, RH Glew. Nutritional analysis of the edible pit of *Sclerocarya birrea* in the Republic of Niger (daniya, Hausa). *J Food Comp Anal* 17:99–111, 2004.

Goldberg T, W Cai, M Peppa, V Dardaine, BS Baliga, J Uribarri, H Vlassara. **Advanced glycoxidation end products** in commonly consumed foods. *J Am Diet Assoc* 104:1287–121, 2004.

Gomez-Alonso S, E Garacia-Romero, I Hermosin-Gutierrez. HPLC analysis of diverse **grape and wine phenolics** using direct injection and multidetection by DAD and fluorescence. *J Food Comp Anal* 20:618–626, 2007.

Gonzalez S, GJ Flick, SF O'Feefe, SE Duncan, E McLean, SR Craig. Composition of **farmed and wild yellow perch** (*Perca flavescens*). *J Food Comp Anal* 19:720–726, 2006. **[proximates, amino acids, minerals, fatty acids]**

Gonzalez-Manzano S, JJ Perez-Alonso, Y Salinas-Moreno, N Mateus, AMS Silva, V de Freitas, C Santos-Buelga. **Flavanol-anthocyanin pigments** in **corn**: NMR characerisation and presence in different purple corn varieties. *J Food Comp Anal* 21:521–526, 2008.

Grzanna R, L Lindmark, CG Frondoza. **Ginger** – An herbal medicinal product with broad anti-inflammatory actions. *J Med Food* 8:125–132, 2005.

Gu L, MA Kelm, JF Hammerstone, G Beecher, J Holden, D Haytowitz, S Gebhardt, RL Prior. Concentrations of **proanthocyanidins** in common foods and estimations of normal consumption. *J Nutr* 134:613–617, 2004.

Guerra NB, E de A Melo, J M Filho. **Antioxidant compounds from coriander** (*Coriandrum sativum* L.) etheric extract. *J Food Comp Anal* 18:193–199, 2005.

Haldimann M, A Alt, A Blanc, K Blondeau. **Iodine** content of food groups. *J Food Comp Anal* 18:461–471, 2005.

Han B-Z, FM Rombouts, MJR Nout. **Amino acid** profiles of **sufu**, a Chinese fermented soybean foods. *J Food Comp Anal* 17:689–698, 2004.

Hanson RM, R-Y Yang, SCS Tsou, D Ledesma, L Engle, T-C Lee. Diversity in **eggplant** (*Solanum melongena*) for **superoxide scavenging activity, total phenolics, and ascorbic acid**. *J Food Comp Anal* 19:594–600, 2006.

Harland BF, S Smikle-Williams, D Oberleas. High performance liquid chromatography analysis of **phytate (IP6) in selected foods**. *J Food Comp Anal* 17:227–233, 2004.

Harnack LJ. Availability of nutrition information on menus at major **chain table-service restaurants**. *J Am Diet Assoc* 106:1012–1015, 2006

Haskell MJ, KM Jamil, F Hassan, JM Peerson, MI Hossain, GJ Fuchs, KH Brown. Daily consumption of **Indian spinach** (*Basella alba*) or **sweet potatoes** has a positive effect on total-body **vitamin A** stores in Bangladeshi men. *Am J Clin Nutr* 80_705–714, 2004.

Hawthorne KM, SA Abrams. Safety and efficacy of **human milk fortification** for very-low-birth-weight infants. *Nutr Rev* 62:482–489, 2004.

He M, K Openo, M McCullough, DP Jones. Total equivalent of reactive chemicals in 142 human food items is highly variable within and between major food groups. *J Nutr* 134:1114–1119, 2004. (**glutathione**)

Heinemann RJB, PL Fagundes, EA Pinto, MVC Penteado, UM Lanfer-Marquez. Comparative study of nutrient composition of comercial **brown, parboiled, and milled rice** from Brazil. *J Food Comp Anal* 18:287–296, 2005. (water, protein, crude fat, ash, 10 minerals)

Hels O, T Larsen, LP Christensen, U Kidmose, N Hassan, SH Thilsted. Contents of **iron, calcium, zinc and beta-carotene in commonly consumed vegetables in Bangladesh**. *J Food Comp Anal* 17:587–595, 2004.

Heo K-S, K-T Lim. Antioxidative effects of **glycoprotein** isolated from *Solanun nigrum* L. *J Medicinal Food* 7:349–357, 2004.

Hidaka S, SY Liu. Effects of gelatins on **calcium phosphate** precipitation: A possible application for distinguishing **bovine bone gelatin** from **porcine skin gelatin**. *J Food Comp Anal* 16:477–483, 2003.

Hidiroglou N, RW Peace, P Jee, D Leggee, H Kuhnlein. Levels of **folate, pyridoxine, niacin and riboflavin** in traditional foods of **Canadian Arctic indigenous peoples**. *J Food Comp Anal* 21:474–480, 2008.

Hoffman LC, K Smit, N Muller. Chemical characteristics of **blesbok** (*Damaliscus dorcas phillipsi*) meat. *J Food Comp Anal* 21:315–319, 2008.

Holden JM, SA Bhagwat, DB Haytowitz, SE Gebhardt, JT Dwyer, J Peterson, GR Beecher, AL Eldridge, D Balentine. Development of a database of critically evaluated **flavonoids** data: Application of USDA's data quality evaluation system. *J Food Comp Anal* 18:829–844, 2005.

Hou C-Y, Y-S Lin, YT Wang, C-M Jiang, M-C Wu. Effect of storage conditions on **methanol** content of **fruit and vegetable juices**. *J Food Comp Anal* 21:410–415, 2008.

Hulshof PJM, T Kosmeijer-Schuil, CE West, PCH Hollman. Quick screening of **maize** kernels for **provitamin A** content, *J Food Comp Anal* 20:655–661, 2007.

Hulshof PJM, T van Roekel-Jansen, P van de Bovenkamp, CE West. Variation in **retinol and carotenoid content of milk and milk products in The Netherlands**. *J Food Comp Anal* 19:67–75, 2005.

Hunt CD, NF Butte, LAK Johnson. **Boron** concentrations in **milk** from mothers of exclusively breast-fed healthy full-term infants are stable during the first four months of lactation. *J Nutr* 135:2383–2386, 2005.

Hunt C, JK Friel, LK Johnson. **Boron** concentrations in **milk** from mothers of full-term and premature infants. *Am J Clin Nutr* 80:1327–1333, 2004. (also includes copper, iron, zinc, and selenium)

Hwant E-S, EH Jeffery. Effects of different processing methods on induction of **quinine** reductase by dietary **broccoli** in rats. *J Med Food* 7:95–99, 2004.

Hymavathi TV, V Khader. **Carotene, ascorbic acid, and sugar** content of **vacuum dehydrated ripe mango powders** stored in flexible packaging material. *J Food Comp Anal* 18:181–192, 2005.

Iacopini P, M Baldi, P Storchi, L Sebastiani. **Catechin, epicatechin, quercetin, rutin, and resveratrol in red grape**: Content, *in vitro* **antioxidant activity** and interactions. *J Food Comp Anal* 21:589–598, 2008.

Ibanez JG, A Carreon-Alvarez, M Barcena-Soto, N Casillas. **Metals** in **alcoholic beverages**: A review of sources, effects, concentrations, removal, speciation, and analysis. *J Food Comp Anal* 21:672–683, 2008. **[Al, CA, Cd, Cu, Fe, Pb, Mg, Mn, Ni, K, Na, Zn]**

Ikeda I, K Tsuda, Y Suzuki, M Kobayashi, T Unno, H Tomoyori, H Goto, Y Kawata, K Imaizumi, A Nozawa, T Kakuda. **Tea catechins** with a galloyl moiety suppress postprandial hypertriacylglycerolemia by delaying lymphatic transport of dietary fat in rats. *J Nutr* 135:155–159, 2005.

Ikem A, NO Egiebor. Assessment of **trace elements** in **canned** fishes (**mackerel, tuna, salmon, sardines, and herrings**) marketed in Georgia and Alabama (United States of America). *J Food Comp Anal* 18:771–787, 2005.

Ilcol YO, R Ozbek, E Hamurtekin, IH Ulus. **Choline** status in newborns, infants, children, breast-feeding women, breast-fed infants, and **human breast milk**. *J Nutr Biochem* 16L489–499, 2005.

Indarti E, MIA Majid, R Hashim, A Chong. Direct FAME synthesis for rapid total **lipid** analysis from **fish oil and cod liver oil**. *J Food Comp Anal* 18:161–170, 2005.

Inoue K, S Murayama, K Takeba, Y Yoshimura, H Nakazawa. Contamination of **xeroestrogens bisphenol A and F in honey**: Safety assessment and analytical method of these compounds in honey. *J Food Comp Anal* 16:497–506, 2003.

Iqbal S, MI Bhanger. Effect of season and production location on **antioxidant activity of *Moringa oleifera* leaves** grown in Pakistan. *J Food Comp Anal* 19:544–551, 2006.

Ishak SA, N Ismail, MAM Noor, H Ahmad. Some physical and chemical properties of **ambarella** (*Spondias cytheres* Sonn.) at three different stages of maturity. *J Food Comp Anal* 18:819–827, 2005.

Issa AY, SR Volate, MJ Wargovich. The role of **phytochemicals** in inhibition of cancer and inflammation: New Directions and perspectives. *J Food Comp Anal* 19:405–419, 2006. [ORAC values for fruits and vegetables]

Iwalewa EO, Co Adewunmi, NOA Omisore, OA Adebanji, Ck Azike, AO Adigun, OA Adesina, OG Olowoyo. **Pro- and antioxidant effects and cytoprotective potentials of nine edible vegetables in southwest Nigeria**. *J Med Food* 8:539–544, 2005.

Jaaarsveld PJ, DW Marais, E Harmse, P Nestel, DB Rodriguez-Amaya. Retention of **β-cartene** in boiled, mashed orange-fleshed **sweet potato**. *J Food Comp Anal* 19:321–329, 2006.

Jakobsen J, I Clausen, T Leth, L Ovesen. A new method for the determination of **vitamin D3 and 25-hydroxyvitamin D3 in meat.** *J Food Comp Anal* 17:777–787, 2004.

Jakszyn P, A Agudo, R Ibanez, R Garcia-Closas, G Pera, P Amiano, CA Gonzalez. Development of a food database of **nitrosamines, heterocyclic amines, and polycyclic aromatic hydrocarbons**. *J Nutr* 134:2011–2014, 2004.

Jalbani N, TG Kazi, MK Jamali, BM Arain, HI Afridi, A Baloch. Evaluation of **aluminum** contents in different **bakery foods** by electrothermal atomic absorption spectrometer. *J Food Comp Anal* 20:226–231, 2007.

Johnson MA. Influence of vitamin K on anticoagulant therapy depends on vitamin K status and the source and chemical forms of vitamin K. *Nutr Rev* 63:91–97, 2005. **[vitamin K in green vegetables, vegetable oils, and nutritional supplements]**

Jonnala RS, NT Dunford, KE Dashiell. **Tocopherol, phytosterol, and phospholipids** compositions of new **high oleic peanut cultivars**. *J Food Comp Anal* 19:601–605, 2006.

Joung H, G Nam, S Yoon, J Lee, JE Shim, HY Paik. Bioavailable zinc intake of Korean adults in relation to the **phytate content of Korean foods**. *J Food Comp Anal* 17:713–724, 2004.

Juarex MD, ME Alfaro, N Samman. **Nutrient retention factors of deep-fried milanesas**. *J Food Comp Anal* 17:119–124, 2004.

Judprasong K, S Charoenkiatkyl, P Susnguag, K Vasanachitt, Y Nakjamanong. **Total and soluble oxalate contents in Thai vegetables, cereal grains, and legume seeds** and their changes after cooking. *J Food Comp Anal* 19:340–347, 2006.

Junhua H, Y Yuexin, C Shruong, W Zhu, W Xiaoli, W Guodong, M Jianhua. Comparison of nutrient composition of **parental rice and rice genetically modified** with cowpea trypsin inhibitor in China. *J Food Comp Anal* 18:297–302, 2005. (macro nutrients, amino acids, fatty acids, thiamin, riboflavin, 9 minerals)

Kabelova I, M Dvorakova, H Cizkova, P Dostalek, K Melzoch. Determination of **free amino acids in beers**: A comparison of Czech and foreign brands. *J Food Comp Anal* 21:736–741, 2008.

Kallithraka S, A A-A Mohdaly, DP Makris, P Kefalas. Determination of major **anthocyanin** pigments in **Hellenic native grape varieties** (*Vitis vinifers* sp.): Association with antiradical activity. *J Food Comp Anal* 18:375–386, 2005.

Kamizake NKK, MM Goncalves, CTBV Zaiz, DAM Zaia. Determination of **total proteins in cow milk powder** samples: A comparative study between the Kjeldahl method and spectrohotometric methods. *J Food Comp Anal* 16:507–516, 2003.

Kano M, T Takayanagi, K Harada, S Sawada, F Ishikawa. Bioavailability of **isoflavones** after ingestion of **soy beverages** in healthy adults. *J Nutr* 136:2291–2296, 2006.

Karabulut I, S Turan. Some properties of **margarines and shortenings marketed in Turkey**. *J Food Comp Anal* 19:55–58, 2005.

Karunaratne AM, PH Amerasinghe, VMS Pamanujam, HH Sandstead, PAJ Perera. **Zinc, iron and phytic acid** levels of some popular foods consumed by rural children in **Sri Lanka**. *J Food Comp Anal* 21:481–488, 2008.

Kawashima LM, LM Valente Soares. **Mineral profile of raw and cooked leafy vegetables** consumed in Southern Brazil. *J Food Comp Anal* 16:605–611, 2003.

Keen CL, RR Holt, PI Oteiza, CG Fraga, HH Schmitz. **Coca antioxidants** and cardiovascular health. *Am J Clin Nutr* 81:298S–303S, 2005.

Kennedy G, O Islam, P Eyzaguirre, S Kennedy. Field testing of plant genetic diversity indicators for nutrition surveys: **Rice-based diet** of rural Bangladesh as a model. *J Food Comp Anal* 18:255–268, 2005.

Kent JA, LR Mitoulas, MD Cregan, DT Ramsay, DA Doherty, PE Hartmann. Volume and frequency of breast-feedings and **fat content of breast milk** throughout the day. *Pediatrics* 117:387–395, 2006.

Khambalia A, ME Latulippe, C Campos, CMS Villalpando, MF Picciano, DL O'Connor. **Milk folate** secretion is not impaired during iron deficiency in humans. *J Nutr* 136:2617–2624, 2006.

Khanizadeh S, R Tsao, D Rekika, R Yang, MT Charles, HPV Rupasinghe. **Polyphenol** composition and **total antioxidant capacity** of selected **apple** genotypes for processing. *J Food Comp Anal* 21:396–401, 2008.

Kidmose U, R-Y Yang, SH Thilsted, LP Christensen, K Brandt. Content of **carotenoids** in commonly consumed **Asian vegetables** and stability and extractability during frying. *J Food Comp Anal* 19:562–571, 2006.

Kim DC, HJ Chae, M-J In. Existence of stable **fibrin-clotting inhibitor in salt-fermented anchovy sauce**. *J Food Comp Anal* 17:113–118, 2004.

Kim S-H, C-B Cui, I-J Kang, SY Kim, S-S Ham. Cytotoxic effect of **buckwheat** (*Fagopyrum esculentum* Moench) **hull** against cancer cells. *J Med Food* 10:232–238, 2007. [minerals Ca, P, Fe, Na, K; fatty acids]

Kim H-K, S-H Ye, T-S Lim, T-Y Ha, J-H Kwon. Physiological activities of **garlic extracts** as affected by habitat and solvents. *J Med Food* 8:476–481, 2005.

Kim M, E-S Kim, M-H Park, S-J Hwang, Y Jeong. **Saengshik**, a formulated health food, decreases blood glucose and increases survival rate in streptozotocin-induced diabetic rats. *J Med Food* 7:162–167, 2004.

Kim M-J, S-J Rhee. **Green tea catechins** protect rats from microwave-induced oxidative damage to heart tissue. *J Medicinal Food* 7:299–304, 2004

Kim M-Y, K Iwai, H Matsue. **Phenolic compositions of Viburnum dilatatum Thunb. Fruits** and their antiradical properties. *J Food Comp Anal* 18:789–802, 2005.

Kim Y-N, DW Giraud, JA Driskell. **Tocopherol and carotenoid** contents of selected **Korean fruits and vegetables**. *J Food Comp Anal* 20:458–465, 2007.

Kiss SA, T Forster, A Dongo. Absorption and effect of the **magnesium** content of a **mineral water** in the human body. *J Am Col Nutr* 23:758S–762S, 2004.

Kiss SA, E Stafanovits-Banyai, M Takacs-Hajos. **Magnesium content of *Rhizobium* nodules in different plants**: The importance of magnesium in nitrogen-fixation of nodules. *J Am Col Nutr* 23:751S–753S, 2004.

Kitta K, M Ebihara, T Iizuka, R Yoshikawa, K Isshiki, S Kawamoto. Variations in **lipid** content and **fatty acid** composition of major **non-glutinous rice cultivars** in Japan. *J Food Comp Anal* 18:269–278, 2005.

Klimczak I, M Malecka, M Szlachta, A Gliszezynska-Swiglo. Effect of storage on the content of **polyphenols, vitamin C, and the antioxidant activity of orange juices**. *J Food Comp Anal* 20:313–322, 2007.

Knize MG, JS Felton. Formation and human risk of carcinogenic **heterocyclic amines** formed from natural precursors in **meat**. *Nutr Rev* 63:158–165, 2005.

Kong L, Y Wang, Y Cao. Determination of *myo*-**inositol and d-*chiro*-inositol in black rice bran** by capillary electrophoresis with electrochemical detection. *J Food Comp Anal* 21:501–504, 2008.

Krawinkel MB, GB Deding. **Bitter gourd** (*Momordica charantia*): A dietary approach to hyperglycemia. *Nutr Rev* 64:331–337, 2006.

Kubo H, K Fujii, T Kawabe, S Matsumoto, H Kishida, K Hosoe. Food content of **ubiquinol-10 and ubiquinone-10** in the Japanese diet. *J Food Comp Anal* 21:199–210, 2008. **(coenzyme Q10)**

Kubo I, N Masuoka, K-I Nihei, B Burgheim. **Manicoba, a quercetin-rich Amazonian dish**. *J Food Comp Anal* 19:579–588, 2006.

Kuda T, M Tsunekawa. H Goto, Y Araki. **Antioxidant properties** of four **edible algae** harvested in the Noto Peninsla, Japan. *J Food Comp Anal* 18:625–633, 2005.

Kuhnlein HV, V Barthet, A Farren, E Falahi, D Leggee, O Receveur, P Berti. **Vitamins A, D, and E in Canadian Arctic traditional food** and adult diets. *J Food Comp Anal* 19:495–506, 2006.

Kuman GS, H Nayaka, SM Dharmesh, PV Salimath. Free and bound **phenolic antioxidants in amla** (*Emblica officinalis*) and **turmeric** (*Curcuma longa*). *J Food Comp Anal* 19:446–452, 2006.

Kumar S, B Aalbersberg. Nutrient retention in foods after earth-oven cooking compared to other forms of domestic cooking. 1. **Proximates, carbohydrates, and dietary fibre.** *J Food Comp Anal* 19:302–310, 2006.

Kumar S, B Aalbersberg. Nutrient retention in foods after earth-oven cooking compard to other forms of domestic cooking. 2. **Vitamins.** *J Food Comp Anal* 19:311–320, 2006. [retinol, beta-carotene, thiamin, riboflavin, niacin, and ascorbic acid]

Kumar V, A Rani, S Solanki, SM Hussain. Influence of growing environment on the biochemical composition and physical characteristics of **soybean seed.** *J Food Comp Anal* 19:188–195, 2006.

Kupper C, Dietary guidelines and implementation for celiac disease. *Gastroenterology* 128:S121–S127, 2005. **[gluten]**

Kuti JO, HB Konoru. **Cyanogenic glycosides** content in two edible leaves of **tree spinach** (*Cnidoscolus* spp.). *J Food Comp Anal* 19:556–561, 2006.

Lamont WH. Concentration of inorganic **arsenic** in samples of **white rice** from the United States. *J Food Comp Anal* 16:687–695, 2003.

Lansky EP. Beware of **pomegranates** bearing 40% **ellagic acid.** *J Med Food* 9:119–122, 2006.

Larsen R, SK Sormo, BT Dragnes, EO Elvevoll. Losses of **taurine, creatine, glycine, and alanine** from **cod** (*Gadus morhua* L.) fillet during processing. *J Food Comp Anal* 20:396–402, 2007.

Ledauphin J, B Basset, S Cohen T Payot, D Barillier. Identification of trace volatile compounds in freshly **distilled calvados and cognac: Carbonyl and sulphur compounds.** *J Food Comp Anal* 19:28–40, 2005.

Ledoux M, J-M Chardigny, M Darbois, Y Soustre, J-L Sebedio, L Laloux. **Fatty acid** composition of **French butters**, with special emphasis on **conjugated linoleic acid (CLA)** isomers. *J Food Comp Anal* 18:409–425, 2005.

Lee H-S, Y-H Cho, S-O Park, S-H Kye, B-H Kim, T-S Hahm, M Kim, JO Lee, C-i Kim. Dietary exposure of the Korean population to **arsenic, cadmium, lead, and mercury.** *J Food Comp Anal* 19:S31–S37, 2006.

Lee J, K-T Hwang, M-S Heo, J-H Lee, K-Y Park. Resistance of *Lactobacillus plantarum* KCTC 3099 from **kimchi** to **oxidative stress.** *J Med Food* 8:299–304, 2005.

Lee K-S, Y-S Choi, J-S Seo. **Sea tangle** supplementation lowers blood glucose and supports antioxidant systems in streptozotocin-induced diabetic rats. *J Med Food* 7:130–135, 2004.

Lee SH, Bh Jung, SY Kim, BC Chung. Determination of **phytoestrogens in traditional medicinal herbs** using gas chromatography-mass spectrometry. *J Nutr Biochem* 15:452–460, 2004.

Leonard SW, CK Good, ET Gugger, MG Traber. **Vitamin E** bioavailability from fortified **breakfast cereal** is greater than that from encapsulated supplements. *Am J Clin Nutr* 79:86892, 2004.

Leskova E, J Kubikova, E Kovacikova, M Kosicka, J Porubska, K Holcikova. **Vitamin losses:** Retention during **heat treatment** and continual changes expressed by mathematical models. *J Food Comp Anal* 19:252–276, 2006.

Levenson CW, DX Axelrad. Too much of a good thing? Update on **fish** consumption and **mercury** exposure. *Nutr Rev* 64:139–145, 2006

Lewis NM, J Ruud. **Blueberies** in the American diet. *Nutr Today* 40:92–96, 2005. [anthocyanins, antioxidant capacity]

Li C, Z Li, M Fa, W cheng, Y Long, T Ding, L Ming. The composition of *Hirsutella sinensis*, anamorph of *Cordyceps sinensis.* *J Food Comp Anal* 19:800–805, 2006. [fungi]

Liang H, QP Yuan, HR Dong, YM Liu. Determination of **sulforaphane in broccoli and cabbage** by high-performance liquid chromatography. *J Food Comp Anal* 19:473–476, 2006.

Lichtenstein AH, NR Matthan, Sm Jalbert, NA Resteghini, EJ Schaeer, LM Ausman. Novel **soybean oils** with different **fatty acid profiles** alter cardiovascular disease risk factors in moderately hyperlpidemic subjects. *Am J Clin Nutr* 84:497–504, 2006.

Lila MA, GG Yousef, Y Jiang, CM Weaver. Sorting out bioactivity in **flavonoid** mixtures. *J Nutr* 135:1231–1235, 2005. [phenolic acids, total phenolics in fruits]

Lin L-Z, S Mukhopadhyay, RJ Robbins, JM Harnly. Identification and quantification of **flavonoids of Mexican oregano** (*Lippia graveolens*) by LC-DAD-ESI/MS analysis. *J Food Comp Anal* 20:361–369, 2007.

Lisiewska Z, W Kmiecik, A Korus. Content of **vitamin C, carotenoids, cholorophylls and polyphenols in green parts of dill** (Anethum graveoleens L.) depending on plant height. *J Food Comp Anal* 19:134–140, 2006.

List GR. Decreasing **trans and saturated fatty acid** content in **food oils.** *Food Tech* 58:23–31, 2004.

Liu X, M Ahzo, J Wang, B Yang, Y Jiang. **Antioxidant activity** of methanolic extract of **embilca fruit** (*Phyllanthus emblica* L.) from six regions in China. *J Food Comp Anal* 21:219–228, 2008.

Lombard K, E Peffley, E Geoffriau, L Thompson, A Herring. **Quercetin in onion** (*Allium cepa* L.) alter heat-treatment simulating home preparation. *J Food Comp Anal* 18:571–581, 2005.

Lombardi-Boccia G, S Lanzi, A Aguzzi. Aspects of meat quality: **trace elements and B vitamins in raw and cooked meats.** *J Food Comp Anal* 18:39–46, 2005. [Fe, Zn, Cu, B1, B2, niacin]

Lopez MJO, M Innocenti, F Ieri, C Giaccherini, a Romani, N Mulinacci. HPLC/DAD/ESI/MS detection of **lignans** from Spanish and Italian *Olea europaea* L. **fruits.** *J Food Comp Anal* 21:62–70, 2008.

Lopez-Amoros ML, T Hernandez, I Estrella. Effect of germination on **legume phenolic compounds and their antioxidant activity.** *J Food Comp Anal* 19:277–283, 2006.

Lopez-Ortiz CM, S Prats-Moya, AB Sanahuja, SE Maestre-Perez, N Grane-Teruel, ML Martin-Carratala. Comparative study of **tocopherol** homologue content in four **almond oil** cultivars during two consecutive years. *J Food Comp Anal* 21:144–151, 2008.

Lorenzo C, F Pardo, A Zalacain, Gl Alonso, MR Salinas. Complementary effect of Cabernet Sauvignon on **Monastrell wines.** *J Food Comp Anal* 21:54–61, 2008. **[polyphenols, anthocyanins]**

Lubetzky R, Y Littner, FB Mimouni, S Dollberg, D Mandel. Circadian variations in **fat content of expressed breast milk** from mothers of preterm infants. *J Am Coll Nutr* 25:151–154, 2006.

Luthria DL, MA Pastor-Corrales. **Phenolic acids** content of fifteen dry edible **bean** (*Phaseolus vulgaris* L.) **varieties.** *J Food Comp Anal* 19:205–211, 2006.

Luthria DL, S Mukhopadhyay, DT Krizek. Content of **total pheonlics and phenolic acids in tomato** (*Lycopersicon esculentum* Mill.) fruits as influenced by cultivar and solar UV radiation. *J Food Comp Anal* 19:771–777, 2006.

Lutter CK, KG Dewey. **Proposed nutrient composition for fortified complementary foods.** *J Nutr* 133:3011S–3020S, 2003.

MacArtain P, CIR Gill, M Brooks, R Campbell, IR Rowland. Nutritional value of edible **seaweeds.** *Nutr Rev* 65:535–543, 2007. **[total, soluble, insoluble fiber; carbohydrate; Ca, K, MG, Na, Cu, Fe, I, Zn; fatty acids; B vitamins, vitamins C and E]**

MacDonald RS, JY Guo, J Copeland, JD Browning, D Sleper, GE Rottinghaus, MA Berhow. Environmental influences on **isoflavones and saponins in soybeans** and their role in colon cancer. J Nutr 135:1239–1232, 2005.

MacLean Jr WC. Use of the **net metabolizable energy** values for labeling of **infant formulas and foods** – potential issues. *J Food Comp Anal* 18:223–239, 2005.

Maisuthisakul P, S Pasuk, P Ritthiruangdej. Relationship between **antioxidant** properties and chemical composition of some Thai plants. *J Food Comp Anal* 21:229–240, 2008.

Makris DP, G Boskou, NK Andrikopoulos. **Polyphenolic content** and in vitro **antioxidant characteristics of wine** industry and other agri-food solid waste extracts. *J Food Comp Anal* 20:125–132, 2007.

Makris DP, S Kallithraka, P Kefalas. **Flavonols in grapes, grape products and wines**: Burden, profile and influential parameters. *J Food Comp Anal* 19:396–404, 2006.

Manach C, A Scalbert, C Morand, C Remesy, L Jimenez. **Polyphenols**: Food sources and bioavailability. *Am J Clin Nutr* 79:727–747, 2004.

Manach C, G Williamson, C Morand, A Scalbert, C Remesy. Bioavailability and bioefficacy of **polyphenols** in humans. I. Review of 97 bioavailability studies. *Am J Clin Nutr* 8:230S–242S, 2005.

Marcason W. What are the facts and myths about **mangosteen**? *J Am Diet Assoc* 106:986, 2006.

Marinova D, F Ribarova. HPLC determination of **carotenoids in Bulgarian berries**. *J Food Comp Anal* 20:370–374, 2007.

Mark BK, JAS Carson. **Vitamin D** and autoimmune disease-Implications for practice from the multiple sclerosis literature. *J Am Diet Assoc* 106:418–424, 2006. [vitamin D and **calcium** in **dietary supplements**]

Martin CL, SP Murphy, DLM Au. Compiling **glycemic index** and **glycemic load** values for addition to a food composition database. *J Food Comp Anal* 21:469–473, 2008.

Martinez-Villaluenga C, A Cardelle-Cobas, N Corzo, A Olano. Study of **galactooligosacharide** composition in commercial **fermented milks**. *J Food Comp Anal* 21:540–544, 2008.

Matloubi H, F Aflaki, M Hadjiezadegan. Effect of **gamma-irradiation on amino acids content of baby food proteins**. *J Food Comp Anal* 17:133–139, 2004.

Mattila P, J Hellstrom. **Phenolic acids in potatoes, vegetables**, and some of their products. *J Food Comp Anal* 20:152–160, 2007.

Mazida MM, MM Salleh, H Osman. Analysis of **volatile aroma compounds** of fresh **chilli (Capsicum annuum)** during stages of maturity using solid phase microextraction (SPME). *J Food Comp Anal* 18:427–437, 2005.

Mazza G, T Cottrell. **Carotenoids and cyanogenic glucosides in Saskatoon berries** (*Amelanchier alnifolia* Nutt.). *J Food Comp Anal* 21:249–254, 2008.

McCabe-Sellers BJ, CG Staggs, ML Bogle. **Tyramine** in foods and monoamine oxidase inhibitor drugs: A crossroad where medicine, nutrition, pharmacy, and food industry converge. *J Food Comp Anal* 19:S58–S65, 2006.

McKay DL, JB Blumberg. **Cranberries** (*Vaccinium macrocarpon*) and cardiovascular disease risk factors. *Nutr Rev* 65:490–502, 2007. [proximates, vitamins, minerals, carotenoids, proanthocyanidins, phenolic compounds]

Melendez-Martinez, AJ, IM Vicario, FJ Heredia. Review: Analysis of **carotenoids in orange juice**. *J Food Comp Anal* 20:638–649, 2007.

Mendez LA, CAS Castro, RB Casso, CMC Leal. Effect of substrate and harvest on the **amino acid** profile of **oyster mushroom** (*Pleurotas ostreatus*). *J Food Comp Anal* 18:447–450, 2005.

Mezadri T, D Villano, MS Fernandez-Pachon, MC Garcia-Parrilla, Am Troncoso. **Antioxidant compounds** and antioxidant **activity** in **acerola** (*Malpighia emarginata* DC.) fruits and derivatives. *J Food Comp Anal* 21:282–290, 2008.

Milinsk MC, R das G Padre, C Hayashi, CC de Oliveira, JV Visentainer, NE de Souza, M Matsushita. Effects of feed protein and lipid contents on **fatty acid profile of snail** (*Helix aspersa maxima*) **meat**. *J Food Comp Anal* 19:212–216, 2006.

Miller-Ihli, NJ, PR Pehrsson, RL Cutrifelli, JM Holden. **Fluoride content of municipal water in the United States**: what percentage if fluoridated? *J Food Comp Anal* 16:621–628, 2003

Misra JB. A mathematical approach to comprehensive evaluation of quality in **groundnut**. *J Food Comp Anal* 17:69–79, 2004.

Mohamed R, M Pineda, M Aguilar. **Antioxidant capacity** of extracts from wild and crop plants of the Mediterranean region. *J Food Sci* 72:S59–S63, 2007

Molldrem KL, J Li, PW Simon, SA Tanumihardjo. **Lutein and beta-carotene** from lutein-containing yellow **carrots** and bioavailable in humans. *Am J Clin Nutr* 80:131–136, 2004.

Monroe D, L Young, JK Wilson, A Chisholm. The **sodium** content of **low cost and private label foods**: Implications for public health. *J NZ Diet Assoc* 58:4–10, 2004.

Monro J. Redefining the **glycemic index** for dietary management of postprandial glycemia. *J Nutr* 133:4256–4258, 2003.

Montealegre RR, RR Peces, JLC Vozmediano, JM Gascuena, EG Romero. **Phenolic compounds in skins and seeds** of ten **grape** *Vitis vinifera* varieties grown in a warm climate. *J Food Comp Anal* 19:687–693, 2006.

Montiel-Herrera M, IL Camacho-Hernandez, A Rios-Morgan, F Delgado-Vargas. Partial physiocochemical and nutritional characterization of the **fruit of** *Vitex mollis* **(Verbenaceae).** *J Food Comp Anal* 17:205–215, 2004.

Moraru C, L Logendra, T-C Lee, H Janes. Characteristics of 10 processing **tomato cultivars grown hydroponically** for the NASA Advanced Life Support (ALS) Program. *J Food Comp Anal* 17:141–154, 2004.

Mosley EE, AL Wright, MK McGuie, MA McGuire. ***Trans* fatty acids in milk produced by women in the United States**. *Am J Clin Nutr* 82:1292–1297, 2005.

Most MM, R Tulley, S Morales, M Lefevre. **Rice bran oil**, not fiber, lowers cholesterol in humans. *Am J Clin Nutr* 81:64–68, 2005. [fatty acids in rice bran oil]

Mourvaki E, G Stefania, R Rossi, S Rufini. **Passionflower fruit** – A new source of **lycopene**. *J Med Food* 8:104–106, 2005.

Mulder TP, AG Rietveld, JM van Amelsvoort. Consumption of both **black tea** and **green tea** results in an increase in the excretion of hippuric acid into urine. *Am J Clin Nutr* 81:256S–260S, 2005. [polyphenols in tea]

Musumeci M, J Simpore, A D'Agata, S Sotgiu, S Musumeci. **Oligosaccharides in colostrum** of Italian and Burkinabe women. *J Ped Gastro Nutr* 43:372–378, 2006.

Nada V, BC Sarkar, HK Sharma, AS Bawa. Physico-chemical properties and estimation of **mineral content in honey** produced form different plants in Northern India. *J Food Comp Anal* 16:613–619, 2003.

Naddeo V, T Zarra, V Belgiorno. A comparative approach to the variation of natural **elements in Italian bottled waters** according to the national and international standard limits. *J Food Comp Anal* 21:505–514, 2008.

Nagao T, Y Komine, S Soga, S Meguro, T Hase, Y Tanaka, I Tokimitsu. Ingestión of a **tea** rich in **catechins** leads to a reduction in body fat and malondialdehyde-modified LDL in men. *Am J Clin Nutr* 81:122–129, 2005.

Nakano S, H Takekoshi, M Nakano. *Chlorella (Chlorella pyrenoidosa)* supplementation decreases **dioxin** and increases **immunoglobulin A** concentrations in **breast milk**. *J Med Food* 10:134–142, 2007.

Nardini M, F Natella, C Scaccini, A Ghiselli. **Phenolic acids** from **beer** are absorbed and extensively metabolized in humans. *J Nutr Biochem* 17:14–22, 2006.

Navarro-Garcia G, L Bringas-Alvarado, R Pacheco-Aguilar, J Ortega-Garcia. **Oxidative resistance, carotenes, tocopherols, and lipid profile of liver oil of the ray** *Rhinoptera steindechneri*. *J food Comp Anal* 17:699–706, 2004.

Ngassoum MB, H Ousmaila, LT Ngamo, PM Maponmetsem, L Jirovetz, G Buchbauer. Aroma compounds of **essential oils** of two varieties of the **spice plant** *Ocimum canum* Sims from northern Cameroon. *J Food Comp Anal* 17:197–204, 2004.

Ngom PT, AC Collinson, J Pido-Lopea, SM Henson, AM Prentice, R Aspinall. Improved thymic function in exclusively breastfed infants is associated with higher **interleukin 7** concentration in their mothers' **breast milk**. *Am J Clin Nutr* 80:722–738, 2004.

Niemenak N, C Rohsius, S Elwers, DO Ndoumou, R Lieberei. Comparative study of different **cocoa** (*Theobroma cacao* L.) clones in terms of their **phenolics and anthocyanins** contents. *J Food Comp Anal* 19:612–619, 2006.

Niewinski MM. Advances in celiac disease and **gluten-free diet**. *J Am Diet Assoc* 108:661–672, 2008.

Niizu PY, DB Rodriguez-Amaya. New data on the **carotenoid** composition of **raw salad vegetables**. *J Food Comp Anal* 18:739–749, 2005.

Nishitani E, YM Sagesaka. Simultaneous determination of **catechins, caffeine and other phenolic compounds in tea** using new HPLC method. *J Food Comp Anal* 17:675–685, 2004.

Nojavan S, F Khalilian, FM Kiaie, A Rahimi, A Arabanian, S Chalavi. Extraction and quantitative determination of **ascorbic acid** during different maturity stages of *Rosa canina* **L. fruit**. *J Food Comp Anal* 21:300–305, 2008.

Normen L, L Ellegard, H Brants, P Dutta, H Andersson. A **phytosterol** database: Fatty foods consumed in Sweden and the Netherlands. *J Food Comp Anal* 20:193–201, 2007.

Oboh G, AA Akindahunsi. **Nutritional and toxicological evaluation of** *Saccharomyces cerevisae* **fermented cassava flour**. *J Food Comp Anal* 18:731–738, 2005.

Oboh G, MM Ekperigin, MI Kazeem. **Nutritional and haemolytic properties of eggplants** (*Solanum macrocarpon*) **leaves**. *J Food Comp Anal* 18:153–160, 2005.

Oboh G, CA Elusiyan. Nutrient composition and antimicrobial activity of **sorrel drinks** (soborodo). *J Medicinal Food* 7:340–342, 2004.

Oboh G. Nutritive value, antioxidant and antimicrobial properties of *Struchium sparganophora* leaves. *J Medicinal Food* 9:276–280, 2006.

Odhav B, S Beekrum, U Akula, H Baijnath. Preliminary assessment of nutritional value of traditional **leafy vegetables** in KwaZulu-Natal, South Africa. *J Food Comp Anal* 20:430–435, 2007.

O'Donnell SI, SL Hoerr, JA Mendoza, ET Goh. Nutrient quality of **fast food kids meals**. *Am J Clin Nutr* 88:13881395, 2008. [**fat, saturated fat, protein, Ca, Fe, vitamin A, vitamin C**]

Oh C-K, M-C Oh, S-H Kim. The depletion of **sodium nitrite** by lactic acid bacteria isolated from **kimchi**. *J Med Food* 7:38–44, 2004.

Ohtsubo K, K Suzuki, Y Yasui, T Kasumi. **Bio-functional components** in the **processed pre-germinated brown rice** by a twin-screw extruder. *J Food Comp Anal* 18:303–316, 2005.

Olguin MC, N Hisano, AE D'Ottavio, MI Zingale, GC Revelant, SA Calderari. Nutritional and antinutritional aspects of an Argentinian **soy flour** assessed on weanling rats. *J Food Comp Anal* 16:441–449, 2003.

Olmez H, F Tuncay, N Ozcan, S Demirel. A survey of **acrylamide** levels in foods from the **Turkish market**. *J Food Comp Anal* 21:564–568, 2008.

Onabanjo OO, CRB Oguntona. **Iron, zinc, copper,** and **phytate** content of standardized **Nigerian dishes**. *J Food Comp Anal* 16:669–676, 2003.

Orban E, M Masci, T Nevigato, G Di Lena, I Casini, R Caproni, L Gambelli, P De Angelis, M Rampacci. Nutritional quality and safety of **whitefish** (*Coregonus lavaretus*) from Italian lakes. *J Food Comp Anal* 19:737–746, 2006. [**proximates, minerals, lipids, fatty acids**]

Ortiz CML, MS P Moya, VB Navarro. A rapid chromatographic method for simultaneous determination of **beta-sitosterol and tocopherol** homologues in **vegetable oils**. *J Food Comp Anal* 19:141–149, 2006.

Ouzouni PK, PG Veltsistas, EK Paleologos, KA Riganakos. Determination of **metal** content in wild edible **mushroom** species from regions of **Greece**. *J Food Comp Anal* 20:480–486, 2007. [Mg, Cr, Mn, Fe, Co, Ni, Cu, Zn, PB, Cd]

Ozcan M. **Antioxidant activities of rosemary, sage, and sumac** extracts and their combinations on stability of natural peanut oil. *J Med Food* 6:267–270, 2003.

Ozcan M. **Mineral composition** of different parts of *Capparis ovata* Desf. var. *canescens* (Coss.) **heywood** growing wild in Turkey. *J Med Food* 8:405–407, 2005.

Ozcan M. Determination of **mineral** contents of **Turkish herbal tea** (*Salvia aucheri* var. *canescens*) at different infusion periods. *J Med Food* 8:110–112, 2005. [**Al, B, Ba, Bi, Ca, Cd, Co, Cr, Cu, Fe, Ga, Ln, K, Li, Mg, Mn, Na, Ni, P, Pb, S, Sr, Ti, V, Zn**]

Ozcan M, J-C Chalchat. Effect of different locations on the **chemical composition of essential oils of laurel** (*Laurus nobilis* L.) **leaves** growing wild in Turkey. *J Med Food* 8:408–411, 2005.

Ozcan MM, LG Pedro, AC Figueiredo, JG Barroso. Constituents of the **essential oil of sea fennel** (*Crithmum maritimum* L.) growing wild in Turkey. *J Med Food* 9:128–130, 2006.

Padovani RM, DM Lima, FAB Colugnati, DB Rodriguez-Amaya. Comparison of **proximate, mineral and vitamin** composition of common **Brazilian and US foods**. *J Food Comp Anal* 20:733–738, 2007.

Pakkala H, H Reinivul, M-L Ovaskainen. Food composition on the World Wide Web: A user-centred (sic) perspective. *J Food Comp Anal* 19:231–240, 2006.

Pallauf K, JC Rivas-Gonzalo, MD del Castillo, MP Cano, S de Pascual-Teresa. Characterization of the **antioxidant composition** of strawberry tree (*Arbutus unedo* L.) fruits. *J Food Comp Anal* 21:273–281, 2008.

Pan American Health Organization and World Health Organization Technical Consultation, October 4–5, 2001. Nutrient composition for **fortified complementary foods**. *J Nutr* 133 (Suppl 9S): 2940S–3020S, 2003.

Parekh PP, AR Khan, MA Torres, ME Kitto. Concentrations of **selenium, barium, and radium in Brazil nuts**. *J Food Comp Anal* 21:332–335, 2008.

Patel S, T Shibamoto. Effect of 20 different yeast strains on the production of **volatile components in Symphony wine**. *J Food Comp Anal* 16:469–476, 2003.

Patthamakanokporn O, P Puwastien, A Nitithamyong, PP Sirichakwal. Changes of **antioxidant activity and total phenolic compounds** during storage of selected **fruits**. *J Food Comp Anal* 21:241–248, 2008.

Pehrsson PR, CR Perry, RC Cutrufelli, KY Patterson, J Wilgler, DB Haytowitz, JM Holden, CD Day, JH Himes, L Harnack, S Levy, J Wefel, J Heilman, KM Phillips, AS Rasor. Sampling and initial findings for a study of **fluoride in drinking water** in the United Status. *J Food Comp Anal* 19:S45–S52, 2006.

Peng L, X Song, X Shi, J Li, C Ye. An improved PHLC method for simultaneous determination of **phenolic compounds, purine alkaloids and theanine** in **Camellia** species. *J Food Comp Anal* 21:559–563, 2008.

Pereira NR, O Ferrarese-Filho, M Matsushita, NE de Souza. **Proximate composition and fatty acid profile of** *Bombyx mori* L. chrysalis toast. *J Food Comp Anal* 16:451–457, 2003.

Perez-Exposito AB, S Villalpando, JA Rivera, IJ Griffin, SA Abrams. **Ferrous sulfate** is more bioavailable among preschoolers than other forms of iron in a **milk-based weaning food** distributed by PROGRESA, a national program in Mexico. *J Nutr* 135:64–69, 2005.

Perez-Prieto LJ, JM Lopez-Roca, E Gomez-Plaza. Differences in major **volatile compounds of red wines** according to storage length and storage conditions. *J Food Comp Anal* 16:697–705, 2003.

Perona JS, R Cabello-Moruno, V Ruiz-Gutierrez. The role of **virgin olive oil** components in the modulation of endothelial function. *J Nutr Biochem* 17:429–445, 2006. [**squalene, β-carotene, β-sitosterol, campesterol, stigmasterol, brassicaterol, tocopherols, phenolic compounds**]

Perring L, D Andrey, M Basic-Dvorzak, D Hammer. Rapid quantification of **iron, copper, and zinc in food premixes** using energy dispersive X-ray fluorescence. *J Food Comp Anal* 18:655–663, 2005.

Peterson JJ, GR Beecher, SA Bhagwat, JT Dwyer, SE Gebhardt, DB Haytowitx, JM Holden. **Flavanones in grapefruit, lemons, and limes**: A compilation and review of the data from the analytical literature. *J Food Comp Anal* 19:S74–S80, 2006.

Peterson JJ, JT Dwyer, GR Beecher, SA Bhagwat, SE Gebhardt, DB Haytowitx, JM Holden. **Flavanones in oranges, tangerines (mandarins), tangors, and tangelos**: A compilation and review of the data from the analytical literature. *J Food Comp Anal* 19:S66–S73, 2006.

Peterson J, J Dwyer, S Bhagwat, D Haytowitz, J Holden, AL Eldridge, B Geecher, J Aladesanmi. **Major flavonoids in dry tea**. *J Food Comp Anal* 18:487–501, 2005.

Philibert A, C Vanier, N Abdelouahab, HM Chan, D Mergler. Fish intake and serum **fatty acid profiles** from **freshwater fish**. *Am J Clin Nutr* 84:1299–1307, 2006.

Phillippy BQ, M Lin, Barbara Rasco. Analysis of **phytate in raw and cooked potatoes**. *J Food Comp Anal* 17:217–226, 2004.

Plessi M, D Bertelli, F Migilietta. Extraction and identification by GC-MS of **phenolic acids in traditional balsamic vinegar from Modena**. *J Food Comp Anal* 19:49–54, 2005.

Polagruto JA, JF Wang-Polagruto, MM Braun, L Lee, C Kwik-Uribe, CL Keen. **Cocoa flavanol-enriched snack bars** containing phytosterols effectively lower total and low-density lipoprotein cholesterol levels. *J Am Diet Assoc* 106:1804–1813, 2006.

Poo-Prieto R, DB Haytowitz, JM Holden G Rogers, S Choumenkovitch, PF Jacques, J Selhub. Use of the affinity/HPLC method for quantitative estimation of **folic acid in enriched cereal grain products**. *J Nutr* 136:3079–3083, 2006.

Prandini A, S Sigolo, G Tansini, N Brogna, G Piva. Different level of **conjugated linoleic acid (CLA) in dairy products from Italy**. *J Food Comp Anal* 20:472–279, 2007.

Pugalenthi M, P Siddhuraju, V Vadivel. Effect of soaking followed by cooking and the addition of α-galactosidase on **oligosaccharides** levels in different *Canavalia* accessions. *J Food Comp Anal* 19:512–517, 2006.

Purchas R, M Zou, P Pearce, F Jackson. Concentrations of **vitamin D3 and 25-hydroxyvitamin D3** in raw and cooked **New Zealand beef and lamb**. *J Food Comp Anal* 20:90–98, 2007.

Puwastien P, N Pinprapai, K Judprasong, T Tamura. International inter-laboratory analyses of food **folate**. *J Food Comp Anal* 18:387–397, 2005.

Qian WL, Z Khan, DG Watson, J Fearnley. Analysis of **sugars in bee pollen and propolis** by ligand exchange chromatography in combination with pulsed amperometric detection and mass spectrometry. *J Food Comp Anal* 21:78–83, 2008.

Qin W, W Dan, D Bin, L Zaijun, H Yanqiang. A spectrophotometric method for determination of **total proteins in cow milk powder** samples using the *o*-nitrophenylfluorone/Mo(VI) complex. *J Food Comp Anal* 19:76–82, 2005.

Raffo An, G La Malfa, V Fogliano, G Maiani, G Quaglia. Seasonal variations in **antioxidant components of cherry tomatoes** (*Lycopersicon esculentum* cv. Naomi F1). *J Food Comp Anal* 19:11–19, 2005.

Raghu V, K Platel, K Srinivasan. Comparison of **ascorbic acid** content of *Emblica officinalis* fruits determined by different analytical methods. *J Food Comp Anal* 20:529–533, 2007.

Raigon MD, J Prohens, JE Munoz-Falcon, F Nuez. Comparison of **eggplant** landraces and commercial varieties for fruit content of **phenolics, minerals**, dry matter and **protein**. *J Food Comp Anal* 21:370–376, 2008. [**P, K, Ca, Mg, Na, Fe, Cu, Zn**]

Ramadan MF, J-T Moersel. Screening of the **antiradical action of vegetable oils**. *J Food Comp Anal* 19:838–842, 2006. [fatty acids of black cumin seed oil, doriander seed oil, and nigver seen oil]

Ramulu P, PU Rao. **Total, insoluble and soluble dietary fiber** contents of **Indian fruits**. *J Food Comp Anal* 16:677–685, 2003.

Rashed MN, ME Soltan. **Major and trace elements** in different types of **Egyptian mono-floral and non-floral bee honeys**. *J Food Comp Anal* 17:725–735, 2004.

Rein D, E Schijlen, T Kooistra, K Herbers, L Verschuren, R Hall, U Sonnewald, A Bovy, R Kleemann. Transgenic **flavonoid tomato** intake reduces C-reactive protein in human C-reactiveprotei transgenic mice more than wild-type tomato. *J Nutr* 136:2331–2337, 2006.

Reinibuo H, L Marjamaki, M Keikkila, SM Virtanen, L Valsta. Revised Finnish **dietary supplement database**. *J Food Comp Anal* 21:464–468, 2008.

Ribarova F, R Zanev, S Shishkov, N Rizov. **Alpha-tocopherol, fatty acids** and their correlations in **Bulgarian foodstuffs**. *J Food Comp Anal* 16:659–667, 2003.

Ribaya-Mercado JD, JB Blumberg. **Lutein and zeaxanthin** and their potential roles in disease prevention. *J Am Col Nutr* 23:567S–587S, 2004.

Ribeiro MLL, JMG Mandarino, MC Carrao-Panizzi, MCN de Oliveira, CBH Campo, AL Nepomuceno, EI Ida. **Isoflavone content and B-glucosidase activity in soybean cultivars** of different maturity groups. *J Food Comp Anal* 20:19–24, 2007.

Rist L, A Muellea, C Barthel, B Snijders, M Jansen, AP Simoes-Wust, M Huber, I Kummeling, U von Mandach, H Steinhart, C Thijs. Influence of organic diet on the amount of **conjugated linoleic acids in breast milk** of lactating women in the Netherlands. *Brit J Nutr* 97:735–743. 2007.

Ritter MMC, GP Savage. **Soluble and insoluble oxalate** content of **nuts**. *J Food Comp Anal* 20:169–174, 2007.

Robbins RJ, A-S Keck, G Banuelos, JW Finley. Cultivation conditions and selenium fertilization after the **pheonlic profile, glucosinolate and sulforaphane content of broccoli**. *J Med Food* 8:204–214, 2005.

Rodriguez-Amaya DB, M Kimura, HT Godoy, J Amaya-Farfar. Updated Brazilian database on food **carotenoids**: Factors affecting carotenoid composition. *J Food Comp Anal* 21:445–463, 2008.

Rodriguez-Bernaldo de Quiros A, HS Costa. Analysis of **carotenoids in vegetable** and plasma **samples**: A review. *J Food Comp Anal* 19:97–111, 2006.

Rodushkin I, A Magnusson. **Aluminium** migration to **orange juice** in laminated paperboard packages. *J Food Comp Anal* 18:365–374, 2005.

Roos N, MM Islam, SH Thilsted. Small **indigenous fish species in Bangladesh**: Contribution to **vitamin A, calcium, and iron** intakes. *J Nutr* 133:4021S–4026S, 2003.

Rodrigues CI, L Marta, R Maia, M Miranda, M Ribeirinho, C Mguas. Application of solid-phase extraction to brewed **coffee caffeine** and **organic acid** determination by UV/HPLC. *J Food Comp Anal* 20:440–448, 2007.

Ross AB, A Kamal-Eldin, P Aman. Dietary **aklylresorcinols**: Absorption, bioactivities, and possible use as biomarkers of **whole-grain wheat- and rye-rich foods**. *Nutr Rev* 62:81–95, 2004.

Roussis IG, I Lambropoulos, P Tzimas, A Gkoulioti, V Marinos, D Tsoupeis, I Boutaris. **Antioxidant activities** of some **Greek wines** and wine phenolic extracts. *J Food Comp Anal* 21:614–621, 2008.

Ruel MT, P Menon, C Loechl, G Pelto. Donated fortified cereal blends improve the **nutrient density of traditional complementary foods in Haiti**, but **iron** and **zinc** gaps remain for infants. *Food Nutr Bull* 25:361–376, 2004.

Ruelas-Inzunza J, G Meza-Lopez, F Paez-Osuna. **Mercury in fish** that are of dietary importance from the coasts of Sinaola (SE Gulf of Califrofnia). *J Food Comp Anal* 21:211–218, 2008.

Rupasinghe HPV, S Clegg. **Total antioxidant capacity, total phenolic content, mineral elements, and histramine** concentrations in **wines** of different fruit sources. *J Food Comp Anal* 20:133–137, 2007.

Russo MV, A De Leonardis, V Macciola. Solid phase extraction - gas-chromatographic method to determine **free cholesterol in animal fats**. *J Food Comp Anal* 18:617–624, 2005.

Rychlik M, K Englert, S Kapfer, E Kirchhoff. **Folate** contents of **legumes** determined by optimized enzyme treatment and stable isotope dilution assays. *J Food Comp Anal* 20:411–419, 2007.

Ryynanen M, A-M Lampi, P Salo-Vaananen, V Ollilainen, V Piironen. A small-scale simple preparation method with HPLC analysis for determination of **tocopherols and tocotrienols in cereals**. *J Food Comp Anal* 17:749–765, 2004.

Saari JT, PG Reeves, WT Johnson, LK Johnson. **Pinto beans** are a source of highly bioavailable **copper**. *J Nutr* 136:2999–3004, 2006

Sabir SM, H Maqsood, I Hayat, MQ Khan, A Khaliq. Elemental and nutritional analysis of **sea buckthorn** (*Hippophae rhamnoides* ssp. *turkestanica*) **berries** of Pakistani origin. *J Med Food* 8:518–522, 2005.

Sahlin E, GP Savage, CE Lister. Investigation of the **antioxidant properties of tomatoes after processing**. *J Food Comp Anal* 17:635–647, 2004.

Salaha M-I, S Kallithraca, I Marmaras, E Koussissi, I Tzourou. A natural alternative to sulphur dioxide for **red wine** production: Influence on colour, **antioxidant activity**, and **anthocyanin content**. *J Food Comp Anal* 21:660–666, 2008.

Saunders D, S Jones, GJ Devane, P Scholes, RJ Lake, Sm Paulin. **Trans fatty acids** in the New Zealand food supply. *J Food Comp Anal* 21:320–325, 2008.

Scherz H, E Kirchhoff. Trace elements in foods: **Zinc** contents of raw foods-A comparison of data originating from different geographical regions of the world. *J Food Comp Anal* 19:420–433, 2006.

Schollenberger M, W Drochner, M Rufle, S Suchy, H Terry-Jara, H-M Muller. **Trichothecene toxins** in different groups of **conventional and organic bread of the German market**. *J Food Comp Anal* 18:69–78, 2005.

Schoppen S AM Perez-Granados, A Carbajal, P Oubina, FJ Sanchez-Muniz, JA Gomez-Geriaue, MP Vaquero. A **sodium-rich carbonated mineral water** reduces cardiovascular risk in postmenopausal women. *J Nutr* 134:1058–1063, 2004.

Schuier M, H Sies, B Illek, H Fischer. **Cocoa-related flavonoids** inhibit CFTR-mediated chloride transport across T84 colon epithelia. *J Nutr* 135:2320–2325, 2005.

Schuppan D, MD Dennis, CP Kelly. Celiac disease: Epidemiology, pathogenesis, diagnosis, and nutritional management *Nutr Clin Care* 8:54–69, 2005. [**prolamines in grains**]

Schwartz H, V Ollilainen, V Piironen, A-M Lampi. **Tocopherol, tocotrienol and plant sterol** contents of **vegetable oils and industrial fats**. *J Food Comp Anal* 21:152–161, 2008.

Schwartz MB, LR Vartanian, CM Wharton, KD Brownell. Examining the nutritional quality of **breakfast cereals** marketed to children. *J Am Diet Assoc* 108:702–705, 2008.

Scott CE, AL Eldridge. Comparison of **carotenoid** content in **fresh, frozen, and canned corn**. *J Food Comp Anal* 18:551–559, 2005.

Seena S, KR Sridhar, AB Arun, C-C Young. Effect of roasting and pressure-cooking on **nutritional and protein quality of seeds of mangrove legume** *Canavalia cathartica* from southwest coast of India. *J Food Comp Anal* 19:284–293, 2006.

Seferoglu S, HG Seferoglu, FE Tekintas, F Balta. Biochemical composition influenced by different locations in Uzun **pistachio** cv. (*Pistacia vera* L.) grown in Turkey. *J Food Comp Anal* 19:461–465, 2006. **[protein, fat, unsaturated and saturated fatty acids]**

Segade SR, ES Vazquez, ED Losada. Influence of ripeness grade on accumulation and extractability of **grape skin anthocyanins** in different cultivars. *J Food Comp Anal* 21:599–607, 2008.

Selli S, T Cabaroglu, A Canbas. **Volatile flavour components of orange juice** obtained from the cv. Kozan of Turkey. *J Food Comp Anal* 17:789–796, 2004.

Sevenhuysen GP. Probability weighting of data in small samples to facilitate nutritional interpretation. *J Food Comp Anal* 17:125–132, 2004.

Sharma S, SP Murphy, LR Wilkens, D Au, L Shen, LN Kolonel. Extending a multiethnic food composition table to include standardized **food group servings**. *J Food Comp Anal* 16:485–495, 2003.

Sharma V, A Gulati, SD Ravindranath, V Kumar. A simple and convenient method for analysis of **tea biochemicals** by reverse phase HPLC. *J Food Comp Anal* 18:583–594, 2005.

Shi J, K Arunasalam, D Yeung, Y Kaduda, G Mittal, Y Jiang. **Saponins** from edible **legumes**: Chemistry, processing, and health benefits. *J Med Food* 7:67–78, 2004.

Shi J, J Yu, JE Pohorly, Y Kakuda. **Polyphenolics in grape seeds** – Biochemistry and functionality. *J Med Food* 6:291–299, 2003.

Shin J-K, G-N Kim, H-D Jang. **Antioxidant and pro-oxidant effects of green tea** extracts in oxygen radical absorbance capacity assay. *J Med Food* 10:32–30, 2007.

Shon M-Y, J Lee, J-H Choi, S-Y Choi, S-H Nam, K-I Seo, S-W Lee, N-J Sung, S-K Park. **Antioxidant and free radical scavenging activity** of methanol extract of *chungkukjang*. *J Food Comp Anal* 20:113–118, 2007. **[fermented soy food]**

Sies H, T Schewe, C Heiss, M Kelm. **Cocoa polyphenols** and inflammatory mediators. *Am J Clin Nutr* 81:304S–312S, 2005.

Sievenpiper JL, JT Arnason, LA Leiter, V Vuksan. Decreasing, null and increasing effects of eight popular types of **ginseng** on acute postprandial glycemic indices in healthy humans: The role of **ginsenosides**. *J Am Col Nutr* 23:248–258, 2004.

Silva TNS, CA Camara, ACS Lins, JM Barbosa-Filho, EMS da Silva, BM Freitas, FAR dos Santos. **Chemical composition** and **free radical scavenging activity** of **pollen** loads from stingles bee *Melipona subnitida* Ducke. *J Food Comp Anal* 19:507–511, 2006.

Simila M, M-L Ovaskainen, MJ Virtanen, LM Valsta. Nutrient content patterns of **Finnish foods** in a food composition database. *J Food Comp Anal* 19:217–224, 2006.

Simsek A, N Artik, E Baspinar. Detection of **raisin concentrate (pekmez) adulteration** by regression analysis method. *J Food Comp Anal* 17:155–163, 2004.

Sin DWM, YC Wong, CY Mak ST Sze, WY Yao. Determination of five **phenolic antioxidants in edible oils**: Method validation and estimation of measurement uncertainly. *J Food Comp Anal* 19:784–791, 2006.

Singh J, AK Upadhyay, K Prasad, A Bahadur, M Rai. Variability of **carotenes, vitamin C, E, and pheolics in** *Brassica* **vegetables**. *J Food Comp Anal* 20:106–112, 2007.

Singletary KW, K-J Jung, M Giusti. **Anthocyanin-rich grape extract** blocks breast cell DNA damage. *J Med Food* 10:244–251, 2007.

Sirichakwal PP, P Puwastien, J Rolngam, R Kongkachuichai. **Selenium content of Thai foods**. *J Food Comp Anal* 18:47–59, 2005.

Sirot V, M Oseredczuk, N Bemrah-Aouachria, J-L Volatier, J-C Leblanc. **Lipid and fatty acid** composition of **fish and seafood** consumed in France: CALIPSO study. *J Food Comp Anal* 21:8–16, 2008.

Slimestad R, K Torskangerpoll, HS Nateland, T Johannessen, NH Giske. **Flavonoids** from **black chokeberries**, *Aronia melanocarpa*. *J Food Comp Anal* 18:61–68, 2005.

Slow S, M Donaggio, PJ Cressey, M Lever, PM George, ST Chambers. The **betaine** content of **New Zealand foods** and estimated intake in the New Zealand diet. *J Food Comp Anal* 18:473–485, 2005.

Somsub W, R Kongkachuichai, P Sungpuag, R Charoensiri. Effects of three conventional cooking methods on **vitamin C, tannin, myo-inositol phosphates** contents in selected **Thai vegetables**. *J Food Comp Anal* 21:187–197, 2008.

Soto-Rodriguez I, PJ Campillo-Velazquez, J Ortega-Martinez, MT Rodriguez-Estrada, G Lercker, HS Garcia. **Cholesterol oxidation** in traditional **Mexican dried and deep-fried food** products. *J Food Comp Anal* 21:489–495, 2008.

Souchet N, S Laplante. Seasonal variation of **Co-enzyme Q10** content in **pelagic fish** tissues from Eastern Quebec. *J Food Comp Anal* 20:403–410, 2007. [mackerel and herring]

Soufleros EH, SA Mygdalia, P Natskoulis. Production process and characterization of the traditional **Greek fruit distillate "Koumaro"** by **aromatic and mineral composition**. *J Food Comp Anal* 18:699–716, 2005.

Sousa WR, C da Rocha, CL Cardoso, DHS Silva, MVB Zanoni, Determination of the relative contribution of **phenolic antioxidants in orange juice** by voltammetric methods. *J Food Comp Anal* 17:619–633, 2004.

Soyer Y, N Koca, F Karadeniz. **Organic acid profile of Turkish white grapes and grape juices**. *J Food Comp Anal* 16:629–636, 2003.

Stadler RH, G Scholz. **Acrylamide**: An update on current knowledge in analysis, levels in food, mechanisms of formation, and potential strategies of control. *Nutr Rev* 62:449–467, 2004.

Staggs CG, WM Sealey, BJ McCabe, Am Teague, DM Mock. Determination of the **biotin** content of **select foods** using accurate and sensitive HPLC/avidin binding. *J Food Comp Anal* 17:767–776, 2004.

Stein LH, A Kiessling, F Manne. Rapid estimation of **fat content** in **salmon fillets** by colour image analysis. *J Food Comp Anal* 20:73–79, 2007.

Storck CR, LP di Sailva, CAA Fagundes. Categorizing **rice cultivars** based on differences in chemical composition. *J Food Comp Anal* 18:333–341, 2005.

Su X, J Duan, Y Jiang, J Shi, Y Kakuda. Effects of soaking conditions on the **antioxidant potentials of oolong tea**. *J Food Comp Anal* 19:348–353, 2006.

Sudhir D, R Karpe, AG Hegde, RM Sharma. **Lead, cadmium, and nickel in chocolates and candies** from suburban areas of Mumbai, India. *J Food Comp Anal* 18:517–522, 2005.

Suetsuna K, K Maekawa, J-R Chen. Antihypertensive effects of *Undaria pinnatifida* (**wakame**) **peptide** on blood pressure in spontaneously hypertensive rats. *J Nutr Biochem* 15:267–272, 2004.

Sultana T, DL McNeil, NG Porter, GP Savage. Inveswtigation of **isothiocyanate** yield from flowering and non-florwering tissues of **wasabi** grown in a flooded system. *J Food Comp Anal* 16:637–646, 2003.

Suresh D, H Manjunatha, K Srinivasan. Effect of heat processing on spices on the concentrations of their **bioactive** principles: **Turmeric** (*Curcuma longa*), **red pepper** (*Capsicum annuum*), and **black pepper** (*Piper nigrum*). *J Food Comp Anal* 20:346–351. 2007.

Sutherland BA, RMA Rahman, I Appleton. Mechanisms of action of **green tea catechins**, with a focus on ischemia-induced neurodegeneration. *J Nutr Biochem* 17:291–306, 2006.

Tabee E, S Azadmard-Damirchi, M Jajerstad, PC Dutta. **Lipids and phytosterol oxidation** in commercial **French fries** commonly consumed in Sweden. *J Food Comp Anal* 21:169–177, 2008.

Tahvonen R, RM Hietanen, J Sibvonen, E Salminen. Influence of different processing methods on the **glycemic index of potato** (Nicola). *J Food Comp Anal* 19:372–378, 2006.

Talpur FN, MI Bhanger, MY Khuhawar. Comparison of **fatty acids and cholesterol** content in the **milk of Pakistani cow breeds**. *J Food Comp Anal* 19:698–703, 2006.

Tang G, J Qin, GG Dolnikowski, RM Russell, MA Grusak. **Spinach** or **carrots** can supply significant amounts of **vitamin A** as assessed by feeding with intrinsically deuterated vegetables. *Am J Clin Nutr* 82:821–828, 2005.

Tang X, DA Cronin, NP Bruton. A simplified approach to the determination of **thiamine and riboflavin in meats** using reverse phase HPLC. *J Food Comp Anal* 19:831–837, 2006.

Tarrago-Trani MT, KM Phillips, LE Lemar, JM Holden. New and existing **oils and fats** used in products with reduced *trans*-**fatty acid** content. *J Am Diet Assoc* 106:867–880, 2006.

Tateo F, M Bononi. Determination of ethylene chlorohydrin as marker of **spices** fumigation with ethylene oxide. *J Food Comp Anal* 19:83–87, 2005.

Tateo F, M Bononi. Determination of **gamma-butyrolactone** (GBL) in foods by SBSE-TD/GC/MS. *J Food Comp Anal* 16:721–727, 2003.

Tateo F, M Bononi, G Andreoli. **Acrylamide** levels in cooked **rice, tomato sauces, and some fast food** on the Italian market. *J Food Comp Anal* 20:232–235, 2007.

Techakriengkrai I, R Surakarnkul. Analysis of **benzoic acid and sorbic acid in Thai rice** wines and distillates by solid-phase sorbent extraction and high-performance liquid chromatography. *J Food Comp Anal* 20:220–225, 2007.

Tesoriere L, D Butera, AM Pintaudi, M Allegra, MA Livera. Supplementation with **cactus pear** (*Opuntia Picus-indica*) fruit decreases oxidative stress in healthy humans: A comparative study with vitamin C. *Am J Clin Nutr* 80:391–395, 2004.

Thanonkaew A, B Soottawat, W Visessanguan. Chemical composition and thermal property of **cuttlefish** (Sepia pharaonis) muscle. *J Food Comp Anal* 19:127–133, 2006.

Thompson CD, A Chisholm, SK McLachlan, JM Campbell. **Brazil nuts**: An effective way to improve **selenium** status. *Am J Clin Nutr* 87:379–384, 2008.

Thompson L, J Morris, E Peffley, C Green, P Pare, D Tissue, R Jasoni, H Jutson, B Wehner, C Kane. **Flavonol content and composition of spring onions** grown hydroponically or in potting soil. *J Food Comp Anal* 18:635–645, 2005.

Toda S. Antioxidative effects of **polyphenols in leaves of** *Houttuynia cordata* on protein fragmentation by copper-hydrogen peroxide *in vitro. J Med Food* 8:266–268, 2005. [**total polyphenol and condensed tannin**]

Toor RK, GP Savage, A Heeb. Influence of different types of fertilizers on the major **antioxidant components of tomatoes**. *J Food Comp Anal* 19:20–27, 2005.

Toor RK, GP Savage, CE Lister. Seasonal variations in the **antioxidant composition of greenhouse grown tomatoes**. *J Food Comp Anal* 19:1–10, 2006.

Topuz A, F Ozdemir. Assessment of **carotenoids, capsaicinoids and ascorbic acid** composition of some selected **pepper cultivars** (*Capsicum annuum* L.) grown in Turkey. *J Food Comp Anal* 20:596–602, 2007.

Tsaanova-Savova S, F Ribarova, M Gerova. **(+)-Catechin and (−)-epicatechin in Bulgarian fruits**. *J Food Comp Anal* 18:691–698, 2005.

Tsiaganis MC, K Laskari, E Melissari. **Fatty acid** composition of *Allium* species lipids. *J Food Comp Anal* 19:620–627, 2006.

Turhan S, NS Ustun, I Bank. Effect of freeze-thaw cycles on **total and heme iron** contents of **bonito** (*Sarda sarda*) and **bluefish** (*Pomatomus saltator*) fillets. *J Food Comp Anal* 19:384–387, 2006.

Turon F, B Rwabwogo, B Barea, M Pina, J Graille. **Fatty acid** composition of **oil** extracted from **Nile perch** (*Lates niloticus*) head. *J Food Comp Anal* 18:717–722, 2005.

Umeta M, CE West, H Fufu. Content of **zinc, iron, calcium**, and their absorption inhibitors in foods commonly consumed in Ethiopia. *J Food Comp Anal* 18:803–817, 2005.

Umphress ST, SP Murphy AA Franke, LJ Custer, CL Blitz. **Isoflavone** content of **foods with soy additives**. *J Food Comp Anal* 18:533–550, 2005.

van Heerden SM, CH Schonfeldt, R Kruger, MF Smit. The nutrient composition of South African **lamb** (A2 grade). *J Food Comp Anal* 20:671–680, 2007.

van Jaarsveld PJ, M Faber, SA Tanumihardjo, P Nestel, CJ Lombard, AJS Benade. **Beta-carotene**-rich **orange-fleshed sweet potato** improves the **vitamin A** status of primary school children assessed with the modified-relative-dose-response test. *Am J Clin Nutr* 81:1080–1087, 2005.

van Jaarsveld PJ, DW Marais, E Harmse, P Nestel, DB Rodriquez-Amaya. Retention of **beta-carotene in boiled, mashed orange-fleshed sweet potato**. *J Food Comp Anal* 19:321–329, 2006.

Vanamala J, L Reddivari, KS Yoo, LM Pike, BS Patil. Variation in the content of **bioactive flavonoids** in different brands of **orange and grapefruit juices**. *J Food Comp Anal* 19:157–166, 2006.

Vargar-Torres A, P Osorio-Diaz, JJ Islas-Hernandez, J Tovar, O Paredes-Lopez, LA Bello-Perez. **Starch digestibility of five cooked black bean** (*Phaseolus vulgaris* **L.**) **varieties**. *J Food Comp Anal* 17:605–612, 2004.

Vasilopoulou E, K Georga, E Grilli, A Linardou, M Vithoulka, A Trichopoulou. Compatibility of computed and chemically determined **macronutrients and energy** content of traditional **Greek recipes**. *J Food Comp Anal* 16:707–719, 2003.

Vicetti R, T Ishitani, A Salas, M Ayala. Use of **alpha-tocopherol** combined with synergists and compared to **other antioxidants** on the oxidative stability of **sardine skin lipids**. *J Food Comp Anal* 18:131–137, 2005.

Vicini J, T Etherton, P Kris-Etherton, J Ballam, S Denham, R Staub, D Goldstein, R Cady, M McGrath, M Luch. Survey of retail **milk** composition as affected by label claims regarding farm-management practices. *J Am Diet Assoc* 108:1198–1203, 2008.

Vilanova M, C Sieiro. Determination of **free and bound terpene** compounds in **Albarino wine**. *J Food Comp Anal* 19:694–697, 2006.

Vlachopoulos C, N Alexopoulos, I Dima, K Aznaouridis, I Andreadou, C Stefanadis. Acute effect of **black and green tea** on aortic stiffness and wave reflections. *Am Col Nutr* 25:216–223, 2006. [**caffeine**]

Vuong LT, AA Franke, LJ Custer, SP Murphy. *Momordica cochinchinensis* Spreng. (gac*)* fruit carotenoids reevaluated. *J Food Comp Anal* 19:664–668, 2006.

Wall MM. **Ascorbic acid, vitamin A, and mineral composition of banana** (Musa sp.) **and papaya** (*Carica papaya*) cultivars grown in Hawaii. *J Food Comp Anal* 19:434–445, 2006. [**beta-carotene, alpha-carotene, beta-cryptoxanthin, lutein, lycopene, P, K, Ca, Mg, Na, Fe, Mn, Zn, Cu, B**]

Wall MM. **Ascorbic acid and mineral composition of longan** (*Dimocarpus longan*), **lychee** (*Litchi chinensis*) and **rambutan** (*Nephelium lappaceum*) cultivars grown in Hawaii. *J Food Comp Anal* 19:655–663, 2006. [**P, K, Ca, Mg, Na, Fe, Mn, Zn, Cu, B**]

Wallingford JC, R Yuhas, S Du, F Zhai, BM Popkin. **Fatty acids in Chinese edible oils**: Value of direct analysis as a basis for labeling. *Food Nutr Bull* 25:330–336, 2004.

Walter M, LP da Silva, CC Denardin. **Rice** and **resistant starch**: Different content depending on chosen methodology. *J Food Comp Anal* 18:279–285, 2005.

Wang D, J Lu, A Miao, Z Xie, D Yang. HPLC-DAD-ESI-MS/MS analysis of **polyphenols and purine alkaloids** in leaves of 22 **tea** cultivars in China. *J Food Comp Anal* 21:361–369, 2008.

Wang J, S Li, Z Wang, B Xin, H Wang. Trophic effect of **bee pollen** on small intestine in broiler chickens. *J Med Food* 10:276–280, 2007. [**9 macronutrients, amino acids, 10 vitamins 9 minerals**]

Wang K-Y, S-N Li, C-S Liu, D-S Perng, Y-C Su, D-C Wu, C-M Jan, C-H Lai, T-N Wang, W-M Wang. Effects of ingesting *Lactobacillus*- and *Bifidobacterium*-containing **yogurt** in subjects with colonized Helicobacter pylori. *Am J Clin Nutr* 80:737–741, 2004.

Wang M-L, J-T Wang, Y-M Choong. A rapid and accurate method for determination of **methanol in alcoholic beverage** by direct injection capillary gas chromatography. *J Food Comp Anal* 17:187–196, 2004.

Wang Q, C Xue, Z Li, J Xu. Analysis of **DHA-rich phospholipids** from **egg of squid** *Sthenoteuthis oualaniensis*. *J Food Comp Anal* 21:356–359, 2008.

Warwick PM. Expression of energy: Commentary on the case for **net metabolizable energy**. *J Food Comp Anal* 18:241–247, 2005.

Weaver KL, P Ivester, JA Chilton, MD Wilso, P Pandey, FH Chilton. The content of favorable and unfavorable **polyunsaturated fatty acids** found in commonly eaten **fish**. *J Am Diet Assoc* 108:1178–1185, 2008.

Weinbrenner T, M Fito, R de la Torre, GT Saez, P Rijken, C Tormos, S Coolen, MF Albaladejo, S Abanades, H Schroder, J Marrugat, M-I Covas. **Olive oils** high in **phenolic compounds** modulate oxidative/antioxidative status in men. *J Nutr* 134:2314–2321, 2004.

Wolever TMS, JC Brand-Miller, J Abernethy, et al (47 additional authors). Measuring the **glycemic index** of foods: Interlaboratory study. *Am J Clin Nutr* 87(suppl):247S–257S, 2008.

Xianquan S, J Shi, Y Kakuda, J Yueming. Stability of **lycopene** during food processing and storage (Review). J Med Food 8:413–422, 2005.

Xin L, H Xiaoyun, L Yunbo, X Guoying, J Xianbin, H Kunlun. Comparative analysis of nutritional composition between herbicide-tolerant **rice** with bar gene and its non-transgenic counterpart. *J food Comp Anal* 21:535–539, 2008. [**proximates, amino acids, fatty acids, 9 minerals, thiamin, riboflavin, vitamin E, phytic acid**]

Xinmin W, Z Ruili, L Zhihua, W Yuanhong, J Tingfu. Determination of **glucosamine and lactose in milk-based formulae** by high-performance liquid chromatography. *J Food Comp Anal* 21:255–258, 2008.

Xu G, X Ye, D Liu, Y Ma, J Chen. Composition and distribution of **phenolic acids** in **Ponkan** (*Citrus poonesis* Hort. Ex Tanaka) and **Huyou** (*Citrus paradisi* Macf. Changsyanhuyou) during maturity. *J Food Comp Anal* 21:382–389, 2008. [**caffeic, p-coumaric, ferulic, sinapic, protocatechuic, p-hydroxybenzoic, and vanillic acids**]

Yen IC, LR de Astudillo, JF Soler, A la Barbera-Sanchez. Paralytic shellfish poisoning **toxin profiles in green mussels from Trinidad and Venezuela**. *J Food Comp Anal* 19:88–94, 2005.

Yilmaz Y, RT Toledo. Oxygen radical absorbance capacities of **grape/wine industry byproducts** and effect of solvent type on extraction of **grape seed polyphenols**. *J Food Comp Anal* 19:41–48, 2005.

Yoshida H, Y Hirakawa, C Murakami, Y Mizushina, T Yamade. Variation in the content of **tocopherols** and distribution of **fatty acids** within **soya bean seeds** (*Glycine max* L.). *J Food Comp Anal* 16:429–440, 2003.

Yoshida H, Y Hirakawa, Y Tomiyama, T Nagamizu, Y Mizushina. **Fatty acid** distributions of **triacylglycerols and phospholipids in peanut seeds** (*Arschis hypogaea* L.) following microwave treatment. *J Food Comp Anal* 18:3–14, 2005.

Yoshida H, Y Tomiyama, Y Hirakawa, Y Mizushina. Microwave roasting effects on the oxidative stability of oils and molecular species of **triacylglycerols in the kernels of pumpkin** (*Cucurbita* spp.) seeds. *J Food Comp Anal* 19:330–339, 2006.

Yu J, M Ahmedna, I Goktepe, J Dai. **Peanut skin procyanidins**: Composition and antioxidant activities as affected by processing. *J Food Comp Anal* 19:3640371, 2006.

Yu L, D Adams, BA Watkins. Comparison of commercial **supplements** containing **conjugated linoleic acid**. *J Food Comp Anal* 16:419–428, 2003.

Yumi AH-YH, M Eng, CIR Gill, H McGlynn, IR Rowland. Components of **olive oil** and chemoprevention of colorectal cancer. *Nutr Rev* 63:374–386, 2005.

Yurchenko S, U Molder. The determination of **polycyclic aromatic hydrocarbons in smoked fish** by gas chromatography mass spectrometry with positive-ion chemical ionization. *J Food Comp Anal* 18:857–869, 2005.

Zaijum L, T Jian, L Huizhen, Z Xia, Y Rui. Determination of trace amounts of **germanium** in food and fruit by spectrophotometry with p-methybenzeneazosalicylflurone. *J Food Comp Anal* 20:1–6, 2007.

Zarnowski R, Y Suzuki. Expedient Soxhlet extraction of **resorcinolic lipids** from **wheat grains**. *J Food Comp Anal* 17:649–663, 2004.

Zhou J, D Han. **Proximate, amino acid, and mineral composition of pupae of the silkworm** *Antheraea pernyi* in China. *J Food Comp Anal* 19:850-593, 2006.

Zmijewski T, R Kujawa, B Jankowska, A Kwiatkowska, A Mamcarz. Slaughter yield, proximate and fatty acid composition and sensory properties of **rapfen** (*Aspius aspius* L) with tissue of **bream** (*Abramis Brama* L) and **pike** (*Esox lucius* L). *J Food Comp Anal* 19:176–181, 2006.

# Index of Food Names for Main Table